Principles of Ambulatory Medicine

Principles of Ambulatory Medicine

Edited by

L. Randol Barker, M.D.

Associate Professor of Medicine,
The Johns Hopkins University School of Medicine;
Director, Division of General Internal Medicine,
Baltimore City Hospitals

John R. Burton, M.D.

Associate Professor of Medicine,
The Johns Hopkins University School of Medicine;
Deputy Director, Department of Medicine,
Baltimore City Hospitals

Philip D. Zieve, M.D.

Professor of Medicine,
The Johns Hopkins University School of Medicine;
Chairman, Department of Medicine,
Baltimore City Hospitals

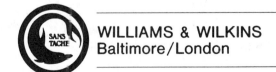

WILLIAMS & WILKINS
Baltimore/London

Made in the United States of America

Reprinted 1983

Library of Congress Cataloging in Publication Data

Main entry under title:

Principles of ambulatory medicine.

Includes bibliographical references and index. 1. Family medicine. 2. Ambulatory medical care. I. Barker, L. Randol (Lee Randol) II. Burton, John R. III. Zieve, Philip D. [DNLM: 1. Ambulatory care.
WE 172 R345]
RC46.P894 1983   616   81-16392
ISBN 0-683-00435-2   AACR2

Composed and printed at the
Waverly Press, Inc.
Mt. Royal and Guilford Aves.
Baltimore, MD 21202, U.S.A.

Preface

This book is directed primarily to the general physician who cares for ambulatory adult patients. The purposes of the book are (a) to provide an in-depth account of the evaluation, management, and long term course of those common clinical problems which are handled by the generalist in the ambulatory setting, and (b) to provide guidelines for recognizing those problems which require either hospitalization or referral for specialized care and for appreciating the expected course of those problems.

For over 60 years, Baltimore City Hospital has offered education to medical students, residents, fellows, and practicing physicians. During the past decade, the full time professional staff of the hospital has developed major teaching and practice initiatives in ambulatory care. The recognition of the need for a clinical textbook which focused upon the ambulatory patient grew directly out of these initiatives. All of the contributors to this text have a present or recent affiliation with Baltimore City Hospital and/ or with The Johns Hopkins University School of Medicine. All have had substantial experience caring for ambulatory patients in their areas of expertise. The editors have worked very closely with all contributors to assure that the material they prepared was focused upon the ambulatory patient.

Three principles have guided the preparation of each chapter:

1. That the physician working in a busy office practice needs to know a great deal about *probabilities* related to his patient's conditions. To address this need, the following types of information are emphasized throughout the book:
   a. Relative frequencies of the conditions which underlie common symptoms.
   b. Distribution of conditions in major subgroups of the population.
   c. The sensitivity, and specificity, and predictive value of diagnostic tests and procedures.
   d. The expected course of conditions, in both treated and untreated patients.
   e. The frequency of the complications of treatment.
2. That the patient, in fact, makes most decisions in ambulatory care and that the physician should emphasize the following aspects of *patient education* to assure that the patient's decisions are appropriate:
   a. Information about the short and long term prognosis of the patient's condition, with special emphasis on the implications of the condition for the patient's usual occupational and recreational activities.
   b. Information about the treatment: *i.e.*, how much the treatment usually helps, the expected duration, the correct schedule for treatment (including options adapted to the patient's life-style), common side effects and cost of the treatment.
   c. Information about the experience the patient will undergo when he is referred for care by a specialist or for diagnostic procedures which require his cooperation.
3. That the physician and the patient should incorporate a *preventive point of view* into all the actions which they take in dealing with a condition. For example, there should be:
   a Primary prevention of certain conditions, in all patients.
   b. Risk reduction, in those patients who already have certain risk factors.
   c. Optimum maintenance of the patient's health, after a symptomatic condition has developed.
   d. Anticipation of and prevention of problems associated with an established condition or with the treatment prescribed for that condition.

In planning the scope of the book, we selected those conditions which most office-based general internists and general or family practitioners encounter in caring for adult patients from the general population. It was clear that the book should include all of the common conditions of the major organ systems which have been the focus of internal medicine. It was equally clear that a large group of conditions outside of the traditional scope of internal medicine should be included because of the importance they assume in everyday office practice. For all of the conditions included, we agreed that there is a special body of information needed for care of the ambulatory patient, as defined in the three principles named above.

An introductory chapter, entitled "The Distinctive Characteristics of Ambulatory Medicine," defines the domain of ambulatory medicine and delineates the knowledge and the skills which are particularly important in the care of ambulatory patients.

There are a limited number of specific references and a few general references at the end of each chapter. These references are included so that interested readers can pursue in greater depth problems of interest to them. Because we have striven to provide the practical information needed to deal with each of the clinical problems included in this book, readers should be able to make practical decisions for their patients without often having to consult the references.

The book is extensively cross-referenced in order both to avoid redundancy and to facilitate access to useful information contained elsewhere in the book.

In addition, for easy reference, the key topics in each chapter are presented in outline form at the beginning of the respective chapter.

ACKNOWLEDGMENTS

The editors wish to acknowledge the helpful suggestions of many colleagues, both generalists and specialists, who reviewed chapters. We are greatly appreciative of the excellent help provided by Mrs. Marjorie Gregerman and her staff in the Department of Art as Applied to Medicine. Two persons, Mrs. Carole Messman and Ms. Susan McFeaters, provided excellent administrative and typographic assistance throughout the preparation of this book.

Contributors

Unless otherwise indicated hospital appointments are at the Baltimore City Hospitals, Baltimore, Maryland, and faculty appointments are at The Johns Hopkins University School of Medicine, Baltimore, Maryland.

Richard P. Allen, Ph.D.
Director, Baltimore Regional Sleep Disorders Center
Assistant Professor of Neurology

Frank C. Arnett, Jr., M.D.
Active Staff
   The Good Samaritan Hospital and
   The Johns Hopkins Hospital
   Baltimore, Maryland
Associate Professor of Medicine

Walter F. Baile, M.D.
Director, Psychiatry Liaison Service
Assistant Professor of Psychiatry and Medicine

L. Randol Barker, M.D., Sc.M.
Chief, Division of General Internal Medicine
Associate Professor of Medicine

Edmund G. Beacham, M.D.
Chief, Division of Geriatrics and Chronic Medicine
Assistant Professor of Medicine Emeritus

Barbara B. Bell, M.D.
Director, Heart Station
Assistant Professor of Pediatrics and Medicine

George E. Bigelow, Ph.D.
Director, Behavioral Pharmacology Research Unit
Associate Professor of Behavioral Biology
   and Assistant Professor of Psychology

Marc R. Blackman, M.D.
Staff Endocrinologist
Assistant Professor of Medicine

Eugene R. Bleecker, M.D.
Chief, Division of Pulmonary Medicine
Assistant Professor of Medicine

John C. Breitner, M.D.
Director, Community Psychiatry
Assistant Professor of Psychiatry

Gary R. Briefel, M.D.
Staff Nephrologist, Director Satellite Dialysis Unit
Assistant Professor of Medicine

Andrew F. Brooker, M.D.
Chief, Division of Orthopedic Surgery
Associate Professor of Orthopedic Surgery

John R. Burton, M.D.
Deputy Director, Department of Medicine
Associate Professor of Medicine

Ronald P. Byank, M.D.
Staff Surgeon
Assistant Professor of Orthopedic Surgery

Edward S. Cohn, M.D.
Chief, Division of Otolaryngology
Assistant Professor of Laryngology and Otology

Peter E. Dans, M.D.
Director, Office of Medical Practice Evaluation
   The Johns Hopkins Hospital, Baltimore
Associate Professor of Medicine

J. Raymond DePaulo, M.D.
Chief, Division of Adult Psychiatry
Assistant Professor of Psychiatry

Burton D'Lugoff, M.D.
Director, Community Health Problems
Assistant Professor of Psychiatry and Medicine

Calvin B. Ernst, M.D.
Surgeon-in-Chief
Professor of Surgery

Robert S. Fisher, M.D., Ph.D.
Fellow in Neurology

Barry Gordon, M.D., Ph.D.
Deputy Chief, Department of Neurology
Assistant Professor of Neurology

Sheldon H. Gottlieb, M.D.
Clinical Director, Division of Cardiology
Assistant Professor of Medicine

Robert I. Gregerman, M.D.
Chief, Division of Endocrinology
Associate Professor of Medicine

Richard J. Gross, M.D.
Associate Director of Primary Care
   Greater Baltimore Medical Center
   Baltimore
Formerly Associate Director, Medical Clinics
Assistant Professor of Medicine and Public Health

Noble M. Hansen, M.D.
Staff Surgeon
Assistant Professor of Orthopedic Surgery

S. Mitchell Harman, M.D., Ph.D.
Staff Endocrinologist
Assistant Professor of Medicine

James Hawthorne, Ph.D.
Director, Southeast Baltimore Drug Treatment Program
Assistant Professor of Medical Psychology

Lorraine F. Josifek, M.D.
Assistant in Neurology

Kripa S. Kashyap, M.D.
Director, Ambulatory Psychiatry Service
Assistant Professor of Psychiatry

Gregory B. Kelly, M.D.
Staff Rheumatologist
Instructor of Medicine

James P. Keogh, M.D.
Chief, Division of Occupational Medicine
Assistant Professor of Medicine

David E. Kern, M.D.
Associate Director, Medical Clinics
Assistant Professor of Medicine

Earl D. R. Kidwell, Jr., M.D.
Chief, Division of Ophthalmology
Assistant Professor of Ophthalmology

Frederick Koster, M.D.
Staff Physician, Infectious Disease Division
  Bernalillo County Medical Center
  Albuquerque, New Mexico
Assistant Professor of Medicine
  University of New Mexico School of Medicine
  Albuquerque, New Mexico

Stanford I. Lamberg, M.D.
Chief, Department of Dermatology
Associate Professor of Dermatology

Bruce S. Lebowitz, D.P.M.
Director, Podiatry Clinic

Ira Liebson, M.D.
Medical Director, Behavioral Pharmacology Research
  Unit
Associate Professor of Psychiatry

Douglas K. MacLeod, D.M.D.
Chief, Department of Dentistry

Clinical Field Instructor
  The University of Maryland Dental School
  Baltimore

Robert L. Marcus, M.D.
Chief, Division of Rheumatology
Assistant Professor of Medicine

Esteban Mezey, M.D.
Chief, Division of Liver Diseases
Professor of Medicine

Louis W. Miller, M.D.
Formerly Assistant Professor of Medicine

Hamilton Moses III, M.D.
Assistant Professor of Neurology

Andrew Munster, M.D.
Director, Baltimore Regional Burn Center
Associate Professor of Surgery and Plastic Surgery

Nathaniel F. Pierce, M.D.
Chief, Division of Infectious Diseases
Professor of Medicine

Robert M. Quinlan, M.D.
Chief of Surgery
  Memorial Hospital
  Worchester, Massachusetts
Associate Professor of Surgery
  University of Massachusetts School of Medicine
  Worcester, Massachusetts

J. Courtland Robinson, M.D.
Director of Obstetrics
Assistant Professor of Gynecology and Obstetrics

W. Robert Rout, M.D.
Staff Surgeon
Assistant Professor of Surgery

R. Bradley Sack, M.D.
Chief, Division of Geographic Medicine
Professor of Medicine

Larry N. Scherzer, M.D.
Director, Behavior Clinic
Assistant Professor of Pediatrics

Chester W. Schmidt, Jr., M.D.
Psychiatrist-in-Chief
Associate Professor of Psychiatry

Marvin M. Schuster, M.D.
Chief, Division of Digestive Diseases
Professor of Medicine and Joint Appointment in Psychiatry

Alfred C. Server, M.D., Ph.D.
Fellow in Neurology

Philip L. Smith, M.D.
Director, Intensive Care Unit
Assistant Professor of Medicine and Instructor of
    Anesthesiology

James K. Smolev, M.D.
Formerly Chief Division of Urology
Assistant Professor of Urology

Everett K. Spees, M.D., Ph.D.
Chief, Division of Transplant Surgery
Associate Professor of Transplantation Surgery

Maxine L. Stitzer, Ph.D.
Associate Professor of
    Behavioral Biology and Assistant Professor of Psy-
        chology

Mahmud A. Thamer, M.D.
Director, Cardiac Rehabilitation Program
Assistant Professor of Medicine

Alexander S. Townes, M.D.
Chief, Medical Services
    Veterans Administration Medical Center
    Memphis, Tennessee

Professor of Medicine
    University of Tennessee School of Medicine
    Memphis, Tennessee

Harold J. Tucker, M.D.
Staff Gastroenterologist
Assistant Professor of Medicine

Martin D. Valentine, M.D.
The Center for Allergic Diseases, The Good Samari-
    tan Hospital
        Baltimore, Maryland
Formerly Director Allergy Clinic
Associate Professor of Medicine

Gustav C. Voigt, M.D.
Director, Emergency Medicine
Associate Professor of Medicine and Assistant Pro-
    fessor of Emergency Medicine

Larry Waterbury, M.D.
Chief, Division of Hematology-Oncology
Associate Professor of Medicine and Assistant Pro-
    fessor of Oncology

Philip D. Zieve, M.D.
Physician-in-Chief
Professor of Medicine

Contents

SECTION 1: Issues of General Concern in Ambulatory Care

SECTION 2: Psychiatric and Behavioral Problems

SECTION 3: Allergy and Infectious Diseases

SECTION 4: Gastrointestinal Problems

SECTION 5: Renal and Urologic Problems

SECTION 6: Hematologic Problems

SECTION 7: Pulmonary Problems

SECTION 8: Cardiovascular Problems

SECTION 9: Musculoskeletal Problems

SECTION 10: Metabolic and Endocrinologic Problems

SECTION 11: Neurologic Problems

SECTION 12: Selected General Surgical Problems

SECTION 13: Gynecologic Problems

SECTION 14: Problems of the Eyes and Ears

SECTION 15: Miscellaneous Problems

SECTION 1

Issues of General Concern in Ambulatory Care

CHAPTER ONE

Distinctive Characteristics of Ambulatory Medicine

L. RANDOL BARKER, M.D.

The fundamental tenet of this book is that ambulatory medicine has a number of distinctive characteristics which should shape the physician's approach to his ambulatory patients. This chapter describes the present domain of ambulatory care in the United States and defines the goals, basic knowledge, and skills which are central in the practice of ambulatory medicine.

THE DOMAIN OF AMBULATORY MEDICINE

The domain of ambulatory medicine comprises a special group of patients with a variety of problems and those physicians and other health professionals who take care of them. Who are the physicians providing ambulatory care? Which patients visit physicians in their offices? What are the problems which these patients present to their physicians? What is the ambulatory care provided for these problems? In order to answer these questions, the United States National Ambulatory Medical Care Survey (NAMCS), started in 1973, has collected information periodically from a representative sample of physician's offices.

Office-based Physicians

Table 1.1 shows the distribution by physician specialty of the 556 million office visits to physicians in the United States during 1979. Of these visits, roughly 35% were to general and family practitioners, and 12% were to internists, the two groups of generalists to whom this book is directed primarily.

Ambulatory Patients

The age and sex distribution of the patients who visit these two groups of generalists is shown in Table 1.2. Approximately 60% of visits to all generalists are made by female patients. The principal

Table 1.1
Number and Percentage Distribution of Office Visits by Physician Specialty: United States, January to December 1979[a]

Physician Specialty	No. of Visits in Thousands	Percentage Distribution of Visits
ALL VISITS	556,313	100.0
PHYSICIAN SPECIALTY		
General and family practice	190,194	34.2
Medical specialties	164,109	29.5
Internal medicine	66,908	12.0
Pediatrics	58,126	10.4
Other	39,075	7.0
Surgical specialists	173,457	31.2
General surgery	33,740	6.1
Obstetrics and gynecology	50,823	9.1
Other	88,894	16.0
Other specialties	28,553	5.1
Psychiatry	17,093	3.1
Other	11,461	2.1

[a] Adapted from *1979 Summary National Ambulatory Medical Care Survey*. Advance data from *Vital and Health Statistics of the National Center for Health Statistics*, No. 66, March 2, 1981.

Table 1.2
Age and Sex of Patients Making Ambulatory Visits to General Family Physicians and Internists, January to December 1975[a]

Age and Sex of Patient	Percentage of Visits	
	To internists	To general and family physicians
Under 15 yr	3.3	14.4
15–24 yr	8.8	16.0
25–44 yr	21.1	24.1
45–64 yr	37.9	27.5
65 yr and over	28.9	18.0
Female	59.9	59.2
Male	40.5	40.8

[a] Adapted from *The National Ambulatory Medical Care Survey: 1975 Summary United States, January–December 1975*, DHEW Publication No. (*PHS*) 78-1784. National Center for Health Statistics, Hyattsville, Md., January 1978.

differences shown in Table 1.2 are that adolescents and young adults account for a larger proportion of visits to general and family physicians than to internists, and that visits by older patients make up a larger proportion of the practice of internists.

The NAMCS definition of an ambulatory patient is "an individual presenting himself for personal health services who is neither bedridden nor currently admitted to any health care institution." We would add to this definition that each ambulatory or homebound patient (or a member of the household) has most of the responsibility for his own care; that is, he must administer most or all of his treatments,

he must monitor his symptoms and functional status, he must adapt his activity to his degree of illness, and he must decide how to deal with new problems when they arise. These characteristics of an ambulatory patient have very important implications for the physician, as discussed below.

Problems of Ambulatory Patients

What types of clinical problems are seen in ambulatory medicine? This question was asked from the point of view of the patient and of the physician in examining a large sample of office visits to generalists participating in the NAMCS. Thus, patients were asked to name the principal reasons for their visits, and physicians were asked to name the principal diagnoses for the problems addressed at the same visits. Tables 1.3 and 1.4 list the most common responses given in the offices of internists and of general and family physicians, respectively. Three points bear emphasis. (a) For internists, 20 diagnoses or problems and for generalists 25 problems or diagnoses accounted for approximately 50% of total visits. (b) There are important differences in the frequency of problems reported by patients and physicians; for example, abdominal pain is fifth among the problems reported by the patients of both types of physicians but does not appear as one of the most common problems reported by either group of physicians. (c) A number of the problems named by patients are symptoms for which a specific diagnosis often cannot be determined.

In this study, physicians were also asked to rate the extent of impairment that might result if no care were available for the patient. The internists rated 70% of problems and the general and family physicians rated 80% of problems as either not serious or only slightly serious in terms of preventable impairment.

Ambulatory Care

The NAMCS defined ambulatory care as "health services rendered to individuals under their own cognizance, any time when they are not in a hospital or other health care institution." Table 1.5 from the 1975 NAMCS report shows the percentage distribution of diagnostic and therapeutic services ordered or provided by internists and general or family physicians for their ambulatory patients. The table also shows the frequency distribution of duration of visit and the prior visit status of patients.

The majority of visits included some type of diagnostic service (for example, over half of the visits included a limited history or physical examination), and the majority of visits included some form of therapy (most commonly a prescription for medicine). At about 18% and 12% of visits, respectively, internists and general/family practitioners devoted a significant part of the visit to medical counseling defined as advice or counsel about diet, change of

Table 1.3
Reasons for Ambulatory Visits to Internists: United States, January to December 1975[a]

	Reasons Named by Patients					Principal Diagnoses Named by Physicians			
Rank	20 Most frequent patient problems, complaints, or symptoms and NAMCS code[b]		Percentage of visits	Cumulative percentage of visits	Rank	20 Most common ICDA 3-digit categories and code[c]		Percentage of visits	Cumulative percentage of visits
1	General and required physical examinations	900, 901	5.6	5.6	1	Essential benign hypertension	401	9.3	9.3
2	Pain in chest	322	4.6	10.2	2	Chronic ischemic heart disease	412	7.9	17.2
3	Problems of lower extremity	400	4.4	14.6	3	Diabetes mellitus	250	4.5	21.7
4	Fatigue	004	4.0	18.6	4	Medical or special examination	Y00	4.1	25.8
5	Abdominal pain	540	3.7	22.3	5	Acute upper respiratory infection	465	2.6	28.4
6	High blood pressure	205	2.9	25.2	6	Neuroses	300	2.3	30.7
7	Problems of back region	415	2.8	28.0	7	Osteoarthritis and allied conditions	713	2.3	33.0
8	Cough	311	2.7	30.7	8	Symptomatic heart disease	427	2.0	35.0
9	Problems of upper extremity	405	2.4	33.1	9	Medical and surgical aftercare	Y10	1.8	36.8
10	Vertigo—dizziness	069	2.3	35.4	10	Rheumatoid arthritis and allied conditions	712	1.6	38.4
11	Shortness of breath	306	2.2	37.6	11	Obesity	277	1.6	40.0
12	Headache	056	2.0	39.6	12	Observation, without need for further medical care	793	1.3	41.3
13	Throat soreness	520	1.8	41.4	13	Emphysema	492	1.3	42.6
14	Diabetes mellitus	991	1.7	43.1	14	Hay fever	507	1.2	43.8
15	Cold	312	1.6	44.7	15	Other eczema and dermatitis	692	1.2	45.0
16	Visits for medication	910	1.4	46.1	16	Other nonarticular rheumatism	717	1.2	46.2
17	Nervousness	810	1.3	47.4	17	Synovitis, bursitis, and tenosynovitis	731	1.1	47.3
18	Problems of face, neck	410	1.2	48.6	18	Arthritis, unspecified	715	1.0	48.3
19	Allergic skin reactions	112	1.2	49.8	19	Symptoms referable to respiratory system	783	1.0	49.3
20	Other symptoms referable to cardiovascular system	220	1.1	50.9	20	Bronchitis, unqualified	490	1.0	50.2

[a] Adapted from *Office Visits to Internists: National Ambulatory Medical Care Survey, United States, 1975*, advance data, No. 16, February 7, 1978.
[b] Symptomatic groupings and code number inclusions are based on a symptom classification developed for use in the NAMCS.
[c] Diagnostic groupings and code number inclusions are based on the *Eighth Revision International Classification of Diseases, Adapted for Use in the United States.*

Table 1.4
Reasons for Ambulatory Visits to General and Family Practitioners: United States, January to December 1975[a]

	Reasons Named by Patients					Principal Diagnoses Given by Physicians			
Rank	Most frequent patient problem, complaint, or symptom and NAMCS code[b]		Percentage of visits	Cumulative percent	Rank	Most common principal diagnosis and ICDA code[c]		Percentage of visits	Cumulative percentage
1	General and required physical examinations	900, 901	4.9	4.9	1	Medical or special examination	Y00	6.3	6.3
2	Problems of back	415	4.1	9.0	2	Essential benign hypertension	401	5.9	12.2
3	Throat soreness	520	3.8	12.8	3	Acute upper respiratory infection, site unspecified	465	3.6	15.8
4	Problems of lower extremity	400	3.8	16.6	4	Diabetes mellitus	250	2.5	18.3
5	Abdominal pain	540	3.1	19.7	5	Medical and surgical aftercare	Y10	2.4	20.7
6	Problems of upper extremity	405	3.1	22.8	6	Acute pharyngitis	462	2.2	22.9
7	Cough	311	3.0	25.8	7	Chronic ischemic heart disease	412	2.2	25.1
8	Visit for medication	910	2.7	28.5	8	Other eczema and dermatitis	692	2.2	27.3
9	Fatigue	004	2.7	31.2	9	Influenza, unqualified	470	2.1	29.4
10	Cold	312	2.6	33.8	10	Obesity	277	2.1	31.5
11	Headache	056	2.5	36.3	11	Neuroses	300	1.8	33.3
12	Pregnancy examination	905	2.4	38.7	12	Bronchitis, unqualified	490	1.7	35.0
13	Pain in chest	322	2.1	40.8	13	Acute tonsillitis	463	1.7	36.7
14	Allergic skin reaction	112	2.0	42.8	14	Arthritis, unspecified	715	1.5	38.2
15	Wounds of skin	116	2.0	44.8	15	Cystitis	595	1.4	39.6
16	High blood pressure	205	1.9	46.7	16	Otitis media	381	1.3	40.9
17	Surgical aftercare	986	1.9	48.6	17	Osteoarthritis	713	1.2	42.1
18	Weight gain	010	1.6	50.2	18	Synovitis, bursitis	731	1.2	43.3
19	Vertigo—dizziness	069	1.5	51.7	19	Other nonarticular rheumatism	717	1.2	44.5
20	Problems of face, neck	410	1.4	53.1	20	Diarrheal disease	009	1.2	45.7
21	Earache	735	1.3	54.4	21	Menopausal symptoms	627	1.1	46.8
22	Fever	002	1.3	55.7	22	Chronic sinusitis	503	1.1	47.9
23	Gynecologic examination	904	1.2	56.9	23	Hay fever	507	1.1	49.0
24	Shortness of breath	306	1.1	58.0	24	Sprains, strains of sacroiliac region	846	1.0	50.0
25	Flu	313	1.1	59.1	25	Inoculations and vaccinations	Y02	1.0	51.0

[a] Adapted from *National Ambulatory Medical Care Survey of Visits to General and Family Practitioners, January–December 1975*, advance data, No. 15, December 14, 1977.
[b] Symptomatic groups and code number inclusions are based on a symptom classification developed for use in the NAMCS.
[c] Diagnostic groupings and code number inclusions are based on the *Eighth Revision International Classification of Diseases, Adapted for Use in the United States.*

Table 1.5
Percentage Distribution of Visits to Office-Based Generalists, by Diagnostic and Therapeutic Services Ordered or Provided, Duration of Visit, and Prior Visit Status: United States, January to December 1975[a]

Diagnostic and Therapeutic Services Ordered or Provided[b]	Percentage of Visits	
	To internists	To general and family practitioners
NO SERVICES PROVIDED	1.3	1.7
DIAGNOSTIC SERVICES PROVIDED		
Limited history or examination	61.4	55.6
Clinical laboratory test	38.5	21.6
X-ray	13.1	6.2
Blood pressure check	61.4	40.2
EKG	14.0	2.3
Hearing test	1.5	0.8
Vision test	2.4	1.4
Endoscopy	1.6	0.6
THERAPEUTIC SERVICES PROVIDED		
Drug administered or prescribed[c]	49.5	55.6
Injection	11.6	21.5
Immunization or desensitization	2.6	3.7
Office surgery	1.5	5.2
Physiotherapy	1.1	3.3
Medical counseling	17.8	11.7
Psychotherapy or therapeutic listening	2.7	2.9
OTHER SERVICES PROVIDED	1.7	3.6
DURATION OF VISIT[d]		
0 min (no face-to-face encounter with physician)	0.7	1.7
1–5 min	5.6	20.5
6–10 min	24.8	34.1
11–15 min	35.6	24.9
16–30 min	24.6	17.0
31 min or more	8.7	1.9
PRIOR VISIT STATUS		
Patient seen for the first time	13.1	12.7
Patient seen before for another problem	20.9	30.5
Patient seen before for current problem	66.0	56.8

[a] Adapted from *Office Visits to Internists: National Ambulatory Medical Care Survey, United States, 1975*, advance data from vital and health statistics of the National Center for Health Statistics, No. *16*, February 7, 1978, and from *National Ambulatory Medical Care Survey of Visits to General and Family Practitioners, January–December, 1975*, advance data from vital and health statistics of the National Center for Health Statistics, No. *15*, December 14, 1977.
[b] Percentage will not add to 100 because most patient visits required the provision of more than one treatment or service.
[c] Includes prescription and nonprescription drugs.
[d] Signifies time spent in face-to-face encounter between physician and patient.

habit or behavior. These data tend to underestimate the amount of time devoted to education of the patient. Observation of office practice has shown that generalists devote about 25% of their patient contact time to patient education and that some patient education in fact occurs during most visits (2).

At 66% of visits to internists and 56% of visits to general and family practitioners, the patient had been seen before for the same problem, and at only 13% (for both groups of physicians) was the patient seen for the first time. These findings point out another distinctive feature of ambulatory medicine—that the decisions made by the generalist usually concern problems already known to him in patients whom he has seen before. The implications of these facts are discussed later in this chapter.

Telephone encounters and *home visits* are two aspects of ambulatory care which have not been studied quantitatively as part of office practice. Nonetheless, both play an important role in the care of ambulatory patients—telephone encounters because they enable physicians and patients to handle many problems efficiently, and home visits, for selected patients, because they enable the physician to provide care to patients who are too frail to make office visits or they enable the physician to learn facts about his patients' home conditions which may facilitate management of their problems at future office visits.

The Domain of Self-Care

Before making visits to physicians, patients usually attempt to diagnose and treat their own symptoms. Studies of the domain of self-care have shown that at any one time approximately 30% of persons are taking nonprescribed medications or are engaged in self-care for a problem for which they have not consulted a physician (8). The frequency distribution of conditions managed by self-care has been estimated by Fry (6) on the basis of many years of general practice in a community well known to him: 25% upper respiratory infections, 20% musculoskeletal symptoms, 20% emotional problems, 10% acute gastrointestinal symptoms, 5% skin rashes, and 20% miscellaneous other symptoms.

The time interval between the onset of symptoms and the decision to go to the physician (*i.e.*, the duration of self-care) is shown for a number of representative conditions in Table 1.6, adapted from NAMCS. Not surprisingly, those acute infections for which self-care failed were mostly seen within a few days, while a majority of subacute problems such as headache and back symptoms were seen after at least 1 week of self-care.

The physician sees only the failures from this informal system of care. As part of his approach to each new problem, he should inquire about the patient's "working diagnosis" and etiological hunches. Such inquiry is often the most efficient way to learn about the roots of a problem, particularly a chronic problem.

Self-care *before* professional care is an important way in which the patient, not the physician, makes the decisions in the domain of ambulatory medicine.

Table 1.6
Percentage Distribution of New Problem Office Visits by Time since Onset of Complaint or Symptom, according to Selected Principal Reasons for Visit: United States; January–December 1977[a]

Principal Reason for Visit	Total	Time since Onset of Complaint or Symptom					
		<1 day	1–6 days	1–3 wk	1–3 mo	>3 mo	Not applicable
		%					
All new problem visits	100.0	8.2	37.3	15.6	10.3	13.9	14.8
Symptoms of throat	100.0	6.9	77.9	10.6	2.3	1.9	0.4
Cough	100.0	3.3	73.0	18.6	2.9	2.1	0.2
Head cold, upper respiratory tract infection	100.0	6.2	72.5	16.5	3.0	1.1	0.7
Fever	100.0	17.6	76.4	4.7	0.2	1.0	
Headache	100.0	5.1	35.6	19.0	16.5	19.7	3.2
Back symptoms	100.0	6.5	37.6	26.4	11.8	16.2	1.5
Chest pain	100.0	7.6	45.8	22.6	9.3	13.6	1.2
Laceration, upper extremity	100.0	70.4	15.4	7.8	3.0	2.1	1.3

[a] From *National Ambulatory Medical Care Survey, 1977, Summary.* National Center for Health Statistics, Hyattsville, Md., 1979.

The patient's primary role in carrying out the plan of care *after* visiting the physician has already been emphasized in the expanded definition of the ambulatory patient given above. These two features combined confirm the primacy of the patient's decisions in influencing the course of events in ambulatory medicine.

The Temporal Dimension in Ambulatory Medicine

The critical temporal dimension of ambulatory medicine cannot be appreciated in the information from NAMCS contained in Tables 1.1–1.6. Table 1.7 shows the 5-year profile of care, mostly ambulatory care, for an elderly woman followed from 1975 through 1979. This patient's story illustrates each of the following important questions for which only the passage of a significant period of time provides the answers:

1. What is the significance of a recent symptom? (e.g., the temporal headache for 1 year reported in 1975, subsequently stable for 5 years.)

2. What is the advisability of initiating a referral for a problem? (e.g., cataract problem identified but asymptomatic in 1975, evaluated when more symptomatic in 1978 and classified as not mature.)

3. How well will the patient (or the patient's family) cooperate with the recommended care? (e.g., the digoxin for heart failure, taken reliably for 5 years.)

4. What is the impact of treatment upon the patient's health? (e.g., adding a diuretic in 1978; heart failure gradually improved during the month following diuretic.)

5. What is the impact of intercurrent medical problems upon the patient's usual activities? (The answer to this question varied over time depending upon intercurrent problems: during the 5 years the patient's ambulation deteriorated greatly; however, other valued activities such as crocheting and canning did not.)

GOALS OF AMBULATORY PATIENT CARE

The Patient's Expectations

The goals of ambulatory patient care are determined by the fact that the patient is residing at home, not in an institution. Residence at home provides a set of expectations which differ greatly from those created by hospital confinement. They are the same expectations that are held by an individual who has not in fact become a patient: that he will play as active a role as possible in the life of his family and community; that he will be as capable as possible of taking care of basic needs such as nutrition, clothing, hygiene, travel, etc.; that on an average day he will be as free as possible of physical and emotional symptoms while engaging in his usual activities; and that he will be generally satisfied with his situation in life. Depending on the severity of his medical problem, an ambulatory patient may be greatly, moderately, or not at all constrained from attaining these expectations. But by virtue of living at home, he will be dealing with these expectations daily, in marked contrast to hospitalized patients for whom these expectations must await return to home.

In ambulatory medicine, then, the ultimate goals of care can be equated with those goals of any individual who is living at home in his community. These goals contain certain implications for the practice of ambulatory medicine.

Implications for Practice

First, in order to decide how any patient is doing, the physician must know about the individual's particular expectations; this usually involves learning about the makeup of the patient's household, about the patient's usual role in the household, and about the patient's usual occupational and recreational activities.

Second, the kind of information described above is particularly important in clinical preventive medi-

**Table 1.7
Profile of 5 Years in the Care of an Elderly Patient (Each Problem *Italicized*)**

Feature	1975	1976	1977	1978	1979
Encounters	Initial visit, 4 office visits, many phone calls	3 office visits, many phone calls	5 office visits, 2 hospital admissions, 1 home visit, many phone calls	4 office visits, many phone calls	4 office visits, many phone calls
Principal medical problems	*Acute myocardial infarction* (mild congestive heart failure; digitalized home management by patient's choice)	Stable (digoxin)	Stable (digoxin)	Congestive heart failure (plus diuretic)	Stable (digoxin, diuretic)
	Degenerative joint disease (knees for years; cervical spine for years)	Waxes and wanes (A.S.A., Motrin)	Same (coated A.S.A.)	Same (coated A.S.A.)	Same (coated A.S.A.)
	Temporal *headaches* for 1 yr (erythrocyte sedimentation rate 30)	Rarely	Rarely	Rarely	Rarely
	Hearing loss (ear, nose, and throat examination: senile high frequency, no prescription)	Stable	Stable	Stable	Stable
	Bilateral cataracts	Stable	Stable	Referred (not mature)	Stable
	Leukoplakia, mouth (biopsy: not malignant)	Stable	Stable	Stable	Referred for change in appearance (biopsy: not malignant)
	Hematocrit 35 (guaiac-negative)	Stable	Stable	Stable	Stable
	Constipation (for years)	Waxes and wanes (over-the-counter) (OTC laxative p.r.n.)	Same (OTC laxative p.r.n.)	Same (OTC laxative p.r.n. and stool softener)	Same (OTC laxative p.r.n. and stool softener)
		Leg cramps (quinine h.s.)	Minimal (quinine h.s.)	Same (quinine h.s.)	Same (quinine h.s.)
		Left cerebral *transient ischemic attack (TIA)*	Left *cerebrovascular accident (CVA)* (hospital, physical therapy)	Stable (right hemiparesis)	Left CVA (home management)
			Dog bite (cellulitis)	No recurrence	No recurrence
			Rectal bleeding (hospital, negative workup)	No recurrence	No recurrence
			Dysuria (culture negative)	*Family* temporarily "exhausted" (Visiting Nurses Association)	Family doing well
				Painful toe	Persists (codeine)
				Appetite lost temporarily	No recurrence
Overall profile	87-yr-old widow living with daughter's family, ambulatory and independent in the home, mentally intact, crochets and cans food; weight 166; multiple medical problems identified at initial visit (above)	88 yr old, status the same; weight 160; 2 new problems (above)	89 yr old, ambulation with walker assistance after CVA; weight 151; 4 new problems (above), hospitalized twice	90 yr old, status the same; weight 140; 3 new problems (above)	91 yr old; ambulation more impaired after second CVA; mentally intact, crochets and cans food; weight 139; no new problem

cine, in which accomplishment is assessed in terms of the patient's degree of *wellness* rather than his degree of sickness. Assessing wellness essentially means determining how successfully patients are meeting their own expectations and determining what health risks they have. For example, a 40-year-old mother who is happily married, free of chronic disease, has stopped smoking, has had periodic negative Pap smears and breast examinations, and drinks alcohol only socially would be assessed as very well. If everything was the same but she smoked three packs of cigarettes daily she would be assessed as only relatively well because of the major risk posed by heavy tobacco exposure. If she was recently divorced, had stopped seeing friends, and was smoking and drinking heavily, she would be assessed as not very well, even though she might not complain of any particular symptoms or have objective evidence of any disease.

Third, knowledge of how well a patient is meeting his expectations is often critical in managing that patient's medical problems. This is because management of an ambulatory patient should be directed not just at physiological disturbances, but also at social disruptions which accompany an illness. This point can be illustrated by a common example, namely, that of the head of a household who has had an uncomplicated myocardial infarction. After 3 months, the patient may be assessed as "status post myocardial infarction—doing well." If he is back at work, then he is indeed "doing well." If he is not back at work and is financially stressed, then he is "not doing well" (even though his cardiovascular status is stable), and he probably needs additional support from his physician.

KNOWLEDGE AND SKILLS CENTRAL TO AMBULATORY MEDICINE

Spectrum of Events in the Care of an Ambulatory Patient

The picture provided by the National Ambulatory Medical Care Survey and other studies of office practice has clear implications for the clinical knowledge and the skills which are most important in the practice of ambulatory medicine. The principal requirements are: knowledge derived from clinical epidemiological studies and skills in communication with patients, in record keeping, and in coordination of care. This can best be illustrated by reviewing the events which may occur whenever an ambulatory patient presents to his physician with a problem (Table 1.8).

First, the physician *reaches a working diagnosis* for the patient's problem. As discussed below, this may vary from a rather nonspecific summary of the patient's situation to a working diagnosis based upon widely accepted criteria.

As a corollary to diagnosing a certain condition,

Table 1.8
Events Which May Occur When an Ambulatory Patient Presents to His Physician with a Problem

Physician reaches a working diagnosis
Physician recognizes the time span during which this problem will be significant for the patient
Actions taken by the physician after the working diagnosis
  Physician initiates management plan
    Patient education
      Prognosis of condition without treatment
      Prognosis with treatment
      Costs of treatment (money, side effects, behavior change)
    Treatment
      Drugs (schedule, dose, when and how to assess impact of drug, when to expect and how to recognize common side effects)
      Activity change
      Diet change
      Rehabilitation service (by referral)
    Referral for expert opinion
Physician monitors response to treatment
Physician monitors for complications of treatment
    Inadequate response
      Patient nonadherence
        Determine reason
      Inadequate drug regimen
        Adjust medication
        Re-evaluate
    Unacceptable side effects
      How to recognize
      How to manage
      When to re-evaluate
Physician monitors for complications of condition, with or without treatment
    New, recurrent, or worsening morbidity which can be managed in ambulatory setting
    New, recurrent, or worsening morbidity requiring hospitalization
      Indications for hospital care
      Special considerations after discharge
        Treatment adjustment anticipated after hospital discharge
        Activity adjustments
        Rehabilitation needs
Physician revises the working diagnosis

the physician usually *recognizes the interval of time over which that condition will be important* for the patient. This requires that the physician be familiar with studies of the condition, treated and untreated, as described below. The projected time interval will determine much of what the physician tells the patient and will indicate how long the condition should be followed. Common examples are (a) conversion to tuberculin positivity, a condition which has implications for the rest of the patient's life, and (b) the development of acute mononucleosis, a condition which usually has implications for only about 1 month.

In ambulatory practice, the majority of the physician's time is devoted to *actions which follow the working diagnosis* (see Table 1.8), *i.e.*, initiating care, managing problems associated with treatment, managing complications of the primary condition, and at times revising the working diagnosis. As discussed below, effective communication, record keeping, and coordination of services are always needed in carrying out these actions.

The *use of diagnostic skill* continues to be very important after the working diagnosis is made; this process is often referred to as "assessment" of the patient's problem. In ambulatory practice, where most visits are for already known conditions (see Table 1.5), the ongoing assessment of the patient is often more challenging than making the initial diagnosis, as illustrated by the following common examples.

Patient Education

A young mother seen in an emergency was given the diagnosis of low back pain. At her physician's office, 1 week later, she reported no improvement. Inquiry indicated that she had continued to lift heavy items at home and was not aware of proper body mechanics (educational diagnosis: patient not aware of appropriate change in activities). In her return phone call 1 week later, she reported that the back pain had resolved after she adopted the correct lifting techniques which were recommended by her physician.

Prescribing Treatment

An elderly woman was prescribed a small dose of digoxin for her congestive heart failure, after her electrolytes and creatinine were checked and found to be normal (assessment: safe to utilize digoxin). Two weeks later, a digoxin level was obtained and found to be in the therapeutic range (assessment: adequate and safe digitalization).

Problems Associated with Treatment

A hypertensive patient, usually well controlled on his medical regimen, had a very high blood pressure at a routine visit. Inquiry about diet and the findings of trace edema plus a 10-pound weight gain suggested the diagnosis: loss of blood pressure control due to excess salt intake.

Complications of an Established Condition

A patient with a history of cerebrovascular accident developed grand mal seizures for the first time 2 months after returning home from the hospital. Evaluation showed no new cause for the seizures. Diagnosis: seizure disorder complicating a stroke.

Revising the Working Diagnosis

A patient with periodic exacerbations of his chronic obstructive pulmonary disease developed an increase in sputum (working diagnosis: exacerbation of chronic obstructive pulmonary disease) which did not show the usual improvement after stopping cig-

arettes for 2 weeks. An x-ray at that time showed a right hilar mass (revised diagnosis: probable bronchogenic carcinoma).

Clinical Epidemiology

Feinstein has defined clinical epidemiology as follows:

"The territory is the clinicostatistical study of diseased populations. The intellectual activities of this territory include the following: the occurrence rates and geographic distribution of disease; the patterns of natural and post-therapeutic events that constitute varying clinical courses in the diverse spectrum of a disease; and the clinical appraisal of therapeutic agents" (5) and of diagnostic tests (*author's addendum*).

Whenever information is available from clinical epidemiological studies of a patient's problem, this information should be used (together with understanding of the patient as a person) to plan care for the patient. The principal uses of clinical epidemiology are (a) making a working diagnosis, (b) understanding the natural history of a condition and the capacity of treatment to alter it, and (c) planning and monitoring treatment.

MAKING A WORKING DIAGNOSIS

In ambulatory medicine, the working diagnosis may range from "healthy without any significant risk factors," to "healthy with risk factors A and B for disease X," to "disease X."

In evaluating a patient for the presence of a risk factor or of an established disease, the physician should be aware of the *prevalence* (i.e., proportion of the population affected at one particular time) and the *incidence* (i.e., proportion of the population newly affected during a specified interval of time) of the suspected condition in the general population and in the particular subgroup(s) to which this patient belongs. This information enables a physician to follow a strategy which is particularly important in reaching a working diagnosis in ambulatory medicine: focusing upon the *probable* and not upon the possible. A familiar example of this strategy is the evaluation of a patient for hypertension. The prevalence of hypertension is 10–20% in adult citizens of the United States. The prevalence of renovascular hypertension is probably less than 0.1% in the population of hypertensive patients. Based on this information, suspicion of and evaluation for hypertension form an appropriate strategy in all adult patients, but suspicion of and evaluation for renovascular hypertension are not appropriate in most hypertensive patients.

Three principal types of clinical data are utilized to reach a working diagnosis:

A single diagnostic test, for example, a biopsy which shows a malignant neoplasm.

A quantitative deviation in a single physiological function, for example, a fasting blood glucose which satisfies a criterion for diabetes.

A cluster of observations which may include symptoms, physical signs, and laboratory test results, for example, criteria for the diagnosis of alcoholism.

There are a number of qualities by which diagnostic and screening tests can be characterized:

The reliability of the test, which is a measure of its repeatability on more than one occasion.

The objectivity of a test, which indicates the repeatability of a test by multiple observers.

The sensitivity of the test, which means the percentage of affected individuals with a positive test (true positive rate).

The specificity of the test, which means the percentage of nonaffected individuals with a negative test (true negative rate).

The predictive value of the test, which means the probability that a specific individual has a suspected condition when the test is positive or does not have the suspected condition when the test is negative. The predictive value of a test is dependent upon the prevalence of that condition in the population being tested. The predictive value is highest when the prevalence of a condition is relatively high and the specificity and sensitivity of the test are also relatively high. As shown in Figure 1.1, the predictive value of a test can be calculated when the prevalence of a condition in the population plus the sensitivity and the specificity of the test are known.

For some conditions, criteria and methods for reaching a diagnosis have been well validated. For many conditions, however, fundamental questions remain unanswered, and diagnosis must be based on what is currently known.

UNDERSTANDING THE NATURAL HISTORY AND THE IMPACT OF TREATMENT

This information is derived from longitudinal studies.

In order to learn the *natural history* of a condition (including a risk factor), a group of patients representative of the population affected by the condition must be followed longitudinally. Ideally the longitudinal study is conducted prospectively, meaning that the questions to be asked and the data to be collected are chosen before subjects are enrolled. In reality, many of the studies of the natural history of conditions have been performed retrospectively (meaning that the primary data were generated before the study was planned and that the patients selected were those available for review at the time the study was planned). At times, a satisfactory "prospective" study can be reconstructed from events which preceded the planning of the study.

In order to delineate the *impact of treatment*, the study design should assure that treated subjects are compared with untreated subjects who are similar in every important characteristic except treatment. These conditions are met best by prospective studies which are designed specifically to evaluate the impact of treatment. Again, ideally, the study is conducted prospectively; participating subjects are allocated randomly to two groups for concurrent study or the same subjects are allocated randomly to study and comparison treatments for cross-over study; the study is double blind, meaning that neither the investigator nor the subjects know who is receiving which

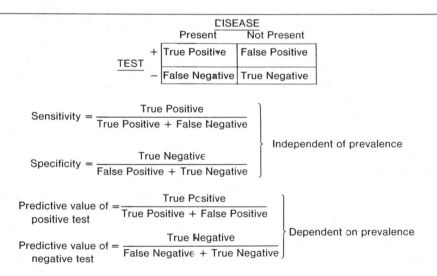

EXAMPLES:				
Prevalence of Condition	Test Characteristics		Predictive Value of a Positive Test	Predictive Value of a Negative Test
	Sensitivity	Specificity		
1%	90%	90%	9%	99.9%
10%	90%	90%	50%	98.7%

Figure 1.1   Methods for determining sensitivity, specificity, and predictive values of a test.

treatment; and a simulation of treatment in the form of a placebo is utilized in the comparison group. For many of the conditions seen in ambulatory medicine, longitudinal studies are either inadequate or have not been conducted at all. One or more of the following flaws are found commonly in existing studies: retrospective methods are used to evaluate treatments; the study group is representative of a narrow subgroup of the range of patients affected by a condition; the comparison group differs significantly from the study group; or the impact of therapy (or of a diagnostic test) on the overall health status of study subjects is not measured.

In the absence of definitive information, the physician must base his decisions upon evaluation of existing information. A good example of this approach is Liang and Fries' (9) discussion of a common problem: the management of asymptomatic hyperuricemia.

Well designed investigations will continue to fill in important gaps in existing information for some common ambulatory conditions. A good example is a cooperative study of the treatment of hypertension in elderly patients currently in progress (1).

PLANNING AND MONITORING TREATMENT

Two questions which occupy most of the physician's time in the care of ambulatory patients are: What treatment shall I recommend? What events related to the treatment should I anticipate after initiating it? The answers to these questions may be found in studies of the effectiveness of a treatment and in studies of the clinical pharmacology of any drug prescribed.

The *effectiveness* of a treatment is a measure of its impact in patients being cared for in the "real world," meaning representative community and practice settings. This concept is different from the familiar concept of the *efficacy* of a therapy, which is a measure of its impact in cooperating patients who belong to formal study groups (described above). For a number of reasons, there are few available studies of effectiveness. In recent years, patient compliance—a major determinant of the effectiveness of treatment in ambulatory patients—has been studied in "real world" settings for a variety of conditions (see Chapter 4). Such studies have generally demonstrated that adherence to a prescribed regimen in ambulatory patients is highly variable, providing insight into the difficulty of achieving expected benefits in individual patients by some of the therapies which are efficacious in study groups.

Clinical pharmacology is the source for the many details needed for appropriate administration of drugs. Apart from the impact of a drug upon a patient's condition, the physician should be aware of the following facts about each drug which he prescribes:

The initial use of the drug: appropriate starting dose and schedule; modifications in dose and sched-

ule dictated by patient age, by concurrently administered drugs, and by the presence of diseases affecting drug metabolism; time interval for the effect of the drug to be apparent; and how to assess the impact of the drug.

The major side effects of the drug: when to anticipate them, and how to detect and manage them.

The major reasons for inadequate response to a drug: nonadherence, insufficient dose of drug, antagonism of the drug by patient behavior or by concurrent drugs, and primary refractoriness to the drug; and how to recognize and manage each of these problems.

There are major gaps in the information needed to provide a complete picture for many drugs even though their efficacy has been confirmed. The following examples illustrate the types of questions which remain only partly answered:

1. Can most antihypertensive drugs be given once or twice daily, instead of 3 or 4 times daily as recommended on the basis of pharmacokinetic studies?

2. What is the minimum duration of antibiotic treatment needed to treat an acute urinary tract infection?

3. What are the minimum aspirin dose and schedule which are beneficial in prophylaxis of transient ischemic attacks?

4. Do patients develop tolerance to the antianginal effects of long acting nitrates? Is there a risk associated with abrupt discontinuation of these drugs?

5. Which diuretic drugs impair glucose tolerance, when does this undesirable effect become apparent, and how reversible is it?

Since drug therapy is the single most common action taken by generalists in ambulatory medicine (see Table 1.5), the answers to such questions are particularly important. However, the physician cannot find definitive answers to many of these questions, and must rely on sources which provide timely critical assessments of drugs* and upon his own judgment.

Communication with Patients

As stated earlier, the goals of care in ambulatory medicine can be equated with the patient's expectations for himself at home and in his community. Attaining these goals is an ongoing process, requiring some measure of continuous care for most patients and recognition that the patient has the major responsibility for carrying out the plan of care. Given these characteristics of ambulatory medicine, skill in interpersonal communication is fundamental to effective practice, for it is in this manner that the

---

* Examples are *The Medical Letter, The American Medical Association (AMA) Drug Evaluation,* and regular reviews such as the "Drugs in Perspective" reports in the *Annals of Internal Medicine* and the "Drug Therapy" reports in the *New England Journal of Medicine.*

physician motivates the patient for his or her role in adhering to the plan of care.

In recent years, the skills in interpersonal communication which are thought to be most valuable in patient care have been delineated, and a few investigations have confirmed the positive impact of these skills on the outcome of care.

PHYSICIAN-PATIENT RELATIONSHIP

A major determinant of communication is the type of relationship which the physician and patient establish. The three major types of relationship have been defined as follows by Szasz and Hollender (10):

Active-Passive. In this relationship, the physician uses all of the authority inherent in his role, while the patient does not actively participate in his treatment. It is generally applicable to emergency situations, such as the care of a severely injured victim of an automobile accident.

Guidance-Cooperation. In this relationship, the physician exercises considerable authority, but the patient is expected to cooperate, with the effectiveness of his cooperation being a factor in determining the outcome. This relationship is particularly applicable in acute diseases such as pneumonia.

Mutual Participation. In this relationship, the patient is expected to be actively responsible for his treatment. The physician works in a collaborative way with the patient and must use persuasion, rather than his authority, to obtain the goals which both he and the patient desire. This relationship is applicable in the management of subacute conditions such as recurrent bronchitis and chronic conditions such as hypertension. The relationship between a physician and a particular patient may vary between these three types depending on changes in the situation. Guidance-cooperation and mutual participation are usually appropriate for achieving desired goals in ambulatory medicine. Both include major participation by the patient, and this participation depends greatly upon the physician's skills in communication with the patient.

THERAPEUTIC COMMUNICATION

The general term for those communication skills which facilitate the process of care is "therapeutic communication." The concept of therapeutic communication embraces skills in history taking as well as skills in communication about treatment, for the manner in which the history is taken will generally influence the patient's degree of cooperation in any plan of care. Inquiry about a patient's problem may be *exploratory* or *directive*. In general, a physician will learn about the problem most efficiently by beginning with exploratory questions and moving to directive questions as his hypothesis for the diagnosis develops. Exploratory inquiry is accomplished by using open ended questions, by allowing adequate time for the patient to respond, and by picking up inportant cues from the patient and inviting the patient to elaborate on them. Directive inquiry is characterized by specific questions, by questions which yield "yes" or "no" responses, and by leading questions which may prompt the patient to give inaccurate answers. These interviewing techniques are illustrated by the following example.

The patient is a nurse who has come for an unscheduled visit because of chest pressure. She has a history of hypertension which is usually well controlled on medicine.

Exploratory Inquiry Progressing to Directive Inquiry

I: Hello, Mrs. Smith. Tell me what the problem is.

P: I am having chest pressure doctor. And I am having funny feelings in this arm (patient pauses).

I: (Interviewer says nothing.)

P: I guess it's nothing but, of course, I was thinking about my heart, with the hypertension and all.

I: Can you tell me what the pressure is like?

P: Well, it is not really pressure. I have nausea and I just feel sick this week (patient pauses again).

I: This week?

P: Yes, it has been a bad week for me (patient gives cue).

I: Oh, bad in what way? (cue followed up).

P: Well, I don't think it's so important, but at work I have been up against it this week.

I: It sounds like something is wrong at work. Do you want to tell me more about that?

P: You see, there is a new supervisor on our ward and (patient pauses) some people think I have got a gripe with her.

I: Oh?

P: You see, I have 5 years seniority over her, and, well, some think I am angry that I did not get promoted.

I: Humm (pauses). Getting back to the problem you came to see about today, can you tell me which day you began to feel sick? (Physician has hypothesis about relationship of symptoms to work stress and will now pursue the hypothesis with more specific questions.)

Directive Inquiry from the Outset

I: Hello, Mrs. Smith. You phoned to say that you are having pressure in the chest this week. Is that right?

P: Yes, doctor.

I: Well, can you please tell me exactly where in your chest you were feeling it?

P: All over my chest, doctor.

I: Show me with your hand please (patient points to entire anterior chest). Tell me how long the pressure lasts when you get it.

P: Oh, it is a problem all of the time now.

I: Is it worse when you are involved in increased physical exercise?

P: Not really.

I: Is it made worse by breathing deeply?

P: No.

I: Have you tried anything for it, for example, aspirin or pain killers?

P: No.

I: You haven't been wakened from sleep with this pressure have you? (This is a leading question.)

P: Oh, yes (pause), yes, I think so.

I: Does this chest pressure of yours go anywhere or just stay in the front of your chest? (Physician has not yet invited the patient to tell her story; no hypothesis has been suggested yet; several of the many possible causes of chest pressure have been tentatively ruled out.)

These two sketches demonstrate that the information a physician obtains and the diagnostic hypothesis which he develops may vary significantly depending on the type of inquiry utilized. As illustrated here, exploratory inquiry may lead more efficiently to the basis for the patient's symptoms than directive inquiry. This is particularly true of the nonspecific symptoms which are so common in ambulatory medicine. Exploratory inquiry, because the patient is invited to tell his story, is usually the best method for detecting the psychosocial stress which underlies many symptoms (see Chapter 9), as these are facets of the patient's experience which are more likely to be revealed in a free flowing account. Last, exploratory inquiry generally indicates genuine interest in the patient and thus promotes patient satisfaction, a powerful determinant of adherence to therapy.

In addition to the form of inquiry, a number of attributes of the interview have been identified as probable determinants of patient satisfaction. Among them are empathy, attention to the patient's privacy, use of language which is clear to the patient, avoidance of complex questions, avoidance of physical barriers between the interviewer and the patient, and maintenance of eye contact with the patient (4).

PATIENT EDUCATION

Interpersonal communication is the principal means by which the physician provides patient education. The results of this important process are delineated best in the *Health Belief Model* (3). They are:

Motivating Factors

1. Belief in the correctness of the diagnosis reached by the physician.

2. Perception that the condition represents a significant threat to the patient's body or to his social role.

3. Perception that treatment will reduce these threats significantly and that the benefits of treatment outweigh its financial, social, and behavioral costs.

Enabling Factors

1. Knowledge of the patient's specific role in treatment.

2. Positive attitude toward adhering to treatment.

Ultimate Educational Outcome: Adherence to treatment.

In planning what to say to a patient and how to say it, the physician should be aware of each of these educational outcomes. The process of educating the patient will differ greatly among individual patients with the same condition. For example, a patient with

newly detected diabetes who has a spouse with diabetes is likely already to be aware of its significance to his health and the value of treatment, and his major educational need may be knowledge of his specific role in treatment. Thus, the physician's first step is identifying the patient's educational needs. The second step is addressing those needs. The third step is assessing how well the patient has met those needs.

Investigations in "real world" practice settings have confirmed the necessity for effective communication of the plan of treatment in achieving adherence to therapy (7). In general, both verbal and written information are important in communicating knowledge of the treatment plan. Table 1.9 lists four factors which have been shown to promote accurate recall of verbally imparted instructions. Table 1.10 summarizes the effect of one of these factors, specific categorization, on recall of the type of information commonly given to patients. The written information needed for effective communication may range from clear instructions transcribed by a pharmacist onto a medication bottle, to a protocol for tapering a drug such as clonidine or prednisone, to detailed information in a brochure which outlines an exercise or diet program.

Follow-up care for ambulatory patients should always include a *careful assessment of adherence to treatment*; in this way, the physician determines the impact of whatever education the patient received about the plan of treatment. Inquiry which invites the patient to produce information will generally yield a more accurate account of what the patient is actually doing than will inquiry leading to a simple "yes" or "no." The following vignettes illustrate the difference:

Patient Asked to Produce Information

I: Now, Mrs. Smith, let's go over the medication which I have prescribed for you. Can you tell me how you are taking it?

P: Well, there is the seizure medicine that I take every day.

I: Yes. Can you tell me how often you take it?

P: Well, I am suppose to take it 3 times daily (pause).

I: Yes?

P: Well, I miss the second pill quite a few times, on the days that I get particularly busy at work and forget....

Patient Asked Yes/No Question

Table 1.9
Factors Which Have Been Shown to Increase Recall of Verbal Information [a]

Use short words and short sentences
Use explicit categorization of information (see Table 1.10)
Use repetition
Use concrete and specific instructions

[a] From P. Ley: "Memory for Medical Information." Paper presented at the Conference on Practical Aspects of Memory, Swansea, Wales, 1978.

Table 1.10
The Effect of Explicit Categorization on Recall of Verbal Medical Information Given to a Layperson[a]

Usual Presentation of Information	Explicit Categorization of Information[b]
1. You have a chest infection.	'I am going to tell you: what is wrong with you
2. And your larynx is slightly inflamed.	what tests we are going to carry out;
3. But I think your heart is all right.	what I think will happen to you;
4. We will do some heart tests to make sure.	what treatment you will need; and
5. We will need to take a blood sample.	what you must do to help yourself'.
6. And you will have to have your chest X-rayed.	First, what is wrong with you . . . (statements 1–3)
7. Your cough will disappear in the next 2 days.	Second, what tests we are going to carry out . . . (statements 4–6)
8. You will feel better in a week or so.	Third, what I think will happen to you . . . (statements 7–9)
9. And you will recover completely.	
10. We will give you an injection of penicillin.	Fourth, what the treatment will be . . . (statements 10–12)
11. And some tablets to take.	
12. I'll give you an inhaler to use.	Finally, what you must do to help yourself . . . (statements 13–15)
13. You must avoid cold draughts.	
14. You must stay indoors in fog.	
15. And you must take 2 hours rest each afternoon.	

[a] Adapted from P. Ley, P. W. Bradshaw, D. Eaves, and C. M. Walker: A method for increasing patients' recall of information presented by doctors. *Psychologic Medicine, 3:* 217, 1973.
[b] When the information in the left column was explicitly categorized (see right column), recall of information was 50% higher.

I: Now, Mrs. Smith, are you taking your seizure medicine 3 times daily as prescribed
P: Oh yes, doctor, I certainly am taking them.
I: Good. . . .

Clinical Records

Clinical records are important to document the course of events. They are valuable chiefly for reference at some later time. For in hospital medicine, since the physician is usually in contact with the patient later the same day or the next day, he can rely on his memory for details he may not have recorded; furthermore, much of the information will have been recorded by the nursing staff. In ambulatory medicine, the time between visits may be days up to months later, so that the physician can rely only upon those facts for which he has written records. The various characteristics of ambulatory medicine which have been discussed earlier point to the critical requirements of such a record, if it is to provide useful points of reference for subsequent care.

As stated earlier, the goal for the patient in ambulatory medicine is attaining and maintaining his expectations in the community despite his medical conditions. To facilitate reaching this ultimate goal, the physician must be aware of three basic sets of information about his patient. These must be recorded for subsequent referral at ambulatory visits:

1. A *social profile*, including information about those family, occupational, and recreational circumstances which determine the patient's expectations.

2. A *problem list*, that is, a list of all medical problems which have been identified in the course of the patient's care.

3. A *preventive care profile* that provides a record of periodic care with the objective of reducing risks of subsequent disease.

Although the patient is responsible for carrying out the plan of care in ambulatory medicine, the physician is responsible for developing the plan and assessing its success at serial visits. Specific recording of clinical evidence, of the interpretation of that evidence, of the specific details of the treatment plan, and of the patient's reported adherence is essential if the record is to provide a reliable reference for serial visits. The writing of problem-oriented progress notes (notes which cover separately each problem being addressed) and the use of the S (subjective) O (objective) A (assessment) P (plan) format (11) for progress notes are recording techniques well suited to these needs. To record observations about adherence to medication or about the course of one or more facets of the patient's condition, separate medication records or flow sheets may also be useful in long term care.

The physician in ambulatory practice is constrained by the limited amount of time he can give to each visit. This has several consequences with respect to what is done and what is recorded at a single visit. First, the physician sets priorities on what should be accomplished at a patient's visit. Second, the physician sifts critical from noncritical information and records only that which is critical, ideally in a format such as SOAP which facilitates efficient review at subsequent visits. Third, the physician uses what he has previously recorded to his best advantage; in particular, he refers to the record briefly to remind him of critical information *before* seeing the patient.

Coordination of Care

The third general skill which is particularly important in ambulatory medicine is skill in coordinating the patient's care. Coordination of care refers to actions which promote appropriate and effective use of services which the patient may need. During the past 20 years, the number of available laboratory services, supportive services, and subspecialty consultative services has grown enormously: there are currently more than 200 health-related professions and occupations; and the ratio of nonphysician health workers to physicians has grown from 10:1 in 1960 to more than 20:1 in 1980. The availability of so many services requires the generalist to be prudent in recommending them, and in utilizing the information or help they provide. The physician should always have information on the cost of a service to his patient, the nature of the experience the patient will undergo, and the likelihood that the service will be of value to the patient.

The services recommended for patients may involve permanent, temporary, or partial transfer of responsibility for the patient's care, or they may be strictly consultative, meaning that they provide information to be utilized directly by the referring generalist (from simple laboratory test results to specific recommendations by a subspecialty consultant).

There are two sets of guidelines which define the role of the general physician in the coordination of services which he recommends for a patient:

1. The physician should begin by ensuring that the patient understands the reason for services which are recommended; he should arrange to obtain information promptly after a service has been performed; and he should assure that the patient learns, as soon as is appropriate, the meaning of this information for the care of his condition.

2. Whenever a physician requests a service for a patient, he should be sure that proper information is given to the person providing the service. For example, there should be a clear indication of what laboratory test is required or of the facts generally needed by subspecialty consultants (see Table 1.11).

Patients sometimes obtain services for medical problems without the intercession of their personal physician. These most often include visits to the emergency room or to specialists such as ophthalmologists. Obtaining information about treatment changes or new diagnoses related to these visits is another way in which the generalist should attempt to coordinate his patient's care.

Containing Costs

In this chapter we have repeatedly emphasized that the patient has a dominant role in ambulatory medicine, particularly with regard to carrying out the plan of care recommended by the physician. However, just as in hospital medicine, the physician in ambulatory medicine is largely responsible for deciding what services the patient should purchase. Although the ways in which patients purchase services in ambulatory care vary from prepayment for all

services to paying out of pocket for each service at the time it is rendered, the impetus for purchasing those services almost always comes from the physician. This is similar to many situations in our society in which the consumer calls upon a professional or expert to make the decision to purchase a particular service.

Owing to the extraordinary increase in available medical services in the past two decades and because of the parallel increase in the cost and the utilization of these services, the containment of the cost of medical care is generally recognized as a national imperative. The need to contain costs has critical implications for generalist physicians in office practice, for it is they who coordinate most of the medical care provided in our society. Table 1.5 above indicates that, in addition to paying for the office visit, the patient, on the recommendation of his physician, purchases one or more discrete services at the majority of office visits (diagnostic testing, office procedures, prescribed medications, consultant opinions, etc.). There is little doubt that many of these services are not necessary for the health of these patients.

There are important ways in which the generalist physician can limit the costs of care. Taking a history carefully and allowing some time to pass before embarking on an extensive diagnostic workup of a new symptom is one way. Keeping himself well informed about the value to the patient's health of a costly diagnostic procedure is a second way. Devoting sufficient time to educating a patient about his condition (especially about conditions which often lead to inappropriate and costly doctor shopping by the patient) is another way. Prescribing only necessary medications and selecting the least expensive preparations (often generic preparations) is a further way. Utilizing home health services and other community services to forestall the need for hospital admission is yet another way. Unhappily, there are powerful incentives in our society for physicians to overutilize technical services, and there are important disincentives for physicians to engage in the inquiry and counseling which might obviate much inappropriate purchasing for patients. It is quite possible that there will be changes in these incentives in the future. In the meantime, the physician who asks routinely "what is the value of this service to this patient?" can identify opportunities to contain costs in his own practice every day.

Table 1.11
Information Which Subspecialty Consultants Generally Need from the Referring Physician

The specific reason for the consultation
Relevant current medical problems
Relevant current medications
What the patient has been told about the referral
The patient's attitude about the problem (if relevant)

References

General

The National Ambulatory Medical Care Survey (periodic publications issued by the Department of Health and Human Services, Washington, DC).

    Nationwide study of a probability sample of office-based physicians from all medical specialty areas, utilizing physician- and patient-generated information to delineate the ambulatory care activities of physicians and patients, started 1973.

Feinstein, AR: Clinical epidemiology. I–III. *Ann Intern Med 69:* 807, 1037, 1287, 1968.

Series of three articles describing lucidly the domain of and the uses of clinical epidemiology.

Fletcher, RH and Fletcher, SW: Clinical research in general medical journals: A 30-year perspective. N Engl J Med 301: 180, 1979.

A critical review of the clinical research methods utilized in studies reported in three general medical journals from 1946 to 1976; it is important to note that a decrease in longitudinal studies was found.

Fries, JF and Vickery, DM (editors): Take Care of Yourself: A Consumer's Guide to Medical Care. Addison-Wesley, Reading, MA, 1976.

Good book to recommend to interested patients; contains sound advice about self-care for most common symptoms.

Fry, J: Common Diseases: Their Nature Incidence and Care, Ed. 2. J. B. Lippincott, Philadelphia, 1979.

Unique account of the longitudinal course of many common diseases, based upon over 25 years of general practice in a single community.

Fuchs, VR (editor): Who Shall Live? Health, Economics, and Social Choice. Basic Books, New York, 1974.

Lucid account of the interrelationship of medical services and the economy.

Griner, PF, Mayewski, RJ, Mushlin, AI and Greenland, P: Selection and interpretation of diagnostic tests and procedures. Ann Intern Med 94: 553, 1981.

Lucid guidelines for appropriate use of diagnostic tests (special supplementary issue).

Mendenhall, RC, Tarlov, AR, Girard, RA, Michel, JK and Radecki, SE: A national study of internal medicine and its specialities: II. Primary care in internal medicine. Ann Intern Med 91: 275, 1979.

Nationwide study of a large sample of internists (including subspecialists), utilizing physician-generated information to delineate the primary care activities of internists.

Noble, J (editor): Primary Care and the Practice of Medicine. Little, Brown, Boston, 1976.

A multiauthored book which discusses in detail many of the relationships between primary care and contemporary society.

Specific

1. Amery A: Antihypertensive therapy in elderly patients: Pilot trial of the European Working Party on high blood pressure in the elderly. Gerontology 23: 426, 1977.
2. Bartlett, EE: The contributions of consumer health education to primary care practice: A review. Medical Care 18: 862, 1980.
3. Becker, MH: The health belief model and sick role behavior. Health Educ Monogr 2: 409, 1974.
4. Bowden, CL and Burstein, AG: Psychosocial Basis of Medical Practice. Williams & Wilkins, Baltimore, 1974.
5. Feinstein, AR: Clinical epidemiology I–III. Ann Intern Med 69: 809, 1968.
6. Fry, J: Common Diseases: Their Nature Incidence and Care, Ed. 2 Chap. 1. J. B. Lippincott, Philadelphia, 1979.
7. Hulka, BS, Cassel, JC, Kupper, LL and Burdette, A: Communication, compliance, and concordance between physicians and patients with prescribed medications. Am J Public Health 66: 847, 1976.
8. Kohn, R and White, KL: Health Care. Oxford University Press, New York, 1976.
9. Liang, MH and Fries, JF: Asymptomatic hyperuricemia: The case for conservative management. Ann Intern Med 88: 666, 1978.
10. Szasz, TS and Hollender, MH: A contribution to the philosophy of medicine—The basic models of the doctor-patient relationship. Arch Intern Med 97: 585, 1956.
11. Weed, LL: Medical Records, Medical Education, and Patient Care. Year Book, Chicago, 1969.

CHAPTER TWO

Preventive Care in Ambulatory Practice

L. RANDOL BARKER, M.D., and LOUIS W. MILLER, M.D.

The practicing physician's task in preventive medicine consists of both disease prevention and the promotion of optimal functioning when disease is present. Therefore, in order to plan preventive care for an individual patient, the physician must know which diseases and disabilities are preventable, and he must have a notion of the level of functioning or "wellness" which it is reasonable to expect for that patient. This important concept is discussed in more detail in Chapter 1.

PRIMARY, SECONDARY, AND TERTIARY PREVENTION

Prevention of disease and disability can be subdivided conceptually into three types according to where in the spectrum of a disease process the preventive intervention occurs (Fig. 2.1).

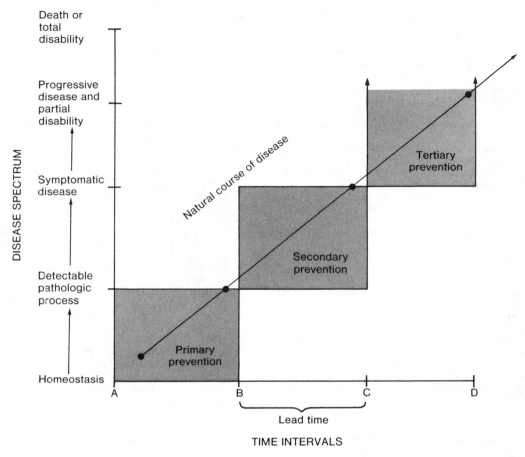

Figure 2.1 Primary, secondary, and tertiary prevention in the spectrum of a disease.

Primary prevention is any intervention which prevents a pathological process from occurring. An example is vaccination with live attenuated rubella virus vaccine which prevents the development of disease by neutralizing the offending agent before the disease process can begin. In a similar fashion, the reduction in a risk factor such as cigarette smoking through a smoking cessation program can be considered primary prevention, because this eliminates a factor known to initiate a number of disease processes. Both are primary preventive interventions since they prevent the disease during the interval *A–B* (Fig. 2.1) before any pathological process can be detected.

Secondary prevention occurs when there is intervention after a pathological process has been initiated but before symptoms occur, during the so-called "lead time" (interval *B–C* in Fig. 2.1). Secondary prevention is of value when two important conditions exist: (a) the pathological process is detectable during the lead time; and (b) treatment initiated before symptoms occur is more beneficial than treatment initiated after symptoms occur. Chemoprophylaxis of tuberculosis is an example of secondary prevention; in this instance, the patient shows evidence of the pathological process by positive delayed skin

sensitivity to tuberculin antigen and, in many cases, X-ray evidence of granuloma formation in the lungs. Behavior modification leading to weight reduction in an obese individual with impaired glucose tolerance would also be considered secondary prevention, since weight loss in such a patient may improve glucose tolerance and forestall or prevent symptomatic diabetes.

Tertiary prevention refers to the prevention of progressive disability in individuals with chronic symptomatic disease (interval *C–D* in Fig. 2.1). Physical and occupational therapy designed to prevent flexion contractures and to restore independent functioning in a stroke victim is an example of tertiary prevention.

THE COMPONENTS OF PREVENTIVE CARE

Periodic Health Assessment

Recommended periodic health assessments for patients in three broad age groups (18 to 35, 36 to 59, 60 or older) are summarized in Tables 2.1 through 2.3. These recommendations are based on a critical review of existing evidence and on recommendations compiled by others. For each recommended health

Table 2.1
Recommended Periodic Health Assessment, Ages 18 to 35

Health Assessment by Generalist	Preventable Condition	Interval (yr)	Type of Prevention	Nature of Action by Generalist	Evidence for Effectiveness of Intervention	Chapter to See for Details
INFECTION						
History of tetanus and diphtheria vaccine in last 10 yr	Tetanus, diphtheria	10	1°	Tetanus-diphtheria vaccine	Established	30
Rubella HI[a] antibody	Congenital rubella syndrome	Once	1°	Rubella vaccine	Fair evidence	30
Assess risk of pneumonococcal pneumonia	Pneumococcal pneumonia	Once	1°	Pneumococcal vaccine	Established	30
Assess risk of influenza	Influenza and complications	1	1°	Influenza vaccine	Established	30
Purified protein derivative (PPD)	Tuberculosis	5	2°	Isoniazid	Established	28
Serologic test for syphilis (STS)	Syphilis	5	2°	Penicillin, report case	Established	29
Gonococcal culture[a]	Gonorrhea	5	2°	Penicillin, report case	Established	26,91
CHRONIC DISEASE						
Weight	Morbid obesity	1	2–3°	Diet, counseling	Not established	73
Blood pressure	Stroke, congestive heart failure, renal failure	1	2°	Confirm high blood pressure, treat	Established	59
Oral examination	Loss of teeth	1	1–2°	Counseling, referral	Fair evidence	98
Hearing and vision	Hearing loss Loss of visual acuity	5	2°	Referral	Established	96
CANCER						
Cervical cytology	Disseminated cervical cancer	3[b]	2°	Referral	Fair evidence	92
Breast exam by physician	Disseminated breast cancer	1	2°	Teach breast examination, referral	Fair evidence	86
Assess breast self-exam						
LIFE-STYLE-RELATED DISEASE						
Smoking	Heart and lung disease	1	1–3°	Counseling	Not established	19
Alcohol abuse	Complications of alcoholism	1	1–3°	Counseling	Not established	20
Drug abuse	Complications of drug abuse	1	1–3°	Counseling	Not established	21
Birth control[a]	Unwanted pregnancy	1	1°	Counseling, prescribing, referring	Established	90

[a] Sexually active women only.
[b] After two negative examinations 1 year apart.

assessment, the tables provide the following information:

1. Preventable conditions for which the assessment is performed.

2. Recommended interval between assessments.

3. Type of prevention indicated (primary, secondary, tertiary).

4. Nature of the action taken by the generalist.

5. Quality of the evidence for improvement in health status through intervention (effectiveness).

6. Location of detailed information elsewhere in this book.

For a number of the health assessments recommended in the tables, the evidence for the effectiveness of intervention is rated as fair or not established. Nevertheless, these are included because the disease consequences related to them are significant and because there is a consensus that preventive intervention is probably effective. For some of these health assessments and for others not yet recommended, future investigations will probably provide more conclusive evidence for the effectiveness of intervention in improving health status. The physician can decide for himself the value of additional health assessments by asking the questions listed in Table 2.4.

Table 2.2
Recommended Periodic Health Assessment, Ages 36 to 59

Health Assessment by Generalist	Preventable Condition	Interval (yr)	Type of Prevention	Nature of Action by Generalist	Evidence for Effectiveness of Intervention	Chapter to See for Details
INFECTION						
History of Tetanus and diphtheria vaccine	Tetanus, diphtheria	10	1°	Tetanus-diphtheria vaccine	Established	30
Assess risk of influenza	Influenza and complications	1	1°	Influenza vaccine	Established	30
Assess risk of pneumococcal pneumonia	Pneumococcal pneumonia	Once	1°	Pneumococcal vaccine	Established	30
Purified protein derivative (PPD)	Tuberculosis	5	2°	Isonioazid	Established	28
Serologic test for syphilis (STS)	Syphilis	5	2°	Penicillin, report case	Established	29
CHRONIC DISEASE						
Weight	Morbid obesity	1	2–3°	Diet, counseling	Not established	73
Blood pressure	Stroke, congestive heart failure, renal failure	1	2°	Confirm high blood pressure, treat	Established	59
Oral examination	Loss of teeth	1	1–2°	Counseling, referral	Fair evidence	98
Tonometry,[a] visual acuity	Loss of vision	5	2°	Referral	Fair evidence	93, 94
Hearing	Hearing loss	5	2°	Referral	Established	93
CANCER						
Cervical cytology	Disseminated cervical cancer	3[b]	2°	Referral	Fair evidence	92
Breast examination by physician	Disseminated breast cancer	1	2°	Teach breast exam, referral	Established	86
Assess breast self-examination						
Mammography (over 50)						
Stool for blood, rectal examination	Disseminated colon or prostate cancer	1	2°	Diagnosis, referral	Not established	34, 35
LIFE-STYLE-RELATED DISEASE						
Smoking	Heart and lung disease	1	1–3°	Counseling	Not established	19
Alcohol abuse	Complications of alcoholism	1	1–3°	Counseling	Not established	20
Drug abuse	Complications of drug abuse	1	1–3°	Counseling	Not established	21

[a] Begin age 45.
[b] After two negative examinations 1 year apart.

The health assessments recommended in Tables 2.1 through 2.3 are guidelines for average adults in the three broad age ranges. Factors which may dictate expanded or more limited health assessment for the individual patient are not included. For many of the conditions named in the tables, there are *subgroups* in the population who are at much higher risk than the average person and who may deserve more frequent or more intensive monitoring. These high risk subgroups are discussed elsewhere in the book. A characteristic which the physician should always consider when planning preventive care is the *expected longevity* of an individual patient. For example, a 55-year-old patient with inoperable lung cancer should receive influenza vaccine but should not receive the other preventive care recommended for patients 36 through 59 years of age. On the other hand, a 50-year-old patient who has survived an uncomplicated myocardial infarction at the age of 48 has a reasonable life expectancy and should be offered all of the preventive care recommended for an individual in his age group.

Preventive Care for Established Conditions

Preventive care pertains to the management of a patient's established condition as well as to early detection and treatment for asymptomatic conditions. In an office practice consisting largely of patients with established conditions such as diabetes, congestive heart failure, and degenerative joint disease, the physician may improve the health of his patients as much by preventive care for these condi-

Table 2.3
Recommended Periodic Health Assessment, Ages 60 or Greater

Health Assessment by Generalist	Preventable Condition	Interval (yr)	Type of Prevention	Nature of Action by Generalist	Evidence for Effectiveness of Intervention	Chapter to See for Details
INFECTION						
History of tetanus diphtheria vaccine in last 10 yr	Tetanus diphtheria	10	1°	TD vaccine	Established	30
Assess risk of influenza	Influenza and complications	1	1°	Influenza vaccine	Established	30
Assess risk of pneumococcal pneumonia	Pneumococcal pneumonia	5	1°	Pneumococcal vaccine	Established	30
Purified protein derivative (PPD)	Tuberculosis	5	2°	Isoniazid	Established	28
Serologic test for syphilis (STS)	Syphilis	5	1°	Penicillin, report case	Established	29
CHRONIC DISEASE						
Weight	Morbid obesity	1	2–3°	Diet, counseling	Not established	73
Blood pressure	Stroke, congestive heart failure, renal failure	1	2°	Confirm high blood pressure, treat	Established	59
Tonometry, visual acuity	Loss of vision	5	2°	Referral	Not established	93,94
Hearing	Hearing loss	5	2°	Referral	Established	93
CANCER						
Cervical cytology[a]	Disseminated cervical cancer	2–3	2°	Referral	Fair evidence	92
Breast examination by physician	Disseminated breast cancer	1	2°	Referral	Fair evidence	86
Assess breast self-examination						
Mammography						
Stool for blood, rectal examination	Disseminated colon or prostate cancer	1	2°	Diagnosis, referral	Not established	34,35
LIFE-STYLE-RELATED DISEASE						
Smoking	Heart and lung disease	1	1–3°	Counseling	Not established	19
Alcohol abuse	Complications of alcoholism	1	1–3°	Counseling	Not established	20
Drug abuse	Complications of drug abuse	1	1–3°	Counseling	Not established	21

[a] Can stop after two consecutive negative smears in this age group.

Table 2.4
Questions to Ask in Evaluating a Recommended Health Assessment

IS THE PREVENTABLE CONDITION IMPORTANT?
  What is the prevalence or incidence?
  What is the size of the attributable morbidity or the mortality?
IS PREVENTIVE INTERVENTION EFFECTIVE?
  Is intervention efficacious in study groups?
  Are compliance levels in nonstudy situations good?
  Are side effects acceptable?
  Is intervention in the asymptomatic stage more beneficial than intervention after symptoms?
DO EFFECTIVE SCREENING TESTS EXIST?
  Do they have acceptable sensitivity, specificity, and predictive value?
  Are they reliable?
  Are they practical and reasonably priced?
  Are the side effects of screening acceptable?

tions as by screening systematically for asymptomatic conditions. Appropriate preventive care for an established disease depends upon the disease, its treatment, and the expectations of the individual patient. This type of care ranges from concrete actions, such as periodic monitoring of the serum potassium in patients taking digitalis and diuretics, to techniques such as short term counseling for a survivor of a myocardial infarction who is showing early symptoms of depression. The strategies for optimal preventive management of specific conditions are emphasized in subsequent chapters of this book. Fundamental to these strategies are the two characteristics they share with early detection and treatment of asymptomatic disease:

1. The physician, not the patient, usually initiates the care.

2. This type of care is designed to protect health

BALTIMORE CITY HOSPITAL
MEDICAL CLINIC
PREVENTIVE CARE AND
FOLLOW-UP CARE FLOW SHEET

	Baseline Information Year						Year					
PREVENTIVE PROFILE	Hx/ PE						Special Senses:					
	Cigarettes						Visual Acuity					
	ETOH/ Drugs						Tonometry/ Discs-Fields					
	Weight						Hearing					
	BP						Dental					
	Hernia											
	Rectal/pelvic prostate						Flu Vacc Pneumovax					
	Pap GC						Tetanus Rubella Titer					
	Breast Exam Mammograph											
	Hct						Breast self exam					
	Guiac						CXR EKG					
	PPD STS											
FLOW SHEET FOR SPECIFIC PROBLEM	Parameter											

A

Figure 2.2 Two examples of preventive care sheets currently in use. *A*, from Medical Clinic, Baltimore City Hospitals; *B*, from Tri-County Family Medicine Program, Dansville, N.Y.

Screening Flow Sheet

TEST	AGE 21	22	23	24	25	26	27	28	29	30	31	32	33	34	35	36	37	38	39	40	41	42	43	44	45	46	47	48	49	50	51	52	53	54	55	56	57	58	59	60	61	62	63	64	65	66	67	68	69	70
Complete History and Physical Examination	●																																																	
History of Rheumatic Fever	●																																																	
Smoking History	●																																																	
History of Alcohol Use	●	●		●		●		●		●		●		●		●		●		●		●		●		●		●		●		●		●		●		●		●		●		●		●		●		●
Blood Pressure	●					●				●				●		●				●				●						●				●						●				●						●
Weight and Height	●			●		●		●		●		●		●		●		●		●		●		●		●		●		●		●		●		●		●		●		●		●		●		●		●
1* Pap Smear	●	●		●		●		●		●		●				●				●				●				●		●				●		●				●										
2* Cholesterol	●			●				●		●		●				●				●				●																										
3* VDRL	●					●												●						●																										
4* PPD	●																																																	
5* Stool for Occult Blood	●									●										●		●		●		●		●		●	●	●		●	●	●	●	●	●	●	●	●	●	●	●	●	●	●	●	●
Teach Self Palpation Breast, Neck, Testes																				●										●										●										
Teach to Report Mouth Sores or Lesions																				●										●										●										
Teach to Report Post Menopausal Bleeding																																																		
B Physician Breast Check	●	●		●		●		●		●		●		●		●		●		●		●		●		●		●		●	●	●		●	●	●	●	●	●	●	●	●	●	●	●	●	●	●	●	●

JCM 471967

prospectively; this is true even when "health" may mean, for an individual patient, a sedentary existence in his own home instead of a hospital admission for a problem (digitalis intoxication, for example, which should have been prevented.)

The General Examination

In addition to the recommendations in Tables 2.1 through 2.3, most physicians will perform a *baseline general examination* (history, physical, and laboratory tests) for some or all of their ambulatory patients. In addition to a baseline examination, some physicians will perform a *periodic general examination* on some or all of their patients. The content of these general examinations will vary from patient to patient and from physician to physician. As contrasted with most of the practices recommended in the tables, there is no firm evidence that general medical examinations benefit the average patient directly. However, general examinations may be advantageous in other ways. For example:

1. A "normal" general examination can provide reassurance, especially to the patient who expressly wants to know if he is in good health.

2. Baseline information is obtained (and documented) which may be of value in assessing symptoms occurring at a later date.

3. Occasionally an asymptomatic condition that can be treated, such as an abdominal aneurysm, is found.

Risk of Labeling

In addition to the benefit which accrues to the patient from appropriate preventive care, there is a risk of creating new morbidity due to the "labeling" which accompanies a positive finding. This risk has been documented for a number of common conditions (1, 3–5). In two ways, the physician can prevent much of the morbidity created by labeling: (a) by confirming that a problem is present, usually by repeat observations, before informing a patient; and (b) by taking the time to explain the meaning of the problem to the patient and to respond to his questions.

Extending Prevention to the Family and the Community

The physician should take action to extend preventive care beyond the individual when this is appropriate. In some instances, he should recommend preventive care for members of a patient's family and an evaluation of the relatives of patients with certain chronic diseases which show a tendency to occur in other family members. γ-Globulin prophylaxis for the family of a patient with infectious hepatitis is a classic example. Equally important is the recommendation of routine breast examination for the daughters of a woman with breast cancer. Prevention should be extended to the community at large when

the physician diagnoses a notifiable communicable disease in an individual patient (see Table 2.5). Similarly, the physician should report to local health authorities any suspected occupational disease in an individual worker. Such reporting may be critical in protecting the health of other workers in that environment (see Chapter 7).

PRACTICING PREVENTIVE CARE

Model approaches to practicing preventive care have been described for a variety of ambulatory care settings (2, 8). It is generally agreed that preventive care must be planned carefully if it is to be offered routinely to patients in a busy practice. Three important considerations in this regard are scheduling of preventive care, documenting of preventive care, and motivating the patient.

Scheduling Preventive Care

In the generally healthy adult who comes for treatment of an acute illness or who calls for a healthy patient examination, a separate visit should be scheduled for preventive care. Thereafter, annual visits should be scheduled. These visits should include those health assessments which are appropriate for the individual patient (see Tables 2.1 to 2.3). In the patient with established chronic disease, periodic preventive care can usually be integrated into follow-up care for the patient's chronic condition, thus obviating the need for separate visits.

Table 2.5
Notifiable Diseases, United States[a]

Amebiasis	Meningococcal infections
Aseptic meningitis	Mumps
Botulism	Pertussis
Brucellosis	Plague
Chancroid	Poliomyelitis
Chicken-pox	Psittacosis
Cholera imported	Rabies
Diphtheria	Rheumatic fever, acute
Encephalitis	Rubella
Gonorrhea	Salmonellosis
Granuloma inguinale	Shigellosis
Hepatitis A	Syphilis
Hepatitis B	Tetanus
Hepatitis unspecified	Trichinosis
Legionellosis	Tuberculosis
Leprosy	Tularemia
Leptospirosis	Typhoid fever
Lymphogranuloma venereum	Typhus fever
Malaria	Murine
Measles	Rocky Mountain spotted fever

[a] Adapted from *Annual Summary 1979 Morbidity and Mortality Weekly Report*. vol. 28, no. 54, September, 1980. *Note*: Many individual states require reporting by physicians of additional diseases, including occupational diseases, food poisoning, animal bites, and regionally significant infectious diseases.

tri county

IMPROVE YOUR CHANCES OF STAYING HEALTHY
BY PERIODIC HEALTH SCREENING

There are many different diseases which can be discovered before they obviously make you ill. The early detection of these diseases is important because the sooner they are discovered the more easily they can be controlled or cured. Discovering these "hidden diseases" by tests, either in the doctor's office or by you at home, is called "periodic health screening".

Family Medicine has a health screening program we want **everyone** involved in. You should have a complete physical examination when you first come to Tri-County so we can get to know your medical problems. You should also definitely have a complete check-up if you are not feeling well or have a medical problem.

On the back of this sheet is a copy of the screening schedule which is in everybody's chart. How often each test should be done depends on how fast the disease progresses. The tests read down the side of the chart and your age is listed across the top. A black circle indicates that a particular test should be done at that age. For example, high blood pressure should be checked for every two years but women should check for breast lumps every month.

Certain problems can be detected or dealt with by you at home. These are:

1. If you smoke - stop.

2. Check for new lumps, especially in the mouth, neck and groin. Report these to your doctor if they persist more than one month.

3. WOMEN! Check your breasts for lumps every month.

4. MEN! Check for lumps on the testicles.

5. Vaginal bleeding after menopause should be reported to the doctor.

6. If you are overweight, now is the best time to start a diet.

Please take a minute to study the chart on the back of this paper; ask the doctor or nurse if you have any questions about it.

The tests are safe, simple and painless, and will only require a few minutes of your time.

Join us in the fight to keep you healthy!

Figure 2.3   Written information about preventive care given to patients in a family practice. From Dr. Paul Frame, Tri-County Family Medicine Program, Dansville, N.Y.

Most scheduled periodic health assessments can be performed by a nurse or a physician's assistant who can often make the practice of preventive care attainable in settings where the physician cannot devote adequate time to this area. However, as noted below, the physician's involvement is particularly important in motivating patient compliance in preventive care.

Documenting Preventive Care

The effectiveness of preventive care depends partly on how well the physician records the periodic assessment of the individual patient, with respect to tests done, drugs prescribed, etc. This is best accomplished by including a separate preventive care sheet in the patient's office folder. Two examples are shown in Figure 2.2. After the preventive care sheet becomes part of the patient's folder, existing information (which may be scattered in records from prior hospital or office care) as well as new information can be recorded to permit an efficient review, and, even more important, prevent unnecessary repetition of tests which have already been done. In designing a preventive care sheet, it is useful to include some unstructured space for recording preventive care information related to established conditions (e.g., serial serum potassium values in a patient with heart failure who is taking diuretics).

Motivating the Patient

Perhaps the most important factor in determining the patient's compliance with preventive care is the patient's motivation to protect his future health. It is probable that motivation to comply with any intervention is enhanced by a trusting patient-physician relationship; such a relationship usually takes time to develop. This relationship would be expected to be particularly important in promoting routine health practices before the onset of symptoms.

A number of specific strategies have been recommended for use in ambulatory practice to motivate patients toward preventive care in a general way; however, none of these has been evaluated with respect to its effectiveness. These strategies range from giving each patient a simple written explanation of screening tests and a list of recommended health-promoting behavior (see Fig. 2.3) to sophisticated methods such as the Health Hazard Appraisal method in which a patient receives a projection of his current expected longevity and the amount by which his expected longevity can be increased by modifying his habits or treating his asymptomatic risk factors (7). A little explored strategy is the use of contract-like agreements to modify behavior, signed by the patient and his physician (6). The effectiveness of such agreements probably depends greatly on the degree of trust existing between patient and physician and on skillful reinforcement by the physician and other persons significant in the patient's life.

References

General

ACS report on the cancer-related health check-up. *Ca-A Cancer J Clin* 30: 194, 1980.

Recommended periodic checkups for early detections of cervical, endometrial, breast, and colon cancer; a very detailed and carefully referenced report.

Barker, WH (ed): *Preventive Medicine in Primary Care.* Springer Verlag, New York, in press.

Proceedings of a 1980 meeting covering the theoretic and practical aspects of incorporating prevention into ambulatory practice.

Breslow, L, Somers, AR: The lifetime health-monitoring program. *N Engl J Med* 296: 601, 1977.

A comprehensive and ambitious plan with heavy emphasis on preventive counseling of patients.

Frame, PS, Carlson, SJ: A critical review of period health screening using specific criteria. *J Fam Pract* 2: 29, 123, 189, 283, 1975.

Extensively referenced review using criteria similar to those in Table 2.4 to evaluate periodic screening for 36 diseases in adults.

Healthy People. The Surgeon General's Report on Health Promotion and Disease Prevention, U. S. Dept. of HEW/Public Health Service (pub. no. 79-55071), 1979.

A philosophical and factual account of the present health status of Americans and of the broad range of specific preventive care and health-promoting actions recommended for the 1980s.

Morbidity and Mortality Weekly Report. Center for Disease Control, Department of Health and Human Services, Atlanta, Georgia.

A weekly report, available without charge, containing very current information about communicable disease incidence (for example, regional incidence of influenza), updated recommendations for communicable disease prevention, and timely reports on outbreaks of a wide variety of preventable diseases.

Specific

1. Bergman, AB and Stamm, SJ: The morbidity of cardiac non-disease in schoolchildren. *N Engl J Med* 276: 1008, 1967.
2. Frame, PS: Periodic health screening in a rural private practice. *J Fam Pract* 9: 57, 1979.
3. Hampton, ML, Anderson, J, Lavizzo, BS and Bergman, AB: Sickle-cell "nondisease," a potentially serious public health problem. *Am J Dis Child* 128: 58, 1974.
4. Haynes, RB, Sackett, DL, Taylor, DW, Gibson, ES and Johnson, AL: Increased absenteeism from work after detection and labeling of hypertensive patients. *N Engl J Med* 299: 741, 1978.
5. Knibbs, S and Jackson, JGL: *Complications of Diabetes,* edited by H. Keen and J. Jarrett, p 265. Year Book, Chicago, 1975.
6. Lewis, CE and Minich, M: Contracts as a means of improving patient compliance. In *Medication Compliance: A Behavioral Management Approach,* edited by I. Barofsky, pp. 69–76. Charles B. Slack, Thorofare, NJ, 1977.
7. Sadusk, JF, Jr and Robbins, LC: Proposal for health hazard appraisal in comprehensive health care. *JAMA* 203: 1108, 1968.
8. Thompson, RS: Approaches to prevention in an HMO setting. *J Fam Pract* 9: 71, 1979.

CHAPTER THREE

Selected Special Services: Disability, Vocational Rehabilitation, and Home Health Services

L. RANDOL BARKER, M.D.

INTRODUCTION

Maintenance of a patient's overall health often requires efforts beyond those of the physician and the patient. Frequently assistance comes from community-based agencies to which physicians may refer their patients. Many of these agencies provide services for patients with specific types of illness; the roles of these "categorical" community services are described in the appropriate chapters in this book. Other services are designed to assist sick persons regardless of their type of illness. This chapter describes the two fundamental services of this kind: (a) Social Security income support programs for disabled persons and (b) home health services. The purposes of the following discussion are to explain eligibility for these services, the nature of the benefits, and the role of the physician in enabling his patients to receive these services.

SOCIAL SECURITY PROGRAMS FOR DISABLED PERSONS

Loss or decrease of a person's ability to earn his living accompanies many illnesses. Beginning with 1954 amendments to the Social Security Act, income support for medically disabled persons has been available in the United States. Further modifications since 1954 have led to the program which exists today. The three fundamental components of the present program are Disability Insurance (DI), Supplemental Security Income (SSI), and Vocational Rehabilitation (VR). Detailed information about each of these services is available from any local Social Security Office.

DEFINITION OF MEDICAL DISABILITY

Under Social Security, disability is defined as "inability to engage in any substantial gainful activity by reason of a medically determinable physical or mental impairment which can be expected to result in death or has lasted or can be expected to last for a continuous period of not less than 12 months...."

Disability Insurance (DI—Title II)

ELIGIBILITY

To be eligible for disability insurance payments, a *disabled worker* must have paid into the Social Security Program for a minimum period of time before becoming disabled; this usually means 5 out of 10 years before the onset of disability. Today, 9 out of 10 workers pay Social Security, meaning that most persons who have worked for more than 5 years are fully insured. For younger workers (up to age 31) there are modified requirements to meet insured status.

The *dependents* of a fully insured worker who is retired, disabled, or deceased may be eligible for disability insurance payments in two situations: (a) a child who became disabled before age 22 (eligible for disability insurance payments at the time that his parent retires, becomes disabled, or dies; payments continue as long as the child's disability lasts); and (b) a widow or widower who did not work under Social Security but who became medically disabled before or within 7 years of the death of a fully insured spouse.

BENEFITS

Disability insurance payments go to disabled workers before the age of 65 (after 65, Social Security Retirement Income replaces disability payments) and to eligible children, widows, or widowers as long as they remain disabled. The first monthly disability insurance check is paid 5 months after a worker's disability has been certified; however, the 5-month "waiting period" begins as of the day the patient was disabled (for example, if a patient is certified as disabled 6 months after he actually became disabled, he receives immediately a check covering the 1 month in excess of the required 5-month wait). Supplemental Security Income (see below) is often awarded to persons who qualify for disability benefits, effective the date they apply for benefits. There is no waiting period. Income for a disabled worker is the same amount as the retirement income the worker would receive if he were 65. The average monthly payment to a disabled worker in 1979 was $370, and to a worker with a wife and dependent children, $728. In that year, DI payment was made to 3 million workers and to 2 million dependents.

In addition to income support, disabled persons under 65 receive Medicare (Social Security Health Insurance) after they have been disabled for 2 consecutive years.

THE PROCESS OF DISABILITY DETERMINATION

There are three basic steps in the process of determining medical disability.

First Step. The patient completes a detailed application at a local Social Security Office. The patient must not be gainfully employed at the time of application. Most patients will initiate disability claims by themselves, but at times the physician may be helpful in suggesting early application to a patient who may not be aware that his medical condition qualifies him for medical disability.

Second Step. The patient's physician receives a request for medical information and returns his report to the state Disability Determination Office. The report sent by the patient's physician should be succinct and precise; and it should provide objective data regarding the condition for which disability is being claimed. It should be divided into the following subheadings: history, physical, laboratory reports, diagnosis, treatment, and response. The information provided should permit the claims reviewers to determine both the severity and the duration of the patient's condition. If malingering is suspected, the report should describe the circumstances that raise doubts rather than recording this assessment without supporting information. In this report the physician is not expected to rate the work disability of the patient. The most helpful guide for completing these medical reports is the booklet entitled *Disability Evaluation Under Social Security: A Handbook for Physicians* (available free from any Social Security Office or the State Disability Determination Services). This guide, updated in 1979, contains the criteria for medical disability for most common conditions. These criteria are the basis for the decisions made by disability claims reviewers. Tables 3.1 through 3.5 contain excerpts from this manual illustrating the criteria for several common conditions: symptomatic ischemic heart disease, chronic obstructive airway disease, cerebrovascular accident, epilepsy due to major motor seizures, and arthritis of a major weight-bearing joint. Since 1980, the Social Security Administration has paid a small fee to physicians for medical reports; previously patients were expected to pay for these reports. In some states, doctors also have access to a free teledictation service for dictating their reports.

Third Step. The information provided by the patient and the physician (the disability claim) is reviewed at the State Disability Determination Office by a team consisting of a disability claims examiner and a physician. If deemed necessary, an independent medical examination is purchased by the Disability Determination Office. By law, a decision about a patient's disability claim must be made within 30 days of receipt of all medical reports at the Disability Determination Office. In keeping with the 1974 Freedom of Information Act, patients may have access to their disability claims files. If an insured worker or a dependent under the age of 22 has an impairment which falls short of the standard criteria for disability but which nevertheless prevents the individual from doing his usual job, other factors (limitations of age, education, training, work experience) may also be considered by the Disability Determination team. Most findings of disability are, however, based on the standard Social Security criteria.

APPEAL PROCESS

If the initial claim of disability has been denied, the claimant may file for reconsideration within 60 days of receiving a denial notice. The case will then be re-evaluated by a different claims examining team. If the claim is denied at this reconsideration, the claimant then has 60 days to file a request for a hearing. Hearings are conducted by administrative law judges or hearing examiners. If, again, the claim is denied, the claimant may make an additional appeal for review by the Appeals Council. After that the case must be taken to the United States District Court.

The patient's personal physician can be instrumental in assuring that his patient gets the fullest consideration in the appeals process. If the physician feels that there are aspects of the patient's illness that make it more severe than the criteria indicate, he should communicate this information in writing, together with support for his opinion, to the Disability Determination Office.

RETURN TO WORK

All claims are reviewed for referral to Vocational Rehabilitation (see below) at the time the disability decision is made. In addition, every person with medical disability is re-evaluated at least every 3 years to determine whether he is still disabled. These two processes and the following conditions are designed to encourage disabled persons to return to work: (a) Disabled beneficiaries may test their ability

Table 3.1
Impairments Qualifying a Person with *Ischemic Heart Disease* for Medical Disability under Social Security[a]

4.04 *Ischemic heart disease with chest pain of cardiac origin as described in §4.00E.*[b] With:

A. Treadmill exercise test (see §4.00F[b] and G) demonstrating one of the following at an exercise level of 5 METs or less:

  1. Horizontal or down-sloping ischemic depression of the ST segment to 1.0 mm or greater, clearly discernible in at least two consecutive complexes which are on a level baseline in any lead; OR

  2. Premature ventricular systoles which are multiform or bidirectional or are sequentially inscribed (3 or more); OR

  3. ST segment elevation to 3 mm or greater; OR

  4. Development of second or third degree heart block; OR

B. In the absence of a report of an acceptable treadmill exercise test (see §4.00G[b]), one of the following:

  1. Transmural myocardial infarction exhibiting a QS pattern or a Q wave with amplitude at least ⅓ of R wave and with a duration of 0.04 second or more. (If these are present in leads III and aVF only, the requisite Q wave findings must be shown, by labelled tracing, to persist on deep inspiration); OR

  2. Resting ECG findings showing ischemic-type (see §4.00F1[b]) depression of ST segment to more than 0.5 mm in either (a) leads I and aVL and V_6 or (b) leads II and III and aVF or (c) leads V_3 through V_6; OR

  3. Resting ECG findings showing an ischemic configuration or current of injury (see §4.00F1[b]) with ST segment elevation to 2 mm, or more in either (a) leads I and aVL and V_6 or (b) leads II and III and aVF or (c) leads V_3 through V_6; OR

  4. Resting ECG findings showing symmetrical inversion of T waves to 5.0 mm. or more in any two leads except leads III or aVR or V_1 or V_2; OR

  5. Inversion of T wave to 1.0 mm or more in any of leads I, II, aVL, V_2 to V_6 *and* R wave of 5.0 mm or more in lead aVL *and* R wave greater than S wave in lead aVF; OR

  6. "Double" Master Two-Step test demonstrating one of the following:

    a. Ischemic depression of ST segment to more than 0.5 mm. lasting for at least 0.08 second beyond the J junction and clearly discernible in at least two consecutive complexes which are on a level baseline in any lead; OR

    b. Development of a second or third degree heart block; OR

  7. Angiographic evidence (see §4.00H[b]) (obtained independent of social security disability evaluation) showing one of the following:

    a. 50% or more narrowing of the left main coronary artery; OR

    b. 70% or more narrowing of a proximal coronary artery (see §4.00H3[b]) (excluding the left main coronary artery); OR

    c. 50% or more narrowing involving a long (greater than 1 cm) segment of a proximal coronary artery or multiple proximal coronary arteries; OR

C. Resting ECG findings showing left bundle branch block as evidenced by QRS duration of 0.12 second or more in leads I, II, or III *and* R peak duration of 0.06 second or more in leads I, aVL, V_5, or V_6, unless there is a coronary angiogram of record which is negative (see criteria in §4.04B7[b]); OR

D. Left ventricular ejection fraction of 30% or less measured at cardiac catheterization or by echocardiography.

[a] From *Disability Evaluation under Social Security: A Handbook for Physicians.* HEW publication No. (SSA) 79-10089, August 1979.
[b] See Handbook for these important details.

to work for 9 months while continuing to receive benefits. After this trial work period, a determination is made whether the work constitutes substantial gainful activity (defined in 1980 as an activity which yields a monthly income of $300 or greater); if it does, benefits are stopped after an additional 3-month adjustment period. (b) If a person who is still disabled becomes unable to work again within the year after Social Security payments have stopped because of substantial gainful activity, the monthly DI benefits can be resumed, usually without a new application. (c) Medicare coverage generally can continue for 3 years after a person's DI benefits stop because of return to substantial gainful activity. If a worker starts receiving DI benefits again within 5 years after the DI was stopped, and if the patient was previously entitled to Medicare, that protection will resume immediately. (d) Work expenses related to the impairment which are paid for by a disabled person can be deducted from the patient's earnings in determining whether these constitute substantial gainful activity. This is true even if these expenses also apply to needs for daily living (such as a wheelchair). (e) In addition to disabled workers, persons disabled before the age of 22 and disabled widows and widowers can also have a trial work period.

Supplemental Security Income

Supplemental security income (SSI) is a federal program which was introduced in 1974. It is paid for out of general funds rather than Social Security funds, but it is administered by the same state agencies which administer the Disability Determination program. The application process is similar to that described above for Social Security Disability Insurance. The same criteria are used to evaluate SSI disability claims as are used for DI claims.

The basic differences between SSI and Social Security benefits are as follows: (a) *Eligibility:* SSI is available for two groups of persons when they are

Table 3.2
Impairments Qualifying a Person with *Chronic Obstructive Pulmonary Disease* for Medical Disability under Social Security[a,b]

Height (inches)	MVV (MBC) Equal to or Less Than (L/min)	AND	FEV$_1$ Equal to or Less Than (L)
57 or less	32		1.0
58	33		1.0
59	34		1.0
60	35		1.1
61	36		1.1
62	37		1.1
63	38		1.1
64	39		1.2
65	40		1.2
66	41		1.2
67	42		1.3
68	43		1.3
69	44		1.3
70	45		1.4
71	46		1.4
72	47		1.4
73 or more	48		1.4

[a] *Chronic obstructive airway disease* (due to any cause). With: Spirometric evidence of airway obstruction demonstrated by MVV (maximum voluntary ventilation) and FEV$_1$ (forced expiratory volume in 1 second), both equal to, or less than, the values specified, corresponding to the person's height. MBC = maximum breathing capacity.
[b] From *Disability Evaluation under Social Security: A Handbook for Physicians*. HEW publication No. (SSA) 79-10089, August 1979.

Table 3.3
Impairments Qualifying a Person with *Cerebrovascular Accident* for Medical Disability under Social Security[a]

Central nervous system vascular accident. With one of the following more than 3 months post-vascular accident:

A. Sensory or motor aphasia resulting in defective speech or communication; OR

B. Significant and persistent disorganization of motor function in two extremities, resulting in sustained disturbance of gross and dexterous movements, or gait and station.[b]

[a] From *Disability Evaluation under Social Security: A Handbook for Physicians*. HEW publication No. (SSA) 79-10089, August 1979.
[b] See Handbook for additional important details.

not insured by Social Security: persons under 65 who are medically disabled and all uninsured persons over the age of 65.* In addition to these two groups, persons who have "presumptive disability" (claim for total disability being processed) and disabled persons who are in the 5-month waiting period for their DI payments to begin may be eligible. Eligibility in all of these groups is based on need (total resources below

Table 3.4
Impairments Qualifying a Person with *Epilepsy Due to Major Motor Seizures* for Medical Disability under Social Security[a,b]

Major motor seizures (grand mal or psychomotor), documented by EEG and by detailed description of a typical seizure pattern, including all associated phenomena: occurring more frequently than once a month, in spite of at least 3 months of prescribed treatment. With:

A. Diurnal episodes (loss of consciousness and convulsive seizures); OR

B. Nocturnal episodes manifesting residuals which intefere significantly with activity during the day.

[a] From *Disability Evaluation under Social Security: A Handbook for Physicians*. HEW publication No. (SSA) 79-10089, August 1979.
[b] See Handbook for additional important details.

Table 3.5
Impairments Qualifying a Person with *Arthritis of a Major Weight-Bearing Joint* for Medical Disability under Social Security[a,b]

Arthritis of a major weight-bearing joint (due to any cause): With limitation of motion and enlargement or effusion in the affected joint, as well as a history of joint pain and stiffness. With:

A. Gross anatomical deformity such as subluxation, contracture, bony or fibrous ankylosis, or instability; OR

B. Ankylosis of the hip outside of the position of function (*i.e.*, at less than 20° or more than 30° of flexion measured from the neutral position) and X-ray evidence of either joint space narrowing with osteophytosis or bony destruction (with erosions or cysts); OR

C. Reconstructive surgery or surgical arthrodesis of a major weight-bearing joint and return to full weight-bearing status did not occur, or is not expected to occur, within 12 months of onset.

[a] From *Disability Evaluation under Social Security: A Handbook for Physicians*. HEW publication No. (SSA) 79-10089, August 1979.
[b] See Handbook for additional important details.

a certain defined level) and the absence of gainful employment (defined as earned monthly income of $300 or more for disability claims). (b) There is *no waiting period*; a person may receive the first SSI payment within 1 month of filing a disability claim. (c) In most states, persons who are approved for SSI are *also eligible for Medicaid* and for other social services provided by their state. (d) All persons receiving SSI are *reviewed once each year* to determine whether they are still eligible.

The maximum monthly income from SSI in 1979 was $238 for an individual and $357 for a couple. In 1979, there were 3.9 million recipients of SSI.

The patient's personal physician plays the same pivotal role in SSI application that he plays in DI application (see above). Until his report is received, no income support can be initiated for his patient.

---

* SSI for persons over 65 is similar to Social Security retirement. These claims are not handled by Disability Determination services.

Vocational Rehabilitation

State Vocational Rehabilitation agencies existed before the federal Disability Determination program was created in 1954. In many states, these agencies administer the Disability Determination program in addition to providing vocational rehabilitation services.

ELIGIBILITY

To be eligible for Vocational Rehabilitation, a person must have a disability which interferes with his capacity to obtain suitable employment or which is a threat to his present career; this does not mean that the person has to meet the criteria for medical disability discussed above. The individual must have a reasonable chance of being able to engage in a suitable occupation after Vocational Rehabilitation services are provided. A suitable occupation would include that of being a housewife provided that Vocational Rehabilitation would enable her to remain in her own home instead of requiring institutional care.

SERVICES

The services provided by Vocational Rehabilitation agencies vary from state to state. However, they usually include the following: (a) *A medical examination.* A complete medical examination is provided to determine the extent of a person's disability. (b) *Counseling and guidance.* A trained rehabilitation counselor is assigned to guide each client through the rehabilitation process. (c) *Physical aides.* Artificial limbs, braces, hearing aids, eye glasses, and wheelchairs are provided if needed. (d) *Job training.* Training for the proper job is provided when necessary. This may be given in a vocational school, college or university, rehabilitation facility, or in the home. (e) *Help with living expenses.* Board, room, transportation expenses, and other necessary expenses may be provided if needed. (f) *Equipment and licenses.* Tools, equipment and licenses necessary for getting started in the right job may be provided. (g) *Job placement.* Placement in the right job is an important part of the rehabilitation process. The abilities of each handicapped individual are carefully matched to job requirements. (h) *Follow-up.* The counselor follows up on each placement to make sure that the client's job is suitable.

THE PHYSICIAN'S ROLE

As noted above, all persons applying for disability benefits are screened for referral to Vocational Rehabilitation. For those persons, the report of the patient's physician (see above) may be utilized by the Vocational Rehabilitation agency. For persons who are not applying for medical disability, the physician will often be asked to provide a general medical report for the Vocational Rehabilitation agency. Perhaps the most important role of the general physician in this regard lies in providing personal encouragement to the patient to apply for Vocational Rehabilitation and his continued interest in the patient's progress. It has been estimated that every 1,000 dollars spent for Vocational Rehabilitation increases by 35,000 dollars the lifetime earnings of those who are rehabilitated. This economic consequence for society, in addition to the benefit to the individual, makes support of the Vocational Rehabilitation a particularly important role for the physician.

HOME HEALTH SERVICES

A consequence of illness as distressing to the patient as the loss of the ability to earn an income is the temporary or permanent loss of the ability to remain at home. Most people will require acute hospital care one or more times in their adult life and a small proportion will also require long term institutional care. The principal objectives of home health services are to minimize the need for admission to either acute or long term care facilities and to decrease the length of stay therein. Numerous studies have shown that these objectives are attained whenever home health services are utilized appropriately; but studies have also shown that home health services are underutilized and that much institutional care could be prevented by broader and more frequent utilization of these services.

The provision of home care services is a long established concept, beginning in this country with a home care program offered by the Boston Dispensary in 1796. A great resurgence of interest in home care began in 1947, with the establishment of the Coordinated Home Care Program at Montefiore Hospital in the Bronx. The provision of a broad array of home health services to a growing number of chronically ill patients caught the imagination of those who recognized the disadvantages and high cost of institutionalization. Home health agencies throughout the country have used Montefiore as a model in developing or expanding home care services. The inclusion of home health services in the coverage provided by Medicare, Medicaid, and other third party insurers has enabled home health agencies to expand greatly in the past two decades.

Range of Services

Health care provided to sick persons at home ranges from basic care provided by nonprofessional family members and friends (at times with the help of Red Cross or similar training in basic care technique), to home food services available at a nominal cost to the patient ("Meals on Wheels"), to care provided by physicians or their associates who make home visits; or by the personnel of certified home health agencies, under the supervision of the patient's physician. When professional help is involved, most of the responsibility for carrying out care is given to the patient or to a member of the patient's family; as noted in Chapter 1, it is this assumption of responsibility by the patient and his family which most clearly distinguishes ambulatory medicine from institution-based medicine.

Today there are approximately 3500 home health agencies in the United States. Agencies may be state and local health departments, nonprofit voluntary agencies, or nominally profitable proprietary agencies. The home care provided by voluntary agencies is coordinated by a visiting nurse. A substantial proportion of the care is often carried out by home health aides, analogous to nursing aides on hospital wards, under the supervision of the nurse. In recent years, nurse practitioners have been added to the staffs of many home health agencies, so that much more sophisticated care can be provided. In addition to nursing, the services may include physical, occupational, and speech therapy, dietary and social work counseling, and homemaker services. Home health agencies also provide the nursing component of hospice programs (see Chapter 18) in many communities.

The types of clinical problems most frequently referred to home health agencies are listed in Table 3.6.

Eligibility

Any patient is eligible for home health services. During the past 15 years, eligibility has been defined principally by the criteria which must be met for reimbursement by third party payors. In general, the following criteria are used: that the patient must have an active medical problem, is under the care of a physician, and requires skilled nursing or other skilled professional help, such as physical or occupational therapy.

The Physician's Role

All physicians should be well acquainted with the home health services available in their community and with the third party coverage which their patients may have for the services (see Table 3.7). Although a patient (or his family) may refer himself for home health services, orders written by the patient's physician are always needed for third party reimbursement.

Table 3.6
Problems Most Commonly Referred for Home Health Services

Postsurgical wound care
Rehabilitation after hospitalization for orthopedic problems
Congestive heart failure (dietary counseling, assessment of medication compliance)
Diabetes (supervise insulin technique, provide dietary counseling, teach urine testing, etc.)
Hypertension (supervise and reinforce compliance with medication, check blood pressure)
Incurable cancer (dietary counseling, psychological, support, hospice)
Stroke and other incapacitating neurologic problems (physical and occupational therapy)
Decubitis and stasis ulcers (supervision of dressing technique)
Dementia and older person living along (assessment of environment for health hazards)
Chronic obstructive pulmonary disease

Table 3.7
Criteria for Third Party Reimbursement for Home Health Services, Current 1981

Part A[a] or Part B Medicare

Part A pays for all covered services (skilled nursing, home health aid, social work, physical, occupational and speech therapy). Care must be provided by a certified Home Health Agency and must be medically necessary. The following conditions must be met:

1. Patient is confined to his home.
2. Need for intermittent skilled nursing, (or nursing aide); physical, occupational or speech therapy; or medical social work.
3. Physician must sign renewal of certification every 60 days.
4. No limit to the number of visits.

Medicaid

Coverage for home health services varies, by state.

Blue Cross and other private health insurance.

Coverage for home health services varies, by plan.

[a] Note that effective July 1, 1981, Part A Medicare, like part B, covers patients even if they have not been recently discharged from a hospital.

The quality of the communication between a patient's physician and the visiting nurse often determines how much the patient will benefit from home health services. When the physician provides clear and thorough initial information, when the physician is accessible to the nurse when needed, and *vice versa*, patients who would otherwise require in-hospital care can receive excellent care in their homes. Some problems are best managed at home, such as adjustment of insulin and diet in a diabetic patient with an intercurrent illness, adjustment of diuretics and diet in a patient with worsening congestive heart failure, assessment of compliance and the response to medication in a patient whose high blood pressure seems refractory to treatment at office visits, and debridement, dressing, and monitoring of a stasis ulcer of the lower extremities.

References

General

Disability Evaluation Under Social Security: A Handbook for Physicians. HEW Publication No. (SSA) 79-10089, August, 1979.
    Gives criteria for impairments which qualify a person for medical disability under Social Security (available free from local Social Security Office and State Disability Determination Service).
Davidson, RC: The future of home health agencies. J Community Health 4: 55, 1978.
    Excellent review of the present and future place of home health agencies in patient care.
Family Health and Home Nursing. Doubleday, Garden City, N.Y., 1979.
    Inexpensive, recently updated Red Cross publication explaining in detail all aspects of caring for sick persons at home.
Brickner, PW: Home Health Care for the Aged. Appleton-Century-Crofts, New York, 1979.
    Extensively referenced resource covering all aspects of home care services for elderly persons.

CHAPTER FOUR

Patient Compliance with Medical Advice

DAVID E. KERN, M.D., and WALTER F. BAILE, M.D.

INTRODUCTION

Common objectives shared by physicians and patients are the relief of symptoms, the improvement of impaired functional status, the prevention of illness, and the increase in meaningful longevity. Most frequently the patient comes to the physician with a problem. The translation of the patient's presenting complaint into a medically intelligible entity involves eliciting and recording an accurate history, the performance of a proper physical examination, ordering of laboratory tests when necessary, and the interpretation of the collected data. This is the role of the clinician as diagnostician. The second function is an educative one, wherein the physician explains the nature of the problem and its management to the patient. The third function is in most cases curative or ameliorative. Up to this point the physician has served to make sense out of an experience which may be novel and disquieting to the patient. From the physician's standpoint there is satisfaction in being able to detect a treatable entity. From the patient's standpoint there may be relief, fear, anxiety, confusion, and/or disbelief. In addition, the patient must now enter into a *therapeutic alliance* with the physician. This involves accepting a treatment which may involve taking medications, keeping follow-up appointments, undertaking preventive health measures, and/or changing deep-seated behavior patterns. The ability of a patient to form a therapeutic alliance with his physician and to share in the responsibility of his illness is in part reflected in his ability to comply with or adhere to medical advice.

From an objective standpoint the sequence of events from history-taking through prescription and patient follow-through is straightforward. Nevertheless, all too often efforts are thwarted owing to the actions of the patient.

Example: Mr. X is a 45-year-old black male who feels dizzy at work. A blood pressure check shows a reading of 180/110. He is told that his "pressure is up" and referred to a physician. Mr. X has never seen a doctor before. After an appropriate physical examination and laboratory work the diagnosis of essential hypertension is confirmed. The physician is happy because he knows that there are efficacious medicines which will prevent complications of hypertension such as stroke and congestive heart failure. The patient is given medication, takes it for a week, feels better, and then stops.

This scenario is common. Physicians, often those who are skillful diagnosticians, are frequently unsuccessful in making their ambulatory patients follow prescribed treatments, even when these are known to be efficacious.

The study of compliance in ambulatory patients is still somewhat in its infancy. Methodological problems exist in the measurement of physician variables and patient variables. Most studies of the factors associated with compliance are cross-sectional rather than prospective, making inferences of causality subject to error. Multiple factors of varying importance are involved, and the independent contribution of each in different settings has been difficult to assess. Furthermore, methods for maintaining improvements in compliance are only just beginning to be investigated. Finally, most studies of compliance have involved hospital-based ambulatory patients, leaving questions about their applicability to office practice.

DEFINITIONS AND CLASSIFICATION

Patient compliance is defined as the extent to which the patient adheres to medical advice. It encompasses taking medications, keeping appointments, undertaking recommended preventive measures, and, with respect to activities such as dieting, exercising, and ceasing to smoke or take alcohol, changing possibly deep-seated behavioral patterns. Some clinicians favor the term *patient adherence* to *patient compliance*, but the latter is more widely used.

Noncompliance can be caused by a failure to understand instructions, *noncomprehension*, or can exist in the presence of adequate understanding, *willful noncompliance*.

Noncompliance in medication taking can be classified as *errors of omission* (a prescribed medicine is not taken), *errors of commission* (a nonprescribed medicine is taken), *dosage errors* (the wrong dose is taken), and *scheduling errors* (the medicine is taken according to the wrong schedule, *e.g.*, once daily instead of twice).

Noncompliance should be viewed as a neutral term with neither negative nor positive connotations. It describes one aspect of patient behavior which may be either appropriate or inappropriate to the patient's best interests. For example, it may be appropriate for a patient with mild chronic obstructive pulmonary disease to be noncompliant in taking a regularly prescribed medicine, such as aminophylline, if it causes more distress (e.g., nausea) than relief. On the other hand, it would be inappropriate for a patient with severe hypertension to stop taking antihypertensive medication because of denial of his medical problem. Finally, it should be realized that responsibility for noncompliant behavior can rest as much with the physician as with the patient. It is not valid, for example, to blame noncompliant patients for failure to understand instructions or to realize the importance of therapy when there has been ineffective communication by the physician.

IMPORTANCE OF COMPLIANCE

Problems Caused by Noncompliance

Patient noncompliance is potentially important from at least three perspectives: individual patient care, public health efforts, and interpretation of the medical literature.

First, patient noncompliance with efficacious therapeutic regimens may thwart the goals of both physician and patient in reducing suffering, preventing illness, improving functional status, and increasing longevity. If the physician is unaware of the patient noncompliance, he may falsely attribute therapeutic failure to inadequate dosage, failure of the regimen itself, or incorrect diagnosis. Any of these conclusions could lead to inappropriate action by the physician. Thus medication might be changed or dosage might be increased, and new diagnoses entertained, so that the patient could be subjected to unnecessary procedures and testing.

Second, noncompliance may increase the cost and reduce the effectiveness of screening, immunization, and disease control programs. For example, a screening program which identifies undiagnosed hypertensives will be less effective and will cost more for each hypertensive complication prevented, if the dropout rate after screening is high or compliance with medication low.

Third, noncompliance may influence the outcome of the therapeutic trials upon which important recommendations are based. Dose-response curves (dose plotted on the abscissa and response on the ordinate) may be shifted to the right by noncompliance, resulting in falsely high estimates for toxic and therapeutic doses. A falsely large response range for a given dose may be reported because of variation in subjects' compliance. In therapeutic trials, noncompliance in the treatment group will reduce the power of the study to detect significant differences between treatment and placebo. Furthermore, differences in compliance among different treatment groups may lead to false conclusions regarding their relative efficacy. Finally, subjects chosen on the basis of proven compliance may not be representative of the population from which they were drawn. Patients with type A (competitive, driving, and independent) personalities, for example, may be less likely to enroll in a coronary prevention program (18), but more likely to have a myocardial infarction. Their under-representation in prevention programs could decrease the overall risk of myocardial infarction for enrollees compared to controls. In the Coronary Drug Project clinical trial of the usefulness of lipid-lowering therapy (2), those subjects who adhered strictly to their regimen of clofibrate had a substantially lower 5-year mortality than did those who did not, but so did those who adhered strictly to their prescribed placebo.

Prevalence of Noncompliance

The prevalence of noncompliance clearly underlines the importance of the problem. Reported noncompliance rates must be viewed critically and compared with caution, because of differences in definition from study to study. Nevertheless, the results of extensive reports are almost unanimous in identifying noncompliance, variably defined, as an extremely prevalent condition. Rates vary from less than 10% to over 90%, depending on the setting. Owing to previous dropouts, cross-sectional studies of patients taking medication chronically tend to underestimate noncompliance, but even then noncompliance is often in the 20% to 70% range. The results of these reports can be summarized as follows:

1. Noncompliance rates tend to be higher for preventive care than for treatment of established illness.
2. There is a marked increase in noncompliance with duration of therapy.
3. Noncompliance is highest for regimens that require significant behavioral change, such as smoking cessation or weight loss.
4. Missed appointments are more common for provider-initiated than patient-initiated visits. Asymptomatic patients are more likely to miss appointments than symptomatic patients.
5. Lack of comprehension of a regimen is a common cause of noncompliance. Unfortunately, most studies do not separate noncomprehension from willful noncompliance, but where studied, noncomprehension has been shown to be responsible for from 20% to 70% of objectively measured noncompliance.

MEASUREMENT OF COMPLIANCE

General Considerations

A variety of methods are available for measuring compliance. Unfortunately, there is no gold standard of validity and each method has strengths and weaknesses. Of general concern are the following issues.

First, it should be recognized that compliance is usually defined arbitrarily. Ideally compliance should be defined in terms of its relationship to therapeutic efficacy. For example, 80% compliance may be required to ensure blood pressure reduction (9), while evidence suggests that consumption of only about one-third of prescribed medicines provides some protection from recurrence of rheumatic fever (14).

Second, compliance reported in terms of percentages does not reflect sequential behavior. For example, omitting medications for 1 week could have an impact on therapeutic efficacy quite different from missing a few doses per week over a much longer period; yet the percentage compliance might be identical.

Third, measuring compliance in populations requires additional considerations. The magnitude of the noncompliance problem will depend upon the choice of denominator, i.e. the definition of the population at risk, which should be clearly stated. Compliance rates will be higher, for example, for a clinic population studied at a single time than for a clinic population studied longitudinally from the inception of therapy, since only the latter approach adequately accounts for patients who completely drop out from care. The compliance distribution (% of patients versus % compliance) should also be reported, since its shape can vary markedly (Fig. 4.1). Reported compliance distribution curves have varied from U-shaped in children given rheumatic fever prophylaxis (6), to skewed bell-shaped for patients taking chronic antacid therapy (19), to relatively uniform for patients

taking antituberculous (12), chronic oral hypoglycemic (4), or psychopharmacological (15) therapy. The shape of the curve may influence the choice of strategies designed to improve compliance. For example, in the case of a U-shaped distribution, attempts to improve compliance might best be directed toward the most noncompliant group of patients, whereas the entire population might be a better target when compliance is normally distributed.

Methods of Measurement

There are several approaches to assessing compliance behavior in patients. Since each method has some limitations it is often necessary for the physician to use several methods to arrive at a reasonably valid estimate of compliance in the individual patient.

ASKING

The simplest and most practical method of assessing compliance behavior is to ask the patient. Self-reports of noncompliance are generally valid. There is even some evidence that patients who admit to being noncompliant may be more amenable to intervention than those who do not (13). Only about 40% to 80% of patients admit their noncompliance, however, so that self-reported compliance cannot be relied upon. In population studies, reported compliance rates have almost always overestimated true compliance rates. Since the manner of asking may influence response, it is generally agreed that patients should be questioned about compliance in a nonthreatening, nonjudgemental way. (See example physician-patient exchange in Chapter 1.)

MEDICATION COUNTING

Medication counting provides a more objective measure of compliance than does simply asking patients, and it has been used to demonstrate the lack of reliability of patient-reported compliance. Results are usually expressed in terms of percentages, which facilitate the construction of distribution curves. The ability to measure sequential behavior depends upon the use of short intervals between counts, which is usually not feasible. While more accurate than reported compliance, medication counts are still not perfect. If the patient is suspicious of being monitored, he can remove medicines from containers without ingesting them. Overestimates of compliance can also occur if other persons are using medicine from the same container. In one study, 10 of 105 patients returned more empty antacid bottles than anticipated from simultaneous monitoring of blood levels of a tracer substance added to the antacid preparation (20). Compliance may be underestimated if the patient is using more than one medication container, but only makes one available for counting. Furthermore, many patients do not bring their medication containers with them to the physician's office,

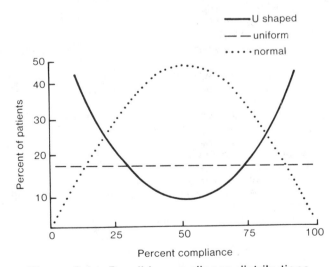

Figure 4.1   Possible compliance distributions.

despite reminders. Finally, some patients might take offense at having their medications counted, resulting in deterioration of the physician-patient relationship. The medication count can be approximated by the more practical and less intrusive method of prescribing quantities of medication which should be consumed within a reasonable interval of time, and then observing the frequency with which prescription renewals are requested.

Ingenious medication dispensers have been devised which monitor not only the amount but also the regularity with which medicine is removed. They are bulky, however, and not commercially available.

ASSAYS

Another objective method of estimating compliance behavior involves testing drug levels in blood, urine, breath or saliva. Drug levels have been shown to correlate with compliance determined by other methods as well as by outcome. Marked variation in drug levels may reflect inconsistencies in medication taking. The monitoring of drug levels and relaying results to the patient may also serve as a stimulus to improve compliance. However, there are limitations to the method. For accurate assessment, multiple measurements are required over an extended period. There is the possibility that, if the patient knows he is being monitored, he may take medicine immediately before the collection of specimens but not at other times. More important may be differences in bioavailability among different preparations of the same medicine and differences in drug absorption, distribution, metabolism, and excretion among individuals, making it impossible in the individual patient to decide whether a low level represents noncompliance or inadequate dosage. The absence of any drug suggests noncompliance, assuming the specimen has been collected appropriately. The physician should have a working knowledge of the pharmacokinetics of the medicine being assayed, so that the collection of specimens can be timed correctly. Compliance with short acting drugs, which are rapidly cleared from the blood and excreted, is difficult to monitor by assay techniques because of the difficulty in collecting specimens at appropriate times. Finally, assays are not available for many medications.

OUTCOME

An even more indirect but objective method of estimating compliance is the monitoring of expected therapeutic or physiological outcome. For example, blood pressure can be followed in a patient taking antihypertensive medication, weight in a patient on a weight reduction diet, and pulse rate in a patient prescribed propranolol. Many of the limitations of drug assays also affect assessment of outcome, which can be influenced by variations in drug bioavailability, absorption, distribution, and excretion; furthermore, multiple measurements are required. Other factors may influence outcome. For example, a reduction in stress may lower blood pressure or the presence of concomitant heart disease might be responsible for bradycardia.

SUPERVISION

An additional approach to assessing compliance is to compare drug levels or outcome of therapy during supervised *versus* unsupervised periods of medicine consumption. Depending upon the pharmacokinetics of the drug, supervision may be accomplished either in the office or in the hospital.

Physicians' Ability to Predict Compliance

The need to measure compliance becomes obvious if one considers that studies have shown that physicians are poor at predicting compliance behavior in their patients, sometimes performing no better than would be expected by chance. Whether physicians can improve their performance by making determined efforts, or by specific training remains to be evaluated.

FACTORS ASSOCIATED WITH COMPLIANCE

Compliance has been associated with factors related to the patient, the disease, the environment, the treatment, and the patient-physician relationship (Table 4.1). Physicians should be aware of the most important of these associations in order to improve their ability to predict noncompliance in their own patients.

Table 4.1
Factors Associated with Compliance

PATIENT CHARACTERISTICS
  Health beliefs (+ or −)[a]
  Previous or concurrent compliant behavior (+)
  Alcoholism and drug addiction (−)
  Psychological factors (+ or −)
DISEASE FEATURES
  Schizphrenia, personality disorders, paranoid disorders, and dementia (−)
ENVIRONMENTAL FACTORS
  Stable family and social support systems (+)
  Waiting time (−)
  Individual *versus* block appointment system (+ vs. −)
  Time between referral and appointment (−)
TREATMENT FACTORS
  Complexity of regimen (−)
  Duration of therapy (−)
  Requirement for behavioral change (−)
FEATURES OF THE PATIENT-PHYSICIAN RELATIONSHIP
  Supervision (+)
  Meeting of patient expectations (+)
  Patient satisfaction (+)
  Effective education (+)
  Continuity of provider care (+)

[a] +, positively associated with compliance; −, negatively associated with compliance.

Patient Characteristics

Surprisingly, sociodemographic variables such as age, sex, race, education, occupation, income, and marital status usually do not correlate with compliance behavior. Elderly patients, however, have been shown to have difficulty in opening childproof medication containers, and thus may not take prescribed medicines. Alcoholism and drug addiction tend to correlate highly with noncompliance. Previous compliance or concurrent compliance with one aspect of treatment usually correlates with adherence to other aspects of the regimen. Psychological factors, such as depression, immaturity, impulsivity, paranoia, hostility, fear of dependence, and type A personality might be expected to correlate with noncompliance, and in some studies such association has been demonstrated. Factors which affect the patient's ability to comprehend, such as dementia or mental retardation, or the presence of a major psychiatric illness, such as schizophrenia which affects the patient's ability to organize and initiate deliberate behavior should also be expected to affect compliance. Moreover, many patients who come to physicians are experiencing considerable anxiety, which may interfere with cognitive functioning of which comprehension is one element. Understanding may be further hampered by the tendency of certain patients, such as blue collar workers, to ask few questions of their physicians even when they desire information (7).

Other important patient characteristics which are often overlooked are "*health beliefs.*" Patient's beliefs about the severity of an illness, their susceptibility to an illness or its complications, the efficacy of treatment, and barriers to therapy have usually been found to be associated with compliance behavior. As distinguished from disease, which is an objective entity based upon the presence of independently verifiable findings, a patient's experience of illness is a subjective state which is shaped by personal, interpersonal and cultural factors. It is the patient's perceptions of disease and treatment that correlate with compliance rather than the objective realities. An extreme example occurs in patients who deny illness. Thus, myocardial infarction patients, who answer "no" or "maybe" rather than "yes" when asked if they have experienced a heart attack, are less likely to comply with physician's instructions for decreased activity and reduced cigarette smoking (3). Patients often have their own models of disease and treatment (8, 22). If this model conflicts with the regimen prescribed for the patient, noncompliance may follow. For example, some patients may change physicians or refuse treatment if they are told that they have both "high blood pressure" and "a low blood count" (anemia). According to some medical beliefs these diagnoses are mutually exclusive, so the physician making them may be regarded as ignorant (22).

Features of the Disease

Unlike severity as perceived by the patient, actual disease severity is usually not associated with compliance behavior. Diagnosis *per se* shows little correlation with compliance, except for patients with schizophrenia and certain personality disorders, especially those with paranoid or antisocial features, who tend to be less compliant.

Environmental Factors

Patients who have stable support systems and stable family situations tend to be more compliant. A spouse's concern about a patient's illness can encourage the patient to make an office visit and thus lead to increased supervision. Appointment keeping has been found to be positively correlated with short office waiting times, individual rather than block appointment systems, and short interval from the time of scheduling to the actual appointment date.

Treatment Factors

The complexity of the medical regimen usually correlates inversely with compliance. In the studies done to date, the number of medications seems more important than the number of daily doses. Side effects of medications are mentioned relatively infrequently in the medical literature, but clearly may cause noncompliance when they interfere with an important function in the individual's life.

The duration of therapy and the requirement of significant behavioral change (e.g., weight reduction or smoking cessation) have been previously mentioned as negatively associated with compliance.

Physician-Patient Relationship

Features of the physician-patient relationship which usually promote compliance include close supervision of the patient by the physician (or his associate), meeting of the patient's expectations, the patient's perception of the physician as friendly, concerned, and empathetic, and continuity of provider.

Effective communication is a prerequisite for several of these features of the relationship. Among the aspects of the communication process which are particularly relevant for the understanding of compliance are the following.

First, *effective transfer of information* is important, since the patient must first understand a regimen before he can be expected to comply with it (5, 10, 23). Yet physicians often do not give sufficient verbal and written information about how often a drug is to be taken, how long it is to be taken, for what purpose, and what side effects might be encountered (23). Failure to test the patient's understanding of the therapeutic regimen may result in failure to detect and correct problems in the instructional process.

Second, *psychological factors* may affect a patient's ability to receive or request information. The physician may be the last resource on a long road of self-medication, lay consultation, and nonprofessional intervention. A patient may have already tried a variety of remedies for his symptoms and may be very concerned at their persistence. Thus there may be factors which interfere with the patient's attention, comprehension, and retention of the physician's message. This has been demonstrated in its most extreme form in studying the family members of patients who have had a myocardial infarction (16). The family tended to retain very little of the explanation of the illness, or of the instructions about postinfarction care given to them by physicians in the hospital. Another example, alluded to above, is that blue collar workers are often reluctant to ask questions which are clearly of concern to them.

Finally, it should be recognized that patients often enter physicians' offices with *half-formed or inaccurate models* to explain their own illness. Discordance between patient and physician models can result in mistrust of the physician and/or noncompliance. For example, some patients with hypertension may feel that they have an intermittent, symptomatic, stress-related condition and take their medicines erratically. Other patients with clearly diagnosable soft tissue injuries may feel that their evaluation was incomplete without an X-ray and therefore mistrust the physician's diagnosis. Mexican-American or Puerto Rican patients who ascribe to the hot-cold theory of health and disease (8) avoid the use of "hot" substances during pregnancy and may, therefore, refuse to take "hot" medications, such as iron and vitamins. Compliance in these cases may only be obtained by encouraging them to "neutralize" the hot properties of these medications with cool substances such as fruit juice or herb tea. Unless patient concerns and beliefs about their illness, evaluation, and treatment are taken into consideration, problems in the patient-physician relationship including noncompliance may ensue.

Understandably, busy practitioners prefer patients who do not ask too many questions about the prescribed treatment and simply follow instructions. While this active-passive relationship may be appropriate for some patients, to be effective with most ambulatory patients the physician must enter into a relationship of mutual participation in which he must listen to the patient, educate and negotiate with him. (see Chapter 1, pages 10–11, for additional description of communication and the physician-patient relationship).

COMPLIANCE-IMPROVING INTERVENTIONS

The techniques designed to improve patient compliance which have been evaluated include organizational, educational, and behavioral interventions. Successful intervention has increased compliance rates by less than 10% to almost 70%, averaging between 25% and 30% (percent change = percent of compliant patients in experimental group minus percent of compliant patients in control group).

Appointment Keeping

A number of factors have been shown to improve appointment-keeping by patients.

Telephone and mail reminders, in which the patient receives a message several days before his scheduled visit informing him of the date and time of the appointment, have consistently improved compliance, usually in the range of 10% to 20%. The introduction of individual, rather than block appointment systems, and the substitution of a single for multiple providers have resulted in decreased waiting time and improved appointment keeping. Individual appointment systems give each patient a precise time for his appointment; block systems schedule several or all patients for one time, usually at the beginning of office hours.

If referral is required, educating the patient about the purpose of referral, secretarial assistance to facilitate scheduling and transportation, and referral to a specific physician and not simply to a specialty group or clinic have also been shown to improve appointment-keeping for diagnostic studies and specialty consultations.

Short Term Therapy

Compliance with short term courses of medication has been increased by the use of verbal and written instructions, the use of long acting parenteral therapy, the use of clearly labeled medication containers, pill calendars (devices on which patients keep track of their medication taking), and special pharmaceutical packaging designed to aid memory.

Although *verbal and written instructions* are clearly important, physicians often communicate poorly both the purpose of a specific regimen and precise directions about how it should be administered. Furthermore, as already noted, psychological factors such as anxiety may interfere with the patient's ability to comprehend initial instructions. Verbal instructions should be brief, clear and explicit, with subsequent repetition and testing of the effectiveness of the communication (also Chapter 1, Table 1.10). Written instructions provide a remedy for forgetfulness and can be reviewed at leisure in the less stressful environment of the patient's home. Interestingly, informing patients of potential drug side effects seems to increase compliance, at least with respect to antidepressant therapy (17).

Long acting parenteral therapy is especially useful in situations where compliance is known to be low. For example, the use of a single intramuscular long acting penicillin rather than 10 days of an oral preparation will improve the effectiveness of therapy.

Chronic Therapy
BEHAVIORAL STRATEGIES

Strategies which incorporate various combinations of increased supervision, tailoring of the medical regimen to individual patient's needs or habits, reinforcement, and patient involvement, have improved compliance with chronic therapy. Instruction alone tends to be less effective in this setting, probably because most patients have already learned their regimen and have been taught something about their disease. Verbal and written instructions, however, would still be important whenever the regimen is changed.

Increased supervision includes scheduling of more frequent provider-patient contacts, the use of reminders, the use of drug assays, and the eliciting of family or community support to assist in administering and monitoring treatment. For example, the physician may request more frequent blood pressure values in a hypertensive patient. The blood pressures can be taken either by a nurse at the physician's office, a nurse at work, by a family member, or by the patient himself.

Tailoring refers to a process whereby the therapeutic regimen is fitted to patient characteristics. Forgetful patients may benefit from linking medication-taking or prescribed activites to other daily behavior, such as eating meals or brushing teeth. In addition, medication should be kept available where it is taken (e.g., at the breakfast table). If possible the patient should avoid taking medication during times of the day when his activities are variable, or when he is likely to be distracted (e.g., at work). Other examples of tailoring include involving patients (especially those who are accustomed to making all of their own decisions) in planning and monitoring their own therapy, substituting liquid medication for tablets in patients who have difficulty in swallowing pills, increasing supervision and peer support for patients who are having difficulty on their own in following a desired regimen (such as a weight reduction diet) and, when possible, prescribing medications which do not contradict the patient's own model of disease.

Reinforcement consists of feedback to the patient of results of drug level assays and therapeutic outcome (e.g., decrease in blood pressure or weight). When the measures indicate compliance, praise or some kind of reward will reinforce desired behavior. When noncompliance is suspected, the problem is discussed with the patient.

Mechanisms of *patient involvement* have included various forms of self-monitoring, such as taking blood pressure at home, and the signing of contracts between patients and physicians. By taking active responsibility for their own care, patients may become more motivated to comply with therapy.

Combination strategies utilize two or more of the above methods. Such a combination strategy utilized to improve behavior in noncompliant postmyocardial infarction patients has been described by Baile and Engel (1). Patient involvement was effected by having patients set their own goals and monitor their own behavior. Frequent contact with the physician allowed reinforcement, modification of goals on a negotiated basis, and discussion of problems with the regimen. Involvement of the spouse also increased supervision.

DIRECT SUPERVISION OF MEDICATION TAKING

Direct supervision of drug intake is especially helpful for ensuring compliance in patients with impaired intellectual or psychological functioning, such as alcoholism, dementia, and schizophrenia. Examples include the use of intermittent supervised oral antituberculosis therapy and the use of long acting parenteral drugs in the ambulatory management of schizophrenia.

MAINTENANCE OF COMPLIANCE

No matter how successful the intervention, compliance tends to decay toward baseline after cessation of the intervention. Hence, there is a need to continue some form of intervention. Unfortunately, there has been little effort to date to study maintenance strategies.

PHYSICIAN EDUCATION AS A COMPLIANCE-IMPROVING STRATEGY

That physicians can bring about improved compliance among their hypertensive patients, after a single tutorial by a physician, was demonstrated in a unique study by Inui et al. (11). Medical residents were presented with information on hypertension, its treatment, and noncompliance together with documentation of the high noncompliance rates among their own patients, and with strategies designed to improve compliance based upon an assessment of patient health beliefs. The physicians were invited to experiment in their own practices with strategies to improve compliance. Follow-up showed improved compliance and blood pressure control among the patients of tutored physicians, but not among patients of untutored physicians.

Ethical Considerations

Sackett points out that the following three conditions should be met before attempting to improve compliance: (a) the diagnosis should be correct, (b) the therapy should be proven efficacious and benefits should outweigh adverse effects, and (c) the patient should be an informed and willing partner in the intervention (21).

While the first two conditions are probably applicable to interventions directed toward populations, they may be too rigid for application to individual patients. Many medicines have not been unequivocally proven to be efficacious, although some evidence supports their usefulness. The physician is justified in encouraging the use of such medications in an attempt to determine whether they relieve symptoms or improve functional status. How else will the physician know whether a given antiarrhythmic or analgesic, for example, is effective for a given patient? In some circumstances, it may be reasonable to prescribe an efficacious medicine as a therapeutic trial, when the diagnosis is in question.

In individual practice, therefore, Sackett's first two conditions might be replaced with the following requirements: (a) that the therapy be rational and based upon sound medical knowledge, and (b) that the potential risks of therapy be small compared to the potential benefits.

The third condition, that of an informed and willing partner in the intervention, is even more difficult to satisfy. In medical practice one may encounter individuals who willfully fail to comply against their own best interest. Is the physician justified in increasing supervision or attempting to elicit familial support in order to improve compliance, without obtaining explicit consent from the patient? On the one hand, the patient has come to the doctor's office and voluntarily entered into the patient-physician relationship, suggesting implicit consent. On the other hand, the patient is willfully noncomplying, suggesting a rejection of this aspect of the relationship. The dilemma may be somewhat artificial since most compliance-improving strategies require participation of the patient and, therefore, implicit consent. Going beyond the patient-physician relationship to enroll family help, however, requires consideration of the patient's feelings with respect to this intervention. The situation becomes more difficult when patients are mentally or psychologically impaired in their ability to make sound decisions. An example might be the symptomatic schizophrenic patient who fails to comply in taking his oral antipsychotic medication, when introduction of long acting parenteral therapy could reduce symptoms, rate of relapse and rehospitalization. There are no definitive guidelines in these situations, but the following suggestions may be helpful: (a) the physician should attempt to determine the patient's own best interest, considering not only the disease but also the patient's desires, psychological makeup, and social environment, and he should use this information as a guide to action; (b) the physician should weigh the relative benefits *versus* risks of intervention (self-monitoring of blood pressure in some individuals, for example, might markedly increase their anxiety); (c) the physician should respect the patient's legal rights; and (d) in particularly difficult situations, such as in the case of mentally incompetent patients, the physician should consult with others before deciding on a course of action. (See Chapter 9 for determination of mental competence.)

Finally, there is the question of at which point the patient's responsibilities begin and those of the physician end. Is the physician ethically bound to identify and treat noncompliance when it compromises the health of his patient? Once a patient-physician relationship has been entered, it is certainly the physician's responsibility to improve the health status of the patient to the best of his ability, taking into consideration the severity of the problem, economic constraints, time constraints, and competing obligations to other patients. To achieve this end a physician should use not only the traditional methods of diagnosis, treatment, and education of patients, but when appropriate, interventions for improving compliance as well.

CLINICAL APPROACH TO NONCOMPLIANCE

In practice, the problem of noncompliance should be handled in the same way as other clinical problems. Whenever possible it should be prevented. When present, it should be diagnosed and treated by accepted diagnostic approaches and treatment modalities.

Noncompliance with Therapeutic Regimens

PREVENTION

It is usually more efficient to use some strategies that will improve compliance with all patients at the inception of treatment, rather than to attempt to identify the noncompliers at a later time. Minimal preventive strategies for all patients would include (a) the use of the simplest possible medical regimen and (b) brief, clear, explicit instructions with subsequent repetition and testing of the effectiveness of the communication.

Tailoring of care to the individual needs of the patient from the outset may increase his satisfaction and improve the chances for compliance. This requires that the physician routinely obtain some of the following facts from most patients: (a) the patient's expectations, motivations, and concerns in seeking care; (b) the patient's explanations for and beliefs about his illness; (c) the patient's need for more or less information about and involvement in his own care; (d) environmental factors, such as work hours, which might influence the patient's ability to follow a therapeutic regimen; and (e) the patient's acceptance and understanding of the physician's explanation and prescription. These facts may be utilized as described above (page 37).

The use of long acting parenteral therapy in lieu of more complicated and prolonged oral regimes (e.g., in the treatment of gonococcal urethritis or streptococcal pharyngitis) will reduce noncompliance and thereby increase the effectiveness of therapy.

DIAGNOSIS (Table 4.2)

The possibility of noncompliant behavior should be considered in all patients, because of its high prevalence and the inability of physicians to predict it intuitively. The failure to see expected therapeutic

Table 4.2
Diagnosis of Noncompliance

SUSPICION
  All patients (special emphasis on patients who fail to achieve expected therapeutic effects or side effects and those with associated risk factors for noncompliance)
MEASUREMENT
  Direct question
  Check frequency of patient-requested prescription renewals or medication count
  Drug assays
  Expected outcomes
  Observation/hospitalization
CAUSE
  Noncomprehension
  Willful noncompliance
    Determine cause of willful noncompliance

Table 4.3
Treatment of Noncompliance

NONCOMPREHENSION
  Verbal and written instructions
    Concise
    Clear
    Explicit
    Repetition
    Testing for comprehension
  Simplification and tailoring of medical regimen
  Supervision of medication taking
WILLFUL NONCOMPLIANCE
  Education and persuasive communication
  Simplification and tailoring of medical regimen
  Increased supervision
  Patient involvement
  Positive reinforcement
  Familial/environmental support
  Supervised medication taking
  Combined interventions
  Need to maintain intervention

or side effects should raise suspicions, as should the presence of other factors known to be associated with noncompliance (see discussion above, p. 34 and Table 4.1).

The first step in diagnosing noncompliance is to ask patients what medicines they are taking, how frequently they are taking them, and how frequently doses are missed. The questioning should be done in an open-ended nonthreatening, nonjudgmental manner (see example, Chapter 1, p. 10). In this way about 50% of noncompliers (and all those who do not comply because they do not understand the requirements) will be identified. If willful noncompliance is suspected despite denial by the patient, medication counts may be instituted but are often impractical as discussed above (p. 33). Instead observations of the frequency of actual *versus* expected prescription renewals may be substituted for formal pill counts. Drug assays and measurement of outcome (e.g., blood pressure in a patient on antihypertensives) can be helpful. The absence of a drug upon assay is virtually diagnostic of noncompliance (assuming that the assay is reliable and the samples have been obtained at appropriate times). The failure to achieve therapeutic drug levels or expected outcomes, however, could be secondary either to noncompliance or inadequate therapy. To distinguish between these two alternatives it may sometimes be necessary to observe drug levels or outcome of treatment during a period in which drugs are taken under direct supervision. This may require a period of hospitalization. In one common condition, hypertension, hospitalization can be avoided by measuring the patient's blood pressure for several hours after supervised ingestion of medication in the office.

Once the presence of noncompliance has been established, its *cause* should be determined. Noncomprehension will be detected by simply asking the patient to describe his regimen. If the patient knows his regimen but does not comply, possible reasons for the noncompliance should be explored (e.g., inappropriate beliefs about the illness or therapy, presence

of side effects, cost of medicines, inconvenience of taking medicines, patient's indifference or depression, etc.) The ways in which these factors may affect compliance behavior has been discussed above (p. 34).

TREATMENT (Table 4.3)

Once noncompliance has been established and it has been decided to try to treat it (after a review of the ethical considerations previously discussed p. 37), several methods are possible. If the problem is noncomprehension, the use of further verbal and written instructions and/or simplification and tailoring of the medical regimen may be indicated. If the patient is still unable to comprehend, supervision of medication taking by family members or by health personnel such as visiting nurses will be required.

When the problem is willful noncompliance, a strategy designed to improve compliance must be tailored to suit each patient's needs. The use of behavioral methods will often be required including further education and persuasive communication, simplifying the medical regimen to fit patient needs (including selecting less costly drugs when indicated), increased supervision, the monitoring and feedback of blood levels or outcome measurements, self-monitoring and patient involvement in planning care, involvement of family members, positive reinforcement, the use of long acting parenteral therapy or other form of supervised medication taking, and the use of special pharmaceutical packaging to aid memory. An effective strategy may have to be continued indefinitely, because compliance tends to decline after the termination of such intervention.

Noncompliance with Appointment Keeping

Missed appointments may be a problem for certain patients. These can be avoided by the techniques described above (pp. 35–36).

References

General

Bartlet, E (editor): *Physician's Patient Education Newsletter* (available by subscription). University of Alabama, Birmingham, AL 35294.

> *Bimonthly newsletter published since 1978. Contains timely accounts and reviews of behavioral approaches to patient compliance.*

Becker, MH and Maiman, RA: Sociobehavioral determinants of compliance with health and medical care recommendations. *Med. Care 13:* 10, 1975.

> *Description of the Health Belief Model and review of its role in explaining compliance behavior.*

Gillum, RF and Barsky, AJ: Diagnosis and management of patient noncompliance. *JAMA 228:* 1563, 1974.

> *Review focusing on psychological factors and the patient-physician interaction.*

Haynes, RB, Taylor, DW and Sackett, DL: (editors): *Compliance in Health Care.* Johns Hopkins University Press, Baltimore, 1979.

> *Excellent comprehensive reference with annotated bibliography. The single best source of information on compliance.*

Imboden, JB and Urbaitis, JC: Patient noncompliance with medical treatment. Contributory factors and management. *J Fam Pract 5:* 888, 1977.

> *Practical suggestions with emphasis on management of patient fear, anxiety, and denial which may contribute to noncompliance.*

Morris, LA and Hapern, JA: Effects of written drug information on patient knowledege and compliance: A literature review. *Am J Public Health 69:* 47, 1979.

> *Review of the effect of written instruction on patient compliance.*

Oppenheim, GL, Bergman, JJ and English, EC: Failed appointments: A review. *J Fam Pract 8:* 789, 1979.

> *Review of the reasons for missed appointments and the methods available to reduce the fail rate.*

Specific

1. Baile, WF and Engel, BT: A behavioral strategy for the treatment of noncompliance following myocardial infarction. *Psychosom Med 40:* 413, 1978.
2. Coronary Drug Project Research Group: Influence of adherence to treatment and response of cholesterol on mortality in the Coronary Drug Project. *N Engl J Med 30:* 1038, 1980.
3. Croog, SH, Shapiro, DS and Levine, S: Denial among heart patients. *Psychosom Med 33:* 385, 1971.
4. Eshelman, FN: Drug compliance in diabetics. *Br Med J 1:* 581, 1978.
5. Francis, V, Korsch, BM and Morris, MS: Gaps in the doctor-patient relationship: Patients response to medical advice. *N Engl J Med 28:* 535, 1969.
6. Gordis, L, Markowitz, M and Lilienfeld, AM: Studies in the epidemiology and preventability of rheumatic fever; IV. A quantitative determination of compliance in children on oral penicillin prophylaxis. *Pediatrics 43:* 173, 1962.
7. Hackett, TP and Cassem, NH: White-collar and blue-collar responses to a heart attack. *J Psychosom Res 20:* 85, 1976.
8. Harwood, A: The hot-cold theory of disease: Implications for treatment of Puerto Rican patients. *JAMA 216:* 1153, 1971.
9. Haynes, RB: Strategies in improving compliance with referrals, appointments, and prescribed medical regimens. In *Compliance in Health Care,* p. 123, edited by RB Haynes, DW Taylor and DL Sackett. Johns Hopkins University Press, Baltimore, 1979.
10. Hulka, BS, Cassel, JC, Kupper, LL and Burdette, A: Communication, compliance, and concordance between physicians and patients with prescribed medications. *Am J Public Health 66:* 847, 1976.
11. Inui, TS: Yourtee, EL and Williamson, JW: Improved outcomes after physician tutorials: A controlled trial. *Ann Intern Med 84:* 646, 1976.
12. Ireland, HD: Outpatient chemotherapy for tuberculosis. *Am Rev Respir Dis 82:* 378, 1960.
13. Johnson, AL, Taylor, DW, Sackett, DL, Dunett, CW and Shimizu, AG: Self-recording of blood pressure in the management of hypertension. *Can Med Assoc J 119:* 1034, 1978.
14. Markowitz, M: Eradication of rheumatic fever: An unfilled hope. *Circulation 41:* 1077, 1970.
15. Mason, AS, Forrest, IS, Forrest, FM and Butler, H: Adherence to maintenance therapy and rehospitalization. *Dis Nerv Syst 24:* 103, 1963.
16. Mayou, R, Williamson, B and Foster, A: Attitudes and advice after myocardial infarction. *Br Med J 1:* 1577, 1976.
17. Meyers, ED and Calvert, EJ: Knowledge of side effects and perserverance with medication. *Br J Psych 132:* 426, 1978.
18. Oldright, NB: Wicks, JR, Hanley, C, Sutton, JR and Jones, NL: Noncompliance in an exercise rehabilitation program for men who have suffered a myocardial infarction. *Can Med Assoc J 118:* 361, 1978.
19. Roth, HP: Accuracy of doctor's estimates and patient's statements on adherence to a drug regimen. *Clin Pharmacol Ther 23:* 361, 1978.
20. Roth, HP, Caron, HS and Hsi, BP: Measuring intake of prescribed medication: A bottle count and a tracer technique compared. *Clin Pharmacol Ther 11:* 228, 1970.
21. Sackett, DL: Introduction, In *Compliance in Health Care,* p. 1, edited by RB Haynes, DW Taylor and DL Sackett. Johns Hopkins University Press, Baltimore, 1979.
22. Snow, LF: Folk medical beliefs and their implications for care of patients: A review based on studies among black Americans. *Ann Intern Med 81:* 82, 1974.
23. Svarstadt, BL: Physician-patient communication and patient conformity with medical advice. In *Health Illness and Medicine. A Leader in Medical Sociology.* Rand-McNally, Chicago, 1979.

CHAPTER FIVE

Adolescent Patients: Special Considerations

LARRY N. SCHERZER, M.D.

INTRODUCTION

As indicated in Chapter 1 (Table 1.2), patients in the age group 15 to 24 account for about 9% of visits to internists and 16% of visits to family or general practitioners in the United States.

From a developmental perspective, adolescence is a time of dynamic changes, with tremendous physical, sexual, intellectual, and psychological growth. This chapter describes the normal changes and the major problems associated with each of these four spheres of development; an understanding of these changes is critical to the proper management of adolescent patients. The last section of the chapter recommends a number of special strategies for conducting ambulatory visits by adolescent patients.

ADOLESCENT MORTALITY AND MORBIDITY

Adolescence is the healthiest period of life; morbidity and mortality rates are low compared with other age groups; but the absolute number of adolescents who die or suffer from chronic illnesses is considerable. Since the number of productive years at stake for a teenager with a significant illness is large, adolescent health deserves a special priority.

Accidents are by far the leading cause of death among adolescents and young adults (see Table 5.1). Preventive measures have, by and large, been bypassed by the victims of accidental death; and, in many instances, behavioral problems underline those deaths. For example, alcohol is implicated in over 50% of automobile accidents, and there may be an element of suicidal intent in many of them.

The second and third leading causes of death in older adolescents (and an important problem in young adolescents) are homicide and suicide, problems that are discussed later in this chapter (page 51).

The fourth leading cause of death among adolescent and young adults is neoplasia. The most frequent diagnoses are acute leukemia (both lymphocytic and myelogenous), lymphomas (including non-Hodgkin's lymphoma and Hodgkin's disease), central nervous system tumors (especially supra- and infratentorial gliomas), bone tumors (especially osteogenic sarcomas and Ewing's sarcomas), and solid organ tumors (especially of genital organs).

As medical treatment improves, conditions that were previously fatal in childhood are being seen more frequently in adolescents and young adults. It is not uncommon that patients with cystic fibrosis, nephritis, congenital heart disease, and leukemia survive into adolescence and young adulthood. The transfer of their care from their pediatrician to an internist may threaten these patients, make it more difficult for them to adapt to their illness, and may even lead to complications requiring hospitalization.

Most visits to a physician by adolescents are for preventive care or are for problems that are relatively minor (Table 5.2). However, a number of more severe medical problems are either limited chiefly to the adolescent period or are problems of adulthood which begin during adolescence (Table 5.3). The data in the tables do not demonstrate the significant distress that many adolescent patients (and their physicians) experience. This distress is often related to the pressures unique to the several chronological stages of adolescence.

The *young teen* (*i.e.,* 11 to 15 years old) with his special concern over physical development, may have anxieties about mutilation and death. Hostility toward an illness may be expressed in a fantasy of invincibility leading to an uncooperative, noncompliant patient. Other young adolescents become greatly depressed by their illnesses and become annoying, complaining, whiny patients, frequently regressing to a childlike dependence on adult caretakers.

The *middle adolescent* (*i.e.,* 14 to 19 years old) who is ill suffers from the loss of valued contact with friends and schools. Important aspirations may be interrupted (and dreams shattered) through illness. Body image is at a critical developmental stage in midadolescence, and the teen may be more worried

Table 5.1
Major Causes of Death Age 15–24: United States 1975[a]

Cause of Death	Rate per 10⁵ Individuals
Accidents	60.3
Homicide	13.7
Suicide	11.8
Neoplasms, malignant and benign	7.1
Cardiovascular disease	4.4
Ill defined conditions	3.8
Infectious illnesses[b]	3.0
All other external causes	2.5
Congenital anomalies	1.6
Gastrointestinal diseases	0.8
Anemias	0.4
Diabetes mellitus	0.4
Complications of pregnancy and childbirth	0.4
Respiratory diseases	0.3
Nephritis and nephrosis	0.3
Nutritional deficiencies	0.1
All other diseases	8.0
Total	118.9
Estimated number of persons (in millions)	39.98
Number of deaths	47,545

[a] Adapted from data presented in *National Center for Health Statistics Monthly Vital Statistic Reports* (Volume 25, No. 10, December 30, 1976 and Volume 25, No. 11, February 11, 1977).
[b] All infectious illnesses including those related to specific organ systems e.g. diarrheal diseases, pneumonia, meningitis, and pyelonephritis.

about a cosmetic defect resulting from an illness than about the disease or its therapy. Such fears need to be faced early and dealt with honestly.

The *older adolescent* (i.e., 18 to 21 years old) shares many adult concerns. For example, anxiety may be expressed over the cost of an illness and the length of hospitalization, and the burdens these place on the family.

An understanding of adolescent development will help the clinician to recognize and deal with these and other special problems.

PHYSICAL DEVELOPMENT

Normal Patterns and Concerns

Physical maturation is an important feature of the second decade of life. Although the rate and the timing of maturation may vary, they follow the hormonal changes of puberty in a given individual.

There is a notable *growth spurt* occurring during the adolescent years, with a 20% to 25% increase in height over a period of 2 to 3 years. This spurt usually occurs earlier in the female than in the male (as does sexual maturation).

During puberty, there is an average twofold increase in both lean and nonlean *body mass*. The ratio of lean to nonlean body mass is greater in males than

Table 5.2
Thirty Most Common Reasons for Physician-Patient Contact for Patients 10–24 Years Old (Based on 2-Year Experience of 118 Family Physicians)[a]

Medical examination for preventive and pre-symptomatic purposes	11,877
Pharyngitis	8,245
Lacerations, contusions, and abrasions	7,714
Prenatal care	4,872
Strains and sprains	4,560
Vulvitis, vaginitis, and cervicitis	2,753
Coryza	2,725
Bronchitis	2,691
Febrile cold	2,388
Menstrual disorders	1,992
Abdominal pain other than colic	1,630
Otitis media, acute	1,561
Headache	1,342
Cystitis	1,313
Contact dermatitis	1,256
Warts	1,032
Sinusitis	1,001
Anxiety neurosis	986
Allergic rhinitis	909
Otitis externa	894
Depressive neurosis	871
Acne	853
Asthma	849
Gonorrhea	780
Acute gastritis or duodenitis	738
Other local infections of skin	730
Specific allergies	717
Physical disorders presumably of psychogenic origin	587
Hypertension	567
Hypochromic anemia	507

[a] Adapted from D. W. Marsland et al. Content of family practice. *Journal of Family Practice*, 3:37–68, 1976.

Table 5.3
Selected Medical Problems Limited to Adolescence or Persisting into Adulthood

Limited Chiefly to Adolescence	Chronic Problems that May Begin in Adolescence
Slipped epiphysis	Obesity
Distortion of body image	Hypertension
Delinquency[a]	Diabetes
Anorexia nervosa	Hypercholesterolemia
Primary amenorrhea	Duodenal ulcer
School or learning problems[b]	Inflammatory bowel disease
	Irritable colon
	Dental caries
	Drug abuse
	Alcoholism
	Personality disorders
	Somatization disorder (hysteria)
	Depressive neurosis

[a] May begin earlier.
[b] Often Develops earlier.

in females. It has been suggested that the greater proportion of fat in females may be related to reserves needed for the onset of menarche and ovulation. Fat accumulation tends to be greatest at the point that growth ceases, and may extend into adulthood.

The *musculoskeletal system* has special characteristics during adolescence. To accommodate growth, the ligaments and tendons become lax and elastic, frequently giving the teen a slouched-over appearance. Similarly, there is an increase in skeletal growth, particularly in long bones; and metaphyseal-epiphyseal junctions remain soft. Thus, the actively growing teen, who may not have developed a muscle mass to correspond to his skeletal growth, may be prone to some special injuries, particularly joint dislocations and fractures along epiphyseal plates.

As with all areas of development, the adolescent may have particular concerns about growth and weight. The principal reason for this is that adolescents often base judgment of each other's adequacy and acceptability on size or (for males) on athletic ability; and adult criteria of social status based on other standards (or prejudices) are of less importance.

Children called "squirt" or "runt" are given various types of parental advice; much of it is not helpful. Some children adapt by engaging in an activity where size is unimportant (e.g., debating, chess, fencing, swimming, body-building, etc.). Occasionally, normal children, with a familial basis of their short stature will require some psychological counseling to promote effective adaptation to their stature. Some individuals who are very sensitive about height and strength limitations may try radical and potentially harmful solutions such as self-injections of purported growth stimulants.

The concern of the adolescent about height may be generalized to many other aspects of appearance, including body habitus, beauty (or lack of beauty), skin condition, etc. The physician should be prepared to recognize when concern about body image is the patient's primary concern and to provide reassurance that he or she is medically and biologically normal. This reassurance can be greatly facilitated at times by suggesting a book in which the adolescent can learn more about normal growth (see p. 53).

Common Problems

SHORT STATURE

(See section on Adolescents with Short Stature and Sexual Maturation Delay, p. 47.)

OBESITY

A practical definition of obesity is a weight of 20% or more over ideal body weight (see also Chapter 73). This can be estimated by determining the weight that corresponds to the growth chart height percentile for the age and sex of the child, and dividing this into the actual weight (see Fig. 5.1). A result of greater than 1.2 would be suspect. This ratio should be compared with the clinical appearance of the child, since the fat distribution changes at puberty in men, when extra weight may be transformed into musculature, and in women, who normally increase their storage of fat. Obesity remains a clinical diagnosis. Adolescent obesity is usually due to overeating. Most estimates place the prevalence between 4% and 10%, with the highest frequency among the lower socioeconomic groups. Frequently, the obesity began in early childhood, but becomes a concern in adolescence because of desires to conform to peer standards.

In order to treat adolescent obesity successfully, the teen himself must be motivated and must accept the physician's assessments and recommendations. Frequently, the patient has attempted to cope with the problem by himself. Certain fad diets, such as fasting, water diets, etc., may yield rapid weight loss, but will deplete the strength of the child. Generally, since no modification of long term eating habits is attempted, the weight is regained upon cessation of the diet. Occasionally, there are serious biological complications to prolonged adherence to highly restrictive diets. Macrobiotic diets have been associated with symptoms of protein and vitamin deficiencies, and liquid protein diets have cardiotoxic effects that have resulted in deaths. Severely calorie-restricted diets will lead to a cessation of linear growth and may cause menstrual irregularities.

Medications have been of no value in weight control. Amphetamines and metamphetamines are contraindicated in adolescents because of their potential for abuse.

Surgical treatment (e.g., jejunal-ileal bypass) of obesity is rarely indicated, particularly in the adolescent years.

One is left with methods of dietary control by modification of behavior together with moderate calorie restriction. These methods, while successful for some are not successful for all. Frequently, the teen who wants to diet is well motivated, if for personal and emotional reasons rather than for reasons of health. A group meeting of obese teens provides a nucleus of peer support, with an opportunity for mutual discussions of problems of dieting and appetite control that may not be aired in a brief office visit. Such a group may also help alleviate home pressures. (Parental coercion and control of diet in the context of a normally antagonistic parent-teen relationship may result in an angry, rebellious youngster who is gaining rather than losing weight.)

For overweight young to midadolescents a reasonable goal is to maintain their current body weight, since excess caloric restriction may result in a loss of lean body weight. For the late adolescent, the goal may be weight loss. For all obese patients, one wishes to achieve a change in long term eating patterns.

Some adolescents overeat because of unresolved psychological difficulties. If there are expressions of

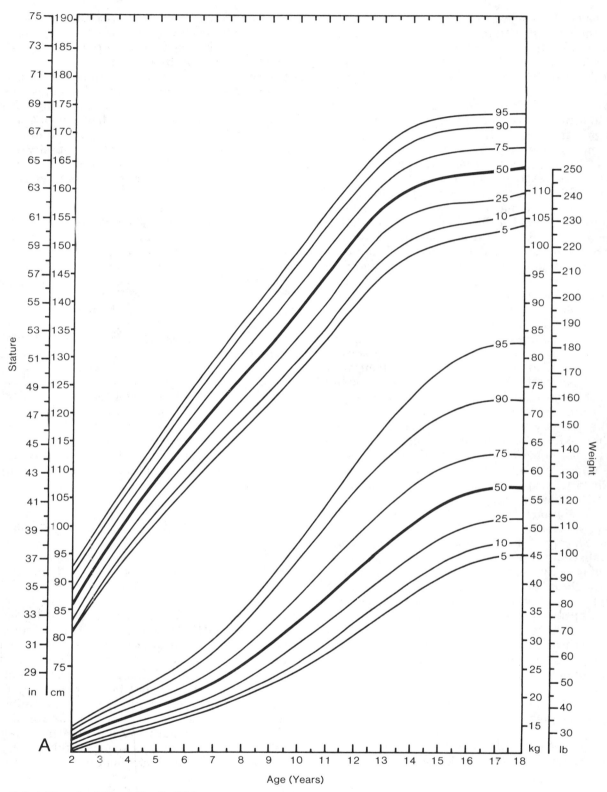

Figure 5.1   Physical Growth: A. Girls
Plot height, weight against chronological age at each encounter. The curve so obtained should parallel percentile lines within clear area (growth patterns of 90% of children/adolescents). If curve deviates from percentile lines, an abnormal growth pattern is likely. The upper series of curves represent the normal range of height at various ages and the lower series of curves, the normal range of weight at various ages. (Source: National Center for Health Statistics: NCHS Growth Charts, 1976. Monthly Vital Statistics Report, Vol. 25, No. 3, Supp. (HRA) 76-1120. Health Resources Administration, Rockville, Md., June 1976.)

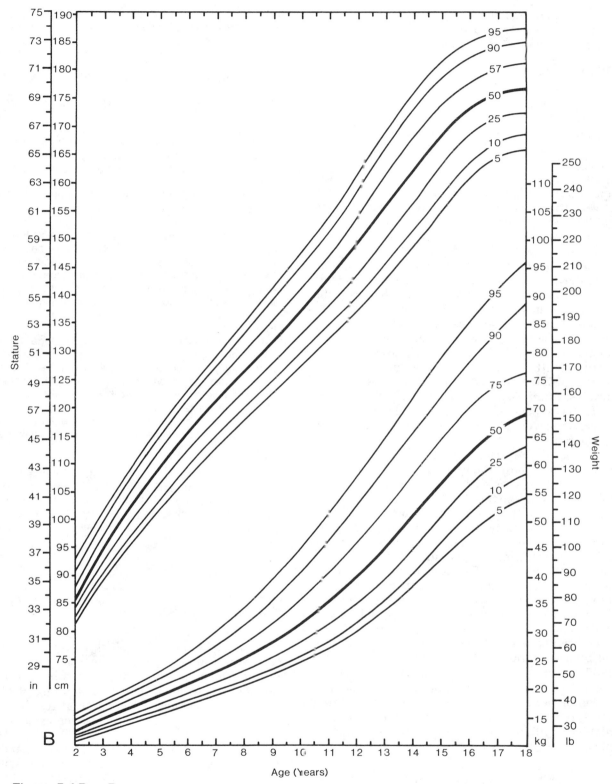

Figure 5.1*B*.   Boys

problems in peer, school, or parental relationships, these should be explored further. Obesity alone, however, is not an indication of psychopathology.

ANOREXIA NERVOSA

Anorexia nervosa is an infrequent but serious disorder of growth in adolescents. It is marked by extreme loss of appetite and of weight (at least 25% of the baseline weight) that is not attributable to a medical or psychiatric illness ordinarily associated with weight loss (*i.e.* inflammatory bowel disease or a major affective disorder). Patients characteristically exhibit an intense fear of becoming obese and, even when very thin, have a distorted body image so that they still consider themselves overweight.

Occasionally, a patient will periodically gorge herself, only to follow this by self-induced vomiting and by further self-reprisals through abstinence from food. As the disease progresses, patients may become withdrawn and depressed, leading to further appetite suppression. Amenorrhea is common in these patients, and it may be the presenting complaint.

Anorexia nervosa is most commonly a disease of young adolescent girls (about 90% of cases); but occasionally it affects males or older females. Most often, the problem develops in children of upper middle class families. Before their illness, the patients typically have been considered "model children," who have done well in school and have been obedient to their parents.

The cause of the disease is unknown. Although there have been many theories proposed to explain it, none is entirely satisfactory. Frequently there has been some stress in the family (divorce, death, change of location) before the onset of the illness.

There is no simple treatment that can be recommended for patients with anorexia nervosa. Help should be sought from a psychiatrist who has experience with the problem. The best results seem to be achieved by involving the patient and her family in an intensive program in which counseling and behavior modification are employed to restructure the patient's eating habits and attitude toward food. Cachectic patients should be hospitalized so that a proper program of nutrition can be instituted.

Complete remission of anorexia nervosa is unusual, but about 75% of patients achieve an acceptable improvement in both their physical and emotional state. The rest remain chronically undernourished and maladapted, and 10% of the total population die of complications of the disease.

SEXUAL DEVELOPMENT

Normal Patterns and Concerns

A major difference between the child and the adolescent is the conversion of the teen into a sexual being. The onset of puberty is associated with an intensification of sexual feelings and desires which

Table 5.4
Typical Progression of Female Adolescent Sexual Development[a]

STAGE 1:
  There is no pubic hair present, and there is no breast enlargement.
  The ovaries have begun to enlarge. The external genitalia are preadolescent or those of a child.
STAGE 2:
  Breast bud formation usually begins before pubic hair growth. A small mound is formed by the elevation of the breast and papilla. Areolar diameter increases. The adolescent height spurt begins, and there is an acceleration in the deposition of total body fat. The adult female habitus emerges as the breasts enlarge and the hips widen.
STAGE 3:
  There is further spread of pubic hair and further enlargement of breasts and areola with no separation of their contours. The vagina enlarges and the vaginal epithelium, responding to estrogen stimulation from the maturing ovaries, increases in thickness, with considerable deposition of glycogen. The height spurt usually reaches a peak early in Stage 3, prior to menarche.
STAGE 4:
  If menarche has not occurred late in Stage 3 it should occur during Stage 4. Axillary hair appears just before or after menarche, usually in early Stage 4. There is a projection of the areola and papilla to form a secondary mound above the level of the breast. The areolar mound may be absent (25% of females). The breasts and pubic hair progress. The ovaries continue to enlarge. Ovulation may occur just after menarche, but it is usually delayed until Stage 5.
STAGE 5:
  Pubic hair and breast development resemble that of the adult female; the areola has recessed to the general contour of the breast. Height increase has decelerated since menarche; height may increase from 2 to 4 inches after menarche. By 2 years after menarche regular ovulation may be expected.
STAGE 6:
  In 10% of females there is a further spread of pubic hair.

[a] From J. M. Tanner: *Growth at Adolescence*, Appleton-Century-Crofts, New York, 1966.

lead to sexual exploration. With the liberalization of sexual mores in recent years, the problems of adolescent pregnancy and veneral diseases have grown to epidemic proportions. An understanding of adolescent sexual development is essential for the practitioner interested in counseling his teenage patients in these areas.

The staging of physical sexual development of adolescents established by Tanner is a widely accepted method of following the physical changes of puberty (Tables 5.4 and 5.5).

As the adolescent enters puberty, he also assumes a role as a sexual being. He must begin to meet expectations of his society, family, and peer group and is pushed into sexual propriety and conformity. These expectations are transmitted to the teen by multiple messages. However, these messages are often conveyed poorly, and many teens remain ignorant and insecure about sexual issues.

Early adolescence is characterized by a bisexual period, in which close friendships are formed with members of the same sex, but heterosexual attitudes develop. One sees young teens developing "best buddy" relationships. The closeness of these relationships may even be on a sexual level, but they are not considered characteristic of adult homosexuality. However, the teen (particularly male) may fear that he is a homosexual; and the frequent name calling of

Table 5.5
Typical Progression of Male Adolescent Sexual Development[a]

STAGE 1:
The male has no pubic hair or increase in size of the penis. This describes the male as a preadolescent or child. However, the testes are beginning to mature. Usually there is considerable acceleration in height and weight gain along with changes in body composition (especially more body fat).

STAGE 2:
There is early growth of the testes and scrotum before pubic hair appears. The height spurt accelerates; the male physique begins to change as fat and muscle are added; and the areola of the breast increases in size and darkens slightly.

STAGE 3:
There is further enlargement of the testes and scrotum, enlargement of the penis (mainly in length), and spreading and darkening of the pubic hair. Facial hair first appears at the corners of the upper lip. The height spurt accelerates further; there is broadening of the shoulders relative to the hips and generalized increased moulding of the body, with considerable increase in muscle mass relative to fat. Hair appears in the perineum. Facial expression is significantly altered and appears more adult. The cartilage of the larynx enlarges, and the voice may begin to deepen. There is transient gynecomastia with a slight projection of the areola.

STAGE 4:
Axillary hair first appears. There is continued enlargement of the scrotum, testes and penis (the last, mainly in breadth). The pubic hair begins to appear adult. Facial hair is still limited to the upper lip and chin. The first ejaculation, indicating considerable growth of the prostate gland, occurs early in Stage 4. Sebaceous glands are approaching adult size and function. The voice deepens further.

STAGE 5:
Genital size and pubic hair distribution are adult in appearance. Hairs are present on the sides of the face. Gynecomastia has disappeared. The height spurt has decelerated and the physique is that of the mature male.

STAGE 6:
Some adolescents have a further spread of pubic hair up the linea alba, which may be described as Stage 6. This later development, often not reached until the early 20s, occurs in 80% of males.

[a] From J. M. Tanner: *Growth at Adolescence*, Appleton-Century-Crofts, New York, 1966.

this period (in which people are called "gay" or "queer" with little provocation) may be taken too seriously. Such individuals need to be reassured of the normality of these concerns. Masturbation tends to be a frequent practice in this period, and there may be associated guilt which increases as the sex drive stimulates the teen to continue the practice. Again, where appropriate, problems associated with masturbation should be met with reassurance of its normality.

In mid- to late adolescence, dating and heterosexual activities begin in earnest. Sorenson (8) found that 52% of all adolescents and 45% of single females have had intercourse by age 19. Frequently, teens rush into sexual activity before they fully understand their own feelings about it. It is often part of the dating relationship; a prerequisite to communication, rather than vice versa. It may be part of thrill-seeking behavior for some teens, and others use it to escape from loneliness and depression. Sexuality may also be used as reward or punishment in some relationships, emulating parental behavior.

Common Problems

SHORT STATURE AND DELAYED SEXUAL MATURATION

A frequent problem that comes to the attention of physicians is the teenager with short stature and/or delayed puberty. These two symptoms are often interrelated, and the medical investigation is similar, so they will be discussed together. However, the presence of one does not necessarily indicate a problem with the other.

Most of these patients simply are at one end of the spectrum of normal development (3). Many teenage boys may not appreciate the fact that some individuals fall into the 10th percentile of a normal curve, and therefore will not respond well to a cursory dismissal of their complaints. Some may be helped by looking at normal growth curves which indicate the predicted ultimate height for persons in their percentile. Detailed discussion may be necessary for patients to comprehend fully and to cope with normal findings.

Assessment of short stature and delayed puberty by the generalist consists of the following steps:

1. A careful history of the onset of puberty and of the height of siblings, parents, and grandparents should be obtained. In particular, it should be noted if there is a history of several short family members (males under 5'6", females under 5'0").

2. Growth records of the patient should be reviewed. Heights and weights should be plotted on an appropriate growth curve (see Fig. 5.1). If a child has followed a single curve throughout life, a significant metabolic reason for his short stature is unlikely. If, however, there is a falling away from a growth line, a metabolic problem is more likely.

3. The medical history should be reviewed, includ-

ing a prenatal and neonatal history. A history of operations, head injuries, or chronic medical conditions that could predispose the individual to failure to thrive should be noted. If the child had a low birth weight, a review of underlying factors may disclose a possible chromosomal abnormality or toxic exposure (e.g., maternal cigarette smoking) that could produce long term growth delay.

4. A developmental and psychosocial history may indicate possible familial problems and/or emotional neglect that could predispose to constitutional growth delay (so-called psychosocial dwarfism).

5. Inquiries into the teen's general health and daily habits may reveal problems needing investigation, such as poor appetite, frequent infections, chronic abdominal pain, or general fatigue and listlessness.

A physical examination is essential, including an accurate height and weight and Tanner stage assessment (Tables 5.4 and 5.5). If the testes are softening and show enlargement, or if breast budding is present, there usually will be a normal sexual development. Unusual facies or ears, unusual hand creases, clinodactyly (deviation or deflection of the fingers), obesity, or delayed intellectual development, may suggest a recognizable hereditary syndrome.

The initial laboratory investigation should include the following: urinalysis; measurement of serum urea nitrogen, creatinine, and electrolytes; hematocrit value and white cell count; as well as X-rays of the hands and wrists to assess skeletal growth (2).

More specific laboratory investigations may be suggested by the history and physical examination. Examples are: (a) thyroid enlargement (testing for hypothyroidism); (b) normal physical examination and appearance but markedly short stature which is falling away from growth lines (testing for growth hormone deficiency); (c) girls with delayed puberty, heights under the 3rd percentile, associated with a short "webbed" neck, a systolic murmur, or widely spaced nipples (buccal smears performed to rule out Turner's syndrome, i.e., X-O chromosomes); (d) striking pubertal delay without a history of similar delay in other family members (testing for gonadal failure: measurement of serum follicle-stimulating and luteinizing hormones, and estradiol and of urinary 17-ketosteroids and 17-hydroxysteroids; vaginal smear for maturation index and buccal smear for chromosome analysis).

Definitive diagnosis and planning for adolescents with suspected endocrine, metabolic, genetic, or psychological reasons for maturation delay requires referral to an appropriate specialist. Patients with hereditary disorders may benefit from genetic counseling, particularly those who will be unable to bear children; for example, patients with Turner's syndrome.

VENEREAL DISEASE

Venereal diseases are epidemic in 15 to 19 year olds. This is partially due to more casual attitudes towards sex, with frequent changes of sex partners.

The diagnosis and treatment of various venereal diseases are discussed elsewhere in this book (see Chapters 26 and 91).

Public health professionals find it disheartening to witness the failure of the medical system in combating the spread of venereal disease. Many teens seem to avoid therapy and continue to pass on their disease. Physicians have not uniformly reported cases of venereal disease, and there has been a tendency to delay treatment and not reach out to case contacts.

Sex education programs have had little impact on the problem. Fear of infection apparently does not deter some teens, who appear irresponsible, impulsive, emotionally insecure, and who appear to have little respect for others. Frequently parents have failed to provide basic information about sex and the risks of infection and pregnancy which accompany it.

In most states, adolescents have a right to receive treatment for venereal disease without their parents' knowledge. The practitioner should be receptive to the teen seeking treatment. Visits for treatment should also be utilized to explain the mechanism of acquiring venereal infection and to explain and encourage the use of condoms to prevent reinfection.

PREGNANCY

Each year over a million women under the age of 20 become pregnant, half of them out of wedlock. Many of these pregnancies are associated with serious medical risks for the mother and the fetus. Mothers under 14 have particularly high risks of toxemia, anemia, prematurity, infants with low birth weight, prolonged labor, and postpartum complications. Many of these problems can be prevented by good obstetrical care, so that the first goal in adolescent pregnancy should be early diagnosis and entry into a comprehensive treatment program.

There are multiple social and behavioral reasons for the high number of teenage pregnancies. For many adolescents, pregnancy may be part of a maladaptive attempt to solve psychological issues, such as independence from a clinging mother, or manipulation of a boyfriend. Such patients may have previously engaged in other maladaptive activities such as drug abuse or delinquency. There may also be an underlying ignorance about methods and availability of birth control (see Chapter 90).

The teenager herself may be ambivalent about her pregnancy. Often, the manipulations that led to the pregnancy in the sense of achieving a prolonged relationship, etc., have not succeeded, and a sense of abandonment is felt. Furthermore, the pregnancy may have resulted in hostility from the family when the teenager is in greatest need of help of her parents.

Clearly the teenager about to make important decisions about herself and her pregnancy requires counseling. It can be provided by the primary physician or by a staff member of a counseling agency such as Planned Parenthood. In either case, the primary physician should be aware of the patient's plan and make himself available for any problems she may wish to discuss. If the teenager decides to continue with the pregnancy, she should be prepared to assume a parenting role. Furthermore, she should be educated about future pregnancies, and given medical assistance for the pediatric care needed for her infant. If possible, day care, vocational, and educational services should be available for the mother so that she may continue her education after the birth of her child. As an integral part of counseling, a stable caring person should be identified (a parent, if possible) who can assist the teen emotionally and financially, and who can help her see the future for herself and her baby in a realistic manner.

RAPE

Rape is a sexual act, usually intercourse, with a nonconsenting victim. The most frequent type of adolescent rape has been called "acquaintance rape," and it is probable that most instances are never reported. In acquaintance rape, the victim is sexually misused by a boyfriend during a date or by a casual friend, or a trusting teen may accompany her friends to a strange place where she is gang-raped.

Teens, in exploring sexuality, may not have set limits to their petting or, if limits have been set unilaterally, they may afford little protection for the victim, especially when the assailant is an adolescent for whom limit-setting has not been successful in other areas. Some teens may also, in their uncertainty, present themselves in provocative, pseudo-mature ways; for example, by wearing outrageous and provocative clothing which may be viewed as sexually inviting by male acquaintances.

There is a tendency in dealing with adolescent rape victims to imply that the assault may have been invited by the victim. Regardless of this possibility, rape should be treated as a very serious problem for the victim who reports it.

Initial care for the rape victim should be handled by a physician, with follow-up by a rape-counseling service if one exists in the community. Often, a physician who is already acquainted with the patient can provide the best care.

There are several important considerations in caring for the rape victim:

1. Rape is a crime of violence, not a sexual act.
2. Above all else, the adolescent reporting rape has usually had a very frightening experience and needs short term counseling (see Chapter 10). She will usually have a number of questions about the physical meaning of her experience, and it is important to provide answers to them.
3. She should be examined carefully for evidence of trauma, both to the pelvic organs and to the rest of her body, and the information should be carefully recorded.
4. She must decide whether she wishes to report the rape to the police. In this instance, it is essential to obtain a wet and fixed smear of the vaginal contents as early as possible to confirm the presence of spermatozoa.
5. Most rape victims will need counseling by their physician and or a counselor for a number of months to discuss persisting anxieties and questions.

PSYCHOSOCIAL DEVELOPMENT

Normal Patterns and Concerns

The major psychosocial developmental task for the adolescent as he approaches adulthood is to increase independence from his parents and to establish a positive identity congruent with social norms.

In early adolescence, the young teen is faced with the dilemma of seeking independence from parents while at the same time relying on them for emotional and physical support. The conflict over independence is evidenced by contradiction and ambivalence. For example, a teen may refuse to listen to parents' suggestions about study habits, but blame mediocre grades on the fact that the parents did not help with homework assignments.

As the teen enters into middle and late adolescence, he demonstrates a remarkable resourcefulness in coping with anxiety over separation and in learning more mature behavior. Much assistance comes through peer relationships. Teens support each other by experimenting with adult roles which mirror societal expectations of behavior; a sense of moral responsibility begins to take shape. In this period, individual identity tends to be blunted by the seeking of independence from the family. Peers tend to look alike, dress alike, date alike, and experiment with drugs and sex alike. Later, as teens address their concerns about careers, a greater differentiation of personalities takes shape, and individual identities emerge.

Normal development also requires the example of secure, healthy parents in an environment in which the teen can feel secure. Thus, parents, who are preoccupied with their own psychological problems at work, in their marriage, or with their own families, may have difficulties helping and coping with the development of their adolescent offspring. Often, such parents have not previously succeeded at their own adolescent tasks and so are unable to proceed with the task of adulthood—they have not developed the ability for intimacy, for close personal feelings, and for the sharing of feelings and thoughts with others.

One clear fact about adolescent development is that its emotional course is variable, even among "normal" adolescents. The idea that adolescence is usually a time of crisis, in which persistent neurotic behavior is essential for development of a personal identity, has not been borne out by longitudinal research. On the other hand, Kysar's study (4) of college freshmen showed that 22% had psychological problems, usually personality disorders of the compulsive, schizoid, or passive-aggressive type expressed as difficulties in academic, social, and psychosexual functioning. Offer's longitudinal study of teenage boys (7) points out that achievement of identity *is* a long term process. His subjects were first studied when they were high school freshmen, and were followed for 7 years. At the end of this interval, most subjects had yet to consolidate their identities to the point where they could develop an intimate relationship, one of the best indicators of progress to adulthood. Despite this, self-satisfaction and parental satisfaction were the norm. For many, adolescence is a crisis but an internalized, noiseless one.

Generally the teen must succeed in the other spheres of development in order to meet successfully tasks in the psychosocial sphere. In retarded children, handicapped children, or chronically ill children, the dependence-independence struggle may persist, impairing the development of self-esteem needed to develop a sense of identity.

Common Problems

JUVENILE DELINQUENCY

Juvenile delinquency is a legal term for youthful behavior that violates the law and would be adjudicated and punished if it had been committed by an adult. It is a major social problem, and will, at times, be brought to the attention of the practitioner who is asked whether there is an underlying psychological cause for the delinquent behavior. In order to deal with this issue, it is necessary to distinguish between three broad categories of delinquency, described by Weiner (9) as sociological delinquency, characterological delinquency, and neurotic delinquency.

Sociological delinquency refers to illegal acts organized by a subcultural group, i.e., street gang. The delinquent acts are adoptive in that the teen receives the approval of his peers. The following four features of the clinical history suggest sociological delinquency: first, the delinquent acts are performed with valued companions, rather than alone or with strangers; second, these teens see themselves as accepted and integral members of their peer group and rarely exhibit feelings of alienation or inadequacy; third, sociological delinquents give little evidence of neurotic symptom formation or basic character flaws; and fourth, these delinquents frequently have had supportive family relationships during early childhood, although there may have been more recent problems which have led to their current activities. Frequently, involvement in other positive group activities will change the delinquent orientation of these teens.

Characterological delinquents reflect a basically antisocial attitude toward life. Their acts do not evoke in them any guilt or remorse. Such teens are frequently loners who have not established a strong relationship of basic trust in their life. Their past history suggests a series of problems, with a flurry of destructive acts, such as fighting, fire setting, and cruelty to animals, preceding their more destructive delinquent activity. Such children often require long term psychiatric treatment.

The *neurotic delinquent* commits destructive acts as an atypical (for him) behavior pattern to illustrate and emphasize certain needs. These acts may reflect feelings of being ignored by family or peers, or indicate that the teen is suffering from some form of psychological distress, most frequently depression. The acts are committed in such a way that the teen will be caught in the process or will give himself away soon after. (Generally, if concealment of illegal acts is repetitive and successful, a neurotic basis of the delinquency is unlikely.) There is rarely a history of early behavioral problems, and typically the delinquent has enjoyed a loving relationship with parents and family members. Occasionally, however, some recent family stress may serve as the trigger for the delinquent act. In general, neurotic delinquency may be treated by the interested practitioner through short term counseling (see Chapter 10).

SUBSTANCE ABUSE

Although substance abuse is a major problem of adult life (see also Chapters 20 and 21), it frequently begins during the adolescent years. Since adolescence is a period of experimentation, it is the rare teen who has not had a drink of alcohol, smoked a cigarette, or tried marijuana. A major concern is to identify the adolescent abuser—one whose life is being disrupted by his aberrant activities. It is this teenager who is most likely to continue to abuse alcohol or drugs in adult life.

The routine examination of a teen, should include direct questioning about his use of alcohol and of drugs. If the use of a substance is excessive and hazardous, the physician should explore the factors that might have led to abuse. Drugs and/or alcohol used to excess are generally an escape from some psychological problem, and it is only by identifying the problem that the abuse may be stopped. Lecturing on the dangers of alcohol, drugs, or tobacco seems to have little impact on adolescents.

Occasionally, the serious abuser of hazardous substances will develop physiological symptoms that are dramatic enough to come to the physician's attention. Hospitalization for observation is almost always indicated for the teenager presenting with drug intoxication, even if emergency room evaluation indicates that there are no immediate medical risks. The possibility of attempted suicide may be real and must be explored. Even if this is not a factor, there is still concern about the teen's ability to control his own drug-abuse behavior.

How and when to intervene in drug-abuse behavior is a difficult question. In part, it is a moral question, where the physician's behavior may be influenced by his own beliefs about the dangers of cigarettes, alcohol, or drugs and about his right to interfere with the actions (albeit dangerous) of an autonomous individual. Furthermore, intervention in this problem is made difficult by the fact that treatment is often ineffective.

DEPRESSION AND SUICIDE

A behavioral hallmark of adolescents is mood shifts, from the peaks of elation to the depths of despair. Depressive symptoms are normal parts of psychosocial development. The quest for identity is balanced by a sense of loss once independence is achieved. Similarly, rejections by peers (e.g., first loves) may be felt very deeply. It is not unusual, as part of these depressions, for the adolescent to contemplate suicide.

Mattsson (5) describes five depressive states of adolescence. Normal *depressive mood swings* represent transient reactions to personal disappointments or family difficulties. They rarely affect other life functions. *Acute depressive reactions* are more severe states, often lasting weeks or months. They are normal reactions, similar to states of grief (See Chapter 18), often related to separation or to loss of a close friend, relative, or teacher. The adolescent who does not successfully work through his grief, and who becomes increasingly depressed and incapacitated by his loss, suffers from a *depressive neurosis*. Such teens withdraw from their normal functioning, are chronically sad, and begin to entertain suicidal ideation. This is a fairly severe level of depression and demands professional intervention. A fourth form of depression, the *masked depressions of adolescence*, can be viewed as a subgroup of the depressive neuroses. Such teens cannot tolerate their painful feelings, and express them through a variety of somatic or behavioral complaints. They may be frequent visitors to the primary care physician, suffering from ill defined, atypical symptoms without clear organic basis. Their behavior may include overeating, delinquent acts, exhibitionist acts resulting in "accidental" self-destruction, drug and alcohol abuse, etc. *Psychotic depressive disorders* are marked by impaired reality testing, thought disorders, paranoia and suicidal intention, in addition to depressive symptomatology.

The primary care physician is sometimes asked to evaluate the depressed or suicidal adolescent. In taking the history, the physician should try to uncover recent events that may have precipitated the depressive disorder: any long-standing family, school, or peer problems; possibilities of organic brain disease or of drug abuse that may mimic depressive symptoms; symptoms of cognitive or reality disturbances, suggesting a psychosis; and symptoms suggesting a masked depression. The physician should not hesitate to talk about depression with the teen. Indeed, such openness may put the adolescent at ease and let him feel that the physician truly understands what he may be feeling. A physical examination will help the physician rule out physical problems, and communication with the school will give the physician some additional observations about the teen in his daily activities.

Most adolescents with depressive symptoms need some counseling. If the primary care physician feels medication is necessary, and is unfamiliar with the use of psychoactive drugs in adolescents, conjoint treatment with a psychiatric consultant may prove helpful. Patients with long-standing depressive symptoms, which suggest thought disturbances, and possible suicide attempts should be referred for psychiatric intervention. Additional details about the office management of depression are contained in Chapter 14.

INTELLECTUAL DEVELOPMENT

Normal Patterns and Concerns

In adolescence, a major change occurs with respect to education and intellect. Schools differentiate students, placing them into vocational or academic tracks. The emphasis shifts from the learning of tasks (e.g., basic reading, writing, and arithmetic) to the accumulation of facts and the ability to think abstractly. As teens prepare for college, learning becomes a competitive task. Career choices become limited as an individual's abilities and talents become manifest. Upon entering college, a greater amount of independence and responsibility is expected. Symbolically, the university begins to resemble the workplace both in terms of potential rewards and of potential pressures.

SCHOLASTIC FAILURE

Academic achievement is strongly related to parental aspirations, socioeconomic status, and intellectual ability. Occasionally, the child cannot meet parental expectations, and the resultant crisis may lead to a visit to the physician's office. Failure in school may also be a symptom of a physical impairment, mental retardation, specific learning disabilities, or emotional stresses. By making an accurate diagnosis of the underlying problem, a caring practitioner may help such children.

First a history is necessary, to determine the nature of the school difficulties. When did they begin—has educational achievement been a problem throughout a school career, as with a global intellectual deficit, or is it specific to certain subjects or tasks, as with learning disorders? Is there a family history of poor school performance, as is seen with familial dyslexics? How does the teen act with his family and peers? Is there evidence of disturbed behavior outside of school as with emotional disorders? Is the family structure stable, or has there been separation, divorce, or death of a parent or grandparent? Is there evidence of substance abuse on the part of the teen, or a member of the family? What has the family done to try to work through problems?

Second, a physical examination, with a careful

neurological examination is indicated, with emphasis on looking for signs of minimal cerebral dysfunction, such as "soft" neurological signs, right-left discrimination or orientation difficulties, or overt signs of cerebral palsy (1). (In such patients, there may be suggestions of a neurological problem in the past medical history; the birth may have been abnormal; or the patient may have shown hyperactivity or attention deficits as a child.) Vision testing and office assessment for slight or moderate hearing loss (see Chapter 93) are also particularly important.

Third, some specific intelligence testing is indicated. Children who are mentally retarded will tend to show low I.Q. scores, and achievement tests will show a delay of several grades in math and reading levels. Children with dyslexia will have a normal I.Q. but will show a wide scatter of scores on subtests, indicating a nonglobal deficit. Achievement tests may also show a difference between abilities in reading and mathematics.

Recent research in learning disabilities indicates that some learning problems may appear relatively late in a school career. The recent criticism of the ability of some college students to write well has given credence to the notion of expressive language disorders, which may not become manifest until adolescence. Some individuals with fine perceptual problems may not reveal difficulties until geometry or drafting is studied in high school.

The Congress, in 1974, passed Federal Law 94-142, assuring a free, appropriate educational placement for all children up to age 21. Thus, adolescents with specific learning problems, retardation, or emotional difficulties are entitled to be placed in a classroom setting where they will learn. If he suspects an unrecognized problem in one of these spheres, the physician may help by referring the patient and his parents for evaluation, usually available through the child's school or the local education system. Unfortunately, problems remain unrecognized for many children, and, out of frustration, they will drop out of school.

A SUGGESTED APPROACH TO THE ADOLESCENT PATIENT IN THE OFFICE SETTING

The physician who deals even occasionally with teens and young adults must be aware of their perspective. Each adolescent approaches the developmental pressures of this period of life with his own particular skills and emotions. From a health perspective, an adolescent can be a responsible partner in maintaining his well being and complying with medical care; or he can be infantile, dependent, uncommunicative, aggressive, or irresponsible. The physician who cares for adolescents must have a temperament equal to coping with them and be a patient and perceptive listener and inquirer.

As shown in Table 5.2, although a general examination is the single most frequent reason for office visits by adolescents, the majority of visits are for specific medical problems. In either of these situations, the practitioner should use appropriate strategies in interviewing and examining the patient and should be alert for clues suggesting problems in any of the major spheres of development described in the preceding sections.

Interviewing Strategies

The physician, in obtaining a history, should interview adolescents in private. The adolescent needs to feel that he is the patient and that his problems are being listened to and taken seriously. Then it is often useful to talk to the parents separately as well.

THE PATIENT

Some adolescent patients are difficult to interview. An uncommunicative patient may have been sent to a physician against his will or may lack verbal skills needed for coherence. The physician must be verbally active with such patients and watch for any nonverbal cues as wedges to try to get the patient to speak. Examples of nonverbal cues are: a look of interest or initiation of eye contact when a subject is mentioned which the patient would like to discuss; a clenched fist when an anger-provoking subject is raised; frequent position change and fidgeting when the patient is anxious about a specific subject or about the visit to the physician in general. Because adolescents are often reticent about their major concerns, an open-minded invitation to share information ("Is there anything else you wanted to talk about?") should be included in each office contact. The initial comprehensive interview may require several sessions. At the first visit, warmth and interest in the adolescent may open the way to better communication in future sessions.

Many adolescents continue to go to their pediatrician for medical care until they enter college, take a job, or marry. Because of this long term association, their relationship may be almost like that of a father and child—warm, intense, and comradely. These feelings cannot be transferred easily to a new physician and it is unwise to attempt to transfer them.

The physician can most effectively surmount such problems by explaining his *modus operandi* in advance, emphasizing that he will be primarily the adolescent's physician, rather than an agent of the patient's parents as had been the case previously. Communications should be adult-to-adult whenever possible.

The internist should encourage the adolescent to initiate patient-doctor contacts, guard against patriarchal advice-giving, and avoid showing disapproval or surprise when the adolescent attempts to impress him with tales of sexual exploits, with the use of vulgar language, etc.

It is wise to establish other ground rules with adolescents. Patient-doctor confidentiality, for example, can be assured to adolescents only in so far as they do not reveal that they are comtemplating harmful acts, such as running away or committing suicide. However, certain privileged communications should be kept confidential from parents. In particular, adolescent minors have the right to be seen for venereal disease or for sex-offense related examinations without the prior consent of a parent. The teen may also wish to keep some health-related or emotional problems, such as drug experimentation, from a parent's knowledge.

THE PARENTS

How does an adolescent's physician communicate with the parent? It is suggested that, whenever possible, a parent should be involved with and concerned about the health of the teen. A separate interview with a parent, immediately before or after the examination, may prove helpful and can emphasize particular concerns downplayed or denied by the patient. The parents of adolescent patients may be useful in aiding treatment, providing emotional support and ensuring compliance with therapy; therefore, informing them about the adolescent's problems and needs is important.

Some parents ask physicians to take on the role of health educator or counselor for their adolescent child. Usually, these requests are for anticipatory guidance about birth control or drug usage. At times, the physician is asked to help the child work through an upcoming family crisis, such as divorce, serious illness, or death. Frequently, adolescents welcome the opportunity to discuss these issues in private. Their knowledge in these areas is often found wanting, and the sensitive physician may help the adolescent grasp realities and make intelligent decisions. A number of books are directed to an adolescent audience in these areas, and it may be useful to make these titles available:

R. A. Gardner: *Boys and Girls Book about Divorce* (*Grades I and Up*), Burtan, New York, 1971.

E. Kay: *Sex and the Young Teenager* (*Grades 7–12*), Franklin-Watts, Inc., New York, 1973.

H. Soethcord: *Sex Before Twenty: New Answers for Young People*, E. P. Dutton, New York, 1971.

K. McCoy and C. Wibbelsman: *The Teenage Body Book*, Pocket Books, New York, 1978.

Parents often have questions about specific adolescent behavior. A particular episode or issue may come to the parents' attention, and they ask the physician whether they should exert control over it. In such instances, the physician should not offer specific advice, but should try to discern any moral or behavioral conflicts between the parents and the adolescent. When the parent's behavior is inconsistent with the parent's own stated values, adolescents will often act in opposition to those values. Miller (6) suggests that parents are not helped in this instance by being told how to behave. Advice either increases the parent's uncertainty when faced with later difficulties or implies that the parent's own opinions are inappropriate. Adolescents probably turn out mentally healthier when presented with models of adult behavior with which their parents are comfortable, whether consistent with societal norms or not. Parents must be prepared, however, to make allowances so that their children have freedom to make their own "mistakes." Family counseling is a technique which the general physician can utilize when several members of a household are involved (see Chapter 10).

Health Assessment

The initial interview(s) should be comprehensive enough to ensure that the adolescent is meeting appropriate developmental tasks. Inquiries should be made into the teens' relationships and functioning with their families, at school, and with peers. It is important to determine whether the teens are establishing positive personal identities (Have they hobbies? Do they voice their own opinions? Can they choose their own friends or must friends be approved by the parents? Do they have plans for the future?); whether they are accepting their sexuality and adjusting to adult sexual roles (Do they date? Are they sexually active? Do they have a knowledge of contraception? Is contraception used?); whether they are establishing independence from the family (Do they drive? Do they earn money on their own? What sort of hours do they keep?); whether they are working toward a career (What are their plans after high school? What subjects in school do they like? What are their grades? Do they plan to go to college? Are their goals realistic and are they supported by the family?); whether they have established good health habits (What are their views about nutrition? Have they experimented with alcohol or drugs? What drugs? Have they ever been drugged or high when driving or when attending school?); and whether affective swings are interfering with functioning (Do they often feel down? What makes them happy? Have sad feelings ever made them consider harming themselves?).

As part of the review of systems before examination, a self-administered medical questionnaire may be useful and time-saving. Such a questionnaire should be brief with language simple enough to be understood by teens with poor reading skills. Positive answers often need to be explored further. A physical examination should be performed in the absence of parents. Teenage girls examined by male physicians may be more comfortable with an adult female in the room with them. Some parts of the physical examination occasionally omitted by physicians but essential for adolescent patients include blood pressure measurement, examination of the entire integument, of the spine (for scoliosis), and of the external genitalia (for signs of venereal disease and for assessment of sexual development using Tanner's staging—see Tables 5.4 and 5.5). All sexually active adolescent girls should have a pelvic examination, including gonorrheal cultures and a Pap smear. If the physician is uncomfortable doing this examination, the teen should be referred to a gynecologist who is used to dealing with adolescents.

There are several useful adjuncts to the physical examination of the healthy adolescent. These include testing for myopia and hyperopia (using a Snellen chart) and screening for deafness (by speaking softly). Adolescence is a period marked by noise pollution, in the form of loud music which can cause permanent damage to the eighth nerve (see Chapter 93). Those adolescents who have difficulty in school should be screened for learning disorders. Having a teenager read a newspaper paragraph out loud, or do some simple arithmetic may reveal a previously undetected learning disability.

Laboratory screening tests for healthy adolescents should include a full urinalysis, a complete blood count, and tuberculin testing. Screening for hyperlipidemias (Chapter 72) is indicated in adolescents with family histories of myocardial infarction or of stroke under the age of 50. Blood chemical screens, chest X-rays, and electrocardiograms are not indicated in healthy adolescents. Specific recommendations regarding periodic health assessment in adolescents and young adults are found in Chapter 2 (Table 2.1).

References

General

Blos, P: *On Adolescence.* The Free Press, New York, 1962.
   A standard treatise on adolescence, with a psychoanalytic perspective.
Erickson, EH: *Identity, Youth, and Crisis.* Norton, New York, 1968.
   The most widely used theoretical model of adolescent psychosocial development.
Gallagher, JR, Heald, FP and Garell, DC (eds.): *Medical Care of the Adolescent,* Ed. 3. Appleton Century-Crofts, New York, 1976.
   An excellent textbook on adolescent medicine. Emphasizes patient-doctor relationship.
Garell, DC (ed.): Symposium in adolescent medicine. *Pediatr. Clin. North Am.* 20: 769, 1973.
   A good series of reviews of clinical problems of adolescents.
Haggerty, RJ: Adolescence, in *Ambulatory Pediatrics,* Ed. 2. W.B. Saunders, Phildelphia, 1977.
   A brief review of adolescent disorders.
Kenniston, K: *Youth, Transition to Adulthood, Vol. II; American Handbook of Psychiatry,* Ed. 2. Basic Books, New York, 1974.
   Another standard text; the perspective is sociological.
Sorenson, RC: *Adolescent Sexuality in Contemporary America.* World, New York, 1973.
   A good overview of sexual problems of adolescents, and proposed social policy approaches.
Tanner, JM: *Growth at Adolescence,* Ed. 2. Charles C Thomas, Springfield, Ill., 1962.
   A classic system for describing the physiological changes of adolescents.

Specific

1. Desmond, MM, Volderman, AL and Fisher, ES: Assessment of learning competence during the pediatric examination. *Curr Prob Pediatr,* **8,** 2, 1978.
2. Greulich, WW and Pyle, SI: *Radiographic Atlas of Skeletal Development of the Hand and Wrist.* Stanford University Press, Stanford, Calif., 1974.
3. Kogut, MD: Growth and development in adolescents. *Pediatr Clin North Am* 20: 789, 1973.
4. Kysar, JR, Zaks, MS, Schuchman, HP, Schon, GL and Rogers, J: Range of psychological functioning in "normal" late adolescents. *Arch Gen Psychiatry* 21: 515, 1969.
5. Mattsson, A: Adolescent depression and suicide. In *Principles of Pediatrics,* pp. 665–669, edited by RA Hockelman, S Blatman, PA Bounell, SB Friedman and HM Seidel. McGraw-Hill, New York, 1978.
6. Miller, D: Adolescent crisis: Challenge for patient, parent, and internist. *Ann Intern Med* 79: 435, 1973.
7. Offer, D, Marcus, D and Offer, JL: A longitudinal study of normal adolescent boys. *Am J Psychiatry* 126: 917, 1970.
8. Sorenson, RC: *Adolescent Sexuality in Contemporary America.* World, New York, 1973.
9. Weiner, IB: Delinquent behavior. In *Psychological Disturbance in Adolescence,* Chap. 8. John Wiley & Sons, New York, 1970.

CHAPTER SIX

Geriatric Patients: Special Considerations

EDMUND G. BEACHAM, M.D.

INTRODUCTION

This chapter will review certain general characteristics of geriatric medicine, and also deal with some specific problems. Where appropriate, reference will be given to other chapters dealing with subjects important to geriatric practice.

There will be an increasing population of elderly patients in the next few decades. In 1900, only 4% of persons living in the United States were 65 or older, compared to more than 10% at the present time. By the year 2000, it is estimated that 12% of the population, or 30 million individuals, will be in this age group (Fig. 6.1). Further it is expected that almost half of this elderly population will be over 75 years of age—the so-called "old old" or the frail elderly (8). In 1900, 29% of persons over 65 years were older than 75; but by 2000 it is estimated that 45% of this population will be older than 75 years. An unrecognized fact is that 95% of all elderly are not institutionalized, but live at home (4), and 30% of these live alone.

A national survey (1) has shown that visits by patients to physicians' offices increase in direct proportion to the patients' age. For the entire population surveyed there were 2.7 visits per year to physicians' offices compared to 4.3 visits per year for elderly patients. The increasing size of the elderly population and the higher rate of office visits by elderly patients will result in an increased geriatric practice for most physicians.

Another survey (2) showed also that 62% of the visits by those over 65 years are for chronic conditions, in contrast to only 31% of visits for those under 65. The survey revealed that elderly patients see physicians mostly for a few relatively common problems (Table 6.1). The problems perceived by the patient, however, are not necessarily the same as the diagnoses established by the physicians (Table 6.2).

DATA BASE FOR THE ELDERLY

Historical Information

Although baseline information about the elderly may be available, it is frequently fragmented at various sites as the patient has moved or changed physicians. Retrieving this information is an important goal in the development of the data base. Before their first visit, it is helpful to ask patients or their relatives, to list their past medical history and sources of medical care so that as much pertinent information as possible may be requested. A simple questionnaire is often helpful in this regard as well as in reporting family, demographic, and social information (Table 6.3). Too complex a questionnaire may frustrate elderly patients and negate its usefulness.

There are several aspects of the history that are particularly important in the elderly population:

NUTRITIONAL HISTORY

The nutritional history in older patients often reveals real or potential problems. Lack of funds may dictate a choice of cheap, poor quality food. Isolation, depression, or a chronic disabling condition of mobility or sight may preclude obtaining or preparing food. Further, poor dentition or absence of teeth may prevent eating certain foods. Much insight into the diet can be gained by having the patient describe the meals eaten on the previous day.

MEDICATION HISTORY

Information about medication is especially pertinent. Frequently elderly patients have over-the-counter medications or outdated prescriptions for

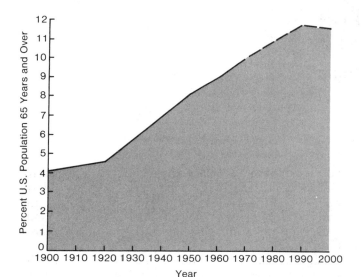

Figure 6.1 Elderly patients in the United States. (Adapted from: U.S. Department of Health, Education and Welfare, prepared by the National Institute on Aging, National Institute of Health: *Our Future Selves: A Research Plan Toward Understanding Aging*, NIH Publication No. 80-1096. National Institute on Aging Information Office, Bethesda, MD., 1980.)

Table 6.1
Most Frequent Reason Given by Patients Over 65 Years for Visits To Physicians' Offices[a]

Patient Problem	Percent of Visits
Musculoskeletal complaints	14.9
Follow-up visits	14.5
Cough or breathlessness	4.7
Fatigue	4.2
Follow-up visits after surgery	4.2
Dizziness and head and neck problems	3.9
Eye problems	3.7
High blood pressure	2.9
Abdominal pain	2.8
Physical examinations	1.9
Visits for medications	1.8
Diabetes mellitus	1.2

[a] Adapted from Advancedata: U.S. Public Health Service Publication No. 22, March 22, 1977 (2). The problems listed above represent approximately two-thirds of total office visits by the elderly.

drugs which may be detrimental to them. It is helpful to have the patient or the patient's family bring all the medications that can be found in the house to the office at the first visit so that they may be reviewed with the physician.

SOCIAL HISTORY

The social history is also of particular importance. Knowing who lives with the older person, or how close to the patient relatives or close friends live, as well as the frequency of their visits will inform the physician of the resources available to the older patient. The physician should also know the physical

Table 6.2
Diagnoses Established by Physicians for Elderly Patients Visiting Their Offices[a]

Diagnosis	Percentage of Visits
Heart disease and arteriosclerosis	10.9
Essential benign hypertension	8.3
Arthritis and allied conditions	6.1
Diabetes mellitus	4.5
Eye problems	4.4
Medical and surgical after care	4.2
Bronchitis and emphysema and upper respiratory infections	3.1
Medical or special examinations	1.4
Neurosis	1.4
Skin problems	1.2

[a] Adapted from Advancedata: U.S. Public Health Service Publication No. 22, March 22, 1977 (2). The above diagnoses accounted for approximately one-half of the problems for which patients saw physicians.

aspects of the elderly patient's dwelling, so that he can make suggestions that may help avert potential dangers. Financial difficulties are also common, and yet the older patient may be embarrassed to raise them as problems.

Evaluating the elderly patient at home at least once is a most productive method of appreciating the patient's environment and social situation.

Physical Examination

In the elderly it is important to provide a careful evaluation of vision, hearing, and dentition, as problems with these functions are very frequent causes of disability. The chapters on cataracts and glaucoma (Chapters 94 and 95), hearing loss (Chapter 93), and dentistry (Chapter 98) discuss the assessment of these problems in some detail.

Evaluation of mobility is also an important part of the initial assessment of an elderly individual. The U.S. Department of Health, Education and Welfare (6) reported that 18% of individuals over 65 years had impaired mobility. Most were hesitant and uncertain in walking, and many required either special equipment or another person to help them ambulate.

Special attention should be directed toward the mental status of the elderly as discussed in the Chapter on Geriatric Psychiatry (Chapter 16). Abnormalities are frequently encountered, and establishment of the mental status initially may help in subsequent management.

Laboratory Data

Since elderly patients have usually been in hospitals, or have been seen by physicians, a data base is often available. It is helpful to collect this information and repeat only that which is necessary. Exhaustive workups or strenuous procedures such as a barium enema, intravenous pyelogram, or pulmonary function studies are often detrimental to older patients and should be selected with care.

Table 6.3
Confidential Health Questionnaire

NAME: _____   DATE OF BIRTH: _____

1. What are your current medical problems or symptoms?
   _____
   _____

2. What medicines do you take every day or often? (Include over-the-counter medication.)
   _____
   _____

3. What medicines or foods are you allergic to?
   _____

4. Do you smoke?   YES_____   NO_____
   If yes, how many packs per day?_____;   for how many years?_____
   How old were you when you started?_____

5. How many cups of coffee and tea do you drink a day?_____

6. How much alcohol do you drink? Daily_____   Weekly_____

7. When was your last tetanus shot?_____

8. Have you lost or gained weight in the past several weeks?_____   How much_____

9. (If female): When was your last Pap test?_____
   Do you examine your breasts regularly?_____

10. Circle any diseases that your blood relatives are known to have:
    Diabetes,   High Blood Pressure,   Cancer,   Heart Attack,   Gout,   Kidney Stones,   Asthma,   Hayfever,   Hives

11. FAMILY HISTORY:

Relations	Medical Problems	Current Age or Age at Death
Mother		
Father		
Brothers and Sisters (list):		
Children:		

12. List hospitalizations in the last 5 years.
    _____
    _____

13. List the names of physicians you have seen in the last 5 years.
    _____
    _____

DIAGNOSIS OF DISEASE IN THE ELDERLY

Disease *versus* Aging

A constant concern of practitioners in dealing with the elderly is the separation of disease from normal aging. Longitudinal studies have demonstrated a gradual decrease in function in many organ systems with advancing age (11). There is, however, great individual variation so that it may be difficult to decide whether any one clinical observation or laboratory value is normal. Figure 6.2 shows several different observations expressed as a percentage of function remaining after age 30, which is arbitrarily taken to represent 100% of function. There is a predictable linear decline which accompanies advancing age in virtually every measurement.

Multiple Pathology in the Elderly

Predictably in the elderly, more often than in the young, multiple organ systems are involved in a variety of disease processes simultaneously. Clustering of problems, especially deafness, diminished vision, heart disease and arthritis is particularly common in older individuals. Since several chronic problems as well as an acute exacerbation of chronic disease, or any combination of acute and chronic illness, are not uncommon, assessment of the elderly patient is difficult.

Altered Reaction to Disease in the Elderly

Elderly patients frequently respond quite differently to disease processes than do younger patients. For example, myocardial infarction may be signaled not by severe chest pain but by congestive heart failure or by changes in mental status. Infection in the elderly is frequently unaccompanied by fever or leukocytosis and may be manifest only by confusion or malaise. In fact acute changes in mental status such as confusion, disorientation, agitation, or delirium all are common manifestations of a variety of disorders in older people, so that a change in behavior in such patients should alert the clinician to the possibility of reversible disease.

MANAGEMENT OF DISEASE IN THE ELDERLY

General

It is clear from the previous sections that the approach to treatment of elderly patients will differ in a number of respects from treatment of younger patients. Limited goals are not only more often appropriate, but limited success is often acceptable. People sometimes have a feeling of hopelessness when dealing with elderly patients, but older people often view their own situations far more optimistically (3). If this is appreciated, the physician may work out with the patient an acceptable goal in the management of a health problem. In general, treatment should be as simple and as singular as possible and as brief and gentle as possible.

Prescriptions

Small doses of medications which are increased as the need indicates minimize the chance of iatrogenic complications. Whenever more than one medication is prescribed to elderly patients, it is almost always necessary that they have supplied to them a "medication" card describing the various medications, the time of their administration, and their use. It is important to minimize the number of doses so that patients will be able to comply.

The effectiveness and toxicity of drugs may be altered in older patients. Decline in total body water and lean mass with advancing age leads to changes

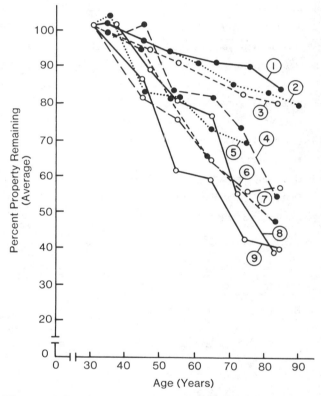

Figure 6.2 Organ system function and aging. *1*, conduction velocity; *2*, basal metabolic rate; *3*, standard cell water; *4*, cardiac index; *5*, standard glomerular filtration rate (inulin); *6*, vital capacity; *7*, standard renal plasma flow (diodrast); *8*, standard renal plasma flow (PAH); *9*, maximal breathing capacity. (Adapted from N. N. Shock: *Scientific American, 206:* 100, 1962 (11).

in distribution of some drugs. Further, drug metabolism may be diminished because of changes in hepatic metabolism or changes in renal function.

DIGOXIN

Digoxin is frequently prescribed for older patients and accounts for almost one-third of all serious adverse drug reactions occurring in the elderly population. Eighty-five percent of the drug is excreted by the kidneys so that the half-life of digoxin increases from about 38 hours in young individuals to approximately 68 hours in older ones. Therefore, the dose needed to maintain an optimal plasma level may be less in the elderly. The concentration of digoxin in the plasma should be measured periodically to ensure that the patient is compliant (level above 0) and is not accumulating the drug to toxic levels. Further, since effectiveness of digoxin in patients who are in sinus rhythm is often limited, the physician will need to review regularly whether digitalis is still required, and to discontinue its use whenever possible (7).

ANALGESICS AND SEDATIVES

Elderly patients are more sensitive to drugs acting on the central nervous system than are younger patients. Morphine and pentazocine (Talwin) have been shown at a given dose to have a greater analgesic effect, and benzodiazepines generally have an increased depressant effect in the elderly. If such agents are prescribed, they should first be given in low doses, with small increments until an effective dose is reached.

PSYCHIATRIC DRUGS

Tricyclic antidepressants have more sedative and anticholinergic effects in older patients. Cardiac arrhythmias, hypotension, confusion, urinary retention, and aggravation of glaucoma are all seen more frequently in elderly patients. A detailed review of these medications in the elderly population can be found in Chapter 16, "Psychiatric Problems of Old Age."

ANTIHYPERTENSIVE DRUGS

Postural hypotension is very common in elderly individuals, particularly in those over 75 (10). This may explain in part their increased sensitivity to antihypertensive drugs. Thus antihypertensive drugs should be used cautiously and the patient should be checked regularly for orthostatic hypotension. Hypertension in the elderly is discussed in more detail in Chapter 59.

PREVENTIVE MEASURES IN THE CARE OF THE ELDERLY

Vaccines

Influenza vaccines should be given yearly to persons over age 65, as well as a recently developed vaccine against the most common strains of pneumococcal bacteria, which is recommended as a single injection (see Chapter 30).

Accidents are common in the elderly (see below). Many older people, especially if they were not in military service may never have received primary tetanus immunization. If it is not clear that a patient has been immunized, primary immunization with tetanus toxoid is appropriate.

Prevention of Accidents

The National Safety Council in 1975 (9) reported 105,000 deaths in the United States directly attributable to accidents. Twenty-four percent of these deaths involved patients 65 years or older. Although the elderly represented 10% of the whole population, they accounted for 71% of fatal falls, 29% of deaths due to fires, and 24% of pedestrian motor vehicle accidents.

Periodic evaluation of hearing and vision is important to detect problems that can be corrected and thus help prevent many of these accidents. When necessary, physicians should emphasize the importance of proper lighting, nonslip floors, railings on steps, and even bedside commodes in the home.

Preretirement Counseling and Planning

Many problems of the elderly can be minimized if they are contemplated before people become old. Not only are books available to help the older person in planning (5), but also large corporations, senior citizen centers, and college centers offer courses in preretirement counseling and planning. Discussion groups cover such topics as anticipated economic changes, changes in tempo and nature of activities, importance of development of hobbies and activities for leisure time.

Community Resources for the Elderly

Physicians working with the elderly should be aware of the resources available to assist in their management. Local or state health departments may have special geriatric divisions. If not, all local or state health departments will have information on availability of nurses, home health care, home-making services, eating together and transportation programs, and other activities of special interest to the elderly. There are also many senior citizen centers available where the elderly can find friends, recreation, and social stimulation.

Finally, detailed planning between the patient and physician before an elderly patient is discharged from the hospital will avert future problems that might otherwise be created by confusion and misunderstanding.

References

General

Adams, GF: *Essentials of Geriatric Medicine.* Oxford Medical Publications, New York, 1977.
> *This short book covers well the process of aging; essentials of clinical practice; common complaints in old age, and use of drugs in geriatric medicine. It includes an excellent table on effects of aging.*

Anderson, WF: *Practical Management of the Elderly.* Blackwell, London, 1977.
> *This internationally known Scottish geriatrician emphasizes day to day care of the elderly person. He stresses preventive aspects of illness as age advances.*

Brocklehurst, JC: *Textbook of Geriatric Medicine and Gerontology,* Ed 2. Churchill Livingstone, New York, 1978.
> *This authoritative British text covers biological gerontology, clinical geriatric medicine, and socio-psychological gerontology, together with organization of medical care for the elderly.*

Cape, R: *Aging: Its Complex Management.* Harper & Row, New York, 1978.

The purpose of this book is to focus attention to clinical problems of the very old. It is well written and covers major problems.

Cowdry, EV and Steinberg, FU: *The Care of the Geriatric Patient,* Ed. 4. C.V. Mosby, St. Louis, 1971.

Comprehensive information about geriatric practice, with more than 50 international contributors.

Freeman, SA, and Steinheber, FU: Geriatric medicine. *Med Clin North Am 60:* No. 6, 1976.

This symposium on geriatric medicine describes the experience of the staff of Coney Island Hospital, New York.

Medical Letter: Drugs in the Elderly, 18 May 1979.

This review discusses analgesics and sedatives; antimicrobials; psychiatric drugs, anticoagulants, antihypertensive and diuretic drugs; digoxin; theophylline and quinidine; and multiple drug regimens.

Reichel, W: *Clinical Aspects of Aging.* Williams & Wilkins, Baltimore, 1978.

This multiauthored book was prepared under the direction of the American Geriatrics Society. It is practical, emphasizes the patient, and was written primarily for continuing education.

Reichel, W: *The Geriatric Patient.* HP Publishing Co., New York, 1978.

This book was based on a collection of Hospital Practice articles. It is directed towards the primary physician caring for the elderly.

Smith, CR: Use of drugs in the aged. *Johns Hopkins Med J 145:* 61, 1979.

This paper discusses reasons for noncompliance of the aged with medication regimens. It reviews pharmacokinetics and aging and reports in detail on digoxin, the benzodiazephines, propranolol, and the opiate analgesics.

Specific

1. Advancedata: U.S. National Center for Health Statistics, U.S. Public Health Service Publication No. 12, October 12, 1977, HRA 77-1250.
2. Advancedata: U.S. National Center for Health Statistics. U.S. Public Health Service, Publication No. 22, March 22, 1977. DHEW publication No. (PHS) 78-1250.
3. Beverly, EV: The beginnings of wisdom about aging. *Geriatrics 30:* 117, 1975.
4. Brickner, PW, Duque, T, Kaufman, A, Sarg, M, Jahre, JA, Maturlo, S and Janeski, JF: The homebound aged. A medically unreached group. *Ann Intern Med 82:* 1, 1975.
5. Buckley, JC: *Retirement Handbook. A complete guide to planning your future,* Ed. 6, edited by H Schmidt. Harper & Row, Hagerstown, Md., 1977.
6. Facts about Older Americans: DHEW Pub. No. (OHDS) 79-20006, 1978.
7. Johnston, GD and McDevitt, DG: Is maintenance digoxin necessary in patients with sinus rhythm? *Lancet 1:* 567, 1979.
8. Kane, R, Solomon, D, Beck, J, Keeler, E and Kane, R: The future need for geriatric manpower in the United States. *N Engl J Med 302:* 1327, 1980.
9. National Safety Council: *Accidents to the Elderly: Age 65 and Over.* National Safety Council, Chicago, Ill., 1975.
10. O'Malley, K and O'Brien, E: Management of hypertension in the elderly. *N Eng J Med 302:* 1397, 1980.
11. Shock, NN: The physiology of aging. *Sci Am 206:* 100, 1962.

CHAPTER SEVEN

Occupational and Environmental Disease

JAMES P. KEOGH, M.D.

INTRODUCTION

Over 100,000 people die each year in the United States as a direct result of occupational disease, and at least 400,000 will develop an occupational disease. Every practitioner will see patients with occupational problems, and he must be prepared to recognize these problems and to provide appropriate care to the patient.

This is an era characterized by an explosive proliferation of new and potentially toxic chemicals which are encountered in homes, schools, the general environment, and especially in the workplace. While this chapter focuses on diseases of the workplace, it should be evident that the chemical era has altered the environment in ways that affect the health of many individuals. Episodes in the past 15 years such as the mercury contamination of Minamata Bay (Japan), the Kepone spill in the James River of Virginia, the contamination of milk and cattle by polybrominated biphenyls in Michigan, and the dioxin contamination of Seveso, Italy, have gained much attention. The extent to which less intense exposure of communities may be causing *unrecognized* problems is an equally grave concern. In the future, few communities in the United States will escape public concern over the health hazards of pesticide spraying, asbestos in school buildings, contaminated drinking water, or toxic waste disposal.

This chapter provides an overview of how occupational diseases occur and outlines an approach to enable the physician to recognize and deal with work-related illnesses. It also provides information about selected occupational diseases and how to obtain more information about them.

THE PATHOGENESIS OF OCCUPATIONAL DISEASE

The pathogenesis of occupational disease is complex and involves not only the interaction between the host and a toxic substance, but a complex set of social interactions.

Toxin-Host Interaction

For an occupational disease to occur, there must be a triad consisting of a toxic agent, a host, and an environment in which the host is exposed (Fig. 7.1). The illness which may result depends on the toxic properties of the substance, its route of entry, the dose received by the host, and the susceptibility of the host to the toxin.

Toxic agents can be inhaled, ingested, or absorbed through the skin. With inhalation, the dose received depends on whether the substance is present as a fume or a dust. Absorption of dust from the lungs depends to a great extent on particle size and distribution, since smaller particles can more easily enter the alveoli and become trapped. The concentration of the substance in the air (which is related to room ventilation, temperature, and humidity), the rate at which the worker is exercising and breathing, protective factors such as special clothing or respirator use are factors which affect the likelihood of illness. Table 7.1 summarizes factors which affect absorption of a toxic substance.

Once the toxic substance is absorbed there may be an instantaneous effect as in the case of carbon monoxide poisoning, a brief latent period, as in the case of occupational asthma, or a latent period of years or decades as in the pneumoconioses. A brief, high dose exposure may cause serious illness and death and be relatively easily recognizable. On the other hand, prolonged exposure to a low dose of a toxin may not cause symptoms at the outset, and identification of remote toxic effects may be quite difficult.

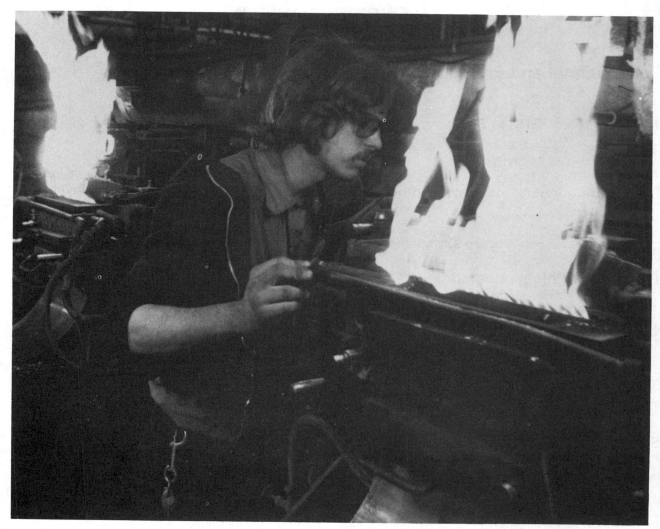

Figure 7.1 Many patients are working in unhealthy and unsafe conditions. Here a worker casts lead plates in an automobile battery plant without protection from fumes. (Photograph courtesy U.S. Department of Labor.)

Table 7.1
Factors Affecting Absorption of a Toxic Substance

CHARACTERISTICS OF THE SUBSTANCE
    Concentration in the air
    Particle size and configuration
    Water solubility
    Taste
    Lipid solubility
CHARACTERISTICS OF THE PATIENT
    Respiratory rate
    Smoking or eating during exposure
    Permeability of clothing
    Sweating
CHARACTERISTICS OF THE ENVIRONMENT
    Ambient temperature and humidity
    Ventilation

Social Interactions Affecting Occupational Disease

Thousands of new chemicals are introduced into industrial processes every year; few have had testing to detect their potential toxicity. Even when toxico-logical screening tests are done on a compound, these may not predict human disease. In all too many cases, the hazardousness of a chemical is recognized only after an outbreak of illness.

Economic factors play a major role in determining how safe a workplace is. Industrial hygiene programs to monitor exposure are common only in the largest plants. Important decisions such as improving ventilation or decreasing exposure to noise may involve significant expense. Therefore management must weigh the benefits of protecting employee health and complying with regulations against the cost of doing so.

The worker may be reluctant to complain about working conditions for fear of losing his job. This is especially marked during periods of high unemployment, when acceptance of unpleasant and potentially unhealthy working conditions may be the price of having a job. The physician who fails to recognize this may be perplexed by his patient's unwillingness to take action to secure better conditions at work.

Even when workers are strongly organized, the desire for a safer workplace may be balanced by a concern that increased production costs may result in a company's decision to relocate its plant to areas where unions are less effective or do not exist.

THE PRIMARY PRACTITIONER'S ROLE

Although episodes of illness caused or exacerbated by the patient's work are frequently seen in ambulatory practice, they are frequently not recognized as such, and even less often are appropriately managed. The practitioner who is prepared to recognize the connection between the patient's symptoms and the patient's work can make a big difference for both the individual and the community. The practitioner who fails to think about the patient's occupation may:

1. Miss the diagnosis entirely and pursue the wrong therapy;
2. Permit continuation of poor working conditions which may subsequently injure others or even result in death.

Two cases illustrate these points:

An 18-year-old woman complained to her physician of a severe cough and some wheezing. He treated her with erythromycin and fluids and advised her to stay in bed for a few days. She recovered and returned to work feeling well. Several days later she had a severe recurrent cough with wheezing and dyspnea and saw her physician again. He again prescribed erythromycin and rest. She remained off work for a week. She felt better and returned to work. After 2 days she became extremely short of breath and was brought to the emergency room. She had severe bronchospasm and was admitted, improving on bronchodilators and steroids after a few days.

History on admission disclosed that her work involved grinding drill bits made of tungsten carbide, a known pulmonary sensitizer. Had the first physician considered the diagnosis of extrinsic asthma he could have prevented the patient's subsequent deterioration.

A 25-year-old man presented to the emergency room of a community hospital with a chief complaint of headache. Physical examination was negative and he was given an aspirin-narcotic compound.

Seen some weeks later, a history of irritability, abdominal pain, insomnia, and constipation was elicited. The patient worked in an automobile assembly plant where he used a grinding wheel to smooth joints filled with a lead-containing solder. His blood lead level was 3 times normal. After therapy with a chelating agent he became symptom-free. Subsequent investigation revealed that most of his co-workers had high blood lead levels; three of them were subsequently treated for lead poisoning. Questioning the patient about his work could have saved him weeks of discomfort and prevented some of his co-workers from being poisoned.

To avoid such mistakes the primary practitioner needs an approach that will work for the whole range of occupational problems. Such an approach has been formulated. Its use requires the practitioner to remember only four important precepts: (a) ask the patient about his job; (b) consider the possibility that the problem may be occupational in etiology; (c) follow up suspicions, others may be in danger; and (d) know that Workmen's Compensation is for the benefit of the patient.

What Is the Patient's Job

The diagnosis of an occupational disease cannot be made unless the physician asks every patient about his job as part of the general medical history (Fig. 7.2). Usually, a brief discussion of the current job including a brief description of how the patient spends his working day is sufficient. Only occasionally is a comprehensive occupational history necessary (Table 7.2).

Inquiring about a patient's job will not only help identify occupational disease, it will provide other useful information. Clearly the physical demands of the job are important when advising a patient about a health problem, as is the working schedule since shift work affects medication schedules, diet, and family life. Financial stress may result from layoffs, whereas regular overtime may bring about psychological stress.

What Is the Possibility That a Problem May Be Occupational in Etiology

The key to identifying occupational disease is to be sure that a toxic/environmental etiology is at least considered. For example, the patient may be asked, "Do you think this problem could have anything to do with your work?" and, "Does anyone else at work have this same problem?" In many cases the patient will say no, which does not exclude the possibility but makes it somewhat less likely. Occasionally, the patient will think that there is a connection, but the physician may recognize that the reasons are invalid. Very often, however, if there is a connection, the patient will be able to identify it. The literature of occupational medicine is replete with episodes where workers knew for months or years of an unusually high incidence of a syndrome and were unable to get their physicians to listen to them.

If neither the physician or the patient know if a syndrome is occupational in origin, there are reference texts available which permit the physician to identify: (a) toxic causes of a given symptom complex (see Levy and Wegman or Proctor and Hughes in the General References), (b) toxic exposures of given professions (see Key et al.) and (c) the effects of exposure to given substances (see Hamilton and Hardy).

Follow Up Suspicions: Others May Be in Danger

If there is suspicion that a patient became ill from an occupational exposure, it is the physician's responsibility to follow up. Not only does diagnosing

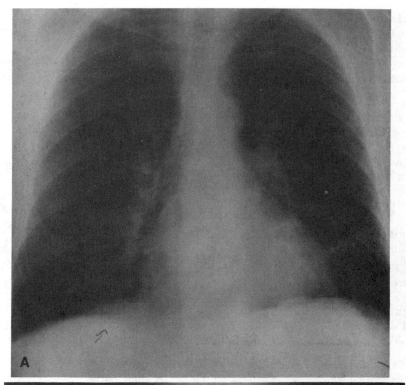

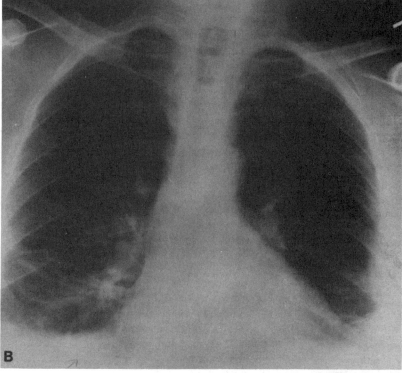

Figure 7.2 *The occupational history is critical.* This 52-year-old man was evaluated for a subendocardial myocardial infarction. His X-ray (*B*) was felt to show bilateral pleural effusions. A film taken 4 years before (*A*) showed only a thin rim of calcification in the diaphragm. After two unsuccessful attempts at thoracentesis, an occupational history was taken which confirmed extensive asbestos exposure ending 10 years before. The presence of pleural thickening, lower lung field interstitial fibrosis, and a calcified pleural plaque is pathognomonic of asbestosis.

an occupational disease affect therapy and eligibility for compensation for a patient, but it may indicate that the health of others is also in danger. Often physicians overcome their own uneasiness about a patient's job by advising the patient to change jobs. Then, instead of the potentially hazardous job being made safe, another unsuspecting person is brought in to take the risk.

There are some circumstances where occupational disease is recognized but the original hazard has been eliminated, for example, a patient with asbestosis who worked in a now closed shipyard. Even in these circumstances, former fellow workers need to be informed of the risk resulting from previous exposure.

The physician should not wait for absolute proof

Table 7.2
How to Take a Comprehensive Occupational History

After completion of comprehensive medical history, then elicit the following information.

Begin with place of birth, community where raised, parents' occupations.

List every job, even brief or part-time jobs, in chronological order.

For each job:

Get a brief description of the patient's actual daily activities.

Ask about exposure to dust, fumes, chemicals, noise, radiation and stress.

Ask about ventilation, protective clothing, respirators, and medical surveillance.

Ask about episodes of work-related illness and whether co-workers have been ill.

Review the details of the current job in depth. Ask about current symptoms and their relationships to work. Are they worse at work, fewer and milder on weekends, worse on a particular day of the week?

List those exposures that may be relevant to the current problem.

Also list those exposures which while not relevant to current symptoms may have implications for health in the future.

of the etiology to begin an investigation of a possible workplace hazard. The least severely affected number of a group of workers may be the one who seeks attention. Moreover, for most occupationally induced diseases, proof of a relationship rests on epidemiological data rather than diagnostic study of the individual patient. Often the most practical way to learn if a patient's problem is caused or exacerbated by his occupation is to find out if fellow workers are similarly affected. Time and again failure of a physician to follow his suspicions has allowed epidemics of occupational disease to continue and expand.

HOW TO FOLLOW UP

In most states, there is a health department unit for investigation of occupational disease. Currently, three states (California, Maryland, and Michigan) require physicians to *report all cases of suspected occupational disease*. Such laws should and probably will become more widespread. Reporting an occupational disease problem to the local health department should be the physician's first resource.

Enforcement of existing workplace regulations is the responsibility of the *Occupational Safety and Health Administration* (OSHA) in the United States Department of Labor (telephone number listed under U.S. Government, Labor Department, OSHA). In some instances there is a state OSHA agency which enforces the federal regulations. In every state, every *employer is obligated to report* workplace injuries and illness to OSHA. In most cases OSHA enforcement officers are able to determine relatively easily if unsafe conditions exist at a workplace, and they will provide a follow-up report to the referring physician. If other workers may be in imminent danger

of being made ill, the physician should communicate this urgently to OSHA to promote an immediate investigation. The physician should request help from OSHA when other workers are in danger or if the local health department is not able to provide help. In instances when OSHA is slow or inept, it is the physician's responsibility to persist with his inquiries so that both the patient and the workplace will get an appropriate evaluation.

Another route for follow-up is to have the patient request assistance from the *National Institute of Occupational Safety and Health (NIOSH)*. This institute is a part of the U.S. Public Health Service's Center for Disease Control which conducts research on occupational disease. An employer, union, or any three employees can request a formal Health Hazard Evaluation (HHE) of a workplace. Furthermore, NIOSH now has Educational Resource Centers where consultants are available to help physicians, employers, and workers, available in each region of the country. These centers can provide literature searches, information on available publications and on current areas of research, and can refer a physician to others who are experts in the field. (Access to regional centers can be provided by the central office.)

NIOSH may be contacted at the following address:

NIOSH
Clearinghouse of Occupational Safety and Health Information
ATTN: Information Retrieval and Analysis Section
4676 Columbia Parkway
Cincinnati, OH 45226.

THE IMPORTANCE OF THE GENERAL PHYSICIAN

It is vitally important that primary practitioners take the time to report and follow up suspected occupational diseases. Although theoretically there is a system of surveillance and inspection of workplaces through OSHA, there are, in fact, only enough inspectors to visit every workplace once in about every 200 years. Furthermore, most workers are unaware of their right to request investigation of potential hazards at work, and corporate medical departments and executives usually do not want government inspectors in their plants. In addition, inspectors who do visit workplaces may lack medical training, so that they often focus on safety, rather than on health issues. For these reasons, if a patient gets an occupational health problem or is exposed to a dangerous situation at work, the physician and his patient need to begin identification of the problem, because it is unlikely that anyone else will do so.

Workmen's Compensation Is for the Benefit of the Patient

Every state has a Workmen's Compensation Act which provides a system of dispensing funds for medical expenses related to occupational disease and injury and for employee's lost earnings. If a physician concludes or even strongly suspects that a patient has an illness caused or made worse by his job, the patient should be encouraged to file for Workmen's Compensation (through his employer, the Workmen's Compensation local office, or his lawyer). There are two reasons for this. First, if a claim is pursued and won (even though it takes time), the patient is usually guaranteed lifetime medical coverage from Workmen's Compensation funds for that illness. Compensation may lift some of the financial burdens from the patient and his family, particularly in chronic or fatal diseases (such as asbestosis). Second, Workmen's Compensation has the potential to encourage safety and to penalize careless employers.

To a great extent, however, Workmen's Compensation has been a failure, chiefly because of inadequate reporting. For example, a 1980 Department of Labor survey showed that only 3% of workers disabled by occupational respiratory disease were receiving compensation. Ninety-seven percent of the disabled workers were not receiving Workmen's Compensation and were living on social security or welfare and their medical bills were being paid by health insurance, Medicare, or state welfare funds. Thus, the economic and social costs of industrial disease are largely borne, not by the companies who may have acted irresponsibly, but by the victims and the taxpayers, including the businesses who are trying to protect their employees properly.

Physicians are often reticent about using Workmen's Compensation, feeling a claim may tie them up in court. This is an unsubstantiated fear since the medical record usually provides sufficient medical evidence and the physician does not have to appear at the hearing. If the record does not provide adequate information, the patient's attorneys will almost always be willing to take a statement from the physician at his convenience.

THE PART-TIME PLANT PHYSICIAN

A primary practitioner may become involved in a workplace at the invitation of the employer or the union representing the employees. Many small and medium-sized workplaces need the assistance of part-time physicians to conduct effective programs to detect and prevent occupational disease. The practitioner should welcome the chance to do something to prevent illness, but needs to take special care to meet the ethical obligations such a role requires. Many physicians in occupational medicine regard themselves as responsible to the management of the company which pays them, rather than to the patients they serve. In some cases, physicians have withheld information from patients about work-related diseases. In other cases, physicians modify their therapy for illnesses and injuries to meet the needs of production rather than the needs of the patient. This role of the "company physician" as servant of

Table 7.3
Responsibilities of the Plant Physician

The primary responsibility of the physician is to the individual patient, no matter who is paying the bill.

The physician may reveal nothing to others, including management, about the patient without his permission. Reports should be limited to a statement on the patient's fitness to work and on any specific limitations of activity.

The physician must acquire all available information about the workplace that may be relevant to a patient's health.

Everything that the physician learns or may deduce about the safety of the workplace must be explained to those whose health may be affected.

The physician should (and is required to in California, Maryland, and Michigan) report occupational disease to the local health department or state OSHA.

The physician should not take sides in any dispute between the management, the workers, or the government, but should only provide accurate information and honest opinion to all concerned.

management and enemy of the patient has had tacit acceptance in the past. In the last decade the American Occupational Medical Association, composed principally of industry-employed physicians, has called for adherence to ethical practice, and many abuses have been ended. Any physician today who practices as a plant physician differently from the way he practices in his own office may face professional disciplinary and malpractice suits. In some plants, workers and management are following the Swedish model of jointly selecting a plant physician. Table 7.3 summarizes the principal responsibilities of a plant physician.

SELECTED OCCUPATIONAL DISEASES

The occupational diseases a physician will encounter depend upon his location in the United States, the industry in the immediate vicinity, and the demographic makeup of the practice. For example, practitioners near retirement communities may see retired workers with previous exposure in all types of industry. Table 7.4 lists selected examples of occupational diseases grouped according to the organ system affected.

Dermatitis and pneumoconiosis are the most frequently reported occupational illnesses. This probably reflects both true incidence (skin and pulmonary epithelium are most in contact with the outside environment) and the greater likelihood of recognition of these disorders as being occupational in origin.

The number of chemicals that are toxic to the liver and kidney is so great that a careful exposure history needs to be taken in all cases of liver inflammation or renal failure. Many chemicals can affect the gastrointestinal tract causing functional disturbances that may be misdiagnosed as peptic disease or irritable bowel disease.

Low level exposure of the respiratory organs to a

Table 7.4
Selected Occupational Problems

Clinical Problem	Causative Agent[a]	Clinical Problem	Causative Agent[a]
CONSTITUTIONAL			Coke oven emissions
Fever	Heat		Cutting oils
	Radiant heated air	**NERVOUS SYSTEM**	
	Microwaves	*Central Effects*	
	Metal fumes:	Altered consciousness	Hundreds of chemicals have central nervous system (CNS)-depressant properties and other CNS effects
	Zinc		
	Copper		
	Magnesium		
	Cadmium	Convulsions	Aldrin
	Dinitrophenol		2-Aminopyridine
	Pentachlorophenol		Camphor
	Dinitro-o-cresol		Chlordane
	Polymer fume (polytetrafluorethylene)		Crag herbicide
			DDT
	Cotton dust		Decaborane
	Bagasse		2,4-Dichlorophenoxyacetic acid
	Moldy hay		Dieldrin
SKIN			1,1-Dimethylhydrazine
Sweating	Organophosphates		Endrin
	Pentachlorophenol		Heptachlor
	Dinitro-o-cresol		Hydrazine
Cyanosis	Methemoglobin formers:		Lindane
	Aniline		Methoxychlor
	Anisidine, ortho- and para-isomers		Methyl bromide
			Methyl chloride
	Dimethylaniline		Methyl iodide
	Dinitrobenzene, all isomers		Methyl mercaptain
	Dinitrotoluene		Monomethylhydrazine
	Monomethylaniline		Nicotine
	p-Nitroaniline		Nitromethane
	Nitrobenzene		Oxalic acid
	p-Nitrocholorobenzene		Pentaborane
	Nitrogen trifluoride		Phenol
	Nitrotoluene		Rotenone
	Perchloryl fluoride		Sodium fluoroacetate
	n-Propyl nitrate		Strychnine
	Tetranitromethane		Tetraethyllead
	o-Toluidine		Tetramethyllead
	Xylidine		Tetramethylsuccinoitrile
Contact dermatitis	Many chemicals with irritant or sensitizing properties		Thallium, soluble compounds
			Toxaphene
Chronic eczematous dermatitis	Solvents	Headaches	Carbon monoxide
	Detergents		Nitrites
Folliculitis	Oil exposure		Nitrates
	Grease exposure		Alcohols
Acne	Polychlorinated biphenyls		Lead
	Chlorinated naphthalenes		Organic lead compounds
	Parafin		Methemoglobin formers (see under cyanosis)
	Coal tar		
	Dioxin	Behavioral change	Mercury
Photosensitization	Coal tar		Lead
	Pitch		Carbon disulfide
	Asphalt		Carbon monoxide
	Anthracene		Methyl chloride
	Creosote		Methyl bromide
	Fluorescein		Manganese
	Phenanthrene	Ataxia, tremor, spasticity	Organic lead compounds
Granulomas	Beryllium		Organic tin compounds
Corns	Asbestos	Hyperreflexia, micrographia	Compounds
	Fiberglass		Mercury
Punctate ulcers	Chromic acid		DDT
Painful burns	Hydrofluoric acid (deep pain out of proportion to appearance of burn)	Peripheral neuropathy	Peripheral neurotoxins:
			Acrylamide
			Arsenic and compounds
Skin cancer	Soots		Calcium arsenate
	Tars		Carbon disulfide
	Arsenic		n-Hexane

Table 7.4—*continued*

Clinical Problem	Causative Agent[a]	Clinical Problem	Causative Agent[a]
	Lead and inorganic lead compounds		Ethanol
	Lead arsenate		Ethylene Gycol
	Dimethylaminoprosionitrile		Lead
	Lucel-7 (2-*t*-butylazo-2-hydroxy 5-methyl hexane)		Methyl bromide
	Mercury		Methyl chloride
	Methyl bromide		Methyl iodide
	Methyl butyl ketone		Triethyl tin
	Thallium, soluble compounds	Eye strain—visual fatigue	Visual display terminals
	2,4,6-Trinitrotoluene	**HEARING**	
	Tri-o-cresyl phosphate	Decreased acuity and tinnitus	Noise exposure especially above 85 decibels
EYE		Acoustic neuritis	Aniline
Conjunctivitis	Ultraviolet radiation (welder's flash)		Arsenic
	Many irritant chemicals		Carbon monoxide
Corneal irritation or scarring	Acids		Hypoxia
	Alkalies		Lead
	Dimethyl sulfate		Organic mercury
	Formaldehyde		Phosphorous
	Methyl dichloropropionate		Sodium nitrate
	Osmic acid	Otitis externa	Contamination of ear plugs used for noise protection
	Sulfur dioxide	Ear pain	Acute shifts in pressure
	1-Butanol	**SMELL**	
	Xylene	Anosmia	Arsenic
	Diazomethane		Benzine
	Dichlorobutenes		Benzol
	Ethylene oxide		Cadmium
	Ethylenimine		Carbon disulfide
	Hydrogen sulfide		Chromium
Corneal edema producing "haloes" around lights	Allyl alcohol		Ethyl acetate
	Amines		Formaldehyde
	Morpholines		Hydrazine
	Diethyldigylocolate		Iodine
	Diisopropylamine		Ketone
	3-Dimethylamino propylamine		Lead
	Ethylenediamine		Mercury
	Tetraethylbutanediamine		Nickel
	Triethylenediamine		Osmium tetroxide
Scarring and discoloration	Benzoquinone		Phosphorous oxychloride
Corneal discoloration as a manifestation of systemic intoxication	Aniline		Phthalic anhydride
	Arsine		Potassium iodide
	Nitrobenzene		Selenium
	Silver		Sulfuric acid
Cataracts	Radiant heat	**TASTE**	
	Microwave exposure	Decreased acuity	Bromine
	Dinitro-o-cresol		Caprolactam
	Dinitrophenol	Alterations in taste	Iodine
Lens deposits and discoloration	Copper		Phosgene
	Iron		Antimony
	Mercury		Arsenic
	Phenylmercuric salts		Bismuth
	Silver		Cadmium
Optic neuritis—visual acuity and visual field defects	Carbon dioxide		Copper
	Carbon monoxide		Gallium
	Carbon disulfide		Lead
	Cyanide		Mercury
	Methanol		Nickel
	Methyl mercury		Nitrogen dioxide
	Napthalene		Selenium
	Thallium		Tellurium
	Lead		Thallium
	Acetylphenylhydrazine		Vanadium
	Benzene		Zinc oxide
	Triethyl tin	**RESPIRATORY**	
	Phosphoros	Nasal septal perforation	Chromic acid and other chromates
	Ethylene glycol	Laryngeal carcinoma	Asbestos
Nystagmus and extraocular muscle palsy	Carbon disulfide	Laryngitis, bronchitis, tracheitis, pneumonitis	Many irritants including:
	Dieldrin		Ammonia

Table 7.4—*continued*

Clinical Problem	Causative Agent[a]	Clinical Problem	Causative Agent[a]
	Chlorine	Benign pneumoconiosis deposits in lung without fibrosis	Aluminum powder
	Oxides of nitrogen		Barium
	Ozone		Graphite
	Phosgene		Iron oxide
	Sulfur dioxide		Tin
	Vanadium pentoxide		Cerium oxide
	Mercury		Silver
	Manganese		Titanium
	Cadmium dust		Ultramarine
Bronchiolitis obliterans	Nitrogen dioxide	Pleural effusion	Asbestos
Allergic alveolitis:			Paraquat
Bagassosis	*Thermoactinomyces vulgaris* and *Micropolyspora* sp.		Talc
		Carcinoma of lung	Arsenic
Bird breeder's lung (pigeon breeder's disease)	Avian proteins		Asbestos
			Bis(chloromethyl)ether
			Chloromethylmethylether
Byssinosis (Cannabosis)	Cotton, flax, and soft fiber hemps		Coke oven emissions
Cheesewasher's lung	*Penicillium caseii*		Chromates
Coffee-worker's lung	Chlorogenic acid	Pleural mesothelioma	Asbestos
Detergents	*Bacillus subtilis*		Zeolite
Farmer's lung	*Micropolyspora faeni* and *Thermoactinomyces vulgaris*	GASTROINTESTINAL	
		Gingivitis and gum pigmentation	Mercury
			Lead
Feathers	Feather proteins		Bismuth
Furrier's lung	Keratinized particles of hair	Dental erosion	Acetic acid
Kapok	*Ceiba pentandra* (fruit) and *Eriodendron anfractuosum* (seedpod)		Hydrochloric acid
			Lactic acid
			Nitric acid
Maltworker's lung	*Aspergillis clavatus*		Nitrogen dioxide
Maple-bark stripper's disease	*Cryptostroma corticale*		Sulfuric acid
Miller's bronchitis	*Aspergillus glaucus* and *Penicillium glaucum*	Tongue paresthesias	Furfural
			Rotenone
			Cresol
Mill fever	*Corchorus capsularis* and *chorchorus olitorius*	Green discoloration	Vanadium
		Esophagitis	Ingestion of a variety of irritants
Mother of pearl (nacre)	Conchiolin	Esophageal carcinoma	Asbestos
Mushroom picker's lung		Nausea and vomiting	Many chemicals including:
Paprika-splitter's lung	*Mucor stolinifer*		Irritants
Sequoiosis	*Graphium* sp.		CNS depressants
Bronchospasm	Pulmonary sensitizers:		Cholinesterase inhibitors
	Castor bean pomace		Methemoglobin formers
	Cobalt, metal fume and dust	Constipation	Lead
	Enzymatic detergents		Barium sulfate
	Grain dusts		Thallium
	Maleic anhydride		Tellurium
	Methylene bisphenyl isocyanate		Vanadium
			Fluorides
	Methyl isocyanate		Nitrous fumes
	Nickel, metal	Hepatomegaly	Hepatoxins:
	p-Phenylenediamine		Acetylene tetrabromide
	Phthalic anhydride		Carbon disulfide
	Platinum salts		Carbon tetrachloride
	Polyvinyl chloride (fume from heated film: meat wrapper's asthama)		Chlorodiphenyl, 42% chlorine
			Chlorodiphenyl, 54% chlorine
			Chloroform
	Toluene 2,4-diisocyanate		p-Dichlorobenzene
	Tungsten carbide		Dimethylacetamide
	Western red cedar dust		Dimethylformamide
	Wood pulp dust		Dioxane
Pulmonary fibrosis	Asbestos		Ethylene chlorohydrin
	Silica		Ethylene dibromide
	Silicates including diatomaceous earth		Ethylene dichloride
			Hexachloronaphthalene
	Beryllium		Kepone
	Talc		Nitroethane
	Coal dust		Octachloronapthalene
	Cobalt		Pentachloronaphthalene
	Hematite		Picric acid
	Kaolin		Tetrachloroethane
	Yttrium		

Table 7.4—*continued*

Clinical Problem	Causative Agent[a]	Clinical Problem	Causative Agent[a]

Jaundice	Tetrachloroethylene
	Tetrachloronaphthalene
	Tetryl
	Trichloroanphthalene
	2,4,6-Trinitrotoluene
	Hepatoxins (see above)
	Hemolytic agents:
	  Arsine
	  Butyl cellosolve
	  Naphthalene
	  Phenylhydrazine
	  Stibine
		Urinary retention
		Urinary frequency
			Benzidine
			β Naphthylamine
			4-Nitrodiphenyl
			Magenta
			Dimethylaminopropionitrile
			Chloroform
			Furfuryl alcohol
			Oxalic acid

Angiosarcoma of liver	Vinyl chloride	REPRODUCTIVE ABNORMALITIES	
Abdominal pain	Antimony Arsenic Bromine Cadmium Lead Mercury Nicotine Organophosphates Thallium Many other chemicals when ingested	Female sterility Male sterility	Arsenic Lead Phosphorous Arsenic Benzene Cadmium Carbon disulfide Carbon monoxide Dibromochloropropane Kepone Lead Manganese Methyl chloride Microwaves to testes (radar workers) Phosphorous Stilbestrol Trichloroethylene
CARDIOVASCULAR SYSTEM *Heart*			

Myocardial damage
 	
Ischemic disease
	Antimony
	Arsine
	Carbon disulfide
	Nitroglycerin
	Nitrogycol
	Other vasodilating nitrates
		Anemia	Lead
			Hemolytic agents:
			  Arsine
			  Butyl cellosolve
			  Naphthalene
			  Phenylhydrazine
			  Stibine

Peripheral Vascular Disease			Marrow depressants: Benzene
Hypertension	Noise exposure Aminopyridine Arsenic Barium Boron hydride Carbon disulfide Cobalt Diphenyl Lead Mercury Thallium	Leukemia	Dinitrophenol Tetryl 2,4,6-Trinitrotoluene Benzene Radiation Styrene-butadiene Ethylene oxide
Vasospastic Disorders "White Finger"	Vibrating tools	Splenomegaly	Beryllium Methyl chloride Naphthalene
Raynaud's Phenomenon	Vinyl chloride		Naphthol Nitrobenzene
GENITOURINARY			Phosphorous

Renal disease	Nephrotoxins:
	  4-Aminodiphenyl
	  Carbon disulfide
	  Carbon tetrachloride
	  Chloroform
	  Dioxane
	  Ethylene chlorohydrin
	  Ethylene dibromide
	  Lead
	  Mercury
	  Oxalic acid
	  Picric acid
	  Tetrachloroethane
	  2,4,6-Trinitrotoluene
	  Turpentine
	  Uranium (natural), soluble and insoluble compounds
		Resorcinol
		
		MUSCULOSKELETAL
		Muscle Cramps
			Boron hydrides
			Camphor
			Chlorobenzenes
			Dinitrophenol
			Hydrofluoric acid
			Lead
			Manganese
			Mercury, organic
			Nicotine
			Ricin
			Tricresol phosphates

Renal carcinoma	4-Aminodiphenyl Auramine	Osteonecrosis Osteomalacia Osteosclerosis Acro-osteolysis	Phosphorous Cadmium Fluorine Vinyl chloride

[a] The types of occupations which most often provide risk of exposures to these agents are most easily identified in Key *et al.* (see General References).

variety of substances may result in the production of nonspecific upper respiratory syndromes which the patient may describe as an intractable cold or as sinus trouble.

Although occupational diseases periodically present with striking and unusual signs, such as acro-osteolysis in vinyl chloride workers or nasal septal perforation in patients exposed to chromates, more commonly, they present with vague systemic symptoms typical of early intoxication.

There are, however, a few specific clinical situations which deserve to be highlighted:

Any Change in Personality or Behavior. Mercury, lead, pesticides and a wide variety of other central nervous system toxins usually present this way.

New Onset of Asthma. Owing to the time lapse when an immunological mechanism is involved, wheezing and dyspnea may not be noted until after the work day is over.

Any Case of Pulmonary Fibrosis. A prolonged latent period between exposure and disease onset means that abnormalities that appear on X-ray may have resulted from a job the patient had decades ago.

Peripheral Neuropathy. A neurologist may immediately recognize a toxic neuropathy by its pattern of presentation, but the primary practitioner may mistake such a pattern for diabetes or alcohol abuse.

Hearing Loss. Noise-induced hearing loss occurs gradually and usually in older workers, so that it is rarely recognized in time to prevent severe damage.

Inability to Conceive. More and more compounds which affect the reproductive system and cause sterility are being identified.

Lung Cancer. Exposure to asbestos and cigarette smoke act synergistically. Such synergism is likely but less established with the other pulmonary carcinogens.

Other Cancers. Specific carcinogens are being identified which definitely have caused human cancers.

References

General

Levy, BS and Wegman, DH (editors): *Occupational Health: Recognizing and Preventing Work-related Disease.* Little, Brown, Boston, 1982.
>*Excellent introductory text for the practitioner.*

Hamilton, A and Hardy, HC: *Industrial Toxicology,* Ed. 3. Publishing Sciences Group, Littleton. Mass., 1974.
>*A short textbook of industrial toxicology.*

Key, MM, Henschet, AF, Butlee, J, Ligo, RN and Tabershaw, IR: *Occupational Diseases: A Guide to Their Recognition.* Rev. Ed. National Institute for Occupational Safety and Health, Washington, 1977.
>*An excellent guide to the hazards of a large number of chemicals.*

Morgan, WK and Seaton, A: *Occupational Lung Disease.* W.B. Saunders, Philadelphia, 1975.
>*This text covers all the pneumoconioses.*

Proctor, NH and Hughes, JP: *Chemical Hazards of the Workplace.* J.B. Lippincott, Philadelphia, 1978.
>*A thorough text on chemical hazards; it includes a section on diagnostic principles.*

Selikoff, IJ and Lee, DH: *Asbestos and Disease.* Academic Press, New York, 1978.
>*An up-to-date monograph.*

CHAPTER EIGHT

The General Physician's Role in the Care of the Patient with Cancer

LARRY WATERBURY, M.D.

In recent years there have been significant advances in the treatment of many different cancers. A massive body of medical literature continues to grow; multidisciplinary cancer treatment centers have arisen around the country; and there has been a marked increase in the amount of basic knowledge pertinent to the diagnosis and treatment of cancer. The general physician may feel overwhelmed by the growing body of specialized knowledge in oncology and inadequate to handle the problems of cancer patients. There is a tendency to relegate the care of all cancer patients to specialists. Although appropriate in certain patients and clinical situations, there are other settings where general physicians should remain active in the cancer patient's care. To the patient with a progressive metastatic tumor, unresponsive or poorly responsive to therapy, the continuing involvement of his personal physician is increasingly important, especially if that doctor-patient relationship has been a longstanding one.

The purpose of this chapter is not to discuss specific cancers, but to examine in a more general way the role of the general physician in the care of patients who have cancer. Common cancers are discussed in other chapters (breast, Chapter 86; lung, Chapter 53; gastrointestinal, Chapter 34; prostate, Chapter 45; gynecologic malignancy, Chapter 92).

Table 8.1 lists a number of nonoperable cancers responsive to modern treatment regimens; patients with such cancers should be referred to cancer specialists. These patients frequently benefit from multimodality treatment. Even within this group of cancers, when specialty help is needed, the general physician will continue to play an important role, especially if the relationship with the patient or the family has been a lengthy one.

INITIAL REFERRAL AND TREATMENT

When possible the general physician should refer patients to specific oncologists whom he trusts and whom he knows to be helpful, considerate clinicians. Multimodality treatment regimens involving the combined efforts of surgical, medical, and radiation oncologists frequently result in a bewildered patient who does not know who the primary responsible physician is. Thus the general physician may need to play a coordinating role or to intercede in order to identify that physician who will be the coordinator for the patient's care and who will be accessible to the patient to answer questions, provide support, improve communications, etc. The general physician should expect to receive up-to-date and complete information about the diagnostic and therapeutic plans and about the patient's current status. His continuing interest in the case is especially helpful if he will be involved in follow-up care after the initial treatment. The general physician may best be able to assess the overall picture and, as time goes on, to identify when problems resulting from treatment (side effects, expense, family disruption, deteriorating psychologic status of patient, etc.) outweigh the likely benefits of continued therapy.

FOLLOW-UP CARE

Many oncologists welcome participation of the primary physician in the patient's follow-up and continuing care. This is particularly important when treatment has been given in an oncology center in a distant city. Some less toxic ambulatory treatment regimens may even be given by the primary physician under the direction of the specialist.

CARE OF PATIENTS UNRESPONSIVE OR POORLY RESPONSIVE TO TREATMENT

Table 8.2 lists a number of cancers less responsive to therapy, where the impact of therapy on survival is unproven or controversial. Diagnosis and initial

Table 8.1
Some Nonoperable Cancers in which Treatment Prolongs Survival[a]

Acute leukemia
Hodgkins disease
Lymphoma
Metastatic testicular cancer
Metastatic ovarian cancer
Small cell carcinoma of the lung
Metastatic breast cancer

[a] Patients with these cancers require specialized treatment, frequently in centers where multimodality therapy is available.

Table 8.2
Some Cancers Where Treatment Provides Palliation in Some Patients
Effects on Survival Unproven or Controversial

Non-oat cell lung cancer (unresectable)
Metastatic large bowel cancer
Metastatic stomach cancer
Metastatic pancreatic cancer
Metastatic malignant melanoma
Hepatoma
Metastatic soft tissue sarcomas
Metastatic cervical cancer
Metastatic endometrial cancer
Metastatic hypernephroma
Metastatic prostate cancer (posthormonal therapy with relapse)

therapy usually require surgery, but when metastasis is proven, the effect of chemotherapy or radiotherapy is at most palliative. In such situations, knowledgeable general physicians may be in the best position to evaluate the total picture and to make recommendations.

1. *Should palliative therapy be recommended?* Although difficult to generalize, a number of factors must be considered in attempting to help patients and their families in deciding whether or not the patient is likely to benefit from palliative therapy. More than age, the functional status of the patient must be considered in such therapeutic decisions. The infirm, ill, poorly functional patient with widely disseminated and rapidly progressive disease may be more harmed by the side effects and discomforts of palliative treatment than benefited, especially if response rates are small and toxicity of treatment is high. Other patients, even if elderly, in good functional status are much more suitable candidates for attempts at palliation. The patient who feels that any chance of response is worth the price of toxicity, and who cannot feel comfortable unless attempting some therapy, should generally be offered treatment.

2. If some attempt at palliative treatment seems worthwhile, *should it be conventional therapy or experimental protocol therapy?* Every oncology center and large cooperative group has a current protocol for the metastatic cancers that are listed in Table 8.2.

Clinical protocols designed to attempt to find improved methods of treatment are important for advances in oncology and to improve the outlook and the comfort of future patients. However, experimental therapy may have less than desirable consequences for the individual patient. Frequently, such protocols involve the investigation of treatments with more toxicity than current conventional therapies. They usually require more frequent visits to the physician as well as more frequent diagnostic tests, because of the necessity to document precisely the objective response. They may therefore also involve increased expense to the patient. Obviously patients agreeing to experimental protocol therapy must be well informed about the implications of the therapy, and that requires that they understand what is to be done. Patients need to realize the differences between experimental treatment and conventional treatment in terms of expense, time, and discomfort. In those diseases where the beneficial effects of therapy remain questionable, the responsible general physician must make sure that both he and the patient are informed about the side effects and likely benefits of therapy. The physician very much needs an experienced and sensitive practical clinical oncologist to give him counsel, including an honest appraisal of effects of treatment in terms of its benefit and toxicity. The helpful consultant must be able to do more than describe the currently popular treatment for the patient's disease; he should be able to tailor the recommendation to the specific patient. No treatment, conventional low dose palliative chemotherapy or radiotherapy, and experimental therapy are all appropriate choices for individual patients in various different clinical situations. In order to make sensitive and responsible recommendations with regard to treatment of patients with metastatic cancer the physician needs to be able to process and integrate a large amount of data of various kinds (Table 8.3). The general physician because of his involvement with the patient and family over a long time may be in the best position to do this.

If he feels therapy is likely to be helpful for the patient, the primary physician must know something about what the patient will experience when he receives radiotherapy or chemotherapy.

RADIOTHERAPY

The patient with cancer frequently has misconceptions about and limited knowledge of radiotherapy. The primary physician at the time that he discusses with the patient possible referral for radiotherapy must spend time in explaining the rationale and hoped for response of the treatment, and he should outline what the patient will experience during treatment. The initial visit usually includes a relevant history and physical examination by the radiotherapist. Further diagnostic tests (X-rays, computerized tomography (CT) scan, etc.) may be obtained. If the therapist agrees that treatment is appropriate, the radiotherapy ports may actually be determined at the first visit; and the patient may receive his first treatment at that time. The patient should be told that skin markings may be placed in order to facilitate the uniformity of subsequent treatments, and that these markings must not be removed. It is important to explain that the therapy machines are bulky and somewhat overwhelming in appearance. Many patients are likely to be frightened by the experience; and if the referring physician appreciates this, it is useful to contact the radiotherapist and to explain the particular fears of the patient ahead of time. Therapists will often give patients and their families a tour of the radiotherapy treatment rooms before starting therapy and will spend extra time answering questions about the treatment and its benefits and complications. The patient should be aware that the treatment itself is *not* painful. The initial consultation is usually time-consuming (several hours), but subsequent treatments are usually scheduled precisely and require only a small amount of time (30 minutes). Treatments are usually given several days a week and the entire course may take several weeks to complete. The patient usually will not see the radiotherapist at the time of each treatment, but will be seen by a radiotherapy nurse or technician. He therefore needs to know precisely with whom to communicate if he has side effects or questions during radiotherapy. The primary physician should be available for phone consultation in order to intercede for the patient should communication problems arise. Also, the follow-up plans after treatment should be outlined. In addition to the timing and types of side effects which the patient may experience, it is important for him to know that the response to treatment is frequently delayed and that sometimes the maximal effect is seen a few weeks after the course of radiotherapy has been completed.

Table 8.3
Factors Affecting Treatment Recommendations in Patients with Cancer

The natural history of the untreated cancer
The proven effect of treatment on the natural history
   Likely effects on survival
   Likelihood of lessening morbidity
Toxicity of treatment
Functional status of the patient
Ability of the patient to comprehend the implications of treatment
Psychological state and philosophical position of the patient
Emotional strength, and attitudes of immediate family
Financial situation, health coverage status

Side Effects

Table 8.4 describes important side effects of radiotherapy. The patient will be most concerned by those

Table 8.4
Important Side Effects of Radiotherapy (9)

Dermatitis (less common with newer high energy machines. Avoid sunlight and extreme cold).

Acute radiation pneumonitis (transient, usually occurring 6–12 weeks after treatment; precipitated by steroid withdrawal, concomitant chemotherapy; usually responds to steroid treatment) (6).

Pulmonary fibrosis (occurs 6–12 months after treatment, not responsive to steroids) (6).

Esophagitis (usually occurs during treatment; particularly severe when radiotherapy and Adriamycin are administered together).

Nausea, vomiting, and diarrhea (occurs during treatment with most abdominal radiotherapy, usually self-limited).

Enteritis (rare, more likely with very high dose treatment; small bowel more sensitive than large bowel and stomach; occurs weeks to years after radiotherapy; manifestations include obstruction, bleeding, perforation) (10).

Pericarditis (occurs months to years after radiation, usually resolves, occasionally progresses to constrictive pericarditis or to tamponade requiring pericardiectomy) (11).

Neurologic side effects (transverse myelitis, very rare; side effects from CNS irradiation in adults are infrequent (2); Lhermitte's sign (the sensation of electric shocks passing down the body when the head is flexed) seen in 10% of patients undergoing mantle irradiation for Hodgkin's disease; after radiotherapy herpes zoster is common).

Hypothyroidism (common in patients treated for Hodgkins disease with mantle field; may develop years after treatment) (9).

Sterility (usually temporary) (8, 9).

Growth retardation in children (occurs both from direct skeletal effects and from hypopituitarism from CNS irradiation) (9).

Dental side effects (severe dental problems are common after head and neck irradiation because of decrease in saliva formation, increased sensitivity to caries, osteonecrosis) (13).

Cystitis (occurs during treatment with pelvic irradiation. Usually self-limited and treated symptomatically with fluids and phenozopyridine (Pyridium), 200 mg q.i.d.).

common side effects which occur during treatment and by those which may remain for a few weeks after treatment is discontinued.

Dermatitis secondary to radiotherapy is less common than it used to be, owing to the use of the modern high energy machines. Severe burning requiring specialized treatment is quite uncommon; however, skin discoloration may occur. The patient should be told that the radiation field should not be exposed to sunlight or extreme cold, and that total, but temporary, hair loss will usually occur in the areas being radiated and that complete return of hair, after high dose radiation, may take many months.

The most troublesome side effects that occur during radiotherapy are *gastrointestinal.* Patients receiving radiation to the chest or upper back frequently experience symptoms of radiation esophagitis (odynophagia and sometimes reflux symptoms which may respond to elevation of the head of the bed and to antacids). Severe esophagitis is more likely to occur when radiotherapy has been used in patients who have had prior chemotherapy with Adriamycin. Superinfection of the irritated esophagus with candida is not unusual, especially in patients who are receiving steroids. This usually responds to treatment with oral Mycostatin (the suppositories seem to work better than the liquid) 4–6 times a day. Occasionally short courses of amphotericin (5–10 mg/day for 14 days) are necessary to cure candida esophagitis but that treatment is best given in the hospital. Abdominal irradiation may cause some troublesome *diarrhea* which may persist to some degree during the entire course of treatment. Other than the importance of replacing fluids and electrolytes, there are some dietary maneuvers which may minimize symptoms; these are listed in Table 8.5. *Nausea and anorexia* are the most troublesome side effects of abdominal irradiation and are discussed separately below.

Patients who receive radiotherapy to the head or neck are subject to special *dental complications.* Before treatment all patients should have a complete dental examination by a dentist experienced in the treatment of patients who have undergone radiotherapy. Damage to the teeth, gums, and bone, plus the xerostomia which results from high dose radiotherapy to the oral mucous membranes and salivary glands may result in severe problems. Many of these can be prevented by appropriate prophylaxis (aggressive treatment of periodontal disease and of infected teeth before radiation) and an ongoing program during and after radiotherapy, which should be strictly followed. The use of artificial saliva may be helpful for patients with xerostomia.

An excellent monograph is available free of charge to patients undergoing radiotherapy (12). Unfortunately not all radiotherapists make this monograph available to their patients. Primary physicians who refer patients for radiotherapy should have this monograph available in their offices and should make sure all patients have access to it before their radiotherapy consultation.

CHEMOTHERAPY

The chemotherapy experience for the patient is so varied (depending on the disease being treated) that it is hard to give a general description. The medical

Table 8.5
Dietary Maneuvers for Therapy-induced Diarrhea (12)

Clear liquids (warm or at room temperature)
Avoid fiber (roughage) in the diet
Take smaller amounts of food more often
Avoid fatty foods
Avoid highly spiced foods
Avoid carbonated drinks, beans, cabbage, broccoli, cauliflower and corn

oncologist giving therapy can best explain to the patient the specifics of treatment, including how it is administered, the frequency of treatment, the hoped for response, and the side effects. The most frequent troublesome side effects for the patient are hair loss and nausea and vomiting. The frequency and degree of hair loss vary with the treatment regimen but it is helpful for the patient to know that hair will regrow once the treatment is discontinued. The treatment of nausea and vomiting is addressed below.

There is an excellent free monograph on chemotherapy written for patients which is available through the National Institutes of Health (1). Primary physicians who refer patients for chemotherapy should have this monograph available for patients, preferably before their first visit with the medical oncologist.

Table 8.6 lists other acute and chronic side effects of various chemotherapeutic agents. Knowledge of the long term side effects of various agents is particularly important for the primary physician who may be responsible for follow-up care of patients with good prognoses following chemotherapy.

NAUSEA, VOMITING, AND ANOREXIA

Nausea and vomiting are by far the most troublesome and common side effects of both radiotherapy and chemotherapy. Unfortunately the symptomatic treatment of nausea is only moderately effective. However there are a number of maneuvers which may help to limit the degree of nausea following chemotherapy or radiotherapy. For example, it is frequently helpful for the nauseated patient to be extremely still, lying down in a quiet room without external stimuli. Antiemetics may help, but unfortu-

nately do not eliminate the nausea completely, especially that associated with intense chemotherapy regimens. However, the use of antiemetics by tablet or by rectal suppository (e.g., prochlorperazine, 10 mg every 6 hours) is recommended. There has been much recent research on the use of oral tetrahydrocannabinol (THC) and other related compounds for the treatment of nausea and vomiting. Results with these compounds have been varied and they are not without side effects (5, 7). Their role in the treatment of therapy-induced nausea and vomiting still remains to be determined.

There are a number of dietary maneuvers which may be helpful to the patient experiencing nausea and vomiting after therapy (Table 8.7). The patient who experiences severe nausea and vomiting after therapy should probably only drink clear liquids until the symptoms are decreased. In general it is more helpful to take smaller portions of food frequently than to take larger meals less often, to take foods that are low in fat, and to avoid overly sweet foods. Mild nausea, especially that experienced before therapy or in anticipation of therapy, may be helped by taking dry toast or crackers in small quantities. It is recommended that patients do not lie down just after eating. Some patients find also that it is helpful not to drink liquids with their food which may increase their feeling of bloating and subsequent nausea. Many patients become nauseated at the smell of food cooking and it may be helpful for them to go to another part of the house or to stay out of the house when food is being prepared. Greasy and fried foods seem to be the worst offenders in this regard and are best avoided.

One of the major problems with intensive cancer therapy is the general *anorexia* which may result in considerable nutritional problems and weight loss. Consultation with a dietitian may be extremely helpful in such a situation. There is an excellent monograph available through the National Institutes of Health which contains all sorts of dietary advice for cancer patients including many recipes (4). It is available free of charge to physicians for their patients and is strongly recommended.

TERMINAL CARE

The primary physician who has participated in various phases of the cancer patient's care and who

Table 8.6
Common Side Effects of Chemotherapy (3, 8, 9)

Hair loss—alkylating agents, vincristine, vinblastine, Adriamycin, mithramycin, daunomycin

Hypercalcemia—estrogens, antiestrogens (tamoxifen).

Fluid retention—estrogens, androgens, steroids.

Skin darkening—Adriamycin (nails), 5-FU, bleomycin.

Dermatitis—Methotrexate, 6-MP, 6-thioguanine

Marrow depression—alkylating agents, vinblastine, nitrosoureas, methotrexate, Adriamycin, cytosine arabinoside, daunomycin, 5-FU, mithramycin, mitomycin C, cis-platinum, procarbazine, hydroxyurea, 6-MP

Neurological—cis-platinum (deafness), vincristine, vinblastine.

Gastrointestinal ulcerations—Methotrexate, 5-FU, bleomycin (mucocutaneous), Adriamycin.

Cardiomyopathy—Adriamycin

Pulmonary fibrosis—bleomycin, alkylating agents

Renal damage—cis-platinum

Red urine—Adriamycin, daunomycin

Hepatic toxicity—mithramycin, methotrexate

Sterility—alkylating agents, combination chemotherapy

Secondary neoplasm—alkylating agents, combination chemotherapy

Table 8.7
Dietary Maneuvers for Therapy-induced Nausea (1, 4, 12)

Smaller portions eaten more slowly
Avoid foods high in fat, and greasy and fried foods
Clear, cool liquids between meals
Crackers or toast
Rest (sitting, not lying) after eating
Avoid food odors (during preparation)

has an ongoing relationship with him and his family is frequently in the best position to help during a patient's terminal illness. The physician who develops some expertise in this regard can find enormous gratification from this role. Chapter 18 deals with many of the issues important to consider in caring for terminal patients.

In the last several years the *hospice concept* has received much support in this country. Central to the concept is the premise that dying patients have specific unique needs which are different from other patients. Although initially hospices were conceived as free standing units separate from acute hospitals, the concept has grown considerably as a general way of caring for terminal patients, rather than as a specific place for their care. One of the primary goals is to provide support for the family so that the patient may be able to spend a large amount of time at home. Many community hospitals are developing hospice programs with coordinated home support services utilizing visiting nurses, volunteers, physical and occupational therapists, home health aids, etc. Such programs can help the primary physician provide physical and emotional support for the patient and his family. An excellent National Institutes of Health publication entitled *Coping with Cancer: A Resource for the Health Professional* is available free of charge from the National Institutes of Health (see General References) which in addition to other useful information, lists organizations and agencies that provide useful services which may aid the physician in his attempt to provide home support for the dying cancer patient.

References

General

Abeloff, M (editor). *Complications of Cancer.* Johns Hopkins University Press. Baltimore, 1979.

A good review of the complications of cancer and of cancer therapy.
Coping with Cancer: A Resource For the Health Professional. NIH Publication No. 80-2080, National Cancer Institute, Office of Cancer Communications, Sept. 1980.

An excellent general review of many aspects of the care of the patient with cancer. Free copies are available by writing the Office of Cancer Communications, Department of Health Education and Welfare, NIH, Bethesda, MD 20205.

Specific

1. Chemotherapy and You: A Guide to Self-help During Treatment. NIH Publication No. 80-1136, Aug. 1980.
2. Deutsch, M, Parsons, JA and Mercado, R: Radiotherapy for intracranial metastases. *Cancer 34:* 1607, 1974.
3. Donaldson, SS and Lenon, RA: Alterations of nutritional status: Impact of chemotherapy and radiation therapy. *Cancer 43:* 2036, 1979.
4. Eating Hints: Recipes and Tips for Better Nutrition During Cancer Treatment. National Institutes of Health Publication No. 80-2079, 1980. (Free copies are available by writing to the Office of Cancer Communications, Dept. HEW, NIH, Bethesda, MD 21205.)
5. Frytab, S, Moentel, CG, *et al.*: Delta-9-tetrahydrocannabinol as an antiemetic for patients receiving cancer chemotherapy. *Ann Intern Med 91:* 825, 1979.
6. Gross, NJ: Pulmonary effects of radiation therapy. *Ann Intern Med 86:* 81, 1977.
7. Laszlo, J: Tetrahydrocannabinol: From pot to prescription? *Ann Intern Med 91:* 916, 1979.
8. Lenhard, RE and Saral, R: Acute complications of chemotherapy. In *Complications of Cancer,* p 357, MD Abeloff (editor). Johns Hopkins University Press, Baltimore, 1979.
9. Meyer, W and Leventhal, B: Late effects of cancer therapy. In *Complications of Cancer,* p. 397, MD Abeloff (editor). Johns Hopkins University Press, Baltimore, 1979.
10. Morgenstern, L, Thompson, R and Friedman, NB: Radiation enteritis. *Am J Surg 134:* 166, 1971.
11. Muggia, EA and Cassileth, PA: Constrictive pericarditis following radiation therapy. *Am J Med 44:* 116, 1968.
12. Radiation Therapy and You: A Guide to Self-Help During Treatment. National Institutes of Health Publication No. 80-2227, 1980. (Free copies are available by writing to the Office of Cancer Communications, Dept. HEW, NIH, Bethesda, MD 20205.)
13. Regeyi, JA, Courtney, RM and Kerr, DA: Dental management of patients irradiated for oral cancer. *Cancer 38:* 994, 1976.

SECTION 2

Psychiatric and Behavioral Problems

CHAPTER NINE

Psychosocial Problems: Evaluation and Case Formulation

CHESTER W. SCHMIDT, JR., M.D. and WALTER F. BAILE, M.D.

Although diagnosis and management are described for a variety of specific conditions in the following chapters, these conditions seldom occur singly or full-blown in medical patients. Rather, these patients will often have some manifestations of one or more behavioral or psychological problems. It is the physician's task to recognize which problem is dominant and to plan the treatment accordingly. Because current psychosocial problems are often predictive of future problems, the physician who provides continuous care can usually anticipate and at times prevent recurrence of these problems.

Given the diverse reasons people visit ambulatory services, the physician needs an efficient method of evaluating the psychosocial symptoms presented by the patient and of collating data into a working diagnosis. Since many patients will be known by the physician, important background information, such as family history, psychosexual development, education, occupational history, marital history, present living conditions, and past psychiatric history, will already be available.

CURRENT EVALUATION

The current evaluation begins with the chief complaint and present history, with an emphasis on the relationship between the *current life situation* and the chief complaint. There are a number of common social factors which may be relevant to the onset of psychological symptoms (see Table 9.1).

In those instances when the patient's behavior is the principal problem and/or when psychologic symptoms are causing a great deal of subjective distress (significant anxiety or depression) or are suggestive of a major psychiatric disorder (schizophrenia or manic depressive illness), the physician should perform a brief mental status examination and should try to identify the patient's dominant personality traits.

Table 9.1
Common Social Factors Related to Psychological Symptoms[a]

1. *Loss*: (a) Personal loss—loss of a loved one through death or desertion; (b) Loss of things—imposed loss of home, cherished possession or job.
2. *Conflict*: (a) Interpersonal—conflict within family, with neighbors or at work, where hostility is recognized; (b) Intrapersonal—role conflict or conflicting demands on the patient (as in a working mother).
3. *Change*: (a) Development—where time of life is the major problem (as in adolescence, menopause, or senescence); (b) Geographic—where a move to an unfamiliar environment is the major problem (as in immigration).
4. *Maladjustment*: (a) Interpersonal—problems between people with no overt conflict (as in failure to achieve a satisfactory sexual relation without hostility between partners); (b) Personal—failure to adjust to the environment (home or job) in the absence of the above mentioned loss, conflict or change.
5. *Stress*: (a) Acute—unexpected event not covered under loss, conflict or change (for example, the sudden illness of a family member or friend); (b) Chronic—long-term situation not included in loss, conflict or change (for instance, the presence of a handicapped child in the family).
6. *Isolation*—not due to any recent loss, change or conflict (as in an elderly widow).
7. *Failure or frustrated expectations*—when the patient's goals in life are not fulfilled and when there is no evidence of an intervening event covered by loss, conflict or change (e.g., failure at school or failure to achieve occupational promotion).

[a] From I.R. McWhinney: Beyond diagnosis, an approach to the integration of behavioral science and clinical medicine, *New England Journal of Medicine, 287*: 384, 1972.

The *mental status examination* is a means of systematically assessing the patient's mental condition. The elements of the mental status examination most useful for the general physician include:

Appearance: Grooming, motor activity (quiet versus agitated.)

General Level of Consciousness: Alert, sleepy, stuporous, obtunded.

Orientation: The patient knows who he is, where he is, and the date (day, month, and year).

Speech: Ability to use customary syntax. Note slurring, inability to find the right word, pressured speech, muteness.

Memory: Recent memory—knowledge of recent events, capacity to remember names of current treating physicians. Remote memory—ability to give history and present illness in proper historical sequence.

Attention and Concentration: Ability to understand and follow directions.

Intelligence: Can be estimated from level of schooling achieved, vocational history, use of words.

Mood: A pervasive, sustained emotion (depressed, euphoric, neutral).

Affect: An observable and immediately expressed emotion (anger, anxiety, fear, humor, etc.). Note whether or not display of affect is consistent with the content of speech, thoughts, and behavior.

Perceptions: Presence of hallucinations (visual, auditory, somatic), delusions, paranoid ideas.

Suicidal Thoughts: Statement or actions that indicate the patient wishes to harm or kill himself.

Homicidal or Violent Thoughts: Statements or actions that indicate patient wishes to harm or kill others.

Judgment: Capacity to understand the situation in which the patient finds himself and a demonstrated ability to comply with instructions and directions for care.

Most of the data required for a complete mental status examination can be obtained from observations made while the patient is giving his history. Only a few sections of the examination require specific questions such as: "Do you hear voices? Have you ever had any visions or seen things that other people don't see? Are you experiencing suicidal thoughts now?"; these questions can be asked at appropriate times during the interview. For the patient in whom the mental status examination suggests a significant cognitive defect, a more formal mental status examination can be administered in a short time (see section on Dementia, Chapter 16 and Table 16.1).

Personality refers to the relatively enduring attitudes and patterns of behavior which typify an individual. Generally a physician becomes acquainted with a patient's personality, particularly the patient's behavior pattern in the face of illness, over a period of months or years. Some patients will exhibit the features of a maladaptive personality (see Table 9.2), and recognition of this may be very helpful in planning the patient's care, as discussed in more detail in Chapter 13.

CASE FORMULATION

After completing the current evaluation, this information should be combined with the prior psychosocial information to provide a formulation of the case. "Case formulation" means a concise summary of the case including the patient's current problem and symptoms, his chief assets and liabilities, the current stresses and/or causes of the symptoms, a

Table 9.2
Maladaptive Personalities Encountered Commonly in Ambulatory Practice (see Chapter 13 for Detailed Descriptions)

The obsessive-compulsive patient
The overly emotional histrionic patient
The overly suspicious querulous (paranoid) patient
The passive-dependent patient
The passive-aggressive patient
The self-sacrificing patient
The patient with exaggerated self-importance

working diagnosis, a treatment plan, and the prognosis.

Example: A 37-year-old married black woman, with four children, working full time, from a stable family known to the physician, is seen for complaints of crampy left upper quadrant pain, abdominal swelling, nausea and vomiting. The pain is described "as if I were having my period." The patient's medical history includes a hysterectomy at the age of 31. She states that her pain had its onset at about the time her husband lost his job and was experiencing impotence. She also reveals that she has been feeling irritable and more short-tempered with her children. She has not been able to discuss either her distress or her husband's problem with him because "he's not the talking type." The problems have reached the point that they are arguing all the time and she is having fantasies of having an affair. Physical examination is essentially negative as is an upper gastrointestinal and gallbladder series. Mental status examination reveals mild anxiety and depression. She is given Donnatol for symptomatic relief and asked to return in a week for further discussion about her difficulties.

The case formulation would be: The patient is a 37-year-old married woman with gastrointestinal symptoms, mild anxiety, and depression (current problem). She is an industrious, stable individual with no evidence of a personality disorder (assets), but when under stress tends to seek magical solutions, at this time sexual fantasies (liability). She is having marital difficulties, secondary to her husband's response to losing his job (current stresses). She is suffering from psychophysiological gastrointestinal symptoms (working diagnosis). The crampy abdominal pain will be treated symptomatically, and the psychological symptoms will be treated with several follow-up visits to help her express her feelings and concerns about her relationship with her husband (treatment plan). Probability of improvement is good (prognosis).

The process of formulating cases in this manner is useful for several reasons: (a) it encourages the physician to relate psychological phenomena to the patient's somatic symptoms; (b) it requires the physician to select a recognized diagnostic category; (c) it leads to treatment which focuses upon both the immediate symptoms and the underlying psychosocial problems; and (d) it gives the physician a reasonable idea of the expected outcome of the problem.

ASSESSMENT OF MENTAL COMPETENCE

Occasionally, the general physician will be expected to assess the mental competence of a patient. Common civil issues of mental competence include: competence to accept or refuse medical care, commitment to hospitals, contesting of wills, and guardianship decisions.

The usual test of the patient's competence in selecting medical care is the determination whether or not the patient understands the nature, benefits, and risks of that care and the consequences of not selecting it. This determination can usually be made without difficulty in patients with mild retardation or dementia and in patients with psychological problems short of frank psychosis. In the ambulatory setting, the major problem presented by such patients is unreliable self-care, particularly medication-taking; here, the assistance of a competent household member may be needed. When the need to determine competence for signing informed consent (for example, consent for an intravenous pyelogram) arises in ambulatory practice, the patient's personal physician is usually the professional who is best qualified to determine whether the patient or his next of kin should sign.

Although commitment laws in most states require examination by a physician and do not specify psychiatric examination, the primary care physician will rarely be required to make commitment determinations. In those instances when a psychiatrist is not available, a complete psychiatric evaluation, including a complete mental status examination, is necessary to determine whether the patient is dangerous to himself or to others, which is the usual test for commitment.

It is even less likely that the primary care physician will be called upon to examine and provide expert testimony in contesting of wills or in determining the need for guardianship for a patient. The ultimate decision in such cases is made by an administrative law judge. These legal proceedings are often adversary in nature, and familiarity with principles of forensic psychiatry and experience as an expert witness are required of the physician participating. Most psychiatrists hesitate to become involved in these proceedings unless they have had special training and experience. Therefore, it is unlikely that the primary care physician will or should be involved unless he, too, has had the necessary training and experience.

General References

Balint, M: *The Doctor, His Patient, and the Illness.* International University Press, New York, 1957.
Engel, GL: The clinical application of the biopsychosocial model. *Am Psychiatry* 137: 5, 1980.
    Both authors explain lucidly the conceptual framework for relating the diagnosis and management of physical symptoms to psychological and social stresses in the patient's life.

CHAPTER TEN

Psychotherapy in Ambulatory Practice

CHESTER W. SCHMIDT, JR., M.D.

Psychotherapy consists of a number of verbal and behavioral processes which are used in the treatment of psychiatric and emotional disorders for the purpose of relieving symptoms and solving intra- and interpersonal problems. Although many different techniques have been described there are fundamental principles which are common to all. Since general physicians have many opportunities to use psychotherapy effectively, either formally or informally, it is important that they have a working knowledge of these principles.

This section will describe: (a) general principles of psychotherapy and (b) specific techniques that are useful in ambulatory practice.

GENERAL PRINCIPLES

Transference

Patients come to physicians for the relief of pain, suffering, and fear associated with illness and disease. They recognize and accept the expertise of the physician and are hopeful and trusting that the physician will relieve their distress. The basic attitudes of hopefulness and trust are positive attributes of the relationship between patient and doctor. There are potent psychosocial roots to the generally positive initial expectations of the patient as he enters into the relationship with the physician. The patient brings with him a history of psychosocial develop-

ment during which time pain, fear, and other forms of distress have been repeatedly relieved by the actions of attentive and affectionate parents. Through these experiences, individuals both consciously and unconsciously come to expect that new people in their lives will behave and interact with them in ways similar to the experiences they had as children with their parents. These expectations are what are known as transference phenomena. Patients will project on to the patient-physician relationship these conscious and unconscious expectations. In fact, at times patients may react to the physician as if the physician were an important parental figure. To the degree that the transference is *positive*, the physician can exercise powerful supportive and healing psychological forces over the patient. Positive transference may explain placebo responses, and its effect must always be kept in mind when evaluating any therapeutic intervention.

Not all transference reactions are positive. Virtually no one comes through their childhood and adolescence without some psychological scars from disappointments, frustrations, and anger that are the results of unmet expectations and other deprivations experienced during the process of growing up. These psychological scars are the historical-developmental roots of maladaptive and negative personality traits such as dependency, passivity, hostility, obsessive-compulsivity, and sociopathy (see Chapter 13). The conscious and unconscious conflicts associated with these traits can also be projected on to the physician-patient relationship. These *negative* transference reactions often cause troubled physician-patient relationships. The more seriously the patient is deprived of parental affection and support during his childhood, the more likely it is that he will manifest these negative traits as an adult, and therefore the more likely it is that negative transference reactions will develop within the patient-physician relationship.

The significance of the transference phenomenon to psychotherapeutic techniques is that it is a basic tool for bringing about positive attitudinal and behavioral change in the patient. For most ambulatory patients psychological distress results from problems within their current relationships with family, friends and associates. The transference will re-create, within a controlled setting, modified but reasonably accurate representations of the patient's current and past relationships. As the patient begins to react to the physician as if he were one of the individuals with whom he (the patient) is having difficulty, the developing relationship and its negative aspects can be examined. Changes in the patient's attitudes and behavior to improve the relationship can then be considered.

The more intense the therapeutic relationship between patient and physician, the more likely it is that both positive and negative transference reactions will appear and become part of the therapeutic effort. Techniques like counseling do not produce intense therapeutic relationships and therefore tend to involve chiefly positive transference.

Counter Transference

Physicians, like their patients, must go through the trials and tribulations of childhood, adolescence, and maturation, and therefore are not immune to the development of negative personality traits. However, society and the medical profession assumes that physicians will not allow these traits to affect the physician-patient relationship. The physician is expected to maintain an objectivity in his relationship with his patients, and to be supportive and empathetic.

When practicing psychotherapy, the physician must be aware of his own idiosyncracies and must keep them under control and out of the therapeutic relationship; i.e., he must avoid counter transference.

The Therapeutic Contract

When a physician and patient agree to engage in counseling, no matter how brief the program, the details of the treatment should be spelled out and agreed to by both parties. That process forms the basis of the treatment contract. The details include frequency of visits, the length of the visits, the fee for the visit, the place in which the treatment is to be conducted, and the approximate length of the treatment program. These details form the boundaries within which the treatment, regardless of specific technique, will take place. The boundaries, although they seem obvious, can become extraordinarily significant during the course of treatment. Patients often react to the boundaries as part of the transference phenomenon by objecting to them, or attempting to change or to violate them. Although there are exceptions, the boundaries should not be modified because of a change in the relationship between the patient and the physician that arises as a result of transference. The contractual agreements are important boundaries and should remain stable throughout the course of the treatment.

Treatment Process

Psychotherapeutic techniques are like all human relationships: they have a beginning, a middle, and an end. The *initial phase* involves continued collection of data about the patient, sharpening of the formulation of the case, and, in collaboration with the patient, development of treatment goals. The initial phase of treatment is like a honeymoon during which the patient's expectations and hopes are expressed by positive transference toward the physician. The *middle phase* of treatment consists of the work of accomplishing the treatment goals agreed to by the patient and the therapist. Efforts to achieve those goals are met with by resistance from the patient as he attempts to avoid making the attitudinal and behavioral changes that are necessary to attain the goals. As the patient's avoidance of doing the work is pointed out or interpreted by the therapist, the patient becomes frustrated and annoyed and may develop negative transference toward the therapist. Recognition of the negative transference reactions and the resolution of them is an important part of the middle phase of treatment.

The *last phase* of treatment is a review of the work accomplished and a preparation for separating the patient from the treatment and the therapist. Separation is an extremely important part of the treatment process. It forces the patient to give up any residual dependency on the therapist. The experience of separating in a constructive fashion strengthens the ego functions of the patient. It is not unusual for the patient to experience a reoccurrence of the symptoms that originally brought him to treatment. However, in order to allow the patient to benefit fully from the separation experience it is important to complete the treatment on schedule as agreed. Inasmuch as general physicians will continue to have a relationship with their patients, separation may not be complete. However, shifting from the psychotherapeutic mode back to the primary care mode (see "Supportive Therapy" below) is a form of separation and contains within it some of the same benefits that would result from a formal psychotherapeutic situation.

PSYCHOSOCIAL TREATMENT TECHNIQUES

Specific management techniques are described for each of the problems covered in subsequent chapters. Here, we describe several general techniques that are useful in managing many of the problems seen in ambulatory practice.

Short Term Counseling

Short term counseling is extremely useful for managing psychosocial problems in an ambulatory setting. It is a *suppressive* form of psychotherapy, meaning that the goals of treatment are to strengthen the defenses of the patient and to relieve symptoms without uncovering the contributions of long-standing intrapsychic conflicts to the current problem.

Short term counseling is ideal for managing transient problems secondary to life stresses and interpersonal difficulties. If more than one or two sessions are judged to be necessary, a specific number of sessions should be planned. Most short term counseling can be accomplished in 5 to 10 weekly sessions, 15 to 30 minutes long.

The physician who engages in counseling should be an observer-participant and should avoid acting as a powerful, all-knowing figure. His general strategy is to help the patient to recognize and make choices that favor resolution of current psychological symptoms. The specific techniques of counseling include the following.

EMPATHIC LISTENING

It is very supportive and reassuring to the patient for the physician to indicate that he is listening and paying close attention to what the patient is saying. Remembering details of the history, responding with appropriate affect to situations described by the patient and indicating to the patient that his feelings have been observed are actions which both demonstrate to the patient that the physician is concerned and which increase the patient's self-esteem.

CLARIFICATION

When a pattern of troubling thoughts or behavior becomes apparent to the physician, he may help the patient by pointing out this pattern. Common examples are (a) the occurrence of psychophysiologic symptoms, such as peptic symptoms, in the face of a variety of psychological stresses; and (b) recurring interpersonal conflicts which are always initiated by some action on the patient's part. By clarifying such patterns for the patient, the physician can help the patient to understand himself better and to discover ways to ameliorate the situation.

VENTILATION OF FEELINGS

Patients who keep to themselves strong feelings about past or current experiences usually feel better by relieving those pent-up emotions. An outpouring of emotion can be elicited sometimes by stating that the patient looks tense, angry or depressed, or by commenting that the experience which the patient has just described must have made the patient feel upset. Encouraging the patient to express feelings and giving the patient permission to vent his feelings may loosen his defenses just enough to allow the ventilation to take place.

ADVICE (PERSUASION)

The physician is considered by the patient to be an expert and should judiciously exercise that expertise. Specific, concrete recommendations are not only useful in a practical medical way, but may also be very helpful for patients who are upset and temporarily unable to use their own coping skills. The physician's advice provides the patient with something to hang on to until he can make decisions himself. Advice may also be used in a confrontational manner, to force the patient to face up to the fact that he is engaging in dangerous or destructive behavior. The

shock value of the confrontation may pierce the complacent defensiveness of the patient, thereby allowing the physician to persuade the patient to change behavior.

EDUCATION

Clear explanation of normal physiology, disease processes, treatment regimens, etc., is often overlooked as a powerful aid in counseling. Besides imparting knowledge, the patient is drawn into a collaborative relationship with the physician.

CONTINGENCY PLANNING

The life situations which create stress for patients are often manageable after even slight changes. Distressed patients often cannot see a means of making those changes. Once the physician has a detailed understanding of the situation, he and the patient can engage in creating plans for improving or coping with the problem. By joining in with the patient in making plans, the physician assists the patient in using his own coping skills and will often evoke from the patient a solution to the problem.

Examples of Short Term Counseling

Example: The mother of an adolescent boy from a family that is known to be stable, without history of significant psychiatric difficulty, reported to her personal physician that her son has been drinking alcohol. The adolescent had no history of antisocial behavior and had a good school record. At a series of 3 weekly visits, 15 minutes in duration, the physician encouraged the mother to express her anxiety and anger about the drinking (empathic listening and encouraging ventilation), supported her concern about the legal implications, and advised her to discuss the matter with her husband for the purpose of setting limits on the drinking (advice). The physician also suggested the mother give him a follow-up call each week for the month following the last session.

Another common example: A middle-aged male with hypertension was not complying with his treatment program. His physician scheduled weekly visits for one month and emphasized having the patient tell his own thoughts about his hypertension (listening) and teaching the patient about the benefits of long term treatment (education and persuasion). Through this process their relationship was strengthened and the patient became willing to follow the treatment program. Counseling in a common situation like this takes advantage of positive transference and requires no change in the physician-patient relationship.

Supportive Therapy

Supportive therapy utilizes the techniques of counseling and, similarly, does not attempt to uncover or resolve psychodynamic issues. Unlike short term counseling, the duration of supportive therapy is open-ended; and it is often incorporated into the routine management of a chronic disease. Patients should participate in the decision about the frequency of visits, and in so doing make a contribution at least to that portion of the treatment contract. This form of psychotherapy is useful, for example, in the long term management of a diabetic patient with a history of poor compliance and multiple family problems. Such a patient is seen once a month for 10 to 15 minutes. The goals of the sessions are:

1. To monitor the patient's diabetic condition.
2. To enhance compliance.
3. To review family problems.

The verbal exchange between the physician and the patient during the visit consists of a review of the therapeutic regimen, an assessment of symptoms, a brief review of what has occurred in the patient's life since the last visit, and a discussion of ways to cope with existing family problems. In this manner, a significant supportive service is provided in the context of management of the patient's organic disease.

Crisis Intervention

Inasmuch as patients often experience major or minor life crises, familiarity with crisis intervention is important for general physicians. Faced with a crisis, patients experience a rise in emotional tension that initiates their usual problem-solving responses. If the crisis is not resolved, however, there is a further rise in tension, accompanied by a state of partial or complete ineffectiveness. If the stress continues with no resolution, further tension is followed by mobilization of internal resources in a final attempt to cope. Finally, if all efforts fail, a breaking point is reached and psychic disorganization results. If feelings of anxiety, depression, hopelessness and helplessness continue, the patient may engage in self-destructive acts or may develop regressive behavior such as uncontrolled crying, muteness and inability to perform basic self-care.

The theoretical basis of crisis intervention includes a focus on the immediate event (stress) accompanied by a recognition that the stress is both a threat to the patient and an opportunity for personal growth if the problem can be overcome. During the initial contact with the patient, the physician's task is to identify the details of the event that has precipitated the crisis. Next, the physician assesses the psychologic effects of the stress on the patient and develops a strategy for reducing the stress. During this phase of intervention, medications may be prescribed to alleviate specific symptoms such as anxiety or sleep loss (see Chapters 12 and 82). When symptoms are partially controlled, discussion of a way of resolving the problem begins. Contingency planning is especially important at this point. If during this phase of treatment the patient experiences strong feelings of rage, anger or guilt, the patient is allowed to ventilate these feelings. However, through his physical presence the physician helps the patient control the level of affect so that the feelings do not generate destructive behavior. The next phase of treatment is the implementation of the specific interventions, mutually agreed upon by the physician and patient, which are expected to resolve the effects of the crisis. The final step of treatment is a review of the entire process to help the patient consolidate the gains made in achieving a resolution of the crisis.

Example of Crisis Intervention: The patient is a 32-year-old mother of 2 young children. Her husband died 2 weeks ago following an industrial accident. She has managed to handle the funeral of her husband with the help and support of several friends. Her own family lives in another part of the country and is not readily available during the crisis. She has been encouraged to come for the evaluation by her friends because of severe headaches and insomnia.

Initial evaluation reveals the patient is in good physical health but she feels abandoned, overwhelmed and grief-stricken. Her headaches and insomnia are adding to the obvious stress of the situation and further sapping her emotional and physical resources. She is judged to be nonsuicidal but even so the analgesics and sedatives prescribed are given in small amounts.

The physician schedules a follow-up visit for *the next day*, which is devoted to a review of her perception of her social and financial situation. The patient gives a reasonable summary of the steps she must take to stabilize her situation but suggests that she might not be up to the task. The physician reviews the effectiveness of the prescribed medicine, makes adjustments as necessary, asks the patient to prepare a list of specific tasks she must accomplish over the next 2 weeks and gives her an appointment *in 2 days*.

During the next visit the patient is asked to review her list. She indicates need to make contact with insurance companies, the personnel office of her husband's employer, Social Security, lawyer, bank, etc. The physician goes over the list with her, encouraging her efforts and calling to her attention that she omitted from the list time to be spent in the company of close friends who might help her with her grief and sense of abandonment.

Subsequent sessions, spaced according to the judgment of the physician, are reviews of the patient's progress in accomplishing the outlined tasks. During one visit the patient becomes very angry, expressing frustration over her inability to contact an insurance agent: "nobody really gives a damn about me." The physician allows the patient to ventilate, is supportive by indicating that people are not always as helpful as they could be, but then continues with the review of the tasks.

Following two or three additional visits the physician judges the patient to be handling her situation competently. The headaches and insomnia have disappeared. He suggests a final visit during which he reviews the process of their meetings and enumerates the steps the patient has taken in order to gain control of her situation. He does not schedule another meeting but offers her future availability if needed.

Family and Marital Counseling

The goals of this form of counseling are: (a) to create effective communications among the family members, (b) to bring to their awareness maladaptive patterns of behavior that may be destructive to one or more members of the family, and (c) to change those maladaptive patterns to constructive patterns of behavior. The specific techniques are similar to those used in individual counseling.

Example of Family Counseling: A couple asked their family physician for help in dealing with their adolescent daughter who was continually misbehaving at school and at home. Evaluation of the problem revealed the parents had not been consistent in their limit-setting for their daughter and the family considered the girl to be "the black sheep" of the family. Counseling for the whole family was recommended. During the first session the family members (parents and children) attacked the daughter, blaming her for all the family's troubles. The physician interrupted the attack by focusing the discussion on the development of a contract between the parents and their daughter designed to define the rules they expected her to follow and the consequences of violating the rules. The next session was a review of the parents' and daughter's adherence to the contract. The parents reported the daughter broke the contract by misbehaving, but one of the older siblings pointed out the parents were inconsistent in their application of the agreed upon limit-setting rules. This revelation confronted the family with the fact that the girl's behavior was a shared responsibility within the family. Over the remaining sessions, the physician continued to encourage the family to establish fair rules to which all could adhere consistently. By focusing on the behavior of the entire family, the pressure on the "bad member" was relieved, destructive patterns of interacting were interrupted, and new, constructive patterns were introduced.

Example of Marital Counseling: A woman reported to her physician on several occasions that she was concerned about her husband's drinking habits. After hearing the complaint several times, the physician decided to evaluate the case further because the husband of the patient was a diabetic who periodically had difficulty following the prescribed program. During the initial meeting the wife re-

stated her concern about the potential ill effects of alcohol on her husband's health and also pointed out that she was helpless to control the drinking. A review of their drinking behavior revealed the wife also drank heavily, although "socially" and that she was responsible for buying and stocking the liquor closet.

On the basis of the evaluation the physician recognized the problems with alcohol were shared by both husband and wife and suggested several visits to help the couple evaluate and possibly modify their drinking habits. During the next meeting the physician taught the couple about diabetes, its treatment and the problems associated with heavy alcohol use. The physician also introduced the concept that they shared the responsibility for the drinking behavior and therefore, control of drinking would require a joint effort. Once the couple was able to agree to this concept, the struggle between them over the drinking was eliminated and they were free to put their energies into a program for modifying both of their drinking habits.

References

General

Cadoret, RJ and King, LJ: *Psychiatry in Primary Care.* C.V. Mosby, Saint Louis, 1974.
Imboden, JB and Urbaitis, JC: *Practical Psychiatry in Medicine.* Appleton-Century-Crofts, New York, 1978.
  Two books containing useful sections on therapeutic techniques appropriate for use in office practice.
Dewald, PA: *Psychotherapy—A Dynamic Approach.* Basic Books, New York, 1969.
  A book which describes the techniques of supportive psychotherapy using the psychoanalytic model of mental functioning.
Frank JD: The influence of patients and therapists expectations on the outcome of psychotherapy. Br J Med Psychol 41: 349, 1968.
  A classic paper on the subject of expectations and treatment outcome.
Jacobson, GF: Programs and techniques of crisis intervention. In *American Handbook of Psychiatry,* Ed. 2, Vol. 2, pp. 811–825, edited by S. Arieti. Basic Books, New York, 1974.
  A concise review of the subject of crisis theory and technique.
Mann, J: The specific limitation of time on psychotherapy. *Semin Psychiatry* 1: 375, 1969.
  A paper which describes how best to structure short term psychotherapy.

CHAPTER ELEVEN

Psychosomatic Conditions

WALTER F. BAILE, M.D.

INTRODUCTION

This chapter describes those emotional and behavioral disturbances which are most often expressed as somatic complaints. Aside from their effects on patients, such disturbances present problems for the physician since patients often present with symptoms which *mimic* those associated with organic disease, *coexist* with organic disease, or serve as "*triggers*" for visits to the physician.

Illness Behavior

The response of a particular individual to a perceived change for the worse in his physiological state is called *illness behavior*. Illness behavior incorporates two independent but complementary concepts: the notion of "illness" (in contradistinction to "disease"), and the notion of an action taken by an individual to deal with his illness.

ILLNESS

It is generally acknowledged that the task of the clinician is not only to treat disease but to alleviate distress (11); this is as it should be, because it is distress which usually brings the patient to the physician in the first place. The patient may be distressed by worry over a painless breast lump or by the pathophysiological changes of a disease process. Moreover, there may be much disease and little illness (e.g., as in a silent myocardial infarction or asymptomatic coin lesion) or much illness and little

disease (e.g., as in severe low back pain). Thus, illness is a *subjective* experience of distress. It is unique to each individual, affects the whole person, is expressed as "symptoms," and may be experienced in the absence of disease. It involves a complex interaction among perceptual, attitudinal, emotional, evaluative, cultural, and physical factors. This is illustrated by the fact that while certain individuals have a tendency to amplify, focus on, and worry about relatively minor changes in their bodily processes (2), others will rationalize and attempt to ignore such alarming bodily changes as the pain associated with a myocardial infarction.

The distinction between disease and illness is not new. Long before scientific principles were applied to the understanding and treatment of disease, ritual and reassurance, empathy and encouragement were the mainstays of healing. Rarely was the course of disease changed. However, if success is measured in terms of relief of distress, the results were often impressive.

Since physicians in ambulatory practice tend to see much distress, the ability to distinguish between illness and disease is crucial. Although the distress may be in response to the pathophysiology of disease, in many situations the severe distress seems out of proportion to the amount of disease, or it may be present even when no disease process can be detected. This often presents a diagnostic dilemma for the clinician. Later on this chapter will illustrate the role that emotional distress plays in the symptoms of many of these patients.

THE DECISION TO SEEK CARE

The patient's decision to seek care is the action by which he brings his illness to the attention of a professional. Studies have shown that the relationship between the presence of symptoms and care-seeking behavior is far from linear. White and his colleagues (12) reviewed English and American studies and calculated that during an average month in a population of 1,000 adults 16 years of age and older, 750 experience what they recognize as an injury or illness on at least one occasion. Among this population, 250 consult a physician, 9 are hospitalized, 5 are referred to another physician; and 1 is referred to a university medical center. In terms of actual disease, there may be little which distinguishes those who come under treatment from those who do not. Thus, in an annual report on health problems in the United States, it was found that about 13% of deaths in 1976 would have been preventable with medical intervention (4), suggesting that patients with obvious signs and symptoms of disease failed to pay attention to their problem. On the other hand, in this report it was also noted that the largest proportion of ambulatory visits were for problems rated as "not serious" by the physician; similar findings have been reported in general practice in England (10).

Many factors determine whether a particular individual seeks medical care at a given time. The simplest assumption is that pain and malaise cause discomfort and distress which interfere with normal functioning or may exceed the individual's threshold for tolerance. Nevertheless many persons avoid medical care despite obvious signs and symptoms of disease, while others appear to overreact to minor problems. Clearly, nonphysiological factors may serve as important "triggers" for utilization of medical care. The importance of these factors is illustrated by the study of Zola and his colleagues (14) who surveyed patients at the time of their first visit to a university medical outpatient clinic to determine why they decided to visit the clinic at that particular time. Extensive interviews and follow-up of the patients indicated that: First, the physical complaints of the patients were often of long duration, and many had tolerated considerable disability before initiating the visit. Second, in most cases the symptom, although it may have caused distress, was related to the person's psychosocial environment. Zola distinguished in his patient population several nonphysiological "triggers" for the decision to seek medical help:

1. The occurrence of an interpersonal crisis (e.g., a young lady who is fighting with her mother over her dating behavior complains of symptoms related to her chronic ear infection).

2. The perceived interference of the symptom with interpersonal or social relationships (e.g., a teenager complains about his acne at a time when his classmates are making dates for the upcoming prom).

3. "Sanctioning"—seeking medical attention because a family member or friend insists (e.g., a woman finally sees a doctor for a painless breast mass after weeks of badgering by her husband).

4. The idea that the symptom will interfere with vocational or physical activity (e.g., a middle-aged man with a long-standing hernia becomes concerned that it will interfere with his sexual performance, soon after he has begun "dating" a year after his wife's death).

5. Providing a time limit for symptoms to abate (e.g., the setting of external time criteria—"if it isn't better in a week, I'll take care of it").

Clearly the interplay between symptoms and care-seeking behavior is complex. In Examples 2 and 3 above, the decision to seek care was prompted by *distress* associated with the symptoms rather than by pain, and there was a direct relationship between the symptoms and the social problem. In Example 1, on the other hand, the symptoms were not directly related to the social problem, but the problem exacerbated existing symptoms of an unrelated illness. Thus visits to physicians may be prompted by psychosocial factors which are related in various ways to concomitant disease.

Somatic symptoms may be the principal symptoms of an acute or chronic psychiatric disorder. *Acute disorders* are often precipitated by discrete environmental stressors, tend to occur in adulthood, and present with symptoms which for the most part are somatic expressions of anxiety and mood disturbance. In many cases the patient has functioned fairly well in job, family, and interpersonal spheres, but a specific event will be associated with the onset of symptoms. The onset of *chronic disorders* may often be traced to adolescence or early adulthood. By the time the patient is seen in later life there is often global disturbance of functioning. These patients are more likely to have severe personality disturbances which are associated with the unconscious use of symptoms and of the sick role to establish some level of functioning, albeit an unsatisfactory one. (See Chapter 13 for an example.)

The various disorders considered in this chapter are disorders in which care-seeking behavior (illness behavior) is disproportionate to the amount of objective evidence for disease. Although these disorders have been separated into discrete categories, there is much overlap among categories.

Prevention of Abnormal Illness Behavior

Given the powerful reinforcers existing in the medical system (e.g. ordering tests, prescribing drugs, inquiring about physical symptoms), the physician who is aware of the role psychosocial problems may play in generating physical complaints and medical visits may be instrumental in preventing abnormal illness behavior. Although it is sometimes difficult to avoid certain tests for fear of missing a diagnosis, the physician must always balance the decision for further workup, on a patient whose history and physical examination are unrevealing, against the knowledge that this may promote excessive physician utilization and prolong the sick role. Questioning the patient briefly about his ability to function in personal, family, and occupational spheres is the most efficient way to determine whether psychosocial factors are involved, and thus to avoid actions which may reinforce illness behavior.

The place of this general preventive approach is pointed out in more detail in the description of each of the specific problems discussed below.

MINOR MOOD DISTURBANCE (DYSPHORIA)

DESCRIPTION

Psychiatric morbidity in general practice most often presents as minor mood disturbance or "dysphoria." These terms refer to symptom complexes which include one or more of the manifestations of anxiety or depression but are less florid than the symptom complexes of full-blown depressive illnesses (see Chapter 14) or anxiety neurosis (see Chapter 12).

Minor mood disturbances usually result from "life crises" reflecting problems in adjusting to demands of the environment (8). In these situations, environmental stressors (physical, interpersonal, economic, etc.) temporarily impair the individual's ability to cope and result in increased tension, worry, demoralization, and irritability. However, the distress may be expressed in somatic terms. Since anxiety and depression cause well known somatic symptoms (13) such as light-headedness, fatigue, gastrointestinal problems, cold intolerance, increased frequency of micturition, palpitations, precordial pain, breathlessness, and flushing, these are often the presenting symptoms of the patient, as seen in the following case.

Example: A 26-year-old, usually shy, parochial school teacher was evaluated for symptoms of dizziness, abdominal cramps, nausea, excessive urination, and a sensation of fullness in the bladder. When physical examination and laboratory tests revealed no physiological disturbance, a more detailed history was taken. It showed that his symptoms began shortly after a confrontation with his school principal over his attempt to organize a teacher's union and his criticism of several school policies. In his ensuing anger he applied for a job which he did not really want. His symptoms prevented him from taking the scheduled examination for the position.

Individuals experiencing similar "distress" are often unaware (or only partially aware) of the relationship between their psychological disturbance and somatic symptoms. Symptoms of anxiety and depression can mimic almost any disease entity. As illustrated in the following example, diagnosis may be particularly difficult when the symptoms of psychosocial distress mimic those of a patient's established disease process.

Example: A 54-year-old widowed white woman recently recovering from a myocardial infarction complained to her physician on several occasions of fatigue, breathlessness, and pleuritic-like chest pain unrelated to exertion. Her physical examination and EKG were unchanged from when she left the hospital. Questioning revealed that she was forced to leave her job after her heart attack and was barely able to afford the $40 per month needed for medication. She tearfully revealed that although her son had offered to help pay for her medication, her daughter-in-law hinted that they could really not afford to help out. This proud and, until recently, self-sufficient woman who was initially reluctant to accept any help was now made to feel like a "charity case" by her son's wife.

In this case anxiety and mild depression produced symptoms, some of which suggested cardiac decompensation. The correct diagnosis was made when psychiatric consultation was eventually requested to rule out "functional" disorder and the appropriate history was elicited.

Distress which is provoked by life crisis is usually *self-limited.* Often the complaints will seem trivial to the physician. The frequency with which episodes of dysphoria occur will depend to a great extent upon the stability of the individual's environment and upon his own internal coping resources. The assumption of the "sick role" on the part of the patient may allow him to relinquish responsibilities temporarily, regroup his forces, and mobilize new resources for coping. A visit to the physician is an attempt to obtain help and it also legitimizes the "sick role."

EVALUATION

In evaluating these patients, the physician should follow two strategies:

1. *To elicit the relevant history.* Asking the patient general questions such as "How are things at home (or at work)?" will generally provide some inkling as to whether there are psychosocial disturbances. If so, diagnosis may be confirmed by a history of sleep and or appetite disturbance, increased irritability, difficulty in concentrating, excess worry, increased tension, and loss of interest in social activities and sexual relations. It is important to allow the patient to expand on his personal history. Although this may lead to the hazard that, once launched, the patient may be reluctant (or difficult) to stop, this does not usually occur. Nor does the patient usually become angry or overwhelmingly emotional which will make the physician feel uncomfortable. Most patients are grateful for a physician's interest in their personal problem, will respect time limits, and with a little advice, reassurance, and encouragement will go on to solve the precipitating problem themselves. Even before the physician has taken a psychosocial history, there may be clues to the diagnosis, such as a bizarre description of the symptoms or failure to respond to previous treatment known to work specifically for a disorder (3).

In some cases, however, patients may be defensive and reluctant to admit any psychosocial problem even when these problems are clearly present. In this case the physician should try to build a trusting relationship, and eventually may be rewarded with the patient's confidence.

2. *To temper the workup.* Obviously the physician should examine the patient and order laboratory tests required to allow him to confirm a diagnosis. However, extensive workups to exclude possible diagnoses may prolong the sick role and run the risk of the patient developing chronic illness behavior. This may occur especially when factors such as compensation claims or other gains are involved or when the stressor is prolonged and beyond the patient's capability to remove, influence, or change it. In these instances unproductive workups and doctor-shopping tend to imbed the patient in the sick role.

MANAGEMENT

Management of patients with minor mood disturbance is based upon several considerations:

1. Patients who are not coping well feel that they have failed. When the physician, in taking the history, explores the possible role of a psychosocial dilemma as an etiological factor in the patient's symptoms, he allows the patient to relinquish his embarrassment and guilt at this perceived failure.

2. Well known psychotherapeutic principles such as catharsis (achieved by ventilation) and transference (see Chapter 10) aid in this process by permitting the patient to discuss his problem in more detail;

3. Explaining the role of emotional factors in eliciting the problem provides a rationale to the patient for his symptoms.

The relief associated with the identification of a psychosocial basis for a patient's somatic complaints is often sufficient to allow him to begin to marshal his own resources for coping (5). However, occasionally patients will need short term counseling (see Chapter 10) to facilitate problem solving.

Drugs Which Exacerbate Dysphoria. In managing medical patients with minor mood disturbances it is important to avoid or to discontinue drugs and other substances which may exacerbate symptoms of dysphoria (see Table 11.1). Sometimes dysphoria may be brought on by the initiation or discontinuation of such drugs, so that the patient's problem may resolve after discontinuation of the offending substance. Two common examples of this situation are (a) the patient with newly diagnosed hypertension who has developed symptoms of depression shortly after beginning treatment with a central acting sympatholytic drug (methyldopa, clonidine, reserpine, propranolol), and (b) the patient who has become tremulous or irritable while taking multiple over-the-counter cold remedies containing sympathomimetic decongestants. Moreover, both excessive use of caffeine and withdrawal of caffeine after habitual use can produce classic symptoms of anxiety; thus management consists chiefly of explaining the role of caffeine in producing symptoms and of having the patient discontinue caffeine use.

SOMATOFORM DISORDERS

Grouped together is a cluster of more serious and often chronic disorders whose essential feature is the presentation by the patient of physical symptoms for which there are no demonstrable findings of organic disease and no known physiological mechanisms to explain the symptom (in contrast with the "dysphorias" in which anxiety and mild depression may produce somatic changes). The patients usually have depression and personality problems, but these may not be readily apparent because of the focus on somatic complaints. For the most part the etiology is poorly understood. Moreover, because most patients are seen by internists and family physicians and do not often come under extended psychiatric observation our understanding of the etiology and natural history of the disorders is incomplete.

Hypochondriasis

DESCRIPTION

Hypochondriasis (see Table 11.2) is a disorder commonly seen in medical practice, the cardinal manifestation of which is an unrealistic interpretation by a patient of normal physical signs or sensations leading him to believe that he suffers from a serious disease. This misbelief is usually refractory to energetic efforts to reassure the patient to the contrary.

Hypochondriasis most commonly has its onset in midlife. It is equally frequent in both sexes and tends to affect all social classes. It usually runs a chronic, fluctuating course. Symptoms and impairment may be severe or mild. Patients often have obsessive-compulsive personality traits, are egocentric and unduly sensitive to criticism, and have difficulty expressing feelings.

In some cases hypochondriasis will dominate the person's entire personality and govern his lifestyle. In others it may exist in milder forms, especially as part of obsessive compulsive personality disorders, and not significantly disturb the individual's functioning. An example of the milder form follows.

Example: A 30-year-old accountant had always been preoccupied about his physical appearance. He attempted to allay this concern by weight lifting and by constantly comparing himself to other individuals. After his father

Table 11.1
Drugs and Other Substances which May Exacerbate (or Produce) Symptoms of Dysphoria

EXACERBATION OF DEPRESSED MOOD
  Antihypertensives
    Clonidine
    Methyldopa
    Reserpine
    Beta Blockers
  Antihistamines
  Anxiolytic drugs
  Neuroleptic drugs
  Sedative-hypnotic drugs
  Alcoholic beverages
EXACERBATION OF SYMPTOMS OF ANXIETY
  Sympathomimetic drugs
    Decongestants (found in most over-the-counter cold remedies)
    Beta-2 bronchodilators
    Weight-reduction agents
  Xanthine-containing drugs, foods, and beverages
    Bronchodilators with theophylline
    Many over-the-counter cold and arthritis remedies
    Use and discontinuation of caffeine
  Thyroid hormone
  Discontinuation of alcohol and sedative-hypnotic drugs.

Table 11.2
Major Features of the Principal Somatoform Disorders

Characteristics	Hypochondriasis (Hypochondriacal Neurosis)	Somatization Disorder (Briquet's Syndrome, Hysteria)	Conversion Disorder (Hysterical Neurosis, Conversion Type)
Essential features	Fear of or belief in presence of serious disease in absence of objective findings; misinterpretation of normal physical symptoms or signs	Multiple somatic complaints without organic pathology; long history of questionable medical treatment, procedures, and surgeries; vague, tangential verbal style	Loss or alteration of sensory or voluntary motor functioning not explained by pathophysiology; usually involves one organ or system
Associated features	May be component of somatization disorder; history of doctor-shopping, anxiety, depression	Interpersonal difficulties; history of depression or suicide attempts or anxiety; lack of insight	May be component of somatization disorder; symptoms often suggest neurological disease
Prevalence	Probably common; equal in men and women	May affect as many as 1% of all women; rare in men	Prevalence in ambulatory practice unknown
Age at onset	Adolescence, 30s or 40s	Adolescence, or young adulthood	Adolescence, early adulthood
Course	Chronic, fluctuating	Chronic, fluctuating	Generally unknown; 50% may recover in 1 year
Impairment and complications	Variable; strained doctor-patient relations	Related to substance abuse, doctor-shopping, medical, surgical procedures; serious depression may lead to suicide attempt	Marked effect on lifestyle; disuse may lead to atrophy; 10–30% of patients develop organic disease related to symptom
Predisposing factors	Psychosocial stressors; (?) previous organic disease	Unknown	Presence of "model," life stress (usually unrecognized by patient)
Familial pattern	Unknown	Occurs with greater than chance frequency in female family members; history of alcoholism and sociopathy in first-degree male relative	Unknown
Differential diagnosis	Physical disorder; psychotic disorders (especially depression)	Physical disorders (e.g., hyperparathyroidism, multiple sclerosis (MS), systemtic lupus erythematosus (SLE); schizophrenia with multiple somatic delusions; major depression; conversion disorder	Physical disorders (e.g., MS, SLE), somatization disorder, hypochondriasis

died of a heart attack he became concerned that he might have heart disease and was fearful about the implication of any insignificant chest pain. He also worried about his blood pressure which was transiently elevated at the time of his yearly physical examinations. His most recent examination revealed insignificantly elevated liver enzymes which he fretted over for weeks. Despite these concerns he rarely missed a day's work. He was not so sure that he did not have a serious disease but thought he had best trust his physician. He was a minor annoyance to his physician because of the difficulty in reassuring him.

While the physician will see patients such as this young man, it is the chronic, older hypochondriac who presents the most difficult management problem. Often he will "doctor shop" because of preoccupation with a single dreaded illness or with a single organ system or several systems. Two striking features of this illness are the amount of worry or concern invested in even a minor symptom such as a scratchy throat or a cough, and the amount of time invested in seeking a diagnosis which may cause extensive doctor shopping and result in unnecessary diagnostic procedures. In severe cases there may be interference with work and the individual may develop the lifestyle of an invalid.

The etiology of this disorder is unknown. Personality traits and psychosocial stressors predispose to its onset as does previous disease in the patient or in a family member who may serve as a "model." The diagnosis is based upon the exclusion of organic causes, the inability to reassure the patient about his symptom and the absence of another mental disorder. The fact that it is usually limited to one organ system, the degree of conviction that the patient expresses in having a disease, and pre-existing obsessive-compulsive personality traits distinguish it from somatization disorder (see description below).

MANAGEMENT

Treatment of the hypochondriac is difficult and frustrating especially when the disorder is chronic and severe. Patients are taxing, demanding, and generally refuse to consider the possibility that they may have an emotional problem.

The viewpoint of Aldrich (1) and the strategy for management he suggests may be useful for both the chronic hypochondriac and for several of the other somatoform disorders mentioned in this chapter. Management of the patient is based upon the following:

1. The symptoms serve a purpose, by means of which a person who is not coping can save face. The sick role exonerates people from normal responsibility.

2. Early learning probably plays a part in the process; persons with chronic hypochondriasis probably were put to bed for minor ailments and had parents who worried excessively about their health.

3. Adults cannot ask for reassurances or nurture unless they are helpless. The health care system is a way to get this support; medicines, examinations, procedures serve to provide attention.

4. New symptoms are ways of assuring attention; intermittent reinforcement by physician, family, etc., strengthen symptom reporting.

5. The motivating forces behind the patient's behavior are beyond his level of awareness.

It follows that: (a) Attempting to reassure the patient of absence of disease will not be effective and will be seen as a rejection. (b) Administration of medicines (especially placebos), tests, and procedures just to "see if there's something we missed" or to prove that the patient is not really sick will reinforce symptoms (this is difficult to avoid in the "age of malpractice"). (c) Referring the patient to a psychiatrist will probably be unsuccessful since it threatens the face-saving purpose of the symptoms. (d) Positive medical diagnoses and specific treatments will not satisfy the patient, and new symptoms will emerge.

Treatment of the hypochondriac, therefore, is based upon the understanding that the patient has learned to cope with everyday problems by avoiding them; this is in part a learned response and has been reinforced by the medical system and the environment. Only by extinction of "illness behavior" and removal of the reinforcers will the patient be able to deal with every day stresses. Treatment must be undertaken by the patient's general physician; the chronic hypochrondriac will not see a psychiatrist since it merely will be interpreted by the patient that "it's all in your head." The following strategy should be utilized:

1. Schedule regular visits (e.g., 15 min every 2 to 4 weeks) so that the patient does not need a new symptom to initiate a visit "only when necessary." The patient is told that his problems are partially due to tension and stress and that visits will focus on these.

2. Stay within the time framework decided even if the patient attempts to prolong the session.

3. Encourage the patient to talk about his or her life situations; clarify alternatives, but remind the patient that the choice among them is his (i.e., avoid giving advice).

4. Downplay the efficacy of medication since it will tend only to reinforce prescription-seeking behavior.

5. Be tolerant of being tested by the patient. At first the patient may telephone between visits with new symptoms; treat new symptoms professionally and detachedly; manage contacts between sessions pleasantly and as quickly as possible; treat frequent between-visit telephone calls with *increased* contact.

Although not always effective, this strategy enables the physician to gain some control in a difficult situation. The greatest danger to its success will be the physician's impatience. The physician should be prepared for improvement to take a long time consistent with the treatment of any chronic physical or psychiatric disorder.

Somatization Disorder (Briquet's syndrome, Hysteria)

DESCRIPTION

This clinical entity, (see Table 11.2) was previously known as "Briquet's syndrome" after the French physician Paul Briquet who first described and categorized the symptoms of more than 400 patients with this disorder. The etiology is unknown; however, it runs in families, affects 1 to 2% of adult women, and the frequency of sociopathy and alcoholism is increased in first degree male relatives of the patient. It is important for the generalist to recognize this entity because it is not uncommon, is often associated with substance abuse, and frequently results in the patient having unnecessary medical and surgical procedures.

The main clinical characteristics of somatization disorder are (a) The patient presents with multiple vague somatic complaints (more than 10) which involve several different organ systems. When seen early in the course, when the patient is usually in her early 20's, the most frequent mode of presentation is with complaints referable to the reproductive tract: painful menstruation, menstrual irregularity, excessive bleeding, severe vomiting throughout pregnancy. Later on there is a shift of symptomatology: headaches, fainting spells, nausea, vomiting, abdominal pains, bowel difficulties, and fatigue predominate. (b) The presenting symptoms have little or no organic basis. One or more symptoms may have the characteristics of a conversion disorder (see below). (c) The patient's medical history will usually include: treatment by a multiplicity of physicians, multiple surgical and medical procedures (laparotomy, removal of "adhesions," and multiple cystoscopies are common) for which there is no organic basis; and possible substance abuse. (d) The mode of presentation of the symptoms is often circumstantial and somewhat incoherent. The physician may feel particularly frustrated and perplexed not only by the variety of somatic complaints, but also because the patient may be unable to give any coherent history of the problems, often interjecting descriptions of how they have affected lifestyle and relationships, relating irrelevant details about treatment, yet being unable to describe the nature, character, location, onset, and duration of the symptoms. (e) Patients often show manifestations of the histrionic personality or the borderline personality (see Chapter 13). (f) Typically the patient's attitude is that she has been sick most of her life, and she has no insight into the true nature of her disorder. (g) There may be a history of a suicide attempt or overt depressive symptoms. (h) The patient often has a history of psychosexual problems—sexual indifference, lack of pleasure during intercourse, painful intercourse. The following case illustrates several of the above points.

Example: The patient was a 53-year-old married white woman who was referred for psychiatric evaluation by her internist who, noting her presentation with "ill defined symptoms" was requesting information about management. She had presented with complaints of generalized muscle aching, and periodic sensations throughout her body described as "what one has when hearing someone scratch his fingers on a blackboard." She also complained of skin lesions on her back and stated she was hypothyroid and suffered from a chronic urinary tract infection. Her past history included tonsillectomy, groin lymph node biopsy (twice), hysterectomy, bladder suspension (twice), rectocele repair, removal of adhesions, multiple cystoscopies, appendectomy, and removal of a tongue papilloma. The patient stated she suffered from Ménière's disease and episodes of hyperventilation. She also carried a diagnosis of "fibrositis" for which she had taken steroids in the past and "restless leg syndrome." Her current medicines were Clinoril, Valium, and Bellergal. She mentioned that she had "always been ill" and that she "hated men." Her psychosocial history included marriage to an alcoholic who abused her, and a positive family history of suicide. In presenting her symptoms, the patient was extremely vague and interjected facts about her emotional life with an inappropriate laugh. She had little insight into the nature of her problem believing her symptoms were due to "food allergy." She had stopped eating everything and at the time of her initial visit to her internist had ingested only distilled water for 4 days. Physical examination and laboratory tests were normal.

Somatization disorder tends to run a chronic but fluctuating course characterized by episodes of aggressive doctor-shopping and interludes in which the patient remains "stably symptomatic." This disorder is not difficult to recognize since the history suggests that it has been present for a number of years. The diffuseness and vagueness of the multiplicity of symptoms, the mode of presentation of complaints, and a past history of doctor-shopping in the context of a mostly negative physical examination and laboratory tests are the essential criteria for making the diagnosis. However, since these patients may indeed experience organic disease, new symptoms need to be evaluated carefully.

MANAGEMENT

Treatment of these patients is difficult because of their lack of insight. To tell the patient "I can't find anything wrong with you" is inviting doctor-shopping. Since many of these patients lead chaotic lives with marital and domestic turmoil, psychosocial crises may precipitate or maintain complaining behavior. The physician, in taking the patient's history, can invite her to talk about her social problems, which may succeed in shifting the focus away from the bodily complaints. An approach similar to that outlined for the treatment of the chronic hypochondriac may succeed in settling the patient down and in stabilizing an emotional crisis. The patient should be prevented from undergoing multiple unnecessary diagnostic procedures and surgery. When the family structure is fairly stable, an attempt may be made to work with family members to achieve limited therapeutic goals for the patient. Prognosis for lasting improvement in this disorder is poor. Some patients may improve with intensive, expert psychotherapy, but for most management consists of careful handling of new complaints as they arise and attempts to help the patients stabilize their living situation.

Conversion Disorder

DESCRIPTION

Conversion disorder (see Table 11.2) or hysterical neurosis, conversion-type, is a disorder in which the patient complains of loss or alteration of voluntary motor function or of some another neurological symptom. The symptom suggests an organic problem, but is instead an expression of an unconscious psychological conflict or need. The symptom can mimic any organic problem or affect any part of the nervous system. The most obvious and classic symptoms are paralysis, aphonia, and seizures.

Example: A 15-year-old girl abruptly lost her voice and developed an unremitting cough for which there was no organic pathology. The symptoms had their onset shortly after her brother had been transferred to the school that she attended. Family counseling by a psychiatrist revealed that the girl's brother had been experiencing emotional problems with which the family had failed to deal, and which recently had been worsening to the point of incipient psychosis. With her brother in the same school, the patient felt even more intensely the burden of keeping the family "secret." By becoming the patient herself she was able to avoid the stressful situation. Her aphonia allowed her to deal with the conflict between her brother's deterioration and the family mores. Family therapy allowed the identification of the real problem and permitted the patient to relinquish her symptom.

Often, as in the above case, the symptom has symbolic value in that it may serve to solve an internal conflict created by a feeling, impulse, or wish which the individual may find morally or ethically unacceptable (primary gain). The conversion may also allow the individual to gain certain support from the environment (secondary gain). A conversion disorder is likely to involve a single symptom during a single episode. Sometimes the symptom mimics those of a previous illness or illnesses of others significant to the patient ("modeling"). The expression of the symptom, however, will often follow the patient's notion of an anatomical distribution or function which will be reflected in the sensory or motor loss.

Conversion symptoms usually have their onset in adolescence or childhood. Their prevalence in ambulatory settings is unknown. Their significance for the generalist is that not only do they mimic organic disease, but also several follow-up studies of hospitalized patients diagnosed as having conversion disorders showed that from 13% to 30% subsequently developed organic disease related to their "conversion" symptoms (6). The organic disorders detected were for the most part neurological. The physician must thus be cautious in his approach to these patients.

The diagnosis is based upon the exclusion of organic pathology and on the presence of several secondary criteria: (a) the pathological process follows the patient's notion of bodily functions; (b) history of previous conversion reactions or undiagnosable physical symptoms is often present; (c) the presence of a symptom "model"; and (d) a temporal relationship between the symptom and an associated life stress is often seen.

The course of the illness is quite variable. The effect on lifestyle may be severe and atrophy from disuse may cause further impairment. Moreover, there is a significant incidence of later organic illness, a high incidence of subsequent major depression or other incapacitating mental illness, and a greatly increased suicide rate.

Conversion symptoms may be distinguished from dysphorias by the "nonphysiological" nature of the symptom, the patient's lack of insight into the relationship of the symptom to the psychosocial precipitant, and the symbolic significance of the symptom.

MANAGEMENT

In general, treatment of conversion symptoms is most likely to succeed in those patients with good premorbid adjustment, where the symptoms were obviously precipitated by a life stress, and where the patient is able to express feelings and to experience distress over the symptoms. A psychiatric consultation may be useful in helping make the diagnosis and in providing suggestions for management, but few patients will comply with long term psychotherapy.

When the diagnosis is made, the physician should avoid confronting the patient about the symptom directly, but should explain to the patient that he is interested in investigating all possible etiological factors, including the relationship of the disorder to stress. This may allow the patient gradually to accept the role of psychological factors and to give up the symptom. The solicitation of the aid of the family is often important. The physician should be aware, however, that conversion symptoms often mask serious psychiatric disorders such as depression. Furthermore, since a significant number of patients do develop organic disease, any changes in symptoms or the development of new symptoms should be taken seriously.

Psychogenic Pain Disorders

DESCRIPTION

Although pain is obviously an important component of organic disease it is just as likely to reflect the presence of a psychiatric disorder. As discussed above, complaints of pain may be part of a psychiatric entity such as Briquet's syndrome in which physical findings to explain the pain are minimal. In Briquet's syndrome, the disorder is chronic, the complaints have been present for an extended period of time, and there are usually other serious psychiatric disturbances such as depression and the presence of severe personality disturbances. Moreover, in Briquet's disorder complaints are multiple, with many organs involved, and previous surgeries frequent.

Probably the most common psychiatric entity which underlies a complaint of pain in general practice is a minor mood disturbance (see above) in which the dysphoric mood lowers the thresholds for both pain tolerance and pain perception; as a result, there will be increased complaints about the normal aches and pains of everyday life or about pain from a coexisting but well controlled condition such as arthritis.

For these patients the pain is in one sense a "ticket" to the doctor. Most of these disorders are acute; there is a detectable stressor in the patient's environment, and the stress will be temporally related to the onset of the symptom. These patients are best described as "temporarily dependent" (10). In the patient who is temporarily incapacitated, once the precipitating stressor is identified it is often not difficult for the physician to shift the focus away from the complaint of pain. This often leads to a marshaling of the patient's own coping resources so that there is some resolution of the crisis and the symptom(s) is alleviated. At times the use of minor tranquilizers and/or hypnotics will be required to reduce anxiety which may interfere with problem-solving or to combat loss of sleep which is sapping the patient's energy.

Sometimes the physician will notice that what began as an acute pain evolves into a chronic pain state, which is undesirable since it often leads to considerable interference with functioning, abuse of analgesics, doctor-shopping, and unnecessary surgery. Often the original mood disturbance deepens as the symptom persists, as iatrogenic factors such as further pain from surgery exacerbate the discomfort, and as the patient's environmental situation deteriorates and his relationship with doctors becomes mutually unsatisfactory.

The evolution of the situation just described is complex and it is only just beginning to be understood. Important are:

1. Certain personality characteristics of the individual, such as inability to express psychological distress in terms of the feelings that are involved. Thus, the patient who may feel angry, helpless, and rejected because of being passed over for a promotion at work may for many reasons find these feelings unacceptable. They may therefore be expressed in physical terms and the physical symptoms become the bodily equivalent of inner feelings which he is unable to express.

2. The failure of the environmental stressor to abate, resulting in continued loss of self-esteem and deepening of the depressive mood, further lowering pain tolerance.

3. The presence of pending litigation involving a compensation claim for the original complaint.

4. Environmental reinforcers which allow the patient to avoid unpleasant or conflicting activities, situations, or feelings by being ill, as well as the advantage of possible increased attention received for being ill.

5. Iatrogenic factors such as unnecessary medical workups or procedures which distract from the primary stressor, further enmesh the patient in the sick role and increase the dependency on the medical system as a way of coping.

In most cases several of these five factors operate at once.

MANAGEMENT

In the patient with pain of relatively recent onset as a primary complaint, and where the physical findings are minimal or do not adquately explain the pain, or where the pain is a symptom of a longstanding but stable disease process which has not recently deteriorated, the physician should attempt to elicit an environmental basis for the patient's distress and treat the disorder as he would a minor mood disturbance (see above).

If patients have difficulty in identifying and expressing their feelings with respect to a definite stressor, the physician should pursue a cautious workup while continuing to take a personal history over a period of several sessions. The establishment of rapport may allow the patient to abandon his defensiveness and gradually express his feelings.

The physician should realize that regardless of the origin of a patient's pain it is often accompanied by emotional disturbance, which frequently leads to a lowering of the threshold for pain. Moreover, anxiety, which is often seen in acute pain states, may evolve into depression if the pain persists. Two axioms follow: (a) The treatment of the anxiety (see Chapter 12) accompanying psychogenic pain may be of significant help both in shortening the time course of the dysphoria and in reducing the need for analgesics and (b) chronic pain is often accompanied by significant depression which may also be treated (see Chapter 14); this may also decrease analgesic use.

When psychogenic pain becomes chronic, the relationship to an environmental stressor may become obscure, depression often occurs, and the patient becomes dependent on analgesics. At this point, referral to a professional who specializes in behavior modification may be helpful. Long term remissions of pain have been obtained by systematically eliminating reinforcers such as sympathy from family over pain and liberal use of analgesics, and by substituting productive behavior incompatible with pain (9).

PSYCHOPHYSIOLOGICAL DISORDERS

DESCRIPTION

At certain times emotional factors may trigger or accompany physiological changes in the body. The resulting symptoms which are called "psychophysiological" are usually not accompanied by significant tissue damage. In the presence of underlying disease, however, the potential for irreversible injury is present. For example, this may occur when strong emotion leads to increased heart rate or coronary vasoconstriction in the presence of underlying atherosclerotic heart disease. A listing of the most common psychophysiological disorders is found in Table 11.3.

Psychophysiological reactions are a normal component of our adaption to our environment. The physiological changes which prepare us for fight or flight when faced with a frightening situation are a good example. Psychophysiological reactions, which are not adaptive, but interfere with functioning, are classified as disorders. The reason that certain individuals react to a stressor with such bodily changes is unknown. Genetic, learning, and personality factors probably all play a part. However, it is clear that the rich connections between the cerebral centers of emotion and arousal on one hand and the autonomic nervous system and the hypothalamic-pituitary neuraxis on the other permit excitation to be transmitted virtually anywhere in the body. Moreover, stimuli which evoke excitation may be a threat to one person or a pleasure to another (for example, the thought of dangling from a cliff at the end of a tether would terrify most people, but might delight a mountain climber). Thus, a key element in the degree of emotional arousal caused by a particular stimulus is its *meaning* to the individual. This should be borne in mind whenever we attempt to assess the relationship

Table 11.3
Common Psychophysiological Conditions [a]

Physiological System	Symptomatic Condition	For Further Information see Chapter
Cardiovascular	Migraine headache	76
	Vasovagal syndrome (fainting)	78
	Tachycardia, palpitations	56
	Angina	54
Gastrointestinal	Irritable bowel	36
	The following symptoms may occur singly or together: anorexia, nausea, vomiting, abdominal cramps, diarrhea, constipation, aerophagia, acid-peptic symptoms	32, 33, 35
Genitourinary	Menstrual disturbances	74
	Difficulties in micturition: frequency (in both sexes); hesitancy (in males)	
	Sexual disorders	17
	Dyspareunia	
	Anorgasmia	
	Inhibited sexual excitement; (impotence, frigidity)	
	Delayed ejaculation; premature ejaculation	
Muscular	Pain secondary to increased muscle tension: occipital or bitemporal headaches, backaches, myalgia in various muscle groups	62, 76
	Fatigue	
	Tremor	79
Respiratory	Hyperventilation syndrome	12
	Bronchospasm	52
	Dyspnea	60
Skin	Hyperhidrosis	97
	Pruritis	97

[a] Modified from J. B. Imboden, in A. M. Harvey, R. J. Johns, A. H. Owens, and R. S. Ross (editors): *The Principles and Practice of Medicine*, Ed. 19, Appleton-Century-Crofts, New York, 1976.

between environmental events and physiological reactions.

Most of the symptomatic conditions listed in Table 11.3 may occur either as psychophysiological disorders or as disorders without a predominantly psychological basis. Diagnostic criteria for most of these conditions are found elsewhere in this book, as indicated in the table. For a patient's symptoms to be labeled as chiefly psychophysiological, there should be both an absence of organic disease and the presence of stressful life situations which bear a temporal relationship to the onset of symptoms. Psychophysiological disorders tend to occur intermittently over a long period of time without evidence of significant

progression in severity, while organic disorders are either self-limited or, if chronic, show progression. Conversion symptoms are differentiated from psychophysiological symptoms by the lack of changes (except for disuse atrophy), and by the fact that the symptom protects the patient from anxiety while in psychophysiological disorders there is often overt anxiety. Psychophysiological disorders are closely related to the dysphorias, but are distinguished from them by the absence of sustained mood change and by the chronicity of symptoms.

MANAGEMENT

Management is based upon identification of an environmental stressor. Investigating the patient's interpersonal relationships for losses, gains, or changes (e.g., an unemployed steelworker's wife gets a job) and looking for "blocked" feelings ("I don't feel like a man anymore," "I'm angry") is a good place to start. Helping the patient to recognize and ventilate his feelings is important. Symptomatic treatment is especially important in some of these disorders (e.g., peptic symptoms, tension headache, bronchospasm) as is the use of minor tranquilizers (see Chapter 12) for a period of time if the patient is experiencing considerable distress.

FACTITIOUS DISORDER WITH PHYSICAL SYMPTOMS (Munchausen Syndrome)

DESCRIPTION

This disorder is characterized by the simulation of a physical disorder in order to obtain hospitalization. Its chronic, more dramatic form, is known as the Munchausen syndrome. It differs from malingering in that for the malingerer, the hospitalization always has a *readily identified* ulterior motive attached to it (e.g., avoidance of jail, debtors, etc.).

Patients with the Munchausen syndrome may simulate almost any physical illness. The illness may be feigned through reporting invented symptoms or by deliberate production of physical signs by injecting noxious substances under the skin to cause abscesses, or by using drugs such as anticoagulants or insulin, etc. Common presenting symptoms in these patients are severe right lower abdominal pain with nausea and vomiting, dizziness and blacking out, massive hemoptysis, generalized rashes, abscesses, and unexplained protracted fever.

In taking the history the physician may note that it is presented with a dramatic flair and that on careful questioning the information given by the patient becomes vague and inconsistent. In its most exaggerated form the patient will tell fantastic stories about prior medical treatment in multiple hospitals, may attempt to impersonate famous individuals, and will have an extensive knowledge of medical history and hospital routines. Often the patient has been a health professional or has been well acquainted with one. Although this disorder is said to be rare in its extreme form, its true prevalence is unknown and it is possible that more subtle forms have yet to be recognized. The etiology is unknown but in many patients there is a strong history of parental abuse and/or deprivation.

MANAGEMENT

Treatment is centered on strategies for keeping the patient out of hospitals. When the syndrome is well recognized, consultation with a psychiatrist when the patient first presents may help in deciding on treatment. Once a patient is admitted to the hospital, treatment must focus on management of physician-staff relations and on persuading the patient to accept psychiatric hospitalization.

References

General

Cadoret, RJ and King, LJ: *Psychiatry in Primary Care.* C. V. Mosby, 1974.
  Excellent account of common problems, emphasizing epidemiology, treatment and outcome; extensively referenced.
Kaplan, HI, Freedman, AM and Sadock, BJ: *Comprehensive Textbook of Psychiatry,* Ed. 3. Williams & Wilkins, Baltimore, 1980.
  Excellent general text.
Reiser, MF (Editor): Volume 4: Organic disorders and psychosomatic medicine. In *American Handbook of Psychiatry,* edited by S. Arietie. Basic Books, New York, 1975.
  Contains excellent reviews of most psychophysiologic conditions.
Diagnostic and Statistical Manual of Mental Disorders, Ed. 3: American Psychiatric Association, 1980.
  Recently up-dated diagnostic criteria and epidemiologic information for all recognized psychiatric disorders.

Specific

1. Aldrich, CK: The severe chronic hypochondriac. *Postgrad Med* 69: 140, 1981.
2. Barskey, AJ: Patients who amplify bodily sensations. *Ann Intern Med* 91: 63, 1979.
3. Drossman, DA: The problem patient: Evaluation and care of medical patients with psychosocial disturbances. *Ann Intern Med* 88: 366, 1978.
4. Health—United States: U.S. Department of Health Education and Welfare, Publication No. (PHS) 78-1237, December 1978.
5. Johnstone, A: Psychiatric screening in general practice. *Lancet* 1: 605, 1976.
6. Lazare, A: Hysteria. In *Massachusetts General Hospital Handbook of Consultation-Liaison Psychiatry,* edited by T Hackett and N Cassem. C. V. Mosby, St. Louis, 1978.
7. Sternbach, RA: Psychophysiology of pain. In *Psychosomatic Medicine. Current Trends and Clinical Applications,* pp. 355–365, edited by ZJ Lipowski, DR Lipsett and PC Whybrow. Oxford University Press, New York, 1977.
8. Stoeckle, J, Zola, IK and Davidson, GE: The quantity and significance of psychological distress in medical patients. *J Chron Dis* 17: 959, 1964.
9. Swanson, DW, Maruta, T and Swenson, WM: Results of behavior modification in the treatment of chronic pain. *Psychosom Med* 41: 55, 1979.
10. Thomas, KB: Temporarily dependent patient in general practice. *Br Med J* 1: 625, 1974.
11. Tumulty, PA: What is a clinician and what does he do? *N Engl J Med* 28: 20, 1970.
12. White, KL, Williams, TF and Greenberg, BG: The ecology of medical care. *N Engl J Med* 265: 885, 1961.
13. Wittenborn, J and Buhler, R: Somatic complaints among depressed women. *Arch Gen Psychiatry* 36: 465, 1979.
14. Zola, IK: Pathways to the doctor—from person to patient. In *Health Illness and Medicine, A Reader in Medical Sociology,* edited by Gl Albrecht and PC Higgins. Rand McNally, Chicago, 1979.

CHAPTER TWELVE

The Anxious Patient

WALTER F. BAILE, M.D.

INTRODUCTION

Anxiety is defined by the American Psychiatric Association as apprehension, tension, or uneasiness that stems from the anticipation of danger, which may be internal or external. Anxiety is a feature common to most psychiatric disorders. That it also occurs periodically as a normal response in many patients seen by the generalist in his practice is not surprising, since the presence of disease almost always represents some threat to an individual's autonomy and present level of functioning. The severity of a patient's anxiety will depend upon one or more of the following factors: (a) situational factors such as unfamiliarity with a new physician or a scheduled visit for a potentially painful procedure; (b) individual factors such as the patient's interpretation of the gravity of his problem, his expectations of disability, and his capacity to assume a certain dependent and trusting relationship with his physician; (c) certain cultural factors which color the meaning of disease and the role of the medical care system in general; and (d) pre-existing psychopathology in the form of anxiety disorders which may be exacerbated by the stress of disease or a concurrent stress in the patient's life. In some instances, anxiety will also be the principal manifestation of organic disorders.

Although this chapter is concerned chiefly with anxiety states indicative of more chronic and severe psychopathology, the presence of moderate degrees of anxiety even in patients who seem to be otherwise functioning well has implications for treatment and care. This is because, as seen in Figure 12.1, anxiety affects performance. At low levels anxiety may actually increase alertness, attentiveness, learning, and comprehension. Beyond a certain point, however, anxiety is no longer adaptive and becomes pathological. It may interfere with a patient's ability to remember certain details relevant to his medical history, to tolerate pain, and to comprehend the physician's message. Thus, it is important for the generalist to be able to detect pathological anxiety in patients and to treat it skillfully, by reassuring the patient, by giving him an opportunity to ventilate his concerns or by providing written information, etc.

SYMPTOMS AND SIGNS OF ANXIETY

In a fairly well functioning individual mild to moderate anxiety is seen frequently as a more or less normal reaction to a threat. The somatic symptoms usually associated with this level of anxiety are increased sweating, tenseness of musculature, and restlessness.

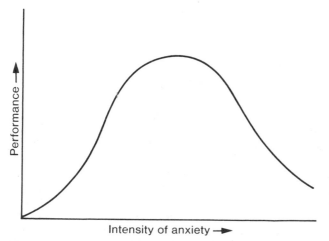

Figure 12.1 Schematic representation of the effect of anxiety on performance.

Table 12.1
Symptoms and Signs of Anxiety[a]

Symptoms	Signs
NERVOUS SYSTEM	**NERVOUS SYSTEM**
Tense, unable to relax	Strained facial expression
Difficulty concentrating, difficulty with memory, loss of interest in usual activities	Stereotypic behavior, e.g., facial tic, nail-biting, chain-smoking
Light-headedness,[b] dizziness,[b] syncope[b]	Cold, clammy handshake
"Bad mood," general irritability, unable to tolerate even mild frustration	Pacing, restlessness
Sleep disturbances: nightmares, difficulty going to sleep[b]	Irritability during physical examination
Ill defined fear of the unknown, terrifying sense of dread	Postural tremor
Fatigue, weakness[b]	Proptosis and stare
Headaches,[b] poor coordination	Dilated pupils
Trembling, numbness and tingling of fingers, toes, and face[b]	Positive Chvostek's sign[b]
Piloerection ("goosebumps")	Carpal-pedal spasm[b]
	Hyperreflexia
CARDIOVASCULAR	**CARDIOVASCULAR**
Palpitations[b]	Sinus tachycardia[b]
Substernal pressure, precordial pain unrelated to exertion[b]	Transient elevated systolic blood pressure
Flushing of face	Functional systolic ejection murmur
PULMONARY	**PULMONARY**
Difficulty breathing adequately[b]	Hyperventilation[b]
Sense of suffocation[b]	Increased frequency of sighing respiration[b]
GASTROINTESTINAL	
Epigastric distress: fullness,[b] belching,[b] heartburn, dyspepsia	
Diarrhea, constipation	
Anorexia, compulsive eating	
GENITOURINARY	
Increased frequency of micturition	
Amenorrhea, excessive menstrual cramps and flow	
Impotence, premature ejaculation	

[a] Adapted from: A. R. Favazza and J. A. Royer: Anxiety, acute and chronic. In *Family Practice*, Ed. 2, edited by R. S. Rakell and H. S. Conn. W. B. Saunders, Philadelphia, 1978.
[b] Denotes symptoms and signs which may be due to hyperventilation.

When anxiety is excessive, however, it may present in a myriad of ways. The symptoms and signs of more severe anxiety are summarized in Table 12.1.

Anxiety has both cognitive and behavioral/physiological aspects (8). On a cognitive level, anxiety is identified with threat, uncertainty, and uneasiness about some future event which is often vague and ill defined. Physiological changes due to both autonomic and somatic arousal often accompany moderate to severe anxiety. At times physiological symptoms (e.g., palpitations) will precede the subjective experience of anxiety. Moreover, such symptoms may intensify anxiety because they frighten the patient, and they may be maintained long after the cognitive distress has been reduced (see discussion of chronic hyperventilation below).

Why a particular individual should be prone to the acute and chronic somatic manifestations of anxiety is not clear. It is possible, however, that chronic hyperventilation may be an important factor in many of the more persistent symptoms such as lightheadedness, paresthesias, precordial pain, chronic breathlessness, and fatigue (10). The hyperventilation paradigm would posit that individuals with anxiety neurosis hyperventilate in response to a variety of emotional or physical stimuli (for example, palpitations) and acquire a habit of breathing which maintains an abnormally low arterial pCO_2. This chronic alkalosis places an individual at or near the threshold for hypocapneic symptoms such as paresthesias and lightheadedness. The symptoms themselves (and perhaps what the patient is told about them) then become a source of increased anxiety for the patient.

SYNDROMES ASSOCIATED WITH PATHOLOGICAL ANXIETY

The distinction between normal and pathological anxiety must of course be arbitrary, and many individuals will experience states of heightened anxiety at one time or another in their lives. When, however, these heights of anxiety are sustained (or when, if intermittent, they are severe enough to interfere with functioning), anxiety may be said to be pathological. Several more or less clearly defined syndromes associated with pathological anxiety have been identified.

Transient Anxiety as a Reaction to Stress

Chapter 11 describes patients who present to the generalist with minor mood disturbances, often manifested by the somatic symptoms of anxiety and mild depression. These are frequently patients who are being followed for long standing but stable disease processes. For the most part minor mood disturbances occur as a reaction to situational stress in patients who are coping well; the emotional disturbance is transient, and brief counseling and appropriate use of psychotropic drugs usually shortens the duration of the disorder (7). The task of the physician in these cases is to recognize and deal with the minor mood disturbance. This will prevent unnecessary procedures and keep the patient from getting enmeshed in chronic illness behavior (see Chapter 11).

Anxiety Neurosis

The main characteristic of this disorder is its chronicity. In some patients the cognitive symptoms of anxiety are dominant while in others the physical or autonomic symptoms predominate. The disorder has important implications for the generalist because afflicted patients not only make increased office visits for trivial complaints (15), but also may present to the physician with a variety of symptoms referable to transient autonomic arousal or to chronic hyperventilation. Often these symptoms become mixed with those of mild depression.

There are two principal patterns in which anxiety is experienced in anxiety neurosis: (a) "trait" anxiety, when anxiety is almost continually present; and (b) "state" anxiety in which anxiety occurs as periodic attacks.

TRAIT ANXIETY

In these patients anxiety can be considered almost part of their character. These are individuals whose everyday baseline level of anxiety is so high that seemingly small crises will often interfere with functioning and lead them to seek reassurance and support. One of the prime sources of support may be the physician. Among the various designations in the medical literature for such patients are "familiar faces," the "worried well," neurotics, or patients with "thick folders." Often they have histories of neurotic symptoms in childhood (enuresis, nail-biting, somnambulism, temper tantrums, separation anxiety when entering school). Frequently they are shy and oversensitive, feel insecure, and become overly concerned with bodily functions. Many have parents who also exhibit anxiety.

ANXIETY STATE

Anxiety "state" is manifested by discrete attacks of anxiety which may range from palpitations to immobilizing panic. Before the recognition of the primary role of anxiety in this disorder, it was known under a variety of names such as Da Costa's syndrome, effort syndrome, neurocirculatory asthenia, cardiac neurosis, and irritable heart (3, 17). Its prevalence in the general population is estimated to be from 2.0 to 4.7%. There are reports of its occurrence in epidemic form in response to an imagined environmental threat (2, 13). Patients with this and related acute anxiety syndromes frequently seek help from generalists because of the predominance of somatic symptoms. In surveys of general medical practice as many as 14% of patients with cardiovascular symptoms have been identified as having the disorder (11).

Anxiety state is primarily a disorder of young adults although it may begin in childhood. Symptoms are usually present in milder forms for some time before the patient consults his physician. Episodes of acute anxiety tend to run in families, as is shown by a high rate of concordance among monozygotic twins.

The principal manifestations of the anxiety state are periodic palpitations, breathlessness, or apprehension, which exist independently of any specific external situation. The most severe episodic attacks are designated *panic attacks*, defined as discreet periods of apprehension or fear and at least four of the following symptoms: dyspnea, palpitations, chest pain or discomfort, choking or smothering sensations, dizziness, vertigo, or unsteady feelings, paresthesias (tingling in hands and feet), hot and cold flashes, sweating, faintness, trembling or shaking, feelings of unreality, fear of dying, going crazy, or doing something uncontrolled during an attack. The patient often never feels quite well between episodes and may be left with a nagging precordial ache, extreme fatigue, or occasional breathlessness.

A large proportion of periodic anxiety attacks are manifested by *hyperventilation* (12). This syndrome is easily recognized when it is full-blown. It is frequently overlooked, however, when the patient overbreathes because of hyperpnea (deep, at times sighing, respiration), which he may not notice, instead of tachypnea, which most patients notice and report. Many of the symptoms and signs characteristic of anxiety may be due to hyperventilation, as indicated by the superscript *b* in Table 12.1. Therefore, complaints of dizziness, paresthesias, breathlessness, and other symptoms for which there are no obvious explanation should be evaluated by having the patient hyperventilate (by breathing rapidly for about 1 min) to determine whether this reproduces his symptoms. Hyperventilation can produce transient T wave inversion and S-T segment depression on the electrocardiogram. Because of this, it is sometimes necessary to exclude coronary artery disease or pulmonary embolism before ascribing a patient's presentation to anxiety-induced hyperventilation.

In addition to periodic attacks, a patient with anxiety neurosis may give a history of a specific *phobia*, defined as a persistent, irrational fear of a specific object, activity, or situation which results in a compelling desire to avoid that stimulus.

COURSE OF ANXIETY NEUROSIS

There are a number of longitudinal studies which illuminate the course of anxiety neurosis. In a 20-year follow-up of 90 patients with the diagnosis of neurocirculatory asthenia, 12% recovered, 35% had continuing symptoms but no disability, 38% had symptoms and mild disability, and 15% were symptomatic with severe disability (16). There was no excess morbidity or mortality in this group of patients. In a 5-year follow-up of 71 patients, 37% still had moderately severe symptoms but few patients were disabled (14); in this study, young age of onset, female sex, shorter duration of illness at time of diagnosis, and a balanced personality were associated with a good outcome.

DIFFERENTIAL DIAGNOSIS

It is important that anxiety neurosis be recognized and distinguished from other conditions for which the treatment and prognosis are very different. Depending upon the symptoms described by the individual patient, the differential diagnosis may include hyperthyroidism, pheochromocytoma, hypoglycemia, sympathomimetic drug side effects, coronary artery disease, pulmonary embolism, temporal lobe epilepsy, and a number of other organic diseases suggested by the symptoms listed in Table 12.1. In most cases an adequate history and physical examination will direct the physician to the appropriate condition; not infrequently, however, some tests will be required before a diagnosis of anxiety neurosis is made. Finally, although anxiety may occur periodically in most psychiatric disorders, it is important to recognize that two disorders for which the mode of treatment is important—schizophrenia and dementia—may initially present with anxiety as the most striking feature. The manifestations of these two disorders are described in Chapters 15 and 16, respectively.

Agoraphobia

Often, although not in every case, the occurrence of severe anxiety or panic attacks will predispose the patient to fear of recurrence of the attack and especially to fear of finding himself in situations where escape might not be available should the attack recur. Initially the individual might avoid tunnels, elevators, crowded areas, bridges, etc.; later he may fear to leave the house altogether. This state of markedly constricted activity is termed agoraphobia. Although the name means "fear of open spaces," this is a misnomer, since it is actually the fear of having a panic attack away from a person or place of help that characterizes the disorder. A state of chronic anxiety may thus develop which leads to incapacitation. Depression often accompanies the disorder as does alcohol or medication abuse with which the patient may indulge himself in an attempt to treat his problem. Little information is available about the proportion of patients with anxiety/panic attacks who develop agoraphobia. Its recognition, however, is extremely important since there are specific behavioral and pharmacological treatments available. When it is suspected, the patient should be referred to a psychiatrist for appropriate management.

Post-Traumatic Stress Disorder

When an individual undergoes a psychologically traumatic event which is outside the range of everyday stressful human experiences (such as divorce, bereavement, etc.), disturbances of mood, autonomic hyperactivity, and impaired cognition may be associated with the re-experiencing of the traumatic event. The trauma may have caused physical harm to the individual (e.g., an assault) or it may not have caused harm but still have been recognized as physically threatening (e.g., an automobile crash). Symptoms may have their onset immediately after the event or they may be delayed for as long as a year. In general the shorter the time between the onset of symptoms and the traumatic event, the better the prognosis.

The main characteristic of the disorder is a recapitulation by the individual of the traumatic event. This may occur in nightmares, intrusive thoughts, or dissociative states in which the person behaves as if he is in the midst of the trauma. Associated with the experience of the stressor there is usually emotional blunting, apathy, autonomic hyperarousal, and difficulty in sleeping. Symptoms may last for periods of 6 months or more. In general, the longer the duration of the disorder, the worse the prognosis. Symptoms may be exacerbated by situations which resemble the circumstances of the original trauma. Associated symptoms of irritability, explosions of aggressive behavior, impulsiveness, inability to concentrate, and, of course, anxiety and depression may occur.

When severe, the disorder may impair functioning considerably. The individual may avoid circumstances which evoke memories of the event. The ability to experience warmth in interpersonal relationships may be impaired. Suicidal behavior and substance abuse are serious complications. Because of these problems, patients with severe post-traumatic stress disorder should be referred to a psychiatrist for expert help.

TREATMENT OF ANXIETY

The treatment of anxiety requires a combination of pharmacological and other approaches. When marked anxiety persists despite the measures described here, referral to a psychiatrist is appropriate.

Counseling

A number of the *counseling techniques* described in Chapter 10 may be helpful in the management of anxiety neurosis, particularly empathic listening and contingency planning. When a patient's anxiety is clearly related to a situational stress, the therapeutic style of interviewing recommended in the discussion of minor mood disturbances (Chapter 11) may greatly alleviate the patient's problems.

Those patients whose symptoms are largely due to *hyperventilation* should be educated about how this symptom is produced, and how breathing can be controlled at the onset of symptoms. If a patient has difficulty learning this, referral to a physical therapist for training in breathing control may help (10). The patient should also be instructed to rebreathe from a bag, which will alleviate symptoms for most patients. The presence of a spouse or friend to hear this information may be very helpful in assisting the patient in handling future attacks.

Pharmacological Treatment

For patients significantly impaired by the symptoms of anxiety, anxiolytic drugs, particularly the benzodiazepines, may be very helpful. A number of other drugs (β-adrenergic blockers, antihistamines, and antidepressants) may be useful in selected patients.

BENZODIAZEPINES

Epidemiology. Although these drugs have a legitimate role in the management of anxiety (6, 18), they are often used indiscriminately. In fact they are the most widely prescribed drugs in the United States. In some communities, up to 20% of the general adult population uses these or related drugs each year; and they are used daily for at least 1 week per year by approximately 10% of adults (18). Physicians may best limit the inappropriate use of these drugs in our society by asking themselves, whenever they consider writing a first prescription for a benzodiazepine, whether the drug is essential to the patient's functioning.

Characteristics. In placebo-controlled trials, benzodiazepines have consistently been found to be effective for the relief of anxiety. Their mechanism of action is still a subject of controversy, but there are indications that they act on multiple sites in the brain including the reticular activating system. The benzodiazepines are less sedating at equivalent doses than barbiturates, are rarely associated with fatalities due to overdose, and have relatively low abuse potential compared with other sedative and hypnotic drugs. Furthermore, physiological dependence is rare, although in patients who have been maintained on high doses for long periods of time, a withdrawal syndrome characterized by insomnia, anorexia, dysphoria, weakness, and (rarely) seizures (4) may occur several days after discontinuation of the drug. Psychological dependence, on the other hand, is a common problem which may be difficult to eliminate in the individual patient. The management of drug dependence is discussed in Chapter 21.

The principal *side effect* of these drugs is drowsiness; ataxia may also occur in a significant proportion of patients, particularly after the first dose. Thus, patients who drive or who operate machinery should be warned of decreased alertness and of possible lack of balance. Drowsiness usually occurs when treatment is first started and when dosage is increased. Older patients and those with liver disease may clear these compounds less efficiently so that a lower dose is required for equivalent anxiolytic action. The small proportion of patients who have suicidal thoughts may experience an increase in this ideation owing to the disinhibiting properties of a benzodiazepine drug. Some individuals who easily become angry may experience increased hostility or even a rage reaction. The evidence concerning the teratogenicity of benzodiazepines is still unclear, but until it is clarified they should not be prescribed for patients in their first trimester of pregnancy.

The benzodiazepines can be divided into different groups (Table 12.2). A therapeutic plasma level is reached in less than an hour after ingestion of all of these drugs. Most produce active metabolites and/or have long half-lives so that they may be administered once a day. Oxazepam and lorazepam have short half-lives and no active metabolites, and must be administered several times a day. Most of the benzodiazepines are excreted by the liver, although oxazepam and lorazepam are conjugated by the liver and then eliminated by the kidneys. Thus individuals with hepatic dysfunction may require smaller doses of the longer acting benzodiazepines. Clorazepate is hydrolyzed to its active metabolite in the stomach; patients with low gastric acidity or taking antacid medication may absorb only minimal amounts of the active metabolite and should not be given this particular drug.

Drug interactions are few. Nevertheless the effects of benzodiazepines are potentiated by other anxiolytics, sedative-hypnotics, and alcohol. For example, most successful benzodiazepine-related suicides occur in persons who are taking one of these central nervous system depressants, especially alcohol, at the same time.

Practical Use of Benzodiazepines. Table 12.2 contains practical information about the available oral preparations of the benzodiazepines commonly prescribed for anxiety. In general, any of these agents can be used, beginning with the minimum daily dose. The principal differences are the shorter duration of action of lorazepam and oxazepam and the low cost of the generic form of chlordiazepoxide.

Benzodiazepines are indicated for the short-term treatment of most patients with generalized anxiety, either acute or chronic. They are also quite useful in treating patients with minor mood disturbances (see Chapter 11) as an adjunct to counseling. They are effective in the treatment of anticipatory anxiety associated with panic attacks (although the attacks themselves are more likely to respond to tricyclic antidepressants) and they may serve as useful adjuncts in the treatment of agoraphobia, although behavioral strategies and tricyclic antidepressants seem to be treatment of choice.

Before prescribing anxiolytic agents, the physician should formulate the patient's problem as clearly as possible. First, he should ask himself several questions: Is this a patient who generally functions well, but is experiencing stress in his environment? Is this patient suffering from chronic anxiety? If so, is there some additional stress which has exacerbated his anxiety? Is the anxiety typical of one of the subsets of anxiety neurosis (panic attacks, agoraphobia)? Second, the physician should attempt to gauge whether the distress is interfering with the patient's

Table 12.2
Usual Dose and Pharmacokinetics of Anxiolytic Benzodiazepines [a]

Drug (Trade Name)	Available Strengths (in mg)	Oral Daily Dose Range, Divided b.i.d. or t.i.d.	Active Metabolites Present	Elimination Half-life (hr)
Chlordiazepoxide (Librium, generic) (Libritabs)	5, 10, 25 (capsules) 5, 10, 25 (tablets)	15–150	Yes	5–30
Clorazepate dipotassium (Tranxene) (Tranxene SD)	3.75, 7.5, 15 (capsules) 22.5 (tablets)	15–60 22.5 (single dose is intended for patients stabilized on 7.5 mg t.i.d.)	Yes Yes	36–200 36–200
(Tranxene SD half-strength)	11.25 (tablets)	11.25 (single dose for patients stabilized on 3.75 mg t.i.d.)	Yes	36–200
Clorazepate monopotassium (Azene)	3.25, 6.5, 13 (capsules)	13–52	Yes	36–200
Diazepam (Valium)	2, 5, 10 (tablets)	4–40	Yes	20–50
Lorazepam (Ativan)	0.5, 1, 2 (tablets)	2–6	No	10–20
Oxazepam (Serax)	10, 15, 30 (capsules) 15 (tablets)	30–120 30–120	No No	5–10 5–10
Prazepam (Verstran)	10 (tablets)	20–60	Yes	36–200

[a] Modified from: S. Zisook and R. DeVaul: Prescribing anxiolytics, *Drug Therapy*, pp. 41–49, November 1979.

functioning (e.g., making him incapable of accomplishing everyday tasks at home or on the job)? Is there significant sleep disturbance?

If the physician at this point decides to prescribe an anxiolytic agent, he should make it clear to the patient that short term treatment is desirable. The following points should be emphasized: (a) significant anxiety is usually periodic; (b) the use of tranquilizers will often allow the patient to mobilize his own resources to cope with precipitating events; (c) the anxiolytic drug should not be taken round the clock on a daily basis, but only as needed in the frequency prescribed; and (d) that most patients do not require more than 2 months of administration. Furthermore, advice, support, and reassurance from the physician will shorten the time that the medication will be required.

In patients with chronic anxiety, where long term use of an anxiolytic drug is a possibility, it is helpful to remember the following:

1. There is often a recent event which has exacerbated the anxiety; for this situation, short term counseling may be the most effective way to reduce anxiety.

2. The patient should be encouraged to use medication only when needed and to have as many periods as possible without drugs.

3. Regular visits (or telephone contacts) to the physician for continued re-evaluation and support are essential.

BARBITURATES

These substances are rarely used for treatment of anxiety today. In addition to the fact that doses that relieve anxiety also produce sedation, these drugs have more side effects, more potential for abuse, and are more lethal when taken in an overdose than the benzodiazepines.

β-ADRENERGIC BLOCKERS

Propranolol and other β-blockers are effective in reducing the marked autonomic symptoms (palpitations, tachycardia, tremor and twitching, cold sweats, and chest constriction) which occur in some anxious individuals (9). Beta-blockers may be particularly helpful prophylactically in individuals with marked autonomic response to particular stresses such as speaking in public. Since these drugs may not eliminate the subjective distress of an anxious person, the patient should be asked whether he feels significantly better after he takes them.

The appropriate dosage of a β-blocking agent can be selected according to the same guidelines and precautions which are given in Chapter 59.

ANTIHISTAMINES

Antihistamines may be prescribed to control anxiety as an alternative to benzodiazepines. They are safer for patients with chronic obstructive pulmonary disease, in whom benzodiazepines may suppress respiration, but their major disadvantage is that they sedate the patient significantly. Hydroxyzine (Atarax, Vistaril), is most frequently prescribed, in doses ranging from 10 to 25 mg three times daily. Antihistamines may also be found in a number of over-the-counter compounds sold for the treatment of anxiety.

ANTIDEPRESSANTS

Tricyclic antidepressants and monamine oxidase (MAO) inhibitors are often effective in the treatment of panic attacks or agoraphobia. These classes of drugs, however, are not effective in the treatment of generalized or anticipatory anxiety. The doses and schedules are similar to those described in Chapter 14.

Relaxation Techniques

As an adjunct to counseling and anxiolytic drugs, techniques for inducing deep states of muscle relaxation may be very helpful in the management of anxiety. Some of these such as zen, yoga, transcendental meditation, and hypnosis have been practiced for centuries. Others such as the relaxation response are new or are variants on the older techniques. As Benson points out in explaining the relaxation response (1), many techniques can decrease sympathetic and somatic activity, resulting in a decrease in heart rate, respiratory rate, and muscle tension. Elements common to these techniques include:

1. Mental Device. There should be a constant stimulus—e.g., sound, word, or phrase repeated silently or audibly, or fixed gazing at an object. The purpose of these procedures is to shift attention from logical, externally oriented thoughts.

2. Passive Attitude. If distracting thoughts do occur during the repetition or gazing, they should be disregarded and attention should be redirected to the technique. The patient should not worry about the quality of his performance.

3. Decreased Muscle Tonus. The subject should be in a comfortable position so that minimal muscular work is required.

4. Quiet Environment. A quiet environment with decreased environmental stimuli should be chosen. Most techniques instruct the subject to close his eyes. A place of worship is often suitable, as is a quiet room.

The general physician may wish to learn some of the simpler techniques and teach them to his patients. He may also purchase or make his own tapes to assist patients with relaxation exercises. A recently published book describes in detail the various techniques and the teaching tapes available for physician and patient alike (5).

PREVENTING ANXIETY

It should be remembered that everyone fears illness and that some anxiety is present in most patients, particularly when they first seek help from a physician. Furthermore, most individuals have their own notions about the cause of their symptoms and its consequences. Frequently, these "belief systems" will have little to do with reality, but they will invariably affect the way the patient perceives procedures and prescriptions administered by the physician. The physician who takes the time to elicit the patient's understanding of his own illness, to correct misconceptions, and to explain the treatment and prognosis can do much to spare the patient needless anxiety.

References

General

Cadoret, RJ and King, LJ: *Psychiatry in Primary Care.* C. V. Mosby, St. Louis, 1974.
    Excellent account of common problems, emphasizing epidemiology, treatment and outcome; extensively referenced.
Diagnostic and Statistical Manual of Mental Disorders, Ed 3: American Psychiatric Association, 1980.
    Recently up-dated diagnostic criteria and epidemiologic information for all recognized psychiatric disorders.

Specific

1. Benson, H, Beary, JF and Carol, MP: The relaxation response. *Psychiatry 37:* 37, 1974.
2. Colligan, MJ, Urtes, M, Wisseman, C, Rosensteel, RE, Anania, TL and Hornung, RW: An investigation of apparent mass psychogenic illness in an electronic plant. *J Behav Med 2:* 297, 1979.
3. Craig, H and White, PD: Etiology and symptoms of neurocirculatory asthenia. *Arch Intern Med 53:* 633, 1934.
4. De la Fuente, JR, Rosenbaum, AH, Martin, HR and Niven, RG: Lorazepam-related withdrawal seizures. *Mayo Clinic Proc 55:* 190, 1980.
5. Gaarder, KR and Montgomery, PS: *Clinical Biofeedback: A Procedural Manual for Behavioral Medicine,* Ed. 2. Williams & Wilkins, Baltimore, 1981.
6. Hollister, L: Benzodiazepines 1980: Current update: A look at the issues. *Psychosomatics 21:* 4, 1980.
7. Johnstone, A and Goldberg, D: Psychiatric screening in general practice. *Lancet 1:* 605, 1976.
8. Lader, M and Marks, I: *Clinical Anxiety.* Grune & Stratton, New York, 1971.
9. Lead Article: Beta-adrenergic blockade and anxiety. *Lancet 2:* 611, 1976.
10. Lum, LC: The syndrome of habitual chronic hyperventilation. In *Modern Trends in Psychosomatic Medicine,* edited by O Hill. Butterworths, Woburn, Mass., 1976.
11. Marks, I and Lader, M: Anxiety states (anxiety neurosis): A review. *J Nerv Ment Dis 156:* 3, 1973.
12. Missri, JC and Alexander, S: Hyperventilation syndrome: A brief review. *JAMA 240:* 2093, 1978.
13. Murphy, LR and Colligan, MJ: Mass psychogenic illness in a shoe factory. *Int Arch Environ Health 44:* 133, 1979.
14. Noyes, R and Clancy, J: Anxiety neurosis: A 5 year follow-up. *J Nerv Ment Dis 162:* 200, 1976.
15. Salkind, MR: Anxiety neurosis in general practice. *Postgrad Med J,* pp. 34, 1972.
16. Wheeler, EO, White, PD, Reed, EW and Cohen, ME: Neurocirculatory asthenia: A 20-year follow-up of 173 patients. *JAMA 142:* 878, 1950.
17. Wood, P: Da Costa's syndrome (or effort syndrome). *Br Med J 1:* 767, 1941.
18. Zisook, S and DeVaul, R: Prescribing anxiolytics. *Drug Therapy,* pp. 41, November 1979.

CHAPTER THIRTEEN

Maladaptive Personalities

WALTER F. BAILE, M.D.

INTRODUCTION

Because of the uniqueness of each individual and the dynamic interaction of the person with his environment, any attempt to classify personality in a systematic way may seem too ambitious. However, as the physician gets to know a patient he will usually detect certain "themes"; these themes comprise relatively consistent attitudes and patterns of behavior, and as such they make up the patient's personality. This chapter describes a number of personality styles which are associated with inflexible or maladaptive behavior. The ability to recognize patients with these personality styles is important, for effective management of medical problems in these patients often requires strategies adapted to their personality.

OBSESSIVE-COMPULSIVE PATIENT

Definition and Recognition

Obsessive-compulsive individuals lead lives characterized by extreme orderliness, adherence to convention, perfectionism, and conscientiousness. On the job they dress very neatly, are always on time, and have a meticulously clean and orderly desk. An over-restrictive conscience provides a strong sense of duty, so that they are blindly loyal and hardworking; they are extremely responsive to the praise of superiors, which inspires in them renewed energy and enthusiasm to tackle new assignments. On the other hand, colleagues or fellow workers will see an obsessive-compulsive person as stiff, formal, inhibited, and dogmatic; they may admire his ability for logical thinking and working with details, but they will be annoyed and frustrated by his rules and regulations. Above average intelligence and a liking for working with factual information will often bring success to the obsessive-compulsive individual in jobs such as accounting; but his dogmatic approach to problem-solving and the tendency to be uncomfortable in situations which are unstructured prevents ascendency to positions of greater responsibility. At home there may be a rigid insistence on following a fixed routine; at times this may provoke anger in the rest of the family who become tired of always going to the same places to eat, for vacations, etc. Excessive frugality may also be a source of friction, and the children may use terms such as "tightwad." A spouse may complain that there is a lack of feeling, an inflexible and uncomprising approach to decisions, and a paucity of imagination. Typically, the obsessive-compulsive will have disdain for others, for no one can do a job as thoroughly as he can.

For the general physician the obsessive-compulsive personality is important for several reasons. First, this personality type has often been found to be associated with classical psychosomatic disorders such as peptic ulcer and ulcerative colitis. Second, because of their conscientiousness, their high standards for performance, and their need to be in control, these individuals may encounter situations at home or at work where their performance needs are frustrated, and they may develop partially decompensated states manifested as somatic symptoms (see Chapter 11). Third, they cooperate well with the management of whatever medical problem they may have if their personality needs are met.

ORIGINS

It is hypothesized that such a rigid overly controlled personality structure results from premature parental insistence on obedience in the child; that is, before the child's intellectual and motor development is up to the task. Thus, as a child the patient may have been expected to be neat at the table, to have been toilet-trained early, and to have controlled his emotions. In submitting to these parental pressures the child must repress strong aggressive and defiant drives which are characteristic of all children. The price paid is an overly strict conscience wherein the traits of obedience and conformity on the one hand, and obstinacy and stubbornness on the other, coexist and mirror the original parental struggle.

Management Strategies

If their personality style is recognized, these individuals can be managed quite easily when medical care is required. Identification with the orderliness and methodical approach of the physician is a source of comfort. Since reliance on factual information and logic are cornerstones of the obsessive-compulsive individual's approach to reality, informing him in detail about his illness and about the rationale for required tests and treatment, etc will be helpful. Such patients also respond to being included in the decision-making process. Because of the need to "do something" to get approval, the patient will often feel better about participating in any treatment plan such as home blood pressure monitoring. However, this must be balanced against his tendency to become overly attentive to detail. He will also respond well to reinforcement and praise.

OVERLY EMOTIONAL HISTRIONIC PATIENT

Definition and Recognition

This personality type is seen mostly in women. Typically, the physician is struck by the patient's excessive preoccupation with her physical attractiveness even when she is in the hospital. This is an attempt to draw attention to herself. Although superficially charming and appealing there will be a lack of emotional balance; thus, behavior is over-reactive and often coquettish. Initial warmth and intensity of emotional expression may mask a tendency toward premature intimacy in relationships, and although at first this may appear charming, the expectation for others to respond in the same eager, warm, and personal way transforms the charm into demanding, egocentric, and inconsiderate actions. Men with this disorder may feel the need to show their manliness, courage, and attractiveness to female doctors and nurses.

These patients are often attractive and seductive. In relationships with the opposite sex there is often an attempt to control or to enter into a dependent relationship. Thus their histrionic behavior may be seen as a way to take care of unmet dependency needs or to counter feelings of helplessness, inadequacy, and anxiety prompted by an interpersonal relationship. Such feelings may also lead to an overly trusting attitude and an initially positive response to the authority of someone whom they believe will provide a magical answer to their problems. Often when these individuals are disappointed, there will be dramatic acting out (including suicide gestures or threats). It is common for patients with this disorder to complain of poor health, such as weakness or headaches. These personality characteristics may be seen in some patients who exhibit conversion disorders and very frequently in patients with somatization disorder (see Chapter 11).

ORIGINS

The principal traits of this personality type are said to be derived from the period of development when the child is between the ages of 3 and 6. During this period, the foundation for sexual identity is laid down when an initially strong attachment to the parent of the opposite sex is relinquished and patterns of identification with the parent of the same sex are strengthened. The superficial warmth, charm, exaggerated emotionality, and sexual provocativeness are hypothesized to be derived from impulses stemming from the early affection for the parent of the opposite sex.

Management Strategies

In dealing with this type of patient, the physician should begin by attempting to answer two important questions: Is this personality part of another entity such as a somatization disorder? Do the physical complaints reflect organic disease?

As mentioned above, these patients may be very seductive and may make the physician uncomfortable. Their overly warm and friendly approach on the other hand may make the physician feel charmed and challenged. However, it is important to remember that underneath this behavior are strong feelings of dependency and desire to control. The physician should therefore avoid getting trapped into an overly familiar relationship with the patient (e.g., by avoiding the use of first names, by assuring a professional posture during office visits, and by having a nurse present when he examines the patient). When these patients do become seriously ill, they may feel that they are unattractive and unsuccessful. During these periods they may become particularly depressed and overemotional or make extra demands on the physi-

cian. When the patient is vulnerable and feeling more helpless, reassurance and explanations about the illness will help the patient distinguish realities from fantasies. At these times it may also be important for the physician to be more supportive, since dependency needs aroused by the illness make the patient more vulnerable to anxiety and depression.

OVERLY SUSPICIOUS QUERULOUS (PARANOID) PATIENT

Definition and Recognition

The characteristic features of this personality type are suspiciousness, hypersensitivity to criticism, and restriction of emotional expansiveness. Thus these individuals tend to be suspicious not only of other people and their motives, but also may show a general cynicism about institutions, about the motives of organizations such as charitable groups whom they may accuse of "ripping off the public," and about legitimate competitions which they will claim are "fixed." Their overall posture toward life is defensive. Such persons question the loyalty of others, exaggerate the need to be self-sufficient, and may be seen by others as guarded and secretive. They may harbor considerable hostility which together with their querulousness leads them to be argumentative, litigious, and to overplay small difficulties with others. Sometimes hypervigilance associated with their defensive attitude toward life will be expressed in tenseness of expression and inability to relax. The individual with a paranoid personality has great difficulty in admitting the possibility that he has made a mistake; thus he will be overly sensitive to criticism and quick to defend himself. Often he will attribute his own failures to the faults of others (projection). At times this need to defend himself from any hint of failure will result in a certain unrealistic self-importance and a disdain for people who are considered as weak, soft, sickly, or defective. Thus, there will be a denial of any passive, soft, or tender feelings in himself; and he will often be seen by others as cold, unemotional, and humorless.

ORIGINS

It is hypothesized that individuals with this personality type have been subjected to excessive parental anger. The features of the personality may be conceptualized as the persistence of childhood defenses against parental anger and rage. The hypervigilance, suspiciousness, and feelings of being taken advantage of are a result of feeling that others will treat him the same way as his parents treated him.

Management Strategies

Two problems confront the physician who manages such patients when they become ill. The first is the meaning of the illness. Because the patient denies being vulnerable and disdains this trait in others, physical disease in himself may arouse strong threats. This can be seen very clearly in illnesses such as myocardial infarction. In this situation, the physician may see "counterphobic" behavior in which the patient struggles to protect himself against the threat of perceived weakness by prematurely engaging in physical activity or avoiding the disclosure of symptoms to the physician. The second difficulty lies in forming a therapeutic alliance. Because of his over-suspiciousness the patient may struggle to stay in charge of his treatment, questioning the physician's diagnosis, reasoning, and the appropriateness of the treatment plan. This may arouse strong competitive urges in the physician, leading to anger toward the patient or refusal to treat the patient. These responses only serve to confirm the patient's view of the world as hostile.

The best approach to management is to provide routinely the fullest possible explanation of the illness and any related procedures. Allowing the patient to share in the treatment plan by exercising options wherever possible will also be helpful. This will help to develop some sense of mastery over a situation in which he feels weak and vulnerable. When symptoms are withheld, or behavior is inappropriate, the physician may sometimes have to confront the patient and to define reality, which may allow the patient to identify with the strength and authority of the physician at a time when he is feeling out of control. A pleading, solicitous approach by the physician, however, will only be seen by the patient as a sign of weakness. A trusting relationship will be developed only with time and patience.

PASSIVE-DEPENDENT PATIENT

Definition and Recognition

Individuals of this type are often unable to make their own decisions, deferring almost all choices to spouses or relatives; they assume passive roles and are convinced that they have very few assets or characteristics which others find admirable. For example, this sense of unworthiness may often result in a man's continually taking jobs which are below his true potential or a woman's willingness to tolerate a husband's abuse rather than leave him. In some cases the individual will attempt to compensate for low self-esteem by investing most of his or her energy in caring for others. As a consequence, the individual with a dependent personality who has invested a strong interest in another person or activity may become anxious or depressed if the situation alters, i.e., if the person leaves or the job changes. In these instances the patient may develop the psychological or somatic symptoms of minor or major mood disturbances (see Chapters 11 and 14) and present symptomatically to the generalist.

In addition these patients may develop various degrees of dependency on the physician. Generally their relationship with him will be "idealized." That is, the physician, in showing warmth, concern, and interest, may elicit emotions related to similar feelings the patient desired in the parent. It is not uncommon in these instances to see affectionate feelings develop in these patients toward physicians of the opposite sex. Sometimes these become overtly sexual, but for most patients they remain on an idealized, platonic level.

On some occasions the physician will meet persons whose anxiety about coping with even the most minimal demands make them into desperate, clinging, dependent individuals. Such persons are overwhelmed with social problems which exacerbate dependency and increase anxiety. These patients may become overdependent on their doctors, behaving like young children who turn to their parents when they are frightened or overwhelmed. They may learn that somatic complaints get attention and medicine and that being sick allows them to avoid feeling that they are not coping (illness behavior, see Chapter 11). These patients may badger their physician with phone calls at the most inopportune times with their worries about nausea or arthritis which is "acting up again."

ORIGINS

An individual's self-esteem is a reflection of his ability to feel competent in roles defined by society and to "feel good" about himself. In general this is a function of the warmth and degree of support a person received from his environment, especially parental figures, as he tackled the developmental tasks which lay on the road to adulthood. A parent overly critical of a child's accomplishments in school and in other spheres because they did not meet his high standards will have seriously undermined the child's morale. This and similar childhood experiences may produce an adult with a predominantly dependent personality style.

Management Strategies

The patient with a very dependent personality who is unable to make his own decisions but whose dependency needs are being met in a reasonable way is unlikely to change; here, in decisions regarding treatment the physician will usually have to include the person responsible for care. This will be especially important in a situation where there is serious illness, in which case the patient may experience further threats to security.

For the dependent patient who still has some capacity for interpersonal growth and is able to develop warm relationships, insight-oriented psychotherapy may be helpful. When the patient's positive feelings toward the physician become an issue in such work, the physician may interpret them by telling the patient that it is not unusual for people to feel warm toward those who take an interest.

The exceedingly clinging individual needs a different management strategy. These persons use their symptoms to get intermittent reinforcement, the most potent kind of reward in operant conditioning. At times they seem to be holding all the cards, since there always lurks the possibility that a new complaint may represent a real change in physical status. The physician is most likely to succeed with these patients when he understands the nature of the process. The patient will not give up his behavior or symptoms until he is sure he does not need them to get attention. Thus an approach such as the one described in the section on hypochondriasis in Chapter 11 will be helpful. Unfortunately, since these individuals do get sick, the physician must stay attentive for new signs and complaints.

PASSIVE-AGGRESSIVE PATIENT AND SELF-SACRIFICING PATIENT

Definition and Recognition

Two other styles of functioning may be seen in patients who, like the passive dependent patient, have difficulty with the responsibilities of adulthood.

The first of these is the *passive-aggressive personality*, in which the maturational block is associated with resistance to demands for adequate performance in both social and occupational spheres. Typically, individuals with this style will demonstrate passive-resistant behavior when required to increase their performance level. Thus they may continually "forget" important tasks such as doctors' appointments, medication administration, etc. They may procrastinate in decision-making until an opportunity has been allowed to slip by, or they may sabotage arrangements made by others to provide them with an opportunity for advancement. Although such a patient rarely expresses anger directly, the physician eventually recognizes that the patient, through forgetfulness, dawdling, stubbornness, and deliberate inefficiency, is actually saying "see if you can get me to do anything—I'm staying right where I am." It is important to recognize that the tendency toward passive-resistant behavior can be pervasive and persistent, in which case it is the hallmark of the passive-aggressive personality, or it can be an isolated regressive phenomenon in an individual who is attempting to cope with an overwhelming stress. Thus it may be seen not infrequently in adolescents who have major illnesses which increase dependency; yet the adolescent will not wish to express his needs, because he is at a stage when increased independence is an important issue.

A similar desire to be taken care of can be seen in the *long-suffering, self-sacrificing* patient. These persons seem always to be subject to some misfortune and disappointment. If examined more carefully, this can usually be shown to be due to an error in judgment made by the patient himself. Furthermore these patients often wear their misfortune as a "badge of courage" and sigh that no matter how much they try, things never seem to work out. Some hint of the problems of these patients may be seen when anger is expressed in statements such as "when things go wrong no one ever seems to be around to help me." Their tendency often to disregard their own comfort and be of service to other people exacerbates the situation.

Management Strategies

It is helpful for the physician to think of both passive-resistant and self-sacrificing behavior as indirect ways of demanding to be taken care of. The physician should avoid getting into a "parent-child" struggle with the patient. For the resistant patient the physician may gently explain the resistant behavior, acknowledge that it is difficult to weather illness alone, and thus acknowledge the patient's dependency needs. With the adolescent patient the approach can be the same; but since the behavior is a reaction to a catastrophic event, the patient can be encouraged to acknowledge his feelings about being ill which can then be explained by the physician.

The self-sacrificing patient may increase his "martyred" behavior when struck by illness. Helpful suggestions and comfort with this patient are usually met with increased complaints, dismissal of evidence of recovery, and accentuation of negative feelings. It is as if the patient is telling those around him that they have to love him because he suffers so much. This often leads to feelings of irritation and anger on the part of the doctor. With such patients the physician may try to explain that improvement in symptoms is an additional benefit for others—emphasizing the patient's important role in assisting others, so that becoming well becomes a route back to his habitual style of coping.

PATIENT WITH EXAGGERATED SELF-IMPORTANCE

Definition and Recognition

Individuals with this personality problem are self-centered, vain, and in need of constant attention and admiration. Their behavior is thus focused on doing the "right things" or being with the "right people" in order to create an "image." An excessive focus on themselves creates a lack of awareness of the feelings of others and in fact often leads to an exploitation of others in order to satisfy needs of self-aggrandizement. As a result relations with others tend to be superficial. Fantasy life also reflects a grandiose sense of self-importance or uniqueness. Thus an overestimation of abilities may lead to fantasies of achieving more power, wealth, brilliance, beauty, or ideal love.

Behind the exaggerated sense of self-importance and the attempt to maintain such an image is a very fragile ego. Thus there is continuous preoccupation with performance, acceptance, and admiration by others. This is revealed best by rage or humiliation in response to even constructive criticism. Normal setbacks are experienced as failures, criticism is poorly tolerated, and unrealistic expectations, exploitativeness, and a sense of entitlement often lead to disappointment. Thus periods of depressed mood and feelings of isolation often result; during severe stress transient psychotic symptoms (e.g., hallucinations or delusion) may be seen.

This personality type is important to the general physician for several reasons. First, because of the inappropriate preoccupation with self, individuals with these characteristics are prone to worry excessively over minor physical symptoms and at times may be refractory to reassurance to the point of hypochondriasis. Second, there may be unrealistic expectations of special consideration from the physician, which often lead to disappointment when these are not met. This is complicated by the fact that the patient's own grandiosity leads him to choose a physician whom he considers to be an eminent expert.

ORIGINS

It is hypothesized that this personality style may reflect an attempt to compensate for loss of self-esteem which occurred early in childhood; for example, the loss of self-esteem in a child who experiences abrupt loss in parental attention because of the birth of a sibling or because of remarriage of a single parent.

Management Strategies

The physician's approach to the patient should be realistic. He must avoid getting into a competitive situation if his competence is challenged, which is especially likely to occur if immediate results are not forthcoming. If the physician is able to acknowledge his own limitations to the patient, the situation may be defused. Furthermore, the physician should try to establish the idea that an illness often does not interfere with achieving goals in life and with being appreciated by others. If the illness is short-lived, reassuring the patient that he will soon return to his usual functional status will be helpful in the overall management.

BORDERLINE PERSONALITY

Definition and Recognition

This personality type has recently received considerable attention in the psychiatric literature as its characteristics have become more clearly defined. It is called "borderline" because it refers to patients whose behavior and sense of reality approach that seen in patients with schizophrenic disorders (see Chapter 15). At one time this disorder was known as "pseudoneurotic schizophrenia" because of the pres-

ence of neurotic phenomena such as phobias and anxiety in these marginally functioning patients. This disorder is more common in women than in men and it may be found in as many as 1 to 2% of the population.

Because his personality organization is impulsive and infantile, the borderline patient will always demonstrate some psychological impairment. When not in the midst of a crisis he may complain of intense emptiness and moods of anger and depression. During a crisis this anger often intensifies and the patient may become argumentative, demanding, and self-destructive. At times conversion symptoms and hypochondriacal complaints may be present (see Chapter 11). In addition, there may be transient psychotic episodes (e.g., paranoid ideation) when the patient becomes frustrated in an interpersonal relationship. Although anger is often a salient feature in these patients, clinging dependency is also prominent. When they feel dependent, a psychological phenomenon called "splitting" may occur, in which people in their environment are categorized either as good persons, who are seen as protective and nurturing, or as bad persons, who are seen as cruel and unsupportive. The borderline patient often turns to alcohol or drug use to control chronic tension and anxiety.

Because these patients may present with neurotic symptoms such as conversion or anxiety, their primary problem may not be recognized unless their overall history is reviewed. A history which includes suicide gestures, pervasive anxiety, mood swings, identity disturbance, and inappropriate anger should suggest borderline personality and should prompt a psychiatric referral.

ORIGINS

It is hypothesized that the borderline personality results from difficulties in the separation phase of human development (which occurs at 16 to 25 months of age) which leave the individual vulnerable to emotional crisis when separation is experienced as an adult.

Management Strategies

In managing the medical problems of a patient with borderline personality, it is important for the physician to realize that he is dealing with an individual who suffers greatly because of his chronic feelings of emptiness, of his fear of being alone, and of the chaos in his interpersonal relationships. Thus, he deserves empathy and understanding. Since this may be difficult when the patient is being demanding, hostile, or manipulative, such a patient is best managed in conjunction with a psychiatrist.

When these patients become seriously ill, their dependency may increase, and the crisis of disease may be enough to trigger transient breaks with reality. At such times, it is particularly important for the general physician to enlist the help of the patient's psychiatrist, especially if the patient requires hospitalization. This is because these patients can present serious management problems in the hospital, characterized by "splitting" the staff into all-good and all-bad, by exhibiting demanding, infantile, and at times hostile behavior, and by threatening self-destructive acts. Ideally the psychiatrist should not wait for a crisis to develop but should see the patient as soon as possible after admission. In this way, he can work with the staff to explain the dynamics and behavior of the borderline personality. Strategies can thus be developed to deal with staff-splitting, acting out, and other disruptive behavior. The occurrence of behavior suggestive of a partial break with reality may necessitate the use of a neuroleptic drug (see chapter 15).

General References

Bowden, CL and Burstein, AG: *Psychosocial basis of Medical Practice.* Williams & Wilkins Co., Baltimore, 1974.

An introduction to human behavior in the clinical setting, with excellent accounts of a number of difficult personality types.
Diagnostic and Statistical Manual of Mental Disorders, Ed. 3. American Psychiatric Association, 1980.
Recently up-dated diagnostic criteria and epidemiologic information for all recognized psychiatric disorders.
Kahana, RG and Bibring, G: Personality types in medical management. In *Psychiatry and Medical Practice in a General Hospital,* pp. 108–123, edited by NE Zinberg. International Universities Press, New York, 1964.
Clear definition of a number of common maladaptive patterns and their management.
Neill, JR, Sandifer, MG: *Practical Manual pf Psychiatric Consultation.* Williams & Wilkins, Baltimore, 1980.
A short, practical text of general hospital psychiatry, particularly useful for managing patients with difficult personalities when they are hospitalized.
Shapiro, D.: *Neurotic Styles.* Basic Books, New York, 1965.
Describes in fine detail the cognitive experiences and behavioral manifestations of the paranoid, hysterical, and impulsive personalities.

CHAPTER FOURTEEN

Affective Disorders

J. RAYMOND DePAULO, M.D.

INTRODUCTION

The most common psychological disturbance in the general population is a disturbance of mood characterized by depression with or without anxiety. The prevalence of this type of disturbance ranges from 10 to 20% for general populations to 20 to 50% for pa-

tients seen in general practice settings to 30 to 60% for general hospital inpatients (4, 5).

Implicit in these figures are two powerful arguments for the diagnosis and treatment of many of these patients by general physicians rather than by psychiatrists: first, there are too many patients for psychiatrists alone to provide the primary care, and second, there is a clear association between these mood disturbances and medical illnesses.

There are five factors which tend to hinder the generalist in helping these patients. These are (a) inadequate detection of a mood disturbance, (b) difficulty in classifying a mood disturbance when it has been detected, (c) difficulty in treating the correctly classified patient because of insufficient knowledge of antidepressant medications or inadequate time to allocate to the counseling of such patients, (d) inadequate knowledge of the prognosis of and the impact of treatment on the various mood disorders, and (e) difficulty in persuading patients with refractory affective disorders to accept referral to a psychiatrist.

The principal mood disturbances are the following:

1. Dysthymic disorder (synonyms: depressive neurosis, characterological depression, minor depression reactive depression)

2. Major affective syndromes (major depression, mania, or manic-depressive disorders)

3. Depression related to recent loss (e.g., grief reaction—see Chapter 18)

4. Depression secondary to medication (See Chapter 11) and to brain disorders (stroke—See Chapter 58 and dementia—see Chapter 16).

5. Temporary minor mood disturbances (see Chapter 11).

DETECTION OF PATIENTS WITH AFFECTIVE SYMPTOMS

Complaints of loss of energy, poor sleep, poor appetite, weight loss, decreased libido, etc., (i.e., vegetative symptoms) should alert physicians to the possibility of depression. However, depressed patients may not complain of those symptoms initially. Studies (10) have shown that these patients, in fact, usually present to generalists with three types of more vague complaints: ill defined functional symptoms, pains of undetermined etiology in a wide variety of anatomical sites, and nervous complaints such as increased tension and feelings of anxiety. Primary complaints about marital distress or job difficulty are also common.

When the physician specifically asks about mood changes and associated symptoms, most depressed patients will acknowledge them. The presence of a mood disturbance should not be taken to explain or to invalidate all physical complaints since coexistence of psychiatric and medical disorders is the rule rather than the exception. Conversely, it is a mistake to conclude that depression (or any other psychiatric illness) is present simply because no objective signs of organic disease can be found. If the patient does suffer from a mood disturbance and if appropriate inquiries are made, it is likely that at least some of the classic features of an affective disorder will be detected.

It is appropriate to ask patients about their mood, their sense of self-esteem and general physical and mental well being, their sleep, appetite, libido, and their feeling about their future. The diagnostic significance of each of these factors is pointed out in the sections on the principal mood disorders below.

Family members, if available, should be asked to confirm and augment the information obtained from the patient. With the patient's agreement, the physician should share with the family his assessment and plans for treatment.

Manic symptoms are usually detected by family members or co-workers. They most commonly include rapid sometimes incoherent speech, insomnia or refusal to sleep, hyperactivity, hypersexuality (often recognized as inappropriate for the particular patient), and hostile aggressive behavior. Manic patients usually feel there is nothing wrong with them and often resist medical attention. If they do bring themselves to ask for medical attention, it is because

they recognize something wrong in their sleep or level of activity, because they feel that others want to hurt them, or because they want the doctor to reassure their "nagging" family that there is nothing wrong with them.

DYSTHYMIC DISORDER (DEPRESSIVE NEUROSIS, CHARACTEROLOGICAL DEPRESSION, MINOR DEPRESSION, REACTIVE DEPRESSION)

Dysthymic disorder is the current name given by the American Psychiatric Association to depressions which lack the severity of major depression (described below). The various designations which have been used for this disorder point out that it is a more-or-less persistent condition (neurosis, characterological). This latter feature distinguishes it from the temporary minor mood disturbances which are seen commonly in medical patients who do not have chronic depression (see Chapter 11).

Patients with minor depression outnumber those with major depressive syndromes by approximately 10 to 1. For reasons that are not clear, neurotic depression is far more common among women than among men. Onset usually occurs around 18 to 30 years, and recurrence during periods of increased stress may characterize the patient's entire adult life. Serious medical illness is likely to precipitate a recurrence.

Diagnosis

The minor depressive disorders are only quantitatively distinct from normal mood responses. The patient's own sense of what is a normal response will often determine why one patient goes to the doctor while another attempts to deal with the perceived problem by other means. However, there is no absolute level of severity which distinguishes normal mood from dysthymic disorder or depressive neurosis.

Minor depression is a disturbance that arises from personality traits which make the patient more susceptible to particular stressful events or environmental demands. Although there is a strong association between certain personality traits (see Chapter 13) and depressive symptoms, different environmental stresses lead to depressive responses in people with different personality traits. For example, a dependent person may be more likely to become depressed when a source of security is threatened than would a relatively independent person. The depressive symptoms in such a patient should concern the general physician when the patient asks for help or when the mood change affects the patient's ability to function effectively.

Presenting or complicating problems associated with depressed mood in these patients include: (a) suicide attempts or self-injurious behavior—usually nonfatal but often requiring heroic medical interventions to prevent a fatal outcome, (b) multiple medical complaints and excessive medical care-seeking behavior or "illness behavior" (see Chapter 11 for additional detail), (c) drug and alcohol abuse, (d) family and marital discord, and (e) job difficulties.

These patients do not usually have the characteristic sustained changes in self-attitude and vital sense (*i.e.*, unwarranted feelings of hopelessness and worthlessness and of bodily deterioration), the psychomotor retardation, or the characteristic early morning awakening with worsening of mood which are seen in patients with major depression (see below). However, difficulty in getting to sleep, lack of appetite, mild weight loss, and loss of energy, and libido are common, as are anxiety symptoms (subjective tenseness, tremulousness, and shortness of breath).

Table 14.1 shows the specific criteria of the American Psychiatric Association (APA) for making the diagnosis of dysthymic disorder.

Management

Detection of the depressed mood and further interviewing to help delineate the external and personal antecedents of the depression is often therapeutic; the interest shown in the patient's story can help to restore lost self-esteem. Whereas occasionally some specific guidance and reassurance will help, more often empathic listening and encouraging the patient to outline his own synthesis of the problem and his approach to solving it provide more durable improvement. Weekly or biweekly visits to the physician for brief supportive psychotherapy for 3 to 6 weeks will often suffice. Useful psychotherapeutic techniques for the generalist are described in more detail in Chapter 10. Occasionally, adjunctive medication may be helpful in more severely affected patients. If generalized anxiety symptoms and/or insomnia predominate, a night-time dose of a benzodiazepine sedative-hypnotic may be helpful (see Chapter 82). If the depressed mood persists or if the patient has panic attacks (see Chapter 12), an antidepressant may be tried. A detailed account of antidepressant drugs is found below in the discussion of the treatment of major depression. It is important to explain to the patient that these are adjunctive treatments so that he does not fear that he is being treated for a major mental disorder. Treatment should be simple, with avoidance of combination preparations and polypharmacy, and relatively brief, *i.e.*, 1 to 6 months. Use of neuroleptics and lithium should not be considered in these patients due to their potentially irreversible side effects. With minor depressive disorders it is equally important to explain and treat concurrent medical conditions and to avoid drugs which may produce or exacerbate depression (see Table 11.1, Chapter 11). If the depression worsens despite treatment, referral to a psychiatrist is indicated.

Table 14.1
American Psychiatric Association Diagnostic Criteria for Dysthymic Disorder (Depressive Neurosis)[a]

A. During the past 2 years (or 1 year for children and adolescents) the individual has been bothered most or all of the time by symptoms characteristic of the depressive syndrome but they have not been of sufficient severity and duration to meet the criteria for a major depressive episode (see Table 14.2).

B. The manifestations of the depressive syndrome may be relatively persistent or separated by periods of normal mood lasting a few days to a few weeks, but no more than a few months at a time.

C. During the depressive periods there is either prominent depressed mood (*e.g.*, sad, blue, down in the dumps, low) or marked loss of interest or pleasure in all, or almost all, usual activities and pastimes.

D. During the depressive periods at least three of the following symptoms are present:
Insomnia or hypersomnia
Low energy level or chronic tiredness
Feelings of inadequacy, loss of self-esteem, or self-deprecation
Decreased effectiveness or productivity at school, work, or home
Decreased attention, concentration, or ability to think clearly
Social withdrawal
Loss of interest in or enjoyment of pleasurable activities
Irritability or excessive anger (in children, expressed toward parents or caretakers)
Inability to respond with apparent pleasure to praise or rewards
Less active or talkative than usual, or feels slowed down or restless
Pessimistic attitude toward the future, brooding about past events, or feeling sorry for self
Tearfulness or crying
Recurrent thoughts of death or suicide

E. Absence of psychotic features, such as delusions, hallucinations, or incoherence, or loosening of associations.

F. If the disturbance is superimposed on a pre-existing mental disorder, such as obsessive compulsive disorder or alcohol dependence, the depressed mood, by virtue of its intensity or effect on functioning, can be clearly distinguished from the individual's usual mood.

[a] Source: *Diagnostic and Statistical Manual of Mental Disorders*, Ed. 3, American Psychiatric Association, 1980. Some of the criteria for children have been omitted from this table.

Prognosis

In contrast to the major affective syndromes, prognosis in dysthmymic disorders cannot be estimated with much confidence. Some general features of outcome have been gleaned from large epidemiological studies. It is probably safe to conclude that *episodes of depressive neurosis usually have a limited course even if untreated*; the best available data suggest an average duration between 1 and 2 years (9). Although short term beneficial effects have been shown with the use of benzodiazepines and tricyclic antidepressants, they are modest at best. Various forms of psychotherapy as well as no treatment have been associated with similarly positive outcomes. Poor outcomes are associated with chronic medical disorders, severe social maladjustments, and coexistent personality disorders (see Chapter 13).

Recurrence of minor depression commonly occurs in the setting of later social stress or of medical illness. This is particularly true during the years of peak risk (*i.e.*, 18 to 30 years).

MAJOR AFFECTIVE SYNDROMES

Mania and major depression are the two syndromes which give the traditional name *manic depressive disorder* to this group of disorders. These disorders are characteristically episodic with complete remissions between episodes. Most patients suffer only recurrent depressive episodes (the unipolar group), a few suffer only manic episodes (they are grouped with bipolar patients), and the remainder suffer both manic and depressive episodes (the bipolar group). In its *Diagnostic and Statistical Manual of Mental Disorders* (see General References), the APA estimates that 18 to 23% of women and 8 to 11% of men experience at least one major depressive episode during their adult life; it may occur at any age. Only 0.4 to 1.2% of adults develop a bipolar disorder; it is equally common in men and women; the first manic episode usually occurs before age 30.

Major Depression

DIAGNOSIS

It is important to differentiate major depression from other major disorders, *i.e.*, schizophrenia and dementia (see Chapters 15 and 16) and from minor or "neurotic" disturbances such as depressive neurosis (see above) and anxiety neurosis (see Chapter 12).

The concept of the "endogenous" depression, although flawed, has provided a durable, usable account of major depressive illness. The fully developed syndrome is characterized by a sustained alteration in mood, self-attitude, and vital sense. The sustained lowering of *mood*, once established, is relatively impervious to environmental influence. A major life stress frequently occurs at the onset of symptoms, but this is not an important criterion for making the diagnosis. The change in *self-attitude* is usually manifested in the development of feelings of guilt, inferiority, uselessness, and hopelessness as the mood descends. The changes in *vital sense* (*i.e.*, the subjective assessment of one's physical and mental functioning) usually include feelings of confusion or poor memory with the inability to concentrate, a lack of energy and easy fatiguability, and occasionally fears or delusions of dying of cancer, losing one's mind, etc.

A patient presenting with a history of an episodic disorder and a fully developed symptom cluster as described is not difficult to diagnose. However, many patients with major depressions present either with few of these characteristic "endogenous" symptoms, with a dominant somatic symptom, or with a clear reason to be depressed, guilty, or hopeless. In such patients, recognition of major depression may be delayed and either the patient may be insufficiently treated or may receive no treatment for this eminently treatable disorder. If the diagnosis is uncertain, the facts should be examined for the specific criteria of the APA for major depressive episode (see Table 14.2). These criteria state that patients with 2 weeks of markedly depressed mood and without characteristic symptoms of schizophrenia who have four of eight symptoms of vegetation and depression should be considered to have a major depressive disorder and treated accordingly. Obviously these criteria will result in some patients being incorrectly classified, even though they would be easily classified with more traditional diagnostic concepts. However, these criteria are useful in supporting the working diagnosis of major depression in order to begin therapy. Recent work suggests that the dexamethasone suppression test may be useful in differentiating a depressive syndrome (plasma cortisol not suppressed by dexamethasone) from a minor affective disturbance (3).

MANAGEMENT

Drugs

For the patient who is maintaining good nutrition and hydration, who is cooperative with treatment, and who is neither overwhelmed with depressive delusions nor suicidal, antidepressant medication is the appropriate initial treatment. Although very useful, the antidepressant drugs, tricyclic antidepressants (TCA) and monoamine oxidase inhibitors (MAOI), are not always effective in eradicating depressive symptoms. Probably only 65% of patients will have a complete remission of symptoms. For most patients, TCAs are more effective than MAOIs and are, therefore, regarded as the drugs of first choice, although MAOIs may be more useful patients with atypical depression with prominent anxiety and panic attacks. The tricyclics derived from amitriptyline (*i.e.*, amitriptyline and nortriptyline) and imipramine (*i.e.*, imipramine and desipramine) are the best studied and most frequently prescribed. Among patients with the syndrome of depression, those with delusions, hallucinations, and profound psychomotor retardation tend to be less responsive to drugs than those without these stigmata; referral for psychiatric consultation and consideration for electroconvulsive therapy is appropriate for such patients. Among patients with suicidal intent (see "Suicide Prevention") the tricyclics should be dispensed in small amounts

Table 14.2
American Psychiatric Association
Diagnostic Criteria for Major Depressive Episode[a]

A. Dysphoric mood or loss of interest or pleasure in all or almost all usual activities and pastimes. The dysphoric mood is characterized by symptoms such as the following: depressed, sad, blue, hopeless, low, down in the dumps, irritable. The mood disturbance must be prominent and relatively persistent, but not necessarily the most dominant symptom, and does not include momentary shifts from one dysphoric mood to another dysphoric mood, e.g., anxiety to depression to anger, such as are seen in states of acute psychotic turmoil.

B. At least four of the following symptoms have each been present nearly every day for a period of at least 2 weeks:
Poor appetite or significant weight loss (when not dieting) or increased appetite or significant weight gain.
Insomnia or hypersomnia (see Chapter 82).
Psychomotor agitation or retardation (but not merely subjective feelings of restlessness or being slowed down).
Loss of interest or pleasure in usual activities, or decrease in sexual drive not limited to a period when delusional or hallucinating.
Loss of energy; fatigue
Feelings of worthlessness, self-reproach, or excessive or inappropriate guilt (either may be delusional).
Complaints or evidence of diminished ability to think or concentrate, such as slowed thinking, or indecisiveness not associated with marked loosening of associations or incoherence.
Recurrent thoughts of death, suicidal ideation, wishes to be dead, or suicide attempt.

C. Neither of the following dominate the clinical picture when an affective syndrome is present (i.e., symptoms in criteria A and B above):
Preoccupation with a mood-incongruent delusion or hallucination (i.e. mood-incongruent psychotic features). Delusions or hallucinations whose content does not involve themes of either personal inadequacy, guilt, disease, death, nihilism, or deserved punishment. Included here are such symptoms as persecutory delusions, thought insertion, thought broadcasting, and delusions of control, whose content has no apparent relationship to any of the themes noted above.
Bizarre behavior.

D. Not superimposed on either schizophrenia, schizophreniform disorder, or a paranoid disorder (see Chapter 15).

E. Not due to any organic mental disorder or uncomplicated bereavement (see Chapter 16 and 18).

[a] Source: Diagnostic and Statistical Manual of Mental Disorders, Ed. 3, American Psychiatric Association, 1980. Special criteria for children have been omitted from this table.

since even a 10-day supply provides a potentially suicidal overdose.

The mechanism of therapeutic action of antidepressant drugs is often explained by the "amine hypothesis." This hypothesis proposes that depression is associated with decreased functional aminergic neurotransmission, specifically that mediated by serotonin and by norepinephrine. It is proposed that antidepressant drugs act by increasing the amount of one or both of these transmitters in the central nervous system. Utilizing this scheme, the TCAs can be divided into two groups (see Table 14.3): the tertiary amines, which inhibit reuptake of serotonin and the secondary amines, which inhibit reuptake of norepinephrine. The MAOIS increase the availability of amine neurotransmitters by blocking their degradation. The clinical evidence to support the amine hypothesis remains scanty.

At the present time, there are no objective criteria for selecting a specific TCA. Hollister (see General References) recommends starting with a tertiary amine, amitriptyline. Another approach would be to start with nortriptyline, a secondary amine, because of its simpler pharmacokinetics (i.e., it has a more predictable dose to blood level relationship than other tricyclics) and because therapeutic response appears clearly linked to a steady-state blood level of 50 to 150 mg/ml of the drug. Combination pills containing TCAs and phenothiazines should not be used in the treatment of depressive disorders, since they carry the risk of side effects from both drugs, and they provide no demonstrated advantage over carefully selected TCAs.

In general, treatment with TCAs should begin at 25 to 75 mg per day (exceptions; 5 to 15 mg for protriptyline and 25 to 50 mg for nortriptyline) and be increased as tolerated to 150 mg per day, the average effective dose for most of these drugs (exceptions: 40 mg for protriptyline and 100 mg for nortriptyline) (see Table 14.3). Starting doses should be reduced by about 50% in older patients (especially those with medical illnesses). TCA dosage may be increased every 2 to 4 days in young physically healthy patients, but weekly increases are safer for older or infirm individuals. Giving the total daily dose at bedtime is desirable for most patients. Since TCAs may interact with a number of commonly prescribed drugs (Table 14.4), simultaneous prescribing with TCAs should be avoided; if this is not possible close monitoring is very important (for example, when a patient is taking antihypertensive drugs and a TCA).

Dosage with MAOIs should begin at 15 mg b.i.d. for phenelzine or 10 mg b.i.d. for tranylcypromine or isocarboxazide, be doubled in a week if tolerated, and then tripled unless therapeutic response or toxicity dictate otherwise (see Table 14.3). The use of MAOIs, particularly tranylcypromine, requires particular caution with respect to diet and the effects of coadministered drugs, in order to avoid a hypertensive crisis (see Table 14.5).

Significant improvement usually occurs after 8 to 10 days of daily administration of a therapeutic dose of any antidepressant; maximum benefit comes after 2 to 6 weeks at this dose. Obtaining TCA blood levels may be helpful if after 2 weeks at a stable dose the patient has shown no response to treatment; either

Table 14.3
Selected Characteristics of Antidepressant Drugs

A. TRICYCLICS

Amine Group	Generic Name	Proprietary Name(s)	Strengths of Oral Preparations (mg)	Usual Effective Dose in mg (Range)	Therapeutic Plasma Level (ng/ml)	Side Effects Antihistamine (sedation)	Side Effects Anti-α-adrenergic (hypotention)	Side Effects Anticholinergic[a]
Tertiary amine	Amitriptyline	Elavil, Endep	10, 25, 50, 75, 100	150 (50–300)	>120[b]	+++	+++	+++
	Doxepin	Sinequan, Adapin	10, 25, 50, 100	150 (50–300)	>90[b]	+++	++	++
	Imipramine	Tofranil, SK-Pramine, Presamine	10, 25, 50	150 (50–300)	>95[b]	++	+++	++
Secondary amine	Desipramine	Norpramin, Pertofrane	25, 50	150 (50–300)	—	+	++	+
	Nortriptyline	Aventyl, Pamelor	10, 25	100 (50–150)	50–150	++	++	++
	Protriptyline	Vivactil	5, 10	40 (15–60)	70–170	+	++	++

B. MONOAMINE OXIDASE INHIBITORS

Generic Name	Proprietary Name	Strengths of Oral Preparations (mg)	Usual Effective Dose in mg (Range)	Side Effects Risk of Hypertensive Crisis	Side Effects Orthostatic Hypotension
Tranylcypromine	Parnate	10	20 (20–60)	++	+
Phenelzine	Nardil	15	30 (30–90)	+	+
Isocarboxazide	Marplan	10	20 (20–60)	+	+

[a] Dry mouth, blurred vision, decreased intestinal motility, decreased bladder tone, tachycardia.
[b] Upper limit not yet established.

noncompliance or rapid metabolism of the drug can be responsible for drug levels below the therapeutic range (Table 14.3). Nortriptyline levels above the upper limit of the therapeutic range may be associated with a loss of therapeutic response (Table 14.3 shows therapeutic ranges).

The antidepressants cause *side effects*, many of which can be grouped according to probable physiological mechanism (see Table 14.3). The physician and the patient must decide which side effects are worth tolerating. Since depressed patients tolerate even mild side effects poorly, the patients should be reassured that the treatment is safe and potentially very helpful. Apart from the specific warnings contained in Tables 14.4 and 14.5, there are no adjunctive measures which are useful in preventing or alleviating the side effects of antidepressant drugs. In addition to the side effects named in Table 14.3, TCAs may produce mild paresthesias, increased appetite with weight gain, granulocytopenia (rarely), anticholinergic delirium (rarely), hypomania, slowed cardiac conduction, and cardiac arrhythmias. Because of the cardiac effects, these drugs should be given cautiously to those patients who have pre-existing conduction abnormalities and to those with unstable cardiac conditions such as a recent myocardial infarction. The major problem associated with the use of MAOIs is acute hypertension caused by foods containing the sympathomimetic agent, tyramine.

Thus, patients taking MAOIs must eliminate certain foods from their diet (Table 14.5).

After recovery from a first or infrequently recurrent depressive syndrome the medication which induced the remission should be continued usually for 3 to 6 months (a period of high risk for relapse); during this interval, dosage should remain at the level which relieved the depression. Occasionally, a lowering of the dose to reduce side effects will be justified. The patient should be told that withdrawal symptoms (nausea, dizziness, headache, increased perspiration, and increased salivation) may occur when tricyclics are discontinued. After electroconvulsive therapy (see below) maintenance treatment with tricyclic antidepressants also reduces the risk of relapse. Exceptions to these guidelines include the occurrence of drug toxicity, the appearance of manic symptoms (which can be induced by the antidepressants), and a history of such regular relapses that indefinite maintenance therapy with a tricyclic or lithium is needed (see section on long term management, p. 117).

Office Psychotherapy

For the first 6 to 8 weeks, the patient with major depression should be seen at least weekly both for adjustment of medication and for brief supportive psychotherapy by the techniques described in Chapter 10. Major life decisions and major shifts in per-

Table 14.4
Drugs which may Interact with Tricyclic Antidepressants (TCA)

Drug	Interaction
Anticholinergic antispasmodics	Enhanced anticholinergic side effects
Antihypertensive drugs	Enhanced orthostatic hypotension
Exception: clonidine and guanethidine	TCA may interfere with antihypertensive effectiveness
Antiparkinsonian drugs (L-dopa and anticholinergic drugs)	Enhanced anticholinergic side effects
Dilantin	May block TCA effectiveness
Methylphenidate (Ritalin)	May increase TCA plasma levels
Monoamine oxidase inhibitors (MAOIs)	Levels of both TCA and MAOI may be increased, enhanced risk of hypertensive crisis
Sedating drugs (alcohol, antihistamines, anxiolytics, hypnotics, neuroleptics)	Enhanced sedation
Sympathomimetics (decongestants, weight reduction agents, stimulants)	TCA may potentiate effects of these drugs

sonal relationships should be gently discouraged until the patient returns to his or her premorbid condition. Frank discussion of suicidal feelings, plans, intentions, risk, and alternatives should be a routine part of each visit (see "Suicide Prevention" below). The patient should be checked routinely for side effects of drugs by being asked about dry mouth, tremor, blurred vision, orthostasis, tachycardia, constipation, and by examining heart rate and rhythm and blood pressure. The more depressed the patient is, the less tolerant he will be of minor adverse drug effects. The support of the doctor in encouraging persistence with drug therapy can be crucial.

Referral for Management

The general physician may choose to manage those patients in whom he diagnoses major depression or he may refer them to a psychiatrist. There are four types of patients who should always be referred for the expertise of a psychiatrist: those who have shown no improvement after 2 to 4 weeks of treatment with therapeutic doses of antidepressant drugs (about one in three patients); those who cannot or will not take antidepressant medications; those who are overtly suicidal; and those who show delusions, hallucinations, or depressive stupor (the patient becomes mute and unresponsive). In these patients, either hospitalization, intensive psychotherapy, more aggressive drug therapy, or electroconvulsive therapy will usually be suggested by the psychiatric consultant. Some

patients will be resistant to the idea of seeing a psychiatrist. The physician can be very persuasive if he explains that additional drug treatments are available, but that their use requires the expert experience of the psychiatrist and that there is an excellent chance of improvement.

Electroconvulsive therapy (ECT) is an effective and rapid treatment for major depressive disorder. This treatment is given only to hospitalized patients; during ECT the patient is anesthetized with a short acting barbiturate anesthetic. There is general agree-

Table 14.5
Restrictions Needed to Avoid Hypertensive Crisis in Patients Taking Monoamine Oxidase Inhibitors

Items To Be Avoided[a]	Comments
FOODS	
Chicken liver	Tyramine content varies from little to 113 mg/g
Pickled herring	Tyramine content reported at 3.03 mg/g
Cheese	Tyramine content may increase with aging. Sharp cheeses, especially cooked and uncooked cheddar, are highly implicated, but no problem with cream and cottage cheese
Yogurt	
Sour Cream	
Beer	
Wine	Not all wines are implicated equally. The problem is noteworthy with Chianti and sherry in small amounts
Broad beans (Fava beans, *Vicia faba*)	Several reported hypertensive crises. These beans are an ingredient in pasta fasula
Canned figs	
Bananas	
Avocados	
Active yeast preparations	No problem with bread
Soy sauce	
Excessive caffeine	
Raisins	
Chocolate	
DRUGS	
Any sympathomimetic drug (decongestants in cold remedies, weight reduction agents, stimulants)	Can lead to hypertensive crisis
Stop monoamine oxidase inhibitors 2 weeks before planned surgery	Hypertensive crisis can occur if sympathomimetic given for vasoconstriction during surgery

[a] As little as 6 mg of tyramine may produce a hypertensive reaction in a patient taking a monoamine oxidase inhibitor.
Source: A. G. Lipman: Interactions between MAO inhibitors and food. *Modern Medicine*, 48: 133–134, 1980.

ment that this treatment is not useful for patients with "neurotic" depression. There is even some evidence that among patients with clear-cut major depression that those with the more severe symptoms will have a better therapeutic response. In a recent double blind, controlled study (in which the control group were treated by sham-ECT) of a large number of patients with endogenous depressions, only a modest, but statistically significant advantage accrued to the ECT-treated patients (6). Failure of drug therapy, the need for a rapid response (as in the starving or suicidal patient), or overwhelming severity of the depression are the prime indications for trying ECT.

The mechanism of action of ECT is unknown, but it appears that the electrical seizure discharge is required for benefit, which comes in an all-or-none fashion after the application of current. There is usually transient memory loss, related to the passage of current through cerebral hemispheres, but therapeutic benefit is not linked to the memory disturbance. Although there are other methods of inducing seizures, the electric current is easiest to control and, therefore, the safest. The normal risk of general anesthesia is the major hazard associated with ECT.

The *adverse effects* which follow ECT primarily involve memory. Commonly, retention of new and occasionally old memories is mildly defective for weeks to several months following a series of ECT treatments. This defect is usually "spotty"—that is, it will be apparent for specific domains of memory, but will not affect many others. Typically, the patient in whom this effect becomes clinically apparent (perhaps 40% of treated patients) will have trouble recalling names of recent acquaintances including doctors, nurses, and other patients. Clinically apparent memory defects typically resolve within a month. More detailed formal testing reveals mild defects up to 6 months—but none at 9 months after treatment.

Patients with brain tumors should not receive ECT. Patients with dementias from neuropathological causes treated with ECT may have temporary worsening of their cognitive impairments, but not infrequently the removal of depression actually helps overall cognitive performance. ECT should be avoided, if possible, within 3 months of myocardial infarction, cerebrovascular accident, or perforated viscus repair.

Mania

DIAGNOSIS

The manic syndrome, like major depression, is defined by a sustained change in mood with parallel changes in self-attitude and vital sense. The manic patient's *mood* may be euphoric or irritable and angry or may alternate between the two. *Self-attitude* becomes one of overconfidence and of an inflated sense of power, position, and importance. *Vital sense* reflects a subjective sense of quickened, acutely accurate thinking, unusual ease in decision-making, a

sense of heightened perception of sounds, colors, tastes, etc. In addition there is usually a sense of increased energy and a decreased need for sleep.

This central triad is often accompanied by parallel psychomotor symptoms. Delusions and hallucinations which are either persecutory or consistent with mood are not uncommon. Occasionally even characteristic symptoms of schizophrenia (see Chapter 15) occur in manic patients, leading to the clinical rule of thumb that so-called "schizophrenic" symptoms are not in themselves diagnostic but should be judged by the company they keep. In the presence of the characteristic manic syndrome and first rank symptoms of schizophrenia some would diagnose "schizoaffective disorder-manic type." Whether or not this is a useful practice, acute treatment and projected outcomes are similar to typical mania. The specific criteria of the American Psychiatric Association for mania are shown in Table 14.6.

MANAGEMENT

Because the disruptive and bizarre symptoms of mania are not seen frequently by the generalist and because it is treated with a drug, lithium, which requires supervision by someone familiar with its use, mania is a problem which should be referred to a psychiatrist. The generalist may play a crucial role in persuading a severely manic patient to accept referral and in following the patient with the psychiatrist if the patient also has a chronic medical problem. Knowledge of lithium treatment and of management techniques for severe mania are therefore important for the generalist.

In its milder form (called hypomania), the manic syndrome may be successfully treated with a neuroleptic (see Chapter 15 for details on neuroleptics) or lithium alone. Since the neuroleptics reduce manic behavior more rapidly, they are often used in combination with lithium in the early phases of treatment. This combined treatment involves greater risk of adverse effects and should be carried out by a psychiatrist. For both short and long term treatment, lithium carbonate is the most useful drug in the manic patient.

LITHIUM (2)

Lithium is given in divided doses. Beginning with 300 to 600 mg on the first day and increasing the dose in small increments every 3 to 4 days to the desired level minimizes nausea (as does taking the dose on a full stomach). The usual maintenance dose is 600 to 1800 mg given in divided doses (three or four times daily with standard preparations and once or twice daily with slow-release preparations). Blood levels, which should be measured 8 to 12 hours after a dose, should be monitored once or twice per week at first. Even when thoroughly stabilized in a compliant patient, lithium levels should be checked at least six times per year. In addition, because of the possibility

Table 14.6
American Psychiatric Association
Diagnostic Criteria for a Manic Episode[a]

A. One or more distinct periods with a predominantly elevated, expansive, or irritable mood. The elevated or irritable mood must be a prominent part of the illness and relatively persistent, although it may alternate or intermingle with depressive mood.

B. Duration of at least 1 week (or any duration if hospitalization is necessary), during which, for most of the time, at least three of the following symptoms have persisted (four if the mood is only irritable) and have been present to a significant degree:

Increase in activity (either socially, at work, or sexually) or physical restlessness

More talkative than usual or pressure to keep talking

Flight of ideas or subjective experience that thoughts are racing

Inflated self-esteem (grandiosity, which may be delusional)

Decreased need for sleep

Distractibility, *i.e.*, attention is too easily drawn to unimportant or irrelevant external stimuli

Excessive involvement in activities that have a high potential for painful consequences which is not recognized, *e.g.*, buying sprees, sexual indiscretions, foolish business investments, reckless driving

C. Neither of the following dominates the clinical picture when an affective syndrome is present (*i.e.*, symptoms in criteria A and B above):

Preoccupation with a mood-incongruent delusion or hallucination (*i.e.*, mood-incongruent psychotic features). Delusions or hallucinations whose content does not involve themes of either personal inadequacy, guilt, disease, death, nihilism, or deserved punishment. Included here are such symptoms as persecutory delusions, thought insertion, thought broadcasting, and delusions of control, whose content has no apparent relationship to any of the themes noted above.

Bizarre behavior

D. Not superimposed on either schizophrenia, schizophreniform disorder, or a paranoid disorder (see Chapter 15).

E. Not due to any organic mental disorder, such as substance intoxication (see Chapters 16 and 21).

[a] Source: *Diagnostic and Statistical Manual of Mental Disorders*, Ed. 3, American Psychiatric Association, 1980. *Note:* A hypomanic episode is a pathological disturbance similar to, but not as severe as, a manic episode.

of long term renal effects, maintenance dosage should be aimed at maintaining the lowest therapeutic level (probably 0.7 to 0.9 meq/liter) and not necessarily the level required for acute anti-manic activity (0.9 to 1.4 meq/liter).

The *adverse effects of lithium* can be divided into three groups: early (associated with rapidly rising blood levels), maintenance (associated with stable levels within the therapeutic range), and toxic (usually associated with high lithium levels). The *early* side effects include nausea and vomiting, diarrhea, mild lassitude, and drowsiness. These effects typi-

cally resolve as the serum level stabilizes in the therapeutic range.

The number of possible side effects from the *maintenance dose* is large enough to warrant a medical review of systems to detect them. The three most important ones are hand tremor, thyroid disturbances, and renal toxicity.

1. An accentuated physiological tremor (see Chapter 79) appears in a large percentage of patients (perhaps 60%), but is rarely severe. A family history of benign essential tremor and of concomitant use of other psychotropic drugs are often associated with more severe tremor.

2. In about 3% of patients, lithium therapy causes nontoxic goiter and mild alterations of thyroid function tests (*i.e.* borderline low thyroxine levels or elevated thyroid-stimulating hormone values). Less frequently, frank hypothyroidism may occur, usually in patients who had subclinical hypothyroidism before receiving lithium. For these reasons thyroid function should be assessed before lithium treatment is begun.

3. Finally, and of greatest concern, long term lithium therapy is associated with renal abnormalities: a renal concentrating defect (partial nephrogenic diabetes insipidus) and mild defects in glomerular filtration rate (GFR). These abnormalities may cause symptoms of diabetes insipidus (polyuria, hypernatremia) in about 10% of patients. The concentrating defect predisposes the patient to dehydration and, therefore, to frank lithium intoxication. Patients must be counseled to maintain good hydration even under circumstances which might inhibit their interest in adequate water intake (including depression) or which would increase water loss (e.g., hot weather). They should also be instructed to report the onset of polyuria at any time in the course of lithium treatment. The GFR should be assessed (see Chapter 44) before lithium is started and reassessed yearly thereafter.

The *toxic* effects of lithium occur uncommonly at normal serum levels, but increase in frequency as serum levels rise past 1.5 meq/liter. Premonitory signs of the central nervous system toxic syndrome are the recurrence of the early gastrointestinal side effects and worsening of polyuria and hand tremor, followed by lethargy and clumsiness. Obvious changes in the level of consciousness are reflected in confusion, delirium, stupor, and finally coma. Focal as well as nonlocalizing neurological signs are often present; occasionally such a patient will have an aphasia. Peak levels near or above 4.0 meq/liter are potentially fatal; death in coma, status epilepticus or due to aspiration pneumonitis can occur. The toxic syndrome is not usually relieved as rapidly as the blood levels, which usually can be reduced rapidly. A rather prolonged 10- to 14-day resolution of the mental state is usual. Management of lithium intoxication begins with an emergency measurement of serum lithium level and the discontinuation of lithium when the early signs of the disorder appear. If the clinical or laboratory evaluations suggest the likelihood of the toxic syndrome, hospitalization is mandatory.

The most important lesson to be learned about lithium intoxication is to prevent it. Overingestion or inadequate renal excretion are the only causes of the disorder.

TREATMENT OF SEVERE MANIA

Severe acute mania requires treatment with both lithium and neuroleptics, which is usually carried out in the hospital. The generalist's role with such patients may include initial diagnosis and then assessment of the acute manic state, persuasion of the manic patient to accept voluntarily hospitalization if needed, assessment of the patient for possible civil commitment, and the management of the acutely manic patient at home or in the office. These last three steps are outlined below.

Relating to the acutely manic patient can be very difficult. The euphoric or irritable manic patient often will not be able to accept the notion that his or her behavior is disturbed and requires inpatient therapy. A rationale for treatment which does not call attention to the obviously disordered behavior is usually more palatable to the patient. Consultation with the family about the plan of treatment should be arranged before, not after, confrontation with the patient. The family should be willing to accept responsibility if they refuse to follow the physician's recommendation.

Although laws on commitment vary from state to state, all states currently have legal provisions to allow the involuntary hospitalization of patients with mental disorders who are clearly dangerous to themselves or others and for whom no less restrictive alternative is appropriate.

For acute manic agitation the use of parenteral haloperidol (Haldol) is usually quite effective. Modest doses (5 to 10 mg intramuscularly) will calm most patients with little or no depression of blood pressure and little sedation. The sedating phenothiazines such as chlorpromazine (Thorazine) are more apt to produce severe orthostatic hypotension, and repeated doses are often necessary to break the agitated manic state. Within 15 to 20 min, intramuscular haloperidol usually brings about a calming trend which lasts for several hours. This period can be used to get the patient admitted to hospital. Even in this short period, however, patients may develop extrapyramidal side effects from haloperidol, most frequently acute dystonic reactions. This condition will be alleviated by 50 mg of intramuscular diphenhydramine (Benadryl).

Prognosis and Long Term Management of Major Affective Disorders

Because of the fundamental similarities, the prognosis of major depression and mania are discussed together. Without modern treatment, patients with these disorders usually recovered spontaneously within 6 to 18 months. With antidepressants, lithium, and ECT, remissions usually can be achieved much more quickly.

A hallmark of the course of affective syndromes is the tendency to relapse. The frequency of relapse is quite variable. However, fewer than 20% of affective syndromes resolve without relapsing at some point. There is a tendency for relapses to become more frequent later in the life of the patient (or later in the course of the illness). There is some evidence that depressions in later life are more severe and treatment-resistant as well. Formerly, this was part of the justification for the now discarded term "involutional melancholia."

The use of lithium and antidepressants has been shown to be beneficial in preventing recurrent affective episodes (8). Depressive relapses which occur in patients taking lithium or tricyclics are usually less severe and of shorter duration. Lithium is the only treatment demonstrated to reduce manic relapses.

The foundations of long term care of patients with bipolar or unipolar affective disorders are the following: a trusting doctor-patient relationship; education and counseling of the patient and his family regarding the course of the illness, the early signs of relapse, and the benefits and hazards of treatment; and maintenance on lithium carbonate or tricyclic antidepressant. Maintenance treatment is usually continued indefinitely for a clearly relapsing disorder. The patient's personal physician can often provide the basic treatment, particularly if he is following the patient for chronic medical problems. Brief visits every 2 to 3 months are sufficient when the patient is well. The objectives of these visits are to monitor the mood state, the drug therapy, and the social progress of the patient. If the patient has a well established trusting and predictable relationship with the doctor, even patients with the most grandiose manic or pessimistic depressive states will be more amenable to accepting necessary additional treatment.

The patient and his family should be educated with respect to the relapsing and remitting course of the illness, which is greatly modified but not usually eradicated by drug therapy. Individual aspects of the illness need to be observed and remembered by patient, family members, and the doctor, in particular, (1) the early symptoms of relapse (which differ from patient to patient); (2) certain signs or symptoms which specifically point to the affective syndrome in contrast to other reasons for changed feelings or behavior; and (3) recognized signs for suicidal or other dangerous behavior, as well as ways to relieve the danger.

CYCLOTHYMIC DISORDER

A bipolar affective disorder which is sufficiently mild or so brief that the episodes fail to meet the

APA Criteria for major depression or mania (Tables 14.2 and 14.5) is categorized as a cyclothymic disorder. These patients must be distinguished from patients with the personality traits of emotional lability and self-dramatization who will often report rapid but unsustained mood changes. The family histories of cyclothymic patients are similar to those of patients with a bipolar affective disorder as is their response to medication. The prognosis is also similar to that of bipolar disorder as 35% of such patients were found to suffer full-blown manic, hypomanic, or depressive episodes in a 2- to 3-year period (1).

SUICIDE PREVENTION

The rate of suicide in most countries is low enough (11 per 100,000 in the United States) that successful prediction of an individual suicide at a given point in time is very unlikely.

Practical strategies in this area are to protect those with relatively high risk in the short term and to reduce the risk in these patients over a longer term. *Risk factors for successful suicide* include older age, male sex, depressive disorder, alcoholism, living alone, previous suicide attempt, and refusal of voluntary psychiatric treatment. Retrospective studies of patient groups with major affective disorders in the era before effective drugs were available suggest that about 15% of the deaths were due to suicide. In addition, clinical observations suggest that the risk of suicide increases when improvement begins (or just after a depressed patient is discharged from hospital) or when the depressive's ruminations become frankly delusional convictions. Retrospective studies also suggest that there are fewer suicides in patients treated with ECT or long term lithium.

In examining information regarding suicide victims, two points stand out: (a) those who die from drug overdose (a large percentage of successful suicides) have usually obtained the lethal dose in a single prescription from a recent visit to a physician, and (b) they have usually communicated their intention before the suicide.

The role of physicians (7) in preventing suicide, therefore, includes: recognition, treatment, and prophylaxis of depression; routine questioning of depressed patients about suicidal ideas, specific plans, and available means; avoiding prescription of potentially lethal amounts of medicines to depressed patients; and short term protection of patients with suicidal intent via hospitalization, including involuntary commitment.

References

General

Brown, JH: Suicide in Britain. *Arch Gen Psychiatry* 36: 1119, 1979.
   An excellent critical review of Britain's experience with suicide and suicidal behavior of the 1960s.
Diagnostic and Statistical Manual of Mental Disorders, Ed. 3: American Psychiatric Association, 1980.
   Recently updated diagnostic criteria and epidemiologic information for all recognized psychiatric disorders.
Hollister, LE: Tricyclic antidepressants. *N Engl J Med* 299: 1106, 1978.
   Good review of the most useful antidepressant drugs.
Jefferson, JW and Griest, JH: *A Primer of Lithium Therapy.* Williams & Wilkins, Baltimore, 1977.
   An excellent book on lithium use and toxicity.

Specific

1. Akiskal, HS, Djenderedjian, AH, Rosenthal, RH and Khani, MK: Cyclothymic disorder: Validating criteria for inclusion in the bipolar affective group. *Am J Psychiatry* 134: 1227, 1977.
2. Baldessarini, RJ and Lipinski, JF: Lithium salts: 1970–1975. *Ann Intern Med* 83: 527, 1975.
3. Carroll, BJ, Feinberg, M, Greden, JF, Tarika, J, Albala, AA, Haskett, RF, McI, JN, Kronfol, Z, Lohr, N, Steiner, M, deVigne, JF and Young, E: A specific laboratory test for the diagnosis of melancholia. *Arch Gen Psychiatry* 38: 15, 1981.
4. DePaulo, JR and Folstein, MF: Psychiatric disturbance in neurological patients: Detection, recognition and hospital course. *Ann Neurol* 4: 225, 1978.
5. Goldberg, DP, Kay, C and Thompson, L: Psychiatric morbidity in general practice and the community. *Psychol Med* 6: 565, 1976.
6. Johnstone, EC, Deakin, JFW, Lawler, P, Frith, CD, Stevens, M, McPherson, K and Crow, TJ: The Northwick Park electroconvulsive therapy trial. *Lancet* 1: 1317, 1980.
7. Murphy, EG: The physician's responsibility for suicide: I. An error of commission; II. Errors of omission. *Ann Intern Med* 82: 301, 305, 1975.
8. Prien, RF, Kle-t, CJ and Caffey, EM, Jr: Lithium carbonate and imipramine in prevention of affective episodes: A comparison in recurrent affective illness. *Arch Gen Psychiatry* 29: 240, 1973.
9. Shepherd, M and Gruenberg, EM: The age for neuroses. *Milbank Mem Fund Q* 35: 258, 1957.
10. Widmer, RB, Cadoret, RJ and North, CS: Depression in primary care—changes in pattern of patients visits and complaints during subsequent developing depressions. *J Fam Pract* 9: 1017, 1979.

CHAPTER FIFTEEN

Schizophrenia

CHESTER W. SCHMIDT, JR., M.D.

Schizophrenia is a mental disorder or group of disorders of unknown etiology. The American Psychiatric Association lists the essential features of the disorder as the presence of certain psychotic features during the active phase of the disease, characteristic chronic symptoms involving multiple psychological processes, deterioration from a previous level of functioning, onset before the age of 45, and duration of at least 6 months. As noted below, none of these symptoms is pathognomonic for schizophrenia and each is seen in other psychotic states associated with both functional and organic mental disorders.

Familiarity with schizophrenia is important to the generalist for two principal reasons: (a) in the prodromal stage, the patient frequently presents first to a general physician, and (b) the generalist can provide most of the care for a patient with this lifelong disorder.

EPIDEMIOLOGY

Schizophrenia has been found in all societies throughout the world. The distribution is assumed to be similar through all populations. Epidemiological studies in Western societies have found the incidence of schizophrenia to range from 50 to 250 cases per 100,000 population per year. Lifetime incidence rates have been reported to range from 0.75 to 2.75%. Studies of incidence and prevalence in Europe using strict and somewhat narrow criteria of schizophrenia have produced case numbers and rates lower than similar studies done in the United States using broader criteria. Currently it is estimated there are 200,000 patients hospitalized in the United States with a diagnosis of schizophrenia. These patients occupy one-half of all the psychiatric beds in the country. In 1943, Lemkau et al. (2) determined that 15 to 25% of patients with schizophrenia never enter the hospital. Developments in psychopharmacology which occurred in the 1950s and the wide availability of ambulatory treatment resources have expanded that number and have greatly reduced the duration of confinement for those schizophrenics who require hospitalization.

Schizophrenia is found with equal frequency in males and females. Onset is usually during young adulthood, with the first hospitalization generally occurring between the ages of 25 and 34 years. Most schizophrenics are single and are found in lower socioeconomic groups. The proposed reason for the clustering of patients in the lower socioeconomic groups is a downward social drift resulting from deterioration of social and vocational function.

ETIOLOGY

The cause or causes of schizophrenia remain unknown. Numerous theories have been offered: constitutional, genetic, neurological, anatomical, biochemical, nutritional, psychosocial, and psychoanalytical. It is known that people related to schizophrenics are at higher risk for the disorder. The increased risk ranges from 3% for second degree relatives, to 7 to 15% for siblings and children of one schizophrenic parent, to 40% for children of two schizophrenic patients. Concordance rates in dizygotic twins are 10 to 15%, and in monozygotic twins 45%. This evidence therefore indicates there is a genetic factor, but such a factor has yet to be defined. A more recent clue to the etiology of schizophrenia has emerged from studies of the pharmacological effects of neuroleptic antipsychotic agents on schizophrenia. These antipsychotic agents have been found to antagonize dopamine-mediated neurotransmission, leading to the speculation that excessive activity of the dopamine systems may be part of a biochemical defect in schizophrenics (3).

NATURAL HISTORY OF SCHIZOPHRENIA

Although the first episode of acute psychosis usually occurs in late adolescence or early adulthood, prodromal manifestations of the disease are often present for years before the acute episode. During the prodromal phase, individuals gradually withdraw from social relationships into their own inner psychological world. They become indifferent to their grooming, develop suspicious attitudes about others, and ignore social graces and social rituals. They appear different, peculiar, and sometimes bizarre. Withdrawal eventually results in a gradual deterioration of scholastic and vocational abilities. In patients who have developed significant social and vocational skills the deterioratiion may be so striking that the patient seems to have a changed personality. In most cases, the patients will have developed only marginal social and vocational skills so that their deterioration appears more insidious.

In one study of the prodromal stage of schizophrenia (5), the majority of patients demonstrated some dysphoria (anxiety or depression) in association with social deterioration; and, it is significant that over half of them developed vague somatic complaints for which they sought help from a general practitioner.

Acute psychotic episodes are marked by the presence of a variety of symptoms: delusions (content of thought); hallucinations (perception); blunted, flattened, or inappropriate affect; illogical thinking and loosening of associations (form of thought); preoccupation with fantasies and an inner psychological world (autism); inability to carry out goal-directed

behavior because of preoccupation with consequences of alternatives (ambivalence); and stereotyped, bizarre, and sometimes rigid posturing. These episodes are often associated with stressful life events. Before neuroleptics were available, these episodes could last from weeks to years. Currently most episodes are brought under pharmacological control within several weeks to 2 months. After treatment, full-blown psychotic symptoms subside and in some cases seem to have disappeared completely. Most patients then resume the withdrawn, distant, odd social manner they manifested before the psychotic episode. Scholastic and vocational ability may slip further. With each subsequent psychotic episode the patients slip further and further into a dependent, regressed state in which they are unable to function and become entirely dependent on family or society. Less than 20% work full-time; the majority are financially supported by welfare programs or by federal disability programs. Institutionalization is required

Table 15.1
Diagnostic Criteria for a Schizophrenic Disorder[a]

A. At least one of the following during a phase the illness:
Bizarre delusions (content is patently absurd and has no possible basis in fact), such as delusions of being controlled, thought broadcasting, thought insertion, or thought withdrawal
Somatic, grandiose, religious, nihilistic, or other delusions without persecutory or jealous content
Delusions with persecutory or jealous content if accompanied by hallucinations of any type
Auditory hallucinations in which either a voice keeps up a running commentary on the individual's behavior or thoughts, or two or more voices converse with each other
Auditory hallucinations on several occasions with content of more than one or two words, having no apparent relation to depression or elation
Inchoherence, marked loosening of associations, markedly illogical thinking, or marked poverty of content of speech if associated with at least one of the following:
    Blunted, flat, or inappropriate affect
    Delusions or hallucinations
    Catatonic or other grossly disorganized behavior
B. Deterioration from a previous level of functioning in such areas as work, social relations, and self-care.
C. Duration: Continuous signs of the illness for at least 6 months at some time during the person's life, with some signs of the illness at present. The 6-month period must include an active phase during which there were symptoms from A, with or without a prodromal or residual phase, as defined below.
Prodromal phase: A clear deterioration in functioning before the active phase of the illness not due to a disturbance in mood or to a substance use disorder and involving at least two of the symptoms noted below
Residual phase: Persistence, following the active phase of the illness, of at least two of the symptoms

noted below, not due to a disturbance in mood or to a substance use disorder
Prodromal or residual symptoms:
Social isolation or withdrawal
Marked impairment in role functioning as wage-earner, student, or homemaker
Markedly peculiar behavior (*e.g.*, collecting garbage, talking to self in public, or hoarding food)
Marked impairment in personal hygiene and grooming
Blunted, flat, or inappropriate affect
Digressive, vague, overelaborate, circumstantial, or metaphorical speech
Odd or bizarre ideation, or magical thinking, *e.g.*, superstitiousness, clarivoyance, telepathy, "sixth sense," "others can feel my feelings," overvalued ideas, ideas of reference
Unusual perceptual experiences, *e.g.*, recurrent illusions, sensing the presence of a force or person not actually present
Examples: Six months of prodromal symptoms with 1 week of symptoms from A; no prodromal symptoms with 6 months of symptoms from A; no prodromal symptoms with 2 weeks of symptoms from A and 6 months of residual symptoms; 6 months of symptoms from A, apparently followed by several years of complete remission, with 1 week of symptoms in A in current episode.
D. The full depressive or manic syndrome (criteria A and B of major depressive or manic episode)[b] if present, developed after any psychotic symptoms, or was brief in duration relative to the duration of the psychotic symptoms in A.
E. Onset of prodromal or active phase of the illness before age 45.
F. Not due to any organic mental disorder or mental retardation.

[a] Adapted from: *Diagnostic and Statistical Manual of Mental Disorders*, Ed. 3, American Psychiatric Association, 1980.
[b] See Chapter 14, Tables 14.2 and 14.6.

in some cases because the patients lose all ability to care for themselves.

Thus, schizophrenia is a lifelong disease consisting of (a) psychotic symptoms which periodically become intense, and (b) an arrest or deterioration of social and vocational functioning probably caused by massive withdrawal of interest in the outside world.

DIAGNOSIS

The diagnosis of schizophrenia, especially during the initial episodes of acute psychosis, is based on clinical judgment and diagnostic criteria which, until recently, were unreliable. There are no pathognomonic symptoms, signs, or laboratory findings which point to the diagnosis. The medical history of the patient does not contribute to the diagnosis and, as discussed above, family history of the disease provides only partial information.

The diagnostic criteria for schizophrenia described in the *Diagnostic Statistical Manual III* of the American Psychiatric Association are an excellent synthesis of several recognized diagnostic schemas (see Table 15.1). Diagnosis rests upon the finding of the symptoms of psychosis elicited by a mental status examination (see Chapter 9) and a history which documents the prodromal phase.

Differential Diagnosis

Any kind of psychotic state may resemble acute schizophrenia. However, differences in symptomatology permit differentiation and diagnosis. *Organic mental disorders* (see Chapter 16) are marked by disturbances in consciousness (delirium), by disorientation with respect to time, place, and person, and by impairment in intellectual functions (memory, calculations, etc.). In addition, especially in persons under 50, there is usually evidence from the history, the physical examination, and laboratory tests of specific organic findings which are etiologically related to the mental condition. *Illicit drugs*, especially amphetamine and phencyclidine (see Chapter 21), may mimic the acute phase of schizophrenia. In addition, a number of *prescription drugs* may occasionally produce hallucinations and other manifestations suggesting psychosis (see Table 15.2). History of drug usage and absence of the prodromal phase help differentiate these conditions from schizophrenia.

The psychotic symptoms of *major affective episodes* (both mania and depression, see Chapter 14) can also be similar to the acute phase of schizophrenia. Affective disorders differ from schizophrenia in that psychotic symptoms (delusions, hallucinations, etc.) appear after the development of the affective disturbance (depression or mania). In schizophrenia, depression or mania may appear, but the affective disturbance occurs after the onset of the psychotic symptoms.

There are several *other functional psychotic conditions* which have symptoms similar to the acute psychotic phase of schizophrenia. However, these psychoses do not include a prodromal phase of withdrawal and deterioration, and patients return to their baseline level of function after recovery from the psychotic episode and do not experience progressive deterioration of function or recurrence of psychotic episodes.

TREATMENT AND PROGNOSIS

Neuroleptic Antipsychotic Drugs

The primary treatment of the acute and chronic psychotic manifestations of schizophrenia in ambulatory or hospitalized patients is with the "neuroleptic" antipsychotic agents (agents which produce symptoms which resemble neurological disease). There are several classes of neuroleptics, with numerous drugs in each class. The common drugs are listed in Table 15.3, together with available strengths and potency equivalents to chlorpromazine.

Although the structures of the various antipsychotics are well known, the pharmacology is not. Dose-response relationships have not yet been worked out for humans. The drugs produce effects

Table 15.2
Prescription Drugs Which Have Been Reported Occasionally to Cause Hallucinations or Other Manifestations of Psychosis[a]

Amantadine (Symmetrel)
Anticonvulsants
Antihistamines
Atropine and anticholinergics
Chloroquine (Aralen)
Cimetidine (Tagamet)
Corticosteroids (prednisone, cortisone, ACTH; others)
Dextroamphetamine
Diazepam (Valium)
Digitalis glycosides
Disopyramide (Norpace)
Disulfiram (Antabuse)
Ethchlorvynol (Placidyl)
Indomethacin (Indocin)
Isoniazid (INH; others)
Levodopa (Dopar; others)
Methyldopa (Aldomet)
Methylphenidate (Ritalin)
Nalidixic acid (NegGram)
Pentazocine (Talwin)
Phenelzine (Nardil)
Phenobarbital
Phenylephrine (Neo-Synephrine)
Procainamide (Pronestyl)
Procaine Penicillin G
Propoxyphene (Darvon)
Propranolol (Inderal)
Quinacrine (Atabrine)

[a] Adapted from Drugs that cause psychiatric symptoms, *The Medical Letter 23:* 9, 1981.

Table 15.3
Available Strengths and Equivalent Doses of Commonly Used Neuroleptic Antipsychotic Agents[a]

Generic Name	Trade Name	Available Strengths of Oral Preparations (mg)	Approximate Equivalent Dose (mg)
Phenothiazines			
Aliphatic			
Chlorpromazine	Thorazine (also generic)	10, 25, 50, 100, 200	100
Triflupromazine	Vesprin	10, 25	30
Piperidines			
Mesoridazine	Serentil	10, 25, 100	50
Piperacetazine	Quide	10, 25	12
Thioridazine	Mellaril	10, 15, 25, 50, 100, 150, 200	95
Piperazines			
Fluphenazine[b]	Prolixin, Permitil	1, 2.5, 5, 10	2
Perphenazine	Trilafon	2, 4, 8, 16	10
Trifluoperazine	Stelazine	1, 2, 5, 10	5
Thioxanthene			
Aliphatic			
Chlorprothixene	Taractan	10, 25, 50, 100	65
Piperazine			
Thiothixene	Navane	1, 2, 5, 10, 25	5
Dibenzazepine			
Loxapine	Loxitane, Daxolin	10, 25, 50	15
Butyrophenone			
Haloperidol[c]	Haldol	0.5, 1, 2, 5, 10	2
Indolone			
Molindone	Moban	5, 10, 25	10

[a] Adapted from R. J. Baldessarini: The neuroleptic antipsychotic drugs, *Postgraduate Medical*, 65: 108, 1979.
[b] Long acting fluphenazine decanoate or enanthate, for injection once weekly, comes in a concentration of 25 mg/ml.
[c] Haloperidol for injection comes in a concentration of 2 mg/ml.

within 1 hr after oral administration and within 10 to 15 min after intramuscular injection. They are lipid-soluble with a high affinity for cell membranes. The drugs and their metabolites are distributed generally throughout the central nervous system with no local or regional accumulation. Metabolites are partially excreted each day with significant portions retained in lipid-rich tissues and connective tissues. As these tissues become saturated the drugs undergo slow turnover. The drugs are detoxified and inactivated mainly through oxidation by hepatic microsomal enzymes, and excreted through both the bile and the urine.

There is no evidence that these agents are addicting, although tolerance to some of the side effects (sedation, hypotension, anticholinergic effects and parkinsonian symptoms) has been reported. The drugs are relatively safe; massive amounts must be taken acutely to produce symptoms of stupor or coma.

The mechanisms of action of the antipsychotics are not fully understood. Although it has been speculated that specific antipsychotic activity may be due to the dopamine antagonistic action of these agents, the drugs have a variety of effects on many metabolic processes.

Treatment of Acute Psychotic Episodes

All of the neuroleptic antipsychotics are equally efficacious for controlling psychotic symptoms as-

sociated with schizophrenia. The choice of one drug over another depends upon predicted differences in side effects, history of a particular patient's response, and the clinician's familiarity with the agent. The treatment of acute psychotic episodes should begin with the equivalent of 300 to 400 mg of chlorpromazine (Thorazine) a day, in divided doses (usually three times daily). Only one antipsychotic should be given at a time because administration of more than one agent increases the probability of side effects.

Combativeness, hyperactivity, and agitation are usually controlled within 24 to 48 hr after beginning treatment. If these symptoms are not modified within that period of time, the dosage should be increased 100 to 200 mg a day, up to the equivalent of 800 to 1000 mg of chlorpromazine. It may be necessary to administer the drugs intramuscularly during the acute phase of agitation if the patient is unable to take oral medication. The butyrophenone, haloperidol (Haldol) 2 to 5 mg, is a good choice for intramuscular injection because of its minimal effects upon circulatory regulation; an equivalent intramascular dose of chlorpromazine (25 mg) can also be used, but the likelihood of orthostatic hypotension (occasionally leading to syncope) is greater.

Delusions, hallucinations, associational defects, negativism, and withdrawal begin to subside within 1 to 2 weeks after treatment begins. Continued improvement of these symptoms may take place over an additional 4- to 8-week period. If very high doses of antipsychotic agents were initially required, the dosage should be reduced to the equivalent of 400 to 600 mg of chlorpromazine as soon as possible. This adjustment in dosage can usually be made 1 to 2 weeks after reaching the peak dose.

EARLY SIDE EFFECTS

Antipsychotic drugs with lower potency per milligram, such as chlorpromazine (see Table 15.3) produce *sedation*, which may be a useful side effect in treating hyperactive or combative patients, but a disadvantage in regressed, withdrawn patients. The *anticholinergic* property of all antipsychotics produces annoying symptoms of dry mouth, stuffy nose, blurred vision, and occasional urinary retention in older patients. These side effects often disappear within 2 to 4 weeks. The most worrisome side effect is *drug-induced parkinson's syndrome*. It occurs with greatest frequency in association with drugs of higher potency per milligram, such as haloperidol (see Table 15.3). The syndrome usually appears within 5 to 30 days of the beginning of treatment and includes tremor, rigidity, bradykinesia, fixed facies, drooling, and stooped posture. Because this problem commonly causes patients to discontinue antipsychotic tretment, it should be managed properly (4). Management consists of: (a) reduction of dosage, if possible; (b) change to another drug; or (c) anti-parkinsonism medication (anticholinergic agent or amantidine, not L-dopa; for details, see Chapter 79). In most cases reduction of dosage and/or addition of small amounts of an antiparkinsonism agent will control these side effects. The parkinsonian effects of neuroleptic drugs tend to decrease after 1 or 2 months. Therefore withdrawal of antiparkinsonism drugs should be attempted after 6 to 12 weeks. Prophylactic treatment of all patients with antiparkinsonism drugs is generally not a good idea because of the additional anticholinergic effects of these drugs.

Acute dystonias occur in occasional patients, within 1 to 5 days of initiating neuroleptic treatment. The symptoms are the sudden onset of severe, tonic contractions of the musculature of the neck (torticollis), of the neck, back, and heels (opisthotonos), of extraocular muscles (oculogyric crises) of the mouth, and of the tongue. These symptoms remit promptly after parenteral injection of either diphenhydramine, (Benedryl, 25 to 50 mg intramuscularly) or benztropine, (Cogentin, 2 mg intravenously). Neuroleptic treatment can be continued in these patients; an antiparkinsonism agent should be added for about 1 month to protect against recurrent dystonia. *Akathisia* may also occur early in treatment. This side effect is marked by motor restlessness with pacing, fidgeting, and "restless legs." Treatment is the same as that prescribed for drug-induced parkinsonism. Diazepam (Valium), 5 mg, two or three times daily, may also help to control this side effect.

A number of non-neurological side effects can result from administration of the antipsychotics. *Cardiovascular* toxicity is usually limited to orthostatic hypotension; frank syncope rarely occurs after intramuscular administration of low potency antipsychotics. Ventricular tachycardia is a very rare side effect. Reversible *cholestatic jaundice* may occur as an allergic response. *Agranulocytosis* is an exceedingly rare side effect.

Since older schizophrenics are more prone to the development of the common side effects, dose levels should be lower by the equivalent of 100 to 200 mg of chlorpromazine. The very high dose range described for treatment of combativeness and hyperactivity should be avoided in elderly patients.

Long Term Drug Treatment of Schizophrenia

The responsibility for the long term care of schizophrenics can be assumed by generalists or by nonmedical mental health professionals under the supervision of a physician.

Pharmacotherapy is the principal mode of long term treatment. Many studies have shown 60 to 70% of schizophrenics relapse within 1 year if they do not receive medication (1). Most patients require antipsychotics indefinitely, but all patients should be treated for at least 2 years following an acute episode.

The goal of long term pharmacotherapy is to minimize psychotic symptoms with the lowest dose of antipsychotic possible. For most patients this dose is the equivalent of 100 to 200 mg chlorpromazine daily. Patients on this dose often continue to have psychotic symptoms but do not seem to be disturbed by them (e.g., "I still hear the voices but they don't seem to bother me").

Some patients temporarily have difficulty maintaining a regular medction schedule because of psychotic disorganization, negativism, or fear of medication. Inability to comply with the medication regimen may signal the onset of an acute episode. With the first indication of a disruption in medication schedule, the patient should be evaluated, frequency of visits increased to at least once per week, and medication increased if warranted. If the patient remains unable to comply, a long acting intramuscular agent fluphenazine (Prolixin), 1 to 2 ml once per week, should be used. The patient can be returned to an oral medication when symptom control is re-established. Long acting intramuscular agents are also useful for new patients for whom no information is available on compliance in aftercare or ambulatory programs.

LATE SIDE EFFECTS

Side effects are rarely a problem for patients on maintenance doses of antipsychotics. When an increase in medication is necessary, drug-induced *parkinsonism* may appear. Patients who experience symptoms of parkinsonism over a long period of time should try other antipsychotic medications until one is found that does not produce the side effect. As noted above, long term use of antiparkinsonism medication is to be avoided if possible (see Chapter 79 for further discussion of drug-induced parkinsonism).

Tardive dyskinesia is an extrapyramidal syndrome which occurs in about 10 to 15% of patients on prolonged (months to years) moderate to high dose antipsychotic chemotherapy. The syndrome consists of involuntary or semivoluntary movements of choreiform, ticlike nature, sometimes associated with a dystonic component which classically involves the tongue, facial, and neck muscles. Younger patients often have significant involvement of the extremities and trunk. Although the syndrome is painless, it can be distressing and can interfere with the patient's ability to feed and care for himself. There is no satisfactory treatment for this problem. Antiparkinsonism medications usually worsen the symptoms. One short term effective treatment is the use of more potent antipsychotics to suppress the symptoms, but this usually requires increasing doses of the suppressing agent, and subsequent withdrawal of antipsychotics often leads to worsening of the symptoms for a period of time. Unfortunately, some patients never completely lose the symptoms.

Overall Management of the Patient

The schizophrenic patient is sensitive to change or instability in any aspect of his life. Therefore one physician or associate should provide continuity and consistency in his relationship with each of these patients so that the clinician becomes a predictable resource for assisting the patient to develop and maintain his social role in the community. Although few schizophrenics work full-time (≤20%), the clinician should refer patients for vocational rehabilitation (see Chapter 3) or sheltered workshops when requested. Most patients determine their own level of social activity and it is fruitless to push them into unwanted activities. The clinician should be available to the patient's family or to foster care providers for periodic review of the patient's progress and expectations.

Recreational or social activities are enjoyed by some patients, but many do not care for them. Ideally, residential facilities are available when there is no family for the patient to live with or when the family has a harmful influence. However, in many communities such facilities do not exist. For some patients the clinican and the ambulatory center itself become the source of the few social contacts which the patient has outside of his home and his inner psychological world.

Office visits should be scheduled on a regular basis, as frequently as once per month, or as infrequently as twice a year. Frequency of visits should be determined on the basis of the current status of the patient, history of the course of the patient's illness, reliability of the patient in taking medication, and the patient's ability to recognize early signs of onset of acute

episodes. Office visits need last only 15 to 20 min and should include an interim history, a brief mental status examination, a review of the effectiveness of medications and of significant side effects, and provision of support or advice regarding the ways in which the patient is dealing with day-to-day matters. In other words these office visits may be defined as supportive therapy, which is described in Chapter 10.

Management is enhanced if the clinician has ready access to social services, emergency mental health services, and psychiatric inpatient services. Social services, especially for financial support (welfare, food stamps, disability payments, etc.) are very important in the management of schizophrenics, because of the usual dependent status of these patients (many acute episodes of psychosis are precipitated by threatened or actual withdrawal of welfare and disability payments).

The generalist caring for a schizophrenic patient may need psychiatric consultation for confirmation of initial diagnosis, for decisions regarding hospitalization, or for treatment recommendations when symptoms respond poorly to antipsychotics or when side effects are intolerable.

Prognosis of the Treated Patient

Schizophrenia is a lifelong disease requiring an open-ended commitment by the clinician. The patient's life is disrupted by periodic psychosis, sometimes necessitating hospitalization, and by an arrest or deterioration of social function. Some patients are able to work and maintain fair levels of interpersonal relationships. Many lead lonely, withdrawn, socially marginal existences. Psychopharmacological treatment is very effective for controlling the symptoms of acute psychosis and for suppressing the intensity of psychotic symptomatology over long periods of time. Suppression of psychosis may permit the patient to use his intellectual and social talents more effectively in developing and maintaining some role in the community; however, the antipsychotics have no direct effect on the deterioration of social function which is so characteristic of schizophrenia.

References

General

Bleuler, E: *Dementia Praecox or the Group of Schizophrenias.* International Universities Press, New York, 1950.
   A classical work on schizophrenia.
Diagnostic and Statistical Manual of Mental Disorders, Ed. 3. American Psychiatric Association, 1980.
   Recently updated diagnostic criteria and epidemiologic information for all recognized psychiatric disorders.
Baldessarini, RJ: Antipsychotic Agents. In *Chemotherapy in Psychiatry.* Harvard University Press, Cambridge, 1977.
   A well referenced primer on the pharmacology and actions of antipsychotic agents.
Tune, LE, McHugh, PR and Coyle, JT: Management of extrapyramidal side effects induced by neuroleptics. *Johns Hopkins Med* 148: 149, 1981.
   Brief, helpful review of current information.

Specific

1. Hogarty, GE, Goldberg, SC, Schooler, NR and Ulrich, RF: Drug and sociotherapy in the aftercare of schizophrenic patients: Two year relapse rates. *Arch Gen Psychiatry 31*: 603, 1974.
2. Lemkau, PU, Tietze, C and Cooper, M: Survey of statistical studies on prevalence and incidence of mental disorder in sample population. *Public Health Rep 58*: 1909, 1943.
3. Snyder, SF: The dopamine hypothesis of schizophrenia: Focus on the dopamine receptor. *Am J Psychiatry 133*: 197, 1976.
4. Van Putten, T: Why do schizophrenic patients refuse to take their drugs? *Arch Gen Psychiatry 31*: 67, 1974.
5. Varsamis, J and Adamson, JD: Early schizophrenia. *Can Psychiatr Assoc J 16*: 487, 1971.

CHAPTER SIXTEEN

Psychiatric Problems of Old Age

JOHN C. BREITNER, M.D.

Psychiatric disorders are twice as common in the elderly as they are in the general adult population. At any one time at least 25% of individuals aged 65 and over have a significant mental disorder (8). Their disorders comprise many different diagnostic entities requiring various approaches to treatment. This chapter summarizes a number of general principles important in geriatric psychiatry, provides recommendations regarding specialty referral for psychiatric disorders in the elderly, and discusses specifically three categories of psychogeriatric disorder that are encountered commonly by the general physician in ambulatory practice: depression, dementia, and delirium.

GENERAL PRINCIPLES

Importance of Diagnosis

Age *per se* does not cause major changes in mental functioning. Instead, the elderly become prone to the development of a host of *specific disorders*. These disorders frequently occur in complex combinations affecting both mind and body, and the reduction of the composite picture to specific diagnostic entities may be challenging. The British geriatrician Sir W. Ferguson Anderson has said, "The greatest gift that a physician can give his elderly patient is a diagnosis ... provided, of course, that it is the right diagnosis." This statement applies with full force to the care of elderly individuals who are mentally ill. Because of the interactions of their multiple disorders elderly patients frequently present a perplexing array of signs and symptoms, often including mental confusion. The clinician must avoid the temptation to group these patients under such noninformative terms as "senile" and must instead evaluate each patient systematically; the goal of this evaluation is a comprehensive and concise diagnostic formulation of the patient's behavioral or mental disorder. Fulfillment of this goal is frequently difficult, and the generalist should not hesitate to seek specialty psychogeriatric or neurological consultation in complicated cases.

Changes in the Epidemiology of Mental Disorders

Although psychiatry in old age deals with the same disorders found in younger adults, important differences exist. New onset of most common psychiatric disorders is uncommon in the elderly (see discussions of the epidemiology in other chapters in this section), except for certain conditions seen more frequently in older people; particularly grief reactions and dementia. Dementia is rare in the young, but it affects 5% of the population over 65 and 20% of those over 80 (6).

Atypical Clinical Presentation

Unusual presentation is common in psychogeriatric disorders, as in many other diseases among the elderly. For example, depressive illness in old age may present initially not with depressed mood but instead with agitation, confusion, or hypochondriasis. The practitioner must consider such atypical presentations in order to include mental disorders among the list of differential diagnostic possibilities.

Interrelationships between Physical Illness and Mental State

These interrelationships are of particular importance in both geriatric psychiatry and geriatric medicine. The following types of problems illustrate this principle:

1. *Idiosyncratic Psychological Reactions of the Elderly to Physical Disorder.* The elderly suffer high rates of physical illness at a time in life when many possess only modest social and financial reserves to deal with illness. It is not surprising, therefore, that many physically ill old people show despondency, anxiety, frustration, irritability, dependency, or other maladaptive attitudes in response to their problems. Such attitudes become an important part of the patient's total problem, since they often exaggerate severity of dysfunction or complicate clinical management.

2. *Specific Psychiatric Complications of Neurological Disease.* Patients with a variety of organic brain diseases have a marked vulnerability to major depressive syndromes. These "organic" depressions respond well to pharmacotherapy with tricyclic antidepressants (see next section), but poorly to counseling and psychotherapy.

3. *Iatrogenic Psychosyndromes.* There is a risk of producing or exacerbating depressive syndromes by the administration of the centrally acting antihypertensive drugs (β-blockers, clonidine, methyldopa, reserpine). Although variable in intensity, such depressions may reach the proportions of a severe affective disorder, and suicides have been reported. A list of these and other drugs which may cause psychiatric disturbance is found in Table 11.1 of Chapter 11.

4. *Dementia Secondary to Primary Medical Problems.* As discussed below, dementia may be a complication, at times reversible, of a variety of primary medical problems.

Importance of the Patient's Social Network

Of special importance when dealing with elderly patients who are ill is awareness of the patient's milieu and social supports. The elderly often suffer financial impoverishment, social isolation, and personal losses, as well as physical illnesses. The ongoing support needed by many elderly individuals in dealing with these problems is provided by family and by other informal sources; the physician must be especially sensitive to the needs of these other caregivers in such cases, as well as to the needs of the patient himself. For patients lacking this informal support system, the physician can make an important impact by referring the patient for help to an effective social worker or to a community agency for the elderly.

SPECIFIC PSYCHOGERIATRIC DISORDERS

Many common psychiatric disorders (e.g., personality disorders, substance abuse) present only subtle differences in diagnosis and treatment in elderly or young patients. Other disorders (e.g., late onset schizophrenia) take special forms in the elderly and should clearly be referred for specialty care. Three categories of mental disorders, depression, delirium, and dementia, are especially common or important in old age; each of these presents practical problems in diagnosis, management, or referral for the general physician.

Depression

Depressed mood is the most common psychiatric symptom in old age. A major reason for the frequency of depression is the fact that it may result from many pre-existing conditions which are themselves common in the elderly.

FORMS OF DEPRESSION

The types of depression seen in the elderly defined by current nomenclature of the American Psychiatric Association are adjustment disorders with depressed mood, dysthymic disorder (depressive neurosis), major affective disorders (major depression and manic-depressive illness), and organic affective syndromes.

An *adjustment disorder* with depression is differentiated from a dysthymic disorder by its relatively acute onset, by the presence of a recent well defined precipitating circumstance (usually death or separation—see Chapter 18), and by the expectation of a fairly rapid and spontaneous recovery. *Dysthymic disorder* implies chronicity and a less well defined or more distant precipitant. Both adjustment and dysthymic disorders are appropriately understood as a reaction of a particular individual to psychosocial threat or loss. While adjustment reactions such as grief after loss of a loved one are commonplace, dysthymic disorders often seem to depend more on vulnerabilities unique to the personality of the affected patient. All but the most severe cases of adjustment disorder are best treated by a general physician who can capitalize on an established relationship with the patient. The techniques of short term and supportive counseling (see Chapter 10) may be applied with good results in such cases. Among individuals with dysthymic disorder a careful history often reveals evidence of life-long personal maladjustment or of previous depressive episodes; management of this disorder is described in Chapter 14.

The multiple forms of the *major affective disorders* are described in Chapter 14. The frequency of major depression increases dramatically among the elderly. Not only do new cases appear quite commonly in late life, but the frequency of recurrence tends to increase with age, and the proportion of depressed (as opposed to manic) episodes increases steadily with aging. The description of this disorder and its treatment, given in Chapter 14, is generally applicable to the elderly, although older victims show agitation more often than retardation, and they almost always show hypochondriacal features. The syndrome is often severe, and this may account for the high rate of completed suicides among old people. Treatment relies mainly on drugs (tricyclic antidepressants) and/or electroconvulsive therapy. The most useful of the tricyclics for the elderly appear to be nortriptyline (Aventyl, Pamelor) and desipramine (Norpramin, Pertofrane). These drugs are given in preference to other agents such as amitriptyline (Elavil, Endep) because of their fewer side effects, particularly anticholinergic effects. These drugs are not without risk (hypotension with dizziness or falling, arrhythmia, urinary retention, delirium), and conservative practice dictates a reduced initial daily dosage in older patients (e.g., 20 mg for nortriptyline, 50 mg for desipramine) and a gradual increase in dosage to the level of therapeutic efficacy.

"Organic" depressions are very similar in appearance to major depressions in patients without organic pathology. The diagnosis is made in the presence of significant symptoms of major depression as well as of evidence of organic neurological disease—e.g., stroke (see Chapter 80), tumor, dementia—judged to be etiologically related to the disturbance (3). Because such organic conditions are common in the elderly, organic depressions are relatively common. Treatment with the tricyclic antidepressants recommended in the preceding paragraph is generally successful, but these drugs must be used cautiously in the brain-damaged patient because of the possibility of provoking delirium.

DEMENTIA SYNDROME OF DEPRESSION (4)

The dementia syndrome (see below) may occur as a manifestation or complication of a depressive illness. Severe depressions can cause reduced mental acumen and performance in any age group, but the depressed elderly individual in particular may show a dramatic decline in intellectual performance. The term pseudodementia has been applied to this condition, implying both that it is not a "true" dementia (based on organic pathology) and that its clinical features differ somewhat from those of dementia syndromes provoked by structural brain pathology. In particular, the dementia syndrome of depression is usually of relatively acute onset, similar to the course of development of the depressive illness; this differs from the more gradual and insidious onset of most dementias caused by structural brain disease. In addition, the patient may complain about his cognitive defect, whereas those with organic dementias show a greater tendency to mask or hide their difficulties. Most important, the patient will show characteristic signs and symptoms of depression, usually a major depression, on both history and examination of the mental state. The importance of diagnosis in this type of dementia syndrome cannot be overemphasized: the disorder is generally reversible and resolves with successful treatment of the underlying affective illness; as such it is probably the most common type of reversible dementia syndrome.

Dementia
(Chronic Organic Brain Syndrome)

DEFINITION AND EPIDEMIOLOGY

Dementia is best defined as a global deterioration in intellectual function(s) which occurs in clear consciousness; and which is of sufficient severity to interfere with social or occupational functioning. That the defect is global, differentiates dementia from pure amnestic syndromes (isolated short and/or long term memory loss), focal aphasic syndromes, or other focal defect states. That it is a deterioration implies a documented reduction in ability from some previously established level, i.e., that it is different from mental retardation. That it occurs in clear consciousness differentiates dementia from delirium (see below). Like delirium, dementia is a clinical syndrome which may have many different etiologies or associated pathologies, some of them treatable. While it is commonly chronic, this is by no means universal. Except for the dementia syndrome of depression discussed above, dementia is almost always due to an organic disease affecting the brain.

Dementia syndromes have become a major public health problem. As mentioned previously, about 5% of the population over 65 is demented. Most dementia occurs, however, among the "very old" or "frail elderly" aged 75 and up. The prevalence of dementia is 20% in persons aged 80 and over; and it is present in approximately one in three persons aged 90 and over. These rates have not decreased in recent years when larger portions of the population have reached advanced age (6). As a result, dementia and its complications have become a leading cause of death, perhaps the fourth or fifth most common cause of mortality in the United States (7).

DIAGNOSIS OF DEMENTIA

The diagnosis of dementia may be simple or quite challenging, depending upon the severity of involvement when the problem is brought to the physician's attention. Two factors commonly delay recognition of dementia by the physician: the tendency for demented patients to attempt to hide their embarrassing problem by rationalization for memory lapses and other defects; and the fact that the earliest changes are often much more apparent in the patient's environment than in a physician's office (for example, leaving a stove burning all night, writing checks inappropriately, forgetting appointments, neglecting personal hygiene or appearance, taking the wrong bus home from shopping, etc.). In order to confirm the presence of dementia, the physician should evaluate the cognitive domain of the patient's mental status. As noted in Chapter 9, this part of the mental status examination is often accomplished through observations made while taking a general medical history, performing a physical examination, and (perhaps most important) obtaining information from the patient's spouse, children, or other close friends. The

Table 16.1
Mini-Mental Status Examination: Instructions for Administration and Scoring[a]

The test takes 5–10 min to administer.

ORIENTATION

1. Ask for year, season, date, day, month. Then ask specifically for parts omitted. One point for each correct. (0–5)

2. Ask in turn for name of state, county, town, hospital or place, floor or street. One point for each correct. (0–5)

REGISTRATION

Ask the patient if you may test his memory. Then say the names of three unrelated objects, clearly and slowly, about 1 second for each. After you have said all three, ask him to repeat them. This first repetition determines his score (0–3) but keep saying them until he can repeat all three up to six trials. If he does not eventually learn all three, recall cannot be meaningfully tested.

ATTENTION AND CALCULATION

Ask the patient to begin with 100 and count backward by 7. Stop after five subtractions (93, 86, 79, 72, 65). Score total number of correct answers, one point for each. (0–5)

If the patient cannot or will not perform this task, ask him to spell the word "world" backward. The score is the number of letters in correct order, e.g., dlrow = 5, dlrwo = 3. (0–5)

RECALL

Ask the patient if he can recall the three words you previously asked him to remember. Score 0–3.

LANGUAGE

Naming: Show the patient a wrist watch and ask him what it is. Repeat for pencil. Score 0–2.

Repetition: Ask the patient to repeat this phrase after you: "No ifs, ands, or buts." Allow only one trial. Score 0 or 1.

Three-stage command: "Take a piece of paper in your right hand, fold it in half, and put it on the floor." Give the patient a piece of blank paper and repeat the command. Score 1 point for each part correctly executed. (0–3)

Reading: On a blank piece of paper print the sentence "Close your eyes," in letters large enough for the patient to see clearly. Ask him to read it and do what it says. Score 1 point only if he actually closes his eyes. (0–1)

Writing: Give the patient a blank piece of paper and ask him to write a sentence for you. Do not dictate a sentence, it is to be written spontaneously. It must contain a subject and verb and be sensible. Correct grammer and punctuation are not necessary. (0–1)

Copying: On a clean piece of paper, draw intersecting pentagons, each side about 1 inch, and ask him to copy it exactly as it is. All 10 angles must be present and 2 must intersect to score 1 point. Tremor and rotation are ignored. (0–1)

Estimate the patient's level of sensorium along a continuum, from alert on the left to coma on the right.

[a] Source: M. F. Folstein, S. E. Folstein, and P. R. McHugh: "Mini-Mental State": A practical method for grading the cognitive state of patients for the clinician, *Journal of Psychiatric Research, 12:* 189, 1975. Total possible score is 30 points. Patients with totals of 20 points or less usually have either dementia, delirium, schizophrenia, or a major affective disorder (pseudodementia).

hallmarks of dementia are evidence of impaired recent memory, judgment, or abstract thinking, and personality change (either alteration or accentuation of premorbid traits).

The "Mini Mental Status Examination," which systematically tests the cognitive domain, is summarized in Table 16.1; this test is useful not only to confirm the presence of significant dementia but to quantify the initial severity of dementia and the changes in severity over time.

ETIOLOGICAL EVALUATION

There are numerous etiologies of the syndrome of dementia. Table 16.2 subdivides them into four groups: Conditions in which dementia is: (a) the only manifestation of neurological disease, (b) associated with other neurological signs and symptoms but not with other medical disease, (c) secondary to a medical disease, and (d) dementia secondary to another psychiatric syndrome (pseudodementia). The frequency of these etiologies is not known; it is likely, however,

Table 16.2
Etiological Classification of Dementia[a]

DEMENTIA THE ONLY MANIFESTATION OF NEUROLOGICAL OR MEDICAL DISEASE:
  Idiopathic degeneration of the cerebral cortex (Alzheimer's or Pick's disease)
DEMENTIA ASSOCIATED WITH OTHER NEUROLOGICAL CONDITIONS:
  Invariably associated with other neurological signs:
    Huntington's chorea (choreoathetosis)
    A large variety of rare degenerative syndromes—most of them of unknown etiology
    Dementia with Parkinson's disease
  Often associated with other neurological signs:
    Cerebral ateriosclerosis
    Brain tumor[b]
    Brain trauma, such as cerebral contusion, midbrain hemorrhage, chronic subdural hematoma[b]
    Low pressure hydrocephalus (always with ataxia of gait and often with sphincteric incontinence)[b]
DEMENTIA SECONDARY TO A MEDICAL CONDITION:
Hypothyroidism[b]
Cushing's disease[b]
Nutritional deficiency states such as pellagra, the Wernicke-Korsakoff syndrome, and subacute combined degeneration of spinal cord and brain (vitamin B_{12} deficiency)[b]
Neurosyphilis: general paresis and meningovascular syphilis[b]
Hepatolenticular degeneration, familial and acquired
Bromidism, chronic barbiturate intoxication[b]
DEMENTIA SECONDARY TO PSYCHOLOGICAL CONDITION:
  The dementia syndrome of depression (pseudodementia)[b]

[a] Adapted from: R. D. Adams: Derangements of intellect, mood, and behavior, In *Harrison's Principles of Internal Medicine*, Ed. 9, edited by K. J. Isselbacher *et al.*, McGraw-Hill, New York, 1980.
[b] Potentially reversible dementia.

that idiopathic degenerative disease of the cerebral cortex explains a sizeable proportion of the cases for which an etiology is not apparent. (Formerly most of these cases were attributed to atherosclerosis.) Recent evidence (2) indicates that a large proportion of these cases may be due to the familial form of the Alzheimer's disease—senile dementia complex. This entity, which appears to be transmitted as an autosomal dominant trait, is identified clinically by prominent aphasic or apractic symptoms.

In evaluating the patient with dementia, the general physician should first determine whether there are manifestations that suggest a certain etiology for the patient's dementia. This evaluation always includes a careful history and physical examination. Laboratory tests should be based chiefly upon the information obtained by history and physical examination.

In some patients the cause of dementia will be quite obvious on the basis of history and physical examination alone; examples include the patient who has had multiple cerebrovascular accidents with simultaneous gradual deterioration in intellectual functioning and the patient who has dementia following severe anoxia or hypoglycemia. In other patients, certain clues suggesting a primary medical or psychological basis for the dementia will enable the general physician to reach a working diagnosis based upon a selective evaluation and to initiate management. Examples are the patient with signs, symptoms, and laboratory confirmation of hypothyroidism (see Chapter 70), vitamin B_{12} deficiency (see Chapter 46), or neurosyphilis (see Chapter 29); or the patient with a prior history of major depression who develops dementia in association with typical symptoms of recurrent depression (see description of the dementia syndrome of depression above).

For a number of patients the probable explanation for dementia cannot be determined by a simple office evaluation. For these patients, radiological or neurological evaluation should be considered especially in the following situations:

1. The patient in whom the evidence suggests a *treatable cause*. Common examples are the patient with findings suggesting brain tumor (relatively rapid progression of symptoms, focal signs—particularly frontal lobe signs, known primary extracranial malignancy such as carcinoma of the lung or breast); the patient with possible subdural hematoma (history of falls and head trauma, anticoagulation therapy); the patient with the syndrome typical of low pressure hydrocephalus (relatively rapid onset, apathy progressing to dementia, bladder and bowel incontinence, gait apraxia—particularly if there is a history of subarachnoid hemorrhage, head trauma, or chronic meningitis).

2. The patient for whom objective diagnosis is important in order to *provide prognostic information* to the family, even though there is nothing to suggest a treatable cause. Common examples are the patient who has responsibility for others and who may need

to have a legal guardian named or the elderly person who is not yet institutionalized or totally dependent at home.

3. The patient in whom dementia appears to be part of a *clinical neurological syndrome*, such as Parkinson's disease or Huntington's chorea, for which a neurologist may provide both diagnostic confirmation and recommendations about prognosis and management.

In the evaluation of demented patients, there is a place for two more general approaches than those just discussed.

The first is the use of laboratory tests to *screen for causes of* dementia. It is reasonable to obtain a small number of screening tests as part of the initial evaluation of most patients. These tests are simple, inexpensive, uninvasive, and they may identify reversible causes of dementia which are not apparent in the history and physical examination. They include a hemogram (if the hematocrit is low and the mean corpuscular volume (MCV) is high, the vitamin B_{12} level should be measured), serum thyroxine, serological test for syphilis, and serum creatinine (uremia). These and other tests utilized in the evaluation of dementia which should not be regarded as screening tests, are summarized in Table 16.3.

The second approach is *to undertake no etiological evaluation* apart from a history and physical examination. This is appropriate in the sizeable proportion of the demented population who are very elderly, have been demented for a number of years, may have coexisting debilitating disease, and are either institutionalized or are getting custodial care at home. For such patients, the possibility of reversing the demen-

Table 16.3
Laboratory Tests Useful in the Etiological Evaluation of Dementia

Test	Etiology
Blood tests:	
Hematocrit and mean corpuscular volume (MCV)[a] (If hematocrit is low and MCV high, measure vitamin B_{12} level)	Vitamin B_{12} deficiency
Thyroid function tests[a]	Hypothyroidism
Serum creatinine[a]	Uremia
Serological test for syphilis[a]	Neurosyphilis
Liver function tests	Hepatolenticular degeneration
Electroencephalogram	Helps confirm cerebral disturbance (if normal, suggests nonorganic diagnosis *i.e.*, depression)
Computerized axial tomography	Identifies atrophy, tumors, subdural hematoma, or hydrocephalus
Lumbar puncture	Confirms neurosyphilis, identify other chronic meningoencephalitis

[a] Reasonable to obtain as screening test for treatable etiology in all patients.

tia is remote, and attention should be focused entirely upon the general measures discussed below.

LONG TERM MANAGEMENT

For most demented patients, a treatable etiology will not be found; or, if found, the treatment may bring only partial improvement. Therefore the major task for the physician is to provide effective help during the patient's progressive decline. Above all, care depends upon the availability of a competent and motivated spouse or other person who supervises the patient from day to day. Through the collaboration of physician, family, and community agencies (e.g. home health services, see Chapter 3), most demented individuals can remain at home for the duration of their lives (usually a number of years after the onset of dementia).

GENERAL MEASURES

Good care for the demented person always requires an awareness of the patient's medical and psychosocial situation, and prompt intervention whenever disruption of these occurs.

The physician should consider particularly the following questions about the *psychosocial situation*: How severely has the dementia syndrome limited the patient in routine daily tasks and abilities for self-care? Does the patient cope effectively when in a thoroughly familiar environment, but falter in unfamiliar surroundings? What measure of ongoing support services are required of family, neighbors, clergy, etc.? What is the patient's attitude toward his illness and toward others in his life? These psychosocial factors are much better indicators of the patient's ability to remain at home than is performance on a mental status examination. Thus, the physician must recognize this fact and be alert for important changes in the patient's social network which may drastically alter the prognosis for remaining in the home.

The careful handling of and anticipation of *medical problems* can also be decisive in attaining the best situation for a demented patient. Prescribed drugs should be kept to an absolute minimum, schedules should be simple for the patient who is still competent to self-administer drugs, and whenever the patient's competence is doubtful, someone else should supervise all medication-taking. An abrupt worsening in the patient's symptoms of dementia should always suggest an intercurrent medical problem, including all of the causes of delirium listed in the next section. The patient's environment should be free of factors which can be hazards to the health of a confused person; particularly common are poor lighting, multiple bottles of medication, potentially toxic household agents stored next to foodstuffs, perishable food kept unrefrigerated or kept refrigerated for prolonged periods (see details in Chapter 25), and difficult-to-operate apparatus which the patient may be expected to use (complicated door locks, appliances with multiple controls, etc).

Competence to manage his own affairs is often a consideration of the demented patient. Guidelines for assessing competence or for obtaining legal guardianship are described in Chapter 9.

Most of these general measures require accurate information about the patient's situation in his home, which can only be obtained adequately by direct observation of the patient at home; ideally such an observation should be made at least once by the physician who is providing long term care. In most communities, a home health agency is available; and assistance from such an agency can be very effective in maintaining the patient at home (for additional detail, see Chapter 3).

SECONDARY PSYCHIATRIC SYNDROMES

In addition to the general measures just described the physician should be alert for three psychiatric problems which occur commonly in demented individuals: *anxiety, agitation, and depression*. To an extent, these symptoms may be comprehended as reactions of demented patients to their disorder. Often, however, the symptoms take on a "free floating" quality and may be attributable to the organic brain disease causing the dementia. The physician must try to ascertain whether such symptoms are strictly psychogenic or indicative of intercurrent illness. For agitation and anxiety, low doses of neuroleptic drugs are usually very helpful—thoridazine (Mellaril), 10 to 25 mg, or haloperidol (Haldol), 1 to 2 mg three times a day (or as single dose treatments, only, when needed). Patients taking these drugs must be monitored for two common side effects—orthostatic hypotension and extrapyramidal symptoms (see details, Chapter 79). Mild depression is best managed with supportive therapy (see Chapter 10).

Major depressions with typical features such as early waking, anorexia, notions of guilt, self-blame, or worthlessness, nihilistic attitudes, or morbid hypochondriasis are also important in patients who have a structural brain disease that has caused dementia (see discussion of treatment of "organic" depression above, p. 127).

Demented patients with at least partial insight into their disability may become profoundly distressed when brought into a situation where they are forced to confront their failing abilities. There often ensues an overwhelming sense of frustration, fear, anger, or anxiety. These poorly controlled emotions further impair the patient's already limited functional ability, and a "positive feedback" effect is created which results in total decompensation of a previously coping individual.

Example: A 72-year-old woman with a history of several small strokes suffered from moderate forgetfulness and confusion but was generally calm and pleasant. Keeping track of the date with a calendar and making copious notes to herself, she managed to maintain an independent existence at home. At the supermarket check-out counter she could not find her wallet but insisted she had money to pay for her food. The clerk grew impatient, and the patient became increasingly agitated, tearful, and accusatory. When the store manager was called, she picked up grocery items and began throwing them.

These *catastrophic reactions* may have an extremely important impact on both the patient and his caregivers. The explanation of their cause and their prevention through avoidance of provoking circumstances can forestall the need for institutionalization. The use of small doses of the neuroleptic drugs haloperidol (Haldol) or thoridazine (Mellaril) may be beneficial in preventing recurrence of these reactions.

DRUGS FOR DEMENTIA

Although statistically significant improvement in mental status and in behavior has been reported (5) in institutionalized demented patients who were treated with an ergot derivative (Hydergine), neither this nor any other drug for dementia has been shown to improve the quality of life for demented persons living in the community. Therefore, there is no basis for recommending such drugs for demented patients followed in ambulatory settings.

Delirium (Acute Organic Brain Syndrome)

DEFINITION AND DIAGNOSIS

The hallmark of delirium is *clouding of consciousness*, with secondary changes in behavior, cognition, or perception. The delirious patient often seems strangely inaccessible or unable to concentrate on his environment or on the task at hand. Bizarre, dreamlike hallucinations may occur. The patient commonly suffers illusions, misinterprets his environment, and may fail to recognize persons well known to him. Because of the bizarre, threatening quality of his perceptions the delirious patient may become wildly

Table 16.4
Diagnostic Criteria for Delirium[a]

Clouding of consciousness (reduced clarity of awareness of the environment), with reduced capacity to shift, focus, and sustain attention to environmental stimuli
At least two of the following:
   Perceptual disturbance: misinterpretations, illusions, or hallucinations
   Speech that is at times incoherent
   Disturbance of sleep-wakefulness cycle, with insomnia or daytime drowsiness
   Increased or decreased psychomotor activity
Disorientation and memory impairment (if testable)
Clinical features that develop over a short period of time (usually hours to days) and tend to fluctuate over the course of a day
Evidence, from the history, physical examination, or laboratory tests, of a specific organic factor judged to be etiologically related to the disturbance

[a] Source: *Diagnostic and Statistical Manual of Mental Disorders*, Ed. 3, American Psychiatric Association, 1980.

Table 16.5
Etiological Classification of Delirium[a]

IN A MEDICAL OR SURGICAL ILLNESS (NO FOCAL OR LATERALIZING NEUROLOGIC SIGNS; CEREBROSPINAL FLUID USUALLY CLEAR):
   Metabolic disorders: hepatic stupor, uremia, hypoxia, hypercapnea, hypoglycemia, porphyria, hyponatremia
   Congestive heart failure
   Typhoid fever
   Pneumonia
   Septicemia
   Rheumatic fever
   Thyrotoxicosis
   Postoperative and post-traumatic states
IN NEUROLOGIC DISEASE THAT CAUSES FOCAL OR LATERALIZING SIGNS OR CHANGES IN THE CEREBROSPINAL FLUID:
   Cerebrovascular disease
   Subarachnoid hemorrhage
   Hypertensive encephalopathy
   Cerebral contusion
   Subdural hematoma
   Tumor
   Abscess
   Meningitis
   Encephalitis
   Postconvulsive delirium
THE ABSTINENCE STATES AND EXOGENOUS INTOXICATIONS (SIGNS OF OTHER MEDICAL, SURGICAL, AND NEUROLOGIC ILLNESSES ABSENT OR COINCIDENTAL):
Withdrawal of alcohol (delirium tremens), barbiturates, and nonbarbiturate sedative drugs, following chronic intoxication
   Drug intoxications due to sedatives, opiates, psychotropic agents, anticholinergics, digitalis, illicit drugs [see Chapter 21], etc.
BECLOUDED DEMENTIA:
   Senile or other brain disease in combination with infective fevers, drug reactions, heart failure, or other medical or surgical disease.

[a] Adapted from R. D. Adams: Delirium and other acute confusional states. In *Harrison's Principles of Internal Medicine*, Ed. 9, edited by K. J. Isselbacher, McGraw-Hill, New York, 1980.

agitated. On the other hand, psychomotor underactivity may dominate the picture. The onset of delirium is acute or subacute, developing over hours or days rather than over weeks or months. The intensity of the disturbance often waxes and wanes through the day and night.

Table 16.4 summarizes the criteria of the American Psychiatric Association for the diagnosis of delirium.

When the manifestations are not florid, the diagnosis of delirium can be missed (1). This error can lead to two catastrophes for the patient—failure of the physician to identify and treat a reversible cause of delirium and, at times, inappropriate commitment to a mental hospital for custodial care. The most helpful data in diagnosing delirium in the patient with less florid symptoms are the duration of behavioral change (obtained from a reliable observer), a careful history of all current drugs or exposure to toxins, new symptoms or signs of physical illness, and the patient's performance in a mental status examination (particularly orientation and recall of events during the past few hours).

Elderly individuals are particularly prone to delirium, probably because (a) the frequency of many of the conditions causing delirium is higher in the elderly, and (b) the aging brain seems particularly susceptible to the development of delirium. In the patient with known dementia, rapid development of clouded consciousness (the feature which distinguishes delirium from dementia) should always prompt evaluation for an intercurrent medical problem. A catastrophic reaction (see above) in the demented patient may resemble delirium; however, as pointed out earlier, a catastrophic reaction always occurs abruptly and in response to an easily identified stressful circumstance.

ETIOLOGICAL EVALUATION

Like dementia, delirium usually has an identifiable cause, a point stressed in the criteria in Table 16.4. Unlike dementia, most causes of delirium are treatable or are self-limited; and the prognosis for return to baseline mental function is good. Table 16.5 subdivides the etiologies of delirium into medical conditions, neurological conditions, drug/toxin excess or withdrawal, and beclouded dementia.

MANAGEMENT

When delirium is diagnosed in the office setting, it is usually necessary to hospitalize the patient for management. However, in some patients, the delirium may be due to a known cause which is brief or which can be readily reversed in the office setting. Examples are the mild delirium which may follow the initial dose of a benzodiazepine or of a potent analgesic such as pentazocine (Talwin); or the delirium accompanying insulin-induced hypoglycemia.

The treatment of delirium begins with diagnosis and *specific treatment* of the underlying disorder. If appropriate treatment is initiated, delirium generally resolves within a period of 24 hr. In a substantial portion of cases, however, exhaustive efforts fail to reveal the etiology. In these instances one can only offer supportive management while awaiting spontaneous resolution of the syndrome.

Delirious patients require *supportive management* in addition to specific treatment. The room should be well lit and stimuli maintained at a moderate level. Frequent reality orientation and reassurance help the patient to remain calm during his frightening ordeal. Extremely disruptive patients may require restraints, but these are rarely required in older patients. Sedation should be given with caution, except in those patients whose delirium is attributable to withdrawal of sedating drugs (e.g., alcohol, sedative-hypnotics). Some agitated elderly delirious patients may respond positively to small doses of haloperidol (Haldol); trial doses of 1 or 2 mg every hour may safely be given for a few hours.

References

General

Birren, JG and Sloane, RB (eds.): *Handbook of Mental Health and Aging.* Prentice Hall, Englewood Cliffs, N.J., 1980.
    Encyclopedic, thorough, and up-to-date.
Isaacs, AD and Post, F (eds.): *Studies in Geriatric Psychiatry.* John Wiley & Sons, New York, 1978.
    A concise, authoritative work with British orientation.

Specific

1. Engel, GL and Romano, J: Delirium: A syndrome of cerebral insufficiency. *J Chronic Dis 9:* 260, 1959.
2. Folstein, MF and Breitner, JCS: Language disorder predicts familial Alzheimer's disease. *Johns Hopkins Med J 149:* 145,1981.
3. Folstein, MF, Maiberger, R and McHugh, PR: Mood disorder as a specific complication of stroke. *J Neurol Neurosurg Psychiat 40:* 1018, 1977.
4. Folstein, MF and McHugh, PR: Dementia syndrome of depression. In *Aging, Vo. 7: Alzheimer's Disease, Senile Dementia and Related Disorders,* edited by R Katzman, RD Terry and KL Bick. Raven Press, New York, 1978.
5. Gaitz, CM, Varner, RV and Overall, JE: Pharmacotherapy for organic brain syndrome in late life: Evaluation of an ergot derivative vs. placebo. *Arch Gen Psychiatry 34:* 839, 1977.
6. Gruenberg, EM: Epidemiology of senile dementia. *Adv Neurol 19:* 437, 1978.
7. Katzman, R: The prevalence and malignancy of Alzheimer Disease: A major killer. *Arch Neurol 33:* 217, 1976.
8. Kay, DWK and Bergmann, K: Epidemiology of mental disorders among the aged in the community. In *Handbook of Mental Health and Aging,* p. 34, edited by JG Birren and RB Sloane. Prentice Hall, Englewood Cliffs, N.J., 1980.

CHAPTER SEVENTEEN

Sexual Disorders

CHESTER W. SCHMIDT, JR., M.D.

The sexual difficulties described by patients to their physicians are evenly divided into sexual problems which accompany physical illness, those which are secondary to side effects of medication or abuse of drugs, and those which are unrelated to physical problems and are purely psychological in origin. Typically the psychologically based sexual problems are related to both psychosocial antecedents and to current stressful life situations which are often self-limited. Those physically related and stress-related problems which are minor and are reversible lend themselves to treatment by counseling techniques which rely heavily on catharsis, reassurance, and education. Although there are limited data to document results of treatment for these types of problems in the ambulatory setting, clinical experience suggests that the outcome for reversible sexual problems is usually good with improvement rates approaching 75%.

THE NORMAL SEXUAL RESPONSE CYCLE

In order to assess these disorders rapidly and accurately it is helpful for the clinician to be familiar with the normal sexual response cycle and the major physiological factors mediating each phase of the cycle. The human sexual response cycle is divided into four phases.

The first phase is one of *desire* and consists of fantasies and wishes to engage in sexual activity. This response is psychic in origin, but the psychic stimulation is mediated by circulating androgens.

The second phase is the *excitement* phase and consists of a number of physiological changes plus the subjective sense of sexual pleasure. In both sexes there is an increase in heart rate, an increase in breathing rate, and development of muscular tension throughout the body, most pronounced in the pelvic area and thighs. For both sexes the major physiological change is the development of vascular congestion in the genital area. For females the manifestations of vasocongestion are vaginal lubrication and swelling of the external genitalia. In males, vasocongestion leads to erection. Vasocongestion may occur via either of two neurological pathways: (a) a reflex pathway initiated by tactile stimulation of the penis or clitoris and mediated by sensory fibers entering the dorsal root ganglia at S_2 through S_4 and by parasympathetic fibers from these ganglia to the perivesicular, prostatic, and cavernous plexuses; postganglionic fibers from these plexuses go to the blood vessels of the corpora cavernosa. (b) A cortical pathway initiated by psychic stimuli and mediated by both parasympathetic and sympathetic fibers. Each of these pathways promotes rapid inflow and retention of blood in the penis and the vulva. In addition to neurological pathways, erection in the male depends upon intact arterial blood flow from the right and left internal pudendal arteries.

The third phase is *orgasm*. Subjectively for both sexes orgasm is a peaking of sexual pleasure accompanied by a sense of release from sexual tension. Physiologically in the male, the most obvious manifestation of orgasm is ejaculation. Ejaculation is mediated by the sympathetic nervous system and consists of two processes: emission, resulting from contraction of the vas deferens, prostate, and seminal vesicles; and ejaculation, resulting from rhythmic contraction of the muscles of the pelvic floor and from closure of the internal sphincters of the bladder (preventing retrograde ejaculation). In the female, the rhythmic contractions take place within the musculature of the outer third of the vagina and in the perineal muscles. The subjective component of orgasm is a cortical sensory phenomenon, purely psychic in origin; it can occur without ejaculation or bladder neck closure.

The fourth phase is called *resolution*, which subjectively is accompanied by a sense of pleasure, warmth, well-being, and relaxation. Physiologically there is a gradual return of heart rate, breathing rate, and muscle tension to the baseline state. Most males are refractory to entering another cycle of sexual activity for some period of time. Women are not subject to this refractory period and may have multiple orgasms following continued or additional stimulation.

Table 17.1
Organic Factors Which May Affect Sexual Response in Both Sexes

Organic Factor	Sexual Disorders
Alcoholic neuropathy	Inhibited excitement, inhibited orgasm
Angina pectoris	Inhibited desire
Any chronic systemic disease	Decreased desire, inhibited excitement
Chronic pain	Decreased desire
Degenerative arthritis and disc disease of lumbrosacral spine	Inhibited desire, inhibited excitement
Diabetes mellitus	Inhibited excitement; retrograde ejaculation, (men) Inhibited orgasm (women)
Endocrine disorders (thyroid deficiency states, Addison's disease, Cushing's disease, hypopituitarism, hyperprolactinemia)	Decreased desire, variable effect on excitement
Multiple sclerosis	Decreased desire, inhibited excitement, inhibited orgasm
Cord lesions:	
Low lesion	Inhibited reflex excitement (psychogenic excitement, and reflex ejaculation may be preserved)
High lesion	Inhibited psychogenic excitement (reflex excitement, and ejaculation may be preserved)
Radical pelvic surgery	Inhibited excitement, inhibited orgasm
Temporal lobe lesions	Decreased or increased desire
Vascular disease:	
Large vessel (Leriche syndrome)	Inhibited excitement
Small vessel (pelvic vascular insufficiency)	Inhibited excitement

Table 17.2
Organic Factors Which May Affect Sexual Response: Men Only

Organic Factor	Sexual Disorders
Dyspareunia (genital pain during intercourse): Disturbed penile anatomy (chordee, Peyrone's disease, traumatic fracture, traumatic amputation) Penile skin infections Prostatic infections Testicular disease (orchitis, epididymitis, tumor, trauma) Urethral infections (gonorrhea, nonspecific urethral infections)	Inhibited desire, inhibited excitement, and inhibited orgasm are disorders which may occur with any of the organic factors listed at the left.
Hypogonadal androgen deficient states (Klinefelter's syndrome, testicular agenesis, Kallman's syndrome, testicular tumors, orchitis, hyperprolactinemia, castration)	Inhibited desire, inhibited excitement, inhibited orgasm
Mechanical problems (inguinal hernia, hydrocele)	Inhibited excitement
Surgical procedures:	
Abdominoperineal bowel resection	Inhibited excitement
Lumbar sympathectomy	Inhibited orgasm
Radical perineal prostatectomy	Inhibited excitement

COMMON SEXUAL DISORDERS

Classification

The nomenclature and criteria used to classify sexual disorders in this chapter are based upon the 1980 edition of the American Psychiatric Association's *Diagnostic and Statistical Manual, DSM III* (2). The assessment and management of the following common sexual disorders are discussed below: inhibited sexual desire (loss of libido); inhibited sexual excitement (impotence); inhibited orgasm; dyspareunia; vaginismus; and premature ejaculation.

As is pointed out below in the criteria for each of these disorders, a physical basis must be excluded before the disorder can be attributed to psychological factors. Since sexual functioning involves neural, vascular, and endocrine physiological mechanisms, there are many physical conditions and drugs which can interrupt normal function. To make matters more complicated these pathological conditions can adversely affect one or more phases of the sexual response cycle (see Tables 17.1–17.4).

General Characteristics
INCIDENCE

The exact incidence of sexual disorders is not known. Estimates of lifetime incidence have ranged from a high of 75% in marriages and other long term relationships to a low of 25%. In all likelihood, the higher estimates include these disorders in their milder and more transient forms. Each type of sexual dysfunction can be found in both hetero- and homosexual couples. The sex ratio varies for the particular dysfunction. For example, inhibited orgasm is more common in females. By definition, premature ejaculation is confined to men and vaginismus is restricted to women.

AGE OF ONSET OF COMMON SEXUAL DISORDERS

Psychological and behavioral antecedents of these disorders can sometimes be found in both adolescent and childhood sexual behaviors and fantasies; however, the common age of onset is early adulthood. Onset can occur at any time during adult life, especially for those dysfunctions which are associated with physical conditions or drugs and for those which are situational or transient.

PREDISPOSING PERSONALITY FACTORS

In general, competent and satisfying sexual function is considered to be associated with a healthy and adaptive personality development. Therefore, defects in personality structure accompanied by maladaptive personality traits or psychopathology may affect sexual function. *Compulsive* traits in men and women

Table 17.3
Organic Factors Which May Affect Sexual Response: Women Only

Organic Factor	Sexual Disorders
Complications of surgery: Ovarian approximation to vagina Posthysterectomy scarring Shortened vagina Dyspareunia (painful intercourse): Agenesis of the vagina Clitoral phymatosis Imperforate hymen, rigid hymen, tender hymenal tags Infections of external genitalia: herpes genitalis, labial cysts, furuncles, Bartholin cyst infections Infections of the vagina: herpes genitalis, *Candida albicans*, Trichomonas Injuries due to birth trauma: episiotomy scars, tears, uterine prolapse Irritations of the vagina: chemical dermatitis (douches), atrophic vaginitis, intercourse with insufficient lubrication Miscellaneous pelvic pathology: Cystitis, urethritis, urethral prolapse Endometriosis, ectopic pregnancy, pelvic inflammatory disease, ovarian cysts and tumors, pelvic tumors Intrauterine device complications	Inhibited desire, inhibited excitement, inhibited orgasm, and vaginismus are disorders which may occur with any of the organic factors listed at the left

Table 17.4
Drugs Which May Affect Sexual Response

Drugs	Sexual Disorders
Alcohol and sedatives (high dose)	Decreased desire, inhibited excitement, delayed orgasm
Androgens	Increased desire (women)
Antidepressants	Decreased or increased desire, inhibited excitement
Antihypertensives: Centrally acting (beta blockers, clonidine, methyldopa, reserpine)	Decreased desire, inhibited excitement, (?) inhibited orgasm
Peripherally acting (guanethidine)	Retrograde ejaculation
Antipsychotics	Decreased or increased desire, inhibited excitement, retrograde ejaculation
Disulfiram	Inhibited excitement, delayed ejaculation
Diuretics (particularly spironolactone)	Inhibited excitement
Estrogens, progesterone Men	Decreased desire, inhibited excitement, inhibited orgasm
Women	Decreased desire
L-Dopa	Increased desire (elderly men)
Marijuana (high dose)	Inhibited excitement (low dose may produce increased desire in men)
Narcotics	Decreased desire, inhibited excitement, inhibited orgasm
Stimulants (high dose) (cocaine, amphetamines)	Decreased desire, inhibited excitement, inhibited orgasm (low dose may produce increased desire)

may be associated with inhibited sexual desire and inhibited sexual excitement. *Passive-aggressive* traits appear to be associated with premature ejaculation. *Histrionic* traits in both men and women may be associated with inhibited sexual excitement and inhibited orgasm. *Negative attitudes toward sexuality* due to particular experience, internal psychic conflicts, or adherence to rigid cultural values can predispose individuals to the development of these dysfunctions.

COURSE

The course of sexual dysfunctions is variable. They may develop after a period of normal functioning or they may be lifelong. They may be generalized, occurring with all partners, or situational, limited to certain partners. There are differing degrees of impairment from partial to total. Usually, early age of onset, and total impairment indicates chronicity and, a poor treatment outcome. Conversely, history of prior adequate sexual function, situational symptoms, and partial impairment indicate a self-limited course and a favorable treatment outcome.

COMPLICATIONS

The major complications are disrupted marital or sexual relationships. In addition, presence of the dysfunction may give rise to a variety of symptoms such as depression, anxiety, guilt, shame, frustration, and anger. These symptoms affect not only the individual but may intrude into most of his or her relationships.

General Approach to the Patient

Since patients often have difficulty discussing sexual problems, the presentation of the chief complaint and history of the present problem may be imprecise. Thus it is important to set aside sufficient time with the patient to achieve a clear statement of the problem. Occasionally, more than one scheduled session may be necessary. The setting for the discussion of the sexual problem should be private. For those patients whose difficulties involve a partner or a spouse, it is important to have the partner's view of the problem. Sometimes the more functional partner will seek help in order to gain support for bringing the less functional partner into the evaluation.

The evaluation should be organized to obtain information about the onset and duration of the problem, about factors that make the problem better or worse, and exploration of concurrent events, such as birth of children, changes in relationships or vocation, onset of physical or emotional illness, and use of new medications. It is always important to elicit from patients their ideas about the etiology of sexual problems and their expectations of treatment.

Inhibited Sexual Desire (Loss of Libido)

DIAGNOSTIC CRITERIA*

Persistent and pervasive inhibition of sexual desire. The judgment of inhibition is made by the clinician's taking into account factors that affect sexual desire such as age, sex, health, intensity, frequency of sexual desire, and the context of the individual's life.

ASSESSMENT

As can be seen from Tables 17.1–17.4 there are many pathological conditions and drugs that have the potential for inhibiting sexual desire. In practice, most of these conditions will be known or easily diagnosed by the physician. Only a few conditions may present with the initial complaint of inhibited desire.

Congenital or acquired *hypogonadism* may be associated with inhibited sexual interest in men (10). Since the testosterone level needed to maintain libido is usually lower than that needed for full stimulation of the prostate and seminal vesicles, the patient should also complain of a decrease or absence of emission when loss of sexual desire is due to hypogonadism. Hypogonadism which occurs before puberty results in eunuchoidism, lack of development

---

* Source: *Diagnostic and Statistical Manual of Mental Disorders,* Ed. 3, page 278. American Psychiatric Association, Washington, D.C., 1980.

of secondary sex characteristics. Similar striking physical findings are not present in patients who acquire hypogonadism after puberty; however, subtle physical changes do occur: decrease in beard growth, tendency to female body habitus, and decreased size of testes. The diagnosis of hypogonadism should be looked for in any male with persistent loss of libido, by obtaining a testosterone level (normal 350 to 800 ng/dl). If the testosterone level is reduced, additional laboratory tests are necessary to differentiate between hypogonadotropic (*i.e.*, hypothalamic-pituitary problem) and hypergonadotropic (*i.e.*, primary testicular failure) hypogonadism. The tests include serum levels of luteinizing hormone (LH) and follicle-stimulating hormone (FSH). Any patient with decreased LH or FSH needs additional evaluation for a pituitary or hypothalamic tumor.

In both sexes *prolactin-secreting microadenomas* of the pituitary can cause loss of sexual interest. In men this is partly due to a prolactin-mediated decrease in gonadotropin output, and the testosterone level is low. Hyperprolactinemia causes amenorrhea and galactorrhea in females, but galactorrhea is rare in affected men. Diagnosis can be made in both sexes by measuring serum prolactin levels (normal less than 15 mg/ml).

In both sexes *alcohol or other substance abuse* can cause inhibited sexual desire. Patients who abuse drugs are usually guarded or untruthful about their habits; therefore, persistence and use of collateral interviews are often necessary in diagnosing the primary problem.

Additional details regarding the assessment of organic causes of inhibited sexual desire are found in Chapter 74.

Depression is a common cause of inhibited sexual desire. Even mild depressive states may result in loss of sexual desire, but in patients suffering from severe depressions this loss is universally observed. The relationship between inhibited sexual desire and the presence of depression may be recognized by noting the patient's mood as well as by obtaining a history of depressive symptoms (see Chapter 14). *Life stresses* (loss of a job, death of a family member or of a friend, birth of a new family member, recent illness such as myocardial infarction, etc.) are common sources of libido loss related to depression or anxiety.

In married couples inhibited sexual desire in one or both partners is often the result of *marital strife*. The differences that arise between the partners create anger which eventually interferes with their sexual relationship. Although spouses may be aware of their anger toward each other, they may fail to draw a connection between loss of sexual interest and their mutual problems, if such problems are not sexual in nature. Assessment requires taking a history from the couple together and from the partners separately. Review of their current life situation will usually elicit the precipitating stresses and highlight the conflicts. The uncovering of extramarital relationships during the assessment requires careful handling by the physician. If both partners are aware of the relationship, then it can be discussed openly. If the extramarital relationship is revealed to the physician during the individual interviews, the physician should ask what the partner intends to do about the relationship, and with the "secret" information now shared with the physician. The responsibility for telling the other partner should be left with the patient. In some cases the extramarital relationship is a peripheral issue, and airing it could be destructive to an otherwise salvageable relationship.

Finally, inhibited sexual desire can be caused by the anxiety and frustration of repeated sexual failure associated with one of the other sexual disorders discussed below.

TREATMENT

Depending upon the etiology, *hypogonadism* in men may be treated by surgery, radiotherapy, hormone replacement, or hormone suppression (in the case of hyperprolactinemia). These treatment modalities are discussed in Chapter 74.

In both sexes, if a *drug* (see Table 17.4) is suspected of interfering with sexual desire, it should be discontinued, if possible, as a diagnostic-therapeutic test. If loss of sexual drive is secondary to alcohol or substance abuse, then treatment should be aimed at controlling the abuse (see Chapters 20 and 21).

Patients with *coronary artery disease*, especially post myocardial infarction, have particular problems associated with sexual function. The management of these patients is discussed as part of the overall approach to rehabilitation after infarction in Chapter 55.

For transient loss of sexual desire secondary to *psychological factors* such as stress, anger, or other interpersonal problems, short term counseling is effective in most instances. The design of the counseling program should include an agreement between the patient or couple and the physician to meet for a specific number of sessions (usually two to five) for approximately 30 min per session.

Example. A couple in their mid-twenties presents with a history of recent loss of sexual desire on the husband's part, and a decrease in the frequency of their sexual relationships. Assessment reveals a past history of mutually satisfying sexual experiences until 1 month ago when the husband was threatened with a job layoff. Although the husband still has his job, the layoff is still a possibility. The wife reports the husband has become quiet, sullen, and has increased drinking of alcohol. They report fighting frequently over small issues. During the initial counseling session the physician suggests that a relationship exists between changes in the husband's behavior and the threatened layoff. The wife indicates that the husband has refused to discuss his concerns because "it is unmanly."

During the next counseling session the physician assists the couple in developing contingency plans to cope with the potential layoff. As they are drawn into the discussions of planning, the couple's anger with each other subsides and a collaborative relationship is re-established. The third session is utilized to review what contingency plans they have made. As an aside, they report that they have resumed their sexual relationship. During the final session the physician (a) reviews the relationship between stress, anger, and the change in sexual functioning; (b) points out that anger subsided when they worked together and that good sex is difficult to experience when they are angry with each other; and (c) encourages them to use what they have learned when stresses arise in the future.

Patients and their physicians often attempt to treat inhibited sexual desire with drugs such as testosterone, alcohol, anti-anxiety compounds, or stimulants. In a recent review (8) it was concluded that there is no scientific basis for prescribing drugs for sexual disorders, except testosterone for the treatment of confirmed hypogonadism and bromocriptine for treatment of hyperprolactinemia, as discussed in Chapter 74.

Inhibited Sexual Excitement (Frigidity, Impotence)

DIAGNOSTIC CRITERIA*

(a) Recurrent and persistent inhibition of sexual excitement during sexual activity manifested by partial or complete failure to attain or maintain erection until completion of the sexual act in males, or partial or complete failure to attain or maintain the lubrication and swelling response of sexual excitement until completion of the sexual act in females.
(b) A clinical judgment that the individual engages in sexual activity that is adequate in focus, intensity, and duration.

ASSESSMENT

In both sexes, partial or complete failure to begin and maintain genital vasocongestion can be caused by a large number of pathological conditions and drugs (see Tables 17.1–17.4). However, the presence of the offending pathological condition will usually be recognized by the physician before the patient complains of inhibited sexual excitement.

In patients with *diabetes mellitus* it is estimated that impotence will eventually affect 25 to 60% of males (3). Because some patients present with impotence as the initial symptom of diabetes, a fasting blood glucose is indicated for any male patient who presents with a chief complaint of impotence. There is no definitive information at this time about the

---

* Source: Diagnostic and Statistical Manual of Mental Disorders, Ed. 3, page 279. American Psychiatric Association, Washington, D.C., 1980.

effect of diabetes on the excitement phase in women; clearly, it can inhibit orgasm in women (7).

There are two conditions in women that may contribute to inhibition of sexual excitement: *vaginitis*, and *atrophic vaginal changes* secondary to menopause. Surprisingly, some women do not associate the presence of vaginitis or atrophic changes with the discomfort or pain these conditions can cause when intercourse is attempted. The history should include questions that determine whether there is pain during intercourse, and the physical examination should include a pelvic examination.

Occlusive vascular disease causing diminished blood flow to the internal pudendal arteries is more likely to affect men than women. Inhibited sexual excitement has been described with large vessel disease (Leriche's syndrome) as well as with medium and small vessel disease. If it is suspected that there is a vascular basis for impotence, the patient should be referred to a urologist for evaluation. The diagnostic techniques which may be employed included angiography of the medium size vessels of the corpus cavernosa, comparison of penile systolic pressures to limb systolic pressures, Doppler measurement of penile blood flow and nocturnal penile tumescence studies (NPT) (5).

The *hypogonadal states* which cause inhibited desire (see above) can also cause inhibited excitement, (10) and the approach to diagnosis is the same (see p. 136).

A stepwise approach to the assessment of impotence can be done in the ambulatory setting in the following manner.

1. *Routine history and physical examination plus fasting serum glucose* (detects or excludes most of the acute or chronic diseases, physical conditions, or offending drugs listed in Tables 17.1–17.4.) If the history indicates that potency is lost or impaired in all sexual experiences (intercourse, masturbation, spontaneous erections, including loss of early morning erections), and potency has diminished in a stepwise fashion over time, suspicion of a covert organic cause should be high.

2. A *testosterone level* should be obtained whenever the history or physical examination suggests an organic basis; if the testosterone level is below normal, referral for an endocrine workup, including evaluation for hyperprolactinemia, is indicated (see p. 136 above).

3. If the assessment does not produce any positive findings at this point, a *psychogenic basis* should be assumed and brief counseling (see below) should be utilized as a diagnostic therapeutic trial.

Inability to attain and maintain levels of excitement that permit a smooth and trouble-free progression from the beginning of a sexual experience to its completion can be caused by any external event or internal psychological event that interferes with the patient's ability to focus on the stimuli which are creating the sexual excitement. A dramatic example of an external event is the ringing of a telephone during the midst of the sexual experience. An internal psychological event might be a recurring thought. The history and assessment should be structured to uncover the presence of external events and the specific content of the psychological events when present. A common finding in many cases is a persistent preoccupation and anxiety about performing successfully. Worry about a successful performance becomes more and more absorbing during the course of the sexual experience so that the psychological activity crowds out the patient's capacity to focus on the sexual stimuli which create the excitement response. When such patients realize they are losing their level of excitement, they try all the harder, shutting off completely their ability to respond to the sexual stimuli. Masters and Johnson have called this process "*spectatoring*" (see General References). The term describes a process whereby the patient, through observation of his performance, psychologically takes himself out of the experience. The mental process is guaranteed to result in loss of sexual excitement. Typically this process may begin after one or two failed performances secondary to external events or stresses. Once the process begins, it becomes internally reinforcing leading to further worry and further failure. When this process is suspected, the history should focus on the patient's mental experiences during sexual intercourse. Such information is difficult for most patients to describe and more than a single interview will be required to obtain it.

Other common causes of psychologically inhibited sexual excitement are *stressful life situations*. Patients who have recently lost a job, have lost a relative, are concerned about retirement, have developed an illness, etc. may not be able to clear their minds of their worries during a sexual experience and therefore cannot respond. Similarly, feelings of anger or resentment directed toward the sexual partner can interfere with the ability to become sexually excited. If the patient with suspected psychogenic impotence does not respond to brief counseling, then referral to a sleep laboratory for nocturnal penile tumescent (NPT) studies (5) should be considered (see Chapter 82). If NPT study indicates organic pathology, additional evaluation for vascular or neurological disorders should be carried out. If a NPT study reveals psychogenic impotence, psychiatric referral is warranted.

TREATMENT

Treatment of *organically based inhibited* sexual excitement *in men* will depend on whether or not the physiological impairment is reversible.

If the disease process has not caused irreversible anatomical or physiological changes treatment of the disease (predominant problem) is dictated. Similarly, side effects of drugs can be reversed by reduction of dosage or, ideally, discontinuation of the drug. Testosterone replacement for hypogonadism produces improvement in sexual excitement within a few weeks (see Chapter 74).

When a disease process has caused permanent impairment of neural, vascular, or anatomical function in males, surgical measures can be considered. Currently there are two types of penile prosthetic devices which allow the impotent male to engage in intercourse. The Small-Carrion (9) prosthesis is a set of semirigid silastic rods which are placed in the penis. The second prosthesis is a hydraulic device (4) which, when implanted, permits voluntary stiffening of the penis. Acceptance and use of both devices is increased if counseling of the patient and his spouse or partner are routine elements of a rehabilitative program before and after surgery.

Little is known about the response to treatment in *women* with disease processes which impair the physiological capacity for sexual excitement. As in men, side effects of drugs can be eliminated by adjustment of dosage or discontinuation of the drug. The management of acute vulvovaginal conditions and atrophic vaginitis is described in Chapter 91.

The strategy for management of *psychologically based* inhibited sexual excitement in both sexes depends on whether the patient has had the dysfunction for a sustained period of time or whether the dysfunction has appeared recently, and there is a prior history of competent sexual functioning. As discussed earlier, transient inhibition of sexual excitement is often secondary to stressful life situations and/or marital discord. These clinical situations often respond to brief counseling. The elements of counseling are similar to those described in the above example of the couple with inhibited sexual desire (see p. 137). The role of the physician is to help the couple recognize the effect of the stress on their relationship as well as the effect of their feelings (often anger) on their ability to relate sexually. Encouragement of collaborative contingency planning for resolving problems reduces anxiety and anger, often helping the couple to return to their baseline level of sexual function. The same principles and steps are applicable to an individual patient.

Patients who have suffered with the dysfunction over a longer period of time or have never functioned competently may be given a trial of short term counseling (Chapter 10). If the counseling does not result in reasonable improvement, referral for more expert help should be considered.

Inhibited Orgasm (Anorgasmia)

DIAGNOSTIC CRITERIA: FOR WOMEN*

Recurrent and persistent inhibition of the female orgasm as manifested by delay in or absence of orgasm following a normal sexual excitement phase

---

* Source: Diagnostic and Statistical Manual of Mental Disorders, Ed. 3, pages 279–280. American Psychiatric Association, Washington, D.C., 1980.

during sexual activity that is judged by the clinician to be adequate in focus, intensity, and duration. Some women are able to experience orgasm during noncoital clitoral stimulation, but are unable to experience it during coitus in the absence of manual clitoral stimulation. There is evidence to suggest that in some instances this represents a normal variation of the female sexual response. The judgment to assign the diagnosis is assisted by a thorough sexual evaluation which may even require a trial of treatment.

DIAGNOSTIC CRITERIA: FOR MEN*

Recurrent and persistent inhibition of the male orgasm as manifested by delay in or absence of ejaculation following an adequate phase of sexual excitement.

ASSESSMENT

The orgasmic response is physiologically governed by the autonomic nervous system in both sexes. The organic conditions which inhibit orgasm are for the most part neurological disorders, drugs which affect the autonomic system, and surgical or traumatic interruption of the involved neural pathways (see Table 17.1–17.4). History-taking and physical examination should focus on these possibilities. In women, diabetic autonomic neuropathy is probably the most common organic cause of inhibited orgasm (7). Men who are experiencing retrograde ejaculation often state they have lost their ability to have orgasms. If history reveals the patient has the subjective sensations of orgasm but has no ejaculate, then the patient should have a urological evaluation of the function of the internal sphincter of the bladder.

Isolated *psychogenic* anorgasmia in men is a rare disorder and is associated with severe personality disturbances. Cases can be divided roughly into two personality types: severe obsessive-compulsive character disorder and severe sadomasochistic character disorder.

Psychologically caused inhibited orgasm is a common problem in *women*. Numerous studies estimate that 10% of the female population is anorgasmic to any stimuli and 30 to 50% of all married women are occasionally anorgasmic with intercourse. Assessment should focus on the duration of the problem, a past history of sexual functioning, the status of relationship to spouse or partner, and the presence of a stressful situation. A history of recent onset, competent past functioning, and identifiable precipitating stresses predicate a good response to treatment. Patients who have been anorgasmic for many years and are seeking help because of a change in their relationship or life situations are more difficult to treat.

Some women will present with a complaint of anorgasmia but evaluation will reveal the patient is actually experiencing inhibited sexual excitement. Since treatment may differ for these disorders, clarification of the phase in which the dysfunction is operating may be important.

TREATMENT (MEN)

It is unusual for men to experience loss of orgasmic capacity due to organic factors while retaining the capacity for erection. In fact it is more usual for men to lose their potency while retaining the capacity for emission and some of the subjective sensations associated with orgasm. Most of the physical conditions, diseases and drugs listed in Tables 17.1, 17.2 and 17.4 will affect the capacity for erection before orgasmic function is impaired. There may be isolated instances of side effects of drugs in which males report loss of ability to experience orgasm, but retain the capacity for erection. In these instances, it is important to distinguish *retrograde ejaculation* from inhibited orgasm. Retrograde ejaculation can occur with some drugs, including thioridazine (Mellaril) and guanethidine (Ismelin) while the other components of orgasm remain intact.

Men who suffer from inhibited orgasm on a psychogenic basis usually have longstanding personality disorders requiring expert psychotherapy to effect improvement.

TREATMENT (WOMEN)

The management of organically caused inhibited orgasm in women is essentially the same as the management of inhibited sexual excitement discussed in the previous section. Except for obvious interruption of critical neural pathways by conditions such as diabetic neuropathy, transection of the cord, pelvic exoneration, cord compression by tumors or other processes, there is little known about the effects of more subtle neuronal or vascular damage on women's orgasmic capacity. There are no known organic therapies for this dysfunction at this time. Therefore, in female patients with known neuronal damage, including diabetic neuropathy, the goal of therapy should be to help the patient adjust to the permanent loss of her sexual responsiveness.

Transient forms of anorgasmia caused by psychogenic factors are amenable to treatment with counseling. A history of previous orgasmic response is a good prognostic indicator. The block in orgasmic response is often due to the process of "spectatoring" already described (see p. 138). The interfering process is usually secondary to stressful life situations and/or marital discord. Counseling for married women and women who have a regular sexual partner should include the partner provided that it is agreeable to the patient. Counseling should be aimed primarily at resolving the dominant problems which are usually life stresses or interpersonal strife. With the single patient, counseling should be directed at helping the patient suppress or remove the psychological events (*i.e.*, spectatoring) which are occurring at a critical time, when the patient has reached a high plateau level of excitement and is prepared for orgasmic release. The interfering psychological events may be removed by having the patient focus to the best of her ability on the physical stimuli which she is experiencing during the excitement phase.

Women with anorgasmia of long duration can be given a trial of counseling. If counseling does not result in substantial improvement, referral for additional evaluation and treatment should be made.

Dyspareunia

DIAGNOSTIC CRITERIA*

Coitus is associated with recurrent and persistent genital pain in either sex.

ASSESSMENT

The common causes of genital pain during intercourse (dyspareunia) are presented in Tables 17.2 and 17.3. In both sexes the complaint of discomfort or pain during intercourse requires a careful history, physical examination, and laboratory testing. The commonest causes are infectious or atropic vaginitis in women, and urethral or prostatic infection in men. Psychogenic dyspareunia is uncommon, and this diagnosis should be made only after organic causes have been excluded.

TREATMENT

The treatment of dyspareunia caused by organic conditions in both men and women is directed at the condition causing the pain (see Chapters 26 and 91). Patients with psychogenic dyspareunia will have many of the features described for those with psychogenic inhibited sexual excitement or inhibited orgasm; that is, the patients will report a prior history of competent sexual function without pain and will have current life stress and/or marital discord. Therefore, the counseling techniques used in the treatment should be very similar to those described for the other two disorders. An important strategy in counseling is to allow the patient a face-saving way of giving up the pain without directly confronting him with the idea that the pain is of psychogenic origin.

A few patients have psychogenic dyspareunia over a sustained period of time. Such patients usually have severe underlying psychiatric conditions and require referral for expert evaluation and treatment.

Vaginismus

DIAGNOSTIC CRITERIA*

A history of recurrent and persistent involuntary spasm of the musculature of the outer third of the vagina that interferes with coitus.

---

* Source: Diagnostic and Statistical Manual of Mental Disorders, Ed. 3, page 280. American Psychiatric Association, Washington, D.C., 1980.

ASSESSMENT

By definition this is a female disorder. There are relatively few causes of organic vaginismus, and they are usually secondary to dyspareunia. Diagnosis of functional vaginismus may be made when pelvic examination is attempted and the physician finds it impossible to pass a finger or speculum into the vagina because of contraction of the musculature around the vaginal outlet.

TREATMENT

The treatment of organic vaginismus is the same as the treatment of the organic causes of dyspareunia.

The treatment of functional vaginismus is based upon *desensitizing* the patient to the experience of penetration. Couples are provided with a series of exercises to be performed in the privacy of their home. Following a relaxing bath, the couple engages in general body touching, excluding the genitals. Next, they repeat general touching but include the genitals, avoiding any touching that is frankly stimulating. At following sessions, they repeat the touching but add the passage of graded sized dilators still avoiding stimulating, touching, or efforts to attain orgasm. When dilators have reached the size approximating the size of the penis then the penis can be substituted as a dilator. The same process can be applied by having the individual woman dilate herself. One problem with the single patient is the possibility that the experience during the sessions at home will not generally apply to a sexual experience with a partner. Should this occur, treatment may have to be delayed until the patient has a regular partner with whom she has a reasonably good relationship and who can participate in the outlined program.

Premature Ejaculation

DIAGNOSTIC CRITERIA*

Ejaculation occurs before the individual wishes it, because of recurrent and persistent absence of reasonable voluntary control of ejaculation and orgasm during sexual activity. The judgment of 'reasonable control' is made by the clinician, taking into account factors that affect duration of the excitement phase, such as age, novelty of the sexual partner, and frequency and duration of coitus.

ASSESSMENT

There are no known organic causes for premature ejaculation; therefore, the assessment of this dysfunction should focus on psychological issues. Whereas some men recognize that orgasm regularly occurs too soon for their partner to enjoy intercourse

* Source: Diagnostic and Statistical Manual of Mental Disorders, Ed. 3, page 280. American Psychiatric Association, Washington, D.C., 1980.

fully, others do not; therefore it is necessary to interview both partners in order to make the diagnosis. Typically the couple will report that the male experiences orgasm as he is attempting to penetrate, just as he has penetrated, or within several thrusts after penetration.

Patients usually have had the dysfunction since they became sexually active. Although occasionally patients may report the recent onset of premature ejaculation, these men have invariably experienced the disorder for a sustained period in the past. Another variation is the patient who reports good control with a girl friend, but premature ejaculation with his spouse.

The personality structure of the premature ejaculator is often passive-aggressive. Evaluation of the relationship usually reveals an ongoing struggle between the couple. The woman is openly angry about some issue (not necessarily the sexual problem); and the man is complacent, content, and puzzled that his partner is upset. Transient episodes of premature ejaculation may be precipitated by marital conflict. Some men who are sufficiently frustrated by the disorder may develop inhibited sexual excitement (impotence) secondarily.

TREATMENT

There are several behavioral methods of treatment which may be adaptable to the ambulatory setting. The key to helping the premature ejaculator is to teach him to become aware of his progression through the sexual response cycle and then, with his partner, to practice one of two control techniques. Patients without regular partners cannot readily use this behavioral method. The techniques are "squeeze technique" and "stop and go." The squeeze technique requires the female partner to place her thumb and first two fingers around the coronal ridge of the penis and press firmly for 10 seconds. The pressure will result in a 10 to 25% loss of erection and a decrease in the subjective sense of arousal. The technique teaches the couple a method of control that can be practiced well before the patient reaches high levels of sexual arousal. The stop and go method accomplishes the same thing by discontinuing all forms of stimulation. The patient and his partner alternately stimulate and practice control with these techniques until they are confident of their ability to exercise control. At this point they progress to coitus, interrupting the experience as necessary with the squeeze or stop and go technique. Additional details can be found in Masters and Johnson's *Human Sexual Inadequacy* (see General References).

HOMOSEXUALITY

General Characteristics

Although homosexuality is no longer classified as a sexual disorder, it is the most common sexual deviation that will be seen by the generalist. Thirty years ago Kinsey (6) estimated that 10% of white American men and one-eighth of white women were predominantly homosexual. Estimates of the prevalence of homosexuality in blacks have not been published. The only disorder including homosexual behavior listed in the DSM III (2) is "ego dystonic homosexuality." The principal feature of this diagnostic classification is a pattern of overt homosexual arousal which is experienced by the individual as unwanted and a source of distress. Further the diagnosis is reserved for those homosexuals for whom changing sexual orientation is a persistent concern.

PREDISPOSING FACTORS

Various attempts to relate homosexuality to abnormal pituitary and sex hormone function have been unsuccessful. There is no evidence to support the contention that homosexuality is genetically determined. Many theories about the etiology of homosexuality involving psychosocial predisposition have been proposed. However, no studies have clearly demonstrated psychosocial etiological precipitants.

COURSE

Most individuals who make a choice of a homosexual orientation continue that orientation as a lifelong pattern. Some homosexuals are socially open about their life style; others are covert.

COMPLICATIONS

In the past, but to a lesser degree at the present time, the principal complication was the social stigma. Bias against homosexuals leads to occupational and other social problems for some, as summarized in Table 17.5. Recently, criminal penalties for homosexuality have been eliminated for consenting adults. The only legal difficulty currently is for those individuals who are promiscuous and who use public facilities for their sexual activities. Homosexuality *per se* is no contraindication for developing sustained, affectionate, long term relationships. There is little evidence to support the contention that homosexual individuals are subject to or manifest greater levels of psychopathology than heterosexual individuals.

Assessment and Management

Assessment of patients who express concerns about homosexual fantasies or experiences should focus on the frequency of the experiences, the patients' decisions to continue with homosexual experiences, and whether they feel comfortable with those decisions. Patients who ultimately choose a homosexual orientation and are comfortable with that choice do not present problems. However, patients who are anxious or depressed about their homosexual inclinations may need therapy. Adolescents or adults who anxiously report isolated epi-

Table 17.5
Influence of Homosexuality on Vocation and Social Life (Results of a Study of 143 Subjects)[a]

	Male Homosexuals N = 86	Female Homosexuals N = 57
	%	%
SOCIAL:		
No negative influence[b]	51	72
Deprived of family life	35	9
Social contacts limited to other homosexuals	14	19
AMBITIONS:		
No negative influence	68	88
Imposed restrictions on choice of work or advancement	32	12
JOB:		
No negative influence	84	88
Reprimanded, fired, or asked to resign because of homosexuality	16	12

[a] Source: M. Saghir and E. Robins; *Male and Female Homosexuality—A Developmental, Psychiatric, and Sociological Investigation.* Williams & Wilkins, Baltimore, 1973.
[b] All negative influences listed are those that subjects felt were specifically a result of being identified as a homosexual.

sodes of homosexual experiences or fantasies may need brief supportive counseling (see Chapter 10).

Homosexuals require special considerations in their *routine medical care*. Those who have multiple partners should always be asked about the presence of symptoms that might be caused by venereal disease and should be screened periodically for type B hepatitis (Chapter 39), syphilis (Chapter 29), and gonorrhea (Chapter 26). Physical examination should include inspection for oral or pharyngeal gonorrhea in addition to a genital examination. Laboratory tests should include stool culture for giardia if there is a history of anal intercourse and of chronic diarrhea.

SPECIAL CONSIDERATIONS FOR SELECTED AGE GROUPS

Elderly Patients

Aging individuals do not lose their capacity for sexual function on the basis of the aging process alone. Elderly patients who have any of the sexual disorders discussed above should be evaluated in the same manner as a younger patient. The changes associated with aging are: slower excitement phase, increased ability to stay at plateau levels of excitement, and, in men, a longer refractory period.

Children

It is unusual for children to complain of sexual difficulties. However, parents will occasionally ask their own physician questions about the developing sexuality of their children. Parents may express concern about the appearance of sexual behavior in children such as mutual exploration of playmates' genitalia or masturbation. The parents can be assured that the behavior is normal and that the behavior should be discouraged in a nonpunitive fashion. Failure to control the behavior may require further evaluation of both the child and the family.

Occasionally the physician may recognize the presence of *sexual abuse* within a family. If the abuse has been committed by someone outside the family, both the child and parents may require supportive counseling to help them vent their fear and anger about the experience. Discovery of sexual abuse within a family needs to be fully evaluated. This should be initiated by reporting the problem to the local department of social services; in each state, this department has a division of protective services to investigate suspected sexual abuse.

Adolescents

Adolescent sexual difficulties (see Chapter 5) may be brought to the attention of the physician either by the adolescent or by the adolescent's parents. Adolescents who are sexually active may have questions about their sexual function, birth control, venereal disease, or abortion. In most states, the physician may provide service for sex-related problems to the adolescent with or without parental consent.

Adolescents may request consultation about isolated homosexual experiences and/or homosexual fantasies. In most cases, the physician's role is to reassure the adolescent that these experiences are normal and are not indicative of the development of lifelong homosexuality. Adolescents who have decided on a homosexual orientation or who are in the process of doing so may be brought to the physician by parents disturbed at the discovery of homosexual activities. In these instances, counseling should be given to the parents in order to help them accept the decision of the adolescent. Older adolescents (above 17 years) are unlikely to change their orientation. Younger adolescents (16 years and below) have not consolidated their personality development and should be referred for psychiatric evaluation and possible treatment.

GENDER IDENTITY DISORDERS

General Characteristics

Gender identity disorders are divided into (a) transsexualism and (b) gender identity disorders of childhood. The essential feature of both disorders is the incongruence between anatomical sex and gender identity.

PREDISPOSING FACTORS

No known genetic or biochemical predisposing factors have as yet been elucidated. There is some evidence that these disorders may stem from faulty parent-child relationships in situations where parents have confused sexual identity, or have a need to raise a child of one sex in the role of the opposite sex.

PREVALENCE

These disorders are apparently rare. Male cases are more common than female, the reported ratio varying from 8 to 1 to as low as 2 to 1.

AGE OF ONSET

For children the initial expression of the wish to be in the cross-gender role may take place as early as the fourth birthday. For adults, the manifestations of this disorder usually become apparent in early adulthood, although the adults usually state that they had been aware of wishes to be in the cross-gender role since childhood or adolescence.

COURSE

The course of the disorder for children is as yet unknown. An undetermined number of affected boys and girls may adopt a homosexual orientation during adolescence or as adults. The course in adults is variable. For some it is chronic and unremitting, with a persistent drive toward attaining surgical reassignment. For others, the intensity of the desire for living and functioning in the cross-gender role waxes and wanes, often associated with current life stress and the appearance of psychiatric symptoms, principally depression. Females who are interested in sexual reassignment are a more homogeneous group than the males, in that they are more likely to have a history of homosexuality and by and large have a more stable course with or without treatment.

COMPLICATIONS

The principal complications are those associated with the desire and attempt to live and function socially and occupationally in the cross-gender role. In addition, there is a moderate degree of associated psychopathology, including episodes of depression and of suicide attempts. In rare instances, affected males may attempt to mutilate their genitals.

ASSESSMENT

The assessment of these disorders in adults is relatively simple in that most individuals will identify themselves as being unhappy with their anatomical sex and interested in a surgical reassignment. No endocrinological studies are indicated and physical findings show that the individuals seeking surgical reassignment are genetically normal men or women. However, the generalist may see rare cases of patients who have a congenital intersexed condition and who are confused about their sexual identification.

TREATMENT

Patients with gender identity disorders should be referred to psychiatrists or to special programs which have the expertise to treat these problems. Transsexuals who are in a cross-gender program and who need continuous administration of cross-gender hormones may be transferred to the generalist. Some physicians may not agree with such treatment, and these patients should be assigned to physicians who are comfortable working with these types of problems.

THE PARAPHILIAS

This is a group of disorders in which sexual interests are directed primarily toward objects other than other human beings, toward sexual acts not usually associated with coitus, or toward coitus performed under bizarre conditions.

Fetishism

Fetishism is the relatively exclusive displacement of erotic interest in sexual satisfaction to an object, or to a body part other than those usually associated with genital sexuality. Common fetish objects are female undergarments (particularly worn or soiled ones), feet, and shoes. Orgasmic release may be achieved by any of the behavior used by adults in sexual activities.

Zoophilia

Zoophilia is the use of animals as a preferred or exclusive method of achieving sexual excitement. The animal may be the object of intercourse or may be trained to excite the human partner sexually by licking or rubbing. The animal is preferred no matter what other forms of sexual outlet are available.

Pedophilia

Pedophilia is a condition in which adults compulsively involve children in their sexual activities. The sexual behavior that results in orgasmic release may be heterosexual or homosexual, and include any behavior utilized by adults in their sexual activities. In the majority of cases, however, the pedophile is concerned with mutual masturbation or fondling rather than coitus.

Exhibitionism

Exhibitionism is the displaying of the genital organs for the purpose of sexual gratification. This perversion is predominantly a male activity. Orgasmic release is usually achieved through masturbation.

Voyeurism

Voyeurism is a deviation in which sexual stimulation and gratification are obtained from looking at the sexual organs of others or from observing their sexual activities. Orgasmic release is usually achieved by masturbating during, or just following, the period of observation.

Sadism and Masochism

Sadism and masochism are deviations in which sexual arousal and gratification are dependent either upon inflicting pain (sadism) or experiencing it (masochism). There is a broad spectrum of behavior ranging from the dim awareness of cruelty or suffering as part of the sexual experience to overt behavior, including extreme physical injury and murder. Aspects of sadism and masochism are usually found in the same individual, even though one or the other behavior appears dominant.

General Characteristics

PREDISPOSING FACTORS

Etiology is unknown. However, history of physical and/or sexual abuse during childhood appears in a modest number of the cases.

PREVALENCE

The disorders are rare. The sex ratio is predominantly in favor of males, with the exception of sexual sadism and masochism.

COURSE

The course of these disorders is usually chronic. Peaks of deviant activity may accompany current life stress or be associated with psychiatric symptomatology, principally depressive episodes. If the deviant behavior brings the individual into conflict with society, the outcome can often include arrest and incarceration. Treatment is difficult because of the egosyntonic nature of the behavior. Anxiety and depression may be associated with the fear of being discovered, arrested, or punished; however, once these dangers have passed, the uncomfortable affect disappears, and the individual has little motivation for treatment.

COMPLICATIONS

Inasmuch as these disorders are often associated with other defects in personality development the capacity for developing long term, affectionate relationships may be impaired. The possibility of being involved in criminal violations has already been mentioned. In some instances the behavior may bring the individual into extremely dangerous situations, resulting in severe injury or death.

ASSESSMENT

It is not difficult to diagnose a specific paraphilia once the history is obtained. No specific laboratory tests are indicated. The physical examination will usually be normal. Sadistic or masochistic behavior may produce physical injuries. Hypersexuality, including some deviant behavior, has been reported to be associated with temporal lobe epilepsy (1). Thus, in cases in which there is suggestion of a seizure disorder, an electroencephalogram is indicated. Psychiatric disorders, principally depression secondary to loss, may precipitate bursts of deviant behavior in paraphiliacs. Abuse of alcohol or of other substances may also increase the behavior.

Stress, anxiety, organic brain syndrome, and mental retardation may lead to episodic deviant behavior, but these episodes are not diagnosed as paraphilia.

TREATMENT

Psychotherapy or other psychological treatment designed to control or eliminate paraphiliac behavior is best provided by a psychiatrist. The general physician's role in the care of these patients is in the management of concurrent medical problems. Of major concern are recognition and treatment of venereal disease in those patients whose sexual behavior is promiscuous, and the possibility of child abuse in families which have paraphiliac members. Many individuals who engage in paraphilias were subjected to physical or sexual abuse as children. The pattern is often passed on from generation to generation.

References

General

Diagnostic and Statistical Manual of Mental Disorders, Ed. 3: American Psychiatric Association, Washington, D.C., 1980
   Recently up-dated diagnostic criteria and epidemiological information for all recognized psychiatric disorders.
Masters, WH, and Johnson, VE: *Human Sexual Inadequacy*. Little, Brown, Boston, 1970.
   The original and still used descriptive work on the behavioral treatment of common sexual disorders.

The Psychiatric Clinics of North America: Sexuality. W. B. Saunders, Philadelphia, 1980.
   A current, concise review.

Specific

1. Blumer, D: Changes of sexual behavior related to temporal lobe disorders in man. *J Sex Res* 6: 173, 1970.
2. *Diagnostic and Statistical Manual of Mental Disorders*, Ed. 3, pp. 261–283. American Psychiatric Association, Washington, D.C., 1980.
3. Ellenberg, M: Impotence in diabetes: The neurologic factor. *Ann Intern Med* 75: 213, 1971.
4. Furlow, WL: Surgical treatment of erectile impotence using the inflatable penile prosthesis. *Sex Disabil* 1: 299, 1978.
5. Karacan, I: Diagnosis of impotence in diabetes mellitus: An objective and specific method. *Ann Intern Med* 92: 334, 1980.
6. Kinsey, AC, Pomeroy, WB, and Martin CE: *Sexual Behavior in the Human Male*, pp. 610–666. W.B. Saunders, Philadelphia, 1948.
7. Kolodny, RC: Sexual Dysfunction in diabetic females. *Diabetes* 20: 557, 1971.
8. Schmidt, CW: Biochemical treatment of sexual disorders. In *The Psychiatric Clinics of North America*. W.B. Saunders, Philadelphia, 1980.
9. Small, MP: The Small-Carrion penile prosthesis: Surgical implant for the management of impotence. *Sex Disabil* 1: 282, 1978.
10. Spark, RF, White, RA, and Connolly, PB: Impotence is not always psychogenic: Newer insights into hypothalamic-pituitary-gonadal dysfunction. *JAMA* 243: 750, 1980.

CHAPTER EIGHTEEN

Dying, Death and Bereavement

KRIPA S. KASHYAP, M.D.

The family physician traditionally took care of his patients from cradle to death, and when they died, he managed the grief and bereavement of the survivors. This situation has changed dramatically in the last 40 to 50 years, in part because of the mobility of the society, in part because of the increased specialization of physicians. Now, 80% of people come to the hospitals to receive terminal care, which cannot be given at home either because of the specialized nature of the care or because of lack of family resources. Up until 40 or 50 years ago a dying patient stayed at home or returned home from the hospital to be with his family when death was imminent. Death was not a taboo and was openly discussed with the patients and their families. The physician had a major role in managing the moment of death. The role of the primary physician has become somewhat limited as the responsibility of this care has shifted to the hospitals.

During the second half of the 20th century interest in the care of dying patients has steadily grown, stimulated in the last decade by the growth of the hospice movement. It is likely that, because of this interest, the general physician again will be able to manage many dying patients in their own homes.

SOCIOPSYCHOLOGICAL ISSUES

Fear of Death

Man is the only creature known who buries his dead; this he has done since the very dawn of human culture, possibly as far back as 50,000 B.C. Before the 11th century, A.D., life after death was seen as a kind of sleep for an indeterminate period. Death was calmly accepted, without fear. Then the concept of the Last Judgment began to be taken seriously. An awe and fear of death became manifest in art and culture. The image of purgatory, heaven, and hell which preoccupied the mind of medieval man continues to exert its influence on a significant sector of society today.

Although aware that death is his ultimate fate, contemporary man is often incapable of facing his own death. In the unconscious, death is always the death of the other. The fear of death is intricately linked with the facing of the finality of one's being and the separation from one's loved ones. Therefore, it is unusual for a person to reflect upon death unless his own life is threatened or unless a close friend or relative is dying.

Fear of Dying

Fear of dying should not be confused with fear of death. Death is the ultimate moment of the cessation of life, and dying is the process whereby that moment is approached. Fear of dying is actually a combination of fear of death and fear of living in dread of death. Whether a man is dying at home or in a hospital, he cannot escape the agony of dying. Writings of doctors who attended many death beds give vivid descriptions of patients ravaged by pain and disease to such a point that they were either beyond caring or were a foul smelling embarrassment to their family and friends. On the other hand, dying in a hospital's impersonal environment surrounded by machines and by unfamiliar staff cannot be glamorized either. The technology which has given us the knowledge and equipment to prolong life is greatly responsible for "the medicalization of death" which we see today. Death is no longer synonymous with the irreversible loss of consciousness. It is a technical phenomenon obtained by cessation of care based upon the decision of the doctor and the family. The management of a dying patient ends with the onset of irreversible coma—and what is left afterward is management of death. Death has been dissected and seen as a phenomenon of several steps—cessation of consciousness, cessation of breathing, and cessation of brain activity, manifested by a flat electroencephalogram. The fear of dying also involves the dread of protracted death.

The fear of dying is further compounded by the following factors: (a) Helplessness over the hopelessness of the treatment; (b) self-blame and guilt feelings; (c) fear of physical injury, mutilation, and crippled existence; and (d) fear of being abandoned.

A dying person continues to hope for a miraculous recovery; but when the hopelessness of the treatment becomes quite evident, a strange sense of helplessness comes over the patient. He starts blaming himself for not having taken good care of himself. He may also feel guilty over his conduct and may see the terminal illness as some kind of punishment. The fear of physical injury and mutilation from a drastic investigative procedure, chemo-, radio- and/or surgical therapy is not to be discounted. Finally, the fear of a crippled existence and of being left alone to die in isolation away from family, friends, and children is present in the back of the mind of every terminal patient.

Emotional Reactions in the Face of Death

Terminally ill patients often go through a series of five stages in accepting the reality of their impending death (4). The duration of these stages and the intensity with which they are experienced are highly variable from one individual to the next. The stages are:

1. Shock and denial
2. Anger
3. Bargaining
4. Depression
5. Acceptance.

During the *first stage*, when the patient is informed of his diagnosis and poor prognosis, he is usually unable to "hear" it. Some patients may be shocked and surprised temporarily, but a profound sense of disbelief in the physician's pronouncements keeps them calm. They may go from physician to physician to find someone to tell them what they would like to hear—that their condition is not serious. This denial of illness can be best summed up in a phrase—"No, not me." Eventually, all such attempts are deemed to be futile and the patient has to face reality.

During the *stage of anger* the patient is often difficult to deal with. He complains about his care and, as a result, he is often avoided by his family, friends, and physicians. This rejection further increases his rage. He is likely to ask "Why me?" He often feels cheated and envious of others. If a person does not feel guilty and lose his self-esteem, he is likely, after this period of anger, to move on to the stage of bargaining. On the other hand, if he feels that he deserves punishment for his past doings as an explanation of his illness, he is likely to become very depressed. From being very "mad" he moves to being very "sad."

During the *stage of bargaining* the dominant theme is—"Yes, it is me, but. . . . " With the realization of an impending death the patient, in exchange for the prolongation of his life, offers to do things which he did not do before or to live his life differently. A number of patients go through a religious experience, and some of them believe that they are "born again." Often at this stage the patient will look comfortable and peaceful, but that sense of well-being is short-lived. As the illness advances and suffering is compounded, the patient becomes depressed.

During the *stage of depression* the reality of death sinks even deeper. The patient may have already gone through many real (and imagined) losses by this time; e.g., he may have lost a body organ, or he may have missed important events in the life of his family, or he may have lost his job or his savings. Depression at this stage is not so much compounded by anger as it is colored with resignation. The patient begins to separate himself from everyone and everything he loved before. At this time he does not want any false hopes. It is a very private and personal time in his life. He may not want any visitors and may not even say much to his own immediate family members. He wants his family's love, affection, and respect but may not be able to give them anything in return. This stage is very difficult for the family.

Finally, when the patient has finished his business—experienced anger and experienced grief—he moves to the *stage of acceptance.* If the patient has the strong support of his family, he will go through all stages to arrive at this final stage of equanimity characterized by tranquility—where the patient is neither happy nor sad. He may simply say "My time is coming close," "It is all right," or "I am ready," etc.

CARE OF A DYING PERSON

Patients are often quite realistically concerned about the impact of their illness and its expensive treatment on their family. The dying person needs to know that he is loved and will always be loved and missed, but at this stage he should not be told how much he is needed for the survival of the family.

Clearly a general physician may see a terminal patient at any moment in the course of the illness, e.g., he may himself diagnose the patient and inform him of the poor prognosis; or he may become involved in the care after the diagnosis has been made at a hospital and the patient has been sent home (or to a hospice) to receive terminal care. In order to provide excellent care for a terminally ill patient, the physician should know his patient as a person. The physician should make a determination not only of the stage of the terminal illness, but also of the patient's psychological stage of accepting impending death (see above). Terminally ill patients' needs differ widely, and every effort should be made to provide care which is adapted to these unique needs.

Often terminally ill patients receive attention during the early stages of their illness, when the diagnosis is first made, but unfortunately attention wanes as their disease progresses. The stages of denial, anger, and depression often cause a withdrawal of family, friends, and physicians which establishes a vicious cycle; i.e., the more the patients are ignored, the more unmanageable and inaccessible they become. For these reasons, the most important principle of the care of a terminal patient is to maintain a *consistency* of involvement. The physician should plan regular contacts with the patient, either by scheduling office visits or making visits to the home. The patient must be reassured that he will continue to get adequate medication to relieve his pain and suffering. However, the most important thing about the continued and consistent involvement in the care of a dying person is that the physician's continued presence gives dignity to the dying person. The patient continues to feel like a *person* till the very end.

Communication

COMMUNICATION OF DIAGNOSIS, TREATMENT PLAN, AND PROGNOSIS

People have different opinions about the need and importance of communication of the diagnosis, treatment plan, and prognosis of terminal patients. A common practice in the past has been to maintain a conspiracy of silence where the physician in collusion with the family members actively has covered up the diagnosis of a terminal illness in order to "protect" the dying man from emotional shock. This practice is now recognized usually to be wrong. Honesty and sincerity in dealing with terminally ill patients make effective management possible. Although patients may get temporarily upset in the beginning, they appreciate the truth in the long run. Moreover, it is then easier for their families to relate to them in an open and honest manner. Families participating in a conspiracy of silence have greater emotional difficulties than do families in situations where truth has prevailed. Occasionally, a patient will indicate that he does not want to know the unpleasant truth; in that case, the physician should respect the patient's wish. However, invariably these patients come to know the nature of their illness even if it has not been expressed to them.

When the physician is ready to discuss the diagnosis and expected course of the illness with his terminally ill patient, he should sit down with the patient and his family in a private place. He should avoid lengthy introductions. He should be precise and concise and should not be hurried. It is important that he pay attention to the emotional reactions of the patient and of the family members. He should also pledge that he will do whatever can be done to reduce suffering as much as possible, and should affirm that he will be involved and supportive to the very end. A majority of patients "do not hear" the bad news when it is first delivered and must be told the truth in small doses in the course of several interviews.

COMMUNICATION OF POSITIVE ATTITUDES OF CARE GIVERS

More important than all the kind words of the physician is the nonverbal message the dying person gets from his caregivers. It is extremely important that the physician and his staff continue to maintain positive and consistent attitudes toward the patient. Genuine *concern* should be visible in both words and deeds as well as *equanimity* on the part of the caregivers, which is often the most reassuring element in the care of the terminally ill. It not only reduces the patient's anxiety, but also makes it easier for him to express his feelings and to ask questions without worrying about the physician's emotional state. It makes honest communication possible.

Special Concerns

RELIEF FROM PAIN

A very basic principle in the care of a terminally ill person is to provide adequate relief of pain. This often requires the administration of narcotics, and because of the physician's fear of inducing addiction, patients may receive doses that are too small or too infrequent to relieve pain adequately. Physicians should be aware that the risk of addiction, in this setting, is slight.

Important considerations in selecting medication for pain are effectiveness, route of administration (e.g., the cachectic patient may have few sites for injections), available forms for oral administration (e.g., some patients may be able to take only liquids easily), and duration of pain relief. Table 18.1 summarizes practical information about a number of narcotics which are used in controlling pain. The synthetic narcotics may cause less nausea and constipation than morphine; however, they may also produce less euphoria than morphine at equivalent analgesic doses. Because of the problem of oversedation and respiratory suppression, it is unwise to use multiple narcotics simultaneously. If one agent is not providing adequate relief, another should be substituted for, not added to, that agent.

Phenothiazines such as fluphenazine 2 to 10 mg daily (see Chapter 15), and tricyclic antidepressants, such as amitriptyline 25 to 100 mg daily (see Chapter 14), used alone or in combination, may provide significant relief from the anxiety and depression accompanying intractable pain; and at times these drugs may diminish the patient's need for narcotic analgesics. Antihistamines may be useful in this situation also, as noted below.

Table 18.1
Selected Drugs for Treating Pain

Constituents	Trade Name	Available Preparations	Usual Dose Range[a]	Peak Effect (hr)	Duration (hr)[f]	Federal Narcotic Schedule
		MODERATELY POTENT				
Codeine sulfate		Tablets 30, 60 mg Injectable 10 mg/5 ml	30–60 mg	2	3–4	II
Codeine-acetaminophen[b]	Tylenol #3	Tablets (30 mg codeine)	1–2 tablets	2	3–4	III
	Tylenol #4	Tablets (60 mg codeine)	1 tablet	2	3–4	
		Elixir (12 mg codeine/5 ml)	15–30 ml			
Oxycodone[c]-aspirin-phenacetin-caffeine	Percodan	Tablets	1–2 tablets	1	3–4	II
Oxycodone[c]-acetaminophen[d]	Tylox	Capsules	1–2 capsules	1	3–4	II
		MOST POTENT				
Morphine sulfate[a]	—	Injectable 10 mg/ml	10–15 mg	1	3–4	II
Methadone[c, f]	Dolophine	Tablets 5, 10 mg Injectable 10 mg/ml	2.5–20 mg	2	4–5	II
Meperidine[c]	Demerol	Tablets 50, 100 mg Syrup 50 mg/5 ml	50–300 mg	2	3–4	II
		Injectable 25 mg/ml 50 mg/ml 75 mg/ml 100 mg/ml	50–100 mg	1	2–4	
Hydromorphone[c]	Dilaudid	Tablets 1, 2, 3, 4 mg	2–8 mg	1	3–4	II
		Suppository 3 mg Injectable 1 mg/ml 2 mg/ml 3 mg/ml 4 mg/ml	1–2 mg	½	3	
Levorphanol[c, f]	Levo-Dromoran	Tablets 2 mg	2–4 mg	2	4–5	II
		Injectable 2 mg/ml	1–2 mg	1	4–5	
Pentazocine[e]	Talwin	Tablet 50 mg	50–150 mg	1		IV
		Injectable 30 mg/2 ml 45 mg/2 ml 60 mg/2 ml	30–60 mg	1	3–4	

[a] Higher doses needed in patients who develop tolerance.
[b] Each tablet contains 300 mg acetaminophen.
[c] Synthetic.
[d] Each capsule contains 500 mg acetaminophen.
[e] A weak narcotic antagonist, may block analgesic effect of simultaneously administered narcotic and may cause abstinence reaction in patient dependent on narcotics.
[f] The plasma half-life of methadone and levorphanol is long (≥ 15 hr) and cumulative effects may occur with continual use of these drugs.

Brompton's mixture, first developed at Brompton Hospital in England, has proved to be useful in treating patients dying of cancer who require analgesia. The preparation, as it is made in this country, contains morphine, prochlorperazine (Compazine), and usually, cocaine. Morphine is relatively long acting when given orally in comparison to other popular narcotics (*i.e.*, meperidine (Demerol), and prochlorperazine reduces somewhat the incidence of anxiety and of nausea and vomiting. Cocaine has been included because it produces euphoria; but tachyphylaxis develops rapidly; and it is not at all clear therefore that it is a necessary ingredient in the mixture. A standard dose of Brompton's is 20 ml every 3 to 4 hr; that amount usually contains 10 mg of morphine, 5 mg of prochlorperazine, and 5 mg of cocaine. It is important, for optimum results, that the mixture be given routinely and not "as necessary."

RELIEF FROM ANXIETY

The physician's concern and accessibility may be all that are necessary to relieve the anxiety of the dying patient. *Tranquilizers* also can be of some help in the management of these patients. Commonly prescribed tranquilizers belong to the benzodiazapine group; their use for the control of anxiety is described in detail in Chapter 12. When insomia is also a major problem, diazepam (Valium), 10 mg, or flurazepam (Dalmane), 30 mg, can be used to induce sleep. Hydroxyzine (Atarax, Vistaril) another important minor tranquilizer, has a number of properties which may make it more beneficial than any of the benzodiazapines (1). It has not only sedative but has antispasmodic, antiemetic, and (when given intramuscularly) analgesic effects. In this regard, hydroxyzine has advantages over phenothiazines, which are not analgesic and which may produce hypotension. Hydroxyzine, 25 to 50 mg by mouth, three times daily is often prescribed to patients who have anxiety as the result of prolonged pain.

RELIEF FROM DEPRESSION

Most of the patients go through the depressive stage without requiring antidepressant medications; although periodically some may require antianxiety medications. The family's and the physician's support is most therapeutic for this kind of depression. Some patients develop severe depression, particularly after a brief stage of anger when they conclude that they are being punished for their sins. Loss of self-esteem, guilt feelings, psychomotor retardation, early morning awakening with a diurnal variation in mood, even suicidal thoughts, may appear in this setting. When five of the eight diagnostic criteria for depression are present (see Chapter 14), tricyclic antidepressants (e.g., amitriptyline (Elavil) 75 mg a day in divided doses) may bring relief. There is a detailed discussion of depression and its treatment in Chapter 14.

GRATIFICATION OF SMALL NEEDS

Removing restrictions from food, alcohol, and cigarettes is not only humane but sensible.

ACCESS TO THE CHILDREN

A dying person has a great need to have access to his children. Likewise, children have a great need to be close to their dying parent. The physician should encourage these necessary contacts.

EMOTIONAL SUPPORT FOR THE FAMILY

The emotional problems of the family of a dying person need attention from the physician. Family members often go through stages of emotional adjustment and have difficulties in accepting the diagnosis and projected course of a terminal illness, just as the patient does. By encouraging honest communication between the patient and his family, the physician can make an important contribution in the care of the dying person. Family members will react differently to the impending death of a person, depending on his age, personality, role and on the status of his relationship with the rest of the family members. To be effective, the physician must be sensitive to these variations and to the needs of individual family members.

The Hospice

In many communities, patients and their families can be cared for by their physician in cooperation with a hospice, a program devised to provide terminal care, including relief of pain, to the dying patient and to provide support to his family. Services are delivered either in the patient's home or in a hospital by a multidisciplinary team under the direction of the physician (see *The Management of Terminal Disease* in the general reference list). A clearing house for information on hospice care in the United States is provided by the National Hospice Organization, 1750 Old Meadow Road, McLean, Virginia, 22102.

THE MANAGEMENT OF GRIEF

If death of a loved one has been unexpected, grief usually begins with an initial stage of shock and disbelief accompanied by a general numbing of all affect. If death has been anticipated, however, this stage is less prominent. There is often a feeling of relief that the dead person's suffering has ended. Soon afterward (within hours to a few days) there is a more demonstrative phase characterized by protest and anguish, often accompanied by tears. These feelings come in waves and may be precipitated by even an indirect reference to the lost person; ordinarily, they do not persist for more than 1 or 2 months. Mourning, however, normally with a slow recovery over a period of a year, is virtually universal. As time passes there often is a preoccupation with memories of the lost person. There may be guilt feelings for not having done enough for the deceased. In some cases, this guilt may be expressed as hostility toward the physician. Bereaved people often have experiences of "seeing" the dead person in a crowd or in some other individual, fleetingly seen, which is then followed by the reality of permanent loss. The bereaved is likely to visit the grave during the first year of loss more frequently than in later years. Sometimes, there is a dramatic change in personality, and the manners and the terminal symptoms of the dying individual are assumed by the bereaved person. This is another way of resolving grief, by attempting to make the lost person a part of the survivor.

Approximately 80% of bereaved people are depressed and have disturbed sleep; and 40% have a poor appetite, weight loss, difficulty in concentrating, and general loss of interest in daily life (2). Depression is especially common in spouses in the middle or later years of their lives. In fact, one-third of this latter group have symptoms which meet the criteria of a diagnosis of a probable affective disorder (Chapter 14) (3). While depression usually lasts for many months, 80% of individuals do show some improvement within 10 weeks (3). However, two-thirds of bereaved spouses at the end of the first year of bereavement continue to have some symptoms of apathy, aimlessness, and a disinclination to look to the future. Only a small fraction of these survivors develop complicated and/or atypical mourning.

The *management of normal grief* during the first year of bereavement has to be individualized by the physician depending on the patient's personal, family, and social background. Patients with only limited psychological insight into their grief process may need medication for the relief of insomnia and anxiety. Flurazepam (Dalmane), 30 mg at bedtime if needed for sleep, and one of the benzodiazapines with a shorter half-life such as oxazepam (Serax), 10 or 15 mg two or three times a day as needed for anxiety, should be considered for 1 to 2 weeks in the management of normal grief. On the other hand, many patients may feel quite satisfied with an empathetic, supportive, and concerned physician. These patients need to be reminded that their grief and its psychophysiological concomitants are normal. This has to be done with special care, acknowledging the irreparable loss while, at the same time, encouraging the bereaved person to pull his life together. The survivors need to be encouraged to lead a full life without feeling guilty. When severe emotional reactions become prolonged, pastoral counseling or psychotherapy may be necessary. Patients with physical symptoms without any clear-cut organic etiology should not be referred to a psychiatrist at first; but they should be seen frequently, examined carefully,

and reassured of their physical health. Extensive diagnostic workups should be avoided as much as possible as they reinforce illness behavior. Furthermore, supportive therapy (see Chapter 10) is more likely to be helpful than is more extensive and complicated psychotherapy. In time, with the completion of their grieving reaction, they will give up their physical symptoms and again become actively engaged in a new life.

During the first year of bereavement special attention should be paid to the patient during holidays, anniversaries, or on other important dates. Some symptoms of acute grief are likely to resurface around these times. Supportive therapy at such times will usually control the symptoms.

The physician is in a good position to detect the early signs of *pathological mourning* when a person either shows no signs of grieving or shows exaggerated features of grieving characterized by excessive and/or prolonged (longer than a year) social isolation, unmoderated guilt or anger, panic attacks, and physical symptoms without any clear-cut organic etiology. In such cases, consultation with a psychiatrist is appropriate to help remove obstacles which have inhibited the mourner from participating in a normal grief reaction (5).

References

General

Bowlby, J: *Separation.* Basic Books, New York, 1973.
  This is the second volume of Bowlby's classic work on attachment and loss, and deals with the issues of anxiety and anger generated in the anticipation of and in the event of separation from a loved one.
Bowlby, J: *Loss.* Basic Books, New York, 1980.
  This is the third and final volume of Bowlby's work on attachment and loss. This is probably the best book ever written on the subject of bereavement.
Kübler-Ross, E: *On Death and Dying.* Macmillan, New York, 1969.
  A classic work on the subject of death and dying.
Saunders, C (ed): *The Management of Terminal Disease.* Year Book, Chicago, 1978.
  This book is an excellent guide to any professional involved in the care of a dying patient; it includes a complete discussion of the hospice concept.

Specific

1. Beaver, WT, and Fleise, G: Comparison of the analgesic effects of morphine, hydroxyzine, and their combination in patients with postoperative pain. In *Advances in Pain Research and Therapy,* Vol. 1, p. 553, edited by JJ Bonica and D Albe-Fessard. Raven Press, New York, 1976.
2. Clayton, PJ, Halikas JA, and Maurice, WL: The bereavement of the widowed. *Dis Nerv Syst* 32: 597, 1971.
3. Clayton, PJ, Halikas JA, and Maurice, WL: The depression of widowhood. *Br J Psychiatry* 120: 71, 1972.
4. Kübler-Ross, E. *On Death and Dying,* Chap. 3-7. Macmillan, New York, 1969.
5. Melges, FT, and DeMaso, DR: Grief-resolution therapy: relieving, revising, and revisiting. *Am J Psychother* 34: 51, 1980.

CHAPTER NINETEEN

Tobacco Use and Dependence*

GEORGE E. BIGELOW, Ph.D., and MAXINE L. STITZER, Ph.D.

Cigarette smoking is the most pernicious of the substance use disorders, representing the single greatest preventable cause of chronic illness in the United States. The perniciousness of the habit relates primarily to the broad social acceptability of smoking and to the general failure to recognize and react to smoking as an activity with significant consequences for health. Physicians will encounter problems with the use of tobacco in their patients principally under two circumstances: (a) self-motivated patients who request aid or advice in quitting smoking or in managing the tobacco abstinence syndrome, and (b) relatively unmotivated patients who are seen by the physician for medical reasons and are recognized as having a smoking habit which increases their risk of illness.

ETIOLOGY

The determinants of tobacco dependence are uncertain. The smoking habit is so widespread that it defies substantial correlation with major environmental and physiological factors. Smoking typically begins in the teenage years or in early adulthood. It appears that social influences are a major factor in sustaining initial smoking experiences. The aversive properties of those experiences (coughing, choking, dysphoric effects) are described even by individuals who subsequently develop into chronic dependent smokers. Nicotine is generally presumed to be the pharmacologically active ingredient which maintains

tobacco smoking, but the evidence on this issue remains equivocal (7, 14).

Whatever the factors that sustain smoking through the period of initial exposure, those individuals who persist are highly likely to become chronic dependent smokers. There is no personality type which is characteristic of smokers, but on the average they tend to be somewhat more extroverted than nonsmokers, and to be somewhat more likely to be adventuresome or risk-taking and to deviate from social norms or rules.

Cigarette smoking runs in families, and this is generally thought to be due to social modeling. An individual with parents and siblings who smoke is 4 times as likely to become a smoker than is a comparable individual from a nonsmoking family. The possibility of genetic or physiological predisposing factors has received little study.

RECOGNITION AND DIAGNOSIS

Only infrequently will patients present with the primary complaint of tobacco dependence, although certainly a small number of patients will initiate requests for advice on how to stop smoking from their physicians. In such cases the physician may generally rely upon patients' reports of the extent of their smoking habit. In cases where there is less motivation, it is wise not to rely completely upon a patient's negative response to the question "Do you smoke?"; some patients, especially those who recognize the ill effects of smoking, will "quit" a few hours or perhaps a day before their appointments. More revealing questions are "Have you ever been a smoker?" and "When did you last have a cigarette?" Under some conditions it may be desirable to assess smoking/nonsmoking status by an objective biological assay. The two most widely used biological procedures are the measurement of thiocyanate levels in blood, urine, or saliva, or of carbon monoxide levels in blood or expired breath. Although neither of these assays is yet routine in medical practice, devices which assay breath carbon monoxide levels and which are suitable for office use are currently available and are widely employed in smoking cessation programs (2). The importance of objective assessment of smoking status is indicated by the fact that up to 20 to 30% of self-reported quitters may show biological evidence that they have continued smoking (9).

* Preparation supported in part by USPHS Research Scientist Development Award DA-00050 and by research grant DA-02599.

COURSE OF THE HABIT

Until recently, the typical course of the habit was one of relatively unabated chronic smoking from the time of initiation throughout the remainder of the smoker's life. In more recent years, as the health hazards of smoking have become more widely recognized and as the social acceptability of smoking has declined, there has been a growing tendency for smokers to discontinue the habit. Now, in the United States there are nearly as many former smokers (approximately 30 million) as there are current smokers (approximately 50 million). Over one-half of current smokers report having made at least one serious attempt to stop smoking, and about 90% of smokers say they would like to quit if there were an easy method to do so. About 30% of smokers report they have made an active attempt to stop smoking within the preceding year. Approximately 60 to 80% of smokers who attempt to quit achieve at least a minimal period of abstinence. However, the relapse rate is high, and approximately two-thirds of quitters resume smoking within 3 to 6 months, often within only a few days. Thus, approximately 15 to 20% of quitters remain cigarette-free for 6 months or more. The probability of relapse following 6 to 12 months of abstinence is relatively small. The vast majority of people who stop smoking permanently do so without formal treatment. Although perhaps half of a population of smokers will indicate an interest in formal programs to help them stop smoking, typically fewer than 10% of them will actually attend a treatment session even when it is conveniently available. Structured cessation programs are, at best, only slightly more successful than self-directed cessation efforts, with approximately 15 to 30% of those enrolled for treatment sustaining long term abstinence.

HEALTH CONSEQUENCES

Risk of Disease

Although smoking increases morbidity and mortality, its effects are unpredictable, and some smokers will escape major health consequences. The overall mortality ratio for all smokers relative to nonsmokers is 1.7; the mortality ratio for the two-pack-a-day smoker is 2.0. Life expectancy is shortened by smoking; it is 8.1 years less for the 30-year-old, two-pack-a-day, smoker than for a comparable nonsmoker. Risk is apparently dose-related, in that it increases with increasing number of cigarettes smoked, with increasing number of years of smoking, with depth of inhalation, and with increasing yield of tar and nicotine of the cigarettes smoked. Smoking is associated with increased risk of cancer (especially of the respiratory tract), cardiovascular disease, chronic obstructive pulmonary disease, and gastric ulcer. Smoking by pregnant women reduces fetal growth, and therefore birth weight, and increases the risk of fetal death; smoking interacts with the use of oral contraceptives by women and increases their risk of myo-

cardial infarction and of subarachnoid hemorrhage. It appears that, in general, smoking cessation results in a decrease in the risk of illness. For example, individuals who stop smoking after myocardial infarction show improved survival rates compared to those who continue smoking (13). Improvements in health are greater for those smokers who quit before the development of symptoms.

Abstinence Syndrome

Upon cessation of smoking, an abstinence syndrome may occur. Physiologically, the tobacco abstinence syndrome is generally inconsequential, consisting of a gradual decline in heart rate and blood pressure. However, the subjective aspects of the syndrome can be very distressing to patients. Symptoms can include irritability, restlessness, sleep disturbances, difficulty in concentrating, anxiety, gastrointestinal disturbances, hunger, weight gain, and, most important, craving for cigarettes (3). Relatively little is known about the nature and course of the tobacco abstinence syndrome, but it appears that patients feel normal again within 1 to 2 weeks of abstinence, except that craving for tobacco may persist for many months (12). There is no commonly accepted treatment for the tobacco abstinence syndrome. Certain characteristics of the syndrome appear to be reactions to nicotine withdrawal and are ameliorated by nicotine administration in experimental studies; however, nicotine administration is not appropriate clinically. It is widely believed, although uncertain at this time, that many aspects of the tobacco abstinence syndrome (especially craving) are not pharmacologically based, but are reactions to the discontinuation of a strongly ingrained habitual behavior. Since the specific signs and symptoms of the abstinence syndrome are quite variable there is no treatment which can be recommended *a priori*. The practitioner may consider symptomatic treatment of those specific problems which arise with each individual patient, but in doing so should weigh the risks and benefits of any therapy against the expected short duration of the tobacco abstinence syndrome.

Passive Smoking

The effects of passive smoking—exposure of nonsmokers to air contaminated by the smoking of others—are not clear at this time, although such exposure is certainly an irritant to many nonsmokers. Young children of smoking parents are more likely to experience respiratory infections than are children of nonsmokers (1), and nonsmokers passively exposed in the workplace show reduction in small airways function (15); the long term relevance to health of these relationships has yet to be determined.

TREATMENT

Role of the Physician

Since most people who stop smoking do so by their own efforts rather than by formal treatment, it is important for the physician to persuade his patients of the importance of stopping. Physicians are in a uniquely effective position to do this. A major reason that patients stop smoking is concern about their health, and smokers cite physicians as the individuals most able to influence their decisions to attempt to stop. The appearance of specific smoking-related health symptoms often serves as the stimulus for efforts to break the smoking habit. Yet few smokers (25% or less) report ever being advised by their physician to stop smoking (9).

The physician has a uniquely persuasive position as an authority figure but has no medically specific skills, techniques, or remedies to offer the smoker who is attempting to quit; he must rely totally upon the patient's disposition to comply with medical advice. It is the physician's responsibility to provide *persuasive advice*. This advice should not rely totally upon fear arousal, but should: (a) point out the association between smoking and the specific symptoms, illnesses, or health risks of the individual patient; (b) point out that stopping smoking can prevent, reverse, or stop the progression of disease (whichever is appropriate); and (c) state clearly and simply the course of action to be taken by the patient. Often, the general statement that "Smoking is bad for your health and you can kill yourself if you continue" is not perceived by patients as an instruction to stop. A more personalized and directive statement can be more persuasive; for example: "I strongly advise you to stop smoking. Especially for people like you who use oral contraceptives the risk of cardiovascular disease or stroke is very substantially increased by smoking"; or, "Your coughing is caused in part by your smoking; I want you to try to give up cigarettes and then we should see some improvement."

It is useful to give patients some brief *printed material* describing techniques of stopping smoking. A variety of such printed materials is available as aids to physicians and can be obtained by contacting local offices of the American Heart Association, American Lung Association, or American Cancer Society, or by contacting the U.S. Public Health Service's Office of Cancer Communications (phone (301) 496-6641) or National Clearinghouse for Smoking and Health (phone (404) 633-3311). The table of contents of the most helpful pamphlet, "Calling it Quits," is shown in Table 19.1. Table 19.2 contains the instructions for a simple 4-week program recommended in this pamphlet. More extensive information is contained in two paperback books which can be recommended to motivated patients (O. F. Pomerleau and C. S. Pomerleau, *Break the Smoking Habit: A Behavioral Program for Giving Up Cigarettes*, Research Press, Champaign, Illinois, 1977; B. G. Danaher and E. Lichtenstein, *Become an Ex-Smoker*, Prentice Hall, Engelwood Cliffs, New Jersey, 1978). All of these published materials are based upon the behavioral principles developed in the most successful formal treatment programs (see below). For patients who will not or cannot utilize written materials the phy-

Table 19.1

Table of Contents of the Pamphlet "Calling It Quits, the Latest Advice on How to Give up Smoking" [a]

An Open Letter From Your Physician	2
When Thinking About Quitting	4
Involve Someone Else	6
Switch Brands	8
Cut Down	10
Just Before Quitting	14
On The Day You Quit	16
Immediately After Quitting	18
Avoid Temptation	20
Find New Habits	22
When You Get The Crazies	24
Marking Progress	26
About Gaining Weight	28
One Popular Four-Week Program	30
Seeking Professional Help	31
When You Have Called It Quits	34
Other Sources Of Information On Quitting	36

[a] Available from the Office of Cancer Communications, Bethesda, Maryland (1979).

Table 19.2

A 4-Week Program Contained in the Pamphlet "Calling It Quits" [a]

These self-help suggestions can be combined into a variety of programs to meet your needs. One popular four-week quitting program is outlined below.

First week: List the positive reasons you want to quit smoking, and read the list daily. Wrap your cigarette pack with paper and rubber bands. Each time you smoke, write down the time of day, what you are doing, how you are feeling, and how important that cigarette is to you on a scale from 1 to 5. Then rewrap the pack.

Second week: Keep reading your list of reasons, and add to it if possible. Don't carry matches, and keep your cigarettes some distance away. Each day, try to smoke fewer cigarettes, eliminating those least or most important (whichever works best).

Third week: Continue with the second week's instructions. Don't buy a new pack until you finish the one you're smoking and never buy a carton. Change brands twice during the week, each time choosing a brand lower in tar and nicotine. Try to stop smoking for 48 hours sometime during the week.

Fourth week: Quit smoking entirely. Increase your physical activity. Avoid situations you most closely associate with smoking. Find a substitute for cigarettes. Do deep breathing exercises whenever you get the urge to smoke.

[a] Pamphlet available from the Office of Cancer Communications, Bethesda, Maryland (1979).

sician should advise that they pick a specific date within the next 3 weeks which will be their personal target date for stopping smoking.

Because the risks of smoking are dose-related, it is reasonable to advise patients that, even in the absence of total cessation, risks are decreased by *reducing the amount of smoking*. If patients do smoke

Table 19.3
Characteristics of Formal Smoking Cessation Programs in the United States[a]

Formal Programs	Brief Description	Duration	Cost[b]
GROUP CLINICS			
America Cancer Society (ACS) American Heart Assoc. (AHA) American Lung Assoc. (ALA)	Physicians, psychiatrists, therapists and ex-smokers provide volunteer services. Positive reinforcement and group interaction are stressed. Participants number 8–18	ACS groups meet approximately 2 hr, twice a week, for 4 weeks. ALA groups meet for 1½ hr, twice a month, for an indefinite period of time	No fee or minimal fee
SmokEnders	Programs are offered in approximately 30 cities. The moderator is an ex-smoker and SmokEnder graduate. The course features a gradual reduction in smoking over the first 5 weeks, followed by 4 weeks of reinforcement after the quit date	SmokEnder participants attend 9 weekly meetings of 2 hr each. Reunions and other reinforcement contacts are provided after the last meeting	Average cost $175 per program
FIVE-DAY PLANS			
Seventh Day Adventist Church	Programs usually include lectures, inspirational messages, films, and group interaction. Some use scare tactics and aversion therapy. Participants are urged to keep personal records, force fluids, Ostay in frequent contact with "buddies," avoid alcohol, caffeine, other smokers, and tension-causing situations. Special diets and exercise programs are often recommended	One and a half to 2 hr for 5 consecutive days	$3.00 to $10.00
Schick Laboratories	Programs are available at 22 cessation centers. Aversion therapy is stressed, which includes methods such as overexposure to smoke, rapid smoking and electric shock applied to the participant's arm	One hour for 5 consecutive days	$450 with a money-back guarantee
FIVE-DAY LIVE-IN PROGRAM			
Seventh Day Adventist Church	At St. Helena Hospital and Health Center in Deer Park, Calif. Individual and group counselling, lectures, films, physical therapy and exercise	One week	$395 which covers room and board, tests, etc.
GRADUATED FILTERS			
Venturi Five-Week Stop Smoking System	Consists of four reusable filters which are reported to reduce tar and nicotine by 95% in the fourth filter	Each filter is used for 1 week	$4.00
Waterpik One Step At A Time	Consists of four reusable filters; reported to reduce tar and nicotine by 90%	Filters are used for 2 weeks	$10.00
Nu-Life Stop Smoking Kit	Consists of 44 disposable filters which are reported to gradually remove up to 96% of cigarette tar and 88% of nicotine	One filter is to be used each day	$10.00
Aqua-Filter	Unlike the other filters, Aqua-Filter makes no claim that its product will assist in gradual smoking withdrawal. The filters are sold 10 to a package and are supposed to eliminate all but an average of 3.15 mg of tar and 0.22 mg of nicotine from each cigarette	Each filter is to be used for 20 cigarettes.	$1.00

[a] Source: "Calling It Quits," Pamphlet available from the Office of Cancer Communications, Bethesda, Maryland (1979).
[b] Costs shown are based on 1979.

fewer cigarettes, they should be cautioned not to increase the number of puffs per cigarette or the depth of inhalation, which results in continued high exposure. Epidemiological data generally indicate that overall risks are lower among individuals smoking so-called "low tar, low nicotine" cigarettes. However, it is not clear at this time whether there is uniformly any benefit to be gained from advising smokers to change to cigarette brands yielding less tar and nicotine. There are several reasons for this. First, it is clear that many smokers who make such a change tend also to change the amount they smoke or the frequency, depth, or duration of inhalation in a compensatory fashion such that they do not reduce their actual exposure appreciably. Second, many so-called low yield cigarettes actually have higher yields of carbon monoxide than do high tar and nicotine cigarettes, and carbon monoxide appears to be one of the smoke constituents related to certain undesirable effects (e.g., impairment of fetal growth and provocation of angina pectoris). The Federal Trade Commission plans to begin publishing data on the carbon monoxide yields of different cigarette brands which, in addition to the currently available data on tar and nicotine yields, may aid in making decisions about brand-switching. Third, biological yield may differ substantially from the published yield. Physicians and patients should understand that these published yields are not the "dosages" delivered by the cigarettes; the yields represent the delivery during standardized machine puffing assays (4, 6). They do not represent either the content of the cigarette or the amount delivered to a smoker. The delivery to the smoker depends upon how the individual smokes. With the recently introduced very low yield cigarettes which utilize ventilated filters to dilute the smoke, it is especially likely that biological delivery will significantly exceed assay delivery since there is partial blocking of the ventilation holes by the smoker (5).

The *outcome of counseling* by physicians varies widely depending upon characteristics of both the patient and the intervention. In unselected general practice, physicians' advice to stop smoking may yield 5 to 25% long term abstinence (9, 11). In patients with specific illnesses the success rate may be much higher; for example, after a first myocardial infarction, simple routine advice to stop smoking will yield 50 to 60% long term abstinence (9).

Organized Treatment

Formal programs (see Table 19.3) to teach people to stop smoking are often available locally at little or no cost through the American Cancer Society, the American Heart Association, the American Lung Association, or the Seventh Day Adventist Church. Commercially available programs such as Smok-Enders appear to be somewhat more comprehensive; however they are more costly and require greater investment of time on the part of the patient. There is little difference in outcome among treatment programs. Most such programs have now incorporated the behavioral principles which have been characteristic of the most successful treatments (self-monitoring, analysis of environmental stimulus factors, and scheduling of rewards).

People who want to stop smoking are often tempted by one of the many fads that advertise effective treatment. In the absence of any established and clearly effective technique one should not denigrate innovations which at least sustain the motivation of some smokers to attempt to abstain. Smokers should, however, be cautioned against excessively costly involvements and against the expectation of any "magic cure" requiring no personal motivation and effort.

Prevention

Given the limited effectiveness of treatment designed to help people stop smoking, *prevention* is clearly most desirable. The prevalence of smoking among adolescent males has been declining in recent years; this is not so for females, who are now as likely to smoke as males. Some progress is being made in developing preventive interventions for preadolescents. These typically involve school-based instruction and practice in resisting social pressures to smoke (8, 10). While these interventions show promise, their active components and long term efficacy are not yet clear.

References

General

U.S. Public Health Service. Smoking and Health: A Report of the Surgeon General. DHEW Publication No. (PHS) 79-50066. U.S. Government Printing Office, Washington, D.C., 1979.
> *The most comprehensive compilation and review of biomedical and behavioral data available.*

Jarvik, ME, Cullen, JW, Gritz, ER, Vogt, TM, and West, LJ (eds): Research on Smoking Behavior. National Institute on Drug Abuse Research Monograph Series No. 17, DHEW Publication No. (ADM) 78-581. U.S. Government Printing Office, Washington, D.C., 1978.
> *Conference proceedings, organized under the topics of epidemiology, etiology, consequences, and behavior change.*

Krasnegor, NA (ed): The Behavioral Aspects of Smoking. National Institute on Drug Abuse Research Monograph Series No. 26, DHEW Publication No. (ADM) 79-882. U.S. Government Printing Office, Washington, D.C., 1979.
> *A discussion of biological, behavioral, and psychosocial issues related to development, treatment, and prevention of the smoking habit.*

Specific

1. Colley, JR, Holland, WW, and Corkhill, RT: Influence of passive smoking and parental phlegm on pneumonia and bronchitis in early childhood. *Lancet* 2: 1031, 1974.
2. Horan, JJ, Hackett, G, and Linberg, SE: Factors to consider when using expired air carbon monoxide in smoking assessment. *Addict Behav* 3: 25, 1978.
3. Jarvik, ME: Biological influences on cigarette smoking. In: The Behavioral Aspects of Smoking. (NIDA Research Monograph Series No. 26, N Krasnegor (ed), pp. 7–45, DHEW Publication

No. (ADM) 79-882). U.S. Government Printing Office, Washington, D.C., 1979.

4. Kozlowski, LT: Tar and nicotine delivery of cigarettes: What a difference a puff makes. *JAMA, 245:* 158, 1981.

5. Kozlowski, LT, Frecker, RC, Khouw, V, and Pope, MA: The misuse of "less-hazardous" cigarettes and its detection: Hole-blocking of ventilated filters. *Am J Public Health 70:* 1202, 1980.

6. Kozlowski, LT, Rickert, WS, Robinson, JC, and Grunberg, NE: Have tar and nicotine yields of cigarettes changed? *Science 209:* 1550, 1980.

7. Kumar, R, Cooke, EC, Lader, MH, and Russell, MAH: Is nicotine important to tobacco smoking? *Clin Pharmacol Ther 21:* 520, 1977.

8. McAlister, A, Perry, C, Killen, J, Slinkard, LA, and Maccoby, N: Pilot study of smoking, alcohol and drug abuse prevention. *Am J Public Health 70:* 719, 1980.

9. Pechacek, TF: Modification of smoking behavior. In: The Behavioral Aspects of Smoking. (NIDA Research Monograph Series No. 26, pp. 127–188, edited by N Krasnegor, DHEW Publication No. (ADM) 79-882). U.S. Government Printing Office, Washington, D.C., 1979.

10. Perry, C, Killen, J, Telch, M, Slinkard, LA, and Danaher, BG:

Modifying smoking behavior of teenagers: A school-based intervention. *Am J Public Health 70:* 722, 1980.

11. Russell, MAH: Smoking problems: An overview. In: Research on Smoking Behavior. (NIDA Research Monograph Series No. 17, pp. 13–34, edited by ME Jarvik, JW Cullen, ER Gritz, TM Vogt, and LJ West, DHEW Publication No. (ADM) 78-581. U.S. Government Printing Office, Washington, D.C., 1977.

12. Shiffman, S.M: The tobacco withdrawal syndrome. In: Cigarette Smoking as a Dependence Process. (NIDA Research Monograph Series No. 23, pp. 158–184, edited by N Krasnegor, DHEW Publication No. (ADM) 79-800). U.S. Government Printing Office, Washington, D.C., 1979.

13. Sparrow, D, Dawber, TR, and Colton, T: The influence of cigarette smoking on prognosis after a first myocardial infarction. *J Chron Dis 31:* 425, 1978.

14. Sutton, SR, Feyerabend, C, Cole, PV, and Russell, MAH: Adjustment of smokers to dilution of tobacco smoke by ventilated cigarette holders. *Clin Pharmacol Ther 24:* 395, 1978.

15. White, JR, and Froeb, HF: Small-airways dysfunction in non-smokers chronically exposed to tobacco smoke. *N Engl J Med 302:* 720, 1980.

CHAPTER TWENTY

Alcohol Intoxication and Alcoholism

IRA LIEBSON, M.D.

Alcoholism, defined as excessive drinking to the point of behavioral or physiological toxicity, afflicts from 5 to 10% of adult males and 2 to 5% of adult females in the United States. The prevalence of alcoholism in a medical practice will vary depending on the population served, but it is likely to be substantially higher than among the general population. There has recently been increased drinking by adolescents and females, and by assimilating ethnic groups in which excessive use of alcohol has traditionally been proscribed. The disorder runs a variable course. At one extreme heavy drinking begins abruptly in adolescence and continues unremittingly, often associated with delinquency in youth and psychopathy in adult life. At the other extreme, and with a much better prognosis, is an apparently "reactive" type of alcoholism, beginning gradually in midlife, often associated with depression, and involving extended periods of abstinence or controlled use. When evaluating therapeutic claims and giving prognoses it is important to keep in mind that in general alcoholism is characterized by a high rate of spontaneous remission, particularly if remission is defined as the resumption of moderate drinking patterns as well as the complete avoidance of alcohol.

Alcoholic beverages can be divided into nondistilled (wine and beer) and distilled varieties. The concentration of alcohol in wine ranges from 10 to 22% by volume and is 12 to 14% in most wines. Beer usually contains 4 to 5% alcohol by volume. The distilled alcoholic beverages are whiskey, brandy, rum, gin, and vodka. Alcoholic fermentation ceases when the concentration of alcohol exceeds 15% by volume, and, therefore, to manufacture more potent beverages distillation is necessary. In the United States, the word "proof" is preceded by a number which is double the percentage of alcohol by volume: thus 90 proof whiskey contains 45% alcohol by volume.

ETIOLOGY

The cause of alcoholism is largely unknown. The disorder runs in families, and this appears to be a function of both genetic transmission and environmental influence. Cross-adoption and twin studies have demonstrated a small but significant genetic component (2), and family studies have revealed familial alcoholism to be associated with criminality and sociopathy amongst nonalcoholic male relatives and with depression in nonalcoholic females. The importance of social and environmental factors is suggested by the normal, or unimodal, distribution of consumption in the population. Thus to the extent that a society supports drinking by its members, there will be more drinking overall, more heavy drinking, and more alcoholism. Groups may foster or proscribe drinking in subtle ways, and this probably accounts for differences in consumption and in rates of alcoholism among various ethnic groups. Not surprisingly specific actions taken by societies to enhance the availability of alcohol, such as lowering the drinking age or making alcohol available at a low price, have resulted in increased drinking in general, and an increased incidence of alcoholism (5).

Psychological theories about the etiology of alcoholism seem to be as numerous as the reasons patients give for their drinking, and are probably just as valid. People seldom know why they behave as they do, but giving a reason for behavior appears to provide comfort. Explaining drinking can also serve to excuse or justify it and may placate the alcoholic's victims or gratify his therapist. When queried by a nonjudgmental physician, however, who keeps his preconceptions about etiology to a minimum, the alcoholic is likely to acknowledge that he has in fact only the foggiest notion of why he drinks. In particular, the tension-reduction hypothesis of addictive drinking has not proved fruitful; although normal drinking may give one a lift, a frequent finding in studies of pathological drinking is that, as with excessive use of other mind-altering drugs, increased use leads to dysphoria. There is no one alcoholic personality type, although impulsive and aggressive people are highly represented among alcoholics. Depression is common, both as an apparent precipitant of drinking and as a consequence; alcoholics have a suicide rate that is 6 times the average, and are particularly at risk while intoxicated.

RECOGNITION AND DIAGNOSIS

All patients should be asked about their drinking, and a nonjudgmental inquiry will be most productive. The physician should not ask merely "Do you drink?" or "How much do you drink?" A detailed inquiry is much more likely to yield significant information about pathological quantities and modes of alcohol consumption. Thus it is useful to ask not only how much, but specifically what beverages are drunk, and when and why they are used. The physician should be aware that severe alcoholism need not present with features of a skid-row adjustment or with physical signs, and he should not assume that alcoholism is not a significant problem among women, adolescents, or elderly individuals. The physician's suspicions should be aroused by the presence of illnesses known to be correlated with drinking and by requests for sedative-hypnotic drugs and antacids. An "alcoholic" odor to the breath during a visit to the doctor's office almost always indicates pathological drinking, and aromatic breath mints are suspicious. A history of difficulty in driving and other accidents, unexplained work absences, domestic discord, tremulousness, or blackouts (memory lacunae) all suggest problem drinking.

BEHAVIORAL COMPLICATIONS

Alcohol Intoxication

The best known acute consequence of alcoholism is alcohol intoxication, which should usually present no diagnostic problem. But just because this condition is so common, diagnostic errors are made when the physician forgets that "drunken behavior"—often with evidence of recent alcohol use—may be caused by a host of conditions, such as infection, metabolic disturbance, neurological disease, or other drug toxicity. Because the alcoholic is especially prone to many disorders that may be manifested as deranged behavior, he should be examined conscientiously before a diagnosis of simple drunkenness is made.

Alcohol intoxication may be characterized by aggressiveness, impaired functioning, paranoia, slurred speech, cerebellar gait, nystagmus, incoordination, loquacity, irritability, euphoria, and depression. "Blackouts," amnesia for events that occurred during the period of intoxication, are common. An initial period of excitement and euphoria is often followed by depression and sleep, or possibly coma. The duration and magnitude of the intoxication depend on dose, the rapidity with which the alcohol was drunk, and on whether the patient drank on an empty stomach (enhancing the rate of absorption). Tolerance is also a significant factor; ethanol is normally metabolized at a rate of 5 to 10 ml per hour, no matter how much is ingested, but an alcoholic may acquire the (reversible) capacity to double his rate of alcohol metabolism. Moreover, alcoholics characteristically develop substantial central tolerance, so that they may appear fairly sober at blood alcohol levels of 150 mg per 100 ml. Most nonalcoholic individuals become intoxicated at levels between 100 and 200 mg per 100 ml, and some, at levels as low as 30 mg per 100 ml. Levels over 400 mg per 100 ml may be lethal, death usually resulting from depressed respiration or aspiration of vomitus.

Alcohol Withdrawal Syndrome

The alcohol withdrawal syndrome is characterized by coarse tremor, nausea and vomiting, malaise, weakness, anxiety, depression, irritability, sleep fragmentation, and signs of autonomic hyperactivity, such as tachycardia, sweating, and hypertension. Symptoms may begin shortly after the cessation of a drinking bout of several days, or may appear during a reduction in drinking. Major motor seizures (rum fits) may occur, usually within the first 48 hr. Seizures may be controlled with intravenous diazepam (Valium), but unless an evaluation reveals seizures unrelated to alcohol withdrawal, chronic anticonvulsant treatment is not effective. Hospitalization is frequently needed to manage withdrawal, especially in patients with complications of addictive drinking such as trauma, infection, or fluid and electrolyte loss.

Alcohol Withdrawal Delirium

When the withdrawal syndrome is complicated by delirium, usually occurring on the second or third day after the cessation of or reduction in drinking, alcohol withdrawal delirium (delirium tremens) is present. This syndrome, which usually occurs in older alcoholics (over 30) who have been drinking addictively for some years, is marked by confusion, disorientation, delusions, vivid auditory and/or visual hallucinations, and, at times, fever. Alcohol withdrawal delirium is both a medical and a psychiatric emergency, which is likely to last a few days. It requires hospitalization, preferably on a medical service.

The alcoholism literature contains many reports of "successful" treatment or prevention of alcohol withdrawal delirium which probably have encouraged indiscriminate drug treatment of uncomplicated alcohol withdrawal. The low incidence of severe withdrawal reactions in these reports is probably a reflection not of the efficacy of the various regimens used, but of the relative rarity of the full-blown withdrawal syndrome (9). Uncomplicated withdrawal should not be treated, but severe withdrawal should be treated as an emergency; where the distinction cannot be made, treatment for severe withdrawal—in hospital—should be instituted.

Alcohol Hallucinosis

Alcohol hallucinosis is a rare withdrawal syndrome distinguished by vivid auditory hallucinations in the context of a clear sensorium. Onset of the syndrome occurs soon after cessation of drinking, usually within the first 48 hr. It lasts from a few hours up to a week; occasionally a chronic form develops. Differentiation from schizophrenia is difficult, and psychiatric consultation is necessary.

Alcohol Idiosyncratic Intoxication

Alcohol idiosyncratic intoxication (pathological intoxication) is also a rare syndrome characterized by an extreme, often aggressive reaction to a low dose of alcohol, which is frequently followed by amnesia for the episode. The behavior is atypical of the person when not drinking. The duration of this condition is brief (hours), and the individual returns to his normal state as the blood alcohol level falls. Temporal lobe epilepsy, sedative-hypnotic abuse, and malingering should be ruled out.

Alcohol Amnestic Disorder (Korsakoff's Psychosis)

Alcohol amnestic disorder is characterized chiefly by short term memory impairment, associated with some loss of long term memory, in the absence of clouded consciousness (delirium) or general loss of intellectual abilities (dementia). (For definitions and detailed discussions of delirium and dementia, see Chapter 16.) In other words, such a patient might be unable to remember new information, such as three objects, several minutes after he was asked to do so (anterograde amnesia). He would show some long term memory loss (retrograde amnesia) with relative sparing of very remote memories, so that he might be able to recall the names of his siblings but not of his children. He might be disoriented but not confused, deluded, or hallucinating. He would be able to carry on a plausibly normal conversation, and to make appropriate deductions from given premises.

Patients with less advanced forms of this disorder may be substantially impaired, but, as the foregoing would suggest, they may appear superficially to be normal, particularly as they frequently attempt to minimize their impairment and to confabulate in order to fill in memory gaps.

The amnestic disorder frequently follows an acute episode of Wernicke's encephalopathy (a syndrome of confusion, ataxia, and impaired eye movement). Parenteral thiamine given during an acute episode of Wernicke's encephalopathy may prevent the amnestic syndrome. Once it develops, no specific treatment is available, and the syndrome usually persists indefinitely, with only slight improvement.

Dementia Associated with Alcoholism

When a more generalized intellectual impairment develops after years of heavy drinking, the diagnosis of dementia associated with alcoholism is appropriate. In advanced cases, where the deficit is substantial, little significant improvement can be expected. Milder forms of this disorder, often difficult to document without neuropsychological testing, are probably common in heavy drinkers, and may respond significantly to abstinence. Since even dried-out alcoholics are likely to show some cognitive impairment for a period of time after cessation of drinking, this diagnosis should not be made unless dementia persists for at least 3 weeks after drinking has stopped (1). Other causes of dementia must be excluded (see Chapter 16).

MEDICAL COMPLICATIONS

Miscellaneous

The deficiencies involved in a diet composed largely of nutritionally empty alcoholic calories (7 cal per g), as well as the direct toxic actions of alcohol itself, have been implicated in the etiology of diseases associated with alcoholism. These disorders are legion, spare no body system, and most are related to the quantity and duration of alcohol consumed (8). Among the commoner findings are the following: gastritis; fatty liver; hepatitis or cirrhosis; pancreatitis; cerebellar ataxia; peripheral neuropathy; unexplained elevation of serum creatine phosphokinase with or without muscle pain and weakness; pulmonary infections suggesting aspiration or impaired defenses (tuberculosis and pneumonia); cancers of the liver and upper digestive tract; unexplained cardiomyopathy; and traumatic injuries.

Fetal Alcohol Syndrome

Because it appears to be both serious and preventable, the fetal alcohol syndrome deserves special mention. The offspring of alcoholic women who continue to drink during pregnancy show an increased incidence of various morphological disorders, as well as impairment of growth, development, and cognition. These abnormalities are nonspecific, and because of the limits to human experimentation, it cannot be determined with certainty to what extent alcohol, as opposed to other drugs or nutritional factors, may be etiologically involved. In any case, it would seem prudent to advise women to drink only minimally, if at all, during pregnancy (7).

TREATMENT OF ALCOHOLISM

The physician will frequently want to refer patients for alcoholism treatment or will be asked to assist in making referrals. Ambulatory alcoholism treatment facilities are ubiquitous, and there should be no difficulty in assisting a sober, motivated patient to apply for treatment.* The intoxicated patient, how-

---

* Beginning with Maryland (1968), most states have recently enacted comprehensive alcoholism laws which define alcohol intoxication and alcoholism as problems to be handled primarily by health care facilities and professionals, not by law enforcement agencies. In response to this legislation, most states have greatly expanded the number of treatment facilities available for the motivated alcoholic.

ever, cannot usually be relied on to initiate ambulatory treatment, and therefore it may be necessary to persuade this type of patient to admit himself briefly to a detoxification facility as the first step in treatment. The acutely intoxicated patient is usually best handled by waiting until the episode subsides. Analeptic drugs such as caffeine are not useful in the stuporous patient, nor is there any practical way significantly to accelerate alcohol metabolism. Restraints should be used judiciously in the agitated patient, as should even the more benign tranquilizers such as diazepam (Valium), because of their synergism with alcohol and with other drugs of abuse which the patient may have ingested. There is no effective therapy for the unmotivated patient, but one should be careful not to prejudge motivation, which is difficult to assess and may vary with time and circumstance. Even if he is unmotivated at one time, the alcoholic patient should be offered treatment at the next opportunity. Many successfully treated patients are those who have been unmotivated earlier in the course of their alcoholism, when the price they were paying for their addictive behavior seemed relatively small and remote.

As is true for other disorders for which no consistently effective treatment exists, there are many therapies for alcoholism. Evidence to date does not demonstrate any superiority for the traditional verbal therapies (group or individual), self-help groups (Alcoholics Anonymous), classical conditioning (e.g., chemical aversion with Antabuse), or operant conditioning methods, although some data have been published to suggest that operant methods might be useful (3). Although a case cannot yet be made for a specific treatment, it is clear that patients who undergo treatment do distinctly better than those who do not, and on this basis treatment should be offered. Since we cannot yet correlate success with certain types of alcoholics with a particular variety of treatment, the selection of therapy may be based on the patient's preference. Thus those alcoholics who indicate that they might find a group approach with a spiritual emphasis acceptable, might best be referred to an Alcoholics Anonymous group in their preferred social stratum, whereas others might be more likely to accept counseling offered in a traditional medical setting. Therapy should be as inexpensive as possible, since the evidence indicates that there is no special advantage to be gained from going to highly sophisticated specialists. Institutionalization should be utilized chiefly for short term detoxification (14 to 21 days); treatment in hospital confers no therapeutic advantage otherwise and is very costly.

As already indicated, drugs have a very limited place in the treatment of alcoholism. In fact the sedative-hypnotics may be dangerous in that they compound the sedating effects of alcohol, and many involve the possibility of abuse. Thus it is probably pointless to attempt to treat alcohol withdrawal with these drugs on an ambulatory basis. If the withdrawal is really serious, the patient belongs in the hospital. It is tempting to medicate the alcoholic with antianxiety agents in the hope that he might substitute controlled use of these drugs for alcohol abuse, but it seldom works that way. If anything, the use of antianxiety drugs on an ambulatory basis may encourage drinking; the drug may lead to drinking just as one drink may lead to another. Although alcoholics are commonly depressed, they usually do not benefit from antidepressant drug treatment, unless they are of the small minority of patients who are experiencing a major affective disorder (see Chapter 14). Because of the seriousness of their disorder, such patients should probably be in a hospital. Disulfiram (Antabuse), taken as a 250-mg tablet daily, can effectively prevent drinking by making the patient subject to an aversive reaction, due to the accumulation of acetaldehyde caused by interference with ethanol metabolism when he drinks while taking the drug. The acetaldehyde syndrome occurs within minutes of drinking, and consists of peripheral vasodilation, throbbing headache, dyspnea, nausea, vomiting, sweating, thirst, chest pain, and potentially dangerous hypotension. The effectiveness of disulfiram as conventionally prescribed has not been established, although there is some evidence that when consistently monitored the drug may be useful as part of a rehabilitation program (4). Its use is contraindicated in patients with significant cardiac, liver, renal, or psychiatric disease.

Surgery in the alcoholic patient can be associated with a number of problems which require astute anticipation, diagnosis, and management. This subject is covered in more detail in Chapter 83.

ALCOHOL-DRUG INTERACTIONS

The general physician should be aware of alcohol-drug interactions, which may involve (a) antagonism, (b) additive and supra-additive (synergistic) effects, and (c) cross-tolerance or synergism (6).

Antagonism between drugs and alcohol, such as occurs with disulfiram, can cause specific, deleterious reactions. Some common drugs in this category are:

Drug	Effect
Chloral hydrate	Generalized vasodilatation
Tolbutamide and other sulfonylureas	Disulfiram-like reaction
Some antimicrobials: chloramphenicol, griseofulvin, isoniazid, metronidazole, and quinacrine	Disulfiram-like reaction

The *additive and synergistic* category of drugs includes agents whose effects may be aggravated by alcohol; for example, in the presence of alcohol, salicylates might be more likely to induce bleeding or

antihypertensive drugs to lower blood pressure. Common drugs in this category are:

Drug	Effect
Tolbutamide and other sulfonylureas	Hypoglycemia
Salicylates	Gastrointestinal bleeding
Antihypertensives, nitroglycerine	Hypotension
Warfarin	Hemorrhage (prothrombin time increased)
Sedative-hypnotics	Central nervous system (CNS) depression
Minor tranquilizers	CNS depression
Major tranquilizers	CNS depression, hypotension, respiratory depression, impaired hepatic function
Antihistamines	CNS depression
Opiates	CNS depression

Either *cross-tolerance or synergism* can occur with some drug-alcohol combinations, depending on the time of drug administration. For example, chronic alcoholics may require an unusually large dose of anesthetic because of cross-tolerance, but at the same time would be susceptible to CNS depression with a low dose of anesthetic when alcohol has been ingested prior to the need for anesthesia. Examples of these drugs include: tolbutamide and other sulfonylureas, phenytoin, anesthetics, warfarin, CNS depressants, and tricyclic antidepressants.

References

General

Criteria Committee, National Council on Alcoholism: Criteria for the diagnosis of alcoholism. *Ann Intern Med* 77: 249, 1972.
   An exhaustive and useful diagnostic scheme which divides alcoholism into physical and psychological-behavioral tracks.
Mendelson, JH, and Mello, NK (eds): *The Diagnosis and Treatment of Alcoholism.* McGraw-Hill, New York, 1979.
   A superior general text.

Specific

1. Allen, RP, Faillace, LA, and Wagman, A: Recovery time for alcoholics after prolonged alcohol intoxication. *Johns Hopkins Med J 128:* 158, 1971.
2. Goodwin, DW: Is alcoholism hereditary? A review and critique. *Arch Gen Psychiatry 25:* 545, 1971.
3. Liebson, IA, Tommasello, A, and Bigelow, GE: A behavioral treatment of alcoholic methadone patients. Ann *Intern Med 89:* 342, 1978.
4. Mottin, JL: Drug-induced attenuation of alcohol consumption: A review and evaluation of claimed, potential, or current therapies. *Q J Stud Alcohol 34:* 444, 1973.
5. Robinson, D: Factors influencing alcohol consumption. In *Alcoholism, New Knowledge and New Responses.* G Edwards and G Grant (Eds). Croom Helm, Ltd., London, 1977.
6. Seixas, FA: Alcohol and its drug interactions. *Ann Intern Med 83:* 86, 1975.
7. Sokol, RJ, Miller, SI, and Reed, G: Alcohol abuse during pregnancy: An epidemiologic study. *Alcoholism Clin Exp Res 4:* 135, 1980.
8. Turner, TB, Mezey, E, and Kimball, AW: Measurement of

alcohol-related effects in man: Chronic effects in relation to levels of alcohol consumption. Part A. *Johns Hopkins Med J* 141: 235, 1977.

9. Victor, M. Treatment of alcohol intoxication and withdrawal syndrome: A critical analysis of the use of drugs and other forms of therapy. In *Treatment Manual for Acute Drug Abuse Emergencies*, PG Bourne (ed). National Clearing House for Drug Abuse Information Pub. No. 16, Washington, D.C., 1974.

CHAPTER TWENTY-ONE

Use and Abuse of Illicit Drugs and Substances

BURTON D'LUGOFF, M.D., and JAMES HAWTHORNE, Ph.D.

DEFINITIONS

Illicit drugs are substances which are taken nonmedically to modify mood or behavior. The use and abuse of such substances dates back thousands of years. Plant alkaloids, alcohol, and an ever increasing array of newly synthesized chemicals have been used in these endeavors. Patterns of use and the social acceptance of use of these agents have differed from time to time and from place to place. Successive generations of a single society have held discordant views about which substance to use, at what age, in what amount, and under which circumstances (as witness the pre- and post-prohibition eras in the United States). Also, in a single historical epoch, neighboring cultures have differed about the sanctioned use of psychoactive substances. Currently, in 20th century Western society the use of illicit substances is expressed in two ways:

1. *Experimental.* The experimental use of illicit substances is sporadic; the initial trial and experience usually are associated with youthful rites of passage. These experiments are of small moment psychologically. Medically they are dangerous only to the extent that possible dosage errors and bizarre or unsterile methods of exposure may occur. Incorrect labeling of such drugs (a common problem), increases the risk of an untoward effect. A 1980 National High School survey (4) revealed that 65% of all respondents had engaged in an experimental trial of an illicit drug (primarily marijuana) and 93% had tried alcohol on at least one occasion.

2. *Social-Recreational.* The social and recreational use of illicit substances suggests that they have been used repetitively but that control has been exerted over the dose and the time of use. The dangers of untoward overdosage, improper exposure, and mislabeling are multiplied by the frequency of use. To the extent that control is effectively exerted to maintain a high degree of social and behavioral function, recreational use also is not psychologically disabling. Most American use of alcohol and marijuana conforms to this pattern of social-recreational use.

Abuse refers to the combination of three characteristics (2):

1. There is a pattern of pathological use of a particular substance. Depending upon the substance, this may be manifested by intoxication throughout the day, inability to cut down or stop use, repeated efforts to control use, continuation of use despite a serious physical disorder which is exacerbated by this substance, need for daily use for adequate functioning, and episodes of a medical complication of substance intoxication.

2. Impairment in social or occupational functioning is caused by the pattern of pathological use of an illicit substance. This refers to failure to meet important obligations to friends and family, to erratic and

impulsive behavior, and to behavior leading to legal difficulties (car accidents, theft).

3. Duration is of at least 1 month. Signs of the drug-abusing pattern do not have to be present continuously throughout the month, but should be sufficiently frequent that a pattern of pathological use causing interference with social or occupational functioning is apparent.

Succeeding sections of this chapter describe the signs and symptoms associated with the substances most frequently abused in the United States today. A cursory listing of all the drugs extant today which have abuse potential would be extremely long. It is possible, however, to group the various substances into broad classes, the members of which share common characteristics and are readily distinguishable from other classes (Table 21.1).

Psychoactive substances may thus be classified as (a) depressants, (b) stimulants, and (c) drugs which alter perception (including hallucinogens).

Table 21.1
Categories of Psychoactive drugs

DEPRESSANTS
  Narcotics:
    Morphine, hydromorphone (Dilaudid), heroin, meperidine (Demerol), codeine, methadone
  Sedative-hypnotics:
    Alcohol, barbiturates, glutethimide (Doriden), methaqualone (Quaalude)
  Minor tranquilizers:
    Diazepam (Valium), chlordiazepoxide (Librium), meprobamate (Equanil or Miltown)
  Inhalants:
    Nitrous oxide, toluene, volatile hydrocarbons
STIMULANTS
  Cocaine, amphetamine methylphenidate (Ritalin), phenmetrazine (Preludin)
DRUGS WHICH ALTER PERCEPTION (INCLUDING HALLUCINOGENS)
  Marijuana, lysergic acid diethylamide (LSD), dimethylamine tryptamine (DMT), psylocybin, phencyclidine (PCP), belladonna alkaloids (atropine, scopolamine)

PREVALENCE

Recent estimates of the prevalence of drug *use* by American's over the age of 12 are summarized in Table 21.2 (8), based on the 1979 National Survey of Drug Abuse. These data were obtained in household interviews, omitting subsets of the population in which drug abuse is probably even more common (*i.e.*, transients, military-base personnel, college dormitory residents, and prisoners).

The 1979 data indicated a number of important long term trends. When compared with similar data from 1972, there was a dramatic increase in reported current use of cocaine and inhalants among young adults (from 9 to 28% and from less than 1 to 17%, respectively). During this interval, there was a slight decrease in the proportion of young adults who reported ever using heroin (from 5 to 4%). When compared with similar data from 1960, there was an increase in the history of marijuana use in the same age group, from 4 to 68%.

Table 21.2
Projected Estimates of the Numbers of People Who Report Having Used Drugs Nonmedically[a]

	18–25 yr (pop. 31,985,000)				Total (pop. 179,358,000)			
	Ever used		Current user		Ever used		Current user	
	%	No.	%	No.	%	No.	%	No.
Marijuana and hashish	68	21,700,000	35	11,200,00	30	54,800,000	13	22,600,000
Inhalants	17	5,400,000	1	300,000	7	12,700,000	1	1,400,000
Hallucinogens	25	8,000,000	4	1,300,000	9	15,800,000	1	1,800,000
PCP	15	4,800,000	—[b]	—[b]	5	8,200,000	—[b]	—[b]
Cocaine	28	9,000,000	9	2,900,000	8	15,100,000	2	4,400,000
Heroin	4	1,300,000	—[c]	—[c]	1	2,600,000	—[c]	—[c]
Stimulants	18	5,800,000	4	1,300,000	8	13,900,000	1	2,100,000
Sedatives	17	5,400,000	3	1,000,000	6	13,900,000	1	2,100,000
Tranquilizers	16	5,100,000	2	600,000	5	9,800,000	—[c]	—[c]
Analgesics	12	3,800,000	1	300,000	5	8,200,000	—[c]	—[c]
Alcohol	95	30,400,000	76	24,300,000	90	160,800,000	61	108,600,000
Cigarettes	83	26,500,000	43	13,800,000	79	142,100,000	36	62,400,000

[a] Estimates are developed from the *National Survey on Drug Abuse: 1979*, by the National Institute of Drug Abuse. The two categories are young adults and the total population over the age of 12. Ever used = used one or more times in a person's life; current user = used at least once in the 30 days prior to the survey.
[b] Not included in the survey.
[c] Amounts of less than 0.5% are not listed.

Table 21.3
Characteristics of Dependence on Depressant Drugs

Drug	Physiological Effect	Withdrawal Symptoms (From 1 to 7 Days after Last Dose)	
Narcotics	Pupillary constriction Analgesia Constipation Respiratory depression	Pupillary dilation Myalgia Diarrhea Stimulation of respiratory centers ("yawning")	
Barbiturate, alcohol, sedative, tranquilizers	Induction of sleep (hypnosis) Sedation Alcohol increases seizure activity	Insomnia Tremulousness Irritability Hyperpyrexia	Minor symptoms for 24 hr to 72 hr
	All other sedatives decrease seizure activity	Delirium Seizures Death	Major symptoms from 72 hr to 2 wk

DEPRESSANT DRUGS

General Characteristics

Central nervous system depressants all share the property of the induction of *psychoactive tolerance*. In this definition tolerance is habituation of the central nervous system to repetitive drug dosages given in a schedule so that there is at all times a measurable level of the drug in the blood. Tolerance results in a diminution or absence of the expected biological effect of a given dose of the drug. Markedly increased amounts of drug are required to achieve the initially desired effect. Psychoactive tolerance is distinguishable from "pharmacological" tolerance, which reflects the induction of catabolic enzymes that metabolize a drug more rapidly on repeated use. Psychoactive tolerance depends upon a change in the neuronal membrane receptors, independent of the rate of metabolism of the drug. Barbiturates induce both pharmacological and psychoactive tolerance. Narcotics produce only psychoactive tolerance.

The time required for the induction of psychoactive tolerance varies from a matter of days following repeated intravenous or intramuscular administration of narcotics, to weeks or months following repeated oral administration of narcotics, barbiturates, alcohol, and other sedatives.

Physiological addiction (dependence) is defined as the point in the induction of tolerance where abrupt cessation of a drug results in withdrawal symptoms (the abstinence state). Withdrawal symptoms are often the mirror image of the biological effects exerted by the drug in question (Table 21.3). As can be seen in the table, narcotic withdrawal, while uncomfortable, is not life-threatening. Sedative withdrawal has both a minor and relatively innocuous symptom complex which occurs initially in all sedative-tolerant individuals and the possibility of a major symptom complex in a smaller fraction of tolerant individuals, which includes seizures and death. This sequence is the same as that referred to as delirium tremens in alcohol withdrawal (see Chapter 20). Alcohol- and sedative-tolerant individuals should have a tapering detoxification in hospital under medical supervision and an absolute prohibition of sudden abstinence or "cold turkey" withdrawal. The inhalants, which also are central nervous system (CNS) depressants, do not usually induce tolerance because their volatility and short term use never leave blood levels sufficiently high long enough to habituate the neuronal membranes.

Prescribing Patterns. An understanding of the induction of tolerance and of physiological addiction should mandate changes in prescribing patterns. Narcotic analgesics, should be given for short term intense pain and sedatives and tranquilizers for emotional crises, with a recognition of the need to limit and taper the drug when the period of intense symptoms is over. Chronic pain, insomnia, chronic anxiety, and emotional distress cannot be treated with a prescribed daily depressant drug without inducing tolerance and physiological addiction. *Intermittent* use is required to avoid addiction. Other modalities, *i.e.*, psychotherapy, relaxation techniques, biofeedback, physiotherapy, and exercise regimens should also be enlisted in treating chronic problems.

A recent change in prescribing patterns de-emphasizing barbiturates and other potent sedatives in favor of the benzodiazepine tranquilizers is to be welcomed for reducing the potential of serious overdosage. The minor tranquilizers, even if attenuated, do, however, induce tolerance and physiological addiction (the shorter acting benzodiazepines are associated occasionally with major withdrawal symptoms). Benzodiazepines are also potentiated by alcohol and other psychoactive substances and must be treated with caution in prescription and use, with adherence to intermittent short term regimens.

Sedative-Hypnotics

USUAL EFFECTS

Intoxication with sedatives is similar to intoxication with alcohol: sufficient amounts are taken to produce a depression of cortical function and to inhibit social and personal inhibitions. This disinhibition is called "a high," a state of euphoria in which mood is elevated and anxiety is reduced. Depending on dose, route of administration, rate of metabolism, and body size, exact effects of the sedative may vary widely from time to time and from individual to individual.

ACUTE ADVERSE EFFECTS

Overshooting the mark may lead to more profound intoxication: slurred speech, impaired judgment, and unsteady gait. Even greater overdose may lead to stupor, coma, respiratory depression, vasomotor collapse, and death. Intoxication from sedatives, as with alcohol intoxication, impairs motor coordination and the ability to make intellectual judgments.

EFFECTS OF CHRONIC USE

A different population of abusers of sedatives is characterized not by the intent to reach disinhibition (a "high") but by the intent to calm anxiety or induce sleep. Physicians will frequently prescribe sedatives (including tranquilizers) without instructions that they should be used only for short term intermittent treatment. Patients will then use the medications on a regular basis, induce tolerance and escalate the dose in order to keep achieving the initially desired end. The seeking of an anxiety-free state may go undetected until the confusion, irritability, slurred speech, and ataxia together are recognized as sedative intoxication. Often the only distinguishing physical features are ecchymoses which result from the patient being uncoordinated during an intoxicated state. Prescriptions and use of individual new sedatives vary widely, almost in a fadlike pattern. Despite assertions to the contrary, all are toleragenic, dangerous when consumed with alcohol or other CNS depressants, and all produce dependency. None should be used in a chronic dosage schedule without serious regard for the possible consequences.

TREATMENT

Sedative overdose is a life-threatening emergency which should be treated in an emergency room.

Because of physiological dependence, patients to be weaned from sedative drugs are at risk of serious withdrawal reactions (including life-threatening seizures). Detoxification should only be attempted in hospital under close medical supervision.

Heroin and Other Narcotics

The heroin addict will not generally be seen in office practice, although he may attempt to obtain prescription drugs when he experiences difficulty in obtaining heroin (diacetylmorphine). Morphine, hydromorphone (Dilaudid), and meperidine (Demerol) are the narcotics that are most preferred by addicts, but they will readily use the whole range of less potent narcotic and non-narcotic analgesics if preferred drugs are unavailable. If analgesics are difficult to obtain, addicts will temporarily use virtually any depressant drug, but will prefer the barbiturates and other potent sedatives such as methaqualone (Quaalude), glutethimide (Doriden), and ethchlorvynol (Placidyl). Alcohol, the benzodiazepines, and promethazine hydrochloride (Phenergan) are often abused by patients maintained on methadone because of their tendency to potentiate the effects of methadone.

USUAL EFFECTS

The acetyl groups on the heroin molecule allow it to penetrate the blood-brain barrier more rapidly than do other narcotics. In the CNS the acetyl moieties are removed, yielding the active compound, morphine. Heroin is usually injected intravenously but can also be injected intramuscularly (skin-popping) or sniffed (snorting). The effects following intravenous injections consist of a brief and intense period of euphoria followed by several hours of a pleasant dreamy state in which the user may slowly nod as if he is falling off to sleep. He may also experience itching of the skin which leads to characteristic scratching movements.

ACUTE ADVERSE EFFECTS

Narcotic overdose is characterized by depressed consciousness and depressed respiration. Pulmonary edema, a common complication of narcotic overdose, contributes to hypoxia and may cause death, even while the needle is still in the vein. Experimental evidence suggests that a massive sympathetic discharge is responsible for this effect.

CHRONIC EFFECTS

The adverse effects of chronic heroin use result from use of dirty needles, the adulterants mixed with the heroin, and the associated life-style (poor nutrition and health care) rather than the drug itself. Heroin generally constitutes only 2 to 5% of the content of a street dose and is usually mixed with milk sugar (lactose) and quinine under nonsterile conditions in which other, more dangerous, adulterants may also be included to mask the dilution of the heroin. Chronic heroin abusers will have needle marks or scars, usually in the antecubital fossae of both arms, on the forearms and wrists, or on the backs of the hands. The presence of abscesses or old abscess scars and of bluish phlebitis scars from past injections also indicates chronic use. Long time users are usually forced to seek out new injection sites as old sites become unusable owing to scarring, and may exhibit fresh needle marks on the legs and neck. In addition to abscesses, chronic intravenous drug use will result in an increased incidence of hepatitis B antigenemia, viral hepatitis, chronic liver disease, cellulitis, endocarditis, and pulmonary hypertension due to microembolization. It has been estimated that at least one-half of all addicts develop chronic liver disease, demonstrated by abnormal liver function tests.

Tolerance to heroin develops quickly and can be demonstrated to some degree after only a few days of administration of the drug. The degree of tolerance and the consequent severity of withdrawal symptomatology will depend primarily on dosage levels, and the frequency and duration of use. However, the severity of a patient's addiction to heroin cannot be defined purely in terms of tolerance or withdrawal symptomatology since heroin addiction is as much a function of psychological and social factors as it is a simple consequence of physical tolerance or of withdrawal symptoms.

Narcotic withdrawal is characterized by anxiety, nausea, yawning, diarrhea, sweating, rhinorrhea, dilated pupils, and pilo erection, ("goose flesh"). In the advanced stages of withdrawal the patient will experience vomiting and muscle spasms which will often appear as jerky "kicking" movements of the legs. Acute narcotic withdrawal may be inadvertantly induced when a narcotic-tolerant individual is given pentazocine (Talwin), an analgesic which is both a narcotic agonist and antagonist. While the untreated addict will experience significant anxiety and discomfort during withdrawal, the process itself presents no serious medical risks. Narcotic addicts tend to confuse anxiety with the early symptoms of withdrawal, so that the diagnosis of withdrawal should be made on the basis of observable symptoms rather than on subjective reports of anxiety and nausea.

TREATMENT

Narcotic overdose must be treated in an emergency room. Emergency treatment requires support of respiratory and cardiovascular functions. A narcotic antagonist (nalorphine, Narcan) is extremely safe and effective in countering the CNS depression caused by narcotic overdose.

As a practical matter, any patient who has been abusing heroin or other narcotics and is willing to accept help should be referred for treatment. The most widely used methods of treatment for narcotic addiction are methadone maintenance and methadone detoxification, both of which are normally administered on an ambulatory basis by specially licensed drug treatment programs. Therapeutic communities offer drug-free residential treatment to highly motivated patients who are able to withdraw from narcotics before entry.

Inhalants: Solvent Abuse

The inhalation of solvents is a form of substance abuse that is most commonly found among young people. Since solvents are easily obtainable and inexpensive, they are likely to be preferred by individuals who lack the money or other resources needed to obtain more desirable drugs. A far from exhaustive list of specific substances subject to this type of abuse includes gasoline, ignition spray, airplane glue, paint thinner, spray paint, lighter fluid, nail polish remover, cleaning fluid, and shoe polish. Inhalation is typically accomplished by saturating a rag with the substance and holding it directly over the face or placing it in a bag which is then placed over the nose and mouth.

USUAL EFFECTS

The effects of solvents are immediate and of short duration usually dissipating in an hour or less. Acute intoxication is similar to alcohol intoxication except for a shorter duration.

ACUTE ADVERSE EFFECTS

A hangover, with symptoms of headache and nausea similar but perhaps milder than the hangover produced by alcohol, has been observed. Some users will experience apparent delirium characterized by tactile hallucinations, spatial distortions, and macropsia or micropsia (body image distortions). Sudden sniffing deaths have been described where inhalants were used during strenuous activity or under conditions where blood oxygen is reduced. Such deaths apparently occur as a result of ventricular fibrillation or of some other arrhythmia. Other deaths have been caused by suffocation when the user loses consciousness with his nose and mouth covered by the bag containing the solvent.

CHRONIC EFFECTS

While current information does not permit clear-cut conclusions concerning the extent of organ damage caused by inhalant abuse, there is cause for concern. The effects of solvents on the CNS, liver, kidneys, and bone marrow are not known. Numerous studies have demonstrated organ damage from long term exposure to relatively low concentrations of industrial solvents, but it is not clear to what extent these findings can be generalized to the short term, high concentration exposures experienced by inhalant abusers. Furthermore in many studies contrasting solvent abusers with control subjects, adverse effects were found in solvent abusers, but the possibility that these were due to factors other than inhalant abuse was not ruled out.

There is evidence that tolerance develops with chronic solvent abuse, but no withdrawal syndrome has been reported, probably because the concentration of the substance in neurons is not sustained.

TREATMENT

Because the acute effects of solvents are usually of short duration, abusers rarely present for medical treatment. On rare occasions a patient may be brought in for treatment of a solvent-induced delirium. Chronic solvent abuse requires the same type of intense counseling and rehabilitative intervention indicated for other forms of self-destructive substance abuse (see below, p. 170).

STIMULANT DRUGS

Cocaine and the amphetamines are the most commonly abused stimulant drugs. Two non-amphetamine stimulants, methylphenidate (Ritalin) and phenmetrazine (Preludin), can produce any of the adverse effects of the amphetamines. Abuse of phenmetrazine appears to be on the rise. While all CNS stimulants, with the exception of cocaine, are available by prescription, it appears that most users do not obtain them through legal channels. Cocaine is by far the most expensive of all of the drugs of this class. Cocaine is generally available as a white powder that is sniffed ("snorted") so that it is absorbed directly into the blood stream through the mucosa of the nose. It is occasionally injected intravenously, swallowed, or smoked. Amphetamines are swallowed or injected intravenously. Methylphenidate and phenmetrazine are swallowed.

Knowing that certain groups are more likely to abuse amphetamines may alert the physician to the possibility of abuse. Such groups include long distance truck drivers, students cramming for examinations, and patients previously treated for obesity with amphetamines or related compounds.

USUAL EFFECTS

Central nervous system stimulants produce euphoria, increased confidence and energy, increased heart rate and blood pressure, dilated pupils, constriction of peripheral blood vessels, and increased body temperature and metabolic rate. All of these effects are caused by a massive sympathetic discharge induced by these drugs. Single doses of amphetamines produce effects lasting 2 to 4 hr. The effects of cocaine are of much shorter duration. When the acute effects of stimulants subside, users often experience lethargy or depression, prolonged sleep, and a voracious appetite.

ACUTE ADVERSE EFFECTS

Extremely large doses of amphetamines may cause hyperpyrexia, hypertension, convulsions, cardiovascular collapse, and death. Large amounts of cocaine, on the other hand, cause depression of the medullary centers, and death may result from cardiac or respiratory arrest. Death from overdose of CNS stimulants is unusual. However, a report (13) suggests that death from cocaine ingestion may be a greater risk than has been previously believed.

CHRONIC EFFECTS

Amphetamines. The chronic amphetamine abuser is typically hyperactive, jittery, and irritable. There is a history of insomnia and anorexia. The patient may be emotionally labile, and his periods of irrita-

bility may alternate with periods of elation and enthusiasm. Physical examination may reveal needle marks, teeth worn from bruxism (grinding of teeth), ulcers on the lips and tongue, tremor, flushing, cardiac arrhythmias, and excessive sweating. Heavy users may exhibit rapid, repetitious, and ritualistic body movements or such movements may be described by companions.

Chronic abusers of amphetamines rapidly develop pharmacological tolerance, so that markedly increasing doses are required to experience effects previously obtained with lower doses.

Repeated exposure to high doses of amphetamines exhausts the supply of preformed noradrenaline, and it has been proposed that the resultant excess in the CNS of other neurotransmitters, notably dopamine and serotonin, explains the development of a reversible organic delusional disorder which closely resembles paranoid schizophrenia (12). Normal subjects, with no previous psychiatric history, developed a delusional disorder following chronic administration of amphetamines (3). Subjects who received high doses (10 mg of dextroamphetamine every hour) developed the disorder within 24 hr. However, the more typical clinical picture is one of gradual onset over a period of days or weeks as the user gradually increases his intake. Initially, the onset of a delusional disorder may be signaled by increased suspiciousness and distrustfulness. In the final stages, patients become markedly paranoid, with delusions of persecution, ideas of reference and, in many cases, visual or auditory hallucination. Displays of aggressiveness, hostility, anxiety, and psychomotor agitation are also commonly observed.

While an amphetamine-induced delusional disorder is difficult to distinguish from paranoid schizophrenia, it may be inferred from (a) a history of recent amphetamine use; (b) intravenous injection sites, malnourishment, bruxism, or other physical symptoms suggestive of amphetamine abuse; or (c) laboratory studies indicating the presence of amphetamines. An amphetamine-induced delusional disorder differs from phencyclidine (PCP)- or lysergic acid diethylamide (LSD)-induced psychosis (see below) in that it begins much more insidiously. Also, the LSD or PCP user may be cognizant of the fact that he is hallucinating, whereas the amphetamine abuser is typically unable to distinguish his hallucinations from reality. Delirium, a common feature of PCP abuse, is a rare consequence of amphetamine abuse.

Amphetamine abusers who abruptly terminate their use of the drug experience a withdrawal reaction (a "crash") characterized by fatigue, depression, and irritability. Patients who develop a high level of pharmacological tolerance for amphetamines may experience severe depression, and therefore may be suicide risks.

Cocaine. People who sniff cocaine no more than 2

or 3 times a week are not likely to experience serious side effects although they do, of course, run the risk of developing psychological dependence. Daily use of substantial doses of cocaine will interfere with normal sleeping and eating patterns and produce irritability, impaired concentration, and weight loss. Chronic users may also exhibit nasal congestion or rhinorrhea, and paranoid or, more rarely, delusional thinking. Occasionally, heavy users will have inflamed, swollen, or ulcerated noses, but perforated septa are quite rare.

The extent to which chronic use of cocaine produces tolerance in humans is unclear. However, cocaine users seem to experience a milder form of the symptoms associated with amphetamine withdrawal, probably as a result of the shorter exposure of the neurons to the drug.

TREATMENT

An organic delusional disorder resulting from stimulant abuse will necessitate hospitalization of the patient for treatment. Assaultive behavior or extreme agitation can be managed with haloperidol (Haldol), 5 to 10 mg intramuscularly. Most amphetamine abusers who have developed tolerance should also be hospitalized. Even where withdrawal does not produce severe discomfort, many patients will experience intense cravings for the drug and hospitalization may be necessary to help them resist the temptation to resume use.

DRUGS WHICH ALTER PERCEPTION

This category encompasses substances which may be CNS stimulants or depressants, but which in their commonly used dose and via their usual route of administration produce exaggerated imaginings, visual hallucinations, altered time perceptions, and subjective feelings of enhancement of sensation.

Marijuana/Hashish

Marijuana consists of the dried leaves of the marijuana (*Cannabis sativa*) plant, which are usually smoked in pipes or cigarettes ("joints"). Hashish is a concentrated resin of cannabis and contains approximately 5 to 10 times as much of the psychoactive ingredient, tetrahydrocannabinol, as does marijuana. The discussion that follows applies to both marijuana and hashish, although the effects associated with higher doses are more likely to occur with hashish than with marijuana.

A 1980 survey (4) suggests that 60% of high school students have used marijuana or hashish by the time they reach their senior year. It appears that experimenting with drugs is a current "rite" of growing up for a majority of adolescents. The same survey indicates that almost half of those who try marijuana do not use other drugs. Unfortunately, there are few published studies to indicate how many users in the "marijuana only" category would be classified as having an abuse problem. Nor is it possible to estimate the incidence of drug abuse problems in those whose drug experimentation goes beyond the use of marijuana. While it can be safely said that only a minority of youthful drug experimenters will develop drug abuse problems, it is less than reassuring that 9.1% of the high school seniors in the study cited above reported daily use of marijuana.

USUAL EFFECTS

The effects of marijuana usually last from 3 to 6 hr. The more common effects are elation, relaxation, an increased tendency to laughter and silliness, a sense of sharpened perception and increased insight, increased vividness and appreciation in all sensory modalities, decreased concentration, loosened associations, increased appetite, tachycardia, mild feelings of paranoia, and a sense of detachment or depersonalization. Lower doses tend to produce relaxation and euphoria, while higher doses tend to result in increasing visual and auditory perceptual distortions. Doses 3 to 5 times higher than those producing relaxation and mild euphoria can result in psychotomimetic effects (depersonalization, auditory, and visual hallucinations). Thus, some of the usual effects of marijuana which might be enjoyable to the experienced user can be frightening to the inexperienced user. The setting is also very important in determining the effects of the drug. Marijuana, when smoked in a pleasant and familiar setting, is less likely to produce a negative response than when used in an unfamiliar or threatening setting. There is substantial evidence that marijuana in dose levels associated with common social usage interferes with intellectual and psychomotor performance. A number of studies indicate that marijuana use will significantly impair driving skills. In the dosage commonly used (10 mg per cigarette), marijuana impairs recent memory, thus interfering with cognition and learning (6).

ACUTE ADVERSE EFFECTS

Considering the large numbers of regular users in the United States it is clear that adverse reactions to marijuana requiring medical treatment are rare. Adverse reactions vary from acute panic lasting for a few hours to an organic delusional disorder which is essentially the same as that produced by a variety of metabolic, toxic, or infectious conditions. Acute panic reactions are most likely to occur in novice users or in users who unexpectedly receive a much higher than usual dose. This reaction is characterized by the appearance of many of the usual effects of the drug in an exaggerated form and by mounting anxiety which often stems from a sense of losing control, which is often expressed as a fear of "going crazy" or, less frequently, of dying. Depression and paranoid feelings have also been reported. Acute panic reactions can vary in intensity and duration but most last only the few hours it takes for the effects of the drug to wear off. Some patients experience persistent anxiety for several days after the initial panic subsides. It has been estimated that 3 intense panic reactions occur per 100,000 exposures (10). Organic delusional disorders are also rare but, again, the probability of such an occurrence increases with higher doses. Reports of enduring psychotic reactions following heavy marijuana use have appeared largely in Eastern literature in countries where marijuana is normally used in much higher doses than in the United States. Reports of psychotic reactions in this country have been rare; moreover that marijuana clearly was the primary etiological agent was not established.

EFFECTS OF CHRONIC USE

It is clear that smoking marijuana, even a few cigarettes daily for only a few weeks, adversely affects pulmonary function (11). It has also been reported that marijuana smoke contains more carcinogens than tobacco smoke (7). There have been conflicting findings concerning possible adverse effects of marijuana on the immune system. Some studies have reported evidence of changes in immunological responsiveness but the practical implications of these changes are not currently known. There is evidence that marijuana reduces testosterone levels in men, although the average level for users remains within normal limits (5). The clinical implications are unclear, but concern has been expressed over possible effects of even small changes in testosterone levels in adolescent males. Animal and human studies have also suggested that chronic marijuana use may have potentially serious effects on female reproductive functions. Years of additional research will be required before adequate conclusions are reached concerning the effects of chronic marijuana use (cf. the 50 years of research to establish some of the long term effects of cigarette smoking).

Marijuana is clearly a CNS depressant. It is cross-tolerant with the barbiturate sedatives; high doses induce psychoactive tolerance and physiological dependence; and it is additive with all other CNS depressants (narcotics, sedatives, alcohol) in depressing the function of the central nervous system. Heretofore, because of the low potency of the marijuana used in the United States (1 to 10 mg per cigarette) these effects were not generally appreciated. With greater potency (new plants yielding 20 mg per cigarette) and greater concentration of the active ingredient in hashish or oil of hashish, users ingesting dosages as high as 30 to 100 mg report more adverse reactions, greater frequency of hallucinations, and more pronounced CNS depression. In one study (9) volunteers who smoked an average of five marijuana cigarettes a day for 64 days exhibited restlessness, sleep disturbance, loss of appetite, and irritability when they stopped using marijuana.

TREATMENT OF ACUTE REACTIONS

Since they must be closely observed and may take several hours to recover, patients suffering from panic reactions are probably best managed in a setting such as a drug abuse program, mental health center, or emergency room where continuing observation and supportive contact can be provided. Generally, these patients require simple reassurance and an explanation that they are experiencing a drug reaction which will dissipate as the drug is eliminated from their bodies. A critical or moralizing attitude will only undermine rapport with the patient, thereby compromising a critical element in management. Delusional patients should be seen in an emergency room since they present more complicated management problems and may require sedation or hospitalization. Furthermore, other causes of organic delusional disorder such as trauma or infection should be ruled out. Restraints should only be used when absolutely necessary for the safety of the patient or of others. Drugs should also not be used unless the patient is extremely agitated and difficult to control. In such cases, diazepam (Valium) is preferred in an initial dose of 20 mg intramuscularly with subsequent doses of 10 mg each hour to a maximum of 60 mg.

Phencyclidine (PCP)

Phencyclidine, a derivative of ketamine, a known barbiturate-like anesthetic, is quite clearly a CNS depressant, capable of inducing psychoactive tolerance. However, PCP exhibits selective action as an anesthetic, appearing to depress sensory tracts including proprioception, pain, touch, and temperature to a greater degree than it depresses cortical function. The resultant state of sensory deprivation and relative cortical wakefulness makes for a peculiar sense of detachment, disembodiment, and weightlessness. These sensations are intensely pleasurable for some, while for others they induce intense anxiety and even panic. Prolonged sensory deprivation, whether chemically induced or provoked mechanically by shielding out visual, auditory, and tactile stimuli, will predictably induce delusions and hallucinations even in normal subjects.

PCP was developed as an anesthetic, but was abandoned for this purpose when it was found to cause disturbing side effects. It continues to be used by veterinarians as an animal tranquilizer or immobilizing agent. Pure PCP is a white powder which dissolves in water. It is usually sprinkled on marijuana, dried parsley flakes, or other organic material and smoked. Less frequently, it is obtained in powder or tablet form and ingested or sniffed ("snorting"). Street names for the drug vary considerably from region to region but it is most commonly known as angel dust, flakes, crystal, hog, or sheets.

USUAL EFFECTS

The effects of PCP tend to be dose-related, although there can be marked differences in the response of different individuals to a given dose or in the response of an individual to the same dose at different times. Individuals who take PCP in the relatively low doses normally associated with street use may experience exhilaration, euphoria, a sense of great strength and power, inebriation, tranquilization, and perceptual disturbances. Some unpleasant effects commonly reported include disorientation, hallucinations, anxiety, paranoia, hyperexcitability, and irritability. At usual street dosages, most users reach peak intoxication in 5 to 30 min and remain "high" for 4 to 6 hr. It may take 24 hr before the user feels completely normal again.

ACUTE ADVERSE EFFECTS

Even in relatively low doses, PCP is capable of occasionally causing severe reactions which may precipitate extreme agitation and acts of violence toward self and others. With higher doses users are more likely to exhibit the symptoms of delirium. The delirious patient can present a bewildering array of symptoms, which can fluctuate markedly over relatively short periods of time. He may be hypervigilant or drowsy, anxious or aggressive, fearful or dauntless. His behavior may fluctuate during the day: alert at times and stuporous at other times.

A cardinal symptom of delirum is clouding of consciousness, defined as a reduction in the clarity of awareness of the environment (2). While obvious in the stuporous or comatose patient, clouding of consciousness will appear in other patients in the form of impairments in concentration, memory, arithmetical ability, orientation, and complex motor functions such as in writing a sentence or drawing an abstract design. Thinking may appear fragmented and disorganized or it may be either unusually accelerated or slowed. Delirious patients may also experience hallucinations, illusions, and delusions. They frequently show a blank stare, and in some instances they may appear almost catatonic. Ataxia, nystagmus, and ptosis are common.

Very high doses of PCP, which are normally the result of oral ingestion rather than of smoking, can result in coma, severe respiratory depression, seizures, and death. There is considerable evidence that PCP will exacerbate an existing psychosis. There have also been reports of psychotic episodes after the use of PCP in patients with no prior history of mental illness.

CHRONIC EFFECTS

Chronic use of PCP may produce persistent changes in personal habits (hygiene or dress), sleep disturbances, mood changes (depression, irritability), paranoid or frankly delusional thinking, and unusual excitability or lethargy (characteristic of sedative abuse, generally). Little is known about long term physical effects.

TREATMENT OF ACUTE REACTIONS

Burns and Lerner (1) reported consistent correlation between the patient's level of consciousness at presentation, the blood level of PCP, and the subsequent response to treatment. Patients who presented with delirium cleared in 3 to 8 hr; patients who remained stuporous or comatose for 1 to 4 hr cleared in 5 to 62 hr; and patients whose stupor or coma lasted 6 hr or more cleared in 75 to 288 hr. Therefore, patients who are delirious at presentation can be treated in an emergency room and do not require hospitalization. Patients who remain comatose or stuporous for more than 2 hr require hospitalization and observation for a minimum of 24 hr.

Lysergic Acid Diethylamide (LSD)

Lysergic acid diethylamide is the prototype of a number of alkaloid substances of such great potency that small doses predictably cause hallucinations. These hallucinogens, including psylocybin, dimethyltryptamine (DMT), and mescaline, are all CNS depressants as well, demonstrably so in higher doses.

LSD ("acid") is sold illicitly in the form of powder, tablets, or capsules. Sugar cubes, small squares of gelatin ("window pane"), or paper ("blotter acid") which have been impregnated with the drug are also available. LSD is usually ingested, and its effects appear within 15 min, reaching a peak at about 90 min, and last for approximately 8 to 10 hr.

USUAL EFFECTS

LSD usually produces some combination of the following subjective effects: depersonalization, altered time perception, labile mood, profound perceptual distortions (usually visual), body image distortion, and feelings of profound insight. Objective effects include tachycardia, palpitations, anorexia, elevated blood pressure, fever, lack of coordination, and dilated pupils.

ACUTE ADVERSE EFFECTS

Inexperienced users may experience an acute panic reaction that occurs because the normal effects of the drug are unfamiliar or unexpected. In more severe reactions, users of LSD may experience hallucinations (usually visual) and delusions which may persist beyond the time during which the drug is circulating in the blood.

Flashbacks, spontaneous recurrences of the original LSD experience, have been estimated to occur in 1 of every 20 users (from days to years later). They are more likely to occur in chronic users. There have also been reports of prolonged psychotic reactions following the use of LSD.

LSD toxicity differs from PCP toxicity and from schizophrenia in several ways: LSD causes dilation of the pupil which is absent in PCP toxicity or in schizophrenia. PCP toxicity usually is characterized by clouding of consciousness, and the patient will often exhibit ataxia, nystagmus, and ptosis, which are not features of LSD toxicity or of schizophrenia.

CHRONIC EFFECTS

Some degree of tolerance develops with repeated use of LSD, but no withdrawal syndrome has been observed.

TREATMENT

Adverse reactions to LSD usually remit in 8 to 24 hr, and hospitalization is usually not necessary. However, the patient will require observation until symptoms clear. Referral to an emergency room or to a drug abuse program which can provide this type of support will usually be necessary. The same supportive measures described earlier for the treatment of adverse reactions to marijuana are appropriate. Extremely agitated patients should be given diazepam (Valium), 20 mg intramuscularly, before being sent to a treatment center.

Belladonna Alkaloids

Belladonna derivatives such as atropine (the active ingredient in Jimson weed) and scopolamine are acetylcholine inhibitors which in high doses will also regularly produce hallucinations, delirium, and varying states of excitement, insomnia and/or amnesia. These effects may be followed by CNS depression and coma. The side effects of these drugs—dryness of the mouth, blurred vision, anhidrosis, photophobia, and tachycardia—limit their appeal as psychoactive agents. Thus, the rare instances of abuse are mostly by youngsters experimenting with Jimson weed in rural areas or, in the past, by use of over-the-counter soporifics which contained scopolamine until banned by the Food and Drug Administration some years ago. Treatment of toxic overdose is a medical emergency requiring gastric lavage and ingestion of activated charcoal to limit intestinal absorption. Physostigmine, 1 to 4 mg, injected intravenously, intramuscularly, or subcutaneously is a specific antidote that abolishes both the peripheral and CNS effects of these alkaloids. Repeated injection at 1 to 2 hr may be necessary.

TREATMENT AND REHABILITATION OF DRUG ABUSERS

All forms of drug abuse require both acute and long term intervention. Acute intervention includes the management of overdose, toxicity and withdrawal, which requires medical treatment and is concerned primarily with the physical effects of drug ingestion. It is important to recognize, however, that when the *immediate* physical consequences of drug abuse have been successfully treated, there remains a critical need to identify and treat the underlying conditions that motivated drug misuse in the first place. Most drug abusers will be found to have significant problems of psychological and social adjust-

ment and will require counseling and rehabilitation over extended periods of time before they are capable of sustained abstinence. If the underlying problems are not addressed, detoxification of the patient, regardless of how it is carried out, is unlikely to result in even brief periods of abstinence.

Insight-oriented psychotherapy has not proven particularly successful in the treatment of drug abusers, particularly those with extensive problems of social adjustment. Preferable approaches stress basic rehabilitation, the development of practical social and vocational skills, and the avoidance of social environments conducive to drug use. In recent years, there has been an increasing recognition that families may actually facilitate or foster drug abuse in one or more of their members. While the few completed studies suggest that family therapy holds considerable promise in the treatment of drug abuse, much more research is required before its effectiveness can be adequately evaluated.

Since many drug abusers suffer from substantial deficits in educational and vocational preparation, lack basic social and recreational skills, and are often handicapped by problems of poor impulse control and low self-esteem, the process of rehabilitation will often take considerable time. As with alcoholics, relapse is not uncommon and intermittent treatment may frequently be required. Although there is evidence that existing treatment shortens the course of the disorder and reduces the amount of injury to both the individual and the community, a definitive treatment for problems of drug abuse does not exist, and those modalities currently available normally require time and patience. Specialized treatment facilities, inpatient, ambulatory, and residential, are now widely available and can be easily located through state and local health departments.

References

General

Bourne, PC (ed): *Acute Drug Abuse Emergencies*. Academic Press, New York, 1976.
> Covers the treatment of overdose and toxic reactions to commonly abused drugs.

Brecher, EM (ed): *Licit and Illicit Drugs*. Little, Brown, Boston, 1972.
> A very readable overview of the history and current status of drug use in the United States.

Dupont, RI, Goldstein, A, and O'Donnell, J (eds): *Handbook on Drug Abuse*. U.S. Government Printing Office, Washington D.C., 1979.
> Provides good coverage of recent trends in drug abuse treatment.

Peterson, RC. *Marijuana Research Findings: 1980*. U.S. Government Printing Office, Washington D.C., 1980
> A comprehensive review of research on marijuana.

Specific

1. Burns, RS, and Lerner, SE: Perspectives: Acute phencyclidine intoxication. *Clin Toxicol 9:* 477, 1976.
2. *Diagnostic and Statistical Manual of Mental Disorders*, Ed. 3. American Psychiatric Association, Washington, D.C., 1980.
3. Griffith, JD, Cavanaugh, JH, and Oates, JA: Psychosis induced

by the administration of d-amphetamine to human volunteers. In *Psychotomimetic Drugs*, edited by DH Efron. Raven Press, New York, 1970.

4. Johnston, LD, Bachman, JG, and O'Malley, PM: Student drug use in American 1975–1980. U.S. Department of Health and Human Sciences, Washington D.C., 1980.

5. Kolodny, RC, Lessin, PJ, Toro, G, Master, WH, and Cohen, S: Depression of plasma testosterone with acute marijuana administration. In *Pharmacology of Marijuana*, edited by MC Braude and S Szara. Raven Press, New York, 1976.

6. Melges, FT, Tinklenberg, JR, Hollister, LE, and Gillespie, HK: Temporal disintegration and depersonalization during marijuana intoxication. *Arch Gen Psychiatry 23:* 204, 1970.

7. Novotny, M, Lee, ML, and Bartle, KD: A possible chemical basis for the higher mutagenicity of marijuana smoke as compared to tobacco smoke. *Experientia 32:* 280, 1976.

8. *The Nation's Health*, official newspaper of the American Public Health Association, p. 1, August 1980.

9. Nowlan, R, and Cohen, S: Tolerance to marijuana. Heart rate and subjective "high." *Clin Pharmacol Ther 22:* 550, 1977.

10. Talbott, JA: Emergency management of marijuana psychosis. In *Acute Drug Abuse Emergencies*, edited by PC Bourne. Academic Press, New York, 1976.

11. Tashkin, DP, Sharpiro, BJ, Lee, YE, and Harper, CE: Subacute effects of heavy marijuana smoking on pulmonary function in healthy men. *N Engl J Med 294:* 125, 1976.

12. Van Kammen, DP: The dopamine hypothesis of schizophrenia revisited. *Psychoneuroendocrinology 4:* 37, 1979.

13. Wetli, CV, and Wright, RK: Death caused by recreational cocaine use. *JAMA, 241:* 2519, 1979.

SECTION 3

Allergy and Infectious Diseases

CHAPTER TWENTY-TWO

Allergy and Related Conditions

MARTIN D. VALENTINE, M.D.

INTRODUCTION

Allergy is a hypersensitive state of altered immunologic activity, resulting from exposure of an animal (the host) to a foreign protein (an allergen). This stimulates production of host proteins (antibodies) which combine with the allergen to inactivate it. During the course of inactivation, reactions occur in the animal to produce the noxious side effects which are recognized as symptoms of allergy.

It is estimated that 17% of Americans suffer from acute and chronic conditions generally considered to be allergic in origin (see Table 22.1); approximately 9% of all office visits to physicians are for one of these conditions (1). The majority of visits are for conditions which are known to be mediated by antibodies of the immunoglobulin E (IgE) class or for conditions which resemble IgE-mediated allergy. Since the symptoms in these patients result from the release or formation of a limited number of chemical mediators, effective pharmacologic treatment may be similar whether or not allergy in the true sense is involved.

It is believed that the ability to synthesize relatively large amounts of IgE with specificity for certain antigens may be inherited. The risk of developing an allergy for a child if one parent is allergic is 1 chance in 3, increasing to 2 out of 3 if both parents are allergic.

This chapter is concerned with IgE-mediated allergy and similar conditions (with the exception of asthma which is discussed in Chapter 52). Other immunopathologic conditions which are not IgE-mediated (drug-induced hepatitis, autoimmune hemolytic anemia, and atopic dermatitis) are discussed elsewhere in this book.

PATHOPHYSIOLOGY

Antibody

Acute allergic reactions are mediated by IgE, which was the fifth class of antibody to be discovered in humans. Never present in large amounts, its level in serum is greatest between puberty and young adulthood. As indicated in Figure 22.1, IgE binds to surface receptors on tissue mast cells and blood basophils. The release of histamine and other chemical mediators from these cells is initiated by the bridging of a pair of IgE molecules on the surface of the cells by an antigen molecule of appropriate specificity.

Allergens

Allergens which have clinical relevance are usually proteins with a molecular weight between 10,000 and 40,000. Low molecular weight substances are gener-

Table 22.1
Estimated Prevalence of Common Allergic Conditions in the General Population[a]

Condition	Prevalence (%)
Allergic rhinitis alone	7
Miscellaneous conditions (eczema, urticaria/angioedema, food/drug/insect allergy)	6
Asthma	4

[a] Source: Asthma and the Other Allergic Diseases: NIAID Task Force Report. NIH Publication No. 79-387, May 1979.

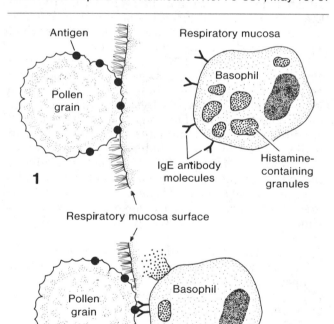

Figure 22.1. Steps in the IgE-mediated response of respiratory mucosa to pollen antigen. *Step 1*, pollen grains containing antigen reach nasal mucosa containing mast cells with IgE antibodies to antigen. *Step 2*, antigen bridges adjacent IgE molecules, initiating histamine release.

ally not allergens unless they, like penicillin for example, are capable of combining as a hapten with a protein.

Mediators

The release or formation of biologically significant chemical mediators is a prerequisite to the development of allergic symptoms. In general, mediators affect smooth muscle contractility and vascular tone and permeability. *Histamine*, released from mast cells and basophils, causes pruritus, flushing, nasal stuffiness, conjunctival injection, bronchoconstriction, uterine contraction, increased permeability of venules, and hypotension. *Anaphylatoxin*, a substance formed during complement activation, induces histamine release. *Bradykinin* and similar polypeptides with potent vasodepressor activity may be responsible in part for the shock of anaphylaxis. *Leukotriene C*, the arachidonic acid metabolite recently identified as slow-reacting substance of anaphylaxis (SRS-A), is a potent bronchoconstrictor.

PHYSIOLOGIC BASIS FOR TREATMENT

Pharmacologic

Drugs can favorably influence the outcome of an allergic condition by acting at various sites in the sequence of the allergic reaction (see Table 22.2). Although no drug prevents antigen-antibody interaction, *disodium cromoglycate* (cromolyn, Intal) prevents mediator release after this interaction has occurred. The formation or release of some mediators is modulated by variation in cellular and tissue levels of cyclic adenosine monophosphate (cAMP), which acts as a "second messenger" for certain energy-requiring metabolic steps. *β-Adrenergic* agonists appear to inhibit mediator release and relax bronchial smooth muscle by increasing cAMP. The *methylxanthines*, such as theophylline, produce similar effects by preventing enzymatic breakdown of cAMP. Con-

Table 22.2
Sites of Action of "Anti-allergic" Drugs

Drug	Action Site	Mode of Action
Cromolyn	Mast cell	Inhibits mediator release
Adrenergics		
α	"Capillary" venules, arterioles	Vasoconstriction
β_2	Mast cell, basophil	Inhibits mediator release (Increases cyclic AMP)
	Bronchial muscle	Relaxes bronchial muscle
Methylxanthines	Mast cell, basophil	Inhibits mediator release (Increases cyclic AMP)
	Bronchial muscle	Relaxes bronchial muscle
Antihistamines	Histamine receptors	Competitive inhibition
Corticosteroids	Not known	Not known

ventional (H-1) *antihistamines* inhibit histamine effects by competing with histamine for H-1 receptor sites. The usefulness of antihistamines is limited by their inability to compete successfully with relatively high tissue concentrations of histamine adjacent to its cellular sites of origin, and also because antihistamines are central nervous system (CNS) depressants. It is unknown why *corticosteroids* exert a beneficial influence in allergic conditions, since in a dose range effective *in vivo*, they seem to have no discernable effect on the events underlying IgE-mediated allergy.

Immunologic

Immunization of humans with extracts of pollens has been shown to result in the appearance in serum of "blocking" antibody (IgG), suppression of specific IgE production, and a reduction in the sensitivity of mediator-containing cells to antigen challenge.

ALLERGIC RHINITIS AND SIMILAR NASAL CONDITIONS

Epidemiology and Natural History

The prevalence of allergic rhinitis in the United States varies from region to region, depending upon the amount and type of pollen in the air. Onset of symptoms is most common between the ages of 10 and 20. The prevalence is approximately 10% in the age group 16 to 64 and may be as high as 20 to 25% in young adults (1).

During the 10 years after onset, about one-third of young adults get better, and almost one-half get worse (1). Some have a permanent remission of symptoms; in the longitudinal study of the Tecumseh population, typical allergic rhinitis remitted entirely in 8% of subjects during a 4-year interval (2). The severity of symptoms tends to decrease in most subjects after the age of 40. Therefore, it is important to consider other causes for apparent allergic rhinitis which begins after age 40. While it is generally thought that asthma develops in many people with allergic rhinitis, in fact only about 10% develop this condition (1).

Differential Diagnosis of Noninfectious Rhinitis

Noninfectious rhinitis refers to those conditions in which there is no purulent discharge from the nose; purulent discharge is typical of nasal and paranasal infections such as viral upper respiratory infection and acute and chronic sinusitis (see Chapter 27). Subjects with noninfectious rhinitis may belong to one of three categories: typical seasonal allergy, perennial (yearround) allergy, and miscellaneous nonallergic causes for nasal symptoms (see Table 22.3). The classification of an individual patient depends chiefly upon information obtained in the history. Some patients may have elements of more than one of these conditions.

Table 22.3
Miscellaneous Nonallergic Causes of Noninfectious Rhinitis

RHINITIS MEDICAMENTOSA
  Antihypertensive medication:
    β-Blockers
    Guanethidine
    Methyldopa
    Reserpine
  Aspirin sensitivity
  Topical decongestant abuse (rebound rhinitis)
ENDOCRINE
  Hypothyroidism
  Pregnancy
  Oral contraceptives
ANATOMIC
  Nasal polyp
  Deviated nasal septum
  Nasal tumor
VASOMOTOR RHINITIS

HISTORY

Symptoms of Noninfectious Rhinitis. The symptoms which trouble patients most are obstruction of nasal airflow, nasal discharge (usually clear), itching of the nose and the soft palate, and sneezing. In addition, discharge, itching, and puffiness of the eyes may occur and there may be periodic loss of smell and taste. Occasionally acute sinusitis (see Chapter 27) or serous otitis media (see Chapter 93) may occur as complications. While these symptoms are not incapacitating, they may interfere significantly with an individual's usual activities and may lead to minor mood disturbance (see Chapter 11) in susceptible individuals. As shown in Figure 22.2, there is considerable day-to-day variability in the severity of symptoms in patients with typical seasonal allergy. Furthermore, the symptoms may vary substantially from year to year.

In nasal allergy due to seasonally prevalent allergens, symptoms will recur each year at approximately the same time. Pollen counts are higher in the morning, and outdoor symptoms are apt to be worse at that time. In nonseasonal allergy, symptoms may be induced by exposure to allergens (such as animal dander) any time during the day. In vasomotor rhinitis (see below), obstructive symptoms are prominent and, in contrast to allergic rhinitis, irritative symptoms (sneezing, itching, and discharge) are usually not pronounced.

Environmental Exposures. In seasonal allergy ("hay fever"), the specific source of the patient's trouble can often be identified by careful history-taking. Skin testing and *in vitro* immunologic tests can be utilized to provide definitive evidence; these measures are appropriate only when an allergen such as dog dander must be identified to assist in environmental treatment or when immunotherapy is being considered (see below). In patients with year-round allergic symptoms, differentiation from nonallergic

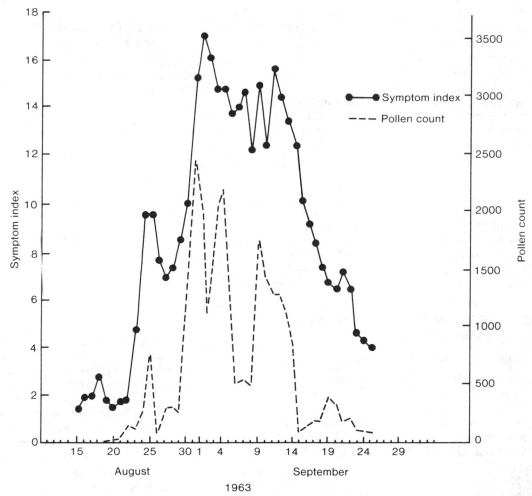

Figure 22.2.   Day-to-day variation in self-reported symptoms during the pollen season, in an untreated patient with allergy to ragweed pollen.

rhinitis may be more difficult. Indirect evidence for an allergic etiology for nasal symptoms includes other manifestations of atopy (see Table 22.1) and a history of typical allergic rhinitis in one or both parents. Blood or nasal eosinophilia (>25% eosinophils in Giemsa-stained nasal smear) may provide additional indirect evidence for allergy.

To a certain extent, even a limited knowledge of local flora will assist the physician in history-taking. The general rule is that plants capable of causing nasal allergy produce copious quantities of pollen in inconspicuous, unattractive flowers which depend on wind for pollination. Therefore, pollen from attractive, pleasantly scented flowers, such as roses is not allergenic, since these flowers depend on insects for pollination. So-called "rose fever" is usually due to allergy to grass pollen, which is prevalent during that period of time when roses are in bloom; the pleasant scent of the rose simply aggravates the patient already irritated by the allergic reaction initiated by grass pollen. In those sections of the country where the seasons are well demarcated, tree pollens are found in early spring, followed in late spring by

grass pollen (Fig. 22.3). Late summer produces ragweed pollen in the east and midwest and cedar pollen in other sections. Mold spores are also prevalent in the fall, but snow during the winter usually prevents further dissemination of spores.

Although *dust* is a mongrel material of uncertain heritage, it may often begin to be irritative during the heating season in northern climes, since all heating systems, but particularly forced air systems tend to disperse dust particles. Among important components of urban dust are the following; fragments of cockroach exoskeleton and excreta; the house dust mite, a nonparasitic organism which exists on human skin scales after they are shed; and aerosolized fragments of the saliva and skin of mammalian pets. Animal hair *per se*, comprising primarily insoluble collagen, is allergenic only by virtue of its burden of dander (shed skin). Symptoms due to animal allergens may be more pronounced in pollen seasons in pollen-sensitive patients and in circumstances when the patient and his pet spend more time indoors, e.g., during the winter months.

Miscellaneous Causes of Nasal Symptoms. As

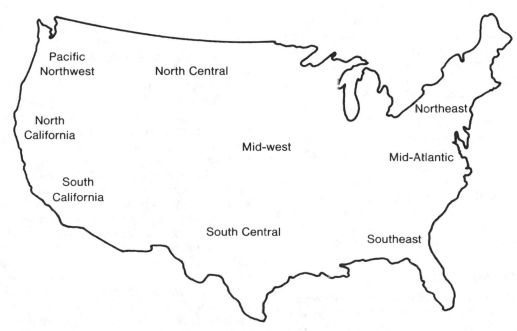

Figure 22.3.   Seasonal occurrence of pollens, selected regions:

Pacific Northwest
Trees: Apr–May
Grasses: Apr–Oct
Weeds: June–Sept
North California
Trees: Feb–May
Grasses: Apr–Sept
Sagebrush: July–Oct
Other weeds: Mar–Oct
South California
Trees: Feb–June
Grasses: Apr–Oct
Sagebrush: July–Oct
Other weeds: June–Oct

North Central
Trees: Mar–May
Grasses: May–Aug
Ragweed: Aug–Sept
Other weeds: June–Sept
Mid-West
Trees: Mar–May
Grasses: May–July
Ragweed: Aug–Oct
Other weeds: July–Oct
South Central
Mountain Cedar: Dec—Feb
Other trees: Feb–Apr
Grasses: Feb–Aug
Ragweed: Aug–Oct
Other weeds: June–Oct

Northeast
Trees: Apr–May
Grasses: May–July
Ragweed: Mid-Aug–Sept
Other weeds: May–Sept
Mid-Atlantic
Trees: Mar–May
Grasses: May–June
Ragweed: Mid-Aug–Sept
Other weeds: May–Sept
Southeast
Trees: Feb–May
Grasses: May–Oct
Ragweed: Aug–Oct
Other weeds: May–Oct

noted above, there are a number of other conditions which may cause symptoms of chronic nasal obstruction. Most of these can be diagnosed or excluded on the basis of the history and physical examination.

Rhinitis medicamentosa refers to symptoms produced by the administration of several sympatholytic drugs (see Table 22.3) or of aspirin, and to symptoms associated with abuse of topical decongestant sprays (abuse refers to frequent use which leads, after 1 to 2 weeks, to tolerance and then to rebound engorgement of submucosal blood vessels as the vasoconstrictive effect of the medication fades). The diagnosis of rhinitis medicamentosa can be made most efficiently by discontinuing the suspected drug. In the case of topical decongestants, the persistence of symptoms after the drug has been stopped suggests allergic or vasomotor rhinitis.

The nasal symptoms, chiefly obstructive, which may accompany *pregnancy, oral contraceptive use,* and *hypothyroidism,* are most readily recognized be-

cause of their temporal association with one of these conditions and their remission when the inciting condition is no longer present.

The recognition of *anatomic causes* for chronic nasal symptoms depends chiefly upon the physical examination (see below). An uncommon problem such as a tumor may be suspected if there are new and progressive symptoms, especially in older individuals. Polyps or deviated nasal septum may produce chronic obstructive symptoms which are difficult to separate from perennial allergy or vasomotor rhinitis. In patients with the combination of aspirin-induced bronchospasm and nasal symptoms (see below, p. 188), polyps are common. Whenever one of these anatomic causes is suspected, the patient should be referred to an otolaryngologist.

In over half of the patients with chronic, nonseasonal nasal symptoms, the clinical evidence will not support the diagnosis of perennial allergy or one of the miscellaneous causes just described. These patients are thought to have the poorly understood condition known as *vasomotor rhinitis* (9). As is true of allergic rhinitis, symptoms of vasomotor rhinitis are also thought to be provoked by environmental stimuli. The pathophysiology of this condition seems to involve inappropriate heightened reactivity of the nasal membranes to a variety of stimuli. Typically the patient awakes in the morning without symptoms but develops nasal congestion, with or without discharge and sneezing, shortly after getting out of bed; moreover, exposure to a cold bedroom or bathroom, particularly to cold bathroom tiles, is frequently identified by the patient as an inciting stimulus. Pleasant scents (in perfumes or in household products such as soaps and detergents), cooking odors, products of combustion, and emotional stress may all precipitate symptoms.

PHYSICAL EXAMINATION

Allergic and vasomotor rhinitis, with or without conjunctivitis, usually presents with swollen nasal membranes and enlarged turbinates which are often described as "pale" or "blue." The usual healthy pink appearance is absent. It may be difficult to differentiate edematous membranes or turbinates from nasal polyps; the appearance of pearly glistening globules, resembling peeled green grapes, in the nasal cavity suggests polyps and requires the opinion of an otolaryngologist. Polyps usually arise from stalks originating in the ethmoid sinuses. They are usually visible on speculum examination; at times, they may fill the nasal cavity.

Management of Allergic Rhinitis

The management of the patient with seasonal or perennial allergic rhinitis is outlined in Table 22.4.

Table 22.4
Management of Allergic Rhinitis

AVOIDANCE AND ENVIRONMENTAL CONTROL
Control dust
Isolate furred animals
Obtain machine-washable polyester pillows
Seal mattress in zippered cover
Close windows, use air-conditioning
Filter air
Electrostatic
HEPA
PHARMACOLOGIC TREATMENT
Antihistamine alone (for discharge, sneezing, itchy eyes)
Decongestant alone (for obstruction)
Antihistamine-decongestant combination
Topical disodium cromoglycate (cromolyn)
Topical corticosteroid
Systemic corticosteroid
IMMUNOTHERAPY
Rational choice of allergens
History
Skin-testing
Adequate dosage essential

AVOIDANCE AND ENVIRONMENTAL CONTROL

The treatment of choice is removal of a suspected allergen from the environment. If this is not possible, other environmental manipulations may be carried out. Since the allergic patient is rarely affected by only one allergen, general control of the environment with respect to removal of as many irritants as possible is often beneficial, even though the irritants play only a contributory role. Thus, the allergic patient will benefit from avoiding smoke in the environment, although smoke is not usually regarded as an antigen-containing substance. Clearly *animal-sensitive* patients will benefit by removing the animal from the home, or attempts to reduce direct contact with it. Improvement of symptoms thereafter is gradual owing to the tendency of microscopic fragments of dander to persist in the environment, even for several months; thorough vacuum cleaning and washing, if feasible, of all fabrics and surfaces are indicated. If it is questionable whether a pet is actually producing allergic symptoms, it is appropriate to send the patient, not the pet, for a short stay away from home. If the symptoms improve outside the home, but recur on return to home, this is presumptive evidence of the presence of allergen(s) in the home, usually from an animal or an unsuspected source of mold or related fungal growth, such as a contaminated humidifier reservoir.

The *quality of the air* in closed environments can have a significant impact on symptoms. Regulation of the relative humidity is useful; it should be maintained between 35 and 40% during the winter. Humidifier reservoirs must be kept clean. Reduction of humidity in warm, humid summer weather may also be beneficial, although this is less critical unless the degree of humidity is such that it supports visible mold growth. Air conditioning and dehumidifiers are thus often necessary where the relative humidity is always high. Any heating, humidifying, or air-cooling device which depends upon the delivery of forced air must have an effective air filter. Two types of air filtration devices may be used. One depends on electrostatic precipitation of particulate matter as it is drawn through a charged field by a blower. The second type depends on the trapping of particulate matter in a specially treated cellulose filter (the so-called HEPA type). Maintenance of the electrostatic filtration devices merely requires cleaning (usually by washing) of the particle-trapping device. With a HEPA type of filter, accessory filters may need to be replaced on a regular basis. These pre-filters are necessary for trapping larger particles which would otherwise impair the efficiency of the unit. In addition to air-filtering devices, the following are desirable: floors which are bare or carpeted with washable rugs; windows that are curtained with washable curtains rather than dust-catching venetian blinds; bedrooms furnished with washable materials and containing a minimum of dust-catching books and brica-brac; and use of pillows of washable polyester and mattresses encased in zippered plastic covers.

DRUG THERAPY

Symptomatic drug treatment of allergic rhinitis is empiric and usually involves striking a satisfactory balance between the beneficial effects of the drug and the undesirable side effects. The goal of therapy is reduction of symptoms to a level which enables the patient to function normally, since complete elimination of symptoms is usually not possible (see Fig 22.4). Antihistamines are the mainstays of empiric therapy. Sympathomimetic decongestants, cromolyn, topical or systemic corticosteroids, and topical ophthalmic agents may be added to antihistamines depending upon the individual patient's needs.

In many patients, an *antihistamine alone* may provide adequate relief most of the time. This is particularly true when irritative symptoms (sneezing, itching, discharge) are the major problems. Many antihistamines are available. Nearly all produce some sedation and drying of the mucous membranes. Ef-

ficacy in suppressing nasal symptoms generally parallels the degree of these two side effects. As indicated in Table 22.5, there are several chemical classes of antihistamines from which to choose in the treatment of allergic rhinitis. Individual patients may respond more readily to a given class, but within classes, differences in efficacy tend to be slight. Once an effective class has been found for a patient, preference within the class will be determined by relative absence of side effects. There is an enormous cost differential between generic and brand name antihistamines, so that once a patient has found an effective product, he should be encouraged to try an equivalent generic. Subtle manufacturing differences between clinically equivalent products may make a particular one more suitable for a given patient. A useful procedure is to choose one drug from each class as a starting point, beginning with the drug named first in each class in Table 22.5. At first it is better to avoid "sustained-release" preparations; they may be used later as a convenience once the right drug is found.

As shown in Table 22.5, antihistamines are avail-

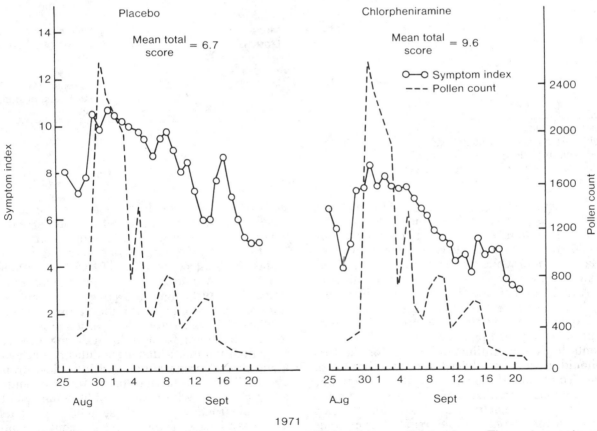

Figure 22.4 Symptom level in patients with allergic rhinitis taking antihistamines. These two sets of data compare the response of carefully matched groups of ragweed-allergic patients either to placebo or to an antihistamine (chlorpheniramine) during the ragwed pollen season. It can be seen that the antihistamine reduces but does not eliminate symptoms (the symptoms recorded by patients were: sneezing, stuffy nose, running nose, red itchy eyes, and cough). (Adapted from M. D. Valentine, P. S. Norman and L. M. Lichtenstein: Evaluation of an antihistamine in ragweed hay fever. In *Evaluation of Gastrointestinal, Pulmonary, Anti-Inflammatory, and Immunological Agents*, edited by F. G. McMahon. Futura Publishing Co., Mount Kisco, N.Y., 1974.)

Table 22.5
Representative Antihistamines Useful in Treatment of Allergic Rhinitis

Generic Name	Trade Name	Duration of Action (hr)	Sedation	Recommended Adult Dose (mg)	Available Preparations (mg)
ETHANOLAMINES					
Diphenhydramine[a]	Benadryl	4–6	Marked	25–50 q.i.d.	Capsule (25, 50), elixir (12.5/5 ml)
Carbinoxamine[b]	Clistin	3–4	Moderate	4 q.i.d.	Tablet, elixir
Doxylamine	Decapryn	4–6	Moderate	12.5–25 q.i.d.	Tablet, syrup
ETHYLENEDIAMINES					
Tripelennamine[b]	Pyribenzamine	4–6	Moderate	50 q.i.d.	Tablet (25, 50), elixir (37.5/5 ml)
ALKYLAMINES					
Chlorpheniramine[a,b,c]	Chlor-Trimeton	4–6	Mild	4 q.i.d.	Tablet (4.8), syrup (2/5 ml)
Dexchlorpheniramine[b]	Polaramine	4–6	Mild	2 q.i.d.	Tablet (4), syrup (2/5 ml)
Brompheniramine[a,b,c]	Dimetane	4–6	Mild	4 q.i.d.	Tablet (4), elixir (2/5 ml)
Triprolidine[a]	Actidil	8–12	Mild	2.5 b.i.d.	Tablet (2.5), syrup (1.25/5 ml)
PHENOTHIAZINES					
Promethazine[a]	Phenergan	4–6	Moderate	12.5–25 q.i.d.	Tablet (12.5, 25, 50), syrup (2.5/5 ml)
Trimeprazine[a,b,c]	Temaril	4–6	Moderate	2.5–7.5 q.i.d.	Capsule (2.5), syrup (2.5/5 ml)
PIPERIDINES					
Azatadine	Optimine	8–12	Moderate	1–2 b.i.d.	Tablet
Cyproheptadine[d]	Periactin	4–6	Marked	4 q.i.d.	Tablet (4), syrup (2/5 ml)
PIPERAZINE					
Hydroxyzine[d]	Atarax, Vistaril	6–12	Moderate	10–25 b.i.d., t.i.d.	Capsule (10, 25, 50, 100), suspension (10/5 ml)

[a] Generic available.
[b] Sustained-release preparation available.
[c] Over-the-counter drug.
[d] More useful in urticaria and pruritus.

able in a variety of strengths and in liquid, tablet, and sustained-released preparations; some are available without prescription. All have their onset of action in 10 to 30 min. Sustained-released preparations generally last 12 hours while standard preparations must be taken at least every 6 to 8 hours for continuous effect. Antihistamines appear to be more effective if dosing is begun in anticipation of symptoms, i.e., before exposure to animals, or before the beginning of the grass or ragweed pollen season.

Patients beginning antihistamine use for the first time should always be advised about the hazard of sedation. To obviate this some patients omit daytime doses and choose to utilize a sustained-release preparation at bedtime, to help assure a good night's sleep and also control adequately the irritative symptoms which are so common upon awakening in the morning.

Sympathomimetic decongestants may add significantly to the beneficial effects of antihistamines. They may be particularly effective in patients who have pronounced obstructive symptoms due to nasal mucosal edema; presumably decongestants work by vasoconstriction which decreases the blood flow to nasal mucosa. A second beneficial property of these agents is that they have a stimulatory effect on the central nervous system, which may counteract antihistamine-induced sedation. Table 22.6 summarizes practical information about a number of commonly prescribed antihistamine-decongestant combinations (all require written prescription). Extendoyl and Histaspan-D incorporate the anticholinergic agent methscopolamine for additional drying effects.

Sympathomimetic decongestants are also available alone in oral preparations and in topical drops and sprays. These forms may be useful in patients with allergic rhinitis whose most troublesome symptom is nasal obstruction or in those who cannot tolerate antihistamines. Decongestant treatment without antihistamine is the treatment of choice in patients with acute sinusitis and serous otitis media, two conditions which may complicate any allergic or nonallergic process producing congestion of the nasal mucosa. Details regarding available decongestant preparations are found in the discussion of serous otitis, Chapter 93.

Table 22.6
Representative Antihistamine-Sympathomimetic Combinations Useful in Treating Allergic Rhinitis

Trade Name	Ingredients	Mg. per Tablet or Capsule	Recommended Adult Dosage	Available Preparations[a]
Pyribenzamine with ephedrine	Tripelennamine	25	1 or 2 tablets q.i.d.	Tablet
	Ephedrine	12		
Co-Pyronil	Thenylpyramine	25	1 capsule t.i.d.	Capsule
	Pyrrobutanine	15		Suspension
	Cyclopentamine	12.5		
Ornade	Chlorpheniramine	8	1 Spansule b.i.d.	Timed release spansule
	Phenylpropanolamine	50		
	Isopropamide iodide	2.5		
Naldecon	Chlorpheniramine	5	1 tablet t.i.d.	Sustained action tablet
	Phenyltoloxamine	15		Syrup
	Phenylpropanolamine	40		
	Phenylephrine	10		
Extendryl or Histaspan-D	Chlorpheniramine	8	1 capsule b.i.d.	Timed action capsule
	Phenylephrine	20		Syrup
	Methscopolamine	2.5		
Isochlor	Chlorpheniramine	4	1 tablet q.i.d.	Tablets
	d-Isoephedrine	25		Syrup
				Sustained release capsule
Dimetapp	Brompheniramine	12	1 Extentab b.i.d.	Extended release tablet
	Phenylpropanolamine	15		Elixir
	Phenylephrine	15		
Actifed	Triprolidine	2.5	1 tablet t.i.d.	Tablet
	d-Isoephedrine	60		Syrup
Disophrol	Dexbrompheniramine	6	1 tablet b.i.d.	Chronotab
Drixoral	d-Isoephedrine	120		Extended release sustained action tablet
Rondec	Carbinoxamine	2.5	1 tablet q.i.d.	Tablet, syrup
	Pseudoephedrine	60		

[a] All require prescription.

In therapeutic doses, sympathomimetic decongestants may cause tachycardia and blood pressure elevation (5). Therefore, it is important to determine the individual patient's blood pressure response before prescribing a sympathomimetic for prolonged use; this can be done within 1 to 3 hours of administration of the drug. Patients with allergic rhinitis should be strongly warned against the routine use of nasal decongestant sprays or drops, as this may lead to rhinitis medicamentosa (see above). Perhaps the best advice for the patient who cannot part with a decongestant spray is that he utilize it only at times when symptom relief is crucial; for example, at bedtime if nasal obstruction makes it difficult to get to sleep (and when the stimulatory effects of oral sympathomimetic decongestants may interfere with sleeping).

For patients whose nasal symptoms are not controlled adequately by antihistamines or decongestants, *topical corticosteroids* may provide excellent relief, at times enabling an almost incapacitated individual to return to normal function. Steroids have a major impact upon obstructive nasal symptoms; simultaneous antihistamine use may, however, be needed to suppress irritative symptoms. Three agents, dexamethasone (Decadron Turbinare), beclomethasone (Vancenase, Beconase), and flunisolide

(Nasalide) have been extensively tested and shown to be effective when administered intranasally as aerosols; they are administered 3 or 4 times daily to both nostrils in metered doses (one or two "puffs" of dexamethasone, one "puff" of beclomethasone, two "puffs" of flunisolide). Each of these agents may cause mild buring; rare side effects include localized Candida, epistaxis, mucosal ulceration, and nasal septal perforation. Patients must be told to expect gradual improvement, over the course of days, in contrast to the immediate response to be expected from a topical vasoconstricter. A disadvantage of flunisolide is that it is packaged in a difficult-to-operate pump-spray device; the other corticosteroids are packaged in easy-to-operate pressurized spray devices. Because topical dexamethasone may cause reversible adrenal suppression after 2 to 3 weeks and beclomethasone rarely does so (11), beclomethasone is now the topical steroid of choice for intranasal use. This agent can be used safely for prolonged periods.

Systemic steroids are occasionally justified in treating seasonal allergy. For example, in a patient who usually requires topical steroids for obstructive symptoms, a 3- or 4-day course of prednisone (20 mg per day) may be needed to relieve nasal obstruction sufficiently so that the aerosol can effectively reach the nasal mucosa. Only rarely should a longer course of steroids (2 to 3 weeks) be utilized to treat allergic rhinitis. The prednisone can usually be tapered rapidly during the last few days of treatment (see further discussion of steroid use in Chapter 71). Although parenteral, "depot," steroid injections are convenient, they are generally contraindicated because they entail greater risk of adrenal suppression.

A possible future adjunct or substitute for antihistamine-decongestant treatment of allergic rhinitis is topical *cromolyn sodium** (4). As indicated in Table 22.2, this agent inhibits mediator release in the mast cells of the nasal mucosa. Aerosolized cromolyn must be administered approximately every 4 hours by metered dose to each nostril in order to prevent symptoms. Mild side effects (chiefly nasal irritation) are common, but they are transient and well tolerated. The disadvantages of this drug are high cost to the patient and the frequent-dose schedule. However, for selected patients with marked seasonal allergy, who get insufficient relief from antihistamines and decongestants, a trial of cromolyn may be appropriate when this drug is available.

MANAGEMENT OF EYE SYMPTOMS

Frequently the nasal symptoms of allergic rhinitis are controlled by one of the above drugs, but the eye symptoms persist. In this situation, any of a number of topical preparations containing α-adrenergic agents such as Vasocon, Prefrin, and Albalon, may be effective; 2 drops should be instilled 3 to 4 times daily. For the patient who is seriously impaired by conjunctival symptoms despite topical vasoconstrictors, either of two relatively weak topical steroids (HMS Liquifilm or FML Liquifilm) may be tried for brief periods; however, an opthalmologist should be consulted, at least by telephone, first. Prolonged use of ophthalmic steroids should be avoided unless the patient has periodic slit-lamp examinations by an ophthalmologist, because of the danger of herpetic keratitis.

REFERRAL TO AN ALLERGIST

If the patient fails to respond to the measures outlined above he should be referred to an allergist for evaluation, to confirm the diagnosis of allergic rhinitis or to disclose any other cause for nasal symtoms, and to determine whether the patient may be a candidate for immunization treatment.

The *immunologic tests* done by an allergist are primarily scratch or intracutaneous tests using solutions of suspected offending allergens. These skin tests are more sensitive, although no more specific, than *in vitro* RAST (RadioAllergoSorbent Test) in which the patient's level of allergen-specific IgE an-

tibody is measured. Moreover, the skin test is far less expensive than the RAST test; therefore, the latter should be reserved for instances where either the skin is not suitable for testing (such as in patients with dermatographism or generalized atopic dermatitis) or where skin reactivity seems to be equivocal when compared to negative and positive controls.

Immunization with sufficient doses of appropriate allergens has been shown to reduce symptoms in 95% of patients with seasonal allergic rhinitis due to ragweed or grass pollens (see Fig. 22.5); however, nearly one-third of patients seem to benefit from a placebo (6). No controlled study has ever demonstrated efficacy of animal dander immunotherapy in patients with perennial rhinitis due to animal exposure. Some allergists, nevertheless, try this mode of therapy in selected hypersensitive patients when manipulation of the environment and pharmacologic control are ineffective.

Because allergic rhinitis is often present in multiple family members, parents may question their physicians about the value of immunotherapy for their affected children. Immunotherapy is rarely indicated in early childhood. Although it may yield apparently good results in the prepubertal child, it should be borne in mind that puberty may also be accompanied by a diminution in symptoms of allergic rhinitis. Therefore, immunotherapy is indicated chiefly in the post-pubertal patient.

Immunotherapy is often arbitrarily recommended for a period of 2 to 3 years. Initially, the patient is given frequent injections of the selected allergen extract, in progressively higher doses until a maintenance dose is selected, after which maintenance injections are given approximately once or twice per month for the duration of immunotherapy. After 2 or 3 years, a decision must be made whether to continue treatment or to stop it and watch for recurrence of symptoms. Some patients who respond well to several years of immunotherapy may continue to enjoy reduced symptoms even after immunotherapy is stopped.

The patient's general physician may at times be asked to administer maintenance subcutaneous allergen injections. There are three types of *untoward reactions* which may occur following allergen injections:

1. An *immediate reaction*, characterized by formation of a wheal and flare at the site of injection. An eruption which is as large as a half dollar is an indication not to increase the dosage of allergen in the subsequent injection. This type of reaction may result from inadvertent administration of the dose too superficially.

2. A *delayed reaction*, which begins 2 to 4 hours after the injection of allergen and reaches a peak at 18 to 24 hours. This is most commonly seen when dust and mold spore antigens are included in the extract, and may be due to nonallergens present in the raw material used to make the extract. This type

---

* This agent is under active review by the Food and Drug Administration but has not yet been approved for intranasal use in the United States.

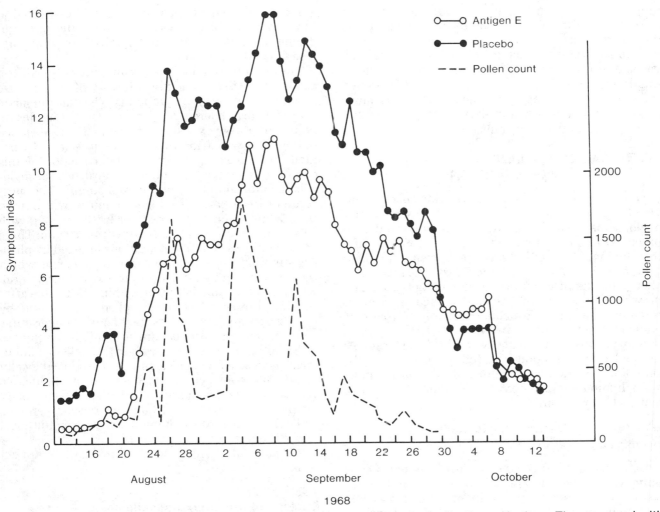

Figure 22.5 Daily symptom scores of patients immunized with a ragweed antigen (Antigen E), compared with matched patients "immunized" with a placebo. (Source: L. M. Lichtenstein, P. S. Norman and W. L. Winkenwerder: A single year of immunotherapy for ragweed hay fever: immunologic and clinical studies. *Annals of Internal Medicine, 75:* 663, 1971.)

of delayed, large local skin reaction may prevent an increase in the dose of allergen because of local discomfort.

3. *Generalized or constitutional reaction.* This may be immediate or delayed; the management of generalized urticaria and anaphylaxis is described below (pp. 185–186).

Management of Rhinitis Due to Topical Decongestant Abuse

Rhinitis medicamentosa of the rebound variety should be suspected whenever there is a history of worsening symptoms of nasal obstruction in association with more than a week of regular (i.e., several times daily) use of a topical deconestant. Management consists of explaining the probable reason for the problem to the patient, discontinuing the topical decongestant, and prescribing a 1- to 2-week course of steroid in aerosol form, which will relieve the symptoms due to rhinitis medicamentosa. The patient

usually has an underlying chronic nasal condition, and appropriate management will be needed when that condition has been identified.

Management of Intranasal Polyps

Polyps may cause symptoms of obstruction to nasal airflow or they may be asymptomatic. They may be seen in association with asthma precipitated by aspirin (see below, p. 188), and there is often associated chronic or acute sinusitis. The treatment of symptomatic polyps consists of topical steroids or polypectomy. When polyps are suspected, the patient should be referred to an otolaryngologist to confirm the diagnosis and to plan appropriate management.

Management of Vasomotor Rhinitis (9)

This nonallergic condition shows little or no response to antihistamines, but symptoms may diminish when the patient is treated with oral decongestants alone (see Chapter 93 for details regarding these preparations). Symptoms may respond to intranasal steroids (see above), which can be prescribed for use during troublesome exacerbations. The most important consideration in management for patients with vasomotor rhinitis is assuring that the patient understands the chronicity of his condition, the limited symptomatic treatment available and the importance of avoiding irritants in his environment and of not abusing topical decongestants.

GENERALIZED ALLERGIC AND ALLERGIC-LIKE REACTIONS

There are two categories of generalized reactions which may be seen in ambulatory settings: urticaria/angioedema (usually not life-threatening) and anaphylaxis/anaphylactoid reactions (often life-threatening). The underlying mechanisms for these generalized reactions are either classic IgE-mediated allergy or one of a number of nonallergic processes in which mediator release and clinical symptoms resemble those in IgE-mediated allergy. These generalized reactions may be precipitated by a wide variety of foreign substances and physical stimuli. At the end of this section, the following five specific causes of generalized reactions are discussed: penicillin, hymenoptera venom, foods, iodinated contrast materials, and aspirin.

Urticaria/Angioedema

DEFINITION AND INCIDENCE

Urticaria and angioedema differ pathologically only with respect to the microscopic depth of the lesion, which consists primarily of the extravascular accumulation of fluid, with no evidence of inflammation. Raised erythematous areas of edema involving only the superficial part of the dermis are urticarial eruptions (hives); while edema extending into the deep dermis and subcutaneous tissue constitutes angioedema. These eruptions usually itch. They may occur anywhere on the body, although angioedema typically occurs on the face and distal portion of the extremities. True urticarial eruptions do not remain in the same area of skin for much longer than 24 hours; persistence of lesions for 72 hours or longer in the same area of skin suggests the possible presence of cutaneous vasculitis as an underlying cause. During a typical episode of acute urticaria, evanescent eruptions may arise in different areas for 1 or more days. Urticaria ceases being acute and becomes chronic after eruptions have continued to appear, recur or persist for 6 weeks or longer.

Urticaria is particularly common in prepubertal females but occurs at some time in approximately one-fifth of the population.

ETIOLOGY AND EVALUATION

A number of etiologies are recognized for urticaria/angioedema. These etiologies are summarized in Table 22.7. Both urticaria and angioedema may occur alone or together in each of the conditions listed in the table; the exception to this rule is the rare syndrome, *hereditary angioedema* (HAE) in which angioedema alone occurs.

The definite (or most likely) cause of *acute* urticaria can often be determined by a history of an exposure preceding the onset of symptoms. The onset of acute urticaria/angioedema may occur from minutes to hours after the exposure to an *inciting substance* (additional discussion of reactions to selected common substances is found in a later section of this chapter). There are a number of urticaria/angioedema states initiated by *physical stimuli*. The most common is dermatographism, a linear wheal with flare which occurs at the site of brisk stroking with a firm object; the eruption fades within 30 min. There are several less common conditions induced by physical stimuli: (a) pressure urticaria/angioedema, which is characterized by local swelling, sometimes painful, which occurs immediately or within 4 to 6 hours after constant pressure has been applied (for example by tight garments); (b) exposure to low temperatures (cold urticaria); (c) exposure to sunlight or intense artificial light (solar urticaria); (d) so-called "cholinergic" urticaria (because it can be reproduced locally in affected subjects by the injection of cholinergic agents) which develops after an increase in core body temperature due to a hot bath, exercise, fever, etc.; and (e) urticaria developing shortly after the local application of heat (heat urticaria).

It is particularly important to consider the rare but

**Table 22.7
Etiology of Urticaria/Angioedema**

ACUTE
  Allergy (IgE-mediated):
    Foods, drugs, insect stings
  Infection:
    Virus (mononucleosis, hepatitis)
    Bacterial (β-haemolytic streptococcus)
  Idiosyncrasy:
    Aspirin
    Iodinated contrast material
    Hereditary angioneurotic edema (HAE)
  Physical agents:
    Dermatographism
    Heat:
      Generalized ("cholinergic")
      Localized
    Cold
    Solar
    Pressure
  Idiopathic
CHRONIC (EPISODE LASTING 6 WEEKS OR LONGER)
  Hepatitis
  Parasitic infestation
  Neoplasm (especially Hodgkins lymphoma)
  Collagen-vascular disease:
  Systemic lupis erythematosus (SLE)
  Polyarteritis
  Idiopathic

potentially life-threatening condition, HAE, in any patient with isolated episodes of angioedema, particularly if there is a history of other family members with angioedema. Onset of symptoms usually occurs before age 20. Typically, the patient does not describe itching. Local trauma may precipitate peripheral attacks. Visceral attacks may occur spontaneously, characterized by abdominal pain. Life-threatening oral or laryngeal edema may occur during any attack. HAE is a nonimmunologic problem, due to deficiency of the inhibitor of the first component of complement. The diagnosis is suggested by a low level of serum C4 and a normal C3 level. Patients with these findings should be referred to an allergist for definitive evaluation, which involves a functional assay for the inhibitor.

It is often difficult to determine the etiology for *chronic* urticaria. The diagnostic workup may include complete blood counts with differential, sedimentation rate, urinalysis, stool examination for ova and parasites and tests for hepatitis antigen (see Chapter 39), cytomegalovirus antibody, heterophile antibody (Mono-spot test, see Chapter 49), cold agglutins, cryoglobulins, C3, C4, or antinuclear antibody. Despite screening tests for underlying conditions, in over 70% of patients with chronic urticaria no etiology is found (so-called idiopathic urticaria).

MANAGEMENT

Many patients with minor episodes of urticaria/angioedema simply tolerate it or learn by trial and error how to eliminate the causative factor(s). Others will seek help from their physician.

The intense *itching* of acute urticaria usually responds promptly to the subcutaneous administration of epinephrine (for adults: 0.2 to 0.5 ml of a 1:1000 solution of aqueous epinephrine, repeated after 15 min if necessary). An antihistamine such as dyphenhydramine (50 mg) or chlorpheniramine (4 mg) orally should be given at the same time. If the parenteral route is used, the initial dose should be reduced 50% to avoid marked sedation.

Additional antihistamines are helpful in preventing prolonged symptoms from urticaria. Hydroxyzine (Vistaril or Atarax) appears to be the most effective for controlling itching (7), particularly in chronic urticaria. A low dose (10 mg every 8 hours) should be tried initially, as the usual dose (25 mg every 8 hours) is much more likely to cause significant sedation. If hydroxyzine is ineffective, cyproheptadine (Periactin) may be tried, beginning with 2 mg every 8 hours and increasing to a maximum of 4 mg, 4 times daily.

These measures are useful in most of the allergic and nonallergic urticaria/angioedema states. There are exceptions, however. Cold urticaria seems to respond best to cyproheptadine (Periactin), 4 mg every 8 hours. Pressure urticaria, when severe enough to require treatment, usually does not respond to antihistamines and may require a short course of corticosteroids. Solar urticaria should be managed with a combination of topical sun screens and hydroxyzine. Finally, HAE does not generally respond well to usual measures, although these may be tried; the mainstay of management is preventive treatment with danazol, a nonvirilizing androgen derivative (3). Life-threatening attacks require admission for observation in an intensive care unit.

Where there is a clear indication that certain conditions promote urticaria, it is important to avoid reexposure since more severe reactions may result. Acute generalized urticaria/angioedema following exposure to a foreign substance signifies that there is a risk of a life-threatening reaction (see below) on reexposure. In addition, in patients with a history of solar, cold, or cholinergic urticaria, there is a small risk of vascular collapse on subsequent exposure. These disquieting facts should be made known to affected subjects and their families in order to emphasize the importance of avoiding exposure, of obtaining immediate medical attention if recurrent exposure occurs, and of administering emergency treatment if there is a severe reaction (anaphylaxis, see next section).

Anaphylaxis/Anaphylactoid Reactions

DEFINITION

Life-threatening acute generalized reactions are not uncommon in ambulatory practice. Table 22.8 lists selected therapeutic and diagnostic substances which have been documented as causes of such reactions; other important causes are insect stings and ingested foods (see below, pp. 187–188).

Anaphylaxis is an immune response to an agent to which an individual has become hypersensitive by

Table 22.8
Selected Therapeutic and Diagnostic Substances Reported to Have Caused Anaphylaxis or Anaphylactoid Reactions[a]

Aspirin (and other nonsteroidal anti-inflammatory agents)
Barbiturates
Blood and blood products
Bromsulfophthalein (BSP)
Cephalosporins
Cyclophosphamide
Dehydrocholate (Decholin)
Diazepam (and other benzodiapeines)
Insulin
Iodinated radiopaque contrast agents
Local anesthetics (procaine, lidocaine)
Penicillins
Phenytoin (and other antiepileptics)
Protamine
Streptomycin
Sulfonamides
Tetanus toxoid
Tetracyclines
Various peptide hormones

[a] Modified from Asthma and the Other Allergic Diseases: NIAID Task Force Report. NIH Publication No. 79-387, May 1979.

prior exposure. A variety of symptoms may occur. Initially, there may be a diffuse erythema of the skin followed by a sense of warmth and then generalized urticaria. Severe and rapidly progressive respiratory distress due to bronchospasm and/or angioedema involving the larynx may follow. Gastrointestinal symptoms may include vomiting, abdominal cramps, and diarrhea (occasionally bloody). Vascular collapse, with or without other symptoms, can occur (anaphylactic shock). Reactions clinically indistinguishable from anaphylaxis can also occur when no allergic basis can be established for the reaction (anaphylactoid reactions).

MANAGEMENT

The recommendations of the National Institutes of Health Task Force on Allergy for the initial management of anaphylaxis and anaphylactoid reactions are summarized in Table 22.9. Because bronchospasm, hypotension, and other hazardous manifestations can recur over a number of hours, the patient should either be hospitalized or kept in an emergency department for observation during the 12 to 24 hours following anaphylaxis.

Avoidance of the offending substance is of course critical in patients with a history of anaphylaxis. The self-treatment kit described below under hymenoptera sting reaction should be prescribed for subjects who are at risk of recurrent accidental exposures.

Table 22.9
Treatment of Anaphylaxis[a]

1. When applicable, place tourniquet above site of injection or sting to obstruct venous return or stop the administration of the causative agent. Remove tourniquet temporarily every 10–15 min
2. Place patient in recumbent position and elevate lower extremities
3. Administer aqueous epinephrine 1:1,000 0.3–0.5 ml subcutaneously or intramuscularly (or if necessary 0.1 ml in 10 ml saline solution given intravenously over several minutes) and repeat as necessary
4. Inject aqueous epinephrine 1:1,000, 0.1 to 0.3 ml at the site of the injection
5. Establish and maintain airway, first with oral airway. If necessary, use endotracheal tube
6. Give oxygen as needed
7. Monitor vital signs frequently
8. If patient is not responding, give diphenhydramine hydrochloride (Benadryl), 60 to 80 mg intravenously over 3 min (maximum, 5 mg per kg in 24 hr)
9. If blood pressure cannot be obtained, give normal saline intravenously and maintain blood pressure with levarternol bitartrate (Levophed), 1 or 2 ampules (8 to 16 mg) in 500 ml 5% glucose in water. Titrate to maintain blood pressure
10. If severe asthma without shock give aminophylline, 500 mg intravenously over 10–20 min
11. While corticosteroids will not be helpful for the acute anaphylaxis, they may prevent protracted anaphylaxis

[a] Modified from: Asthma and the Other Allergic Dieases: NIAID Task Force Report. NIH Publication No. 79-387, May 1979.

Selected Causes of Generalized Reactions

PENICILLIN

Penicilin allergy is a common concern in ambulatory practice, where short courses of penicillin or one of the semisynthetic penicillins are frequently prescribed. The physician may be confronted with either of two problems.

The commonest problem is the patient who needs penicillin and gives a *history of penicillin "allergy."* For the infections treated in ambulatory practice, there is almost always a suitable alternative to a penicillin (throughout this volume, the appropriate alternative is named wherever a penicillin is recommended). The most prudent strategy is to select an alternative drug whenever there is a possibility of prior penicillin allergy, even though this will lead to some unneccessary substitution, as almost half of patients giving a history of penicillin allergy do not in fact show allergic reactions when rechallenged with penicillin (10). In an ambulatory patient who has been labeled "allergic to penicillin" on the basis of an atypical "allergic" reaction, genuine penicillin allergy can be confirmed or excluded by skin-testing, ideally utilizing both major and minor determinant penicillin antigens (10); this may be particularly desirable in a young adult who may be denied access to penicillin throughout his life on the basis of unsubstantiated "penicillin allergy." When such a patient is seen in ambulatory practice, the best plan is to select alternatives to penicillin when antibiotics are needed and to refer the patient to an allergist or dermatologist for administration and interpretation of these critical skin tests.

Approximately half of patients with confirmed penicillin allergy also have positive skin tests to cephalosporin antigens (10). Therefore, cephalosporin antibiotics should not be given to persons allergic to penicillin, and *vice versa.*

Less commonly, the physician in ambulatory practice will have to manage a *first reaction to penicillin.* Table 22.10 shows the approximate incidence of each of three types of allergic reactions (immediate, accelerated, late) following either parenteral or oral administration of penicillin. The management of the more common late reactions (usually nonurticarial morbilliform rashes) is reassurance and a short course of an antihistamine if itching is a problem. The acute management of accelerated and immediate reactions is described in the preceding sections on urticaria and anaphylaxis. Long term management requires assuring that the patient and his immediate family know that all forms of penicillin and the related cephalosporin antibiotics should be avoided.

AMPICILLIN RASH

Ampicillin commonly causes a nonallergic maculopapular rash which is not pruritic. It occurs in approximately 9% of all patients given ampicillin and as high as 50% of patients with mononucleosis (1). The risk of developing this type of rash is also higher

Table 22.10
Estimated Incidence of Allergic Reactions to penicillin[a]

Type of Reaction	Manifestations	Time of Occurrence after First Dose of Penicillin	Percentage of Treated Patients Showing Reaction
Late reactions	Skin rash	≥72 hr	1.4
Accelerated reactions	Urticaria	1–72 hr	0.3
Immediate reactions	Generalized urticaria	2–30 min	0.3
	Anaphylaxis	2–30 min	0.04
	Anaphylactic deaths[b]	—	0.001

[a] Modified from Asthma and the Other Allergic Diseases: NIAID Task Force Report. NIH Publication No. 79-387, May 1979. Results are based upon 70 to 80 million therapeutic courses of penicillin or semisynthetic penicillin or cephalosporin given per annum in the United States.
[b] From 400 to 800 deaths per year in the United States.

in patients with lymphatic leukemia, hyperuricemia, and those taking allopurinol. Rechallenge with ampicillin at a later time often causes no recurrence of the rash or other adverse reactions; therefore, a well documented history of this kind of ampicillin rash is not a contraindication to subsequent ampicillin (or other penicillin) treatment.

HYMENOPTERA VENOM

Stings by yellow jackets, hornets, honeybees, and wasps result in generalized allergic reactions of varying severity in approximately 0.4% of the population (1).

IgE-mediated hypersensitivity to these insect venoms may be confirmed by skin testing with suitable dilutions of available venoms; this is most appropriately done by an allergist. Since victims, unless already familiar with the distinguishing features of the various hymenoptera, are often unable to tell bees from yellow jackets, hornets, or wasps, skin testing with individual venoms is particularly important. After a generalized allergic reaction to an insect sting has been treated (see above) the general physician should immediately initiate a plan to protect the patient's future health. Avoidance of recurrent exposure is critical. In particular, wearing shoes at all times is the single most important safeguard to the patient. However, because of the possibility of unavoidable re-exposure, despite the patient's best efforts, the patient (and ideally a companion whenever the patient is out of doors) should know both the early signs of a generalized reaction and how to administer emergency treatment. An *emergency self-treatment* kit containing syringes preloaded with epinephrine should be prescribed. An example is the Ana-Kit (Hollister) which contains a two-dose syringe which allows administration of two measured doses (0.3 ml each) of epinephrine; two 4-mg tablets of chlorpheniramine; two sterile swabs; tourniquet; and instructions. The Epi-Pen (Center Laboratories) provides a single 0.3 mg dose of epinephrine in an automatic injector which some patients may prefer. The general physician should familiarize himself with one of these kits, keep one in his office, and review its use with any susceptible patient.

Any patient with sensitivity to one of these venoms confirmed by skin test who has had a past history of a potentially life-threatening reaction has a greater than 50% chance of a similar reaction if stung again and should therefore be offered *immunization* with those venoms to which he is reactive. Such treatment is analogous to that described above (p. 182) for seasonal allergy; it reduces the likelihood of a future severe reaction to less than 5%. Once immunotherapy is instituted for insect venom hypersensitivity, it must be maintained through the use of booster injections at 4- to 6-weekly intervals indefinitely.

Even patients who do not have life-threatening reactions (i.e., those who have urticaria/angioedema or other cutaneous symptoms), may be at increased risk of a more severe reaction on re-exposure; therefore, such patients also should be referred to an allergist for skin-testing and for a careful explanation of the available methods of protection (immunization or an emergency self-treatment kit). Patients whose reactions have been local (confined to an area contiguous to the site of the sting) are not considered candidates for immunotherapy, even if the reaction is large.

FOOD

The gastrointestinal tract is sufficiently permeable to antigens found in food that some individuals experience one or more manifestations of allergy after the ingestion of a food to which they have become sensitive. Clinically apparent food allergy is much more common in young children than in adolescents or adults. In adults food allergy usually manifests as urticaria/angioedema or anaphylaxis. In children (particularly those sensitive to cow's milk), rhinitis, eczema, asthma, and colic may also occur. The most common causes of food allergy are listed in Table 22.11 Allergy to shellfish has nothing to do with susceptibility to the nonimmunologic reactions to iodinated contrast materials seen after administration of these materials (see below).

Evidence of sensitization to food antigens can be confirmed by skin testing. It has been established, however, that many subjects exhibit positive skin tests to certain foods but have no clinically relevant symptoms; because of these "false positives," skin tests are not useful in the routine evaluation of food allergy. At present, the only ways of *establishing* that a certain food is a cause of allergic manifestations are

Table 22.11
Foods Which Most Often Cause Allergic Reactions

MOST COMMON:
  Seafood
  Eggs
  Nuts
  Seeds
OTHERS:
  Milk
  Chocolate
  Grains (barley, rice, wheat)
  Fruits (citrus, melons, bananas, strawberries)
  Vegetables (tomatoes, spinach, corn, potatoes, soy bean)

by elimination diets or by blind challenge and objective evaluation of the results. A blind challenge should not be carried out when an anaphylactic reaction is thought to be due to a particular food, because of the potential danger of the reaction.

There is no good evidence for nonantibody-mediated food hypersensitivity, although many practitioners claim to be able to use various techniques to substantiate food sensitivity. A variety of symptoms including hyperactivity, depression, difficulty in concentration, and memory loss have all been blamed on food "allergy." Evidence to support such notions consists of uncontrolled observations by physicians who strongly believe in the existence of such entities.

The management of food allergy is avoidance and, in selected instances, prescription of and education about self-treatment kits (see above). No evidence exists that food sensitivity can be "neutralized" by injections of food extracts.

IODINATED CONTRAST MATERIALS

Patients receiving intravenous iodinated contrast materials may develop one of three reactions which resemble allergic reactions. Neither IgE-mediated allergy nor other immunologic mechanisms have been found to explain these reactions, although complement activation may be shown *in vitro*. The three types of reaction are:

1. *Rash.* Onset of urticaria/angioedema, usually accompanied by generalized itching.

2. *Anaphylactoid.* Cough, dyspnea, wheezing, syncope, with or without urticaria/angioedema.

3. *Vasomotor.* An exaggerated response to dye injection, with more than the usual amount of flushing and nausea, frequently accompanied by a sensation of numbness and tingling of the extremities and transient hypotension of a mild degree.

It is estimated that there is a 1 to 2% risk of developing one of these reactions in the general population and an approximately 35% risk in patients with a prior history of a reaction (1). At the present time, there is no method such as a skin test or a small trial dose to identify prospectively the patient at risk.

Management of the acute reaction is similar to that described for generalized allergic reactions above.

The patient should be carefully educated about the risk of recurrence; and repeat studies with iodinated contrast materials should be avoided whenever possible. In the event that a patient with a history of a reaction (either urticaria/angioedema or anaphylactoid) must undergo a later study, the following regimen should be followed (12): a total of 150 mg of prednisone given in divided doses (30 mg orally every 6 hours for 3 doses before dye administration and for 2 doses afterward), and 50 mg of diphendydramine intramuscularly 5 or 10 min before the procedure. This regimen reduces, but does not eliminate entirely, the risk of recurrent reaction.

ASPIRIN

Aspirin (acetylsalicylic acid) can produce either urticaria/angioedema or an anaphylactoid reaction

Table 22.12
Aspirin Preparations and Aspirin-containing Products

Alka-Seltzer[a]
Anacin[a]
Arthritis Pain Formula[a]
Ascodeen-30
Ascriptin[a]
Aspergum[a]
Bayer Aspirin[a]
Bufferin[a]
Cama Inlay-Tabs[a]
Cirin
Congespirin[a]
Cope
Coricidin[a]
Dristan[a]
Duradyne DHC Tablets
Duragesic Tablets
Ecotrin[a]
Empirin
Emprazil
Excedrin
Fiorinal
Goody's Headache Powders[a]
Measurin
Midol[a]
Momentum Muscular Backache Formula
Pabirin
Panalgesic[a]
Percodan
Persistin
Phenaphen
Quiet World Analgesic/Sleeping Aid[a]
Rhinex
St. Joseph Cold Tablets for Children[a]
Sine-off Tablets-Aspirin Formula[a]
Stanback[a]
Stero-Darvon
Supac
Synalgos
Triaminicin[a]
Vanquish[a]
Viro-Med[a]

[a] Over-the-counter.

in susceptible subjects. These reactions usually occur in patients with a prior history of some type of allergy. It is estimated that this type of aspirin sensitivity may develop in up to 10% of asthmatics (1); the problem is particularly common in patients with both bronchial asthma and nasal polyps.

IgE-mediated allergy to aspirin has not been demonstrated. Further evidence against an allergic basis is the fact that affected individuals may show similar reactions to analgesic drugs not related antigenically to aspirin (indomethacin (Indocin), mefanemic acid (Ponstel)) and to the food-coloring yellow dye, tartrazine, utilized in some foods, beverages, and medication coatings.

The first generalized reaction to aspirin usually occurs in adulthood, most typically a number of years after the onset of asthma (8). Symptoms may occur immediately after aspirin ingestion or a number of hours later. Because of this delay, the role of aspirin may be overlooked by the patient; therefore, it is important to question any patient with an unexplained generalized reaction about the use of aspirin or one of the other agents known to produce these reactions.

The management of the generalized reactions in these patients is the same as that described earlier for urticaria/angioedema and for anaphylaxis. Avoidance of products containing aspirin (see Table 22.12) and the other agents which may induce these symptoms is essential after the diagnosis has been established. Affected patients should be instructed explicitly to use only acetaminophen (Tylenol or a noncoated generic) when they need a mild analgesic or antipyretic.

References

General

Middleton, E, Reed, CE and Ellis, EF (eds): *Allergy; Principles and Practice.* C.V. Mosby, St. Louis, 1978.

  A two-volume compendium with chapters by many recognized authorities on various topics. It is worthwhile to read about a subject in both this and in Samter (see below), since the discussions are often complementary, and at times contradictory.

Mygind, N: *Nasal Allergy.* Blackwell Scientific Publications, Oxford, 1978.

  Recommended for the physician who has more than a superficial interest in nasal problems. One author, one style, clearly written and reasonably concise.

Samter, MD (ed): *Immunological Diseases,* Ed. 3. Little, Brown, Boston, 1978.

  Two-volume work containing more detail on treatment of general problems in immunology than in Middleton et al.

Specific

1. Asthma and the Other Allergic Diseases: NIAID Task Force Report, NIH Publication, No. 79-387, May 1979.
2. Broder, I, Higgins, MW, Mathews, KP and Keller, JB: Epidemiology of asthma and allergic rhinitis in a total community, Tecumseh, Michigan. *J Allergy Clin Immunol* 54: 100, 1974.
3. Gelfand, JA, Sherins, RJ, Alling, DW and Frank, MM: Treatment of hereditary angioedema with danazol: reversal of clinical and biochemical abnormalities. *N Engl J Med* 295: 1444, 1976.
4. Handelman, NI, Friday, GA, Schwartz, HJ, Kuhn, FS, Lindsay, DE, Koors, PG, Moyer, RP, Smith, CS, Kemper, CF, Nagel, JF, Rosch, J, Murphey, S and Miller, DL: Cromolyn sodium nasal solution in the prophylactic treatment of pollen-induced seasonal allergic rhinitis. *J Allergy Clin Immunol* 59: 237, 1977.
5. Horowitz, JD, Howes, LG, Christophidis, N, Lang, WJ, Fennessy, MR, Rand, MJ and Louis, WJ: Hypertensive responses induced by phenylpropanolamine in anorectic and decongestant preparations. *Lancet* 1: 60, 1980.
6. Norman, PS: Specific therapy in allergy. *Med Clin North Am* 58: 111, 1974.
7. Rhoades, RB, Leifer, KN, Cohan, R and Wittig, HJ: Suppression of histamine-induced pruritis by three antihistamine drugs. *J Allergy Clin Immunol* 55: 180, 1975.
8. Samter, M and Beers, Jr, RF: Intolerance to aspirin. Clinical studies and consideration of its pathogenesis. *Ann Intern Med* 68: 975, 1968.
9. Stewart, Jr, TW: Vasomotor rhinitis: Neglected cause of nasal congestion. *Postgrad Med* 67: 171, 1980.
10. Sullivan, TJ, Wedner, HJ, Shatz, GS, Yecies, LD and Parker, CW: *Skin Testing to Detect Penicillin Allergy.* C.V. Mosby, St. Louis, 1981.
11. Tarlo, SM, Cockcroft, DW, Dolovich, J and Hargreave, FE: Beclomethasone dipropionate aerosol in perennial rhinitis. *J Allergy Clin Immunol* 59: 232, 1977.
12. Zweiman, B, Mishkin, MM and Hildreth, EA: An approach to the performance of contrast studies in contrast material-reactive persons. *Ann Intern Med* 83: 159, 1975.

CHAPTER TWENTY-THREE

Undifferentiated Acute Febrile Illness

NATHANIEL F. PIERCE, M.D.

INTRODUCTION

Acute febrile illnesses are encountered frequently in medical practice. Such episodes have many possible causes and range in significance from trivial to life-threatening. For those which require treatment, accurate diagnosis is obviously needed to guide the choice of therapy. In most instances, fever is accompanied by localizing complaints or physical findings which suggest specific diagnoses and guide the selection of diagnostic laboratory studies. Such episodes can usually be diagnosed promptly and appropriate management readily instituted. Thus, for example, fever plus dysuria suggests the diagnosis of urinary tract infection, indicates the need for a urinalysis and urine culture, and is likely to require antibiotic therapy.

A more difficult problem may be posed, however, when fever occurs as an isolated complaint or is accompanied only by nonspecific constitutional symptoms, such as chills, malaise, anorexia, or modest weight loss. Such episodes of acute undifferentiated febrile illness are the subject of this chapter. Although they may raise the fear of serious illness in the minds of both patient and physician, most of these illnesses are benign and resolve spontaneously in 2 weeks or less, without a specific diagnosis being made. In only a very few instances do undifferentiated febrile illnesses persist and remain unexplained despite continued careful observation of the patient and the performance of routine diagnostic laboratory tests. Only when fever has lasted at least 3 weeks in such patients should it be designated "fever of unknown origin" (FUO). Patients with FUO usually require hospitalization for more extensive diagnostic evaluation, whereas unexplained febrile illnesses of shorter duration are usually managed on an ambulatory basis. The aim of this chapter is to describe a rational approach to the diagnosis and management of such acute undifferentiated febrile episodes, emphasizing a careful balance between cautious observation and active investigation.

ETIOLOGIC CONSIDERATIONS

Infections

Infection is undoubtedly the most common cause of acute undifferentiated fever. An abrupt onset of fever is especially suggestive of infection; however, other causes are possible. The majority of episodes of undifferentiated fever due to infection are self-limited, eventuate in complete recovery without treatment, and are likely to be of viral etiology. The viral agents which cause these episodes are rarely identified and attempts to identify causative viruses by cultural or serologic methods are not usually warranted.

Certain infections may also begin as undifferentiated fever but develop diagnostic signs or symptoms after 1 or several days. These account for only a small portion of the episodes of acute undifferentiated fever, but include serious, sometimes potentially lethal, infections which require prompt diagnosis and treatment. Most common among these are viral infections, such as infectious mononucleosis, viral hepatitis, chicken pox (varicella), and German measles (rubella), rickettsial infections, such as Rocky Mountain spotted fever and Q fever; a variety of localized bacterial infections, such as those involving the pleura, biliary tract, retroperitoneum, kidney, liver, and spleen; and several bacteremic infections, especially acute bacterial endocarditis and salmonella bacteremia. If there has been recent travel to appropriate developing countries the list of etiologic considerations should include malaria, dengue fever, scrub typhus, and leptospirosis, and the possibility of viral hepatitis and salmonella bacteremia is increased.

Drugs

A small portion of acute undifferentiated febrile episodes is caused by drugs. Almost any drug can cause fever in a sensitized individual. Those most frequently responsible are listed in Table 23.1. Fever may begin promptly after starting the drug or may be delayed by several weeks; it may be low grade, or may exceed 104°F (40°C). Chills are uncommon with drug fever, but their presence does not exclude this diagnosis. A maculopapular skin rash or eosinophilia occurs in a minor proportion of cases. Removal of the offending drug is usually followed by defervescence in 1 to 2 days; however, fever may last several days, or up to 2 to 3 weeks, if the drug is eliminated slowly, e.g., iodides.

Other Causes

Other acute processes which may cause undifferentiated fever include vascular occlusive and/or inflammatory events such as deep vein thrombophlebitis, minor pulmonary emboli, and asymptomatic myocardial infarction. Similarly, fever may be the only manifestation of acute hemolytic episodes, such as occur in acute autoimmune hemolytic anemia, hemolytic anemia due to glucose-6-phosphate dehydrogenase (G6PD) deficiency, and the painless crises of sickle cell disease.

Special Risk Patients

In patients with certain preexisting conditions, serious infections play an increased role in causing acute undifferentiated fever. Patients with lymphomas, especially Hodgkin's disease, or receiving therapeutic doses of corticosteroids (more than 20 mg daily of hydrocortisone or an equivalent dose of another steroid), especially if combined with other immunosuppressive agents, are at increased risk of developing primary or reactivation tuberculosis, acquiring or reactivating certain fungal infections (e.g., cryptococcosis, histoplasmosis, and coccidioidomycosis), reactivating certain viral infections (e.g., herpes zoster, or cytomegalovirus infections), or developing infections due to *Pneumocystis carinii* or toxoplasma. Patients with established rheumatic valvular disease, certain types of congenital heart disease (e.g., ventricular septal defect, patent ductus arteriosus, or coarctation of the aorta), or prosthetic heart valves or vascular grafts are at increased risk of bacterial endocarditis (acute or subacute) or endovascular infection. Patients with multiple myeloma, or surgical splenectomy or autosplenectomy due to sickle cell disease, are at increased risk of

Table 23.1
Important Causes of Drug Fever

Sulfonamides	Phenolphthalein
Nitrofurantoin	Thiouracils
Antibiotics[a]	Procainamide
Barbiturates	Quinidine
Diphenylhydantoin	Atropine
Iodides	Methyldopa
	Hydralazine
INH	Ethambutol
(isoniazid,	
isonicotinic	
acid hydrazide)	

[a] Especially penicillins and cephalosporins.

serious spontaneous bacteremia, due especially to *Streptococcus pneumoniae, Haemophilus influenzae* or salmonellae. Persons with advanced hepatic cirrhosis, especially when it is accompanied by ascites, may develop spontaneous bacterial peritonitis, often without localizing signs or symptoms. And persons who administer illicit drugs to themselves intravenously are at risk of developing bacterial sepsis due to contaminated needles or nonsterile technique.

In other patients, especially elderly people and chronic alcoholics, the usual signs and symptoms of some acute bacterial infections may be diminished or absent. Fever may be the only manifestation of pneumonia, empyema, or localized intra-abdominal infection in such persons.

Chronic Fever

The major causes of unexplained fever lasting more than 3 weeks (FUO) differ appreciably from those described above. The most common causes are (a) chronic infections, especially tuberculosis, subacute bacterial endocarditis, chronic osteomyelitis, occult intra-abdominal abscesses, and brucellosis; (b) collagen-vascular or rheumatic diseases, especially systemic lupus erythematosus, temporal arteritis, rheumatic fever, and rheumatoid arthritis; (c) certain neoplasms, especially lymphoma, acute leukemia, reticulum cell sarcoma, hypernephroma, hepatoma, pancreatic carcinoma, carcinoma of the lung, and malignancies involving bone, and (d) miscellaneous disorders such as alcoholic hepatitis, hyperthyroidism, drug fever, inflammatory bowel disease, sarcoidosis, thyroiditis, and recurrent pulmonary emboli.

Early diagnosis of these chronic disorders is sometimes possible, especially when localizing symptoms or signs are present. Otherwise, these diagnoses are usually considered only when fever has been unexplained for at least 3 weeks and preliminary diagnostic studies have been unrewarding.

DIAGNOSTIC APPROACH

There are two major goals in managing patients with acute undifferentiated fever; first, early diagnosis in those few instances of serious illness which require specific treatment, and second, the avoidance of unnecessary and expensive diagnostic studies and "blind therapy" for the majority of patients whose course will prove benign and self-limited. The key to achievement of these goals is careful, repeated evaluation of the patient's history and physical findings and judicious use of diagnostic tests. A sequential evaluation process, which emphasizes frequent reevaluation combined with increasing diagnostic studies, is summarized in Table 23.2 and described below.

Normal Temperature Range

The normal temperature range varies from person to person, and at times an individual will be concerned about a temperature reading which seems higher than "normal." The oral temperature of most

Table 23.2
Acute Undifferentiated Febrile Illness: Summary of Sequential Evaluation Process

Evaluation Process	Comment
INITIAL EVALUATION	
1. History, physical examination; if negative and not seriously ill, observe 7–10 days; frequent phone contact	Spontaneous defervescence common, benign illness common
2. More thorough evaluation of "special risk" patients, including laboratory studies	Increased risk that fever is caused by serious illness, usually infection
3. If seriously ill: more extensive laboratory studies; may need hospitalization and treatment	
REPEAT EVALUATIONS (AT WEEKLY INTERVALS)	
1. Carefully repeated history and physical examination, expanded laboratory evaluation	Thorough re-evaluation often detects cause of fever
2. Discontinue recent drugs, document fever	
AFTER 3 WEEKS	
1. Begin evaluation for true FUO, usually requires hospitalization	Spontaneous defervescence uncommon, fever usually due to serious illness with substantial risk of mortality

Table 23.3
Signs or Symptoms to Be Sought During the Initial Evaluation of Patients with Acute Undifferentiated Fever

Anatomical Site	Symptom	Sign
Ear, nose, throat	Ear pain	Red eardrum
	Sinus pain	Sinus tenderness
	Sore throat	Injected pharynx
	Toothache	Tooth tenderness
Eyes	Visual impairment	
Lower respiratory tract	Dyspnea	Abnormal breath sounds
	Cough	Pleural rub
	Shortness of breath	
Cardiac	Chest pain	New or changing murmur
		Pericardial rub
Gastrointestinal	Abdominal pain	Abdominal tenderness
	Nausea, vomiting	Hepatic enlargement
	Diarrhea	Jaundice
Genitourinary	Hematuria	Costovertebral angle
	Dysuria	tenderness
	Flank pain	
Muscle, bone, joint	Myalgias	Arthritis
	Arthralgias	Focal bone tenderness
Skin		Rash
		Boils
		Venipuncture marks
Neurological	Severe headache	Meningismus
	Neck pain	Lethargy, coma, disorientation
	Seizures	
Lymphoid		Splenomegaly
		Tender, enlarged lymph node(s)

healthy individuals remains within the range 96.5°F (35.8°C) to 99°F (37.2°C). There is a diurnal variation as great as 2°F in many individuals, the lowest temperature occurring between 2 a.m. and 4 a.m. and the highest between 6 p.m. and 10 p.m. In very hot weather, an individual's temperature may be 0.5°F to 1°F higher than usual. Very vigorous exercise such as marathon running will cause the temperature to rise as high as 105°F.

Whenever a slightly higher temperature is reported, in the absence of any symptoms of infection, the patient should be asked to keep a 2- or 3-day record of morning and evening temperatures. This record will usually indicate temperature variations within the normal range, and the patient can be reassured that he does not have a fever.

Initial Evaluation

The initial evaluation of most patients with an acute undifferentiated febrile illness requires about 15 minutes. A febrile illness is present if an oral temperature exceeding 99.5°F (37.6°C) is found on examination or by history. The evaluation of such patients should aim to detect the signs, symptoms, or historical background which localizes the cause of fever or suggests specific diagnoses as indicated in Table 23.3. A history of similar symptoms among others at home or work suggests an infectious process. Fever with no other signs or symptoms in a patient recently started on a new drug suggests drug fever. If no localizing signs or symptoms are found and the patients does not seem seriously ill, no further evaluation is needed. The patient should be reassured and instructed to keep a record of morning and evening temperatures at home if the fever persists. A telephone call should be scheduled after 1 or 2 days, as a simple means of following the course of the illness, detecting new complaints, and providing reassurance. If undifferentiated fever persists for 7 to 10 days, the patient should return for a thorough re-evaluation.

Exceptions to this pattern of management are patients whose constitutional symptoms are severe, who have those underlying conditions which predispose to serious infections or mask their manifestations (see above), who have been recently hospitalized or have undergone invasive diagnostic studies, or who describe fever of at least 2 weeks duration when first seen. The initial evaluation of such patients should be expanded to include a thorough history and physical examination, as described below under "Re-evaluation," and the following laboratory studies: chest X-ray with posteroanterior (PA) and lateral views, complete blood count with differential, erythrocyte sedimentation rate, liver function tests, blood cultures (aerobic and anaerobic) from at least two sites, urinalysis, and quantitative urine culture, if the urinalysis reveals pyuria or bacteriuria. Positive findings should be used to guide further studies or treatment. Patients with severe constitutional symptoms may require hospitalization and prompt antibiotic therapy for possible bacteremia, especially if underlying conditions predisposing to bacteremia are present and/or hematologic findings suggestive of bacteremia are found (e.g. Döhle bodies or vacuoles in polymorphonuclear neutrophilic leukocytes (PMNs), or increased numbers of PMN band-forms with an elevated or depressed total white count). If not hospitalized, such patients should be re-evaluated daily by telephone or by an office visit until severe symptoms subside or the cause is determined.

Reevaluation

Patients with unexplained fever lasting a week or more after the initial evaluation should be thoroughly re-evaluated. *The history* should be carefully reviewed, including a history of recent travel (especially to areas of poor sanitation), contact with persons with infectious or febrile illnesses (especially hepatitis or mononucleosis), drug use (including recently prescribed drugs, over-the-counter medications, and illicit drugs), alcohol abuse, and familial disorders associated with fever or infection. The past medical and surgical history should be thoroughly explored. The review of systems should be repeated to detect any new complaints or subtle complaints missed at the initial evaluation. Trivial symptoms, such as vague abdominal discomfort, may prove of great value in localizing the cause of fever.

The *physical examination* should be meticulously reperformed. As with the history, subtle findings may prove invaluable. Essential procedures sometimes ignored, but which must be included, are funduscopic examination of the eyes (after dilating the pupils, if necessary), examination for a tender or enlarged temporal artery, search for a new or changing heart murmur, detection of enlargement or tenderness of the thyroid gland, search for pericardial, pleural, or hepatic friction rubs, search for hepatomegaly or splenomegaly, detection of subtle abdominal or hepatic tenderness, examination of the rectum and prostate, pelvic examination, thorough search for lymphadenopathy including epitrochler nodes, and examination of skin and mucus membranes (including conjunctivae) for petechiae, and of nail beds for splinter hemorrhages.

Laboratory studies should also be initiated. A complete blood count, differential count, and urinalysis should be performed. Additional studies should include a chest X-ray (PA and lateral views), erythrocyte sedimentation rate, serum alkaline phosphatase, SGOT, SGPT, and a test for occult fecal blood. At least two blood cultures (each cultured aerobically and anaerobically) should be obtained. The urine should be cultured if pyuria or bacteriuria is observed. An intermediate strength PPD test should be applied. If there has been travel within 6 months to an area where malaria is endemic, appropriate blood smears should be examined. Any medications started during the previous 2 months should be discontinued or, if that is not possible, replaced by substitutes. This is especially important for those drugs listed in Table 23.1. (Digitalis preparations do not cause drug fever and need not be discontinued.)

Patients should then chart their temperature at least twice daily for another full week. If unexplained fever persists, the history and physical examination should again be reviewed with great care. Additional laboratory studies and tests should include skin tests for cutaneous anergy (if intermediate purified protein derivative (PPD) was negative), an electrocardiogram, serum calcium determination, serum titers of antistreptolysin O, rheumatoid factor and antinuclear antibody, and a monospot test. The complete blood count, differential count, and urinalysis should be repeated.

If fever is still unexplained, temperature should again be charted for a full week. Documentation of temperature recordings by an independent observer is important to rule out factitious fever. Patients remaining febrile for at least 3 weeks and lacking a recognized cause or provisional diagnosis despite the evaluations described above should be hospitalized for more extensive studies.

MANAGEMENT OF FEVER

Fever is not usually harmful and antipyretic therapy is not often needed. Moreover, such treatment may confuse the clinical picture by altering the temperature pattern. In certain circumstances, however control of fever is desirable. These include, (a) persons with severely compromised cardiac function in whom fever-associated tachycardia further impairs cardiac output, and (b) persons such as alcoholics or those with senile dementia who develop increasing confusion or delerium when febrile.

Aspirin is usually effective as an antipyretic, but may cause an uncomfortable diaphoresis or actually precipitate shaking chills. These side effects can be minimized by giving the dose of 0.3 to 0.6 g regularly at 3- to 4-hour intervals. Acetaminophen, in similar dosage, may be used in patients allergic to aspirin, with hemorrhagic diatheses, or with a history of gastrointestinal bleeding, or poor tolerance of aspirin.

Antibiotics have no place in the treatment of patients with acute undifferentiated fever, except in patients who apper dangerously ill or who have seriously compromised defenses against infection. The premature use of antibiotics serves only to confuse interpretation of the patient's clinical course, add unnecessary expense, and risk the addition of drug toxicity to the patient's complaints. In most instances, antibiotics should be withheld until a diagnosis for which they are indicated is made.

The daily activities of febrile patients need not be severely restricted, but should be moderated to provide additional rest, light meals, and the avoidance of strenuous or tiring tasks.

References

Cluff, LE and Johnson, JE: Drug fever. *Prog Allergy* 8: 149, 1964.
A thorough review of the features of drug fever and the most common causative agents.
Esposito, AL and Gleckman, RA: A diagnostic approach to the adult with fever of unknown origin. *Arch Intern Med* 139: 575, 1979.
This article includes initial evaluation of patients with acute undifferentiated fever as well as those with true fever of unknown origin.
Petersdorf, RG and Beeson, PB: Fever of unexplained origin: Report on 100 cases. *Medicine* 40: 1, 1961.
A classic description of true fever of unknown origin.
Vickery, DM and Quinnell, RK: Fever of unknown origin: An algorithmic approach. *JAMA* 238: 2183, 1977.
A useful example of a systematic approach to evaluation of fever.

CHAPTER TWENTY-FOUR

Bacterial Infections of the Skin

NATHANIEL F. PIERCE, M.D.

INTRODUCTION

Skin infections are extremely common. Although most are trivial in nature and are managed at home without medical assistance, each year about 5% of the population develops skin infections which require medical attention; these are usually caused by *Streptococcus pyogenes* or *Staphylococcus aureus*. The seriousness of these infections depends upon the nature of the infecting organism, especially its array of virulence factors such as proteolytic enzymes and toxins, and upon the condition of normal host defense mechanisms. Thus, cutaneous infections due to *S. pyogenes* or *S. aureus* in otherwise healthy persons usually cause only modest morbidity and respond rapidly to appropriate treatment. However, the same organisms can cause serious infections in diabetics, in persons with impaired blood supply to, or lymphatic or venous drainage of, the infected site, or in patients with defects in leukocytic or immunologic defense mechanisms. Serious infection is also more likely when other bacteria, or combinations of bacteria, are involved such as occurs in bites, or wounds contaminated with fecal material, animal products, or soil.

This chapter has two aims: first, to aid recognition and guide treatment of those skin infections which can be readily managed on an ambulatory basis, and second, to describe those infections which require more intensive management, either in hospital or by specialists.

SUPERFICIAL INFECTIONS CAUSED PREDOMINANTLY BY *STREPTOCOCCUS PYOGENES*

Impetigo, ecthyma, and erysipelas are due largely to *S. pyogenes*, although *S. aureus* may play a causative role in some instances. These infections are all superficial, arising from breaks in the skin which are often so minor that they are unnoticed.

Impetigo

Impetigo occurs mostly among preschool children, especially in warm humid climates and when personal hygiene is poor. Under these conditions, the disease is highly contagious and distinct outbreaks may occur. Older children and adults are only occasionally affected. Although *S. pyogenes* is usually the causative agent, *S. aureus* is often present and sometimes appears to play a pathogenic role. Impetigo begins as a pruritic focal superficial eruption of small 1- to 2-mm vesicles, often on the face near the nares, or on the chin. There is usually no history of preceding trauma. In several days the vesicles change to pustules which break, become crusted, and have an erythematous base. Regional lymphadenopathy is common, but there are no constitutional symptoms. Without treatment, the process persists; it may spread due to scratching, or remain localized. Healing occurs without scarring. Streptococcal impetigo may recur if personal hygiene is not improved.

A bullous form of impetigo is caused by *S. aureus*. It can cause epidemics among newborns, but occurs only sporadically among children; adult cases are uncommon. The process begins as a macular erythematous rash. The characteristic thin walled, fluid-filled, superficial bullae appear within 1 to 3 days and range from 1 to several centimeters in diameter. These rupture, desquamation occurs, and healing without scarring follows in about 7 days. In its most dramatic form, this process causes the "scalded skin" syndrome, a disease of small children in which there is extensive superficial desquamation.

Ecthyma

Ecthyma occurs under the same conditions of poor hygiene that promote streptococcal impetigo. It is characterized by discrete ulcerating lesions (3 to 10 mm diameter) with an adherent necrotic crust and surrounding erythema; a small amount of pus often underlies the crust. The ulcer is sufficiently deep to cause permanent scarring. Lesions are most common on the anterior tibial surface at sites of minor trauma or insect bites. Untreated, the lesions tend to spread centrifugally and there may be associated lymphadenopathy; systemic symptoms, however, are lacking. Cultures of pus may yield both S. pyogenes and S. aureus, but the former appear to play the major pathogenic role.

Erysipelas

Erysipelas involves progressive, often rapid, spread of infection through superficial layers of skin and lymphatics. It may occur after a minor wound in normal skin, but is more likely when prior injury or disease has impaired the lymphatic or venous drainage of the skin or left extensive scarring, as for example in a patient with chronic venous insufficiency of the lower extremities or with a radical mastectomy. The infection is characterized by a rapidly spreading area of marked erythema with warmth, local pain, a sharp margin between involved and uninvolved skin, and firm edema which gives the skin a typical "orange peel" appearance. Fluctuation and dermal necrosis are lacking, although there may be seropurulent drainage at the inoculation site. Erythema frequently extends centrally along superficial draining lymphatics; regional lymph nodes are often enlarged and tender. Systemic toxicity, chills, and fever are common. If untreated, metastatic infection may occur, and there is appreciable mortality. Facial infections are dangerous because of possible intracranial spread via draining lymphatics or veins. Extensive involvement of the trunk causes increased morbidity and a risk of mortality. Almost all episodes of erysipelas are due to S. pyogenes, although a very few are due to S. aureus and these cannot always be distinguished clinically. Infections resembling erysipelas may also be caused by Pasteurella multocida or Erysipelothrix rhusiopathiae (see Table 24.4).

Management

Bacterial cultures of the lesions of impetigo, bullous impetigo, and ecthyma are not usually helpful. Impetigo and ecthyma may reveal mixed cultures of S. pyogenes and S. aureus, whereas lesions of bullous impetigo are frequently sterile. Similarly, cultures of early and mild erysipelas are unnecessary. In contrast, blood cultures should be obtained when erysipelas is extensive or associated with marked systemic toxicity (e.g., temperature greater than 102°F, shaking chills, patient feels "sick"). Should there be seropurulent drainage at the site of inoculation, this should be cultured as well. Placing the culture swab in a transport medium, such as Carey-Blair medium, preserves the specimen until it reaches the diagnostic laboratory. Attempts to isolate the organism by culturing sterile saline injected and withdrawn at the edge of the lesion are usually unsuccessful.

Systemic antibiotic therapy is required for all streptococcal and related skin infections (Tables 24.1 and 24.2). In general, an oral penicillin is adequate except

Table 24.1
Antibiotic Selection for Skin Infections Due to Streptococcus pyogenes or Staphylococcus aureus

Infection	Antibiotic[a]	
STREPTOCOCCAL INFECTIONS		
Impetigo	Benzathine penicillin	(i.m.)
	Penicillin V	(oral)
	Erythromycin	(oral)
Ecthyma	As for impetigo	
Erysipelas—mild	Penicillin V	(oral)
	Erythromycin	(oral)
Erysipelas—severe	Penicillin G	(i.m. or i.v.)
STAPHYLOCOCCAL INFECTIONS		
Folliculitis	None	
Furunculosis, boils	Dicloxacillin	(oral)
	Erythromycin	(oral)
Bullous impetigo	As for furunculosis	
Carbuncle	Dicloxacillin	(oral)
	Nafcillin	(i.v.)
	Vancomycin	(i.v.)
Cellulitis	As for carbuncle	

[a] A single antibiotic is given. Choices are in order of preference and include an alternate choice for patients allergic to penicillin. See text for duration of therapy and adjunctive treatment. Dosage recommendations are in Table 24.2.

Table 24.2
Antibiotic Dosage for Skin Infections Due to Streptococcus pyogenes and Staphylococcus aureus in Adults[a]

Antibiotic	Dosage
AMBULATORY TREATMENT: MILD INFECTION	
Benzathine penicillin	1,200,000 units i.m., once
Penicillin V	500 mg p.o. 4 times/day
Erythromycin	250–500 mg p.o. 4 times/day
Dicloxacillin	250 mg p.o. 4 times/day
PARENTERAL TREATMENT: SEVERE INFECTION	
Penicillin G	600,000–2,000,000 units i.v. every 6 hr
Nafcillin	1.0–1.5 g i.v. every 4 hr
Vancomycin	0.25–0.5 g i.v. every 6 hr

[a] Choice of antibiotics for specific infections is described in the text and summarized in Table 24.1.

in persons with suspected penicillin allergy, with disease likely to be due to S. aureus (e.g., bullous impetigo), or with extensive infection associated with systemic toxicity. To eradicate completely group A streptococci, antibiotic treatment should routinely be given for 10 days, even though marked improvement may occur earlier.

Streptococcal impetigo and ecthyma are treated similarly. Penicillin V given orally is adequate. A single parenteral injection of benzathine penicillin is also effective and assures adequate duration of therapy. Oral erythromycin is a satisfactory alternative. Adjunctive therapy includes careful daily soaking of lesions to remove crusted debris using warm water with an iodophor (a soap which releases iodine in a nontoxic, nonstaining form) or with a soap which contains hexachlorophene. Topically applied antibiotics are of little value and should not be used. Prevention depends primarily upon improved personal hygiene; the most important preventive measure is careful frequent skin cleansing with soap and water.

Treatment of bullous impetigo is directed at penicillin-resistant staphylococci. The same treatment should be used for the small portion of patients with impetigo which does not respond to treatment with penicillin V; in such patients S. aureus appears to play a pathogenic role and antistaphylococcal therapy is usually effective. Oral dicloxacillin is suitable with erythromycin as an effective alternative.

Minor episodes of erysipelas may be treated with oral penicillin V or erythromycin. Careful local application of moist heat to the affected area appears to hasten clearing of the infection. Serious episodes are those with marked systemic toxicity, extensive lesions, facial lesions, or those occurring in compromised hosts, e.g., diabetics. Such patients usually require hospitalization and more intensive antibiotic treatment (Tables 24.1 and 24.2). Special attention should also be paid to patients with atherosclerotic peripheral vascular disease who have infections of their lower extremities. In such patients, the affected leg should be rested and elevated; sustained pressure on any part of the leg or foot should be avoided.

Persons with preexisting damage to the veins or lymphatics of an extremity may experience repeated episodes of erysipelas which cause further damage. Patients who have recurrent infections should receive continuous antibiotic prophylaxis with penicillin V (250 mg twice daily), benzathine penicillin (600,000 units intramuscularly monthly), or erythromycin (250 mg twice daily). Reduction of chronic edema by fitted pressure stockings or by diuretics helps to reduce susceptibility to this infection.

Superficial skin infections respond rapidly to appropriate therapy. Systemic toxicity and erythema associated with erysipelas usually abate within 3 or 4 days, and discrete skin lesions show marked healing within 10 days. During this period, activity should be restricted in accord with the extent of morbidity.

Minor lesions require no restrictions. Persons with any form of impetigo should avoid contact with infants and small children until lesions heal.

Complications

Streptococcal skin infections do not cause rheumatic fever but may cause acute glomerulonephritis if the streptococcal strain is nephritogenic. Nephritis is not prevented by antibiotic therapy. If a nephritogenic strain is known to be present in the community, initial and 14-day follow-up evaluation should include a urinalysis. Otherwise, nephritis will first be suggested by gross hematuria, acute hypertension or signs of salt and water retention, such as dependent edema or congestive heart failure.

Bacteremia with metastatic infection may complicate neglected or severe episodes of erysipelas. Metastatic infection should be considered in patients with severe disease who respond poorly to treatment or develop findings suggestive of distant localized infection. Possible metastatic infections include meningitis, endocarditis, septic arthritis, infection of preexisting pleural effusions or ascites, or solid organ abscesses, e.g., in the liver or spleen.

PUSTULAR INFECTIONS CAUSED BY *STAPHYLOCOCCUS AUREUS*

These infections include folliculitis, furunculosis, hydradenitis suppurativa, and carbuncles. They represent increasingly severe results of the infection of hair follicles, sebaceous glands, or sweat glands by S. aureus, the end result being inflammation and abscess formation.

Folliculitis

Folliculitis involves minor inflammation of individual hair follicles, often with formation of small superficial pustules. There is little pain or surrounding erythema. In some persons, lesions may recur for months or even years. A common area of involvement is the bearded part of the face in which minor trauma from shaving may be a contributing factor.

Furunculosis

Deeper infection of follicles or cutaneous glands leads to formation of pustular furuncles (boils are large furuncles). These lesions range in diameter from about 5 mm to 2 to 3 cm and occur most commonly on hairy areas exposed to friction, trauma, or maceration, e.g., the buttocks, neck, face, axillae, groin, forearms, thighs, and upper back. Furunculosis may also complicate the acne of adolescence. Furuncles begin with pruritus, local tenderness and erythema, followed by swelling and marked local pain. As pus forms in the center of the lesion, the overlying skin becomes thin, the lesion becomes elevated, pain increases, and spontaneous drainage of pus ultimately occurs, usually with prompt relief of pain and rapid healing. Furunculosis may be a recurrent problem in some persons, especially diabetics and persons who are chronic nasal carriers of S. aureus.

Hydradenitis Suppurativa

This is a particular form of furunculosis due to obstruction of apocrine sweat glands, usually in the axilla, perineum, or groin. The process is chronic, perpetuated in part by the scars, abscesses, and the sinus tracts which develop in the involved skin.

Carbuncles

A carbuncle is a coalescent mass of deeply infected follicles or sebaceous glands with multiple interconnecting sinus tracts and cutaneous openings which drain pus ineffectively. Carbuncles usually occur in the thick skin on the back of the neck or the upper back. Once formed, the lesions steadily worsen, with increasing pain, erythema, swelling, purulent drainage, and lateral enlargement; they vary in diameter from 3 to 10 cm, or larger. Fever and systemic toxicity are common. Carbuncles occur with increased frequency in diabetics. Once established, they may recur in the damaged area of skin.

Management

Bacterial cultures of typical lesions are usually unnecessary since virtually all are caused by S. aureus and most isolates will prove resistant to penicillin G.

Minimal lesions, such as *folliculitis*, require little therapy. Careful twice daily cleansing with a mild soap, preferably one containing hexachlorophene, and avoidance of minor trauma and irritants such as cosmetics or abrasive soaps are usually sufficient.

Furuncles should be managed initially by application of warm moist heat (either as moist compresses or baths) for about 30 min, 4 times a day. Small lesions, i.e., those less than 1 cm in diameter, will often drain spontaneously after 1 to 3 days and require no further treatment. Larger lesions, painful lesions, or lesions which do not drain spontaneously should be drained surgically when they feel fluctuant or contain visible pus. This can be done in the office by making a single incision into the abscess with a scalpel, after the skin has been anesthetized with a topical spray such as ethyl chloride. Antibiotic therapy is not required except for more extensive lesions such as multiple furuncles, carbuncles, or lesions associated with marked surrounding inflammation, in which case oral dicloxacillin or erythromycin (Tables 24.1 and 24.2) should be given until signs of inflammation completely subside, which may take 2 weeks or longer. *Carbuncles* require extensive surgical drainage which is best done in a hospital. Patients with severe systemic toxicity, such as diabetics with carbuncles, require parenteral therapy with a penicillinase-resistant penicillin; vancomycin is an effective alternative for those allergic to penicillin.

Recurrent furunculosis may prove a frustrating problem. Management of individual episodes is as described above, but other steps should also be taken. The anterior nares should be cultured to determine whether this is the likely source of the reinfecting staphylococci. Patients with positive nasal cultures should be treated by application of bacitracin ointment to the anterior nares 3 or 4 times daily for 14 days. Prolonged therapy with bacitracin ointment may be needed if cultures become positive upon cessation of treatment. Bacterial contamination of skin should be meticulously controlled by bathing and shampooing 3 times daily with hexachlorophene soaps, and daily changes of bed and bath linens.

Recurrent furunculosis may occur in certain disorders which impair host defenses. Tests for diabetes mellitus should be made; if positive, strict control of hyperglycemia may prove beneficial. Defects in polymorphonuclear leukocyte function are a rare cause of recurrent furunculosis, but should be considered in patients who show an increased incidence or severity of infections due to staphylococci, Gram-negative bacteria, and fungi.

Hydradenitis suppurativa is an extremely difficult problem which requires prolonged, often lifelong, treatment by multiple methods. These include selective surgical drainage of abscesses, elimination of irritants such as tight clothing, antiperspirants, and shaving of the axillae, careful frequent cleansing of skin with antiseptic agents, local application of heat, intermittent or chronic systemic antibiotic therapy, and in some cases local irradiation or excisional surgery. Management of such patients is best done by physicians especially skilled in the treatment of skin disorders.

Complications

Staphylococcal skin infections may disseminate to other sites. This is especially true in patients with extensive inflammation and systemic toxicity, such as those with carbuncles, in whom bacteremia is common. However, even an innocent appearing furuncle may cause metastatic infection, especially in patients with foci of increased susceptibility, such as ventricular septal defect, valvular heart disease, or arthritic joint. Patients with demonstrated bacteremia who have such preexisting susceptible foci, or whose systemic complaints (fever, focal pain) persist despite antibiotic treatment, should be carefully examined for metastatic infection.

WOUND INFECTIONS

Any break in the skin may become infected. This includes not only obvious trauma, such as lacerations, burns, abrasions, and animal or human bites, but also minor defects such as scratches and insect bites. The features of the resultant infection vary widely; they depend upon the nature of the wound, the type of infecting organism(s), and the defensive responses of the infected person. In many instances, early appropriate management given on an ambulatory basis is sufficient. In others, recognition of serious infection and prompt hospitalization for vigorous medical and/or surgical treatment is of prime importance. Table 24.3 describes findings which require hospitalization and/or surgical intervention. Specific wound infections which can often be managed on an ambulatory basis are discussed below.

Cellulitis

Acute cellulitis (Table 24.4) is a spreading infection of skin and subcutaneous tissues. The involved area,

Table 24.3
Skin Infections: Findings which Necessitate Hospitalization and/or Surgical Intervention

Finding	Comment
Extensive cellulitis or erysipelas with toxicity	Needs parenteral antibiotics, close observation
Diminished arterial pulse in cool, swollen, pale, infected extremity	Possible fasciitis, a surgical emergency
Cellulitis with cutaneous necrosis and/or subcutaneous gas	Needs parenteral antibiotics and possible surgical drainage/debridement
Closed space infections of the hand	Needs surgical drainage

Table 24.4
Important Causes of Bacterial Cellulitis

Cause	Important features
Streptococcus pyogenes or *Staphylococcus aureus*	See text
Gram-negative enteric bacilli, especially *Escherichia coli*	Occur in fecally contaminated wounds; gas may be present; surgical drainage required for gas or pus
Mixed anaerobic and enteric aerobic bacteria	Occur in fecally contaminated wounds; gas may be present; surgical drainage required
Bacillus anthracis	Causes anthrax when minor wound is inoculated by contaminated animal products; local chancre-like lesion develops followed by systemic toxicity
Erysipelothrix rhusiopathiae	Erysipelas-like lesion with central clearing; due to wound contamination with fish or meat products; treated with penicillin V or tetracycline
Pasteurella multocida	Erysipelas-like lesion which follows a dog or cat scratch or bite; treated with penicillin V or tetracycline
Marine vibrios	Necrotizing cellulitis after minor wound is contaminated by sea water or shell fish
Aeromonas hydrophila	Wound contaminated by fresh water swimming

which enlarges steadily, is painful, tender, and intensely erythematous. Chills and fever are common and bacteremia may occur. The lesion differs from erysipelas in that its margin is not as sharply demarcated nor is it elevated. There may be purulent or serous drainage at the inoculation site; in severe cases, patches of involved skin may become necrotic.

The most common causes of acute cellulitis are *S. pyogenes* and *S. aureus*. Presence of Gram-positive cocci in drainage from the wound is presumptive evidence that they are causative. Infection due to these agents may progress rapidly, especially when it involves an area of chronic edema. Lower extremity infection in persons with peripheral arterial insufficiency may precipitate tissue necrosis and secondary infection. Management should include culture of any wound drainage (as described for erysipelas) and prompt antibiotic therapy. In mild cases, treatment may be given on an ambulatory basis. The treatment selected should be effective for infections due to penicillin-resistant staphylococci, as well as penicillin-sensitive streptococci. Oral dicloxacillin is adequate for infections due to either type of organism; erythromycin is suitable for patients allergic to penicillin (Tables 24.1 and 24.2). Local application of moist heat is a useful adjunct to antibiotic treatment; care should be taken, however, to avoid burns, especially in persons with impaired sensitivity to pain. Improvement is usually apparent in 3 or 4 days; during this period, patients should rest the involved area and be told to report promptly any worsening of the infection or of constitutional symptoms. Severe infections require hospitalization and parenteral treatment with a penicillinase-resistant penicillin or vancomycin. This includes patients with extensive lesions, lesions of the face, or serious toxicity.

Secondarily Infected Ulcers

Cutaneous ulcers are caused by a wide variety of conditions including peripheral vascular disease, arterial insufficiency, pressure sores, neurologic disorders, etc. Management of the ulcer is generally aimed at the underlying cause and seeks to improve blood flow, reduce edema, and avoid pressure and trauma (see Chapter 85). Control of secondary infection is also of considerable importance. Superficial colonization with a variety of bacteria is unavoidable and without consequence; however, infection which is deeper or laterally invasive prevents healing and may interfere with other treatments, such as skin grafting. Infection is best controlled by repeated careful cleaning and local debridement. Systemic antibiotics should be used only when all other methods fail to control surrounding infections. The choice of antibiotic should be based on cultures of the wound, obtaining purulent material if possible. Local antibacterials are sometimes helpful. Those effective against a broad spectrum of bacterial agents include polymyxin-bacitracin-neomycin ointment and topical furacin; these should be applied 3 times daily until healing occurs or it is apparent they are ineffective. Soaking with 3% acetic acid 3 to 4 times daily, is helpful in controlling bacterial growth in ulcers colonized with *Pseudomonas aeruginosa*.

Cutaneous Diphtheria

Cutaneous ulcers or other skin lesions may become secondarily infected with *Corynebacterium diphtheriae* causing cutaneous diphtheria. Although the cutaneous lesion may appear benign, myocarditis or neuropathy develops in about 3% of cases. Outbreaks have occurred in the northwest and southwest parts of the United States, primarily among Native Americans or urban indigents. The presence of cutaneous diphtheria in a community should increase suspicion that skin wounds may harbor this agent. The diagnosis should be suspected when existing wounds develop a gray-yellow or gray-brown covering membrane and surrounding erythema (1). Typically, the membrane can be easily removed to reveal a clean base. Other minor skin lesions may also become infected. Typical organisms can be seen in methylene blue stains of smears from the wound and confirmed by culture on Loeffler's or tellurite agar. Presumptive cases should be reported to public health officials and treated with equine diphtheria antitoxin (20,000 to 40,000 units intramuscularly or intravenously after testing for hypersensitivity to horse serum) and either erythromycin (2 g/day, orally) or procaine penicillin (1.2 million units/day, intramuscularly) for 7 to 10 days.

Bites

Bite wounds become infected with the oral, salivary, or dental flora of the biting person or animal and may cause serious local or systemic infections. Initial management before signs of infection appear is of primary importance in preventing certain infections. Appropriate prophylaxis for tetanus is required for all bite wounds (2) (see Chapter 30).

Human bites are contaminated with a complex variety of aerobic and anaerobic oral bacteria. Without treatment, a severe necrotizing cellulitis frequently results. Minor lesions that break the skin should be washed thoroughly and treated with a combination of dicloxacillin (250 mg, 4 times/day) and ampicillin (500 mg, 4 times/day) given orally; oral clindamycin (150 to 300 mg 4 times/day) is appropriate for patients allergic to penicillin. More severe wounds, including wounds of the hands and knuckles, require meticulous debridement and possible tendon repairs. These should be referred for surgical management.

Dog bites carry the risk of local soft tissue infection and raise the threat of rabies. Minor abrasions, shallow punctures, or superficial lacerations require no therapy for local infection other than thorough cleansing with soap and water. More extensive or deeper bites require surgical management for debridement and, in some cases, primary closure; ampicillin (500 mg by mouth 4 times/day) should also be given. Rabies precautions should be taken with all dog bites, no matter how minor. This includes bites by domestic pets, even though the risk of rabies among them is very small. The dog should be quarantined for 10 days; if it is a pet, it may be observed at its home. If it remains well, there is no risk of rabies. If the dog develops suspicious symptoms or dies, its brain should be examined immediately; prophylaxis is required if evidence of rabies is found. If the dog escapes after biting, and especially if the bite was unprovoked, rabies prophylaxis with rabies immune globulin and human diploid cell rabies vaccine is usually indicated (3).

Bites by *other domestic animals*, e.g., cats, should be managed as described for dogs. Bites by *wild animals* carry a greater risk of rabies and are treated similarly, except that rabies prophylaxis is usually required (unless the animal's brain can be examined). Wild animals with the greatest risk of carrying rabies include raccoons, skunks, foxes, coyotes, and bats.

Guidance on the use of rabies prophylaxis, management of the biting animal, and the risk of rabies among various animal species should be sought from local or state health authorities.

Puncture Wounds

Most puncture wounds involve the feet or hands and carry the risk of introduction of infecting bacteria which cannot be removed by washing or debridement. In all instances, patients should receive appropriate prophylaxis for tetanus (3). Low risk wounds, i.e., those not likely to be contaminated by soil or fecal material and in which the wound site is healthy well vascularized tissue, need only be thoroughly washed and observed for several days for signs of developing infection. Should infection develop, any wound drainage should be cultured and treatment begun with dicloxacillin (250 mg, 4 times daily) or erythromycin (250 to 500 mg, 4 times daily) for presumptive staphylococcal or streptococcal infection; the wound site should also be soaked in warm soapy water for 30 min at least 4 times a day. Higher risk wounds, i.e., those likely to be contaminated with fecal material, soil, or foreign debris, or occurring at susceptible sites such as in a diabetic or an extremity with an inadequate blood supply, should be treated with one of the above antibiotics from the outset and the wound site should be rested and treated with warm soaks as above. The patient should promptly report any evidence of inflammation, swelling, or persisting pain. If purulent drainage develops, this should be cultured. Antibiotic management may need to be altered if Gram-negative bacilli are isolated. If pus develops, surgical drainage is probably required.

References

General

Causey, WA: Staphylococcal and streptococcal infections of the skin. *Primary Care* 6(1): 127, 1979.

A good general review of the features and treatment of these infections.

Koblenzer, PJ: Common bacterial infections of the skin in children. *Pediatr Clin North Am* 25(2): 321, 1978.
  A useful review of the subject with excellent pictures of typical lesions.

Musher, DM and McKenzie, SO: Infections due to *Staphylococcus aureus. Medicine* 56(5): 383, 1977.
  With a section on staphylococcal skin infections, including those which resemble erysipelas.

Peter, G and Smith AL: Group A streptococcal infections of the skin and pharynx. *N Engl J Med* 297: 311, 365, 1977.
  An excellent, thorough review of basic and clinical features of streptococcal skin infections.

Wannamaker, LW: Differences between streptococcal infections of the throat and of the skin. *N Engl J Med* 282: 23, 78, 1970.
  A scholarly discussion by an expert on the subject.

Specific

1. Belsey, MA, Sinclair, M, Roder, MR and LeBlanc, DR: *Corynebacterium diphtheriae* skin infections in Alabama and Louisiana: A factor in the epidemiology of diphtheria. *N Engl J Med* 280: 135, 1969.
2. Center for Disease Control: Diphtheria and tetanus toxoids and pertussis vaccine. *Morbidity and Mortality Weekly Reports* 26: 401, 1977.
3. Center for Disease Control: Rabies prevention. *Morbidity and Mortality Weekly Reports* 29: 265, 1980.

CHAPTER TWENTY-FIVE

Acute Gastroenteritis and Associated Conditions

R. BRADLEY SACK, M.D., and L. RANDOL BARKER, M.D.

INTRODUCTION

Acute symptoms of gastroenteritis may follow the ingestion of a wide variety of infectious and chemical agents. Ingestion may occur because of direct person-to-person contact or, more commonly, via food or water. With several important exceptions, the acute illnesses caused by these agents are characterized by diarrhea, with or without other gastrointestinal symptoms (nausea, vomiting, abdominal pain) or systemic symptoms (anorexia, fever, malaise, orthostatic hypotension, neurologic symptoms).

Diarrhea is defined as an increase in frequency and/or amount of fecal evacuations, which are usually fluid (see Chapter 35). The diarrhea of gastroenteritis usually begins abruptly, sometimes preceded by systemic symptoms, and the hour of onset can usually be documented by the patient. With few exceptions, the illness is self-limited and will terminate within 1 to 5 days.

Table 25.1 (infectious agents) and Table 25.2 (chemical agents) summarize the etiologic agents, the pathophysiology, clinical and epidemiologic features, and principles of treatment for those conditions which may occur in the United States.

EPIDEMIOLOGY

The *incidence* of the conditions listed in Tables 25.1 and 25.2 varies from year to year; and the true incidence is never known since a large proportion of cases are not reported to physicians or health authorities. Even when outbreaks of gastroenteritis involving multiple persons are fully investigated, the *etiology* can be established with relative certainty only 50 to 75% of the time. Based upon annual surveillance by the United States Center for Disease Control (CDC), it is known that the majority of reported outbreaks (and therefore probably the majority of cases) are due to *Staphylococcus aureus,* followed by *Salmonella* species, and *Clostridium perfringens.* Physicians and patients frequently call an illness "viral gastroenteritis," although viral agents probably account for only a modest proportion of acute gastrointestinal illness in adults (15, 23). Studies

Table 25.1
Characteristics of Acute Illness Due to Ingestion of Infectious Agents

Agent	Pathogenesis	Usual Clinical Features	Frequency in USA	Epidemiologic Features				Diagnosis	Specific Therapy
				Usual pattern[a]	Source (reservoir)	Transmission to man	Incubation period		
BACTERIA									
Bacillus cereus	Enterotoxin produced in food or in intestine	Vomiting if preformed toxin in food, diarrhea	Not common	CSO	Soil	Foodborne	2–16 hr	Culture suspected food	None
Campylobacter jejuni	Invasion of large and small intestine	Fever, abdominal pain, diarrhea	Probably relatively common	S or CSO	Animal feces	Foodborne or waterborne	? (probably 24–48 hr)	Culture stool, blood	Erythromycin (see text)
Clostridium botulinum	Neurotoxin produced in food	Vomiting, diarrhea, symmetric motor paralysis: cranial nerves, respiratory paralysis, death	Uncommon	CSO	Animal feces, soil	Foodborne (canned, low pH, anaerobic)	12–36 hr	Culture food, identify toxin in food, blood, stool	Polyvalent antitoxin
Clostridium difficile	Cytotoxic enterotoxin produced in large intestine secondary to overgrowth	Fever, abdominal pain, diarrhea (often bloody) in a patient currently or recently on antibiotics	Uncommon	S	Humans (normal intestinal flora)	Probably not necessary but may occur	After several days of antibiotics	Culture stool, identify enterotoxin in stool	Vancomycin (see text)
Clostridium perfringens	Enterotoxin released during sporulation in large intestine	Diarrhea, occasionally vomiting	Relatively common	CSO	Human feces, animal feces, soil	Foodborne (meats)	12–24 hr	Culture suspected food	None
Escherichia coli: Enterotoxigenic	Enterotoxin produced in small intestine	Voluminous watery diarrhea without fever (traveler's diarrhea)	Relatively common (travelers)	CSO, S	Human feces	Foodborne	24–48 hr	Culture stool, identify enterotoxin in stool	None
Invasive	Invasion of large intestinal mucosa	Fever, diarrhea (often bloody)	Rare	CSO, S	Human feces	Foodborne (cheeses)	24–48 hr	Culture stool	Same as Shigella (see text)
Salmonella (many species)	Invasion of small and large intestine	Fever and diarrhea (see Table 25.3)	Relatively common	CSO	Animal feces	Foodborne (many foods, see text) person-to-person	12–48 hr	Culture stool	Selected cases only (see text)
Salmonella typhi	Invasion of small intestine mucosa, systemic dissemination	Protracted illness: fever, malaise, headache, constipation more often than diarrhea, splenomegaly, occasionally intestinal perforation	Uncommon	S	Human feces	Person-to-person, foodborne	4 days–3 weeks	Culture blood, stool, antibacterial antibodies	Chloramphenicol
Shigella species	Invasion of large intestine	Fever, diarrhea (often bloody) (see Table 25.3)	Relatively common	S	Human feces	Person-to-person	12–48 hr	Culture stool	Ampicillin (see text)
Staphylococcus aureus	Enterotoxin produced in food	Vomiting dominates, diarrhea (see Table 25.3)	Very common	CSO	Human skin, nares, mouth	Foodborne (many foods, see text)	2–8 hr	Culture food, and foodhandlers	None

Table 25.1—continued

Agent	Pathogenesis	Usual Clinical Features	Frequency in USA	Usual pattern[a]	Source (reservoir)	Transmission to man	Incubation period	Diagnosis	Specific Therapy
					Epidemiologic Features				
Streptococcus group A	Invasion of upper respiratory tract	Streptococcal pharyngitis syndrome (see Chapter 27)	Uncommon (by this mode of transmission)	CSO	Human pharynx, skin lesions	Foodborne	1–3 days	Culture throat, food, skin lesions of foodhandlers	Penicillin (see Chapter 27)
Vibrio cholerae	Enterotoxin produced in small intestine	Voluminous watery diarrhea without fever	Rare	CSO, S	Human feces	Waterborne and foodborne	12 hr–5 days	Culture stool, antibacterial and antitoxic antibody	Tetracycline
Vibrio parahaemolyticus	Probably both invasion and enterotoxin production; exact mechanism unknown	Diarrhea, abdominal cramps	Uncommon	CSO, S	Seawater	Foodborne (various types of seafood from estuary and seawater)	15–24 hr	Culture stool	None
Yersinia enterocolitica	Invasion of small and large intestine	Fever, abdominal pain, may suggest appendicitis, diarrhea	Uncommon	CSO, S	Animal feces	Foodborne, person-to-person	Probably 3–7 days	Culture stool	Probably tetracycline or trimethoprim–sulfamethoxazole
VIRUS									
Parvovirus-like agents (Norwalk agent)	Invasion of small intestine	Vomiting and diarrhea (see Table 25.3)	? (may be relatively common)	CSO	Human feces	Waterborne, person-to-person (secondary cases)	1–3 days	Rise in antiviral antibody (not generally available)	None
Rotavirus	Invasion of small intestine	Severe gastroenteritis in young children, mild in adults	Relatively common	S	Human feces	Person-to-person (secondary cases)	1–3 days	Rise in antiviral antibody	None
PROTOZOA AND HELMINTHS									
Entamoeba histolytica	Invasion of large intestine	Diarrhea, often chronic and bloody	Uncommon (travelers)	CSO, S	Human feces	Waterborne, person-to-person	Few days to months	Examine stool for trophozoites	Quinacrine (see text)
Giardia lamblia	Colonization and occasional invasion of small intestine	Diarrhea, flatulence with foul-smelling stools	Uncommon (travelers)	CSO, S	Human feces	Waterborne, Person-to-person	1–4 weeks	Examine stool for trophozoites	Metronidazole (see text)
Trichinella spiralis	(a) Encysted trichinae mature, mate, reproduce in small intestine; (b) Larvae penetrate intestine, migrate to muscles where they cause inflammation and become encysted	Diarrhea, puffy eyes, muscle aching, fever, occasionally severe heart failure; eosinophilia typical	Uncommon	CSO, S	Animal muscle (Swine, many wild animals)	Foodborne	2–28 days	Skin tests, antibody, muscle biopsy	Thiabendazole, occasionally steroids (see text)

[a] CSO, common source outbreak; S, sporadic.

Table 25.2
Characteristics of Acute Illness Due to Ingestion of Chemical Agents

Agent	Pathogenesis	Clinical Features	Frequency in USA	Pattern[a]	Epidemiologic Features		Incubation period	Diagnosis	Specific therapy
					Source	Transmission to man			
SEAFOOD									
Ciguatoxin	Toxin with character of cholinesterase inhibitor	Vomiting and diarrhea, paresthesia (warmth, extremities), metallic taste, blurred vision, sharp pains in extremities, respiratory paralysis	Uncommon (Florida)	CSO, S	Food chain of bottom-dwelling fish caught in Florida, Hawaii (red snapper, barracuda)	Foodborne	1–6 hr	Clinical and epidmiologic features	None (sensory symptoms may last days to months)
Scombrotoxin	Toxin with properties of histamine	"Histamine reaction" (flushing, headache, dizziness, burning of mouth and throat; urticaria, pruritus, and bronchospasm)	Uncommon (Florida, California)	CSO, S	Bacteria acting on fish flesh (tuna, mackerel, bonito, skipjack)	Foodborne	Minutes to 1 hr	Clinical and epidemiologic features	None (lasts few hours–few days)
Paralytic shellfish toxin	Neurotoxin causing motor paralysis	Paresthesia (warmth, extremities), floating sensation, dysphonia, dysphagia, weakness and respiratory paralysis	Uncommon	CSO, S	Toxic dinoflagellates concentrated in filter feeding bivalves (mussels, clams, oysters, scallops)	Foodborne	<30 min	Clinical and epidemiologic features	None (lasts few hours–few days)
MUSHROOMS									
Muscarine	Muscarinic cholinergic response	Colicky abdominal pain, nausea, vomiting, diarrhea, salivation, miosis, blurred vision, bradycardia, hypotension	Uncommon	CSO, S	Amanita muscaria	Foodborne	Few minutes—few hours	Clinical and epidemiologic features	Atropine 0.1–0.5 mg s.c. or i.v.
Phalloidin (and other toxins)	Diverse cytotoxic effects, multisystemic	Stage 1: nausea, abdominal pain, vomiting, bloody diarrhea, marked weakness, hypotension (shock) Stage 2: Clinical improvement (day 2 or 3) Stage 3: Severe hepatic failure, delirium, frequent fatal outcome		CSO, S	Amanita phalloides and other Amanita species	Foodborne	6–15 hr	Clinical and epidemiologic features	None
MISCELLANEOUS									
Heavy metals (antimony, cadmium, copper, iron, tin, zinc)	Upper gastrointestinal irritation	Metallic taste to food, nausea, vomiting, or diarrhea	Uncommon	CSO, S	Containers made of alloy which includes a heavy metal	Foodborne (food prepared in, stored in, or eaten from a container from which heavy metal leached)	5 min to 8 hr	Clinical and epidemiologic features	None
Monosodium glutamate (MSG)	Idiopathic reaction	Burning sensation in chest, neck, abdomen, extremities	Relatively common	S	Foods prepared with large amounts of MSG	Foodborne (Chinese restaurant foods)	3 min to 2 hr	Clinical and epidemiologic features	None

[a] CSO, common source outbreak; S, sporadic.

of outbreaks of viral gastroenteritis in adults have shown that the symptoms it produces overlap with the symptoms produced by several common bacterial pathogens (see Table 25.3). A viral etiology is more likely when secondary cases develop in a household, a pattern which suggests person-to-person spread rather than one-time exposure to a common food.

The *sources and modes of transmission* of the etiologic agents causing foodborne illness are summarized in Tables 25.1 and 25.2. These features of the three most common etiologic agents illustrate the diverse ways that foodborne disease is acquired (7):

1. Humans whose skin or nasal mucosa is colonized are almost always the source of *S. aureus*. Contamination of food with small numbers of staphylococci is undoubtedly very common. Staphylococcal food poisoning occurs when contaminated foods are allowed to stand long enough for organisms to multiply and produce enterotoxin. The principal foods in which this occurs are those high in protein (ham, pork, beef, poultry, either cooked or in salads, and cream-filled cakes and pastries) and those with a relatively high salt or sugar content (ham, salads, and custards).

2. Animals are the source of most of the *Salmonella* serotypes causing most human disease; only *Salmonella typhi* and *Salmonella paratyphi* are carried by humans. Transmission from animal to man occurs chiefly by fecal contamination of equipment and personnel involved in the packaging and preparing of foods—most commonly poultry, red meats, and eggs or their byproducts.

3. *C. perfringens* is a ubiquitous organism found in human and animal feces and in soil. Meats are the most frequently contaminated foods; transmission of enough organisms to produce illness occurs typically with inadequately heated or reheated meats (spores may survive at normal cooking temperatures and then germinate and multiply while foods are being held at warm temperatures or being rewarmed at temperatures that do not inhibit bacterial growth).

The vast majority of episodes of foodborne illness follow the ingestion of *normally safe foods* which have been rendered unsafe owing to one (or more) of the following factors (6): failure to refrigerate foods properly or to heat foods thoroughly, preparing foods a day or more before they are served, allowing foods to remain at warm temperatures, failure to reheat or cook foods at temperatures that kill vegetative bacteria, incorporating raw (contaminated) ingredients into foods that receive no further cooking, failure to clean and disinfect kitchen or processing plant equipment, and contamination by infected food handlers who practice poor personal hygiene. A small minority of foodborne illnesses is due to the ingestion of *foods which are always unsafe* owing to the presence of toxins which cannot be rendered innocuous by cooking or other means, *i.e.*, ciguatoxin, scombratoxin, amanita toxins, paralytic shellfish toxin, mushroom toxin, and heavy metals (11, 14).

The *place of ingestion* of the etiologic agent is usually the patient's home or a restaurant, and, less commonly, a social gathering or an institutional eating place.

For most of the conditions listed in Tables 25.1 and 25.2, *individuals are at risk at all ages*, and a single episode does not confer protective immunity against a later episode. A particularly high rate of diarrheal illness occurs in people who travel to developing countries.

PATHOGENESIS

As indicated in Tables 25.1 and 25.2, the majority of the etiologic agents produce symptoms due either to inflammation of the gastrointestinal tract or to physiologic events related to one or more toxins.

In recent years, the common bacterial diarrheal syndromes have been separated into invasive and enterotoxigenic syndromes (see Table 25.4) (18, 20), an important advance because of the implications for antibiotic treatment. In *invasive disease*, the etiologic agent enters the intestinal mucosal cells, often destroying them, and the diarrhea is a result of this destructive process with its accompanying inflammatory response. This usually occurs in the large bowel and produces systemic symptoms (particularly fever), local symptoms (tenesmus, abdominal discomfort), and frequent small amounts of stool which contain pus cells and often blood. Shigellosis is the prototype of this syndrome (16). In *enterotoxigenic diarrhea*, the organisms do not invade tissue, but colonize and multiply on the small bowel mucosal surface; during this process they produce enterotoxins which act as chemical mediators and cause hypersecretion of fluid and electrolytes by the small bowel. Little tissue damage is produced, and inflammation of the mucosa is minimal. Symptoms consist of simple watery diarrhea (which may be volumi-

Table 25.3
Comparison of Symptoms of Viral and Bacterial Gastroenteritis in Adults

Symptom	Percentage with Symptom				
	Viral gastroenteritis		Bacterial gastroenteritis		
	Rotavirus[a]	Norwalk agent[b]	Salmonella[b]	Shigella[b]	Staphylococcus aureus[b]
Nausea	2	85	50	45	62
Vomiting	9	84	23	39	86
Abdominal cramps	26	62	78	60	86
Diarrhea	33	44	73	100	67
Fever	5	32	49	72	10
Headache	NR[c]	37	33	6	8

[a] Source: W. M. Wenman, D. Hinde, S. Feltham, and M. Gurwith: *New England Journal of Medicine, 301:* 303, 1979.
[b] Source: J. L. Adler, and R. Zickl: *Journal of Infectious Disease, 119:* 668, 1969.
[c] Not reported.

Table 25.4
Characteristics Distinguishing Invasive and Enterotoxigenic Diarrhea

Feature	Invasive Diarrhea	Enterotoxigenic Diarrhea
History	Fever, abdominal pain, tenesmus, may have blood in stool	Watery diarrhea with little or no fever or other systemic symptoms
Physical examination	Fever, abdominal tenderness; proctoscopy may be indicated	May be signs of salt and water depletion
Laboratory studies	Stool culture (may be diagnostic) Fecal leukocytes in large numbers[a] White count may be elevated	Stool culture usually negative unless special culture techniques available White count usually normal, but may be elevated
Therapy	Oral fluids and electrolytes (usually only small quantities needed) Antimicrobials often indicated[b]	Oral fluids and electrolytes (substantial quantities may be needed) Antimicrobials not indicated
Course	Improvement in 1–2 days, particularly if appropriate antimicrobials used	Duration of 1–2 days usually; may last up to 5 days

[a] Use a drop of methylene blue stain with liquid stool.
[b] See text for recommendations for specific bacterial pathogens.

nous), accompanied by minimal systemic signs, unless dehydration becomes significant. The prototypes of this syndrome are diarrheas caused by *Vibrio cholerae* and by enterotoxigenic *Escherichia coli* (9, 22).

PATIENT EVALUATION

Historical Information

In addition to a history of the specific symptoms the most useful information will be:

1. A history of *food intake* within the past 48 hours, particularly noting any deviation from the patient's usual pattern, such as eating an unusual food (e.g., a special fish), attending a picnic or potluck dinner, or preparing food in an unconventional container (e.g., in a copper pot).

2. A history of a *similar illness in others* (family members or members of a group who ate with the patient). This will be helpful in suggesting a common source outbreak.

3. The probable *incubation period*. This may be helpful in suggesting the most likely etiology for a patient's illness (see Tables 25.1 and 25.2). For example, the onset of symptoms immediately after ingestion almost always indicates chemical food poisoning; onset of symptoms within a few hours of eating strongly suggests staphylococcal food poisoning; and onset of symptoms after 1 or more weeks of exposure suggests uncommon problems such as giardiasis.

4. Is the patient currently taking antibiotics (particularly clindamycin) or has he taken them in the last 2 weeks? This could suggest the possibility of antibiotic-associated diarrhea which, when severe, is most commonly due to *Clostridium difficile* (4).

5. A history of *neurologic symptoms* following ingestion of canned foods should always suggest botulism or one of the other sources of neurotoxins (all rare) listed in Table 25.2.

Physical Examination

The physical examination is usually of minimal help in establishing an etiologic agent. Probably the most important observation is the temperature: fever or significant abdominal tenderness in association with diarrhea suggests an invasive organism. Poor skin turgor and postural hypotension suggest significant salt and water deficits, (relatively uncommon in adults with diarrhea in the United States). Infrequently occurring conditions in which the physical findings may be very helpful are botulism and other neurotoxic forms of food poisoning, and trichinosis (see Tables 25.1 and 25.2).

Laboratory Studies

In the majority of patients with acute gastrointestinal illness, no laboratory studies are indicated. If there is a suggestion of a common source outbreak, however, special cultures and tests for toxins in stools and in food, primarily for epidemiologic purposes should be obtained.

In patients with a combination of diarrhea for more than 24 hours, fever, and blood in the stool or significant dehydration, a minimum number of laboratory studies is indicated (17), i.e., (a) stool culture for *Salmonella, Shigella, Campylobacter* (8) and *Yersinia* (5) (unfortunately enterotoxigenic *E. coli*, invasive *E. coli*, vibrios, and viral agents cannot be identified in routine laboratories because of the special techniques required); (b) a white blood cell count (an elevated count and/or shift to younger polymorphonuclear forms supports the diagnosis of invasive diarrheal disease); and (c) serum electrolytes (if significant dehydration is found).

In suspected cases, the laboratory should be asked to examine the stool for *Giardia lambia* or *Entamoeba histolytica* (Table 25.1). For optimal identification of trophozoites of these organisms, fresh stools should be examined immediately by an experienced observer. For the diagnosis of giardiasis, stools may need to be examined repeatedly. *E. histolytica* trophozoites are best identified from the mucus taken from the base of ulcerations seen at proctoscopy.

Additional laboratory tests should be ordered for certain conditions (see Tables 25.1 and 25.2).

MANAGEMENT

In all patients with acute diarrhea, symptomatic treatment is of primary importance. In addition, some patients may require specific therapy (*i.e.*, antibiotics), usually indicated on the basis of the history and physical examination. Most episodes of acute diarrhea are self-limited, lasting 1 to 2 days, or occasionally as long as 5 to 10 days. Resolution of illness is thought to be due to the local secretory immune response of the gastrointestinal tract.

Symptomatic Treatment

FLUID THERAPY

With the exception of giardiasis, amebiasis, and the more severe cases of shigellosis and salmonellosis, practically all acute diarrheal disease seen in the United States can be treated with only symptomatic therapy, the mainstay of which is the replacement of fluids and electrolytes lost in the stool. Since in most patients the disease is mild, and the amount of stool is small, replacement is relatively simple. Patients should be encouraged to drink lots of fluids, to avoid spicy foods, and otherwise to eat what they like.

In patients who have a *very large loss of stool* and who experience weakness and a feeling of being "washed out" with or without signs of dehydration, replacement should consist of fluids containing electrolytes and glucose. In many parts of the world, an oral glucose-electrolyte replacement solution is available commercially for this purpose (19). It contains the following (in mEq/liter): sodium, 90; potassium, 20; chloride, 80; and bicarbonate, 40, in addition to 2 g of glucose per 100 ml of fluid. A reasonable approximation of this solution can be made by mixing the following ingredients found in most homes (13):

Prepare two separate glasses of the following:

GLASS 1

Orange, apple, or other fruit juice (rich in
   potassium) . . . . .8 ounces
Honey or corn syrup (contains glucose
   necessary for absorption of essential
   salts) . . . . 1/2 teaspoon
Table salt (contains sodium and chloride) . . 1 pinch

GLASS 2

Water. . . . . .8 ounces
Baking soda (contains sodium bicarbonate) . 1/4 teaspoon

The patient should be instructed to drink alternately from each glass, taking in an amount that approximates his stool loss (on the average one glass per bowel movement).

Patients experiencing *severe diarrhea or vomiting* which precludes easy ingestion of oral replacement fluids and those who have evidence of moderate to severe salt and water depletion should be hospitalized for initial intravenous fluid replacement with Ringer's lactate or its equivalent.

OTHER SYMPTOMATIC MEASURES

Two medications are commonly used to treat the diarrhea of gastroenteritis. Diphenoxylate with atropine (Lomotil) causes a decrease in intestinal motility and stool frequency; it may be very useful to the patient at times when frequent defecation would be embarrassing. Since this drug does not alter the natural course of the disease, however, and is potentially harmful if invasive pathogens such as *Shigella* are causing the diarrhea, it should only be used infrequently. The dose is 1 to 2 tablets every 6 hours. *Kaolin and pectin mixtures* (e.g., Kaopectate) have primarily a placebo effect. They add to the bulk of the stool, and thus the stools appear to be less watery; actual fluid loss, however, is not affected by these agents.

In patients with *severe vomiting*, commonly seen in staphylococcal food poisoning, the antiemetic drug Prochlorperazine (Compazine) may be very helpful, given as a 25-mg rectal suppository 2 or 3 times daily.

Specific Treatment

In patients in whom *shigellosis* is strongly suspected, or from whom the organism has been cultured in the stool, appropriate antibiotic treatment should be given as this will shorten the illness from 3 to 7 days to 1 to 2 days (12). Ampicillin, 500 mg 4 times a day for 5 days, is adequate therapy. For patients allergic to penicillin, or those in whom an ampicillin-resistant organism is isolated, trimethoprim-sulfamethoxazole is a suitable alternative. The dose is 2 tablets every 12 hours for 5 days.

If *Salmonella* is isolated from diarrheal stool, patients should *not* be given antibiotics unless there is evidence of systemic disease, such as high fever or other signs of toxicity, lasting more than 1 day. It has been found that routine treatment of *Salmonella* gastroenteritis with antibiotics leads to a prolongation of the carrier state in some individuals (1). Even without antibiotic treatment, patients may excrete *Salmonella* in the stool for several weeks to months after their acute illness has terminated. If there is systemic disease, ampicillin (as for shigellosis) or chloramphenicol, 500 mg 4 times daily for 1 week, is adequate.

Patients infected with *Campylobacter* (8) probably will benefit from antibiotic therapy, but there are no controlled studies to confirm this. Erythromycin, 500 mg 4 times a day for 7 days, seems to be the drug of choice; most strains are also sensitive to similar doses of tetracyclines.

In patients who develop significant *diarrhea related to antibiotics*, the antibiotic should be stopped and another substituted if antibiotic therapy must be continued. In the majority of cases, however, which are usually due to *C. difficile*, oral vancomycin, 500 mg 4 times a day for 5 days, will usually shorten the illness (4).

Patients with *giardiasis and amebiasis* definitely require appropriate therapy. For giardiasis, the drug of choice is quinacrine hydrochloride, 100 mg 3 times a day, for 5 days. Metronidazole (Flagyl), 750 mg 3 times a day for 5 to 10 days is also effective. For moderate to severe amebic dysentery, metronidazole, should be administered, 750 mg 3 times a day for 5 to 10 days, plus diiodohydroxyquin (Diodoquin), 600 mg 3 times a day for 3 weeks, to prevent the carrier state.

Trichinosis is treated with thiabendazole, 25 mg per kg twice a day for 5 to 7 days. High doses of prednisone (e.g., 30 to 50 mg daily) should be given simultaneously if symptoms are pronounced (see Table 25.1).

Patients with *suspected botulism* should be hospitalized in an intensive care unit immediately and should be given polyvalent antitoxin, which must be obtained through the local health department.

Patients with mushroom poisoning due to *Amanita muscaria* should be treated with atropine (see Table 25.2).

The Patient's Role in Therapy

Acute gastroenteritis, like the common cold, is an illness which is often diagnosed and handled by the patient without contacting a physician. In some instances, the patient will contact the physician by telephone, and a working diagnosis and plan of therapy can be established without an office visit. This is particularly true for healthy patients with typical symptoms of staphylococcal food poisoning. In all situations, whether the patient is examined by the physician or not, it should be stressed to the patient that care of gastroenteritis requires the regular taking of fluids, at times supplemented by an oral electrolyte solution (see above), and by oral antibiotics if prescribed. The patient will be expected to estimate the severity of his diarrhea in order to plan fluid replacement. He should be advised to notify his physician if his diarrhea becomes worse or if he feels increasingly ill with systemic symptoms such as fever, nausea, and vomiting. He need not return for a follow-up visit unless his symptoms persist beyond 2 to 3 days, or unless stool cultures have been taken and reveal that antibiotic therapy is indicated. Limitation of activity should be dictated entirely by how the patient feels and by his proximity to toilet facilities.

Course of Illness

The dehydrated patient will feel almost immediate improvement when adequate oral replacement fluids are given. When the patient is given antimicrobial therapy for an invasive pathogen, there should be a noticeable decrease in diarrhea and fever within 24 to 36 hours.

An *atypical course* will occasionally occur after initial diagnosis and treatment. Any patient may develop an increase in diarrhea after being initially seen, which could result in unanticipated significant dehydration. An increase in severity of symptoms could also occur if the patient were developing antibiotic-associated enterocolitis. An initial episode of ulcerative colitis could be misdiagnosed as shigellosis, in which case antibiotic therapy would not result in improvement; and the occasional patient with antibiotic-resistant *Shigella* may not respond to initial therapy, indicating the need for an alternative drug.

PREVENTION

Primary Prevention

Primary prevention of the diseases discussed above can theoretically be accomplished by these measures: (a) reduction of the agent's presence in the environment, (b) increasing resistance of the host (by immunization or prophylactic antibiotics), and (c) environmental measures which block the transmission of the agent (2). Regulations governing sewage treatment, water purification, and food processing, packing, and preparation provide the principal protective barriers to foodborne disease *outside the home. In the home*, almost all forms of foodborne disease can be prevented if several measures are followed routinely (see Table 25.5). Many people do not realize that some of the food they prepare each day is contaminated before cooking, and that proper cooking and storing, not absence of contamination, is the way in which most food is rendered safe to eat. Whenever food known to be contaminated is eaten raw, the risk of foodborne disease is present; this is particularly important with respect to shellfish, which concentrate microbial organisms from the wa-

Table 25.5
Measures to Prevent Foodborne Disease in the Home

1. Refrigerate all foods which are capable of supporting microbial growth (perishable foods)
2. Avoid keeping perishable foods for long periods even in refrigerator
3. Cook all foods at sufficiently high temperatures before serving (212°F (100°C) or higher for all oven-cooked meats and at least 15 minutes boiling time for all boiled foods. Same procedure when foods are reheated)
4. Avoid preparing perishable foods a day or more before they are to be served
5. Avoid allowing foods to stand at warm temperatures for several hours before being served
6. Avoid incorporating raw (contaminated) ingredients into foods that receive no further cooking
7. Thoroughly clean kitchen equipment after it has been in contact with perishable foods
8. Avoid using utensils that may contain toxic metals
9. Avoid foods which are unsafe no matter how they are processed (see text, p. 204)

ters in which they are grown; routine surveillance of these waters by public health authorities is the major mode of protecting persons who eat raw shellfish (14).

Secondary Prevention

After an outbreak of an acute enteric illness, appropriate measures should be taken to prevent additional cases.

In the household, any foods suspected of transmitting illness should be thrown away (in the event that an epidemiologic investigation is warranted, a sample should be submitted to the local health department). An error in storage or cooking of the suspected food will often be evident; the patient's physician should point out this error and, most important, review the standard precautions as listed in Table 25.5 to prevent repeated episodes of foodborne illness. When a member of a household has an enteric infection which is transmissible from person-to-person (see Table 25.1), this individual should be instructed to wash his/her hands frequently *especially* before preparing food for others. When shigellosis or salmonellosis occurs in a person involved in food-handling, it is critical to obtain three negative stool cultures, assuring eradication of the carrier state, before the individual returns to food-handling.

When exposure *outside the home* is suspected by the physician, the problem should be reported immediately to the local health department; it is the health department's responsibility to undertake an epidemiologic investigation in order to protect others. Each year, investigations of 400 to 500 outbreaks of foodborne illness are reported to the Center for Disease Control, and many lead to measures that interrupt potentially widespread outbreaks of diseases, some of them particularly hazardous (3).

Prophylaxis for Short Term Travelers to the Developing World

These individuals should be advised of the high risk of developing diarrhea during their visit and should take precautions to ensure that safe water is used and that eating uncooked vegetables or unpeeled fruits is avoided. Even with these precautions, the risk of developing diarrhea is sizable. The problem may be prevented effectively (about 70 to 90%) in persons traveling for up to 1 month by oral doxycycline, taken 100 mg per day (1 capsule) with food (21). This may be particularly important in elderly travelers or in those with known medical problems in whom diarrhea with accompanying dehydration would pose a significant health hazard. Another prophylactic measure for short term travelers is the taking of bismuth-subsalicylate (Pepto-Bismol), 8 ounces per day (10). This will prevent about 65% of traveler's diarrhea; however, it does require a large volume of medication, and the patient ingests the salicylate equivalent of 2.6 g of aspirin each day,

which is potentially hazardous in patients who may already be taking aspirin.

Travelers with diarrhea should be advised to treat themselves symptomatically as described above. When packets of glucose-electrolytes (mentioned previously) become commercially available, it would be ideal to take a few of these along. There are no controlled studies of the use of antibiotics in the treatment of traveler's diarrhea. It is presumed, however, that either doxycycline (if not already being used prophylactically) given as 100 mg twice a day for 2 to 3 days or trimethoprim-sulfamethoxazole given as 1 tablet twice a day for 2 days would be adequate.

References

General

Benenson, AS (ed.): *Control of Communicable Diseases in Man,* ed. 12. American Public Health Association, Washington, D.C., 1975.

    A concise summary of epidemiology, management, and prevention of communicable diseases, updated periodically.

Blacklow, NR and Cutzor, G: Viral gastroenteritis. *N Engl J Med* 304: 397, 1981.

    Excellent review of the role of viruses in gastroenteritis.

Center for Disease Control: Foodborne Disease Outbreaks, Annual Summary, Atlanta, Ga.

    This report, published annually, provides the most current overview of foodborne disease epidemiology; it includes detailed reports on important new problems each year.

Health Information for International Travel: U.S. Department of Health and Human Services, Center for Disease Control (CDC), Atlanta, Georgia.

    This booklet, which is updated yearly, contains recommendations for vaccination and prophylaxis against communicable diseases throughout the world. Available free.

Hughes, JM, Horwitz, MA, Merson, MH, Barker, WH, Jr and Gangarosa, EJ: Foodborne disease outbreaks of chemical etiology in the United States, 1970–1974. *Am J Epidemiol* 105: 233, 1977.

    Excellent review of epidemiologic and clinical features of foodborne illness due to toxic and chemical agents.

Specific

1. Aserkoff, B and Bennett, JV: Effect of antibiotic therapy in acute salmonellosis on the fecal excretion of salmonellae. *N Eng J Med* 281: 636, 1969.
2. Barker, WH: Perspectives on acute enteric disease epidemiology and control. *Bull Pan Am Health Org* 9: 148, 1975.
3. Barker, WH, Weissman, JB, Dowell, VR, Jr, Gutmann, L and Kautter, DA: Type B botulism outbreak caused by a commercial food product. *JAMA* 237: 456, 1977.
4. Bartlett, JG: Antibiotic-associated pseudomembranous colitis. *Rev Infect Dis* 1: 530, 1979.
5. Black, RE, Jackson, RJ, Tsai, T, Medvesky, M, Shayegani, M, Feeley, JC, MacLeod, KI, and Wakelee, AM: Epidemic *Yersinia enterocolitica* infection due to contaminated chocolate milk. *N Engl J Med* 298: 76, 1977.
6. Bryan, FL: Emerging foodborne diseases; II. Factors that contribute to outbreaks and their control. *J Milk Food Technol* 35: 632, 1972.
7. Bryan, FL: Emerging foodborne diseases; I. Their surveillance and epidemiology. *J Milk Food Technol* 35: 618, 1972.
8. Butzler, JP and Skirrow, MB: Campylobacter enteritis. *Clin Gastroenterol* 8: 737, 1979.
9. Cholera and Related Diarrheas, 43rd Nobel Symposium, edited by O. Ouchterlony and J Holmgren. S. Karger, Basel, Switzerland, 1980.
10. DuPont, HL, Sullivan, P, Evans, DG, Pickering, LK, Evans, DJ,

Vollet, JJ, Ericsson, CD, Ackerman, PB and Tjoa, WS: Prevention of travelers' diarrhea (emporiatric enteritis): prophylactic administration of subsalicylate bismuth. *JAMA 243:* 237, 1980.

11. Gosselin, RE, Hodge, HC, Smith, RP and Gleason, MN: *Clinical Toxicology of Commercial Products*, ed. 4. Williams & Wilkins, Baltimore, 1976.

12. Haltalin, KC, Kusmiesz, HT, Hinton, LV and Nelson, JD: Treatment of acute diarrhea in outpatients. *Am J Dis Child 124:* 554, 1972.

13. Health Information for International Travel 1978: HEW Publication No. (CDC) 78–280. U.S. Department of Health, Education, Welfare, PHS, Center for Disease Control, Atlanta, Georgia.

14. Hughes, JM and Merson, MH: Current concepts: fish and shellfish poisoning. *N Engl J Med 295:* 1117, 1976.

15. Kapikian, AZ, Yolken, RH, Wyatt, RG, Kalica, AR, Chanock, RM and Kim, HW: Viral diarrhea: etiology and control. *Am J Clin Nutr 31:* 2219, 1978.

16. Keusch, GT: Shigella infections. *Clin Gastroenterol 8:* 645, 1979.

17. Koplan, JF, Ferraro, MJ, Fineberg, HV and Rosenberg, ML: Value of stool cultures. *Lancet*, August 23, 1980.

18. Pierce, NF: Infections of the gastrointestinal tract. In *Principles and Practice of Medicine*, ed. 20, edited by AM Harvey, RJ Johns, VA McKusick, AH Owens, RS Ross Appleton-Century-Crofts, New York, 1980.

19. Pierce, NF and Hirschhorn, N: Oral fluid-a simple weapon against dehydration in diarrhoea: How it works and how to use it. *WHO Chronicle 31:* 87, 1977.

20. Plotkin GR, Kluge, RM and Waldman, RH: Gastroenteritis: etiology, pathophysiology and clinical manifestations. *Medicine 58:* 95, 1979.

21. Sack, DA, Kaminsky, DC, Sack, RB, Itotia, JN, Arthur, RR, Kapikian, AZ, Orskov, F and Orskov, I: Prophylactic doxycycline for travelers' diarrhea: results of a prospective double-blind study of Peace Corps Volunteers in Kenya. *N Engl J Med 298:* 758, 1978.

22. Sack, RB: Enterotoxigenic *Escherichia coli*: identification and characterization. *J Inf Dis 142:* 279, 1980.

23. Wenman, WM, Hinde, D, Feltham, S and Gurwith, M: Rotovirus infection in adults. Results of a prospective family study. *N Engl J Med 301:* 303, 1979.

CHAPTER TWENTY-SIX

Genitourinary Infections

JOHN R. BURTON, M.D., and JAMES K. SMOLEV, M.D.

INTRODUCTION

Urinary tract infection (UTI) is one of the commonest disorders seen by the primary care physician. Although most of these infections are uncomplicated and easily treated, some of them pose a threat to the kidneys and, sometimes, to life itself. This chapter provides a practical approach to the diagnosis, classification, evaluation, management, and follow-up of patients who have urinary tract infections.

PATHOGENESIS—GENERAL CONDITIONS

Gram-negative bacteria, particularly *Escherichia coli* account for the vast majority of UTIs. There are over 100 serotypes of *E. coli*, differentiated by the character of the "O antigen (a component of the cell wall), but only 8 of these commonly cause infection. Other Gram-negative bacteria, such as *Enterobacter*, *Klebsiella*, *Proteus* species, and *Pseudomonas*, and Gram-positive bacteria, such as *Streptococcus faecalis*, also cause UTIs, although less commonly than *E. coli*. Viruses, mycobacterium, fungi and parasites cause UTIs very rarely.

In women, it is clear that the major cause of UTI is invasion of the urinary tract by bacteria which have ascended the urethra from contamination of the introitus. Women who are prone to infection have colonization of the vaginal introitus with the same serotypes of *E. coli* found in the fecal flora. There is evidence that this colonization is favored by a pH of the introitus greater than 4.4, by the absence of the production of cervicovaginal antibody (a surface antibody produced by the local tissues) to the colonizing bacteria (17), and by urethral trauma (e.g., during intercourse).

Infection of the bladder and kidneys *in men* is unlikely in an anatomically normal tract (as opposed to its common occurrence in women). The much lower incidence of urinary tract infection in men has been attributed to the long male urethra, to the absence of colonization of bacteria near the meatus, and to an antibacterial factor—*prostatic antibacterial factor* (PAF)—which is present in prostatic fluid (and is markedly diminished in some men with recurrent prostatic infection).

The bladder has unique *intrinsic defenses* against infection. The washout of bacteria by periodic voiding is probably one important defense mechanism. The bladder mucosa also removes surface organisms (perhaps by phagocytosis, the secretion of mucus, surface antibody production, or all of these); this defense mechanism is severely limited if residual urine is present.

Urinary tract infections occur more regularly and persistently in both men and women who have a structural abnormality of the urinary tract (such as an obstruction) or who have been catheterized or instrumented. Vesicoureteral reflux (the retrograde flow of urine from the bladder to the ureters) may be associated with, but is not necessarily a cause of, ascending infection. Infection in women also occurs more frequently in pregnancy 4 to 6% incidence) especially if they also have sickle cell trait (10 to 15% incidence). Diabetes mellitus in women, but not in men, is associated with an increased prevalence (2 to 3-fold) of urinary tract infections, especially pyelonephritis.

GENERAL DIAGNOSTIC CONSIDERATIONS

The diagnosis of urinary tract infection is suggested by the history and physical examination and confirmed by examination of the urine. Sometimes, X-rays and instrumentation of the urinary tract are necessary ancillary procedures. The symptoms and signs of UTI are discussed below in sections that describe the specific classes of these disorders, but the process of obtaining and evaluating a urine specimen and the radiological assessment of the urinary tract are the same, regardless of the pattern of infection, and are discussed below

Urine Examination

There are three reasons why the urinalysis is the most important study in the evaluation of the patient suspected of having UTI:

1. A negative urinalysis makes a UTI unlikely; approximately 30% of women with symptoms of "urinary tract infection" have sterile urine (10). Unfortunately, a great many of these women have been inappropriately labeled as having a UTI, because a urinalysis or urine culture has not been done.

2. An abnormal urinalysis and a positive culture may be found even in the absence of symptoms.

3. Urinalysis may aid in the localization of an infection within the urinary tract (see below).

The urinalysis should, therefore, always be performed and followed with a culture if there is evidence of infection (see below).

COLLECTION

Collection of the urine specimen requires special attention since bacteria and cells on the skin near the urethra may contaminate the urine. However, a carefully instructed patient can usually obtain a *clean caught midstream specimen*.

Men can easily obtain an uncontaminated specimen by cleansing the glands of the penis using one or two 4 × 4-inch gauze wipes containing liquid detergent followed by rinsing with gauze soaked in tap water. In uncircumcised males the foreskin must be retracted. After initially voiding a small amount of urine into the toilet (except when a segmental collection is obtained, p. 212) a midstream specimen is collected into a sterile container.

In *women*, the procedure is more difficult and careful instructions are necessary. While sitting on the toilet with one leg swung fully to the side, the vulva are separated and the area around the urethra is cleansed 2 or 3 times with a 4 × 4-inch gauze soaked with liquid detergent and rinsed with two or three gauzes soaked with tap water. The initial portion of urine is voided into the toilet and a midstream specimen is then collected in a sterile container. Commercial urine collection kits are available but often are expensive and sometimes contain small cotton-balls which may be hard for many patients to use. Kunin (see "General References") has published specific instructions on the collection of specimens which may be helpful for patients. The "clean caught" procedure may be impossible in women who are very obese or who have other disabilities. The finding of more than an occasional vaginal squamous cell in the urine specimen indicates that contamination has occurred. In this instance, urine must be obtained by either bladder catheterization or by suprapubic tap.

Catheterization of the urinary bladder is accomplished by using a No. 14 catheter, inserted through the urethra into the bladder and removed when the specimen has been obtained. This requires careful preparation and cleansing of the urethra (with an aseptic solution such as Betadine) to minimize the risk of introducing an infection. Alternatively, a *suprapubic* tap may be done by the general physician if certain precautions are taken. The patient must have a full bladder—uncomfortable to the patient, with palpable suprapubic tenderness on examination, although often in women the bladder is not felt—and the lower abdomen should not have surgical scars. Two to five hours after the ingestion of 200 to 300 ml of fluid to the point of having a full bladder, the patient should lie supine for the procedure. The skin is cleansed with a sterilizing solution and the skin above the symphysis pubis is anesthetized with 1% Xylocaine. Then a 21–22-gauge 3½-inch spinal needle is gently inserted into the bladder, and a urine specimen is aspirated with a syringe. This procedure is, within the limits described above, preferable to bladder catheterization which has 1 to 2% risk of introducing infection. With experience, and when the patient comes to the office well hydrated, this procedure takes actually less time than catheterization, and tolerated as well, if not better, by the patient.

URINALYSIS

If the urine specimen cannot be processed within 10 to 15 min of obtaining it, it must be refrigerated (and transported to a laboratory in this manner). The *uncentrifuged* specimen can be examined microscopically under a coverslip with use of the oil immersion lens. The finding of bacteria by this method has a 90% correlation with the subsequent culture of over one million bacteria per ml of urine. The number of white cells in the uncentrifuged urine can be roughly quantitated microscopically in a counting chamber by the use of the low powered lens. The finding of more than three white cells per cubic mm is abnormal (although not specific for infection). The finding of three or less white cells per cu mm suggests that infection is not present (13).

The urine is more easily analyzed, however, after it is *centrifuged*: a drop of the sediment is examined by use of the high dry lens of the microscope. If bacteria are seen, infection is likely. Quantitation of white blood cells after centrifugation is not very reliable; however, the identification of *white cell casts* is diagnostic of pyelonephritis. Red blood cells are often present in the urine in association with infection but may reflect a number of other processes as well (see Chapter 41).

The urine may also be analyzed by a multiple reagent *dipstick*. There may be a nonspecific positive test for blood and/or protein, but the most important measurement is the urinary pH. In an infected patient, a pH greater than 7.0 (if the patient is not a vegetarian) suggests the presence of infection by a urea-splitting organism, usually a *Proteus* species. The recent addition of the nitrite test to the multiple reagent dipstick should not lead the physician to use it as a reliable method to rule out bacteruria in a symptomatic patient or in a random urine specimen. The use of the nitrite test for the purpose of detecting infection is most valuable when used in mass screening. Bacteria in the bladder reduce nitrate to nitrite and the latter can be measured colorimetrically using a dipstick. Because the generation of nitrite from nitrate by bacteria requires time, the test is best performed on the first voided morning specimen and is most sensitive when repeated on three different morning specimens.

CULTURE

When UTI is suspected and before therapy is given, a culture should always be obtained. Culture of the urine must be performed within a few minutes after it is collected. Bacteria multiply logarithmically if urine is incubated at room temperature; and, for this reason, the urine should be plated on a dip agar transport device (Uricult, bacteriuria screening test, or Bacturcult—available from commercial laboratories) or it should be refrigerated until it reaches the laboratory. (The physician should be certain that there is a refrigerator in the motor veichle transporting the specimen to the laboratory.) The physician should not process cultures or perform sensitivity testing in his office unless a single individual can be dedicated to this task and quality control measures can be maintained.

Traditionally, 10^5 colonies of bacteria per ml have been considered indicative of significant infection; most patients with UTIs have bacterial counts above this level. However, any number of bacterial colonies may be significant if they represent a single species and are present in association with symptoms suggesting an infection.

When urine specimens are contaminated by surface bacteria, cultures may yield bacterial counts of less than 10^5 organisms per ml, or they may yield multiple species. In the latter situation, a carefully obtained clean caught urine specimen should be obtained or, if this is difficult, a specimen should be obtained by catheterization or by suprapubic aspiration of the bladder (see above). Not infrequently, a presumptive diagnosis of UTI has been made and antimicrobials have been prescribed by the time the laboratory reports that multiple organisms have been cultured. In this instance, the patient should be contacted by telephone to inquire about symptoms. If improvement has occurred, the antimicrobial course should be completed it it has not been and a repeat culture obtained at follow-up (see below, p. 213). If there has not been a significant response to the prescribed therapy, another urine specimen should be obtained for urinalysis and culture either by a very careful repeated clean caught collection or preferably by a suprapubic aspiration or catheterization.

Localizing the Site of Infection

There are several techniques which may localize infection in selected cases. *The antibody-coated bacteria test* (21) takes advantage of the host immune response to invasion by bacteria of tissue, such as kidney, bladder wall, or prostate. The bacteria may be identified in the urine by the use of fluorescent antibodies against the immune globulins (generated by the host) which coat the bacteria. This test, while helpful in differentiating bladder bacteriuria from pyelonephritis, is not yet widely available commercially. Furthermore, because it reflects tissue invasion anywhere in the urinary tract, it is not specific for pyelonephritis (15). Currently, its use is limited to the evaluation of patients with frequently recurrent UTIs or of pregnant patients with bacteriuria (see below).

Urinary tract infection may also be localized by the *catheterization of the ureters* by a urologist. In this manner infected urine in the upper tracts can be demonstrated. This technique, however, is rarely done except when it is necessary to demonstrate that infection is localized to one kidney (*e.g.*, for consideration of removal of a chronically infected nonfunctioning kidney). A third method of localization, the *bladder washout technique* (5), is too cumbersome for routine office practice.

In the *male patient*, infection of the prostate and/or bladder can be confirmed by comparison of quantitative bacterial counts on the first 10 ml of voided urine (urethral specimen—voided bladder specimen 1, VB_1), the midstream urine specimen (bladder specimen—voided bladder specimen 2, VB_2), a drop of expressed prostatic secretion (EPS), and the first 5 to 10 ml of urine voided after prostatic massage (prostatic specimen—voided bladder specimen 3, VB_3) (Fig. 26.1). Prostatic massage is accomplished by firm rolling pressure and working from the superior and lateral margin toward the midline and inferior margin. The seminal vesicles should be stripped also. If no secretions result, stripping the bulbar portion of the urethra may provide several drops of prostatic fluid.

In the performance of this *segmented collection technique*, it is important that the patient have some urine in the bladder at the time of the prostatic massage. Occasionally the prostate gland is too tender to massage, in which case a specimen may be obtained by having the patient masturbate and by culturing the ejaculate. To conclude that an infected EPS, VB_3, or ejaculate represents prostatitis alone, the bladder urine (VB_2) should show no or very few colonies.

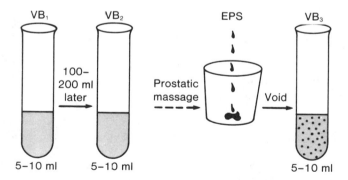

Figure 26.1 Segmented culture of the lower urinary tract in the male patient. VB_1, first voided urine; VB_2, midstream urine; EPS, expressed prostate secretions; VB_3, first voided urine after massage. (After T. A. Stamey: *Pathogenesis and Treatment of Urinary Tract Infections*, Williams & Wilkins, Baltimore, 1980.)

Table 26.1

Indications for Obtaining an Intravenous Pylogram (IVP) in Patients with Urinary Tract Infection

Acute pyelonephritis in male patients
Acute pyelonephritis in women when symptoms worsen or fail to improve after 2 or 3 days of antibiotic treatment
Renal colic (see Chapter 43)
Palpable bladder or renal mass
Evidence of a neurogenic bladder
Urea-splitting organism—usually *Proteus* species
Frequently recurrent urinary tract infections in women (more than three or four per year)
Failure to eradicate infection with appropriate therapy
Patients with newly recognized renal failure (an infusion IVP should be performed in the presence of renal failure)

Radiography

The intravenous pyelogram (IVP) is not necessary in the vast majority of patients with uncomplicated UTI. It may help, however, in the evaluation of certain patients (Table 26.1) who are suspected of having structural abnormalities, the correction of which may prevent recurrence or may even be lifesaving. In addition to identifying problems which predispose to infection (such as reflux, a stone, or obstruction), an IVP will help to identify changes in the upper tract, such as scarring or caliectasis, which represent loss of renal parenchyma as well as abnormalities in the lower tract, such as bladder diverticula.

The voiding cystourethrogram may show abnormalities of the bladder outlet and urethra and may demonstrate urethral reflux. In adult patients this procedure is rarely necessary and it is not recommended without a urologic consultation.

CLASSIFICATION OF AND APPROACH TO PATIENTS WITH URINARY TRACT INFECTION

Infections in Women

In most practices, several women with urinary infections will be seen weekly. The patients can be classified into several subgroups.

FIRST INFECTION, OCCASIONAL INFECTION, OR UNCOMPLICATED INFECTION

Women with this very common problem account for the vast majority of patients who have a UTI. The problem is characterized by symptoms of bladder irritation (frequency, urgency, and dysuria) and occasionally by hematuria. Chills and fever almost always indicate pyelonephritis, but the absence of these symptoms does not rule out that condition (6). The diagnosis of a UTI is confirmed by urinalysis and urine culture, as discussed above (p. 211). The infection will often clear spontaneously in time, but treatment dramatically shortens the symptomatic period and should be given.

TREATMENT

Usually uncomplicated UTIs are sensitive to multiple antibiotics. Traditionally a 7- to 10-day course of antimicrobials has been given; but, recently, a single dose of a parenteral antimicrobial (7, 14) or a single dose or a 3-day course of an oral antimicrobial (1, 4) has been shown to eradicate approximately 90 to 95% of uncomplicated cystitis in young women. There have been several complementary studies which indicate that the single oral dose now can be recommended in preference to the traditional 7- to 10-day course since the single dose is associated with significantly fewer side effects, is less expensive, and assures compliance (20). To maximize the efficacy of this regimen, certain precautions are necessary: single dose oral therapy should not be used when renal parenchyma infection is suspected (e.g., if fever or chills are present), during pregnancy, if follow-up is uncertain, or if there is any suggestion of an underlying systemic problem (such as diabetes mellitus) or a urologic problem (such as a history of stones, severe reflux, or renal failure). One of the following single dose oral regimens is acceptable: amoxicillin, 3 g (available as 500-mg capsules generic); sulfisoxazole, 2 g (available as 500-mg tablets, Gantrisin or generic); trimethoprim 160 mg with sulfamethoxazole 800 mg (available in tablets, Bactrim DS or Septra DS). Other antimicrobials should not be used for single dose therapy.

When this regimen is initiated the patient should return in approximately 1 to 2 weeks so that a repeat urinalysis and urine culture may be obtained. By this method most of the few patients who experience a relapse can be recognized early and be given a more prolonged course of therapy. Although the length of this more prolonged course of therapy has not been defined precisely, a reasonable approach when early relapse is identified after a single dose is to administer a 7 to 10-day course of an antimicrobial selected on the basis of the results of the initial urine culture and reassess the patient again in 4 to 6 weeks. Also this follow-up visit will provide the opportunity for the physician to educate the patient about UTIs (see below, "Follow-Up").

Since the single dose therapy is only recently gaining acceptance, and since more extensive and long term follow-up studies performed in a typical practice environment are not yet available, the well proven traditional course of a 7 to 10-day oral antimicrobial may be preferred by some physicians. However, there is no evidence that treatment beyond 7 to 10 days is beneficial. The selection of antimicrobial should be based on cost and avoidance of any drug to which the patient is allergic. The results of culture sensitivity testing will ultimately guide the choice of therapy for patients with infections with more resistent organisms, but these results often are not available for 48 to 72 hours. Prompt initiation of therapy is appropriate, before the culture report, to control the patient's symptoms (Table 26.2). Sulfonamides are prescribed more often than are other agents and are recommended except when prior resistance has been noted, in which case either ampicillin, nitrofurantoin, or tetracycline are reasonable alternatives. The urinary analgesic phenazopyridine (Pyridium) is not required when antimicrobials are prescribed.

A useful way to spare patients the expense of purchasing additional medication when a change in medication is indicated is to provide the patient with a 3-day supply of antimicrobial from the office stock. The patient is instructed to telephone the office after 3 days, to obtain a prescription to complete the 7 to 10-day course of this or another appropriate, antimicrobial. This practice also provides an efficient follow-up at which time a patient with uncomplicated infection should be nearly symptom-free. If the symptoms have not significantly diminished, persistent bacteria may be present, and the patient should be re-evaluated (see below, "Persistent Bacteriuria"). Recurrences after the eradication of bacteria and after the patient is no longer taking an antimicrobial are common, however, and follow-up is necessary

FOLLOW-UP

It is usual that the first office visit is taken up in establishing the diagnosis and initiating therapy. As cited above, phone follow-up will occasionally identify the need for prompt re-evaluation. If the symptoms have cleared, re-evaluation of the patient in the office in to 4 to 6 weeks is recommended, in order to educate the patient about UTI (Table 26.3) and to reassess the urine. Many patients who have a persisting nidus of infection and who have received only a 10-day course of antimicrobials will have evidence

Table 26.2
Antimicrobial Agents which May Be Used in Uncomplicated Urinary Tract Infection

Agent	Dose
FIRST CHOICE	
Ampicillin	250–500 mg 4 times a day
Amoxicillin	250–500 mg every 8 hours
Nitrofurantoin (Furadantin or Macrodantin)	100 mg 4 times a day
Sulfonamides (Gantrisin)[a,b]	500 mg 4 times a day
Trimethoprim[c] and sulfamethoxazole[b] (Bactrim or Septra)	2 tablets twice a day or 1 double strength (DS) tablet twice a day
SECOND CHOICE	
Cephalosporins[d] (cephalexin)	250–500 mg 4 times a day
Tetracycline[c]	250–500 mg 4 times a day

[a] Resistance may occur after frequent episodes of urinary tract infection.
[b] Avoid in women who are breast feeding.
[c] Avoid in pregnancy.
[d] Often more costly.

Table 26.3
Points to Consider in Educating Women Who Have Had an Uncomplicated Infection

Infections are often recurrent. However, the following measures may decrease the recurrence rate:

Avoid a full bladder. This is an especially important reminder during travel

High fluid intake (1 liter in 2–3 hr) may eradicate an infection that has just become symptomatic

Many infections result from the presence of bacteria (identical to bacteria in the feces) near the opening of the urethra. Therefore after a bowel movement the anus should be wiped in the direction of anterior to posterior

Irritation to the urethra, as occurs with sexual intercourse, is associated with the movement of bacteria into the bladder. Voiding after intercourse, therefore, may help in preventing recurrent infection

Infections in the absence of structural urologic disorder is rarely, if ever, associated with the development of chronic renal failure

Prompt recognition and treatment will help control symptoms

Even if recurrent infections are frequent, there is much that can be done to control symptoms (see discussion of prophylaxis under "Recurrent Infection—Reinfection Type")

of a *relapse* (see p. 218) by this time (bacteriuria and pyuria), although it is frequently asymptomatic.

RECURRENT INFECTION—REINFECTION TYPE

The vast majority of women with recurrent urinary tract infections have become reinfected (rather than an exacerbation of a smoldering quiescent infection). While the infections are symptomatic and occasionally may be associated with pyelonephritis, recurrent reinfection in whom with structurally normal urinary tracts rarely, if ever, leads to the development of chronic renal failure.

Treatment. The approach to women with anatomically normal urinary tracts and the syndrome of reinfection has been vastly improved by the understanding of the pathogenesis of UTI in women. In the past, these women are often treated with a variety of painful manipulations, such as urethral dilatation, urethral incision, transurethral resection of the bladder neck, installation of a variety of intravesicle agents, and other inappropriate and ineffective maneuvers. Instead each episode of bacterial infection should be treated as outlined above in the section on first infections (p. 213). If there are frequent recurrences, such as three or four or more in a year, prophylactic antimicrobials should be used.

Prophylactic Antimicrobials. After eradicating a recurrent infection, a prophylactic antimicrobial may be initiated.

A number of studies have confirmed the efficacy of prophylaxis in reducing the number of urinary tract reinfections in women (8, 16). The agents which have been used are effective when given as a single

small dose at bedtime. A dose taken after sexual intercourse is also effective. Since the dose is small treatment is inexpensive, the patient acceptance is good, and side effects are uncommon.

Many agents have been shown to be effective prophylactically, but nitrofurantoin (Furadantin) 50 mg at bedtime, trimethoprim-sulfamethoxazole (Septra, Bactrim) 40/200 mg, half tablet at bedtime, and cephalexin (Keflex or generic) 250 mg, half tablet at bedtime, are used most commonly and are recommended. However, even with low doses of nitrofurantoin there has been some evidence of serious adverse effects (20), especially in older women; this agent is therefore best avoided in women over approximately age 30 to 35. Prophylactic therapy should be continued for 6 months. During prophylaxis, the patient should have a urinalysis performed every 3 to 4 months to ensure that there is no pyuria or bacteriuria. If after the cessation of prophylaxis there are still frequent recurrences, prophylaxis for a longer period (such as a year) should be tried (after a course of appropriate eradicative therapy). Prophylactic therapy has improved dramatically the lives of many women with distressingly frequent UTIs.

ASYMPTOMATIC BACTERIURIA

Associated with Pregnancy. Asymptomatic bacteriuria in pregnancy is relatively common, affecting up to 4 to 6% of women in the first trimester. Recognition of this fact is important, since eradication of this bacteriuria will reduce the high incidence of symptomatic UTI that will subsequently occur during pregnancy and may reduce the risk of immature and premature birth which occurs in women with antibody-coated bacteria in the urine.

Unassociated with Pregnancy. When asymptomatic bacteriuria is identified in women who are not pregnant, the management is uncertain. While a few women will eventually develop symptomatic infection, the likelihood is very much less than it is in pregnant women; in most the bacteriuria will clear spontaneously. Since, if asymptomatic bacteriuria is treated repeatedly, recolonization with another species may occur, asymptomatic bacteriuria in nonpregnant women should be treated only with a single course of therapy; if it recurs, a structural problem should be sought. If found, persistent infection may be present (see p. 218). If, on the other hand, no structural problem is found, the bacteriuria is best left untreated unless symptoms develop. Thus, screening for asymptomatic bacteriuria in nonpregnant adult women is not recommended.

CLINICAL SYNDROMES WHICH MIMIC "CLASSICAL" URINARY TRACT INFECTION

Two clinical syndromes in women which mimic "classical" UTI (*i.e.,* > 10⁵ bacteria per ml of urine) are analogous to prostatodynia in men (see p. 217) and because of their high prevalence deserve special attention. They are the urethral syndrome and interstitial cystitis.

URETHRAL SYNDROME (DYSURIA-PYURIA SYNDROME)

This syndrome is characterized by bladder irritation, frequency, urgency, and dysuria without "significant" (greater than 10^5) bacterial colonies per ml on culture. With the increased ability to define bacteria and other infectious agents in the urinary tract (see above), a new understanding of the syndrome has evolved.

Etiology. Dysuria-pyuria syndrome may be the better term since dysuria is invariable and pyuria (greater than 8 white blood cells per cu mm of clean uncentrifuged urine) has important etiologic implications (18). Studies (2, 3, 18) have shown that many women with the syndrome have bacterial infection. Patients may have cultures that show fewer than 10^5 colonies of bacteria (especially of *E. coli*, but occasionally of other bacteria) and yet respond to appropriate antimicrobial eradicative therapy. Also in many women urine cultured by the usual bacteriologic techniques appears sterile, but when the urine is cultured by use of special methods it will grow infectious agents such as *Mycoplasma hominis, Ureaplasma urealyticum,* herpes simplex virus, cytomegalovirus and, especially, *Chlamydia trachomatis.* These infections usually will clear spontaneously although some of the nonviral agents can be eradicated more quickly by tetracycline.

Approach to patient. Based on these observations, the following approach to women with symptoms of dysuria is suggested. The patient should have a urinalysis and urine culture and, if pyuria is present, an antimicrobial drug should be given. If the culture of the urine is sterile and symptoms persist, the patient should return to the office for a pelvic examination if it was not done initially (see below). On the other hand, if pyuria is present, but the culture did not show bacterial growth, chlamydia or other agents that are difficult to culture may be present and a 7- to 10-day course of tetracycline, 250 mg 4 times a day, should be given. Follow-up thereafter should be the same as that described for women with bacterial cystitis (see above).

It is important, in the initial evaluation of sexually active women, to ask them if they have a vaginal discharge. If so, a pelvic examination and examination of the vaginal discharge should be done because vulvovaginitis from candidiasis, trichomoniasis, herpes, or even gonorrhea may be present and account for the symptoms of dysuria (see Chapter 91) (3).

Five to ten percent of women who have the urethral syndrome do not have a demonstrable infectious agent even if special cultural methods are used; most often these patients do not have pyuria. The cause of the syndrome in these instances is not known. In this group, treatment with reassurance, sitz baths, and the urinary analgesic phenazopyridine (Pyridium), 200 mg 3 times a day for 5 to 10 days, will provide some relief. The patient should be informed that the medication often causes the urine to appear orange. If symptoms persist, referral to a urologist is indicated.

INTERSTITIAL CYSTITIS

Interstitial cystitis is an occasionally seen disorder which early in its course may be confused with the urethral syndrome. Interstitial cystitis causes symptoms of suprapubic discomfort, especially when the bladder is full, and symptoms are relieved by voiding. The patient may experience progressive urinary frequency and eventually patients may have to void 4 to 6 times per hour, often throughout the night. This disease is difficult to diagnose, and therapy is often unsatisfactory. If suspected on the basis of the history, referral to a urologist is indicated. The urologist will perform a cystoscopy in order to establish the diagnosis and exclude other causes of the symptoms (bladder tumor, for example). No definitive therapy has yet been developed for treatment of this condition.

Infections in Men

BACTERIAL CYSTITIS

This infection is similar in presentation to that in a female patient and is diagnosed by the same method (see above). It suggests the presence, however, of an underlying structural problem, such as prostatic hypertrophy, and a diagnostic workup including a prostatic examination, assessment of renal function by a determination of serum creatinine or creatinine clearance, and an IVP and a urologic consultation for consideration of cystoscopy are appropriate.

The treatment of bacterial cystitis should be similar to the traditional 7- to 10-day course described above, page 213 and in Table 26.2. The treatment course may need to be prolonged further, however, if the workup reveals a structural problem (see below, "Persistent Infection" and "Recurrent Infection—Relapse Type"). A single dose of an antimicrobial as described for use in female patients with uncomplicated infection should never be used in men.

Men with bacterial cystitis should be followed carefully even if the initial evaluation was unrevealing as many will be found to have recurrent infection—relapse type (see below). Many men with relapse infection have bacterial prostatitis; therefore, a follow-up visit in 4 to 6 weeks after the initial infection should include a segmented urine collection.

PROSTATITIS

Prostatitis is classified as bacterial prostatitis, nonbacterial prostatitis (prostatosis), or the much less common prostatic infections due to a virus, a parasite, tuberculosis, a fungus or to nonspecific granulomatous changes (12).

Acute Bacterial Prostatitis. Acute bacterial prostatitis is characterized often by an abrupt onset of fever, chills, low back pain and perineal pain with irritative urinary tract symptoms, although on some occasions systemic symptoms are not pronounced. Perineal discomfort may be worsened by defecation. In addition, the patient may have initial, terminal, or occasionally, total hematuria (see Chapter 41). Rectal examination usually discloses a tender, swollen, and boggy prostate. The urinalysis, as well as expressed prostatic secretions (EPS) (see above p. 212), contain leukocytes, and culture will often grow the responsible bacterial pathogen. The prostate may be too tender to massage and an EPS or VB_3 (see above p. 212) specimen cannot be obtained. Almost always in this situation the urethral (VB_1) or bladder urine (VB_2) specimen will contain bacteria; and sensitivity testing can be performed on bacteria grown from these specimens. If bacteria are not seen in the urine, material for culture may be obtained by having the patient masturbate as discussed above (p 212).

When the diagnosis is made, the patient may occasionally require hospitalization, although if systemic symptoms are minimal, ambulatory therapy is appropriate. Trimethoprim (Proloprim or Trimpex), 100 mg twice a day, trimethoprim-sulfamethoxazole (Bactrim or Septra), 2 tablets twice a day, carbenicillin (Geocillin) 2 tablets 4 times a day, clindamycin (Cleocin), 150 to 300 mg every 6 hours, or erythromycin, 250 to 500 mg twice a day, achieve a high level of tissue concentration in the prostatic fluid and can be prescribed to an ambulatory patient. Trimethoprim-sulfamethoxazole (Bactrim or Septra) is suggested as initial therapy until culture sensitivity tests are available and then an adjustment in antimicrobial selection is made if necessary (trimethoprim holds promise as the agent of first choice but further clinical trials are necessary). Therapy with antimicrobials should be continued for 2 weeks.

Bed rest and sitz baths for 20 to 30 min 2 or 3 times a day may provide comfort. Occasionally, prostatitis results in acute urinary retention, which requires hospitalization and urgent urologic consultation. The palpable irregularity of the prostate gland following acute infection may persist for several months. The acute infection is readily controlled but recurrences may occur, especially in older individuals.

Men below 50, the age where benign prostatic hyperplasia (BPH) occurs, do not need a urologic evaluation if the acute prostatitis responds within several days. Men older than 50 should be referred routinely to a urologist because of the likelihood of associated BPH and the high recurrence rate.

Chronic Bacterial Prostatitis. The organisms that cause chronic bacterial prostatitis most often are Gram-negative bacilli, *E. coli* being the most common organism, followed by *Enterococcus*, *Proteus*, and *Klebsiella*. Most patients with chronic bacterial prostatitis present with mild symptoms of irritative voiding such as frequency, urgency, and dysuria, and occasionally there is urethral discharge. Fever is absent. Patients may also have painful ejaculation with hematospermia (see Chapter 41). On rectal examination the prostate gland feels somewhat irregular and may be mildly tender, although the signs are often unremarkable.

The diagnosis is confirmed by the presence of greater than 10 to 20 while blood cells per high power field in the prostatic fluid or by the isolation of bacteria from expressed prostatic secretions (EPS) or from the urine voided after prostatic massage (VB_3); at the same time the bladder urine (VB_2) is sterile or contains only a few colonies of bacteria and often a small number in the urethral specimen (VB_1) (see p. 212). Obstructive symptoms are rare. Most often the patients have intermittent symptomatic episodes which have been controlled with a 10- to 14-day course of antibiotics. Unfortunately, however, recurrent infection is frequent owing to persistence of bacteria within the urinary tract (see p. 218). Chronic prostatitis may also be a reservoir for acute symptomatic cystitis or pyelonephritis.

If the infectious organism is sensitive to trimethoprim-sulfamethoxazole (Bactrim or Septra), a 12-week course consisting of 2 tablets twice a day in patients with chronic prostatitis does offer a 30% chance of a long term cure (12). For any chance of such a cure, a repeat culture of the expressed prostatic secretions and of the urine voided after prostatic massage should be sterile after 4 weeks of treatment. If the culture at 4 weeks is not sterile, continued therapy will fail and should be stopped. Some patients in whom oral therapy has failed may be cured by the administration of an aminoglycoside antibiotic parenterally for 7 days, but this requires hospitalization and careful monitoring of renal function to avoid renal injury.

If all efforts to eradicate infection fail, symptoms usually can be controlled with very low dose trimethoprim-sulfamethoxazole, one-half tablet nightly indefinitely. The only way to effect a cure is by radical prostatectomy, but the morbidity of this procedure precludes its use for benign disease. Repeated prostatic massage has not been shown to be effective. It is important that patients with refractory chronic bacterial prostatitis be evaluated for the presence of *prostatic stones* by an X-ray of the kidney, ureters, and bladder (KUB) and, if stones are seen, the patient should be referred to a urologist. Patients with prostatic stones are often infected with a *Pseudomonas* species. Patients, on the other hand, who are not infected and incidentally found to have prostatic calculi do not need to be referred to a urologist as the stones are frequently of no significance.

Nonbacterial Prostatitis (Prostatosis). A certain group of patients have all the symptoms of chronic bacterial infection of the prostate, but no organism can be demonstrated; *i.e.,* they have nonbacterial prostatitis (prostatosis). These patients have mild perineal pain and irritative symptoms on urination, as well as white cells in the smear of the expressed prostatic secretions (EPS) or in the third voided urine (VB₃); yet, no organisms are cultured. Culture of the secretions and urine by special techniques occasionally reveals infectious agents such as mycoplasma, *Gardernella vaginali*, *U. urealyticum*, or *Chlamydia* species; the significance of these findings is unknown. It is very difficult to cure patients with this syndrome but they should be given an antibiotic such as trimethoprim (Proloprim or Trimpex), 100 mg twice a day, erythromycin, 250 mg 4 times a day, or trimethoprim-sulfamethoxazole (Bactrim or Septra), 2 tablets twice a day, for a 2-week course; if there is no response to the therapy or if the syndrome recurs, no subsequent antibiotics should be prescribed. Instead, an antispasmodic agent such as oxybutynin (Ditropan), 5 mg 2 to 3 times a day should be tried.

Interstitial cystitis and *in situ* bladder cancer may mimic symptoms of nonbacterial prostatitis; both conditions require cystoscopic examination for confirmation. Therefore, if the symptoms of nonbacterial prostatitis recur after a single course of treatment, a urologic consultation should be requested to exclude these conditions and to educate the patient about the benign nature of prostatosis.

Prostatodynia. Patients with a syndrome called prostatodynia have symptoms suggesting prostatic inflammation, but have no evidence of inflammation on physical examination, have no white blood cells in the urine or expressed prostatic secretions, and have sterile segmented urine cultures. There is some evidence that the syndrome may be due to a neurologic disorder and that muscle relaxants or α-sympathetic blocking agents such as phenoxbenzamine (Dibenzyline) are effective. If this syndrome is suspected, urologic consultation is suggested to confirm the diagnosis, rule out interstitial cystitis and bladder cancer, and to initiate therapy.

EPIDIDYMITIS

Epididymitis is a common intrascrotal infection which affects adult male patients. Organisms are thought to reach the epididymis through the lumen of the vas deferens from infected urine, posterior urethra, or seminal vesicles. Epididymitis is manifest as an abrupt swelling of the epididymis which rapidly spreads, presenting often as a generalized inflammation of the entire hemiscrotum and making the differentiation from an acute orchitis impossible. Frequently, fever, chills and irritative bladder symptoms are also present. The differential diagnosis includes torsion of the testicle, acute orchitis, and tumor of the testicle with hemorrhage or hydrocele. Several observations help differentiate torsion from epididymitis: torsion occurs in young boys and epididymitis occurs after sexual activity begins; the urinalysis is normal in torsion but usually shows pyuria and may show a

urethral discharge in epididymitis; elevation of the scrotum often relieves the pain of epididymitis, but intensifies the discomfort in torsion. Occasionally, however, it is not possible to distinguish torsion from epididymitis in which case the patient should be referred to a urologist for emergency evaluation.

Although epididymitis may be distinguished from orchitis in its early stages; by physical examination, this is impossible when it has developed substantially. However, the presence of a urethral discharge or pyuria suggests epididymitis. A tumor of the testis is usually identified by its hardness and insensitivity to pressure. A hydrocele is usually easy to identify as it is painless and transluminates light. While gonococcus causes some episodes of urethritis, chlamydia has been found to be a common cause of epididymitis in men less than 50 years; while in older men who have benign prostatic hypertrophy, the coliform organisms are more common. In some instances no infectious agent can be identified. Once the diagnosis of epididymitis is made on clinical grounds, it should be confirmed by culture of the urine and expressed prostatic secretions which usually demonstrate an infectious agent.

Treatment with ampicillin, 500 mg 4 times a day, or tetracycline, 500 mg 4 times a day, in addition to scrotal support, bed rest, and sitz baths will usually control infection within several days. Treatment should be continued for 14 days, and the patients should be informed that induration and edema in the region of the epididymis may persist for as long as 6 to 8 weeks. In the older patient with acute epididymitis, a search for obstruction at the bladder outlet (see Chapter 45) should be done as soon as the acute symptoms are controlled. On rare occasions, continued pain from chronic epididymitis may occur and, if it does, a urologist should be consulted since some of the patients so affected may require an epididymectomy.

URETHRITIS (9)

Urethritis is an acute inflammation of the urethra which may be classified as gonococcal or nongonococcal. Nongonococcal urethritis is more common and the most common cause for it is *C. trachomatis*. Symptoms of urethritis in the male patient include a discharge from the urethra, dysuria, and a sensation of itching at the distal end of the penis. There is no associated fever. Diagnosis of urethritis depends on the examination and culture of the urethral discharge. Material from the male urethra is best obtained using a sterile calcium alginate swab (Caligiswab, Type 1), available from physician supply stores. The Caligiswab is much smaller than the usual cotton swab and, for this reason, it is much less distressing to the patient.

A culture of the urethra using a calcium alginate swab or a culture of the discharge should always be done by plating the swab on Transgrow, which must be at room temperature. Approximately 40% of men with gonorrhea are asymptomatic and swabbing the urethra for a culture of *Neisseria gonorrhea* is appropriate whenever there is a history of exposure.

Swartz and co-workers (19) have pointed out the usefulness of counting the white blood cells after staining the discharge with gram stain. A Caligiswab is passed into the urethra then rolled over a 1 × 2-cm area on a slide, which is stained by gram stain. Gonococcal urethritis is almost always associated with greater than 50 white blood cells per high power field compared with less than 2 in normal men and a count of between 4 and 50 per high power field in patients with nongonococcal urethritis.

Gonococcal urethritis is diagnosed by the presence on Gram stain of many white blood cells and of extra- or intracellular Gram-negative diplococci; the treatment is either with parenteral penicillin and oral probenecid or oral ampicillin, or tetracycline or parenteral spectinomycin (Table 26.4).

In *nongonococcal urethritis* the discharge continues for a longer period and is more mucoid, and the smear has fewer white blood cells and no stainable bacteria. Treatment of nongonococcal urethritis is with tetracycline or erythromycin (Table 26.4). The treatment is usually effective but recurrences develop commonly.

Since all of the forms of urethritis must be assumed to be sexually transmitted, the patient's partner or partners should be treated with a regimen appropriate for the urethritis and the patient should use a condom until the infection has been controlled.

When patients continue to have recurrences of nongonococcal urethritis or have persistent symptoms unresponsive to antimicrobial agents, they should have bacteriologic studies to evaluate the possibility of a chronic bacterial prostatitis and they should also undergo urologic investigation for evaluation of possible urethral stricture, foreign bodies, or other intraurethral lesions.

Gonorrhea in women is discussed in Chapter 91.

Table 26.4
Management of Urethritis in Men

Gonococcal urethritis (one of the following treatments):
  Procaine penicillin, 4.8 million units intramuscularly plus 1.0 g probenecid orally 30 min before injection
  Ampicillin, 3.5 g orally in a single dose plus 1.0 g probenecid orally
  Tetracycline, 500 mg orally 4 times a day for 5 days
  Spectinomycin, 2.0 g intamuscularly for penicillin-resistant gonococci or for patients allergic to penicillin or intolerant of tetracycline
Nongonococcal urethritis (one of the following treatments):
  Tetracycline, 500 mg orally 4 times a day for 7 days
  Erythromycin, 500 mg orally 4 times a day for 14 days
Treat partner(s) appropriately
Follow-up for recurrence, complications (sticture, prostatitis, epididymitis), or, especially in gonococcal urethritis, infection elsewhere (oropharyngeal, arthritis)
Report to state health department as required

Table 26.5
Differential Diagnostic Possibilities when Urinary Tract Infection Is Not Eradicated by Therapy

Use of an antimicrobial to which the infectious agent lacks sensitivity
Failure of the patient to take the antimicrobial
Presence of an underlying structural problem such as an obstruction, diverticulum, or stone
Renal failure (inadequate urinary concentration)

Persistent Infection

As noted above, treatment in the male or female patient of infection in a normal urinary tract with an appropriate antimicrobial should result in the sterilization of the urine within 72 hours. By this time, symptoms should have abated or, at least, markedly diminished. If symptoms continue, a persistent infection may be present, and it should be established by a repeat urine culture. If any growth of the bacterial species present in the urine before treatment occurs, further evaluation is necessary. Several causes (Table 26.5) should be considered. A test of renal function (determination of a serum creatinine level or of creatinine clearance) and an IVP are suggested if infection persists in a patient who has taken the appropriate antimicrobial therapy.

Recurrent Infection—Relapse Type

Recurrent infection with the same organism is called relapse infection and implies the persistence of bacteria in tissue within the urinary tract. Relapse infection is, in fact, very similar to persistent infection except that in relapse bacterial sterility has been demonstrated either while the patient is on or has completed antimicrobial therapy, whereas sterility is never demonstrated with persistent infection. Relapse occurs most often within 6 weeks of completion of a course of antimicrobial therapy. An underlying structural problem is often present in both men and women with this problem. In women it is very much less common than reinfection (see above p. 214), but it is quite difficult to document because most infections are a result of *E. coli* which has many serotypes and these cannot be differentiated by routine bacteriologic laboratory techniques. Therefore, recurrent UTI due to *E. coli* may be either relapse (same serotype) or reinfection (different serotype). On the other hand, relapse of infection with organisms other than *E. coli* may be diagnosed by routine bacteriologic culture. In women, if *recurrent* infection with *E. coli* occurs 3 times in a 12-month period, or if *relapse* infection with other species occurs, evaluation as outlined above in the section on "Persistent Infection" to exclude the possibility of structural abnormality is appropriate. If a structural abnormality is identified, it should be corrected if possible; if relapse infection is documented and there is no structural abnormality, a more prolonged course (6 weeks) of an appropriate antimicrobial agent should be prescribed.

If a woman or man has a structural abnormality of the urinary tract that cannot be corrected, sterilization of the urinary tract usually is not possible. However, *suppressive therapy* may decrease the frequency of symptomatic exacerbations or of episodes of sepsis. Suppressive therapy (as opposed to eradicative or prophylactic therapy) is accomplished for sensitive organisms by the use of sulfisoxazole (Gantrisin), 500 mg twice a day or trimethoprim-sulfamethoxazole (Bactrim or Septra), 1 tablet twice a day. An alternative to these agents is methenamine hippurate (Hiprex or Urex), 1 g twice a day, or methenamine mandelate (such as Mandelamine or Thiacide), 1 g 4 times a day. However, for these latter agents to be active the urine pH must be below 5.5, so that acidifying agents such as ascorbic acid must be used and the patient must test the urine regularly and adjust the dose of vitamin C accordingly (often several grams/day are required) to assure the acidification of the urine. Thus these agents are unacceptable for most patients.

Acute Pyelonephritis

Pyelonephritis is a bacterial infection of the kidney that most often results from an ascending infection. It is suggested by the presence of bladder irritative symptoms, in addition to flank pain, fever and, frequently, abdominal pain. Bacterial infection of the kidney may also be present without any of these signs or symptoms or with only bladder irritation (6). The urinalysis will show changes as outlined above (p. 211), but only the presence of white blood cell casts are diagnostic of pyelonephritis. "Glitter cells" (white blood cells that glitter upon microscopic evaluation because of granules in the cytoplasm) are often touted as diagnostic, but they are not specific (11).

Clinically apparent acute pyelonephritis is men suggests the presence of a structural problem predisposing to infection and is an indication for immediate hospitalization, parenteral antimicrobial therapy, and an urgent IVP. In a women, an underlying structural problem is much less likely to be present. Therefore, the decision for hospitalization and evaluation requires careful consideration. The patient can be managed at home if she does not appear severely ill or exhibit sepsis, is reliable, is able to take oral antimicrobials, and if access to the physician is guaranteed, should symptoms worsen. If a patient is managed at home, follow-up by the physician in 24 hours by phone is necessary. If there has not been significant improvement during that time, the physician should consider the possibility of an undrained infection (due to obstruction or abscess, for example) and arrange for prompt hospitalization for parenteral antibiotics, IVP, and emergency urologic consultation.

The initial antimicrobial for the patient who is managed at home can be any of the agents listed in Table 26.2 with an appropriate adjustment based on the results of the urine culture and on sensitivity testing (see above). Forcing fluid is not necessary, and may theoretically be detrimental, as the concentration of antimicrobials in the urine and in the renal tissue may be diluted (22). However, intake should be adequate to replace fluid losses, including the additional fluid lost by fever or by vomiting.

If the acute episode of pyelonephritis promptly resolves, then follow-up at 1 month is appropriate (see above, p. 213). An IVP, unless indicated for evaluation of a nonresponsive patient, should not be done until that time. An IVP performed during the acute state sometimes shows a nonspecific diffuse or segmented decrease in the concentration of dye, a delay in the nephrogram on the affected side, distortion of the collection system, and mild urethral reflux. Also, the kidneys may be enlarged. These changes will reverse in several weeks as the infection subsides. Therefore, to avoid being misled by these transient changes and thus to avoid repeating studies, an elective IVP should be postponed until several weeks after the acute episode has abated.

References

General

Kunin, CM: *Detection, Prevention and Management of Urinary Tract Infection*, Ed. 3. Lea & Febiger, Philadelphia, 1979.
   A very well written comprehensive monograph covering all aspects of urinary tract infections.
Stamey, TA: *Pathogenesis and Treatment of Urinary Tract Infections.* Williams & Wilkins, Baltimore, 1980.
   A comprehensive, well-referenced monograph.

Specific

1. Bailey, RR and Abbott, GD: Treatment of urinary tract infection with a single dose of trimethoprim-sulfamethoxazole. *Can Med Assoc J* 118: 551, 1978.
2. Brooks, D and Mauder, A: Pathogenesis of urethral syndrome in women and its diagnosis in general practice. *Lancet* 2: 893, 1972.
3. Dans, PE and Klaus, B: Dysuria in women. *Johns Hopkins Med J* 138: 13, 1976.
4. Fair, WR, Crane, DB, Peterson, LJ, Dahmer, C, Tague, B and Amos, W: Three-day treatment of urinary tract infections. *J Urol* 123: 77, 1980.
5. Fairley, KF, Bond, AG, Brown, RB, et al.: Simple test to determine the site of urinary tract infections. *Lancet* 2: 7513, 1967.
6. Fairley, KF, Carson, NE, Gutcj, RC, Leighton, P, Grounds, AD, Lird, EC, Malcum, PHG, Sleeman, RL and O'Keefe, CM: Site of infection in acute urinary tract infection in general practice. *Lancet* 2: 615, 1971.
7. Fang, LST, Tolkoff-Rubin, NE and Rubin, RH: Efficacy of single-dose and conventional amoxicillin therapy in urinary tract infection localized by the antibody-coated bacterial technique. *N Engl J Med* 298: 413, 1978.
8. Harding, GKM and Ronald, AR: A controlled study of antimicrobial prophylaxis of recurrent urinary infection in women. *N Engl J Med* 291: 597, 1974.
9. Jacobs, NF and Kraus, SJ: Gonococcal and nongonococcal urethritis in men. *Ann Intern Med* 82: 7, 1975.
10. Kraft, JK and Stamey TA: The natural history of symptomatic recurrent bacteria in women. *Medicine* 56: 55, 1977.
11. McGuckin M, Cohen, L and McGregor RR: Significance of pyuria in urinary sediment. *J Urol* 120: 452, 1978.
12. Mears, EJ: Prostatitis. *Annu Rev Med* 30: 279, 1979.
13. Musher, DM, Thorsteinsson, SB and Airola, VM: Quantitative urinalysis, *JAMA* 236: 2069, 1976.
14. Ronald, AR, Boutros, P and Mourtada, H: Bacteriuria locali-

zation and response to single-dose therapy in women. *JAMA* 235: 1854, 1976.

15. Rumans, LW and Vosti, KL: The relationship of antibody-coated bacteria to clinical syndromes. *Arch Intern Med* 138: 1077, 1978.
16. Stamey, TA, Cindy, M and Mihara G: Prophylactic efficacy of nitrofurantoin macrocrystals and trimethoprim-sulfamethoxazole in urinary tract infections. *N Engl J Med* 296: 780, 1977.
17. Stamey, TA and Sexton, CC: The role of vaginal colonization with enterobacteriaceae in recurrent urinary infections. *J Urol* 113: 214, 1975.
18. Stamm, WE, Wagner, KF, Ansel, RL, Alexander, ER, Turek, M, Courts, GW and Holmes, KK: Causes of the acute urethral

syndrome in women. *N Engl J Med* 303: 409, 1980.
19. Swartz, SL, Kraus SJ, Hermann, KL, Stargel, MD, Brown, WS and Allen, SD: Diagnosis and etiology of nongonorrhea urethritis. *J Infect Dis* 138: 445, 1978.
20. The Medical Letter of Drugs and Therapeutics: Treatment of urinary tract infections 23: 69, 1981.
21. Thomas, VL, Forland, M and Shelkov, A: Proteinuria and antibody-coated bacteria in the urine. *N Engl J Med* 297: 617, 1977.
22. Whelton, A and Walker WG: An approach to the interpretation of drug concentrations in the kidney. *Johns Hopkins Med J* 142: 8, 1978.

CHAPTER TWENTY-SEVEN

Respiratory Infections

FREDERICK KOSTER, M.D.

UPPER RESPIRATORY INFECTIONS

Magnitude of the Problem

Upper respiratory infections (URI) are the most common acute illnesses in the United States and the industrialized world. Although these infections are the most common causes of absences from school or work, the vast majority are self-diagnosed and self-treated and do not come to the attention of a physician (Americans spend $500 to $700 million annually for over-the-counter medications for the relief of upper respiratory symptoms). However, 6% of visits to office-based internists are for URI complaints (cough, sore throat, or a cold—see Table 1.2).

Principal Syndromes

THE COMMON COLD

The common cold is a mild, self-limited syndrome caused by viral infection of the upper respiratory tract mucosa and characterized by one or more of the following symptoms: nasal discharge and obstruction, sneezing, sore throat, cough, and hoarseness.

Epidemiology and Transmission

The common cold syndrome is caused by a variety of viruses which are clinically indistinguishable from each other, yet have distinct seasonal peaks for unknown reasons. Rhinoviruses constitute the etiologic agent in 25 to 30% of colds, with seasonal peaks in early fall and mid-to-late spring. Coronaviruses account for another 10 to 15% of annual colds, with a seasonal peak in midwinter. Influenza, parainfluenza, respiratory syncytial viruses, and adenovirus are etiologic agents for another 10 to 15% although this group more commonly presents with the typical influenza syndrome as discussed below.

On the average, adults have two to four colds per year; children have six to eight (13). Since person-to-person spread of colds occurs mainly in the home and at school, school children usually serve as carriers for introducing colds into the family. Thus mothers tend to have higher secondary attack rates than do fathers. Transmission of rhinovirus is most efficient by direct physical contact (14). Frequent, unconscious touching of virus-contaminated nasal mucosa contaminates the subject's hands. Infectious material can survive on the hand for as long as 4 hours, during which time hand-to-hand contact with susceptible subjects serves to transmit the virus. Exposure to susceptible subjects across even short distances of air is an inefficient method of transmission of rhinoviruses, although aerosol transmission of particles effectively transmits some viruses (e.g., Coxsackie, influenza, and adenovirus). Thus transmission of colds may be low even in congested offices if hand-to-hand contact is avoided.

Clinical Characteristics

The correct diagnosis of the common cold is readily made by the patient. After an incubation period of 48 to 72 hours, the syndrome begins with mild malaise, rhinorrhea, sneezing, and scratchy throat, and increases to maximum severity on the 2nd to 4th day. Viral excretion and communicability are maximal during the period of severest symptoms. Fever is usually not present but, if present, rarely exceeds 1°F elevation. Cough and hoarseness may begin later, and their severity and duration are increased in cigarette smokers. Conversely, neither cigarette smoking nor exposure to cold appear to increase the attack rate of colds. Rhinovirus colds usually last 1 week but in one-quarter of cases last up to 2 weeks.

Identification of the causative virus by clinical observation is not possible, nor is it necessary for management. The primary challenge for the physician is to identify the cases with complicating secondary bacterial sinusitis (see below) and otitis media (see Chapter 93), for whom antibiotics will be beneficial. The physical examination should therefore include the pharynx, nasal cavity, ears, and sinuses. The value of sinus transillumination and radiography, pneumatic otoscopy, and throat culture are discussed in sections on sinusitis (p. 226), otitis (Chapter 93), and pharyngitis (p. 224), respectively.

Treatment

In view of the absence of specific antiviral therapy for the uncomplicated common cold, symptomatic treatment is the only treatment available. Aspirin is the best drug for relief of fever and myalgias, but may increase viral excretion, a finding of unknown epidemiologic significance (23). Bed rest is not necessary to facilitate recovery. Steam or cool mist helps liquefy secretions. Sipping hot chicken soup (the only soup studied) increases the clearance of nasal mucus, although it is not clear whether the benefit of this timeless remedy is mediated exclusively through inhaling water vapor or through an additional effect of an aromatic compound (22). There is no symptomatic remedy for hoarseness, which is due to inflammation and edema of the vocal cords; the patient should, however, be advised to rest his voice as this may shorten recovery time.

Nasal congestion is best relieved by *topical decongestants*; sprays rather than drops are preferred for ease of administration. Most over-the-counter short acting (3 to 4 hours) sprays contain 0.5% phenylephrine; some patients prefer the milder effect of 0.25% phenylephrine (sold as Neo-Synephrine). Longer act-

ing topical decongestants (8 to 10 hours) are 0.1% xylometazoline (Otrivin) or 0.05% oxymetazoline (Afrin); they may occasionally produce a stinging sensation when first used. Patients should be cautioned against using drops or sprays for more than 5 days to avoid the rebound effect, defined as an increase in nasal congestion when decongestant medication is discontinued. (See additional discussion of topical decongestants, Chapter 22.)

Oral decongestants, phenylpropanolamine (contained in a large number of over-the-counter products) and pseudoephedrine (Sudafed 30 mg over-the-counter or 60 mg by prescription; also available as Sudafed S.A., a sustained-action preparation containing 120 mg of pseudoephedrine, taken every 12 hours) are somewhat helpful but must be used judiciously because they may cause elevation of blood pressure.

Antihistamines have a marginal effect in attenuating cold symptoms (17). The combination of decongestant and antihistamine, while often helpful in allergic rhinitis (see Chapter 22), is a more expensive, less effective alternative to topical decongestants; this is also true of the many cold remedies containing antihistamines, decongestants, analgesics, caffeine, and a variety of other ingredients (19).

A large number of over-the-counter *cough* remedies are available. These contain various combinations of cough suppressants, expectorants, decongestants, analgesics, and alcohol (28). There is no evidence that any expectorant is effective in URIs and it is more rational and far less expensive to utilize the other ingredients individually in appropriate doses (see additional discussion of cough suppressants below, page 228).

Antibiotics are useless in the uncomplicated cold.

Prevention and Patient Education

Future vaccines are unlikely, especially since at least 89 different serotypes of rhinoviruses have been confirmed and since infection occurs despite the presence of specific serum antibody. Since transmission occurs chiefly by physical contact, it is reasonable to counsel patients and those around them that transmission can be minimized by handwashing, reduced finger-to-nose contact, and reduced exposure to the cold sufferer. Physicians should be particularly vigilant to avoid contact with the patient's secretions and should wash their hands carefully after examining the infected patient. Although physicians with common colds may examine patients if they wash their hands and avoid sneezing on the patient, physicians with the flu syndrome should avoid patient contact (see below).

Prophylactic and therapeutic properties of large doses of *vitamin C* have been examined in a number of trials, and no consistent beneficial effect has been found (4). In those studies suggesting a benefit, the placebo effect could not be excluded since subjects could identify the vitamin C capsule by taste. In doses above 4 g per day, vitamin C may cause diarrhea and has the potential of precipitating urate, oxalate, and cystine stones in susceptible individuals. Other uncommon effects include diminishing the anticoagulant effect of warfarin, and confusing urine glucose tests, causing a false negative glucose oxidase (Dextrostix, Tes-Tape) or a false positive copper reduction test (Clinitest tablets).

FLU SYNDROME

Although there is considerable overlap in the two syndromes, the flu syndrome is sufficiently distinct from the common cold syndrome, especially in terms of potential complications, that the two are discussed separately. Flu presents as the abrupt onset of malaise, myalgia, headache, and fever, and substantial morbidity (including prostration in severe cases) persists for 1 to 2 weeks. In two small studies as many as 85% of cases of flu syndrome were due to the influenza virus during an epidemic (12). Other viruses, especially parainfluenza, respiratory syncytial and adenovirus, are agents that produce the same clinical syndrome.

Epidemiology

Epidemic spread of the influenza virus is a function of the appearance of new antigenic variations of the virus in nonimmune populations. Antigenic variations occur almost annually in influenza serotype A, whereas variation occurs much less frequently in influenza B. Major variation is called antigenic shift and results in *pandemic spread* of a new strain, almost always type A, throughout regions of the world where there is little natural immunity. The most recent pandemics were in the winters of 1957–1958, 1968–1969, and 1977–1978 and they varied considerably in severity. In between pandemics, minor antigenic variations occur frequently, resulting in nearly annual epidemics during the winter months. Such *interpandemic spread*, although less dramatic,

occurs frequently and therefore accounts for greater cumulative morbidity and mortality than pandemic spread. In some years there are no influenza epidemics, for example in the winters of 1976–1977 and 1978–1979, as measured by excess mortality due to pneumonia or influenza reported to the Center for Disease Control (Fig. 27.1). Although it is often not possible clinically to separate infections due to type A or B, influenza A is responsible for greater excess mortality than type B.

Influenza virus appears to be transmitted by virus-containing small particle aerosols dispersed by sneezing, coughing, or talking. The incubation period is 18 to 72 hours. Viral shedding persists for 5 to 10 days, but virus is present in high titer in secretions for only 48 hours after the onset of clinical illness. In the community, person-to-person transmission is rapid, with spread initially among children, then adults. In local epidemics the incidence of cases reaches a peak in 2 to 3 weeks and persists for only 5 to 6 weeks.

Clinical Characteristics

Uncomplicated influenza, type A or type B, has an abrupt onset of systemic symptoms including fever, chills, headache, myalgias, and malaise. The fever, which may rise to 106°F (41°C) in some cases, typically lasts 3 days, although frequently it persists for 5 to 7 days. Headache and myalgias, involving the back, arms, legs and occasionally the eyes, are the predominant symptoms, persisting as long as the fever. Respiratory symptoms such as cough, nasal discharge, hoarseness, and sore throat appear as systemic symptoms wane. Cough and weakness may persist for 2 or more weeks.

Physical findings include general toxicity, flushed face, hot skin, watery red eyes, clear nasal discharge, tender cervical lymph nodes and, occasionally, localized rales in the chest. The white cell count and differential count demonstrate mild neutropenia and

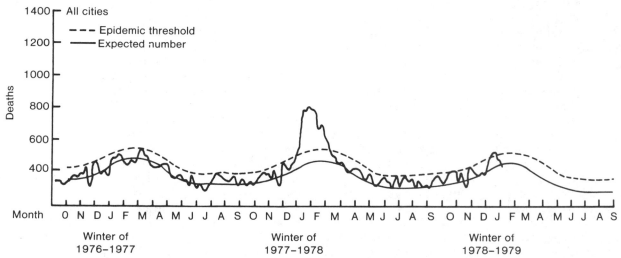

Figure 27.1 Reported pneumonia-influenza deaths in 121 U.S. cities, September 1976 to August 1979. (Source: *Morbidity and Mortality Weekly Report*, Vol. 28, No. 54, September 1980.)

relative lymphocytosis, due to absolute granulocytopenia.

Treatment

One antiviral agent, *amantadine* (Symmetrel), is approved for treatment of type A influenza infections. Amantadine attenuates clinical disease in all patients with influenza A by reducing the fever by 50% and by shortening the duration of illness by 1 or 2 days; these benefits are seen only if the drug is administered within 24 to 48 hours of onset of illness. Side effects, which include insomnia, nervousness, dizziness, and difficulty in concentrating, occur in about 7% of adults, appear a few hours after the first dose, tend to diminish after repeated doses, and disappear upon discontinuation of the drug. The cost of a therapeutic course (200 mg loading dose followed by 100 mg twice a day for 5 days) is approximately 5 dollars, in contrast to the more costly prophylactic course (6) discussed in Chapter 30. Treatment with amantadine should be seriously considered for patients at high risk of morbidity and mortality who develop an influenza-like illness in a community where the state or local health department has reported influenza A. Groups at high risk include:

1. Unvaccinated children and adults with chronic diseases including pulmonary, cardiovascular, metabolic neuromuscular, or immunodeficiency diseases.

2. Adults whose activities are vital to community function, including selected hospital personnel.

3. Patients with life-threatening primary influenzal pneumonia, although the efficacy of amantadine in such patients has not been demonstrated.

Because of the side effects, only partial effectiveness, difficulty of identifying influenza A infections in the individual, and difficulty in initiating therapy early in clinical illness, amantadine has not achieved widespread use. The physician must balance benefits and side effects in each case.

Supportive measures are important for symptomatic relief. Bed rest and adequate fluid intake should be advised. Aspirin, 600 to 900 mg every 3 to 4 hours, or acetaminophen if aspirin is contraindicated, reduces headache, fever, and myalgia. Sponging with tepid water is effective in lowering high fever, whereas sponging with isopropyl alcohol only increases the patient's discomfort. Relief of nasal discharge may be obtained by agents discussed in the section on the common cold (p. 221). Relief of cough with cough suppressants is discussed in the section on acute bronchitis (p. 228).

Complications

Patients should be advised that dyspnea, hemoptysis, wheezing, purulent sputum, fever persisting more than 7 days, and, rarely, dark urine, severe muscle pain and tenderness, herald complications that demand prompt medical attention and usually hospitalization.

Pulmonary complications exhibit a continuous spectrum of severity, from mild airway hyper-reactivity without pulmonary infiltrates, to segmental influenza pneumonia or secondary bacterial pneumonia, to fulminant bilateral influenza pneumonia with the adult respiratory distress syndrome (ARDS).

Airway hyper-reactivity is most common after influenza, but may occur in less severe form following many viral upper respiratory infections (15). It appears to be caused by destruction of epithelial cells secondary to viral invasion and may result from heightened sensitization of afferent cholinergic irritant receptors in the respiratory mucosa. Exposure to inhaled irritants induces a vagally mediated increase in airway resistance, manifested clinically by bronchospasm, coughing, or both; cough may also be due to direct stimulation of cholinergic irritant receptors as these are the receptors which mediate the cough reflex (for additional details, see Chapter 50). Patients with asthma or chronic bronchitis have even greater bronchoconstrictor responses because of their underlying bronchial smooth muscle hyperreactivity. Airway hyperreactivity can be demonstrated for 3 to 8 weeks after influenza and other viral infections, and occasionally it may last for 4 to 6 months even in nonatopic patients.

The relationship between airway hyper-reactivity and *persistent symptoms following influenza* is not entirely clear; however, it is likely that nonproductive cough, wheezing, and dyspnea on exertion are related to airway hyper-reactivity. These postflu symptoms seem to be particularly common in urban areas during periods of high air pollution. Chest roentgenograms are clear. Both cough and wheezing, following an otherwise uncomplicated flulike infection, may be treated with a trial of a bronchodilator (see Chapter 52) as needed and at bedtime. Patients troubled particularly by nighttime cough will obtain additional relief with 15 to 30 mg of codeine at bedtime.

During influenza epidemics, there is a 2- to 3-fold increase in the incidence of *pneumonia* (11). The incidence of postinfluenzal bronchitis and pneumonia varies with age: low (5%) below age 50 and very high (60 to 70%) over age 70. Mortality from pneumonia during influenza epidemics clearly increases for those with chronic pulmonary disease and congestive heart failure.

Primary influenza viral pneumonia is a rare complication occurring predominantly among persons with cardiovascular disease, but occasionally in healthy young adults. After several days of typical influenzal symptoms, fever, cough, and dyspnea rapidly progress to cyanosis and delirium, often developing into adult respiratory distress syndrome. Immediate hospitalization and intensive care are required, but mortality remains high.

Milder influenza pneumonia may be restricted to a single lobe. Patients present with persistent fever, cough and dyspnea, localized rales, normal white blood cell count, and subsequently experience a benign course.

Secondary bacterial pneumonia and bronchitis complicate up to 10% of influenza A illness, depending on age group and chronic pulmonary or cardiac disease. Pneumonic complications of influenza B are less common but are becoming increasingly recognized (1). The presentation is typically biphasic: the initial influenzal illness is followed by several days of clinical improvement, and then there is an exacerbation of fever with production of purulent or bloody sputum. The predominant bacterial pathogen is *Streptococcus pneumoniae*, but *Haemophilus influenzae* and *Staphylococcus aureus* are also common; the last mentioned has a mortality rate of approximately 50% in this setting. The diagnosis and management of pneumonia are discussed below (p. 229).

Nonpulmonary complications of influenza are unusual. Myositis, with thigh pain and inability to walk, occurs occasionally in children and adolescents. Severe myositis with myoglobinuria and acute renal failure has been observed in adults after both influenza A and B. Guillain-Barré syndrome, encephalitis, and transverse myelitis are neurologic complications associated with influenza A, and rarely B, infection, but no firm causal relationship has been established. Reye's syndrome, on the other hand, is a rare but severe complication of influenza, usually type B, presenting as a change in mental status and progressing to coma and hepatic failure. Although the mean age of attack is 6 years, occasional cases of Reye's syndrome have occurred in adolescents. With the exception of mild myositis, all of the nonpulmonary complications of influenza require hospitalization for differential diagnosis and management.

Prevention. The use of influenza vaccine and amantadine prophylaxis in ambulatory practice are discussed in Chapter 30.

PHARYNGITIS

Sore throat is the fourth most common symptom seen in medical practice (5). The physician's most important task in the evaluation of pharyngitis is to identify and treat group A streptococcal infections in adults, especially those with a history of prior rheumatic fever, and to recognize less common causes of pharyngitis associated with more serious systemic illness.

Etiologic Subgroups. Streptococcal pharyngitis cannot be identified by observing the appearance of the pharynx alone, since a number of other causes for sore throat produce similar changes.

Nonexudative pharyngitis is usually due to rhinovirus, coronavirus, and respiratory syncytical, parainfluenza, and influenza viruses. *Exudative pharyngitis* is seen in some or most patients with infection due to group A β-hemolytic streptococcus, mixed anaerobic infections, *Neisseria gonorrheae*, adenovirus, herpes simplex, and Epstein-Barr virus (infectious mononucleosis). In addition, diphtheria may present early as a simple exudative pharyngitis before pseudomembrane formation, but sore throat is usually not the presenting complaint. Pharyngeal

gonorrhea, usually asymptomatic but occasionally exudative and associated with cervical adenitis, is common in partners practicing orogenital sex and may be particularly common in pregnant women. Infectious mononucleosis (see Chapter 49) is characterized by the clinical triad of sore throat, fever, and lymphadenopathy with or without mild tenderness; it can be distinguished with certainty from streptococcal infection on clinical grounds only when hepatosplenomegaly and a maculopapular skin rash (similar to a drug eruption or rubella) are present. Palatal petechiae may be seen in mononucleosis but may also occur with rubella and streptococcal pharyngitis. Pharyngoconjunctival fever is usually accompanied by influenza-like symptoms and can be distinguished by concurrent conjunctivitis in one-third of cases and a history of swimming pool exposure 1 week prior to onset. Herpes simplex, herpangina and aphthous stomatitis are distinguished by the presence of mucosal vesicles or ulcers (see additional details in Chapter 98). Finally, agranulocytosis and leukemia are rare causes of persistent sore throat.

Diagnosis, Management, and Course

1. *Group A Streptococcal Pharyngitis:* Diagnosis relies on the throat culture. Office throat culture kits are inexpensive and offer rapid diagnosis and high sensitivity (approximately 95%). Although the technique may appear simple, some physicians use inadequate plating technique, leading to false negatives; these could be avoided by instruction of the physician in the bacteriology department at any local hospital. Many physicians prefer to send throat swabs or transport media to state or regional laboratories. Rapid diagnosis using Gram stain of pharyngeal swab material yields variable results even with skilled observers and is thus not recommended.

The standard approach is to make culture studies of all febrile patients with pharyngitis and to treat subsequently only those patients found to be positive for group A streptococcus. If cultures are made from only febrile patients, less than 10% of cases with positive infection will be missed and only 30% of all sore throats will be cultured (9). All patients with a history of rheumatic fever must be tested by culture whether or not fever is present. In three situations in which group A streptococcus is suspected, antibiotic treatment should be started before throat culture results are known: (a) patients with a past history of rheumatic fever not currently on prophylaxis, (b) young patients with a strong family history of rheumatic fever, and (c) all cases of pharyngitis in an explosive epidemic in semiclosed populations. Local health authorities should be notified immediately in this situation.

Symptomatic *family contacts* of patients with streptococcal pharyngitis as well as asymptomatic contacts in families with a history of rheumatic fever or in poor families living in crowded conditions should have cultures made and, should be treated if the cultures are positive. It is not clear whether asymptomatic contacts in families living in uncrowded conditions should be tested by culture.

In adults over the age of 15 without a prior history of acute rheumatic fever (ARF), first attacks of ARF are extremely rare. Therefore the principal goals of treatment for streptococcal pharyngitis are the amelioration of symptoms, the prevention of local suppurative complications, and the prevention of spread. Since early therapy (in the first 2 or 3 days) is required for symptomatic relief, most physicians do not wait for culture results in patients with severe pharyngitis. In patients being treated to prevent recurrence of ARF, therapy within 7 days of onset is sufficient.

The preferred therapy is parenteral benzathine penicillin, 1.2 million units given once, because it obviates noncompliance. If oral therapy is given, the recommended regimen is penicillin V 250 mg, 3 times a day, for 10 days. For patients allergic to penicillin erythromycin, 250 mg, every 6 hours for 10 days, is recommended.

2. *Gonococcal Pharyngitis:* Gonococcal pharyngitis is diagnosed by throat culture. Special culture techniques should be used to detect gonorrhea in specimens from patients practicing orogenital sex. Gram stain of direct pharyngeal smear is insensitive and nonspecific. Calcium alginate swabs should be used, as ordinary cotton swabs contain inhibitory fatty acids. The swab should be immediately plated on a modified Thayer-Martin medium which is incorporated in a number of inexpensive kits for office culture. For throat cultures, however, N. gonorrhoeae must be distinguished from *Neisseria meningitidis* and *Neisseria lactamicus* by carbohydrate fermentation and serology; therefore, cultures should be sent to state or regional laboratories. Effective treatment is either procaine penicillin G, 4.8 million units, divided between two intramuscular sites, plus 1.0 g of oral probenecid, or tetracycline in a 1.5-g loading dose followed by 0.5 g 4 times daily for 4 days. Ampicillin and spectinomycin are associated with unacceptable failure rates in the treatment of pharyngeal gonorrhea. A follow-up culture 7 days after completion of therapy should be done as a test of cure.

3. *Diphtheria:* This diagnosis should be suspected when there is a grayish membrane in the anterior nares, or on the tonsils, uvula, or larynx (infectious mononucleosis and "strep throat" display a creamy white exudate and do not involve the uvula). Treatment must begin before bacteriologic confirmation and requires hospitalization for bed rest, close observation, antitoxin, and penicillin. Management of contacts is discussed in Chapter 30.

4. *Other Bacteria:* Throat cultures often grow staphylococci, group B streptococci, and various Gram-negative enterobacteria. None of these species colonizing the pharynx has been shown to be an etiologic agent in pharyngitis and patients who harbor them should not be treated with antimicrobial agents.

ACUTE SINUSITIS

This is a bacterial infection of one or more paranasal sinuses which complicates about 0.5% of viral upper respiratory infections. Sinusitis may also be a complication of noninfectious rhinitis, polyps, foreign bodies, or anatomic nasal obstruction of sinus drainage. Up to 10% of cases of acute sinusitis are an extension of dental abscess. Nursing home or homebound patients with nasogastric tubes occasionally have occult sinusitis as a cause of persistent fever.

Diagnosis

Acute sinusitis in the autumn, winter, and spring usually develops during the course of a viral upper respiratory infection. Sinusitis in the summer often is associated with swimming and diving or with allergic rhinitis (see Chapter 22).

The *pain* of sinusitis is due to periosteal reaction secondary to an expanding purulent inflammation behind an outlet obstruction. The pain is dull in the early stages, but becomes throbbing in later stages. Coughing, dependency, and percussion over the involved sinus exacerbate the pain. Percussion of the teeth is often painful in maxillary sinusitis. The facial pain associated with the noninfectious causes of nasal congestion (see Chapter 22) may resemble the early pain of acute sinusitis, but it is less localized and does not become progressively worse. Other causes of facial pain to be distinguished from sinusitis are dental abscess (Chapter 98), migraine, cluster headache, and trigeminal neuralgia (Chapter 76) (25).

Nontender edema of the eyelids, seen predominantly in children, may occur with uncomplicated ethmoid and maxillary sinusitis. Acute sinusitis may present without pain as in subacute sinusitis (see below), usually in the guise of a cold persisting for more than 7 weeks and accompanied by cough due to postnasal drip, purulent nasal discharge, and headache.

Examination should include the pharynx, nose, ears, and teeth. Transillumination can be a helpful office procedure. In a completely darkened room a small strong light (an ordinary flashlight is not sufficient) is placed under the supraorbital ridge to illuminate the frontal sinuses and through the patient's pursed lips to illuminate the maxillary sinuses. Complete opacification is strong evidence for infection. Complete light transmission rules out active infection. Usually diminished light transmission is seen; one-quarter of this group of patients will have active infection. Proper interpretation of transillumination findings requires training, preferably in cooperation with an otolaryngologist.

Radiologic examination of the sinuses, comprising four views to visualize all paranasal sinuses, is the most sensitive diagnostic test in acute sinusitis. This procedure is not necessary in patients with typical signs and symptoms. It is most helpful in the diagnostic workup of headache and in those patients who do not respond to therapy or who are toxic and require accurate diagnosis early.

Most cases of acute sinusitis can be treated without culture. Nasopharyngeal swabs are usually contaminated with normal flora and are of no use. Studies employing antral puncture (8) indicate that *S. pneumoniae* and unencapsulated *H. influenzae* are the bacterial agents in 60% of acute infections and probably in most acute exacerbations of chronic sinusitis. Anaerobes, *Streptococcus pyogenes, Neisseria catarrhalis* α-hemolytic streptococci, and Gram-negative aerobes each cause a small percentage of infections. *S. aureus* causes less than 5% and tends to be associated with pansinusitis and general toxicity.

Management and Course

Antibiotics. Ampicillin or amoxicillin provides the best coverage of the two most common bacterial agents, in a dose of 500 mg, 4 times daily for 10 days. In penicillin-allergic patients, trimethoprim-sulfamethoxazole (Bactrim or Septra), 2 tablets twice a day for 10 days, or erythromycin, 500 mg 4 times a day for 10 days, are good alternatives.

Symptomatic therapy to improve sinus drainage is important. A decongestant spray, such as Neo-Synephrine 0.25 or 0.5%, is most convenient, administered as an initial squirt to decrease congestion in the membranes of the anterior nares, followed 5 to 10 min later by a second squirt delivered deeper to the middle meatus. This is repeated every 4 hours for 2 to 4 days and followed by oral decongestants (see details on common cold, p. 221) for an additional 2 weeks. Steam inhalation is often helpful. Pain relief is important, and codeine may be required. Patients who plan to fly, especially in nonpressurized aircraft, should take an oral decongestant before takeoff, supplemented with topical decongestant spray every 4 hours.

Resolution of facial pain, headache, and fever is expected by 5 to 7 days. If no response occurs by this time, referral to an otolaryngologist for radiography, antral puncture, or surgical drainage is advisable. Toxic patients, especially those with frontoethmoid sinusitis, should be referred at initial presentation for hospitalization, drainage, and definitive parenteral antibiotics. Patients whose symptoms worsen during the first 48 hours of vigorous ambulatory therapy should be referred. Many patients with severe facial pain are benefited by early antral puncture for pain relief.

Complications of acute sinusitis are unusual, but present as medical emergencies and consist of direct extension of infection to adjacent orbits, bone, blood vessels, and central nervous system. Nontender periorbital edema represents restriction of orbital venous outflow through congested ethmoid veins, is not associated with decreased visual acuity, and is appropriately managed with vigorous medical therapy. However, tender periorbital swelling, associated with proptosis and chemosis, represents orbital cellulitis and requires immediate referral to an otolaryngologist. Subsequent progression of cellulitis to subperiosteal or orbital abscess, associated with ophthalmoplegia and loss of vision, requires emergency surgical drainage. Osteomyelitis is most often a complication of frontal sinusitis. Cavernous sinus thrombosis should be suspected in the patient with signs of orbital complications plus extreme toxicity. Intracranial extension is rare, but life-threatening, presenting most commonly as meningitis. Abscesses in the brain and epidural and subdural spaces present more insidiously. Frontal lobe abscess may present as mild headache, low grade fever, malaise, and personality change. In poorly controlled diabetics and immunocompromised hosts rhinocerebral mucormycosis begins in the nose and maxillary sinuses and may be recognized by a black eschar on the nasal turbinates.

SUBACUTE AND CHRONIC SINUSITIS

When the symptoms of acute sinusitis, especially pain and fever, subside with therapy, but purulent nasal discharge continues, this stage is called *subacute sinusitis.* Despite persistence of radiologic changes, this stage usually resolves after an additional 2 to 3 weeks of conservative management, including antibiotics and oral decongestants.

Chronic sinusitis resists accurate definition, but appears to result from episodes of prolonged, repeated, or inadequately treated acute sinusitis. This results in the loss of normal ciliated epithelial lining of the sinus cavity, which becomes populated by anaerobic and Gram-negative bacteria. Acute exacerbations occur, due primarily to the common organisms of acute sinusitis (*H. influenzae* and *S. pneumoniae*). Chronic sinusitis commonly complicates certain systemic diseases, such as sarcoidosis, Wegener's granulomatosis, and allergic rhinitis with asthma. In allergic rhinitis, control of asthma is often facilitated by treatment of the sinusitis.

Diagnosis and Management

Persistent purulent nasal discharge despite adequate medical therapy is the primary feature of chronic sinusitis. Facial pain and tenderness are minimal or absent. The sinuses transilluminate light poorly. Radiologic examination usually reveals clouding of the cavities and thickening (greater than 5 mm) of the mucosal lining. For this reason sinus films are of limited value in acute exacerbations superimposed on chronic sinusitis.

Referral to an otolaryngologist for appropriate surgical drainage is recommended.

PHARYNGEAL ABSCESS

Occasionally, after several days of symptoms due to an upper respiratory tract infection, the patient will develop a complicating infection of one of the closed compartments adjacent to the pharynx. The most common of these pharyngeal abscesses are peritonsillar abscess and retropharyngeal abscess. When one of these conditions is suspected, the patient should be referred immediately for evaluation and management by an otolaryngologist.

Peritonsillar Abscess. Patients with this condition develop severe odynophagia; they are not only unable to take liquids but, they may be unable to swallow their own saliva, resulting in early dehydration. The voice acquires a muffled quality, and trismus may be present. Fever, malaise, and systemic toxicity are typical. Dramatic relief may occur if the abscess drains spontaneously before the patient seeks medical attention. On physical examination, there is a swelling of the anterior tonsilar pillar at its superior pole. The involved tonsil itself may or may not be enlarged, but it is displaced medially. This condition is almost always unilateral.

Retropharyngeal Abscess. The symptoms of this condition are similar to those of peritonsillar abscess. In addition, there may be respiratory embarrassment if the process extends inferiorly toward the larynx. Trismus is not common. On examination, a swelling in the posterior oropharynx is readily seen. Lateral soft tissue X-rays of the neck may disclose expansion of the soft tissue density in the posterior pharyngeal space.

Management. Incision and drainage, either using an 18-gauge needle or a surgical blade, is the treatment of choice for both of these conditions. This should be performed by an otolaryngologist or an oral surgeon. Antibiotics and warm saline gargles should follow drainage.

EPIGLOTTITIS

Acute epiglottitis is a fulminant, life-threatening, but curable condition. The epiglottis serves as a valve which closes over the proximal portion of the trachea during swallowing, to prevent aspiration. When the epiglottis becomes inflamed, the resultant edema causes it to curl posteriorly and inferiorly, thereby reducing the glottic aperture. Inspiration, which draws it down, further reduces the effective airway.

Epiglottitis is an extremely rare complication of upper respiratory infections. Most cases occur in children, although the condition may occur in adults.

The diagnosis of epiglottitis should be suspected in patients presenting with a sore throat, dysphagia, and progressive respiratory distress, all of short duration. On physical examination, stridor may be noted in inspiration. The patients are usual febrile. The oropharynx may be erythematous, but an important clue to the diagnosis is the relatively uninvolved appearance of the oropharynx found in some patients. Soft tissue X-rays of the neck may show edema of the epiglottis and narrowing of the aperture. The diagnosis is confirmed by indirect laryngoscopy which

reveals marked edema of the epiglottis; this procedure must be performed cautiously as it may induce additional obstruction.

Management requires immediate admission to an intensive care unit, where close observation is essential since a number of patients with acute epiglottitis will require emergency tracheotomy.

Telephone Assessment and Self-Care for Upper Respiratory Infection

Most physicians welcome the opportunity to assess URI symptoms initially by phone. The phone assessment should accomplish the following:

1. Differentiate between infectious and allergic problems.

2. Among the patients with acute infections, distinguish those with possible bacterial infections or superinfections who should be examined to decide whether antibiotics should be prescribed.

3. Identify those who may be suffering from complications of a URI which require office evaluation. The following symptoms and signs should be sought: (a) symptoms lasting more than 3 weeks; (b) fever lasting more than 1 week, or associated with delirium; (c) purulent nasal discharge with sinus pain; (d), purulent sputum, chest pain, dyspnea, or hemoptysis; (e) ear pain or discharge; (f) sore throat and a history of rheumatic fever; (g) the combination of cough and fever over 102°F (39°C) or fever for more than 4 days; (h) hoarseness more than 1 month; (i) pleuritic chest pain; and (j) marked odynophagia; (k) the combination of dysphagia, stridor, and difficulty in breathing.

4. For those patients not needing a visit, provide simple instructions for self-care based upon the measures described earlier (see p. 221).

Increasing numbers of patients will be consulting self-care algorithms (28). The book *Take Care of Yourself* by Vickery and Fries (see "General References") is one of the most widely distributed collections of algorithms. In one evaluation (3), strict adherence to the algorithms for colds, influenza, cough, and sore throat would have increased the number of patient visits to a physician. Thus, this standard set of instructions exhibited sensitivity, missing few people who need to be examined, yet lacked specificity and led to unnecessary visits. This study points to the need to search for symptom complexes which identify patients likely to be helped by a visit to a physician.

LOWER RESPIRATORY INFECTIONS

Acute Bronchitis

CLINICAL CHARACTERISTICS

Acute bronchitis is an inflammatory condition of the tracheobronchial tree that results from respiratory infections with common cold viruses, influenza, adenovirus, *Mycoplasma pneumoniae*, and rarely *Bordetella pertussis*. The role of secondary bacterial invasion is not clear. The illness is characterized by cough, with or without sputum production, persisting longer than expected (usually 1 to 2 weeks) after the onset of an acute URI.

Rhinovirus and coronavirus, by virtue of their high prevalence, are common etiologic agents for mild bronchitis of short duration and without fever. Influenza, adenovirus, and *M. pneumoniae* cause a more severe bronchitis associated with fever and burning substernal pain. Mucoid sputum production develops in half of all cases and is not helpful in distinguishing etiologic agents. Frequency and duration of cough are increased in young adult cigarette smokers.

The patient presenting with a cough as the predominant or only respiratory symptom may have either pneumonia, bronchitis, or a variety of noninfectious conditions associated with persistent cough. Diagnostic efforts should be directed at identifying those patients with pneumonia and with noninfectious causes of cough, leaving acute bronchitis as a diagnosis of exclusion.

The diagnosis of pneumonia is discussed below (p. 230). Approaching the patient who has a persistent cough without apparent infectious etiology, the physician should consider the anatomy and physiology of the cough reflex (Chapter 50). Airborne irritants, especially smog containing sulfur dioxide, and allergens cause bronchitic symptoms. Repeated small aspiration of oral and upper airway secretions, especially in the elderly and the alcoholic with incompetent glottic function, is associated with nighttime cough.

Identification of the agent in most episodes of acute bronchitis is not possible. Bacterial cultures of sputum are useless, since the contribution of bacteria to acute bronchitis is unclear and sputum is readily contaminated by nasopharyngeal flora. Culture facilities for viral agents and *M. pneumoniae* are not widely available. *M. pneumoniae* may be implicated if bullous myringitis is observed, or suggested if (a) the patient is a young adult, (b) similar cases are occurring in the family or in close contacts, and (c) the case occurs in the summer or early fall season. The diagnosis can be confirmed by a 4-fold rise in complement fixation titer in convalescent serum.

Pertussis, rare in adults, is characterized by initial nonspecific symptoms of malaise and rhinorrhea followed by 1 to 4 weeks of severe paroxysms of repetitive coughs without inspiration. The paroxysm is terminated by an inspiratory whoop. The clinical symptoms are attenuated in previously immunized adults and children, who act as reservoirs of infection for nonimmune infants. *B. pertussis* is identified by culture of nasopharyngeal swab on special media, or more rapidly by direct immune fluorescent staining of organisms on smear of nasopharyngeal secretions.

TREATMENT

It is standard practice to prescribe an antibiotic such as ampicillin if persistent purulent sputum is associated with acute bronchitis. Only one properly controlled trial has evaluated the efficacy of antibiotic therapy in acute bronchitis in patients without asthma or chronic bronchitis; no difference in resolution of symptoms was found between the antibiotic and placebo groups (24). Therefore, more studies must be performed before firm recommendations can be offered. If epidemiologic evidence for infection with *M. pneumoniae* exists (see p. 230), a 2-week course of erythromycin, 500 mg 4 times a day, or tetracycline, 250 mg 4 times a day, is indicated. *B. pertussis* infection is treated with erythromycin.

Treatment is usually symptomatic. Many patients will have tried an over-the-counter cough suppressant containing dextromethorphan without relief. Cough suppression, primarily to get a good night's sleep, is best obtained with preparations containing codeine, although in titrating up to an effective dose, patients should be warned of problems with drowsiness and constipation. Both codeine (15 to 60 mg single dose, 45 to 160 mg total daily dose) and dextromethorphan (15 to 20 mg single dose) have histamine-releasing properties and should be used cautiously in asthmatics. Except in allergic rhinitis with postnasal drip, antihistamines, present in many combination cough remedies, should be avoided because they dry out secretions. There is no consistent evidence that expectorants or glyceryl guaiacolate alter the course of bronchitis. Maintaining hydration with oral fluids is a reasonable approach to preventing mucous plugs. Inhaled steam and cool mist provide symptomatic relief, but fail to deliver water droplets into the smaller airways. Some physicians fear that use of cool mist may contaminate airways with Gram-negative aerobic bacteria that inhabit some home humidifiers and that improperly used steam may cause burns. Patients should be strongly encouraged to stop smoking at least for the duration of the acute illness. Those smokers with a history of chronic cough before their bronchitis may be more motivated to discontinue smoking permanently in the face of the acute illness. In 50% of those who discontinue smoking, the chronic cough will resolve completely within 1 month.

Acute Exacerbations of Chronic Bronchitis

CLINICAL CHARACTERISTICS

Respiratory infections contribute to the episodic worsening of cough and increased sputum production in the patient with chronic bronchitis, and they are the most common identifiable causes of death in these patients. Evidence that infections in adulthood play an independent role in the deterioration of pulmonary function, however, is lacking (26).

The most important indicator of intercurrent infection is the patient's report of a change in color, consistency, and amount of sputum. Patients who consistently produce purulent sputum may notice increasing cough, dyspnea, and fatigue. Systemic toxicity with fever and chills is generally absent unless pneumonia is present.

The role of bacteria in acute exacerbations of chronic bronchitis is difficult to assess. The bronchial secretions of patients with chronic bronchitis contain pneumococci, unencapsulated *Haemophilus* species, and normal pharyngeal flora, which persist through asymtomatic intervals. The development of purulent sputum is not correlated with the presence of one or more specific bacterial species. These bacteria appear *de novo* during acute exacerbations in only a small percentage of uncolonized patients. Similarly, the acquisition of a new *serotype* of either pneumococci or encapsulated *Haemophilus* species is usually *not* followed by a clinical exacerbation. In summary, a primary role for these bacteria in the pathogenesis of clinical exacerbations remains unclear, and performing Gram stain and a culture of the sputum during acute exacerbations will not provide useful information.

Viruses (influenza, parainfluenza, respiratory syncytial, rhinovirus, and coronavirus) may cause up to 50% of acute infectious exacerbations. *M. pneumoniae* may be the agent in up to 10% of episodes.

TREATMENT

Acute exacerbations of chronic bronchitis should always be managed with more vigorous applications of routine therapy for chronic symptoms. Clearance of secretions should be promoted with postural drainage and therapeutic doses of bronchodilators, (see Chapter 52). Cough suppressants and sedatives should be avoided. Smokers should be strongly counseled to discontinue cigarettes at least until their acute symptoms have resolved. As noted earlier (p. 228), chronic cough will resolve completely within 1 month in half of those patients who are motivated by an acute illness to discontinue cigarettes permanently.

Antibiotic prophylaxis is commonly used in the management of chronic bronchitis, but the efficacy of this practice is not yet convincingly demonstrated (26). Many studies have suggested that continuous prophylaxis with tetracycline in low doses reduces the frequency of exacerbations during the winter months. The conclusions of most studies, however, do not stand up to rigorous statistical analysis. In addition, there is considerable concern that such widespread use of prophylactic antibiotics without clear effectiveness may promote emergence and dissemination of antibiotic-resistant strains in the community.

Efficacy of *short term antibiotic therapy* given for acute exacerbations is unclear due to the difficulty in assessing therapeutic benefits. For the individual patient, efficacy appears to be based primarily on the patient's reported response to antibiotics during previous exacerbations. A common approach is to provide reliable patients who have three or more acute exacerbations per year with a prescription for tetra-

cycline, 250 mg 4 times daily for 7 to 14 days. Ampicillin 250 to 500 mg 4 times daily, and trimethoprim-sulfamethoxazole 2 tablets twice daily, are alternatives. The patient is instructed to begin the antibiotic within 24 hours of the first sign of a "chest cold," since earlier onset of therapy may be more effective in alleviating symptoms and preventing lost time from work (26). Oral penicillin V and chloramphenicol are not appropriate alternatives, since penicillin is not effective against the *Haemophilus* species; and there are many safer alternatives to chloramphenicol. Sputum purulence, spirometry, and chest roentgenogram often will not improve, but subjective measures of well-being may improve.

Some patients managed at home for acute exacerbations will not improve by any criteria or will deteriorate after self-initiated therapy. The patient should be asked to keep in touch by phone during the acute episode so that symptoms indicating pneumonia will be detected early.

Pneumonia

There are over 3,000,000 episodes of pneumonia annually in the United States, responsible for over 30 million days of disability requiring bed rest. With influenza, pneumonia ranks fifth as a cause of death and first among infectious diseases (5).

DEFINITION

Bronchitis and pneumonia represent a continuum of lower respiratory infection. Aspirated pathogens including bacteria, mycoplasma, and viruses invade the bronchial epithelium. The extent of involvement of adjacent lung parenchyma determines whether or not there is an infiltrate on chest roentgenogram. The alveolar inflammation spreads like a grass fire, and the advancing edge of edema and leukocyte infiltration are not radiologically apparent. Patients seen early and those with emphysema and reduced parenchyma may fail to show any infiltrate or may show a patchy infiltrate on their chest film despite the presence of considerable inflammation. Thus the clinical distinction between acute bronchitis and acute pneumonia is often an arbitrary radiologic distinction. Early management and the decision for hospitalization must focus on the overall condition of the patient in terms of signs and symptoms of systemic toxicity as well as of localized pulmonary infection.

The clinical presentation of pneumonia can be divided into two categories: "bacterial pneumonias" and "atypical pneumonias." "Atypical" historically referred to cold hemagglutinin-positive pneumonias which have more recently been identified as being due to *M. pneumoniae*. Atypical pneumonias due to a variety of other viral, bacterial, and chlamydial agents may be clinically indistinguishable from mycoplasmal pneumonia until definitive diagnostic studies are done. The usefulness in separating "bacterial" from "atypical" pneumonia lies in predicting outcome and need for hospitalization, at the time of initial presentation in the office. Thus only a small proportion of cases of mycoplasmal and viral pneumonia require hospitalization, whereas probably 80 to 90% of pneumococcal and other bacterial pneumonias require hospitalization. The following discussion is restricted to the recognition of patients requiring hospitalization for pneumonia and to the management of pneumonia in the ambulatory patient.

CLINICAL FEATURES

Bacterial pneumonias comprise half of all adult pneumonias, and 60 to 90% of these are due to *S. pneumoniae*. Pneumococcal pneumonia may occur in a previously healthy adult, or following an upper respiratory infection, usually with the abrupt onset of a single shaking chill, fever, pleuritic chest pain, and cough productive of purulent or rusty sputum. In the setting of compromised pulmonary clearance of secretions (depressed consciousness, morbid obesity, abdominal surgery, chronic bronchitis, congestive heart failure, and alcoholism) which predisposes to pneumococcal and other bacterial pneumonias, onset of clinical symptoms may be more insidious. Other types of bacterial pneumonias are more common in different clinical settings: staphylococcal and *H. influenzae* following influenza A or B; *Haemophilus*, *Klebsiella*, and anaerobic pneumonias in alcoholics; anaerobic and Gram-negative pneumonias in nursing home residents or recently hospitalized patients.

The *atypical pneumonia* syndrome comprises the majority of pneumonias in persons under 40. *M. pneumoniae* is the agent in 60 to 90% of pneumonias in this age group (10). A number of viruses (influenza A and B, respiratory syncytial virus, parainfluenza, adenovirus), chlamydia (psittacosis), rickettsia (Q fever), and bacteria (tularemia and legionnaires' dis-

ease) present as a pneumonitis which clinically is indistinguishable from mycoplasmal pneumonia. The onset is a flulike illness, with fever, headache, myalgias, and malaise. At onset or several days later a nonproductive hacking cough and substernal chest pain appears, accompanied by dyspnea and respiratory distress in more severe cases. Pleuritic chest pain and hemoptysis are unusual.

Complications of *M. pneumoniae* are more common in severely ill patients who probably require hospitalization, but may appear in patients initially managed at home. These complications include sinusitis, otitis media, myringitis (diagnostic if bullae seen), erythema multiforme or erythema nodosum, intravascular hemolysis, meningoencephalitis, toxic psychosis, myocarditis, and pericarditis. Persistent hacking cough, lasting as long as 6 weeks despite therapy, is common and requires symptomatic relief with codeine (see p. 228). Relapse of the primary disease occurs in up to 10% of cases, usually 2 to 3 weeks after the initial illness, and is probably related to the persistence of mycoplasma in bronchial epithelium for up to 14 weeks.

Diarrhea, relative bradycardia, abdominal pain, liver enzyme elevations, and hematuria may occur in *legionnaires' disease* but can accompany pneumonia due to viruses and mycoplasma (16). Signs of encephalopathy (confusion, delirium, stupor) are clearly more common in legionnaires' disease.

EPIDEMIOLOGY

Important clues for diagnosis may be obtained from a knowledge of seasonal, environmental, and occupational predilections of the different etiologic agents. Epidemiologic clues for 10 types of atypical pneumonia are listed in Table 27.1.

Table 27.1
Epidemiologic Clues for the Presumptive Diagnosis of Atypical Pneumonia

Organism or Disease	Peak Seasonal Incidence	Incubation Period (days)	Epidemiologic Setting
Mycoplasma pneumoniae	Summer, early fall	14–28	Family—3 weeks between onset among individuals
Respiratory syncytial virus	Late winter and spring	2–8	Bronchiolitis in children < 5 years. Mild upper respiratory infection in adult contacts, with mean symptomatic period of 9 days. More severe in elderly
Influenza A and B	Winter epidemics	1–2	Adult cases follow school absenteeism
Parainfluenza 1 + 2	Fall	3–8	Croup in children, unusual in adults
Parinfluenza 3	All year	3–8	Family—mild upper respiratory infection in adults, more severe in elderly
Adenovirus (type 4, 7)	Winter	4–5	Military recruits
Psittacosis	All year	6–15	Occupational or household exposure to birds, especially parrots, turkeys, and pigeons (20% have no bird exposure)
Tularemia (pulmonary)	All year	2–4	Handling infected rodents and rabbits
Q fever	All year	14–28	Contact with sheep, goats, cattle
Legionnaires'	Outbreaks in summer, sporadic through year	2–10 (epidemic cases)	Contact with construction sites and stagnant water in air-cooling apparatus (some reports)

PHYSICAL EXAMINATION

The physical examination does not usually distinguish between bacterial and atypical pneumonia syndromes. Crepitant rales that do not clear with cough are suggestive of pneumonia of either type. Signs of consolidation (bronchial breath sounds, dullness to percussion, and egophony) are more common in bacterial pneumonia. In early stages of pneumonia the examination may be normal, despite an infiltrate on X-ray. On the other hand, rales and rhonchi may indicate pneumonia before the appearance of an infiltrate.

LABORATORY EXAMINATION

Although *routine laboratory examinations* are not helpful in identifying the etiology of pneumonia, every patient suspected of having pneumonia should have a chest X-ray, peripheral blood white cell count and differential count, and two blood cultures when possible. A white cell count over 15,000 is usually associated with bacterial pneumonia. Although the X-ray is essential for the diagnosis of pneumonia, it does not necessarily rule out pneumonia and is not specific in terms of etiologic agent. For example, in one study (27) in which diagnosis was attempted by six radiologists from the chest film alone, mycoplasmal pneumonia was incorrectly identified as bacterial in a significant proportion of patients.

If the chest X-ray or clinical findings indicate pneumonia, a *sputum Gram stain* is often instrumental in directing initial therapy; and cultures of sputum and blood should be obtained. The rapid Gram-stain technique requires only 1 to 2 min: (a) heat fixation; (b) 5 seconds crystal violet, water rinse; (c) 5 seconds Gram's iodine, water rinse; (d) decolorize thin part of the smear with 4.5 drops of 95% alcohol, water rinse; (e) 5 seconds safranine, water rinse; (f) blot dry. The sputum sample is probably of lower respiratory tract origin if there are fewer than 10 squamous epithelial cells, and more than 25 polymorphonuclear leukocytes, per high dry (100×) field, except in leukopenic patients. The appearance of columnar ciliated epithelial cells assures lower tract origin. Sputum smears positive for pneumococci (Gram-positive lancet-shaped diplococci) are helpful in directing therapy (21). Sputum, often foul-smelling, containing mixed flora with pleomorphic Gram-negative bacilli and tiny or pleomorphic Gram-positive cocci is consistent with anaerobic aspiration pneumonia. Pneumonia due to *Staphylococcus* or *Haemophilus* organisms usually is accompanied by sputum containing abundant large Gram-positive cocci, or small Gram-negative coccobacilli, respectively.

Sputum samples from patients with atypical pneumonia presenting as a flulike illness characteristically contain few bacteria and only modest numbers of leukocytes. On the other hand, sputum from some mycoplasmal and viral pneumonias contains abundant leukocytes but few bacteria. Many patients produce no sputum, including one-half of patients with *legionella pneumophila*. If such patients are toxic they may require hospitalization for more invasive diagnostic studies such as transtracheal aspiration.

Unlike sputum Gram stains, *sputum cultures* have limited utility in the management of ambulatory pneumonias, since sputum samples are often contaminated by oral pneumococci. Moreover, pneumococci fail to grow in 45% of cultures from cases of pneumococcal pneumonia (2). In view of the confusing data, routine sputum cultures are not recommended, with the following important exceptions: patients, such as nursing home residents or those recently discharged from a general hospital, who are at greater risk for nonpneumococcal pneumonia; and patients with sputum Gram stains demonstrating a predominance of nonpneumococcal bacterial pathogens.

The majority of pneumonias, which cannot be diagnosed by blood or sputum culture, do not require definitive diagnosis by *serology*. If, however, the patient fails to respond to 3 to 5 days of therapy and has been ill less than 14 days, an acute serum sample should be obtained and stored. After 3 weeks of illness, a convalescent serum sample should be obtained and both samples submitted to a state or regional health laboratory for diagnostic serology. Guided by epidemiologic clues (Table 27.1), complement fixation titers for *M. pneumoniae*, Q fever, psittacosis, influenza, respiratory syncytial and parainfluenza viruses, and adenovirus may be requested. An indirect immunofluorescent assay on paired sera is available to diagnose legionnaires' disease. Tularemia is usually diagnosed by an agglutination assay.

The presence of serum *cold agglutinins* is often used as a rapid diagnostic test for mycoplasmal pneumonia. This test, however, has several drawbacks. The sample must be maintained at close to 37°C for delivery to the laboratory. In addition, the test is not very sensitive; (only about half of patients with mycoplasmal infection are positive), and not very specific (half of all positive tests are due to other diseases, including pneumococcal and adenovirus pneumonia).

MANAGEMENT: HOSPITALIZATION

The need for hospitalization must be individually determined for each patient, but in general is based on how sick the patient is and what underlying diseases are present. Patients who are toxic, diaphoretic, dyspneic, cyanotic, fatigued from respiratory effort, have hemoptysis, or have difficulty clearing secretions should be hospitalized.

Underlying problems which predispose the patient to more serious disease, and would best be managed in the hospital, are the following:

1. Age over 50 years, obstructive or bronchospastic lung disease, congestive heart failure, diabetes, renal insufficiency, malignancy, postsplenectomy, sickle cell anemia, alcoholism, drug abuse, or concomitant tuberculosis.

2. Peripheral white cell count <5000, ileus, or abdominal distention.

3. Suspicion of recent major aspiration due to history of head trauma, sedative use, acute alcoholism, seizures, dental anesthesia, loss of consciousness, or esophageal motility disorder.

4. Extrapulmonary complications (large pleural effusion, meningitis, septic arthritis, peritonitis, metastatic abscesses, etc.).

5. Hospitalization within the last 4 weeks, or residence in nursing home, increasing chance of a Gram-negative or a resistant nosocomial pathogen.

6. Inability to care for self if living alone.

MANAGEMENT: AMBULATORY

Initial Management. If the clinical presentation supports the diagnosis of pneumococcal pneumonia, the antibiotic of choice is penicillin, 600,000 units of procaine penicillin administered intramuscularly in the office, followed by oral penicillin V, 250 mg every 6 hours for 10 days. If the clinical presentation suggests the atypical pneumonia syndrome and an adequate sputum smear is nondiagnostic, or if there is no sputum, or if the patient is allergic to penicillin, erythromycin, 500 mg 4 times daily for 14 days, is recommended. Patients with persisting cough or slow resolution of symptoms may benefit from an additional week of erythromycin. Patients receiving erythromycin should be advised that crampy abdominal pain is a frequent benign side effect which often can be ameliorated by taking the medication with meals (without impairing its absorption) or by lowering the dose. Erythromycin can raise blood theophyllin levels, occasionally into the toxic range, and doses of the latter drug should be monitored and adjusted. Many physicians treat *all* ambulatory patients with pneumonia with erythromycin. The advantage is coverage for pneumococcal and mycoplasmal infections, as well as legionnaires' and many milder anaerobic infections. Since up to 10% of pneumococcal isolates are resistant to tetracycline, this drug is reserved for the occasional patient who fails to respond to erythromycin or in whom tularemia or Q fever is suspected epidemiologically. In these situations, a 2- to 3-week course of tetracycline, 500 mg 4 times daily, is appropriate.

Follow-up. The patient should be advised to keep in close contact by phone, maintain good hydration with oral fluids, use aspirin or acetaminophen to control fever and headache, and avoid cough suppressants and cigarettes. A phone call to the patient 24 hours after the initial visit provides a check on antibiotic compliance and side effects and on the status of symptoms; also it reassures the acutely ill patient that he has access to the physician should his condition worsen or fail to improve.

A follow-up visit to the office 3 to 4 days later will help assess response to therapy. Uncomplicated pneumococcal pneumonia in the uncompromised host will respond to penicillin completely in 48 to 72 hours. Erythromycin will substantially reduce fever and systemic symptoms in most patients with mycoplasmal pneumonia by 3 to 6 days. Therefore if substantial clinical response to penicillin has not occurred, either switching to erythromycin or hospitalizing the patient for further diagnostic studies should be contemplated.

Early follow-up chest X-rays are mandatory in patients who fail to show clinical improvement by 5 to 7 days of therapy, or who have a later relapse. Since 3% of patients who have a bronchogenic carcinoma (see Chapter 53) initially present with a typical pneumonitis with or without consolidation (7), all patients over 40 and all smokers should have a test-of-cure chest X-ray at 4 to 6 weeks, the interval in which radiologic clearing is expected for uncomplicated cases of pneumococcal and mycoplasmal pneumonia (18). Old age, chronic obstructive lung disease, and alcoholism may delay radiologic clearing for an additional 2 to 6 weeks (18).

PREVENTION

Polyvalent pneumococcal vaccine and influenza vaccines are discussed in detail in Chapter 30. No special precautions to isolate the ambulatory pneumonia patient need to be taken. Household contacts of pneumonia patients need no special surveillance, with the exceptions of pneumonic disease due to tuberculosis d(see Chapter 28), tularemia, plague, and meningococci.

References

General

Benenson, AS (ed.): *Control of Communicable Diseases in Man,* Ed. 12. American Public Health Association, Washington, D.C., 1975.
  A concise summary of epidemiology and management of communicable diseases.

Mandell, GL, Douglas RG, Jr and Bennett, JE (eds.): *Principles and Practice of Infectious Diseases.* Wiley, New York, 1979.
  The standard textbook of infectious diseases.

Vickery DM and Fries, JF: *Take Care of Yourself. A Consumer's Guide to Medical Care.* Addison-Wesley, Reading, Mass., 1976.
  Simple algorithms for self-care of common medical problems.

Specific

1. Baine, WB, Luby, JP and Martin, SW: Severe illness with influenza B. *Am J Med 68:* 181, 1980.
2. Barrett-Connor, E: The nonvalue of sputum culture in the diagnosis of pneumococcal pneumonia. *Am Rev Resp Dis 103:* 845, 1971.
3. Berg, AO, and LoGerfo, JP: Potential effect of self-care algorithms on the number of physician visits. *N Engl J Med 300:* 535, 1979.
4. Chalmers TC: Effects of ascorbic acid on the common cold. An evaluation of the evidence. *Am J Med 58:* 532, 1975.
5. Current estimates from the Health Interview Survey: United States—1976. Vital and Health Statistics, Series 10, Number 119, DHEW publication No. (PHS) 78-1547, 1977.
6. Delker, LL, Moser, RH, Nelson JD, Rodstein, M, Rolls, K, Sanford, JP and Swarts, MH: Amantadine: does it have a role in the prevention and treatment of influenza? A National Institutes of Health Consensus Development Conference. *Ann Intern Med 92:* 256, 1980.

7. Drevvatne, T and Frimann-Dahl, J: Peripheral bronchial carcinomas: a radiological and pathological study. *Br J Radiol 34:* 180, 1961.
8. Evans, Jr, FO, Sydnor, JB, Moore, WEC, Moore, GE, Manwaring, JL, Brill, AH, Jackson, RT, Hanna, S, Skaar, JS, Holdeman, LV, Fitz-Hugh, GS, Sande, MA and Gwaltney, Jr, JM: Sinusitis of the maxillary antrum. *N Engl J Med 293:* 735, 1975.
9. Feinstein, AR, Spagnuolo, M, Wood, HF, Taranta, A, Tursky, E and Kleinberg, E: Rheumatic fever in children and adolescents. *Ann Intern Med 60:* 68, 1964.
10. Foy, HM, Kenny, GE, McMahan, R, Mansy, AM and Grayston, JT: *Mycoplasma pneumoniae* pneumonia in an urban area. *JAMA 214:* 1666, 1970.
11. Foy, HM, Cooney, MK, Allan, I and Kenny, GE: Rates of pneumonia during influenza epidemics in Seattle, 1964 to 1975. *JAMA 241:* 253, 1979.
12. Fry, J: Influenza A cases in 1957: clinical and epidemiological features in a general practice. *Br Med J 1:* 250, 1958.
13. Gwaltney, Jr, JM, Hendley, JO, Simon, G and Jordan, Jr, WS: Rhinovirus infections in an industrial population. 1. The occurrence illness. *N Engl J Med 275:* 1261, 1966.
14. Gwaltney, Jr, JM, Moskalski, PB and Hindley, JO: Hand to hand transmission of rhinovirus colds. *Ann Intern Med 88:* 463, 1978.
15. Hall, WJ and Douglas, Jr, RG: Pulmonary function during and after common respiratory infections. *Annu Rev Med 31:* 233, 1980.
16. Helms, CM, Viner, JP, Sturm, RH, Renner, ED and Johnson, W: Comparative features of pneumococcal, mycoplasmal, and Legionnaires' disease pneumonias. *Ann Intern Med 90:* 543,

1979.
17. Howard, JC, Kantner, TR, Lilienfield, LS, Princiotto, JV, Krum, RE, Crutcher, JE, Belman, MA and Danzig, MR: Effectiveness of antihistamines in the symptomatic management of the common cold. *JAMA 242:* 2414, 1979.
18. Jay, SJ Johanson, Jr, WG and Pierce, AK: The radiographic resolution of *Streptococcus pneumoniae* pneumonia. *N Engl J Med 293:* 798, 1975.
19. Oral cold remedies: *Med. Lett. 17:* 89, 1975.
20. Over-the-counter cough remedies: *Med. Lett. 21:* 103, 1979.
21. Rein, MF, Gwaltney, JM, O'Brien, WM, Jennings, RH and Mandell, GL: Accuracy of Gram's stain in identifying pneumococci in sputum. *JAMA 239:* 2671, 1978.
22. Saketkoo, K, Januszkiewicz, A and Sackner, MA: Effects of drinking hot water and chicken soup on nasal mucus velocity and nasal airflow resistance. *Chest 74:* 408, 1978.
23. Stanley, ED Jackson, GG et al.: virus shedding with aspirin treatment of rhinovirus infection. *JAMA 231:* 1248, 1975.
24. Stott, NV: Randomized controlled trial of antibiotics in patients with cough and purulent sputum. *Br Med J 2:* 556, 1976.
25. Strome, M: Rhino-sinusitis and midfacial pain in adolescents. *Practitioner 217:* 914, 1976.
26. Tager I and Spiezer, FE: Role of infection in chronic bronchitis. *N Engl J Med 292:* 563, 1975.
27. Tew, J, Colenoff, L and Berlin, BS: Bacterial or nonbacterial pneumonia: accuracy of radiographic diagnosis. *Radiology 124:* 607, 1977.
28. Wood, RW, Tompkins, RK and Wolcott, BW: An efficient strategy for managing acute respiratory illness in adults. *Ann Intern Med 93:* 757, 1980.

CHAPTER TWENTY-EIGHT

Tuberculosis in the Ambulatory Patient

R. BRADLEY SACK, M.D., and FREDERICK KOSTER, M.D.

DEFINITION OF THE PROBLEM

Epidemiology

Tuberculosis, though steadily decreasing in frequency in the United States, is still a disease with which all practitioners need to be familiar because of its diverse clinical presentations, most of which are first seen in an ambulatory setting. Approximately 28,000 new cases of tuberculosis, mostly in adults, are diagnosed annually in the United States (data for 1979); many of these are in subpopulations (blacks and indians) and geographic areas (large urban centers) with case rates considerably higher than that of the rest of the population. Table 28.1 summarizes recent national statistics on tuberculosis and the important trends in incidence and mortality from tuberculosis during the past 40 years.

Table 28.1
Summary of National Tuberculosis Statistics, Showing Long Term Trends and Recent Statistics[a]

	Incidence and Mortality Trends				
	1949	1959	1969	1974	1978
Reported new cases	134,865	57,535	39,120	30,122	28,521
Reported mortality	NA[b]	NA	5,567	3,513	2,914

	Distribution of New Cases by Age, 1979				
Age range	0–4	5–14	15–24	25 and over	Total
Reported new cases	989	631	2,158	23,848	27,669

Distribution of New Cases by Region and State, 1979

New England	835	Mo.	500	*Western South Central*	3,471
Maine	56	N. Dak.	22	Ark.	382
N.H.	25	S. Dak.	55	La.	647
Vt.	29	Nebr.	30	Okla.	352
Mass.	476	Kans.	104	Texas	2,090
R.I.	80	*South Atlantic*	6,033	*Mountain*	919
Conn.	169	Del.	63	Mont.	39
Mid Atlantic	4,238	Md.	648	Idaho	21
NY (excl. NYC)	699	D.C.	324	Wyo.	19
N.Y.C.	1,530	Va.	747	Colo.	170
N.J.	933	W. Va.	221	N. Mex.	153
Pa.	1,076	N.C.	990	Ariz.	417
Eastern North Central	4,075	S.C.	483	Utah	46
Ohio	764	Ga.	929	Nev.	54
Ind.	509	Fla.	1,628	*Pacific*	4,543
Ill.	1,540	*Eastern South Central*	2,580	Wash.	321
Mich.	1,052	Ky.	635	Oreg.	179
Wis.	210	Tenn.	748	Calif.	3,642
Western North Central	975	Ala.	644	Alaska	90
Minn.	190	Miss.	553	Hawaii	311
Iowa	74				

[a] Source: *Morbidity and Mortality Weekly Report*, Vol. 28, No. 54, September 1980.
[b] NA, not available.

Reactivation and Primary Tuberculosis

The majority of the sporadic new cases of tuberculosis are due to *reactivation* of a remote primary infection; patients in this situation are those who have had untreated or inadequately treated active tuberculosis and those with positive tuberculin reactions who have neither a past history of active tuberculosis nor documented conversion from tuberculin negativity during an interval of 1 year or less (11). *Primary* tuberculosis means newly acquired evidence for infection (either recent conversion to tuberculin positivity or the onset of active disease shortly after exposure to a patient with known active disease). Persons at highest risk of developing primary tuberculosis are those living with, or having close contact with, a person who has undetected, and therefore untreated active disease.

Most patients with tuberculosis are minimally symptomatic or are asymptomatic, which is why public health screening programs are critical for case detection. General physicians, although usually not involved in mass screening efforts, will see patients for routine examinations who have positive skin tests or patients who have specific signs or symptoms suggestive of tuberculosis. This chapter is concerned largely with the detection of the disease in such patients and with the treatment given them in the ambulatory setting.

Etiology

The etiology of tuberculosis in the United States is almost always *Mycobacterium tuberculosis*. In some parts of the world other strains (such as bovine and avian strains) may also be important in human disease. Atypical mycobacteria such as *Mycobacterium kansasii* and *Mycobacterium intracellulare*, and certain fungi such as *Cryptococcus neoformans* and *Histoplasma capsulatum* may produce disease indistinguishable from tuberculosis, and should be considered in the differential diagnosis.

DIAGNOSIS

History

Tuberculosis, when symptomatic, almost always presents with signs and symptoms of weeks' to months' duration. Almost the only time it presents as acute disease is in rare cases of acute meningitis or tuberculous pneumonia. The history should be directed toward both defining the symptom complex and determining possible exposure to known sources of disease.

Since tuberculosis has multiple presentations (12), the physician should be suspicious about anyone with chronic unexplained symptoms. Weight loss (documented over a defined period of time), fever (particularly in the late evenings), night sweats (to be differentiated from environmentally induced sweats), decreased appetite, and the loss of a sense of well-being are the most important nonspecific symptoms. Persistent cough (usually with sputum production), hemoptysis, and pleuritic chest pain are more specific findings suggestive of pulmonary involvement.

It is important to know if the patient has previously had tuberculosis, if the patient has previously been skin-tested for tuberculosis (and if so, when he was tested and what the results were), and when the patient has had previous chest films (and where they can be obtained).

Possibly significant history also includes any family member or close friend with known tuberculosis, any person in school or at work with known disease, and any recent history of travel to the developing world, where tuberculosis is common.

Physical Examination

The physical examination often may be entirely negative, even with obvious evidence of pulmonary disease on the chest film. The following positive findings, when present, may be of considerable help in suggesting the diagnosis: auscultatory evidence of pulmonary cavitation (bronchovesicular breathing and whispered pectoriloquy); evidence of pleural effusion; supra- and infra-clavicular retraction; lymphadenopathy; evidence of weight loss, as indicated by loose skin folds of the upper arms; and fever. Although rare in the United States, large matted, nontender cervical lymph nodes (at times with draining sinuses) are almost diagnostic of *scrofula*, a form of tuberculous adenitis (which may also be due to atypical mycobacteria) seen primarily in children.

Tuberculin Skin Tests

If the patient has previously had a negative skin test or has not had a skin test at all, a test with intermediate strength PPD (purified protein derivative) (5 tuberculin units, Tween-stabilized) should be applied intradermally on the volar skin of the forearm. Ideally, a control test should be placed on the opposite arm, containing a ubiquitous antigen, such as candida or mumps. The reactions should be read at 48 hours. A practical method for determining the diameter of the indurated area is the ball-point pen method (10): a line is drawn from a point 1 to 2 cm away from the margin of a positive reaction; when the pen tip reaches the margin of the indurated area,

definite resistance is felt; this is repeated on the opposite side, and the diameter of the indurated reaction is measured. The interpretation and significance of tuberculin tests are summarized in Table 28.2.

A person with a known positive tuberculin skin test does not need to have one repeated; if the test is repeated, there is a small risk of producing a very *strong positive reaction* characterized by tender induration, axillary adenopathy, and temperature elevation (as high as 102°F (38.5°C)), and slough of the epidermis after a week. This problem is best treated with a sterile gauze dressing inpregnated with a topical steroid such as 0.1% triamcinolone.

First strength and second strength tuberculin tests are rarely if ever useful in the diagnosis of tuberculosis. The tests are used as screening tests, and positive tests should be confirmed by an intermediate PPD.

M. tuberculosis shares antigens with related mycobacteria, and therefore a positive skin test is not completely specific. However, most cross-reactions will be less than 10 mm in diameter. Skin-testing with specific atypical mycobacterial antigens is not possible, since the antigens are not available for general use.

It should be remembered that a negative tuberculin skin test does not rule out the diagnosis of tuberculosis; intercurrent febrile illnesses, skin-testing within 30 days of vaccination with a live virus, underlying disease or immunosuppressive drugs which may suppress delayed hypersensitivity reactions, and errors in administration of the test material may explain these false negative reactions.

In persons such as hospital employees who are skin-tested frequently, a *booster phenomenon* may interfere with the interpretation of the test (13). Persons with a remote tuberculous or atypical mycobacterial infection who have become skin test-negative may, upon repeat skin-testing, develop a positive response owing to this boosting effect. The booster effect can best be evaluated by administering a second tuberculin test 1 week after the first test in persons who initially have a negative response. If the second response is positive, these persons can be said to have had past infection, but are not considered to have a recently acquired infection. The boosting effect is only of importance in persons who are repeatedly skin-tested.

Laboratory Examination

CHEST X-RAY

Both posteroanterior (PA) and lateral views should be obtained. In the patient with strongly suggestive clinical evidence for tuberculosis, an apical lordotic view should also be obtained when the PA and lateral views appear to be normal. The radiological findings typical of TB (apical scarring, hilar adenopathy with peripheral infiltrate, upper lobe cavitation, miliary

Table 28.2
Evaluation of Tuberculin Skin Tests (5 Tuberculin Units)

Reaction[a]	Associated Features	Significance	Therapy[b]
Positive	Unknown duration:		
	Chest film negative	Probably old infection unless recently acquired disease	Consider INH treatment for 1 yr, if under age 35 yr
	Chest film positive	Old tuberculous disease, at risk for developing reactivation	Consider INH treatment for 1 yr
	Close contact of patients with tuberculosis	May represent recent disease	Consider INH treatment for 1 yr
Positive	Recent development (<1 yr)	Recent acquisition of tuberculosis	INH treatment for 1 yr
Positive	In patient beginning long term course of corticosteroids	Patient at increased risk of developing clinical tuberculosis	Consider INH treatment for duration of steroid course or for 1 yr
Negative	In patient also negative to ubiquitous antigens	Anergic, noninterpretable	Repeat PPD; follow with chest X-ray if necessary
Negative	In patient with recent close contact with tuberculosis patient	Does not rule out early tuberculous infection	Treat with INH; retest in 3 months. If positive continue for 1 yr. If still negative may stop INH
Negative	In patients taking high dose corticosteroids or immunosuppressives	Uninterpretable	Follow with chest X-rays; treat with INH if disease proved or highly suspected

[a] Interpretation of readings:
Negative:　5 mm induration or less. (A booster response may be seen in persons who have repeated tuberculin skin tests; this can be detected by repeated skin testing 1 week after an initial negative test. Positive booster responses do not indicate recent conversion.)
Intermediate: 5–10 mm induration (needs to be repeated; consider atypical mycobacterial disease).
Positive:　10 mm induration or more.
[b] INH, isoniazid; PPD, purified protein derivative.

infiltrate, etc.) are not specific; however, a negative chest film rules out pulmonary tuberculosis (with the rare exception of early miliary disease), making the chest film a very sensitive test.

CULTURES AND SMEARS

Sputum, for smear (acid-fast stain) and culture, should be obtained at least 3 times. A positive sputum smear is highly suggestive of tuberculosis (not absolutely diagnostic because of the possibility of atypical infection or of contamination); and a positive culture is diagnostic. If sputum is difficult to obtain, one can try to induce sputum production with nebulization of hypertonic saline, or one can obtain morning gastric aspirates, which contain the swallowed sputum (6). Gastric samples should not be examined by acid-fast stain and should be sent for culture only, as smears of gastric contents frequently show commensal acid-fast organisms and are not useful for diagnosis.

In a patient having a positive PPD and persistent pyuria without bacteriuria, three urine samples should be obtained for tuberculosis culture (again a positive acid-fast urine smear is only suggestive, since there are commensal acid-fast organisms such as *Mycobacterium smegmatis* that inhabit the urinary tract; therefore, only cultures are of diagnostic value).

The initial positive cultures from any source should be tested for sensitivity to drugs used to treat tuber-

culosis since resistant organisms may necessitate a change in treatment.

MISCELLANEOUS LABORATORY TESTS

Complete Blood Count. The hematocrit value may be normal or low; the anemia due to tuberculosis is normochronic and normocytic, the so-called anemia of chronic disease (see Chapter 46). The white blood cell count and differential count are usually normal; occasionally a monocytosis is seen in persons with severe disease.

Urinalysis. This should be obtained routinely; if sterile pyuria is found it is suggestive of renal TB and cultures should be sent as described above.

Liver Function Tests. Tests for serum glutamic-oxaloacetic transaminase (SGOT), serum glutamic-pyruvic transaminase (SGPT), alkaline phosphatase, and bilirubin may be helpful if disseminated disease or liver involvement is suspected.

Other Procedures. Other procedures, such as thoracentesis, lumbar puncture, and liver biopsy are indicated only when specific organ involvement is suspected. These are best done in hospitalized patients.

Presumptive Diagnosis

The *presumptive diagnosis of active tuberculosis* can be made when any of the following is found:

1. A typical chest X-ray.
2. A positive sputum smear.
3. A biopsy showing caseating granulomas with or without acid-fast organisms.
4. A recent change (within 1 year) of the tuberculin skin test from negative to positive, associated with other characteristic systemic symptoms/signs.

The diagnosis of active tuberculosis is *confirmed* by a positive culture from any body fluid or biopsy specimen.

COURSE AND MANAGEMENT

Overview

Most persons infected with *M. tuberculosis* are unaware that they have it; only 5 to 10% of infected persons become ill, and a positive PPD or calcified nodes on chest film may be the only indicators of the past disease. Individuals in the latter group are at continual risk of reactivating their disease, however, since it is known that live *M. tuberculosis* may persist in the tissues of an infected individual for a lifetime. In fact, such individuals have a much higher rate of development of clinical disease than do people not previously infected.

Table 28.3
Drug Regimens for the Ambulatory Treatment of Tuberculosis

LONG TERM THERAPY
Preferred: (a) Isoniazid, 300 mg, plus ethambutol, 15 mg/kg, given once a day for 18 months
or
(b) Isoniazid, 300 mg plus rifampin, 600 mg, given once a day for 18 months
Alternative (in Isoniazid, 15 mg/kg, plus rifampin, 600 mg, given twice a week under supervision for 18 months
noncompliant patients)
SHORT COURSE THERAPY (now considered an acceptable alternative for compliant or noncompliant patients with uncomplicated pulmonary tuberculosis)
9-Months Course: Isoniazid, 300 mg, and rifampin, 600 mg, given daily for first 4 weeks; then twice weekly isoniazid, 15 mg/kg (usually 900 mg for adults) and rifampin, 600 mg with supervision; or the daily doses can be continued in compliant patients. Ethambutol can be added if primary drug-resistance is suspected; treatment should be given at least 6 months after sputum cultures become negative, so it may need to be extended beyond 9 months in some patients. Patients should be followed closely for 1 year after completing therapy, for relapse

Table 28.4
Oral Antituberculous Drugs: Dosage and Important Side Effects

Drug	Daily Dose	Available Strengths (mg)	Side Effects
FIRST LINE DRUGS			
Isoniazid	300 mg	100, 300	Hepatitis, peripheral neuropathy, increases Dilantin level
Ethambutol	15 mg/kg	100, 400	Optic neuritis
Rifampin[a]	600 mg	300	Hepatitis, hemolytic reactions, hypersensitivity; drug interaction important[a]
SECOND LINE DRUGS			
p-Aminosalicylic acid (PAS)	12–15 g	500	Gastric irritation, hepatitis
Ethionamide	0.75–1.0 g	250	Gastric irritation, hepatitis
Cycloserine	0.75–1.0 g	250	Seizures, psychosis
Pyrazinamide	20–35 mg/kg	500	Hepatic toxicity

[a] Accelerates the metabolism of coumarin-type anticoagulants, oral contraceptives, corticosteroids, digitoxin, methadone, and oral hypoglycemic agents.

When tuberculosis is diagnosed in association with systemic signs or symptoms, there is no question that the patient should be treated. Persons with positive tuberculin reactions as the only manifestation of disease constitute a more difficult problem (see Table 28.2 and "Isoniazid Prophylaxis" below).

Once the diagnosis is strongly suspected or made, the question arises of how best to initiate therapy. Since it may take 4 weeks before cultures of *M. tuberculosis* become positive, therapy must usually be initiated on the basis of the chest film, sputum smears, and/or a strong clinical suspicion.

If the patient is well enough to care for himself, can take oral medications regularly, and has no extrapulmonary disease, he can be successfully treated without hospitalization.

Treatment

CHEMOTHERAPY (Tables 28.3 and 28.4)

To treat active tuberculosis, only *two oral drugs* are necessary unless the organisms are drug-resistant, as shown by *in vitro* testing; a single drug should never be used, because it increases the risk of the emergence of resistant organisms during therapy. The two-drug combinations most commonly used are: isoniazid (300 mg/day, adult dose) and ethambutol (15 mg/kg/day, adult dose), or isoniazid and rifampin (600 mg/day, adult dose).

The standard period of recommended treatment, until very recently, has been 18 months; this has resulted in the cure of nearly all patients. There is now good evidence that treatment for 9 months with the combination of the two bacteriocidal drugs, isoniazid and rifampin, is perfectly adequate (see Table 28.3). This short course chemotherapy has been accepted as an alternative to the long established treatment regimen of 18 months by the Center for Disease Control and the American Thoracic Society (1).

Regimens containing *second line drugs* need to be considered only in patients who have developed adverse reactions to the standard drugs, which is uncommon, or in patients with drug-resistant tuberculosis. This latter group is usually composed of people who have been treated previously for tuberculosis, or who have acquired tuberculosis in Southeast Asia or Mexico.

Pregnant women can receive isoniazid and ethambutol, since they are both known to be tolerated well by the fetus.

Patients with *impaired renal function* should be treated with isoniazid and rifampin, since ethambutol is excreted mainly by the kidneys, and its dosage would have to be adjusted.

SYMPTOMATIC THERAPY

Usually no symptomatic therapy is required, except that patients should be encouraged to eat an adequate diet. If a patient has symptoms that require special management (such as high fever and toxicity for which steroids may be helpful, or a pleural effusion that needs draining), hospitalization is necessary.

If the patient is eating poorly, the physician should add pyridoxine (5 mg/day) to the regimen to prevent the peripheral neuropathy that can be seen with isoniazid administration. This is not necessary if the patient is able to eat normally.

Course in Treated Patient

FOLLOW-UP SCHEDULE

After treatment has been initiated, the patient should be seen or contacted at least once per month, chiefly to assure drug compliance (see below) and to monitor for drug side effects (see below). For the first 3 months, sputum cultures should be obtained; and at 3 months and 6 months to 1 year a chest X-ray should be obtained. Sputum culture should be negative after 3 months of therapy, although occasionally nonculturable acid-fast organisms will be seen on smear for longer periods. A test-of-cure culture should be done on all patients at 5 or 6 months. Resolution of pulmonary infiltrates is often slow; the former practice of monthly chest films is therefore not warranted. Chest films are most helpful in excluding progression of disease and in documenting the patient's status when the tuberculosis is cured.

At the cessation of traditional chemotherapy regimens (18 months) prolonged follow-up is not necessary. After alternate-course or short-course chemotherapy (Table 28.3), it is recommended that close follow-up be continued for another 12 months to detect relapses by symptoms and sputum cultures.

USUAL RESPONSE

Patients diagnosed as having tuberculosis who comply with therapy have an excellent prognosis. The only exceptions are the rare patient with organisms resistant to the usual antituberculous drugs, or the patient who develops adverse effects from the antituberculous therapy. These problems are discussed in more detail below.

The patient should show some symptomatic improvement within 1 week of being started on antituberculous therapy. Improvement is usually indicated by an increased sense of well-being, an increase in appetite, and a decrease in cough, fever, and night sweats; temperature should be normal within 10 days of initiating treatment. The patient is usually back to his usual state of health in 1 to 2 months.

The improvement is secondary to the antibacterial effects of the drugs, which leads to a decrease in the inflammatory response of the host. After 1 week of therapy, the patient can be considered noninfectious.

POSSIBLE COMPLICATIONS

A number of problems may complicate the management of tuberculosis. The patient may have disease due to *drug-resistant M. tuberculosis* (7). This may occur in 5% of newly diagnosed cases in the United States (4% for isoniazid; 1% for ethambutol or rifampin); but at a much higher frequency if the disease was acquired abroad, particularly in Southeast Asia (15%) and Mexico. In this case, the patient may show a delayed clinical response during the first few weeks of therapy. Since the laboratory may take 8 to 10 weeks to provide the sensitivity data on the original bacteriologic isolates, it may be difficult to detect this problem early. If resistance is strongly suspected (as in a patient with previously treated tuberculosis) or documented, the drug regimen should consist of two antituberculous drugs which the patient has not taken before; ideally these drugs should be selected on the basis of the sensitivity pattern of the organism. It is suggested that consultation be obtained before embarking on a course of therapy with second-line, less effective drugs, however.

The patient may *comply poorly* with the daily medication regimen (see below).

The patient may develop *drug toxicity* from the antituberculous medication (Table 28.4).

Isoniazid. Hepatic toxicity is the most common adverse reaction; it occurs at a biochemical level in approximately 20% of persons who take the drug (3); the incidence of toxicity increases with age and with excessive alcohol intake (5, 8). Laboratory evidence of mild injury to the liver is not in itself a reason to stop the drug, however, since in most subjects the SGOT level returns to normal while the drug is being continued. If the patient develops clinical jaundice or develops fever and elevated liver enzymes, the drug should, of course, be stopped. The liver injury is usually reversible, and will correct itself without further therapy. In some persons, however (elderly men and particularly those with chronic alcoholic-related liver disease) the liver injury may be severe and sometimes fatal. Isoniazid liver toxicity most often occurs early in therapy, so that the first 2 to 3 months are the most critical in the detection of adverse drug reactions. Specific guidelines for monitoring for isoniazid hepatitis are contained in the section on prevention (below, p. 240). Peripheral neuropathy is an uncommon complication of isoniazid therapy which occurs only in persons on an inadequate diet and can be prevented by taking 5 mg of pyridoxine every day.

Ethambutol. The most serious side effect of ethambutol is optic neuritis, resulting in decrease of visual acuity and in inability to distinguish the color green. This problem was seen frequently when the drug was given in a dose of 25 mg/kg. It is extremely uncommon at the recommended daily dose of 15 mg/kg.

Rifampin. Serious allergic complications of rifampin therapy, including thrombocytopenia manifested by purpura, petechiae, and hematuria, and a "flu syndrome," occur in approximately 1% of patients, and necessitate cessation of therapy. There is a modest increase in hepatic toxicity which may be additive to isoniazid toxicity so that patients on the short course intermittent rifampin-isoniazid protocol should be closely supervised. Patients should be warned that rifampin may result in an orange-red color in secretions such as urine, saliva, etc. Rifampin accelerates the metabolism of other drugs (Table 28.4) and may necessitate an increase in the dose of these drugs.

Problems Requiring Hospitalization. Ambulatory patients started on treatment should not require hospitalization. The few possible exceptions are: (a) the development of progressive and debilitating disease, due either to resistant organisms or to poor compliance by the patient, and (b) severe toxic reactions to drugs, particularly isoniazid.

The Patient's Role in Therapy

The patient's role is of the utmost importance to the successful treatment of tuberculosis, since he must faithfully administer the drugs daily for a period of 9 or 18 months and return for regular follow-up visits.

Because noncompliance accounts for most therapeutic failures, the most important function of monthly visits is the documentation and reinforcement of compliance (see Chapter 4). When therapy is begun, the patient should be thoroughly educated about the course and therapy of his disease, so that the illusion of health when symptoms disappear will not cause premature cessation of therapy. The physician should help the patient design techniques to avoid missing daily medication due to forgetfulness.

Pill counts at follow-up visits may be helpful. In noncompliant patients, the modified regimen (shorter duration and twice weekly medication) summarized in Table 28.3 may be particularly useful. If there are problems with compliance which cannot be solved by the physician, the patient should be referred to public health authorities for supervision of long term care. Such authorities will provide home visits if necessary and will ensure that the patient is not lost to follow-up.

The patient should be advised about the communicable nature of his disease, which is particularly important until he has been on therapy for at least a week. During that first week, he should minimize his contact with others, and be advised simply to cough into tissue which then can be incinerated. After 1 week, he should be considered not contagious, and his activities can be dictated solely by his sense of well-being. Patients taking isoniazid should be given specific advice and monitored for hepatitis as outlined in the following section.

PREVENTION OF TUBERCULOSIS

Case Detection among Known Contacts

An integral part of initiation of care in any patient with active tuberculosis is case-reporting to the local health authority and investigation of contacts. This entails tuberculin-testing of all household and intimate "nonhousehold" contacts, and retesting of nonreactors in 2 to 3 months. Reactors are examined by chest X-ray and if free of active disease are given chemoprophylaxis with isoniazid for 1 year. With the exception of evaluating family members this type of investigation is usually impossible for a physician to carry out alone and should be done by the local city or county health department. Such departments have trained personnel who are available to visit homes and work places in order to detect cases in contacts. In many states, it is required by law that persons with newly diagnosed tuberculosis (or with a strongly suspected diagnosis) be reported to the public health authorities.

Tuberculin Testing in Prevention

(See method, p. 235 above, and interpretation, Table 28.2.)

Ideally the tuberculin skin test status of all individuals should be determined at some time in their early adult life. In almost all school age children, screening for tuberculin positivity is coordinated with school health programs. In adult populations, a number of factors such as urban residence, the presence of chronic disease, a history of residence in underdeveloped countries, and health care occupation increase the importance of periodic tuberculin testing. This is particularly true for those individuals for whom isoniazid is recommended if the PPD is positive (see next section).

Because of the increased risk of contact with unrecognized cases of tuberculosis, physicians and hospital personnel have an increased chance of acquiring infection (twice the risk of the general population). Both for personal protection and because of the risk of transmitting tuberculosis to patients, physicians and other health workers should have annual tuberculin testing and should take isoniazid chemoprophylaxis if they convert from negative to positive.

Isoniazid Prophylaxis

Isoniazid prophylaxis (300 mg daily for 1 year) has been shown to be of marked value in preventing new cases of active tuberculosis among special groups of persons at high risk. Because of the recognition of isoniazid-induced hepatitis, however, the indications for the use of isoniazid have narrowed somewhat in recent years. At the present time the following groups of persons are felt to have a risk-benefit ratio high enough to be treated prophylactically with isoniazid (2, 4, 9): (a) close contacts of active infectious cases; (b) persons with recent skin test conversion (not those with booster responses, see above, p. 235); (c) persons with positive skin tests and an abnormal chest X-ray suggestive of old tuberculosis; (d) persons with a known history of old tuberculosis who have never been given antibacterial treatment; (e) persons with positive skin tests who will be given corticosteroid or immunosuppressive therapy; and (f) persons with a positive skin test only, who are under the age of 35 years.

The guidelines recommended by the American Thoracic Society for monitoring patients taking isoniazid are the following (2).

Individuals receiving preventive therapy or a responsible adult in a household with children on preventive therapy should be questioned carefully at monthly intervals for the following:

1. Symptoms consistent with those of liver damage or other toxic effects; that is, unexplained anorexia, nausea, or vomiting of greater than 3 days duration, fatigue or weakness of greater than 3 days duration, persistent paresthesias of the hands and feet.

2. Signs consistent with those of liver damage or other toxic effects; that is, persistent dark urine, icterus, rash, elevated temperature of greater than 3 days' duration without explanation.

Monitoring by routine laboratory tests (e.g., SGOT, SGPT, serum bilirubin, and alkaline phosphatase) is not useful in predicting hepatic disease in isoniazid recipients and therefore is not recommended. However, in evaluating signs and symptoms such tests are mandatory. Preventive therapy should be reinstituted only if biochemical studies are normal and signs and symptoms are absent.

Because it has been recognized that this monitoring plan may fail to detect an occasional patient with severe hepatitis (3), monthly measurement of the SGOT level is recommended by some authorities. This would detect the transient SGOT elevation which occurs in approximately 20% of subjects taking isoniazid; a cut-off level, such as a level 3 or 5 times normal, is recommended as the criterion for discontinuing isoniazid. Glassroth (see "General References") suggests monthly measurement of the SGOT level in those patients who are in the groups at the highest risk of developing isoniazid hepatitis; i.e., those over 35 years of age, daily "drinkers," patients concomitantly taking other potentially hepatoxic drugs, and patients with a history of liver disease.

References

General

Byrd, RB, Horn, BR, Solomon, DA, Griggs, GA and Wilder, NJ: Treatment of tuberculosis by the nonpulmonary physician. *Ann Intern Med 86:* 799, 1977.
   Useful summary of the most common mistakes made by general physicians treating patients for tuberculosis.
Glassroth, MD, Robins, AG and Snider, DE, Jr: Tuberculosis in the 1980s. *N Engl J Med 302:* 1441, 1980.
   Extensively referenced and up to date review.

Specific

1. American Thoracic Society and Center for Disease Control: Guidelines for short-course tuberculosis chemotherapy. *Am Rev Respir Dis 121:* 611, 1980.
2. American Thoracic Society, Medical Section of the American Lung Association: Preventive therapy of tuberculous infection. *Am Rev Respir Dis 110:* 371, 1974.
3. Byrd, RG, Horn, BR, Solomon, DA and Griggs, GA: Toxic effects of Isoniazid in tuberculosis chemoprophylaxis. *JAMA 241:* 1239, 1979.
4. Comstock, GW and Edwards, PQ: The competing risks of tuberculosis and hepatitis for adult tuberculin reactors. *Am Rev Respir Dis 111:* 573, 1975.
5. Garibaldi, RA, Drusin, RE, Ferebee, SH and Gregg, MD: Isoniazid-associated hepatitis: report of an outbreak. *Am Rev Respir Dis 106:* 357, 1972.
6. Houk, VH, Kent, DC, Baker, JH, Sorense, K and Hanzel, GD: In-depth analysis of a micro-cutbreak of tuberculosis in a closed environment. *Arch Envirn Health 16:* 4, 1968.
7. Kopanoff, DE, Kilburn, JO, Glassroth, JL, Snider, DE Jr, Farer, LS and Good, RC: A continuing survey of tuberculosis primary drug resistance in the United States: March 1975 to November 1977. A United States Public Health Service cooperative study. *Am Rev Respir Dis 118:* 835, 1978.
8. Maddrey, WC and Boitnott, JK: Isoniazid hepatitis. *Ann Intern Med 79:* 1, 1973.
9. Moulding, T: Chemoprophylaxis of tuberculosis: when is the benefit worth the risk and cost? *Ann Intern Med 74:* 761, 1971.
10. Sokal, JE: Measurement of delayed skin-test responses. *N Engl J Med 293:* 501, 1975.
11. Stead, WW: Pathogenesis of the sporadic case of tuberculosis. *N Engl J Med 277:* 1008, 1967.
12. Stead, WW, Kerby, GR, Schlueter, DP and Jordahl, CW: The clinical spectrum of primary tuberculosis in adults: confusion with reinfection in the pathogenesis of chronic tuberculosis. *Ann Intern Med 68:* 731, 1968.
13. Thompson, NJ, Glassroth, JL, Snider, DE Jr and Farer, LS: The booster phenomenon in serial tuberculin testing. *Am Rev Respir Dis 119:* 587, 1979.

CHAPTER TWENTY-NINE

Syphilis

PETER E. DANS, M.D.

EPIDEMIOLOGY

Syphilis was a major medical and social scourge until the advent of penicillin. The combination of effective therapy and contact tracing brought the incidence of new infections to a low point in the 1950s (see Table 29.1). Since the 1960s, the number of early cases has increased, but the prevalence of late and late latent syphilis has continued to decline.

While the occurrence is usually sporadic, there have been explosive outbreaks. These are increasingly being traced to male homosexuals or bisexuals. In 1969, approximately one-fourth of the male patients acquiring the disease were homosexuals or bisexuals; currently this percentage is about 50%—whereas the proportion of men in the population estimated to be homosexual is approximately 10%.

STAGES OF THE DISEASE (see Table 29.2)

The acquired form of the disease evolves through different stages: primary, secondary, early and late latent, and tertiary or late syphilis.

Primary Syphilis

Primary syphilis is characterized by the development of a lesion at the site of inoculation of *Treponema pallidum*, the etiologic organism. This "chancre" appears 10 to 90 days (average 21 days) following infection as a single painless papule which, when it ulcerates, becomes highly infectious. It can vary in size from a few millimeters to a few centimeters in diameter. There is associated regional lymphadenopathy. Major considerations in the differential diagnosis are summarized in Table 29.3. The diagnosis at this stage is made definitively by darkfield examination of the fluid overlying the ulcer. Serologic tests for syphilis are positive in approximately 75 to 80% of patients at this stage (see "Serodiagnosis").

Secondary Syphilis

Secondary syphilis occurs 6 weeks to 6 months after initial contact. The most characteristic finding is a nonpruritic rash which is usually maculopapular, but not vesticular or bullous. It can involve all areas of the skin, including the palms and soles. Scalp and eyelash involvement may lead to alopecia. Lesions can be present in the mucous membranes of the mouth (gray patches on an erythematous base) and in warm, moist areas such as the axillary and genital regions. A flat, wartlike lesion, condyloma latum, is diagnostic but must be distinguished from the more common pointy, fleshy, genital wart (condyloma acuminatum). The lesions of the mucous membranes and the skin lesions in moist areas are highly infectious.

Constitutional symptoms such as fever, headache, malaise, and general lymphadenopathy are common. Less commonly there is iritis, deafness, or signs and symptoms of hepatitis, of immune-complex nephropathy or of meningitis. Darkfield examination of moist lesions is positive; however, it should not be performed on oral lesions because of the presence of spirochetes that are part of the normal mouth flora. Serologic tests for syphilis are positive in virtually 100% of patients at this stage. The major considerations in differential diagnosis are infections, exanthematous conditions, drug reactions, and pityriasis rosea, a seasonal disease (spring and fall) characterized by a single, large initial lesion called the herald patch and subsequently by a pruritic erythematous, maculopapular rash which develops along the lines of skin cleavage on the trunk (see Chapter 97).

Secondary syphilis may *relapse* if untreated or inadequately treated. Relapses are clinically identical to initial episodes although condyloma latum may be more common. Relapse occurs in about 25% of untreated persons at some time during the first 4 years after infection (90% within 1 year of infection). There is always a rise in STS titer during relapse. Treatment is the same as that for an initial episode of secondary syphilis.

Approximately 1% of patients in the secondary stage may develop frank *meningitis*, and as many as half of these patients may not have skin lesions. This syndrome is characterized by headache, stiff neck, cranial nerve lesions, and sometimes papilledema or seizures. The cerebrospinal fluid (CSF) is diagnostic (increased mononuclear cells and protein plus spirochetes on darkfield examination and an abnormal serologic test).

Latent Syphilis

Latent syphilis is, as the name implies, the period after infection with *T. pallidum* when there are no manifestations of the disease. This stage is divided into *early* latent (less than 1 year's duration) and *late* latent (greater than 1 year's duration). The only way such patients come to diagnosis is through routine serologic testing which shows positive nontreponemal and treponemal tests (see "Serodiagnosis"). Detection early in this stage is important not only to prevent further complications in the one-third of untreated patients who go on to develop late manifestations of syphilis, but also for contact tracing. Contact tracing is usually performed only in contacts of patients with infectious or early latent syphilis.

Tertiary Syphilis

Tertiary or late disease is divided into three principal forms: late benign syphilis, cardiovascular syphilis, and neurosyphilis.

Table 29.1
Annual Reported Cases of Syphilis in the United States[a]

Stage	1943	1956	1965	1980
Infectious (primary and secondary) syphilis	82,204	6,392	23,338	27,204
Early latent <1 year duration	149,390	19,783	17,458	20,167
Late and late latent	251,958	95,097	67,317	20,976
Total	483,552	121,272	108,113	68,132

[a] Source: J. Blount, Center for Disease Control, Department of Health and Human Services, Atlanta, Georgia (personal communication).

Table 29.2
Outline of Clinical Stages of Syphilis (See Details in Text)

Stage	Characteristic Findings	Usual Onset after Exposure	Persistence of Stage in Untreated Patients	Darkfield	Sensitivity of Serologic Tests (%)[a]		
					VDRL	FTA-ABS	RPR
PRIMARY	Chancre—may be absent or not visible (*e.g.*, in vagina or mouth)	10–90 days (average 21 days)	2–6 wk	+ (chancre, lymph nodes)	78[b]	85	80[b]
SECONDARY	Rash, condyloma latum, lymphadenopathy	6 wk to 6 mo	2–6 wk; recurrences in 25% over 2-yr period	+ (especially moist lesions)	97	99	99
ACUTE SYPHILITIC MENINGITIS	Headache, cranial nerve lesions, papilledema	6 wk to 2 yr	Not applicable	+ CSF	97	99	99
LATENT			May be life-long 1/3 of untreated patients develop tertiary syphilis	−	74	95	70–92
Early	None	≤1 yr after infection					
Late	None	≥1 yr after infection					
LATE (TERTIARY)							
Benign	Gumma	2–10 yr	Indolent	−	77	95	
Cardiovascular	Aortic aneurysm Aortic insufficiency Coronary artery disease	10–30 yr	Progressive; may be fatal	Aorta may be +	77	95	92
Neurosyphilis		5–35 yr	Progressive; may be fatal	Brain may be +	77	95	92
Asymptomatic	None						
Meningovascular	Signs of infection depending on area involved	2–5 yr					
Paresis	Minor personality change to frank psychosis	≥20 yr					
Tabes dorsalis	Signs of posterior column degeneration	≥25 yr					

[a] Performed on blood specimens from untreated patients.
[b] May not become positive until 1–2 weeks *after* appearance of chancre.

Table 29.3
Differential Diagnosis of a Genital Sore

PRIMARY SYPHILIS (CHANCRE)
Incubation period 10–90 days (average, 21 days)
Usually painless (in absence of secondary infection)
Not vesicular
Usually single indurated ulcer
Spirochete on darkfield examination
Nontender inguinal adenopathy
HERPES SIMPLEX
Incubation period 24–48 hr
Usually painful
Vesicular
Usually multiple ulcers
Multinucleated giant cells on Giemsa stain plus virus on culture
Tender inguinal adenopathy
CHANCROID
Multiple soft superficial erosions
Nontender adenopathy. *Hemophilus ducreyi* on Gram stain of dried smear (small Gram-negative bacillus)
GRANULOMA INGUINALE
Soft occasionally raised, granular lesions in inguinal area; Donovan bodies on smear (histiocytes with intracytoplasmic encapsulated Gram-negative bacilli)
OTHER CONSIDERATIONS
Trauma, carcinoma, scabies, lichen planus, psoriasis, fixed drug eruption (especially phenolphthalein), fungus infection, folliculitis

Late benign syphilis is rare today. The usual lesion is a gumma (a lesion which may be microscopic or several centimeters in size). It is a hypersensitivity reaction to the organism and does not usually contain viable organisms. A gumma usually occurs within 2 to 10 years of infection. It occurs most commonly on the skin (ulcerative or nodular-ulcerative), in bone, or in the liver; it can be very destructive if it occurs in the brain, liver, or heart. Confirmation of diagnosis may be made on the basis of dramatic healing of visible gummas following treatment.

Cardiovascular syphilis is estimated to occur in about 12% of untreated men and 5% of untreated women from 5 to 30 years after initiation of the disease. Aortitis is the commonest cardiovascular manifestation. The organism destroys the elastic tissue of the media of the aorta and produces an endarteritis of the vasa vasorum. Clinical manifestations include aneurysm of the ascending aorta and progressive dilatation of the aortic ring, resulting in aortic insufficiency and heart failure. When the coronary ostia are involved, angina pectoris may result. Linear calcification of the ascending aorta is a common radiologic finding in syphilitic aortitis; it may precede clinical symptoms and signs of aortic involvement.

Asymptomatic neurosyphilis is defined as a positive cerebrospinal fluid serologic test for syphilis (CSF-STS) in an untreated patient who has no manifestations of symptomatic neurosyphilis; a pleocytosis and an elevated protein are usually present in the CSF. The magnitude of the risk of acquiring this form of syphilis after initial infection is unknown but is probably very low.

Symptomatic neurosyphilis occurs in a minority of patients (about 10 to 20%) with untreated syphilis. The risk of developing symptomatic neurosyphilis after a primary infection appears to be greater in men than women and in whites than blacks. Symptomatic neurosyphilis is divided into various types depending upon the site of major involvement:

1. *Meningovascular syphilis* usually occurs within 2 to 5 years after primary infection. Common manifestations include headache, irritability, and personality changes. Focal neurologic signs often develop as clinical consequences of syphilitic vasculitis involving small end arteries. The severity of the patient's functional disability depends upon the extent and location of the accompanying cerebrovascular inflammation and occlusion.

2. *Tabes dorsalis* usually occurs 25 to 30 years after infection. It is characterized by symptoms and signs of posterior column degeneration (ataxia, areflexia, broad-based gait, incontinence, impotence, visceral pain crises, and paresthesias or "lightning" pains in the extremities). Characteristic findings also include trophic joint changes (Charcot's joints), the Argyll Robertson pupil (small, irregular pupil which accommodates but does not react to light), and optic atrophy (in about 10% of patients).

3. The syndrome of *general paresis* usually occurs 20 or more years after infection. It is due to destruction of the parenchyma of the cerebral cortex. It consists of personality changes, irritability, poor judgment, insomnia, and memory loss. The progressive dementia in these patients may be characterized by periodic euphoria and delusions of grandeur.

The definitive diagnosis of neurosyphilis is based upon cerebrospinal fluid findings: elevated protein and mononuclear cells, as well as a positive serologic test for syphilis (see "Serodiagnosis").

SERODIAGNOSIS

Characteristics of Tests

Serologic tests are of two basic types: (a) *nontreponemal* serologic tests for syphilis or STS (e.g., Venereal Disease Research Laboratory slide test, VDRL; and rapid plasma reagin, RPR) which detect nonspecific (nontreponemal) antibody called reagin; and (b) *treponemal* tests (e.g., the fluorescent treponemal antibody-absorption, FTA-ABS) which detects specific antibodies to *T. pallidum*. Figure 29.1 shows the patterns of these serologic tests during the course of untreated syphilis. The sensitivity of these tests (the percentage of infected patients with reactivity) varies at each stage of the disease (see Table 29.2).

NONTREPONEMAL TESTS

The RPR and VDRL tests have a specificity (percentage of negatives that are true negatives) of 60 to

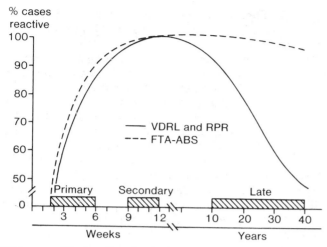

Figure 29.1 Serology of untreated syphilis. (Adapted from A. L. Wallace and L. C. Norins: Syphilis serology today. *Progress in Clinical Pathology, 2:* 198, 1969.)

95%, depending upon the prevalence of conditions causing false positivity in the test population. *Acute false positive* reactions lasting less than 6 months occur in viral and bacterial pneumonia, hepatitis, pregnancy, mononucleosis, measles, malaria, and following smallpox vaccination. *Chronic biologic false positive* reactions (lasting greater than 6 months) occur in diseases of disordered immunity such as systemic lupus erythematosus, rheumatoid arthritis, and Waldenström's macroglobulinemia as well as in persons with chronic liver disease, heroin addicts, elderly persons (approximately 1% of persons over 70 and 10% of persons over 80), and in a few patients on a hereditary basis. Because of the possibility of biologic false positives and because of occasional laboratory reporting errors, the STS should be repeated whenever it is positive in a person who is unlikely to have acquired syphilis.

The *CSF-VDRL* is a sensitive test for the detection of neurosyphilis, although it can occasionally be negative in patients with tabes dorsalis. The VDRL is almost 100% specific for CNS syphilis. (There have been case reports of a false positive CSF-VDRL due to traumatic lumbar puncture, CNS tumor, or systemic inflammatory conditions.) Because the experience with CSF FTA-ABS is limited, the VDRL test is the test of choice when the CSF is being evaluated for evidence of neurosyphilis (7).

TREPONEMAL TESTS

When properly performed the FTA-ABS has a specificity of 99.5%. *False positive reactions* do occur, however, in patients with lupus erythematosus, rheumatoid arthritis, chronic liver disease, some infections and in other patients for unexplained reasons. Since small errors in laboratory technique can affect the results of the FTA-ABS test more than the nontreponemal tests, this test should be utilized selectively, *i.e.* only in patients with a reactive VDRL or

RPR test except when tertiary syphilis is strongly suspected. (1), Both the RPR and the VDRL test may be negative in the peripheral blood in up to 30% of patients with tertiary syphilis. Using FTA-ABS test in these ways converts the population in which the test is used from one of low prevalence (less than 1%) of syphilis to one of high prevalence i.e., 60 to 95%. Consequently, the ratio of true positives to false positives will be very high. Furthermore, the FTA-ABS test should not be repeated in known positives, since the antibody rarely disappears even after therapy (Fig. 29.1). *Borderline FTA-ABS results should be considered neither reactive nor nonreactive.* Although a follow-up FTA-ABS should be done, most patients with borderline reactions do not have syphilis.

Use in Screening

A nontreponemal serologic test for syphilis should be used as a screening test in patients who are sexually active with multiple partners and thereby at increased risk for acquisition of syphilis. Since the proportion of homosexuals among patients with infectious syphilis is disproportionately high, particular attention should be given to case detection and education in this group. In addition to patients currently having sex with multiple partners, all adults who may have acquired syphilis earlier in their lives should be screened at least once in order to exclude latent syphilis. In most hospital settings an STS should be done routinely on a patient's first admission. In subsequent admissions, a repeat STS should be done only in those patients deemed to be at risk of acquiring a new infection. Middle aged and older persons with a positive test usually have a low reactivity in the nontreponemal test and fall into the category of late latent or adequately treated serofast syphilis.

Pattern after Treatment

The VDRL reverts to negative in greater than 90% of patients treated for primary or secondary syphilis, but the FTA-ABS remains positive in most (Fig. 29.2). In patients treated for early latent syphilis the VDRL becomes negative within 5 years of treatment in approximately 75%, while only about 25% of patients with treated late latent syphilis will be seronegative in 5 years (6).

TREATMENT

Regimens

The treatment of choice for primary, secondary, and early latent syphilis, as well as for known contacts of a patient with infectious syphilis, is 2.4 million units of benzathine penicillin G (LA Bicillin) intramuscularly. Alternatives for persons allergic to penicillin are total doses of 30 g of oral tetracycline or erythromycin (2 g a day for 15 days). For persons treated for gonorrhea, the usual antimicrobial regi-

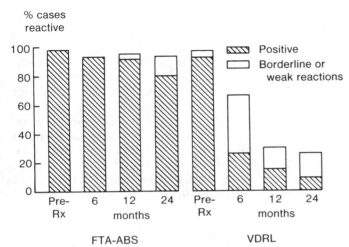

Figure 29.2 Serologic reactivity of 80 patients treated for darkfield positive primary or secondary syphilis and observed for 2 years, with use of FTA-ABS and VDRL tests. (Adapted from A. L. Schroeter et al.: *Journal of the American Medical Association,* 221: 471, 1972. © American Medical Association.)

mens for this disease (see Chapters 26 and 95) are also effective against incubating syphilis which may have been acquired simultaneously with the gonorrhea.

For patients with late syphilis or latent syphilis of greater than 1 year's duration, or for patients who have not had a spinal fluid examination to exclude asymptomatic neurosyphilis, the regimen of choice is 2.4 million units of benzathine penicillin G (LA Bicillin) weekly for 3 weeks or in patients allergic to penicillin, 60 g total dose of tetracycline or erythromycin (2 g a day for 30 days).

In patients who have confirmed neurosyphilis, recommended therapy consists of 12 to 24 million units of intravenous aqueous crystalline penicillin G daily for 10 days. This is based on recent case reports of the failure of the usual benzathine penicillin therapy to eradicate the organism and to arrest the disease (3, 4). Because of uncertainty about the effectiveness of alternatives to penicillin in patients with neurosyphilis, patients giving a history of penicillin allergy should be evaluated by skin testing (Chapter 22) before using an alternative treatment.

Effectiveness

Long term follow-up studies have shown that the results of treatment vary depending upon the stage of syphilis which is treated.

In a recent study of patients with primary and secondary syphilis treated with the usual doses of benzathine penicillin G, 5% required retreatment, and approximately 10% of those treated with the usual doses of tetracycline and erythromycin required retreatment (10). The criteria for retreatment in this study were recurrence or persistence of clinical manifestations or failure of the VDRL titer to decrease 4-fold within 1 year.

The effectiveness of treatment in the patient with latent syphilis is difficult to assess because of the absence of any markers to follow. In a recent review, all of 469 patients with late latent syphilis accumulated from various sources were symptom-free during a 12-year follow-up after treatment (5).

The effectiveness of treatment of cardiovascular syphilis has been debated (2). Most investigators feel that treatment may arrest the disease, but does not reverse it. In fact, there is evidence that, because of the weakening of the media of the aorta, aneurysms will continue to enlarge even after adequate treatment.

The results of treatment for neurosyphilis vary directly with the extent of the disease and inversely with the duration of the disease. Thus treatment appears to be helpful in reversing the signs and symptoms of acute meningovascular syphilis and in stabilizing tabes dorsalis, but is less helpful in generalized paresis, especially if given late in the course of the disease (12).

Jarisch-Herxheimer Reaction (8, 9, 11)

The Jarisch-Herxheimer reaction is usually characterized by mild temperature elevation within 6 to 8 hours of administration of penicillin. It occurs several hours afer the *first* injection of penicillin and it appears to be caused by microbial lysis and the release of endotoxin. It does not occur after subsequent injections. It is estimated that this reaction occurs, usually in a mild form, in 50% of patients with primary syphilis, 75 to 90% of patients with secondary syphilis, and 30% of patients with late disease. When it occurs during treatment of secondary syphilis, skin lesions become more prominent. The reaction lasts for a few hours and should be treated with mild analgesics.

Occasionally the Jarisch-Herxheimer reaction can be quite severe and include fever, chills, headache, muscle and joint pains, sore throat, and hypotension.

PRACTICAL APPROACH TO THE PATIENT

Patients in whom syphilis must be considered usually present to their physicians because (a) they have a "sore" or rash, (b) they have been referred as a known contact of a patient with infectious syphilis, (c) they are worried about a recent sexual liaison, or (d) a routine premarital, prior blood donor, or health screening serologic test is reported to be positive. The diagnosis of syphilis must be made carefully, as it can have a major impact on the relationships of patients with their contacts and on how they view themselves. A systematic approach to diagnosis and management is outlined here.

Evaluation

The *history* should include a description of a sore or rash if present; determination of whether the patient has had a previous history of syphilis; review of previous serologic tests for syphilis as far back as the last negative one; history of the patient's type of sexual practices (to guide the physical examination); and information about recent partners and their disease status.

The *physical examination* should include a careful search of the areas where sexual contact has occurred (especially the anogenital area and the mouth), inspection of any skin lesions, search for regional and generalized lymphadenopathy, examination of the liver, and brief neurologic, psychiatric, and cardiovascular evaluations whenever late disease is a concern.

Laboratory data should include darkfield microscopy (if available) of all suspicious lesions and serologic testing for syphilis (see "Serodiagnosis"). Cerebrospinal fluid (CSF) examination is mandatory in patients with psychiatric or neurologic signs or symptoms. In asymptomatic patients who have had syphilis for more than 1 year, the Center for Disease Control recommends a lumbar puncture (to exclude asymptomatic neurosyphilis). Most patients with low STS titers ($\leq$1:2) either have latent disease or have been adequately treated in the past without being aware of it, since the CSF examination is almost always negative; it is therefore reasonable to treat patients with low titers for latent syphilis without performing a lumbar puncture. Asymptomatic patients with STS titers of 1:4 or higher should have a CSF examination in order to exclude neurosyphilis.

The diagnosis of syphilis rests on the positive finding of darkfield microscopy or the combination of a positive nontreponemal test and treponemal test. When the diagnosis of syphilis is made, it should be staged appropriately according to the stages outlined above.

Management

The management plan is contingent on the appropriate diagnosis. The most common error occurs in formulating the assessment and plan e.g., "positive VDRL-treat with penicillin." Treatment of syphilis of a given stage is indicated, treatment of a positive VDRL *per se* is not.

ANTIBIOTIC THERAPY

This is described for each stage of syphilis above (p. 245).

FOLLOW-UP

In follow-up of the patient, the titer of the nontreponemal test remains the most useful index of the effectiveness of treatment. A high titer is more likely to occur in early syphilis or in active late disease; where this is present, a VDRL or RPR should be obtained every 3 months for a year to see if the patient has a 4-fold or greater fall in titer (for example a 1:32 titer which falls to 1:2). If the expected fall in titer does not occur within 1 year, the patient should be re-treated. It is important to use the same nontreponemal test on all serial specimens from the same patient since the RPR is a more sensitive test than the VDRL; and titers obtained with these two techniques cannot be compared in follow-up assessment. Patients with persistently high titers after 1 year (1:4 or higher) should be given one further treatment course—after a CSF examination if that has not been done. Patients who have a 4-fold or greater rise in titer during follow-up should be considered to be reinfected and staged and treated accordingly. In patients with very low titers, as is usually the case in the late latent stage, there is no practical way of assessing the adequacy of therapy.

CONTACT TRACING

Contact tracing is mandatory in all patients who have had syphilis for less than 1 year. In most cases this is handled through proper reporting of the patient to local public health authorities and through venereal disease investigators. Because of rapport with the patient, the physician may choose to coordinate contact-tracing himself. In this era of freer discussion of human sexuality, this poses less of a problem; however, the physician may encounter a situation where the patient does not wish to be straightforward with partners about outside liaisons. Such contact-tracing often requires ingenuity on the part of the physician and close work with the patient to respect his wishes without harming the partner. In most jurisdictions, the physician is obligated by law either to find and treat the contacts of patients with infectious syphilis or to report the patient so that contact detection will be accomplished. Contacts of patients with infectious syphilis seen during the incubation period (10 to 90 days, average 20 days) should receive prompt treatment for primary syphilis without waiting for clinical manifestations or laboratory results. Contacts seen after the incubation period should be thoroughly evaluated for infectious syphilis; if syphilis is present, they should be treated and their contacts should be located.

EDUCATION

This should focus on prevention, with a brief description of other sexually transmitted diseases for which the patient is at risk. If patients have sexual relations with multiple partners and plan to continue this pattern, they should be cautioned to have periodic cultures for gonococcus and also periodic serologic tests for syphilis. The use of the condom as a protection against venereal disease transmission should be recommended strongly.

References

General

Clark, EG and Danbolt, N: The Oslo study of the natural course of untreated syphilis. *Med Clin North Am 48*: 613, 1964.
  Long term study of the natural history of syphilis in 1404 subjects.

Jaffee, HW: The laboratory diagnosis of syphilis—new concepts. *Ann Intern Med* 83: 846, 1975.
    Critical review of syphilis serology.
Rosebury, T. *Microbes and Morals.* Vebany Press, New York, 1971.
    Fascinating account of the history of sexually transmitted disease.
Symposium on venereal disease and gay men: *Sex Transm Dis* 4: 41, 1977.
    Useful summary of the problem of syphilis in homosexuals.
Fiumara, NJ, Shinberg, JD, Byrne, EM and Fountaine, J: An outbreak of gonorrhea and early syphilis in Massachusetts. *N Engl J Med* 256: 982, 1957.
    Detailed account of the spread of syphilis and of contact-tracing in a local outbreak.

Specific

1. Dans PE: FTA-ABS tests. A diagnostic help or hindrance? *South Med J 70*: 312, 1977.
2. Dunlop, EMC: Penicillin and the control of syphilis. *Am Heart J 88*: 395, 1974.
3. Greene, BM, Miller, NR and Bynum, TE: Failure of penicillin

G benzathine in the treatment of neurosyphilis. *Arch Intern Med 140*: 1117, 1980.
4. Hooshmand, H, Escobar, MR and Kopf, SW: Neurosyphilis, a study of 241 patients. *JAMA 219*: 726, 1972.
5. Idsoe, G, Guthe, T and Willcox, RR: Penicillin in the treatment of syphilis. The experience of three decades. *Bull WHO* Supplement to Vol. 474, 1972.
6. Fiumara, NJ: Serologic responses to treatment of 128 patients with late latent syphilis. *Am Vener Dis Assoc 6*: 243, 1979.
7. Jaffe, HW, Larsen, SA, Peters, M, Jove, DF, Lopez, B and Schroeter, AL: Tests for treponemal antibody in CSF. *Arch Intern Med 138*: 252, 1978.
8. Jarisch Herxheimer Reaction: Editorial. *Br Med J 1*: 384, 1967.
9. Putkonen, T, Salo, OP and Mustarallio, KK: Febrile Herxheimer reaction in different phases of primary and secondary syphilis. *Br J Vener Dis 42*: 181, 1966.
10. Schroeter, AL, Lucas, JB, Price, EV and Volume, VH: Treatment for early syphilis and reactivity of serologic tests. *JAMA 221*: 471, 1972.
11. The Jarisch-Herxheimer Reaction: *Lancet 1*: 340, 1977.
12. Wilner, G and Brody, JA: Prognosis of general paresis after treatment. *Lancet 2*: 1370, 1968.

CHAPTER THIRTY

Immunization to Prevent Infectious Disease

R. BRADLEY SACK, M.D., and L. RANDOL BARKER, M.D.

Protection against infectious diseases can be conferred by *active immunization* with vaccines, and by *passive immunization* with immune globulin preparations. As newly purified antigens become available, and as the mechanisms of the immune response become better understood, there will continue to be new vaccines available for protection against important infectious diseases. Immunization is most often used in adults in the United States to protect against the following diseases: hepatitis, influenza, mumps, pneumococcal disease, rabies, rubella, and tetanus. This chapter describes available vaccines and immune globulin preparations utilized to prevent these diseases, focusing upon the two critical questions commonly considered in practice: (a) Who should receive immunization? and (b) When should they receive it?

PATIENT ASSESSMENT

History

There are a number of questions that should be asked whenever immunization is contemplated.

The *history of previous immunizations* should be determined. In young adults, this may be readily known; in older persons, this information is often obscure. Patients may or may not keep personal records which can be of use. For example, persons who have served in the military will have received a large number of immunizations. They and persons who frequently travel abroad may have this information recorded on their International Vaccination Card Immunization history is particularly important in determining (a) whether to give tetanus toxoid or antitoxin following an injury, (b) whether diphtheria should be seriously considered in the diagnosis of acute pharyngitis (see Chapter 27), and (c) what immunizations to give to patients traveling outside the United States.

A *history of prior allergic reactions* or other untoward reactions to vaccines or their components should always be excluded before giving an immunization. Most vaccines are now highly purified, and allergic reactions following their use are rare. However, persons allergic to eggs, for instance, should not receive vaccines made in eggs. Some persons experience unusually severe reactions to bacterial vaccines such as typhoid and cholera vaccines. A history of a previous severe response to a vaccine is a contraindication to its use. Some antiviral vaccines contain trace amounts of antibiotics (used often in tissue culture preparations) to which the patient may be hypersensitive; this information should be determined from the package insert before administration of vaccine to susceptible patients.

The following conditions are those for which use of a live virus is contraindicated: patients with either a known *immunodeficiency disease* or recent treatment with an immunosuppressive drug, and *pregnant* women, in whom the live virus vaccine might pose a possible risk to the developing fetus.

A *recent injection of* γ-*globulin* (within 3 months) requires that use of live virus vaccines be postponed, since there may be interference with the antibody response. For the same reason, γ-globulin should not be administered earlier than 2 weeks following live virus vaccine.

Finally, a patient with an *acute febrile illness* should generally not be immunized until after the illness has resolved, because any side effects might add to the patient's morbidity, and because the effectiveness of the vaccination may be diminished.

Physical Examination

When immunization is contemplated, the physical examination usually adds little to the assessment of the patient. Pregnancy or an active infection (see above) may be confirmed on examination. In one instance, smallpox vaccination, the finding of significant eczema is a contraindication to vaccination because of the risk of dissemination. However, since smallpox has been eradicated, this precaution is only relevant to laboratory workers who are studying the smallpox virus and who should therefore be vaccinated.

Immunologic Testing

Immunologic tests are useful in deciding about immunization in two situations: (a) in considering the use of hyperimmune globulin preparations for protection against hepatitis B; if the exposed person already has antibody to hepatitis B surface antigen, additional protection is unnecessary (see Chapter 39);

and (b) when considering the use of rubella vaccine for a woman of childbearing age; if she already has antibodies to rubella, further immunization is unnecessary.

IMMUNIZATION PROCEDURES

The physician should always be familiar with the information contained in the *package insert* when giving a vaccine. This information includes dose, route of administration, common and uncommon side effects, contraindications, whether there is contamination with antibiotics, interval between immunizations, and additional detail.

Many of the widely used vaccines can be *given simultaneously.* The Center for Disease Control lists the following guidelines for simultaneous vaccine administration: (a) Inactivated vaccines can be administered simultaneously at separate sites (at the same site in the case of widely used combination vaccines such as tetanus and diphtheria toxoids). However, when vaccines commonly associated with side effects are given together (e.g., cholera, typhoid, plague) the side effects may be accentuated; and consideration should be given to vaccinating on separate occasions. (b) an inactivated vaccine and a live, attenuated virus vaccine can be administered simultaneously at separate sites.

Patients should be told at the time of immunization that they may experience some local soreness and possibly fever and malaise during the following 24 to 48 hours. They can be instructed to take aspirin or acetaminophen (Tylenol) if these symptoms are bothersome. Because of the rare possibility of anaphylactic reactions, persons receiving any immunization should wait in the office where they can be observed for about 15 minutes. Finally, patients should be clearly informed of the name of the immunizations they have received and be encouraged to keep a written record of them.

SPECIFIC VACCINES AND IMMUNE GLOBULIN PREPARATIONS

Table 30.1 summarizes information on all of the major available vaccines and immune globulin preparations. The following sections provide practical information on problems which are most likely to be encountered in ambulatory practice.

Hepatitis (5, 12)

At present, only passive immunization with preparations of gamma globulin is used widely in the prevention of hepatitis. A vaccine which stimulates active immunity to hepatitis B is now available. Because of its high cost, it is recommended chiefly for persons at increased risk, especially those who handle blood and blood products, dialysis unit patients and staff, and male homosexuals. Persons who have HBs antibody do not require vaccination.

Table 30.1
Identity, Characteristics, and Administration of Available Vaccines and Immune Globulin Preparations

Vaccine or Immune Globulin (References)	Type Preparation	Population to Be Immunized	Age at Which Immunization Usually Done	Immunization Schedule	Possible Adverse Reactions	Contraindications
FOR USE IN UNITED STATES POPULATIONS						
Diphtheria vaccine (7, 11)	Killed bacteria and toxoid	All	Child or adult	Series of three primary injections with boosters every 10 yr if known risk exists[a]	Local pain and swelling	None
Tetanus toxoid (11)	Toxoid	All	Child or adult	Series of three injections with boosters every 10 yr as necessary following injury[a]	Local pain and swelling	None
Tetanus immune globulin	Human antiserum	Unimmunized person with dirty wound	—	Single injection for prophylaxis	Not significant	None
Pertussis vaccine	Killed bacteria	All children	Child only	Series of three injections with boosters to age 6	Fever, occasionally severe neurologic reactions	Adulthood (>6 yr)
Polio vaccine (6) Oral	Live attenuated virus	All	Child	Primary series of three oral preparations	Not significant, rare clinical disease	Immunodeficiency disease and pregnancy
Parenteral	Killed virus	All	Child	Primary series of four injections	Not significant	None
Measles vaccine (9)	Live attenuated virus	All children	Child (>12 months of age)	Single injection	Fever	Immunodeficiency disease and pregnancy
Rubella vaccine	Live attenuated virus	All children and female adolescents	Child and adolescent females	Single injection	Arthralgias, fever in young women	Immunodeficiency disease and pregnancy (immunization not indicated if antibody titre is ≥1:8)
Mumps vaccine	Live attenuated virus	All children and young adults without history of mumps	Child	Single injection	Not significant	Immunodeficiency disease
Influenza vaccine (4, 8, 13, 15)	Killed virus (whole virus and "split virus preparations") preparations of virus change yearly	Persons at risk, chronic illness	Child or adult	Adults: Single injection (whole virus) repeated yearly. Children under 13: split virus preparation, two doses	Mild fever, allergic reactions Guillain-Barré syndrome rarely	Allergy to eggs
Hepatitis B vaccine[b]	Inactivated viral constituents from infected humans	Health workers and others at increased risk	Usually adults	Three injections (0 time, 1 month, 6 months)	Not significant	Known HBsAb positivity (not needed)
Hepatitis globulin (5, 12) Pooled (ISG)	Pooled human γ-globulin	Persons exposed to hepatitis A (and B)	Usually adults	Hepatitis A: 0.02 ml/kg, once Hepatitis B: 0.06 ml/kg, twice	Not significant	None
High titred (HBIG)	Hepatitis B immune globulin	Persons exposed to hepatitis B only	Usually adults	0.06 ml/kg at time of exposure and again 1 month later (see details, Table 30.2)	Not significant	None (not necessary if contact has antibodies to hepatitis B surface antigen)
Meningococcal vaccine (14)	Purified polysaccharide (serogroups A and C)	Only during epidemic disease. Persons at high risks (military)	All ages; young adult military	Single injection	Erythema at injection site; not significant	None
Rabies vaccine (1, 3)	Killed virus (human diploid vaccine)	Persons bitten by possible rabid animal	All ages—postexposure	Multiple injection of vaccine (four) plus rabies immune globulin	Pain, rare neurologic reactions	None
Pneumococcal vaccine (2)	Polyvalent purified polysaccharides	Persons with asplenia or splenic dysfunction. Persons with chronic illness	Any age (over 2 yr)	Single injection, not repeated	Erythema at injection site	Pregnancy
Bacillus Calmette and Guerin (BCG) vaccine (10)	Live attenuated bacteria	Used to immunize newborns in developing countries and persons with excessively high risk of developing tuberculosis		Single injection, intradermal	Prolonged granuloma or ulcer at injection site, lymphadenitis	Immunodeficiency disease and pregnancy

Table 30.1—continued

Vaccine or Immune Globulin (References)	Type Preparation	Population to Be Immunized	Age at Which Immunization Usually Done	Immunization Schedule	Possible Adverse Reactions	Contraindications
FOR TRAVELERS TO DEVELOPING COUNTRIES[a]						
Smallpox vaccine	Live attenuated virus	Only lab workers handling small-pox virus. Disease is eradicated	Child (in past)	Single vaccination repeated at 3-yr intervals	Dissemination in persons with eczema (1 death/10^6 vaccinations)	Eczema, immunodeficiency disease and pregnancy
Yellow fever vaccine	Live attenuated virus	Travelers to endemic areas	Any age	Single injection, repeated at 10-yr intervals	Fever, lymphadenitis	Immunodeficiency disease and pregnancy
Cholera vaccine	Killed bacteria	Travelers, only if countries to be visited require it	Any age	Two injections, 1 week apart; repeat booster after 6 months	Fever, pain at injection site	None
Typhoid vaccine	Killed bacteria	Travelers to developing world	Any age	Series of two injections, 1 month apart; booster every 3 yr	Fever, pain at injection site	None
Hepatitis A globulin pooled (ISG)	Human serum, pooled	Travelers, long term, to developing world	Any age	Single injection (0.06 ml/kg) with repeat every 5 months for persons living abroad	Not significant	None
Typhus vaccine	Killed Rickettsia	Travelers to endemic areas only	Any age	Two injections given 1 month apart	Fever, pain at injection site	Allergy to eggs
Plague vaccine	Killed bacteria	Travelers to endemic areas only—certain parts of Southeast Asia	Any age	Three injections	Fever, pain at injection site	None

[a] Boosters of diphtheria and tetanus are particularly important for those traveling to underdeveloped countries.
[b] Licensed 1981. Duration of immunity not known.

Pooled human γ-globulin (immune serum globulin, ISG) is 80 to 90% effective in preventing *hepatitis A* in exposed persons. It should be given to the following: (a) Close contacts of persons with known hepatitis A (family members or intimate friends, but not schoolmates or fellow workers unless some unusually high possibility of fecal-oral transmission is suspected). ISG should be given as soon as possible after the known exposure, certainly within 1 week. The usual adult dose is 0.02 ml/kg (intramuscularly). (b) Persons traveling to the developing world for more than a few weeks and planning to live in the community rather than in tourist facilities (this includes diplomatic personnel, missionaries, business persons, and Peace Corps Volunteers). The usual dose is 0.02 ml/kg for persons who will be at risk for 2 to 3 months and 0.06 ml/kg every 5 months for persons living in high-risk areas for longer periods.

Pooled γ-globulin (ISG) in relatively large doses (0.06 ml/kg intramuscularly in two doses 4 weeks apart) may also be useful in preventing *hepatitis B*. However, a costly, globulin preparation of high titer (hepatitis B immune globulin, HBIG) is available and is approximately 75% effective in preventing hepatitis in those persons known to have direct exposure to hepatitis B virus. Exposure usually occurs through accidental needle pricks, handling of infected blood, or through sexual exposure to a person known to be infected. As mentioned above, exposed persons who are known to have antibody to the surface antigen do not need postexposure prophylaxis.

Table 30.2 summarizes the recommendations of the Center for Disease Control for the postexposure prophylaxis of persons exposed to blood from patients who may have hepatitis B. Although the question has not been adequately studied, it is likely that the measures outlined in Table 30.2 are also effective following sexual exposure to persons with hepatitis B.

There is no immune globulin preparation known to be protective against non-A, non-B hepatitis, which is most frequently seen following multiple blood transfusions.

Hepatitis in ambulatory patients is discussed in Chapter 39.

Tetanus (11)

Each year, over 100 cases of tetanus are reported in the United States. There is no known subclinical "natural" immunity to tetanus, so that every person is susceptible unless he has been actively immunized. Tetanus usually follows penetrating wounds due to accidents and animal bites (see Chapter 24). In persons who have been actively immunized at any time in their life, injection of toxoid once every 10 years is necessary to boost their antitoxin titers to protective levels. If a person at risk of developing tetanus from a wound has received a toxoid booster in the last 10 years, no additional toxoid is required; if such a

Table 30.2
Summary of Postexposure Prophylaxis of Acute Exposures to Blood which May Contain Hepatitis B Virus[a]

Exposure	HBsAg[b] Testing of Source	Recommended Prophylaxis
HBsAg positive	—	HBIG[c] (0.06 ml/kg) immediately and 1 month later
HBsAg status unknown, source known:		
High risk[d]	Yes	ISG[e] (0.06 ml/kg) immediately, and a) if source is HBsAg positive HBIG (0.06 ml/kg) immediately and 1 month later or b) if source is HBsAg negative, nothing
Low risk[f]	No	Nothing or ISG (0.06 ml/kg)
HBsAg status unknown, source unknown	No	Nothing or ISG (0.06 ml/kg)

[a] Source: *Morbidity and Mortality Weekly Report*, Vol. 30, No. 34, p. 433, 1981
[b] Hepatitis B surface antigen.
[c] Hepatitis B immune globulin.
[d] Exposure to patient with acute, unconfirmed viral hepatitis; patients institutionalized with Down's syndrome; patients on hemodialysis; persons of Asian origin; male homosexuals; users of illicit, intravenous drugs.
[e] Immune serum globulin.
[f] Exposure to the average patient.

person has never received toxoid immunization or is unsure about it, passive immunization with tetanus antitoxin (250 units) should be given. This preparation is made from human sera, and therefore hypersensitivity reactions are not a problem, in contrast to the previous situation when horse serum preparations were used. Persons who require tetanus antitoxin should at the same time (but at a different site) be given their first dose of toxoid, followed by repeat doses of toxoid 1 month and 8 to 12 months later. If these persons have never been immunized against diphtheria, they should be given tetanus and diphtheria toxoids, adult type (Td), as discussed in the next section.

Diphtheria (7,11)

Each year, 200 to 300 cases of diphtheria are reported in the United States. Although subclinical infection may occur and confer immunity in unimmunized persons, it is recommended that all persons who have never been given diphtheria toxoid should receive it. This is particularly important for unimmunized persons at increased risk of exposure to diphtheria (*i.e.*, physicians, nurses, other hospital personnel, teachers, and staff and patients of institutions for the mentally handicapped). For unimmunized school age children and adults, tetanus and diphtheria toxoids, adult type (Td) are used. This preparation contains only about 25% of the diphtheria toxoid contained in the DPT (diphtheria-pertussis-tetanus) combined vaccine utilized in infants; this minimizes the risk of severe reactions in adults, previously a significant problem. Primary immunization consists of an initial dose, a 1-month dose, and a third dose at the 6th to 12th month; a booster is recommended every 10 years to assure protection. In adults, there is a high incidence (25 to 50%) of local soreness, swelling, and itching following Td injections; fever occurs in less than 10% and urticaria in approximately 2% of individuals. Serious reactions (massive swelling of the whole arm, abscess, or anaphylaxis) occur rarely (11).

For asymptomatic unimmunized contacts of patients with diphtheria, management includes: (a) prophylactic antibiotics (600,000 units of benzathine penicillin intramuscularly or a 7-day course of erythromycin 250 mg, 4 times daily); (b) primary vaccination as outlined above; and (c) daily surveillance for 7 days for clinical evidence of diphtheria (see Chapter 27).

Influenza (4,8,13,15)

Killed virus vaccines have been available for the prevention of influenza for many years. Earlier preparations contained nonspecific protein which frequently led to fever and malaise after the vaccine had been administered. Preparations now available are highly purified, and reaction rates are very low. Each year's vaccine is polyvalent, containing antigenic material from the type A and type B strains which are expected to prevail in a given year.

Influenza vaccine is recommended annually for those persons in whom influenza causes the highest morbidity and mortality: all individuals over 60 years and individuals of all ages with significant heart, lung, or chronic debilitating disease. The vaccine is also recommended for those involved in critical jobs where their absence may be highly detrimental (e.g., firemen, policemen, selected hospital personnel).

Influenza vaccine is about 70% protective, as determined in a number of experimental trials involving healthy adults and in retrospective studies involving young and elderly individuals (3, 10). The antigens in the vaccine must, of course, be appropriate for the prevailing influenza virus strain. The vaccine should be given in the fall, before the influenza season, which usually occurs between December and April.

During confirmed local outbreaks of influenza A, the antiviral drug *amantadine* (Symmetrel) can be utilized prophylactically as well as therapeutically (see Chapter 27 for a discussion of therapeutic use). Amantadine prevents clinical disease due to influenza A viruses in approximately 70% of subjects. The prophylactic use of this drug has been recommended (11) for the following groups of subjects:

1. Unvaccinated children and adults at high risk of serious morbidity and mortality because of underlying diseases, which include pulmonary, cardiovascular, metabolic, neuromuscular, or immunodeficiency diseases. Note that dosage regimens have not been well defined in patients with renal insufficiency; hence, its use in this group of patients should be cautious.

2. Adults whose activities are vital to community function and who have not been vaccinated with an appropriate contemporary influenza vaccine: for example, policemen, firemen, selected hospital personnel. Such persons are in frequent contact with others who may have influenza and should be considered at higher risk of contracting influenza than the general population.

3. Persons in semiclosed institutional environments, especially older persons, who have not received the current influenza vaccine.

The drug should be taken once daily (200 mg) during the local outbreak (usually a period of 2 to 3 months). Subjects should be warned of the following transient central nervous system side effects, which may occur during the first few days in 5 to 10% of subjects: insomnia, light-headedness, nervousness, drowsiness, difficulty in concentrating.

Clinical influenza in ambulatory patients is discussed in Chapter 27.

Pneumococcal Disease (2)

A purified polyvalent polysaccharide vaccine is available for the prevention of pneumococcal disease in persons at high risk, including persons who have had a splenectomy, those with sickle cell anemia, and adults with chronic lung disease. The vaccine is about 80% protective against the pneumococcal serotypes which it contains (14 serotypes which are responsible for approximately 80% of pneumococcal disease in the United States). The vaccine produces very few untoward effects and can be given as a single injection. Because of a high incidence of adverse reactions to reinjection of pneumococcal vaccine, second or "booster" doses should not be given.

Clinical pneumococcal pneumonia in ambulatory practice is discussed in Chapter 27.

Rubella

In the decade 1970 to 1980, the number of cases of rubella reported annually in the United States fell from approximately 55,000 to approximately 4,000. The number of reported cases of congenital rubella syndrome remained unchanged during this decade, however (27 to 50 cases per year).

Since about 1970, immunization against rubella has been administered routinely to children between ages 1 and 2. The major rationale for this vaccine is to prevent the spread of rubella to pregnant women and thereby to reduce the incidence of the congenital rubella syndrome.

Adolescent females and women in the child-bearing age group should be offered immunization also. However, they should first have their rubella antibody titer checked to determine whether they are already immune, owing to prior infection or immunization. A titer of 1:8 or greater indicates immunity. Since it is not clear that receiving rubella vaccine as a child will offer protection 10 to 30 years later, an antibody test is recommended even for women immunized in the distant past. The reason for determining immunity status before vaccination is that the rubella vaccine may occasionally cause significant fever and arthralgias in adults; thus the vaccine should not be given if it is not necessary. Before the vaccine is given, a woman should be cautioned against becoming pregnant (see Chapter 90, "Birth Control") for the 3 months immediately following the immunization since there is the possibility of fetal damage by the live virus.

Mumps

In the decade 1970 to 1980, the number of cases of mumps reported annually in the United States fell from approximately 100,000 to approximately 15,000. This decline is probably in part due to the use of mumps vaccine during this interval.

Live attenuated-virus mumps vaccine is now recommended routinely for children and for those young adults with no history of mumps; most people over the age of 25, however, can be considered immune. Since in susceptible adults the mumps virus can cause severe symptoms (orchitis, meningitis, or pancreatitis), there is good reason to provide this protection. Unimmunized persons may have had an immunizing subclinical infection, since only one out of every three cases of mumps in childhood is symptomatic. Unlike rubella, there is not a reliable test for prior immunity to mumps. However, there are no serious side effects from the vaccine, making prior determinations of immunity less important.

Rabies (1, 3)

In the past 10 years, one to four cases of human rabies has been reported each year in the United States. Theoretically all of these cases are preventable if protective treatment is given promptly.

In June 1980, killed virus rabies vaccine produced in human diploid cells was licensed for use in the United States. This vaccine has two major advantages over the previously used duck embryo vaccine: (a) higher levels of antibody are stimulated with fewer doses; and (b) fewer adverse reactions occur. For individuals who are at risk of developing rabies (see Chapter 24), the recommended treatment schedule is as follows: on day 1, simultaneous administration of antirabies globulin (as human rabies immune globulin, HRIG, if available; otherwise as heterologous antiglobulin) and the first dose of rabies vaccine; vaccine is repeated on days 3, 7, 14 and 30. The effectiveness of this vaccine in stimulating antibody and in protecting patients from rabies has been well established (3). Adverse reactions (urticaria, anaphylaxis, transient headache, and fever) occur in less than 0.5% of persons receiving this vaccine (1). The vaccine and antiglobulin are available from local health departments.

Measles (9)

Measles is a moderately severe illness in most persons and has a case fatality rate of 1:1,000. Since 1963, measles vaccines have been available (initially, killed virus vaccines, and since 1968, attenuated live virus vaccines). In the interval 1960 to 1980, during which measles vaccination of children was introduced generally in the United States, the number of cases reported annually fell from over 400,000 to less than 15,000.

In 1978, the Secretary of Health Education and Welfare announced the eradication of measles as the goal of the national measles immunization effort. The principal strategy for accomplishing this goal is immunization of all children at approximately 15 months of age. Since the introduction of immunization of this age group, the largest proportion of measles cases has occurred in adolescents and young adults, the subgroups most likely to have missed both live virus immunization and exposure to natural measles. Because neither serologic testing nor history of childhood measles is a reliable method to assess immunity to measles, it is difficult to provide a general recommendation for measles protection of this age group. Diminishing the risk of exposure to nonimmune adults by thorough immunization of children is the most practical approach.

Tuberculosis (10)

Efforts to control tuberculosis in the United States are based upon early identification of active disease and upon isoniazid prophylaxis of the contacts of tuberculous patients and other groups at increased risk (see Chapter 28). Because the incidence of new tuberculosis is low in this country (approximately 28,000 cases per year) and because most new cases are due to reactivation of disease in older individuals who acquired their infection in an era when the risk of infection was much higher, the indications for immunization with BCG (bacillus of Calmette and Guérin) vaccine are very limited. The specific recommendations of the U.S. Public Health Service (10) are as follows:

1. BCG vaccination should be seriously considered for persons who are tuberculin skin test-negative and who have repeated exposure to persistently untreated or ineffectively treated, sputum-positive pulmonary tuberculosis.

2. BCG vaccination should be considered for well defined communities or groups if an excessive rate of new infections can be demonstrated and the usual surveillance and treatment programs have failed or have been shown not to be applicable. Such groups might exist among the socially disaffiliated and those without a regular source of health care, possibly including some alcoholics, drug addicts, and migrants. Groups such as health workers who may be at particular risk of exposure to unrecognized pulmonary tuberculosis should, where possible, be kept under surveillance for evidence of newly acquired tuberculous infection. It must be recognized that only the occurrence of new infections reflects whether transmission is actually occurring.

The recommended route of administration for the BCG strain utilized in this country is intradermal or subcutaneous. If after 2 or 3 months the patient's tuberculin skin test remains negative, vaccination should be repeated. Contraindications to BCG vaccine are compromised immunity due to malignancy or immunosuppressive therapy and pregnancy. After BCG immunization, it is not possible to distinguish between a positive tuberculin skin test resulting from infection with virulent *M. tuberculosis* and one resulting from the BCG vaccine. Because the protective efficacy of BCG vaccine is not absolute, tuberculosis should be included in the differential diagnosis of any tuberculosis-like illness occurring in vaccinated individuals.

References

General

Benenson, AS (ed.): *Control of Communicable Diseases in Man*, Ed. 12 American Public Health Association, Washington, D.C., 1975.
   A concise summary of epidemiology, management, and prevention of communicable diseases, updated periodically.
Health Information for International Travel: U.S. Department of Health and Human Services, Center for Disease Control (CDC), Atlanta, Georgia.
   This booklet, which is updated yearly, contains recommendations for vaccination and prophylaxis against communicable diseases throughout the world. Available free.
The Immunization Practices Advisory Committee: Recommendations appear periodically in the *Morbidity and Mortality Weekly Report*, published by The Center for Disease Control.
   These recommendations are also published periodically in the Annals of Internal Medicine and The Medical Letter.
Morbidity and Mortality Weekly Report, Annual Summary 1979: U.S. Department of Health and Human Services, Vol. 28, No. 54, September 1980.
   This annual report summarizes the incidence of reportable diseases for the current year and for previous years and decades (beginning with 1940).

Specific

1. Adverse Reactions to Human Diploid Cell Rabies Vaccine: *Morbidity and Mortality Weekly Report* 29: 609, December 19, 1980.
2. Austrian, R, Douglas, RM, Schiffman, G, Coetzee, AM, Koornhof, HJ, Hayden-Smith, S and Reid, RDW: Prevention of pneumococcal pneumonia by vaccination. *Trans Assoc Am Phys* 89: 184, 1976.
3. Bahmanyar, M, Fayaz, A, Nour-Salehi, S, Mahammadi, M and Koprowski, H: Successful protection of humans exposed to

rabies infection: postexposure treatment with the new human diploid cell rabies vaccine and antirabies serum. *JAMA 236:* 2751, 1976.

4. Barker, WH and Mullooly, JP: Influenza vaccination of elderly persons: reduction in pneumonia and influenza hospitalizations and deaths. *JAMA 244:* 2547, 1980.

5. Grady, GF, Lee, VA, Prince, AM, Gitnick, GL, Fawaz, KA, Vyas, GN, Levitt, MD, Senior, JR, Galambos, JT, Bynum, TE, Singleton, JW, Clowdus, BF, Akdamar, K, Aach, RD, Winkelman, EI, Schiff, GM and Hersh, T: Hepatitis B immune globulin for accidental exposures among medical personnel: final report of a multicenter controlled trial. *J Infect Dis 138:* 625, 1979.

6. Horstmann, DM: Viral vaccines and their ways. *Rev Infect Dis 1:* 502, 1979.

7. Middaugh, JP: Side effects of diphtheria-tetanus toxoid in adults. *Am J Public Health 69:* 246, 1979.

8. Parkman, PD, Galasso, GH, Top, FH and Noble, GR: Summary of clinical trials of influenza vaccines. *J Infect Dis 134:* 100, 1976.

9. Rand, KH and Reuman, PD: Measles: ready for eradication? *Ann Intern Med 90:* 978, 1979.

10. Recommendation of the Public Health Service Advisory Committee on Immunization Practices: BCG vaccines. Center for Disease Control, Morbidity and Mortality (US DHEW), February 22, 1975.

11. Recommendation of the Immunization Practices Advisory Committee (ACIP): Diphtheria, tetanus, and pertussis: guidelines for vaccine prophylaxis and other preventive measures. *Morbidity and Mortality Weekly Report 26:* 401, 1977.

12. Seeff, LB and Hoofnagle, JH: Immunoprophylaxis of viral hepatitis. *Gastroenterology 77:* 161, 1979.

13. Symposium: Amantadine: Does it have a role in the prevention and treatment of influenza? A National Institutes of Health Consensus Development Conference. *Ann Intern Med 92:* 256, 1980.

14. Wahdan, MH, Rizk, F, El-Akkad, AM, Ghoroury, AA, Hablas, R, Girgis, NI, Amer, A, Boctar, W, Sippel, JE, Gotschlich, EC, Triau, R, Sanhorn, WR and Cvjetanovic, B: A controlled field trial of a serogroup A meningococcal polysaccharide vaccine. *Bull WHO 48:* 667, 1973.

15. Wright, PF, Dolin, R and LaMontagne, JR: Summary of clinical trials of influenza vaccine II. *J Infect Dis 134:* 633, 1976.

SECTION 4

Gastrointestinal Problems

CHAPTER THIRTY-ONE

Disorders of the Esophagus: Dysphagia and Gastroesophageal Reflux

HAROLD J. TUCKER, M.D.

DYSPHAGIA

Difficulty in swallowing, dysphagia, is an extremely reliable indicator of disturbance in oropharyngeal or esophageal function. It should never be dismissed as an "emotional" problem or a symptom of "globus hystericus" (see p. 262). The patient frequently says that food is sticking in his chest, often pinpointing the involved area. Occasionally, dysphagia may be accompanied by pain on swallowing, *odynophagia*, but the two symptoms are quite distinct and may occur independently.

Physiology of Swallowing

Normal swallowing requires the coordination of the skeletal muscles of the pharynx, the cricopharyngeus muscle (the upper esophageal sphincter) and the proximal one-third of the esophagus, with the smooth muscle of the distal body of the esophagus and the lower esophageal sphincter. Thus, the initiation of swallowing is voluntary, but involuntary processes subsequently propel the swallowed bolus through the esophagus into the stomach. The following sequence of events occurs during normal swallowing: relaxation of the upper esophageal sphincter to permit entry of the bolus into the esophagus; closure of the sphincter to prevent esophageal-pharyngeal regurgitation and aspiration; propulsion of the bolus distally by esophageal peristalsis; relaxation of the lower esophageal sphincter (LES), to allow easy entrance of the bolus into the stomach; and prompt closure of the LES to prevent reflux of gastric contents.

Dysphagia may occur from a disturbance of any of the anatomic structures or of the physiologic events involved in normal swallowing.

Clinical Evaluation

HISTORY

Because of the complexity of the swallowing mechanism, the causes of dysphagia are quite varied. Certain aspects of the history are very helpful in elucidating the underlying disorder. Difficulty in swallowing solids strongly suggests an anatomic obstruction—such as carcinoma, stricture, or esophageal ring, whereas difficulty in swallowing solids and liquids suggests a motility disturbance—such as achalasia, scleroderma, or diffuse esophageal spasm.

The history may also be useful in identifying the region of abnormal function as either *pre-esophageal* (oropharyngeal) or *esophageal* (Table 31.1). Symptoms suggestive of pre-esophageal dysphagia include regurgitation of liquid through the nose, aspiration with swallowing, and an inability to propel a bolus of food into the pharynx. The most common causes of this type of dysphagia are neuromuscular conditions, such as bulbar palsy due to brainstem infarcts or tumors, pseudobulbar palsy (usually from bilateral cerebral vascular accidents which have compromised cortical function), polymyositis, and myasthenia gravis. Patients with esophageal dysphagia complain of retrosternal fullness after swallowing and of the feeling that food is stuck at a certain point in the esophagus—often relieved by regurgitation. Esophageal dysphagia is most commonly caused by narrowing of the lumen by either inflammatory or neoplastic strictures. The history, then, indicates whether the dysphagia is due to an anatomic obstruction or to a neuromuscular disturbance, and focuses attention on the region of involvement.

Mild *weight loss* may be described by patients with any type of chronic dysphagia, due to voluntary decrease in intake of food which often accompanies their symptoms. More severe weight loss, plus anorexia, suggests carcinoma.

SPECIAL STUDIES

To delineate the cause of dysphagia, one or more of the following procedures should be employed: radiologic studies; esophagoscopy; and esophageal motility studies.

Consultation with a gastroenterologist is recommended for most patients with dysphagia, both for evaluation of the clinical problem and for the performance of esophagoscopy and motility studies.

Radiology. The initial study in most patients with dysphagia should be a *barium swallow*, a procedure which can identify motility disturbances as well as anatomic deformities, and is the easiest procedure for the patient to tolerate (it takes only 15 to 20 min and is associated with essentially no discomfort). As with all radiologic studies, the radiologist should be informed about the specific disorders that are most suspected. Without this communication, the radiologist may perform a routine barium swallow looking for only carcinoma, stricture, hiatal hernia, or reflux and may not pay specific attention to the motility pattern. Proper radiographic evaluation of esophageal motility requires that the patient be placed in the recumbent position and that the flow of the barium column be monitored. In this way, normal peristalsis can be seen to propel the bolus of barium distally, while in motor disorders the barium may not move distally until the patient is tilted upright. In addition, to observe the rapid activity of pharyngeal contractions and to detect abnormal esophageal contractions, the barium swallow should be recorded on cine film (a cine esophagogram). In this fashion, barium studies often can detect both organic and functional abnormalities leading to dysphagia. However, a negative study does not exclude either anatomic or motor disorders of the esophagus and a positive study seldom permits a specific diagnosis to be made; therefore, a barium swallow should always be followed by endoscopy.

Endoscopy. Esophagoscopy is an essential part of the evaluation of dysphagia. Because of the insensitivity of the barium swallow, endoscopy should be performed in all patients with persistent dysphagia, particularly in those with persistent difficulty in swallowing solid food. Esophagoscopy is complementary to the radiographic examination. The procedure is well tolerated, and can generally be performed on an ambulatory basis. When a lesion is detected by the radiographic test, endoscopy provides the most direct approach to establish the nature of the lesion, whether inflammatory or neoplastic. Biopsies and brushings for cytologic evaluation can be obtained under visual guidance. Further, the instrument may disrupt esophageal webs or rings that are causing the dysphagia, and thus may be both a diagnostic and a therapeutic tool. Inability to pass the endoscope through the esophagus into the stomach confirms an anatomic cause of the dysphagia, and rules out a motor disturbance (e.g., achalasia). The patient's experience with upper gastrointestinal endoscopy is described in Chapter 32.

Recording of Esophageal Motility. Esophageal manometry is the best procedure for the evaluation of esophageal motor function. This study measures the strength, function, and coordination of both the upper and lower esophageal sphincters and of the

Table 31.1
Types of Dysphagia

	Symptoms	Common Causes
Pre-esophageal (oro-pharyngeal)	Regurgitation of liquid through the nose, aspiration with swallowing, inability to propel a bolus into the pharynx	Neuromuscular conditions: brainstem lesions, polymyositis, myasthenia, pseudo-bulbar palsy
Esophageal	Retrosternal fullness after swallowing	Strictures: inflammatory or neoplastic
	Sticking of a bolus at a certain point	Motor disturbance (e.g., achalasia)

body of the esophagus in response to a swallow (Fig. 31.1A). The procedure is well tolerated, takes only about 20 min, and involves the passage of a narrow triple lumen catheter either through the nose or the mouth into the stomach. Recordings are made of the amplitude and coordination of contractions within the pharynx and esophagus as the catheter is withdrawn. Various motility disturbances can be diagnosed by use of this technique (Table 31.2). Esophageal manometry should be performed in all patients for whom a structural cause for the dysphagia cannot be found.

Specific Causes of Dysphagia
CARCINOMA OF ESOPHAGUS

Cancer of the esophagus should always be suspected as the cause of dysphagia in a patient over the age of 40. The incidence of esophageal carcinoma in the United States is approximately 7500 cases per year. Men, especially black men, are more likely to develop esophageal cancer than are women. Predis-

posing factors include cigarette smoking, heavy alcohol use, lye strictures, achalasia, Plummer-Vinson syndrome (see below, p. 261), and Barrett's mucosa.

In the vast majority of cases, esophageal cancer is of the squamous cell type. These tumors are most common in the middle third of the esophagus. Adenocarcinoma is more likely to be seen when the normal squamous cells of the esophagogastric junction are destroyed by reflux (see below) and are replaced by columnar cells (Barrett's mucosa). Carcinoma of the cardia of the stomach may directly extend into the lower esophagus and obstruct the esophageal lumen.

Diagnosis. The diagnosis of esophageal cancer is generally made only after symptoms have developed, by which time the lesion is already advanced, with involvement of regional lymph nodes. In patients with predisposing conditions, such as achalasia or Barrett's mucosa, earlier detection of the cancer may be achieved by regular (exact frequency yet to be determined) esophagoscopy with cytologic brushings of the entire esophagus. Most patients present with

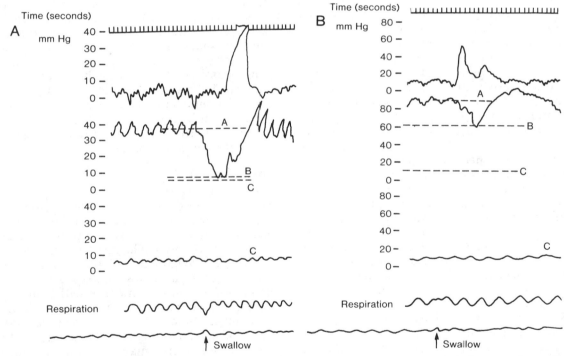

Figure 31.1   *A*, esophageal manometry tracing in a normal subject demonstrating the esophageal response during a single swallow. Pressure recordings are obtained at 5-cm intervals from the esophagus, lower esophagus, lower esophageal sphincter (LES), and stomach. Prior to the swallow, the LES maintains a high pressure (*A*) compared to intragastric pressure (*C*). With a swallow, there is prompt relaxation of the LES (*B*) toward gastric pressure (*C*). An esophageal contraction occurs in the esophageal body in response to a swallow (primary peristalsis). The LES returns to its basal level as the esophageal contraction reaches the LES. *B*, esophageal manometry tracing in a patient with achalasia. The basal LES pressure (*A*) is abnormally high (>80 in tracing). With a swallow, there is incomplete relaxation of the LES (*B*), leaving a residual high pressure compared to gastric pressure (*C*). In the esophageal body nonperistaltic, repetitive contractions may be found, but there is no normal peristalsis. (Adapted from S. Cohen and W. Lipshutz: Lower esophageal sphincter dysfunction in achalasia. *Gastroenterology, 61:* 814, 1971.)

Table 31.2
Esophageal Motility Study

	Normal Response to Swallow	Achalasia	Diffuse Spasm	Scleroderma	Dermatomyositis
Pharynx	Normal contraction at nadir of relaxation of upper esophageal sphincter	Normal	Normal	Normal	Low
Upper esophageal sphincter	High pressure zone with complete relaxation	Normal	Normal	Normal	Low pressure with partial relaxation
Midbody of esophagus	Peristaltic wave of contraction	Aperistalsis; occasional simultaneous contractions	Some peristalsis with frequent repetitive and simultaneous contractions	Proximal esophagus—normal; distal—loss of amplitude progressing to aperistalsis	Proximal esophagus—low amplitude waves; distal esophagus—normal
Lower esophageal sphincter	High pressure zone with complete relaxation	Hypertonic—incomplete relaxation	Usually normal but may be high with incomplete relaxation	Low pressure	Normal pressure and relaxation

dysphagia for several months and with progressive weight loss. Odynophagia (pain on swallowing) may accompany the dysphagia. Occult blood loss is common but hematemesis is unusual.

The diagnostic workup includes a barium swallow and upper endoscopy. After the barium swallow, endoscopy should be performed in all patients. Even if the X-ray is negative, the endoscope can still detect mucosal lesions. When the tumor is already defined by X-ray, endoscopy can supply a tissue diagnosis, which is important in deciding whether surgery or radiation is indicated. Multiple biopsies and directed brush cytologies obtained via the endoscope provide a positive tissue diagnosis in over 95% of cases. However, radiologic evaluation remains important as it provides useful information concerning the degree of esophageal obstruction, the length of the tumor, and the appearance of the fundus of the stomach. With the combined use of these two techniques, differentiation can be made between cancer of the esophagus and other esophageal lesions—such as peptic stricture of the esophagus, achalasia, severe esophagitis, and esophageal varices.

Therapy. Therapy for esophageal cancer is generally surgery or radiation. The choice between these two forms of therapy depends generally on the cell type and the location of the neoplasm. Adenocarcinoma is less radiosensitive, usually occurs in the distal one-third of the esophagus, and therefore, is better suited for a surgical approach. Squamous cell carcinoma is relatively radiosensitive, and numerous studies suggest that radiation of the lesions in the distal and middle thirds of the esophagus is as effective as is surgery (4) (see Chapter 8 for a discussion of radiotherapy in the treatment of cancer). Surgical resection is more extensive and less well tolerated, the more proximal the tumor. Combination radiotherapy and resection have been reported to improve

survival but greater experience with this approach is needed. With either approach, the prognosis is very poor: 75% are dead within 1 year of diagnosis; and 95%, by 5 years. Palliation, i.e., maintenance of an open esophagus so that the patient can swallow food and saliva, should be the minimal aim of therapy. At times, passing dilators through the tumor and inserting prosthetic tubes into the esophageal lumen, are helpful adjuncts to provide some degree of palliation.

Therapeutic decisions are best made together by the general physician, the gastroenterologist, the surgeon, and the radiation therapist.

ACHALASIA

Achalasia (spasm of the lower esophageal sphincter) is a motor disorder of the distal esophagus causing dysphagia for solids and liquids. The condition occurs in all age groups, with a peak incidence in the 4th and 5th decades. The incidence of this disorder is about 1 per 100,000 population per year. Men and women are equally susceptible to the disease. Patients present most commonly with progressive dysphagia for both solids and liquids and, frequently, with regurgitation of ingested material. Pulmonary symptoms such as nocturnal coughing and even aspiration pneumonia may be the initial mode of presentation. Occasionally, substernal chest pain is associated with the dysphagia.

Pathogenesis. The pathogenesis of achalasia is not known. There have been several studies that have described abnormalities in the myenteric ganglion cells in the distal esophagus (LES zone) and in the body of the esophagus, as well as abnormalities in the vagal nucleus and its peripheral fibers. However, these findings have not been consistent. Pharmacologic studies have further supported the concept of denervation of the esophagus. There is an exaggerated response of the LES and of the body of the esophagus to cholinergic stimulation (e.g., in the Mecholyl test) and to the hormone gastrin, consistent with the concept of denervation hypersensitivity. The cause for the neuropathic injury is unknown.

Diagnosis. The routine chest X-ray frequently suggests the diagnosis. The normal gastric air bubble is absent, and an air fluid level in the dilated esophagus is sometimes seen behind the heart. With a very dilated and tortuous esophagus, the mediastinum appears widened. The typical features on barium esophagogram (Fig. 31.2) include (a) smooth tapered narrowing of the distal end of the esophagus that fails to open properly, (b) retention of barium and secretions in the more proximal esophagus, and (c) absence of peristalsis. The distal narrowing is often described as a "bird beak" or "pen quill" deformity. It is important that the patient be examined while he is supine (see above), to evaluate peristalsis, and while he is upright, to demonstrate the height of the retained barium-filled column.

Esophageal manometry has demonstrated three distinct abnormalities in patients with achalasia: (a) hypertonicity of the LES, (b) failure of the LES to relax following a swallow, and (c) absence of peristalsis of the entire esophagus. This procedure should be done, if possible, in every patient with the disease so that the results of treatment can be measured against the baseline pressures. In achalasia, the basal LES pressure is elevated, at times to very high levels, and the degree of relaxation is incomplete, generally less than 50% (Fig. 31.1B). Thus, there is a constant high pressure zone that impedes the passage of the esophageal contents. Peristalsis is also absent, further impairing the propulsion of the bolus distally. At times the esophageal contractions, while not peristaltic or propagative, are of high amplitude and simultaneous, resulting in the chest pain. Injection of a cholinergic agent (Mecholyl test) has been shown to cause a marked increase in the LES pressure in patients with achalasia. However, since this test is not specific for achalasia, is uncomfortable for the patient, and provides little additional information, there is no need to perform it.

Differential Diagnosis. Achalasia must be differentiated from other disorders that lead to obstruction of the passage of food into the stomach. Esophageal strictures, both peptic and neoplastic, and carcinomas at the esophagogastric (EG) junction may result in symptoms and even in a radiographic and manometric picture similar to that of achalasia (6). Thus, it is important that all such patients be evaluated with endoscopy. Failure to pass the endoscope into the stomach indicates an anatomic obstruction (such as carcinoma or stricture) rather than a functional one (such as achalasia). Scleroderma (see below) with its associated esophageal motility disturbance may result in dysphagia with diminished peristalsis seen on X-ray. However, generally by the time patients with esophageal scleroderma develop stricture and dilation of the esophagus that may mimic achalasia,

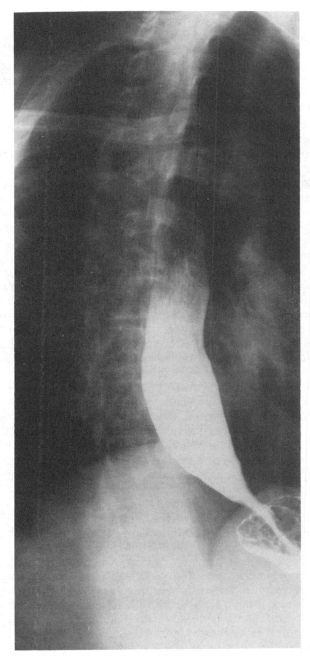

Figure 31.2   Barium swallow in a patient with achalasia. The esophagus is dilated, and the tapered distal segment never opens normally. Under fluoroscopy, no peristalsis is seen, but simultaneous contractions are noted.

they usually have other obvious stigmata of scleroderma (particularly tight skin of the face and hands or Raynaud's phenomenon). Further, on esophageal manometry the LES pressure in scleroderma is low rather than high as it is in achalasia (Table 31.2), and the disorder of motility is confined to the smooth muscle portion (distal two-thirds) of the esophagus, with a normally functioning proximal segment. In patients from South America, Chagas' disease may result in a megaesophagus, and present with mano-metric patterns identical to that of achalasia.

Therapy. There are two types of therapy for achalasia: pneumatic dilation and surgery. Both forms of therapy are aimed at reducing the pressure gradient between the esophagus and the stomach, thus decreasing the severity of the dysphagia. The aperistalsis and impaired sphincter relaxation persist after therapy. *Pneumatic dilation* is performed by a gastroenterologist in the hospital. The esophagus is aspirated completely prior to the dilation. After premedication with analgesics and sedatives, a bag dilator is passed into the stomach. The dilator is a weighted tube, the distal portion of which includes an inflatable balloon. Under fluoroscopic guidance, the balloon portion is positioned across the area of the LES. It is then inflated for 30 sec to 2 min, causing a forceful disruption of the LES muscle. The dilator is then removed and can be expected to be blood streaked. The patient usually experiences chest pain during the procedure. The major risk of the procedure is esophageal perforation which occurs in 1 to 5% of dilations. The day following the dilation, the LES pressure may be recorded manometrically to document that the dilation has indeed lowered the basal LES pressure significantly. Satisfactory results, *i.e.,* improvement in dysphagia, weight gain, and decrease in retention of barium, can be expected in about 75% of cases. In successful cases, there is immediate relief of symptoms. The patient is then observed overnight and is discharged the following day. Dilation can be repeated if symptoms of dysphagia recur or worsen, but most patients have only minimal symptoms for many years after therapy.

Surgical therapy involves a thoracotomy with transection of the circular muscle of the LES zone to the level of the mucosa, the Heller myotomy. This surgical approach provides similar satisfactory results, with a success rate of 75 to 80%. The procedure may cause significant reflux esophagitis in as many as 25% of patients. As a result of this troublesome complication, some have advocated combining a fundoplication with the myotomy. Because of the ease to the patients of pneumatic dilation compared to a thoracotomy, and because of the high incidence of reflux after surgery, pneumatic dilation is generally the initial procedure of choice. Surgery should be reserved for (a) failure of repeated dilations to provide symptomatic relief, (b) esophageal perforation secondary to pneumatic dilation, (c) inability to perform dilation because of the shape of the esophagus or the presence of an epiphrenic diverticulum, and (d) inability to exclude carcinoma.

Complications. A major complication of achalasia is esophageal cancer. The incidence of this complication ranges from 6 to 29% in various series (2). The development of cancer in patients with achalasia should not be confused with cancer of the esophagogastric junction presenting with an achalasia-like picture. The cancer that develops in patients with primary achalasia usually occurs many years after the diagnosis of achalasia has been established, is of the squamous cell type, and generally occurs in the midportion of the esophagus. There is no evidence that successful therapy of achalasia prevents the development of cancer. Thus, all such patients should be under surveillance with periodic endoscopy with esophageal cytology (exact frequency yet to be determined but probably of the order of every 1 to 3 years).

DIFFUSE ESOPHAGEAL SPASM

Clinical Presentation. Symptomatic diffuse esophageal spasm (SDES) is a disorder characterized by nonperistaltic esophageal contractions, often of high amplitude, that result in dysphagia and substernal chest pain. The disorder is seen equally in both sexes and at all ages (although it appears to be rare in children). The dysphagia is intermittent and is experienced for both solids and liquids. The pain also is intermittent, and may, at times, be provoked by certain foods, particularly hot and cold beverages. At other times, the pain occurs spontaneously and may even awaken the patient at night. The pain is highly variable in quality, sometimes described as knifelike; sometimes as dull and crushing; it may radiate to the neck, back, or arms. It may be brief, or it may last for hours. Because of its location, radiation, and "crushing" quality, it is frequently confused with the pain of ischemic heart disease. When no cardiac disease is found, many of these patients are believed to have a psychogenic disturbance. Thus, this condition is often underdiagnosed and is easily confused with other conditions.

Diagnosis. The procedures for the diagnosis of this condition include radiographic studies and esophageal manometry. The *barium swallow*, or preferably the cine-esophagogram, may demonstrate nonperistaltic spontaneous and simultaneous contractions (tertiary waves). These abnormal contractions are frequently encountered during routine barium swallow, especially in the elderly and by themselves do not make a diagnosis of esophageal spasm without the appropriate clinical history. Further, as SDES is an intermittent condition, the barium swallow may be normal or may be too insensitive to detect the motility disturbance. *Esophageal motility* studies are more sensitive (Table 31.2). Provocative agents (Mecholyl, pentagastrin) can be employed during the motility studies to identify more clearly those patients who develop chest pain associated with abnormal esophageal contractions. In patients who are considered to have angina but are found to have normal coronary arteries, esophageal motility studies can demonstrate an esophageal cause for the chest pain in a significant number of patients, as high as 50% in some studies (1). Patients with typical symptoms of SDES in whom abnormal contractions are demonstrated on a barium swallow do not need esophageal manometry.

Esophageal Spasm Induced by Reflux. In some patients, the esophageal spasm and its symptoms are induced by reflux of gastric acid into the esophagus (see below, p. 262); such patients may present with symptoms only of chest pain and/or dysphagia, without any history of heartburn. It is important to recognize acid-induced esophageal spasm, as the therapy for this condition will vary from that of the primary form of SDES. The acid-induced spasm can be suggested by the presence of a low LES pressure on esophageal manometry. During an esophageal motility study, the esophagus can be perfused over a 20-min period with 0.1% hydrochloric acid (Bernstein test). The patient's subjective sensation in response to the acid infusion is evaluated at the same time as his esophageal contractions are measured. A positive study is characterized by the occurrence of the patient's typical symptoms during the acid perfusion, in association with abnormal esophageal contractions (ideally in the absence of electrocardiographic changes), and by the relief of these symptoms when the acid is cleared from the esophagus by saline infusion. Therapy should be directed at the gastroesophageal reflux primarily (see below, p. 264). Therapy for the esophageal spasm (see below) may actually worsen the condition by further lowering LES tone, thus promoting more reflux.

Therapy. Therapy for SDES is aimed at reducing the amplitude and frequency of the abnormal contractions. The patient should first be reassured that there is an organic cause for this discomfort, but that it is not of cardiac origin. Identification and avoidance of precipitating factors, such as cold beverages or emotional reactions, should be recommended. Pharmacotherapy also can be very helpful. Nitroglycerin, a smooth muscle relaxant, has been shown manometrically to reduce spasm and clinically to relieve symptoms (5). A long acting nitrate should be used (e.g., isosorbide dinitrate 5 to 10 mg sublingually or orally), especially prophylactically, such as before meals. Anticholinergics (e.g., propantheline bromide, Probanthine, 15 mg orally before meals) also reduce the amplitude of the spastic type contraction and may be useful. If these efforts fail, forceful dilation may be recommended. Dilation is most successful in patients with elevated LES pressures and with dysphagia as the predominant symptom. Chest pain on the other hand appears to be less likely to respond to dilation. A long myotomy, cutting the esophageal muscle from the esophogogastric junction to the aortic arch, has been advocated for the rare patient refractory to all of the above measures. Although the reported results of this procedure are impressive, the potential complications are significant and very difficult to manage. Myotomy should be reserved for those few patients with well documented esophageal spasm that is severely disabling and truly intractable. The majority of patients have attacks episodically, learn to avoid precipitating causes, and can be managed successfully medically.

SCLERODERMA OF THE ESOPHAGUS

The esophagus is involved in as many as 80% of patients with scleroderma. At times the esophageal symptoms are the presenting complaint which lead to the diagnosis. Indeed, the esophagus may demonstrate the characteristic abnormalities even before skin changes occur. The main symptoms of esophageal scleroderma are heartburn and dysphagia. The cause for these symptoms can readily be appreciated by examining the esophageal motility (Table 31.2). In esophageal scleroderma the LES pressure is very low, resulting in free gastroesophageal reflux. In addition, the peristaltic waves initially are of reduced amplitude, progressing later to complete aperistalsis in the smooth muscle portion of the esophagus, sparing the skeletal muscle portion. As peristalsis is impaired, the refluxed acid remains abnormally long in the esophagus, perhaps accounting for the frequent development of an esophageal stricture in this disorder. Thus, the dysphagia may be due to the primary motor abnormality or may signify the development of a peptic stricture.

The pathogenesis of scleroderma is unknown. In the esophagus, the disorder is not simply secondary to replacement of muscle fibers with collagen, since the motility dysfunction can be demonstrated in the absence of histopathologic changes. Several studies have suggested a neural defect rather than a primary myogenic disorder.

Scleroderma is a chronically progressive disease for which no specific treatment exists. Therapy of esophageal manifestations is directed at symptomatic relief and prevention of strictures.

Patients with scleroderma, whether or not they have dysphagia or heartburn, should be referred to a gastroenterologist for evaluation of esophageal motility, and to diagnose reflux esophagitis and stricture formation. If reflux is present, the patient should be treated intensively with cimetidine and antacids (see p. 264) to try to prevent stricture formation (see below, p. 262). Strictures should be dilated by bougienage (see below, p. 264). Stimulation of the smooth muscle by bethanechol (Urecholine) or metoclopramide, to enhance LES tone and improve peristaltic contractions also may be tried (see below, p. 264). If muscle atrophy is already present, however, these agents may not be helpful. Antireflux surgery should be avoided if at all possible because the motility disorder may lead to significant dysphagia after fundoplication.

ESOPHAGEAL WEBS AND RINGS

Dysphagia for solid foods may be caused by esophageal webs or rings. An esophageal *web* is a mucosal structure that protrudes into the lumen, most commonly in the proximal esophagus. The association of an iron deficiency anemia with a proximal esophageal web constitutes the *Plummer-Vinson syndrome.* Esophageal *rings* are located in the distal esophagus and may be either mucosal or muscular; rings can be demonstrated in up to 10% of the population, but rarely cause symptoms.

The ring that occurs at the gastroesophageal junction is referred to as *Schatzki's ring*. The origin of these lesions is unclear, some being congenital and others probably acquired. They are often found in asymptomatic individuals. There is no evidence that gastroesophageal reflux is associated with the development of the Schatzki ring, even in the presence of a hiatal hernia.

Symptoms arise when the ring narrows the esophageal lumen to less than 13 mm. A typical presenting symptom of a patient with an esophageal ring is intermittent dysphagia for solid foods. The patient may point to the area of the ring. At times a bolus of food may become impacted; the patient then regurgitates and subsequently may be able to resume eating without further difficulty. The intermittency of the dysphagia, the chronicity of the condition, and the difficulty in making the diagnosis unless specifically suspected often results in misdiagnosis and inappropriate therapy.

The diagnosis of esophageal ring is best made by *barium swallow*. The lower esophageal ring is best detected when the lower segment of the esophagus is distended as it is during a Valsalva maneuver. Endoscopy is sometimes helpful to differentiate rings from annular strictures secondary to either reflux esophagitis or carcinoma. Cervical webs are frequently missed on conventional radiography, but may be detected with cine studies. The webs are usually detected on the anterior surface of the esophagus and lateral and oblique films are needed to demonstrate these lesions. *Endoscopy* frequently fails to visualize cervical webs, but may disrupt the lesion during blind passage of the instrument into the esophagus. The endoscope may well demonstrate an esophageal ring during air insufflation of the distal esophagus.

Therapy generally involves reassurance with recommendation to chew food well and slowly, as well as mechanical disruption of the ring or web. If the webs are associated with iron deficiency, the treatment of the anemia is believed to cause rapid regression of the web. Bougienage with a large caliber dilator frequently disrupts the lower esophageal ring with complete relief of the dysphagia. The procedure causes transient discomfort but much less pain than does pneumatic dilation. It is ordinarily done by a gastroenterologist in his office. Rarely symptoms may persist after bougienage, and pneumatic dilation (see above) or even surgery may be necessary.

GLOBUS HYSTERICUS

Globus hystericus is a diagnosis frequently made in patients with dysphagia who have no demonstrable organic disease. However, this condition does not produce dysphagia and should not be used to explain away the symptom of dysphagia. Patients with globus describe the sensation of a "lump" in the throat, but they do not actually have difficulty swallowing. At times, these symptoms may be more pronounced with eating. However, when specifically questioned, patients will deny dysphagia, or food "sticking" or being "held up" in this region; and they will state that the symptom is present even when they are not eating. The pathogenesis of this condition is unknown, but hypertonicity of the upper esophageal sphincter, as a primary disorder or as a consequence of esophageal reflux has been suggested. A psychophysiologic disturbance may also be the cause as this symptom is usually seen in anxious patients (see Chapter 12). Reassurance and an explanation of the problem form the basis for treatment. Mild sedation may be helpful. The significance of this disorder is mainly its differentiation from other conditions that produce true dysphagia.

GASTROESOPHAGEAL REFLUX

Symptomatic gastroesophageal reflux is a common clinical condition that may lead to significant morbidity. It is now well established that competency of the LES is the major deterrent against reflux. The presence of a hiatal hernia is not a factor in gastroesophageal reflux as it does not affect the strength of the LES. Therefore, whether or not a hiatal hernia is present, therapy, whether it be medical or surgical, should be directed toward restoration of LES competency.

Pathophysiology

Several abnormalities in LES function have been observed in patients with gastroesophageal reflux. First, the basal LES tone is lower than in normals. Second, the hypotensive LES fails to rise in pressure appropriately with increases in intragastric pressure. Third, in patients with reflux, the response of the LES to a meal is low compared to that of normal subjects (3). These pathophysiologic abnormalities help explain the occurrence of reflux under basal conditions, during periods of increased intra-abdominal pressure, and postprandially when acid secretion is stimulated.

Etiology

Gastroesophageal reflux may occur in several different conditions. *Idiopathic hypotension* of the LES is the most common cause of reflux. The sphincter tone is low and responds poorly to physiologic excitatory stimuli. The etiology is unknown, but defects in myogenic, neurogenic, and hormonal function of the LES have been suggested. Patients with *scleroderma* frequently complain of reflux, or present with stricture formation even in the absence of reflux symptoms. *Pregnancy* is a condition that is commonly associated with reflux, with 30 to 50% of pregnant women experiencing heartburn, usually during their third trimester. Estrogen and progesterone are known to reduce LES tone; and, with increase in intra-abdominal pressure during gestation, reflux frequently results. *Hypothyroidism* may also cause decreased LES tone and reduced peristaltic force, but rarely is a cause of symptomatic gastroesophageal reflux. *Iatrogenic causes* of reflux are common: anticholinergics, nitrites, tranquilizers, and β-adrenergic agents are all capable of reducing LES pressure. Also smoking cigarettes and eating *certain foods* (e.g., fatty foods and chocolate) reduce LES pressure and may induce symptomatic reflux, usually within an hour of ingestion. Other foods like coffee, alcohol, and citrus fruits may induce similar symptoms without affecting LES pressure.

Diagnosis

HISTORY

Heartburn is the classic symptom of gastroesophageal reflux. Most patients complain of burning substernal pain that radiates upward, often aggravated by meals and by lying down and relieved by sitting up. The exact cause of the pain is not known. A sour taste is another common complaint. *Dysphagia* suggests the presence of a motor abnormality or a stricture (see above). *Odynophagia*, or pain on swallowing, is an infrequent complaint with reflux esophagitis and usually signifies severe disease.

TESTS

A variety of tests are available to confirm the clinical diagnosis. As no single test provides complete information about the cause and consequences of reflux, judicious selection among these tests is required. A comparison of all tests indicates that the combination of esophageal biopsies or acid infusion tests with acid reflux measurements gives about a 90% positive diagnosis. This yield is higher than that of any single test for this disorder.

Performance and selection of these various tests will generally require consultation with a gastroenterologist. For the majority of patients with classic symptoms of gastroesophageal reflux, empiric therapy can be instituted before performing any of these diagnostic procedures. However, in cases with an uncertain diagnosis, or in patients who fail to respond to standard therapy (see below), one or more of these esophageal function tests may be indicated to document the presence and degree of reflux. Certainly before antireflux surgery is performed, unequivocal evidence should be obtained that gastroesophageal reflux is causing the patient's symptoms.

The *acid reflux test* involves the placement of a pH probe in the esophagus several centimeters proximal to the LES and documenting the drop of intraesophageal pH with the occurrence of reflux. The experience of the patient during the passage of this probe is the same as it is during the passing of a nasogastric tube. A pH of less than 4 is considered a positive test, documenting the reflux of acid into the esophagus.

Similarly *esophageal manometry* (see p. 256) can determine the strength of the LES (normally 12 to 30 mm mercury). In over 80% of patients with reflux, the LES pressure will be low. Abnormal motility can be documented at the same time and scleroderma can even be diagnosed as a cause for the gastroesophageal reflux via this technique. During the motility study, the *Bernstein (acid perfusion) test* can be performed. Reproduction of the patient's symptoms via infusion of acid and relief of the symptoms with infusion of distilled water is considered a positive test (see p. 261). This study confirms that the patient's symptoms can be produced by acid. The patient's experience during the performance of the test, which takes 30 min or less, is essentially the same as it is during the measurement of esophageal motility (see p. 257) except that heartburn may be produced by the infusion of acid.

Radiologic studies are useful in identifying the complications of reflux such as esophageal ulcers or stricture, but are too insensitive to be relied on to confirm the presence of reflux. As stated above, the presence of hiatal hernia on barium swallow does not diagnose gastroesophageal reflux and should not be incriminated as the cause for the patient's symptoms. Also, the demonstration of reflux by barium swallow does not establish that the patient's symptoms are due to reflux; therefore the barium swallow cannot be relied upon as a single test to make the diagnosis of reflux. *Endoscopy* may detect ulceration and esophageal strictures. Mucosal biopsies can provide histologic evidence of acute esophagitis and of the chronic effects of reflux, even when the endoscopic appearance of the esophagus is normal. Characteristic microscopic changes secondary to reflux include increased thickness of the basal cell zone and proximity of the dermal papillae to the epithelial surface. The presence of polymorphonuclear leukocytes in the squamous lining indicates acute inflammation.

Complications

The complications of reflux include hemorrhage, ulcerations, stricture formation, and development of Barrett's epithelium. Esophagitis is the cause of 5 to 10% of all cases of upper gastrointestinal hemorrhage. Peptic ulcers and strictures must be differentiated from malignancy and from caustic ingestion. The presence of a midesophageal ulcer or stricture should raise the suspicion of Barrett's epithelium (columnar type mucosa that replaces the squamous mucosa damaged by chronic reflux). This type of columnar mucosa contains several differing cell types, including parietal cells capable of secreting acid. Of further significance is that this mucosa is a metaplastic response to inflammation and thus may progress to the development of adenocarcinoma. Patients with this type of mucosa should therefore be under surveillance for the development of cancer. There are reports of regression of this abnormal mucosa following successful antireflux surgery.

Therapy

The therapy for gastroesophageal reflux is aimed at reducing the volume and acidity of the gastric contents and at restoring LES competence. The vast majority of patients can be managed successfully with relatively simple therapy. The *initial step* (Table 31.3) consists of dietary and mechanical maneuvers, antacids, and discontinuance of drugs, when possible, and foods that reduce LES tone. Certain foods, such as coffee, citrus juice, and spices which further irritate the inflamed esophagus and provoke pain, should also be restricted. Patients should be instructed not to lie down after a meal as this promotes greater reflux. Elevation of the head of the bed 6 to 8 inches (not just sleeping on more pillows) and avoidance of tight garments that increase intra-abdominal pressure are also helpful. Antacids, when given in effective doses (see Table 31.3), improve symptoms in 70% of cases. These compounds not only neutralize the acidic gastric contents but, by alkalinizing the stomach, may also increase LES pressure, thus decreasing the frequency of reflux. A combination of antacid plus alginic acid (Gaviscon) is reported to be especially helpful because of the ability of the alginic acid to form a foamy gel-like layer on top of the gastric fluid.

The *second stage* of therapy, if necessary, involves the use of drugs that inhibit gastric acid secretion or increase LES pressure. These medications should be instituted if initial measures fail to relieve symptoms. Cimetidine (Tagamet), the H_2 receptor antagonist, markedly reduces acid secretion but has no effect on LES tone in man. Reflux symptoms are greatly decreased with this drug compared to placebo. The required duration of therapy with cimetidine is not established; 4 to 6 weeks of therapy is a reasonable course. Occasionally, in patients with persistent symptoms, it is useful to give 300 mg of cimetidine at bedtime indefinitely. Cholinergic drugs, such as bethanechol (Urecholine), increase LES tone and speed the rate of gastric emptying. Symptoms are improved even though cholinergic agents stimulate gastric secretion. Metoclopramide (Reglan), a smooth muscle stimulant, also increases LES tone and may be useful in the treatment of patients with reflux. These agents should be employed in a stepwise fashion before declaring the patient's symptoms refractory to medical management.

Surgery is indicated in only 3 to 10% of patients with gastroesophageal reflux. The indications are (a) stricture, (b) hemorrhage secondary to erosive esophagitis, (c) peptic ulcer of the esophagus, (d) recurrent aspiration pneumonia secondary to reflux, and (e) intractability of symptoms. Before surgery is considered, however, the diagnosis of gastroesophageal reflux should be unequivocal and the patient should have received maximum medical therapy. Operations incorporating a fundoplication around the distal esophagus provide symptomatic improvement in about 90% of patients. Simple repair of a hiatus hernia

Table 31.3
Management of Gastroesophageal Reflux

STAGE I:
General recommendations:
　Elevate head of bed
　Avoid fatty foods, chocolate, alcohol
　Avoid citrus fruit juices, smoking, coffee
　Avoid tight-fitting garments or activities that increase intra-abdominal pressure
　Lose weight
　Avoid late night snacks or lying down shortly after a meal
　Discontinue medications that lower the lower esophageal sphincter pressure
Medications: Antacids—30–45 ml 1 hr *after* meals and at bedtime or antacids plus alginic acid—2 tablets after meals and at bedtime
STAGE II:
　Cimetidine (300 mg) *before* meals, and at bedtime
　Bethanechol (25 mg) or metoclopramide (10–20 mg) before meals and at bedtime
STAGE III:
　Surgery: Fundoplication

has not been equally effective nor is the benefit long lasting. The fundoplication procedure recreates an effective barrier to reflux. Several variations of the fundoplication are available and local surgical expertise generally dictates the specific type of operation that is performed. Complications include dysphagia, which is often only transient, and the "gas-bloat" syndrome from the inability to belch. Antireflux surgery for patients with scleroderma is potentially hazardous as it may markedly exacerbate dysphagia (see above, p. 261). Vagotomy is not indicated in the treatment of gastroesophageal reflux.

References

General

Cohen, S: Motor disorders of the esophagus. *N Engl J Med* 301: 184, 1979.
　Excellent review of classification and evaluation of this topic.
Snape, WJ, Jr, and Cohen, S: Gastroesophageal reflux: Advances in medical and surgical treatment. In *Progress in Gastroenterology, Vol. III*, Chap. 25, p. 695, edited by GB Jerzy Glass. Grune & Stratton, New York, 1977.
　Thorough review of pathophysiology and therapy.

Specific

1. Brand, D, Martin, D and Pope, C: Esophageal manometrics in patients with angina-like chest pain. *Am J Dig Dis* 22: 300, 1977.
2. Just-Viera, J, and Haight, C: Achalasia and carcinoma of the esophagus. *Surg Gynecol Obstet* 128: 1081, 1969.
3. Farrell, RL, Gastell, DO and McGuigan, JE: Measurements and comparisons of lower esophageal sphincter pressures and serum gastrin levels in patients with gastroesophageal reflux. *Gastroenterology* 67: 415, 1974.
4. Parker, E and Moertel, C: Carcinoma of the esophagus: is there a role for surgery? *Am J Dig Dis* 23: 730, 1978.
5. Swamy, N: Esophageal spasm: clinical and manometric response to nitroglycerin and long acting nitrites. *Gastroenterology* 72: 23, 1977.
6. Tucker H, Snape, WJ, Jr and Cohen, S: Achalasia secondary to carcinoma: manometric and clinical features. *Ann Intern Med* 89: 315, 1978.

CHAPTER THIRTY-TWO

Abdominal Pain

MARVIN M. SCHUSTER, M.D.

Abdominal pain is one of the most common presenting complaints of patients to their physicians. In ambulatory practice, it is the fifth most common symptom generally, and the second most common symptom of women (Chapter 1). Many patients complain of having chronic persistent or recurrent pain; and in this population, it is important to consider functional as well as organic causes for the symptom. Acute abdominal pain (occurring within 24 hours of the patient seeking help) almost always reflects an organic process. In any case, whether chronic or acute, abdominal pain due to an organic cause is more often a symptom of gastrointestinal disease than nongastrointestinal disease.

The physician's response to the patient with abdominal pain will be influenced by its rapidity of onset, its apparent severity, its location, and by accompanying signs and symptoms (fever, gastrointestinal bleeding, diarrhea, etc.) that may suggest a specific process. Although there is no information about the relative frequency of the various causes of abdominal pain, experience suggests that, most often, acute pain is self-limited (abates within hours), and that the pain is usually attributed, without proof, to viral gastroenteritis or to dietary indiscretion. Chronic pain, if associated with an organic process, is most often due to peptic disease, gallbladder disease, chronic relapsing pancreatitis (primarily in alcoholics), or carcinoma (most commonly pancreatic or colonic). The other symptoms and signs that ac-

company these processes are discussed in a general way in this chapter and more specifically in the various chapters devoted to these conditions.

The significance of pain is determined by two major factors—the characteristics of the pain, and the characteristics of the patient. The relative significance of pain to the patient depends on its severity and frequency, the degree to which it interferes with his daily life or sleep patterns, and its meaning to him, both implied and symbolic. Even severe pain can be tolerated for brief periods if it appears infrequently whereas less severe pain may be less tolerable if it interrupts important activities or disturbs sleep. Pain which has no anticipated end is generally less well tolerated than pain which, even though intense has a predictable span. The threshold of pain tolerance varies considerably from one individual to another, because of both neurologic and psychologic factors When pain suggests to the patient a serious underlying disorder such as cancer, this concern itself may decrease his tolerance for pain. Also, pain which is primarily organic may be reinforced by the secondary psychosocial gains that it provides.

Management of any type of pain can be significantly improved by consideration of certain general principles. For example, reassurance that pain can be relieved by medication or surgery can significantly raise the threshold of tolerance. On the other hand the existence of severe pain sensitizes patients to additional, less intense pain (such as lumbar puncture or venipuncture) and the patients "over-reaction" to the second pain should not be taken to imply that the primary pain is psychogenic. Another common misconception is that alleviation of pain by placebo implies psychogenic origin; in fact, organic pain may be more readily relieved by placebo than is psychogenic pain. A post hoc rationalization which accounts for this phenomenon views the patient with organic pain as a person who wants desperately to get rid of his pain, whereas the person with psychogenic pain may be unwilling "to give it up" because of secondary gain.

TYPES OF ABDOMINAL PAIN

A few general concepts concerning abdominal pain are reviewed here, since their understanding can be quite helpful diagnostically. Pain involving the digestive system can be visceral, parietal, referred, or psychogenic. Metabolically associated and neurogenic pain (see below) are presumed to operate through one or more of these mechanisms.

Visceral Pain

Visceral pain can result from spasm or stretch of the muscle wall of a hollow viscus, from distension of the capsule of a solid organ such as the liver, or from inflammation and ischemia of a visceral structure. Tenderness associated with visceral pain (including sometimes rebound tenderness) is often felt directly over the part of the digestive system that is involved although (except for the terminal ileum) small bowel tenderness is usually not well localized. Abdominal viscera are insensitive to cutting, tearing, crushing, and burning.

Parietal Pain

The parietal peritoneum, mesentery, and posterior peritoneal covering are sensitive to forces similar to those that affect the viscera, but the omentum and anterior abdominal wall are less sensitive. Parietal tenderness is more localized than visceral tenderness, and rebound tenderness is experienced over the involved area. Parietal pain that is the result of generalized inflammation (peritonitis) encompasses a large area of the peritoneum. A rigid abdomen, associated with pain, usually means that the inflammation is severe.

Referred Pain

Both visceral and parietal pain may be referred to a remote site along shared nerve pathways (dermatomes). Gallbladder pain, for example, typically radiates to the infrascapular area, and right diaphragmatic pain, to the right shoulder. The more severe the visceral pain, the more likely it is to be referred to the back, as for example with esophageal spasm or with cholecystitis. The skin overlying the dermatome to which the pain is referred may be hypersensitive. Deep palpation of the primary site of the painful organ may intensify the pain, not only locally, but at its referred site, whereas the reverse is not true: deep palpation over the referred site does not usually enhance pain over the primary site.

Abdominal Pain Caused by Metabolic Disease

Metabolic disease may produce intestinal pain by a direct effect on the alimentary tract, as, for example, when intestinal spasm is induced by porphyria, lead poisoning, or familial Mediterranean fever. In hereditary angioneurotic edema, C-1 esterase deficiency may produce intestinal swelling which can result in pain due to partial obstruction or to intestinal spasm. On the other hand, metabolic disorders may secondarily produce gastrointestinal pain; for example, hyperparathyroidism may produce a painful peptic ulcer or pancreatitis. Hyperlipidemia also may evoke pancreatitis, but may be associated with abdominal pain in the absence of this entity.

Neurogenic Pain

Neurogenic abdominal pain (causalgia) is experienced by the patient as a burning sensation along the route of distribution of the nerve, and is sometimes associated with hyperesthesia. Usually the spinal root is involved by Herpes zoster, carcinoma, or arthritis, etc., but peripheral neuropathies due to operative trauma or to diabetes may also produce neurogenic abdominal pain. There is no relationship of neurogenic pain to digestive function (e.g., eating or defecating).

Psychogenic Pain

Psychogenic pain may represent a conversion reaction which results in the perception of pain where no organic dysfunction exists; or it may result from psychophysiologic reactions characterized by pathological or physiologic responses to psychologic events (see Chapter 11). For example, emotional stress can lead to painful intestinal spasm in patients with irritable bowel syndrome (Chapter 36). This spasm is a measurable physiological event. Similarly, stress may lead to gastric hypersecretion which also can be quantitated. Pain or tenderness that represents a conversion reaction (emotions converted into somatic complaints) may disappear during periods of distraction. Such pain may be inconsistent and incompatible with known neuroanatomy and neurophysiology.

HISTORICAL CLUES TO DIAGNOSIS AND MANAGEMENT

Although the successful diagnosis of conditions that present with abdominal pain depends on meticulous pursuit of leads that are provided by history and physical examination, familiarity with standard questions and examination techniques assists in ensuring completeness. Questions relating to local features include the nature and quality of pain, its location, radiation, intensity, timing, duration, course and the factors which precipitate, aggravate, and alleviate it. Associated symptoms and signs include tenderness, fever and chills, anorexia, nausea and vomiting, diarrhea and constipation, obstruction, borborygmus, rectal bleeding, passing of mucus, jaundice, and genitourinary symptoms.

Rapidity of Onset of Pain

The temporal development of abdominal pain is an important factor which guides the physician in the urgency and direction of the evaluation. In particular, pain that develops abruptly within minutes and becomes rapidly severe is very ominous (Table 32.1).

In addition, situations in which a silent period follows the initial symptoms are notoriously deceptive problems for the primary physician. For example, a perforated viscus or an intestinal infarction may be characterized by resolution of the intense initial pain hours after perforation first occurs and

Table 32.1
Causes of Acute Abdominal Pain According to Rapidity of Onset[a]

Intestinal Causes	Extraintestinal Causes
ABRUPT ONSET (INSTANTANEOUS)	
Perforated ulcer	Ruptured or dissecting
Ruptured abscess or hematoma	aneurysm
Intestinal infarct	Ruptured ectopic pregnancy
Ruptured esophagus	Pneumothorax
	Myocardial infarct
	Pulmonary infarct
RAPID ONSET (MINUTES)	
Perforated viscus	Ureteral colic
Strangulated viscus	Renal colic
Volvulus	Ectopic pregnancy
Pancreatitis	
Biliary colic	
Mesenteric infarct	
Diverticulitis	
Penetrating peptic ulcer	
High intestinal obstruction	
Appendicitis (gradual onset more common)	
GRADUAL ONSET (HOURS)	
Appendicitis	Cystitis
Strangulated hernia	Pyelitis
Low small intestinal obstruction	Salpingitis
Cholecystitis	Prostatitis
Pancreatitis	Threatened abortion
Gastritis	Urinary retention
Peptic ulcer	Pneumonitis
Colonic diverticulitis	
Meckel's diverticulitis	
Crohn's disease	
Ulcerative colitis	
Mesenteric lymphadenitis	
Abscess	
Intestinal infarct	
Mesenteric cyst	

[a] Adapted from L. W. Way: Abdominal pain and the acute abdomen. In *Gastrointestinal Disease*, p. 405, edited by M. Sleisenger and J. Fordtran, W. B. Saunders, Philadelphia, 1978.

by a recurrence of pain several hours later when peritonitis and volume depletion are well established.

Almost always, therefore, if the patient complains of an abrupt onset of severe abdominal pain on the day that he visits the physician, even if the pain has resolved and the abdominal examination is unrevealing, a complete blood count, urinalysis, chest X-ray, plain and upright films of the abdomen, and close surveillance over several hours are imperative and are usually best accomplished in an emergency room.

When the onset of pain is more gradual, there are many more possible causes, and considerable judgment is necessary in deciding about the urgency and direction of the evaluation. The physician will need particularly to be guided by the patient's history, the nature and location of the pain (see below), and by the examination (see below). In all cases follow-up examination is warranted. Newly experienced abdominal pain should never be dismissed, even if it is felt to be innocuous, without follow-up, at least by phone, within a few days. In this way, any important new symptoms will not be missed. It is best for the physician to initiate this follow-up since it will obviate the need for the patient to decide whether a change in symptoms is important enough to trouble the physician.

Nature and Location of Pain (Tables 32.2 and 32.3)

Esophageal pain is generally described as pressing, constricting, or burning. It is usually located in the substernal area and, when severe, radiates through to the back. The location of the pain is a good clue to the location of the underlying disease. Although pain from the lower esophageal region may be referred higher, lesions high in the esophagus do not refer to the lower part of the esophagus.

Gastric pain is usually experienced in the subxiphoid area or the left upper quadrant. Although gastritis is perceived as a true pain (often burning or cramping in quality), the distress caused by both duodenal and gastric ulcer is experienced as a gnawing discomfort or as a hunger sensation rather than as pain. The discomfort caused by peptic ulcer is felt on an empty stomach and is relieved by eating. Thus nocturnal pain of peptic ulcer usually awakens the patient between 1 and 3 a.m. In contrast, pain of gastritis may be aggravated by eating or relieved only momentarily and then subsequently intensified over a period of 10 to 15 min. A change from ulcer distress to a burning, boring, or knifelike pain (especially when there is radiation through to the back) is an indication of a complication of ulcer—namely penetration. Pain that is precipitated by meals suggests gastric outlet obstruction (often due to pyloric channel ulcer) or high intestinal obstruction.

Duodenal pain is felt also in the epigastric area or slightly to the right of it; and it too may radiate through to the back. When perforation of an ulcer occurs the pain appears abruptly in the epigastric region and later settles into the right lower quadrant as gastric contents are spilled into the right gutter.

Small intestinal pain is generally diffuse and poorly localized. It is experienced in the periumbilical area, and when severe, radiates through to the back. Pain deriving from the terminal ileum may be localized to the right lower quadrant. Uncommonly it may radiate down the leg. Small intestinal pain is generally crampy, sharp, or aching. Bloating, distension, and dull ache are terms that frequently describe prolonged mechanical obstruction or reflex ileus, whereas more acute forms may be manifested by sharp steady pain. Associated fever and chills suggest inflammatory bowel disease.

Table 32.2
Nature and Location of Gastrointestinal Pain

Organ Involved	Nature of Pain	Location of Pain
Esophagus	Burning, constricting	Upper lesions → high substernal Lower lesions → low substernal or referred upward Severe → back
Stomach	Gnawing discomfort, pain	Epigastric Left upper quadrant
Duodenum	Gnawing discomfort, hunger, pain	Epigastric
Small intestine	Ache, cramp, bloating, sharp	Diffuse Periumbilical Terminal ileum → right lower quadrant
Colon	As above	Lower abdomen Sigmoid → left lower quadrant Rectum → midline and sacrum
Pancreas	Excruciating, constant	Upper abdomen radiating to back
Gallbladder	Severe, later dull ache	Right upper quadrant Radiates to right scapula or interscapular area
Liver	Ache, occasionally sharp	Right lower rib cage Right upper quadrant if liver is enlarged

Colonic pain is better localized, often to the lower abdomen. Sigmoid pain is felt in the left lower quadrant, and rectal pain is often described by the patient as being located over the rectum, usually in the midline. Colonic pain generally is crampy or of an aching quality unless perforation occurs, and then it is frequently severe and constant. Although aggravation of pain by emotional tension is seen with functional disorders such as irritable bowel syndrome, the pain of many organic disorders can also be accentuated by stress. Associated fever and chills suggest diverticulitis, diverticular abscess, or ulcerative colitis.

Pancreatic pain is excruciating and constant and usually is located in the upper abdomen with radiation through to the back, but may be felt in almost any area of the abdomen. Pancreatitis is almost invariably associated with vomiting. If vomiting is not present, other diagnoses such as pancreatic carcinoma should be considered.

Appendicitis often begins as diffuse abdominal pain that intensifies over a period of hours as it settles in the right lower quadrant. The pain of appendicitis is frequently aggravated by extension of the right leg.

Gallbladder pain generally begins in the right upper quadrant or epigastrium and radiates to the interscapular area or to the right infrascapular area. It is excruciatingly severe, may be aggravated by deep inspiration, and is replaced by a dull, aching sensation that persists for hours after the severe pain subsides. Tenderness can often be elicited by deep palpation under the rib in the area of the gall bladder, especially during deep inspiration. Gallbladder pain often appears several hours after a heavy dinner. Associated fever and chills suggest ascending cholangitis.

Hepatic pain localizes over the liver, and a tender liver can be demonstrated by palpating the edge during deep inspiration or by fist percussion over the lower right rib cage anteriorly (or over the right upper quadrant if the liver is enlarged).

PHYSICAL EXAMINATION

The patient's *general appearance* provides clues concerning the severity, the duration, and frequently the cause of the underlying condition. The cold, sweat, and pallor of shock along with the marble skin (superficial vessels seen over blanched skin) indicating vasoconstriction are signs of significant hemorrhage. Tachycardia and perspiration are seen in both shock and sepsis, but the skin in shock is cold and clammy while in sepsis it is warm and moist. Signs of sepsis suggest bacterial enteritis, inflammatory bowel disease, intra-abdominal abscess, cholangitis, pancreatitis, peritonitis, or pyelonephritis.

The position assumed by the patient may be characteristic of a particular disorder. A position of truncal flexure often typifies patients with pancreatitis, while patients with gallbladder colic tend to pace or writhe about and appear restless in their unsuccessful attempt to find a comfortable position. This is in sharp contrast to the immobile position assumed by patients with peritonitis who attempt to avoid even the slightest jarring movement.

Inspection of the abdomen is facilitated by using incident lighting to visualize abdominal asymmetry and to outline masses and pulsations. In thin patients with partial obstruction peristaltic intestinal movement may be seen through the abdominal wall, and churning peristalsis may coincide with reports of crampy abdominal pain. Flank discoloration (Gray-Turner sign) or periumbilical discoloration (Cullen sign) results from retroperitoneal or intra-abdominal

Table 32.3
Differential Diagnosis of Abdominal Pain Due to Gastrointestinal Disorders [a]

A. Character, Location, Production or Relief

Disorder	Character	Location	Produced or Relieved by
Peptic ulcer	Gnawing hunger discomfort, occasionally burning, gastric—within minutes after meals, duodenal—usually several hours after meals	Subxiphoid, may radiate to back	Produced by empty stomach, relieved by food, antacids or cimetidine
Penetrating ulcer	Severe boring constant pain	Subxiphoid radiating to back	May awaken patient in early morning hours, may be relieved by antacids or cimetidine.
Perforated ulcer	Abrupt, severe pain followed within 6 hr by deceptive refractory period with diminishing of pain	Initially epigastric—then right lower quadrant (right gutter)	Initial pain spontaneous, peritonitis aggravated by movement
Small bowel obstruction	Crampy severe pain with partial obstruction, constant pain develops with complete obstruction or strangulation	Generalized periumbilical or localized over strangulation	Relieved by intubation decompression
Large bowel obstruction	Crampy pain initially, constant pain with subsequent distension or strangulation, onset less sudden than upper intestinal obstruction	May be localized or generalized	Occasionally relieved by intubation decompression
Intestinal infarct	Severe, excruciating, abrupt onset	Generalized	Relieved only by surgery
Intussusception	Sudden onset severe crampy pain	Periumbilical	Temporary relief may occur with emesis
Appendicitis	Initially colic then continuous with varying intensity	Initial colic in periumbilical area, subsequently continuous in right lower quadrant, occasional testicular radiation	Aggravated by extension of right leg
Pancreatitis	Severe constant pain	Epigastric, radiation to back or lower abdomen	Often initiated by alcoholic binge or eating after binge, by common duct obstruction, penetrating ulcer, or blunt trauma
Cholecystitis	Constant, severe pain preceding nausea and vomiting; subsidence of pain followed by aching	Right upper quadrant radiating to infrascapular region	Precipitated by heavy meal and aggravated by deep inspiration
Biliary colic	Crampy, severe pain	Epigastrium, radiating to right upper quadrant and subscapular region	Precipitated by heavy meal within 1–3 hr
Diverticulitis	Crampy or continuous pain	Left lower quadrant, may radiate to back	Relieved by anticholinergics and antibiotics
Crohn's disease	Crampy with partial obstruction and continuous pain with inflammatory mass	Periumbilical or right lower quadrant, may radiate to back	May be precipitated by milk. Relieved by defecation or intubation decompression
Ulcerative colitis	Crampy pain usually, may be constant with toxic dilation	Often left lower quadrant or any area of colon, generalized with toxic megacolon or perforation	Precipitated by emotional stress or infection. Toxic megacolon by opiates or enemas. Relieved temporarily by defecation

(continued on page 270)

hemorrhage dissecting into the subcutaneous tissues and may indicate hemorrhagic pancreatitis. A strangulated hernia may protrude visibly from ventral defects, the inguinal area, or into the scrotum where peristaltic contractions may occasionally be appreciated. Patients with subphrenic abscess or gallbladder disease may have inspiratory pain that results in splinting and in avoidance of deep inspiration.

Auscultation should always be performed before palpation so that abdominal sounds may be evaluated before they are altered by palpation. At times borborygmus will be audible without the stethoscope. Specifically one should search for hyper- or hypoperistaltic sounds, the high tinkles of obstruction, and for bruits suggesting vascular distortion from aneurysms, compression of blood vessels, or invasion of blood vessels (as for example invasion of the splenic artery in advanced pancreatic carcinoma). Although a silent abdomen implies reflex ileus, bowel sounds may also be quiet or markedly diminished late in the course of mechanical obstruction. Whenever obstruction (especially gastric outlet obstruction) is considered, the physician should try to elicit a succussion splash. This is done by placing the stethoscope over the area (e.g., the stomach) and shaking the patient gently but abruptly. The sloshing sound indicates the presence of air and fluid. This finding in the stomach 3 or more hours after eating or drinking indicates delayed gastric emptying or, rarely, marked hypersecretion.

Gentle *percussion* should precede palpation and is an excellent means for detecting rebound tenderness, masses, and tympany (either generalized or localized) over an area of ileus or obstruction. Since air will rise

Table 32.3 (*continued*)
Differential Diagnosis of Abdominal Pain Due to Gastrointestinal Disorders[a]
B. Abnormal Physical Findings, Associated Signs, and Laboratory Features

Disorder	Abnormal Physical Findings	Associated Signs and Symptoms	Laboratory Features
Peptic ulcer	Subxiphoid tenderness	Nausea, vomiting, retrosternal burning; weight gain with duodenal ulcer; weight stable or loss with gastric ulcer	Endoscopic or X-ray demonstration of ulcer, possible occult blood in stool or melena and iron deficiency anemia
Penetrating ulcer	Marked subxiphoid tenderness	Writhing, clutching abdomen	Amylase may be elevated
Perforated ulcer	Initially rigid with rebound, during refractory stage tenderness disappears to return later, absence of liver dullness with intraperitoneal air	Patient lies rigidly still, pale, perspiring; emesis may be present	Upright film shows free air under diaphragm, leukocytosis
Small bowel obstruction	Borborygmus, high pitched sound with rushes initially; later quiet abdomen; tenderness may be mild or rebound tenderness may be present	Emesis (may be feculent with lower obstruction), obstipation, may be weak with shocklike appearance	Plain film of abdomen showing air fluid levels, may show stepladder pattern.
Large bowel obstruction	Initially hyperperistalsis with high pitched rushes, subsequently distension and decrease in bowel signs	Nausea but less vomiting than with high obstruction, obstipation or marked constipation	Large bowel distension with air fluid levels and no air demonstrated distal to obstruction
Intestinal infarct	Quiet bowel sounds, tenderness present but not commensurate with pain, later rebound tenderness	Shock, bloody diarrhea, melena, vomiting; history of intestinal angina	Leukocytosis, hemoconcentration; bloody fluid on paracentesis; plain film of abdomen may reveal normal gas pattern or no gas due to fluid filled loops
Intussusception	Tender mass in abdomen, high pitched peristaltic rushes	Initially normal stool after onset, then bloody mucus and constipation; vomiting is late; fever after strangulation	Barium enema demonstrates coiled spring appearance of invagination; with ileocecal intussusception, small bowel loop is in colon
Appendicitis	Localized rebound tenderness, hyperesthesia over area	Initially diarrhea, then constipation; nausea, vomiting may be present; fever, tachycardia; rectal tenderness in right perirectal area	Leukocytosis
Pancreatitis	Marked epigastric tenderness, guarding and upper abdominal distension	Emesis almost invariable, fever, with hemorrhagic pancreatitis purple color in flank or periumbilical region	Marked leukocytosis, hyperamylasemia; serum calcium depression on days 2 and 4, toxic psychosis on days 2 and 4; X-ray may show calcification, localized ileus, or colon cut-off sign; upper gastrointestinal series demonstrates pancreatic enlargement and spicules in C loop of duodenum; may have left pleural effusion
Cholecystitis	Tenderness over gallbladder area especially on deep inspiration, Murphy's sign may be positive	More common in obese women 40 years or older or after pregnancy, high incidence among some American Indian populations	Leukocytosis; plain film may show calcified stone; oral cholecystogram nonvisualized during attacks, TcHIDA nonvisualized; cholangiograms may show radiopaque stones
Biliary colic	As above	As above; jaundice may be present	Radiopaque stones may be seen on plain film; nonvisualization on cholecystogram during colic; subsequently may show radiolucent stones; i.v. cholangiogram may show dilated duct; bilirubin, alkaline phosphatase increase; may have hyperamylasemia
Diverticulitis	Guarding and tenderness in left lower quadrant	Constipation, fever, tachycardia; rectal tenderness on left; may have urinary frequency or dysuria from pericolonic involvement	Leukocytosis, barium enema shows diverticula but may not visualize during acute episode, may show partial obstruction
Crohn's disease	Tender mass in right lower quadrant, borborygmus	Nausea, vomiting, diarrhea, fever; may have perirectal fistula; tender mass in right rectal area, occasional clubbing	Anemia, elevated sedimentation rate; small bowel series shows cobblestone appearance or string sign
Ulcerative colitis	Tender over involved area, distended especially over transverse colon with toxic megacolon	Frequent passage of small amounts of bloody liquid stool; tenesmus with rectal involvement; fever, tachycardia, arthralgia, erythema nodosa; proctoscopy reveals bleeding and friability	Anemia; elevated sedimentation rate; barium enema demonstrates ulcerations, shortening, effacement of colon

[a] Modified from: *Handbook of Differential Diagnosis*, Vol. 2, Part I. The Abdomen. Rocom Press, Nutley, N.J., 1974.

to the area between the liver and the abdominal wall, absence of liver dullness with the patient in a recumbent position is an important finding indicating the presence of free air in the abdominal cavity.

Before *palpation*, it is wise to ask the patient to point to the site of maximum pain. Gentle palpation should at first avoid that site to minimize the chances that muscle guarding will interfere with the examination. Preferably the patient should be lying perfectly flat on his back with knees flexed to facilitate relaxation of abdominal muscles. Guarding may be localized over specific lesions (often inflammatory) or there may be marked rigidity if pain is severe, as in perforation or penetration. Subxiphoid tenderness suggests an active ulcer. Tenderness over the liver, especially when the liver edge is brought down against the examining finger by deep inspiration, suggests inflammation in this organ. With gallbladder disease tenderness is localized to the region of the gallbladder and with cystic or common direct obstruction a distended viscus can sometimes be felt as well. Right lower quadrant tenderness is found with appendicitis as well as with Crohn's disease involving the ileum or the ileocecal area. A left lower quadrant tender sigmoid cord is felt most commonly with irritable bowel syndrome, but can also indicate diverticular disease. A distinct tender mass in the right lower quadrant suggests inflammation (usually Crohn's disease) extending beyond the bowel; a similar finding in the left lower quadrant is suggestive of diverticulitis. Boardlike rigidity indicates an intra-abdominal catastrophe such as perforation or infarction. Pulsatile masses should be differentiated from laterally expansile masses since the former can represent a mass overlying an artery, whereas the latter implies aneurysmal dilation. When localized perforation has occurred, rebound tenderness may be localized over the area. Hyperesthesia may exist over the segmental distribution of the spinal nerve that innervates the particular area of the viscus. This finding is detected by gently rubbing the fingers over the skin of the involved dermatome.

Rectal examination can be extremely helpful in localizing areas of tenderness as well as in palpating masses through the rectum. Periappendiceal abscesses can sometimes be identified in this manner as can a perforated diverticulum. On digital examination the finger should circumscribe a complete circle examining the entire perirectal area.

Genital and pelvic examination, like the rectal examination, should be performed in all patients with abdominal pain since it can detect hernias as well as genitourinary and other pelvic problems.

If analgesic drugs have been administered, it is useful to re-examine the patient after pain has been relieved to identify masses or localized tenderness that may have been obscured by guarding and rigidity.

LABORATORY TESTS

A complete blood count, urinalysis, and test for occult blood in the stool are required in every person with serious acute abdominal pain (see above), as are a chest X-ray and a plain and upright film of the abdomen. Other laboratory tests should be ordered as indicated by the specific findings.

A low hematocrit value or hemoglobin concentration can call attention to intraperitoneal or retroperitoneal bleeding, while hemoconcentration raises consideration of mesenteric vascular occlusion. High white count and high erythrocyte sedimentation rate suggest inflammation or infection. Blood in the urine points to kidney stones as a possible source of pain, while white cells point to infection. Glycosuria may arouse suspicion of a diabetic crisis.

The presence of occult blood in the stool reinforces concern about the gastrointestinal tract as a source of painful symptoms, and may be an early sign of vascular ischemia or intussusception, or a sign of more common lesions such as peptic ulcer, polyp, or inflammatory bowel disease.

RADIOLOGY

Plain and upright films of the abdomen are helpful in delineating gas patterns which may demonstrate displacement of intestine by intra-abdominal masses or may show localized loops of ileus, such as one sees with pancreatitis or pyelonephritis. Air is distributed more widely in the small bowel in reflex ileus and in intestinal obstruction. In the latter the typical stepladder pattern is often encountered, with slight separation of the loops due to edema of the wall of the small bowel; an upright film demonstrates air fluid levels in the dilated loops. Absence of air distal to a specific point suggests obstruction at that point. Volvulus can be diagnosed on the plain film which demonstrates a sausage-shaped air or air-fluid filled viscus coming to an apex. In gastric volvulus the greater curvature is seen above the lesser curve; and a double air fluid level is a classic finding, one level being in the lesser curvature of the fundus; the other in the antrum (because of the inverted U-shaped stomach under these conditions). Free air under the diaphragm on the upright film indicates a perforated viscus unless the patient has had recent surgery (at which time air was introduced) or has pneumatosis cystoides intestinalis, in which case a large amount of air may appear subdiaphragmatically from ruptured pseudocysts. The important clue to pneumatosis cystoides intestinalis is the presence of free air in the absence of signs or symptoms of perforation or peritonitis. Radiopaque gallbladder or kidney stones or pancreatic calcification seen on plain film may help corroborate a suspected diagnosis or point attention toward one of these organs.

Contrast studies are performed for specific indications. For example, an upper gastrointestinal series (see "Patient Experience," p. 276) can be performed instead of upper endoscopy (see below) when the history is typical of peptic ulcer and not suggestive of esophagitis, gastritis, or duodenitis (diagnoses which are not well demonstrated by X-ray examination). An upper gastrointestinal series is also helpful when pancreatitis or pancreatic pseudocyst is thought to be the basis of the pain, since the compression on the C loop of the duodenum may suggest these diagnoses. Barium enema (see "Patient Experience," in Chapter 34) can be useful, not only in demonstrating a low site of obstruction but also in reducing an intussusception. When pain is thought to result from gallbladder disease (see Chapter 87), and opaque stones are not visible on plain abdominal film, an oral cholecystogram may demonstrate radiolucent stones; if the gallbladder fails to be visualized with reinforced dosage, a diseased gallbladder is quite likely. *TcHIDA or PipHIDA radioisotopic studies* may demonstrate obstruction of the common or cystic duct. This technique requires injection of isotope and serial views for 1 hour, while the appearance of isotope in the gallbladder is examined (a sonogram is usually performed beforehand to localize the gallbladder).

Ultrasonography is an excellent means of demonstrating stones in the gallbladder, but is not reliable in detecting ductal stones. Ultrasonography is also useful in showing pancreatic edema or pseudocysts, in evaluating a suspected abdominal aortic aneurysm, and in evaluating a patient who is difficult to examine for an intraabdominal mass; this technique has the advantage of avoiding irradiation. Sonography is often unsatisfactory in obese persons and in persons with metal abdominal sutures because adipose tissue and metal reflect sound.

Computerized tomography (CT) is a sensitive means of demonstrating masses, infarcted tissue, and cysts, but is expensive and exposes the patient to irradiation.

Table 32.4 compares the ultrasound and CT technique and the patient experience.

Selective *mesenteric angiography* should be performed in patients suspected of having mesenteric vascular ischemia (particularly in elderly persons with postprandial abdominal pain), or mesenteric vascular occlusion (e.g., in women taking contraceptive medication). This is particularly helpful in older patients since normal arteriographic findings rule out mesenteric vascular disease; on the other hand, occlusion even of two of the three major aortic branches (celiac, superior mesenteric, and inferior mesenteric arteries) may occur without symptoms of mesenteric vascular disease. The patient experience is similar to that described for renal arteriography (Chapter 59).

ENDOSCOPY

Upper gastrointestinal endoscopy requires referral to a gastroenterologist (see below). It should be considered as an ambulatory procedure to clarify or confirm findings in upper gastrointestinal series or to obtain a biopsy for diagnosis (e.g., when cancer is suspected). Endoscopy should be one of the first diagnostic procedures performed when abdominal pain is associated with upper gastrointestinal bleeding (see Chapter 34), but these patients should be hospitalized (see below).

Proctoscopy should be performed in any patient with abdominal pain and rectal bleeding or a change in bowel habits or in any patient in whom inflammatory bowel disease (proctitis, ulcerative colitis, Crohn's disease) is suspected. Moreover, anal lesions such as hemorrhoids and fissures are best demonstrated by proctoscopy. The procedure routinely should precede roentgenographic examination of the lower bowel since the barium enema does not visualize the lower rectum.

Colonoscopy, like upper endoscopy, requires referral to a gastroenterologist (see below). It should be considered in patients with abdominal pain who have occult rectal bleeding (see Chapter 34), in those with suspected diffuse colonic inflammatory disease (ulcerative colitis, Crohn's disease), or suspected ischemic colitis, and in patients with polypoid lesions on barium enema who require biopsy or, often, resection of the lesion. Colonoscopy cannot be performed within a day or two of a barium X-ray of the lower or upper gastrointestinal tract.

Patient Experience. In addition to concerns about facts relating to endoscopy, many patients have specific apprehensions and misconceptions which can only be managed

Table 32.4
Ultrasound and Computerized Tomography (CT) Scanning: Comparison of the Technique and the Patient Experience [a]

Characteristic	Ultrasound	CT
Basis of tissue attenuation	Tissue elasticity, acoustic impedance	Electron density; linear attenuation coefficient
Radiation dose or toxic effect	None known at diagnostic energy levels	8–10 R (skin exposure)
Morphologic detail	Good	Excellent
Contrast medium useful	None	Iodinated intravascular agents; diatrizoate meglumine (Gastrografin)
Time for examination	½–1 hr	½–1 hr
Operator skill	Substantial	Minimal
Ease of interpretation	Complex—many artifacts	Straightforward
Preparation	Nothing by mouth after midnight (for pelvis, three glasses of water 1 hr before study and do not void)	Evacuate barium from recent gastrointestinal studies (or wait 1 week)
Cooperation	Lie still, supine	Lie still, supine

[a] Adapted from: J. T. Ferrucci, Jr.: Body ultrasonography (first of two parts). *New England Journal of Medicine, 300:* 538, 1979.

appropriately if the patient is encouraged to express them. The most common questions concern the indication for the procedure and the anticipated benefits, and technical details about the procedure itself, including prior preparation, side effects, and risks. Much of the patient's anxiety can be allayed if the referring physician can answer these questions appropriately. The physician may find it helpful to emphasize that recent scientific and technical advances have improved instrumentation so that the new fiberoptic instruments can be passed with little discomfort and that photographs can be taken for detailed study, as well as brushings for cytology and biopsy for histology.

Upper Endoscopy (Esophagoscopy, Gastroscopy, Duodenoscopy): Preparation varies, but usually the patient will be asked to fast for 8 hours before the procedure and will be given a topical anesthetic by gargle or atomizer spray and also an intravenous or intramuscular sedative or tranquilizer. It is often helpful to reassure patients that the procedure can be and in fact often is performed without any premedication, as for example in patients with massive bleeding. Moreover, although the swallowing of tubes sounds like an awesome task, the knowledge that endoscopy is performed in patients of all ages and that children as well as elderly people tolerate the procedure well is also reassuring. The instrument is about the diameter of the fifth finger and introduction produces discomfort rather than pain. The entire procedure seldom lasts more than 20 min. Instillation of air, which is necessary to distend the organ so that it can be well visualized, tends to produce a sensation of bloating. This air can be aspirated at the end of the procedure.

The discomfort from upper endoscopy is usually much less than that from a barium enema, and biopsies are painless. A topical anesthetic is administered initially to minimize gagging. During the procedure, the patient experiences the sensation of having something in his throat that he cannot swallow. Bleeding and perforation, the most serious complications, are extremely rare. The procedure is usually performed on an outpatient basis, and since sedation is generally employed, the patient should be accompanied by someone who will be able to take him home following the procedure.

Proctosigmoidoscopy: Whether or not prior preparation is appropriate depends on the suspected pathology. If proctoscopy is performed to detect or biopsy a mass lesion, a laxative is used the day before and a cleansing enema is given on the morning of the procedure. On the other hand, mucosal lesions (such as inflammatory bowel disease) are best demonstrated without preparation (other than a natural bowel movement the morning of the procedure). Most enema preparations tend to produce some mucosal edema that may obscure mucosal lesions. Proctosigmoidoscopy is not painful, but there is an uncomfortable sensation produced by the distention of the rectosigmoid region by the instrument and by air.

Fiberoptic Sigmoidoscopy and Colonoscopy: Fiberoptic sigmoidoscopy can generally be performed if a laxative is administered the day before the procedure and if an enema is given on the morning of the procedure. Colonoscopy requires further cleaning, usually necessitating a liquid diet 2 to 3 days before the procedure in addition to laxatives and enema. Good cleansing is especially important if polypectomy is contemplated. For colonoscopy premedication similar to that used in upper endoscopy (see above) is appropriate, as well as an intravenous analgesic such as Demerol to minimize the discomfort and crampy pain commonly associated with insufflation of air and negotiation of curves. The procedure may take from 30 min to over 1 hour. Polypectomy adds additional time as well as additional risk, but generally does not increase discomfort nor involve the additional recovery time that would be required after an abdominal operation to remove polyps.

TREATMENT

The treatment of patients with abdominal pain depends on the severity of the pain, its rapidity of onset, and on the nature of the underlying condition, if known. Severe pain, with an abrupt or rapid onset frequently reflects a gastrointestinal disorder that will require surgical intervention (see Table 32.1). Hospitalization and consultation with a gastroenterologist and a surgeon should be requested immediately in almost all cases. Less severe pain (pain that does not prevent the patient from ambulating, talking normally, thinking coherently, etc.) should not be treated aggressively with analgesic drugs until an attempt has been made to establish a diagnosis, since the pain will often abate spontaneously within minutes or hours and will not recur. In such circumstances, no further evaluation is indicated. If the pain recurs or persists and the cause is not obvious, the screening tests described on page 271 should be done. If these tests do not provide a diagnosis, referral to a gastroenterologist is indicated.

As a general rule, analgesic drugs may be prescribed to patients with persistent pain, but opiates should be avoided if possible, because they may aggravate the underlying condition. (For example, morphine may aggravate pancreatitis by producing duodenal and ampullary spasm, thus enhancing pancreatic duct obstruction; and opiates or anticholinergics may produce toxic megacolon in patients with active ulcerative colitis. Furthermore, there is a risk of narcotic addiction in any patient whose pain is likely to be of prolonged duration.)

References

Ferrucci, JT, Jr: Body ultrasonography (first of two parts). N Engl J Med 300: 538, 1979.
   Good review of the clinical uses of sonography, with useful comparison of computerized tomography scanning.
Handbook of Differential Diagnosis, Vol. 2, Part I. The Abdomen. Rocom Press, Nutley, N.J., 1974.
   Excellent illustrations by M. F. Netter and good tables.
Hendrix, TR and Cameron, JL: Abdominal pain. In Principles and Practice of Medicine, Ed. 20, edited by AM Harvey, RJ Johns, VA McKusick, AH Owens and RS Ross. Appleton-Century-Crofts, New York, 1980.
   Excellent chapter written by a gastroenterologist and a surgeon, organized for the most part as a problem-solving approach for ambulatory and hospitalized patients.
Way, LW: Abdominal pain in the acute abdomen. In Gastrointestinal Disease, edited by MH Sleisenger and JS Fordtran. W. B. Saunders, Philadelphia, 1978.
   Very good discussion organized along classical rather than problem-oriented lines: written by an experienced surgeon.

CHAPTER THIRTY-THREE

Peptic Ulcer Disease

HAROLD J. TUCKER, M.D.

EPIDEMIOLOGY

Peptic ulcer disease is a common clinical entity. However, for unknown reasons the incidence of peptic ulcer disease, both duodenal and gastric, has been declining for the last 20 to 30 years. The current incidence of new cases of duodenal ulcer disease is about 2 per 1000 men and 0.8 per 1000 women per year. For gastric ulcer, the incidence is only 0.5 and 0.3 per 1000 per year, respectively. The highest incidence is between the ages of 45 and 65 in men and over the age of 55 in women. The overall prevalence of the disease in the general population remains high (about 10%).

RISK FACTORS

Certain factors are associated with an increased risk of developing peptic ulcer disease (Table 33.1). Genetic factors appear to play an important role. Men (see above) are more prone to both duodenal and gastric ulcers than are women. Duodenal ulcer is 3 times more common in first degree relatives of a patient with a duodenal ulcer than in the general population. Furthermore, certain genetic markers, such as pepsinogen I, HLA-B5, and red blood cell acetylcholinesterase, can identify groups at increased risk. With the aid of such markers, peptic ulcer disease has been shown to be genetically heterogeneous. In certain families there appears to be an autosomal dominant mode of inheritance, while in others no discernible pattern is found.

The role of *stress* in the pathogenesis of peptic ulcer disease is well recognized but difficult to quantitate. Nevertheless, it is clear that threats to the psychological or physical well-being of some people appear to predispose them to peptic ulceration. Why some people react to stress by developing peptic disease, others by developing another disease (e.g., inflammatory bowel disease, asthma, or hypertension) is unknown (see Chapter 11 for a discussion of psychosomatic illness).

Cigarette smoking has been repeatedly demonstrated to be associated with an increased frequency of duodenal ulcer disease with frequencies ranging between 33 and 100% above that of nonsmokers (3). In addition, there is some evidence that cigarette smoking may delay the healing rate of both gastric and duodenal ulcers. There is no epidemiologic evidence that alcohol is ulcerogenic, although it is a known cause of acute gastritis. Coffee, both caffeinated and decaffeinated, is a mild stimulant of gastric acid secretion. Symptoms may be exacerbated by coffee but a definite causal relationship with ulcer disease has not been demonstrated.

Certain disease states have been associated with an increased frequency of peptic ulcer disease. Evidence for such associations must be carefully evaluated in light of the high prevalence of ulcer disease in the general population and the frequent use of ulcerogenic drugs. There is, however, good evidence linking duodenal (but not gastric) ulcer disease with chronic obstructive pulmonary disease, alcoholic cirrhosis, and chronic renal failure. Peptic ulcers occur in 10 to 25% of patients with hyperparathyroidism.

Table 33.1
Risk Factors for Peptic Ulcer Disease

Male sex
First degree relative with duodenal ulcer
Genetic markers:
　Elevated levels of pepsinogen I
　Presence of HLA-B5 antigen
　Decreased red blood cell acetylcholinesterase
Stress
Cigarette smoking
Zollinger-Ellison syndrome
Chronic renal failure—for duodenal ulcer disease only
Chronic obstructive pulmonary disease—for duodenal ulcer
　disease only.
Alcoholic cirrhosis—for duodenal ulcer disease only
Drugs: Aspirin—for gastric ulcer disease only

Conditions that lead to increased gastric acid secretion also predispose to ulcer disease. The Zollinger-Ellison syndrome, or gastrinoma (see below), is the best example of such a condition. Extensive small bowel resection may also lead to hyperplasia of antral gastrin-containing cells and result in ulcer disease. Retained antrum following gastric surgery is yet another example of uninhibited acid production associated with recurrent ulcerations.

Many drugs are reputed to be ulcerogenic although the evidence is not well established for most of them. Aspirin is one drug that does appear to cause gastric (but not duodenal) ulcers. Experimentally, aspirin disrupts the gastric mucosa both physiologically and anatomically, leading to ulcer formation. Chronic aspirin use has been shown epidemiologically to be linked to an increased frequency of gastric ulceration. Aspirin use also increases the risk of bleeding from peptic lesions (see Chapter 48). Enteric coated or buffered aspirin has no advantage over regular aspirin with respect to these untoward effects.

There is no evidence that other anti-inflammatory agents cause ulcers. Corticosteroids have frequently been linked to the formation of ulcers and to the complications of hemorrhage and perforation. Prospective and retrospective studies of this issue have concluded that steroids do not increase the prevalence of peptic ulcer disease or of its complications (2). The same statement can be made for agents like indomethacin, phenylbutazone, and other anti-inflammatory agents.

NORMAL GASTRIC FUNCTION

The two primary functions of the stomach are the secretion of various substances that are important in digestion and absorption and the movement of gastric contents downstream into the small intestine. There are four primary classes of secretory cells: mucus-secreting cells of the cardia, hydrochloric acid-secreting parietal cells of the body (which also secrete intrinsic factor—see Chapter 46), pepsinogen-secreting chief cells of the body, and gastrin-secreting G

cells of the antrum. Gastric function is regulated by neural and hormonal influences which determine the rate and amount that the various cells secrete and the rate at which the stomach empties its contents into the duodenum. During the *cephalic phase* of gastric activity, the anticipation of eating initiates cholinergic impulses which, via the vagus nerve, stimulate parietal cell secretion of acid and G cell secretion of gastrin (which then also stimulates acid secretion). During the *gastric phase*, distention of the stomach by food causes local nerve endings to stimulate acid and gastrin secretion further—the G cells are also directly stimulated by protein and protein breakdown products and inhibited by acid. During the *intestinal phase* of gastric activity, intestinal hormones (secretin, cholecystokinin, and probably others), the secretion of which is stimulated directly by gastric acid, inhibit the action of gastrin on the parietal cells.

PATHOPHYSIOLOGY

The pathophysiology of duodenal ulcer disease differs from that of gastric ulcer disease.

Duodenal Ulcer

Simplistically, duodenal ulcer disease can be viewed as the result of an imbalance between the normal duodenal defense mechanisms and the amount of acid delivered to the duodenum from the stomach. Multiple abnormalities have been identified that result in this imbalance (Table 33.2): (a) increased parietal cell mass, (b) increased capacity of parietal cells to secrete acid, (c) increased vagal "drive" to secrete acid, (d) defective inhibition of gastrin release and of gastric secretion following gastric acidification or following a meal (these first four abnormalities result in a considerably increased acid production compared to normal), (e) abnormally rapid gastric emptying, and (f) altered duodenal defense mechanisms.

Duodenal defense mechanisms include neutralization of acid by pancreatic bicarbonate and absorption of acid by duodenal contents. There are some data to suggest that pancreatic bicarbonate secretion is decreased by nicotine. This observation may provide an explanation for the association between smoking and ulcer disease, but its true significance is still

Table 33.2
Pathophysiology of Duodenal Ulcer

Increased mass of parietal cells
　increased number of parietal cells
　increased capacity of cells to secrete acid
Increased sensitivity of parietal cells (*e.g.*, to food, histamine and gastrin)
Increased activity of stimulators of parietal cell secretion (*e.g.*, gastrin or the vagus nerve)
Increased rate of emptying of the stomach
Decreased duodenal defense mechanisms

uncertain. Pancreatic secretion is otherwise normal in peptic ulcer disease and there is no increased risk in patients with chronic pancreatitis.

Gastric Ulcer

The current understanding of the pathogenesis of gastric ulceration is less clear. It is generally believed that the basic defect in gastric ulcer formation is the disruption of the gastric mucosal barrier. It has been shown that this barrier can be broken by such irritants as bile, alcohol, and aspirin. These experimental observations help explain the epidemiologic data associating alcohol with acute gastritis, and aspirin with gastric ulcers and erosions. Furthermore, in patients with gastric ulcers, radiologic and manometric studies have suggested that there is an increased duodenal gastric reflux. This reflux of bile across an incompetent pyloric sphincter results in the disruption of the mucosal barrier. Once the barrier is broken, hydrogen ion may diffuse back into the gastric cells leading to ulceration via local histamine release, vasodilation, and tissue damage. Thus, according to this concept, gastric ulcer formation requires injury to the gastric mucosal barrier and the presence of some, but not necessarily an excessive amount of, acid.

Another factor that may be involved in the formation of some gastric ulcers is pyloric stenosis, which most commonly occurs secondary to a chronic duodenal ulcer that antedates the formation of a gastric ulcer. With pyloric deformity there may be poor gastric emptying resulting in stasis and antral distension. This distension leads to increased gastrin release and increased gastric acid production. This hypothesis is supported by the frequent association radiographically of both duodenal and gastric ulcerations. In the Veterans Administration (VA) Cooperative study of gastric ulcer, over 40% of patients had radiographic evidence of concurrent duodenal ulcer disease (5). Furthermore, patients with gastric ulcers just proximal to the pylorus are frequently found to produce increased amounts of acid, just as patients with duodenal ulcers do.

DIAGNOSIS

History

The most common symptom of peptic ulcer disease is epigastric distress—vague discomfort or a feeling of gnawing hunger—usually in the midline. If actual pain occurs, it is typically aching or burning.

Classically, the distress of duodenal ulcers occurs several hours after a meal, and may awaken the patient from sleep; it is relieved within minutes by food, antacids, or vomiting. Typically distress is not present before breakfast. In patients with gastric ulcers, the history is more variable. In some, a similar distress-food-relief pattern exists, while in others there is no relationship with food. Occasionally, the distress is actually exacerbated by food.

Other less frequent symptoms of ulcer disease include nausea, vomiting, and heartburn. However, in some patients with ulcers one or more of these symptoms may occur in the absence of typical ulcer pain. Weight loss occurs in up to 50% of patients with a benign gastric ulcer (and is therefore not a helpful feature in distinguishing a benign from a malignant ulcer). Patients with duodenal ulcer often gain weight because they eat more in an attempt to control their pain.

The history may also suggest certain complications. Pyloric obstruction presents first with early satiety and then with persistent vomiting, frequently of undigested food. A change in the quality of the pain or radiation of the pain to the back or shoulder, suggests penetration of the ulcer. A history of melena suggests bleeding.

Physical Examination

The physical exam may provide supportive, although nonspecific information. Localized epigastric tenderness is common. The presence of a succussion splash 4 hours postprandially is evidence of gastric outlet obstruction. Rectal examination should be included in the initial physical examination to obtain a stool specimen for testing for occult blood.

Radiologic Studies

Confirmation of the presence of peptic ulcer disease can be made with barium studies or with endoscopy. The patient should be told that the upper gastrointestinal series requires him to have a series of X-rays taken after he swallows a bolus of barium, that peristalsis is monitored fluoroscopically during the procedure, and that to coat as much of the stomach and duodenum as possible, he will be photographed while he is prone. The entire procedure takes about 20 to 25 min. Endoscopically demonstrable duodenal or gastric ulcers are visible by barium X-ray in up to 80% of cases.

DUODENAL ULCER

The radiographic diagnosis of duodenal ulcer disease depends upon the detection of an ulcer crater. Associated findings include edema and radiation of the duodenal folds adjacent to the ulcer, deformity of the bulb, and spasm. Occasionally the ulcer crater may not be detected because of overhanging edematous folds which prevent filling of the crater with barium, shallowness of the ulcer crater, or an inadequate technique. Air contrast studies enhance the detection rate of shallow ulcers and erosions. Ulcers greater than 3 cm are classified as giant duodenal ulcers. Duodenal ulcers do not carry the risk of malignancy that gastric ulcers do and therefore follow-up X-rays to confirm healing are generally not needed. In patients with chronic ulcer disease with severe deformity of the bulb, distinction radiographically between old scarring with deformity and new active ulcerations is often very difficult. Comparison with previous films and correlation with the clinical state is needed in these cases.

In the postoperative patient, barium studies are often difficult to evaluate. With conventional studies, anastomotic ulcers are detected in only 50% of cases. The air contrast technique may be of more value in this situation. Distinction between surgical deformity and recurrent ulcerations is often difficult without a previous postoperative study for comparison.

GASTRIC ULCER

Radiologic studies are valuable in the detection and evaluation of gastric ulcers. The radiographic features characteristic of a benign gastric ulcer include (a) penetration of the ulcer crater beyond the expected course of the gastric lumen; (b) radiating gastric folds converging on the ulcer reaching right up to the ulcer margin; (c) smooth appearance of surrounding mucosa; (d) central location of the ulcer, surrounded by a smooth mound of edematous mucosa; and (e) smooth and round or oval margins of the ulcer crater. The radiation of the gastric folds up to the thin overhanging margin of the ulcer is probably the most reliable sign of benignity. Appreciation of the surrounding gastric mucosa and the radiation of the folds is best achieved with good air contrast technique (Fig. 33.1). (The air contrast study causes distention of the stomach but no real pain.) The size of the ulcer is not helpful as a differential point in an individual case, except that the incidence of malignancy in gastric ulcers increases with increasing size of the ulcer crater. Similarly, location of the ulcer is not of predictive value. Coexistent duodenal ulcer disease (seen in 40% of gastric ulcer patients) considerably decreases the likelihood that a gastric ulcer is

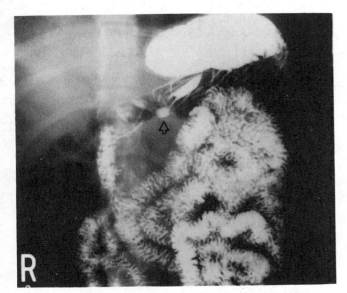

Figure 33.1 X-ray study in a patient with a benign gastric ulcer. The presence of gastric folds radiating to the edge of the ulcer, with no distortion of the surrounding mucosa is characteristic of a benign gastric ulcer.

malignant, but does not rule it out. Multiple ulcers need to be evaluated and followed individually.

In evaluating a gastric ulcer, the radiologist generally describes it as benign, malignant, or indeterminant. As many as 10% of gastric ulcers may be classified in this last category. Although the radiographic impression of a benign or malignant ulcer is generally very accurate, discrepancies still occur. The incidence of malignancy in an ulcer diagnosed radiographically as benign ranges from 3 to 7% with higher frequencies when "indeterminant" lesions are included. Air contrast techniques may decrease this error rate. Furthermore, barium studies may miss lesions, particularly when multiple ulcers are present. Carefully performed radiography may detect 90% of ulcers seen by endoscopy. Thus, while a barium study is frequently the initial procedure of choice for gastric ulcers, it must be recognized that its sensitivity is less than that of endoscopy and that it is associated occasionally with erroneous results.

Endoscopy

Endoscopy is of value in the diagnosis of both duodenal and gastric ulcers. It has the advantages of increased sensitivity, the opportunity for obtaining biopsies, and the avoidance of radiation. In certain situations endoscopy may be the preferred initial mode of examination rather than X-ray (see p. 273 for a description of the patient's experience with endoscopy).

DUODENAL ULCERS

Indications for endoscopy for duodenal ulcer disease include: (a) abdominal pain suggestive of peptic ulcer disease with negative X-ray studies, (b) refractory or recurrent ulcer symptoms despite appropriate medical therapy of radiologically visible ulcers, (c) evaluation for anastomotic ulcers, (d) differentiation between old scarring and new active ulcer craters seen on X-ray, (e) acute pyloric obstruction, and (f) upper gastrointestinal bleeding. Routine duodenal ulcers do not require endoscopic evaluations with biopsies, as the risk of malignancy is extremely low, nor do they need to be followed endoscopically until they heal. In the patient known to have peptic ulcer disease who presents with recurrent typical symptoms, the indications for repeat X-ray studies, endoscopy, or empiric therapy have not been established. The advantages and disadvantages of the various alternatives should be considered for each individual patient.

GASTRIC ULCER

There is considerable controversy over the role of endoscopy in patients with gastric ulcer. Clearly in the patient whose clinical condition or whose radiographic studies suggest a gastric malignancy endoscopic evaluation is indicated. Adenocarcinoma of the stomach, lymphoma, metastatic carcinoma to the stomach (e.g., malignant melanoma) and leiomyosarcoma all may be ulcerated and may be differentiated by endoscopy and biopsy. Even in patients with a benign appearing ulcer, early endoscopy is frequently recommended because of its increased accuracy in distinguishing benign *versus* malignant disease and its increased sensitivity in demonstrating multiple ulcers, gastritis, and coexisting duodenal ulcer disease. Endoscopy with multiple biopsies and directed brushings for cytology can accurately diagnose gastric ulcers in 97 to 99% of cases. However, it can also be argued that routine early endoscopy is unnecessary because (a) newer air contrast radiographic techniques may provide similar degrees of accuracy, (b) the incidence of gastric carcinoma is decreasing, (c) the prognosis of patients found to have a gastric malignancy may be unaltered even with earlier detection, and (d) patients are frequently elderly and the risk of endoscopy may outweigh the benefit. In addition, as the ultimate determinant of the benign nature of an ulcer is that it heals completely and resolves, some would argue that a late endoscopic evaluation to determine whether there has been complete resolution of the ulcer is the most important one.

It is apparent that judgment and individualization are important. Endoscopy is the most accurate means of distinguishing a benign from a malignant ulcer. In the elderly patient with severe cardiac or pulmonary disease in whom gastric surgery would be almost unthinkable, even for malignant disease, endoscopy for an ulcer that appears benign is unwarranted. Otherwise endoscopy should be performed routinely soon after diagnosis. The mode of follow-up frequently depends on the individual evaluation. In the patient with an ulcer that appears benign by X-ray and by endoscopy, radiologic follow-up to complete healing is generally satisfactory. Clearly if the initial ulcer cannot be well visualized on X-ray, endoscopy should be used to follow the healing of the ulcer. In the patient with a suspicious or "indeterminant" lesion by X-ray but without initial endoscopic evaluation, endoscopy should be performed subsequently to confirm complete healing of the ulcer. Malignant ulcers have been found to have resolved on radiographic studies but not on endoscopic evaluation. Finally, ulcers that fail to heal after an appropriate interval should be re-evaluated endoscopically. It should be recognized that, because of greater sensitivity of the procedure, the healing rate shown by endoscopy is probably slower than the generally accepted healing rate, defined radiographically as 50% reduction in size of ulcer at 6 weeks and complete healing at 12 weeks.

Gastric Analysis

Gastric secretory studies have enhanced the understanding of the pathophysiology of ulcer disease, but are of limited clinical usefulness. While many patients with duodenal ulcer disease can be shown to hypersecrete acid, over one-half of such patients actually have normal levels of acid production. The presence of hypersecretion, furthermore, does not predict the development of ulcer disease in an individual patient. Dyspepsia with a negative X-ray is not an indication for gastric analysis.

In patients with gastric ulcers, gastric analysis is only rarely helpful. Persistent achlorhydria despite stimulation (with Histalog or pentagastrin) strongly suggests that the ulcer is malignant; but on the other hand, over 80% of patients with malignancies will have demonstrable acid production following stimulation.

The main indications for gastric analysis are for preoperative evaluation of patients with suspected Zollinger-Ellison syndrome (see below) or in the postgastrectomy patient with recurrent ulcer disease. However, gastric analysis is not useful as an indicator of the type of surgery needed—more acid production does not necessarily require more gastric resection (6).

Gastric analysis requires gastric intubation for about 2 hours. The procedure is performed in the gastrointestinal laboratory of most hospitals (not in the general physician's office). During the first hour, the volume and hydrogen ion activity of gastric secretions are measured and are reported as the basal acid output (BAO) in milliequivalents per hour. Secretion is then stimulated, usually with pentagastrin or Histalog. The former, a synthetic analogue of gastrin, is generally recommended as it has fewer side effects than Histalog (a histamine analogue) and causes peak secretion earlier. Volume and hydrogen ion activity are again measured for the next hour and reported as maximal acid output (MAO). Peak acid output (PAO) is similar to MAO, but refers to the highest acid output following stimulation rather than the total acid output. Mean basal secretion and maximal acid secretion in normals are 2.4 and 25 meq per hour, respectively, while in patients with duodenal ulcers the mean values are 5 and 43 meq per hour, respectively.

Serum Gastrin Measurements

Measurements of the level of gastrin in the blood are now readily available and are of use in the evaluation of patients with peptic ulcer disease. The fasting basal serum gastrin level is normal (i.e., <150 pg/ml) in patients with duodenal and gastric ulcer disease but is elevated, often to very high levels (usually 1000 pg/ml or more), in patients with the Zollinger-Ellison syndrome (see below). Therefore, fasting gastrin determinations are very useful in screening for this condition. In patients with frequently recurrent ulcers, and in patients refractory to conventional therapy—features suggestive of the syndrome—several (two or three) fasting serum gastrin determinations should be made to rule out this condition since the levels may fluctuate. Also, in all patients undergoing elective ulcer surgery, a preoperative gastrin level should be measured, (see p. 288 for discussion of hypergastrinemia).

NATURAL HISTORY

Both duodenal and gastric ulcers recur extremely frequently. In multiple series, using periodic endoscopic examination after healing of the initial ulcer and cessation of medical therapy, the recurrence rate for duodenal ulcer disease has been 50 to 77% within the first 6 months (8). Some of these recurrences are asymptomatic and detected only endoscopically, but the majority are associated with typical ulcer symptoms. Similarly, for gastric ulcers, the recurrence rate is also high with 30 to 56% recurring within a 2-year period. In the VA cooperative study 11% had two recurrences within a 2-year interval. In patients whose index ulcer healed slowly (persisting for over 3 months), the recurrence rate was even higher—67% within 2 years (5). Although first recurrence of a gastric ulcer does not increase the risk for subsequent recurrences, the rate remains high (30 to 40%).

Complications of peptic ulcer disease are also common. *Hemorrhage* occurs in about 15 to 20% of patients over a 15- to 25-year follow-up, somewhat more frequently in patients with duodenal ulcers than in patients with gastric ulcers. Recurrent hemorrhage is also common, occurring in 30 to 50% of patients with duodenal ulcer disease. The incidence of recurrent hemorrhage after the first, second, or third hemorrhage remains constant at 30 to 50%. In gastric ulcer disease, a second hemorrhage occurs up to 40% of the time and subsequent bleeding occurs in 25% of cases. The age of the patient or the severity of the index hemorrhage does not predict the likelihood of subsequent hemorrhage. *Perforations* occur in 5 to 10% of patients with peptic ulcer disease, more commonly in patients with duodenal ulcers. *Pyloric outlet obstruction* is the least common major complication of peptic ulcer disease, occurring in less than 5% of patients, the vast majority of whom have duodenal ulcer disease.

DYSPEPSIA WITHOUT ULCERATION

A large group of patients have vague epigastric discomfort, including mild nausea, without radiographic or endoscopic evidence of ulceration. These patients ordinarily do not have the typical symptoms of a peptic ulcer described above (p. 276). If they do have such symptoms, they should be treated medically in the same way that they would were an ulcer demonstrable (see below). If their symptoms are atypical, another process should be considered (e.g., gallbladder disease, see Chapter 87) as should the somatization of an emotional problem (see Chapter 11).

MEDICAL THERAPY

Medical therapy includes dietary manipulations and restrictions, antacids, and antisecretory agents. Its purpose is to relieve pain, promote healing, and to prevent recurrences and complications. Surgical therapy is aimed at reducing the capacity of the stomach to secrete acid and at treating severe complications of the disease (massive bleeding, perforation, obstruction).

Diet and Related Restrictions

There is no evidence that modification of the diet is helpful in the treatment of peptic ulcer disease. Bland diets and increased milk consumption have not been shown to be of any benefit. It is more important to identify specific foods, if any, that seem to exacerbate symptoms in the individual patient. For example, caffeinated beverages may mildly stimulate acid secretion and may aggravate symptoms. However, in the absence of such aggravation, there is little benefit from restricting coffee or caffeine as these agents are not usually related to ulcer formation. Patients should be advised to eat regularly, but not to increase the frequency of meals or to use "bedtime snacks" habitually.

Avoidance of alcohol is frequently recommended. However, while alcohol has been shown to cause acute gastritis it is not directly related to ulcer disease. Restriction of alcohol is advisable for the general health of the patient but not specifically because of ulcer disease.

Aspirin, however, should be avoided in all patients with ulcers, or a history of ulcers. Aspirin is associated with gastric ulcer formation and may promote bleeding from both duodenal and gastric lesions. Similar restrictions are often imposed on other anti-inflammatory agents such as indomethacin but with less supportive evidence. While it is unclear what effect these agents have in the presence of an acute ulcer, their use is not contraindicated by the simple history of past ulcer disease.

Patients should be strongly advised to discontinue cigarette smoking. Its use has been associated with duodenal ulcer disease and may decrease the healing rate of both duodenal and gastric ulcers.

Antacids

Antacids have long been the mainstay of ulcer therapy. With appropriate dosage, antacids have been shown to be superior to placebo in promoting healing of duodenal ulcers. Although a relatively high percentage of ulcers do heal with placebo therapy over a 4-week period (45%), complete healing with antacid use was found in 78% of patients in one study (10). Interestingly, it does appear that despite its positive effect on ulcer healing, antacid therapy is no better than placebo in relieving symptoms of duodenal ulcer. Despite widespread acceptance, there is

Table 33.3
Comparison of Various Antacids[a]

Brand Name	Contents			One Dose[b]		Cost (¢)
	Al	Mg	Ca	Vol (ml)	Na (mg)	
Mylanta II	+	+		30	47.9	20
Maalox	+	+		48	53.8	25
Mylanta	+	+		52	40.6	23
Riopan	+	+		56	7.9	22
Amphojel	+			64	77.0	28
Gelusil	+	+		93	132.7	37
Camalox	+	+	+	35	17.8	16

[a] From A. Ippoliti, and W. Peterson: The pharmacology of peptic ulcer disease. *Clinics of Gastroenterology, 8:* 54, 1979.
[b] Dose defined as volume of antacid with neutralizing capability equivalent to 30 ml (1 oz) of Mylanta II.

little evidence that antacids relieve symptoms or promote healing of gastric ulcers.

Despite their widespread use, antacids are frequently misused in terms of proper dosage and optimal timing of administration. A wide variety of antacid preparations are commercially available, but not all antacids are the same. Preparations differ in their ability to neutralize acid, in their composition, and in their cost. Table 33.3 lists a comparative analysis of the doses, costs, and sodium content of commonly used antacids based on the acid neutralization effect of 30 ml (1 ounce) of a potent antacid, Mylanta-II. For example, 30 ml of Gelusil provides only one-third of the neutralizing effect of the same volume of Mylanta-II. It is clearly important, therefore, to know which antacid is being used by the patient and to prescribe the appropriate dose. Ideally that dose of antacid should be based on the patient's acid secretory status with hypersecreters (greater than 25 meq per hour MAO—see p. 278) requiring more antacids than hyposecreters. For the majority of patients with duodenal ulcers a dose equal to the neutralizing effect of 1 ounce (30 ml) of Mylanta-II provides effective acid neutralization. Antacid tablets are less effective in their acid-buffering capacity than are the liquid forms.

The timing of the antacid dose is also of importance in achieving optimal acid neutralization. In patients with duodenal ulcer disease, there is exaggerated and prolonged secretion of acid in response to a meal. Thus, while a meal may buffer the acid, gastric emptying of the meal may be rapid, so that high levels of acid are left to bathe the duodenum. For this reason, frequent meals are also ineffective, and may even be harmful, as the postprandial hypersecretion actually exacerbates the ulcer condition. It has been shown, however, that adequate doses of antacid (1 ounce of Mylanta-II or an equivalent), given at 1 and 3 hours following a meal can effectively neutralize gastric secretion for about 4 hours. Giving this dose of antacid at these intervals following a meal and at bedtime results in the high rate of ulcer healing described

above. Antacid therapy should be continued for a 4- to 6-week period, after which it may be stopped completely if the ulcer has healed or used on an "as needed" basis if occasional symptoms recur.

Antacids have a number of potential side effects. The most common side effect is *alteration of bowel habits*—an effect that is predictable and inevitable at the doses recommended, depending on the composition of the antacid. Magnesium-containing antacids (e.g., Maalox) result in diarrhea, while aluminum-containing compounds, (e.g., Amphojel) are constipating. Most antacids attempt to balance these two ingredients, but invariably the effect of one predominates. Alternating doses between two different antacids (Mylanta-II and Amphojel) can prevent this problem. It is important to recommend this pattern at the outset rather than run the risk of a patient discontinuing the antacid because of resultant diarrhea or constipation. The patient should be instructed about the rationale for alternating the antacids, and he should balance the frequency of alternating the antacids with the stool pattern desired.

Electrolyte problems have also been noted when antacids are used. *Hypermagnesemia* can occur in patients with renal failure. *Hypophosphatemia* may result from aluminum hydroxide-containing compounds that bind intraluminal phosphate causing severe muscle weakness and hemolysis of red cells. *Hypercalcemia*, with its consequences, can be seen after prolonged use of calcium-containing antacids (Tums). These latter antacids are very potent but are not recommended, not only because of the extraintestinal complications of hypercalcemia, but also because of the stimulant effect of hypercalcemia on gastric acid secretion. Thus, although these antacids transiently and effectively neutralize gastric acid, the absorbed calcium subsequently creates a rebound phenomenon of gastric hypersecretion which may exacerbate the ulcer diathesis. For similar reasons, consumption of large quantities of milk is generally not recommended.

A well confirmed problem with antacid therapy is poor compliance, in part because of the high frequency of daily doses, the inconvenience of liquid preparations, and the high cost of recommended antacid regimens (see Table 33.3). Furthermore, since antacids are not prescription drugs, the patient may not have explicit written instructions on the bottle (recommendations on the bottle are often quite different from those needed for ulcer healing). Clearly, when antacids are selected for ulcer therapy, the physician should write down the regimen and should take the time to explain the rationale for what may seem to the patient a very large amount of antacid. As noted below, cimetidine has important advantages over antacids in facilitating patient compliance.

Cimetidine

Cimetidine (Tagamet) is a competitive antagonist for the histamine (H_2) receptor site of the gastric mucosa cells. It effectively blocks acid secretion in response to a wide variety of stimuli—including food, cholinergic agents, pentagastrin, histamine, and hypoglycemia. It is unquestionably superior to placebo in healing of duodenal ulcers, with a 70 to 80% success rate at 4 to 6 weeks. In addition, it is effective in controlling the symptoms and the ulcer diathesis in patients with the Zollinger-Ellison syndrome (see below). At a dose of 300 mg, there is marked supression of acid production for about 4 hours. The drug should be given 4 times a day, before meals (to block postprandial acid hypersecretion) and at bedtime (to decrease nocturnal acid secretion). The dose should be modified in patients with renal failure and given every 8 hours in patients with moderate renal impairment (creatinine clearance of 19 to 35 ml per min) and only every 12 hours with severe renal insufficiency (creatinine clearance less than 10 ml per min).

Cimetidine is similar to antacids in its effectiveness. There appears to be no difference in the relief of symptoms or in the rate of healing of duodenal or gastric ulcers when cimetidine is compared to intensive antacid therapy (e.g., Mylanta-II, 210 ml per day). It is not clear that cimetidine (or antacids—see above) is superior to placebo in healing gastric ulcers. In addition there are no data to show that the combination of cimetidine and antacids is more effective than either alone in the treatment of duodenal ulcer. Cimetidine has one advantage over antacids which may influence the choice of initial therapy for many patients, i.e., it is far more convenient to take. The cost of 1 month's course of cimetidine is comparable to that of intensive antacid therapy (about $36 to $38 per month). Current evidence does not support the concept of a rebound phenomenon after cessation of cimetidine therapy or the need for tapering of the dose.

Cimetidine appears to have few significant *side effects*. Most studies of toxicity have been linked to short term administration of the drug, and therefore the safety of long term use of cimetidine has not been clearly established. Several potential side effects have received particular attention. Neutropenia has been of considerable concern, since a previous investigational H_2 receptor antagonist, metiamide, was associated with this potentially life-threatening complication. However, in the making of cimetidine, the thiourea group contained in metiamide and thought to be the cause for the bone marrow toxicity, was replaced with a cyanoguanidine group. There are no experimental data to indicate that cimetidine is toxic to leukocytes. Since its widespread use over the past several years, there have been several isolated case reports of neutropenia, often not secondary to bone marrow suppression, and of thrombocytopenia associated with concomitant cimetidine use. In the majority of these reports, a direct causal relationship between cimetidine and the hematologic abnormality was not established. Thus, there is little evidence that cimetidine is a bone marrow suppressant, and follow-up white blood cell counts and platelet counts are not recommended during cimetidine therapy.

An antiandrogenic effect of cimetidine has been demonstrated in several animal species. Prostatic weight and the size of the testis, prostate, and seminal vesicles have decreased in animals given this drug. In humans, gynecomastia has occurred, most frequently in patients taking high doses and/or prolonged therapy, as in patients with the Zollinger-Ellison syndrome. Blood levels of testosterone, luteinizing hormone, and follicle-stimulating hormone are normal, but prolactin levels are elevated. With discontinuation of cimetidine, the gynecomastia generally has slowly resolved.

Numerous nonspecific side effects have been reported during cimetidine usage. These have included diarrhea, headache, fatigue, and dizziness. In a group of patients taking placebo or antacids as necessary, the frequency of these side effects was similar. Mental confusion has been reported, generally in elderly patients with some degree of renal impairment. Cimetidine may also interfere with the metabolic clearance of certain drugs such as diazepam (Valium), chlordiazepoxide (Librium), warfarin (Coumadin), and propanolol (Inderal).

Anticholinergics

The role of anticholinergic drugs in the treatment of duodenal ulcer is uncertain. These agents are capable of reducing basal acid secretion by 50% and reducing stimulated acid secretion by 30 to 50%, with an inhibitory effect lasting 4 to 5 hours. Recent data have suggested that it is not necessary to give near toxic doses of anticholinergics to reduce acid secretion effectively but that a single standard dose of 15 mg of propantheline bromide (Pro-Banthine) achieves an optimal result. Despite this potentially beneficial function, the data on the relief of ulcer symptoms and on the ulcer healing rates with anticholinergics have been conflicting. Currently, anticholinergics are not recommended as first line therapy for duodenal ulcer disease. Rather their main use has been as an adjunct to antacids or to cimetidine. Anticholinergics can enhance the inhibitory effect on acid secretion of cimetidine, and prolong the hypochlorhydric state for over 5 hours. Thus, these agents are recommended as additional therapy in patients unresponsive to cimetidine or to antacids, in patients with nocturnal pain, and in patients with gastrinoma (Zollinger-Ellison syndrome—see below). If relief of nocturnal pain or prolongation of the effect of antacids or cimetidine is the aim, it seems reasonable to use an anticholinergic drug that may provide a longer duration of effect. Glycopyrrolate (Robinul), 1 to 2 mg is a typical long acting anticholinergic that may be most appropriate at bedtime.

There is no indication that anticholinergics are helpful in the treatment of gastric ulcer. Indeed, these drugs may inhibit gastric emptying which may prolong gastric ulcer disease. In addition, anticholinergics may impair pyloric sphincter function, resulting in an increased reflux of bile. Thus, in patients with gastric ulcers, these drugs may actually be harmful and should not be used.

The side effects of anticholinergic therapy include dry mouth, urinary retention, constipation, and aggravation of glaucoma. Gastroesophageal reflux (see above) may also be aggravated. In patients with marked pyloric deformity secondary to chronic ulcer disease, anticholinergic therapy may decrease gastric motility and cause gastric outlet obstruction.

Other Agents

Carbenoxalone, bismuth, and prostaglandins are additional drugs, not yet licensed for routine use in this country, that may have some beneficial effect on ulcer healing. *Carbenoxalone* has been extensively studied in Europe with improved healing rates of both duodenal and gastric ulcers. Aldosterone-like side effects have limited its usefulness. *Bismuth* has been demonstrated to be equally effective in a small number of studies. Its mode of action, like carbenoxalone, is unknown, but binding of pepsin or improvement in mucosal resistance to ulceration are possible mechanisms. *Prostaglandins* are currently being investigated for their protective effect against gastric erosions and ulcerations.

Summary of Medical Therapy: Recommendations

DUODENAL ULCER

Therapy for acute duodenal ulcers involves the following: (a) avoidance of cigarette smoking; (b) intensive antacid therapy (equivalent to 30 ml of Mylanta-II, given at 1 and 3 hours following meals and at bedtime) or cimetidine 300 mg q.i.d., preferably before meals and at bedtime. For the patient with nocturnal pain, adding an anticholinergic agent such as glycopyrrolate (Robinul, 1 mg) or propantheline bromide (Pro-Banthine, 15 mg) at bedtime may be beneficial. Doubling the dose of antacids at night may also be helpful. This therapy should be continued for 4 to 6 weeks (even if all symptoms have been relieved earlier) by which time ulcers will have healed in over 80% of patients. Follow-up X-ray or endoscopy is generally not indicated, and therapy can be discontinued at this time.

Peptic symptoms are usually relieved by antacids or cimetidine within 2 or 3 days. If the patient has failed to respond, re-evaluation is important to be certain that the symptoms are indeed due to ulcer disease. The addition of antacids with cimetidine, or the addition of an anticholinergic drug may be helpful to patients who have continuing peptic disease. Identification of potentially aggravating factors such as stress or continued cigarette smoking should be made. The value of supportive counseling (Chapter 10) and of the short term use of drugs to relieve anxiety (Chapter 12) also should not be forgotten.

GASTRIC ULCER

There is less evidence in general that the recommended medical therapy is more helpful than placebo in the treatment of patients with gastric ulcers. Patients should be instructed to discontinue cigarette smoking and the use of aspirin. Other gastric irritants such as alcohol should also be avoided. Antacids or cimetidine should be used in the same doses as recommended for the treatment of duodenal ulcer. Therapy should be continued until complete healing of the ulcer has been documented. Evaluation (X-rays or endoscopy) should be made at 6 weeks following initial identification of the ulcer, and if the ulcer persists, again at 12 weeks. If the ulcer persists despite 3 months of medical therapy, the physician should again make certain, by endoscopy, that the lesion is benign. If the ulcer is felt to be benign, the decision to continue medical therapy is generally based on the patient's clinical condition, the degree of healing that has already occurred, and the risks of complications and recurrences *versus* the risk of surgery.

Maintenance Therapy

Patients with peptic ulcer disease should be made aware that ulcers frequently recur, and that the propensity to form new ulcers persists for a long, but probably not indeterminate, period of time. Theoretically, if one could safely reduce the frequency of these recurrences, one could markedly reduce the morbidity and complication rates of ulcer disease. Cimetidine and anticholinergics have both been investigated in this regard. Several studies have confirmed the preventive role of maintenance cimetidine therapy in doses ranging from 400 mg at bedtime to 400 mg twice a day. The cumulative recurrence rate for patients maintained on placebo, after documented healing of the index duodenal ulcer, was 83% over a 1-year period compared to 18% on cimetidine maintenance therapy (1). Thus, both symptomatic and asymptomatic, but endoscopically identified, recurrences can be markedly reduced in frequency by such therapy. The long term benefit and safety of the therapy remains unresolved. Anticholinergics, given at full doses, also reduce the incidence of symptomatic recurrences.

Even though maintenance therapy is effective, the indications for it are still unclear. In most studies, patients with recurrent ulcers tend to have severe long standing ulcer disease. It is certainly possible that in many other patients, the risk of recurrence is relatively low, and the need for preventive measures may not be as great. Long term safety of treatment is still of some concern. Thus, maintenance therapy is probably not indicated in all patients after their first ulcer but should be reserved for the patient with severe disease judged by frequent complications (e.g., recurrent hemorrhage) or frequent symptomatic recurrences. In such patients, maintenance therapy with cimetidine, 400 mg at bedtime or twice a day for 1 year, may be indicated. Further evaluation of this problem is still needed.

SURGICAL THERAPY

Surgery is effective therapy for the relief of ulcer symptoms and for the prevention of ulcer recurrence. While certain postoperative problems are common, the vast majority of patients feel significantly better after surgery. Thus, in the appropriate setting, surgery should be considered as a good and effective alternative form of therapy, rather than as a punishment for failure to respond to medical therapy.

Indications

The indications for ulcer surgery are perforation, hemorrhage, gastric outlet obstruction, and intractability. At times, obviously, surgery is performed as an emergency, but often it is performed after a prolonged period of symptomatic ulcer disease. Intractability is probably the weakest indication for ulcer surgery, although it may be the one most commonly used. It should be recognized that intractability may be due to the disease itself, to the patient's noncompliance with an appropriate medical regimen, or to insufficient medical therapy provided by the clinician. Thorough review with the patient of maximal medical therapy as outlined above will help delineate the cause for the refractoriness of the medical therapy.

Prior to surgery, except for emergency situations, some preoperative assessment should be made to rule out Zollinger-Ellison syndrome (see below) and hypercalcemia.

Types of Operations

A variety of operations are available for the treatment of ulcer disease. The physician should discuss with the surgeon the various alternatives and reach an agreement about which operation may be best suited for the individual patient. Of course, the final decision is generally made by the surgeon in the operating room after he has evaluated the gastroduodenal area. The patient should also be educated about the rationale for the planned surgical approach and what the expected outcome is.

DUODENAL ULCER

For duodenal ulcer disease, surgery involves a vagotomy plus either a drainage procedure or a concomitant gastric resection. Vagotomy is indicated as it reduces basal acid secretion and reduces the sensitivity of the parietal cells to various stimuli, including gastrin. There are three types of vagal resections; (a) truncal, (b) gastric (selective), and (c) proximal gastric (parietal cell or superselective). *Truncal vagotomy* involves division of the main vagal fibers as they pass through the esophageal hiatus. All other abdominal organs that are innervated by the vagus nerve, in addition to the stomach, are therefore affected by this form of vagotomy. In addition, the vagotomy interferes with antral motility and gastric emptying. Thus, to prevent gastric stasis, a drainage procedure (pyloroplasty) is required in conjunction with this type of operation.

Selective or gastric vagotomy was introduced in order to avoid the unnecessary effect of the truncal vagotomy on extragastric sites. Selective vagotomy is effective in reducing acid secretion. However, as it impairs gastric emptying, a drainage procedure must be employed with this operation also. The loss of control of gastric emptying and the ablation of the pyloric sphincter are themselves major causes for various postgastrectomy complications. As a result the usefulness of this form of vagotomy is limited.

Proximal gastric or parietal cell vagotomy is an attempt to inhibit acid secretion only, and to avoid significant disruption of normal gastric motility. The operation involves cutting of the vagal branches innervating the body of the stomach, but preserving the antral fibers. Thus, with a properly performed operation a drainage procedure is believed to be unnecessary. As a result, this type of operation, which does not involve any gastric resection or formation of an anastomosis, has a very low mortality rate, avoids early postoperative complications such as suture breakdown and fistulization, and significantly reduces postgastrectomy complications such as diarrhea and the dumping syndrome (see below). Early experience, or perhaps inexperience, with this procedure has resulted in an ulcer recurrence rate that approaches that of a truncal vagotomy and pyloroplasty—about 6 to 8%—and in some cases even exceeds that level. However, it certainly appears that as surgeons become more experienced and skilled with this procedure, parietal cell vagotomy will become the procedure of choice for ulcer disease.

Currently, two of the most commonly employed operations are *vagotomy plus pyloroplasty* (V + P), and *vagotomy plus antrectomy* (V + A). Some surgeons extend the antrectomy (distal 20% of the stomach) to a hemigastrectomy (resection of 50% of the stomach). The advantages of V + P are that it is technically an easier procedure and is associated with a lower mortality (less than 1%). The major disadvantage is a higher ulcer recurrence rate (6 to 8%). Vagotomy plus resection is technically more time-consuming and involves formation of an anastomosis; therefore, it may cause a higher immediate postoperative morbidity, as well as a higher mortality rate. However, when performed by an experienced surgeon electively on a stable patient, the reported mortality is only 1% and the recurrence rate is also 1% or less. Thus, in the elderly unstable patient, V + P may be the most appropriate procedure. However, in the young patient, the concern over the rate of recurrent disease is an important consideration, and V + A may then be the most appropriate form of surgery.

GASTRIC ULCER

For gastric ulcers the type of surgery is less certain, as our understanding of the condition is less clear. In contrast to duodenal ulcer disease a vagotomy may not be indicated in all patients with a gastric ulcer undergoing surgery. However, in patients who have evidence of concomitant duodenal ulcer disease (approximately 10 to 40% of patients with gastric ulcers) and in patients who have pyloric ulcers, which generally behave as duodenal ulcers, a vagotomy is clearly indicated. If the ulcer is within the antrum, an antrectomy or hemigastrectomy which includes the ulcer is frequently the preferred operation. When the ulcer cannot be included in the gastric resection, a full thickness biopsy of the ulcer should be taken for frozen section to rule out malignancy. The recurrence rate for gastric ulcers after these types of operation is very low (1 to 2%).

Following antrectomy or hemigastrectomy, the stomach may be anastomosed to the duodenum (Bilroth I anastomosis) or to the jejunum (Bilroth II). The type of anastomosis is determined by the surgeon based on the degree of duodenal deformity and on technical considerations.

Postgastrectomy Syndromes

A wide variety of problems develop in the postgastrectomy state (Table 33.4). In 10% of patients, the postgastrectomy complications are severe. Many of these conditions result from the altered physiology created by the surgery. An appreciation of the pathophysiology of these problems is important to their overall management.

POSTCIBAL SYMPTOMS: PAIN; VOMITING; EARLY SATIETY; AND THE DUMPING SYNDROME

The most common complaints of the postgastrectomy patient are early satiety and postcibal vomiting, frequently accompanied by epigastric pain. These complaints occur commonly (25 to 60% of patients in

Table 33.4
Range of Reported Prevalence (Percent) of Various Problems after Ulcer Surgery[a]

Problem	V + P	V + A	STG-BII	STG-BI
Gastrointestinal symptoms (excluding diarrhea)	25–65	34–63	3–51	40
Hypoglycemic symptoms	6–12	4–16	1–12	—
Diarrhea	16–30	1–43	2–17	18
Weight loss	5–39	10–42	25–44	36
Anemia	3–18	7	9–44	17
Bone disease	—	—	1–13	—

[a] From J. Meyer: Chronic morbidity after ulcer surgery, p. 960, in *Gastrointestinal Disease*, edited by M. Sleisenger and J. Fordtran. W. B. Saunders, Philadelphia, 1978.
[b] V + P, vagotomy plus pyloroplasty; V + A, vagotomy plus antrectomy; STg-BII, subtotal gastrectomy with Bilroth-II anastomosis; STg-BI, subtotal gastrectomy with Bilroth-I anastomosis.

various series, usually within 3 or 4 months) in both vagotomized and nonvagotomized patients who have undergone either simple drainage procedures or more extensive gastric resections. The exact cause of these problems is not known.

There is evidence to suggest that postcibal complications are related to the entry of fluid into the small bowel. The timing of these symptoms occurs at periods coincident with the transit of solutions from the stomach into the intestine (first 30 min following a meal). Distension of the proximal bowel may produce many of the same symptoms. Vomiting, when it occurs, is usually of small volume and is bile-stained. Vagotomy inhibits the fundic relaxation that occurs with swallowing food. As the stomach fails to distend, liquids in particular, are emptied into the small bowel more rapidly, resulting in distension of the intestine as well as in a rapid delivery of hypertonic fluids.

The postprandial complaints may be associated with vasomotor phenomena, such as light-headedness, diaphoresis, and postural hypotension. The combination of these vasomotor conditions and the above alimentary complaints is commonly referred to as "the dumping syndrome." The pathogenesis of this syndrome is unknown. However, current concepts center around the effect of various hormones (serotonin, gastric inhibitory peptide) which can induce experimentally similar vasomotor phenomena. These hormones may be released by intestinal distension and/or the influx of hypertonic solutions into the jejunum. In addition, hypertonic solutions may draw excess fluid into the intestinal lumen, causing hypovolemia. However, the role that transient hypovolemia plays in the dumping syndrome is uncertain as prevention of it does not regularly prevent symptoms of the syndrome.

Management of this condition is aimed at slowing gastric emptying and avoiding hypertonic solutions and overdistension of the intestine. The patient should be instructed to eat frequent small meals that are high in protein and low in carbohydrates. It is important that patients do not drink while eating a meal, as liquids accelerate gastric emptying. Lying down after a meal may be helpful as it slows down gastric emptying and may also reduce the intensity of the vasomotor symptoms.

The postcibal complaints must be differentiated from other postoperative causes of epigastric pain and vomiting. Afferent loop obstruction, gastric outlet obstruction, recurrent ulcerations at the anastomosis, and reflux gastritis all must be considered in the patient who complains of postprandial pain and vomiting. *Partial afferent loop obstruction* is an uncommon complication but deserves special attention as it is surgically remediable. Pain occurs as the obstructed afferent limb distends with pancreatic and biliary secretions that are increased in volume following a meal. Vomiting is typically bilious and contains little if any food. The diagnosis can be made by the radiographic demonstration of a dilated limb that is slow to empty. During endoscopy it may be impossible to pass the endoscope into the afferent loop. When the diagnosis is established, surgical revision is necessary.

Gastric outlet obstruction on the other hand is usually associated with vomiting of a large volume of undigested food. X-ray studies and endoscopy can demonstrate the nature of the obstruction. It may be caused by scarring or by surgical deformity at the anastomosis as well as by recurrent ulcerations.

Anastomotic ulcers should clearly be considered as a potential cause for postprandial pain and vomiting. They may occur at any time after the operation—even years later. The preoperative history of pain-food-relief no longer applies to anastomotic ulcers. Conventional X-ray studies in the postgastrectomy state usually do not identify these marginal ulcers. Air-contrast studies and, preferably, endoscopy are more sensitive in the detection of these recurrent lesions (see p. 277).

With loss or bypass of the pyloric sphincter, bile can reflux freely into the stomach, an event that is routinely seen on endoscopy in the patient after gastrectomy. It is believed, with some experimental data as support, that chronic perfusion of the gastric mucosa with bile leads to acute and possibly chronic *gastritis*. However, the correlation between the severity of the symptoms and the severity of the gross and microscopic appearance of the gastritis is very poor. Perianastomotic gastritis is commonly seen on endoscopy whether or not the patient has symptoms. Thus, it is sometimes very difficult to be certain that the symptoms of epigastric pain and bilious vomiting are due to the gastritis seen on endoscopy. When the gastritis is severe as judged by endoscopy and histologic evaluation, and no other cause or explanation for the symptoms is apparent, the diagnosis of bile gastritis (alkaline or reflux gastritis) is usually made. Various kinds of treatment have been proposed for this difficult condition. Medical therapy is of unproven value. Most patients are hypochlorhydric and further effort to reduce acid secretion by cimetidine or antacids is rarely helpful. Amphojel, an aluminum hydroxide-containing antacid (Table 33.3), binds bile salts and has been advocated as potentially useful in this condition but there are few data to support that contention. Similarly, cholestyramine, a resin which binds bile salts, is of no benefit. In isolated reports, some patients are said to have benefited from metaclopramide (Reglan) a smooth muscle stimulant, which improves gastric emptying, but again, value of this drug for this condition is uncertain. Surgery has provided the most consistently beneficial results in patients with bile gastritis. Formation of a Roux-en-Y anastomosis with diversion of the bile away from the stomach, is often very effective. Thus, in the select patient with a troublesome condition, a second operation to divert the bile downstream may be necessary.

DIARRHEA

Chronic diarrhea occurs in 10 to 40% of patients following ulcer surgery, usually within 3 to 4 months of the operation. It is much less common when only a parietal cell vagotomy is performed. In some studies, the severity and prevalence of the diarrhea has decreased with time after the initial surgery, but in the prospective VA study on ulcer surgery there was no difference in the prevalence of the diarrhea at 2 and 5 years postoperatively (11). Multiple factors have been suggested as causes for the diarrhea, and in some patients, several factors may be working in concert. Causes for the diarrhea that are related to the ulcer surgery include (a) increase in fecal bile acids, (b) rapid gastric emptying, (c) rapid intestinal transit, (d) lactose intolerance, (e) development of malabsorption, (f) gastrocolic fistula, (g) Zollinger-Ellison syndrome, and (h) inadvertent gastroileal anastomosis. The evaluation of chronic diarrhea in general is discussed in Chapter 35.

Increased loss of bile acids into the colon has been reported in a number of series of patients after gastrectomy. Bile salts, when they reach the colon, may promote mucosal secretions which lead to diarrhea. Clinically, many postgastrectomy patients with diarrhea have responded to cholestyramine, which binds bile salts. This abnormality in the handling of bile salts has been attributed to the vagotomy and therefore is often referred to as "postvagotomy diarrhea." The mechanism by which the vagotomy alters bile salt absorption or secretion is unknown.

Rapid gastric emptying may contribute to the diarrhea in several ways. The effects of the delivery of the hypertonic volume to the small intestine have been discussed above in association with the dumping syndrome. In addition, patients with latent lactose intolerance may develop diarrhea as their low level of the intestinal enzyme, lactase, is overwhelmed by the rapid delivery of a lactose load. Thus, lactose-restricted diets may also be beneficial in such patients.

Significant *malabsorption* (greater than 12 to 15% fecal fat excretion) is a rare complication of the postgastrectomy state. Mild degrees of steatorrhea are common, however, resulting from poor mixing of food with pancreatic and biliary secretions, rapid transit, and maldigestion of food stuffs. Additionally, bacterial overgrowth may occur in the afferent loop. Rarely, a patient with latent celiac disease may be revealed by ulcer surgery.

The evaluation of malabsorption and diarrhea is discussed in detail in Chapter 35. Pancreatic insufficiency may be difficult to diagnose in the setting of a Bilroth II operation and therapeutic trials of pancreatic enzymes may be needed. X-ray studies may disclose a gastrojejunal-colonic fistula that leads to diarrhea and, frequently, to feculent vomiting. The Zollinger-Ellison syndrome (see below) should be considered in any patient with coexisting ulcer disease and diarrhea. When significant malabsorption is present a bile salt breath test and small bowel biopsy are indicated to look for bacterial overgrowth and for primary small bowel disease such as sprue (see Chapter 35).

Therapeutically, any or all of the following may be beneficial, depending on the results of evaluation of the diarrhea: (a) lactose-restricted diet, (b) treatment for dumping syndrome and rapid gastric emptying with small frequent feedings and with liquids taken only between meals, (c) trial of cholestyramine—one scoop (4 g) q.i.d. which often can be reduced to a lower dosage once the diarrhea is controlled, and (d) antidiarrheal medications, like Lomotil or Imodium taken with meals to decrease the intestinal rush. The symptomatic treatment of diarrhea is discussed also in Chapter 35.

WEIGHT LOSS

Weight loss occurs in 30 to 40% of patients after ulcer surgery. While it is generally believed that weight loss is more common or more significant after subtotal gastrectomy than after vagotomy and drainage, the results of prospective surgical series are conflicting. It is important to recognize, however, that as with most postgastrectomy problems, weight loss is not strictly correlated with a reduction in the size of the stomach.

The most common cause of weight loss is a reduction in caloric intake. Patients may eat less following surgery because of: (a) early satiety, (b) symptoms of the dumping syndrome, (c) postprandial abdominal pain, and (d) attempts to avoid postprandial diarrhea. The mechanisms and management of these postprandial problems are discussed above. It is important to review these aspects of the postgastrectomy state with the patient to identify the factors contributing to the weight loss. Encouraging the patient to consume small feedings and even to supplement his diet with high caloric additives, such as Ensure or Precision, may be helpful.

Other causes for significant weight loss include (a) malabsorption, (b) development of gastro-jejunal-colic fistula, and (c) development of carcinoma in the gastric remnant. While malabsorption is common following ulcer surgery, it is usually minimal. Fecal excretion of fat rarely exceeds 15% of oral intake after V + P or even after subtotal gastrectomy with gastrojejunostomy. Nitrogen loss also does not play a significant role. An increase in oral intake by 10% would compensate for the degree of fecal loss of fat and nitrogen. Infrequently, the steatorrhea exceeds 15% and contributes to significant weight loss. Causes for this degree of malabsorption include (a) celiac sprue unmasked by the gastric surgery, (b) pancreatic insufficiency, and (c) bacterial overgrowth. As these conditions require specific therapy, in the patient with significant weight loss (greater than 10% preoperative weight), malabsorption should be docu-

mented by measurement of fecal fat excretion over a 72-hour period. When greater than 12 to 15% excretion is found, patients should be evaluated for these specific causes of malabsorption. Consultation with a gastroenterologist is recommended under these circumstances. A small bowel biopsy and evaluation for bacterial overgrowth (bile salt breath test (Chapter 35), Schilling test (Chapter 35), or quantification of intestinal bacteria) will usually be performed.

ANEMIA

Anemia may occur following any of the traditional operations used in treatment of peptic ulcer disease; the prevalence is somewhat higher after gastrojejunostomy (9 to 44%) compared to other operations (less than 20%). The anemia occurs gradually, usually several years postoperatively. By far the most common cause is iron deficiency due to chronic blood loss, secondary to recurrent ulcer disease or, more often, to stomal gastritis. Much less commonly, macrocytic anemia, due to folate or vitamin B_{12} deficiency, occurs: folate deficiency because of poor intake in anorectic patients or to malabsorption (see above); B_{12} deficiency because of loss of intrinsic factor-secreting parietal cells in patients with high subtotal gastrectomies or because of malabsorption due to bacterial overgrowth in the small intestine. (The diagnosis and treatment of macrocytic anemia are discussed in Chapter 46.)

RECURRENT ULCER

Recurrent ulceration following ulcer surgery is uncommon. However, management of this complication is often difficult and frequently requires a second operative procedure. Recurrences commonly occur within the first 2 years after the initial surgery but may occur many years later. The type of initial surgery influences the rate of recurrence, with less than a 1% recurrence rate after vagotomy and resection, 6 to 8% after vagotomy plus pyloroplasty, and up to 36% after resection of less than two-thirds of the stomach without vagotomy. Recurrence rate after parietal cell vagotomy is reported to be anywhere from 0 to 25%. The recurrent ulcers occur near the anastomosis, most commonly on the intestinal side.

The cardinal features of recurrent ulcer are abdominal pain, weight loss, and gastrointestinal bleeding. The pain is often in the left upper quadrant or to the left of the epigastrium. The relationship of the pain to meals is variable; it may actually be exacerbated by eating so that food is avoided and marked loss of weight ensues. Bleeding occurs in two-thirds of patients and may present as an overt gastrointestinal hemorrhage. Nausea and vomiting are frequent nonspecific findings. The recurrent ulcer with its attendant edema may lead to gastric outlet obstruction or even to afferent loop obstruction. A dramatic presentation is that of feculent vomiting with severe diarrhea, indicative of the formation of a gastrojejunal-colic fistula.

The diagnosis can be confirmed by radiographic and endoscopic studies. Single contrast upper gastrointestinal series, however, reveals anastomotic ulcers in only 50% of cases in which they are present. Air contrast X-rays may improve this yield. Endoscopy is the most sensitive technique and distinguishes between recurrent ulcerations and severe gastritis.

An evaluation must be made of the underlying cause of the recurrent ulcer. The most common cause is an inadequate surgical procedure (12). In some patients, an incomplete (or no) vagotomy was performed, while in others inadequate gastric resection was done. In cases where the recurrent ulcer develops on the gastric side of the anastomosis, inadequate drainage or gastric emptying should be considered. Zollinger-Ellison syndrome (see below) should always be considered, as over one-fourth of patients with this syndrome have already undergone at least one ulcer operation before the appropriate diagnosis is made.

In patients with a recurrent gastric ulcer, special consideration should be given to the possibility of a gastric malignancy and endoscopy should be performed routinely.

Both medical and surgical therapy have their place in the management of the postoperative recurrent ulcer. Therapy with antacids is not very successful. Recently however, cimetidine has been demonstrated to heal anastomotic ulcers effectively in a small group of patients (4); the long term course of these patients is still unknown.

To the dismay of the patient, a second operation is at times required to control the ulcer disease. The type of reoperation is frequently determined by the initial operation, with risk of recurrences still a problem. As a general rule, repeat vagotomy and gastric resection are required, with more limited operations resulting in a high frequency of a second recurrence. For patients with an initial adequate resection (two-thirds gastrectomy), a repeat abdominal or even a thoracic vagotomy may be all that is needed.

Gastric irradiation may be an alternative for the inoperable patient as it may result in reduction in acid secretion for about 6 months and allow one ulcer to heal. The consultant gastroenterologist should advise the generalist in this regard.

BONE DISEASE

Defects in bone formation and metabolism may occur after ulcer surgery. Osteomalacia and osteoporosis have been reported, but are thought to be rare following vagotomy and drainage procedures. Fractures are more common in the postgastrectomy patient. Malabsorption of vitamin D and/or calcium are believed to be responsible for the bone disease. Patients generally present with recurrent fractures or with back pain due to a collapsed vertebra. Therapy includes supplemental calcium or vitamin D. While the incidence of symptoms is low, this problem may accentuate other conditions that also lead to osteoporosis such as in postmenopausal women or in patients taking corticosteroids.

CARCINOMA IN THE GASTRIC REMNANT

The development of gastric carcinoma years after ulcer surgery has only recently been recognized. In reported series, the carcinoma develops more than 15 years following the initial surgery (7). It is difficult to ascertain the true risk of this rare complicaton as many of these patients are now elderly and are therefore at an age when the incidence of gastric carcinoma in the general population is at its peak. It is believed that as a result of gastric surgery, there is constant free reflux of bile into the stomach. This enterogastric reflux has been shown in animals to result in alterations in the gastric mucosa, gradually evolving from chronic to atrophic gastritis and then to neoplastic changes. Similarly, in patients, one can demonstrate chronic gastritis around the anastomosis. It is in this area that most of the gastric remnant carcinomas develop. The clinical features include abdominal pain, weight loss, and bleeding. The diagnosis is often difficult as the radiographic appearance of the "normal" gastric remnant frequently consists of hyperplastic folds and irregularity of the anastomosis. Endoscopy with biopsy may be the most helpful means of recognizing the carcinomatous changes. The prognosis is reported to be poor in this type of gastric cancer.

ZOLLINGER-ELLISON SYNDROME

The Zollinger-Ellison syndrome represents a prototype of the relationship of gastrin, acid secretion, and ulcer formation. The syndrome results from a non-beta-islet-cell tumor of the pancreas that autonomously secretes gastrin, and is therefore called a *gastrinoma*. In the majority of cases there are multiple tumors, most commonly found in the head of the pancreas. They vary considerably in size from several millimeters, often undetectable at surgery, to huge masses that may even be palpable through the abdominal wall. Approximately two-thirds of gastrinomas are malignant in their biologic behavior and histologic appearance; they can metastasize and be a cause of death, although generally they are slow growing.

With the introduction of readily available measurement of gastrin, the concept of the clinical features of the Zollinger-Ellison syndrome have begun to change. The original description of the syndrome focused on the virulent nature of the ulcer diathesis and on the atypical location for the ulcers. It is now recognized, however, that 75% of ulcers in patients with Zollinger-Ellison syndrome occur in the duodenal bulb and appear as routine single duodenal ulcers. The finding, however, of postbulbar and jejunal ulcerations should alert the physician to the possibility of the syndrome. Over one-quarter of patients undergo ulcer surgery before the diagnosis of the syndrome, which is usually made only when anastomotic ulcers develop. Diarrhea is another frequent symptom, occurring in more than one-third of patients, which may precede the formation of ulcers by several years; however, 7% of patients have diarrhea and never develop an ulcer.

Diagnosis

The diagnosis of the Zollinger-Ellison syndrome should be suspected under the following conditions: (a) failure of medical therapy, resulting in the need for ulcer surgery; (b) giant ulcer; (c) multiple ulcers; (d) postbulbar or jejunal ulcers; (e) anastomotic ulcer; (f) ulcer disease in association with diarrhea (but not diarrhea secondary to drugs); and (g) radiographic or secretory evidence of gastric hypersecretion.

The diagnosis of the Zollinger-Ellison syndrome is usually based on the fasting serum gastrin concentration. Elevations greater than 1000 pg/ml in association with the typical clinical picture are nearly diagnostic of a gastrinoma.

However, in patients with mild elevations of the serum gastrin concentration (*i.e.*, between 150 and 300 pg/ml), and in postoperative patients, differentiation between Zollinger-Ellison syndrome and other causes for hypergastrinemia is important. Consultation with a gastroenterologist is advisable. Other conditions that may lead to hypergastrinemia include (a) retained antrum, (b) G-cell hyperplasia, (c) postvagotomy plus pyloroplasty, (d) small portion of population with routine duodenal ulcer disease, and (e) pernicious anemia.

Differentiation of these disorders from the Zollinger-Ellison syndrome requires the use of provocative tests, the secretin and calcium infusion tests, generally performed by a gastroenterologist. The secretin test is preferred as it is more reliable and is safer. In both tests, the response of the serum gastrin level to the infusion of a stimulating substance is monitored. In the *secretin test*, the serum gastrin level rises, usually within the first half-hour, after the injection of secretin in patients with Zollinger-Ellison syndrome, whereas in all other disorders, the gastrin level falls or is unchanged.

In the *calcium infusion test*, serum gastrin determinations are made immediately before and then repeatedly for 4 hours after the intravenous administration of calcium. In all conditions, the gastrin level increases. However, in the Zollinger-Ellison syndrome, the response is exaggerated with a greater than 50% rise over basal levels.

Gastric analysis (see above, p. 278) may provide further supportive data. Marked hypersecretion is found in both the basal state and following pentagastrin stimulation. Since the stomach is being influenced by an autonomous tumor, further stimulation with exogenous pentagastrin provides little additional stimulation to secretion. Thus, the BAO/MAO ratio is 0.6 or greater in this syndrome. However, there is considerable overlap with normal values so that the gastric secretory data alone cannot be used to make the diagnosis.

A variety of attempts have been made to localize the gastrinoma in the hope that excision of an isolated tumor would be curative. Unfortunately, such efforts have not been successful as multiple tumors are frequently present; small lesions are undetectable by surgical inspection of the pancreas; and these tumors frequently have metastasized by the time surgical exploration is performed. The recent use of selective pancreatic venography with measurements of gastrin levels from each venous site may provide an improved method to localize the gastrinoma.

Therapy

Because the tumor mass is rarely localized and curable by local resection, therapy has been directed at the end organ. Total gastrectomy has been the procedure of choice. While there is little evidence to suggest that gastrectomy alters the biologic behavior of the gastrinoma, it does prevent the consequences of the hypersecretion of acid. In the past, patients died from this condition most often because of the virulent nature of the ulcer diathesis, including frequent recurrences, diarrhea, and even malabsorption, as well as multiple operations. Complete removal of the end organ prevents these complications.

More recently, medical therapy has been successful in controlling the ulcer disease and the diarrhea. Cimetidine, a histamine (H_2) receptor antagonist, is capable of inhibiting gastric acid secretion in response to a variety of stimuli (see p. 280). For most patients with gastrinoma, the standard dose of cimetidine, 1200 mg per day, is sufficient to control acid production. In a small percentage, increased doses of cimetidine or the addition of an anticholinergic drug is needed. Such medically treated patients are, obviously, required to take medications frequently and for many years, probably the rest of their lives. Thus, while this may be a major disadvantage in some patients, it is important to recognize that medical therapy can provide an effective alternative to total gastrectomy (9). Even if surgery is performed, medical therapy can provide time to stabilize the patient, to correct nutritional deficiencies, and to allow the surgery to be performed on an elective basis.

References

General

Ippoliti, A and Peterson, W: The pharmacology of peptic ulcer disease. *Clin. Gastroenterol.* 8: 53, 1979
   Recent update on use of various medications. Provides good comparative analysis.

Specific

1. Bodemar, G and Walan, A: Maintenance treatment of recurrent peptic ulcer by cimetidine. *Lancet* 1: 403, 1978.

2. Conn, HO and Blitzer, BL: Non-association of adrenocorticoid therapy and peptic ulcer. *N Engl J Med 294:* 473, 1976.
3. Friedman, G Siegelaub, AB and Seltzer, C: Cigarettes, alcohol, coffee, and peptic ulcer. *N Engl J Med 290:* 469, 1974.
4. Gugler, R, Lindstaedt, H and Miederer, S: Cimetidine for anastomotic ulcers after partial gastrectomy. *N Engl J Med 301:* 1077, 1979.
5. Hanscom, D and Buchman, E: The follow-up period (V.A. Cooperative Study on Gastric Ulcer). *Gastroenterology 61:* 585, 1971.
6. Johnston, D, Pickford, IR, Walker, BE and Goligher, JC: Highly selective vagotomy for duodenal ulcer: do hypersecretors need antrectomy. *Br Med J 1:* 716, 1975.
7. Kobayashi, S, Prolla, J and Kirsner, J: Late gastric carcinoma developing after surgery for benign conditions. *Am J Digest Dis 15:* 905, 1970.
8. Korman, MG, Hetzel, D, Hansky, J, et al.: Relapse rate of duodenal ulcer after cessation of long-term cimetidine treatment. A double blind controlled study. *Digest Dis Sci 25:* 88, 1980.
9. McCarthy, D: The place of surgery in the Zollinger-Ellison syndrome. *N Engl J Med 302:* 1344, 1980.
10. Peterson, WL, Sturdevant, RAL, Frankl, HD, et al.: Healing of duodenal ulcer with an antacid regimen. *N Engl J Med 297:* 341, 1977.
11. Postlethwait, RW: Five year followup: results of operation for duodenal ulcer. *Surg Gynecol Obstet 137:* 387, 1973.
12. Stabile, B and Passaro, E: Recurrent peptic ulcer. *Gastroenterology 70:* 124, 1976.

CHAPTER THIRTY-FOUR

Gastrointestinal Bleeding

HAROLD J. TUCKER, M.D.

The presence of blood in the stool is always a significant finding that requires thorough investigation. Gastrointestinal bleeding may present as (a) occult blood, (b) melena (black stool) or intermittent hematochezia (the passage of overtly bloody stool), and (c) massive hemorrhage. The last situation requires immediate hospitalization and, often, emergency diagnostic procedures. (The vomiting of blood, also, almost always dictates immediate hospitalization.) Otherwise, the evaluation of gastrointestinal bleeding often can be performed in an ambulatory setting. Table 34.1 shows the common conditions associated with gastrointestinal bleeding.

TESTS FOR DETECTION OF BLOOD IN STOOL

A variety of tests are available to detect blood in the stool. These tests differ in sensitivity and specificity and therefore differ in their value as indicators of disease. The three commonly used tests for fecal occult blood are the orthotolidine tablet test (Hematest); the dilute alcoholic solution of guaiac test (guaiac); and the modified guaiac slide test (Hemoccult). These tests depend on the enzymatic peroxidase activity of hemoglobin and reflect the concentration of hemoglobin in the stool. In "normal" subjects, the hemoglobin concentration of the stool is less than 2 mg of hemoglobin per gram of stool as measured by tagged red cell assay. Both the guaiac and Hematest assays are extremely sensitive and may be positive at this normal level of fecal hemoglobin concentration. As a result, the false positive rate for these tests is excessively high, 60 and 30%, respectively; that is, evaluation of a patient with a positive stool guaiac test, for example, will be negative 60% of the time.

However, the Hemoccult slide test, because it is less sensitive, has reduced the false positive rate to as low as 1 to 2% (3). If multiple slides (three pairs) are evaluated, the false negative rate for Hemoccult is similar to that of the other tests, approximately 15 to 20%. Therefore, a positive test for occult blood, with the Hemoccult slide test, is highly specific for significant bleeding although only moderately sensitive. Since colonic cancers and polyps may bleed intermittently, multiple specimens should be evaluated. In patients over the age of 40 with at least one positive slide test, about 15% have carcinoma, and another 30% have polyps greater than 5 mm in length (2). In asymptomatic patients with a positive slide

Table 34.1
Common Causes of Gastrointestinal Bleeding

OCCULT BLEEDING
  Colonic polyps
  Colonic cancer
  Peptic ulcer disease
  Gastric cancer
MELENA
  Duodenal ulcer
  Gastric ulcer
  Gastritis
  Gastric carcinoma
  Esophagitis
HEMATOCHEZIA
  Rectal outlet disorders (hemorrhoids, cryptitis, fissures)
  Colonic polyps
  Colonic cancer
  Diverticulosis
  Inflammatory bowel disease
  Angiodysplasia

test who have carcinoma, over 80% have lesions limited to the bowel (2). Thus, a positive Hemoccult test for occult blood in the stool requires further investigation.

Laxatives increase both the number of positive and false positive results of the Hemoccult test (probably by an irritant effect on the normal colonic mucosa and on colonic lesions—such as cancer). For this reason, many screening programs have recommended a high bulk diet for several days before the stool is tested in the hope of maximizing the discovery of occult lesions. False negative results are more likely in patients taking high doses of vitamin C. Oral iron therapy may cause black stool but does not alter the results of the Hemoccult test.

EVALUATION OF PATIENTS WHO HAVE GASTROINTESTINAL BLEEDING

Choosing Appropriate Tests

The history and physical examination direct the sequence of the various tests used to investigate a patient with gastrointestinal bleeding. The patient's age, the nature of associated symptoms, and the severity of bleeding are all important factors. For example, patients with peptic symptoms (Chapter 33) require an initial evaluation of their stomach and duodenum, while patients with a change in bowel habits require an initial evaluation of their colon. In general, patients under the age of 35 are less likely to have a colonic lesion than are patients over 35. Peptic disease and benign rectal lesions are more evenly distributed in adults of all ages.

In asymptomatic patients with occult fecal blood or in patients with hematochezia but with no other symptoms, the lower bowel should be investigated first. In patients with melena but with no other symptoms, the upper gastrointestinal tract should be investigated first. The more precise sequence in which the tests are done is described below.

Lower Gastrointestinal Tract

Proctosigmoidoscopy should always be the first test done in the evaluation of the lower bowel; it should be followed by an air-contrast barium enema (see below). In patients over the age of 35, colonoscopy should be the next test, even if the barium enema is negative.

The finding of hemorrhoids, polyps, or even a rectal cancer on proctoscopy does not obviate the need for a barium study. However, if the pattern of bleeding is consistent with rectal disease (see Chapter 88), if a rectal lesion is seen during proctoscopy, and if the colonic mucosa is well visualized by barium enema and is normal, colonoscopy is not necessary. Also, diverticulosis (see Chapter 37), found on barium enema, should not be considered the cause of intermittent mild hematochezia until colonoscopy has failed to provide another explanation.

PROCTOSIGMOIDOSCOPY

Anorectal lesions either cannot be visualized or are poorly visualized by barium enema. Cryptitis, bleeding hemorrhoids, fissures, and proctitis can only be seen by proctoscopy; and rectal polyps or cancer are much better seen by proctoscopy than by a barium enema. The preparation of the patient for this procedure and the patient's experience during the procedure are described in Chapter 32.

Flexible sigmoidoscopy is a relatively new procedure used to evaluate the descending colon. It has limited value, however, in patients with gastrointestinal bleeding, as colonoscopy is still required to evaluate the possibility of more proximal colonic lesions.

RADIOLOGIC STUDIES

The barium enema is a valuable test in the detection of colonic lesions. Even in patients with suspected anorectal disease, the barium enema is indicated to rule out other lesions, particularly in patients at high risk for polyps and cancer. The barium enema may also detect diverticula, inflammatory bowel disease, strictures, extraluminal masses or intramural filling defects from endometriosis or from metastatic tumor.

The *double (air) contrast barium* technique is preferred in the search for a colonic source of bleeding. This technique has the advantage over the conventional single contrast barium enema in providing much better detail of the mucosa. One study showed that single contrast technique missed as many as 45% of polyps compared to 12% missed by air contrast (7). Early changes of inflammatory bowel disease are also detectable by this technique. However, because of the risk of perforation, the double contrast barium enema should not be requested in patients suspected of having an obstructing lesion or diverticulitis.

Patient Experience. The patient's colon must be cleaned before the study can be performed satisfactorily. A reasonable regimen is the ingestion of 2 to 3 liters of liquids as well as a low residue diet (see Table 35.2, Chapter 35) the day before the examination and administration of a laxative, such as 2 to 4 tablespoons of milk of magnesia at night; on the morning of the examination, a sodium phosphate enema (Fleet) is self-administered. This preparation will be effective in about 90% of patients. Patients who are chronically constipated may need 2 days of preparation.

The patient should be told that the barium will be introduced into his rectum, while he lies on his left side, through a lubricated plastic enema tip; often a balloon is then inflated around the tip to seal the rectal ampulla. He will then be told to lie on his back while the barium is allowed to flow in, intermittently, under fluoroscopic observation. Frequently, cramping is experienced during this process. After the colon is filled, several films will be taken, with the patient in various positions. The barium will then be evacuated. The films will be developed and an additional film will be taken after evacuation. The entire procedure takes 45 to 60 min.

The *air contrast barium enema* differs from the standard technique in that a smaller amount of very dense barium is introduced followed by insufflation of air. All patients experience cramping during this procedure (usually more than is experienced during the standard barium enema), and atropine may be given to inhibit cramping. The patient will be flatulent for several hours after the procedure.

COLONOSCOPY

Colonoscopy is indicated in patients with gastrointestinal bleeding of suspected colonic origin in whom proctosigmoidoscopy and barium enema have not provided an unequivocal diagnosis. In patients with polyps, colonoscopy may also provide a way in which the polyps can be removed without major surgery (see below). An experienced endoscopist can reach the cecum in over 90% of cases. The complications from the procedure are mainly perforation and hemorrhage; the overall complication rate for diagnostic colonoscopy is 0.3 to 0.4%, with a mortality rate of 0.02%. If polypectomy is performed, the morbidity rate increases to 1 to 2%, but the mortality rate remains the same (5).

The sensitivity of colonoscopy in experienced hands is much higher than that of even an air contrast barium enema (see above): only 2% of polyps are not diagnosed. In anemic patients with occult bleeding Tedesco *et al.* (6) showed that colonoscopy revealed polyps (greater than 5 mm) or cancer in 15% of patients with negative barium enema examinations and that, in patients with rectal bleeding, 34% had a significant lesion (including 11% with cancer) when the barium enema was reported as negative or simply as showing diverticulosis.

Patient Experience. Preparation for colonoscopy usually includes a liquid diet for 2 or 3 days and laxatives and enemas (prescribed by the consultant gastroenterologist). Before the procedure, the patient is sedated intravenously (usually with Demerol and Valium). During the procedure, the patient may experience some discomfort when the bowel is distended with air for inspection and as the colonoscope is maneuvered through the bowel lumen. The duration of the procedure is variable, depending on the tortuosity of the colon, the presence of disease, and on the skill of the endoscopist; but, on the average it lasts from 30 to 60 min.

Upper Gastrointestinal Tract

The sequence of tests performed in the evaluation of the upper gastrointestinal tract depends on the diagnosis that is suspected. Usually an upper gastrointestinal series is done first—especially in patients with suspected peptic disease or carcinoma. On the other hand, if an inflammatory process is suspected (esophagitis or gastritis), endoscopy might be done preferentially. If the patient has melena and an upper gastrointestinal series is negative, or reveals a gastric ulcer (Chapter 33) or a tumor, endoscopy should be the next routine procedure. If the upper and lower gastrointestinal tract have been evaluated in a patient with gastrointestinal bleeding, and the studies have been negative, a small bowel series should be considered to investigate the possibility of Crohn's disease and other disorders that affect mainly the small intestine.

RADIOLOGIC STUDIES

The *upper gastrointestinal series* is valuable in the detection of mass lesions in the esophagus and stomach and in identifying gastric and duodenal ulcerations. It is well tolerated, serves as a permanent guide for follow-up evaluation, and is relatively inexpensive. The air contrast technique affords better mucosal detail than the standard study and should be used in the evaluation of gastric and esophageal erosions. The patient's experience during the performance of an upper gastrointestinal series is described in Chapter 33.

The conventional *small bowel series* is very poor at detecting small lesions of the intestine (such as cancer or a leiomyoma). Disorders like Crohn's disease or lymphoma are more likely to be revealed by X-ray (although a definitive diagnosis will only be made by biopsy). These sources of bleeding are relatively uncommon and should be suspected only when the more frequent conditions (peptic ulcer disease, colonic polyps) have been excluded. The patient should be warned that the small bowel series will require him to spend 1 to 5 hours in the radiology waiting room during which time films will be taken every 30 min.

ENDOSCOPY

Upper endoscopy is now a widely used and readily available means of investigating gastrointestinal blood loss. This technique not only is more sensitive than are X-rays but also provides a direct means of obtaining specimens for histologic examination. Because of the increased sensitivity, endoscopy is indicated even if barium studies have been negative. Endoscopy is usually recommended only after barium X-rays have been done, however, because it is less well tolerated, is associated with more risk, is more costly than X-rays, and it can be avoided if a diagnosis can be made radiologically. Further, it is technically easier to perform endoscopy if the location of a lesion has already been identified by X-ray studies.

Patient Experience. Upper endoscopy is an outpatient procedure that usually takes less than 15 min. The patient fasts overnight before the procedure. He is sedated with intravenous medication (Valium and Demerol) and his throat is anesthetized with a topical anesthetic. Some gagging is common during passage of the endoscope into the esophagus. Under direct vision, biopsies and cytologic brushings can be obtained from suspicious lesions and for histologic confirmation. Complications include perforation and bleeding but are extremely uncommon. Use of the "pediatric" endoscope has become increasingly popular as it is very well tolerated by patients and still provides good visualization of the mucosal detail.

SELECTED LESIONS THAT BLEED

The commonest cause of upper gastrointestinal bleeding—peptic disease—is discussed in Chapter 33. Several common causes of lower gastrointestinal bleeding are discussed in other chapters: benign anorectal disorders (Chapter 88), inflammatory bowel disease (Chapter 35), and diverticulosis (Chapter 37).

Colonic Polyps

Colonic polyps should be suspected in any patient over 30 years of age who has gastrointestinal bleeding. Bleeding may be occult or may occur as intermittent hematochezia. The patient is often totally asymptomatic but may complain of a change in bowel habits, abdominal pain, or of passing mucus per rectum. It is believed that all cancers of the colon (excluding those associated with ulcerative colitis, see Chapter 35) arise from these benign epithelial tumors (4). Thus, the way to prevent colonic cancer is to discover and remove polyps before they have become malignant. Although polyps are most common in the rectosigmoid region, they may be found anywhere in the colon. The detection of a polyp on proctoscopy or on barium enema is an indication for referral to a gastroenterologist.

The risk of polyps becoming malignant is related to their histologic type and size. Hyperplastic polyps, the most common type in adults, have no malignant potential. Villous and tubular adenomas, however, carry a definite risk of malignant transformation that increases as they increase in size. The risk that a villous adenoma over 2 cm is cancerous is over 50% (4) (Table 34.2). Fortunately, if the cancer remains confined to the mucosa of the polyp (*carcinoma in situ*), colonoscopic polypectomy is curative. Once the cancer has infiltrated the stalk of the polyp, surgery is indicated. Since the cancerous change in the polyp may be focal, single biopsies of a polyp are not sufficient to exclude the presence of a malignancy.

Table 34.2
Polyps: Relationship of Size, Histological Type, and Risk of Carcinoma

Histological Type	Size		
	Under 1 cm	1–2 cm	Over 2 cm
Tubular adenoma	1.0%	10.2%	34.7%
Intermediate type	3.9%	7.4%	45.8%
Villous adenoma	9.5%	10.3%	52.9%

Once a polyp has been detected, surveillance for additional polyps is essential. In 30% of patients more than one polyp is present at the time of initial investigation. Subsequent development of new polyps occurs in at least 10% of patients. The patient should continue to have yearly tests for occult blood in the stool. The finding of a single positive test is an indication for a repeat evaluation. Even when the stools are negative for blood, periodic evaluation of the colon is still recommended. Colonoscopy or air contrast barium enema should be repeated every 3 to 4 years to detect early lesions.

Multiple polyposis syndromes are rare inherited abnormalities which are significant for their malignant potential. Familial polyposis, Gardner's syndrome, and Turcot's syndrome all are associated with multiple adenomatous polyps of the colon (Fig. 34.1) and therefore carry a high risk of the development of carcinoma. Gardner's syndrome includes osteomas and soft tissue tumors, and Turcot's syndrome, tumors of the central nervous system. Familial polyposis and Gardner's syndrome are inherited as an autosomal dominant defect; Turcot's syndrome, as an autosomal recessive. The diagnosis of a polyposis syndrome is usually made when the patient is in his 20s, with cancer developing some 20 years later. There is considerable controversy about the therapy of these conditions. Colonic resection is indicated but its extent and timing are not uniformly agreed upon. Ideally, when rectal polyps are present, a proctocolectomy should be performed to eliminate the risk of cancer. However, as the patients are generally quite young, the prospect of an ileostomy (see Chapter 38) and of potential sexual dysfunction is often overwhelming to them. Subtotal colectomy with ileal-rectal anastomosis is better tolerated by the patient, but requires frequent evaluations of the rectum with removal of all new polyps. Even then, the risk of rectal carcinoma remains high. Newer operations involving ileorectal pull-through procedures are being studied with early encouraging results. Consultation with a gastroenterologist and gastrointestinal surgeon is recommended as soon as the diagnosis is made.

Colonic polyposis syndromes should be distinguished from conditions associated with juvenile polyps or hamartomas that are of low malignant potential. The *Peutz-Jegher's syndrome* consists of multiple hamartomas, predominantly of the small intestine, associated with buccal and cutaneous pigmentation.

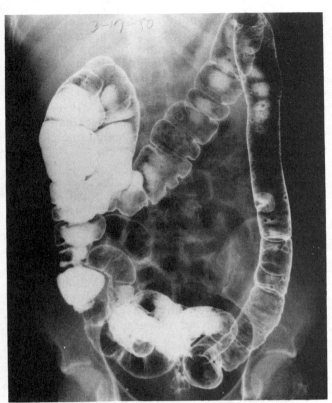

Figure 34.1 Double (air) contrast barium enema performed in a patient with familial polyposis. With this technique, numerous polyps, of varying sizes, may be seen throughout the colon.

While the malignant potential of the hamartomas is low, duodenal and ovarian carcinomas have been reported in 2 to 5% of patients. Rarely *juvenile polyps* may occur throughout the gastrointestinal tract. In the absence of associated extracolonic manifestations, this syndrome is called *generalized juvenile polyposis*; when accompanied by alopecia, nail bed changes, hyperpigmentation, and malabsorption, it is called the *Cronkhite-Canada syndrome*.

Colonic Cancer

EPIDEMIOLOGY AND ETIOLOGY

Colonic carcinoma is one of the most common causes of death from cancer in this country. Its incidence is second only to skin and lung cancer. In an attempt to reduce the high incidence and mortality rate of this cancer, efforts are being directed toward identification of risk factors and toward earlier detection of the lesions.

Colon cancer occurs with increasing frequency in older age groups, with a peak incidence in the 6th and 7th decades. Geographic differences in the mortality rates due to this neoplasm have suggested an etiologic role for dietary and environmental factors. The three main predisposing causes of large bowel cancer are colonic polyps, familial polyposis, and ulcerative colitis (see above and Chapter 35). The

presence of these conditions dictates the need for a strict surveillance program in patients with these conditions, and even, at times, prophylactic surgery to prevent the development of large bowel cancer. (See p. 292 for cancer-polyp association, and p. 306 for risk of cancer in ulcerative colitis.)

SCREENING TESTS

Because of the high incidence of colon cancer, and its precursor, the colonic polyp, screening tests should be performed routinely in all patients over 30 years old The most important and cost effective is the *testing of stool for occult blood*. Six stools should be tested consecutively for occult blood annually by use of the Hemoccult slide test, the most reliable technique (see p. 289). The Hemoccult-II provides a convenient method of checking two different parts of a stool at one time. These slides or cards are convenient for the patient because they can be mailed to the physician's office without a significant loss in the rate of positive reactions. In one study, 80% of patients ultimately found to have colonic cancer after detection of occult blood in their stool in a screening program had disease limited to the bowel (and therefore had a good prognosis) (2).

In addition to multiple tests for occult blood, a *yearly rectal examination* should also be performed in patients over the age of 40. Proctosigmoidoscopy should also be performed in two consecutive years to ensure a normal rectum and rectosigmoid area. Subsequently, proctoscopy can be performed every 3 to 5 years in the asymptomatic patient who has negative tests for fecal blood. Yearly proctoscopy has not proved to be of sufficient additional value to warrant its cost and discomfort.

DIAGNOSIS

History. Unfortunately, most patients with adenocarcinoma of the colon are diagnosed only after symptoms have developed. Less than 5% are asymptomatic at time of diagnosis, and it is in this group, that the highest chance for cure exists. The major symptoms are abdominal pain (25 to 75%) and a change in bowel habits (20 to 50%), either constipation or diarrhea. Abdominal pain is least common in patients with cancer of the rectum, where even large lesions can be accommodated without producing symptoms. Gross blood in the stool is another common complaint, occurring in 75% of patients with rectal cancer and in 30 to 40% of patients with colonic cancer above the rectum. Unfortunately, this hematochezia is frequently mistakenly attributed to hemorrhoids.

Physical Examination. The findings on physical examination vary according to the location and extent of the lesion. The primary tumor may be palpable as an abdominal mass, particularly in lesions of the right colon where lesions can remain "asymptomatic" for long periods of time., Metastatic disease may be suggested by the presence of a large, hard nodular liver, ascites, peripheral adenopathy, or by palpating a mass in the cul-de-sac on rectal exam. Signs of anemia may be present, particularly in cecal and ascending colon lesions that may bleed occultly for months or even years before the diagnosis is made. Most patients will have a positive test for occult blood (at least one) sometime during their course of illness.

Radiologic Studies. The diagnosis of colon cancer is made most often on barium enema. Findings may include a polypoid mass, stenosis, either as a stricture or with an "apple-core" appearance, distortion of the mucosa, and localized rigidity of the bowel wall. At times, distortion or fixation of adjacent structures may be seen. The development of a gastrocolic fistula, best seen on barium enema, is also suggestive of a primary colonic neoplasm.

The accuracy of the radiographic diagnosis of colon cancer is excellent, except at opposite ends of the large bowel. The cecum is often difficult to evaluate because of the inability to cleanse the region completely and, at times, to distinguish a "prominent" ileocecal valve or a sphincter from a mass. The rectum is also difficult to visualize optimally, as frequently it is obscured by the balloon through which the barium is administered. Thus, proctoscopy is essential in any patient suspected of having a colorectal carcinoma.

Endoscopy. The role of endoscopy varies depending on the location of the tumor. Proctosigmoidoscopy with biopsy is the best and most direct method of diagnosing rectal carcinoma. For lesions above the reach of the sigmoidoscope, the accuracy of a well performed barium enema is so high that colonoscopy to obtain preoperative histologic diagnosis is not generally needed. However, it should be recognized that spasm, benign strictures, and even stool can be confused with cancer on radiographic examination and that some polypoid lesions, even if large or sessile, can be removed via the colonoscope.

In addition, colonoscopy does have an important role in the evaluation for other colonic lesions (see p. 291). The prevalence of coexistent polyps in patients with colon cancer is high, ranging from 10 to 30%. These residual polyps may develop later into carcinoma, accounting for the incidence of a second colon cancer in 5 to 10% of patients with cancer of the colon who have been followed for up to 25 years (4). In addition, synchronous colon carcinomas occur in 3 to 5% of patients. Thus, colonoscopy is helpful in ensuring that the rest of the colon is free of neoplastic lesions. Optimally, colonoscopy should be performed preoperatively; otherwise, it should be done within the first year postoperatively.

CARCINOEMBRYONIC ANTIGEN

Carcinoembryonic antigen (CEA) is a normal fetal antigen that is found in the blood of many patients with carcinoma of the colon (about 50% of patients with local disease and about 80% of patients with metastatic disease). It also is found sometimes in the blood of patients with other malignancies or with a variety of benign conditions (including heavy cigarette smoking). Therefore CEA titers are not useful screening tests for the presence of colon cancer.

The assay is helpful, however, in the postoperative management of patients who have CEA in their blood at the time of diagnosis. Persistently elevated CEA levels postoperatively suggest metastatic disease; falling levels that then rise on follow-up evaluation suggest the re-emergence of the malignant tumor, usually at a remote site.

THERAPY

Surgery is the most effective therapy for colon carcinoma. Inoperable low rectal and anal lesions may be treated with radiation. Chemotherapy provides little additional benefit at the present time.

PREOPERATIVE EVALUATION

Prior to surgery, most patients should undergo evaluation for metastatic disease. Liver function tests should be performed routinely. The role of routine liver scan, computerized tomography, and ultrasound of the liver in the diagnosis of hepatic metastasis remains to be determined. In patients with bowel obstruction or bleeding, surgery may still be needed as palliation, despite the presence of liver metastases. In patients asymptomatic from their bowel lesions, the presence of hepatic metastases should deter surgical intervention. However, abnormal liver function tests alone should not be considered absolute evidence of metastatic disease. A histologic diagnosis should be made, if possible. (Needle liver biopsy is a simple way to obtain tissue.) A preoperative CEA level should also be determined as a baseline (see above).

For patients requiring an ostomy, preoperative evaluation by an enterostomal therapist is very helpful, not only to discuss with the patient problems and concerns about the ostomy, but also to mark the proper location of the ostomy preoperatively.

PROGNOSIS

The prognosis for colon carcinoma is based on several variables. The major variable is the extent of the tumor, in terms of its invasion through the bowel wall and of its lymph node involvement (Table 34.3). Vessel invasion and the degree of differentiation of the tumor histologically also affect survival. The pathologist's interpretation of the resected specimen is

Table 34.3
Colon Carcinoma

Classification	Staging and 5-Year Survival	
	Microscopic findings	Percent 5-year survival
A	Disease limited to mucosa	95
B	Tumor extends to serosa	60–70
C	Tumor extends to serosa and nodes involved	<40
D	Distant metastases	<5

much more meaningful than the surgeon's estimation of "curable."

FOLLOW-UP CARE

Most patients undergoing resection of colon cancer do well in the early postoperative period. Diarrhea may be present early, but it is usually transient and is easily controlled with antidiarrheal medication if needed. The patient with a colostomy needs continued follow-up care by the surgeon and the enterostomal therapist to ensure proper functioning and handling of the ostomy (see Chapter 35).

The long term follow-up is aimed at detection of recurrence or spread of the cancer and at continued surveillance for new colonic lesions. Most commonly, metastases occur in adjacent nodes with spread to the liver. Thus, physical examinations, and liver function tests should be performed once a year for several more years. CEA levels should be obtained at similar intervals.

To evaluate for new colonic lesions, or for the infrequent occurrence of tumor at the anastomosis, colonoscopy should be performed within the first 6 to 12 months postoperatively. If no lesions are found, repeat colonoscopy or air-contrast barium enema should be performed about every 3 years. In the interim, yearly evaluation for occult fecal blood loss should be performed with three to six Hemoccult slides. Should any of these slide tests be positive, colonoscopy should be repeated.

Arteriovenous Malformations of Colon

Arteriovenous malformations of the colon may be a source of gastrointestinal bleeding, most often in the elderly. A variety of terms have been used to describe these abnormalities including angiodysplasia, hemangioma, and vascular ectasia. The etiology of the disorder is unknown. While the lesions may occur throughout the gastrointestinal tract, they are found most commonly in the mucosa of the cecum and ascending colon where multiple lesions are often found, ranging in size from 1 mm to over 1 cm. An association of angiodysplasia of the colon with aortic stenosis has been observed repeatedly (1).

The prevalence of angiodysplasia and the frequency with which it causes bleeding is still uncertain. With increasing utilization of selective angiography, the disorder is being recognized more frequently. In one study of patients over the age of 60 without even a history of gastrointestinal bleeding, submucosal vascular ectasis was detected in 53%

and mucosal lesions in 27% (1). It was suggested, therefore, that angiodysplasia may be the most common cause of bleeding from the right colon, and may be the most common cause of major lower intestinal bleeding in the elderly.

These dysplastic lesions, when they bleed, usually produce hematochezia. The bleeding is often brisk, and may be massive, but occult blood loss also may occur. Bleeding often stops spontaneously, but commonly recurs. The *diagnosis* is best made by selective arteriography (by which a malformation can be visualized even when the bleeding has stopped) or by colonoscopy. The lesions cannot be detected by barium enema, are not recognizable from the serosal surface by the surgeon, and are often overlooked by the pathologist. Lesions that have bled should be excised, preferably by surgical resection of the involved colon. However, colonoscopic removal of discrete mucosal lesions can be performed by an experienced gastroenterologist.

The generalist should be aware of this disorder, especially in elderly patients who present to him with gastrointestinal bleeding in whom initial evaluation (see above) is unrevealing; but the diagnosis will be made only after consultation with a gastroenterologist and a radiologist.

References

General

Winawer, S and Sherlock, P: Approach to screening and diagnosis in colorectal cancer. *Semin Oncol* 3: 387, 1976.
    Reviews value of various screening tests and provides useful recommendations.

Specific

1. Boley, SJ, Sammartano, R, Adams, A, DeBrase, A, Kleinhaus, S and Sprayregen, S: Nature and etiology of vascular ectasias of the colon. *Gastroenterology* 72: 650, 1977.
2. Bond, J and Gilbertson, U: Early detection of colonic carcinoma by mass screening for occult stool blood: a preliminary report. *Gastroenterology* 72: A8, 1977.
3. Morris, D, Hansell, J, Ostrow, JD and Lee, C: Reliability of chemical tests for fecal occult blood in hospitalized patients. *Am J Digest Dis* 21: 845, 1976.
4. Muto, T, Bussey, HJ and Morson, BL: The evolution of cancer of the colon and rectum. *Cancer* 36: 2251, 1975.
5. Silvis, SE, Nebel, O, Rogers, G, et al.: Results of the 1974 American Society for Gastrointestinal Endoscopy Survey. *JAMA* 235: 928, 1976.
6. Tedesco, F, Waye, J, Raskin, J, et al.: Colonoscopic evaluation of rectal bleeding—a study of 304 patients. *Ann Intern Med* 89: 907, 1978.
7. Thoeni, RF and Menuck, L: Comparison of barium enema and colonoscopy in the detection of small colonic polyps. *Radiology* 124: 631, 1977.

CHAPTER THIRTY-FIVE

Constipation and Diarrhea

HAROLD J. TUCKER, M.D.

CONSTIPATION

Definition

Constipation is often defined as the infrequent, difficult passage of stool. However, it may mean different things to different people: that the stools are too infrequent, too difficult to expel, too hard, too small, or that there is a sensation of incomplete evacuation. Of these, frequency of bowel movements is the most readily measured aspect. Several studies have identified that there is a wide variation in the frequency of bowel movements among normal subjects of both sexes and of all ages, ranging from three per day to three per week. Therefore, someone who has less than three bowel movements per week is constipated, by definition. On the other hand, a change in frequency of movements from, say, two per day to three per week, may also signify constipation.

Almost always, constipation is due to a delay in transit within the colon. A wide variety of conditions may affect colonic transit (Table 35.1). There may be structural abnormalities that obstruct the passage of intraluminal contents, or there may be conditions that alter colonic motility. Evaluation of patients with constipation must therefore include consideration of a wide variety of possible etiologies. Although it is difficult to be precise about the relative frequencies of these etiologies, in general, chronic constipation (months or longer) is most commonly due to an idiopathic motility disorder (such as in sedentary old people eating a low fiber diet or in patients with an irritable bowel syndrome), to the use of constipating drugs, and to local rectal problems (fissures, hemorrhoids, and tumors).

Evaluation

HISTORY

The history provides the most useful information about the etiology of constipation. It may reveal a gross misconception about normal bowel habits, or a neurotic preoccupation with bowel function. It is important to determine whether there is a history of, or suggestion of, a systemic process (e.g., hypothyroidism or scleroderma), a neurologic disorder (e.g., cerebrovascular disease or Parkinson's disease) or the taking of drugs (e.g., anticholinergics or antidepressants), all of which are known to affect colonic motility. Most systemic or neurologic diseases are almost certain to affect organs outside the gastrointestinal tract so that, in addition to constipation, patients have symptoms that reflect extraintestinal dysfunction. On the other hand, local processes (e.g., strictures or tumors), which produce symptoms in addition to constipation, cause primarily gastrointestinal symptoms, such as abdominal pain or rectal bleeding. In this regard bleeding per rectum is surprisingly common in patients with chronic constipation and must be thoroughly investigated (see Chapter 35) since, although it usually is caused by perianal disease (fissures, hemorrhoids, or cryptitis), it is occasionally caused by carcinoma of the colon.

PHYSICAL EXAMINATION

The physical examination should be focused on the identification of underlying causes of constipation. Rectal examination should be done routinely to look for fissures, hemorrhoids, and inflammation as well as anal stenosis or stricture, secondary to previous surgery or inflammation. The anal sphincter normally is closed. A gaping anal opening, or asymmetry of the anal opening may indicate a neurologic disorder (spinal cord trauma, peripheral neuropathy) that impairs sphincteric function. After inspection, a careful digital examination should be performed to evaluate the strength of the anal sphincters, the presence of masses, the consistency of the stool, and the presence of any painful or tender areas.

Table 35.1
Various Causes of Constipation

IDIOPATHIC (POSSIBLE MECHANISMS):
  Dietary factors—low residue
  Motility disturbances—colonic inertia or spasm (irritable bowel syndrome)
  Sedentary living combined with a low residue diet
STRUCTURAL ABNORMALITIES:
  Tumors
  Strictures
  Anorectal disorders—fissures, thrombosed hemorrhoids
ENDOCRINE/METABOLIC:
  Diabetes mellitus
  Hypothyroidism
  Hypercalcemia
  Pregnancy
  Hypokalemia
NEUROGENIC:
  Hirschsprung's disease
  Trauma
  Spinal cord tumors
  Cerebrovascular events
SMOOTH MUSCLE/CONNECTIVE TISSUE DISORDERS:
  Scleroderma
  Amyloidosis
DRUGS:
  Narcotics
  Anticholinergics
  Antacids—aluminum, and calcium-containing compounds
  Antidepressants (e.g., amitriphylline—Elavil and imipramine—Tofranil)
PSYCHOGENIC

ENDOSCOPY

Anoscopy and *proctosigmoidoscopy* should be performed routinely in constipated patients. Proctosigmoidoscopy can be performed in the office, often without a prior enema. In fact, when the appearance of the mucosa is important (as it is in patients with suspected ulcerative colitis), an enema should be avoided. In contrast, if exophytic bleeding lesions (i.e., polyps) are suspected, a cleaning enema (e.g., Fleet enema) is desirable and is usually self-administered by the patient at home before the office visit. Anoscopy may be needed to search properly for hemorrhoids or fissures. Proctosigmoidoscopy can be performed with the patient in the knee-chest position on a routine examining table, or in the left lateral position. Sigmoidoscopy should be performed to the highest level possible, with limitations imposed by the patient's tolerance of the procedure, the presence of stool, and the length of the instrument (a rigid scope extends to 25 cm while a flexible instrument can be passed to 60 cm). It is important to recognize that even a good air-contrast barium enema is not a substitute for sigmoidoscopy as the most distal 15 to 20 cm of the colon are notoriously difficult to evaluate radiographically. The patient's experience during proctosigmoidoscopy is described in Chapter 32.

Inflamed hemorrhoids and fissures, found during sigmoidoscopy, may be caused by constipation, but may also cause pain on defecation, and thus may promote constipation. These are also common causes of bleeding in the chronically constipated patient. A spotty brown pigment, *melanosis coli*, is indicative of chronic laxative abuse (see below, p. 303), particularly of the anthraquinone family (e.g., cascara). An obstructing lesion, such as a carcinoma or polyp, may also be identified by proctosigmoidoscopy.

A *rectal biopsy* may diagnose amyloidosis, ulcerative colitis, or Crohn's disease, and a deeper, suction biopsy of a rectal valve may diagnose Hirschsprung's disease. Biopsies of the rectal mucosa can be taken safely below the peritoneal reflection (about 12 cm proximal to the anus in man, 8 cm in women). Punch biopsies can be performed by a general physician who has had appropriate training and experience. Suction biopsies should be performed only by a surgeon or gastroenterologist. Rectal biopsy should be painless unless a tender inflamed lesion is biopsied and, if done properly, the risk of bleeding and perforation, the major complications, is very low.

RADIOGRAPHIC STUDIES

Radiographic examination is primarily helpful in the detection of obstructing lesions and should be performed in all adult patients who complain of constipation of relatively recent onset (within the preceding 6 months). The plain film of the abdomen may occasionally diagnose an obstructing carcinoma before a barium study has been done. The presence of a megacolon or a volvulus, either of the sigmoid or cecum, also may be easily diagnosed by a plain film. The more recent the onset of constipation, the more likely it is that the *barium enema* (see patient experience, Chapter 34) will yield positive results. Obstructing neoplasms and strictures can be identified by barium studies. Sometimes, patients with Hirschsprung's disease reach adolescence or adulthood without the diagnosis having been made. A narrowed rectal segment on X-ray is a clue to the diagnosis in such cases; it can be best seen when the patient is in the lateral oblique position, and the X-ray is taken just as the barium is being instilled. The radiologist may also comment on the motility of the colon, particularly if there is significant spasm or if haustral markings are absent, seen in patients who use laxatives chronically or who have an atonic megacolon. Repeated barium studies are rarely helpful unless some aspect of the history or physical examination suggests a new development.

MANOMETRY

In patients suspected of having Hirschsprung's disease, *anal manometry* is a very simple and useful test. It is generally available in most medical centers and may be performed by either a gastroenterologist or a surgeon. The test involves insertion of balloon-tipped catheters into the anorectal region. Pressure measurements are made of the internal and external anal sphincter as well as within the rectum. Normally, with sudden distension of the rectum, the internal anal sphincter relaxes; and the external sphincter contracts. In Hirschsprung's disease, this rectal anal inhibitory reflex is abnormal and the internal anal sphincter fails to relax with rectal distension. This test is especially useful in cases of short segment or ultrashort segment Hirschsprung's disease in which the diagnosis is very difficult to establish by rectal biopsy.

OTHER STUDIES

Colonic motility tests and transit studies are additional procedures that may provide insight into the pathophysiology of constipation. These studies are generally available only in selected centers where there is specific interest in this problem. They should be performed in the few patients who are severely impaired by constipation and who are refractory to conventional therapy.

Colonic motility studies are generally performed by placing catheters, which monitor intracolonic pressures, in the rectal and sigmoid regions. The study can identify various patterns of colonic activity in patients with constipation. In some, high amplitude phasic contractions are seen spontaneously as well as in response to stimulation. This type of segmental activity is sometimes associated with pain and is believed to cause constipation by impeding the distal flow of luminal contents. In other patients an atonic pattern is found, characterized by a decreased response to stimulation and a loss of resistance to distension (4).

Colonic transit time can be measured by plotting the expulsion of radiopaque markers after ingestion. Daily plain films of the abdomen demonstrate the course of these markers through the gastrointestinal tract. In almost all normal subjects, 20 radiopaque markers will be evacuated within a week. Retention of these markers beyond that time period confirms the presence of constipation. Moreover, the distribution of these markers may have a relationship to the underlying motility disturbance (5).

Treatment

The treatment for constipation should, if possible, be based on the correction of the underlying abnormality. For example, if there is a systemic disease that can be treated (e.g., hypothyroidism) or a constipating drug that can be stopped, this is an ideal situation since it can easily be corrected. The simple use of laxatives as a reflex response to this symptom should be discouraged. Successful therapy must include an open discussion with the patient about the broad limits of normal bowel function and about the patient's own concepts of normal bowel activity.

BOWEL RETRAINING

Bowel retraining is an important initial aspect of therapy for those patients whose constipation does not have an identifiable and remediable cause. The patient should be encouraged to have a regular daily routine with time set aside for having a bowel movement, preferably within 5 to 10 min after a meal, to take advantage of the strong stimulus of the gastrocolic reflex. This behavior modification program allows the patient to become more aware of and responsive to the normal urges to defecate. Patients should be advised always to respond to such urges. In the severely constipated patient, a bowel-retraining program may be initiated with the use of enemas or suppositories to enhance bowel activity at the desired time. For enemas, lukewarm tap water should be used since all other solutions may be irritating if used repetitively. The enema should be given within an hour of eating a meal to take advantage of the gastrocolic reflex. For suppositories, glycerin or bisacodyl (Dulcolax) should be used, again just after eating; however, they should not be used for more than a few days because they may eventually be irritating.

DIET

Diet is an important factor in bowel function. Numerous studies have indicated that high fiber diets speed the transit of material through the gastrointestinal tract and increase stool frequency. Several mechanisms may account for this observation: (a) fiber may act as a bulk-forming agent, (b) fiber may increase the concentration of fecal bile salts which have a pronounced cathartic effect, and (c) fiber, metabolized by colonic bacteria to nonabsorbable volatile fatty acids, may act as an osmotic cathartic. Thus, the low fiber diet generally consumed in this

Table 35.2
Foods High in Fiber Content [a]

Type of Food	Grams of Fiber per Average Serving
CEREAL	
Bran, prepared	1.70
Bran, flakes	1.53
Grape nuts	0.72
Shredded wheat	0.78
BREAD	
Rye	0.36
Whole wheat	0.36
VEGETABLES	
Peas	1.65
Squash (winter)	1.40
Sweet potatoes	1.00
Broccoli	1.30
Brussel sprouts	1.30
String beans	1.05
FRUITS	
Blackberries	4.1
Black raspberries	3.5
Red raspberries	2.8
Apples	1.0
Pears	1.4
Strawberries	1.2

[a] Adapted from J. L. Kantor and L. F. Cooper: The dietetic treatment of constipation with special reference to food fiber. *Annals of Internal Medicine, 10:* 965, 1937.

country may account for the large number of patients who complain of constipation. As an initial step, the patient should be placed on a diet rich in fiber content. As listed in Table 35.2, there are a variety of foods high in fiber suitable for the patient's daily diet.

LAXATIVES

Despite numerous warnings, laxatives are still popular in the treatment of constipation. The presence of an estimated 700 or more commercially available laxatives and enema preparations attests to the widespread use of these agents. The mechanism of action for most laxatives is poorly understood, and the potential for toxicity is often underestimated (Table 35.3). Few data are available for comparison among the various laxatives, and the decision to use a particular laxative often is determined by individual preference rather than by objective evidence of efficacy or safety.

Different categories of laxatives act by different mechanisms. *Bulk-forming agents* are natural or synthetic polysaccharides or cellulose derivatives that exert their laxative effect by absorbing water and increasing fecal mass. Methycellulose, psyllium seed, and bran are examples of such laxatives. In addition to their hydrophilic properties, these agents are metabolized by colonic bacteria, resulting in accumulation of osmotically active metabolites. These laxatives are extremely effective in increasing stool frequency. There have been isolated reports of obstruction secondary to hydrophilic agents in patients with esophageal or small bowel strictures. In the majority of cases, however, this type of laxative is highly effective and the potential for adverse effects appears to be low. However, in patients with an atonic form of constipation, particularly with megacolon, these agents are often ineffective and produce an uncomfortable sensation of bloating and gaseousness at high doses.

Dioctyl sodium sulfosuccinate (Colace) is frequently labeled as a *stool softener* or a wetting agent. Its use as a softener rather than as a true laxative may well be a function of the dosage. The safety of this commonly used agent has been questioned, as the drug has been associated with enhancement of hepatotoxicity when combined with other potentially hepatotoxic agents. As its clinical efficacy as a laxative is uncertain and as it has the potential of serious toxicity, this drug should not be used routinely in the treatment of constipation.

The *saline laxatives* are generally magnesium or sodium salts that are poorly absorbed and therefore

Table 35.3
Laxatives

Classification and Active Ingredient	Examples	Dose	Average Onset of Action	Potential Adverse Effects
BULK			12–24 hr or more	Increased gas and bloating sensation; bowel obstruction if stricture present
Psyllium seed	Konsyl Effersyllium	1 tsp to 2 tbsp/day		
Plus Dextrose	Metamucil L.A. Formula			
Bran		4+ tbsp/day		
EMOLLIENT (SOFTENERS)			24–48 hr	Electrolyte imbalance; may potentiate hepatotoxicity of other agents
Dioctyl sodium (or calcium) sulfosuccinate	Colace	1–3 caps/day		
	Surfak	1 cap/day		
SALINE			3–6 hr or less	Hypermagensemia, hypocalcemia, hyperphosphatemia in chronic renal failure
Magnesium salts	Milk of magnesia, magnesium citrate,	2–4 tabs		
Sodium salts	Effervescent sodium phosphate			
STIMULANT			6–8 hr	Dermatitis; electrolyte imbalance, melanosis coli
Phenolphthalein	Correctol, Ex-Lax	1–2 tabs (100–200 mg)		
Disacodyl	Dulcolax	2–3 tabs (10–15 mg)		
Senna	Senokot	1–4 tsp or 2–4 tabs		
Cascara	Various	1 tab or 1 tsp		
Ricinoleic acid	Castor oil	1–2 tsp		
OSMOTIC				Excessive gas production
Lactulose	Cephulac, Chronulac	1–2 tbsp/day		

act as hyperosmolar solutions. It has been suggested that these compounds (e.g., magnesium sulfate, milk of magnesia, and sodium phosphate) also release cholecystokinin, a hormone which is known to stimulate colonic motility. Complications include hypermagnesemia in patients with renal failure and hypocalcemia from phosphate overdoses.

Stimulant laxatives such as anthraquinone derivatives (senna, cascara) and diphenylmethane compounds (phenolphthalein, bisacodyl) exert their effects primarily by altering electrolyte transport by the intestinal mucosa and intestinal motor activity. The effect of these agents is claimed to be more specific on the colon. Phenolphthalein, an ingredient found in many over-the-counter preparations, has been associated with severe allergic dermatitis. The chronic use of the anthraquinone derivatives has also been reported to induce damage to the intramural plexus, and thus actually to worsen bowel motility. Agents, such as these that affect electrolyte transport, may result in significant hypokalemia, factitious diarrhea, protein-losing enteropathy, and salt overload. While these agents are undoubtedly effective, their chronic use may lead to significant side effects and should be avoided when possible.

Castor oil, previously thought to be a stimulant laxative, is now understood to exert its cathartic effect by alteration of intestinal fluid and electrolyte secretion. Ricinoleic acid, the active ingredient of castor oil, has effects on the small and large intestine similar to that of bile acids: it inhibits absorption of sodium and glucose, and stimulates fluid and electrolyte secretion by increasing cellular cyclic adenosine monophosphate (AMP) and by inhibiting sodium-potassium adenosine triphosphatase (ATPase). This increase in intraluminal fluid content may then secondarily affect intestinal motility.

Lactulose (Cephulac or Chronulac syrup) is a semi-isynthetic disaccharide that is not metabolized by the intestinal enzymes. As a result, water and electrolytes are retained within the intestinal lumen by the osmotic effect of this undigested sugar. In addition, this agent is converted by colonic bacteria to organic acids which may further alter electrolyte transport and/or affect colonic motility. Lactulose is commonly used in patients with hepatic encephalopathy. It has also been shown to be an effective laxative in patients with chronic constipation. There is little current information on the relative merits of lactulose *versus* bulk laxatives except that lactulose is relatively expensive and requires 24 to 48 hours to achieve its effect.

Surgery is rarely necessary in the treatment of constipated patients. It is, however, required for resection of an obstructing lesion, and myectomy may be needed for treatment of Hirschsprung's disease. Various procedures have been recommended for patients with megacolon who suffer from recurrent volvulus, ranging from simple tacking down of the loose mesentery to resection of bowel. Finally, in severe cases of intractable constipation, extensive surgery has been advocated varying from resection of redundant sigmoid loops to subtotal colectomy with ileal-proctostomy. The exact role and precise indication for this type of surgery remain to be more clearly defined.

DIARRHEA

Diarrhea is a troublesome problem which almost everyone has experienced. In the vast majority of cases, the diarrheal illness begins abruptly, lasts only a day or two, and resolves without serious sequelae (see Chapter 25). Only occasionally does the illness continue for more than a week or do symptoms recur after the initial attack. The task facing the clinician is to identify the few patients with a significant underlying disorder that may require a specific therapeutic approach.

Definition

Patients complaining of diarrhea generally have an increase in the frequency and fluid volume of the bowel movement. Stool weight is the best objective measurement of diarrhea, with mean weights in this country ranging normally between 100 and 200 g per day. The patient should be given a preweighed clean paint can so that he can collect his stool. It is important that the measurement be made in all patients who have chronic diarrhea in whom the cause is not clear. Most cases of significant diarrhea will have in excess of 250 g of stool per day. There is a subset of patients with diarrhea who present with the frequent passage of small volumes of liquid stool. Patients with inflammatory conditions or space-occupying lesions of the rectum may present in this fashion.

Pathophysiology

There are several basic causes of diarrhea: (a) osmotic load within the intestine resulting in retention of water within the lumen, (b) excessive secretion of electrolytes and water into the intestinal lumen, (c) exudation of protein and fluid from the intestinal mucosa, and (d) altered intestinal motility.

Osmotic diarrhea occurs when poorly absorbable material retains fluid within the intestinal lumen. This mechanism operates in patients with malabsorption or with lactose intolerance in which poorly absorbed sugars accumulate within the intestinal lumen and exert a considerably osmotic load. Magnesium-containing laxatives and some magnesium-containing antacids (e.g., Maalox) probably produce diarrhea through a similar mechanism.

Secretory diarrhea is perhaps the best studied pathophysiologic type of diarrhea. In such cases, the intestinal mucosa secretes increased amounts of water and electrolytes, under the stimulation of a variety of substances, of which cholera toxin is the prototype (some enterotoxigenic *Escherichia coli* produce diarrhea in the same way (see Chapter 25); other substances include bile acids and long chain fatty acids (postileal resection, Crohn's disease, or a malabsorption syndrome), certain gastrointestinal hormones, and anthraquinone laxatives (see above, p. 300). Many of these stimulating agents have been shown to increase intracellular cyclic AMP and to inhibit sodium potassium ATPase. The increase in cyclic AMP leads to increased secretion.

Exudative diarrhea results from the outpouring of protein, blood, or mucus from an inflamed or ulcerated mucosa. Ulcerative colitis, Crohn's disease, salmonellosis, and infiltrative disorders like Whipple's disease and lymphoma are examples of this mechanism.

Motility disorders may lead to diarrhea, although the exact correlation between the abnormal motility and the diarrhea is not completely understood. The *irritable bowel syndrome* (see Chapter 36) is generally believed to be a motor disorder that causes abdominal pain and altered bowel habits, with diarrhea predominating in many patients. Diabetes mellitus may also lead to diarrhea due to neurogenic dysfunction. Other conditions, like scleroderma, can lead to stasis of the bowel with resultant bacterial overgrowth, steatorrhea, and diarrhea.

It is not always possible to identify one particular mechanism to account for diarrhea in a given patient; sometimes more than one mechanism is operative. However, an appreciation of pathophysiology enables the physician to understand better the clinical features of a diarrheal illness and to select appropriate therapy.

Evaluation of Acute Diarrhea

(Acute diarrhea due to infectious agents is discussed in greater detail in Chapter 25.) The vast majority of patients who present to the physician with a sudden onset of diarrhea generally have a benign, self-limited illness. These patients will not require an extensive evaluation and can be simply reassured. It is important, however, to recognize that a small percentage of such patients may actually have a significant underlying illness for which specific therapy is needed.

If diarrhea persists for more than 72 hours or if there is gross blood in the stool, an evaluation is indicated. In any case, the patient should always be' evaluated (if possible) before medicine is prescribed, since in certain situations even nonspecific antidiarrheal therapy may actually be harmful.

HISTORY

The history clearly reveals whether the illness is acute or chronic and also provides major clues to the underlying cause. The sudden onset of loose watery stool is most commonly due to an infectious process, and much less often due to ingestion of drugs or poisons. Infectious diarrhea is likely to affect more than one person. Frequently, no specific bacterial agent is identified and the syndrome is labeled "viral

gastroenteritis." Bacteria may cause diarrhea by a direct effect on the bowel or by elaboration of a toxin that produces intestinal dysfunction. Toxin-induced diarrhea, often associated with vomiting, begins within 6 hours of ingestion of contaminated food, whereas bacteria-induced diarrhea does not begin for 12 to 24 hours. Bloody diarrhea should never be ascribed to "viral" or to toxin-mediated diarrhea; it is more likely to be due to bacterial infection (*Shigella*, *Campylobacter*, *Yersinia*, and *Salmonella*), or to ulcerative colitis, or ischemic bowel disease. Information about recent travel should include not only trips out of the country but also camping or fishing trips. Giardiasis, for example, may be carried by beavers who contaminate water supplies and cause both epidemic outbreaks as well as individual cases of acute diarrhea among campers and back packers. Recent use of drugs is a common cause of new onset diarrhea (Table 35.4), which is often overlooked by both the physician and the patient. Some antihypertensives (e.g., methyldopa, hydralazine, reserpine, and guanethidine), magnesium-containing antacids, broad spectrum antibiotics, and quinidine are commonly used drugs that can lead to diarrhea.

PHYSICAL EXAMINATION

Physical examination is generally unremarkable. The patient's state of hydration should be estimated, as it is an important measure of the severity of the diarrhea and of the need for hospitalization. Abdominal examination may reveal mild diffuse tenderness. The bowel sounds are clearly active or hyperactive. Rectal examination is essential since diarrhea may be the initial manifestation of obstructing rectal carcinoma; furthermore in the geriatric population, fecal impactions may result in "overflow" diarrhea so that constipating agents may be mistakenly recommended.

STOOL EXAMINATION

If diarrhea has lasted for more than 72 hours, the stool should be examined for the presence of blood, fecal leukocytes, and enteric pathogens. Blood in the stool suggests mucosal disruption and is not a feature of osmotic or secretory diarrhea. Inflammatory conditions like ulcerative colitis and pseudomembranous colitis frequently present with bloody diarrhea.

Fecal leukocytes are best seen by microscopic examination of the liquid portion of the stool after staining with methylene blue or Gram's stain (3). They are not seen in infectious processes that do not invade the mucosa such as "viral enteritis," toxin-mediated diarrhea, cholera, or infection with noninvasive E. coli (see Chapter 25). *Salmonella*, *Shigella*, amoebae, and *Campylobacter*, which are invasive organisms, typically lead to exudation of fecal leukocytes, as does chronic inflammatory bowel disease. In these conditions, in which the mucosal barrier is broken, the course of the diarrheal illness is unpredictable and may even become life-threatening. The absence of fecal leukocytes or blood is, therefore, very reassuring and, in these cases, the disease is usually transient.

Stool cultures for bacterial pathogens should be obtained on all patients who have fecal leukocytes. Specific isolation techniques are needed to diagnose *Yersinia* and *Campylobacteria*, common causes of acute diarrhea, and should be requested. The differentiation on clinical grounds between acute infectious diarrhea secondary to *Salmonella* or *Shigella* and nonspecific acute inflammatory bowel disease is extremely difficult without a stool culture. In the absence of fecal leukocytes, stool cultures are generally negative and are not useful. Gram stain of the stool is not helpful except in cases of suspected staphylococcal enterocolitis or gonococcal proctitis.

Examination of the stool for parasites such as amoebae and *Giardia* is very important even in the absence of a history of travel since the organism may be passed by personal contact with a carrier. Microscopic examination of the inflammatory exudate of a patient with acute amebic colitis will almost always demonstrate motile trophozoites. Rectal biopsy may identify the organisms in the exudate. Giardiasis can be detected on examination of fresh stool in only about 50% of patients. If the physician is not proficient in the identification of protozoons in the stool, he must refer the patient to a medical center or must rely on serology or rectal biopsy to diagnose amoebiasis or duodenal aspiration or biopsy to diagnose giardiasis.

ENDOSCOPY

Proctosigmoidoscopy is important in patients with acute diarrhea associated with fecal leukocytes or fecal blood. The proctoscopy should be performed without a prior enema, as enemas may alter the appearance of the mucosa and reduce the chance of detecting intestinal pathogens like amoebae.

Many acute diarrheal illnesses produce a similar, nonspecific mucosal appearance on proctoscopy but certain findings are suggestive of specific diseases. In viral enteritis, giardiasis, toxin-mediated diarrhea, drug-induced diarrhea, and other conditions not accompanied by fecal leukocytes or blood loss, the proctoscopy is normal. In ulcerative colitis the rectal mucosa is involved in at least 95% of cases, and the mucosa is uniformly abnormal with bleeding and a granular friable appearance. Uncommonly, Crohn's disease affects the rectum and causes discrete aphthoid ulcers with normal intervening mucosa. Amebiasis classically produces flask-shaped ulcers that may be single or multiple, with normal intervening mucosa; more often, however, it produces a pattern very similar to ulcerative colitis. In shigellosis, multiple small superficial ulcers may be seen, but the appearance may also be indistinguishable from ulcerative colitis. Pseudomembranous colitis is identified by the presence of numerous raised yellow plaques covering an inflamed mucosa. Occasionally a carcinoma or large villous adenoma may be de-

tected by sigmoidoscopy. Proctoscopy also provides an extremely opportune time to obtain samples of stool and exudate for culture and microscopic examination. The patient's experience with proctosigmoidoscopy is described in Chapter 32.

RADIOGRAPHIC STUDIES

Radiography is of very limited value in evaluation of acute diarrhea and may, in fact, be confusing. In patients suspected of having inflammatory bowel disease or ischemic colitis, plain films of the abdomen may demonstrate an irregular appearance to the bowel wall secondary to mucosal edema, often described as "thumb-printing." In the gravely ill patient with fulminant colitis, the X-ray may confirm the presence of "toxic megacolon." In the vast majority of cases of acute diarrhea, a plain film is not needed. Barium studies during the acute phase of the diarrhea are likewise not needed and in certain conditions may even be hazardous, as in patients with severe colitis or ischemic bowel disease. Similarly, a small bowel series during acute "vital enteritis" may be frighteningly abnormal, resembling sprue, and yet may rapidly return to normal after resolution of the acute illness.

Evaluation of Chronic Diarrhea

The approach to patients with either acute diarrhea which lasts longer than 72 hours or chronic diarrhea (lasting longer than 2 weeks) is very much the same. While the *physician* may be reassured, knowing that the majority of such patients do not suffer from any serious aggressive or disabling disease, the *patient* requires a specific diagnosis and effective therapy. The differential diagnosis is so varied, and the available tests are so numerous, that the diagnostic workup of chronic diarrhea poses a difficult problem. The following discussion provides a practical approach to this problem.

HISTORY

The history is often very helpful in differentiating organic from "functional" diarrhea—i.e., irritable bowel syndrome and painless ("nervous") diarrhea (see Chapter 36). If organic diarrhea is suspected, the physician must determine whether the pathogenic mechanism is osmotic, secretory, motor, or exudative (see above). In patients with so-called "functional diarrhea," the history of diarrhea often dates back many months or years, although occasionally it can be traced to a specific acute diarrheal illness. Despite the chronicity, no sequelae, such as weight loss, anemia, or hypoalbuminemia have occurred. The patient typically complains of several watery, at times explosive, bowel movements early in the morning, and then no subsequent movements the rest of the day. Nocturnal bowel movements are rare. The total stool output is usually small, however—often less than 200 g per day and rarely if ever greater than 500 g per day. Mucus is present frequently. There is no blood in the stool unless secondary conditions, such as anal fissures, have developed. Postprandial pain is a feature of irritable bowel syndrome, but is absent in patients with "nervous" or "painless" diarrhea. The condition frequently waxes and wanes in severity, and stress often exacerbates the symptoms.

The most common cause of chronic secretory diarrhea is *laxative abuse*. It should be suspected in apparently healthy patients with large volume diarrhea, especially if they have *melanosis coli* on proctoscopic examination (see above, p. 302). Although such patients may have emotional problems with which the physician must deal (see Chapter 11), often the abuse simply reflects an individual's misconception about how often he should have a bowel movement and his attempt to adhere to that standard.

In patients with organic disease, the history may indicate the part of the intestinal tract that is involved. The passage of a large volume of frothy, malodorous stools without blood suggests small bowel diarrhea, often secondary to malabsorption. The frequent passage of small volumes of poorly formed bloody stools suggests inflammatory, exudative disorders of the colon like ulcerative colitis. The presence of recognizable fat droplets (oil) suggests malabsorption, frequently secondary to pancreatic insufficiency. (Floating stools and undigested food in the stools are not helpful observations as they may be seen in both organic and functional diarrheal states.) The association of diarrhea with the ingestion of certain dietary products (milk, hyperosmolar solutions) may go unrecognized by the patient unless he is specifically asked. A detailed drug history (see below) is also important since many drugs may cause diarrhea.

Other symptoms may help the physician to arrive at a specific diagnosis. *Arthritis and arthralgias* may suggest the presence of one of several uncommon bowel diseases, *e.g.*, inflammatory bowel disease and Whipple's disease; conversely diarrhea may be an important feature of Reiter's syndrome (Chapter 8). *Weight loss*, in the absence of anorexia, should suggest malabsorption, hyperthyroidism, or a hypermetabolic tumor. *Abdominal pain* may reflect the irritable bowel syndrome (Chapter 36), in which case it is generally in the left lower quadrant or in the suprapubic region, or a disease of the small bowel (e.g., Crohn's disease) in which case it is periumbilical.

PHYSICAL EXAMINATION

The physical examination may reveal additional information about the etiology of the diarrhea. Patients with malabsorption may have evidence of weight loss, peripheral neuropathy (secondary to vitamin deficiency), and carpopedal spasm (secondary to hypocalcemia). Erythema nodosum and pyoderma gangrenosum may be seen in some cases of inflammatory bowel disease. Hyperpigmentation is a feature of Whipple's disease and Addison's disease. Diabetic diarrhea is frequently associated with other evidence of autonomic dysfunction such as postural hypotension. Nondeforming arthritis is a feature of Whipple's disease and inflammatory bowel disease. Hepatosplenomegaly and lymphadenopathy suggest lymphoma or Whipple's disease. The abdominal examination may reveal an arterial bruit or an aortic aneurysm which suggests ischemic bowel disease. A rectal examination may disclose perianal disease (e.g., abscesses or fistulas, secondary to Crohn's disease) a rectal tumor, or a fecal impaction.

ENDOSCOPY

Proctoscopy should be performed during the initial visit without a prior cleansing enema. Proctoscopic exam of the rectal mucosa and a rectal biopsy (see p. 297) may suggest specific etiologies—ulcerative colitis, Crohn's disease, amebiasis, pseudomembranous colitis, Whipple's disease, or amyloidosis. The finding of *melanosis coli* in a patient complaining of diarrhea indicates laxative abuse. At the time of proctoscopy, stool specimens are obtained for microscopic evaluation and culture. Gonococcal proctitis appears similar to ulcerative proctitis (see below) and requires direct plating on a warm special culture medium (Thayer-Martin) with prompt incubation. Routine stool cultures should be made as well. The stool should be examined for pus cells, blood, fat (Sudan stain), and parasites (see p. 302).

After this initial evaluation, the etiology of the chronic diarrhea in most patients is either evident or strongly suspected. It is usually possible to distinguish functional from organic diarrhea; to detect evidence of inflammatory or infiltrative disease; to suspect the presence of malabsorption; to characterize the diarrhea as "small bowel" or "large bowel"; and even to suggest the underlying pathophysiology. Further evaluation is then dictated by the results of this initial workup.

LABORATORY STUDIES

Laboratory studies should be selected to support the clinical impression but rarely are able to make or exclude a specific diagnosis. For example, the erythrocyte sedimentation rate (ESR) may be elevated in a variety of inflammatory diseases that cause diarrhea, but a normal ESR does not exclude inflammatory bowel disease or a connective tissue disorder.

RADIOLOGIC STUDIES

A plain film of the abdomen may reveal pancreatic calcifications (indicative of chronic pancreatitis) or a dilated small bowel or an abnormal bowel contour (such as in inflammatory bowel disease).

In the patient over 40 years old, with chronic or recurrent diarrhea, a *barium enema* is indicated during the initial evaluation. In younger patients, barium studies are unlikely to be useful unless a specific disorder is suspected. The presence of blood in the stool, at any age, is a clear indication for a barium enema, regardless of the presence of hemorrhoids or fissures. Neoplastic and inflammatory conditions may be diagnosed in this way and ulcerative colitis and Crohn's disease of the colon can be differentiated in about 90% of cases. When the barium enema is introduced, an attempt should be made to reflux barium into the terminal small bowel to rule out Crohn's disease of the ileum.

The timing of the barium study is important. Barium will interfere with the collection of stool for measurement of volume and fat and with the detection of parasites. A barium enema should be delayed for 1 week following a rectal biopsy to prevent colonic perforation. The patient's experience with the barium enema is discussed in Chapter 34.

A *small bowel series* (see Chapter 34 for a discussion of the patient's experience with this procedure) is helpful in distinguishing mucosal disease (celiac sprue), inflammatory conditions (Crohn's disease), and infiltrative processes (Whipple's disease or amyloidosis). In addition, a small bowel series is indicated in postsurgical patients to clarify the anatomy (e.g., a blind loop or fistulas) and to detect localized areas of dilation and stasis.

OTHER STUDIES

A *quantitative stool collection*, while regarded as unpleasant by both the patient and laboratory personnel, is a very informative test. It should be employed early in the evaluation of patients in whom the initial routine workup does not suggest a diagnosis. The test can be performed in the ambulatory setting by having the patient collect all of his stool in a preweighed container (such as a paint can), usually supplied by the clinical laboratory. The test should be performed before barium studies or other invasive tests in these patients. As mentioned previously, the normal stool weight is less than 250 g per day (or less than 250 ml per day). Most patients with the irritable bowel syndrome will have stool volumes within this range. A stool volume of greater than 1000 ml per day suggests a secretory diarrhea.

The *osmolality and electrolyte* concentration of the specimen can also be measured. In osmotic diarrhea, the measured fecal osmolality is greater than twice the sum of fecal sodium and potassium. In secretory diarrhea, the calculated and measured osmolality are the same. *Fecal fat* should also be measured during this collection. Normally less than 7% of ingested fat is secreted in the stool per day (6 to 7 g on an average American diet containing 70 to 100 g of fat). The presence of steatorrhea dictates a different approach to the remainder of the workup (see below). In the absence of excessive fat excretion, or of evidence of an exudative process (e.g., inflammatory bowel disease), high volume diarrhea suggests a secretory process.

In patients suspected of having a secretory diarrhea, further evaluation will generally require hospitalization and consultation with a gastroenterologist. In secretory diarrhea, having the patient ingest nothing by mouth for 48 hours will not alter the volume of diarrhea, whereas in osmotic diarrhea the stool volume will significantly decrease. Causes of chronic secretory diarrhea include hormone-secreting tumors and surreptitious laxative abuse. Evaluation of such patients frequently requires availability of various hormone assays. Familiarity with these uncommon conditions is needed to approach the differential diagnosis judiciously.

EVALUATION OF MALABSORPTION

When the quantitative fecal collection demonstrates steatorrhea, the evaluation of the diarrhea should be focused on the cause of malabsorption. Basically malabsorption can result from (a) small intestinal disease, (b) pancreatic disease, (c) hepatobiliary disease, and (d) gastric disease. A series of diagnostic studies is utilized initially to define the organ involved and then to diagnose the specific disease. Consultation with a gastroenterologist is generally recommended to help perform and analyze these various tests.

The *d-xylose test* measures the absorptive capacity of the proximal small bowel. Normally, the sugar is absorbed passively by the intact small intestinal mucosa, enters the blood, and is excreted in the urine. The test is performed in the same manner as an oral glucose tolerance test, and can be performed in the ambulatory setting by most clinical laboratories. A 25- or 50-g oral dose of xylose is given, and the patient's urine is collected over the next 5 hours. Blood samples are collected at 1 and 2 hours after ingestion. In disorders of the intestinal mucosa (sprue, Whipple's disease) xylose is poorly absorbed and low levels are found in the serum and urine. Uncommonly, massive bacterial overgrowth may also produce an abnormal d-xylose test that reverts to normal with treatment. Since an abnormal xylose test suggests mucosal disease, a small bowel biopsy should be performed next.

If the *d-xylose* test is normal, pancreatic insufficiency is the most likely cause of steatorrhea. In this case pancreatic calcifications may be seen on an abdominal plain film, and diabetes mellitus is frequently present. Pancreatic insufficiency can be confirmed by measuring pancreatic secretions (secretin test) or by measuring intraluminal contents after a test meal. These tests, performed usually in the gastroenterology laboratory of a medical center, involve intubation of the duodenum with collection of intraluminal contents. Often, however, if a presumptive diagnosis of pancreatic insufficiency is made, the patient is treated empirically with pancreatic enzymes; diagnostic and therapeutic decisions should be made in consultation with a gastroenterologist.

Suction biopsy of the small intestine is often useful in the detection of various disorders that may cause malabsorption and/or diarrhea. The procedure can be performed by a gastroenterologist in an ambulatory setting. The biopsy instrument, a small caliber tube, is passed by mouth through the stomach, and positioned fluoroscopically at the duodenal-jejunal junction. The patient is given prior mild sedation

(Valium intravenously) and a topical anesthetic is sprayed onto the back of the pharynx. The procedure may last from 15 min to 2 or 3 hours depending on the ease of passage of the tube (usually the tube can be passed rapidly). Complications (including perforation and bleeding) are extremely rare. Disorders that may be diagnosed by small bowel biopsy include sprue, Whipple's disease, intestinal lymphoma, amyloidosis, lymphangiectasia, and eosinophilic gastroenteritis. Giardiasis also can be diagnosed by examination of the intestinal mucosa and of the intestinal mucus or fluid by the pathologist or the consulting gastroenterologist.

Disorders of the terminal ileum (Crohn's disease, ileal resection) may also lead to diarrhea and malabsorption. Evaluation should include a *Schilling test* or a *bile salt breath test*. The Schilling test measures vitamin B_{12} absorption, which is abnormal in disorders of the terminal ileum, the site of B_{12} absorption. Absorption is impaired despite the presence of intrinsic factor (see Chapter 46) or the administration of antibiotics.

Similarly, the bile salt breath test measures bile acid absorption which is also abnormal in disorders of the terminal ileum. The patient is given orally a radiolabeled (^{14}C) bile salt. In the presence of terminal ileal disease, the bile salt is malabsorbed, and excess acid reaches the colon, where bacteria deconjugate it and release $^{14}CO_2$ which diffuses across the colon and is excreted in the breath. Therefore, in ileal disease, the level of $^{14}CO_2$ in the patient's expired air is abnormally high. The same abnormality can be seen when there is bacterial overgrowth in the small bowel, so that the bile acid is deconjugated and metabolized there instead of in the colon. Bile acid malabsorption due to bacterial overgrowth is reversed when the patient is given antibiotics. Both the Schilling test and the bile salt breath test are performed by nuclear medicine specialists.

Specific Causes of Chronic Diarrhea

LACTOSE INTOLERANCE

Lactose intolerance is the most common form of carbohydrate malabsorption. It results from a deficiency or total absence of the enzyme lactase in the brush border of the intestinal mucosa, which causes maldigestion and therefore malabsorption of lactose. The unabsorbed carbohydrate exerts an osmotic effect which draws water into the intestinal lumen. In the colon, the lactose is metabolized by bacteria to organic acid, CO_2, and hydrogen. The acid contributes to the diarrhea by both an osmotic effect and an irritating effect on the colonic mucosa. Thus, the unabsorbed carbohydrate if present in sufficient quantities (the critical amount varies widely) may cause diarrhea, gaseousness, bloating, and abdominal cramps.

Lactose intolerance may be present either as an inherited condition or one that develops because of damage to intestinal epithelium (e.g., due to infectious enteritis or sprue). Even in patients with a genetic disorder the onset of the disease is unpredictable and may not occur until adult life. The secondary cases are usually, but not always, reversible if the underlying disease is successfully treated. The severity of the clinical symptoms is highly variable.

In some patients even small amounts of lactose produce severe symptoms while in others large quantities may be consumed with no or only minimal symptoms. Isolated lactose deficiency is most common in blacks (70 to 75% prevalence), and in many Asians (87% prevalence among Chinese), but may also be found in 5 to 20% of the white population in this country (2). The condition is more pronounced in certain clinical settings: when superimposed on another diarrheal disorder, most commonly irritable bowel syndrome; after gastric surgery, which permits rapid delivery of lactose to the small bowel; and when a patient consumes extra amounts of milk as part of therapy for ulcer disease.

The *diagnosis* of lactose intolerance is suggested by the history and by the response to a lactose-free diet. Nearly a third of patients with symptomatic lactose intolerance, however, may not have made the correlation between the dietary intake and the resulting symptoms, as a wide variety of foods, ranging from bread to instant coffee, contain lactose.

Specific tests for the diagnosis of lactose intolerance include the lactose tolerance test and the hydrogen breath test. The *lactose tolerance test* measures changes in the concentration of serum glucose after ingestion of 50 g of lactose. A rise in glucose of 20 mg/100 ml above fasting is normal. The test has about a 30% false positive rate, and its validity depends on a variety of factors besides simply the presence of the lactase enzyme. The *hydrogen breath* test is easier to perform and is more accurate. Unabsorbed lactose is fermented by colonic bacteria and the resultant hydrogen is absorbed and expired in the breath. In normal subjects after a lactose load, there is only a trace amount of hydrogen in the expired air, whereas in lactose-deficient patients substantial levels are recorded. This test is widely available; it is usually performed by a nuclear medicine specialist and requires only 1 or 2 hours of the patient's time.

Ordinarily, a 3-week trial of a diet that is free of milk and milk products is a satisfactory therapeutic trial to test the diagnosis of lactose intolerance. The other tests are indicated only in equivocal cases.

FECAL IMPACTION

Although it is the result of chronic constipation, fecal impaction commonly causes diarrhea. The adults most at risk for impaction are elderly sedentary people—often bedridden. The feces are usually impacted in the rectum or in the rectosigmoid region, but occasionally may extend high up into the colon (rarely, even to the cecum). The leaking of colonic fluid around the impaction, resulting in the passage of frequent small volume watery bowel movements, accounts for the diarrhea. Other symptoms are common but are usually nonspecific: a sense of fullness in the rectum, vague lower abdominal pain, nausea, and headache. On *physical examination*, the firm stool is palpable in the left lower quadrant of the abdomen, which is best examined bimanually (a finger of one hand in the rectum and the other hand on the abdomen). The impaction is *best removed* manually, if it is low enough, or through the sigmoidoscope, if it is not. Enemas are of no help in this regard. Common *complications* of impaction include recurrent urinary tract infection (because of compression of the ureters—more common in women), intestinal obstruction, perforation of the colon, and local ulceration.

ULCERATIVE COLITIS

Ulcerative colitis is a chronic inflammatory disorder of colonic mucosa; its cause is unknown. It is recommended that patients with this condition be followed by the general physician in consultation with a gastroenterologist. The disorder may affect patients of any age, including the elderly, with a peak incidence in the 3rd and 4th decades.

The clinical picture of ulcerative colitis is highly variable. The disorder may be limited to the rectum (ulcerative proctitis) or may involve the entire colon. Symptoms may range from occasional rectal bleeding, even without diarrhea, to profuse watery and bloody diarrhea. The severity of the initial presentation and the extent of the disease at the time of the initial attack have been shown to be useful predictors of the eventual course of the disease. Most patients (about 60%) have mild disease, *i.e.*, less than four bowel movements a day without fever, weight loss, or hypoalbuminemia. The vast majority of these patients will have colitis limited to the rectosigmoid region or to the colon. About 10 to 15% of patients with ulcerative colitis develop severe pancolitis with accompanying deterioration in their general health. Another 25% have moderate disease with more troublesome diarrhea, often containing blood, accompanied by crampy lower abdominal pain. Patients with moderate or severe disease may also have systemic symptoms of fever, fatigue, and weight loss. The clinical course is characterized by periodic exacerbations which in general respond well to adjustments in medical therapy. The smallest group of patients with ulcerative colitis is that with severe disease. This group includes the 1% of patients who present initially with fulminant colitis. In patients with severe colitis, symptoms may suddenly worsen with profuse diarrhea, rectal bleeding, and high fevers. Plain films of the abdomen may demonstrate a dilated bowel ("toxic megacolon"). Mortality is high in this group of patients.

As there is no specific test for or histopathology of ulcerative colitis, the diagnosis depends on the constellation of symptoms, on the appropriate endoscopic and histologic appearance of the colonic mucosa, on the exclusion of other inflammatory conditions, and on the natural history of the disorder. Patients with acute presentations, depending on the circumstances, must be differentiated from patients with bacterial diarrheas (see Chapter 25), amebiasis (see above, p. 302), Crohn's disease (see below), and ischemic colitis (ischemic colitis presents with acute abdominal pain and the passage of bloody stool; this is a disease of middle-aged or older people who usually have evidence of generalized atherosclerosis).

Treatment. Medical therapy for ulcerative colitis generally includes corticosteroids and sulfasalazine (Azulfidine). Steroids are particularly useful for acute exacerbations, but are not helpful in preventing relapses. Conversely, sulfasalazine is of limited value in the treatment of acute attacks, but has been shown to reduce the frequency of exacerbations and may allow reduction of the dosage of steroids. A minority of patients with ulcerative colitis need continuous steroid therapy. Other drugs, such as cytotoxic agents, require further evaluation before they can be recommended.

Surgery in ulcerative colitis is curative and patients should be counseled early in their course about the role of surgery in the treatment of this disorder. Patients should be informed about the indications for surgery and the types of operations that are available. Early attention to this issue will enable the patient to accept an operation more readily if it is needed. Surgery for ulcerative colitis involves a proctocolectomy with an ileostomy to which a stomal appliance is attached to assure continence. Construction of a continent ileostomy, a relatively new procedure, avoids the need for a stomal appliance, but the procedure is technically difficult and, in 30% of cases, requires at least one revision. However, as experience with this operation increases, it may become more popular. Also, early experience with ileorectal pull-through operations suggests that continence can be preserved after this procedure as well and this operation too may be offered more frequently in the future.

Cancer of the Colon. The risk of cancer of the colon is increased 5 to 10 times in patients with ulcerative colitis. The major risk factors are (a) duration of disease—risk increases significantly after 8 to 10 years of disease; (b) extent of colonic involvement—pancolitis carries the highest risk, while the risk in patients with ulcerative proctitis is similar to that of the general population; and (c) age of onset of disease—patients under the age of 25 at the time of onset have the highest risk, independent of the extent of disease. The cancer may be found anywhere in the colon although most commonly it is within the rectum or rectosigmoid. It may be multicentric. It is important that the patient know about the risk of cancer since it may influence his decision to undergo colectomy. After they have had the disease for 7 years, high risk patients should have yearly evaluations of the colon by either colonoscopy or air contrast barium enema. In addition, since dysplastic changes of the colonic mucosa have been identified as "precancer" and have been shown to correlate closely with the development of cancer elsewhere in the colon, serial colonic and rectal biopsies should be obtained in high risk patients.

CROHN'S DISEASE

Crohn's disease or regional enteritis is a chronic inflammatory condition of unknown cause involving all layers of the intestine. The condition most commonly affects the terminal ileum, but any area from the esophagus to the anus can be involved. The onset of the disease most commonly is in adolescence and young adulthood.

Presentation. Crohn's disease may be localized initially to the small bowel, involve small bowel and colon, or be confined to the colon only. The inflammatory process usually remains confined to the initial site of involvement unless surgery is performed. Recurrence is the rule following surgery, and the condition may then involve additional segments of bowel. As the inflammatory process persists, the bowel wall becomes thickened and stenotic leading to bowel obstruction. Fistula formation is characteristic and may spread to involve any contiguous structure. As a result, abscess formation and infection may complicate the clinical course. Diarrhea, abdominal pain, and weight loss are the common symptoms. Unlike the symtomatology in ulcerative colitis, persistent rectal bleeding is not a prominent feature.

The *differential diagnosis* includes disorders of both the small and large bowel. Occasionally the patient presents with fever and acute right lower quadrant pain resembling acute appendicitis. When there is terminal ileal involvement, Crohn's disease must be distinguished from lymphoma and tuberculosis. Colonic involvement may suggest ulcerative colitis (see above), ischemic colitis, or carcinoma (see Chapter 34). The predominant involvement of the distal small bowel and the right colon, the presence of characteristic skip areas, stricturing of the bowel, and fistula formation are helpful diagnostic features that suggest Crohn's disease.

Treatment. Therapy for Crohn's disease is similar to that for ulcerative colitis, depending heavily on corticosteroids and sulfasalazine (Azulfidine). These agents may be effective in treating the recurrent attacks that characterize Crohn's disease, but neither agent has been shown to be effective in preventing relapses. Metronidazole (Flagyl), may prove to be effective for perirectal fistulas. Immunosuppressants, like azathioprine (Imuran) have produced variable results, and their use in this condition must be considered experimental.

Surgery is sometimes necessary in Crohn's disease to treat the complications of the inflammatory process. Surgery is indicated for (a) resection of fibrotic obstructing lesions, (b) drainage of abscesses, and (c) resection of complicated fistulas. Occasionally the disease is refractory to medical therapy, and the diseased bowel must be resected. It must be recognized that surgery is not intended to be curative, so that removal of normal bowel to achieve wide "disease-free' margins is generally not indicated. Bypass surgery is being performed less often, as there appears to be an increasing frequency of the development of cancer in bypassed segments. In the rare patient whose disease is extensive and unresponsive to medical and surgical intervention, or in whom a short bowel syndrome has developed secondary to the disease and to repeated surgery, long term home parenteral hyperalimentation can be beneficial in providing good nutritional support and even in ameliorating symptoms.

Course. Despite its chronicity and tendency for recurrence, Crohn's disease takes a highly variable course. Prolonged relatively asymptomatic periods occur, even after years of disease activity and after multiple operations. There is a poor correlation between the clinical severity and the radiologic appearance of the disease. Mortality from the disease is low. As the natural history is so variable, the physician should approach the patient with Crohn's disease in a positive and hopeful fashion, yet be aware of the potential for significant morbidity. All patients should be followed in close consultation with a gastroenterologist.

DRUG-INDUCED DIARRHEA

A variety of commonly used medications may cause diarrhea (Table 35.4). The diarrhea may be a direct result of the pharmacologic activity of the drug (e.g., magnesium-containing antacids or colchicine); or the mechanism for the induction of diarrhea may

Table 35.4
Common Drugs That May Induce Diarrhea

ANTIBIOTICS:
  Clindamycin
  Ampicillin
  Cephalosporin
ANTACIDS: Magnesium-containing
ANTIHYPERTENSIVE AGENTS:
  Guanethidine
  Hydralazine
  Methyldopa
  Propranolol
  Reserpine
CARDIOVASCULAR AGENTS:
  Digitalis
  Quinidine
ANTIMETABOLITES: Colchicine
ALCOHOL
NUTRITIONAL SUPPLEMENTS: Hyperosmolar solutions
  (enteral feedings)
POTENT DIURETICS:
  Furosemide
  Ethacrynic acid

be unknown (e.g., hydralazine or propranolol). The diarrhea may also signify drug toxicity (e.g., digitalis). Certain drugs have repeatedly been associated with diarrhea (antibiotics, antacids, quinidine, digitalis, alcohol) while in other cases (hydralazine, propranolol) the relationship is not well established (1).

Diarrhea associated with antibiotics may range from a mild increase in the frequency and volume of stools to a toxic, life-threatening condition. Diarrhea may develop during the course of antibiotic therapy, after either parenteral or oral use, but may also occur up to 3 weeks after discontinuation of the drugs. The antibiotics most commonly associated with diarrhea are ampicillin, tetracycline, clindamycin, and the cephalosporins.

In the more severe forms of antibiotic-associated diarrhea the diarrhea is bloody and is accompanied by abdominal cramps and fever. Proctoscopy may reveal pseudomembranes which appear as raised plaques on edematous friable mucosa. Histologically these pseudomembranes are collections of fibrin, mucin, and leukocytes. The etiology of pseudomembranous colitis is now believed to be due to the proliferation of *Clostridium difficile* and the elaboration of its toxin. This organism accounts for the vast majority of cases of pseudomembranous colitis and for about 20% of antibiotic-associated diarrhea in general.

Therapy involves discontinuation of the antibiotics and, in cases of pseudomembranous colitis, administration of oral vancomycin (see Chapter 25). This antibiotic is effective against clostridial organisms, and the response is fairly rapid. Relapses after discontinuation of vancomycin have been reported. Oral cholestyramine has also been used effectively to bind the toxin. Antidiarrheal medications are contraindicated as they may actually prolong the duration of the disease.

POSTSURGICAL DIARRHEA

A variety of surgical procedures may result in diarrhea. Obviously, *extensive small bowel resections*, e.g., for mesenteric vascular occlusions, result in severe diarrhea and steatorrhea. Management of such patients requires careful attention to nutritional factors and often requires narcotics for control of the diarrhea. Long term home hyperalimentation (currently available only through a few university centers and requiring special equipment and specially trained personnel) has allowed patients to overcome the severe malabsorption that would accompany massive small bowel resection.

Resection of the ileum is less well tolerated than is resection of the jejunum since the ileum serves as the only site for absorption of bile acids. When the ileal resection is limited (less than 100 cm) the total bile acid pool remains sufficient to prevent significant steatorrhea. However, there is still an excessive loading of bile salts into the colon where they stimulate mucosal secretion and result in diarrhea. Therapy for this form of diarrhea is aimed at binding the fecal bile acids with an agent such as cholestyramine. The dose is 4 g (usually provided by one package or scoopful), given before meals and at bedtime. When ileal resection is more extensive, (greater than 100 cm) the total bile acid pool becomes diminished below the critical level needed for proper digestion and absorption of fat, and steatorrhea develops. The use of cholestyramine in this situation only further depletes the bile acid pool and worsens the steatorrhea and diarrhea. Therefore, dietary fat should be supplied in the form of medium chain triglycerides which do not require bile salts for absorption. Commercial preparations are available (e.g., Portagen) and consultation with a nutritionist as well as a gastroenterologist is recommended.

Diarrhea may also follow *gastric surgery*. At times the vagotomy causes diarrhea by altering intestinal motility, and for unclear reasons, by increasing the concentration of fecal bile salts. Therapy with cholestyramine has been successful in this postvagotomy syndrome. Gastric surgery may also unmask a latent lactase deficiency, or rarely, a latent celiac sprue. The blind loop syndrome with resultant bacterial overgrowth, dumping syndrome, inadvertent gastroileal anastomosis, and gastrocolic fistula are all complications that may result in diarrhea in patients after gastrectomy (see Chapter 33).

Diarrhea occurs rarely following routine cholecystectomy, but, when it does occur, it has been associated with an increased concentration of fecal bile salts. Therapy with cholestyramine is effective. Subtotal colectomy, with an ileal-rectal anastomosis, (e.g., for multiple polyposis) frequently results in diarrhea which is usually easily controlled by antidiarrheal medication (see below) and diminishes with time. Segmental colonic resection usually does not result in diarrhea.

Symptomatic Antidiarrheal Therapy

Diarrhea is, after all, merely a symptom, and therapy, if possible, should be directed at the primary underlying process. However, a wide variety of agents are available for symptomatic control of diarrhea. The efficacy of these agents is highly variable, and the mechanism of action of many is poorly understood. Symptomatic treatment should be avoided (except in minimal doses to prevent marked discomfort) in acute infectious diarrhea, since early suppression of diarrhea in these conditions prolongs the diarrhea.

Hydrophilic bulk-forming agents, like psyllium seed (Metamucil, Konsyl), have been shown to improve the consistency of ileostomy and colostomy effluent. These agents, which paradoxically are also used in treating constipation (see p. 299), are particularly useful in patients with painless diarrhea and in patients with irritable bowel syndrome (Chapter 36).

Another group of antidiarrheal medications are classified as *adsorbents* on the premise that these agents adsorb factors within the intestinal lumen which cause diarrhea. Medications of this group include kaolin and pectin (Kaopectate), bismuth salts (Pepto-Bismol), aluminum hydroxide (Amphojel), and cholestyramine (Questran). These agents are generally available over the counter, but their value is not well established. Pepto-Bismol has been shown, however, to be effective in controlling the symptoms of traveler's diarrhea (see Chapter 25). Cholestyramine, as previously mentioned, is effective in treating bile acid-induced diarrhea as in patients after ileal resection, vagotomy, or cholecystectomy. This drug also may bind other compounds, like digoxin and warfarin, and thereby decrease their absorption.

Opiate and opioid derivatives are probably the most effective antidiarrheal medications. Opiate drugs delay the transit of intraluminal contents through the small and large intestine. A possible central effect cannot be excluded. In patients with extensive small bowel resection tincture of opium or codeine may be the only effective form of therapy. The synthetic agents, diphenoxylate-atropine (Lomotil) and loperamide (Imodium) are effective also and generally are very well tolerated. The atropine in Lomotil contributes little to its antidiarrheal effect, but may cause significant toxicity. Imodium has the theoretical advantages of a more favorable ratio of gastrointestinal effects to central nervous system effects and a longer duration of action. Imodium has the practical disadvantage of being relatively expensive, costing about $25.00 per 100 tablets compared to approximately $18.00 for Lomotil. The development of megacolon, prolongation of symptoms, and worsening of pseudomembranous colitis have all been linked to the injudicious use of these agents in patients with bacterial diarrhea. The potential risk for abuse is theoretically less for Imodium, but has probably been overemphasized for Lomotil.

Another class of drugs that is under intensive investigation is classified as "*antisecretory.*" Some of these drugs inhibit the synthesis of prostaglandins, ubiquitous fatty acids which increase intestinal secretion by stimulating adenylate cyclase activity within intestinal cells. (Adenylate cyclase is the enzyme which catalyzes the formation of cyclic AMP, the concentration of which influences certain transport systems in cell membranes.) Other drugs of this class inhibit adenylate cyclase directly. For example, indomethacin (Indocin) inhibits prostaglandin synthesis and has been shown experimentally to inhibit the effect of enterotoxin; and propranolol (Inderal), an inhibitor of adenylate cyclase, suppresses bile acid-induced fluid accumulation in intestinal loops. Certain diuretics, like ethracynic acid (Edecrin), which act on electrolyte transport, also have been shown to be effective enterotoxin antagonists. While these antisecretory agents are not now recommended for use in antidiarrheal therapy, investigation into their mechanism of action may lead to the development of new effective forms of therapy against diarrhea.

Since there are few data to allow an objective comparison of the various antidiarrheal medications, the choice of drug must be based on efficacy, safety, and cost. For acute self-limited illnesses, drugs like kaolin-pectate, and bismuth salts are often tried by patients, even before a physician is consulted. For such patients, diphenoxylate-atropine or loperamide are highly effective. Patients should be instructed to use medication after a diarrheal movement, not to exceed eight tablets per day. Loperamide may provide longer diarrhea-free intervals with fewer side effects (6).

For patients with chronic diarrhea, the choice of medication is based on the severity of the diarrhea and on its cause. In patients with the diarrhea-predominant form of the irritable bowel syndrome (Chapter 36), hydrophilic agents may be useful. The dose should be titrated to the desired bowel habits, with doses ranging from one teaspoon to two tablespoons per day mixed in 8 oz of juice or water. In patients with diarrhea from other causes diphenoxylate-atropine or loperamide should be tried. These medications can be given in divided doses throughout the day. Diarrhea can also be prevented by taking one or two tablets before engaging in an event associated with diarrhea (meals, examinations, etc).

In more severe cases of diarrhea, narcotics are necessary. Tincture of opium is convenient because it can easily be titrated (by the drop) to control diarrhea at the lowest possible dose. A recommended starting dose is 6 drops every 4 to 6 hours, to be adjusted by one or two drops per dose depending on the patient's response. Codeine, at a dose of 15 to 30 mg, may also be used with the same dosage schedule.

References

General

Matseshe, J and Phillips, S: Chronic diarrhea: a practical approach. *Med Clin North Am* 62: 141, 1978.
    Provides clear guidelines to the evaluation of this problem and indications for various tests.
Schuster, MM: Constipation and anorectal disorders. *Clin. Gastroenterol* 6: 643, 1977.

Specific

1. Deren, JJ: Iatrogenic diarrhea. *Pract Gastroenterol* 4: 25, 1980.
2. Gray, GM: Intestinal disaccharidase deficiencies and glucose-galactose malabsorption. In *Metabolic Basis of Inherited Disease*, Ed. 4, p. 1526 edited by JB Stanbury, JB Wyngaarden and DS Fredrickson. McGraw-Hill, New York, 1978.
3. Harris, JC, DuPont, HL and Hornick, RB: Fecal leukocytes in diarrheal illness. *Ann Intern Med* 76: 697, 1972.
4. Kaufman, N and Schuster, M: Colonic motility studies differentiate three types of constipation. *Gastroenterology* 76: 1166, 1979.
5. Martelli, H, Devroede, G, Arhan, P, et al.: Some parameters of large bowel motility in normal man. *Gastroenterology* 75: 612, 1978.
6. Palmer, KR, Corbett, CL and Holdsworth, CD: Double blind cross-over study comparing loperamide, codeine, and diphenoxylate in the treatment of chronic diarrhea. *Gastroenterology* 79: 1272, 1980.

CHAPTER THIRTY-SIX

The Irritable Bowel Syndrome

MARVIN M. SCHUSTER, M.D.

DEFINITION AND EPIDEMIOLOGY

Irritable bowel syndrome (IBS) is the most common gastrointestinal condition encountered in medical practice. The syndrome is diagnosed on the basis of: (a) abdominal pain, (b) altered bowel habits, and (c) the absence of detectable organic pathology. A related condition, *painless (or "nervous") diarrhea*, should be considered either as a separate entity, or at best a variant of IBS, because it affects persons with different personality profiles, is more directly and immediately related to emotional stress, and has a different course and prognosis. Symptoms of IBS generally appear during late teenage or in the early 20s and more commonly afflict women than men, the disorder having a female to male predominance of 2:1. The symptoms rarely appear for the first time after the age of 50, and therefore the physician should be extremely reluctant to make this diagnosis in the older patient who has had a recent onset of symptoms. There is some question about whether recurrent abdominal pain of childhood is a form of IBS or leads to IBS in later life.

There are many other terms by which irritable bowel syndrome is known. These include mucus colitis, nervous colitis, spastic colon, nervous colon, irritated colon, and unstable colon. The term "colitis" is especially inappropriate since no inflammation is present and since it is frightening to the patient, who easily confuses it with ulcerative colitis. This misconception imposes unnecessary stress on patients whose condition is readily aggravated by stress. The term irritable bowel syndrome is more appropriate than other terms because it refers to general gastrointestinal irritability, indicating that areas other than the colon may be involved, and it also emphasizes that this is a syndrome and not a specific disease.

PATHOPHYSIOLOGY

The signs and symptoms of irritable bowel syndrome appear related predominantly to exaggeration of normal intestinal motility patterns. In normal subjects the dominant type of motor activity is that of segmenting contractions, which tend to retard the forward movement of intraluminal contents. This impeding activity represents about 90% or more of the wave types recorded in normal individuals. When this type of activity is excessive, constipation ensues. In diarrheal states this activity is markedly diminished or abolished and is replaced by infrequent mass propulsive movements (which may occur 5 or 6 times a day during episodes of diarrhea). The symptoms of irritable bowel syndrome (abdominal pain, constipation, diarrhea) are related to excessively strong, spastic contractions of either the segmenting (impeding) or of the propulsive type. The motility pattern of IBS has been described as the paradoxical motility of constipation and diarrhea, but the paradox is a spurious one, if these basic principles are understood.

Motility can be influenced by a number of factors such as meals, emotionally stressful situations, anxiety, and various drugs (e.g., opiates). In IBS, exacerbation of symptoms by meals is thought to be related to an exaggeration of the normal biphasic postprandial response—the gastroileocolic response, which consists of an early neurogenic (reflex) component during the first 15 to 30 min postprandially, and hormonally stimulated contractions that appear after 40 min. The hormonal phase may be initiated by gastrointestinal hormones released during feeding. For example cholecystokinin, which is released as food enters the duodenum, can reproduce postprandial symptoms in some patients with IBS, and these symptoms are associated with increased motility. Whether this or other hormones of this type are clinically important is unknown.

DIAGNOSIS

History

Most patients with IBS come to medical attention after their symptoms have been present for months or years. Major complaints are those of pain and altered bowel habits. Which of these two components is emphasized depends on which is the more disturbing to the patient. This, in turn, is determined by the intensity of each symptom, by the patient's reaction to it, and by the disruptive effects of the symptom on the patient's function and activities. For example, some patients are less bothered by abdominal pain which can be hidden from others but are perturbed by urgent diarrhea which interferes with their job or social functions. The pattern of symptoms varies considerably from person to person but remains fairly consistent for a given individual, with changes for an individual occurring predominantly in intensity or frequency of occurrence. Typically, symptoms are intermittent with symptom-free periods lasting days, weeks, or, rarely, months. An occasional patient will have symptoms every day.

PAIN

The quality of pain may be described by one patient as crampy, by another as sharp or burning. For most, the pain is relieved temporarily by a bowel movement. One of the most important features that differentiates functional from organic pain is that the pain does not awaken the patient from sleep. It is important that the question concerning this feature is carefully phrased, since there is an important distinction between awakening with pain and being awakened by pain. Patients with IBS who are depressed have early morning awakening, and, after awakening, experience pain; but close questioning can determine that the patient was not awakened by the pain. The location of pain may vary from person to person, but is fairly consistent for a given person. Pain may be localized to any quadrant, although it is more commonly in the lower abdomen than anywhere else and in the left lower quadrant more commonly than in the right. Although the pain usually does not radiate, some patients describe transmission into the lower back or down the legs. The distribution of the pain is generally over a wide enough area so that the patient, when asked to point to the location of the pain, does so with the flat of his hand rather than with a finger, and often makes a circular motion covering a broad area. More often than not, the onset of pain does not appear to correlate with any known precipitating stressful event; instead, periods of illness may correlate with general periods of stress over months or years. It is important to determine what life experiences or interpersonal relationships constitute stress for a particular person so that this can be taken into account when establishing a treatment program.

ALTERED BOWEL HABITS

The altered pattern of defecation in patients with irritable bowel syndrome may consist of constipation, diarrhea, or more commonly, alternating constipation and diarrhea, with one of the two predominating (Chapter 35 discusses these symptoms in detail). As with pain, the altered pattern of defecation, though variable from person to person, is fairly consistent for a given individual, changing only in periodicity and intensity.

Not infrequently the major disordered bowel function occurs in the morning, with the first stool being normal in consistency followed in rapid succession by increasingly loose stools, sometimes associated with flatulence and sometimes also precipitated by meals. The bowel movements are accompanied by a great deal of urgency and are preceded by cramps which are relieved by defecation. Formed stools are often compressed and of narrow pencil-sized diameter because of the molding effect of rectosigmoid spasm. In other instances spasm of the colon results in the passage of scybalous stools described by the patient as dehydrated pellets. Mucus may cover the stools or be passed separately. Stools may mistakenly be referred to as diarrheal when they consist of frequently passed small quantities of soft fragments that are narrow in caliber. Explosive defecation may result from evacuation of gas along with the stool.

Painless Diarrhea. Patients who present with diarrhea but do not have abdominal pain generally are thought to have a disorder that is different from irritable bowel syndrome, although sometimes painless diarrhea is classified as a variant of the irritable bowel syndrome. Compared to patients with IBS their symptoms are more directly related to a stressful event, follow more immediately upon that stress, and respond more readily and dramatically to alleviation of stress. Also the prognosis is generally better than it is in classical IBS.

RELATIONSHIP OF SYMPTOMS TO MEALS

Some, but not all patients with IBS, experience exacerbation of their symptoms postprandially. They appear to be a special subset of patients; there is some indication that postprandial exacerbation may be related to gastrointestinal hormones (such as cholecystokinin) that are released as food enters the alimentary canal. Some patients report intolerance of specific foods, most commonly milk, caffeine, fried foods, and red wine.

GAS

Intestinal gas derives either from swallowing of air, from bacterial breakdown of poorly digested foods, or from diminished absorption of gas (which may occur during the rapid transit which accompanies diarrhea). Aerophagia is aggravated by frequent swallowing while chewing gum and during nervous states and is induced by a dry throat or by the excessive intake of carbonated beverages including beer. Increased gas production follows eating of legumes (beans, for example) which contain stachyose and raffinose, substances that can only be digested by colonic flora, resulting in release of large amounts of hydrogen in the colon. If patients have milk intolerance because of lactase deficiency, undigested lactose enters into the colon where it is broken down by colonic bacteria, also resulting in gaseous distension.

Although gaseous distension is a frequent complaint, actual measurements have demonstrated that patients with IBS have no more gas than do normal subjects. Instead, they have a decreased tolerance to distension from normal amounts of gas, a factor which may be related to hypermotility of their bowel and to the lowered threshold for distension-induced spasm. Gas, because it tends to rise, usually forms pockets under the splenic flexure, which is the highest portion of the colon in the upright position. This entrapment of air is further facilitated by distal rectosigmoid spasm which impedes its passage. The *splenic flexure syndrome* which ensues is experienced as chest pain that may mimic the pain of myocardial ischemia. A similar *hepatic flexure syndrome* can accompany gas trapped on the right side and may mimic the pain of cholecystitis.

Studies in which air has been instilled into the small bowel have demonstrated that patients with IBS tend to reflux gas more readily into the stomach than do normal subjects, which may explain their complaint of increased belching. This complaint too seems to result from abnormal intestinal motility.

UPPER GASTROINTESTINAL SYMPTOMS

One-fourth to one-half of patients with IBS complain of dyspeptic symptoms such as heartburn, "indigestion," pain, and nausea (but rarely vomiting). These upper gastrointestinal symptoms reinforce the concept that the motor abnormality is not restricted to the colon alone.

SIGNIFICANCE OF WEIGHT LOSS AND BLEEDING

Irritable bowel syndrome *per se* is not associated with either weight loss or gastrointestinal bleeding, and the appearance of either of these two symptoms in patients with IBS should alert the physician to another disorder. However, significant depression accompanying irritable bowel syndrome may explain substantial weight loss, just as anal fissures or hemorrhoids resulting from the altered bowel habits of the syndrome may explain bright red rectal bleeding. Nevertheless, either of these two symptoms warrants a meticulous search for other disorders including cancer. A sudden change in symptom pattern after a period of many years also warrants a search for a new disorder.

Table 36.1
Psychological Features of Irritable Bowel Syndrome[a]

Psychopathology	Diagnostic Features	Treatment
Depression	Sad, tearful, hopeless, fatigue, loss of interest, early morning awakening	Antidepressant medication, environmental manipulation
Anxiety	Symptoms increased by stress	Relaxation training. Environmental manipulation. Learn coping techniques
Gratification from illness behavior	Symptoms often interfere with work or socializing	Treat as a physical deformity. Encourage maximum activity. Discourage talking to others about illness. Recognize chronic nature of disorder
Cancerphobia	Patient or family reports fear. Patient describes similarity of his symptoms with a known cancer victim	Adequate early workup; then limit further investigation. Discuss openly with patient

[a] After W.E. Whitehead and M. M. Schuster: Psychological management of irritable bowel syndrome *Practical Gastroenterology, 3:* 32, 1979.

PSYCHOLOGICAL FACTORS (see Table 36.1)

Seventy percent of patients with IBS have abnormal scores on psychological testing. The psychologic disturbances that most commonly accompany irritable bowel syndrome are hysteria, anxiety, depression, and cancerphobia. Of these, anxiety is the most readily detected and perhaps the easiest to treat by pharmacological means, by psychologic approaches, or by environmental manipulation. Depression is generally masked, and is commonly overlooked by patient and physician alike (see Chapter 14). This is in part because somatization, a common manifestation of depression, results in a focus upon complaints that may misdirect the physician's attention from underlying psychologic factors. Depression should be suspected in patients who appear preoccupied or sad or who by their report or the report of family members have lost interest in matters that formerly interested them. Cancerphobia may be suggested when the patient compares his symptoms with those of a relative or friend who has had cancer. In addition to determining whether or not the patient has an unwarranted and excessive fear of cancer the physician should also seek to elicit from him and from other informants any other fears or concerns that the patient has with respect to himself and his illness.

Physical Examination

Except for an anxious demeanor, patients with IBS usually look remarkably healthy, and physical examination is correspondingly normal with the frequent exception of mildly increased tympany to percussion over one or more areas of the colon and a tender cordlike sigmoid palpable in the left lower quadrant. A palpable sigmoid itself is not an unusual finding, even in normal people, because firm stool may be present in this area, but tenderness is significant. Tenderness may be present in other areas also, particularly in the right lower quadrant, where a squishy cecum may be palpated.

Digital rectal examination is usually unremarkable, but may reveal excessive tenderness. Proctoscopic examination should demonstrate no structural abnormality, but often does reveal rectal and rectosigmoid spasm and excessive tenderness, that precludes advance beyond 12 or 13 cm. At times excessive mucus is encountered.

In patients with symptoms of IBS, the physician should look for signs of hyperthyroidism, masses, adenopathy, and partial intestinal obstruction as well as for abdominal bruits which might signal ischemic intestinal angina in the elderly.

Laboratory Tests

Basic laboratory tests should be carried out to demonstrate the absence of anemia, normal white blood cell count and sedimentation rate, the absence of blood, ova, and parasites on three stool examinations, a negative sigmoidoscopy, and (when symptoms are severe enough or prolonged enough to warrant the study) a barium enema negative except for spastic contractions. Effacement of haustra may be seen in the barium enema if there has been prolonged laxative abuse (see Chapter 35). Occasionally a small bowel series will be necessary to rule out Crohn's disease, especially when diarrhea predominates. Painful splenic flexure symptoms sometimes require studies to rule out coronary artery disease (see Chapter 54).

The basic principle in the selection and timing of laboratory tests is to perform as early as possible those tests which are necessary to convince both the physician and the patient that organic disease has been ruled out. It is generally imprudent to postpone some tests for a later date or to repeat tests continually, since this behavior arouses the suspicion that the diagnosis is uncertain, that the disease might be progressive, or that a new and more dire consequence such as cancer or colitis may be developing.

Differential Diagnosis

Many of the symptoms of irritable bowel syndrome are nonspecific and can be produced by other disorders. A careful travel history should be obtained relative to possible bacterial infection or parasitic infestation including giardiasis and amoebiasis.

Since patients with lactose intolerance often do not associate their symptoms with milk, the failure to find a direct relationship between milk intake and diarrhea should not dissuade the physician from testing for milk tolerance. Lactose intolerance is best ruled out by a therapeutic trial on a lactose-free diet for 3 weeks, eliminating all milk and milk products

including butter, cottage cheese, yogurt, and soft cheeses. Aged cheeses such as Swiss cheese and Jarlsberg are permissible since most of the lactose in them has been eliminated. Acidophilus milk (cultured with Lactobacillus acidophilus), contrary to popular misconception, contains the same amount of lactose as does regular milk. However lactose can be eliminated from milk by adding two packets of lactase (Lactaid, Maxilact, or a similar preparation) to a quart of milk, which is then permitted to remain overnight in the refrigerator; this procedure reduces, but does not eliminate entirely, the symptoms of lactose intolerance (3). Otherwise, nondairy (lactose-free) substitutes such as Coffeemate, Cremora, or Mocha Mix may be used. Margarine may be substituted for butter. If all symptoms disappear on a lactose-free diet, then the diagnosis is that of lactose intolerance. Partial improvement implies that, in addition to irritable bowel syndrome, the patient has lactose intolerance and that some of the symptoms (usually those of gaseous bloating and diarrhea) are due to the intolerance. The therapeutic dietary trial is more useful than a lactose tolerance test, which simply tests the patient's response to a given amount of lactose in a single dose at a particular time.

Among the other disorders which can mimic symptoms of diarrhea-predominant irritable bowel syndrome are hyperthyroidism, nontropical sprue, carcinoid, Zollinger-Ellison syndrome, medullary carcinoma of the thyroid, diabetic autonomic neuropathy, Addison's disease, and Whipple's disease. Constipation-predominant IBS may be mimicked by hypothyroidism, hyperparathyroidism, diverticular disease, intestinal obstruction, and colon cancer. Suspicion of any of these disorders justifies the appropriate tests to rule them out. Further evaluation of patients with atypical symptoms of irritable bowel syndrome should be done in consultation with a gastroenterologist

THERAPY

Natural History

There is evidence that approximately 10 to 15% of the general adult population who have not sought medical attention for irritable bowel complaints have symptoms which are sufficiently precise to qualify for the diagnosis of irritable bowel syndrome (4). It is currently uncertain whether patients who seek medical attention are different from those who do not, and whether this difference, if it exists, is based on the severity of symptoms or on their effect on a particular person. Approximately one-fourth of patients who seek medical treatment for IBS ultimately have a permanent remission. It is unclear whether this represents the natural course of the disease or a response to early treatment of mild disease. The patient who is referred for gastroenterological consultation often has correspondingly more severe and chronic symptoms and generally experiences a more prolonged course.

Although there is little information concerning patients with IBS who present to the primary care physician, it has been shown that the course of patients seen by gastroenterologists follows a fairly consistent pattern that is characteristic for the given individual. In fact the pattern is so consistent that any significant change should be accepted as a warning of a new superimposed problem warranting further investigation.

General Principles

Since the underlying etiology of IBS is unknown, treatment is symptomatic and relies on education, reassurance, diet, supportive and behavioral therapy, and pharmacotherapy aimed at both the underlying motor disorder and its psychologic concomitants. Successful management requires an interest in the patient and his disorder, an understanding on the part of both patient and physician of what is known about IBS and, above all, a recognition of the chronic nature of the disorder, which implies acceptance of a prolonged cooperative therapeutic endeavor.

Education and Reassurance

Treatment begins with the first interview and physical examination, which should be designed to begin to establish a relationship of mutual interest and confidence and which should be thorough enough to demonstrate to the patient that the physician has taken seriously the complaints and is performing all the necessary maneuvers to rule out organic causes. At the same time attention to the details of all the contributing factors, including diet, emotional reactions, interpersonal relationships, social interactions, and the patient's fears and concerns, provides ample evidence to the patient that these are important factors for him to consider and with which he must deal. The worst mistake that a physician can make is to downplay the symptoms on the grounds that they exist only in the patient's mind. This is incorrect physiologically and therapeutically; a definite motor disorder exists and can be demonstrated by both myoelectric and motility recordings.

It is important to take the time to explain to the patient the present understanding of the disordered motility (see p. 310) and the factors influencing it, to emphasize that although the disorder is chronic, it can be managed by appropriate cooperation between patient and physician. The demonstrated ability of the physician to predict the course establishes that he is knowledgeable and promotes confidence. Furthermore, if the patient knows what to anticipate and understands that treatment can be expected to ameliorate rather than eliminate the disorder, he is better prepared to face recurrence, which otherwise might be disappointing and frightening. Labeling and un-

derstanding the abnormal motor activity can be reassuring to the patient and may provide him with the patience required to wait for gradual improvement. At the same time the positive implications of the diagnosis should be underscored, emphasizing that IBS, though often persistent, does not lead to cancer, colitis, or ileitis and does not alter life expectancy.

Diet

Even when the patient keeps a meticulous daily log relating onset of symptoms to life events (including activities, interpersonal relations, and food intake), it is often difficult to make direct associations with any degree of specificity. It is best to explain to those individuals who have postprandial distress that, although some foods may be bothersome, it is usually the act of eating (rather than a specific food) that aggravates the symptoms. Since a lactose-free diet can provide dramatic relief for patients who are lactose-intolerant, it is worthwhile trying such a diet in every patient (as stated above). Otherwise the most that can be said about food intolerance is that some people react badly to coffee, carbonated beverages, and spicy sauces, although no convincing evidence exists in this regard. Therefore patients may wish to abstain from these foods for a period, noting whether symptoms recur on at least two occasions when each substance is reintroduced. Any food that is definitely associated with precipitation of symptoms should obviously be avoided, but one should be careful not to create a dietary cripple.

Although the therapeutic role of bran in the treatment of IBS has not been established, some patients with constipation-predominant IBS do derive benefit from a diet comprising at least 14 g of bran. This can be administered as 2 tablespoons of miller's unprocessed bran 3 times daily. Bran can be obtained from a health food store. Since it looks and tastes like sawdust, it can be camouflaged in cereal, baked in cookies, or taken with a beverage. Studies in another disorder, diverticular disease, show that the effect of bran on transit and motility appears to be specific and is not common to all fibers (1). Therefore lettuce, celery, and fruits may not produce similar results. Bran has been shown to increase the size of stool and the frequency of its passage. Patients should be warned that there might be some increase in flatulence when bran is first administered, but that it will wear off by the end of 3 weeks in 80% of patients. However, 15 or 20% of people find these side effects intolerable even after 3 weeks. Dosage should be titrated for each patient, weighing the beneficial effects against the annoying side effects.

The hydrophilic colloids (bulk agents such as Metamucil, Konsyl, or L.A. Formula containing psyllium seed) may be especially useful in those patients who have alternating constipation and diarrhea. Because of their hydrophilic qualities they tend to bind water and therefore decrease the fluidity of diarrheal stools, while preventing excess dehydration in constipated patients. Initially, 1 to 2 tablespoons of hydrophilic powder are prescribed in conjunction with a meal 2 to 3 times a day, and the dose is gradually diminished to once a day (adjusting to the patient's response). It is better to prescribe the agent before or after a meal rather than at bedtime, so that it becomes mixed with the meal as it traverses the gastrointestinal tract. When taken at night the medication can result in the passage of rock-hard stool followed by a gelatinous mass. Patients who are thin should take the bulk agent after meals, since it tends to suppress appetite, whereas obese patients may derive benefit from taking it before meals, thus achieving satiation without caloric content.

Drugs

Although there are ample theoretical grounds for prescribing antispasmodic medication, clinical experience with spasmolytic agents has been disappointing. Nevertheless some patients improve with antispasmodic drugs, particularly those whose symptoms are induced by meals and those who complain of tenesmus. Well controlled studies are needed to determine whether anticholinergic medication has more than a placebo effect. When used for those whose symptoms are related to meals, anticholinergics should be prescribed 30 to 45 min before meals so that the major benefit of the drug will be available at the time of anticipated symptoms. Patients with tenesmus should take the drug on a regular basis, timing the dose so that it is given as close as possible to 1 hour before anticipated symptoms. There is no evidence that one anticholinergic is better than another, but it seems logical to use drugs which have the highest ratio of antispasmodic to antisecretory effect, so that a large dose can be administered to suppress spasm without producing undesirable side effects such as dry mouth. Mebeverine, a spasmolytic agent with little or no antisecretory effect, is available in most countries outside the United States and is prescribed in doses of 100 to 200 mg q.i.d. (half an hour before meals if symptoms are meal-related). In this country dicyclomine hydrochloride (Bentyl) is given in dosages of 20 to 40 mg, 4 times a day, as tolerated. The major side effects are tachycardia and orthostatic hypotension. Thus, baseline and follow-up recordings of pulse rate and blood pressure, with the patient seated and standing are very important. Dicyclomine should be prescribed in small quantities to elderly people who are susceptible to orthostatic changes; for example, 10-mg doses on a divided basis, gradually increasing to reach the desired effect as tolerated. If improvement ensues, long term medication for months or years is warranted. Tolerance usually does not develop but change to a different anticholinergic may be helpful if benefit decreases. A therapeutic trial should be carried out for at least 3 weeks to test the efficacy of the drug.

Significant diarrhea may respond to diphenoxylate (Lomotil) 1 to 2 tablets every 6 hours while diarrhea persists The related drug, loperamide (Imodium) has a longer duration of action and 1 to 2 tablets every 8 hours may be given. Care should be taken to discontinue medication as soon as the diarrhea is controlled in order to avoid inducing constipation, especially in those patients who are prone to have alternating diarrhea and constipation. Patients who have strongly diarrhea-predominant IBS and who do not respond to the above medications may benefit from codeine 30 to 60 mg every 6 hours especially if pain is disabling. Because of its potential addicting qualities, codeine should be prescribed with caution, although addiction is rare when codeine is taken for diarrhea. This is partially because intestinal tolerance to the drug does not develop. The same dose that controls diarrhea at one stage continues to control it subsequently, and escalating doses are not required as they are in patients who have developed central nervous system addiction.

Analgesic medication should be avoided if possible, and when needed should be prescribed in the mildest form and lowest dose possible. Aspirin and acetaminophen, however, are rarely effective. Pentazocine (Talwin), 50 to 100 mg, can be given every 6 hours as needed for severe pain, but the number of tablets taken should be monitored. Morphine and codeine (see above) generally should be avoided, especially when constipation exists, because they tend to aggravate spasm; and Demerol should be reserved for extreme pain on unusual occasions.

GAS CONTROL

Most medications designed to alleviate gaseous distension have proven disappointing. However, simethicone (Mylicon), 2 to 4 tablets with meals, or activated charcoal, four tablets with meals and at bedtime, can be prescribed as a therapeutic trial. Phazyme 95, 1 to 2 tablets with meals and at bedtime, or similar enzymes such as Ilozyme, Pancrease, Viokase. Cotazym etc., can also be tried.

Psychologic Management (see Table 36.1)

Psychologic management begins with the recognition of depression, anxiety, and somatization of affect. Symptoms of IBS often are anxiety-provoking and frequently are perpetuated by social reinforcement (secondary gain). Psychologic evaluation and management usually can be effectively performed by the interested physician without the need for psychiatric referral. The condition itself is not an indication for psychiatric consultation. Referral should be reserved for those patients who would need expert psychotherapy whether or not they have irritable bowel syndrome.

Psychologic management is dictated by answers to the following questions:

1. Is there evidence of anxiety and are the symp-

toms aggravated by stress? If so, what are the specific stresses? Stress-induced anxiety can be handled by avoiding or modifying situational factors, and by teaching relaxation techniques (using audiotapes).* Occasionally mild tranquilizing agents are indicated (see Chapter 12).

2. Is the patient depressed? As with anxiety, attempts should be made to determine specific depressing situations and especially to determine whether simple maneuvers can alter them. If not, the patient sometimes can learn new ways of handling situations which cannot be avoided. Tricyclic antidepressants (see Chapter 14) prove helpful in depression.

3. Does gratification from illness behavior (see Chapter 11) reinforce the illness? Evidence that this is so derives from the history that the illness keeps the patient from job-related or social discomfort and stress. The spouse, family, or friends respond sympathetically to the patient's symptoms, providing further reinforcement. The patient's motivation is generally unconscious, and it is a strategic error to accuse a patient of trying to derive benefit from the illness. Treatment is designed to reduce the amount of gratification that illness behavior evokes. The patient is asked not to discuss his illness with family members, but instead to reserve his complaints for his physician. In return family members are instructed to help the patient by discouraging excessive discussion of his illness and by avoiding overly sympathetic responses. The patient is instructed to view the illness as he would a physical disability which he would like to overcome by pushing his performance to maximum capacity.

4. What misconceptions does the patient have about his illness? The answer to this question can be obtained from questions directed to the patient as well as to his family who may provide information that the patient is reluctant to give. A rational explanation of the patient's disorder is necessary, but the physician should also listen attentively to the patient's irrational fears (of cancer, for example), and he should deal with them as well. Patience is required since these issues may need to be worked through repetitively. A steady, supportive approach is most desirable, as well as a clear demonstration that the physician is acquainted with and sensitive to the patient, his disorder, and his needs. Regular (although not necessarily frequent) follow-up visits supply reassurance to the patient while "p.r.n." (as the need arises) visits are often viewed as abandonment or an indication of impotence on the part of a physician who feels incapable of providing further help. Furthermore, p.r.n. visits lend themselves to greater

abuse by the patient who is seeking secondary gains (see also Chapter 11).

PROGNOSIS

Whether treatment alters the prognosis or simply affects the patient's ability to accept or deal with his symptoms has not been established. It is difficult to determine the impact of a specific form of treatment on the natural course of irritable bowel syndrome for a number of reasons: First, each patient is different; some have milder symptoms, some more severe; some have frequent reccurrences, some infrequent. Second, patients with painless diarrhea (see p. 310) have been included in some of the studies and excluded from others. Prognosis for this group is better than that of IBS patients with pain; and the number of such patients included in any given study markedly influences the results of a particular treatment program. Third, the more serious the associated psychologic factors, the more prolonged the course of IBS, no matter what the underlying precipitating factors and presentation. Fourth, physicians are different in their training, interest, background, and approaches. Fifth, a variety of treatment programs have been fashionable from time to time and none has undergone systematic, long term evaluation in a manner that provides useful scientific data. All of these factors underscore the need for organized, individualized, multifaceted management by a physician who is interested, educated, skillful, and compassionate.

References

General

Chaudhary, NA and Truelove, SC: The irritable colon syndrome. A study of the clinical features, predisposing causes, and prognosis in 130 cases. Q J Med 31: 307, 1962.
  Good clinical review based on analysis of personal experience in a large number of patients.
Schuster, MM (Ed.): Irritable bowel syndrome. Pract Gastroenterol 3: 3, 4, 5, 6 (May–Dec), 1979.
  In-depth and up-to-date symposium consisting of fifteen articles by leading experts, each focusing on a specific clinical aspect of irritable bowel syndrome.
Thompson, WG: The Irritable Gut. University Park Press, Baltimore, 1979.
  A delightfully written overview of functional disorders of the gut including irritable bowel syndrome.

Specific

1. Eastwood, MA, Smith, AN, Brydon, WG and Pritchard, J: Comparison of bran, ispaghula and lactulose on colon function in diverticular disease. Gut 19: 1144, 1978.
2. Eastwood, MA, Smith, AN, Brydon, WG and Pritchard, J: Colonic function in patients with divericular disease. Lancet 1: 1181, 1978.
3. Reasoner, J, Maculan, TP, Rand, AG and Thayer, WR: Clinical studies with low-lactose milk. Am J Clin Nutr 34: 54, 1981.
4. Whitehead, WE, Winget, C, Fedoravicius, A, Wooley, S and Blackwell, B: Learned illness behavior in patients with irritable bowel syndrome and peptic ulcer. Dig Dis Sci 27: in press.

---

*An excellent program was developed by Brudzinski and is sold by BMA Audio Cassettes, 200 Park Ave. South, New York, NY 10003.

CHAPTER THIRTY-SEVEN

Diverticular Disease

HAROLD J. TUCKER, M.D.

DEFINITIONS

The term "diverticular disease" encompasses a variety of clinical states that may differ in their etiology and prognosis. The nomenclature of diverticular disease of the colon is listed in Table 37.1. As can be seen from this classification, *diverticulosis* simply refers to the presence of diverticula (actually, since they contain no muscular wall, pseudodiverticula). *Symptomatic diverticular disease* refers to diverticulosis associated with pain and altered bowel habits in the absence of evidence of diverticular inflammation. *Diverticulitis* is the occurrence of inflamed diverticula, generally implying perforation of a diverticulum. The *prediverticular state* is characterized by the radiographic, pathologic, and often clinical features of diverticulosis without the formation of diverticula. The distinction between these entities is more than semantic as the pathophysiology and natural history of each of these conditions probably vary.

EPIDEMIOLOGY AND PATHOGENESIS

The prevalence of diverticular disease in the United States, although extremely low before the age of 30, increases considerably thereafter so that, currently, 20% of men and women over 40, and 50% over 60, have diverticulosis of the colon. These figures reflect a striking rise in the frequency of the condition over the last 70 years (5% of people over 60 were affected in the early years of this century) that is paralleled by a 25% decrease in total crude fiber in the average American diet. This association has lead to the hypothesis that a low fiber diet increases intraluminal pressure and that the increased pressure leads to herniation of the mucosa through weakened or porous parts of the colonic muscle. In support of this hypothesis is the demonstration of exaggerated contractile responses of the sigmoid colon which contains diverticula, in response to meals and cholinergic stimulation. Thus, both a low fiber diet and disordered colonic motility have been implicated in the pathogenesis of diverticulosis.

This "dismotility" hypothesis, however, has not proved to be applicable to all cases of diverticulosis. It is now recognized that the abnormal motor response of the sigmoid colon is more closely associated with the symptoms of lower abdominal pain than with the presence of diverticula. Indeed, in patients with asymptomatic diverticulosis, the sigmoid motility pattern is normal, while many subjects with similar symptoms but with no diverticula have an abnormal motor response. The history of symptoms of abdominal pain in many patients with diverticular disease is short and does not suggest the presence of any prolonged motility disturbance. Thus, while a motility disturbance may account for some of the symptoms associated with diverticulosis, it alone cannot account for the development of diverticulosis.

Another aspect in the pathogenesis of this condition is the weakness in the colonic wall through which the mucosa herniates to form the diverticulum. The site of herniation occurs at areas of least resistance, most often at points of penetration of intramural vessels through the circular muscle layer. The association of colonic diverticula with scleroderma and with Marfan's and Ehlers-Danlos syndromes

Table 37.1
Nomenclature of Diverticular Disease of Colon[a]

DIVERTICULOSIS (presence of multiple diverticula):
  Asymptomatic
  Symptomatic (pain, bowel irregularity)
  Complicated by hemorrhage
DIVERTICULITIS (necrotizing inflammation in one or more
    diverticula):
  With microperforation (local inflammation)
  With macroperforation, manifested by abscess, fistula,
  peritonitis, obstruction, or hemorrhage
PREDIVERTICULAR STATE: Muscular thickening and
    shortening of colonic wall without recognizable diverticula

[a] Adapted from: T. Almy and D. Howell: Diverticular disease of the colon. *New England Journal of Medicine, 302:* 324, 1980.

suggests that loss of muscle mass or defects in collagen may be important factors. (The diverticula associated with these diseases are actually "true" diverticula in that the muscle of the bowel wall is also involved.) Changes in collagen synthesis are known to occur with aging and may explain the increased prevalence of diverticular disease in elderly people. Thus, the formation of diverticula may also involve a degenerative process of the colonic muscle with a change in tensile strength of the colon wall.

ASYMPTOMATIC DIVERTICULOSIS

The majority of patients with diverticulosis detected on barium enema are entirely asymptomatic. The diverticula may be localized to the rectosigmoid junction or may involve the entire colon diffusely. The sigmoid colon is involved almost always (95% of the time). Rectal diverticula rarely occur, because of the muscular wrapping of the rectum.

The natural history of diverticulosis is variable. The majority of patients are asymptomatic; however, diverticulitis does occur in 10 to 25%, and bleeding, somewhat less often. In some patients, symptoms develop similar to those of the irritable bowel syndrome. The association between the irritable bowel syndrome (IBS) and diverticulosis is unclear. One study demonstrated an increase in the development of diverticulosis in patients with IBS (1). However, in most patients with diverticulosis, there is no history of antecedent IBS (see Chapter 36).

There is little evidence that therapy for asymptomatic diverticulosis is of any value. If the development of diverticulosis is really related to low fiber intake with resultant increased intraluminal pressure during segmental activity, then a high fiber diet may be beneficial. However, there is no evidence that such therapy prevents or even delays the occurrence of symptomatic diverticular disease, or of complications such as diverticulitis or hemorrhage. Maintenance of regular bowel habits without the use of laxatives is probably the best advice for these patients. It is also prudent to alert them to the manifestations of symptomatic diverticular disease (see below) and to urge them to seek medical care promptly should such symptoms develop.

SYMPTOMATIC DIVERTICULAR DISEASE

Diagnosis

Diverticular disease may at times cause abdominal pain and an alteration in bowel habits. The crampy pain is generally in the left lower quadrant, made worse by meals (presumably due to gastrocolic reflex) and at least partially relieved by having a bowel movement or by passing flatus. Bowel habits, usually during the painful episodes, become irregular, with development of constipation, diarrhea, or both in an alternating fashion. These painful attacks are usually episodic rather than continuous.

Physical examination reveals tenderness, at times marked, in the left lower quadrant. A tender sigmoid loop may be palpable, but there is no other palpable mass. The stool should be negative for occult blood, but rectal bleeding may be found due to coincidental rectal outlet disorders such as fissures or hemorrhoids. Fever is not present.

Proctosigmoidoscopy, if performed during an attack, will show a normal colonic mucosa. However, considerable pain and spasm may be caused by the procedure.

The *barium enema* (see Chapter 34, "Patient Experience") is essential both for the diagnosis of diverticulosis and for excluding other reasons for symptoms. Spasm may be a feature of diverticular disease, but fistulae or a mass suggests either diverticulitis, carcinoma, or Crohn's disease.

Therapy

The therapy for symptomatic diverticular disease is based on the assumption that low fiber diets and increased colonic pressure are important pathogenetic factors. Diets high in fiber (see Table 35.2, Chapter 35) are prescribed and have been shown to be effective in improving bowel transit and in relieving symptoms. Commercial preparations of hyrophilic colloids made from vegetable fiber are available and convenient, but are expensive compared to dietary sources (see Table 35.3, Chapter 35). Thus, patients should be instructed about high fiber diets, and, if necessary, be given hydrophilic agents, such as Metamucil, 1 tablespoon per day in a glass of water or juice.

In addition to dietary maneuvers, anticholinergic drugs or antispasmodic drugs may also be helpful. While these agents are not of proven value for this condition, some patients do respond. Dicyclomine (Bentyl), at a dose of 10 to 20 mg before meals and at bedtime is an often used initial drug. Other more potent anticholinergics may produce adverse side effects and may aggravate the constipation.

The patient should be told that the course of the disease is unpredictable and that attacks will probably be experienced at irregular intervals (months to years) for the rest of his life. There is no reason for the patient to continue to take medication for the condition between attacks, but maintenance of a high fiber diet is reasonable.

DIVERTICULITIS

In general, diverticulitis results from perforation of a diverticulum. The perforation may be grossly evident with fistulization and abscess formation, or it may be only microscopic, and well confined. As noted previously, diverticulitis occurs in less than one-quarter of all patients with diverticulosis. Even this estimate is probably exaggerated, as convincing evidence for the presence of inflammation is often lacking. The recurrence rate for diverticulitis treated medically or surgically is about 25% (2).

Diagnosis

The cardinal symptoms of acute diverticulitis are pain and fever. The pain may be severe and abrupt in onset. Complete obstruction may occur with resultant abdominal distension and nausea. Urinary tract symptoms and purulent vaginal discharge may occur because of fistula formation or because of inflammation of contiguous structures. The severity of the symptoms depends on the extent of the peridiverticular inflammation.

Abdominal tenderness and fever are found on *physical examination*. Localized peritonitis may be noted by the marked direct and rebound tenderness over the involved area, generally most pronounced in the left lower quadrant. Rectal bleeding occurs in about 25% of patients, and is usually occult. A pelvic mass may be felt on rectal and vaginal examination.

Leukocytosis is almost always present. Pyuria and/or hematuria may be found owing to contiguous involvement with the bladder or ureter.

The *differential diagnosis* includes painful diverticular disease, carcinoma of the colon, and inflammatory or ischemic bowel disease. The presence of peritonitis, fever, and leukocytosis rules out simple symtomatic diverticular disease. The other conditions are distinguished from diverticulitis by their clinical course and by proctoscopy and barium enema.

Proctoscopy (see "Patient Experience," Chapter 32) can be performed in patients with acute diverticulitis if the diagnosis is in doubt. The rigid proctosigmoidoscope will, in general, not reach the area containing the diverticula, but can exclude ulcerative colitis and rectal carcinoma. (The consultant gastroenterologist usually will not perform flexible sigmoidoscopy because of the risk of converting a confined infection to an open perforation.)

The timing of the *barium enema* depends on the clinical setting. In general, the barium enema should be delayed for 3 to 6 weeks to allow resolution of the acute inflammation and thereby to reduce the risk of perforation. The X-ray should be performed at this time not so much to make the diagnosis of diverticulitis but to exclude other conditions, such as carcinoma or Crohn's disease.

The barium enema can be performed earlier if the diagnosis is uncertain. In such cases, the radiologist must be informed of the potential diagnosis, and he should perform as limited a study as needed to make the definitive diagnosis. The diagnosis of diverticulitis is based on the finding of a mass effect on the contour of the bowel or the extravasation of the barium outside a diverticulum. The presence of spasm, or thickening of the bowel wall are not, by themselves, radiographic evidence of diverticulitis.

Therapy

Patients with diverticulitis should be hospitalized, placed on bowel rest, and given analgesics and antibiotics (preferably, a combination to which normal aerobic and anaerobic bacteria are sensitive).

For the vast majority of patients, this medical therapy will be successful; and in 75% of cases, there will be no recurrence over the next 10 years. However, failure to resolve the acute inflammatory process, recurrent attacks of diverticulitis, and obstructive stricture formation are indications for surgical intervention. It seems reasonable, although not established, that patients should be placed on a high fiber diet following recovery from an acute episode of diverticulitis.

DIVERTICULAR BLEEDING

Diverticulosis is the most common cause of massive lower gastrointestinal bleeding in adults. However, failure to distinguish diverticular hemorrhage from bleeding secondary to *angiodysplasia of the colon* (Chapter 34) has resulted in an overestimate of the incidence of diverticular bleeding. Both diverticulosis and angiodysplasia occur commonly in the older population, and frequently occur in the ascending colon, a common site of massive lower gastrointestinal bleeding. The exact mechanism for initiating diverticular bleeding is uncertain. There is no evidence that dietary therapy reduces the risk of hemorrhage. Most instances of bleeding occur in patients who are otherwise asymptomatic.

Massive hemorrhage is the most common mode of presentation for diverticular bleeding. However, massive lower gastrointestinal bleeding in a patient known to have diverticula should not automatically be ascribed to diverticulosis; in 30% of cases colonoscopy detects a second lesion (cancer, angiodysplasia) equally capable of causing bleeding (3). Occult bleeding should only be ascribed to diverticulosis after other causes have been excluded by a thorough evaluation (see Chapter 34).

Patients with diverticular hemorrhage require hospitalization for hemodynamic stabilization, diagnosis, and therapy. About 80% of patients will stop bleeding, and only 20 to 25% will bleed a second time during a several year follow-up study.

References

General

Almy, T and Howell, D: Diverticular disease of the colon. *N Engl J Med 302*: 324, 1980.
   A good discussion on pathophysiology and classification of diverticular disease. Well referenced.

Specific

1. Havia, T and Manner, R: The irritable colon syndrome. A follow-up study with special reference to the development of diverticula. *Acta Chir Scand 137*: 569, 1971.
2. Larson, D, Masters, S and Spiro, H: Medical and surgical therapy in diverticular disease. A comparative study. *Gastroenterology 71*: 734, 1976.
3. Tedesco, F, Waye, J, Raskin, J, et al.: Colonoscopic evaluation of rectal bleeding—a study of 304 patients. *Ann Intern Med 89*: 907, 1978.

CHAPTER THIRTY-EIGHT

Care of Patient Who Has a Colostomy or Ileostomy

MARVIN M. SCHUSTER, M.D.

INTRODUCTION

Ostomies are openings of a portion of the gastrointestinal tract—usually the ileum or the colon—which have been surgically diverted to the abdominal wall. It is estimated that there are in excess of one million ostomates (the preferred term for people with ostomies) in North America. Unfortunately the amount of time devoted in medical curriculum and postgraduate training to the care of ostomies is not commensurate with these impressive numbers, and therefore few physicians have the necessary background to be appropriately helpful to the ostomate. This is particularly unfortunate in light of the fact that the partial or total colectomy that results in an ileostomy or colostomy often cures the underlying condition, leaving a healthy patient who is capable of normal function, assuming that he receives appropriate preoperative preparation and postoperative ostomy care.

Ninety percent of ileostomies are performed for ulcerative colitis. Less often, other conditions such as Crohn's disease of the colon or familial polyposis require this operation. Most of the patients are young, 75% or more being between the age of 20 and 45 years of age.

In contrast, colostomies are usually performed for cancer of the rectum, and less often for diverticulitis, or for neurologic impairment or gunshot wounds which have led to incontinence. Both children and young adults with congenital disorders such as imperforate anus may have colostomies, but 80% of patients who have colostomy surgery are over the age of 50.

Appropriate management of the stoma begins before surgery, and continues for a short period after successful surgery and for a longer period when old problems persist or new ones arise.

PREOPERATIVE CARE

Ostomy management should begin as soon as ostomy surgery is seriously considered. For preparation of the patient to be most effective, family members should be included, since the approach is best tailored to meet the needs of the patient and the family. Preparation should encompass a brief description of the surgery, emphasizing the benefits to be derived, and of the stoma, stressing the fact that the stoma itself need not interfere with any aspect of future life except for vigorous body contact sports. Emphasis is placed on the fact that modern developments in appliances permit normal functioning and that there is no way that anyone will be able to tell that the patient has an ostomy. After these brief introductory comments the patient and family should be given an opportunity to voice their concerns and to ask questions, both during this first discussion and later, when the initial shock has worn off.

Many resources are available during the preoperative stage: the informed physician or surgeon, specially trained stoma nurses or enterostomal therapists (most of whom are nurses who have had specialized training at one of the schools of enterostomal therapy), and members of the visiting committee of the local chapter of the United Ostomy Association. The latter are usually lay ostomates trained as members of the visiting committee, who are specifically selected whenever possible to match the patient in age and sex (and frequently in socioeconomic status), so that the patient can identify readily with the visitor. The benefits to be derived from the visiting team cannot be overemphasized; for even the most comforting of professionals cannot be as reassuring to the patient as some kindred soul who has undergone similar surgery, has adjusted to it, and is leading a healthy, productive and joyful life.

Pamphlets, available through the local ostomy chapters, can assist the patient in his acceptance of the procedure, provide an optimistic projection for the future, and educate him in the use of ostomy appliances and in colostomy irrigation. In addition, films on preoperative preparation are available; these can be shown in portable projectors so that they can be viewed in the doctor's office, hospital clinic, or the patient's home.* These films are particularly useful when viewed by the patient after the first discussion of the topic, because they not only depict healthy ostomates who discuss their initial and subsequent adjustment, but also provide minimal basic anatomical information and information concerning appliances. Such information not only allays fears and misconceptions, but also provides the basis for logical questions.

What to Tell the Patient about Conventional Ileostomy

Conventional ileostomies require that the patient continuously wear a pouch which is applied to the body using a skin barrier (a wafer-like adhesive) that provides a water-tight seal. In this manner the intestinal contents (a better term than stool or waste material) discharge into the pouch, which can be emptied into the toilet simply by unclipping the end of the pouch 4 or 5 times a day. The contents are liquid and usually odorless. The pouch is flat and cannot be detected through the clothing or even in a bathing suit. The seal is tight enough so that persons can swim, dive, and participate in dancing and in sports such as skiing or baseball. Modern materials are so effective that the pouch can be worn for a week at a time without being removed.

What to Tell the Patient about a Kock, or Internal Pouch

The Kock pouch or internal pouch (sometimes called "continent ileostomy") consists of several loops of small intestine sutured to each other and opened so that they form a reservoir pouch (artificial rectum) within the abdomen. This reservoir is connected to the abdominal wall with a short segment of ileum and opens into the abdominal wall much as a conventional ileostomy does, except that it can be placed much lower on the abdomen since it will not require a pouch if it performs well. Between the pouch and the short ileal conduit, a nipple valve is constructed by inverting the ileum into the pouch in such a manner that it prevents leakage and therefore provides continence. In order to evacuate the contents of the pouch the patient inserts a silastic catheter into it through the ileostomy and the nipple valve. The ileal contents then drain through the catheter into the toilet bowl. Although frequent drainage is necessary initially, eventually most patients drain 3 or 4 times a day. Because it does not require an external appliance the stoma can be placed near the

groin, permitting the wearing of brief attire such as a bikini.

This type of surgery is not recommended for patients who have Crohn's disease involving the ileum. Moreover, one-third of the operations are not initially successful in providing total continence and therefore require revision, and in some instances more than one revision. These factors need to be taken into consideration when deciding the appropriate form of surgery for the specific patient, especially when patients with conventional ileostomies ask about the advisability of converting their conventional, well functioning ileostomy to the "continent ileostomy." This operation is also not appropriate for people who have neurologic disorders that impair manual dexterity and interfere with insertion of the silastic catheter.

What to Tell the Patient about Colostomy

There are basically four different types of colostomies: the dry colostomy, the wet colostomy, the loop colostomy, and the continent colostomy utilizing the magnetic cap. Most permanent colostomies are *dry sigmoid colostomies* which result from rectal resection, usually for cancer of the rectum. Since only the rectum has been removed, there is no alteration of the usual stool consistency. This is an important feature since it means that patients who have frequent and erratic bowel habits, as for example with irritable bowel, will continue to have these bowel habits and therefore will have unpredictable evacuation. They will most likely have to wear an appliance. Patients who have more regular bowel habits can often develop controlled evacuations by use of irrigation (enemas) which they administer initially daily for proper control, and later in most instances every 2 days. Some colostomates simply wear a small adhesive Band-Aid or gauze pad, although most prefer to wear a small appliance (stoma cap) to protect them against incontinence during those few days a year when they develop the same episodes of diarrhea that affect the general population. Patients who suffer from irritable bowel syndrome (see Chapter 36) or nervous diarrhea before surgery will continue to have similar symptoms after surgery and therefore may not achieve continence during intervals between irrigations.

The *wet colostomy* refers to loose stool that occurs when a colostomy is situated proximal to the splenic flexure. This type of colostomy is usually performed as a temporary bypass and is generally less desirable, since evacuations are more frequent and cannot be controlled by irrigation, and since the contents are malodorous because of colonic bacterial action. A permanent ileostomy is generally preferable to a permanent wet colostomy. The wet colostomy requires an appliance large enough to contain the colonic evacuations.

Loop colostomies and *double barrel colostomies*

---

* One such film is *Ostomy a New Beginning.* Available from Milner Fenwick, 2125 Greenspring Dr., Timonium, MD 21093. Cost $250.00.

are performed as (usually temporary) diverting procedures in the proximal colon. The loop is brought over a glass or plastic rod, and the resultant irregular oblong shape may make a water-tight appliance fit difficult.

Research is currently underway toward perfecting a magnetic cap which covers the colostomy in order to provide continence. It is held in place by a magnetic ring sutured around the stoma. The cap is removed when evacuation is desired. At present the procedure is available only at selected centers since there are many complications, and the success rate is less than 50%.

Informed consent for colostomy requires that the patient be made aware of possible postoperative impotence. If impotence does occur, psychologic adjustment to it is improved with preoperative counseling. Impotence is uncommon among ileostomates, but some degree of sexual impairment occurs in 80% of colostomates, 50% of whom are totally impotent after surgery. This is due to the wide resection that is necessary for rectal cancer surgery, the major indication for a colostomy, as well as to the advanced age of the colostomate compared to the ileostomate. Patients may be reassured that sexual counseling is available if problems arise and that many couples have found alternative satisfactory means of sexual gratification. In selected patients, it may be appropriate to offer the possibility of penile implants (see Chapter 17). Obviously these concerns are less significant for the female ostomate who does not suffer from impaired performance, although impaired gratification may still be an important factor.

POSTOPERATIVE MANAGEMENT

Only late postoperative problems will be discussed here since the early problems will be managed in hospital. Four major categories of problems are (a) psychologic adjustment, (b) sexual adjustment, (c) appliance management, and (d) local and physiological problems. Again, all can be minimized by appropriate preoperative preparation and counseling of the patient and the patient's family by an informed physician working with the appropriate members of the health team.

Psychologic Adjustment

A concerted effort should be made postoperatively by the medical team as well as by the family, and particularly the spouse, to restore self-esteem and foster independence. During the early postoperative months men tend to depend on their wives for nursing care, but women seem to prefer help from other women (daughters, mothers, sisters) rather than from husbands. This is explained by the fact that wives express more concern about being physically unacceptable to the husband than vice versa. On the other hand, one-fifth of wives have been reported to react by vomiting, fainting, or showing frank expressions of disgust when first exposed to their husband's stoma. This obviously engenders a sense of rejection, degradation, and loss of self-esteem. All too often little consideration is given by the physician to the possibility of such exaggerated responses or their consequences. Attendance at meetings of local ostomy chapters is a good way of preparing the family during the postoperative period. Formal psychotherapy may be needed when depression is severe, when suicidal inclinations appear prominent, or when behavior is bizarre.

Sexual Adjustment

When debilitating illnesses, such as inflammatory bowel disease, have led to decreased libido and impaired sexual function, ileostomy may lead to improved postoperative sexual function and more satisfactory sexual relations. This is less often true when colostomies, performed with proctectomy and radical pelvic dissection, lead to neurologic impairment of potency. Even in these circumstances psychological factors may play a major role, as demonstrated by a survey (1) which reported that all men who had had extramarital affairs before surgery terminated these relationships postoperatively feeling that only their wives would accept them. Also, cessation of relationships involving a female colostomate was invariably initiated by the female and was never reported to be a result of rejection by the husband.

In general, impaired sexual relationships may result from neurologic impairment, depression with loss of libido, inhibitions due to a sense of humiliation and embarrassment, or in some unfortunate instances, from rejection by the spouse. An awareness of these possibilities will prepare the physician to assist with preventive or corrective measures. Frank discussions with the male patient may in some instances indicate the advisability of urologic referral for prosthesis. Sexual counseling by the attending physician or specially trained counselors may assist in adjustment to alternate forms of sexual gratification.

Appliance Management

Modern improvements have impressively decreased the number of problems that are directly attributable to the appliance.

SKIN PROBLEMS

Skin breakdown, a problem which used to plague 50% of ileostomates, is now uncommon because of effective skin barriers which have replaced the old cement adhesives. Hypersensitivity to adhesives or the pouch can be diagnosed when the contour of skin reaction conforms to that of the adhesive or the pouch. If hypersensitivity is suspected, a patch test utilizing the arm or trunk distant from the stoma may confirm the suspicion. Skin problems are more common among ileostomates than colostomates because ileostomy effluent contains digestive enzymes. Skin that has been excoriated by ileal leakage should be treated with a cortisone spray such as Kenalog and an antifungal powder such as Mycostatin, neither of which interferes with adherence of the appliance. Ointments and creams should be avoided because they do prevent adhesion. More serious skin problems should be referred to gastroenterologists and to enterostomal therapists experienced with ostomy care. Skin complications for proximal colostomies may be similar to those of ileostomies.

ODOR

Odor problems are more commonly encountered by colostomates than ileostomates because of putrefactive bacteria present in the colon. Some bacterial colonization of the ileum takes place after colectomy, but odor problems occur only occasionally in 50% of ileostomates and more often in about a third. Sudden increase in gas and odor may signify partial intestinal obstruction. Dietary factors such as oils, fat-soluble vitamins, eggs, and onions may be associated with offensive odors and may be diagnosed by careful dietary history or by use of elimination diets. Odors may also be due to malabsorption resulting from small bowel disease or resection. A number of deodorants are available that can be placed into the pouch, (Nilodor, Banish, Aspirin and Ostoban powder) and additonally bismuth subcarbonate orally may be helpful. Marlen opaque double lined odor-free pouch is an effective barrier for most odor problems. Proper cleaning and drying of appliances between uses is also important in discouraging odor-forming bacteria.

LEAKAGE

Under ordinary circumstances leakage is rarely seen with new appliances, but may become a problem if pregnancy or postoperative weight gain (as for example when patient has been emaciated from inflammatory bowel disease) may change body contour requiring refitting of the appliance. The stoma may shrink during the first 6 to 8 weeks after surgery and good follow-up care is vital for at least the first postoperative year. Minimal bleeding at the stoma may occur occasionally and is no cause for alarm. A soft wet cloth should be used to clean the stoma, since dry materials may stick to the surface and cause bleeding. Skin excoriation can occur as a result of perspiration under the pouch, particularly in hot weather. This can be prevented by wearing a cover over the pouch and also by powdering the skin liberally.

Local and Physiologic Complications

Ileostomates are much more likely to experience complications of this type than are colostomates and most of these complications appear within the first year after surgery. Obstruction due to volvulus, herniation, or adhesions is the most commonly encountered problem, while prolapse, retraction, and fistula formation are seen less frequently. These problems usually require consultation with a surgeon or gastroenterologist and often need surgical correction. Crampy abdominal pains, abdominal distension, vomiting, and excessive diarrheal discharge suggest the presence of obstruction. Gastroenteritis may mimic some of these symptoms but persists only for several days.

Because of the absence of normal colonic absorptive function, ileostomates may be susceptible to dehydration or electrolyte imbalance (particularly salt depletion), especially in hot weather because of sweating and increased incidence of infectious diarrhea. For this reason ileostomates should be encouraged to increase water and salt intake during the summer unless there are medical contraindications. Antidiarrheal agents such as deodorized tincture of opium, Lomotil, or Imodium may be needed during these periods and also should be available during travel to foreign countries where traveler's diarrhea may be a problem.

With these minimal precautions neither ileostomy nor colostomy imposes any dietary restrictions, except that ileostomates should avoid excessive quantities of peanuts or fibrous foods such as bean sprouts, which have been reported to be associated with obstruction. Taken in modertion, however, these foods usually present no problem.

Colostomy Irrigation

Although a few colostomates (having distal colostomy) find that they can have controlled bowel movements by careful dietary manipulations, the vast majority use irrigation to control evacuation. This simply involves the instillation of 1 liter of warm tap water through the colostomy. The replacement of the old irrigating catheter with the blunt cone (which is placed against the stoma to prevent backflow) has virtually eliminated the problems of perforation. Although tepid water is preferred in order to avoid cramping, some patients find cold water more effective. It is normal for patients to have an initial evacuation followed within a half an hour by further excretion; for this reason the patient should be advised to continue wearing the irrigation sleeve (long pouch) with the end closed for a half an hour after irrigation. Cramps experienced during the irrigation may be due to rapid instillation of water, air distension of the bowel resulting from failure to expel the air from the irrigating tip, or from obstruction. Constipation and diarrhea should be handled much in the same fashion as with patients who have intact colons (see Chapter 35), relying on dietary manipulations as much as possible (prunes and bran for constipation and hard cheeses and rice for diarrhea).

References

General

Kretschmer, KP: The intestinal stoma. *Major Probl Clin Surg 24,* 1975.
    Valuable for both physicians and patients.
Schuster, MM and Bengel, JR: Management of ileostomy and colostomy. In *Clinical Medicine,* edited by R. G. Farmer. Harper & Row, New York (in press).
    A comprehensive review directed primarily at physicians.

Sparberg, M: *Ileostomy Care.* Charles C Thomas, Springfield, Ill., 1971.
Walter, FC: *Modern Stoma Care.* Churchill Livingstone, New York, 1976.
    The above two references are useful texts for both physicians and patients.

Specific

1. Dyk, RB and Sutherland, AM: Adaptation of spouse and other family members to the ostomy patients. *Cancer 9:* 123, 1956.

CHAPTER THIRTY-NINE

Diseases of the Liver

ESTEBAN MEZEY, M.D.

HEPATITIS

Hepatitis is an inflammatory condition which may be localized in the liver or may be part of a generalized systemic process. Acute hepatitis is usually a self-limited disease. The principal causes of acute hepatitis are viruses, drugs, and alcohol. Chronic hepatitis refers to unresolved hepatitis which has persisted for a period longer than 6 months. Cirrhosis is often the principal consequence of chronic hepatitis.

Acute Hepatitis

VIRAL HEPATITIS

Viral hepatitis is a systemic infection whose principal manifestations are hepatic. The two principal types of viral hepatitis which are well defined separate entities are type A and type B. The term non-A, non-B hepatitis refers to those cases which cannot be identified as either hepatitis A or B and are not caused by other viruses (such as cytomegalic virus or Epstein-Barr virus).

The characteristic features of type A, B and non-A, non-B hepatitis are shown in Table 39.1. Type A hepatitis, previously known as infectious hepatitis, is more common than the other types. It is usually transmitted by the fecal-oral route and has a particularly high incidence wherever persons come in close contact under poor hygienic conditions. A number of epidemics have been described after fecal contamination of the water or food supply. Ingestion of contaminated shell fish has been associated with sporadic cases as well as with epidemics.

Type B hepatitis, previously named serum hepatitis, is usually transmitted by the parenteral route from blood, blood products, or contaminated needles. However, it has also been shown to be transmitted by the ingestion of contaminated blood, by sexual contact, and from the mother to the fetus.

Type non-A, non-B hepatitis is principally acquired by the parenteral route from blood transfusions or from intravenous drug abuse (5). The importance of nonparenteral routes of infection remains to be determined. Non-A, non-B hepatitis is currently responsible for 90% of transfusion-transmitted hepatitis. The use of commercial blood appears to be the most significant factor in the transmission of this type of hepatitis.

Clinical Presentation. The clinical symptoms of the various types of hepatitis are similar. However, viral hepatitis, type B and type non-A, non-B, is usually more severe, and is associated with a higher incidence of morbidity and mortality and late sequelae. The majority of cases of hepatitis are anicteric; patients have a few nonspecific symptoms such as

Table 39.1
Comparison of Characteristics of Various Types of Viral Hepatitis

Characteristic	Type A	Type B	Type Non-A Non-B
Hepatitis A antibody	Appearance or increase in titer	Absent No change in titer	Absent No change in titer
Hepatitis B surface antigen	Absent	Present in early stage of illness	Absent
Incubation period	15–50 days	50–160 days	15–160 days
Route of infection	Oral and parenteral	Usually parenteral, also oral or sexual	Usually parenteral
Age preference	Children	Any age	Any age
Seasonal incidence	Autumn-winter, epidemic outbreaks	All year	All year
Severity	Usually mild	Often severe	Often severe
Mortality	0.1%	1.0%	1.0%
Prophylactic value of γ-globulin	Good	Good with hyperimmune hepatitis B globulin	Good

fatigue and nausea; and the disease is often misdiagnosed as a flulike illness. The correct diagnosis, if suspected, is made by demonstrating bilirubin in the urine and an increase in serum transaminases. In icteric disease the symptoms which usually precede jaundice are anorexia, fatigue, abdominal discomfort, and nausea. Erythematous skin rashes, urticaria, and arthralgias may also appear. These initial symptoms are followed within 10 days by the appearance of dark urine, often pruritus, and jaundice. It is at this stage that most patients seek medical attention. On physical examination a tender palpable liver is found in about 70% of the patients. Posterior cervical lymphadenopathy and splenomegaly may also be present. Jaundice usually increases in intensity in the first few days and then begins to decrease, disappearing completely by 2 to 8 weeks after onset.

Laboratory Features. A mild degree of transient anemia, granulocytopenia, lymphocytosis with the appearance of atypical lymphocytes, and mild hemolytic anemia, with an increase in the reticulocyte count, are commonly found in patients with viral hepatitis. Both direct and total fraction of serum bilirubin rise, the height reached by the total bilirubin being an indication of the severity of the disease. However, total serum bilirubin levels greater than 30 mg/dl are almost invariably due to complicating hemolysis. The serum transaminases generally rise before the onset of detectable jaundice, may reach levels as high as several thousand units, and may remain elevated for several weeks. The height reached by the transaminases in the serum provides only a rough estimate of the degree of hepatocellular injury and is of no prognostic value. However, a rapid fall in transaminases from a high peak value to normal in less than 1 week may be an indication of fulminant hepatitis with massive necrosis and collapse of liver parenchyma. The serum alkaline phosphatase usually rises in the early cholestatic phase of hepatitis, remains elevated throughout the illness, and is often the last serum enzyme to return to normal levels after clinical recovery. The serum al-

bumin is normal in acute hepatitis. Serum γ-globulins are frequently transiently elevated. The prothrombin time is usually normal and, if prolonged, is usually responsive to the administration of vitamin K. Prolongation of the prothrombin time with no response to vitamin K administration suggests severe hepatitis; and if the prolongation increases, it is indicative of fulminant hepatitis.

Immunological Features. A marked advance in the diagnosis of hepatitis occurred with the discovery in 1964 of an antigenic substance in the blood which was later documented to be associated only with type B hepatitis. This antigen, initially named Australian antigen because it was first detected in the serum of an Australian aborigine, is now designated hepatitis B surface antigen. In 1973 the hepatitis A antigen was discovered, and the determination of serum antibodies to this antigen began to be used for the identification of type A hepatitis. At present there is no marker available for the identification of non-A, non-B hepatitis.

In acute type A hepatitis fecal excretion of hepatitis A antigen (HA Ag) can be demonstrated a few days before the increase in serum transaminase, rising to a peak during maximum serum transaminase elevation, and then falling as jaundice appears. Antibody to hepatitis (anti-HA, predominantly IgM) appears in the serum as HA Ag disappears from the stool, and rises rapidly to high levels. Afterwards antibody titers (predominantly IgG) remain detectable for at least 10 years, conferring immunity against reinfection. Since hepatitis A infection is very common, many healthy individuals have detectable anti-HA in the serum. The prevalence of positive anti-HA is about 30% in the United States and as high as 90% in certain areas of Latin America and Asia (22). Hence, identification of an acute episode of hepatitis as type A requires a high titer of anti-HA of the IgM class or the appearance of or a rise in anti-HA titer in the serum collected during the convalescent as compared with the acute stage of hepatitis.

The hepatitis B virus by electron microscopy appears as a double shelled 42 nm spherical particle originally called the Dane particle. The outer shell of this particle is hepatitis B surface antigen (HB$_S$Ag), while the inner core contains an antigen which has been designated the hepatitis B core antigen (HB$_C$Ag). The inner core also contains double stranded DNA and DNA polymerase activity. In acute type B viral hepatitis HB$_S$Ag first appears in the blood 1 to 2 weeks before, and usually disappears by 2 months after, the onset of clinical symptoms (Fig. 39.1). Radioimmunoassay and reverse passive hemagglutination are the only reliable procedures for detection of HB$_S$Ag. (The hemagglutination technique is slightly less sensitive than the radioimmunoassay.) Antibody to hepatitis B core antigen (anti-HB$_C$) appears in the serum at the onset of clinical symptoms, reaches a peak soon after the maximal level of serum transaminases is reached, and then falls gradually, becoming undetectable 1 to 2 years after the infection. Antibody to the hepatitis B surface antigen (anti-HB$_S$) usually appears during the convalescence when HB$_S$Ag is no longer detectable and then persists for many years. The presence of HB$_S$Ag, anti-HB$_C$, or a rise in anti-HB$_S$ titer during the acute illness is evidence that the hepatitis is due to the hepatitis B virus (9). Persistence of HB$_S$Ag in the serum beyond 3 months after the infection suggests that the patient has become a chronic carrier of the hepatitis B virus (14). High titers of anti-HB$_C$ but absent anti-HB$_S$ are usually found in association with HB$_S$Ag in the carrier state. The presence of anti-HB$_S$ indicates that the patient has had a prior infection with type B hepatitis and now is immune to reinfection. In 1972 a new antigen termed e antigen was discovered in HB$_S$Ag-positive sera. The e antigen (HB$_e$Ag), although associated only with type B hepatitis, is immunologically distinct from HB$_S$Ag and HB$_C$Ag. HB$_e$Ag appears transiently in the serum during the early phase of acute type B hepatitis. In chronic carriers of HB$_S$Ag the presence of HB$_e$Ag is a marker of active virus replication and correlates with infectivity of the carrier (7). Some studies suggest that the presence of HB$_e$Ag in the chronic carrier is an indicator of progression of acute hepatitis B to chronic hepatitis or cirrhosis.

Hepatitis non-A, non-B has been transmitted to chimpanzees by serum derived from patients with acute and chronic non-A, non-B hepatitis suggesting that patients can become carriers of the agent responsible for this type of hepatitis. Since there are no serologic markers for this hepatitis, the diagnosis remains one of exclusion (5).

At present the practical diagnostic usefulness of the immunologic markers for hepatitis is as follows: hepatitis A infection is confirmed by the demonstration of a rise in anti-HA titer in the serum collected during convalescence as compared with the acute stage of hepatitis, or preferably the presence of anti-HA of the IgM class. Infection with hepatitis B is usually confirmed by the presence of HB$_S$Ag; but if

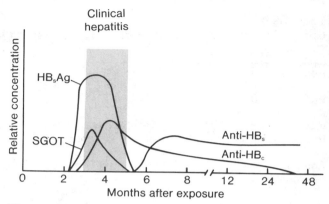

Figure 39.1   Pattern of appearance of hepatitis B surface antigen (HB$_S$Ag) and antibodies to hepatitis B surface antigen (Anti-HB$_S$) and to hepatitis B core antigen (anti-HB$_C$) in acute hepatitis B infection. (From E. Mezey: Specific liver diseases, in *The Laboratory in Clinical Medicine*, Ed. 2 edited by J. A. Halsted and C. H. Halsted, W.B. Saunders, Philadelphia, 1981, with permission.)

the antigen is absent and it is clinically indicated, the diagnosis can be confirmed by demonstrating anti-HB$_C$. The determination of anti-HB$_S$ is useful to find out whether or not a person is immune to hepatitis B and a candidate for prophylaxis, a subject which is discussed later in this chapter (p. 328).

Management. Acute viral hepatitis usually resolves completely in 1 to 3 months. There is no specific therapy. Bed rest is indicated initially in the symptomatic patient because it often alleviates the symptoms, although there is no evidence that it changes the overall course of the illness (13). As the patient's symptoms improve, a gradual increase in activity is allowed as tolerated by the patient. Intake of a normal calorie, high protein diet should be encouraged, although it is often difficult for the patient to eat because of nausea and anorexia. However, these symptoms are usually minimal in the morning and hence, the patient should be encouraged to eat a large breakfast. Strict isolation of the patient to his own room and bathroom is often impractical and probably unnecessary. General hygienic measures such as washing the hands after contact with the patient and careful handling of stool and blood samples are mandatory.

Hospitalization is indicated in patients in whom the diagnosis is uncertain, and in those who have severe symptoms of nausea and vomiting, changes in mental status, or a prothrombin time that is prolonged more than 4 seconds above the control value. In addition, it is usually advisable to admit to the hospital patients over the age of 50 years, who tend to have a more severe course of hepatitis than do younger patients, as well as those patients who do not have somebody at home who can observe and help them.

Nausea can be controlled with oral Benadryl 25 mg

3 times a day without danger of central nervous system depression. No sedatives or tranquilizers should be given because they may precipitate hepatic encephalopathy. Corticosteroids are of no value in the treatment of acute viral hepatitis.

Patients should be followed at intervals varying from 1 to 3 weeks and should not be discharged from ambulatory care until all symptoms have disappeared, and all laboratory tests have returned to normal. Patients are advised not to ingest alcoholic beverages until 1 month after all laboratory tests have returned to normal.

Liver Biopsy. Liver biopsies are only indicated if the diagnosis is uncertain or if the clinical course of the disease is prolonged beyond 6 months. A specialist in liver disease should be consulted to evaluate the patient and to perform the liver biopsy.

For liver biopsy the patient is admitted to the hospital. Before admission for this procedure the patient should be demonstrated to have a history of normal hemostasis, a prothrombin time less than 4 seconds above control, and a platelet count greater than 80,000 per cu mm. A liver biopsy is contraindicated if there is an infiltrate in the right lower lung, or a right-sided pleural effusion, absent hepatic dullness to percussion, suspected liver hemangioma or abscess, massive ascites, extrahepatic obstruction or severe anemia (hemoglobin less than 10 g/dl). After application of local anesthesia the liver biopsy is performed by the intercostal right subcutaneous route using suction with a needle 1.6 mm in diameter. It entails minimal risk when done by a skilled operator. The most common complication is pleuritic pain lasting a few hours after the biopsy which is noted in about 5% of the cases. The most serious complications are bleeding and bile peritonitis, which occur in less than 1% of cases. The incidence of mortality from liver biopsy is 0.2%.

Prognosis. The majority of patients with acute viral hepatitis recover from their illness without any sequelae. The mortality rate from all types of hepatitis is less than 0.1%. The principal cause of death is the development of fulminant hepatitis which is more common in type B hepatitis. Fulminant hepatitis, which is rare, usually overcomes the patient within 10 days of the onset of the symptoms of hepatitis. Older patients and patients with other medical illnesses such as diabetes are more likely to have a prolonged course and higher mortality. Indications of a poor prognosis are changes in mental status, a nonpalpable liver which is also small on hepatic scan, or a liver that decreases rapidly in size, and a prothrombin time that is prolonged more than 4 seconds above normal.

Chronic hepatitis and cirrhosis occur in approximately 3 to 5% of patients with type B and non-A, non-B hepatitis. They do not occur after type A hepatitis. These complications should be suspected in patients who continue to have clinical and laboratory evidence of liver disease 6 months following the onset of acute hepatitis (18). Most patients clear the HB$_S$Ag from their serum within 3 months of the onset of the illness. About 10% of patients with type B hepatitis become chronic carriers of HB$_S$Ag. Chronic carriers of HB$_S$Ag with abnormal serum transaminases should be evaluated for the development of chronic active hepatitis by liver biopsy. An increased incidence of hepatocellular carcinoma has been found in carriers of HB$_S$Ag.

Differential Diagnosis. A number of other viruses have been reported to cause hepatitis. *Cytomegalic inclusion infection,* usually clinically inapparent in the adult, can present with manifestations of hepatitis in patients being administered immunosuppressive therapy or following blood transfusions in healthy subjects; the diagnosis is made by culture of the urine. *Mononucleosis* (caused by the Epstein-Barr virus) frequently is associated with hepatocellular dysfunction with mild transient jaundice in 5 to 10% of patients. The presence of a heterophil antibody, which is not absorbed by guinea pig kidney, or a positive mononucleosis spot test, confirms the diagnosis (see Chapter 49).

Hepatitis due to *leptospirosis* should be suspected in patients who have been in close contact with rodents; the diagnosis is established by recovery of leptospiras in culture of the blood or by a rise in antibodies in the course of the disease. *Drug hepatitis* (p. 328) presents with clinical features which are indistinguishable from viral hepatitis, and a history of drug intake is a most important clue in suspecting the diagnosis. *Alcoholic hepatitis* (p. 329) usually develops after recent heavy alcohol ingestion; the serum transaminases are rarely elevated more than 10 times above normal and the elevation is primarily in the serum glutamic oxalacetic transaminase (SGOT). In patients with marked cholestasis as evidenced by persistent elevation of the bilirubin, high serum alkaline phosphatase, and pruritus in association with persistent dark urine and light stools, the diagnosis of extrahepatic biliary obstruction should be entertained. An abnormal sonogram may provide a clue to extrahepatic obstruction if the biliary ducts are found to be dilated, and the patient should then be referred to a specialist in liver diseases for further evaluation.

Prevention and Prophylaxis of Viral Hepatitis. General hygienic measures such as washing the hands after contact with the patient are the most effective means of preventing the spread of hepatitis from patients to other persons. The patient's dishes and eating utensils can be shared by other persons only if cleaned by heating above 120° C for 15 to 20 min in a dishwasher, after the patient has used them. Assignment of the patient to a separate bathroom is ideal, but often impractical. The viruses are present in feces, blood, and other body fluids of the patients. The handling of all of these materials should be done with care. Since the virus appears in the stool during the prodromal period of hepatitis, the precautions mentioned should be taken routinely in environments where there is a high risk of development of hepatitis, such as in institutions for the mentally retarded. The screening of blood for HB$_S$Ag for transfusion has virtually eliminated the development of type B hepatitis following blood transfusions. Hence 90% of post-transfusion hepatitis at present is type non-A, non-B. The development of post-transfusion hepatitis can be reduced further by using voluntary rather than commercial blood donors. Other sources of type B and non-A, non-B which can easily be controlled are contaminated needles, pins used to test sensation, and dental and surgical instruments. All used needles or pins should be discarded in specially labeled bottles containing 40% formalin, which is known to inactivate the hepatitis virus. The preferred method for cleaning surgical and dental instruments is by heat sterilization. The risk that most health workers who are HB$_S$Ag-positive pose to their patients is minimal if high standards of hygiene are maintained (10). The exceptions are dentists and surgeons who often develop cuts on their hands while operating. Dentists are urged to wear gloves regardless of whether or not they are HB$_S$Ag-positive to protect themselves and their patients. Patients who have had hepatitis B or hepatitis non-A, non-B and have recovered (clinically and, in the case of hepatitis B, serologically) may be infectious for many years and therefore should not be allowed to donate blood.

Standard immune serum globulin is known to prevent the clinical manifestations of hepatitis A in 80 to 90% of persons when administered early after exposure. However, it does not prevent subclinical infection. It is indicated for close personal contacts of patients with known hepatitis A, inmates of institutions during an epidemic of hepatitis A, and travellers to areas where hepatitis is endemic. It is not indicated for casual acquaintances or co-workers of the patient or for persons who are known to have anti-HA antibody in their serum. The recommended dose of standard immune globulin is 0.02 ml/kg. For continuous protection of persons in hepatitis-endemic areas repeated doses of standard immune, serum globulin, 0.06 ml/kg, should be given every 6 months.

The role of standard immune serum globulin in the prevention of type B hepatitis is uncertain. *Hepatitis B immune globulin* (containing a high titer of anti-HB$_S$) prevents approximately 75% of cases of type B hepatitis in people who have been stuck with needles contaminated by HB$_S$Ag-positive patients, in spouses of HB$_S$Ag-positive individuals, in newborns of HB$_S$Ag-positive mothers, and in the staff of dialysis units (16). It is not indicated for casual or work contacts of patients with type B hepatitis or for persons who have been demonstrated to have anti-HB$_S$. Testing for anti-HB$_S$ should be done routinely before administration of hepatitis B immune globulin provided that the results of the tests can be obtained

within 1 week of exposure to the virus. The recommended dose of hepatitis B immune globulin is 0.06 ml/kg which corresponds to 4 ml for an adult, with the dose repeated in 1 month. An initial dose should be given immediately after a person has been stuck with a contaminated needle and as soon as possible to spouses of HB$_S$Ag-positive individuals. Patients and staff of dialysis units should be given 2 ml every 4 to 6 months, and 4 ml after exposure to contaminated blood.

Table 30.2 (Chapter 30) summarizes recommendations for hepatitis prophylaxis for persons exposed to the blood of patients whose hepatitis status is unknown.

The incidence of post-transfusion non-A, non-B hepatitis is decreased by the administration of 10 ml of standard immune serum globulin if given before or immediately after the transfusion. However, elimination of commercial blood donors seems to be a more practical way of preventing post-transfusion non-A, non-B hepatitis.

DRUG-INDUCED HEPATITIS

The liver is the principle organ concerned with drug metabolism; and, hence, it is not surprising that it is also a principal target for drug toxicity. Every drug has the potential for producing hepatocellular damage. Drug-induced hepatitis results either from direct hepatotoxicity or from an idiosyncratic reaction (host hypersensitivity). *Hepatotoxic reactions* caused by direct toxins such as carbon tetrachloride and inorganic phosphorus are dose-dependent and reproducible with a brief interval after exposure to the drug. *Idiosyncratic reactions* are the more common response to drugs. Characteristically, they are not dose-dependent, occur in only a small number of individuals who are exposed, and are preceded by a sensitizing period of 1 to 4 weeks of exposure or a history of prior exposure. Drug reactions may be cholestatic, simulate viral hepatitis, or combine features of both processes.

Cholestatic Reactions. Cholestasis is due to a direct dose-related effect of the administration of anabolic steroids and oral contraceptives. Cholestasis occurs in 1 to 2% of patients receiving anabolic steroids, but occurs less frequently after the ingestion of oral contraceptive drugs. Jaundice and pruritus are prominent symptoms. The elevated serum bilirubin is composed principally of the direct fraction. Serum alkaline phosphatase and cholesterol are elevated, while serum transaminases are normal or only slightly elevated. Cholestasis disappears soon after withdrawal of the offending drug.

A much larger number of drugs cause cholestasis due to hypersensitivity. Examples are phenothiazine derivatives such as chlorpromazine, antibiotics such as erythromycin, antithyroid drugs such as propylthiouracil and methimazole, hypoglycemic agents such as tolbutamide and chlorpropamide, and cytotoxic drugs such as chlorambucil. Common clinical features of these drug reactions are fever, right upper quadrant abdominal pain, pruritus, skin rash, and eosinophilia. Serum transaminases are moderately elevated (less than 10 times above normal). The clinical and laboratory abnormalities usually subside between 2 to 4 weeks after discontinuation of the drug, although on occasion cholestasis persists for months to years. Severe pruritus is treated with cholestyramine (Questran) given in a dose of 4 g 3 times a day before meals. Relief of pruritus is obtained in 4 to 7 days after starting this medication. Patients with cholestasis should be hospitalized whenever the jaundice persists unchanged or increases 2 to 4 weeks after discontinuation of the drug.

Hepatocellular Reactions. Most agents that produce direct hepatocellular damage are toxins rather than drugs. Acetaminophen, however, is a drug that produces hepatic necrosis in all individuals if ingested in a large dose (greater than 10 g), usually in a suicide attempt. Shortly after ingestion the patient develops nausea and vomiting, but evidence of hepatocellular damage often does not become apparent until 48 hours later when serum transaminases rise and the prothrombin time becomes prolonged. The patient's condition then deteriorates; jaundice appears and central nervous system depression may occur. The mortality rate of patients who took an overdose of acetaminophen was found to be 3.5% in one large study (8). Thus patients who are known or are suspected of ingesting toxic amounts of acetaminophen should be hospitalized.

Idiosyncratic hepatocellular reactions have been reported after the administration of a number of drugs, the most common of which are isoniazid, α-methyldopa, phenylbutazone, 6-mercaptopurine, and halothane. Asymptomatic increases in serum transaminases, which subside despite continued administration of the drug, have been reported in 5 to 10% of patients taking isoniazid or α-methyldopa (11). Because of the frequent transient nature of the serum transaminase elevations, there is no need to monitor this test in asymptomatic patients. However, the development of symptoms of fatigue and anorexia or of nausea and general malaise is an indication for determination of serum transaminases; and if transaminase activity is increased, the drug should be discontinued immediately because this often heralds the onset of severe hepatocellular damage. The incidence of acute hepatitis in patients taking the drugs listed above is 0.1 to 0.3%. Women and older patients are more likely to be affected. The onset of the reaction is between 1 and 10 weeks after the start of therapy. The symptoms, laboratory tests, and findings on liver biopsy are indistinguishable from those of viral hepatitis (see p. 324). The hepatitis usually resolves after the drug is discontinued. However, a mortality rate as high as 12% has been reported for severe hepatitis due to isoniazid. Moreover, chronic active liver disease can develop if the drug responsible for the hepatitis is continued. Administration of corticosteroids is not indicated in drug-induced hepatitis.

ALCOHOLIC HEPATITIS

This condition is seen most frequently after prolonged heavy alcohol intake. Women are more susceptible to alcoholic liver disease than men. This lesion usually does not develop in men who drink less than 80 g of ethanol per day or in women who drink half this amount (equivalent to 8 and 4 ounces of 86 proof whiskey, respectively). Many of the presenting clinical characteristics of patients with alcoholic hepatitis (such as anorexia, marked fatigue, jaundice, and tender hepatomegaly) are indistinguishable from those of viral hepatitis (see pp. 324–325). However, patients with alcoholic hepatitis are more likely to have fever and leukocytosis. The elevation of the serum transaminases is rarely 10 times above normal, and frequently there is a prolongation of the prothrombin time. The elevation of SGOT is characteristically higher than that of serum glutamic pyruvic transaminase (SGPT). Patients with alcoholic hepatitis should be admitted to the hospital, and a definite diagnosis established by liver biopsy, if not contraindicated by abnormal hemostatic function. Liver biopsy differentiates alcoholic hepatitis from drug-induced hepatitis and viral hepatitis and gives an indication of any underlying chronic liver disease. The illness is often more severe than in patients with viral hepatitis, and decompensation with hepatic encephalopathy and death can occur. About one-third of patients with alcoholic hepatitis have been shown to progress to cirrhosis, often in a short period of 6 months (6).

Chronic Hepatitis

Chronic hepatitis refers to chronic inflammation of the liver detected by abnormal liver tests or by abnormal liver histology which has persisted for longer than 6 months. The spectrum of chronic hepatitis varies from a benign reversible process to an unrelenting process which often progresses to cirrhosis. Liver histology is essential both for the diagnosis and to establish the severity of the disease and the need for treatment. Two types of chronic hepatitis are recognized by the examination of tissue obtained on liver biopsy: chronic persistent hepatitis which is a self-limited disease and does not require therapy; and chronic active hepatitis which is a progressive process associated with increased morbidity and mortality, and which often improves with therapy. In chronic persistent hepatitis liver biopsy reveals portal inflammation often with expansion of the portal areas and focal parenchymal necrosis with preservation of the lobular architecture and slight or absent fibrosis; whereas in chronic active hepatitis there is extension of inflammation and necrosis from the portal area to the hepatocytes adjacent to it (piecemeal necrosis), disruption of the lobular architecture, and increased fibrosis with the formation of intralobular septa of fibrous tissue (bridging) (1).

The principal causes of chronic hepatitis are infection with hepatitis viruses, both type B and type non-A, non-B (not type A), idiopathic (formerly called lupoid hepatitis), and drugs such as isoniazid, α-methyldopa, and oxyphenacetin. In addition, Wilson's disease, α_1-antitrypsin deficiency, and primary biliary cirrhosis may present with clinical and histologic features of chronic hepatitis.

CHRONIC PERSISTENT HEPATITIS

Patients with chronic persistent hepatitis are either asymptomatic or have mild nonspecific symptoms such as fatigue. On physical examination there are no peripheral manifestations of chronic liver disease, but there may be mild hepatomegaly. Laboratory tests show mild elevation of serum transaminases (2 to 5 times normal) but the remainder of the liver tests are usually normal. Forty percent of the patients have detectable HB$_S$Ag in the serum. The diagnosis is established by liver biopsy and the patient is then reassured about the benign course of his condition. If symptoms and elevation of the transaminases persist, a liver biopsy is indicated after 2 to 3 years to rule out a sampling error on the initial liver biopsy. Patients with persistent hepatitis have been shown to have elevated serum transaminases for over 10 years without any evidence of progression of the disease.

CHRONIC ACTIVE HEPATITIS

The onset of chronic active hepatitis is usually insidious. The patient may be asymptomatic and liver disease may be detected by transaminase elevations done on routine testing or he may present symptoms of general malaise, fatigue, abdominal discomfort, anorexia, and jaundice. In about a third of the patients the disease evolves from a clinically overt episode of acute hepatitis. Physical examination in patients with chronic active hepatitis reveals hepatomegaly, and often peripheral manifestations of chronic liver disease such as spider angiomas, palmar erythema, and gynecomastia. Elevations of serum bilirubin, transaminases, and globulins are the most sensitive indicators of the activity of the hepatocellular damage, while decreases in serum albumin and prolongation of the prothrombin time reflect loss of hepatocellular function and a poor prognosis. Older male patients are more likely to have HB$_S$Ag in the serum and to present with an acute onset of illness (15). On the other hand, HB$_S$Ag-negative patients are more likely to be women and to present with systemic symptoms of acne, amenorrhea, arthralgia and arthritis, pleurisy, or intermittent fever. In addition, they may have associated thyroiditis, Sjögren's syndrome, ulcerative colitis, glomerulonephritis, or hemolytic anemia. Laboratory tests on these patients show evidence of immunologic hyperactivity: serum

γ-globulin is often markedly elevated; lupus erythematosus (LE) cells are present; and there is an increased incidence of elevation of the titer of antinuclear antibodies and smooth muscle antibodies. In addition, antimitochondrial antibodies are found in 15% of these patients.

The clinical course of patients with chronic active hepatitis is quite variable. Patients can be asymptomatic for a long time, have periods of intermittent worsening and remission, or have a progressive course to cirrhosis and death if untreated (17).

Differential Diagnosis. The diagnosis of *Wilson's disease* should be considered in all patients, particularly those under 25 years who present with clinical and laboratory features of chronic hepatitis (20). Wilson's disease is discussed in more detail in the section on cirrhosis (p. 332). The diagnosis of *chronic hepatitis due to α_1-antitrypsin deficiency* is suggested by the finding of an absent or low α_1-globulin on serum protein electrophoresis (4). The diagnosis is established by demonstrating a low value of α_1-antitrypsin in the serum by quantitative measurement and by protease inhibitor (Pi) typing (4). The common allele is PiM, while liver disease occurs in about 20% of individuals who are homozygous for the allele PiZ. Liver biopsy reveals PAS-positive cytoplasmic inclusions which are resistant to diastase in both homozygous and heterozygous individuals for the allele PiZ. There is no known therapy for this deficiency which is transmitted by codominant inheritance. The diagnostic characteristics of *primary biliary cirrhosis* are discussed in the section on cirrhosis (p. 332). The diagnosis of *drug-induced chronic hepatitis* (p. 328) is dependent on a careful history and on the demonstration of improvement of the patient after discontinuation of drugs which are known to produce this illness. In most cases chronic active hepatitis due to drugs will revert to normal after discontinuation of the offending drug (8).

Therapy. Corticosteroids have been shown to be beneficial in symptomatic patients with chronic active hepatitis who are HB$_S$Ag-negative. Clinical, biochemical, and histologic improvement and even remission have been observed; and mortality has been reduced after therapy with corticosteroids (19). Prednisone or prednisolone, 40 to 60 mg, is given initially to suppress the activity of the disease and then tapered slowly, usually over a period of 1 to 3 months to a maintenance dose of 15 to 20 mg. Symptomatic improvement followed by a fall in serum transaminases occurs in the first few weeks. Histologic transformation to a lesion of persistent hepatitis will occur in some patients within a 2-year period. Treatment with corticosteroids is discontinued in patients who attain remission. In the remainder of the patients it is not continued beyond 4 years because the prospect of remission diminishes while the risk of side effects increases (2). Asymptomatic patients with chronic active hepatitis who are HB$_S$Ag-negative are usually only treated if they have marked elevations of serum transaminases (greater than 10 times above normal) and histologic evidence of severe liver disease (marked multilobular necrosis and bridging). Patients with chronic hepatitis who are HBsAg-positive are much less responsive to corticosteroid therapy (15); only symptomatic patients are treated, and if there is no response to the therapy within a year, the steroids should be discontinued.

UNEXPLAINED ELEVATIONS OF SERUM ENZYMES

Elevations of serum transaminases and alkaline phosphatase are occasionally found in normal subjects or in patients not suspected of having liver disease. In such a situation the abnormality should first be confirmed by repeat testing. Next, it is important to remember that elevated serum transaminases and alkaline phosphatase do not necessarily originate from the liver. For example, elevated serum transaminases can be due to injury to the heart and striated muscle; if the source of the serum transaminases is muscle, the more specific creatine kinase will also be elevated. An isolated increase of serum alkaline phosphatase can originate from liver or bone. The hepatic origin of alkaline phosphatase can be confirmed by demonstration of an elevated 5'-nucleotidase, which, unlike alkaline phosphatase is present only in the liver and in the epithelium of the bile ducts. By contrast, an elevated serum alkaline phosphatase accompanied by a normal serum 5'-nucleotidase is almost invariably due to bone disease; a very common cause of such an occurrence is a recent bone fracture. Any persistent elevation of serum transaminases for longer than 6 months which remains unexplained is an indication for liver biopsy to rule out chronic hepatitis. A persistent elevation of serum alkaline phosphatase in the absence of an elevated serum bilirubin can occur in fatty liver, which is common in the diabetic and obese patient or can be the result of space-occupying lesions, such as granulomas or occasionally metastatic carcinoma. A liver scan is recommended in these cases to rule out metastatic carcinoma, but a liver biopsy is indicated only if the scan shows a space-occupying lesion or if there is clinical suspicion of diseases such as tuberculosis and sarcoidosis that result in hepatic granuloma.

ALCOHOLIC FATTY LIVER

Fatty liver is due to alterations of lipid metabolism caused by alcohol, and therefore occurs in all persons ingesting alcohol in excessive amounts. It is manifested mainly by a feeling of abdominal fullness due to hepatomegaly and mild elevation of the serum transaminases (rarely more than 2 times above normal). On occasion marked fatty infiltration is associated with symptoms of malaise, weakness, anorexia, tender hepatomegaly, and even jaundice. These symptomatic patients require admission to the hospital and a liver biopsy to distinguish fatty liver

from alcoholic hepatitis and cirrhosis. The treatment of fatty liver consists of bed rest and abstinence from alcohol. With abstinence the abnormal accumulation of fat will disappear in a period of 4 to 6 weeks. As the patient improves, the liver decreases in size and becomes nontender. Serum bilirubin and transaminases promptly return to normal. Recurrent episodes of symptomatic fatty liver are common after heavy alcohol ingestion, but there is no evidence that this lesion in itself leads to cirrhosis.

CIRRHOSIS

Cirrhosis is a chronic diffuse liver disease, characterized by widespread hepatic fibrosis and nodule formation. The fibrosis is the result of extensive destruction of liver cells, and the nodularity represents regeneration. For clinical purposes cirrhosis can be classified into the following major categories: alcoholic (micronodular), postnecrotic (macronodular), cardiac, biliary, Wilson's disease, hemochromatosis, and schistosomiasis. The two major types of cirrhosis are alcoholic, which is characterized by regular small nodules, and postnecrotic, in which there is extensive scarring of the liver and the presence of irregular nodules of various sizes (21). On occasion cirrhosis of the alcoholic is of the macronodular type; this is more common in chronic alcoholics who no longer drink alcohol. The onset of cirrhosis is usually insidious and associated with nonspecific symptoms such as fatigue, anorexia, weight loss, nausea, and abdominal discomfort. As the disease progresses, signs of hepatocellular failure become prominent: jaundice, edema, ascites, electrolyte abnormalities, bleeding tendencies, spider angiomas, palmar erythema, gynecomastia, impotence, and loss of axillary and pubic hair. Hepatomegaly and portal hypertension resulting in splenomegaly and a venous collateral circulation are common. The most severe complications of cirrhosis are hepatic encephalopathy, bleeding from esophageal varices, and infection. Patients with alcoholic cirrhosis often present with recurring episodes of hepatocellular failure, precipitated by hepatocellular necrosis and fatty infiltrations induced by alcohol ingestion, which is reversible with clinical improvement after abstinence from alcohol, and after bed rest and optimal nutrition. By contrast, patients with postnecrotic cirrhosis are more likely to present insidiously with evidence of portal hypertension. When hepatocellular failure occurs in these patients, it is usually a terminal event because it is the result of excessive fibrosis and reduced hepatic parenchymal mass rather than of reversible lesions such as necrosis and fatty infiltration found in alcoholic cirrhosis. Rapid deterioration of patients with cirrhosis should raise the suspicion of a complicating hepatocellular carcinoma. Common laboratory findings in patients with cirrhosis include anemia, a normal or slightly decreased white blood cell count, and moderate thrombocytopenia. The most frequent abnormal liver tests are hyperbilirubinemia, a depressed serum albumin, elevated serum globulins, and a prolonged prothrombin time. Liver biopsy is indicated to establish a firm diagnosis in all cases where hemostatic function allows this procedure to be done (see p. 327).

Differential Diagnosis

The diagnostic characteristics of some of the other types of cirrhosis are as follows: (a) *Cardiac cirrhosis* develops only after prolonged and severe cardiac failure, usually due to valvular disease, particularly in patients with tricuspid incompetence or in patients with constrictive pericarditis. Jaundice, hepatomegaly, and ascites are prominent features, but the diagnosis can only be established with certainty by liver biopsy. Treatment of cardiac failure, in particular of constrictive pericarditis by pericardiectomy, results in improvement of liver function. (b) *Primary biliary cirrhosis* (3) is a chronic disease of unknown cause which is characterized by progressive intrahepatic cholestasis and is most frequently seen in middle-aged females. The principal manifestations are jaundice with pruritus, hepatomegaly, hypercholesterolemia with the formation of xanthoma and xanthelasma, and steatorrhea due to the decreased delivery of bile acids to the intestine. Antimitochondrial antibodies are found in 95% of these patients, and their presence is virtually diagnostic. Liver biopsy in the early stages reveals injury to the septal and large intralobular bile ducts with surrounding accumulation of the inflammatory plasma cells and lymphocytes and with granuloma formation. In the end stages of the disease cirrhosis develops which is nearly indistinguishable from postnecrotic (macronodular) cirrhosis. (c) *Wilson's disease* is a rare disorder of copper metabolism which is inherited as an autosomal recessive (20). Its symptoms are due to hepatic and neurologic dysfunction. In children the principal symptoms are due to liver involvement, while in adults neurologic symptoms tend to predominate. The diagnosis should be suspected in all children or young adults who develop cirrhosis since treatment with copper-chelating agents can arrest the disease and alleviate all symptoms. A characteristic finding which is virtually diagnostic is the presence of Kaiser-Fleischer rings, which are greenish brown rings found in the posterior surface and periphery of the cornea. Since these rings cannot often be seen by the naked eye, it is important to refer all suspected patients to the ophthalmologist for slit-lamp examination of the cornea. Serum ceruloplasmin, the copper binding protein, is reduced in most but not all cases. Histologic examination of a liver biopsy is not diagnostic. However, quantitative determination of copper with finding of more than 250 µg per g of dry liver weight or the urinary excretion of more than 50 µg per 24 hours is diagnostic. Hospitalization is not required for treatment of Wilson's disease with d-penicillamine. (d) *Hemochromatosis* is an inherited disorder of iron metabolism, resulting in excessive body iron which is principally characterized by cirrhosis, diabetes mellitus, and grayish pigmentation of the skin. Other symptoms are cardiac failure and arrhythmias, peripheral neuritis, arthritis, and testicular atrophy. The iron overload appears to be due to an increased absorption of dietary iron and the mode of inheritance is autosomal recessive. The disease usually appears in persons over 40 years of age and develops earlier in males, probably because of the menstrual loss of iron in females. The diagnosis is made by demonstrating a high serum iron (greater than 150 µg/dl), a high saturation of iron binding protein (greater than 50%), and increased serum ferritin, usually in a patient with a family history of the disease (12). (e) *Hepatic schistosomiasis* may occur in persons from tropical areas who have been infected by schistosome cercariae while swimming or walking in infested water. The liver disease is due to the deposition of ova of *Schistosoma mansoni* in the portal areas, with the development of an inflammatory reaction, often with granuloma formation and periportal fibrosis. Jaundice is uncommon in these patients on presentation. The most common laboratory abnormalities are increases in serum alkaline phosphatase and mild elevations of serum bilirubin and transaminases. The diagnosis of active infection is made by demonstrating mobile schistosoma ova on fresh examination of rectal biopsy, and the diagnosis of liver involvement is made by showing the presence of ova capsules on liver biopsy.

Management

The treatment of uncomplicated cirrhosis consists of voluntary restriction of activity if the patient has weakness and fatigue, a diet high in protein but low in salt, and abstinence from alcohol. This regimen almost invariably results in improvement of hepatocellular function in patients with alcoholic cirrhosis and occasionally in patients with postnecrotic cirrhosis. Tranquilizers and sedatives should be avoided. Infection and gastrointestinal bleeding, which in addition to alcohol ingestion are frequent precipitating factors of decompensation, should be searched for and treated. Vitamin K, 15 mg parenterally, may improve abnormal prolongation of the prothrombin time. Multivitamins and folic acid, 1 mg a day, may be given if the patient's dietary intake does not appear to be adequate or if there is evidence of vitamin deficiencies. Potassium deficiency is frequent and may contribute to the precipitation of hepatic encephalopathy, but its extent is difficult to assess because serum potassium concentration is a poor reflection of the total body potassium. However, when serum potassium falls below 3.5 meq/L, the deficit of body potassium is approximately 300 to 500 meq. This can be replaced over a period of a few days with oral solutions of 10% potassium chloride which provides 40 meq of potassium per ounce. Fluid retention is treated with sodium restriction (500 mg of sodium chloride per day) and diuretics. The induced diuresis should be slow and result in a loss of no more than 2.27 kg (5 lb) of weight per week because of the danger of precipitating electrolyte depletion and hypokalemia. Diuresis can be initiated by Aldactone, 25 mg orally 3 times a day. The development of acute hepatic encephalopathy manifested by asterixis or by changes in mental status is an indication that the patient should be hospitalized for evaluation and treatment. However, patients with chronic hepatic encephalopathy can be treated with protein restriction and lactulose in daily doses of 60 to 100 g a day on an ambulatory basis. Lactulose usually is not effective unless it also increases the frequency of bowel movements. Acute and chronic gastrointestinal bleeding is an indication for hospitalization.

References

General

Dienstag, JL: Hepatitis A virus: identification, characterization, and epidemiologic investigations. Prog Liver Dis 6: 343, 1979.
  Excellent review of all aspects of hepatitis A virus, including clinical characteristics of hepatitis A infection and prophylaxis.
Hoyumpa, AM Jr, Greene, HL, Dunn, GD and Schenker, S: Fatty liver: biochemical and clinical considerations. Am J Dig Dis 20: 1142, 1975.
  Discusses various causes, clinical presentation, and management of fatty liver.
Leevy, CM, Popper, H and Sherlock S: Diseases of the liver and biliary tract. Standardization of nomenclature, diagnostic criteria and diagnostic methodology. Fogarty International Center Proceedings No. 22, DHEW Publication No. (NIH) 76-725, 1976.
Sherlock, S: Long incubation (virus B, HAA-associated) hepatitis. Gut 13: 297, 1972.
  Reviews characteristics of the hepatitis B virus and clinical characteristics of hepatitis B virus infection.
Sherlock, S: Hepatic reactions to drugs. Gut 20: 634, 1979.
  Good basic review of drug hepatitis. Discusses mechanisms of drug injury.

Specific

1. Boyer, JL: Chronic hepatitis—a perspective on classification and determinants of prognosis. Gastroenterology 70: 1161, 1976.
2. Davis, GL and Czaja, AJ: Prolonged steroid therapy for severe chronic active liver disease (CALD): a diminishing return? Gastroenterology 78: 1153, 1980.
3. Dickson, ER, Fleming, CP and Ludwig, J: Primary biliary cirrhosis. Prog Liver Dis 6: 487, 1979.
4. Fagerhol, MK and Laurell, CB: The polymorphism of "preal-

bumins" and α_1-antitrypsin in human sera. Clin Chim Acta 16: 199, 1967.
5. Feinstone, SM and Purcell, RH: Non-A, non-B hepatitis. Annu Rev Med 29: 359, 1978.
6. Galambos, JT: Alcoholic hepatitis: its therapy and prognosis. Prog Liver Dis 4: 567, 1972.
7. Grady, GF and the U.S. National Heart and Lung Institute Collaborative Study Group: Relation of e antigen to infectivity of HBsAg-positive inoculations among medical personnel. Lancet 2: 492, 1976.
8. Hamlyn, AN, Douglas, AP and James, O: The spectrum of paracetamol (acetaminophen) overdose: clinical and epidemiological studies. Postgrad Med J 54: 400, 1978.
9. Krugman, S, Overby, LR, Mushahwar, IK, Ling, CM, Frösner, GG and Deinhardt, F: Viral hepatitis, type B. Studies on natural history and prevention re-examined. N Engl J Med 300: 101, 1979.
10. LaBrecque, DR and Freeman, R: Risk of transmitting hepatitis B from staff to patient in a renal dialysis unit. Gastroenterology 75: 972, 1978.
11. Maddrey, WC and Boitnott, JK: Drug-induced chronic liver disease. Gastroenterology 72: 1348, 1977.
12. Powell, LW and Halliday, JW: The detection of early hemochromatosis. Am J Dig Dis 23: 377, 1978.
13. Repsher, LH and Freebern, RK: Effects of early and vigorous exercise on recovery from infectious hepatitis. N Engl J Med 281: 1393, 1969.
14. Sampliner, RE, Hamilton, FA, Iseri, OA, Tabor, E and Boitnott, J: The liver histology and frequency of clearance of the hepatitis B surface antigen (HBs Ag) in chronic carriers. Am J Med Sci 277: 17, 1979.
15. Schalm, SW, Summerskill, WHJ, Gitnick, GL and Elvebach, LR: Contrasting features and responses to treatment of severe chronic active liver disease with and without hepatitis Bs antigen. Gut 17: 781, 1976.
16. Seeff, LB and Hoofnagle, JH: Immunoprophylaxis of viral hepatitis. Gastroenterology 77: 161, 1979.
17. Sherlock, S. Chronic hepatitis. Gut 15: 581, 1974.
18. Sherlock, S. Predicting progression of acute type-B hepatitis to chronicity. Lancet 2: 354, 1976.
19. Soloway, RD, Summerskill, WHJ, Baggenstoss, AH, Geall, MG, Gitnick, GL, Elveback, LR and Schoenfield, LS: Clinical, biochemical, and histological remission of severe chronic active liver disease: A controlled study of treatments and early prognosis. Gastroenterology 63: 820, 1972.
20. Sternlieb, I and Scheinberg, IH: Chronic hepatitis as a first manifestation of Wilson's Disease. Ann Intern Med 76: 59, 1972.
21. Summerskill, WHJ, Davidson, CS, Dible, JH, Mallory, K, Sherlock, S, Turner, MD and Wolfe, SJ: Cirrhosis of the liver. A study of alcoholic and non-alcoholic patients in Boston and London. N Engl J Med 262: 1, 1960.
22. Szmuness, W, Dienstag, JC, Purcell, RH, Harley, EJ, Stevens, CE and Wong, DC: Distribution of antibody to hepatitis A antigen in urban adult populations. N Engl J Med 295: 755, 1976.

SECTION 5

Renal and Urologic Problems

CHAPTER FORTY

Proteinuria

JOHN R. BURTON, M.D.

Proteinuria is frequently encountered in ambulatory practice. It may signify a serious underlying disorder or it may be simply an abnormal laboratory finding in an asymptomatic individual with little or no effect on his present or future health.

This chapter will discuss the methods of detection of protein in the urine and describe an approach to the evaluation and management of this problem.

METHODS FOR DETECTING PROTEINURIA

Normally a small amount of protein is present in the urine. There is limited glomerular filtration of albumin and relatively greater filtration of lower molecular weight proteins, with nearly complete tubular reabsorption or digestion of filtered proteins. There is some tubular secretion, especially of a heavy molecular weight protein called the Tamm-Horsfall protein. The Tamm-Horsfall protein is the only protein identified in the urine that is not found in the plasma, and it forms the matrix that is seen in all urinary casts (4). The quantity of protein in the urine is normally less than 150 mg per 24 hours. While this is a small quantity, it may be detected by sensitive screening tests when the urine is physiologically concentrated.

Certain disease states affect the glomeruli and/or the tubules resulting in increased amounts of proteins in the urine. Office screening for proteinuria is easily accomplished by several accessible and inexpensive semiquantitative methods described in detail below.

All methods have some limitations as shown in Table 40.1 which provides a summary of the false results that are obtained under different conditions. It is clear that a combination of the dipstick test and one of the others may be required for diagnosis. Moreover, *all* methods are sensitive (dipstick detects 20 to 30 mg protein per dl, sulfosalicylic acid and heat and acetic acid, 5 to 10 mg per dl) so that false positive results may be obtained on concentrated urine.

Table 40.1
Urinary Constituents which Alter the Results of Protein Screening Tests

Urinary Constituents	Dipstick	Sulfosalicyclic Acid	Heat and Acetic Acid
Radiographic contrast media	No effect	False positive	False positive
Tolbutamide metabolites	No effect	False positive	False positive
Sulfisoxazole metabolites	No effect	False positive	False positive
Highly alkaline urine	False positive	False negative	False negative
High salt concentration	False negative	No effect	No effect
Vaginal or prostatic secretion	No effect	False positive	False positive

DIPSTICK

This is the most practical and easiest test for semiquantitation of urinary proteins. When moistened with urine, the stick becomes yellow when protein is absent. As protein concentration increases, interference with the dye-buffer combination results in an increasingly green color. While simple and inexpensive, the technique has several limitations: (a) the dipstick method is primarily *sensitive to albumin.* Therefore, globulins or parts of globulins (heavy or light chains—Bence-Jones protein) may be missed; (b) since the color raction is pH-dependent, false positive reactions may be observed if the *urine is alkaline* (pH greater than 7.5). This error can be avoided by adding a drop of strong acid (*e.g.*, 1 N HCl) prior to testing to assure that the pH in the urine is less than 7.0; and (c) *high concentrations of salt* in the urine will reduce the quantitative estimate of protein. This effect should be considered if the reaction is 1+ or 2+ and the patient is known to eat large quantities of salt. (The dipstick technique is not affected by urine turbidity or by drugs.) Because of these limitations, an alternative method of screening for proteinuria should be available in the physician's office. Either of the methods described below is satisfactory.

SULFOSALICYLIC ACID (SSA)

Another relatively easy and inexpensive semiquantitative test for proteinuria is protein precipitation with a 3 to 10% solution of sulfosalicylic acid. This solution is added to the urine in an approximate ratio of 8 ml to 2 ml of urine. After inversion and incubation at room temperature for a few moments flocculation is graded on a 0 to 4+ basis. The SSA test is important since it will precipitate globulins and light chains and, therefore, can reliably detect Bence-Jones protein.

SSA is used most frequently in two situations: as a check when the dipstick is negative, if there is a large quantity of salt in the urine or when globulins or light chains are being sought. False positive test results occur, however, if the urine is turbid and in this situation the urine must be filtered before it is tested. False positive results also occur when the test is done within 3 days of the administration of iodinated radiological contrast media or administration of some drugs (Table 40.1). In addition, the SSA test will detect proteins of prostatic and vaginal origin. The physician should take care to avoid these contaminants by not palpating the prostate before collecting urine from men and by obtaining a clean voided urine specimen from women, which should show no or only a few vaginal cells microscopically.

SSA is available from some pharmacies or from hospital laboratories. It is also marketed as Bumintest tablets by the Ames Company and is available through physician or surgical supply stores. When dissolved in water as directed the tablets will provide a solution containing about 5% SSA.

HEAT AND ACETIC ACID

This method is more time-consuming and is recommended as a second method of urine protein testing only when SSA is not available. Glacial acetic acid may be purchased at a photography store, and must be diluted for accurate results. The diluted solution, 1 volume of glacial acetic acid to 2 volumes of water, may be stored and used as necessary. The test is performed by heating the top of a test tube containing approximately 10 ml of urine. After the top of the urine begins to boil rapidly, 3 or 4 drops of the diluted acetic acid are added. Reheating to boiling causes a white precipitate to form if protein (either globulin or albumin) is present in the urine specimen. False positive results occur if the specimen is contaminated with prostatic or vaginal secretions or in the presence of certain drugs or radiographic contrast media (Table 40.1). Further, the rapid boiling may mask the visualization of a transient precipitation of Bence-Jones protein.

OFFICE ASSESSMENT OF PATIENTS WITH PROTEINURIA

When proteinuria is identified and confirmed, much can be done in the office to diagnose the problem and to minimize referral. First, it is important to define as closely as possible the *onset of proteinuria* by reviewing results of previous urinalyses done for insurance, school, military, employment, or previous health examinations. Occasionally, the patient may notice a foaming of the urine upon voiding when proteinuria is massive. Further, the onset of edema, nocturia, or hypertension may date the onset of a disease associated with proteinuria.

Second, *the physical examination* should be reviewed for the presence of signs which may be associated with the cause of renal disease (such as diabetic retinopathy or large polycystic kidneys) or which may result from renal disease (such as edema) or both (such as hypertension).

Third, a *microscopic urinalysis* should be done. The presence of other abnormalities such as hematuria, casts, and/or inflammatory cells will suggest specific patterns of renal disease of which proteinuria may be just a concomitant.

Fourth, an *assessment of renal filtration function* by measurement of serum creatinine or of creatinine clearance is the most important assessment of renal function (see Chapter 44, "Chronic Renal Failure").

Fifth, it is important to *quantitate the proteinuria* by examining a 24-hour urine sample as this will help to classify the disorder (see below) and assist in the development of the differential diagnosis. The patient will need precise instructions, verbal as well as written, to ensure adequacy of a 24-hour urine collection.

Twenty-Four Hour Urine Collection for Protein

A container without preservatives, usually a gallon jug, is given to the patient with instructions about the collection process. The 24-hour collection is best done on a day when the patient will be using one toilet; and it is helpful for the patient to place a note on the toilet on the day of collection to remind him to collect all required specimens. On the day of collection the first voided morning specimen is discarded; and then all urine in the next 24 hours, including the *next* morning's first voided specimen, is collected in the container. Once collected, it is not necessary to cool the urine; and it is not critical when the protein determination is done.

Quantitation of urine protein is a precise measurement in a well-controlled laboratory, and any value greater than 150 mg per day is considered abnormal. The simultaneous measurement of urinary creatinine is an index of the adequacy of collection and is helpful. Most individuals who are not wasted and are of average body mass produce between 800 and 1500 mg of creatinine per day. The determination of urine protein/creatinine ratio may be useful and eliminates the need for precise volume or time measurements. A ratio of greater than 0.1 mg of protein per mg of creatinine is considered abnormal. Proteinuria is classified as *non-nephrotic* if the excretion is between 150 mg and 3500 mg in 24 hours and classified as *nephrotic* when the excretion is greater than 3500 mg in 24 hours, regardless of the presence or absence of other manifestations of nephrotic syndrome (low serum albumin, edema, high serum cholesterol).

NON-NEPHROTIC PROTEINURIA

A physician considering the differential diagnosis of patients with this range of proteinuria should first rule out physiological explanations or problems that are not primarily renal. These are listed in Table 40.2

Table 40.2
Causes of Proteinuria Not Due to a Primary Renal Disease

Congestive heart failure
Epinephrine administrtion
Exercise
Fever
Stress resulting in catecholamine release

Table 40.3
Selected Investigations which May be Appropriate in the Dignosis of Proteinuria That is not Isolated or That is Nephrotic

Antinuclear antibody, if systemic lupus erythematosus (SLE) is suspected
Antistreptolysin (ASO) titer, if there is a possibility of post streptococcal glomerulonephritis
Complement (C_3, C_4), if glomerulonephritis is suspected
Complete blood count, to provide a baseline evaluation for subsequent use and to provide a clue for a systemic illness (such as leukemia)
Erythrocyte sedimentation rate, if collegen vascular disease is suspected
Fasting blood sugar, to consider the possibility of diabetes mellitus
Hepatitis B surface antigen, if hepatitis associated vasculitis may be present
Intravenous pyelogram, to provide evidence for structural renal disease (such as papillary necrosis)
Lupus erythematosus (LE) prep, if SLE is suspected
Serum albumin, if nephrotic range proteinuria is present
Serum electrolytes (Na^+, K^+, Cl^-, HCO_3^-, Ca^{2+}, PO_4^{2-}), to provide a screen for abnormalities subsequent to renal disease
Serum and urine protein electrophoresis, if multiple myeloma is suspected
Uric acid, to screen for urate-related renal disease
Urine culture, if pyuria present
X-ray of chest, to provide evidence for a systemic disease, for example sarcoidosis

and can be eliminated by brief questioning and repeat semiquantitative assessment of urine protein. A variety of primary renal and systemic diseases may be associated with non-nephrotic range proteinuria. Also most, if not all, causes of nephrotic range proteinuria (see below) may be associated with non-nephrotic range protein excretion at some time in their course.

Non-isolated Proteinuria

If an abnormality related to proteinuria is discovered during initial evaluation (e.g., hypertension, hematuria or renal failure) further investigation may be necessary. The direction and extent of the investigation depend on the nature of the abnormality. Renal biopsy may be indicated especially if there is hematuria, red blood cell casts, mild renal failure, or evidence of systemic disease (e.g., systemic lupus erythematosus (SLE)). Table 40.3 lists some additional investigations which may be indicated to evaluate abnormalities associated with proteinuria. A telephone consultation with a nephrologist may be helpful in deciding the need for further evaluation.

Isolated Proteinuria in Apparently Healthy Persons

If the initial evaluation is negative except for the presence of isolated proteinuria, the proteinuria may be further classified as persistent (25 to 30% of patients) or intermittent (70 to 75% of patients) (7). The physician can determine which pattern is present by obtaining multiple specimens over several months. The 24-hour urine protein excretion is almost always less than 1 g in patients with isolated proteinuria.

PERSISTENT PROTEINURIA

Patients with protein in greater than 80% of urine specimens are defined as having persistent proteinuria. The disorder may be further classified by evaluating the effect of posture. Constant persistent proteinuria is present when the patient is recumbent and on quiet ambulation; and fixed and orthostatic persistant proteinuria is present when the patient is in the upright position only (see below).

Constant Proteinuria. In most patients with constant proteinuria, diverse morphologic changes are identified in kidney biopsy specimens. Few long term studies of these patients have been made but their course is likely to be indolent. Renal failure develops very rarely, although most patients develop abnormal urine sediment, and 50% develop hypertension (1). It is not necessary to perform renal biopsy when there are no other findings, but yearly re-evaluation is appropriate and should include blood pressure measurement, urinalysis, and determination of 24-hour protein excretion and of serum creatinine and creatinine clearance.

Fixed and Orthostatic Proteinuria. The phenomenon of regularly reproducible postural proteinuria has been clarified largely by the work of Robinson *et al.* (6) who have followed for several years a number of male military recruits who have had this problem. Orthostatic proteinuria is defined as proteinuria only in the upright position. Its pathogenesis is not known. A simple method of determining the presence of this phenomenon is to have the patient collect two urine specimens. The patient rests quietly for 2 hours and then voids just before retiring in the evening. The patient does not get out of bed for 8 hours, and then upon arising voids completely into a container labeled "recumbent urine." The patient then stays up but is not vigorously active and collects all subsequent urine over the next 8 hours and then voids fully at the end of this collection period. This specimen is labeled "ambulatory urine." The protein concentrations in the urine specimens are then compared. An alternative to this method requires less time but is less quantitative. When this latter test is conducted during moderate fluid restriction, the results are reproducible. On the morning after overnight fluid deprivation, two or more urine specimens are collected consecutively during each of two se-

quentially assumed body postures: recumbence and quiet ambulation. A semiquantitative test and a measurement of urine concentration to confirm antidiuresis are performed on each sample (7). In patients with orthostatic proteinuria the "recumbent" protein excretion is negligible, whereas proteinuria is found when the patient assumes upright posture.

A renal biopsy is not necessary in the evaluation of a patient with this problem; but, when done as part of a research protocol, minor abnormalities have been defined in approximately half of the individuals while the others have had a biopsy that appeared normal on light microscopy (studies utilizing electron and/or immunofluorescent microscopy have not been done). It would, however, be prudent to follow the patient by measuring urinary protein excretion and serum creatinine or creatinine clearance on a yearly basis.

If fixed and orthostatic proteinuria is documented, then the prognosis seems to be excellent. Military recruits with this problem have been followed for 10 years (6). None have developed renal failure, and approximately half are no longer proteinuric. Patients who have been free of protein in the urine at 5-year follow-up have remained protein-free after 10 years. (A 20-year follow-up of this group of patients is planned) (7). Also, a small number of patients re-evaluated 42 to 50 years following the establishment of the diagnosis of postural proteinuria manifest an excellent prognosis (8).

INTERMITTENT PROTEINURA

A study of individuals with intermittent isolated proteinuria (protein in less than 80% of specimens) revealed definite abnormalities by light microscopic analysis of renal tissue in approximately 60% of patients while approximately 40% had a normal or nearly normal biopsy (5). The significance of these findings is unclear, however, in light of an independent study which retrospectively analyzed the prognostic significance of proteinuria in male college students and found there was no excess mortality 37 to 45 years later; morbidity not studied (3).

In any case, patients who are found to have asymptomatic intermittent proteinuria and who have no evidence of systemic or renal disease can be given an optimistic prognosis. It is not necessary to perform kidney biopsy in these individuals, but it would be prudent to follow them yearly with measurement of urine protein excretion, a urinalysis, and determination of serum creatinine and creatinine clearance. Should deterioration in function, significant increase in protein excretion or new abnormalities occur, then reassessment and possibly a renal biopsy are necessary.

NEPHROTIC PROTEINURA

When a 24-hour protein quantitation reveals greater than 3.5 g of protein, nephrotic range protein-

Table 40.4
Causes of Nephrotic Syndrome in Adults [a]

MOST COMMON
    Diabetes mellitus—most common
    Idiopathic membranous glomerulopathy—second most common
    Idiopathic lipoid nephrosis—third most common in adults (most common in children)
LESS COMMON
    Focal glomerular sclerosis
    Proliferative glomerulonephritis
    Membranoproliferative glomerulonephritis
    Collagen vascular disease
    Amyloidosis

[a] An extensive list of potential causes of nephrotic syndrome can be found in L. E. Early and M. Foreland: Nephrotic syndrome. In *Strauss and Welt's Diseases of the Kidney*, Ed. 3, edited by L. E. Early and C. W. Gottschalk, Little Brown & Co., Boston, 1979.

uria is established by definition, and is indicative of glomerular disease. There are many causes of nephrotic syndrome, but there are relatively few conditions which are seen with significant frequency in a general medical practice (Table 40.4). When nephrotic range proteinuria develops in a patient who has been diabetic for over 10 to 15 years, the renal lesion is almost always diabetic glomerulosclerosis, particularly if the patient also has diabetic microaneurysms in the retina. In this setting, a renal biopsy is usually not necessary. On the other hand, a biopsy is usually necessary to diagnose a specific primary renal disease or if a diagnosis cannot be made by other tests (e.g., detection of Bence-Jones proterinuria or rectal biopsy for amyloid), or it may be needed to guide therapy or to help determine prognosis (e.g., SLE). Table 40.3 lists some of the laboratory evaluations which may be helpful in determining the cause of renal disease. Renal biopsy is helpful in classifying the pathologic process, and thereby aids in the determination of the patient's prognosis and in deciding about therapy. A consultation with a nephrologist may be appropriate to help decide the need for biopsy as well as to provide suggestions for treatment.

Renal Biopsy

Patient Experience. Renal biopsy requires hospitalization for 24 to 48 hours. Generally, in patients without renal failure and no bleeding abnormality, percutaneous biopsy is performed under local anesthesia with fluoroscopic or sonographic guidance. This technique permits the nephrologist to sample the lower portion of the kidney and to avoid the hilar vessels and the renal collecting system. With percutaneous biopsy the patient usually experiences minimal discomfort and is able to be out of bed in 12 hours.

The biopsy core is approximately 1 mm in diameter and approximately 10 to 20 mm in length. Usually two such tissue cores are obtained. The risk associated with percutaneous renal biopsy is small if performed by an experienced physician.

COMPLICATIONS

Microscopic hematuria is almost inevitable, and usually there is a small hematoma at the biopsy site on the surface of the kidney. It is, however, usually of no clinical consequence. Gross hematuria occurs in approximately 5 to 10% of patients, but less than 5% require a transfusion to replace blood loss. Less than 1 in 1,000 patients requires nephrectomy because of continued massive bleeding, and mortality from biopsy is very rare. A renal arteriovenous fistula may develop after biopsy, but it usually closes spontaneously. Rarely this complication may require treatment if bleeding continues or if hypertension develops (2). Even more rarely, there may be perforation of another viscus.

When percutaneous biopsy is not feasible, open biopsy can be obtained; some surgeons perform this procedure under local anesthesia in selected patients.

Regardless of the technique of obtaining the biopsy, the evaluation of tissue by the pathologist should include light, immunofluorescent, and electron microscopy and it should be done by a pathologist experienced in preparation and interpretation of renal biopsy material.

The physician who has referred a patient to a nephrologist for percutaneous biopsy or to a surgeon for open biopsy should expect communication on the following: the probable diagnosis, based upon all aspects of the microscopic assessment; whether or not specific therapy for the condition is indicated; and what prognostic judgement can be made. Knowledge that guides therapy in disease associated with nephrotic syndrome is continually developing, and current information should be expected from the consultant.

MANAGEMENT OF PATIENTS WITH PROTEINURIA

Non-nephrotic proteinuria requires no special treatment. The physician's major effort is directed at diagnosis, education, surveillance, and at treatment of any underlying disease.

Some patients with nephrotic range proteinuria are asymptomatic and require no therapy unless the results of the renal biopsy dictate that treatment be given. When either edema or hypoalbuminemia is present, special therapy may be indicated. (In the absence of renal failure, albumin synthesis is either increased or normal in patients with the nephrotic syndrome.) Generally, assurance of an *adequate protein intake* is accomplished in patients who have nephrotic range proteinuria by the daily administration of 2 to 3 g of protein per kg dry weight (estimated or actual weight before edema developed). This can be accomplished with protein supplements such as eggnog, milkshakes, or meat protein supplements. High protein intake can be discontinued if remission is obtained.

In the presence of edema, *salt restriction* to a tolerable level such as a no-added-salt diet (approximately 3 to 4 g of Na) is appropriate. If the edema is more severe and is unresponsive to sodium chloride restriction, then the *cautious use of diuretics* may be helpful, beginning with thiazides and then substituting loop diuretics (furosamide, ethacrynic acid) if necessary. There should not be an attempt to rid the patient entirely of edema which could risk contraction of the circulating volume with serious consequences; the patient may benefit from alternate-day diuretics which will diminish the risk of inducing serious volume contraction. Potassium-sparing diuretics (spironolactone or triamterene) may be added if renal failure is absent and if loop diuretics have not been entirely adequate. If acceptable control is still not achieved, consultation with a nephrologist is appropriate. Prediction of the course and selection of specific therapy in patients with nephrotic range proteinuria depend on the pathologic pattern that is identified in the biopsy. Patients with nephrotic range proteinuria will need regularly scheduled office visits at 1 to 4 month intervals. Usually this follow-up is done by the primary physician and the patient will see the nephrologist only once a year. The office visit provides an opportunity to review the patient's symptoms and to perform a limited physical examination (which, at a minimum, should include weight, volume assessment, and blood pressure) as well as to evaluate the 24-hour urine protein excretion, the renal function (creatinine or creatinine clearance), and the serum electrolytes if diuretics are being used. Less frequently an assessment of the serum albumin may be necessary.

References

General

Pesce, A and First, MR: Proteinuria: An integrated review. In *Kidney Disease*, Vol. 1, JS Camerson, RJ Glassock, and C Van Ypersele de Strihov. Marcel Dekker, New York, 1979.

    A valuable monograph which provides a thorough review of the mechanism and pathophysiology of proteinuria as well as a discussion of disease states.

Specific

1. King, SE: Diastolic hypertension and chronic proteinuria. *Am J Cardiol 9*: 669, 1962
2. Leiter, E, Gribetz, D and Cohen, S: Arteriovenous fistula after percutaneous needle biopsy—surgical repair with preservation of renal function. *J Engl J Med 287*: 971, 1972
3. Levitt, JI: The prognostic significance of proteinuria in young college students. *Ann Intern Med 66*: 685, 1967.
4. McQueen, EG and Sidney, M: Composition of urinary casts. *Lancet 1*: 397, 1966.
5. Muth, RG: Asymptomatic mild intermittent proteinuria. *Arch Intern Med 115*: 569, 1965
6. Robinson, RR, Thompson, AL and Durrett, RR: Fixed and reproducible orthostatic proteinuria; VI. Results of a 10-year follow-up evaluation. *Ann Intern Med 73*: 235, 1970
7. Robinson, RR: Isolated proteinuria in asymptomatic patients. *Kidney Int 18*: 399, 1980.
8. Rytand, DA and Spreiter, S: Prognosis in postural (orthostatic) proteinuria. Forty- to fifty-year follow-up of six patients after diagnosis by Thomas Addis. *N Engl J Med 305*: 618, 1981.

CHAPTER FORTY-ONE

Hematuria

JAMES K. SMOLEV, M.D.

INTRODUCTION

Hematuria is a common finding and it is of particular importance to the ambulatory physician because of the proportion of office visits related to genitourinary problems—approximately 7% (5). This chapter reviews the significance of hematuria including problems that may be confused with this condition, provides a differential diagnosis of hematuria, and suggests guidelines which will help determine the need for and type of consultation that may be appropriate.

SIGNIFICANCE OF HEMATURIA

Normally 1 to 2 million red blood cells are lost in the urine every 24 hours. However, when studied microscopically in centrifuged urine, this amounts to only 1 to 2 red blood cells per high power field. Therefore, the finding of more than 3 or 4 red blood cells per high power field should be considered abnormal, and requires an explanation. Under certain conditions, however, hematuria may be considered normal; for example it will often be found just after pelvic or prostatic examination, bladder instrumentation, catheterization, or a prostate or renal biopsy or even after vigorous exercise. Therefore, in these situations repeat urinalyses should be done before other causes of the problem are considered. Also, if a female patient is menstruating or a male patient has a lesion on his foreskin, an evaluation for hematuria should not be undertaken unless bleeding persists after menstruation stops or after the lesion is treated.

Hematuria may be a manifestation of a serious disease, which may be otherwise asymptomatic. For example, Golin and Howard (3) and Carson and co-workers (2) found a tumor of the genitourinary tract in 10% and 12.5%, respectively, of patients studied because of microscopic hematuria. On the other hand, the finding of red urine or red blood cells in the urine may not be significant. For example, as mentioned above the remarkable increase in the number of red blood cells in the urine after vigorous exercise may not be abnormal unless a repeat urinalysis under resting conditions also shows hematuria. Certain urinary pigments and other chemicals may simulate hematuria but may be excluded by the demonstration of a *normal* microscopic urinalysis and a *negative dipstick* test for blood. Common examples of these agents are anthocyanins (beets), phenolphthalein (laxatives such as Correctol, Feen-A-Mint, Ex-Lax, Phenolox), phenazopyridine (Pyridium), and porphyrin. Moreover when urine pH is low, crystals of uric acid have a reddish hue but these can be seen by microscopic examination, and both crystals and color will disappear by the addition of alkali (such as a drop of ammonia water) to the urine specimen.

Hematuria is alarming to a patient, who is frequently concerned about the amount of blood that is lost. Excessive blood loss is unusual and the patient will benefit from reassurance about this; nevertheless, it is important for the physician to appreciate that the amount of hematuria has no correlation with the seriousness of the underlying cause of the problem.

PATTERNS OF HEMATURIA

Hematuria may be gross or microscopic, and may occur intermittently or continuously. Intermittent hematuria should not, however, be dismissed as relatively insignificant since most serious disorders—including neoplasia—frequently are characterized by intermittent hematuria. Moreover hematuria from any cause may manifest as gross hematuria on some occasions and at other times as microscopic hematuria.

Microscopic

Microscopic hematuria is generally identified by microscopic examination of the urine or by observation of a positive dipstick test for blood in the urine.

DIPSTICK SCREENING TEST

Most multipurpose reagent strips have a colorimetric test for pigments; this test may often be the first clue to the presence of hematuria. The test detects hemoglobins and myoglobins, but it is not specific, therefore requiring caution in interpretation (Table 41.1). Hemoglobin from intravascular hemolysis and myoglobin released from injured muscles both produce a positive reaction. Furthermore, since the test

Table 41.1
Limits of Dipstick Method for Detection of Blood in the Urine

REASONS FOR A POSITIVE TEST
  Hematuria—greater than approximately 10 red blood cells per high power field
  Hematuria with red blood cell lysis
    From hypotonic urine (specific gravity less than 1.008)
    From highly alkaline urine (pH greater than 6.5–7.0)
  Hemoglobinuria—from intravascular hemolysis
  Myoglobinuria—from muscle injury
  False positive reactions
    From hypochlorite (bleach) contamination of container
    From peroxidase (from heavy growth of bacteria)
REASONS FOR A FALSE NEGATIVE TEST
  Vitamin C—ingestion by the patient of large amounts of vitamin C (>200 mg per day) results in diminished oxidation potential of the test material. The dipstick test may miss trace quantities of blood, although usually there is a quantitative decrease in the estimate of blood (such as 3+ to 2+) (6). (This is of concern only if red blood cells are observed but the dipstick test is negative).
  Formaldehyde—ingestion of bacterial suppressant agents (such as Mandelamine or Hiprex) which produce formaldehyde in acid urine or contamination of the container with formaldehyde will diminish the oxidizing potential of the reagent strips. This results in a quantitative estimate error or, if hematuria is minimal, false negative results.

requires an oxidation reaction, false positive results may occur in the presence of oxidizing agents such as hypochlorite (contamination from bleach *in vitro*) or peroxidases (from bacteria when the urine is heavily infected). In addition, false negative reactions may occur because of reduction of the oxidizing potential of the strip if the patient has ingested large amounts of vitamin C, or agents which form formaldehyde in the urine (such as Mandelamine or Hiprex), or if the urine specimen container has been contaminated with formaldehyde. For these reasons the dipstick screening technique should not be taken as diagnostic but should always be confirmed by a microscopic urinalysis.

The dipstick test is not a useful way to quantitate hematuria. The test is more sensitive to free hemoglobin than to hemoglobin contained in red blood cells. The lower limit of sensitivity is approximately 30 μg per dl of hemoglobin (approximately equivalent to 10 red blood cells per cu mm of urine (the approximate volume in one high power field). Therefore, with fewer than about 10 red blood cells per high power field, the dipstick test may be negative. On the other hand, if the cells in the urine have lysed because

the urine is hypotonic (specific gravity less than 1.008) or because of the presence of highly alkaline urine (greater than pH 6.5 to 7.0), the dipstick will then be more sensitive than the microscopic assessment; however, hemoglobin can still not be differentiated from myoglobin under these circumstances.

Gross

The pattern of gross hematuria is helpful in identifying its cause. *Initial hematuria* is the appearance of blood just as urination is initiated, with clearing as voiding continues. It is due to a disease in the urethra. *Terminal hematuria* is the appearance of hematuria just at the conclusion of voiding, and it indicates a disease near the bladder neck or the posterior urethra. *Total gross hematuria* is the appearance of blood throughout most of the urinary stream and may result from a disease process in any portion of the urinary tract.

When evaluating patients who have gross hematuria, it is helpful to note any associated symptoms which help delineate the underlying problem. For example, colic suggests a renal calculus; and irritative symptoms (frequency, urgency and dysuria) suggest urinary tract infection.

Hematuria confirmed as indicated above should always be considered abnormal and a thorough evaluation should be planned.

CAUSES OF HEMATURIA

Evaluation of hematuria results in the establishment of a specific diagnosis in 50 to 80% of patients (2,3). Table 41.2 provides a selected list of causes of hematuria arranged according to the presence of associated findings on urinalysis and Table 41.3 is a selected list of common causes of hematuria that might be suspected based on the patient's age and sex.

APPROACH TO EVALUATION OF PATIENTS WITH HEMATURIA

Using Tables 41.2 and 41.3 as a guide, the physician should review the patient's history, perform a physical examination, and review the urinalysis to determine the direction for subsequent evaluation.

Isolated

Isolated hematuria is best evaluated by obtaining a complete blood count, including a platelet count, and in Black patients, a hemoglobin electrophoresis (see Chapter 46). Renal function should be assessed by the measurement of serum creatinine or by creatinine clearance to establish associated renal failure (see Chapter 44). In an individual who is over the age of 30, a neoplastic process should be considered and urine cytology studies should be made. Approximately 30% of tumors in the upper urinary tract and

Table 41.2
Selected Causes of Hemturia and Associated Findings in Urinalysis

Hematuria Alone	Hematuria and Pyuria with Little or No Proteinuria	Hematuria with Casts and/or with Significant Proteinuria (Greater than 1 g/24 hr)

Disorders anatomically adjacent to the urinary tract:
  Aortic aneurysm
  Renal artery aneurysm
  Pelvic or retroperitoneal disease (e.g., lymphoma)
Anticoagulant drugs (an underlying cause unmasked by anticoagulants is present in 80%) (1)
Arteriovenous fistula (kidney)
Benign prostatic hypertrophy
Calculi (see Chapter 43)
Diverticula:
  Calyceal
  Urethral
  Bladder
Emboli
Glomerulonephritis—e.g., IgA nephropathy
Hereditary disorders:
  Alport's disease
  Cystic disease:
    Polycystic disease
    Medullary cystic disease
    Medullary sponge kidney
  Hemoglobinopathy (SS, SA, SC, S Thal)
  Hemangioma
  Arteriovenous malformation
Neoplasia (benign or malignant)
Telangiectasia
Thomrombocytopenia
Trauma
Urethritis
Varicosities
  "Benign essential hematuria"—see text
	Infection (anywhere in the genitourinary tract):
	  Bacterial
	  Fungal
	  Mycobacterial
	  Viral
	  Helminthic (schistomiasis)
		Hypertension—especially accelerated
		Emboli
		Glomerulonephritis:
		  Primary:
		    IgA nephropathy
		    Membranoproliferative
		    Focal
		  Systemic:
		    Systemic lupus erythematosus
		    Polyarteritis nodosa
		    Henoch-Schölein
		    Goodpasture's syndrome
		Leukemia (acute)
		Nephrotoxins—examples:
		  Anti-inflammatory agents
		  Lithium
		  Penicillin and its derivatives
		Thrombosis of the renal vein

approximately 50% of bladder tumors will result in positive cytology. It is best to obtain specific information from the laboratory about the proper method for collection and transfer to the laboratory and about whether the patient should be hydrated or dehydrated for the procedure. Three separate specimens obtained on different days are considered an adequate initial screen.

If after this evaluation no diagnosis is established, an intravenous pyelogram (IVP) should be performed. If the IVP is normal, a urologist should be consulted for consideration of further evaluation using cystoscopy or a computerized tomography (CT) scan. Based on this initial assessment the urologist may suggest sonography, nephrotomogram, renal scan, or angiography.

If the patient is having gross hematuria, it is a particularly opportune time for the urologist to perform endoscopy as it may allow him to visualize the site of the blood loss which then can become the focus of more definitive evaluation. Cystoscopy is not contraindicated in patients with hematuria who also have a coagulopathy (iatrogenic or otherwise), but biopsy should not be done.

Should this entire evaluation be negative, then a nephrologist should be consulted for consideration of percutaneous renal biopsy (see Chapter 40).

Association with Pyuria

If a patient is found to have hematuria associated with pyuria (with or without irritative symptoms), an infectious cause is likely and routine bacterial cultures should be obtained. If a specific infection is identified, appropriate antimicrobial therapy should be begun (see Chapter 26), after which the patient should be follow up to ensure that hematuria has been eradicated and does not recur. If irritative symptoms (frequency, dysuria, and urgency) suggesting infection have been present and the routine culture is sterile, viral infection or tuberculosis may be present. However, because noninfectious disorders of

Table 41.3
Common Causes of Hematuria Arranged by Age and Sex[a]

Age (yr)	Sex	Causes
0–20	Male and female	Acute glomerulonephritis
		Acute urinary tract infection (viral, bacterial)
		Congenital urinary tract anomalies
20–40	Male and female	Acute urinary tract infection
		Calculus
		Sickle cell disease
		Tumor
40–60	Male	Bladder tumor[b]
		Calculus
		Infection
		Renal tumor[b]
	Female	Infection
		Stone
		Bladder tumor[b]
		Renal tumor[b]
Over 60	Male	Benign prostatic hyperplasia; prostate carcinoma[b]
		Bladder tumor[b]
		Renal tumor[b]
	female	Bladder tumor[b]
		Infection
		Renal tumor[b]

[a] Adapted from A. W. Wyker and J. Y. Gillenwater: *Method of Urology*, Williams & Wilkins, Baltimore, 1975.
[b] Tumor will account for 50% of patients with gross hematuria that are over 50 years old.

the bladder (including malignancies) may produce similar symptoms, the physician should ensure that symptoms have abated and that urinalysis is normal on two or three subsequent occasions. Viral infections should be short lived and nonrecurrent. The confirmation by culture of the diagnosis of tuberculous infection of the urinary tract requires several weeks; an acid-fast stain of the urine is not a reliable indicator because of the regular presence of acid-fast material from smegma bacilli.

Associated with Urinary Casts or Significant Proteinuria

In a situation where hematuria is associated with urinary casts or significant proteinuria (greater than 1 g per 24 hours), evaluation for glomerular disease is indicated (see Chapter 40). Direct referral to a nephrologist for consideration of renal biopsy is often appropriate.

SURVEILLANCE OF PATIENTS

By following this approach, a cause for hematuria will be identified in approximately 50 to 80% of patients (2, 3). However, even when this evaluation has not revealed the underlying cause, the physician

should not presume the situation to be innocuous, as serious problems (such as tumor) may be identified at follow-up (3). If the complete initial workup is negative, it therefore would be prudent to see these patients every 3 to 6 months. On these occasions the history, physical examination, and urinalysis should be reviewed; in patients over 30, a urine specimen should be sent for cytologic examination. If there is continued hematuria that has not been explained after 1 year, the IVP should be repeated and consultation with a urologist should be arranged for consideration for a repeat cystoscopy.

The diagnosis of *benign essential hematuria* has no meaning. When the initial evaluation fails to reveal a cause of the hematuria, that hematuria should be labeled "unexplained" and it should not be considered benign until no cause has been identified after 2 years of follow-up.

HEMATOSPERMIA (4)

The presence of blood in the ejaculate of males is an alarming but usually innocuous symptom. This problem occurs most often in men over 40, and most often the episodes recur over several weeks or months. When it occurs in an otherwise asymptomatic man who has a normal physical examination (including rectal examination of the prostate and seminal vesicles) and a normal urinalysis, the patient should be reassured that it is innocuous and that no further workup is necessary. If there is any abnormality, further evaluation for benign prostatic hypertrophy or cancer of the prostate, seminal vesicles, bladder, or urethra should be considered and a urologist consulted.

References

General

Wyker, AW and Gillenwater, JY: Signs and symptoms of urological disorders and differential diagnoses. In *Method of Urology*. Williams & Wilkins, Baltimore, 1975.
    A concise text covering all aspects of urology.

Specific

1. Antolak, SJ and Mellinger, GT: Urologic evaluation of hematuria occurring during anticoagulant therapy. *Urology* 101: 111, 1969.
2. Carson, CC, Sergura, JW and Greene, LF: Clinical importance of microhematuria. *JAMA* 241: 149, 1979.
3. Golin, LA and Howard, RS: Asymptomatic microscopic hematuria. *Urology* 124: 389, 1980.
4. Leary, FJ, Aguilo, JJ: Clinical significance of hematospermia *Mayo Clin Proc* 49: 815, 1974.
5. National Ambulatory Medical Care Survey: Series 13, No. 33; D.H.E.W. Publication No. (PHS) 78-1784. U.S. Department Health, Education and Welfare, January 1978.
6. Smith, BC, Peake, MJ and Fraser, CG: Urinalysis by use of a multitest reagent strip; two dipsticks compared. *Clin Chem* 23: 2337, 1977.

CHAPTER FORTY-TWO

Hypokalemia

JOHN R. BURTON, M.D.

Low levels of potassium in the serum are frequently encountered in ambulatory practice. The consequences are often trivial, but occasionally are life-threatening. Loss of potassium through the gastrointestinal tract and by use of diuretics account for the majority of patients with hypokalemia seen in an ambulatory practice, but there is an extensive differential diagnosis with which the practitioner must be familiar in the event of one of the more common causes is not present. This chapter will review the physiological background, outline the symptomatic consequences of potassium depletion, develop an approach to the differential diagnosis, and discuss the management of patients with hypokalemia.

PHYSIOLOGICAL BACKGROUND

Total body potassium is approximately 50 meq per kg body weight. For example, a 70-kg (144 lb) person would have approximately 3500 meq of total body potassium. Serum potassium reflects, but does not indicate with certainty, total body potassium. Generally a decrease of 1.0 meq of potassium in the serum reflects approximately a 10 to 20% deficiency of total body potassium.

The balance of potassium is zealously guarded during health. This balance is schematically represented in Figure 42.1. It can be seen from the figure that a relatively small amount of potassium (approximately 2%) exists outside body cells and a large amount (approximately 98%) exists inside cells. This asymmetry of distribution of potassium is determined by (a) the relative permeability of cell membranes to sodium and potassium, (b) sodium-potassium-ATPase activity within membranes, (c) electrochemical forces, (d) hydrogen ion activity of extracellular fluid, (e) insulin independent of glucose transport, (f) epinephrine, and (g) aldosterone. The electrocardiogram is a useful way of assessing the relative intra- to extracellular potassium ratio. Figure 42.2 schematically represents changes in the electrocardiogram as potassium concentration is changed.

The delicate balance of potassium is largely modulated by the excretion of potassium by the kidneys. Ninety percent of ingested potassium is excreted in the urine; the remainder is excreted in the intestinal tract. The skin is usually an insignificant site of potassium loss. In temperate climates less than 5 meq/day of potassium are lost in sweat. However, with profuse sweating dermal losses of potassium may approach 25 to 30 meq/day.

Renal potassium excretion is a distal tubular function since potassium is freely filtered by the glomerulus and then nearly completely reabsorbed by the proximal tubule. Excretion is regulated by (a) the rate of urine flow bathing the distal tubular cells; (b) the concentration of potassium in the distal tubular cells; (c) the level in the blood of aldosterone, a hormone which stimulates excretion of potassium, increasing its concentration in the tubular cells; and (d) the relative electrochemical forces between tubular fluid and tubular cells. (The more negative the charge of the urinary fluid the greater the electrochemical force attracting potassium from the cells to the tubular fluid.) Although potassium balance is delicate, conservation is not nearly as efficient as it is with respect to sodium. Generally, up to 15 meq of potassium per day are lost in the urine even with no potassium intake.

Although the intestinal tract accounts for approx-

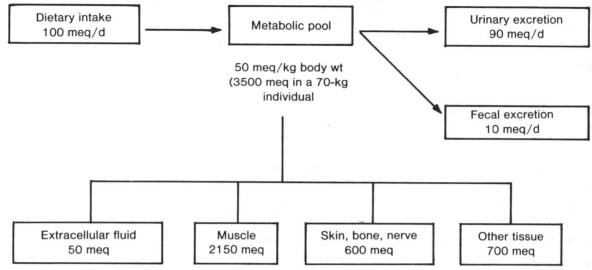

Figure 42.1 Balance of potassium. (Adapted from Kliger and Hayslett: Disorders of potassium. In *Acid-Base and potassium Hemostasis*, edited by B. M. Brenner and J. H. Stein, Churchill Livingstone, New York, 1978.)

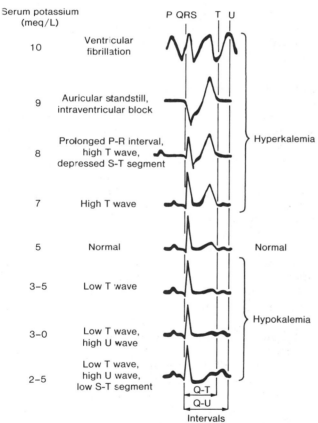

Figure 42.2 Electrocardiogram in assessment of potassium. (Adapted from G. E. Burch and T. Winsor: *A Primer of Electrocardiography*, Ed. 6, p. 128, Lea & Febiger, Philadelphia, 1972.)

imately 10% of potassium excretion normally, when uremia is present, the gastrointestinal tract excretes increased amounts of potassium and may account for 1/3 of the total potassium excreted by the uremic individual.

SYMPTOMATIC CONSEQUENCES OF POTASSIUM DEPLETION

Most often the practitioner detects mild hypokalemia in an asymptomatic individual. Almost as often the symptoms of the problem which has led to potassium depletion are prominent; for example, vomiting or diarrhea. However, there are a variety of less frequent symptomatic, and potentially serious, consequences of severe potassium depletion with which the practitioner should be familiar.

Skeletal muscle, which has a very high cellular potassium content, manifests potassium depletion by symptoms ranging from mild weakness to paralysis, including failure of respiratory musculature. Muscles depleted of potassium are also at risk from an ischemic insult. For this reason a potassium-depleted individual performing physical exercise may develop myonecrosis and occasionally myoglobinuric acute renal failure.

Cardiac muscle may show patchy microscopic necrosis in states of chronic potassium depletion; and, as a result, not infrequently conduction abnormalities develop. Myocardial cells are also more sensitive to digitalis preparations in the face of potassium depletion. Digitalis toxicity may occur at nontoxic plasma levels when hypokalemia is present (1). Postural hypotension is seen with severe potassium depletion and may develop after only several days of potassium deficiency.

Potassium depletion affects the musculature of the *gastrointestinal tract* resulting in decreased motility with clinical manifestations of ileus.

In the *kidney*, *chronic* potassium depletion results in microscopic changes of vacuolar formation in the distal nephron. Renal function is impaired with *severe* potassium deficiency, and mild degrees of renal failure occur. The patient with chronic potassium depletion is also unable to concentrate and acidify the urine normally, although this condition takes several weeks to manifest maximally.

A variety of *vague symptoms* have been attributed to hypokalemia including muscular cramps, agitation, depression, fatigue, and weakness. Chronic potassium deficiency may be associated with *carbohydrate intolerance*. Potassium depletion also is associated with precipitation of *hepatic encephalopathy* in patients with severe liver disease and a tendency to hepatic failure.

DIFFERENTIAL DIAGNOSIS

The four mechanisms which may lead to hypokalemia are listed in Table 42.1. Gastrointestinal potassium loss and diuretics account for the vast majority of patients seen in ambulatory practice with low plasma potassium.

These problems will be discussed in detail, and the remainder of the chapter will provide a brief approach to the less common causes of hypokalemia.

Gastrointestinal Losses Resulting in Potassium Deficiency

Excessive loss of potassium from the gastrointestinal tract is overall the most frequent cause of hypokalemia. This is usually associated with clinical contraction of the extracellular fluid volume which will be readily detected on physical examination with evidence of weight loss, a lower than usual jugular venous pressure, a decrease in skin turgor and, frequently, orthostatic hypotension and tachycardia. The urinary potassium level is helpful in identifying the site of gastrointestinal potassium loss. Urinary potassium would logically be expected to be low when potassium deficiency results from gastrointestinal losses and the kidney attempts maximally to conserve potassium. That is true, however, only if potassium is lost from the intestinal tract distal to the stomach. Gastrointestinal fluid losses because of vomiting or nasogastric suction result in urinary potassium wasting and associated metabolic alkalosis.

CHLORIDE DEPLETION

The gastric juices are rich in hydrochloric acid and losses from the stomach because of vomiting or nasogastric suction result in the loss primarily of hydrogen and chloride. These losses induce a metabolic alkalosis (hydrogen ion deficiency) and chloride deficiency. The chloride deficiency results in an inadequate reabsorption of sodium by the renal proximal tubules since sodium in the proximal tubule is reabsorbed with chloride. Consequently, because of chloride deficiency, an excess amount of sodium is delivered to the distal tubules of the nephron. There, sodium is reabsorbed under the influence of aldosterone, and potassium and hydrogen ions are excreted. The result of loss of chloride from the stomach, therefore, is loss of potassium and hydrogen by the kidney, with subsequent hypokalemia and metabolic alkalosis, and the urine will show relatively high concentrations of potassium, usually greater than 40 meq per liter, and an acid pH.

BICARBONATE DEPLETION

Fluid loss from the gastrointestinal tract below the stomach results in a low urinary potassium and frequently a systemic acidosis secondary to gastrointestinal bicarbonate loss. This situation is commonly seen in patients who have acute and chronic diarrhea or who have malabsorption syndromes.

The colon may excrete large quantities of potassium. Usual colonic content contains approximately 40 meq/L, but on occasion colonic mucus may contain up to 90 meq/L . There are isolated reports of diarrhea secondary to *laxative abuse* resulting in potassium depletion, but there are no data available to indicate how commonly this occurs. Most practitioners will witness it only occasionally. *Enemas* also may result in significant potassium depletion but only if patients are receiving multiple enemas frequently.

Patients with a *villous adenoma* of the colon often develop hypokalemia because of excess excretion of potassium by the tumor. They usually notice the passage of large quantities of mucus with their bowel movements although the stool itself may appear normal. Therefore, the diagnosis of villous adenoma should be considered when loss of potassium from the gastrointestinal tract is suspected, but there is no immediately obvious historical explanation.

Diuretics

Diuretics that act proximally in the nephron accelerate potassium excretion by increasing the amount of sodium that is delivered to the distal tubules. There, sodium is reabsorbed but, as a result, increased amounts of potassium and hydrogen ions are excreted. Furosemide and ethacrynic acid, as well as the thiazides and chlorthalidone, are diuretics that act in this way.

DIURETICS IN NONEDEMATOUS PATIENTS

Patients who take diuretics but who are not edematous (for example, a patient with mild hypertension who is being treated with a thiazide diuretic) are not usually potassium-depleted. When studied prospectively, less than 5% of such individuals develop a deficiency of total body potassium (3). Frequently, however, the serum potassium level only falls 0.3 to 1.2 meq/L below the normal level in the absence of diuretics, representing an insignificant change in total body potassium. Significant hypokalemia (levels be-

Table 42.1
Basic Mechanisms of Hypokalemia

Excessive gastrointestinal loss of potassium
Excessive renal loss of potassium
Diminished potassium intake
Maldistribution of extracellular and intracellular potassium

low 3.0 meq/L) is encountered only occasionally and when confirmed should alert the practitioner to two possible explanations: (a) *Excess salt intake.* A high intake of sodium chloride in a patient who is taking a potassium-wasting diuretic will increase the amount of sodium delivered to the distal nephron, accelerating potassium excretion, and leading to potassium depletion. Moderate salt restriction during diuretic treatment precludes increased distal delivery of sodium and thereby protects against this mechanism for excessive potassium loss. (b) An unrecognized *potassium-wasting state.* Both primary and secondary aldosteronism may be revealed as excessive hypokalemia following the introduction of potassium-wasting diuretics. These states should be suspected particularly if the potassium value of the untreated individual was in the low or low normal range. Additional discussion of these states is found later in this chapter (p. 350).

Metabolic alkalosis is seen in nonedematous patients who are taking diuretics. Many of the potent potassium-wasting diuretics induce a net loss of hydrogen ion, causing a rise in serum bicarbonate. Further, the excretion of urine containing relatively large amounts of sodium and chloride and relatively little bicarbonate contracts the extracellular fluid and results in a rise in plasma bicarbonate concentration. Alkalosis develops which then is propagated by chloruresis and subsequent chloride deficiency and which can be corrected only by a chloride-containing salt as discussed below (p. 349).

DIURETICS IN EDEMATOUS PATIENTS

Edematous patients receiving diuretics frequently develop a serious depletion of total body potassium, because of a high rate of secretion of aldosterone and enhanced reabsorption of sodium by the kidney. This situation most commonly occurs in patients with congestive heart failure, cirrhosis with ascites, or the nephrotic syndrome. Metabolic alkalosis is also very frequently present and in this instance, just as in the situation associated with hydrochloric acid loss from the stomach, it is impossible to correct the potassium deficiency without correction of the associated chloride deficiency (see p. 347). That may be done only by providing potassium chloride. Potassium deficiency in the edematous patient cannot be corrected by administration of potassium salt that does not contain chloride, such as gluconate or citrate.

MONITORING POTASSIUM IN PATIENTS RECEIVING DIURETICS

Before administration of oral diuretics, serum potassium should be measured. If it is normal, serum potassium should be measured approximately 1 month after the initiation of or increase in dose of the diuretic. Most of the occasional patients who tend to develop hypokalemia will have done so by this time. Subsequent to that initial follow-up, a yearly assessment is probably adequate in the nonedema-

tous patient unless other indications for measurement of serum potassium arise. In edematous patients with associated secondary hyperaldosteronism there is a greater stimulus for potassium depletion, and monitoring should be more frequent.

Table 42.2
Some Common Potassium-Rich Foods

Food Source	Average Portion	Potassium (meq)	Sodium (meq)
VEGETABLES			
Artichoke	1 large	22.0	3.7
Beans			
Cooked dried	½ cup	10.7	—
Lima	⅝ cup	10.8	—
Brussels sprouts	7 medium	7	—
Corn	1 ear	5.0	—
Potato			
White	1 boiled	7.3	—
Sweet	1 boiled	7.7	—
Tomato	1 medium	9.4	—
Fresh			
Canned	½ cup	5.6	3.3
Squash—winter	½ cup boiled	11.9	—
MEATS			
Hamburger	1 patty	9.8	1.7
Rib roast	2 slices	11.2	2.5
Fish, *e.g.* haddock	1 medium fillet	8.0	7.7
Clams	4 large	6.0	1.7
Oysters	6 medium	3.1	3.1
FRUITS			
Apple	1 medium	2.8	—
Applesauce	⅓ cup	1.7	—
Apricots	3 medium	7.2	—
Avocado	½ pitted	15.5	—
Banana	1–6 inch	9.5	—
Cantaloupe	¼ medium	6.4	—
Dates	10 pitted	16.6	—
Fruit cocktail	½ cup	4.3	—
Grapefruit	½ medium	3.5	—
Melon	¼ small	6.4	—
Orange	1 small	7.7	—
Peach	1 medium	5.2	—
Pear	1 medium	6.7	—
Plum	2 medium	7.7	—
Prunes, dried	10 medium	17.8	—
Raisins	1 tablespoon	2.0	—
Strawberries	10 large	4.2	—
Watermelon	1 slice	15.4	—
JUICE			
Grapefruit	1 cup	10.4	—
Orange	1 cup	12.4	—
Pineapple	1 cup	9.2	—
Prune	1 cup	15.0	—
Tomato	1 cup	13.7	20.9
Vegetable	1 cup	14.1	21.7
NUTS			
Peanuts—roasted	1 tablespoon	3.0	—
Peanut butter	2 tablespoons	2.0	—
Mixed nuts	3½ oz	2.0	—
MILK			
Buttermilk	8 oz	8.0	14
Skim milk	8 oz	8.5	6
Whole milk	8 oz	9.0	5

DIET AND POTASSIUM SUPPLEMENTS IN PATIENTS TAKING POTASSIUM-WASTING DIURETICS

Potassium deficiency, when it occurs in patients who are receiving diuretics, is a result of increased urinary loss of potassium. It occurs rarely in nonedematous patients as potassium is widely available in foods. A typical daily diet in the United States contains 60 to 100 meq of potassium. When initiating diuretic therapy in the presence or absence of edema, it is sensible for the practitioner to suggest that the patient ingest approximately 100 meq of potassium per day. There are a variety of foods relatively high in content of potassium (Table 42.2). Many have found it helpful to issue a patient, who has just been started on diuretics, a list of such foods to assure that the patient knows how to plan a 100 meq per day intake. The current admonishment to take diuretic tablets with a glass of orange juice (12 meq of potassium) or a banana (9 meq of potassium) is relatively insignificant dietary advice.

It has been estimated that nearly one-third of patients who take diuretics receive potassium supplements (3). For the most part, this is inappropriate and is associated with approximately a 6% incidence of toxicity from hyperkalemia and from gastrointestinal disturbances; moreover it is an unnecessary expense.

Supplementation with potassium salts is needed in less than 5% of patients who are receiving diuretics, and who are not edematous, unless there is an associated risk of toxicity from even slight degrees of potassium depletion. Predisposition to hypokalemic toxicity most commonly occurs in ambulatory practice in two situations. First, it occurs in patients who are simultaneously receiving digitalis. Slight degrees of potassium depletion may be associated with digitalis intoxication even when digitalis levels are in the nontoxic range. Second, toxicity from hypokalemia may occur in patients who have liver disease because of the development of hepatic encephalopathy. Other people at high risk are those that have problems that in themselves may be associated with potassium depletion such as malabsorption syndromes and exogenous or endogenous mineralocorticoid or glucocorticoid excess.

In the nonedematous patient who is not predisposed to toxicity, potassium supplements are not necessary, except in the occasional individual whose plasma potassium falls below 3.0 meq/L. In this instance a coexisting condition associated with excess loss of potassium should be suspected. When the potassium level is between 3 and 3.5 meq/L it is reasonable to prescribe potassium salts if the patient manifests any symptoms or signs suggestive of potassium deficiency. If the symptoms abate, then potassium supplement should be continued.

The practitioner is frequently faced with patients who having started on diuretics, complain of minor symptoms such as fatigue and muscular aches or weakness and who have a very slight fall in their potassium levels. Studies have failed to relate such symptoms to potassium deficiency. Potassium supplements are, however, often prescribed in this situation as a trial and discontinued if symptoms do not abate.

The volume depletion and loss of potassium that may complicate diuretic therapy often can be minimized or eliminated by using diuretics every other day. The regimen has value when the diuretics are administered for control of edema. Their effectiveness as antihypertensive agents requires that they be administered daily.

If prescription of potassium is indicated, a variety of potassium salts are available (Table 42.3). When potassium salts are given prophylactically as in the nonedematous patient who has some risk of potassium depletion any potassium salt may be prescribed selected on the basis of palatability and cost.

On the other hand, in the patient who has developed hypokalemia after taking diuretics, potassium supplementation must be provided by administration of potassium chloride. Volume contraction and chloride depletion with high aldosterone production increase avidity of the distal nephron for sodium so that there is increased excretion of potassium and hydrogen ions. The potassium deficiency cannot be corrected until the chloride depletion is corrected exactly analogous to the situation in which hypokalemia is associated with vomiting or nasogastric suction. Potassium chloride is available in 10 to 20% solutions.

In the 10% solution, each 15-ml dose contains 20 meq of potassium. The aim should be to administer 40 to 60 meq of potassium supplement per day. Potassium chloride is a relatively inexpensive medication with minimal side effects, except for hyperkalemia when it is inappropriately prescribed. Its palatability is its greatest limiting factor. Often, patients find potassium salts more tolerable when chilled and taken with tomato juice (100 ml contain 8 meq sodium).

Table 42.3
Commonly Available Potassium Salts

Source	Potassium Concentration
SOLUTIONS[a]	
Potassium chloride	
10%	20 meq/15 ml
15%	30 meq/15 ml
20%	40 meq/15 ml
Potassium citrate	30 meq/15 ml
Potassium gluconate	20 meq/15 ml
EFFERVESCENT GRANULES OR TABLETS	
Potassium chloride	20 meq/packet
TABLETS	
Potassium chloride in wax matrix	6, 7, and 8 meq/tablet
Potassium gluconate	5 meq/tablet

[a] Available with or without sugar and in different flavors. Taste generally improved by chilling.

Potassium chloride inbedded in wax matrix tablets (such as Slow-K) does not have the bad taste that limits the use of the liquid by many patients. Although more costly, it is safe and has only occasionally been reported to be associated with small intestinal ulceration and bleeding. In the past these latter complications occurred frequently with enteric coated potassium chloride tablets and led to their disuse.

In edematous patients potassium depletion is much more common than it is in patients without edema so that supplementation at the initiation of diuretic therapy is indicated.

After initiating the administration of potassium salts, the potassium level should be checked in 2 to 4 weeks and then, if normal, at 3-month intervals in the edematous patient and approximately at 6- to 12-month intervals in the nonedematous patient.

POTASSIUM-SPARING DIURETICS

If potassium salts are not effective in correcting the potassium depletion associated with the administration of potassium-wasting diuretics, then the addition of potassium-sparing diuretics such as spironolactone, triamterene, or amiloride is indicated. This situation mostly occurs in patients who have primary or secondary aldosteronism. The potassium-sparing agents prevent the distal tubular excretion of large quantities of potassium. The dose of each drug is adjusted according to the response of the serum potassium. Their maximum activity is generally seen 2 or 3 days after their initiation, so that dose adjustments can be made every 3 or 4 days until a dose is obtained which controls the serum potassium. Careful surveillance of the serum potassium, once stable, at approximately 4- to 12-week intervals, is important, to avoid the dangerous complication of hyperkalemia.

Less Common Causes of Hypokalemia

The less common causes of hypokalemia seen in ambulatory practice are dietary deficiency, excess urinary potassium loss due to one of a number of syndromes, and maldistribution of body potassium. The approach to diagnosing one of these mechanisms is based upon historical information, physical examination, urinary potassium levels, acid-base status, and activity of renin in the peripheral blood. An unexpected low serum potassium value should always be confirmed by repeat testing 2 or 3 times before initiating a further workup.

DEFICIENT POTASSIUM INTAKE

There is a wide distribution of potassium in foods. Therefore, it is unusual for dietary potassium deficiency to occur unless the patient fails to eat adequately for a prolonged interval. Alcoholic patients and patients with terminal malignancy may become hypokalemic in this manner. Also, if a patient is catabolic with an excess loss of tissue potassium, an unsupplemented diet may be relatively deficient in potassium. Dietary deficiency is established by history, clinical evidence of malnutrition, the absence of other obvious causes of hypokalemia, and correction of the deficiency with a balanced diet with or without potassium supplements. In such patients, the urinary output of potassium should be less than 10 to 20 meq per day when they are hypokalemic; there is usually an obligate loss of up to 15 meq per day.

EXCESSIVE LOSSES OF POTASSIUM IN URINE

An unexplained excessive loss of potassium in the urine (greater than 20 meq/L) is a diagnostic challenge encountered occasionally in ambulatory practice. The differential diagnosis in this situation is complex, but can be simplified by assessing the acid-base status of the patient as outlined in Table 42.4.

EXCESSIVE PRODUCTION OF MINERALOCORTICOID HORMONES

This complex problem underlies the majority of etiologies encountered in the hypokalemic patient who does not have a more common problem. It is

---

Table 42.4
Hypokalemia Secondary to Renal Loss

Determine that patient is not using a potassium-losing diuretic

Consider when there is no suggestion of dietary inadequacy or gastrointestinal symptoms suggesting potassium loss

Document by identifying a spot urine potassium concentration of greater than 20 meq/L or urine potassium excretion of greater than 20 meq/24 hr

Classify on the basis of the plasma bicarbonate concentration

HIGH BICARBONATE
Measure peripheral renin under proper conditions:

Low Renin	*High Renin*
1. Primary aldosteronism (occasional)	1. Secondary aldosteronism (common)
a. Adenoma	a. Associated with edema-forming state
b. Bilateral adrenal hyperplasia	b. Diuretic use associated with volume depletion
c. Congenital block	c. Renovascular hypertension
d. Exogenous hormone—gluco or mineralocorticoid	d. Accelerated hypertension
2. Licorice excess (rare)	e. Renin-excreting tumor
3. Liddle's syndrome (very rare)	2. Bartter's syndrome (rare)

LOW BICARBONATE
  Renal tubular acidosis (occasional)
  Diabetic ketoacidosis (common)
NORMAL BICARBONATE
  Magnesium deficiency (occasional)
  Osmotic diuresis (occasional)
  Leukemia (rare)

imperative in this situation to have the support of a laboratory experienced in hormonal measurement; otherwise definitive workup is impossible. Certain basic diagnoses may be made in an office, however, which may minimize the need for referral of patients to a center experienced in evaluation of abnormalities of aldosterone production.

Table 42.4 outlines the diagnostic possibilities related to the concentration of serum bicarbonate and of renin in the serum. Before approaching the diagnostic possibilities the practitioner needs to obtain an accurate history, identify normal or high blood pressure, and establish the presence or absence of edema.

It is mandatory to measure plasma renin under

Table 42.5
Drugs Known to Affect Peripheral Renin Activity[a]

DRUGS CAUSING AN INCREASE IN PERIPHERAL
      ACTIVITY:
  Alpha blockers
  Anesthetics
  Beta blockers
  Caffeine
  Chlorpromazine
  Converting enzyme inhibitors such as captopril
  Diuretics
  Estrogen[b]
  Glucagon
  Glucocorticoids[b]
  Mineralocorticoid antagonists
  Saralasin[c]
  Theophylline
  Vasodilators
    Hydralazine
    Minoxidil
    Diazoxide
    Nitroprusside
    Bupicomide
DRUGS CAUSING A DECREASE IN PERIPHERAL
      ACTIVITY:
  Alpha agonists
  Alpha-methyldopa
  Beta blockers
  Carbenoxalone
  Clonidine
  Ganglion blockers
  Labetalol
  Prazosine
  Prostaglandin inhibitors
    Aspirin
    Ibuprofen
    Indomethacin
  Reserpine
  Saralasin[c]
  Somatostatin
  Vasopressin

[a] Adapted from M. Schambelan and J. R. Stockigt: Pathophysiology of the renin-angiotensin system. In *Hormonal Function and the Kidney*, edited by B. M. Benner and J. H. Stein. Churchill Livingstone, New York, 1979.
[b] Effect is on renin substrate with resultant increased renin activity.
[c] Effect dependent on sodium status and renin level.

defined conditions of salt balance and position, and since many medications influence peripheral venous activity (Table 42.5), all such drugs should be discontinued for 2 weeks before the plasma renin is measured. Further, spironolactone is particularly potent, and has been documented to interfere with renin measurement for as long as 6 months after it has been discontinued (4).

A number of protocols have been developed to effect a mild stimulation of renin production to assess the true suppression that is characteristic of primary aldosteronism (Table 42.6). Hyperaldosteronism is suggested also by the failure to suppress aldosterone production after loading the patient with sodium chloride.

In physician's offices, protocols to measure renin are frequently not practical, but the peripheral plasma renin may be obtained if measured under proper conditions. A useful procedure for mild stimulation of renin production is outlined in Table 42.7.

If the peripheral renin is low, indicating suppression, further evaluation of a sophisticated nature is required to establish and to localize excess primary aldosterone or other corticoid hormone production. For this, referral to a center experienced in these measurements is suggested. If, on the other hand, a high peripheral renin is found, then secondary hyperaldosteronism is present.

Primary Hyperaldosteronism. The symptomatic findings of primary hyperaldosteronism—in addition to hypertension—are related to potassium depletion and occur only when such depletion is severe: weakness, paralysis, tetany, arrhythmias, polyuria, polydipsia. Patients with primary hyperaldosteronism almost always have spontaneous hypokalemia. Less than 10% have transiently normal levels of potassium; and these few patients will manifest hypokalemia, often profound, if potassium-wasting diuretics or large amounts of sodium chloride are administered. Both of these circumstances result in increased delivery of sodium to the distal nephron where, under the influence of excessive aldosterone, sodium is reabsorbed and potassium and hydrogen ions are excreted, resulting in hypokalemia and metabolic alkalosis.

Attempts to uncover patients with primary aldosteronism should be limited to situations in which—if the condition is found to be present—surgery would be undertaken. Such cases include young individuals (less than age 40) and those with hypertension that is not easily managed medically. It must be borne in mind, however, that most patients with primary aldosteronism can be treated with the aldosterone antagonist, spironolactone (Aldactone), or with spironolactone in combination with a diuretic (see below).

Initial screening for primary aldosteronism is best performed by careful determination of serum potassium on multiple (at least three) occasions. During these times the patient should not have received

Table 42.6
References for Protocols for Evaluation of Renin-Aldosterone Axis

First Author	Reference	Comment
Brunner, H. R., et al.	Circulation Research, 33 (suppl. 1), 1–99, 1973	Emphasizes moderate sodium restriction so urine excretion is < 100 meq/day
Wallach, K., et al.[a]	Annals of Internal Medicine, 82: 27–34, 1975	Renin activity stimulation with intravenous furosemide followed by 4-hr ambulation
Kowarski, A. A., et al.	Johns Hopkins Medical Journal, 142: 35–38, 1978	Measured 24-hr integrated concentration of aldosterone and renin. Emphasizes wide minute to minute swings of hormone and the importance of the aldosterone renin ratio
Brunner, H. R., et al.	New England Journal of Medicine, 286: 441–449, 1972	Emphasizes the effect of upright posture on renin activity and relates this to 24-hr sodium excretion
Kaplan, N. M., et al.	Annals of Internal Medicine, 84: 639–645, 1976	Short protocol with furosemide administration and 30 min upright posture

[a] Reference 5.

Table 42.7
Protocol for Mild Stimulation of Renin Production

1. Discontinue medications known to affect renin
2. No-added-salt diet for 1 week
    a. If there is doubt concerning dietary compliance, a 24-hr urine Na should confirm less than 100 meq excretion/24 hr[a]
3. On day of study:
    a. The patient should take furosemide (Lasix) 40 mg orally at 6–8 a.m.
    b. The patient may rest for 1–2 hr and then assume the upright posture (slow walking) for an additional 2–3 hr
    c. Collect the peripheral venous specimen in an EDTA tube while patient is standing
    d. The specimen should be quickly taken to the laboratory or chilled in the refrigerator (4–5°C) if there will be a delay before delivery to the laboratory (a delay beyond overnight should be avoided)
    e. In the laboratory the plasma is separated and frozen to −20°C until the assay can be performed

[a] Reference 2.

diuretics for at least 2 to 3 weeks and should not be ingesting a low sodium diet. If definite hypokalemia is shown to be present, plasma renin should then be measured. Plasma renin is suppressed in primary aldosteronism, but it is also low or undetectable in many normal persons. Suppressed renin is not demonstrated unless the value remains low following a stimulation test. Screening for suppressed renin is performed as outlined in Table 42.7. If hypokalemia and low renin coexist, further evaluation will include determination of urinary or plasma aldosterone. Referral to an endocrinologist or nephrologist with expertise in this area should be made at this point. The results of determinations of aldosterone under nonstandardized conditions (lack of control of sodium intake) are uninterpretable. Further, some commercial laboratories are unreliable.

When hypokalemia, suppressed renin, and aldosterone excess have been unequivocally established, localization procedures are undertaken by the consultant (selective arteriography; retrograde venography with selective venous sampling for aldosterone; adrenal scanning with radioiodine-labeled cholesterol). These procedures also serve to distinguish adenomas from nodular hyperplasia. Adenomas as small as 0.5 cm have been localized in this way, their excision has led to cure of hypertension. If evidence for bilateral nodular hyperplasia is found, surgery is usually not undertaken, since in such cases bilateral adrenalectomy is necessary, despite which most patients do not experience relief of hypertension. These patients are best managed medically. After obtaining a renin determination in the workup (see above), a trial of spironolactone (Aldactone) is useful with all patients. Large doses (400 to 600 mg daily) are necessary and several weeks may be needed for a response. Failure of spironolactone to normalize the blood pressure while normalizing the hypokalemia strongly suggests that—regardless of the anatomic basis for the aldosterone excess—surgery would not be curative of the hypertension. Such a situation is to be expected in nodular hyperplasia and in a minority of cases of solitary adenoma.

Secondary Hyperaldosteronism. Hypokalemia is often associated with secondary hyperaldosteronism. Secondary hyperaldosteronism is characterized by a large potassium deficiency with metabolic alkalosis, excess urinary potassium loss, and high peripheral renin.

Secondary hyperaldosteronism is most often seen in *edema-forming states* in patients with heart failure, cirrhosis, or nephrotic syndrome.

Accelerated hypertension is associated with hypokalemia and metabolic alkalosis in approximately 20% of patients, due to high renin production from the bilateral renal ischemia.

Fifteen percent of patients with *renal vascular hypertension* have hypokalemia. The hypokalemia is secondary to unilateral renal ischemia and high renin production with secondary hyperaldosteronism. Similarly, but rarely, *renin-secreting renal tumors* may result in hypokalemic metabolic alkalosis from renal potassium losses and are associated with a high peripheral renin and thereby a secondary high aldosterone concentration. These conditions will need to be considered in hypertensive patients when secondary hyperaldosteronism is felt to be the cause of hypokalemia after congestive heart failure, ascites, and nephrotic syndrome are ruled out.

Bartter's Syndrome. This rare disorder is characterized by marked elevation of production of aldosterone and renin with severe hypokalemic metabolic alkalosis and excess urinary potassium and chloride losses, but with normal blood pressure and absence of edema.

MALDISTRIBUTION OF POTASSIUM

Alkalosis is associated with a shift of potassium from extracellular fluid into cells. This shift occurs regardless of whether the alkalosis is induced on a metabolic or respiratory basis. It is not associated with severe total body potassium depletion but is nevertheless associated with sensitivity to digitalis. *Hypokalemic periodic paralysis* is a rare disorder characterized by episodes of paralysis precipitated by a variety of stimuli including the administration of insulin, glucose, or ACTH. Although a fall in serum potassium is regularly demonstrated during the paralysis, balance studies indicate an increase in total body potassium, implying a shift of potassium from extracelluar to intracellular fluid.

Vitamin B_{12}, when administered initially in the therapy of anemia due to vitamin B_{12} deficiency, may cause severe shifts of potassium as metabolic activity is increased in platelets and red blood cell precursors. When unrecognized and untreated, fatal hypokalemia has been demonstrated in this setting. Careful observation of serum potassium in this situation will alert the practitioner to appropriate therapy.

Soluble barium salts. (carbonate, chloride, hydroxide, nitrate, acetate, sulfide) are associated with hypokalemia by creating a maldistribution of potassium. This is extraordinarily rare, but occurs episodically with poisoning from some rodenticides, depilatories, and fireworks. Epidemics secondary to barium chloride contamination of table salt have occurred in two recorded instances. Barium sulfate is not soluble and is not a cause of hypokalemia.

References

General

BM Brenner, and Stein, JH (eds): *Acid-Base and Potassium Homeostasis*. Churchill Livingstone, New York, 1978.
   Provides a well referenced update on disorders of potassium metabolism.
Kassirer, JP and Harrington, JT: Diuretics and potassium metabolism: a reassessment of the need, effectiveness and safety of potassium therapy. *Kidney Int* 11: 505, 1977.
   A scholarly, thoroughly referenced, overview of potassium balance in diuretic therapy.
Nardone, DA, McDonald, WJ and Girard, DE: Mechanisms in hypokalemia: clinical correlation. *Medicine* 57: 435, 1978.
   This paper presents a logical approach to the diagnosis of hypokalemia based on the site of potassium loss and the associated acid-base status.
Schultze, RG: Potassium metabolism. In *Current Nephrology, Vol. 3*, pp. 41–62, edited by HC Gonick. Houghton Mifflin, Boston, 1979.
   An extensively referenced update covering many aspects of potassium metabolism.
Streeten, DHP, Tomycz, N and Anderson GH: Reliability of screening methods for the diagnosis of primary aldosteronism. *Am J Med* 67: 403, 1979.
   Reviews the methods for screening for primary aldosteronism in 1036 consecutive referred hypertension patients.

Specific

1. Aronson, JK, Grahame-Smith, DG and Wigley, FM: Monitoring digoxin therapy: the use of plasma digoxin concentration measurements in the diagnosis of digoxin toxicity. *Q J Med* 47: 111, 1978.
2. Laragh, JH, Baer, L, Brunner, HR, Buhler, FR, Sealey, JE and Vaughan, Jr, ED: Renin angiotensin and aldosterone system in pathogenesis and management of hypertensive vascular disease. *Am J Med* 52: 633, 1972.
3. Lawson, DH: Adverse reactions to potassium chloride. *Q J Med* 43: 433, 1974.
4. Lowder, SE and Liddle, GW: Prolonged alteration of renin responsiveness after spironolactone therapy. *N Engl J Med* 291: 1243, 1974.
5. Wallach, L, Nyarai, I and Dawson, KG: Stimulated renin: a screening test for hypertension. *Ann Intern Med* 82: 27, 1975.

CHAPTER FORTY-THREE

Urinary Stones

JAMES K. SMOLEV, M.D., and JOHN R. BURTON, M.D.

Urinary stones are very common in the United States, affecting up to 6% of the population. The physician will encounter such patients frequently and will therefore need to be familiar with the evaluation and management of this common problem. Although urologic intervention or nephrologic consultation may occasionally be required, the vast majority of patients with stones can be evaluated, treated, and followed by the primary care physician. This chapter will review the various manifestations of stone disease; the types of urinary stones; the evaluation of patients with stones; the acute and chronic management of patients with urinary stones and finally, when to obtain consultation in these patients.

PRESENTATION OF URINARY STONE DISEASE

Physicians will encounter patients who have urinary stone disease in one of five clinical settings: (a) in a patient with acute colic, (b) a patient with persistent or recurrent urinary tract infection, (c) a patient with isolated hematuria, (d) a patient with no symptoms in whom a stone is discovered incidentally on an X-ray taken for other purposes, or (e) a patient who gives a history of having had a stone.

Acute Colic

PRESENTATION

Most patients with urinary stones will have at some time an acute episode of colic. The stone, if obstructing, causes ureteral spasm resulting in severe intermittent pain. The location of the pain depends on the location of the stone in the ureter but is most often felt in the flank; and then as the stone moves distally, pain radiates in a characteristic pattern around the groin and into the testicles in the male or the labia majora in the female. Nausea, vomiting, paralytic ileus, and other gastrointestinal symptoms which often suggest a primary gastrointestinal problem may be associated with pain. Examination reveals a uncomfortable, restless patient. There may be costovertebral tenderness as well as deep tenderness in the abdomen. More important, there are no signs of peritoneal irritation present (guarding, rebound, or rigidity). Fever is not present unless urinary tract infection has developed in the obstructed urinary tract.

Urinalysis almost always demonstrates microscopic (or gross) hematuria. The presence of pyuria is important since chronic bacterial infection may be associated with the development of urinary stones; however, pyuria may be absent even if infection is present during complete ureteral obstruction.

MANAGEMENT

The aim of management of a patient with colic should be (a) relief of discomfort, (b) surveillance for infection, and (c) determination whether stones will pass spontaneously or will require surgical removal. The abdominal X-ray is useful in monitoring the site and progression of the stone. Approximately 90% of renal stones are radiodense and will be seen on a good quality X-ray. The size and position of the stone will help decide the urgency of subsequent studies such as an intravenous pyelogram. In general, stones that are less than 5 mm will pass spontaneously; those between 5 and 10 mm have a 50% chance of passing spontaneously; and those greater than 10 mm usually require surgical removal. The common sites where stones become lodged are (a) the renal calyx, (b) the ureteral pelvic junction, (c) in the ureter at the pelvic brim where the ureter begins to pass over the iliac vessels, (d) in the lower third of the ureter, and (e) at the ureterovesical junction. If there is doubt about whether calcification seen on the plain X-ray is within the urinary tract, an oblique view may help. It is also important to review old abdominal films taken for any reason to see if a stone was present at that time. An intravenous pyelogram should also be obtained as soon as possible in the patient with colic, as it will help establish the diagnosis especially in patients with radiolucent stones and it will provide certain important information (see below) that will aid in management.

Several factors will help the physician decide whether to hospitalize a patient with renal colic, to obtain urgent urologic consultation, or to manage the patient at home. First, the patient with nausea and vomiting cannot be assured of an adequate fluid intake or of adequate oral analgesic and should be admitted to a hospital. Second, fever suggests infection proximal to an obstructing stone and urgent urologic consultation should be obtained. Third, if an intravenous pyelogram (IVP) reveals any of the following findings, urgent urologic consultation should be obtained: (a) a nonfunctioning kidney (completely obstructed ureter), (b) a partially obstructed ureter from a solitary kidney, and (c) urine extravasation. Fourth, if the stone is greater than 10 mm, spontaneous passage is very unlikely and urologic consultation should be obtained.

Most patients can be managed at home by the general physician. Forced hydration of 2 to 3 liters of fluid per 24 hours is necessary to maintain a good urinary flow and help in moving the stone. When the patient is voiding, all of the urine should be strained through an old stocking or a filter so that the passed stone may be saved and analyzed. It is important to prescribe analgesic medication such as meperidene (Demerol) 50 to 100 mg every 4 to 6 hours to control the discomfort. A phenothiazine (e.g., Phenergan 25 mg) given with the Demerol will provide additional relief. The patient should be instructed to contact his physician should fever, intractable pain, or vomiting develop. The physician will want to follow the patient by arranging for a weekly X-ray of the abdomen to determine the progression of the stone. If by 6 weeks the stone has not passed it is unlikely that spontaneous passage will occur and urologic consultation should be obtained. Because of the demands of their occupation or social reasons, some patients will want to consider surgical removal of the stone earlier, and therefore request urologic consultation sooner.

Stones which pass from the ureter into the bladder generally pass with ease through the urethra. In the event of a bladder outlet obstruction, a stone may be retained in the bladder (bladder stone) where it may grow and in time become an infection stone.

An occasional patient who has acute ureteral colic will give a history of allergy to radiologic dye. In this instance, an ultrasound study of the collecting system of the kidney may help in deciding about the presence of obstruction or the presence of a solitary kidney. If this is unavailable, then urologic consultation should be obtained so that either an antegrade or retrograde pyelogram can be considered. These methods are also available for individuals who have given a history of allergy to IVP dye. It is important for the physician to recognize that occasionally a patient with a history strongly suggestive of renal colic may have another cause for the pain. A dissection of the aorta, acute back strain or lumbar disc disease, the passage of blood clots in the ureters as in sickle cell disease or renal infarct, as well as malingering should be considered. A malingerer will give a classic history of acute renal colic to a physician seen for the first time and will also relate a history of allergy to IVP dye. Often these patients will have blood (obtained from a fingerstick or oral injury) in the urine specimen they give to the physician.

When a patient is referred to a urologist for stone removal, there are several options. Lower ureteral stones may be removed using a basket which is inserted through a cystoscope. This procedure is very similar to cystoscopic examination but requires general or spinal anesthesia and hospitalization. Stones located more proximally may require removal by open ureterolithotomy, open pyelolithotomy or, in the case of a staghorn calculus, nephrolithotomy. These techniques all require hospitalization and are performed under general anesthesia.

Other Patterns of Stone Presentation

Urinary stones usually produce symptoms that suggest acute colic, at least at some time in their course. If stones are discovered in patients who do not have colic (see p. 354), they demand the same evaluation and management (see below) as does the patient who has passed a stone after acute colic.

TYPES OF STONES AND THEIR CAUSES

There are four main types of urinary calculi: (a) calcium, oxalate or phosphate, (b) uric acid, (c) struvite—triple phosphate—(magnesium, ammonium phosphate), and (d) cystine. Calcium stones are by far the most common. Table 43.1 shows the classification of stone-forming patients by the type of stone passed.

It is important for the clinician caring for a patient with stone disease to be familiar with the metabolic associations these patients may have. This understanding will be helpful in planning a diagnostic evaluation and specific therapy (see below). This is particularly true in the most prevalent stone type—calcium.

Calcium Stones

Table 43.2 shows the metabolic and clinical disorders in calcium stone formers. This table shows that in almost 80% of patients who have had a calcium

Table 43.1
Classification of Stone-forming Patient by Type of Stone Passed[a]

	Coe Series 519 Patients	Combined Series 1870 Patients
Calcium oxalate (with or without phosphate)	88.6[b]	63.2[b]
Calcium phosphate	2.1	7.4
Calcium and uric acid	4.2	—
Uric acid	1.5	5.4
Cystine	0.6	2.5
Struvite	3.0	21.5

[a] From F. L. Coe: *Nephrolithiasis Pathogenesis and Treatment*, Year Book Medical Publishers, Inc., Chicago, 1978.
[b] All values expressed as percentages of patients in each category.

Table 43.2
Metabolic and Clinical Disorders in 460 Consecutive Calcium Stone Formers[a]

	No. of Patients	(%)
Idiopathic hypercalciuria	95	(20.7)
Marginal hypercalciuria[b]	53	(11.5)
Hyperuricosuria[c]	67	(14.6)
Hypercalciuria and Hyperuricosuria[d]	54	(11.7)
Hyperuricemia	26	(5.7)
Primary hyperparathyroidism	24	(5.2)
Renal tubular acidosis[e]	17	(3.7)
Inflammatory bowel disease[f]	21	(4.6)
Medullary sponge kidney	7	(1.5)
Sarcoidosis	3	(0.7)
No disorder found	93	(20.2)
Total	460	

[a] From F. L. Coe: *Nephrolithiasis Pathogenesis and Treatment*, Year Book Medical Publishers, Inc., Chicago, 1978.
[b] Urine calcium > 140 mg/g creatinine but less than in hypercalciuria (250 mg/24 hr in women and 300 mg/24 hr in men).
[c] Urine uric acid above 800 mg (men) and 750 mg (women), in at least one of two 24-hr urine collections.
[d] Marginal hypercalciuria not included.
[e] Distal, hereditary form.
[f] Regional enteritis, ulcerative colitis, granulomatous ileocolitis.

stone the cause is known. The approach to these disorders is discussed below.

Uric Acid Stone

Uric acid stones are caused by the high insolubility of undissociated uric acid (pK of 5.7—i.e., 50% of uric acid undissociated at pH 5.7, 90% is undissociated at pH 4.7). Three factors are associated with uric acid stone formation: (a) hyperuricosuria, (b) highly acid urine, and (c) low urinary volume. The prevalence of uric acid stones in the general population is very low (Table 43.3). On the other hand, uric acid stones are very prevalent in patients who have gout, asymptomatic hyperuricemia, or hyperuricosuria. Many patients will have passed uric acid stones long before a

gouty attack has occurred. It is known that many patients with gout produce an abnormally high fraction of their daily acid load as titratable acid rather than as ammonium and therefore have an unusually low average urinary pH. Further, patients with chronic diarrhea, or patients with excessive fluid loss from the skin may have highly concentrated urine which will predispose to uric acid calculus formation. Patients who have myeloproliferative disease and those that have solid tumors that are undergoing lysis may have excessive uric acid excretion, which may be associated with uric acid stones and tubular plugs of urate. Patients with gout also have more calcium stones than the general population (11). The association may result from crystallization of uric acid which then forms a nidus for calcium deposition.

Struvite Stones (Infection Stones)

It is generally believed that infection stones form primarily as a consequence of the hydrolysis of urea and the production of ammonia by the bacterial enzyme urease. The production of ammonia leads to a highly alkaline urine which promotes the precipitation of magnesium, ammonium, and phosphate. These are the components of the infection-induced or struvite stone. The majority of urea-splitting organisms are of the *Proteus* species; however, *Pseudomonas*, *Klebsiella*, *Staphylococcus* and some *Escherichia coli* strains are capable of producing urease. Struvite stones do not form *de novo* but almost always are a complication of another primary stone disease where infection has become superimposed,

Table 43.3
Prevalence of Uric Acid Stones in Various Populations

Population	Prevalence (%)
General population	0.01
Patients with gout	22
Hyperuricemia in men[a]:	
7–8 mg/dl	12.7
8–9 mg/dl	22
> 9 mg/dl	40
Hyperuricosuria in primary gout[b]:	
< 300 mg/24 hr	11
300–699 mg/24 hr	21
700–1100 mg/24 hr	35
> 1100 mg/24 hr	50

[a] A. P. Hall, P. E. Barry, T. R. Dawber, and P. M. McNamarea: Epidemiology of gout and hyperuricemia. *American Journal of Medicine*, 42: 27, 1967.
[b] T. Yü and A. B. Gutman: Uric acid nephrolithiasis in gout. *Annals of Internal Medicine*, 67: 1133, 1967.

Table 43.4
Urinary Cystine Excretion

Normal individuals	< 100 mg
Heterozygotes for cystinuria	150–300 mg
Homozygotes for cystinuria	> 600 mg

and especially are likely to grow into *staghorn calculi* (large stones which cannot pass the uretopelvic junction and which form a cast of all or a portion of the pelvicocalyceal system).

Cystine Stones

Cystine stones are the least common type of urinary calculi, and the general physician will encounter this problem only rarely and then most likely in young patients. The stone forms because of crystallization of cystine when the urine is supersaturated with this substance, which occurs when there is a defect in renal tubular reabsorption of filtered cystine. This is a particularly virulent form of stone disease and may be associated with staghorn calculi. In addition to cystinuria, there is usually urinary loss of other basic amino acids including ornithine, lysine, and arginine. The disorder is an inherited autosomal recessive trait although some heterozygous patients have excess cystine excretion as is shown in Table 43.4. Cystine is much less soluble in acid urine than it is in alkaline urine, and cystine stones generally, therefore, will form when urine is acid and cystine excretion is greater than 400 mg per 24 hours.

NATURAL HISTORY OF URINARY STONE DISEASE

Urinary calculus disease is a chronic illness. Once a stone has formed, there is a tendency for recurrence and management (see below) will be tailored to the stone activity, the type of stone, and any associated metabolic abnormality.

Stone activity—the number of stones formed and the change in size of existing stones—is an important, although at times difficult, determination to be made. It requires a yearly review of stones passed and removed, as well as an evaluation by abdominal X-ray of increase in size of known stones or the appearance of new stones. The activity of urinary calculi depends on a number of factors: stone type, associated metabolic abnormality, treatment received (both specific and nonspecific), and age. Precise rates of recurrence therefore cannot be given with real accuracy.

Since calcium stone formers make up the largest population of patients with stones, there is more information about recurrences in this group. In solitary calcium stone formers (history of passing a single stone) there is a recurrence in half of the patients by 5 years and in two-thirds of the patients within 9 years, with a peak recurrence at about 2 years and a second smaller peak at 8 years after passage of the initial stone (Fig. 43.1).

Because of this high recurrence rate it is suggested that evaluation for associated metabolic abnormalities be undertaken in each patient who has formed a calcium stone. Also since approximately 80% of stones are calcium, an evaluation is suggested if the stone type is unknown. If a passed stone is known to

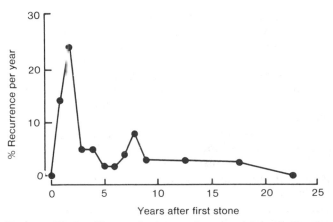

Figure 43.1   Rate of stone recurrence in patients who have formed a single calcium stone. (From F. L. Coe: *Nephrolithiasis Pathogenesis and Treatment*, Year Book Medical Publishers, Inc., Chicago, 1978.)

be uric acid, struvite, or cystine, recurrence is also likely and a metabolic evaluation should be undertaken; and since calcium stones may be mixed with these types, the evaluation should be comprehensive.

DIAGNOSTIC WORKUP OF PATIENTS WITH URINARY STONE DISEASE

Evaluation of patients with stone disease can be accomplished entirely in an ambulatory setting. This evaluation depends on history, physical examination, and certain laboratory measurements.

History

A history is important in determining the activity of stone disease (see above) as well as in providing clues to the nature of the stone. *Family history* may provide a clue to cystine stones, uric acid stones (gout), and some calcium stones (*e.g.*, those associated with renal tubular acidosis). *Dietary history* may reveal a gluttony of calcium, purine, and/or oxalate (see below). The *eating habits* are important. For example, if a patient takes only one large meal a day, there may be a sudden wave of uric acid that requires excretion in a highly acid urine resulting in predisposition to uric acid calculi. High protein meat diets may be associated with excess ingestion and excretion of acid and thereby may be connected with stone disease. An approximate daily fluid intake is also an important part of the history. Some individuals may ingest as little as 500 to 700 ml per day and thus have concentrated urine most of the day. *Medication history* is important. For example, aspirin in high doses (more than 5 g/day, especially if the urine is also alkaline) and probenecid are associated with increased uric acid excretion and may be a predisposition to uric acid calculi. Further, calcium-containing antacids (*e.g.*, Camalox, Bisodol, Titralac, or Tums) as well as vitamin D may be associated with hypercalciuria and calcium stone formation. Acetazolamide (Diamox) may be associated with development of chronically alkaline urine and a higher incidence of calcium calculi. Triamterene and its metabolites have been found in urinary calculi and may be the only ingredient. For this reason, a history of the use of triamterene preparations (Dyazide or Dyrenium) should be sought (5) and its use discontinued in patients with a history of urinary calculus. Moreover, certain medications such as thiazides or allopurinol will interfere with calcium and uric acid excretion, respectively, and interfere with results of testing in a patient who is being evaluated for renal stone disease. *Occupational history* is important in that the environmental temperature (and therefore fluid losses) and/or the accessibility to fluids are factors influencing stone formation by promoting decreased output of highly concentrated urine.

Physical Examination

Physical examination (when there is no colic) occasionally will give clues to specific problems. For example, band keratopathy may be seen in hyperparathyroidism, or there may be signs of sarcoidosis, hyperthyroidism, inflammatory bowel disease, neoplasia, or gouty arthritis. Most often, however, the examination is normal.

Urinalysis

The urinalysis provides a simple assessment that may give specific direction to the determination of the cause of the urinary calculus. It is important that urinalysis is complete, including the determination of pH. The pH is usually acid in patients with a uric acid or a cystine stone and is invariably alkaline in patients with struvite stones. The pH may suggest the presence of renal tubular acidosis (RTA). The first voided morning urine is usually acid, so that finding a urine pH > 6.0 in this specimen suggests the possibility of RTA. The microscopic analysis may show crystals or evidence of infection. Crystals of cystine have the appearance of a benzene ring and are highly suggestive of cystinuria. Other crystals are more variable and are not diagnostic. Oxalate crystals appear in urine normally and their identification should not suggest a disorder.

Stone Analysis

If a stone is available it should be analyzed as the stone type will determine the approach to evaluation and treatment. Stones can be analyzed inexpensively at commercial laboratories and stones may be mailed without preservative for this purpose.

Laboratory Assessment (Table 43.5)

A thorough laboratory analysis as described in this section is important even in patients where a stone has been available for analysis. This evaluation is necessary because there are many causes of stone formation: for example, struvite stones often start as

Table 43.5
Laboratory Assessment of Patients with Urinary Calculi[a]

Measurement	Day of Testing			
	1	2	3	4
24-hr urinary volume	√	√	√	√
24-hr urinary calcium[b]	√			√
24-hr urinary uric acid[c]		√	√	
24-hr urinary creatinine	√			√
Urinalysis	√			
Urine cystine screen	√			
Urine culture (if pyuria)	√			
Urine pH (taken on first voided morning specimen collected under mineral oil)	√			
Serum calcium	√			
Serum phosphorus	√			
Serum uric acid	√			
Serum chloride	√			
Serum bicarbonate	√			
Serum creatinine	√			
Serum urea nitrogen	√			

[a] During evaluation patient should follow their usual diet and life habits except on day 4 (second urinary calcium determination) when a 1-g calcium intake should be ensured (see text p. 359).
[b] The 24-hr urine container should contain 15 ml of concentrated HCl (with warning to avoid contact).
[c] The 24-hr urine container should contain a few crystals of thymol to retard bacterial overgrowth.

some other primary stone type—most often calcium; and patients with pure uric acid or cystine stones occasionally have other stone types as well. Patients will usually comply with the testing necessary for proper evaluation of a metabolic disorder if they understand the relative ease with which it may be accomplished, the high rate of recurrent calculi, and the importance of specific therapy for different metabolic problems (see below).

Laboratory assessment of patients who have formed urinary calculi is relatively simple and noninvasive and can be easily performed in the office. It is important that this initial evaluation be accomplished *without* the patient modifying his diet or habits so that an underlying process associated with urinary calculus disease will not be masked.

An *intravenous pyelogram* if not done previously as part of the evaluation of an episode of acute colic should be done in an attempt to search for underlying structural disease (such as anatomic abnormality of the lower tract or medullary sponge kidney).

In addition to the laboratory assessment outlined in Table 43.5, *parathyroid hormone* should be determined if hypercalcemia and hypercalciuria are documented and if other causes of hypercalcemia are ruled out (see Chapter 71). *Oxalate* should also be determined when hyperoxaluria is expected clinically (Table 43.6), although oxalate determination is

Table 43.6
Situations Where Hyperoxaluria May Be Expected

Hereditary overproduction—unusually virulent stone disease with frequent recurrences and nephrocalcinosis often occurring before age 12 years
Methoxyflurane anesthesia—immediately following
Ethylene glycol ingestion—immediately following
Chronic inflammatory bowel disease, ileal resection, or small bowel bypass
Cellulose phosphate ingestion—during entire period of ingestion
Oxalate gluttony (tea, spinach, rhubarb).

Table 43.7
Causes of Hypercalciuria That May Not Be Associated with Hypercalcemia

Idiopathic hypercalciuria
Furosemide and ethacrynic acid administration
Excessive salt ingestion
Exogenous adrenal corticosteroids
Cushing's syndrome
Paget's disease of bone
Immobilization
Progressive bone disease
Malignant tumors
Hyperthyroidism
Sarcoidosis
Renal tubular acidosis
Other causes of metabolic acidosis
Medullary sponge kidney
Severe phosphate deprivation

not always a reliable analysis and hyperoxaluria is uncommon; therefore, it is not a routinely performed measurement.

HYPERCALCIURIA

While calcium excretion varies somewhat with intake of calcium and of protein, generally the upper limits of calcium excretion for individuals eating a normal diet are 250 mg/24 hours for women and 300 mg/24 hours for men. Patients with hypercalciuria without hypercalcemia deserve special attention because they are seen quite commonly and because of the variable pathogenesis of their stones. Table 43.7 lists the causes of hypercalciuria that may be unassociated with hypercalcemia.

Most patients will have idiopathic hypercalciuria either from a *renal leak* (renal hypercalciuria) or *excessive gastrointestinal absorption* (absorptive hypercalciuria) of calcium. In the latter, which occurs more commonly, there is excess gastrointestinal absorption (and then excretion) of calcium after the ingestion of calcium. The differentiation of renal from absorptive hypercalciuria requires the use of an *oral calcium tolerance test* (1, 7) which, because of its complexity, is not routinely recommended in an office practice. However, it is important to be aware

that some patients with absorptive hypercalciuria may have normal calcium excretion if they inadvertently restrict their calcium intake on the day of the urine collection. Therefore, it is advantageous to ensure the patient has at least 1-g intake of calcium on the 4th day of urine collection (second urine calcium determination)—Table 43.5. This calcium intake may be ensured by having the patient drink 1 quart of whole milk (approximately 250 mg of calcium per 8 ounces) or, if milk is not tolerated, calcium glubionate (Neo-Calglucon Syrup, available from a pharmacy without a prescription), 1 tablespoon 3 times a day (345 mg of calcium per tablespoon). Some patients with hypercalciuria, especially the absorptive type, will benefit by restriction of calcium in the diet (see below).

PREVENTIVE TREATMENT OF URINARY CALCULUS DISEASE

General Measures

It is important to educate patients who have formed stones about the nature of urinary calculi, their natural history, the importance of regular surveillance, and the effectiveness of therapy.

DIET

Specific diet restriction is discussed under the various stone types (see below).

FLUID INTAKE

Regardless of the type of stone that has been formed, a patient should maintain a high intake of fluids to ensure a urinary output of 3 to 4 liters per day. This high urinary output prevents supersaturation of urine by material which may form calculi and the high flow rate may wash out small crystalline formations before they produce any obstructive symptoms.

Patients with recurrent stone disease require a high fluid intake throughout the day and night (8). This can be accomplished by having the individual drink 3 liters through the day and then take 1 or 2 glasses of water before retiring. This should result in a nocturnal diuresis necessitating voiding 3 to 4 hours later at which time a further ingestion of 1 or 2 glasses of water will continue the diuresis until morning. Although annoying to the patient, once the habit is formed it is a small nuisance compared to the benefit of preventing subsequent stone formation.

HABITS

Patients should be counseled to avoid dehydration and consequently concentrated urine when participating in sports, during travel, or at work.

Specific Therapy for Hypercalciuria

Hypercalciuria is the most frequent disorder uncovered during the evaluation of patients with urinary calculus disease. In addition to the general measures described above there are several specific therapies.

The decision, however, to use specific therapy (especially pharmacologic therapy) must be made on an individual basis. The rate of stone recurrence for a large population of patients may not apply to an individual patient. It is prudent to use only general therapeutic measures until there is an increase in stone activity. At this time a decision should be made about adding such specific therapy as might be appropriate from the workup.

RESTRICTED CALCIUM DIET

This is suggested in the patient who has been found to have hypercalciuria. A severely calcium-restricted diet is not generally advocated and may have limitations because of the induction of chronic negative calcium balance and its potential for subsequent bone disease. Generally a calcium-restricted diet is obtained by limiting intake of milk and milk products, in which case the calcium intake may fall from 1500 to 2000 mg to 400 to 700 mg/24 hours.

THIAZIDE DIURETICS (10)

Thiazide administration has been shown to cause a fall in urinary calcium excretion by as much as 50–60%. It also increases (by action on the tubular transport mechanism) magnesium and zinc excretion, which may be important in the inhibition of calcium crystallization. Thiazides are useful in the treatment of many types of calcium stone formers and are an ideal choice in the treatment of renal hypercalciuria. Thiazides should be administered in a dose equivalent to hydrochlorothiazide, 50 mg twice a day.

ORTHOPHOSPHATE (INORGANIC PHOSPHATE) (4)

The use of inorganic phosphate is still controversial. Its method of action may be to decrease calcium absorption directly by forming unabsorbable complexes in the gastrointestinal tract (therefore making it apparently ideal for treatment of patients with absorptive hypercalciuria), but also to some extent by increasing plasma phosphate. This, in turn, leads to a fall in the ionized calcium, resulting in increased parathyroid hormone production, a subsequent fall in the glomerular filtration rate, and an increase in renal tubular calcium absorption. Further, the increased plasma phosphate may inhibit the renal production of 1,25-dihydroxyvitamin D_3, a substance which increases calcium absorption. Increased phosphate absorption may also decrease stone formation by increasing urinary pyrophosphate which inhibits crystal formation.

There are risks associated with using orthophosphates. The excess stimulation of parathyroid hormone could result in bone disease and increase in plasma phosphate concentration could lead to renal disease. Further, many patients have had intolerable diarrhea, nausea, or vomiting. The inorganic phosphate salts are prescribed primarily as a mixture of sodium and potassium phosphate (e.g., K-Phos) 1 g 4 times a day. The administration of these agents however is not recommended without at least a telephone consultation with a nephrologist or urologist.

CELLULOSE PHOSPHATE (6)

This an ion exchange resin which is frequently described in the medical literature, but is not available in this country, presumably because it has not been considered to be sufficiently marketable. It is available in other countries. It is administered with meals (5 to 10 g, 3 times a day). Its use is especially promulgated for the treatment of absorptive hypercalciuria because it increases the fecal excretion of calcium by binding dietary calcium and also by binding calcium that has been secreted by the gastrointestinal tract. The decreased absorption of calcium by the bowel results in a fall in urinary calcium excretion with an associated increase in urinary phosphate excretion. This agent may result in chronic negative calcium balance and subsequent bone disease. Its use, because of the quantity required, may be unacceptable to many patients and it frequently causes unacceptable diarrhea and/or occasional offensive stools.

Patients with Calcium and Uric Acid Stones Who Are Found to Have Hyperuricosuria

If purine gluttony is present hyperuricosuria can be modified by dietary restriction of purine-rich food such as liver, kidney, and fish roe. Gluttony, however, is not often the problem, and other means are necessary.

Uric acid stone formation can be markedly modified by increasing the urinary pH. Figure 43.2 shows the dissociation curve of uric acid, and it can be seen that increasing the pH of the urine from 4.5 to 5.5 or 6.5 increases uric acid dissociation, resulting in an

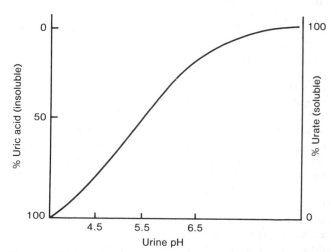

Figure 43.2 Dissociation curve of uric acid over physiologic range of urine pH.

increase from 15% to 40% and 80% dissociation, respectively. This alkalinization can be accomplished by the administration of sodium bicarbonate several times a day. However, because sodium bicarbonate frequently causes gas and gastrointestinal discomfort, citrate salts (Polycitra, 15 ml, 4 times a day) is more palatable, and therefore preferable. The metabolism of citrate results in the generation of bicarbonate. During the initial week of treatment and periodically thereafter, the patient should be taught to measure his urinary pH several times a day to ensure proper alkalinization (urine pH > 6.0). If either citrate or bicarbonate is not practical, the urine pH may be increased by using acetazolamide (Diamox), 250 to 500 g, 4 times a day.

Should these agents not be effective in controlling recurrence of uric acid stones, if the urine pH cannot be kept above 6, or if uric acid excretion is above 650 mg, allopurinol (which decreases uric acid production) may be used. Allopurinol (Zyloprim) should be initiated at a dose of 200 mg once a day and raised to a level that controls uric acid excretion to below 500 or 600 mg/24 hours (doses greater than 300 mg are divided in two daily doses). Complications from allopurinol are common. Although usually minor, including minor skin rash, drug fever, or precipitation of an acute gouty attack, the drug should be discontinued whenever a skin rash or fever occurs because diffuse fatal systemic vasculitis has been reported. Allopurinol also has been reported to be associated, although rarely, with the acceleration of cataract formation, with cholestatic hepatitis, and with leukopenia. The use of allopurinol is especially important as a preventive measure in patients who have excess uric acid excretion because of a myeloproliferative disease or in anticipation of tumor lysis.

Hyperoxaluria

In this group of patients the aim is to lower oxalate excretion. Treatment depends to some extent on the cause of the hyperoxyluria and frequently a telephone consultation with a nephrologist may be helpful in managing a patient with this complex problem. The consultant may consider the use of cholestyramine in the dose of 8 to 16 g per day, in adddtion to increased calcium supplementation and a low oxalate diet. In patients who have had ileal resection, when hyperoxaluria is associated with pyridoxine deficiency, the use of this vitamin (150 to 400 mg every 24 hours) may provide benefit.

Cystinuria

This group of stone formers generally have particularly virulent disease and are best managed in consultation with a nephrologist. Generally it is necessary to raise urinary pH in a manner similar to the method used in patients with uric acid stones (see above) and, if stone activity continues, to use d-penicillamine, which forms complexes with cystine and prevents its precipitation.

Struvite or Infection Stones

Infection stones are particularly virulent. Untreated patients with infected staghorn calculi frequently develop sepsis and require urgent nephrectomy. Further, when the disease is bilateral there is an associated 25% mortality rate in 5 years (9). In view of this morbidity and with the recent advance in surgical techniques for controlling infection stones, early urological referral is suggested. The goal of surgery in such patients is to remove the stone totally. This may be done by a variety of surgical approaches. The operative mortality for these procedures in skilled hands is less than 1%. Application of hypothermia combined with a technique permitting the kidney to be bivalved has permitted great success in total stone removal with preservation of renal function. There is however still a relatively high recurrence rate. In another treatment the stone may be perfused and dissolved by an acid solution (Renacidin) using a percutaneous catheter placed antegrade into the pelvis of the kidney (3).

In addition to the surgical treatment of stone disease, medical therapy is an important adjunct. Associated metabolic abnormalities should be sought and treated. Specific antimicrobial therapy is necessary in conjunction with surgery and, where stones cannot be removed surgically, suppressive therapy with antimicrobials may decrease the incidence of septicemia. Experimentally, the use of oral agents which prevent infecting bacteria from splitting urea (urease inhibitors), have been shown to decrease recurrence of some struvite stones by preventing the formation of highly alkaline urine resulting from the ammonium produced by urea-splitting organisms. Acetohydroxamic acid, and hydroxyurea are currently under evaluation. These agents may be available to the physician in the near future but their use should be coordinated by a urologist.

Urinary Calculi in Patients Without an Identifiable Metabolic Disorder

Approximately 10 to 15% of stone formers found after evaluation to not have a metabolic disorder may respond to thiazides and/or allopurinol as outlined above (2).

References

General

Coe, FL: *Nephrolithiasis Pathogenesis and Treatment.* Year Book Medical Publishers, Chicago, 1978.

    An excellent 230-page monograph which covers all aspects of urinary calculus disease.

Coe, FL. (guest ed.): Nephrolithiasis. In *Contemporary Issues in Nephrology, Vol. 5,* edited by BM Brenner and JH Stein. Churchill Livingstone, New York, 1980.

    This is a review monograph covering all aspects of urinary stone disease and provides an extensive documentation of the literature.

Pak, CYC: *Calcium Urolithiasis.* Plenum Medical Book, New York, 1978.

    This 160-page monograph provides a detailed review of cal-

cium stone disease and practical guidelines for evaluation, treatment, and follow-up.

Wickman, JEA (ed.): *Urinary Calculus Disease.* Churchill Livingstone, New York, 1979.

A 200-page multiauthored monograph covering all aspects of urinary calculus disease and especially the surgical treatment.

Specific

1. Broadus, AE, Dominguez, M and Bartter, FC: Pathophysiological studies in idiopathic hypercalciuria: use of an oral calcium tolerance test to characterize distinctive hypercalciuria subgroups. *J Clin Endocrinol Metab 47:* 751, 1978.
2. Coe, FL: Treated and untreated recurrent calcium nephrolithiasis in patients with idiopathic hypercalciuria, hyperuricosuria, or no metabolic disorder. *Ann Intern Med 87:* 404, 1977.
3. Dretler, SP, Pfister, RC and Newhouse, JH: Renal stone dissolution via percutaneous nephrostomy. *N Engl J Med 300:* 341, 1979.
4. Ettinger, B: Recurrent nephrolithiasis: natural history and ef-

fect of phosphate therapy. A double-blind controlled study. *Am J Med 61:* 200, 1976.
5. Ettinger, B, Oldroyd, NO and Surgel, F: Triamterene nephrolithiasis. *JAMA 244:* 2443, 1980.
6. Pak, CY, Delea, CS and Bartter, FC: Successful treatment of recurrent nephrolithiasis (calcium stones) with cellulose phosphate. *N Engl J Med 290:* 175, 1974.
7. Pak, CYV, Kaplan, RA, Bone, H, Townsend, J and Waters, O: A simple test for the diagnosis of absorptive, resorptive and renal hypercalciurias. *N Engl J Med 292:* 497, 1975.
8. Pak, CY, Sakhaee, K, Crowther, C and Krinkley, L: Evidence justifying a high fluid intake in treatment of nephrolithiasis. *Ann Intern Med 93:* 36, 1980.
9. Wojewski, A and Zajaczkowski, T: The treatment of bilateral staghorn calculi of the kidneys. *Int Urol Nephrol 5:* 249, 1974.
10. Yendt, ER: Renal calculi. *Can Med Assoc J 102:* 479, 1970.
11. Yü, T and Butman, AB: Uric acid nephrolithiasis in gout. Predisposing factors. *Ann Intern Med 67:* 1133, 1967.

CHAPTER FORTY-FOUR

Chronic Renal Failure

GARY R. BRIEFEL, M.D.

Each year increasing numbers of patients are referred to "end stage renal programs" for treatment with dialysis or transplantation (Fig. 44.1). In 1978 approximately 80 patients per million population were referred. Many other patients with less advanced disease can be treated without dialysis or transplantation, and the majority of these patients can be managed by the physician in an ambulatory setting.

This chapter will review the evaluation, clinical course, manifestations, and management of patients with chronic renal insufficiency in its predialysis stages.

DIAGNOSIS OF CHRONIC RENAL INSUFFICIENCY

Presentation and Estimation of Severity

Owing to the remarkable reserve and adaptive capabilities of the kidney, symptoms of uremia do not appear until renal function is reduced to 10 to 15% of normal. Therefore, unless clearly recognizable signs of renal involvement are present (Table 44.1) many patients will progress to renal failure asymptomatically. Often these patients are detected during the evaluation of nonspecific symptoms or of unrelated disorders.

The detection of significant renal impairment

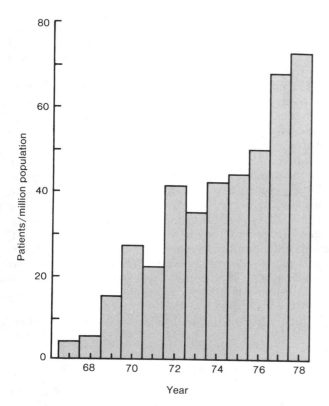

Figure 44.1 Patients referred for dialysis or transplantation in the United States. Each bar indicates the number of new patients per million population who entered the program per year. Since 1970 the average annual increase in new patients has been 17% per year. (From R. V. M. Cestero, O. Jacobs, and R. B. Freeman: A regional end-stage renal disease program; twelve years experience. *Annals of Internal Medicine, 93:* 494, 1980.)

Table 44.1
Common Clinical Presentations of Renal Disease

Hematuria
Proteinuria
Urinary tract infections
Nephrolithiasis
Obstruction
Hypertension
"Uremic" symptoms
Asymptomatic

should initiate a series of investigations which establish the chronicity of the disease, the rate of progression, and the potential responsiveness to specific therapy. The estimation of severity of renal disease is best accomplished by obtaining a serum creatinine and/or creatinine clearance. The *serum creatinine* is a better indicator of renal function than is blood urea nitrogen (BUN) since the latter is affected by nonrenal factors such as diet, intestinal bleeding, liver function, and protein catabolism. The general relationship between serum creatinine and glomerular

filtration rate (GFR) is shown in Figure 44.2 which illustrates several important points. In the early stages of renal insufficiency the serum creatinine is an insensitive indicator of functional impairment since it may remain in the "normal" range (less than 1.5 to 1.8 mg/dl) until GFR has decreased by as much as 50%. During the period when creatinine rises from 2 to 4 mg/dl, GFR falls from 50 to 25% of normal. Therefore, most of the loss of functioning nephrons occurs at levels of creatinine which might be considered to be only modestly elevated. Once GFR is reduced to 20 to 30% of normal, the curve rises steeply and deterioration appears to be rapid. Absolute changes in serum creatinine at low levels of GFR are, therefore, relatively less significant than those seen in early renal insufficiency. For example, in a patient with advanced renal failure (creatinine > 7 mg/dl) a change in serum creatinine of up to 1 mg/dl could be due to minor daily fluctuations in renal function and might not reflect true progression of renal disease.

The amount of muscle mass (muscles produce creatinine) must also be taken into account in evaluating the serum creatinine. For example (as shown in Fig. 44.2), a muscular patient who produces 1.5 g of creatine per day will have a GFR of 30 ml/min when his serum creatinine is 5 mg/dl; while an emaciated patient who produces only 0.5 g of creatinine per day will have a creatinine clearance of only 10 ml/min at the same level of serum creatinine. In addition, serum creatinine concentrations may underestimate the severity of the disease since in advanced renal insufficiency, creatinine production may be decreased and extrarenal routes of creatinine excretion become significant.

For these reasons, calculation of the *creatinine clearance* provides a more accurate reflection of renal function than does the serum creatinine. The creati-

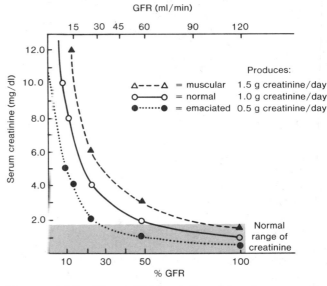

Figure 44.2 Theoretical relationship of serum creatinine to glomerular filtration rate.

nine clearance is a close approximation of glomerular filtration rate. The formula used for calculating clearance is $UV/P \div 1440$ where U is urine creatinine in mg/dl, V is urine volume in ml/day, and P is plasma creatinine in mg/dl; 1440 is the number of minutes in 24 hours. The result is expressed in ml/min, and normal creatinine clearance is approximately 100 to 140 ml/min in men and 85 to 120 ml/min in women. A correction can be made for body surface area, but this is not needed for clinical purposes. A 24-hour urine collection is used to determine daily creatinine production(UV). To confirm the adequacy of this collection the daily creatinine production may be estimated by multiplying body weight in kilograms by 20 for men and by 15 for women. This estimation, however, will no longer be valid when severe chronic renal failure (GFR < 20 ml/min) causes a fall in the production of creatinine. A urine sample collected over a shorter interval (e.g., 2 to 4 hours) may also be used for calculation of the clearance (using the same formula but altering the minutes of collection) when a 24-hour collection is impractical; but inaccuracies in determining the creatinine clearance may result from incomplete collection and from variation in endogenous creatinine production. The patient should be instructed to choose a convenient time to begin the collection—usually upon rising in the morning. At this time he voids and discards the urine but collects all subsequent urine until the same time the following day when he again voids and adds that specimen to the collection. The patient should be instructed to report an incomplete collection. The blood sample for measurement of creatinine is generally obtained at the end of the collection period but may be obtained at any time during the collection.

It is important for the physician to understand that changes in GFR (reflected by an increasing serum creatinine or a falling clearance) are not necessarily related to changes in intrinsic kidney function and may be due to other factors (see below p. 372). A gradual reduction of GFR with age has been well documented and occurs even in the absence of overt renal disease (11). Thus, at age 80 years, for example, an individual may have "physiologically" lost 30 to 50% of his previous GFR.

Search for Reversible Disease and Determination of Prognosis

Although many forms of renal disease have no specific therapy, the serious physical, psychological, and economic impact of chronic renal failure makes it important to detect those processes which are treatable or have reversible components. A list of those illnesses known or thought to respond to therapy are listed in Table 44.2. In those instances in which therapy is not available, or is of questionable utility, the physician must temper his desire to intervene with potentially toxic drugs (prednisone, azathioprine, cyclophosphamide) with the likelihood of

producing further harm, particularly in those whose renal disease is advanced. Therapeutic decisions of this nature should be made in conjunction with a nephrologist.

The establishment of the etiology of renal disease helps to determine prognosis. The specific pathological processes leading to progressive renal loss may have characteristic rates of progression which are useful in planning management (Table 44.3). For example, patients with polycystic kidney disease have the most indolent courses; and some never progress to the point of chronic renal failure. More aggressive courses, with advanced renal failure developing within several months to a year, are more likely to occur in patients with diseases such as, so-called, idiopathic rapidly progressive glomerulonephritis, systemic lupus erythematosus (SLE), or accelerated hypertension. Most renal diseases fall, however, into an intermediate group with renal failure developing within 1 to 5 years.

Since 5 to 20% of renal diseases which may cause

Table 44.2
Potentially Reversible Renal Disease and Therapy

Acute tubular necrosis—supportive treatment and dialysis if necessary
Arterial occlusions—surgery
Drug-induced renal disease—withhold drug
Exogenous poison, heavy metal—avoid further exposure
Hypercalcemia—correct chemical imbalance
Hypertensive nephropathy—antihypertensive drugs
Hyperuricemia—correct chemical imbalance
Hypokalemia—correct chemical imbalance
Lipoid nephrosis—prednisone
Neoplastic (myeloma)—chemotherapy
Obstruction—surgery
Pyelonephritis—antibiotics
Sarcoidosis—prednisone
Systemic lupus erythematosus (SLE)—steroids and azathioprine or cyclophosphamide
Wegener's granulomatosis—cyclophosphamide

Table 44.3
Estimated Time for the Progression to End Stage of Selected Renal Diseases[a]

RAPID (less than 1 yr)
    Rapidly progressive glomerulonephritis (GN)
    Scleroderma, Goodpasture's syndrome
    Accelerated hypertension, systemic lupus erythematosus (SLE)
MODERATE (1–5 yr)
    Diabetes mellitus (after the onset of proteinuria)
    Membranous glomerulonephritis
    Membranoproliferative GN, focal sclerosis, SLE
SLOW (greater than 5 yr)
    Polycystic kidney disease, hereditary nephritis
    Chronic hypertension, SLE

[a] Times provided are only estimates due to variability within each class.

Table 44.4
Selected Hereditary Diseases Resulting in Renal Insufficiency

Polycystic kidney disease—autosomal dominant (AD)
Hereditary nephritis (Alport's syndrome)—AD
Medullary cystic disease—AD or autosomal recessive (AR)
Cystinuria—AR

renal insufficiency have genetic components (if diabetes is included, the number exceeds 30%) important family planning may be indicated after a diagnostic evaluation (Table 44.4). Both genetic factors and the presence of systemic illnesses may affect decisions relating to management by dialysis or to transplantation of patients with chronic renal insufficiency. The decision to transplant may have to be modified in those patients where the renal disease is known to recur in the kidney transplant (for example, focal sclerosis or mebranoproliferative glomerulonephritis).

Methods of Evaluation

Since many patients with chronic renal insufficiency are now detected early in their course by routine screening, specific findings on history and physical examination are often absent. Routine and special laboratory testing in these cases frequently permit establishment of a definitive diagnosis. The complete evaluation may be rather brief as in the patient with advanced renal insufficiency and markedly shrunken kidneys; or extensive in the patient who has potentially reversible disease of presumed recent onset. As a rule, the entire renal workup can be performed on an ambulatory basis.

HISTORY AND PHYSICAL EXAMINATION

Findings in the history and physical examination can be useful both in establishing the nature of the renal disease and in determining its effect on the patient. In evaluating the new patient it is helpful to differentiate between those with renal disease secondary to involvement from systemic illnesses and those with primary forms of kidney disease. The relationship between kidney disease in patients with a history of longstanding diabetes mellitus, collagen vascular disease, or pelvic carcinoma is usually obvious. A history of hypertension is harder to interpret since it may be either the cause or result of renal disease. The use or abuse of certain drugs (Table 44.5) may be either responsible for the production of renal damage (heroin, analgesics, etc.) or for the aggravation of preexisting insufficiency (diuretics, aminoglycosides) (3). A detailed family history, as already mentioned, may suggest the presence of a genetically related disorder.

When a history of systemic illness or of familial disorders is absent, the physician must try to establish the nature of the primary renal disease. A history

Table 44.5
Some Commonly Used Drugs Which May Adversely Affect Renal Function[a]

ANTIBIOTICS
  Aminoglycosides—(ATN)
  Penicillins—(IN)
  Cephalosporins—(ATN and IN)
  Tetracyclines—(increased acidosis and azotemia)
ANALGESICS
  Aspirin—(PN and increased serum creatinine by decreasing GFR and renal blood flow)
  Acetoaminophen—(PN)
  Phenacetin—(PN and IN)
  Nonsteroidal analgesics—(IN and increased serum creatinine by decreasing GFR and renal blood flow)
DIURETICS
  Furosemide—(rare IN and by volume depletion)
  Thiazides—(rare vasculitis and by volume depletion)
MISCELLANEOUS AGENTS
  Radioiodinated contrast materials—(ATN)
  Methysergide—(retroperitoneal fibrosis causing obstructive uropathy)
  Penicillamine—(NS)
  Gold—(NS)
  Intravenous heroin—(NS)
  Lead—(nephrosclerosis and IN)
  Cimetidine—(increased creatinine by unknown mechanism)
  Sulfinpyrazone—(precipitates nephrolithiasis)
  Propranolol—(unknown mechanism, ? incidence)

[a] ATN, acute tubular necrosis; PN, papillary necrosis; IN, interstitial nephritis; NS, nephrotic syndrome.

of hematuria, edema, renal colic, urinary tract infection, or of difficulty voiding may suggest a particular class of renal disorder which will require further investigation by specific laboratory procedures.

Since symptoms do not appear until late, in many patients, it is often difficult to pinpoint the onset of disease. Important clues can sometimes be found when records of physical examinations performed for work, insurance, or military purposes are reviewed.

The physical examination should likewise be directed at looking for signs of systemic illnesses with renal involvement. These might include high blood pressure, hypertensive or diabetic retinopathy, adenoma sebaceum (tuberous sclerosis), vasculitic skin rash, or sclerodactyly (scleroderma). Enlarged kidneys may be found in polycystic disease or in hydronephrosis. A pelvic or rectal exam should be performed to look for lesions causing lower urinary tract obstruction. A residual urine volume after voiding that is larger than approximately 100 ml should raise concern for bladder outlet obstruction (see Chapter 45) or neuropathic bladder (most commonly in diabetes). The discovery of signs or symptoms of heart failure, pericarditis, or neuropathy are related to the stage of renal failure and are not helpful in establishing an etiology.

LABORATORY INVESTIGATIONS

The basis of any renal evaluation is the urinalysis. Although red blood cells can be seen with any renal disorder, when associated with casts, they are most indicative of a glomerular or vascular lesion. White blood cells, with or without casts, are found in the interstitial nephritides including, but not limited to, bacterial pyelonephritis. Hyaline or granular casts carry less diagnostic information and can be seen in a variety of renal disorders. The urine dipstick is only a rough guide to the amount of proteinuria. A 24-hour urine specimen should be obtained to quantify proteinuria and to calculate the creatinine clearance. The finding of nephrotic range proteinuria (greater than 3.5 g/day) usually indicates a glomerular lesion, whereas lesser amounts are seen in some glomerular or vascular disorders and in most interstitial forms of nephritis (Chapter 40).

Other studies with possible diagnostic significance in glomerulonephritis are the test of serum complement (C3 and C4), antistreptolysin-O titer, antinuclear antibody, lupus erythematosus preparation, rheumatoid factor, and cryoglobulins. These tests should be ordered when an immunologic disease is being considered or when the diagnosis is completely obscure. The test for hepatitis B surface antigen should be performed as its presence may be associated with certain forms of renal disease; and also because in any patient being referred for chronic dialysis or transplantation, precautions will need to be taken to prevent hepatitis infection in other patients and personnel.

The severity of anemia very roughly parallels the blood urea nitrogen as shown in Figure 44.3. The absence of anemia in patients with renal insufficiency should suggest either recent onset, the presence of polycystic kidney disease, or hydronephrosis. A peripheral smear should be examined carefully for abnormalities suggesting specific renal problems.

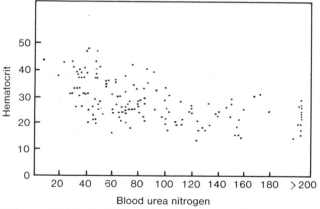

Figure 44.3 Relation of blood urea nitrogen to hematocrit. (From A. J. Erslev: Erythrocyte function of the kidney. In *Physiology of the Human Kidney*, p. 521, edited by L. G. Wesson, Grune & Stratton, New York, 1969.)

Rouleux formation suggests the diagnosis of multiple myeloma, while leukopenia may be associated with collagen vascular diseases. A microangiopathic hemolytic anemia can be seen in patients with thrombotic thrombocytopenic purpura, hemolytic uremic syndrome, accelerated hypertension, or scleroderma.

Measurements should be made of serum chemistries including fasting glucose, electrolytes (Na, K, Cl, CO_2, Ca, PO_4), liver function tests, and uric acid. Hypercalcemia may suggest the presence of a tumor or hyperparathyroidism. The uric acid level is usually elevated in patients with chronic renal insufficiency, but a uric acid level greater than 12 mg/dl may indicate the presence of primary hyperuricemia or of a myeloproliferative disorder.

RENAL IMAGING TECHNIQUES

Anatomic and functional evaluation of the kidney can be obtained by a variety of tests, all of which need not necessarily be performed on any individual patient. Renal imaging techniques in chronic renal failure should be used to: (a) establish renal size, (b) detect remediable lesions, and (c) determine etiology.

An *abdominal X-ray* (kidney, ureter, bladder (KUB)), with tomograms if necessary, is the simplest and least expensive test for estimating renal size. Normal kidney size is approximately 12 to 13 cm or 3 to 4 lumbar vertebrae. The left kidney is usually 0.5 cm larger than the right. *Sonography* is an alternative noninvasive means of estimating renal size and will also detect significant hydronephrosis. On sonography, the kidneys appear smaller (normal 9 to 10 cm) than on X-ray examinations owing to the lack of a projection effect. Small kidneys by either technique usually indicate advanced chronic renal disease. However, normal or large kidneys may be seen in chronic renal failure. Hydronephrosis due to obstruction should be ruled out in every patient with chronic renal insufficiency. If the screening sonogram, for example, suggests the presence of hydronephrosis, an intravenous pyelogram (IVP) with delayed films should be ordered to delineate the problem further. Adequate anatomic detail can be obtained even when the creatinine is 10 mg/dl or greater. Subsequent evaluation of the obstructed kidney may include a retrograde pyelogram or sonographically controlled percutaneous antegrade pyelograms. The advantage of the latter technique is that it allows placement of a simultaneous percutaneous nephrostomy tube for drainage. Patients with late stage renal failure who have small kidneys generally require no further radiologic evaluation.

The IVP may be useful in delineating the etiology of renal failure, particularly in those diseases which produce gross anatomic abnormalities such as pyelonephritis, nephrolithiasis, polycystic kidneys, obstruction, or papillary necrosis. The IVP is much less useful in patients with evidence of parenchymal disorders such as glomerulonephritis since it cannot resolve such fine anatomical details. Although IVPs can be performed in advanced renal failure by combining the use of high dose contrast materials with tomography (6), there is a significant risk of producing acute renal failure, particularly in elderly or diabetic patients. The use of radiocontrast materials, of any kind, cannot be recommended in these patients unless specific information which cannot be obtained by other means is needed. Further, since the decline in renal function appears to be partially preventable by avoiding volume depletion, patients should be instructed to maintain fluid intake both before and following examination.

The *renal angiogram* or *computerized tomography* are not routinely performed in patients with chronic renal failure and contribute mainly to the evaluation of vascular or of mass lesions. The *renal radioisotope scan* is of limited usefulness in evaluating chronic renal insufficiency, as it provides functional rather than anatomical information. The data provided are dependent on the radioisotope used. The technetium scan, which allows for estimation of renal perfusion, may however be useful to determine the viability of an obstructed kidney or one with staghorn calculi.

RENAL BIOPSY

Once the baseline data have been accumulated, a nephrologist should be consulted, at least by telephone, to help in interpreting the information and to decide whether a renal biopsy is indicated. The renal biopsy provides direct information and for most disease entities is the most specific diagnostic test available. The biopsy should be performed when the diagnosis is uncertain, to estimate prognosis, and to help demonstrate renal involvement of a systemic illness. Renal biopsies can be performed safely percutaneously (see Chapter 40). However, if the kidneys are very small or if renal failure is advanced, a biopsy is usually not done.

Following the initial establishment of an actual or presumptive diagnosis, laboratory measurements, in conjunction with clinical findings, will be utilized as a guide to subsequent management.

THERAPY

General Considerations

In addition to its role in maintaining water and electrolyte balance, the kidney has important endocrine and metabolic functions. It produces or degrades hormones responsible for normal bone formation (parathyroid hormone, 1,25-dihydroxyvitamin D_3), red blood cell production (erythropoietin), and blood pressure control (renin and prostaglandins). The proximal tubular cell of the kidney is also responsible for the degradation of many other polypeptide hormones, including insulin, which is of clinical relevance in the diabetic patient with incipient renal failure. Since the kidney is a major excretory route for a variety of drugs, a reduction in dosage is often necessary to compensate for the prolongation of half-life which occurs in renal failure (2). The physician should always review the appropriate dose and frequency of administration before any drug is prescribed to a patient with renal failure. Before the kidney fails to perform its combined excretory and metabolic functions, many adaptive changes occur which help maintain relative homeostasis and are important in understanding the management of patients with chronic renal insufficiency.

Much of our understanding of the adaptation to the progressive loss of functioning nephron units has been generated by Bricker, Bourgognie, and their co-workers (4). Briefly, the diseased kidney behaves as though each remaining nephron is functionally intact (maintains glomerulotubular balance) and retains its ability to regulate individually the many solutes for which it is responsible. In advanced renal failure this occurs despite a reduction of total nephrons from one million to one hundred thousand per kidney. This means that, for continued homeostasis, each remaining nephron must excrete 100 times the amount of solute excreted in the healthy person. Because each remaining nephron is functioning close to its maximum capacity, the failing kidney's ability to increase or reduce excretion of many solutes is limited. Clinically, this observation relates to the need to adjust intake of salt, water, potassium, and acid so as not to exceed or fall below the upper and lower limits of excretory capacity. The control systems regulating solute balance in chronic renal failure have been best worked out for calcium, phosphorus, and sodium. The adaptive effort developing as a result of kidney failure at times has harmful effects on other organ systems and has been termed the "trade-off" hypothesis. This is best exemplified by the development of secondary hyperparathyroidism as a consequence of the impaired ability of the kidney to excrete phosphate as glomerular filtration rate is diminished (see below). Some investigators believe that other uremic complications result from similar changes in other as yet unidentified control systems.

During the course of progressive renal insufficiency, certain functions fail before others, in a predictable fashion; and each stage will result in a unique constellation of signs and symptoms. Therapy, therefore, must be based on the degree of renal insufficiency rather than on treating all patients with renal failure alike. To illustrate this point, the following discussion on the management of chronic renal insufficiency will be related to the degree of renal failure.

Since many of the problems which plague the dialysis population have their onset in less advanced stages of renal insufficiency, an aim of management of patients with any renal disease is to minimize the factors which lead to long term complications. Therapy in the later stages of renal failure is aimed at alleviating symptoms and preparing patients for timely dialysis or transplantation.

Mild to Moderate Renal Insufficiency

The term *mild* renal insufficiency will include patients with GFRs between 50 and 30 ml/min or a serum creatinine of approximately 2 to 5 mg/dl. Patients with *moderate* renal insufficiency have GFRs between 30 and 15 ml/min or a serum creatinine between 5 and 10 mg/dl.

Unless specific renal syndromes (e.g., nephrotic syndrome) or sysemic illness (e.g., SLE) are present, most cases of mild renal insufficiency are detected by abnormal blood chemistry determinations or urinalysis. Symptoms are more likely to be present in moderate renal insufficiency and include impaired mental concentration, sleep disturbance, polyuria, fatigue, anorexia, edema, or metallic taste.

DIETARY MANAGEMENT

Dietary management in mild to moderate renal insufficiency is primarily directed at maintaining adequate volume by manipulating salt intake. As function declines, the ability of the kidney to balance salt intake at the extremes becomes limited. Volume overload or depletion may develop if this range is exceeded. Most patients with chronic renal insufficiency maintain balance on a 4- to 6-g salt intake unless congestive heart failure or hypertension is present, when salt intake should be reduced to 2 g or less per day. Rarely patients will require salt supplements of up to 20 g per day to prevent volume depletion and are termed "salt wasters." Modification of salt prescription should be based on serial measurements of weight, blood pressure, and the physical examination. When salt restriction alone is insufficient, furosemide (Lasix) can be used and is generally successful at increasing salt excretion. The dose required, however, is generally greater than that in patients with normal renal function. The dose range for furosemide is 40 to 400 mg/day given as a single dose. Ethacrynic acid in high doses may cause more side effects and is not recommended. Decreased salt intake or excess losses may occur during intercurrent illness associated with vomiting or diarrhea. Since the diseased kidney is not able acutely to conserve sodium normally, volume depletion and thereby reduction of GFR may result. Sodium losses can be replaced either orally or intravenously.

Potassium restriction is generally unnecessary at this level of chronic renal failure, except in the subgroup of patients with hyporeninemic-hypoaldosteronism (see below), but careful monitoring of serum levels is indicated. Although diluting and concentrating ability is reduced in renal failure, most patients do not require specific instructions regarding water intake, unless they develop hyponatremia. Prolonged periods of dehydration are to be avoided.

Protein restriction, important in managing the patient with advanced renal failure (see below), is generally not needed in mild or moderate renal failure.

CALCIUM AND PHOSPHORUS

Renal osteodystrophy is a general term which encompasses osteitis fibrosa, osteomalacia, osteosclerosis, and osteoporosis occurring in uremic patients. The pathophysiologic factors resulting in osteodystrophy originate in the early stages of renal failure, although clinical manifestations generally do not develop until the patient is on dialysis.

Secondary hyperparathyroidism resulting in osteitis fibrosa has multiple etiologies (5). Renal phosphate excretion diminishes as GFR falls, resulting in small increments of serum phosphorus and a reciprocal fall in calcium levels. Parathyroid hormone (PTH) secretion increases as a response to these stimuli and remains elevated to maintain calcium-phosphorus balance. The inverse relationship between PTH and GFR is sufficient to maintain normal calcium and phosphorus levels until the creatinine clearance falls below 30 ml/min. Serum levels of 1,25-dihydroxyvitamin D_3, as well as calcium absorption by the gut, are normal in patients with mild to moderate renal insufficiency, but fall as renal failure becomes more advanced. This fall results in hypocalcemia and a further stimulus to PTH secretion. Skeletal resistance to the effects of PTH on calcium reabsorption have also been described in patients with mild to moderate renal failure and may contribute to hyperparathyroidism. Osteomalacia in renal insufficiency is partly due to the failure by the diseased kidney to convert 25-hydroxyvitamin D_3, to its more active form, 1,25-dihydroxyvitamin D_3. Abnormal collagen synthesis has also been implicated as the cause of osteomalacia in uremia. Chronic metabolic acidosis resulting in titration of bone buffers may also contribute to the pathogenesis of renal osteodystrophy.

The typical clinical features of renal osteodystrophy, including bone pain, fractures, and proximal myopathy, are not often seen in the predialysis patient. While not necessary to make initial management decisions, it may be of value to obtain in patients with renal failure a base line radiological bone survey (skull, pelvis, hands) for evidence of renal osteodystrophy and for later comparison should the disease progress. Routine PTH levels will be high in azotemic patients since the most commonly available assays measure the carboxyl-terminal fragment, which depends on renal excretion, and, therefore, does not accurately reflect actual parathyroid gland activity. Therefore, determination of PTH level, when it is necessary, should be by an assay which measures the intact or N-terminal hormone.

The therapy for renal osteodystrophy in its preclinical stages is under considerable investigation and is debated. Animal studies have shown that phosphate restriction in early renal failure can prevent the rise of PTH levels. Although a proportionate reduction of phosphate intake as renal function declines may eventually prove beneficial in the long term prevention of osteodystrophy, human data to support this method of treatment are lacking. In addition, chronic phosphate depletion may predispose patients to the development of osteomalacia. The role of bicarbonate therapy in countering the effects of chronic acidosis on bone is also unknown.

Once serum phosphorus becomes elevated in moderate renal failure (e.g., greater than 5.5 mg/dl), therapy should be started in order to restore the levels to normal. This is best accomplished by having the patient take *phosphate binders with* his meals. Oral antacids containing aluminum hydroxide (Alterna Gel or Amphojel) or aluminum carbonate (Basaljel) bind phosphate in the intestine into insoluble salts and are effective at reducing phosphate absorption. The binders come in liquid, tablet, or capsule forms. The liquid is the most effective but the least well tolerated. Patients should be aware that they may become nauseated, bloated, or constipated. Stool softeners or sorbitol can be used to counter the constipation. Other medications (Table 44.6), such as digoxin, should not be given simultaneously with phosphate binders since their absorption can be adversely affected. The initial dose should be 1 or 2 tablespoons or tablets/capsules given with meals, and can be increased until serum phosphorus is normalized (4.5 to 5.5 mg/dl). Serum phosphorus concentration should be monitored every 1 to 2 months to avoid the syndrome of phosphate depletion (low serum phosphorus) which may result in osteomalacia and bone fractures. Aluminum-containing antacids should also be used for the treatment of gastritis or ulcers since magnesium toxicity can occur in a patient with chronic renal failure taking magnesium-containing antacids. Aluminum accumulation has been implicated in the development of the dialysis encephalopathy syndrome. To date, however, there is no satisfactory alternative treatment for hyperphosphatemia.

After normalization of serum phosphorus, subsequent therapy is directed at maintaining normal serum calcium levels to avoid further stimulation of parathyroid hormone secretion. If the calcium level is low the diet should be supplemented with *calcium carbonate* tablets 600 mg 4 times a day (1 g of ele-

Table 44.6
Drugs Whose Bioavailability Is Altered by Phosphate Binders

DECREASED
Digoxin
Oral anticoagulants
Tetracycline
Anticholinergics
Aspirin
Chlorpromazine
INCREASED
Penicillin
Pseudoephedrine

mental calcium per day) to assure an adequate intake and provide sufficient calcium for bone mineralization. Calcium lactate may also be substituted if carbonate is not tolerated (see below, p. 370).

The indications for *vitamin D sterols* have not been entirely established. An important role for vitamin D deficiency in the pathogenesis of uremic osteodystrophy during early renal insufficiency has not been unequivocally established. Therefore, the use of vitamin D sterols for the prophylactic control of osteodystrophy in patients with early to moderate renal failure is not recommended. In more advanced stages of renal failure both intestinal calcium absorption and serum levels of 1,25-dihydroxy vitamin D_3, are reduced. Therefore, in these patients, when hypocalcemia is resistent to calcium supplementation or when evidence of secondary hyperparathyroidism exists, vitamin D should be given.

The form of vitamin D used is important since preparations (e.g., vitamin D_3) requiring final activation by the kidney have proven to be ineffective in the usual doses. Dihydrotachysterol (DHT) is a synthetic analogue of 1,25-dihydroxyvitamin D_3 and does not require renal activation. When given in oral doses of 0.125 to 0.5 mg per day, it has been effective in normalizing calcium absorption and serum calcium levels in azotemic patients. Recently available preparations such as 1,25-dihydroxyvitamin D_3 (Rocaltrol) are effective in low doses because they do not require renal activation. Direct comparisons between DHT and Rocaltrol have not been performed; however, episodes of hypercalcemia are seen in almost 50% of patients receiving the latter form. On the other hand, Rocaltrol does have the advantage that, should hypercalcemia develop, it is of short duration once the vitamin D is stopped. None of the vitamin D sterols have been consistently shown to heal the osteomalacic lesions. Despite the theoretical advantage of 1,25-dihydroxyvitamin D_3, the generalist should begin therapy with DHT because of the greater experience accumulated with this drug. The more potent preparations should be reserved for patients who are refractory to treatment with DHT. These patients should be referred to a nephrologist or someone else familiar with the treatment of renal osteodystrophy. Vitamin D therapy should not be used when calcium levels are greater than 9.5 mg/100 ml or when serum phosphorus is greater than 6 mg/100 ml because of the possibility of metastatic calcification. Monitoring of serum calcium (every month once stable) is important in patients taking vitamin D to detect the development of hypercalcemia. Serum phosphorus will often rise following institution of vitamin D therapy because both calcium and phosphorus absorption are thereby increased. Avoidance of hypercalcemia or hyperphosphatemia by careful monitoring should prevent the fall in GFR reported in some patients with advanced renal insufficiency taking vitamin D.

ACIDOSIS

A mild hyperchloremic metabolic acidosis may be seen in patients with early renal insufficiency as the ability of the kidney to produce ammonia is lost. However, the process is generally not serve enough to warrant therapy. The association of hyperkalemia and hyperchloremic metabolic acidosis in mild renal insufficiency should suggest the syndrome of *hyporeninemic-hypoaldosteronism* (9). This syndrome occurs most frequently in azotemic patients with hypertension, diabetes mellitus, or interstitial nephritis. This disorder probably has multiple causes but is due in most to a depression of the renin-angiotensin-aldosterone axis. The diagnosis is supported by the finding of a plasma renin concentration which is low and fails to increase following an acute challenge with furosemide (Lasix) e.g., 40 mg orally and upright posture for 2 to 4 hours. The patient should have no evidence of glucocorticoid deficiency (random cortisol concentration of 15 to 25 ng/dl; see also Chapter 71). These patients are at risk of developing severe hyperkalemia during salt restriction or periods of volume depletion. Treatment of nonhypertensive patients may be attempted with mineralocorticoids (fludrocortisone; Florinef, 0.05 to 0.1 mg/day), or with a combination of furosemide plus salt (NaHCO₃). Because therapy is frequently complicated, these patients are best managed in conjunction with a nephrologist or endocrinologist.

Patients whose level of serum bicarbonate falls below 15 meq/L have reduced buffer reserves and run the risk of severe acidosis during periods of stress induced by infection or volume depletion. If protein restriction (see below, p. 371), which reduces exogenous acid load is insufficient to restore buffering capacity, base in the form of sodium bicarbonate (NaHCO₃), 300 to 600 mg, 4 times a day may be given, provided sodium excess (edema) is not a problem. Should NaHCO₃ not be tolerated because of gastrointestinal complaints (belching and bloatedness), calcium lactate, 300 to 600 mg 4 times a day, may be given (lactate will generate bicarbonate as it is metabolized by the liver).

HYPERTENSION

Hypertension (see also Chapter 59) may result from, or cause, renal failure and always requires therapy. Antihypertensive therapy in patients with mild to moderate renal insufficiency is similar to that of patients with normal renal function and hypertension. A salt-restricted diet may be attempted as a first step. Loop diuretics can be added when salt restriction is insufficient or when vasodilating drugs lead to secondary salt retention. Thiazides are generally avoided in patients with moderate renal insufficiency as they lose their diuretic effect when GFR is reduced below 30 ml/min. Methyldopa, clonidine, hydralazine, prazosin, and propranolol are all useful in patients with chronic renal insufficiency. Reports of

irreversible reductions in glomerular filtration rate in normal subjects who are taking propranolol and who have normal or abnormal renal function suggest that renal function should be carefully monitored at frequent intervals (1). As renal function deteriorates, the use of larger doses of diuretics will often be necessary to control hypertension. There is often a fine line between effective blood pressure control and hypotension when potent diuretics and antihypertensives are being used; therefore, careful monitoring of the blood pressure (both resting and orthostatic) and serum creatinine are necessary. It is not unusual for patients with hypertensive renal disease to show a temporary decrease in renal function when blood pressure control is instituted, followed by improvement in function. An occasional patient receiving regular dialysis has regained sufficient function to discontinue dialysis for up to several years with continued control of blood pressure. Nephrectomy, although usually leading to improved blood pressure control, can generally be avoided with the use of potent drugs such as minoxidil or captopril (for detailed discussion of this drug, see Chapter 59). Long term control of hypertension is important in reducing the risk of accelerated atherosclerosis seen in patients on dialysis.

ANEMIA

A mild normochromic normocytic anemia is generally present and its severity is proportional to the degree of renal insufficiency (Fig. 44.3). The anemia results mainly from shortened red blood cell survival and an inability to compensate because of decreased erythropoietin production. Other causes of anemia must, of course, be ruled out. Patients generally tolerate this degree of anemia well and transfusions are not necessary unless symptoms related to congestive heart failure, cardiac ischemia, or syncope occur.

HYPERURICEMIA

As discussed below (p. 373) the only indication for treating hyperuricemia in chronic renal disease is to treat gout; there is no evidence that hyperuricemia *per se* causes or worsens chronic renal failure.

PATIENT EDUCATION

Following development of the data base, the patient should be informed about the nature, etiology, and expected course of his renal disease. Generally, once the patient has reached moderate renal insufficiency, in the absence of specific therapy, further progression should be expected. The patient should be aware that, although his therapy is geared to slowing the progression of his disease, he may eventually require dialysis or transplantation. The primary physician, if he is familiar with the techniques and expectations of hemodialysis and transplantation (discussed later), can be most helpful in advising the patient. At this stage of renal insufficiency, little or no change in life-style is expected, particularly if anemia is mild and coexisting illnesses are absent. Patients who work in extremely hot environments where fluid loss is significant should be advised to find less strenuous occupations.

MONITORING THE PATIENT

The patient should have scheduled office visits every 3 or 4 months early in the course for monitoring of weight, serum creatinine, blood urea nitrogen (BUN), electrolytes, creatinine clearance, urinalysis, and complete blood counts. As renal failure progresses, visits will neeed to be spaced more closely, usually at 1-month intervals until dialysis becomes necessary. Drug dosage should be periodically reviewed and adjusted for the degree of renal dysfunction. If not already done, the patient should be referred to a nephrologist associated with a dialysis or transplant center. Placement of vascular access, usually an arteriovenous fistula, should be completed when the GFR reaches 15 ml/min, particularly in those patients with rapidly progressive courses or poor vasculature. Discussion of transplantation from living relations at this point will provide time for identification and evaluation of potential donors.

Advanced Renal Failure

Advanced renal failure is defined as GFR of less than 15 ml/min or a serum creatinine of greater than 10 mg/dl. At this level of renal function most patients will manifest symptoms of uremia. These symptoms are often vague and nonspecific. Initially there is weakness, lassitude, and somnolence. Gastrointestinal symptoms (anorexia, nausea, vomiting, hiccoughs, and metallic taste) are common once the clearance falls below 10 ml/min. Salt retention may result in hypertension or congestive heart failure, both of which may also be presenting features of advanced renal failure. Less commonly patients will present with signs of more advanced uremia such as seizures, pericarditis, bleeding, or coma. It is in these patients that the differentiation between acute and chronic renal failure is often most difficult to make.

During this period, each of the management plans described above should be followed with special considerations in dietary management and in handling of anemia and the patient should be prepared for dialysis or transplantation. It is important that a nephrologist be intimately involved in planning care for the patient at this stage of renal failure.

DIET

The major adjustment for patients progressing to advanced renal failure is the imposition of dietary restrictions. Patients who develop uremic symptoms should be placed on a protein-restricted diet. Although the exact nature of uremic toxins is unknown, they are related, in part, to the end products of protein metabolism. Therapy initially consists of re-ducing protein intake to 40 to 60 g per day. Caloric intake in the form of carbohydrates and fat is increased in order to prevent the patient from developing negative nitrogen balance from protein restriction. Total caloric intake should be maintained between 2 and 3 thousand calories per day. Consultation with a dietitian familiar with the management of renal failure will help assure that an appropriate diet is provided. An order for a "renal failure diet" is meaningless and may often be harmful since this is often interpreted as including severe salt restriction and can lead to prerenal azotemia. In general, if symptoms persist and the creatinine clearance falls below 5 ml/min, dialysis should be instituted. If dialysis is unavailable or if the patient must wait for vascular access to be prepared, a more severe form of protein restriction is often necessary. This should include a 20-g protein diet containing protein of high biologic value (mostly containing essential amino acids, e.g., eggs) or using essential amino acid supplements. The more severe the protein restriction, the more important it is to assure adequate caloric intake to prevent nitrogen wasting, a consequent rise in BUN and potassium concentration, and a fall in bicarbonate concentration. If dialysis is available, there is nothing to be gained by maintaining a patient on severe protein restriction, particularly since these diets are unpalatable and noncompliance is common.

If hyperkalemia develops, *potassium restriction* is necessary and intake should be limited to between 2 and 2.2 g (40 to 50 meq) per day (see Chapter 42 for a table of potassium content of common foods). Patients who are on salt restriction must be instructed that salt substitutes are not acceptable since they are usually in the form of potassium salts.

ANEMIA

The hematocrit value will generally fall to between 15 and 25% in a patient with advanced renal insufficiency. Most patients are placed on a multivitamin regimen, including folate to replace the vitamins lacking in the restrictive diets. Anabolic steroids which stimulate erythropoietin production have been shown to be useful in improving hemoglobin levels in patients on dialysis. Although anabolic steroids may increase the red blood cell mass slightly in uremic patients not yet on dialysis, they also lead to significant side effects such as salt retention and are not recommended. Blood transfusion, when necessary, should not be withheld for fear of sensitizing a potential transplant recipient. Studies indicate that transplanted patients with multiple blood transfusions have higher success rates than those not receiving transfusions (8). The use of washed, leukocyte-poor, packed red blood cells is recommended. Iron deficiency is almost universal in patients on hemodialysis but may also occur in the pre-dialysis patient, particularly if multiple blood samples have been taken. Iron deficiency is best diagnosed in chronic renal failure by demonstrating a low serum ferritin level.

TIMING OF DIALYSIS

The goal of dialysis is to maintain health at a level consistent with a relatively normal life-style. It is not advisable, therefore, to wait for signs and symptoms, such as pericarditis, seizures, coma, or bleeding before initiating dialysis. Although there is no absolute level of serum creatinine at which dialysis should be initiated, a creatinine clearance of less than 5 ml/min or a serum creatinine of greater than 10 to 12 mg/dl are the usual criteria. Delay in starting dialysis can lead to severe peripheral neuropathy, malnutrition, or pericarditis from which total recovery may not be possible. Sometimes, particularly when living related donor transplantation is possible, a patient may receive a kidney transplant without ever requiring dialysis therapy. This might be particularly advisable in patients with diabetes mellitus or in young children, as both groups of patients tend to have a poor prognosis on dialysis. Further discussion on the relative merits of dialysis and transplantation is found below (p. 373).

MONITORING THE PATIENT

As GFR falls and the serum creatinine rises, the likelihood of finding significant metabolic acidosis or electrolyte disturbances increases. Therefore, office visits should be more frequent. Patients who have bicarbonate levels <15 meq/dl or potassium levels >5.5 meq/dl should be seen at 1 to 2-week intervals, whereas others without these problems may be seen monthly. With proper planning, it should be possible to begin dialysis without the patient ever requiring admission to the hospital.

Uremia and Coexisting Disorders

Nonrenal diseases often occur in patients with uremia and complicate management. In some, such as patients with SLE or diabetes mellitus, the renal disease is part of a systemic illness which affects many organ systems. Others may have disease unrelated to the kidney problem, such as coronary artery disease, chronic obstructive pulmonary disease, or malignancy. Interaction of the components of the uremic syndrome with other illnesses is important in managing these patients.

Diabetes mellitus. Up to 50% of insulin-dependent diabetics and a substantial proportion of patients with non-insulin-dependent diabetes develop chronic renal insufficiency, and patients with diabetes account for up to 30% of many dialysis populations. The mechanism whereby diabetes affects the kidney is predominantly through a microvasculopathy producing nodular glomerulosclerosis. A relationship between poor glucose control and the progression of renal disease has not been unequivocally established, although much evidence is accumulating to suggest that microvascular disease is related to hyperglycemia (Chapter 68). The onset of renal disease usually develops after 10 to 15 years of diabetes and initially is manifest by proteinuria. Azotemia soon follows, and there is usually a rapid decline in renal function leading to renal insufficiency within another 1 or 2 years. Renal disease may reduce insulin requirement, an effect related at least in part to decreased hormone degradation in the renal tubules as renal failure progresses. Some oral hypoglycemic agents are excreted by the kidney. Therefore, the physician should regularly reassess the insulin or oral hypoglycemic dose in patients whose renal function is failing. Although diabetics are clearly more difficult to manage than patients with renal disease alone, diabetes *per se* is not a contraindication to dialysis or transplantation. The form of therapy which is best suited to patients with diabetes and renal failure (hemodialysis, peritoneal dialysis, or transplantation) is yet to be determined. The diabetic patient should be reminded that dialysis or transplantation are supportive therapies for renal dysfunction and will not improve their diabetes. The referring physician should also remember that the course of these patients is less favorable than is that of patients with kidney disease without diabetes.

Heart Disease. Heart disease often exists in patients with renal insufficiency, particularly those with diabetes or hypertension. These patients respond, as do others, to salt restriction, diuretics, and digitalis. The maintenance dose of digoxin needs to be adjusted in patients with renal insufficiency since the kidney is responsible for 85% of digoxin metabolism. A nomogram (7) can be used for calculating the approximate dose. More practically, a dose of digoxin of 0.125 mg is initiated and then adjusted according to the serum digoxin level, unless atrial fibrillation is present when the ventricular rate can serve as a guide to therapy.

ASSESSMENT OF DETERIORATION OF RENAL FUNCTION

The significance of changes in serum creatinine depends on the degree of renal insufficiency. In general, small changes in serum creatinine are more significant at higher levels of GFR than are those occurring at low GFRs. Once serum creatinine exceeds 5 mg/dl, a change in 1 mg/dl from visit to visit may not be related to real changes in renal function. Before any change in renal function can be attributed to the natural progression of the underlying renal disease, several alternative possibilities should be considered (Table 44.7).

Volume depletion is probably the most common nonrenal cause for a fall in GFR. It may be related to an intercurrent illness associated with anorexia, fever, gastrointestinal losses of sodium and water, overexcessive salt restriction, or diuretic use. Clinical signs of volume depletion may be absent, and a therapeutic trial may be required to establish the diagnosis. Weight loss between office visits may be the most important diagnostic clue to the presence of

Table 44.7
Causes of Renal Function Deterioration

Volume depletion
Congestive heart failure
Drug nephrotoxicity
Ureteral or urethral obstruction
Crystal deposition
Hyperphosphatemia—hypercalcemia
Hypertension
Radiocontrast materials (oral and parenteral)
Pyelonephritis (bacterial, mycobacterial or fungal)

volume depletion. The urinary sodium concentration (if low) or osmolality (if high) may be helpful in establishing the diagnosis of volume depletion; but since concentrating and salt-conserving ability in these patients is often impaired, the values may not be diagnostic in spite of the presence of significant volume depletion.

Patients with decompensated *congestive heart failure* may also present with superimposed prerenal azotemia. Treatment with pre- and after load reducers, digoxin, and diuretics may often improve renal function (see Chapter 58).

Drugs given for treatment of various disorders can be related to decreases in renal function (Table 44.5). A careful review, therefore, of the patient's medication is necessary to rule out deterioration of renal function caused by drugs.

Obstruction, because of its reversibility, should always be considered in patients with falling GFR. This is particularly true in elderly men predisposed to prostatic hypertrophy or in diabetics who may have autonomic neuropathy affecting bladder emptying. Drugs which reduce bladder tone (particularly antidepressants, antispasmodics, and antiparkinsonian drugs with anticholinergic properties) should always be considered as a cause of obstruction.

Crystal deposition in the kidney has been suggested by some as a cause of progressive renal deterioration in patients with azotemia. Elevation of the serum uric acid is common in advanced renal insufficiency. The relationship between elevated uric acid, urate deposition in the kidney, and the development of gouty nephropathy in patients with clinical gout has, however, been questioned (12), and there is no convincing evidence that normalizing serum uric acid in patients with chronic renal insufficiency is useful in preventing further deterioration. Allopurinol is not used, therefore, unless it is needed to control clinical gout.

Several studies performed in rats have shown that *restriction of phosphate* intake may prevent progression of renal insufficiency by preventing renal calcification. Similar studies in humans have not been performed, however. Phosphate should be controlled, therefore, as outlined above (p. 369) bearing in mind the real possibility of developing osteomalacia due to phosphate depletion if phosphate intake is too severely restricted.

Urinary tract infections may also be related to deterioration of renal function, so that urinalysis and, if this is abnormal, urine culture are indicated when creatinine concentration begins to rise. Other infections, including viral illnesses, may also cause serum creatinine to rise.

Hypertension is also a cause of renal damage and should be treated even though transient decreases in renal function may occur.

Only after the above causes have been excluded is it reasonable to assume that the change in renal function is related to the underlying disease process.

DIALYSIS AND TRANSPLANTATION

Provisions for dialysis should be concluded months in advance of need. Deciding on the most appropriate form of therapy should follow discussions between the patient, family, primary physician, and nephrologist. The following is an outline of the procedures and expectations involved in dialysis or transplantation and should be helpful in reaching the most appropriate decision for an individual patient.

Dialysis

In 1980 over 50,000 patients were being maintained on dialysis in the United States. Either hemodialysis or peritoneal dialysis may be performed in a center or at the patient's home. Most patients will receive dialysis either as a continued form of therapy or temporarily while awaiting transplantation. Although dialysis does not correct all the metabolic abnormalities of chronic renal failure it has enabled thousands of patients to lead productive lives.

The decision to dialyze a patient with a malignancy or with other advanced systemic illnesses such as scleroderma or diabetes is often difficult and requires in-depth discussion with the patient, family, primary care physician, and nephrologist before the actual need for dialysis is at hand. The duration and quality of life and the patient's will to live are some of the factors which must be considered. Many of the patients with extensive multisystem illnesses require extra medical, psychological, and social support. The absence of strong family support is often a critical factor resulting in poor medical outcome. Denial of dialysis for patients with renal failure and multisystem disorders, without individual consideration and evaluation, is no longer justifiable.

HEMODIALYSIS

The first step requires the creation of vascular access to allow for the repeated venipunctures necessary for this form of dialysis. The preferred access is usually an arteriovenous fistula which is located at the wrist of the nondominant arm. The creation of an arteriovenous fistula can be performed, in most instances, under local anesthesia and often as an outpatient. Vascular access should be created 2 to 3 months in advance of the need for dialysis to allow for adequate maturation. The most common complications of vascular access are clotting and infection.

Hemodialysis is performed 2 or 3 times per week; each session lasts approximately 5 hours. Hospital-based dialysis should always be utilized for those patients who require intensive monitoring for medical reasons. Home dialysis is encouraged in those patients with a good home situation and a willing partner. Home patients have the most flexible schedules and a greater sense of control than do hospital-based patients and, therefore, have the greatest chance of maintaining their previous life-style. The remainder of the patients can be treated at satellite centers or self-care units which allow patients to take a major responsibility for their care under supervision, and which also result in reduced costs.

As a group, hemodialysis patients have a 10% mortality rate per year. Home dialysis patients, who are generally healthier, do better than those with coexistent illnesses or than the elderly. The development of some long term complications of chronic renal failure including progressive neuropathy, renal osteodystrophy, cardiovascular disease, and endocrine disturbances reflect the fact that dialysis does not correct all the metabolic abnormalities of uremia.

PERITONEAL DIALYSIS

Peritoneal dialysis is an acceptable mode of chronic dialysis. Its drawbacks (low efficiency and increased dialysis time) are offset by its simplicity, safety, and application to patients with inadequate vascular access. The use of a chronic peritoneal catheter obviates the need for repeated punctures and decreases the rate of infection. Patients often find home dialysis with chronic peritoneal dialysis, because of its technical simplicity, more acceptable than hemodialysis. Generally, 36 hours per week of peritoneal dialysis are needed but this may be divided into two or three sessions which often can be maintained overnight using an automated peritoneal dialysis cycler. The peritoneal catheter is placed at the time of the initial dialysis and does not require a maturation period. The major drawback to peritoneal dialysis is peritoneal infection. The incidence is one episode of peritonitis every 6 to 8 dialysis months (these are generally controlled with antibiotics). Further, a peritoneal catheter will need to be replaced about once a year. A variation of chronic peritoneal dialysis has become increasingly available: *continuous ambulatory peritoneal dialysis* (CAPD). This technique requires that the patient constantly carry 2 liters of peritoneal dialysate in his abdomen. The fluid is changed approximately every 4 hours but this technique allows the patient to be free from mechanical fluid cycling devices. The initial results suggest improved patient freedom and impressive control of metabolic abnormalities and blood pressure (10). If the infection rate can be reduced, CAPD may prove to be a major advance in the treatment of end stage renal failure.

Patient survival statistics with chronic peritoneal dialysis are difficult to interpret because the populations used to generate these statistics are not comparable to the patients on hemodialysis. Whether hemodialysis or peritoneal dialysis will be used partly depends on the center to which the patient is referred and on that center's familiarity or preference for either therapy.

RENAL TRANSPLANTATION

The promise of renal transplantation is tantalizing since theoretically it allows for the complete restoration of lost renal function, including not only fluid and electrolyte balance, but excretion of all metabolic toxins and return of normal hormonal and metabolic function. This promise is frustrated by the transplantation surgeon's inability to guarantee a successful outcome, as a result of immunologic rejection or technical failures. The success of renal transplantation depends greatly on the degree of antigenic similarity between donor and recipient. Except in the case of identical twins (when no rejection occurs) the best results occur in living related donor, HLA identical, sibling transplants with kidney survival rates of greater than 90% at 1 year (75% at 5 years). More commonly performed are 2 antigen matched transplants from sibling to sibling or parent to child with a 75% success rate at 1 year (55% at 5 years). The majority of patients do not have the potential of living related donors and must await a cadaveric transplant which, despite the best tissue typing, has a significantly lower success rate of about 55% at 1 year (25% at 5 years). Patient survival on the other hand, either living related or cadaveric transplants, approximates that of good hemodialysis.

Uncomplicated kidney transplants require at least a 3- to 4-week hospitalization and often longer until the kidney has stabilized and immunosuppressant drugs have been tapered. After kidney transplantation, the patient requires lifelong immunosuppression, usually with prednisone and azathioprine. He must also learn to live with the risk of potential rejection and a return to dialysis. Although successful renal transplantation may entirely correct the uremic syndrome, patients run the risk with long term immunosuppression, including the development of steroid complications, malignancies, or infections.

Since the primary physician often knows the patient exceptionally well, he can be of great value in advising which forms of therapy might coincide best with the patient's expectations. Frequently, patients will have a better understanding of their choices if they visit a dialysis or transplant unit and talk with patients and staff before this treatment is necessary for them. The decision to transplant is the most clear-cut in adolescent or young adult patients who wish to pursue an active, vigorous life, to have a job and to have intact sexual functions, particularly if a living related donor transplant is available. Elderly patients or those with extensive multisystem organ disease may not benefit by renal transplantation. For others, a period of dialysis and assessment of the patient's adjustment to this therapy will often help in determining whether to continue dialysis or to attempt transplantation. It is often important for the primary physician to take part in this decision, since the nephrologist or transplant surgeon may have a vested interest in which therapy he recommends. The patient who adjusts well to dialysis can often be fully rehabilitated and maintain a job as efficiently as the patient with successful renal transplant does. At the present time it appears that quality of life is the most important criterion determining therapy, since the survival rate appears to be similar in patients undergoing either transplantation or dialysis.

Conclusion

The financial impact of chronic renal failure and the cost of hemodialysis and transplantation, which initially were prohibitively expensive, have been minimized by the extension of the Medicare Program to patients with chronic renal failure under the age of 65. Nevertheless, patients often have to quit their jobs because of chronic illness or because of the time requirements of dialysis. Living with a chronic disease often affects the entire family. Despite theoretical advances in dialysis and transplantation, great improvement in the quality of life of patients with chronic renal failure has not occurred in recent years. The best hope, therefore, for the treatment of renal failure lies in the prevention of and early treatment of reversible renal disease (Table 44.2) rather than in the treatment of the end stage. The role of prevention lies mainly with the primary physician seeing patients in an ambulatory care setting.

References

General

Campbell, JD and Campbell, AR: The social and economic costs of end-stage renal disease. N Engl J Med 299: 386, 1978.
   A patient's view of the effects of living with renal failure.

Friedman, EA (ed): *Strategy in Renal Failure.* John Wiley & Sons, New York, 1978.
   Readable and comprehensive review of the management of uremic patients. Sections on dialysis and transplantation of patients with systemic diseases.

Guttmann, RD: Renal transplantation I, II. N Engl J Med 301: 975, 1038, 1979.
   A complete discussion of transplantation.

Massry, SG Goldstein, DA and Molluche, HH: Current status of the use of 1.25-(OH)$_2$-D$_3$ in the management of renal osteodystrophy. Kidney Int 18: 409, 1980.
   An excellent editorial review on renal osteodystrophy and the rationale and method of treatment.

Roxe, DM: Toxic nephropathy from diagnostic and therapeutic agents. Am J Med 69: 759, 1980.
   This article provides a brief review of diagnostic and therapeutic drugs which have nephrotoxicity, and reviews the mechanism of toxicity.

Specific

1. Bauer, JH and Brooks, CS: The long-term effect of propranolol therapy on renal function. Am J Med 66: 405, 1979.
2. Bennett, WM, Muther, RS, Parker, RA, Feig, P, Morrison, G, Golper, TA and Singer, I: Drug therapy in renal failure: dosing guidelines for adults. Part I and Part 2. Ann Intern Med 93: 62 and 286, 1980.
3. Bennett, WM, Plamp, C and Porter, GA: Drug-related syndromes in clinical nephropathy. Ann Intern Med 87: 582, 1977.
4. Bricker, NS, Bourgoignie, JJ and Weber, H: The renal response to progressive nephron loss. In The Kidney, Vol. 1, edited by BM Brenner and FC Rector. W.B. Saunders, Philadelphia, 1976.
5. Coburn, JW: Renal osteodystrophy. Kidney Int 17: 677, 1980.
6. Cunningham, JJ: Excretory urography in acute and chronic renal failure. Current concepts and techniques. Urology 5: 303, 1975.
7. Jelliffe, RW and Brooker, G: A nomogram for digoxin therapy. Am J Med 57: 63, 1974.
8. Opelz, G and Terasaki, PI: Prolongation effect of blood transfusions on kidney graft survival. Transplantation 22: 380, 1976.
9. Phelps, KR, Lieberman, RL, Oh, MS and Carroll, HJ: Pathophysiology of the syndrome of hyporeninemic hypoaldosteronism. Metabolism 29: 186, 1980.
10. Popovich, RP, Moncrief, JW, Nolph, KD, Ghods, AJ, Twardowski, ZJ and Pyle, WK: Continuous ambulatory peritoneal dialysis. Ann Intern Med 88: 449, 1978.
11. Rowe, JW, Andres, R, Tobin, JD, Norris, AH and Shock, NW: Age-adjusted standards for creatinine clearance. Ann Intern Med 84: 567, 1976.
12. Yu, T, Berger, L, Dorph, DJ and Smith, H: Renal function in gout Factors influencing the renal hemodynamics. Am J Med 67: 766, 1979.

CHAPTER FORTY-FIVE

Bladder Outlet Obstruction

JAMES K. SMOLEV, M.D.

INTRODUCTION

The bladder, bladder outlet, prostate, and urethra may be affected by a wide variety of conditions which result in symptoms of urinary obstruction or bladder irritability. These disorders are very common. Annually, there are 5.6 office visits per 100 population for diseases of the urinary system, and the frequency of these visits increases with age to approximately 10 visits per 100 population of those over 65 years of age (1). A significant proportion of these visits are for various infections of the urinary tract which are discussed in detail in Chapter 26. This chapter will provide a practical approach to patients with bladder outlet obstruction.

Bladder outlet obstruction is characterized by symptoms of urinary hesitancy, diminished force and caliber of the stream, and postvoid dribbling. Urinary frequency and nocturia result from a diminished bladder capacity caused by bladder muscle hypertrophy. The hypertrophy results in increased intravesical pressure during voiding thereby providing compensation for the obstruction. In time however, the bladder will decompensate which will lead to the presence of residual urine, infection, hematuria, hydronephrosis, and renal failure.

Benign prostatic hyperplasia (BPH) is the commonest cause of bladder outlet obstruction in males over 50 years of age. Autopsy studies have shown that 50 to 60% of men over 50 have significant enlargement of the prostate due to BPH and the prevalence increases with age. A number of other conditions may also cause symptoms of bladder outlet obstruction in the male: urethral stricture; carcinoma of the prostate; neurogenic bladder; bladder calculus; prostatitis (which may be repressed with antibiotics—see Chapter 26); bladder neck contracture; and carcinoma of the bladder. Also, functional obstruction, seen in both women and men, may result from chronic bladder distention, debilitating disease, psychogenic retention, or medications.

The primary physician can usually arrive at a working diagnosis and determine the need for a referral—either urgently or electively—by reviewing the patient's history, physical examination and performing several laboratory tests.

HISTORY

Patients with urethral stricture usually have a history of prior urethral trauma, instrumentation (most commonly, indwelling Foley catheter), or urethritis and, in association with symptoms of bladder outlet obstruction, may notice a split urine stream. Carcinoma of the prostate may present with obstructive symptoms which are often of a shorter duration than those seen in patients with BPH. Furthermore, symptoms of back or bone pain, anorexia, or weight loss suggest malignancy. Neurogenic bladder should be suspected when other symptoms of neurologic disease are present, when disorders of bowel or sexual function coexist with bladder outlet obstruction, or when a systemic disease which causes neurologic bladder dysfunction (such as diabetes mellitus or tabes dorsalis) exists.

A history of current and recently used medications (Table 45.1) is mandatory in the evaluation of the patient with symptoms of bladder outlet obstruction. Anticholinergic agents (antispasmodic and antiparkinsonian drugs) as well as many antidepressant drugs depress bladder muscle contractility; sympathomimetic agents (such as ephedrine) increase bladder outlet resistance. A diuresis (such as from a diuretic, glucosuria, or a large, brisk fluid intake) may overstretch a partially compensated detrusor muscle and cause acute urinary retention.

It is important to distinguish *bladder outlet obstructive symptoms*—hesitancy, decreased stream, postvoid dribbling, from *irritative bladder symptoms*—frequency, urgency, nocturia. Although anatomic or functional obstruction may produce both types of symptoms, only irritative symptoms are seen with cystitis (see Chapter 26), bladder stones (see Chapter

Table 45.1
Pharmacologic Agents with Known Influence On Bladder Function

DRUGS WHICH INCREASE BLADDER TONE AND CONTRACTILITY:
   Bethanecol (Urecholine)
DRUGS WHICH DECREASE BLADDER CONTRACTILITY:
   Anticholinergic drugs (e.g., Pro-Banthine or Donnatal)
   Antidepressent drugs (e.g., Elavil or Tofranil)
DRUGS WHICH INCREASE BLADDER OUTLET RESISTENCE:
   Antiparkinson drugs (e.g., Levodopa or Sinemet)
   Sympathomimetic drugs (e.g., Actifed, Brethine, Dexedrine, Isuprel, Novafed, Sudafed, Triaminic)
DRUGS WHICH INCREASE URINARY VOLUME:
   Diuretics

43), and bladder carcinoma. Finally, the differentiation of polyuria from urinary frequency, and nocturia from enuresis (bedwetting) can be made by appropriate questioning.

PHYSICAL EXAMINATION

The physical examination of the patient with symptoms of bladder outlet obstruction should be thorough, with special emphasis on the urinary tract.

The *abdominal examination* may reveal several findings: a distended bladder from retention, renal tenderness (from infection or hydronephrosis) or a renal mass (from hydronephrosis), inguinal herniae from straining at urination when outlet obstruction is present. In the male, the *examination of the penis* may reveal phimosis or urethral meatal stenosis which could cause obstruction. The *examination of the epididymides* may show evidence of acute or chronic infection which is a complication of bladder outlet obstruction. A brief *neurologic examination*, particularly of the anal sphincter tone, genital and perineal sensation, and motor, sensory, and reflex activity of the lower extremities may disclose abnormalities which would suggest a neurogenic bladder as the cause of the patient's symptoms.

A careful *rectal examination* of the prostate is important in evaluating the patient with suspected BPH or prostate carcinoma even though there are certain limits: rectal palpation permits examination only of the posterior lobes of the prostate and BPH most commonly involves the unpalpable lateral and median lobes; moreover, the size of the prostate gland as estimated by rectal examination is not directly related to the degree of urinary obstruction.

The most important information obtained from the rectal examination is the *consistency* of the prostate gland. In patients with prostate enlargement, BPH can be differentiated from prostatic carcinoma with over 75% certainty based on the rectal examination. The patient may be examined in the decubitus, knee-chest, or standing-bending position. The patient should void as fully as possible before the examination since a full bladder will distort the size of the prostate. To prevent anal sphincter spasm, appropriate time should be used to explain the procedure to the patient. Using ample lubricant, the anal sphincter should be slowly and gently dilated by gradual insertion of the finger through the anus asking the patient to bear down slightly. This examination will permit the determination of shape and consistency of the prostate as well as the presence of tenderness and of the adequacy of sphincter tone.

The normal prostate is palpable 2 to 5 cm from the anal verge through the anterior rectal wall. The examining finger can normally reach over the top (base) of the prostate, as well as over each lateral border. A median sulcus is appreciated in the midline. The posterior lobes of the prostate can be compared in size, configuration, and consistency with the tip of the nose.

BPH not only often results in obliteration of the median sulcus, but also the examining finger may not reach the base of the gland. The consistency of the gland in BPH is smooth, and rubbery—very similar to the thenar eminence of the hand. The gland is not tender unless prostatitis is present. BPH may be characterized by symmetrical or asymmetrical enlargement and by distinct nodules called spheroids. The clinical differentiation between carcinoma and asymmetric or nodular BPH is based on the degree of induration or hardness of the gland.

Classically, prostatic carcinoma is characterized by a rock hard nodule or mass involving one or both posterior lobes. Palpation of the zygomatic arch of the face offers a similar consistency to prostatic carcinoma. However, not all hard nodules will be found on biopsy to be cancer. In approximately 30 to 40%, there will be granulomatous prostatitis, prostatic calculi, spheroids of BPH, or nodularity resulting from transurethral prostatic resection.

If the physician is suspicious of prostatic carcinoma it is important to determine the extent of the local lesion—single nodule, diffuse involvement, or extension outside the capsule and to refer the patient to a urologist.

PRELIMINARY LABORATORY ASSESSMENT

At this juncture in the evaluation of the patient who has symptoms of bladder outlet obstruction which are felt to be due to BPH, the general physician must determine the need and urgency for urological consultation. A urinalysis, urine culture (if pyuria is present), and a measurement of serum creatinine or creatinine clearance will provide the information necessary to make this decision.

If the patient does not have hematuria, urinary tract infection, or renal failure and if the diagnosis of BPH is likely, further evaluation will depend on whether the patient is a candidate for surgery (Table

Table 45.2
Indications for Surgery in Patients Who Are Thought to Have Benign Prostatic Hyperplasia

Acute urinary retention[a]
Epididymitis (especially if recurrent)
Hematuria
Recurrent urinary tract infections
Renal failure[a]
Chronic symptoms which are intolerable.

[a] Necessitate urgent urologic referral.

45.2). If there is no indication for surgery, then no further evaluation is, at this juncture, necessary.

UROLOGIC INVESTIGATION

When surgery is a consideration and a patient is referred to a urologist, several further assessments are frequently made.

Radiology

Intravenous pyelography (IVP) is usually performed in order to determine whether there is hydronephrosis or other structural disease of the urinary tract. Besides assessing the upper urinary tract, this study may demonstrate bladder trabeculations or significant residual urine. The pelvic and vertebral bones can also be evaluated and may provide a clue to the presence of metastatic prostatic cancer.

If a patient has a history of an allergic reaction to intravenous contrast material, there are several alternative methods for studying the urinary tract. *Renal ultrasound* is useful in the detection of significant obstruction. Depending on the agent used, a *renal scan* may be used to demonstrate renal blood flow or delayed excretion suggesting obstruction. A *retrograde pyelogram* done in conjunction with cystoscopy (see below) will provide visualization of dilated ureters. The dye used during this procedure is not absorbed and can be used safely in allergic patients.

If an IVP is felt to be mandatory in a patient with a history of previous mild to moderate reaction, there is approximately a 35% chance of reaction. A decision to perform a study in this instance must be made on an individual basis and in consultation with the radiologist and urologist and the guidelines suggested in Chapter 22 should be followed. If the history suggests a urethral stricture, a *retrograde urethrogram* may be performed. This procedure requires urethral catheterization, instillation of contrast material, and then the obtaining of an X-ray while the patient is voiding. There is no need for anesthesia during this procedure, and there is only minimal discomfort during insertion of the catheter.

Instrumentation

A urologist will gain considerable information in the evaluation of a patient with symptoms of bladder outlet obstruction by performing several invasive procedures. Because these procedures may be associated with the development of infection they should not be done casually.

BLADDER CATHETERIZATION FOR POSTVOID VOLUME

Inserting a urethral catheter immediately after a patient has voided will determine the amount of residual urine (greater than 100 ml is abnormal), as well as help determine if there is a urethral stricture. (While it is possible for the general physician to perform this procedure no information will be obtained which would then lead to a decision to refer the patient.) If a neurogenic bladder is suspected as a cause of the patient's symptoms, a cystometrogram may be done by the urologist using the same catheter. These procedures can be accomplished in 15 min in an office or outpatient department with minimal discomfort and few complications.

CYSTOURETHROSCOPY

Patient Experience. Cystoscopy may easily be done in a urologist's office using local anesthesia. When performed under these conditions, the patient will often perceive a feeling of suprapubic pressure as the bladder is being filled with the irrigating fluid, but the degree of discomfort is usually slight. Examination of the entire urethra, prostate, and bladder takes just a few minutes. However if a retrograde pyelogram is performed, another 15 min may be required. Following cystoscopy, patients will often experience marked dysuria. The patient should have been advised about this and informed that it may be relieved by voiding while sitting in a bath tub filled with warm water or by taking phenazopyridine (Pyridium) 100 mg 3 to 4 times a day. Hematuria following cystoscopy is also common and may persist for 2 or 3 days. The patient should be informed of this possibility, reassured that it is benign, and advised to force fluids (2 to 3 liters/day) should it occur. Infection in the urinary tract occurs only rarely following cystoscopy. Occasionally, acute urinary retention occurs from edema of the prostate subsequent to instrumentation. If this complication occurs, the insertion of an indwelling catheter and hospitalization are necessary. An uncommon long term complication of cystoscopy is urethral stricture. The use of newer, smaller instruments is likely to eliminate this complication.

The urologist learns a great deal from the cystoscopic examination. The entire urethra is seen. The size of the prostate, the degree of occlusiveness, trabeculation in the bladder, and diverticula are all directly visualized. This information is most important in helping the urologist decide the need for and the type of surgery.

TREATMENT OF BLADDER OUTLET OBSTRUCTION

Benign Prostatic Hypertrophy

The only currently available treatment for BPH is prostatectomy. In the future, pharmacological therapy which diminishes the size of an obstructing gland may be available.

The urologist removes the obstructing prostatic tissue either transurethrally (TURP), or by one of the open operative approaches (suprapubic or perineal). The particular approach used will depend on a combination of the condition of the patient, the size and configuration of the prostate gland, and the urologist's experience. In general, glands which are very large are removed by open prostatectomy and smaller glands by TURP.

TRANSURETHRAL RESECTION OF THE PROSTATE

TURP is the most commonly used procedure in the treatment of BPH.

Patient Experience. TURP requires hospitalization for 4 to 7 days; general or spinal anesthesia is used and the procedure is usually well tolerated.

Complications have been minimized by the use of smaller more efficient instruments, and improved lighting and irrigating fluids. Nevertheless, bleeding, infection, and hyponatremia (from absorption of irrigation fluid) occur. Long term complications or TURP include *urethral stricture* (see below), *bladder neck contracture*, and *incontinence* (see below). A frequent consequence of TURP is *retrograde ejaculation*—a situation characterized by the ejaculation of semen into the bladder rather than externally through the urethra. This phenomenon occurs because the bladder neck is resected as part of the TURP and, therefore, cannot subsequently contract as is necessary to produce antegrade ejaculation. This consequence should be discussed with sexually active patients and their partners before prostatectomy. TURP should not produce organic erectile impotence; however, psychologic impotence may follow genitourinary surgery.

After TURP most patients can resume normal physical and sexual activity after 4 weeks of convalescence. Complete healing of the prostatic fossa, however, usually takes 2 to 3 months.

OPEN PROSTATECTOMY

Open prostatectomy requires a slightly longer hospitalization and recovery period. This approach is used when, in addition to having a large prostate, the patient has a coincidental bladder condition which can be repaired at the same time (*e.g.*, bladder diverticulum or bladder stone). Organic erectile impotence occurs occasionally, especially when the perineal approach has been used. If this complication occurs an evaluation should be performed (see Chapter 17) before attributing the impotence to the surgery and presuming it to be irreversible.

It is very important for a patient undergoing any form of prostatectomy for BPH to understand that the entire prostate gland is not removed. Because of the presence of residual prostate tissue, these patients remain at risk equal to the general population, of developing prostatic carcinoma. Rectal examinations

should be done every 12 months, therefore, to detect changes which may suggest malignancy. Also, because residual prostatic tissue remains, there may develop later recurrent symptoms or complications from prostatic hypertrophy.

Urethral Stricture

A urethral stricture may be treated either with urethral dilation, transurethral incision of the stricture, or open urethral surgery. The method will be individualized depending on the length and location of the stricture, the patient's overall health, and the urologist's experience.

Prostatic Carcinoma

The therapy of prostatic carcinoma is somewhat controversial but may be approached based on the stage of the disease (Table 45.3).

Stage A prostatic carcinoma is disease unsuspected on rectal examination of the prostate, but which is discovered at the time of prostatectomy done for obstructive symptoms. In this instance, the urologist will initiate a metastatic evaluation for carcinoma of the prostate by obtaining a serum acid phosphatase determination, bone scan, and intravenous pyelogram.

In the situation of Stage A disease, controversy exists regarding the most accurate method of further classification. Studies (5) have shown that first level lymph nodes (the obturator and iliac nodes) are positive in from 12 to 50% of prostatic cancers which are found only on pathologic examinations. Because of this, the procedures of lymphangiography, computerized tomography (CT) scanning, and open surgical lymphadenectomy all have advocates as well as detractors.

If there is no evidence for lymph node involvement, the prostatic tissue that has been resected should be re-examined to determine the percentage of the tissue involved by carcinoma. If less than 5% of the available tissue is cancer—and if it is well-differentiated—then *Stage A₁ disease* is present, and no further therapy is required. Careful follow-up by a urologist every 3 to 6 months for 3 years and then yearly is necessary, to determine recurrence by performing

Table 45.3
Staging of Prostatic Carcinoma

Stage	Description
A	Clinically undetectable; found on pathologic examination after prostatectomy
A₁	Focal; well-differentiated
A₂	Diffuse; poorly differentiated
B	Limited to prostate on rectal examination
B₁	Solitary nodule; <1.5 cm; one lobe
B₂	One whole lobe or both lobes
C	Locally extending outside of prostatic capsule or seminal vesicles
D	Distant metastases

Table 45.4
Survival with Prostatic Carcinoma with Treatment Except as Noted

Stage	% Survival	
	5-Year	15-Year
A_1	Normal life expectancy	
A_2	50%	
$B_1{}^a$	85–90%^{c}	50%
$B_2{}^b$	20%	1%
C	50%	
D	50% (3 yr)	

^{a} Radical surgery.
^{b} Untreated.
^{c} Survival is better than Stage A_2 probably because the cancer can be detected on examination and may be therefore detected earlier; also A_2 is a larger more poorly differentiated cancer.

rectal examination and perhaps cytoscopy. If a larger percentage of the tissue is cancer, or if it is less well differentiated, the classification is *Stage A_2* and most authorities recommend definitive radiotherapy as the treatment (6). Radiation cystitis and proctitis occur with this form of treatment in approximately 30% and 25%, respectively; but frequently symptoms can be controlled with treatment.

Stage B carcinoma is defined as disease limited to the prostate gland and is detected clinically either as a nodule or as diffuse hardness of a lobe. If less than one lobe is involved and if the patient is under 70 years of age and has no contraindicating medical diseases, he is a candidate for curative radical prostatectomy. In the hands of a urologist experienced in this type of surgery, the operative complication of incontinence can be minimized. However, impotence invariably accompanies radical prostatectomy and the patient will need ultimately to be treated with a penile prosthesis if he and his partner desire. An alternative treatment is curative radiotherapy when surgery is unacceptable or not possible.

Most extensive localized prostatic cancer, Stage C, is best treated by definitive radiotherapy (5). If bladder outlet obstruction is also present, the patient may also need a TURP and this occasionally will need to be repeated.

Metastatic or *Stage D* prostatic cancer is best managed by hormonal therapy when symptoms require treatment. Studies by the Veterans Administration Cooperative Urological Research Group (VACURG) have shown that hormonal therapy initiated at the time of diagnosis does not prolong survival compared to hormonal therapy initiated only in response to symptoms (such as bone pain) (3, 4). Diethylstilbestrol (1 to 3 mg/day) and orchiectomy give similar results, producing a 85 to 90% partial symptomatic response rate in previously untreated patients. The duration of response is on the average 18 months although prolonged remissions have been documented. There is no advantage to combining orchiectomy and estrogen therapy. Generally, estrogen therapy, which causes salt and water retention, should be avoided in patients who also have an edema-forming illness not controlled by diuretics. Investigation is under way to evaluate cytotoxic chemotherapy in all stages of prostatic carcinoma (2).

Much of the controversy in the diagnosis and treatment of prostatic cancer results from the inability to assess accurately the influence of prostate cancer on longevity. Prostate cancer occurs in older men who often have coexisting diseases which influence longevity. Also, the natural history of the disease is not well understood. The best estimates for survival with various stages of prostatic cancer with the treatments discussed above are listed in Table 45.4.

References

General

Catalona, WJ and Scott, WW: Carcinoma of the prostate. In *Campbell's Urology*, Ed. 4, edited by JH Harrison, RF Gittes, AD Perlmutter, TA Stamey and PC Walsh. W. B. Saunders, Philadelphia, 1979.

Walsh, PC: Benign prostate hyperplasia. In *Campbell's Urology*, Ed. 4, edited by JH Harrison, RF Gittes, AD Perlmutter, TA Stamey and PC Walsh. W. B. Saunders, Philadelphia, 1979.

   Both chapters provide an in-depth review of their respective subjects.

Specific

1. *Advancedata: U.S. Dept. of Health and Human Services. No. 63 Nov. 3, 1980.*
2. Anderson, T: Chemotherapy of urologic cancer—principles and practice. In *Principles and Management of Urologic Cancer*, edited by N. Javadpour. Williams & Wilkins, Baltimore, 1979.
3. Bailar, JC and Byar, DP: Estrogen treatment for cancer of the prostate: early results with three doses of diethylstilbestrol and placebo. *Cancer 26*: 257, 1970.
4. Byar, DP: The Veterans Administration Cooperative Urologic Research Group's studies of cancer of the prostate. *Cancer 32*: 1126, 1973.
5. Catalona, WJ and Scott, WW: Carcinoma of the prostate: a review. *J Urol 119*: 1, 1978.
6. Whitmore, WF, Jr, Batata, M and Hilaris, B: Prostate irradiation: iodine-125 implantation. in *Cancer of the Genitourinary Tract*, edited by DE Johnson and ML Samuels. Raven Press, New York, 1979.

SECTION 6

Hematologic Problems

CHAPTER FORTY-SIX

Anemia

LARRY WATERBURY, M.D.

GENERAL CONSIDERATIONS

Anemia, a reduction of the proportion of red cells or of hemoglobin in the blood, is a condition, like hypoxia or jaundice, which always reflects a primary underlying disease. Although there are sometimes symptoms (e.g., shortness of breath on exertion) or signs (e.g., pallor) which are associated with anemia, the diagnosis of the condition is essentially dependent on one or more laboratory measurements—such as the hematocrit value (the proportion of centrifuged packed red cells in a volume of blood) or the hemoglobin concentration. In general, anemia is defined in a man as a condition in which the hematocrit value is less than 42% or the hemoglobin concentration less than 14 g/100 ml and in a woman as a hematocrit value less than 37% or a hemoglobin concentration less than 12g/100 ml. When anemia is diagnosed, other measurements, described below, are important in establishing the cause of the process and in leading the clinician to appropriate therapy.

Most of the routine complete blood counts (CBC) obtained in clinical practice in this country are determined by automated counting methods (Table 46.1). The CBC usually reports the hemoglobin concentration (Hgb), hematocrit value (Hct), red blood cell count (RBC), white cell count, mean corpuscular volume (MCV), mean corpuscular hemoglobin (MCH), and mean corpuscular hemoglobin concentration (MCHC). One commonly used automated system (Coulter) measures the hemoglobin, RBC, and MCV, and from these variables calculates the hematocrit value, MCH, and MCHC. With the use of the automated counters the indices (MCH, MCHC, MCV), especially the MCV, are precise, accurate measurements which can be utilized in approaching the diagnostic workup of anemia. The calculated Hct value is a few percentage points lower than that obtained by centrifugation (packed cells trap plasma, distorting the ratio of red cells to plasma).

Table 46.1
Representative Normal Values (Coulter S)

	Men	Women
Hemoglobin (Hgb), g/dl blood	14–18	12–16
Hematocrit (Hct), %	42–54	37–47
Mean corpuscular volume (MCV), fl	82–98	82–98
Mean corpuscular hemoglobin (MCH), pg	27–32	27–32
Mean corpuscular hemoglobin concentration (MCHC), g/dl red blood cells	31.5–36	31.5–36

APPROACH TO EVALUATION OF ANEMIA

The routine data base which should be obtained on every anemic patient includes the hematocrit value, hemoglobin concentration, MCV, MCHC, and reticulocyte count. A smear of the peripheral blood should be obtained by fingerstick or from unanticoagulated blood on the tip of a venipuncture needle. (Anticoagulants distort the morphology of the blood cells.) The smear may be stained in the physician's office or transported to an outside laboratory to be stained and interpreted. On the basis of all of these data, and a complete history and physical examination, the physician can progress a long way toward an etiologic diagnosis of the anemia. Three questions should be asked:

1. *What is the MCV?* With the use of the automated counters the MCV is a direct measurement of red cell size. The normal range varies with individual laboratories but is approximately 82 to 98 femtoliters (fl). Actually it is helpful to use a broader normal range of 80 to 100 fl to classify the anemia as microcytic (MCV less than 80 fl), normocytic (MCV 80 to 100 fl), or macrocytic (MCV greater than 100 fl). Microcytic and macrocytic anemias have very limited differential diagnoses, and therefore by simply noting the MCV the physician can limit greatly the diagnostic approach when the anemia is microcytic or macrocytic.

2. *What is the Basic Mechanism of the Anemia?* There are only three ways patients become anemic: (a) decreased effective production of red cells by bone marrow, (b) bleeding, or (c) hemolysis. The most helpful laboratory measurement in defining the mechanism of anemia is the reticulocyte count. The *reticulocyte count* is used to assess the appropriateness of the response of the bone marrow to anemia. The normal reticulocyte count is approximately 1%, representing the 1% of new cells which are released into the circulation from the bone marrow daily (the ordinary red cell life span being in the range of 100 days). Under the stimulus of erythropoietin, in the anemic patient the bone marrow should be able to triple acutely its output of new cells; when anemia is chronic and severe, the bone marrow may be able to increase its output of cells to 8 to 10 times normal.

This increased bone marrow activity is reflected in an appropriately elevated reticulocyte count. The reticulocyte count must be adjusted for the level of anemia to obtain a value known as the *reticulocyte index* (Table 46.2), a more accurate reflection of erythropoiesis. In patients with bleeding or hemolysis the reticulocyte index should be at least 3%, whereas in patients with anemia due to decreased production of red cells the reticulocyte index is less than 3%, and usually less than 1.5%.

In addition to the reticulocyte index serial hematocrit values over a few days or weeks may provide the physician with clues to the mechanism of the anemia. Total shutdown of production in the marrow in the absence of bleeding or hemolysis will result in a fall in the hematocrit value of only 3 or 4 percentage points per week. If the value has fallen more rapidly, bleeding or hemolysis must have taken place. Anemia with an appropriate reticulocyte response in the absence of bleeding usually means hemolysis.

3. *Does the Patient Have Another Problem that Is Commonly Associated with Anemia?* Table 46.3 lists anemias commonly associated with various clinical characteristics and diseases. For this purpose race and sex are also taken into consideration. Women are more frequently iron deficient than are men and black patients are more likely than are whites to have hemoglobinopathies or glucose-6-phosphate dehydrogenase deficiency.

In summary, the initial data base should enable the physician to classify the anemia on the basis of the MCV, to categorize the basic mechanism of the anemia, and to consider possible causes based upon the patient's problem list. This initial assessment should then suggest the appropriate further diagnostic workup.

ANEMIA WITH A LOW MCV

Table 46.4 lists those anemias commonly associated with a low MCV. For the most part the diagnosis rests between iron deficiency anemia and thalassemia. Occasionally the anemia of chronic inflammation and, even more rarely, sideroblastic anemia are microcytic, although more often they are normocytic or, in the case of sideroblastic anemia, sometimes macrocytic.

Iron Deficiency Anemia

Although dietary iron deficiency does occur in the infant and during the rapid growth phase of adoles-

Table 46.2
Reticulocyte Index

$$\text{Reticulocyte index} = \text{reticulocyte count} \times \frac{\text{patient hct}}{\text{normal hct}}$$

Example: reticulocyte count 6%, hematocrit 15%

$$\text{Reticulocyte index} = 6 \times \frac{15}{45} = 2\%$$

Table 46.3
Anemias Associated with Various Clinical Characteristics

FEMALE: Iron deficiency

BLACKS: Glucose-6-phosphate dehydrogenase (G-6-PD) deficiency, hemoglobinopathies, thalassemia

MEDITERRANEAN ORIGIN: G-6-PD deficiency, thalassemia

FAR EAST ORIGIN: Hemoglobinopathies

VIRAL INFECTIONS: Immune hemolysis. Decreased production

BACTERIAL INFECTION:
  Anemia of inflammation
  Microangiopathic hemolysis
  Oxidative hemolysis (G-6-PD deficiency)
  Other hemolytic mechanisms

MALIGNANCY:
  Microangiopathic hemolysis
  Immune hemolysis
  Decreased production

ALCOHOLIC LIVER DISEASE:
  Bleeding
  Hypersplenism
  Folate deficiency
  Decreased production
  Sideroblastic anemia
  Iron deficiency
  Hemolysis

HYPER-HYPOTHYROIDISM:
  Decreased production
  Pernicious anemia
  Iron deficiency

RENAL FAILURE:
  Decreased production
  Hemolysis
  Bleeding

AORTIC VALVE REPLACEMENT: Microangiopathic hemolysis

MALIGNANT HYPERTENSION: Microangiopathic hemolysis

RHEUMATOID SYNDROMES:
  Anemia of inflammation
  Iron deficiency
  Immune hemolysis

COLLAGEN VASCULAR DISEASE:
  Immune hemolysis
  Anemia of inflammation

DRUGS:
  Aldomet: Immune hemolysis
  Quinine/quinidine: Immune hemolysis
  Penicillin: Immune hemolysis (rare)
  Butazolidin/Chloramphenicol: Dose related marrow depression; Idiosyncratic aplastic anemia
  Gold: Aplastic anemia
  Antituberculosis drugs: Sideroblastic anemia
  Dilantin: Megaloblastic anemia (folate). Pure red cell aplasia
  Sulfa: G-6-PD hemolysis

cence, in this country iron deficiency generally occurs only as a result of bleeding. Iron deficiency from menstruation and from pregnancy is extremely common in women; but iron deficiency in a man or in a postmenopausal woman should be considered to be due to gastrointestinal bleeding until proven otherwise.

DIAGNOSIS

The history and physical examination may yield information that suggests the presence of iron deficiency. Such information includes a history of multiple past pregnancies in a woman; strange dietary habits such as the eating of ice, starch, or clay (pica); any past history of gastrointestinal bleeding, a sore tongue, brittle and ridged fingernails, spoon nails, and cheilosis. The physical findings are seen only after iron deficiency has been long standing and severe.

Most of the body's iron is incorporated in hemoglobin, but approximately one-third of it is stored in reticuloendothelial sites, primarily in the spleen, liver, and bone marrow. In patients with slow continued bleeding the reticuloendothelial iron stores supply the bone marrow's requirement for iron until the stores are depleted. It is at this point that iron deficiency anemia begins to develop. In iron deficiency cell size (MCV) correlates with the degree of anemia, so that very mild iron deficiency anemia may be associated with normal sized cells (8). The MCV progressively decreases as the anemia becomes more severe, but the mean corpuscular hemoglobin concentration (MCHC), usually remains normal until the hematocrit value falls below 30%. As the anemia becomes more marked, the red cells also become progressively more distorted (poikilocytosis). Table 46.5 illustrates the relationship between the hematocrit value, the MCV, and the degree of red cell distortion (poikilocytosis) seen in iron deficiency anemia.

Often the diagnosis of iron deficiency is obvious after the initial history, physical examination, and standard laboratory evaluation. If not, a number of other tests may be useful: The *reticulocyte index* is inappropriately low for the degree of anemia. The *serum iron* concentration (SI) is low but is usually low also in patients with acute and chronic inflammation and malignancy. Furthermore, an acute infectious process such as pneumococcal pneumonia will cause an immediate drop in the serum iron even though the patient is not iron-deficient. Classically, the *total iron binding capacity* (TIBC) is elevated. It is a measure of the serum transferrin, the iron transport protein which supplies bone marrow reticulocytes with iron. However, many iron-deficient patients have a normal TIBC, and it may be low in cases of chronic inflammation or of malignancy whether or not iron deficiency is present. The *bone marrow iron stain* is the most definitive way to prove a diagnosis of iron deficiency, since iron stores are

Table 46.4
Causes of Anemia with Low Mean Corpuscular Volume (MCV)

Iron deficiency
Thalassemia
Anemia of chronic inflammation (occasionally)
Sideroblastic anemia (rarely)

Table 46.5
Representative Data Base at Various Stages in the Slow Development of Severe Iron Deficiency Anemia[a]

Hct	42	42	35	27	19
MCV (82–98 fl)	92	88	82	75	68
MCHC (32–36 g/dl)	33	33	33	31	29
SI (65–175 µg/dl)	70	60	35	20	20
TIBC (250–375 µg/dl)	300	300	300	400	450
Serum ferritin (10–200 µg/ml)	60	30	5	3	1
Peripheral smear	Normal	Normal	Normal	1+ poikilocytosis 1+ hypo-chromia	4+ poikilocytosis 4+ hypo-chromia
Bone marrow iron stores	Present	Absent	Absent	Absent	Absent

[a] Hct, hematocrit; MCV, mean corpuscular volume; MCHC, mean corpuscular hemoglobin; SI, serum iron; TIBC, total iron binding capacity. Numbers in parentheses are the range of normal values.

Table 46.6
Inappropriately Normal or Elevated Serum Ferritin Levels

Acute liver disease
Cirrhosis
Hodgkin's disease
Acute leukemias
Solid tumors (occasional)
Fever
Acute inflammation
Renal dialysis patients
Recent treatment with iron

depleted when iron deficiency anemia is present and are normal or elevated in patients with microcytic anemia due to other causes.

Recently, *serum ferritin* has become very helpful in the assessment of body iron stores (12). Ferritin is a water-soluble complex of iron and a binding protein, apoferritin. In general, the serum ferritin concentration reflects the status of the reticuloendothelial stores. A low serum ferritin almost always reflects iron deficiency. A very elevated serum ferritin usually signifies iron overload, as in the patient who has received multiple transfusions. There are, however, a number of clinical situations in which the serum ferritin may be spuriously normal or even elevated in the presence of iron deficiency anemia (Table 46.6). In these situations it may be difficult to make a definitive diagnosis of iron deficiency without a bone marrow iron stain.

TREATMENT

After institution of oral iron therapy, the reticulocyte response is maximal at around 7 to 10 days. The hematocrit value begins to rise after about 1 week, and in the uncomplicated case a normal hematocrit value is reached in a few weeks. However, it takes many months of therapy for patients subsequently to replete their iron stores. In the menstruating woman with iron deficiency anemia, treatment for a year may be necessary; and in the man with iron defi-

ciency anemia, treatment for 6 months is frequently indicated. Iron deficiency is very common in the menstruating woman, especially in those with heavy menstrual periods and a history of multiple pregnancies. Some may require constant iron therapy to maintain a normal hematocrit value. Standard treatment with oral iron consists of 1 tablet of iron (e.g., ferrous sulfate, 300 mg which contains 60 mg of elemental iron) 3 times daily on an empty stomach (1 hour before meals). If it is difficult for patients to take the noontime dose, it is reasonable to omit it. There are numerous preparations of iron other than ferrous sulfate, but there is usually no justification for recommending any of them unless a reduction in the dose of elemental iron is required (see below). It is especially important to avoid time release spansules and enteric coated preparations. They are costly, and absorption is variable. Preparations containing iron, including ferrous sulfate, can be obtained without prescription. The most vigorously promoted iron preparation, Geritol, costs the patient approximately 5 times as much as ferrous sulfate. The addition of ascorbic acid to iron preparations to increase absorption is not worth the cost.

Approximately 15% of patients have gastrointestinal side effects from oral iron, most commonly constipation, but abdominal cramping and diarrhea are also seen. When such side effects develop, the physician may elect to administer iron only once a day, or he may instruct the patient to take his iron with meals instead of on an empty stomach. Taking iron with food will decrease iron absorption by approximately 50%, but absorption will still be sufficient to replenish the body's iron if treatment is continued long enough. If symptoms still continue after these alterations in dose and schedule, it is helpful to decrease the individual dose of oral iron. If the dose is decreased to less than 40 mg of elemental iron, symptoms will frequently abate. This can be done by using pediatric liquid preparations which are usually well tolerated. If these adjustments in the dosage and schedule of oral iron administration are made, *parenteral iron* is rarely indicated. Parenteral therapy is indicated, however, in patients with small and large bowel inflammation, rapid gastrointestinal transit, or malabsorption, and when the patient has severe iron deficiency and noncompliance has been repetitively proven. Guidelines for the dosage of parenteral iron are provided in the insert that accompanies each vial. Side effects from parenteral iron include pain and rash at the injection site, staining of the skin, fever, and rare anaphylactoid reactions.

Thalassemia

In the normal adult there are three hemoglobins present in mature red cells: A, the major component, and two minor components, A_2 and F (fetal). Each hemoglobin molecule consists of four heme groups and four globin chains; the globin chains in each molecule are of two different types. All three hemoglobins have two α-globin chains but differ in the second set (β, δ, γ) of globin chains (Table 46.7).

Thalassemia is an inherited defect in either α or β chain production. β-Thalassemia (16) is seen in the United States primarily in black patients or those of Mediterranean (Greek and Italian) origin; the genetics of α-thalassemia are more complicated, and the disorder appears to have a wider racial distribution than does β-thalassemia. Most patients have inherited only one defective gene (heterozygotes) and are clinically asymptomatic but have marked red cell microcytosis. The diagnosis is important as the entity is frequently confused with iron deficiency anemia resulting in life-long repetitive workups for gastrointestinal bleeding and inappropriate treatment with iron. Patients with homozygous β-thalassemia usually do not survive into adulthood; homozygous α-thalassemia is not compatible with life.

DIAGNOSIS

Table 46.8 lists the typical routine data base for the patient with heterozygous α- or β-thalassemia. The combination of a low MCV and a mild anemia should alert the physician to the diagnosis since in iron deficiency the degree of microcytosis parallels the severity of the anemia (see above). This discrepancy between the MCV and the Hct value, plus the frequent presence of coarsely stippled red cells on peripheral smear should result in the presumptive diagnosis of heterozygous thalassemia.

In the forms of β-thalassemia most commonly seen in the United States there is a decreased production

Table 46.3
Heterozygous Thalassemia: Typical Data Base[a]

Hct	37%
MCV	69 fl
MCH	20 pg
MCHC	32 g/dl
Reticulocyte count	2.5%
Red blood cell morphology	Microcytosis, poikilocytosis, stippling
Ferritin	Normal or increased

[a] Abbreviations as in Table 46.5.

of β chains with a compensatory increase in the production of δ chains resulting in a decreased production of hemoglobin A and an increased production of hemoglobin A_2. This increase can be assessed by electrophoresis of the hemoglobin, and is a definitive diagnostic test for β-thalassemia. Less commonly, in this country, increases in hemoglobin F may be seen in patients with β-thalassemia. Hemoglobin F must be assayed by a separate special technique (alkali denaturation test for hemoglobin F).

The α-thalassemias are more difficult to diagnose, since a decreased production of α chains will affect the production of all three of the normal types of hemoglobin. A definitive diagnosis of one of the α-thalassemia syndromes may be quite difficult and may require family studies or techniques available only in research laboratories. However, the diagnosis of presumptive α-thalassemia in the setting of an appropriate data base (hematologic values consistent with the diagnosis in the absence of iron deficiency and of β-thalassemia) is reasonable even in the absence of laboratory confirmation.

PATIENT EDUCATION

It is important for the physician to explain to patients with heterozygous thalassemia that the clinical features of their condition mimic iron deficiency. The patient should be put on guard against repetitive diagnostic workups for iron deficiency. The physician should emphasize the benign nature of the illness and that the anemia, being mild, usually does not cause any symptoms. He should caution the patient against taking oral iron since thalassemic patients actually have an increase in iron stores. Genetic counseling is important; a couple, both heterozygous for β-thalassemia, have a 25% chance of having a child with homozygous thalassemia. Furthermore, the genetic defect for thalassemia and those for hemoglobin S and C are alleles. Hemoglobin S-thalassemia may be a severe disease.

Miscellaneous

The *anemia of chronic disease* and the *anemia of malignancy* may be associated with a low MCV (although the MCV is usually normal). These entities are discussed below in the section dealing with normocytic anemia (p. 394). *Sideroblastic anemias* (char-

Table 46.7
Globin Chain Composition of Normal Adult Hemoglobins

		% of Total in Normal Adults
Hgb A	$\alpha_2\beta_2$	97%
Hgb A_2	$\alpha_2\delta_2$	2%
Hgb F	$\alpha_2\gamma_2$	1%

acterized by increased iron stores and by ringed sideroblasts in the bone marrow) are occasionally microcytic, and some hemoglobinopathies are associated with a low MCV (hemoglobin E). The former are best treated in consultation with a hematologist; the latter are rare in this country.

ANEMIA WITH HIGH MCV

The physician should recognize that an MCV greater than 100 fl is abnormal and an attempt should be made to explain the abnormality. Table 46.9 lists conditions associated with an elevated MCV (6). For the most part, the diseases associated with an elevated MCV are liver disease, the megaloblastic anemias (including drug-induced megaloblastosis), and the refractory anemias with hypercellular bone marrows (preleukemia, sideroblastic anemia). Occasionally an elevated MCV measured by the automatic counter is *spurious*, caused by red cell antibodies or by marked rouleaux formation in patients with a very high erythrocyte sedimentation rate. Since young red cells are large, patients with a marked *reticulocytosis* may have an elevated MCV.

Liver Disease

Chronic hepatocellular and obstructive liver disease results in loading of cholesterol in the lipid portion of the red cell membrane, so that the cell increases in size. Thus the MCV is frequently elevated but is usually not greater than 110 fl. On smears, cells appear to be round and centrally targeted, without significant variation in shape. This morphologic abnormality is not a cause for anemia. However, patients with liver disease frequently have other reasons to be anemic (bleeding, hemolysis, folic acid deficiency). The severe alcoholic often has an elevated MCV even in the absence of overt liver disease or of marked megaloblastosis (7). Presumably the elevated MCV results from either periodic episodes of alcoholic liver disease, or from folic acid deficiency, or both. Owing to poor diet, the alcoholic frequently becomes folic acid-depleted. In addition, alcohol interferes with folic acid metabolism.

Table 46.9
Differential diagnosis of Mean Corpuscular Volume (MCV) Greater Than 100 fl

Spurious
Reticulocytosis (marked)
Liver disease
Alcoholism
Refractory anemia (preleukemia, sideroblastic anemia)
Drugs
Megaloblastic anemias
Normal variant

Table 46.10
Causes of Vitamin B_{12} and Folic Acid Megaloblastosis

B_{12}
  Pernicious anemia (acquired and congenital)
  Gastrectomy
  Ileal resection
  Crohn's disease and tropical sprue
  Fish tapeworm infestation
  Blind loop syndrome
  Nutritional deficiency (vegans diet, rare)
  Familial selective malabsorption (Imerslund's syndrome)
FOLIC ACID
  Dietary (old age, the alcoholic, chronic disease)
  Malabsorption (sprue)
  Hemodialysis
  Severe exfoliative skin disease (*e.g.*, psoriasis)
  Drugs:
    Interference with absorption or utilization (Dilantin, alcohol)
    Dihydrofolate reductase inhibitors (methotrexate, trimethoprim)
  Increased requirements:
  Pregnancy
  Infancy
  Hemolysis (*e.g.*, sickle cell anemia)

Megaloblastic Anemia (11)

Table 46.10 lists the various etiologies of megaloblastic anemia related to vitamin B_{12} or folic acid deficiency. The body's stores of B_{12} are such that a diet without B_{12} (one in which animal protein was completely excluded) would not result in B_{12} induced megaloblastosis for several years; therefore dietary B_{12} deficiency is extremely rare. By far, the most common etiology of B_{12} deficiency is pernicious anemia, an acquired defect of the gastric mucosa resulting in deficient formation of intrinsic factor, a substance which binds ingested B_{12} and allows its absorption in the terminal ileum. Patients with pernicious anemia are usually elderly and complain of sore mouth, indigestion, and constipation or diarrhea. Neurological problems including peripheral neuropathy, dorsal column dysfunction (loss of vibratory and position sense in the lower extremities), and changes in affect are common. The anemia develops so slowly that patients frequently present with very low hematocrit values and yet remarkably good cardiovascular compensation for their anemia. Such patients usually have an expanded total blood volume and are prone to develop heart failure if given transfusions. B_{12} deficiency from other causes (Table 46.10) is less common. Patients who have had total gastrectomy or ileal resection or who have ileal disease (Crohn's disease, tropical sprue) are likely to develop B_{12} deficiency and should receive prophylactic B_{12}. B_{12} deficiency after partial gastrectomy is uncommon.

In contrast to B_{12} the body's stores of folic acid are depleted rapidly when patients eat a diet deficient in folate (the main sources of folate in the diet are leafy vegetables, fruits, nuts, and liver). Folic acid deficiency therefore is most often dietary. For example, pregnant women have an increased need for folate, and without prenatal care may develop folate deficiency, as may patients whose dietary intake is severely restricted because of chronic disease or multiple surgical procedures. Intestinal malabsorption due to any cause is also a common cause of folate deficiency. Finally, a number of drugs may be associated with folate deficiency: Dilantin interferes with folate absorption; alcohol interferes with folate utilization; and methotrexate and trimethoprim-sulfamethoxazole (Bactrim, Septra) interfere with folate metabolism. Also some chemotherapeutic agents used in the treatment of cancer cause megaloblastosis (e.g., hydroxyurea, cytosine arabinoside, 6-mercaptopurine, Imuran) by inhibiting the synthesis of nucleic acids.

DIAGNOSIS

The morphology of the peripheral blood and bone marrow is the same in patients with folic acid and B_{12} deficiencies. With a severe megaloblastic anemia the MCV is frequently markedly elevated. An MCV of greater than 120 fl is almost always due to a megaloblastic anemia. The red cells in the peripheral blood are characterized by marked variation in size and shape. The common cell is a macro-ovalocyte (large egg-shaped cell). One may also see Howell-Jolly bodies (nuclear fragments), Pappenheimer bodies (iron granules), and nucleated red blood cells. The nuclei of the neutrophils are frequently hypersegmented, and commonly there is a neutropenia and thrombocytopenia. The bone marrow is typically markedly cellular revealing characteristic megaloblastic changes of all cell lines. The bone marrow iron stain usually reveals increased numbers of iron-containing nucleated red cells (sideroblasts).

Folic Acid and B_{12} Assay. Classically in B_{12} deficiency (pernicious anemia), the serum B_{12} level is quite low (less than 100 pg/ml) and the serum folate level is high. However, with the currently used radioimmune dilution assays the serum B_{12} level is a less reliable index than in former days when a microbiologic assay was used. Up to 10% of patients with pernicious anemia may have B_{12} levels in the normal range with this technique. In folic acid deficiency typically the serum folate level is quite low (usually less than 2 ng/ml). The serum B_{12} level is usually normal, but, for reasons that are not entirely clear, it may be slightly reduced in up to 50% of patients. Such patients do not need supplementary B_{12}. Table 46.11 lists some important points to remember about serum B_{12} and folic acid assays.

The Schilling Test. The Schilling test is a measure of B_{12} absorption and requires the measurement of total radioactivity excreted during a 24-hour period

Table 46.11
B_{12} and Folic Acid Assays

RADIOIMMUNE SERUM B_{12} ASSAYS
  Technical problems result in false negative and false positive assays
  Perhaps 10% of patients with pernicious anemia will have a normal assay
  The serum B_{12} level is increased in myeloproliferative diseases (polycythemia vera, chronic myeloid leukemia)
  The assay may be unreliable for weeks after parenteral B_{12}
SERUM FOLATE ASSAY
  In dietary folic acid deficiency the folate level is normalized by transfusion or even by eating a few good meals
  The level may become normal if the serum is left with the red cells for several hours because of leakage of folate out of the cells
  If assayed by microbiologic techniques the folate level will be spuriously low if the patient is taking antibiotics

after the ingestion of radioactive B_{12}. This test is primarily useful in cases where the data are confusing, and/or in cases already treated with folate or B_{12}, where the serum levels are no longer helpful. The Schilling test requires a cooperative patient who is able to collect a 24-hour urine sample. The test includes the following steps: After voiding, the patient takes 0.5 μcurie of ^{60}Co or ^{57}Co cyanocobalamine by mouth. A 24-hour urine collection is initiated; at 2 hours 1 mg of B_{12} is given by injection (the flushing dose) and the percentage of the radioactive B_{12} excreted in 24 hours is determined. Normally 7% or more of the dose is excreted in 24 hours. Incomplete collection will result in a spuriously low Schilling test and a false diagnosis of B_{12} malabsorption. In addition, if there is severe megaloblastic anemia, there are changes in the gastrointestinal mucosa which will affect B_{12} absorption. For example, the Schilling test may be abnormal in folic acid deficiency until the megaloblastic process is treated for a week or two.

Other Laboratory Features. Megaloblastic anemias are essentially hemolytic in that there is marked destruction of abnormally formed cells within the marrow (ineffective erythropoiesis) which frequently results in indirect hyperbilirubinemia and an elevated serum lactate dehydrogenase. The serum iron is usually elevated and the reticulocyte index is inappropriately low.

Gastric achlorhydria is present in pernicious anemia, and antibodies to gastric mucosal cells and to intrinsic factor are frequently present, as are other autoantibodies, especially antithyroid and antiadrenal antibodies. There is an increased prevalence of thyroid disease (hypo- and hyperthyroidism and euthyroid goiter) in patients with pernicious anemia.

TREATMENT

The usual treatment for B_{12} deficiency is monthly intramuscular administration of 100 μg of B_{12} for the rest of the patient's life. Many physicians will treat patients daily while they are in the hospital, particularly if they have neurologic signs; however, there is little evidence that this practice is more efficacious.

One to 5 mg of folic acid daily is adequate treatment for patients with folic acid deficiency. Treatment should be given at least until a normal hematocrit level is reached and continued if the patient is not eating an adequate diet or if the underlying disease persists (malabsorption, for example). Patients with a chronic hemolytic state, such as sickle cell anemia, patients on hemodialysis (folic acid is dialyzable), and pregnant patients, should receive prophylactic treatment. Whether or not patients are hospitalized, depends on the severity of their symptoms and signs, the severity of their anemia, and in the case of folate deficiency, the nature of their underlying disease.

With appropriate treatment of megaloblastic anemia there is a rapid reticulocytosis which reaches a peak at about 7 to 10 days; the hematocrit begins to rise in about 1 week; and in uncomplicated cases will rise at a rate of 4 to 5 percentage points per week. The leukopenia and thrombocytopenia respond dramatically and white blood cell and platelet counts may return to normal in a day or two. There is a variable response of the neurologic complications of B_{12} deficiency. "Megaloblastic madness" usually abates dramatically. Dorsal column problems and peripheral neuropathies will usually improve, but more slowly. Cortical spinal tract signs are usually refractory to treatment.

The serum potassium frequently falls with treatment of megaloblastic anemia, and there are case reports of fatal cardiac arrhythmias because of hypokalemia. Therefore it is important to monitor the serum potassium and to supplement it as needed (see Chapter 42).

Refractory Anemia with Hyperplastic Bone Marrow (14)

This uncommon syndrome is an acquired disorder of bone marrow stem cells seen in elderly patients and in many ways may mimic megaloblastic anemia. However, the morphologic features of the bone marrow and usually the peripheral smear, are different (Table 46.12). There are characteristic morphologic white cell changes, the serum B_{12} and folic acid levels are high, and the patients do not respond to folic acid or B_{12}. In the bone marrow ringed sideroblasts (red cell precursors containing granules of iron which form a ring around the nuclei) are common as are megaloblastoid changes. Approximately 25% of patients develop acute nonlymphocytic leukemia, usually within a year, but sometimes only after several years.

ANEMIAS WITH NORMAL MCV AND APPROPRIATE RETICULOCYTE INDEX (HEMOLYSIS AND BLEEDING)

Anemias due to bleeding and hemolysis are associated with an appropriate bone marrow response manifested by an appropriate reticulocyte index. The MCV is usually normal; however, if the reticulocyte count is high, the MCV may be slightly elevated. The diagnosis of hemolysis is suggested by an anemia with a reticulocyte index of at least 3% in the absence of overt bleeding. It should be remembered that bleeding is far more common than hemolysis and that bleeding in certain body sites (e.g., retroperitoneal bleeding in patients taking anticoagulants or bleeding into the site of a hip fracture) may be associated with a marked drop in hematocrit value and a high reticulocyte count, without external evidence of blood loss. Furthermore, the correction of anemias which are due to decreased bone marrow production

Table 46.12
Laboratory Features in Three Conditions Associated with an Elevated Mean Corpuscular Volume (MCV)

	Liver Disease	Megaloblastic Anemia	Refractory Anemia ("Preleukemia")
MCV	Usually <110 fl	Maybe >110 fl	Usually <110 fl
White blood cells (WBCs)	Variable	Frequently decreased	Frequently decreased
Platelets	Variable	Frequently decreased	Frequently decreased
Red blood cell (RBC) morphology	Targets, no anisocytosis and poikilocytosis	Marked anisocytosis and poikilocytosis, macro-ovalocytes	Marked anisocytosis and poikilocytosis, may mimic megaloblastic anemia
Nucleated RBCs	Not common	Common	Common
WBC morphology	Normal	Hypersegmented nuclei of neutrophils	Abnormal mononuclear cells, no nuclear hypersegmentation of neutrophils
Platelet morphology	Normal	Normal	Frequently large and degranulated
Serum folate	Depends on diet	Decreased in folate deficiency, elevated in B_{12} deficiency	Normal or elevated
Serum B_{12}	Normal	Decreased in B_{12} deficiency, may be slightly decreased in folate deficiency	Normal or elevated

may also give a data base which mimics hemolysis (e.g., patients with an appropriate reticulocyte response after being treated with iron, folic acid, or B$_{12}$, or after alcohol withdrawal).

Approach to Hemolysis (10)

It is appropriate to attempt to prove that hemolysis is occurring before obtaining diagnostic tests for specific etiologies. The diagnostic approach to hemolysis varies, depending upon whether hemolysis is primarily *intravascular* or *extravascular*.

INTRAVASCULAR HEMOLYSIS

Table 46.13 lists hemolytic mechanisms associated with intravascular destruction of red cells. Almost all of them require that the patient be hospitalized and that, if possible, diagnostic testing and treatment be planned in consultation with a hematologist. In intravascular hemolysis red cell lysis occurs within the vascular space, resulting in hemoglobinemia. The plasma becomes visibly red or brown (methemoglobin) at a low concentration of hemoglobin (around 30 mg/100 ml). Free hemoglobin initially binds to haptoglobin (a binding protein produced in the liver). Once haptoglobin is saturated, free hemoglobin passes through the glomerulus and hemoglobinuria occurs. Some of the hemoglobin in the renal tubules is absorbed by the renal tubular cells which slough into the urine several days later and stain positively for iron (urine hemosiderin). The latter test, therefore, is helpful in documenting the presence of intravascular hemolysis several days after it has occurred. Table 46.14 suggests an appropriate data base when

Table 46.13
Clinical States Associated with Intravascular Hemolysis

Acute hemolytic transfusion reactions
Severe and extensive burns
Physical trauma (*e.g.*, march hemoglobinuria)
Severe microangiopathic hemolysis (*e.g.*, aortic valve prosthesis)
Acute glucose-6-phosphate dehydrogenase deficiency hemolysis
Paroxysmal nocturnal hemoglobinuria
Clostridial sepsis

Table 46.14
Appropriate Further Data Base when Intravascular Hemolysis Is Suspected

Observation of the serum/plasma
Observation of the urine
Measurement of free plasma hemoglobin
Heme pigment test of the urine if there are no red cells in the urine sediment
Measurement of serum haptoglobin
Iron stain of urine sediment for hemosiderin several days after a presumed hemolytic event

Table 46.15
Most Common Causes of Extravascular Hemolysis

Autoimmune hemolysis
Delayed hemolytic transfusion reactions
Hemoglobinopathies
Hereditary spherocytosis
Hypersplenism
Hemolysis with liver disease

hemolysis is suspected in those clinical states associated with intravascular hemolysis.

EXTRAVASCULAR HEMOLYSIS

Most hemolysis occurs extravascularly within cells of the reticuloendothelial system. A diagnosis of extravascular hemolysis is more difficult to prove than that of intravascular hemolysis. There is no hemoglobinemia, hemoglobinuria, or hemosiderinuria. Haptoglobin is partially saturated because there is a slight leakage of free hemoglobin into the circulation. There may be indirect hyperbilirubinemia, but this is an extremely insensitive sign of hemolysis. There is an increase in fecal and urine urobilinogen, but these substances are also difficult to quantitate. Other tests of hemolysis such as red cell survival are difficult, and the results are not known for several days. The physician must frequently be satisfied with only a presumptive diagnosis of extravascular hemolysis. Therefore, when extravascular hemolysis is suspected, it may be appropriate to obtain tests diagnostic of specific disease states based on a knowledge of the patient's other problems and on the baseline data base (Table 46.15).

Information from the Peripheral Smear. In hemolytic states the peripheral smear frequently reveals only evidence of the response of the bone marrow to hemolysis (large polychromatophilic or finely stippled red cells). It does not, as many physicians believe, always reveal fragmented red cells. Occasionally, however, the smear may give further clues about the specific etiology of the hemolysis as indicated below.

Spherocytes. Spherocytes are seen in small numbers in many hemolytic states. When present in large numbers they suggest either hereditary spherocytosis, autoimmune hemolysis, or one of the hemoglobin C hemoglobinopathies.

Elliptocytes. In large numbers these suggest a diagnosis of hereditary elliptocytosis.

Fragmented cells (schistocytes). Sharply pointed fragmented cells (helmet cells, spiculated cells, triangle cells) are seen in microangiopathic states (see p. 391).

Spiculated Cells. Sometimes these cells are seen in patients with severe liver disease and hemolysis (usually in a terminal stage of liver disease). Spiculated cells are also one type of schistocyte found in the blood of patients with microangiopathic hemolysis.

"Bite" Cells (Blister Cells). Such cells are sometimes seen in patients with oxidative hemolysis (glucose-6-phosphate dehydrogenase deficiency). In "bite" cells all the hemoglobin appears to be pushed to one side of the cell.

Poikilocytosis and the Hemoglobinopathies. In patients with sickle cell disease and in the various other sickle cell syndromes the peripheral smear is frequently diagnostic (see below).

Hemolysis with a Positive Coombs' Test (15)

Once the physician suspects hemolysis, the diagnostic testing should be guided by the patient's problem list. Because of the relatively common occurrence of immune hemolysis and the important therapeutic implications of such a diagnosis, it is desirable to obtain a Coombs' test at this stage in the workup.

POSITIVE DIRECT COOMBS' TEST

The direct Coombs' test is done by mixing the patients cells with Coombs' antiserum containing antibody to IgG and to complement. If the test is positive, the physician should first ascertain from the laboratory personnel that the positive result is attributable to antibody and/or complement on the red cell surface. If this is the case, it is important to determine whether the antibody is an *isoantibody* or an *autoantibody.*

Isoantibodies are antibodies induced by prior transfusion or, in a woman, by placental transfer of fetal red cells. The antibodies are directed against specific minor red cell antigens and it is important to identify them in the event that future transfusions are necessary. Ordinarily the antibody is primarily present in the patient's plasma and is identified by an antibody screen (indirect Coombs' test). However, a direct Coombs' test would also be positive due to the presence of isoantibodies if the patient had recently been transfused with cells that were still circulating and sensitized by the antibody.

In a patient with hemolysis, if there has not been a recent transfusion, a positive direct Coombs' test generally implies the presence of an autoantibody. In this situation the antibody may be present in the serum as well as on the surface of the red cells. Table 46.16 describes the differences between iso- and autoantibodies. Autoantibodies are classified as either

Table 46.16
Comparison of Isoantibody and Autoantibody

	Isoantibody	Autoantibody
Direct Coombs'	Frequently negative. May be positive if sensitized foreign red cells are still circulating	Positive
Indirect Coombs' Antibody screen (panel)	Positive Specificity is seen	Positive or negative Panagglutination, no specificity seen

Table 46.17
Autoimmune Hemolysis Due to a "Warm Antibody": Differential Diagnosis

IDIOPATHIC
SECONDARY
  Infection (particularly viral)
  Drugs:
    Aldomet
    Penicillin
    Quinine/quinidine
  Collagen vascular disease (systemic lupus erythematosus)
  Lymphoproliferative disorders
  Miscellaneous (thyroid disease, malignancy, etc.)

warm antibodies or *cold antibodies.* Warm antibodies are usually IgG and cannot be identified by direct agglutination of red cells, but require a Coombs' test. Cold antibodies, however, are usually IgM, cause direct agglutination of red cells in the cold and result in a positive Coombs' test because of fixation of complement to the red cell which is identified by nonspecific Coombs' antiserum.

HEMOLYSIS DUE TO WARM ANTIBODIES

Table 46.17 lists the conditions commonly associated with autoimmune hemolysis resulting from a warm antibody. Patients may develop such antibodies secondary to one of a number of conditions, including infections (particularly viral), collagen vascular disease (systemic lupus erythematosus, SLE), lymphoproliferative diseases, other malignancies, and secondary also to the effect of drugs. The most common drug causing a positive Coombs' test is α-methyldopa (Aldomet) (19). A positive Coombs' test is not usually observed unless the patient has been taking high doses of Aldomet for a long period of time; in such circumstances a positive Coombs' test is not uncommon but hemolysis is rare.

Idiopathic autoimmune hemolysis is a relatively infrequent disease; sometimes it precedes the development of SLE or lymphoma. Patients usually present with anemia, which may be severe. On physical examination the spleen is slightly enlarged in 50% of patients, and mild jaundice and fever are not uncommon. The peripheral smear shows a marked polychromatophilia, spherocytosis, and, frequently, a markedly elevated reticulocyte count. Autoimmune hemolysis which is temporary, e.g., caused by drug administration or by viral infections, usually requires no treatment (although if a drug is implicated, it should be discontinued). The process gradually remits over the course of 3 to 4 weeks. Patients receiving Aldomet, who do not have hemolysis but do have a positive Coombs' test, need not discontinue use of the drug. Patients with chronic primary autoimmune hemolysis should be referred to a hematologist, who usually prescribes corticosteroids, which are usually effective if first given in reasonably high doses and slowly tapered as the anemia improves. Occasionally splenectomy is required for refractory cases. In patients with secondary chronic autoimmune hemolysis treatment of the underlying disease is the most important therapy.

COLD AGGLUTININ HEMOLYSIS

The most common etiology of autoimmune hemolysis due to a cold antibody is viral or mycoplasma pneumonia (13). Severe hemolysis is rare. Chronic cold agglutinin hemolysis secondary to a collagen vascular disorder or to a lymphoproliferative disease is frequently more refractory to treatment with steroids and splenectomy than is the case with warm antibody hemolysis. Transfusion therapy may be a problem in such cases since the antibody is a pan-agglutinin and reacts with all blood types; therefore, a compatible cross match may be impossible to obtain. Ordinarily the IgM antibody in cold agglutinin hemolysis is not significantly hemolytic, and transfusions may be attempted cautiously when absolutely necessary (17).

Hemolysis with Fragmented Red Cells on Peripheral Smear (3)

Table 46.18 lists those conditions associated with hemolysis and the presence of fragmented red cells on peripheral smear. The peripheral blood is characterized by the presence of sharply pointed poikilocytes (schistocytes). Such cells are quite characteristic and are clearly differentiated from abnormally shaped red cells seen in other conditions. The hemolysis may be severe, and in such cases is usually intravascular, resulting in hemoglobinemia, hemoglobinuria, haptoglobin saturation, and, subsequently, hemosiderinuria (see p. 389). Red cell fragmentation may occur after insertion of a prosthetic aortic valve. Rarely this may be associated with clinically significant hemolysis. More frequently red cell fragmentation is due to arteriolar lesions (fibrin, inflammation, etc.) which cause damage to red cells as they pass through the damaged vessel. When fragmented red cells are accompanied by thrombocytopenia, one should consider the possibility of *disseminated intravascular coagulation* (Chapter 47) and of the syndrome known as *thrombotic thrombocytopenic pur-*

Table 46.18
Hemolysis with Fragmented Red Cells on Peripheral Smear: Differential Diagnosis

Aortic valve prosthesis
Arteritis (malignant hypertension, polyarteritis, etc.)
Disseminated intravascular coagulation (DIC)
Thrombotic thrombocytopenic purpura (TTP)
Hemolytic uremic syndrome
Malignancy
Giant hemangiomas
Renal transplant rejection
Eclampsia

pura. This latter syndrome is usually accompanied by fever, by neurologic defects which characteristically fluctuate, and by some degree of renal failure. The mortality rate is high, and patients suspected of suffering from this condition should be hospitalized immediately and treated in consultation with a hematologist. The hemolytic uremic syndrome is a related (perhaps identical) syndrome, more common in children, characterized by the prominence of renal failure over other organ dysfunction.

Hemolysis with Enlarged Spleen (Hypersplenism) (5)

It is important to remember that not all large spleens cause "cytopenias" and that the degree of cytopenia does not necessarily correlate with the size of the spleen. Thrombocytopenia and leukopenia are more common than is anemia. Splenomegaly, from almost any cause, may result in hypersplenism but the syndrome is seen most often in patients who have chronic liver disease and congestive splenomegaly. Splenomegaly is sometimes seen in patients with hemolysis from other mechanisms such as autoimmune hemolysis or hereditary spherocytosis. Rarely, splenectomy is necessary because of severe cytopenias resulting from hypersplenism. Occasional patients with Felty's syndrome (see Chapter 67) are benefited by splenectomy as are some patients with chronic leukemia or lymphoma.

Glucose-6-Phosphate Dehydrogenase (G-6-PD) Deficiency (2)

G-6-PD deficiency is seen primarily in black patients in the United States. Inheritance is sex-linked. Ten percent of black males are affected (hemizygotes) as are 20% of black females (heterozygotes). In the affected black patients hemolysis due to G-6-PD deficiency is an acute intravascular hemolytic event usually precipitated either by infection or by an oxidant drug. Drugs known to precipitate hemolysis include sulfonamides, nitrofurantoin, and primaquine. Caucasian-type G-6-PD deficiency is seen primarily in patients from Mediterranean countries and usually is more severe than the African type, sometimes causing chronic persisting, partially compensated, hemolysis.

Diagnosis after a hemolytic event may be difficult, especially in the female heterozygotes. G-6-PD deficiency screening tests (available from most commercial and hospital laboratories) may be normal at this time and even the affected hemizygote black male may have a normal screening test for several weeks after hemolysis (young cells have more G-6-PD activity). Occasionally a characteristic cell ("bite cell") is seen in the peripheral blood during a hemolytic event.

Although the frequency of the genetic defect is high, the incidence of severe hemolysis with provocation (infection, drugs) is low. Ordinarily routine screening before treatment with a known oxidant drug (e.g., sulfonamide) is not advocated.

Sickle Cell Disorders (1)

Approximately 10% of the black population in the United States carry the sickle cell gene. The gene is also present to a lesser extent in Greeks, Italians, Arabians, and persons from India. Hemoglobin S results from a mutation in the β-globin chain in hemoglobin which, when oxygen tension is reduced, causes the formation of rigid elongated tactoids which distort red cell shape and increase red cell rigidity. The clumping together of sickled cells leads to tissue ischemia and infarction. A number of common inherited disorders involving hemoglobin S are listed below.

SICKLE CELL TRAIT

Most people who are heterozygous for hemoglobin S (sickle cell trait) are completely well and are not anemic. The peripheral smear appears normal, although sickling is seen if the blood is deoxygenated. Hemoglobin electrophoresis reveals approximately 40% hemoglobin S and 60% hemoglobin A, whereas hemoglobinS, A_2, and F are present in normal concentration.

Most patients with sickle trait lead a normal life. However, rare clinical events attributable to the presence of sickle cell hemoglobin do occur. For example, splenic infarction at high altitudes (>10,000 feet) has been reported. (Oxygen pressures in commercial aircraft are high enough that individuals with sickle cell trait may fly with impunity.) Occasionally infarctions occur in other more vital organs during vigorous exercise. All individuals with sickle cell trait have renal tubular dysfunction resulting in hyposthenuria; and on occasion severe hematuria may occur due to hypertonicity in the renal medulla, resulting in sickling and leading to ischemia and tubular infarction. Persons with sickle cell trait have a higher incidence of renal infections, especially during pregnancy.

It is important to identify patients with sickle cell trait so that they may be given genetic counseling. A couple, both heterozygous for hemoglobin S, should be informed that they have a 25% chance of having a child with sickle cell anemia. There are a few centers in this country where prenatal diagnosis of sickle cell anemia by amniocentesis is now possible; presumably the technique will be more widely available in the near future.

SICKLE CELL ANEMIA (HEMOGLOBIN SS) (18)

Sickle cell anemia exists in approximately 0.25% of the black population in the United States. The disease is usually severe, resulting in significant morbidity as well as in a shortened life expectancy. One of the most disturbing features of the illness is the painful ("thrombotic") crisis, a recurrent episode of severe pain, usually in the limbs and the abdomen, due to small infarctions in multiple sites. Patients have a lifelong, often severe, anemia, with hematocrit values which range from the high teens to the mid-30s (average—mid-20s). The primary mechanism of the anemia is extravascular hemolysis, so that there is a chronic reticulocytosis and a chronic indirect hyperbilirubinemia. The patients usually have a leukocytosis, the white count rising occasionally as high as 30 to 40,000/ml during a painful crisis. A mild thrombocytosis is also common. The peripheral smear shows markedly distorted red cells including characteristically sickled cells. Upon electrophoresis only hemoglobin S with a variable amount of hemoglobin F (no hemoglobin A) is detected.

The multiple and repetitive episodes of organ ischemia due to sickling result in a host of abnormalities. The bones characteristically appear abnormal on X-ray, revealing areas of old infarction which mimic the changes of osteomyelitis. The medullary spaces are usually widened due to the marked compensatory expansion of bone marrow. The spine frequently takes on a distorted appearance, and aseptic necrosis of the femoral (and, rarely, humeral) head is common, sometimes requiring joint replacement. Many adult patients are tall with long, thin extremities. Puberty is frequently delayed. Splenomegaly usually disappears by age 8 due to repeated infarctions of the spleen. An adult with sickle cell anemia is essentially autosplenectomized. This lack of splenic function contributes to the propensity for infections, related especially to a decreased ability to resist pneumococcal infections. *Gallstones* (pigment stones) are common, and sicklers do develop cholecystitis which may be extremely difficult to differentiate clinically from a syndrome of intrahepatic cholestasis secondary to sickling in the hepatic sinusoids. There is some hazard to *surgery* (see Chapter 87), but patients with recurrent abdominal pain consistent with cholecystitis, who have gallstones, should probably have elective cholecystectomy. *Pregnancy* in women with SS disease is complicated by increased risk of pyelonephritis, pulmonary infarction, antepartum hemorrhage, prematurity, and fetal death. With time, patients develop *cardiomegaly* and chronic myocardial disease related to repetitive microinfarctions of the heart. Murmurs are frequent and may suggest rheumatic or congenital heart disease. Patients with sickle cell anemia develop *venous thromboses* and pulmonary embolism. They also develop thromboses *in situ* in the lungs followed, after many years, by chronic scarring and fibrosis. Pulmonary thrombosis/embolism may lead to pulmonary hypertension and heart failure. Cerebral vascular accidents are common, including infarction and intracerebral and subarachnoid hemorrhage. Seizures are frequent as well. Up to 75% of patients with sickle cell anemia develop *leg ulcerations* which may be chronic and extremely difficult to heal. Sickle cell patients are very prone to serious *retinopathy*, which rarely may lead to blindness, due to plugging of small retinal capillaries and subsequent neovascularization. It is important for these patients to be examined yearly by an ophthalmologist as some of the retinopathy problems can be prevented by photocoagulation of abnormal new retinal vessels.

SC DISEASE

The genes which code for hemoglobin S and hemoglobin C are alleles. The C hemoglobin mutation is relatively common in blacks (about 2% prevalence), and patients doubly heterozygous for S and C constitute approximately 0.15% of that population. The syndrome is very similar to that of SS disease but is usually somewhat more mild. In contrast to sickle cell anemia, the spleen is palpable in 50% of adult patients.

S-THALASSEMIA

Patients doubly heterozygous for hemoglobin S and thalassemia trait have a syndrome similar to sickle cell anemia but usually much more mild. Characteristically the MCV is low and target cells are more prominent on smear than they are in SS disease. The speen may be palpable, and the hemoglobin electrophoresis reveals 70 to 80% hemoglobin S and smaller amounts of hemoglobin A and F (the reverse of the pattern in sickle cell trait).

TREATMENT

Painful "Thrombotic" Crisis. Painful crises are frequently severe and may last for a few hours to several days and occasionally for several weeks. They may be associated with high fever, and with neutrophilia, which makes it difficult but important to differentiate crises from infection. There is no specific therapy. The patient is usually treated with narcotics and with hydration. Since patients can become addicted to narcotics because of the repetitive episodes of severe pain, it is important to limit strictly the amount of narcotics given them in ambulatory practice. When pain is severe and persistent, hospitalization is indicated.

Infection. As mentioned above, patients with sickle cell anemia are prone to infections, especially with the pneumococcus. Patients with sickle cell anemia should receive pneumococcal vaccine (see Chapter 30) and should be encouraged to seek medical help at the first evidence of infection or fever.

Hemolytic and Aplastic Crises. Acceleration of hemolysis is quite unusual. If hematocrit values drop significantly below baseline, it is most likely to be because of decreased marrow production, associated with infection. Such episodes are much more common in children. If they occur, hospitalization and transfusion are often necessary. Patients with chronic severe hemolysis have an increased requirement for folic acid, and folic acid deficiency may occur resulting in reticulocytopenia and more severe anemia. Therefore, daily folic acid therapy (1 mg) is reasonable for all patients with sickle cell anemia.

Thrombosis/Embolization. When patients with sickle cell disease develop deep vein thrombosis or pulmonary embolism, they should be treated with anticoagulants as would any patient with such problems (see Chapter 48). However, venography should be avoided because of the danger of the development of leg ulcers in any patient with SS hemoglobin whose lower extremities are traumatized. It is frequently difficult to distinguish pulmonary thrombotic/embolic problems from pneumonia.

Leg Ulcers. Leg ulcers are often large and are particularly refractory to treatment. Skin grafting is usually only temporarily helpful and frequently does not seem to be worth the time and discomfort involved. It is important to keep the ulcers clean, to elevate the legs frequently, and to use surgical stockings and elastic wraps.

Hematuria. Patients with sickle cell trait, sickle cell anemia, SC disease, and sickle cell-thalassemia all are prone to bouts of severe hematuria related to sickling and to medullary ischemia precipitated by the hypertonicity of the renal medulla. Bleeding can occur for days or even weeks. Maintenance of a high urine flow is important and usually successful in stopping the hematuria.

Priapism. Priapism is common in SS and SC disease and usually results in permanent impotence once it has resolved. If urologic intervention is to be attempted, it must be done within a few hours of the onset of the priapism. It is frequently only temporarily helpful. Once impotence has occurred, penile prostheses are sometimes quite helpful.

RECOMMENDATIONS FOR PREVENTIVE CARE

1. *General.* It is important to remember that patients with sickle cell disorders have a lifelong chronic illness and will require frequent and recurrent use of the health care system. The patient needs one general physician who is familiar with the case, and needs access to a physician 24 hours a day. The availability of emergency care 24 hours a day is also exceedingly important.

2. *Infection.* There should be rapid medical evaluation of fever, chills, or other signs of infection. The patient should be immunized with the pneumococcal vaccine (see Chapter 30). Because heart murmurs and cardiomegaly are common, it is often difficult to know if a patient with sickle cell anemia has rheumatic heart disease. If the physician is in doubt, it is reasonable for him to prescribe prophylactic antibiotics before dental procedures, etc. (see Chapter 83)

3. *Narcotic abuse.* As mentioned above, analgesics should be given in doses sufficient to relieve pain during a thrombotic crisis. However, the use of narcotics on an ambulatory basis should be avoided if at all possible, since addiction can occur. Easy access to the physician should obviate the need to give the patient a supply of narcotics to take in case of pain.

4. *Folic Acid.* Patients should receive 1 mg of folic acid daily.

Table 46.19
Anemia with a Normal Mean Corpuscular Volume (MCV) and Low Reticulocyte Index: Differential Diagnosis

Renal failure
Anemia of chronic disease (inflammatory disease and malignancy)
Anemia of hypoendocrine states (hypothyroidism, etc.)
Mild (early) iron deficiency
Combined iron deficiency and megaloblastic anemia
Sideroblastic anemia
Aplastic anemia
Bone marrow infiltration (myelophthisis)
Bleeding or hemolysis plus one of the above

ANEMIAS WITH NORMAL MCV AND AN INAPPROPRIATELY LOW RETICULOCYTE INDEX

Mild normocytic anemias without appropriate reticulocyte responses are among the most common problems seen in clinical practice. Before considering possible etiologies and embarking on a diagnostic workup, it is important for the physician to be sure that the hematocrit value/hemoglobin concentration is reproducibly low. Moreover, the normal values for the laboratory should be known. For example, in some laboratories an hematocrit value of 35% in a woman is normal. One should also consider the variation in normal values related to age, sex, pregnancy, etc. Finally one should be sure that volume overload is not the etiology. Marked volume shifts may result in swings in hematocrit value of 6 or 8 percentage points. Table 46.19 lists the differential diagnosis of a normocytic anemia with an inappropriately low reticulocyte count.

Anemia of Renal Failure (9)

Patients with uremia are anemic primarily because of decreased production of erythropoietin. The red cell morphology on smear is usually normal, but occasionally spiculated cells (burr cells) may be seen. An occasional patient may have a microangiopathic peripheral smear (see p. 391). There may be a mild thrombocytopenia, and the nuclei of the neutrophils may be hypersegmented even in the absence of folic acid deficiency. The hematocrit value depends on the degree of renal failure (see Fig. 44.3 in Chapter 44). Anemia is unusual if the creatinine is less than 3 mg/100 ml. The hematocrit value seen in patients with renal failure on dialysis is extremely variable (from the low teens, requiring transfusion, up to the mid-thirties). It is important to remember that patients in renal failure may also be anemic because of iron deficiency (secondary to blood loss) or because of folate deficiency (since folic acid is dialyzable). Some patients with glomerulonephritis or arteritis may have a microangiopathic hemolytic anemia.

Anemia of Chronic Disease (4)

Any chronic inflammatory disease (e.g., rheumatoid arthritis) or malignant neoplastic disease may cause mild to moderate anemia, unrelated to blood loss or hemolysis. (If the hematocrit value is less than 25%, another explanation should be sought.) Red cell morphology is usually normal but occasionally the MCV may be less than 80 fl, requiring differentiation of the process from other causes of a microcytic anemia (see p. 382). The serum iron and the total iron binding capacity are low; the percent saturation may be just as low as it is in iron deficiency ($\leq$10%). The serum ferritin is normal or elevated, and bone marrow iron stores are normal or increased.

In addition to chronic infections, an *acute* infection or inflammation will cause a drop in serum iron, reticulocytopenia, and a decrease in bone marrow red cell production. If present for 1 week or more, therefore, an acute inflammatory process may result in a fall in the hematocrit value of several percentage points.

Mild Early Iron Deficiency

Although severe iron deficiency results in a microcytic anemia (see pp. 382–385), in the early stages mild iron deficiency may result in anemia with a normal peripheral smear and a normal MCV. Diagnosis can usually be made by measurement of serum ferritin or by a bone marrow iron stain. In addition, a patient with severe iron deficiency, when it accompanies a macrocytic anemia such as a megaloblastic anemia (as in an alcoholic patient with iron deficiency and folic acid deficiency) may have a severe anemia which is normocytic. The reticulocyte count is inappropriately low until alcohol is withdrawn and iron and folate are administered.

Anemia in the Elderly

Old age *per se* is not an explanation for a significant normocytic anemia. Hematocrit values in healthy patients in their 70s are only slightly lower than they are in the normal general adult range (Table 46.1). However, it is in elderly patients that frustrating, mild, unexplained, normocytic anemias occur. In such patients the following possible explanations should be considered: (a) fluid overload, (b) blood loss from phlebotomy if the patient has been hospitalized recently, and (c) any recent inflammatory disease (viral or bacterial infection, inflammatory joint problem) which may depress bone marrow production and, if present for several days, may result in a drop in hematocrit value. If none of the above explanations seems appropriate, and there is no reason to suspect an underlying problem to explain the hematocrit value, it is reasonable simply to follow the hematocrit value without further diagnostic workup. If it is known that the anemia is relatively recent (e.g., if there is a record of a normal hematocrit value 3 months previously), then other efforts should be made to explain the anemia. For example, the possibility of occult gastrointestinal bleeding with early iron deficiency, and of the anemia of chronic disease (has there been a recent weight loss, fever, etc?) should be entertained.

References

General

Williams, WJ, Beutler, E, Erslev, AJ and Rundles, RW (Eds.): *Hematology.* McGraw-Hill, New York, 1977. *The currently standard text.*

Specific

1. Abramson, H, Bertles, JF and Wethers, DL (Eds.): *Sickle Cell Disease,* C.V. Mosby, St. Louis, 1973.
2. Beutler, E: Glucose-6-Phosphate dehydrogenase deficiency: diagnosis; clinical and genetic implications. *Am J Clin Pathol 47:* 303, 1967.
3. Brain, MC: Microangiopathic hemolytic anemia. *N Engl J Med 281:* 833, 1969.
4. Cartwright, GE: The anemia of chronic disorders. *Semin Hematol 3:* 351, 1966.
5. Dameshek, W: Hypersplenism. *Bull NY Acad Med 31:* 113, 1955.
6. Davidson, RJL and Hamilton, PJ: High mean red cell volume: its incidence and significance in routine hematology. *J Clin Pathol 31:* 493, 1978,
7. Eichner, ER: The hematologic disorders of alcoholism. *Am J Med 54:* 621, 1973.
8. England, JM, Ward, SM and Down, MC: Microcytosis, anisocytosis and the red cell indices in iron deficiency. *Br J Haematol 34:* 589, 1976.
9. Erslev, AJ: Management of anemia of chronic renal failure. *Clin Nephrol 2:* 174, 1974.
10. Hillman, RS and Finch, CA: *Red Cell Manual,* pp. 7–12, 18–19, and 40–46. F.A. Davis, Philadelphia, 1978.
11. Hoffbrand, AV (Ed.): Megaloblastic anaemia. *Clin Haematol 5:* 1976.
12. Halliday JW and Powell, LW: Serum ferritin and isoferritins in clinical medicine. *Prog Hematol 11:* 229, 1979.
13. Jacobson, LB, Longstreth, GF and Edgington, TS: Clinical and immunologic features of transient cold agglutinin hemolytic anemia. *Am J Med 54:* 514, 1973.
14. Linman, JW and Saarni, MI: The preleukemic syndrome. *Semin Hematol 11:* 93, 1974.
15. Pirofsky, B: Clinical aspects of autoimmune hemolytic anemia. *Semin Hematol 13:* 251, 1976.
16. Rawley, PT: The diagnosis of beta-thalassemia trait: a review. *Am J Hematol 1:* 129, 1976.
17. Rosenfield, RE and Jagathambal, Transfusion therapy for autoimmune hemolytic anemia. *Semin Hematol 13:* 311, 1976.
18. Sergeant, GR: *The Clinical Features of Sickle Cell Disease.* North-Holland, Amsterdam, 1974.
19. Worlledge, SM: Immune drug-induced hemolytic anemias. *Semin Hematol 10:* 327, 1973.

CHAPTER FORTY-SEVEN

Disorders of Hemostasis

PHILIP D. ZIEVE, M.D.

HEMOSTATIC FUNCTION

In healthy man a number of different processes interact to ensure that blood is maintained in a fluid

Table 47.1
Laboratory Evaluation of Hemostatic Function

System	Screening Tests	Specific Tests
Blood vessels	None	Depends on suspected underlying disorder (see text)
Platelets— quantitative	Scanning of a stained smear of the peripheral blood	Platelet count
Platelets— qualitative	Bleeding time	Platelet aggregation Platelet release reaction
Coagulation	Partial thromboplastin time, Prothrombin time	Factor assays

state until the integrity of a blood vessel wall is compromised; at that point, a plug is rapidly formed to prevent exsanguination. Three major systems are involved in this regard: the vasculature itself, the blood platelets, and the coagulation system (Table 47.1).

Blood Vessels

Trauma to blood vessels is by far the commonest cause of untoward bleeding. If blood vessels are abnormal because of inherited or acquired defects, excessive bleeding is more likely in response to trauma. There is no good screening test to evaluate blood vessel integrity so the demonstration of an abnormal vasculature must first depend on a strong suspicion generated by the history and physical examination.

Blood Platelets

Platelets provide a cellular defense against the loss of blood from traumatized vessels, especially where blood flow is relatively rapid as it is on the arterial side of the circulation and in the left heart. Platelets are particularly effective in sealing leaks from small arterioles and capillaries; and when platelets are abnormal, either quantitatively or qualitatively, it is these vessels which bleed most prominently. The platelet plug is initiated by the exposure of platelets to subendothelial collagen which is exposed by injury to the vascular intima. Thereafter, aggregating agents such as thrombin and adenosine diphosphate cause the accretion of platelets at that site, eventually forming an adhesive plug which within minutes prevents the further flow of blood. Eventually the plug is replaced by fibrin laid down by the activation of the coagulation mechanism, which occurs simultaneously with the initiation of platelet plug formation. The best screening test for the evaluation of the numbers of platelets in the blood is observation of a stained smear of the peripheral blood. With relatively little experience it is easy to determine whether the platelet count is unusually low or high. In un-anticoagulated blood, at least one clump of platelets should be seen, on the average, in every oil immersion field. In anticoagulated blood, one platelet should be seen for every 10 to 20 red cells. If a quantitative

abnormality is suspected, a precise platelet count can be obtained. Tests such as the bleeding time and the measurement of clot retraction are much less useful as screening tests for detecting *quantitative* abnormalities of platelets. However, the bleeding time, despite its limitations, is still the best screening test to evaluate *qualitative* abnormalities of platelet function (see below, p. 401).

Coagulation

The generation of a solid fibrin clot from circulating soluble fibrinogen is the body's major defense against the loss of blood from the vasculature, especially from blood vessels larger than the capillary, arteriole, and venule. Coagulation is initiated by the exposure of proteins to an altered blood vessel surface, most commonly after trauma, and to thromboplastic substances to which the blood is exposed normally also when blood vessels are injured. Thereafter a series of enzymatic reactions occur which result in the conversion of fibrinogen by the proteolytic enzyme, thrombin, to fibrin. There are two converging pathways of coagulation which are important in this mechanism: the first, the so-called intrinsic pathway, which begins with surface activation of coagulation proteins, and the second, the so-called extrinsic pathway, which begins with the exposure of the blood to tissue thromboplastin. The best screening tests to detect abnormalities of clotting are the partial thromboplastin time, which tests the intrinsic and the final common pathway and the prothrombin time, which tests the extrinsic and the final common pathway. Both of these tests are reliably performed by hematology laboratories. The clotting time is an insensitive test and should not be relied upon as a screening procedure to detect abnormalities in this system.

There are enzymatic mechanisms which oppose coagulation and which prevent unwarranted widespread clotting of the blood when a blood vessel is injured. These mechanisms, although clearly important physiologically, are rarely recognized clinically; but a few cases have been reported of patients with an increased tendency to thrombosis and low levels of antithrombin activity. The fibrinolytic system generates the proteolytic enzyme, plasmin, which adsorbs to the clots and results in their ultimate dissolution. Bleeding as the result of increased endogenous fibrinolytic activity is essentially unheard of and the practicing physician need not be concerned with this possibility. Moreover, although there has been some interest in recent years in stimulating fibrinolysis by the infusion of activating enzymes in the treatment of thrombotic disease, the therapy, which may result in bleeding, requires hospitalization and in any case is not widely practiced.

EVALUATION OF PATIENTS

The history is the most important aid in determining whether or not a patient has a hemorrhagic diathesis. Patients with either congenital disorders of hemostasis or acquired disorders of long standing will almost certainly have had unexpectedly excessive bleeding in response to minor trauma or to surgery. The clinician should ask specifically whether the patient has required transfusion following an operative procedure or a seemingly minor trauma.

Bleeding due to trauma to the vasculature is overwhelmingly more common than bleeding due to defective hemostasis. Therefore, patients who present, for example, with gastrointestinal or genitourinary hemorrhage are more likely to have a lesion, such as a peptic ulcer, a carcinoma, a diverticulum, or a renal calculus, that has bled than a disorder of hemostasis. Similarly, nose bleeds, bleeding gums, or excessive menstrual flow most likely reflect local (usually benign) problems. Futhermore, even if patients have hemostatic dysfunction, they are likely to bleed from local lesions, the propensity to bleed of which has been accentuated by the hemostatic abnormality.

Specific disorders of hemostasis may be suspected strongly on the basis of the patient's history and because of characteristic findings on physical examination (see Fig. 47.1 and below), but in almost all instances laboratory tests are required before a specific diagnosis can be made. Screening tests, procedures which are extremely sensitive to alterations in hemostasis, are ordinarily relied upon first in a patient with a suspected hemorrhagic diathesis. If any of these tests is abnormal, or if the clinician strongly suspects that a disorder of hemostasis exists even if the tests are not abnormal, more specific tests are indicated; these are best performed in consultation with a hematologist. A number of years ago, the bleeding time and the clotting time were the most common tests performed to screen patients for possible disorders of hemostasis. Although both of these have lost favor because of their lack of sensitivity, the bleeding time, as mentioned above, despite its limitations is still the only readily performed procedure to detect *qualitative* abnormalities of blood platelets (see p. 401).

DISORDERS OF BLOOD VESSELS

Vascular disease (Table 47.2) is diagnosed uncommonly as a cause of a hemorrhagic diathesis, in part because, except for trauma, disorders of the vasculature that result in untoward bleeding are relatively rare (1), and in part because there is no reliable test to detect generalized vascular dysfunction. The primary hemorrhagic manifestation of vascular disease is purpura, a confluent purplish discoloration of the skin due to extravasation of blood from cutaneous and subcutaneous blood vessels. Although patients with an abnormal vasculature may occasionally experience bleeding from relatively large blood vessels, most commonly they bleed into the skin or mucous membranes. Because purpura is a common response to minor trauma, it cannot in itself be taken as evidence of an underlying hemorrhagic diathesis.

Cutaneous Lesions

Unexplained bruises, especially in the lower extremities, are common and usually are not associated with an underlying disease process. A history of "easy bruisability" therefore is not likely, in itself, to lead to a diagnosis of a disorder of hemostasis. Similarly, *senile purpura*, which occurs characteristically on the dorsum of the hand and the extensor surfaces of the forearms, does not represent a generalized hemorrhagic diathesis, but results from the loss of connective tissue support to intracutaneous blood vessels which then are easily traumatized and bleed

Table 47.2
Bleeding Due to Vascular Disease

Cutaneous	Mucocutaneous
Senile purpura	Amyloidosis
Steroid purpura	Myeloma
Autoerythrocyte sensitization	Macroglobulinemia
Cryoglobulinemia	Vitamin C deficiency
Hyperglobulinemia of Waldenström	Hereditary hemorrhagic telangiectasia

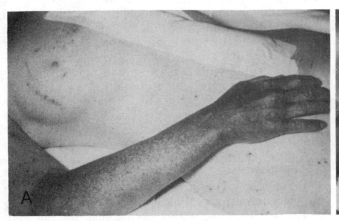
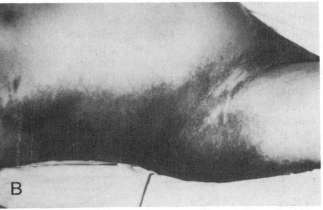

Figure 47.1   Bleeding due to thrombocytopenia compared to bleeding due to abnormal coagulation: *A*, immune thrombocytopenic purpura; *B*, hemophilia A. (Reproduced from P. D. Zieve and J. Levin (see "General References").)

within the substance of the skin. Identical lesions are seen sometimes in patients with *Cushing's syndrome* or in patients who have received corticosteroid therapy.

Allergic purpura (Henoch-Schönlein purpura) (2) represents a hypersensitivity reaction to an antigenic stimulus which usually cannot be identified (although occasionally a drug or a bacterial infection can be incriminated as a provocative agent). Characteristically patients develop a symmetrical petechial rash, most prominent on the extremities. The lesions are slightly raised, distinguishing them from the petechiae of thrombocytopenia. No hemostatic dysfunction is associated with this condition; the cutaneous manifestations of the disorder are part of a widespread vasculitis, the manifestations of which also may include arthralgias (sometimes with evidence of joint effusions) fever, malaise, abdominal pain, gastrointestinal bleeding, and renal disease due to a focal glomerulonephritis which occasionally may progress to chronic renal failure. There is no specific treatment for this condition although if the patient is taking a drug that is suspected to be a sensitizing agent, it should be discontinued. Most patients recover spontaneously within 3 or 4 weeks, but sometimes signs and symptoms of the disease continue for up to a year. Patients should be reassured while they are symptomatic that unless they have evidence of progressive renal disease, they will recover ultimately.

Autoerythrocyte sensitization (13) is a disorder characterized by apparently spontaneous painful ecchymoses, usually on the lower extremities and anterior trunk. The disorder is named as it is because of a belief at one time that it arose as the result of a hypersensitivity response to the patients' red cells or red cell stroma, and in fact the lesions can sometimes be produced by injection of red cells into the skin of these patients. It has become apparent, however, that virtually all patients with the disorder, most of whom are women, are severely psychoneurotic and in some instances frankly psychotic; and many people believe now that the lesions are self-inflicted (13).

Cryoglobulinemia (4) either as a special feature of dysproteinemia, (see below) or as a benign primary abnormality, sometimes associated with immune complex disease, may also cause purpuric bleeding especially on the lower extremities, the ear lobes, or the tip of the nose. Patients with immune complex disease may have associated renal failure.

The diagnosis of cryoglobulinemia may be made by placing a sample of the patients serum in a refrigerator overnight and then inspecting the serum to see whether a white gel or precipitate has formed which disappears when the specimen is warmed. The blood for this test should be drawn in a warm syringe, and then it should be allowed to clot and retract in a 37°C water bath.

Hyperglobulinemic purpura of Waldenström (7) is a rare condition characterized by purpura, especially of the lower extremities, an elevated erythrocyte sedimentation rate, mild anemia, and a polyclonal increase in the blood of a mixture of IgG and anti-IgG immunoglobulins. The disease is more common in women and, particularly after the age of 40, may be associated with an underlying collagen vascular disorder. The primary condition is untreatable, but is generally benign.

Mucocutaneous Lesions

Some patients with vascular disease are prone to bleed from the oral, nasal, or gastrointestinal mucosa, as well as from the skin. Such patients may present to their physicians, not only with cutaneous hemorrhage, but with bleeding gums, epistaxis, hematemesis, or melena.

Primary Amyloidosis (3). Mucocutaneous bleeding may be a symptom of primary amyloidosis because of the deposition of amyloid within the walls of blood vessels. Periorbital bleeding and bleeding in skin folds are especially common. The skin in the areas of hemorrhage sometimes appears thickened because of palpable amyloid deposits within it. Patients suspected of having this disorder should have skin biopsies with appropriate staining as well as serum and urine electrophoresis in an attempt to make a specific diagnosis.

Dysproteinemia (12). Either myeloma or macroglobulinemia, may be associated with untoward bleeding, either because of increased viscosity of the blood or because the coating of blood vessels and platelets with the abnormal protein interferes with normal hemostatic function. Abnormal coagulation is also common in patients with these disorders. Patients suspected of having dysproteinemia should have samples of their serum and urine examined by electrophoresis in an attempt to demonstrate a monoclonal protein. If the diagnosis of dysproteinemia seems likely on the basis of this test and of the clinical presentation, consultation with a hematologist or oncologist is appropriate.

Vitamin C Deficiency (5). There are three situations in which symptomatic vitamin C deficiency (scurvy) might be seen in this country: in chronic alcoholics, food faddists, and in chronically ill or debilitated patients. Since humans, unlike most animals, are unable to synthesize vitamin C, they are dependent upon exogenous sources such as fruits or leafy vegetables. People who cannot or will not eat an adequate diet of foods which contain the vitamin are subject to the manifestations of scurvy. The signs and symptoms of scurvy are largely attributable to the formation of defective connective tissue, because of the human body's absolute dependence on vitamin C for the synthesis of normal collagen. Mucocutaneous bleeding is common in patients with vitamin C deficiency, who present characteristically with large ecchymoses on their extremities, with bleeding gums, and, very suggestive of this disorder, perifollicular hemorrhages which appear commonly on the lower extremities and anterior trunk. Sometimes patients with vitamin C deficiency develop hemarthroses similar to those seen in patients with severe coagulation disorders. All of the manifestations of scurvy are readily reversed by administration of vitamin C, so that although the disorder is uncommon it should be considered in patients with compatible signs and symptoms. Vitamin C deficiency can be confirmed by assay of the blood, but this is usually unnecessary since, if the diagnosis is suspected, a therapeutic trial of vitamin C is innocuous.

Hereditary Hemorrhagic Telangiectasia (11). This is an inherited abnormality of blood vessels (an autosomal dominant condition) in which there is dilation of abnormally thin walled venules and capillaries. The dilations result in characteristic telangiectases which are small, flat, red or purple lesions which blanch on pressure. They occur throughout the body but can be seen externally most commonly on the lips, the tongue, the mucous membranes of the nose, and on the hands. Lesions of larger blood vessels also occur in this disease, most commonly pulmonary arteriovenous fistulas which develop in up to one-third of patients and which may cause "high output" heart failure. The mucocutaneous lesions may bleed excessively when traumatized. Recurrent epistaxis is the most common symptom of patients with the disorder, but the most troublesome problem is recurrent gastrointestinal bleeding which is notoriously difficult to manage. Accessible lesions can ordinarily be treated by local compression. There is no pharmacologic agent which will alter the course of the condition, but symptoms are quite variable; and many patients experience relatively little difficulty during the course of their life.

DISORDERS OF PLATELETS

Thrombocytopenia is one of the most common acquired disorders of hemostasis. The normal platelet count is between 150,000 and 400,000/cu mm, but the platelet count ordinarily must be reduced below 50,000/cu mm before untoward bleeding is observed. Even then symptoms are usually not observed unless the patient is traumatized. So-called spontaneous bleeding is unlikely unless the platelet count is reduced below 20,000/cu mm. The characteristic lesion of thrombocytopenia is the petechia, a small purpuric hemorrhage occurring on the skin or mucous membranes, especially at sites of elevated capillary pressure, such as the lower extremities, the forearm after inflation of a blood pressure cuff, or the face after prolonged crying or coughing. In fact if capillary pressure is raised high enough, or if capillaries are damaged after sunburn, for example, petechiae may be seen in otherwise normal people. Although cutaneous bleeding may be the first clue to the diagnosis of thrombocytopenia, morbidity from the disorder is more likely to result from gastrointestinal or genitourinary hemorrhage. As previously mentioned (see p.

397) if bleeding from these sites occurs, the patient should be examined at an appropriate time to determine whether an organic lesion such as a carcinoma of the colon or of the kidney has bled in association with defective hemostasis. The most feared complication of thrombocytopenia is intracerebral bleeding which, although it occurs infrequently, is still one of the major causes of death in patients with the disorder.

Evaluation of Thrombocytopenic Patient

The most common reasons for the development of thrombocytopenia are decreased production and increased sequestration of platelets. In ambulatory practice, however, the physician will most often encounter patients with platelet counts lower than normal in whom the precise pathophysiology of thrombocytopenia is not clear.

Many patients are found to have thrombocytopenia during the course of routine hematologic studies performed to obtain baseline data, or as part of an evaluation of an apparently unrelated condition. If the platelet count is over 50,000/cu mm in such circumstances, and the history, physical examination, and other hematologic evaluation, do not suggest that an underlying disease is present which urgently requires diagnosis and treatment, the clinician is probably justified in simply following the patient with serial platelet counts (performed monthly until it is determined how stable the counts are). If the counts do not decrease further, and if no other evidence of a disease process emerges, there is no need to stress the patient with further diagnostic procedures.

Symptomatic thrombocytopenia due to *decreased production* of platelets is usually observed in conjunction with processes, such as aplastic anemia, leukemia, or disseminated tuberculosis, that affect other hematologic cell lines. In contrast, severe thrombocytopenia due to *increased destruction* of platelets does not necessarily indicate the presence of a disease process that is affecting parts or systems of the body other than the blood platelets or their precursors. In order to be reasonably certain, however, about the pathophysiology of thrombocytopenia it is necessary to perform an aspiration of the bone marrow and to evaluate the numbers of megakaryocytes on a properly stained smear. That requires referral to a hematologist. Patients who have thrombocytopenia because of diseases involving the bone marrow will have reduced numbers of megakaryocytes; if the underlying disease process is severe, it is likely that abnormalities of production of, or qualitative changes in, other cell lines also will be noted. On the other hand it the patient is thrombocytopenic because of increased destruction of platelets, the numbers of megakaryocytes will be increased and the marrow will otherwise appear normal (although increased erythroid activity might be seen in those patients who are bleeding). If the practitioner decides that a bone marrow aspirate is indicated because of the severity of the thrombocytopenia (ordinarily less than 20,000 to 30,000 platelets/cu mm), because of evidence of a hemorrhagic diathesis at higher platelet counts, or because of a suspicion of a generalized underlying disease affecting the bone marrow, referral to a consultant in hematology is warranted. Depending on the nature of the underlying disease, it would then be appropriate for the hematologist to initiate and maintain therapy, or to refer the patient back to the primary physician.

Decreased Production of Platelets (Table 47.3)

Decreased production is a common mechanism for thrombocytopenia in ambulatory patients. Suppression of thrombopoiesis is often associated with *viral infections*, such as benign upper respiratory infections, infectious mononucleosis, and childhood exanthems. In most cases, bone marrow aspirates show megakaryocytes in normal or reduced numbers, although they sometimes appear morphologically abnormal. At other times increased numbers of megakaryocytes have been seen, suggestive of a destructive process (perhaps immunologic) to which the marrow has responded with increased production of platelets. In general, patients with benign viral infections are not likely to have severe thrombocytopenia and so are not at major risk of bleeding. The process ordinarily dissipates as the infection resolves.

Certain *drugs* predictably produce thrombocytopenia by affecting thrombopoiesis. Among these, cytotoxic agents are unlikely to be administered by the general internist. Chloramphenicol suppresses hematopoiesis and if given for a long period of time (usually more than a few weeks) may produce pancytopenia. It is unlikely that the practitioner would prescribe chloramphenicol for long periods in ambulatory practice, but if he does, he should be aware that the process is reversible when the drug is discontinued, in contrast to the much rarer cases of aplastic anemia caused by chloramphenicol which do not appear to be dose-related and are probably not reversible.

Although thiazide diuretics have been reported to produce mild to moderate thrombocytopenia commonly, in fact a clear-cut cause and effect relationship has not been demonstrated unequivocally. In the reported studies platelet counts have fallen several weeks after the beginning of therapy, sometimes associated with morphologically abnormal megakaryocytes. Rarely, however, thiazides have been clearly implicated in immunologically induced destructive thrombocytopenia (see below). Thiazide diuretics also are a common cause of allergic purpura (see p. 398), but patients with this condition have normal platelet counts.

Conceivably a large number of drugs are capable of producing thrombocytopenia by suppressing thrombopoiesis. Therefore, if patients are symptomatic from thrombocytopenia or have counts below 50,000/cu mm and the cause of thrombocytopenia is not known, the practitioner would be advised to discontinue administration of all drugs that are not considered absolutely essential.

MANAGEMENT

Unless thrombocytopenia is severe or unless patients have demonstrated a hemorrhagic diathesis, treatment is not necessary. Clearly, if drugs are incriminated in the process, they should be discontinued, if possible. If it is expected that thrombocytopenia will be transient, (as, for example, in patients being treated with cytotoxic therapy for an underlying malignancy), treatment with platelet transfusions sometimes is indicated. Also, some patients with chronic diseases of the bone marrow such as aplastic anemia may require more regular platelet transfusion. In any event, patients who are considered candidates for platelet transfusions should be followed by hematologists or oncologists as well as by the primary physician.

Increased Destruction of Platelets (Table 47.4)

Destruction of platelets as a cause of thrombocytopenia is infrequently seen in ambulatory practice but, when seen, is most likely to have an immunologic basis. *Autoimmune thrombocytopenia* (10), the most common of the antibody-induced disorders associ-

Table 47.3
Thrombocytopenia Due to Decreased Production of Platelets

GENERALIZED DISORDERS OF HEMATOPOIESIS
  Aplastic anemia[a]
  Invasive processes: leukemia, metastatic carcinoma, disseminated infection (*e.g.*, tuberculosis)[a]
  Folate or vitamin B_{12} deficiency[a]
  Drugs: cytotoxic agents, chloramphenicol
SPECIFIC DISORDERS OF THROMBOPOIESIS
  Certain infections (usually viral)[b]
  Certain drugs (in most cases, cause and effect have not been demonstrated)

---

[a] Not discussed in text.
[b] Processes most likely to be seen in ambulatory practice.

Table 47.4
Thrombocytopenia Due to Increased Destruction of Platelets

IMMUNOLOGIC
  Autoimmune[b]
  Isoimmune: neonatal and post-transfusion[a]
  Drug-induced: quinidine, quinine, gold, heroin
NONIMMUNOLOGIC
  Infections[a]
  Drug-induced: alcohol[b]
  Mechanical injury[a]

---

[a] Not discussed in text.
[b] Processes most likely to be seen in ambulatory practice.

ated with a low platelet count, is a diagnosis made in a practitioner's office by exclusion. Such patients characteristically present with petechial bleeding. Physical examination reveals no other evidence of disease; in particular, the spleen is usually not palpable. An acute disease, often preceded by benign viral infection, is seen more commonly in children and, by definition, lasts less than 6 months. The chronic illness (formerly called ITP, idiopathic thrombocytopenic purpura) lasts longer than 6 months and is seen more often in women than men (ratio of 3 or 4 to 1). The chronic disorder sometimes is associated with an underlying lymphoproliferative disorder, a collagen vascular disease, especially systemic lupus erythematosus and, more rarely, with autoimmune hemolytic anemia. The disease has been shown to be due to an antibody adsorbed to the surface of circulating platelets which results in their premature destruction by the reticuloendothelial system.

A large number of drugs (9) have been associated with thrombocytopenia on an immunologic basis. The most common are quinidine and quinine, but even these agents are implicated rarely. However, if a patient presents to the practitioner with severe thrombocytopenia due to increased destruction of circulating platelets, it is important to ask what drugs the patient is taking and to consider stopping them if there is any question of their being involved in the process. In recent years it has been demonstrated that occasional patients with rheumatoid arthritis treated with gold salts will develop thrombocytopenia that has an immunologic basis; in fact this process appears to be much more common than the generalized suppression of hematopoiesis occasionally associated with the administration of gold. In addition, several cases have been reported where heroin addicts have thrombocytopenia of an immune type, apparently produced by heroin (or an adulterant used with it).

It is not unusual for *alcoholics* to develop thrombocytopenia, usually to a moderate degree, after a binge. Alcohol appears to damage platelet membranes causing their premature destruction and also to inhibit compensatory increase in platelet production by marrow megakaryocytes. Once the binge is over, the platelet count returns to normal (or transiently higher than normal) in 4 to 5 days. Alcoholics of long standing who have developed cirrhosis of the liver and portal hypertension may have chronic thrombocytopenia because of increased sequestration of platelets in their spleens.

MANAGEMENT

Patients who are thrombocytopenic because of increased destruction of platelets also should be treated in consultation with a hematologist. If the patient presents with untoward bleeding, or if platelet counts are lower than 20,000/cu mm and immediate consul-

tation is not available, the practitioner would be justified in beginning treatment with the equivalent of 60 mg of prednisone a day and hospitalizing the patient while awaiting expert advice. Modification of the steroid dose, and decisions about splenectomy or other kinds of therapy should be made in conjunction with an experienced hematologist.

After treatment, approximately 90% of patients with chronic autoimmune thrombocytopenia ultimately have a permanent remission to the point where their platelet counts are high enough to support normal hemostasis without continued therapy. The rest require the continuing care of a hematologist.

Increased Sequestration of Platelets

Patients with large spleens often have thrombocytopenia because of redistribution of platelets within a larger splenic pool, most commonly because of congestive splenomegaly associated with portal hypertension. Splenectomy reverses thrombocytopenia, but should only be considered if there is a clear-cut hemorrhagic diathesis and if the underlying disease responsible for the enlarged spleen permits an operation to be performed.

Increased Utilization of Platelets

Patients with disseminated intravascular coagulation (8) characteristically have thrombocytopenia almost always in association with multiple defects in coagulation. Such patients often present acutely ill because of the underlying disease which has incited the hemostatic disorder. For example, in patients with various complications of pregnancy, disseminated carcinoma, or in some patients with septicemia, hemostatic mechanisms have been activated because of exposure of the circulating blood to thromboplastic material. The hemorrhagic diathesis is manifest most commonly by widespread bruising, petechiae, and mucous membrane bleeding, occasionally but not often associated clinically with evidence of venous or arterial thrombosis. In addition to thrombocytopenia patients present with disordered coagulation, which can be identified by measuring the prothrombin time, the partial prothromboplastin time, the concentration of fibrinogen in the plasma, and by the demonstration of increased titers of fibrinogen and fibrin degradation products in the plasma or serum. These products are formed by the fibrinolysis of fibrin by plasmin, the major proteolytic enzyme of the blood. Patients who are strongly suspected of having disseminated intravascular coagulation or in whom the diagnosis has been made, should be hospitalized for further treatment and to identify and treat the underlying disease.

Qualitative Disorders of Platelets (14)

A number of inherited abnormalities of platelets have been identified which result in impaired hemostasis even though platelet counts are usually within normal limits. In general the hemorrhagic diathesis associated with these conditions is milder than it is in patients with severe thrombocytopenia. Practitioners are unlikely to see these patients in their practice, but in patients who have unexplained bleeding, such as frequent epistaxis or recurrent gastrointestinal hemorrhage, with apparently normal coagulation and normal platelet counts, it is reasonable to perform a bleeding time, which is almost always abnormal in patients with qualitatively abnormal platelets. Similar abnormalities may be acquired in patients with various disease states, most commonly uremia; in fact, patients with chronic renal failure who have a tendency to bleed often improve after hemodialysis. Perhaps the most common acquired qualitative disorder of blood platelets occurs after the ingestion of small doses of aspirin which regularly prolongs the bleeding time and interferes with platelet aggregation and with the release of certain intracellular platelet constituents. Although untoward bleeding is unusual in patients who have taken aspirin, the drug may intensify a pre-existing tendency to bleed.

Thrombocytosis

Platelet counts above 400,000, unless associated with a myeloproliferative disorder such as polycythemia vera, myeloid metaplasia, or chronic granulocytic leukemia, are not in themselves associated with an increased risk of morbidity from excessive bleeding or clotting. They may, however, signify the presence of an underlying disease which requires attention. If on a routine evaluation there are a large number of platelets on the patient's peripheral blood smear, the practitioner should ask for a platelet count. If thrombocytosis exists, the most common causes are inflammatory disease and solid tumor malignancies. Since there are, however, a large number of conditions that have at least on occasion been associated with an elevated platelet count there is no reason for the practitioner to perform more than his usual comprehensive history and physical examination and any laboratory tests suggested by these examinations in attempts to explain the thrombocytosis.

Patients with myeloproliferative disorders, if they have thrombocytosis, almost always have also large distorted platelets on smear and other hematologic abnormalities typical of the particular disease. The great majority of those patients will also have splenomegaly. The treatment of thrombocytosis associated with myeloproliferative disease should be made in consultation with a hematologist.

COAGULATION DISORDERS

Patients who have a deficiency of one or more of the coagulation proteins are more likely to have extensive soft tissue bleeding or major hemorrage in response to trauma than are patients with disorders of the vasculature or of blood platelets (petechiae (see p. 399) are never a sign of abnormal coagulation). Congenital disorders of coagulation are relatively rare; the most common of them is hemophilia A (Factor VIII deficiency) an X-linked disorder that affects only 1 out of 10,000 males in the population. Congenital disorders are ordinarily readily diagnosed because of the history of lifelong bleeding and because, in the case of hemophilia, a history of characteristic hemorrhage into joints and soft tissues. Patients who have a severe hemorrhagic diathesis because of a congenital abnormality of clotting almost always have markedly low levels of the deficient coagulation protein. Therefore screening tests such as the partial thromboplastin time are almost always abnormal and provide clues to the presence of the disorder. It is unlikely that the practitioner will encounter such patients since most of them are diagnosed in childhood and are treated by experienced hemotologists thereafter. If the clinician should encounter such a patient, however, whom he suspects of having a congenital disorder of coagulation, but who has not previously been diagnosed, referral to an appropriate center would be warranted.

Von Willebrand's Syndrome (6) is an inherited abnormality of hemostasis (autosomal dominant) in which there is a reduction in antihemophilic globulin as well as a qualitative disorder of platelets which results in a prolonged bleeding time and decreased platelet adhesiveness. The platelets of these patients characteristically do not aggregate *in vitro* when exposed to the obsolete antibiotic ristocetin. The course of the disease as well as the extent of the laboratory abnormalities are quite variable from one patient to another, but in general the hemorrhagic diathesis is milder than it is in hemophilia A. Patients bleed most commonly from their gastrointestinal tract; it is not unusual that symptoms of the disease are not apparent until the patient is an adult. The bleeding time and the partial thromboplastin time are useful screening tests, but any patient suspected of having the disorder should have plasma Factor VIII assayed as well. The syndrome differs from true hemophilia in that after transfusion there is a more gradual, but often greater, rise in Factor VIII activity than would be anticipated on the basis of the amount of Factor VIII infused. Therefore, bleeding patients usually require fewer transfusions than do patients with true hemophilia. The diagnosis and treatment of patients with von Willebrand's syndrome, however, require the ongoing participation of a qualified hematologist.

Acquired disorders of coagulation are more common than congenital ones. By their nature they are more likely to be associated with multiple defects in hemostasis such as are seen in patients with disseminated intravascular coagulation (see above, p. 401) or in patients taking anticoagulant drugs (see Chapter 48). The diagnosis and management of these problems are discussed on those pages.

Table 47.5
Advice to Be Given Patients with a Disorder of Hemostasis

Take only medicine prescribed by your doctor. Do not take aspirin or cold remedies. You may take Tylenol instead of aspirin for pain, colds etc.

Do not drink any alcoholic beverage

Avoid any activity that might expose you unnecessarily to trauma; for example, contact sports

Wear a bracelet (provided by the physician), identifying you as a "bleeder" and giving the name of your disorder

Call your physician whenever:

You experience any abnormal bleeding (including excessive menstrual bleeding)

Before you visit your dentist

Before seeing any other physician

If you are hospitalized for any reason, without his knowing it

ADVICE TO PATIENTS WHO HAVE A DISORDER OF HEMOSTASIS

Table 47.5 lists some rules to give patients who have hemostatic dysfunction (also see Table 48.2, Chapter 48). It is also important that the patient knows the name of his disease and its clinical manifestations.

References

General

Williams, WJ, Beutler, E, Erslev, AJ and Rundles, RW (Eds): *Hematology*. McGraw-Hill, New York, 1977.
The currently standard text.

Zieve, PD and Levin, J: *Disorders of Hemostasis*. W.B. Saunders, Philadelphia, 1976.
A concise practical approach.

Specific

1. Bick, RL: Vascular disorders associated with thrombohemorrhagic phenomena. *Semin Thromb Hemostas* 5 (3): 167, 1979.
2. Cream, J, Gumpel, JM and Peachey, RDG: Schönlein-Henoch purpura in the adult. A study of 77 adults with anaphylactoid or Schönlein-Henoch purpura. *Q J Med* 39: 461, 1970.
3. Glenner, GG: Amyloid deposits and amyloidosis. *N Engl J Med* 302: 1283 and 1333, 1980.
4. Grey, HM and Kohler, PF: Cryoimmunoglobulins. *Semin Hematol* 10: 87, 1973.
5. Hodges, RE, Hood, J, Canham, JE, Sauberlich, HE and Baker, EM: Clinical manifestations of ascorbic acid deficiency in man. *Am J Clin Nutr* 24: 432, 1971.
6. Hoyer, LW: Von Willebrand's disease. *Prog Hemostas Thromb* 3: 231, 1976.
7. Kyle, RA, Gleich, GJ, Bayrid, ED and Vaughn, JH: Benign hypergammaglobulinemic purpura of Waldenström. *Medicine* 50: 113, 1971.
8. Merskey, C, Johnson, AJ, Kleiner, GJ and Wohl, H: The defibrination syndrome: clinical features and laboratory diagnosis. *Br J Haematol* 13: 528, 1967.
9. Miescher, PA: Drug-induced thrombocytopenia. *Semin Hematol* 10: 311, 1973.
10. Mueller-Eckhardt, C: Idiopathic thrombocytopenic purpura (ITP): clinical and immunologic considerations, *Semin Thromb Hemostas* 3 (3): 125, 1977.
11. Osler, W: On multiple hereditary telangiectases with recurring haemorrhages. *Q J Med* 1: 53, 1907.
12. Perkins, HA, MacKenzie, MR and Fudenberg, HH: Hemostatic defects in dysproteinemias. *Blood* 35: 695, 1970.
13. Ratnoff, OD: The psychogenic purpuras: a review of autoerythrocyte sensitization, autosensitization to DNA, "hysterical" and factitial bleeding, and the religious stigmata. *Semin Hematol* 17: 192, 1980.
14. Weiss, HJ: Platelet physiology and abnormalities of platelet function. *N Engl J Med* 293: 531 and 580, 1975.

CHAPTER FORTY-EIGHT

Thromboembolic Disease

PHILIP D. ZIEVE, M.D.

Patients with acute vascular occlusions, whether they be venous or arterial, almost always require hospitalization for initial diagnosis and treatment. The responsibility of the clinician in his office, therefore, is initially to recognize the problem and arrange for hospitalization in an appropriate facility and ultimately to manage the patients once discharged from the hospital.

VENOUS THROMBOEMBOLISM

Presentation

The majority of patients who present to the physician with symptoms and signs of venous occlusion have formed clots in the veins of the lower extremities. The primary pathologic process is stasis of blood (such as might be seen in people who are chronically ill, obese, or for other reasons lead sedentary lives). Patients usually present with swelling, pain, and tenderness of the affected extremity, although swelling alone and, more rarely, pain or tenderness alone may be the presenting symptom. Embolism to the lungs of clots from veins of the lower extremities is the major complication experienced by patients with this problem and is the primary reason why diagnosis and treatment are urgent. On the basis of history and physical examination alone it is virtually impossible to distinguish thrombosis of the deep veins of the lower extremities from other processes. Since it is clots in the deep veins that impose the risk of pulmonary embolism, it is extremely important to make this distinction so that rational treatment can be instituted. Therefore, patients suspected of having thrombosis of the deep veins, or of having had pulmonary embolism without clinical evidence of peripheral thrombosis *must* undergo specific diagnostic studies so that appropriate therapy for venous thromboembolism may be instituted. The most reliable diagnostic test is contrast venography. If characteristic filling defects are seen in radiographs of the veins after injection of contrast material, the diagnosis is established (Fig. 48.1). However, because of the potential morbidity of the procedure (see below), other tests have been recommended. The three most popular are impedance plethysmography, Doppler ultrasonography, and scanning of the extremities after injection of radioiodinated fibrinogen. The latter, because it is not very sensitive to clots in proximal veins, is not recommended for routine use. Both plethysmography and ultrasonography may be falsely positive in patients with venous stasis. These tests may be substituted for venography if the following conditions are met: (a) thrombophlebitis is suspected on clinical grounds, and plethysmography or ultrasonography is positive; and (b) the vascular laboratory has established that the results of the procedure have a high correlation with those of venography. If thrombophlebitis is suspected but plethysmography and/or ultrasonography is negative, ven-

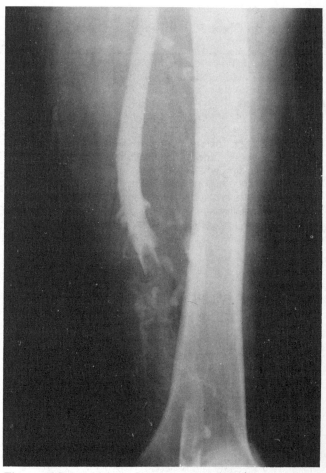

Figure 48.1   Venogram showing clots of deep veins of thigh.

ography must be done. Once a definite diagnosis of deep venous thrombosis is made, the patient must be hospitalized for treatment.

Patient Experience. Impedance plethysmography is performed by inflating a pneumatic cuff at the mid-thigh to occlude venous return, and then rapidly deflating it. The changes in blood volume are measured by changes in electrical resistance detected by a pair of electrodes attached to the cuff. There is no discomfort associated with this procedure other than the mild transient sensation of increased pressure during the few seconds of inflation.

Venography is performed after injection of a contrast medium into a dorsal vein of the foot (2). The patient should be warned that the procedure commonly is associated with unpleasant burning or cramping in the lower extremity while the dye is being injected. In addition, up to one-quarter of patients develop a painful swelling of the leg and ankle which begins 2 to 12 hours after the study, intensifies for 12 to 24 hours, and then begins to subside. The pathogenesis of this delayed reaction is unclear; no specific therapy, therefore, is indicated. There is a risk that venography itself will cause thrombosis; the incidence of deep vein thrombosis, proved by repeat venography, is probably in the range of 3 to 13%, and of superficial thrombosis, 6 to 25%.

If patients present with signs and symptoms of pulmonary embolism (see Chapter 50), the first diagnostic procedure should be a ventilation/perfusion scan of their lungs. If the scan is negative or read as "low probability" and the patient has signs and symptoms of venous occlusion of the lower extremities, further diagnostic studies should be done, as described above, to establish that diagnosis. If the lung scan is interpreted as indeterminate or high probability, the patient should be hospitalized—in the first instance for pulmonary angiography and in the second, for treatment. In many instances, however, the clinician will elect to admit the patient to the hospital on the basis of the clinical presentation and then obtain all necessary diagnostic procedures.

Treatment

The most important therapy for patients with thromboembolic disease of the lower extremities is anticoagulation. That is usually instituted in the hospital with heparin which is administered on the average for 10 days. Heparin is utilized because its onset of action is immediate and because of an unsubstantiated impression that it is a more effective anticoagulant than are coumarin compounds, the other major class of available anticoagulant drugs.

COUMARIN COMPOUNDS

Coumarin compounds are the drugs commonly used, however, in the anticoagulation of ambulatory patients. Ordinarily patients who have been hospitalized for diagnosis and initial treatment of venous thromboembolic disease are given a coumarin compound while heparin is being administered so that by the time that drug is discontinued, the full effect of the coumarin has become established. Coumarins interfere with the synthesis of vitamin K-dependent clotting factors (Factors II, VII, IX, and X) by the liver. Their effect is not fully realized, therefore, until they have been given for approximately 5 days. The administration of warfarin, the commonly used coumarin, usually is initiated in doses of 10 mg a day and then adjusted depending upon the therapeutic response, which is monitored by use of the prothrombin time, a reproducible, dependable test performed reliably by most clinical laboratories. The goal of anticoagulant therapy with coumarin is to maintain the prothrombin time 1½ to 2½ times the control value since it is within this range that a reasonable therapeutic effect is achieved and the risk of untoward bleeding is relatively small. During the first several weeks of administration of warfarin, the prothrombin time should be measured at least every few days until it is determined that the proper dosage schedule has been achieved. Thereafter it is appropriate to measure the anticoagulant response

monthly. At the same time it is prudent to examine the patient's urine and stool for occult blood and to assess his hematocrit value or hemoglobin concentration.

During the course of anticoagulation with coumarin compounds patients should be instructed to avoid predictable trauma such as might be expected from playing contact sports or from working in an environment associated with a high risk of injury. The physician should not give intramuscular injections to the anticoagulated patient; subcutaneous injections, done properly, are safe. Venipunctures are also safe, but the wound should be compressed for 10 to 15 min after the needle is withdrawn. Arterial punctures are contraindicated as outpatient procedures, where prolonged compression and observation of the puncture site are impractical.

Factors Affecting Response. There are a number of factors that might alter the patients responsiveness to warfarin following a period of stability (Table 48.1). Rarely the amount of vitamin K ingested in the patient's diet might be altered drastically, increasing the potency of warfarin if less vitamin K is ingested and decreasing it if considerably more is ingested. Significantly decreased ingestion of vitamin K is almost always associated with a markedly decreased intake of food, for example, in patients who are anorexic because of illness or who have instituted severe dietary restrictions in an attempt to lose weight. The effect of reduction in intake of vitamin K will be most pronounced in those patients who are concomitantly receiving antibiotics, which will inhibit the synthesis of vitamin K by normal flora of the intestinal tract. Because the vitamin K-dependent clotting factors are synthesized in the liver and because coumadins are metabolized by the liver, patients who develop intercurrent hepatic illness (hepatitis, for example) should be watched carefully for enhanced effective anticoagulation. In such a circumstance, the clinician would be wise to measure prothrombin times more frequently, but would not be required to discontinue warfarin unless bleeding ensued or the prothrombin time became significantly prolonged over the baseline therapeutic control.

One of the major problems confronting the clini-

Table 48.1
Some Factors That May Affect a Patient's Response to Warfarin

Enhanced Response	Reduced Response
Vitamin K deficiency	Barbiturates
Liver disease	Glutethimide
Drugs:	Griseofulvin
Chloral hydrate	Spironolactone
Cimetidine	
Phenylbutazone	
Quinidine	
Anabolic steroids	
Heparin	

cian in dealing with a patient taking coumarin anticoagulants is the possibility of drug interaction. A number of pharmacologic agents will potentiate the anticoagulant effect of coumarins and a few will inhibit it. The major drugs implicated are listed in Table 48.1. The clinician should be cautious, however, when initiating any new forms of therapy, or discontinuing old ones, in a patient who is receiving coumarin anticoagulants. Prothrombin times should be checked more frequently for several weeks to be sure that the pharmacologic response to coumarin has not been altered. In general, the likelihood of a potentiated response is much higher than that of an inhibitory one, so that there is greater risk of an increased susceptibility to bleeding than of an inhibition of anticoagulation. The clinician should also be careful about the use of drugs, such as aspirin, which have an effect on hemostasis that might be enhanced by warfarin or that may produce bleeding by injuring the gastric mucosa (Table 48.2).

Complications. It has been reported recently that there is a major risk in the use of coumarin compounds (and/or heparin) in pregnant patients (8). Major hemorrhagic complications occur in the fetus as well as teratogenic effects unrelated to the anticoagulant action. It has been recommended, therefore, that pregnancy be avoided in women who are being treated with anticoagulant drugs since a normal infant can be expected in only about two-thirds of such pregnancies.

By far the major complication experienced by patients taking coumarin anticoagulants is hemorrhage (5,6). Minor episodes such as small bruises and bleeding gums following brushing of the teeth are relatively common, but ordinarily do not require a change in the dose schedule of the anticoagulant. Occult rectal bleeding, minor bleeding from hemorrhoids, microscopic hematuria, and menorrhagia will be encountered in less than 10% of patients. When bleeding

Table 48.2
Advice to Be Given Patients Taking a Coumarin Anticoagulant

Take *only* medicines prescribed by your doctor. Do not take mineral oil, laxatives, aspirin, vitamins, or cold remedies. You may take Tylenol instead of aspirin for pain

Take your coumadin at the same time each day

Do not eat fish, broccoli, spinach, cabbage, kale, or cauliflower

Do not drink beer or any alcoholic beverage

Avoid any activity that might expose you unnecessarily to trauma, for example, contact sports

Call your doctor immediately whenever:
  You experience any abnormal bleeding
  Before you visit your dentist
  Before seeing any other physician
  If you cannot keep your scheduled appointment
  Before leaving on a trip
  If you are hospitalized, for any reason, without his knowing it

of this kind is observed, it is essential to make every attempt to establish the site of bleeding by the use of appropriate diagnostic studies. If prothrombin times have been maintained within the therapeutic range, the rapidity and extent of bleeding will dictate to the clinician whether or not the anticoagulant drug should be discontinued, at least temporarily. Major genitourinary or gastrointestinal bleeding sufficient to lower the hematocrit value or hemoglobin concentration, or bleeding of any degree in the central nervous system, dictates prompt discontinuation of the anticoagulant and immediate hospitalization for further diagnosis and treatment. It would be prudent for the physician to administer 25 to 50 mg of vitamin K_1 (AquaMephyton) intravenously at a rate no greater than 5 mg per min while arranging for hospitalization. (The prothrombin time will begin to shorten in 4 to 6 hours and, in most patients, will be in a safe range in 12 to 24 hours.) Major hemorrhage is often associated with an independent organic process such as a peptic ulcer, a carcinoma of the colon, or a cerebrovascular lesion; bleeding of this kind is likely to occur even when the prothrombin time is in the so-called therapeutic range.

It has been noted repeatedly that elderly patients, especially women, are more likely to have enhanced bleeding in response to coumarin anticoagulation; that experience, however, has not been universal.

Rarely, patients administered a coumarin anticoagulant will develop, within 10 days, hemorrhagic infarcts in their skin (often in women's breasts) with eventual sloughing of necrotic tissue. Under such circumstances, the drug must be stopped immediately.

Table 48.2 provides information useful for patients at the onset of anticoagulation or at the time that the patient is discharged from hospital. Selection of patients who are able to follow these rules will diminish considerably the incidence of hemorrhagic complications in patients taking anticoagulant drugs (also see Table 47.5, Chapter 47).

HEPARIN

Since heparin must be administered parenterally it is not a drug that can be conveniently used by outpatients. If, because of unacceptable side effects unrelated to its anticoagulant effect, a coumarin cannot be used, the practitioner must decide whether or not the risk of administration of heparin is greater than the risk of no anticoagulation at all. Full dose heparin, administered in an outpatient setting for the minimum 3 months necessary to achieve the kind of prophylaxis required, must be considered dangerous because of the relatively high incidence of untoward bleeding associated with its use. Moreover the effects of the drug when it is administered subcutaneously (the only practical route in nonhospitalized patients) will be much less predictable than they are when the drug is administered intravenously by use of a constant infusion pump. The practitioner would be faced both with the possibility of undertreatment and of overtreatment, with its accompanying risk of major bleeding. Therefore, except in extraordinary circumstances, the practitioner should avoid the use of full dose heparin in treating outpatients.

There have been two studies to date that have examined the effectiveness of a so-called low dose heparin regimen (5000 units twice a day intramuscularly) *versus* warfarin in preventing recurrence of deep venous thrombosis or of pulmonary embolism in patients who have recovered from an acute thromboembolic event (3,10). The studies are conflicting and therefore it is difficult to be enthusiastic in recommending this approach. However, if a patient has had a major thromboembolic event and *cannot* be treated with warfarin anticoagulants, a low dose regimen might be tried—for example, 5000 units administered intramuscularly twice a day for a 3-month period. Either the practitioner or one of his health extenders would instruct the patient, or a member of his family, about the proper way to administer the drug. Even with the low dose regimen the major complication from the use of heparin is bleeding. The risk is quite small, however, especially compared to the full dose regimen, so that untoward bleeding is expected only in those patients who already have a propensity to bleed because of an underlying disorder of hemostasis or because of a local lesion, such as a peptic ulcer, that is susceptible to hemorrhage. Because the effect of heparin in low doses is not reflected by a consistent abnormality of any of the usual tests of coagulation, there is no means by which the clinican can monitor this regimen.

ASPIRIN

Although aspirin (see below, p. 408) has been recommended in the prophylaxis of venous thromboembolism, there is no consensus that it is useful; and there is no justification for prescribing it as treatment of venous thrombosis.

Course

Patients who are being treated with coumarin anticoagulants have a recurrence rate of venous thromboembolism of between 10 to 40 episodes per 1000 patient months (4). One month after discharge from hospital, the rate stabilizes at approximately 10 episodes per 1000 patient months and remains in that range or slightly lower thereafter. The beneficial effect of anticoagulant therapy in such patients is most pronounced during the first 2 months after discharge from hospital; after 3 months the recurrence rate is the same whether the patient is anticoagulated or not, thereby providing a rationale for discontinuing therapy after 3 months in patients who are not at high risk because of continuing stasis (4). Patients who maintain risk factors for thromboembolic disease (chronic venous stasis for whatever reason) may,

barring complications of drugs, be considered for more prolonged periods of treatment. Although there is no reliable information in this regard, it is reasonable to continue therapy for high risk patients indefinitely unless a contraindication—such as major bleeding—develops.

Patients who have sustained thromboses of the deep veins of the lower extremities should be advised by their physicians to avoid prolonged sitting or standing in one position, should be encouraged to elevate their legs for 2 to 3 periods of 30 min each day, and to wear elastic stockings to promote venous return. Although the effectiveness of these maneuvers has not been established, there is little or no risk associated with any of them, and they may be of some value. At such time when a decision is made to discontinue anticoagulation therapy, it may be terminated abruptly without fear of an increased risk of early recurrence of venous thrombosis; the so-called "rebound phenomenon" has never been demonstrated.

Some patients, after repeated attacks of thrombosis of the veins of the lower extremities, will develop chronic changes in those veins with loss of competence of the valves and hemorrhage of small tributary veins leading to chronic edema and discoloration of the legs and ankles. Sometimes painful stasis ulcers also will develop that make it very difficult for the patient to move about. The treatment of this postphlebitic syndrome is the promotion of venous return from the lower extremities by the use of support stockings during the day and by elevation of the lower extremities for several hours each day. In those patients who have developed ulcers, bed rest with persistent elevation of the extremity above the level of the heart is recommended and, if necessary, administration of appropriate antibiotics. On such a regimen, the ulcers will invariably heal although they may recur if the patients are not careful to continue to follow prescribed conservative therapy (see chapter 85).

ARTERIAL THROMBOEMBOLISM

Unlike clots that form in the venous circulation, arterial thrombosis is primarily initiated by platelet plug formation, begun by the adherence of ambient platelets to altered surfaces in arterial vessels or in the left heart. Symptoms and signs of thrombosis appear more abruptly than do those of venous occlusion and commonly are associated with necrosis of tissue that had been fed by the now obstructed vessel. Heparin and coumarin anticoagulants, both experimentally and clinically, are of little use in preventing the formation of such clots or in preventing their propagation. There is a great deal of interest, therefore, in the use of drugs that interfere with platelet plug formation and that might be useful in the prophylaxis of arterial thromboembolism. Although a number of agents have been tested, only three—aspirin, dipyridamole, and sulfinpyrazone—can reasonably be expected to be efficacious and even these agents have not been clearly established as useful.

Aspirin

This drug, the most commonly used therapeutic agent in the world, has for some years been recognized to interfere with platelet function and therefore to inhibit platelet plug formation. It is now recognized that aspirin interferes with the formation of a very potent aggregating substance, thromboxane A_2, formed in platelets by the metabolism of prostaglandins. Aspirin inhibits the rate-limiting enzyme in this reaction, cyclooxygenase; as the result, the aggregation of platelets by collagen or connective tissue is inhibited and the release of substances, which themselves stimulate platelet aggregation, is impaired. Presumably as a result of the impairment, the bleeding time in patients taking even a single tablet of aspirin a day is prolonged.

Unless aspirin is administered to patients with an underlying hemostatic disorder (including the administration of an anticoagulant drug—see above) a hemorrhagic diathesis is unusual. However, it has been well established that aspirin has a toxic effect on the mucosa of the gastrointestinal tract which may result in bleeding or may increase the likelihood of hemorrhage from pre-existent peptic ulcerations.

There have been a number of studies performed to assess the efficacy of aspirin as a prophylactic agent in patients with atherosclerotic heart disease and cerebrovascular disease. To date there is no conclusive evidence that the drug is of any use in patients who have sustained a myocardial infarction in preventing either reinfarction or death (1). There is information, however, to suggest that aspirin reduces the incidence of transient ischemic attacks in men only when given in doses of 1200 mg a day (13); a single study suggested that the incidence of major stroke and death from cerebrovascular disease was also reduced considerably in men who had had transient ischemic attacks if they were given similar doses of aspirin (7). Finally, there is suggestive but inconclusive evidence of a positive effect of aspirin in preventing embolization in patients who have undergone implantation of prosthetic heart valves.

One of the problems in evaluating all of the studies that have been performed is that there is no good information on the proper dose of aspirin to be administered to achieve a maximum effect. There is some suggestion, however, that a relatively small dose (150 mg a day) might be optimal since larger doses inhibit the formation by blood vessels, of a prostaglandin metabolite, prostyclin, which appears to be a natural inhibitor of platelet aggregation (9). Until the problem is resolved, and more definitive studies are performed, it would be reasonable for the clinician to administer aspirin indefinitely to men who have experienced transient ischemic attacks.

Since the best studies have utilized 1200 mg of the drug a day, and since there is no definite information to suggest currently that a different dose would be more beneficial, such a dose would be reasonable. Currently there is no other indication for the prescription to patients of aspirin in the prophylaxis of atherosclerotic vascular disease.

Dipyridamole

Dipyridamole (Persantine) was developed as a vasodilating agent, but subsequently was discovered to interfere with platelet plug formation *in vivo*. The drug can be shown *in vitro* to inhibit phosphodiesterase, the enzyme which breaks down cyclic adenosine monophosphate (AMP) within blood platelets and other cells. Cyclic AMP is a potent inhibitor of platelet aggregation and dipyridamole presumably exerts its effect by maintaining higher levels of cyclic AMP within platelets. There is no evidence *in vitro*, however, that dipyridamole inhibits the aggregation of platelets or the release reaction nor is the bleeding time *in vivo* prolonged by this drug. Experimental studies have revealed no evidence that dipyridamole is of use in patients with ischemic heart disease or cerebrovascular disease. In patients who have prosthetic heart valves there is some suggestion that embolization may be prevented by dipyridamole, but few data have been obtained. At present, therefore, there is no justification for the use of dipyridamole in clinical practice to prevent arterial thrombembolism. In some studies dipyridamole and aspirin have been administered together and it is conceivable that some synergism may be attained in this manner since the drugs have different mechanisms of action. However, again there is no information to recommend the use of this combination.

Sulfinpyrazone

Sulfinpyrazone (Anturane) was developed as a uricurosuric agent but, like aspirin, has been discovered to inhibit prostaglandin (and therefore thromboxane A_2) synthesis *in vitro*. Unlike aspirin this biochemical effect is quite transient and is therefore dependent upon continued administration of the drug. Sulfinpyrazone has no effect on the aggregation of platelets or on the bleeding time. There has been no demonstration of a positive effect of this drug as a prophylactic agent in patients with cerebrovascular disease (13); neither is there any study to indicate that sulfinpyrazone is of use in patients with prosthetic heart valves. However, a large collaborative randomized double blind study has been reported demonstrating that sulfinpyrazone reduces considerably the incidence of sudden death for 7 months after myocardial infarction (12). Thereafter no effect of the drug could be demonstrated. The design of this study has been challenged by the Food and Drug Administration, and the data are being analyzed by an independent group (11). Additional experiments will undoubtedly

Table 48.3
Evidence of Effects of Drugs on Thromboembolic Disease

Drug	Ischemic Heart Disease	Prosthetic Heart Valves	Cerebrovascular Disease
Aspirin	Inconclusive	Suggestive but inconclusive evidence of positive effect in preventing embolization only	Positive effect in men only (see text)
Dipyridamole	Not yet demonstrated	Few data; may prevent embolization	No effect
Sulfinpyrazone	Unclear	No data	No effect

be necessary to establish definitively the efficacy of sulfinpyrazone in patients who have had an acute myocardial infarction. If sulfinpyrazone is administered, the most common adverse reactions of which the clinician should be aware are "peptic" symptoms best treated by administering the drug concomitantly with antacids.

SUMMARY

Table 48.3 summarizes the evidence for the use of agents which interfere with platelet function in the treatment and prophylaxis of thromboembolic disease.

References

General

Deykin, D: Warfarin therapy. N Engl J Med 283: 436, 1970.
   A sensible comprehensive review—not at all outdated.
Mammen, EF (Ed): Venous thromboembolism. Semin Thromb Hemostas 2: No. 4, 1976.
   A well referenced series of articles.
Wautier, JL and Caen, JP: Pharmacology of platelet suppressive agents. Semin Thromb Hemostas 5: 293, 1979.
   A well referenced noncritical review.
Weiss, HJ: Antiplatelet therapy. N Engl J Med 298: 1344 and 1403, 1978.
   A critical review.
Zieve, PD and Levin, J: Bleeding induced by anticoagulant drugs. In Disorders of Hemostasis. W. B. Saunders, Philadelphia, 1976.
   A readable summary of the problem.

Specific

1. Aspirin Myocardial Infarction Study Research Group: A randomized controlled trial of aspirin in persons recovered from myocardial infarction. JAMA 243: 661, 1980.
2. Bettman, MA and Paulin, S: Leg phlebography: the incidence, nature, and modification of undesirable side effects. Diagn Radiol 122: 101, 1977.
3. Bynum, LJ and Wilson JE III: Low-dose heparin therapy in the long-term management of venous thromboembolism. Am J Med 67: 553, 1979.
4. Coon, WW and Willis, PW III: Recurrence of venous thromboembolism. Surgery 73: 823, 1973.
5. Coon, WW and Willis, PW III: Hemorrhagic complications of anticoagulant therapy. Arch Intern Med 133: 386, 1974.
6. Davis FB, Estruch, MT, Samson-Corvera, EB, Voigt, GC and Tobin, JD: Management of anticoagulation in outpatients. Arch Intern Med 137: 197, 1977.
7. Fields, WS, Lemak, NA, Frankowski, RF and Hardy, RJ: Controlled trial of aspirin in cerebral ischemia. Stroke 8: 301, 1977.
8. Hall, JG, Pauli, RM and Wilson, KM: Maternal and fetal sequelae of anticoagulation during pregnancy. Am J Med 68: 122, 1980.
9. Harter, HR, Burch, JW, Majerus, PW, Stanford, N, Delmez, JA, Anderson, CB and Weerts, CA: Prevention of thrombosis in patients on hemodialysis by low-dose aspirin. N Engl J Med 301: 577, 1979.
10. Hull, F, Delmore, T, Genton, E, Hirsch, J, Gent, M, Sackett, D, McLoughlin, D and Armstrong, P: Warfarin sodium versus low-dose heparin in the long-term treatment of venous thrombosis. N Engl J Med 301: 855, 1979.
11. Relman, AS: Sulfinpyrazone after myocardial infarction: no decision yet. N Engl J Med 303: 1476, 1981.
12. The Anturane Reinfarction Trial Research Group: Sulfinpyrazone in the prevention of sudden death after myocardial infarction. N Engl J Med 302: 250, 1980.
13. The Canadian Cooperative Study Group: A randomized trial of aspirin and sulfinpyrazone in threatened stroke. N Engl J Med 299: 53, 1978.

CHAPTER FORTY-NINE

Infectious Mononucleosis

LARRY WATERBURY, M.D.

Table 49.1
Signs and Symptoms of Infectious Mononucleosis

Common Symptoms		Common Signs		Less Common Signs and Symptoms	
Malaise	100%	Adenopathy	100%	Jaundice	10%
Sore throat	85%	Fever	90%	Arthralgia	5%
Warmth, chilliness	70%	Pharyngitis	85%	Skin rash	5%
Anorexia	70%	Splenomegaly	60%	Diarrhea	5%
Headache	50%	Bradycardia	40%	Photophobia	5%
Cough	40%	Periorbital edema	25%		
Myalgia	25%	Palatal enanthem	25%		

SIGNS AND SYMPTOMS

Infectious mononucleosis is an acute febrile illness seen primarily in teenagers and young adults. Classically patients present with pharyngitis, lymphadenopathy, splenomegaly, and marked atypical lymphocytosis seen on peripheral smear. Table 49.1 lists the relative frequency of the characteristic signs and symptoms associated with the illness. Pharyngitis can be extremely severe and is frequently accompanied by an exudate which may be foul smelling. Rarely it may be so severe that it leads to respiratory obstruction. Many of the relatively few patients who do not present with pharyngitis simply have a nonspecific febrile illness associated with malaise. Other patients present with mild jaundice and a syndrome that mimics infectious hepatitis. Posterior cervical adenopathy is characteristic of almost all patients, and there is frequently generalized lymph node enlargement as well. Some patients may experience a protracted course with nonspecific symptoms, lymphadenopathy, and splenomegaly persisting for weeks. Most patients are significantly improved by the end of 3 weeks.

Patients usually present to the physician at the end of the first week of a nonspecific illness characterized by malaise, and perhaps by anorexia, mild headache, and low grade fever. Adenopathy, splenomegaly, and pharyngitis usually appear at about this time and slowly resolve over the following weeks. However, as noted below, the classical laboratory features of the illness may not be present until the second or third week of the clinical illness.

LABORATORY FEATURES

The hematocrit value is usually normal, although mild hemolysis is seen on occasion. Rarely, a severe autoimmune hemolytic anemia is seen. The peripheral white cell count is usually elevated with the maximal elevation occurring during the 2nd or 3rd week of the clinical illness. Early in the course there may be a severe absolute neutropenia. Occasionally the absolute neutrophil count is less than 500/cu mm. The differential count of the white cells is characterized by an absolute lymphocytosis with large numbers of atypical lymphocytes. The platelet count is normal to slightly decreased in the majority of the patients. Severe thrombocytopenia may occur, but is rare. Liver function tests are usually mildly abnormal. Slight increases in the activity of hepatic enzymes are common, and up to 50% of patients may show slight hyperbilirubinemia. Enzyme levels never reach the height seen in viral hepatitis.

Serologic Features

Diagnosis is based upon the presence of typical clinical features and characteristic serologic tests. Epidemiologic data strongly implicate the Epstein-Barr (EB) virus (a herpes virus) as the etiologic agent in infectious mononucleosis (2). Antibody titers to EB virus rise early in the course of the illness and then fall slowly over several weeks, although never back to normal (3). Heterophil antibodies are elevated in most patients and are maximally positive during the 3rd week of clinical illness. Differential absorption studies are necessary to identify the presence of those heterophil antibodies which are specific for infectious mononucleosis (the antibodies are absorbed by bovine red cells but not by guinea pig kidney). A number of rapid macroagglutination slide tests are commercially available (4). Most utilize horse red cells which are more sensitive than sheep red cells in the detection of heterophil antibodies. Some kits utilize differential absorption techniques as well. In general, the slide kits are quite sensitive to the detection of heterophil antibodies but may yield positive results also in other conditions associated with such antibodies (serum sickness, viral hepatitis, cytomegalovirus infections, other viral illnesses, leukemia).

In patients with classic symptoms of infectious mononucleosis a positive mononucleosis slide test is sufficient serologic confirmation for the diagnosis for clinical purposes. Some 5 to 10% of patients with clinical infectious mononucleosis and appropriate changes in the titer of EB virus antibody are heterophil antibody-negative. Another 5 to 10% of patients with clinical features of infectious mononucleosis have another illness (cytomegalovirus infection, toxoplasmosis, etc.)

DIFFERENTIAL DIAGNOSIS

The differential diagnosis of infectious mononucleosis includes a number of other infectious processes and even malignant conditions. An occasional case associated with bizarre lymphocyte morphology and thrombocytopenia may mimic acute leukemia. Perhaps most confusing are infections due to the cytomegalovirus (CMV). In such infections pharyngitis and lymphadenopathy are much less common. CMV infections probably account for the majority of cases of seronegative mononucleosis. Acute toxoplasmosis may also mimic infectious mononucleosis, but pharyngitis is less common. The diagnosis can usually be established by the demonstration of a rising IgM toxoplasmosis titer.

The pharyngitis in infectious mononucleosis may closely resemble that of exudative streptococcal pharyngitis and all patients should have throat cultures to rule out bacterial infection.

COMPLICATIONS (1)

Severe complications of infectious mononucleosis are rare, but do occur. They include neurologic problems (encephalitis, meningitis, peripheral neuropathy, Guillain-Barré syndrome), bacterial superinfection, and splenic rupture. The latter has accounted for a number of deaths, especially since the diagnosis is easily missed. The physician should be suspicious of such a diagnosis if there is a recent history of sudden, brief, sharp abdominal pain. Occasional deaths have been seen also with severe pharyngitis and airway obstruction.

TREATMENT

There is no specific treatment for infectious mononucleosis, and all that is usually necessary is supportive care. There is no evidence that prolonged bed rest is helpful. It is reasonable for patients to avoid strenuous activities until they feel strong enough to participate Contact sports should be avoided if the spleen is tender or significantly enlarged. Since splenomegaly may persist for months, however, it seems unreasonable to avoid contact sports until the spleen is no longer palpable. Although contacts do occasionally develop infectious mononucleosis there is no evidence that the disease is highly infective and patients should not be rigidly restricted from interpersonal contacts.

Surgery, of course, is indicated for splenic rupture (5). Corticosteroids are usually reserved for patients with severe pharyngitis and impending airway obstruction in which situation they are usually dramatically effective. Ordinarily a high dose (such as 40 to 60 mg prednisone daily) is given initially, with rapid tapering of treatment by 1 week to 10 days.

References

General

Carter, RL and Penman, HG (Eds): *Infectious Mononucleosis.* Blackwell Oxford, 1969.

Hoagland RJ: *Infectious Mononucleosis.* Grune & Stratton, New York, 1969.

Shurin, SB: Infectious mononucleosis. *Pediatr Clin North Am* 26: 315, 1979.

Specific

1. Dorman, JM, Glick, TH, Shannon, DG, et al.: Complications of infectious mononucleosis. *Am J Dis Child* 128: 239, 1974.
2. Evans, AS, Niederman, JC and McCollum, RW: Seroepidemiologic studies of infectious mononucleosis with EB virus. *N Eng J Med* 279: 1121, 1968.
3. Henle, W, Henle, GE and Horwitz, CA: Epstein-Barr virus specific diagnostic tests in infectious mononucleosis. *Hum Pathol* 5: 551, 1974.
4. Rippey, JH and Bowman, HE: Infectious mononucleosis test performance on CAP survey specimens. *Am J Clin Pathol* 72: 363, 1979.
5. Rutkow, IM: Rupture of the spleen in infectious mononucleosis *Arch Surg* 113: 718, 1978.

SECTION 7

Pulmonary Problems

CHAPTER FIFTY

Common Pulmonary Problems: Cough, Hemoptysis, Dyspnea, and Chest Pain

PHILIP L. SMITH, M.D., and EUGENE R. BLEECKER, M.D.

Patients with acute respiratory diseases usually develop symptoms that result in the rapid diagnosis and treatment of the underlying disorder. On the other hand, chronic diseases of the lung, that cause slowly progressive symptoms, may go undetected unless incidentally discovered as part of a general medical evaluation that includes routine chest roentgenogram and screening pulmonary function tests. This chapter will discuss three common pulmonary symptoms with which the general physician is often confronted: cough, hemoptysis, dyspnea, and noncardiac chest pain.

COUGH

Cough is an important defense mechanism that clears the airways of secretions and inhaled particles. In association with other respiratory symptoms, cough frequently causes the patient to consult with a physician. Cough is composed of three phases: a deep inspiration, closure of the glottis accompanied by a rapid increase in pleural pressure, a final opening of the glottis, and an explosive release of pressure.

A brief understanding of the anatomy of the cough reflex will aid in the evaluation and treatment of cough. Coughing is initiated by stimulation of mucosal neural receptors located primarily in the nasopharynx, larynx, trachea, and bronchi to the level of the terminal bronchioles. Stimulation of the receptors in the nasopharynx also may cause sneezing, whereas stimulation of tracheal and bronchial receptors also may cause bronchospasm. After activation of the receptors, impulses are conducted along afferent pathways in the 9th and 10th cranial nerves to the cough center in the medulla. The cough reflex is completed through efferent pathways which cause forceful contraction of the diaphragm and other expiratory muscles. There are many different stimuli that activate these receptors, but all essentially initiate cough by some form of mechanical or chemical irritation. Acute inflammation of the airways found in bronchitis and tracheitis may disrupt the bronchial mucosa, increasing its permeability, and possibly exposing the receptors. Furthermore, the accompanying increases in respiratory secretions will lead to cough. Environmental pollutants, such as cigarette smoke, can directly stimulate the receptors without necessarily provoking an inflammatory reaction. Finally, although reflex bronchoconstriction may be caused by stimulation of irritant receptors, bronchospasm itself stimulates irritant receptors, leading to cough.

Acute Cough Syndromes

Table 50.1 shows the common and uncommon causes of cough. Cough that occurs as a symptom of acute inflammatory disease, such as tracheitis and tracheobronchitis secondary to upper respiratory infection, usually is limited by the length of the illness. However, cough that is triggered by mild bronchospasm may persist for weeks to months following a viral upper respiratory tract infection (see below). Usually viral infections and atypical pneumonias are associated with nonproductive coughs, while bacterial infections are associated with significant sputum production. Younger patients tend to have a more productive cough associated with pneumonia while older individuals, especially those with chronic obstructive pulmonary disease, may retain secretions because of airway collapse during coughing. When a productive cough follows a typical viral syndrome, it may also signal the development of a superimposed

**Table 50.1
Causes of Cough**

Causes	Examples
COMMON CAUSES	
Acute	
Inflammation	Tracheitis, bronchitis, pneumonia
Irritation	Air pollutants
Bronchospasm	Postrespiratory infections
Chronic	
Inflammation	Bronchitis, pollution, cigarettes, bronchiectasis
Irritation	Cigarettes, cancer
Bronchospasm	Asthma, postrespiratory infection
LESS COMMON CAUSES	
Irritation	Aortic aneurysm, chronic aspiration, auditory canal stimulation (cerumen, hair)
Inflammation	Sarcoid, alveolitis
Psychogenic	

bacterial bronchitis or pneumonia. High concentrations of industrial pollutants, such as insoluble gases (for example, SO_3 or NO_2) which are not removed in the upper airway can cause either a nonproductive or a productive cough secondary to chemical irritation.

Chronic Cough Syndromes

Coughing that is persistent is more bothersome than the acute cough syndrome described above. Clearly the most common cause of coughing is cigarette smoking. Such coughing is usually dry and hacking, and is worse in the morning. The number of cigarettes smoked bears little relationship to the development of cough except at very high levels of cigarette consumption (three to four packs per day) (15). Perhaps because they inhale deeply, smokers of marijuana may complain of a cough after smoking only one to two cigarettes daily. By definition, all patients with bronchitis have productive coughs. While cough is a prominent symptom in patients with bronchogenic and mediastinal tumors, patients with metastatic tumors or with nodules that arise peripherally outside of the airways or beyond irritant receptors seldom present with cough. In nonsmokers, the most common cause of chronic cough is postnasal drip resulting from chronic sinusitis or allergic rhinitis (15). It is very important to recognize that airway obstruction in smokers and in nonsmokers can be associated with a chronic dry cough. This may be the only manifestation of obstructive airway disease and need not be associated with dyspnea, wheezing, or with large changes in pulmonary function.

Other less common causes of chronic cough include any process that stimulates the neural receptors in the pleura and pericardium (5). Even impacted cerumen in the external auditory canal can elicit a chronic cough. If a complete history and physical examination have revealed no positive findings, it is often tempting to attribute chronic cough to a psychogenic etiology; however, this is an extremely rare cause of coughing and has most often been reported in children. Psychogenic cough is not productive; it subsides during sleep, and is clearly related to emotional stress (7).

Evaluation

Evaluation of the acute and chronic cough syndromes is similar. Usually a history and physical examination will yield a presumptive diagnosis. Information should be obtained about the circumstances surrounding the development and duration of the cough, environmental exposure, smoking history, and any past history of obstructive airway disease. A history of constant swallowing or of throat-clearing suggests postnasal drip, even though the patient may deny many other symptoms associated with sinusitis.

Although the physical examination seldom provides a specific diagnosis, it may provide important clues. Careful examination of the ear, nose, throat, and lower respiratory tract is of paramount importance. Cobblestoning in the oropharynx represents lymphoid hyperplasia that is commonly seen in patients with chronic sinusitis, but this is a nonspecific finding that can be found in other conditions not necessarily associated with cough. Examination of the chest may reveal rhonchi caused by the loose secretions that result from acute or chronic infection. Occasionally a localized wheeze suggests a bronchogenic tumor, whereas generalized wheezing at end expiration confirms the diagnosis of obstructive lung disease. (However, a normal physical examination cannot exclude a diagnosis of airway obstruction.) Finally, the physical examination allows the physician to observe the quality and severity of the cough. A harsh cough associated with loose secretions is characteristic of tracheobronchitis resulting from viral upper respiratory infection. When little or no coughing occurs in the course of a visit to the physician, the patient should be asked to cough to see whether the cough is productive or is associated with wheezing. This is also useful since some patients, especially women, refuse to admit to expectoration of sputum and often unconsciously swallow their secretions.

If a diagnosis is not obvious after a history and physical examination, laboratory testing is indicated. A complete blood count and microscopic examination of the sputum should be performed. Sputum with eosinophilia, as seen in asthma, may appear purulent; thus if it is not examined microscopically, the patient may be treated inappropriately with antibiotics. A chest roentgenogram will demonstrate virtually all acute infections that involve the pulmonary parenchyma as well as some of the rarer causes of chronic cough such as aortic aneurysm and sarcoidosis. Patients with coughing due to viral and bacterial tracheobronchitis, asthma, or to cigarette smoking will usually have a normal chest roentgenogram or may have changes that suggest underlying obstructive pulmonary disease (hyperinflation). A spirogram should also be obtained to document airway obstruction (see below). Patients with reversible obstruction may have only intermittent bronchospasm, and between attacks their pulmonary function may be normal.

If no specific diagnosis has been made after this evaluation, the patient should be seen periodically for 1 to 2 months before other invasive diagnostic procedures are attempted. When the chest roentgenogram is normal, bronchoscopy, for example, seldom provides a specific diagnosis. Although a proximal bronchogenic tumor can be hidden on a chest roentgenogram by the mediastinal shadows, patients with these tumors often not only have a chronic cough but also have associated hemoptysis (see below) (15).

Confirmation that bronchospasm and hyper-reactive airways are the causes of persistent coughing can be obtained by bronchoprovocation tests either with pharmacologic agents, such as histamine and methacholine or with exercise, although these tests are not always essential (see Chapter 52). The tests are not routine, and the patient will need to be referred to a pulmonary subspecialist who has special laboratory facilities available to perform bronchoprovocation. These procedures should be done only after a medical history, physical examination, and laboratory studies, including routine spirometry, have been completed since they are not indicated in patients with obvious spasmodic asthma or with significant obstructive airway disease. The main purpose of such testing is to confirm the presence of hyper-reactive airways in patients with an equivocal history and laboratory studies. If bronchoprovocation is not readily available, then routine spirometry that is consistent with early airways obstruction (see Chapter 52) may provide adequate supporting evidence for the physician to initiate a diagnostic trial with bronchodilators.

Therapy

The specific therapy of the various acute inflammatory and irritating processes likely to cause coughing is discussed in detail in individual chapters dealing with these topics.

In general, viral tracheobronchitis requires only symptomatic therapy since coughing will usually spontaneously subside in 2 to 4 weeks. Patients with bacterial bronchitis or pneumonia require antibiotics (Chapter 27). Patients with persistent coughing and a history compatible with allergic airways disease (rhinitis, extrinsic asthma), intermittent (intrinsic asthma) or chronic obstructive airways disease, as well as those with bronchospasm and coughing following a viral upper respiratory tract infection should

have a diagnostic and therapeutic trial with bronchodilators. Therapy with bronchodilators should be started after a spirogram is obtained to document airflow obstruction or after appropriate bronchoprovocation studies (see above). Treatment should begin with an inhaled long acting specific β_2-sympathomimetic agonist (metaproterenol, terbutaline, fenoterol) and later, if necessary, an oral methylxanthine can be added. A detailed therapeutic approach to the pharmacologic treatment of bronchospasm is presented in Chapter 52.

The cessation of cigarette smoking and the avoidance of a polluted environment will improve an acute cough. Chronic coughing also responds to symptomatic treatment although the response is often not as dramatic. The patient who continues to smoke and to complain of cough is particularly frustrating. It is often difficult to convince these patients that as few as one to two cigarettes per day cause airway irritation and inflammation. In one study of 200 patients with a chronic cough, 50% had relief within 1 month of cessation of cigarette smoking while eventually 77% of these patients had complete resolution of their cough (14).

If a patient has impacted cerumen in the auditory canal, removal of the irritation provides immediate relief. On the other hand if a patient has an aortic aneurysm or a bronchogenic tumor, therapy must be directed at these underlying etiologies.

After specific therapy has been initiated, the use of *antitussives* should be considered. In spite of the enormous demands made for antitussives, there are few situations in which these preparations are absolutely necessary. Moreover, the expectoration of sputum is a major goal in the therapy of inflammatory lung disease. Therefore, when antitussives are needed in patients with productive coughs, it is usually better to attempt cough reduction (not total suppression), primarily to allow the patients to sleep. In the United States there are several hundred cough and decongestant preparations, sold usually as combination products. Understandably, the Federal Drug Administration has made efforts recently to eliminate many of these preparations from the marketplace.

Antitussives act on the cough reflex either by anesthetizing the peripheral irritant receptors or by increasing the threshold of the cough center. Table 50.2 summarizes the most useful active non-narcotic oral antitussives, their site of action, and their recommended dosages.

Probably the two most effective "non-narcotic" antitussives are dextromethorphan and benzonatate. Dextromethorphan is chemically derived from the opiates; however, it is classified as non-narcotic because it has no sedative or analgesic effects and, therefore, has little potential for abuse. Dextromethorphan is the most commonly used antitussive and suppresses cough centrally. It is metabolized by the liver and should be avoided in patients with signifi-

Table 50.2
Non-Narcotic Antitussives

Drug	Brand Name	Usual Dose	Site of Action	Comment
Benzonatate	Tessalon	100–200 mg q.i.d.	Peripheral	Considered most effective peripheral agent
Dextromethorphan	Many preparations	15–30 mg q.i.d.	Central	Considered most effective central agent
Noscapine	Tusscapine	15–30 mg q.i.d.	Central	
Levopropoxyphene	Novrad	100 mg q.i.d.	Central	

cant hepatic insufficiency. Occasionally, the drug will cause nausea or dizziness, and overdosages of more than 200 mg will lead to central nervous system depression. Benzonatate is a peripherally acting anesthetic similar to tetracaine. Its only side effects are mild dizziness, vertigo, and occasional nausea. If the drug is accidentally chewed, both unpleasant taste and prolonged oral anesthesia result. Overdosage has been associated with central nervous system stimulation resulting in tremors followed by profound central nervous depression. It is reasonable to treat patients initially with dextromethorphan and, if intolerable cough persists, to substitute benzonatate. Two other useful oral antitussives, noscapine and levopropoxyphene, are less commonly used but are useful alternatives if neither dextromethorphan nor benzonatate can be taken.

If non-narcotic antitussives are ineffective, then codeine should be tried. Many clinicians will in fact prescribe codeine preferentially to patients with persistent cough because it is a more potent cough suppressant than the non-narcotic agents. Codeine is effective in doses of 10–20 mg administered every 3–6 hours. The common side effects—nausea, vomiting, constipation, dry mouth, and sedation—are usually not experienced when these recommended doses are employed.

Topical anesthetics can be used as cough suppressants but they are weak, usually ineffective, and may cause hypersensitivity reactions. These weak anesthetics primarily anesthetize the irritant and pain receptors in the oral pharynx and are contained in many over-the-counter gargles and throat lozenges. If they are abused and used in excessive doses, the gag reflex will be abolished and the risk of pulmonary aspiration will be increased.

The use of expectorants and humidification of the airways in patients with respiratory disease is discussed in Chapter 52.

HEMOPTYSIS

Hemoptysis is defined as the expectoration of blood; it can range from the coughing of minimal amounts of blood-tinged sputum to the coughing of large amounts of blood with clots. Distinguishing between hemoptysis and hematemesis is not difficult since expectorated blood usually is bright red, frothy, has an alkaline pH, and is often mixed with sputum containing macrophages and white blood cells. Frequently, patients with hemoptysis will complain of a tickling or bothersome irritation in their chest and be able to localize these sensations to one lung. On the other hand, hematemesis is characterized by blood that is darker brown, has an acid pH, and is mixed with food particles; often there is a history of alcoholism, drug abuse, or of previous gastrointestinal disease. In massive hemoptysis or hematemesis, the distinction is not difficult since the physician can easily differentiate coughing from vomiting. However, blood originating in the sinuses or in the upper airway can be aspirated and later expectorated. Thus, a careful history and physical examination must be performed in this situation to avoid inappropriate evaluation and treatment. The patient should be instructed always to collect and save his bloody sputum so that the hemoptysis can be quantified. A history of hemoptysis should not be ignored if a patient cannot produce a specimen on command since the symptom can be intermittent.

The various pulmonary causes of hemoptysis are summarized in Table 50.3. Published reports about the relative probabilities of the various causes of hemoptysis reflect the type and location of the institution providing the report. Studies from large urban centers report a greater incidence of infectious etiologies such as tuberculosis (8); those from the Veteran's Administration find primarily lung cancer and bronchitis; and studies from predominantly referral institutions present unusual causes. The etiology of hemoptysis found in an ambulatory setting will also depend on the type and location of the medical practice.

If there is blood streaking of the sputum, bronchitis or bronchiectasis is the cause 30 to 60% of the time, and lung cancer is responsible 20 to 30% of the time. When the entire sputum is bloody, carcinoma or bronchiectasis is more likely than bronchitis. However, with the more liberal ambulatory use of antibiotics and the appropriate decline in the use of diagnostic bronchography, structural bronchiectasis resulting from recurrent infection is probably underdiagnosed while bronchitis (chronic productive cough) is overdiagnosed. Active cavitary tuberculosis is now a less common cause of hemoptysis than it once was although "dry" bronchiectasis from old tuberculous infection is still frequently found. Bronchogenic carcinoma that originates in major bronchi

Table 50.3
Pulmonary Causes of Hemoptysis

COMMON	
Inflammatory	Bronchitis, bronchiectasis, tuberculosis, pneumonia, lung abscess
Neoplasm	Lung cancer
Vascular	Pulmonary embolus/infarction
LESS COMMON	
Inflammatory/ Immunologic	Goodpasture's syndrome, idiopathic pulmonary hemosiderosis, cavitary disease (with a "fungus ball"), parasites, broncholithiasis, cystic fibrosis
Neoplasm	Bronchial adenoma, metastatic cancer
Vascular	Arteriovenous malformation, sequestration, mitral stenosis, anticoagulation
Chest trauma	

often presents with hemoptysis resulting from an associated infection, erosion of the tumor through the bronchial mucosa, or from actual bleeding from a friable cancer. Usually blood originating from pneumonia or a lung abscess is mixed with "pus," and the sputum appears red-brown or red-green. Hemoptysis from pulmonary emboli occurs in approximately 30% of cases of documented emboli associated with an infarction of the lung (1). Interestingly, even with the advent of the fiberoptic bronchoscope, the cause of hemoptysis remains undiagnosed 5 to 15% of the time (16).

Less common causes of hemoptysis are also listed in Table 50.3, but again this ranking reflects to some extent the location of a practice since mycetomas within fungus cavities (6) and parasitic diseases that cause hemoptysis, for example, will be much more frequently seen in endemic areas of the country. While the more common presentation of bronchial adenomas is atelectasis with cough and fever, bleeding does occur since these tumors are vascular. Metastatic tumors tend to enlarge within the lung parenchyma; thus bleeding as the initial presentation is exceedingly rare. Chronic mitral stenosis with poorly controlled congestive heart failure and pulmonary hypertension will lead to bleeding of the bronchial veins and to blood-tinged sputum. Hemoptysis can occur in patients treated with warfarin or heparin, especially those who have associated lung disease such as bronchitis or cancer, even if the anticoagulation is carefully controlled. Occasionally blunt chest trauma will produce hemoptysis in an otherwise healthy individual.

Evaluation

The diagnostic evaluation of hemoptysis is aimed at localizing the site and quantifying the amount of bleeding, beginning with a history and physical examination, followed by an examination of the chest roentgenogram. Every patient should be asked to try to identify whether the bleeding stems from extrathoracic sites, including the gastrointestinal tract, or from the lungs. If the source of hemoptysis is an intrathoracic structure, the patient should be asked to localize the site of bleeding to a specific area or at least to the right or left lung. An attempt should then be made to quantitate the amount of hemoptysis since patients who have expectorated more than 25 to 50 ml of bright red blood during a 24-hour period require immediate hospitalization. Although rare, massive hemoptysis of more than 600 ml of blood during a 24-hour period represents a medical emergency since survival of the patient is dependent on rapid diagnosis and on surgical therapy (10). Other useful data that should be elicited during a medical history include a prior history of tuberculosis, chronic bronchitis, evidence of systemic symptoms compatible with a pulmonary neoplasm, or a recent history of an acute pulmonary infectious process or chest trauma. A history of mitral valvular heart disease or of travel with exposure to parasitic agents should alert the physician to these rare causes of bleeding. During the physical examination, extrathoracic sources of bleeding from structures such as the nasal passages, sinuses, and pharynx should be sought.

Localized wheezing or rales suggest disease confined to one side of the chest, information that may be particularly useful when the chest roentgenogram is normal. Next, sputum should be repeatedly collected and examined to quantify the severity of the hemoptysis (8). The presence of clots suggests slower bleeding.

Evaluation of the chest roentgenogram is critical since all acute inflammatory diseases such as active tuberculosis, pneumonia, and lung abscess will produce obvious pulmonary infiltrates. In addition, 85% of neoplasms and most pulmonary emboli with an associated infarction will also show localized pulmonary lesions. However, localization of the bleeding source is frequently precluded by bilateral aspiration of blood or by the presence of bilateral pulmonary disease on chest roentgenogram. Patients with bronchitis or bronchiectasis often have normal films. If the bronchiectasis is a result of old tuberculosis, however, apical scarring may suggest the diagnosis; otherwise, there may be increased lower lobe markings or infiltrates if there is recurrent infection. Bronchitis is a clinical diagnosis made in patients with a productive cough, although differentiation of bronchitis from bronchiectasis is difficult by history and chest roentgenogram alone. Bronchography can be used to distinguish these entities, but the complications of this procedure do not warrant its diagnostic use unless bleeding is recurrent and severe, and surgical resection is being considered. Furthermore, the medical management of both diseases is the same.

The primary diagnostic entity that must be excluded in patients with the first episode of hemoptysis is lung cancer (see Chapter 53). Tumors that cause hemoptysis typically arise in central bronchi, and the diagnosis is usually made with a chest roentgenogram and bronchoscopy. Since 15% of patients with lung tumors who present with hemoptysis may have a normal chest roentgenogram (16), most pulmonologists recommend bronchoscopy, bronchial brushings, and bronchial washings in patients presenting with their first episode of hemoptysis. However, some have advocated simply observing patients less than 40 years old who have a normal chest roentgenogram and hemoptysis of less than 1 week duration since they have a relatively small chance of a pulmonary malignancy (11). Unfortunately, the published series supporting this approach are small, but this argument may be more compelling considering the recent spiraling costs of health care. An alternative is to obtain three sputum cytologies followed by bronchoscopy if the cytologies are negative. Bronchoscopy is possible in selected ambulatory patients (see Chapter 53 for a description of the patient's experience during this procedure). In patients with positive sputum cytologies or with an abnormal chest roentgenogram consistent with lung cancer, the evaluation should proceed as outlined in Chapter 53.

Rare vascular causes of hemoptysis should be considered when common causes seem unlikely. Mitral stenosis causes hemoptysis only after years of pulmonary hypertension, venous congestion, and gross cardiomegaly; therefore, the physical examination and chest roentgenogram provide useful diagnostic clues. Usually arteriovenous malformations can be diagnosed with a chest roentgenogram that demonstrates two visible vessels feeding the malformation. A tomogram, computerized axial tomography (CT) scan, or angiogram may be necessary to confirm the diagnosis of a vascular malformation.

If the evaluation, including history and physical examination, sputum cytology, chest roentgenogram, and bronchoscopy, is unrevealing, additional procedures, such as whole lung tomography or computerized axial tomography, will add little to the diagnostic evaluation. In such cases, further evaluation will depend on the severity of the process, its duration, and on clues to the presence of relatively rare conditions.

Therapy

Not every patient with hemoptysis needs admission to the hospital for diagnosis and treatment. Nevertheless, all patients over 40 years old with their first episode of hemoptysis do need a thorough investigation. Also, patients with significant hemoptysis (8, 10) (more than 25 to 50 ml of blood per day) require hospitalization and rapid diagnostic evaluation. If there is evidence of airways obstruction, treatment with bronchodilators may relieve coughing and reduce hemoptysis. Patients with the diagnosis of bronchitis or of bronchiectasis can usually be treated on an ambulatory basis with antibiotics, such as tetracycline or ampicillin, 1 to 2 g a day for 10 days. Blood

streaking of the sputum usually resolves within 2 to 3 days, but a full course of antibiotic therapy should be completed. When hemoptysis is due to pneumonia, lung abscess, or tuberculosis, no specific therapy is needed other than treatment of the underlying condition (see Chapters 27 and 28). Arteriovenous malformations often stop bleeding spontaneously; but if the bleeding persists, angiography will be necessary to document the extent of the malformation followed by either therapeutic embolization (13) or surgical removal. Mitral stenosis that results in hemoptysis indicates severe pulmonary hypertension and is often too far advanced to allow surgical correction, but cardiologic consultation should be obtained in order to evaluate and to maximize the medical therapy of left heart failure. In this situation, palliation and cough suppressant therapy should be attempted.

Careful cough suppressant therapy can be an important treatment in the acute phase of hemoptysis since this allows clots to form and to occlude the area of bleeding. However, it must be cautioned that oversedating the patient can lead to aspiration and asphyxiation if significant bleeding persists. Cough suppressants are primarily needed when there is active bleeding and clots are being expectorated regularly. On the other hand, blood streaking of the sputum does not require cough suppressant therapy. Furthermore, in patients with pneumonia or lung abscess, where blood is mixed with purulent expectorations, cough suppressant therapy is contraindicated because pulmonary drainage is an important part of treatment.

DYSPNEA

Breathing is an unconscious act that usually occurs effortlessly; yet even a normal person becomes aware of his breathing during deep sighs or during moderate to severe exercise. Dyspnea, the abnormal uncomfortable sensation of breathlessness, is difficult to define since patients often cannot accurately perceive or quantitate this feeling. Similar to an individual's threshold for the recognition of pain, the complaint of dyspnea is dependent both on the individual's limit for discomfort and on the specific circumstances which provoke shortness of breath. Thus, dyspnea must be defined in terms of what is abnormal for a particular individual in the context of his level of fitness and the amount of activity that is associated with breathlessness. Some patients become dyspneic with relatively small measurable alterations in ventilation, while others, such as patients who are hyperventilating with Kussmaul breathing, may not complain of dyspnea. Fortunately, a reasonable correlation exists between the degree of dyspnea and objective measurements of physiologic dysfunction.

Often the actual complaint of dyspnea may not be expressed as such and it may vary depending on the type of precipitating illness as well as on whether it developed abruptly or over a longer period of time. Thus, the asthmatic may complain of acute shortness of breath or of a "tightness" in his chest, while the patient with an acute pulmonary embolism may state that his breath has suddenly been taken away, and he cannot "get enough air" even though he ventilates easily. In contrast, the patient with emphysema who has modified his life-style may dismiss the sensation of breathlessness as part of his advancing age.

Normal Ventilation

There is no single mechanism responsible for dyspnea. Since dyspnea is the result of a variety of diverse influences acting alone or together, a brief discussion of the control of ventilation may help the practicing physician understand the complexity of dyspnea and why this sensation often does not immediately respond to correction of obvious physiologic abnormalities. Normally ventilation is coupled to the individual's metabolic demands as reflected in the oxygen consumption and carbon dioxide elimination necessary to meet a given level of activity. These needs are sensed by peripheral (carotid and aortic bodies) and central (medullary) chemical chemoreceptors that respond to the O_2, CO_2, and pH of blood and cerebral spinal fluid. The acute stimulation of these receptors provokes changes in minute ventilation. In addition, the control and regulation of the rate and pattern of breathing are influenced by the reflex effects of activation of neural receptors that lie in the lung parenchyma, airways, blood vessels, respiratory muscles (diaphragm), and chest wall. For example, receptors in the chest wall and diaphragm will respond to increased stiffness (decreased compliance) in the lung that occurs with fluid accumulation or with interstitial fibrosis. In addition, interstitial edema may activate "J" receptors located in the alveolar interstitium and may reflexly cause dyspnea in patients with pulmonary edema. Other receptors located in the airway epithelium cause rapid, shallow breathing, coughing, and bronchospasm when irritating substances are inhaled. Finally, the central nervous system alone can cause large alterations in breathing leading to hyperventilation in association with anxiety attacks (see Chapter 12). This discussion should help in understanding, for example, why the correction of arterial hypoxemia alone in a patient with an asthmatic attack usually does not relieve the sensation of breathlessness. In this situation, dyspnea results from the complex interaction of both chemical and neural stimuli to breathe, coupled with an individual's response to these signals. Correction of only one of these problems, therefore, is not sufficient to abolish dyspnea.

Evaluation

The causes of dyspnea are diverse and include essentially all diseases that result in significant functional impairment of either the respiratory system (gas exchange and/or pulmonary mechanics) or the cardiovascular system (circulatory and/or cardiac function) as well as any hematologic abnormality that impairs oxygen delivery. Table 50.4 summarizes the general disease categories that are likely to cause abnormal breathlessness.

In ambulatory practice the major causes of dyspnea are obstructive airways disease and arteriosclerotic and hypertensive heart disease, either alone or in combination. The prevalence of symptomatic lung disease in a specific geographic region or socioeconomic group is further modified by the prevalence of cigarette consumption, urban pollution, and occupational exposure to inhaled toxic substances. Further-

Table 50.4
Causes of Dyspnea

Dyspnea	Acute	Chronic
COMMON		
Pulmonary:		
Obstructive airways disease	Asthma, bronchitis	Bronchitis, emphysema
Restrictive lung disease	Pneumothorax	Pleural effusions, cancer
Inflammatory	Pneumonia	
Vascular	Pulmonary embolism	
Cardiac	Left heart failure, acute myocardial infarction	
Other	Psychogenic	Obesity, anemia
LESS COMMON		
Pulmonary:		
Upper airway obstruction	Epiglottitis, aspiration (foreign body)	
Restrictive lung disease		Diffuse, interstitial lung disease, diaphragm paralyses, kyphoscoliosis
Cardiac		Pericarditis
Other		Anemia, thyrotoxicosis

more, the clinical circumstances and sequence of events in which dyspnea occurs will aid in its evaluation. For example, the etiology of dyspnea is obvious in a teenager with seasonal asthma who develops shortness of breath and wheezing during a picnic in late summer (ragweed season). Often an upper respiratory tract infection will trigger pulmonary decompensation and dyspnea in patients with long-standing chronic obstructive lung disease. Upper respiratory airway obstruction in epiglottitis or foreign body aspiration can lead to acute severe dyspnea. Pleural effusions commonly occur with advanced lung cancer or as a complication of pulmonary infections and will cause dyspnea when they are large and involve more than half of one hemothorax. Congestive heart failure is often associated with typical anginal chest pain, and dyspnea will develop slowly or rapidly depending on whether there is acute or chronic cardiac decompensation. Psychogenic dyspnea or the hyperventilation syndrome has a rapid onset and is usually found in emotionally disturbed or anxious patients (see Chapter 12). Patients with severe chronic anemia tend to complain of dyspnea more often than patients with anemia secondary to acute blood loss, in which orthostatic dizziness and syncope are more common.

One of the first steps in evaluating a patient who complains of dyspnea is deciding whether the symptoms reflect an acute or chronic event since the more serious causes of dyspnea tend to present abruptly. In general, dyspnea of sudden onset is easier to evaluate, but the evaluation must proceed quickly to determine whether the patient should be admitted to the hospital for more extensive evaluation and therapy. On the other hand, the evaluation of chronic dyspnea can usually be accomplished more slowly in an ambulatory setting.

EVALUATION OF DYSPNEA OF SUDDEN ONSET

In a young patient, the medical history and physical examination alone will often suggest a presumptive diagnosis such as asthma, pneumonia, or pneumothorax. These diseases present with clinical findings including wheezing, localized rales and rub, evidence of pulmonary consolidation, or a unilateral decrease in breath sounds. In general, bronchitis does not cause dyspnea in a healthy individual unless bronchospasm, as manifested by wheezing, is also present. Acute left ventricular failure or angina with cardiac decompensation will cause acute dyspnea and may be associated with distended neck veins, an S3 gallop, diffuse or basalar rales, wheezing, and pedal edema (see Chapter 58). Unfortunately, some of these clinical findings, such as distended neck veins and wheezing, can be observed in patients with acute exacerbations of obstructive airways disease. Frequently, patients with cardiopulmonary disease present with a mixture of these physical findings; therefore, further laboratory examination is necessary. The chest roentgenogram and electrocardiogram are the two most useful tests that help distinguish acute cardiac from pulmonary disease. Also, if available, a spirogram can be used to document the presence and severity of functional pulmonary disease and serves as a guide in the therapy of bronchospasm (see Chapter 52). All acute inflammatory pulmonary disease causing significant dyspnea will appear as localized or diffuse parenchymal infiltrates on a chest roentgenogram. A significant pneumothorax can be easily missed and diagnostic accuracy will be improved with an expiratory film. The development of acute hyperinflation on a chest roentgenogram indicates severe bronchospasm. In contrast, congestive heart failure will produce interstitial or alveolar fluid accumulation often associated with an increase in size of cardiac silhouette. Besides the chest roentgenogram an electrocardiogram must be examined for cardiac arrhythmias or ischemic changes. Even without a history of chest pain, an electrocardiogram still should be obtained to exclude the diagnosis of a silent myocardial infarction.

PULMONARY EMBOLISM

Pulmonary embolism is a major cause of acute dyspnea, but the diagnosis can be difficult. Its evaluation requires a systematic approach with a logical sequence of diagnostic testing.

The incidence of pulmonary embolism is high in patients with a recent history of peripheral venous disease, prolonged immobilization, chronic obstructive lung disease, or congestive heart failure. In a multicenter study (1) 60% of patients with pulmonary embolism were men; of the women who had pulmonary emboli under age 45, 75% were found to be using oral contraceptives (see Chapter 90). In this same study, the most frequent symptoms present at the time of diagnosis were dyspnea and chest pain. These two symptoms were found in over 80% of patients; hemoptysis, cough, and apprehension were seen less frequently. The physical examination is usually not helpful in the diagnosis, especially since many of the patients have underlying respiratory and cardiovascular diseases which, in themselves, produce abnormal physical findings: tachycardia, tachypnea, an accentuated second pulmonic heart sound, etc.

Most laboratory tests are not useful in the diagnosis of pulmonary embolism (12). Chest roentgenograms are frequently abnormal, but the findings are non-specific (localized infiltrates, atelectasis, an elevated hemidiaphragm, or a pleural effusion). The arterial gas tensions are also often abnormal (reduced PaO_2 and $PaCO_2$), but are not helpful diagnostically, in part because of considerable variation and in part because of the high prevalence of cardiopulmonary diseases that alter both the PaO_2 and $PaCO_2$.

The most useful procedure in the screening of patients for pulmonary embolism is a ventilation/perfusion (V/Q) scan of the lungs. (A perfusion scan alone will not always permit the probabilities of embolism to be established accurately.) Whether or not the patient is hospitalized before having the scan depends on the severity of the presentation. There is little discomfort associated with a lung scan. The patient should be instructed that he will inhale an oxygen and xenon mixture for 3 to 4 min, followed by a venous injection of radioactive labeled technetium. Several different projections are then recorded on a scanner while the patient is lying on a table.

The V/Q scan is 100% sensitive, but can be nonspecific depending on the configuration, location, and number of perfusion defects seen (9). If the V/Q scan is normal, the diagnosis of an acute pulmonary embolus is excluded. In general, 5 to 7% of patients with a low probability V/Q lung scan have an associated pulmonary embolus, while 20 to 30% of patients with moderate probability, and 80 to 90% of patients with high probability scans have a pulmonary embolism. However, it must be emphasized that the use of these probabilities is dependent on strict adherence to accepted published criteria for interpreting lung scans (2) and on the experience of the individual nuclear medicine laboratory. Patients with low, moderate, or high probability scans should be hospitalized for further diagnostic studies (angiography) and/or anticoagulation with heparin (see Chapter 48). Patients with acute dyspnea and simultaneous symptoms and signs of peripheral venous thrombosis (less than 40% of patients with pulmonary emboli) should undergo venography to confirm the diagnosis (see Chapter 48). If venography is positive, the patient should be hospitalized for initiation of anticoagulant therapy.

The resolution of pulmonary emboli varies and can occur as early as 1 to 2 weeks after small emboli. With larger emboli and in those patients with underlying cardiopulmonary disease, there may be angiographic evidence of emboli persisting for 2 or 3 months (3). If chest pain occurs after discharge, a repeat lung scan (and perhaps, depending on the results, angiography) is necessary to determine whether embolization has recurred.

Evaluation of Chronic or Progressive Dyspnea

The evaluation of chronic, progressive dyspnea can be a simple or complicated process depending on the responsible disease. In contrast to acute dyspnea, chronic dyspnea usually is more difficult to diagnose and often requires more extensive diagnostic procedures; therefore, the evaluation should proceed in a logical sequence to avoid initially expensive and invasive laboratory testing. The first step is a careful history. Because shortness of breath is appropriate to certain levels of activity depending on the fitness of the individual, the physician must decide whether the patient's symptoms are abnormal, and if so, over what period of time they have developed. Many patients with chronic cardiopulmonary disease adapt to the insidious onset of dyspnea by subconsciously changing daily habits and avoiding physical activity. To quantitate the degree of dyspnea, the physician must determine what specific activity causes dyspnea and compare the patient's abilities to perform work with an appropriate peer group and with his baseline performance. Thus, the complaint of dyspnea in a 35-year-old who normally runs 5 miles and now becomes short of breath after running only 2 miles should not be ignored.

Initial laboratory testing should include a chest roentgenogram, which may reveal advanced degrees of obstructive pulmonary disease, the presence of diffuse interstitial lung disease, or cardiovascular disease manifested by either cardiomegaly or by signs of congestive heart failure. An electrocardiogram is necessary to document the presence of typical ischemic electrocardiographic abnormalities, arrhythmias, and hypertrophy of cardiac chambers. Pulmonary function should be assessed initially with a spirogram, because this test categorizes the two most common pulmonary diseases—namely obstructive or restrictive lung disease (see Chapter 52). If airflow obstruction is present, the response to bronchodilators aids in predicting the response to therapy. A normal spirogram virtually excludes significant parenchymal or airways disease. Although patients with classic asthma may have a normal spirogram during symptom-free periods, they can be diagnosed by their characteristic clinical history. Additional specialized procedures that aid in the diagnosis of asthma are discussed in Chapter 52. Finally, initial laboratory testing should include a hemoglobin determination or hematocrit value to determine whether a patient is severely anemic or polycythemic.

If an obvious cause of dyspnea is not found after these initial investigations, the next step will include more specialized testing procedures that may not be readily available to all physicians. Nevertheless, it is important to understand when these tests are appropriate and how they are performed. For the most part, these tests are available for ambulatory patients by referral to hospital pulmonary function or cardiac diagnostic laboratories, and through consultation with pulmonary or cardiac subspecialists.

1. *Complete Pulmonary Function Tests:* In addition to baseline spirometry (see Chapter 52) other pulmonary function tests include the measurement of total lung capacity and functional residual capacity. These tests quantitate the degree of hyperinflation or restriction that results from either obstructive airways disease or restrictive lung disease. The single breath diffusion capacity measures the amount of alveolar capillary surface area for gas exchange. Thus, the diffusion capacity is reduced when emphysema destroys the alveolar capillary surface area and when pulmonary emboli or other vascular occlusive disease decreases the pulmonary capillary surface area. An elevated diffusion capacity is found in conditions that elevate the pulmonary blood volume—for example, erythrocytosis or early congestive heart failure. These additional tests should only be consid-

ered if spirometry is abnormal. The experience of the patient during the performance of these tests is described in Chapter 52.

2. *Arterial Blood Gas Analysis*: Initially, an arterial blood gas determination should be performed to document the presence of hypoxemia or hypercapnia and to characterize the acid-base status. Several general points require emphasis: First, a normal resting arterial blood gas does not exclude significant pulmonary disease. In fact many patients with severe chronic obstructive lung disease have normal resting arterial $PaCO_2$ and pH with only a slight reduction in PaO_2. Therefore, during an evaluation for dyspnea, a blood gas should always be used in conjunction with other assessments of pulmonary function. Second, arterial blood gases drawn after completion of exercise in a dyspneic patient may not provide useful information about exercise-induced changes in blood gases since abnormalities in gas exchange that occur during exercise usually reverse immediately. Third, for reasons discussed above, measurement of blood gases should not be used as a definitive screening procedure to exclude the diagnosis of pulmonary embolism.

3. *Cardiovascular Testing*: The use of specialized noninvasive cardiovascular evaluation including echocardiograms and gated heartpool nuclear scanning to assess right and left ventricular function or the presence of valvular heart disease is discussed in the cardiovascular section (Chapter 57).

4. *Exercise Testing*: If a patient is dyspneic on exertion, and baseline testing of cardiopulmonary function, as described above, is normal or only mildly abnormal, exercise testing should be considered.

In general, there are two types of exercise tests available. The first is a standard *cardiac stress test* where the patient exercises and is then observed for the development of chest pain and for electrocardiographic ischemic changes (Chapter 54). In referral centers, this cardiac stress test has been modified recently to permit functional evaluation of cardiac performance during exercise by using radioisotope scanning techniques with thallium (Chapter 54). The second type of exercise testing is a *cardiopulmonary stress test* in which cardiac function, pulmonary gas exchange, ventilation, and physical fitness are quantitated at specific work loads. As far as the patient is concerned, the only difference between this test and the standard cardiac stress test is that he may have an arterial line in place and that he always will be breathing into a mouthpiece. Such complicated invasive cardiopulmonary stress testing is justified and useful in order to determine whether dyspnea is due to either (a) cardiac or pulmonary disease, (b) exercise-induced asthma, or (c) poor physical fitness. One can use this test to evaluate the results of treatment regimes, such as the efficacy of anti-inflammatory drugs (e.g., corticosteroids) for the therapy of acute interstitial lung disease or the effects of supplemental oxygen in patients with severe hypoxemia. Further-

more, the test can measure the ability of a patient with underlying cardiopulmonary disease to achieve work loads appropriate for activities of daily life. This type of testing is particularly useful in evaluating patients for disability, since static pulmonary function and noninvasive cardiac testing may not accurately estimate the functional state of a given patient during actual working conditions. These tests are not office procedures and require expert interpretation by cardiologists or pulmonologists. Most cardiologists do not perform full cardiopulmonary stress tests. Cardiac stress testing will relate information on the presence of angina, arrhythmias, or myocardial ischemia during exercise. On the other hand, most pulmonologists may not be well trained in the sophisticated interpretation of electrocardiographic changes during exercise. Usually, it is possible for the referring physician to determine the most likely etiology for dyspnea and to make the appropriate referral. In large hospital centers with combined cardiopulmonary laboratories, simultaneous consultation and exercise testing by cardiologists and pulmonologists may be available.

This approach will almost always answer the questions necessary for the evaluation and establishment of a therapeutic regimen in patients with dyspnea. At times, a patient with circulatory abnormalities may need a brief hospital admission for additional invasive cardiac catheterization studies to assess the state of the pulmonary vasculature or the degree of cardiac dysfunction. For example, it may be necessary to insert a Swan-Ganz catheter into the pulmonary circulation and to measure directly pulmonary arterial pressures and pulmonary capillary wedge pressures to learn whether a patient with severe obstructive lung disease and cor pulmonale also has significant functional left ventricular failure which requires treatment.

Therapy

There are no specific therapeutic modalities for treatment of dyspnea. Treatment of this symptom is primarily aimed at therapy of the underlying cardiac, pulmonary, or hematologic disorders that cause abnormal breathlessness.

NONCARDIAC CHEST PAIN

Chest pain is a particularly frightening symptom because of the widespread knowledge and concern about heart disease; however, nonspecific musculoskeletal pain is more common than angina, especially in patients less than 40 years old. Most patients with chest pain can be evaluated and treated in an ambulatory setting; a few patients require referral to a specialist. The common noncardiac cause of chest pain will be discussed in this section which should be read in conjunction with Chapter 54.

Afferent neural impulses responsible for thoracic pain are carried by the sympathetic chain, vagus, and

Table 50.5
Causes of Chest Pain

COMMON CAUSES	
Chest wall (musculo-skeletal)	Nonspecific (smokers, non-smokers with increased exertion)
	Costochondritis (Tietze's syndrome)
Cardiac	Angina
Pulmonary	Tracheitis, cough, pleuritis, pneumonia
LESS COMMON CAUSES	
Chest wall (musculo-skeletal)	Thoracic outlet syndrome, herpes zoster, fractured rib, tumor
Cardiac	Aneurysm, pericarditis
Pulmonary	Pneumothorax, pulmonary embolus, pulmonary hypertension, cancer
Gastrointestinal	Stomach disease, duodenal ulcer, abdominal infection, peritonitis, esophageal reflux
Neurologic	Radicular pain of cervical spine disease

phrenic nerves. Visceral structures which include the lung, diaphragm, heart, and esophagus all lie within the thoracic cage and have overlapping innervation. Chest pain arising from these different organs will often have similar referral patterns; therefore, irritation of the diaphragmatic pleura, diaphragm, or pericardium, due to either thoracic or abdominal disease, causes chest pain radiating to the shoulder. In addition, the patient may have more difficulty localizing pain from the deeper anatomic structures within the chest, while diseases involving the superficial structures, muscles, and ribs will be more easily localized. Since the lung parenchyma has no innervation, alveolar or interstitial disease does not cause chest pain unless the pulmonary vasculature, bronchi, or pleura are involved.

Table 50.5 lists selected common and less common causes of chest pain. Fleeting, sharp, or lancelike chest pain is probably the most common complaint in patients who do not have evidence of organic heart disease. Smokers complain more frequently than nonsmokers of both angina-like and non-angina-like chest pain. This has resulted in use of the term "tobacco angina" to describe two distinct types of chest pain in smokers (4). First, there are some smokers with pre-existing angina who clearly have their pain precipitated by smoking. There is also a second larger group of smokers who have normal or diseased hearts, and complain of intermittent chest pains with anginal and nonanginal characteristics that are not necessarily associated with smoking of a cigarette. This chest pain is not relieved by nitroglycerin or provoked by exercise. It gradually disappears within weeks to months, sometimes years after the cessation of smoking; and it is assumed that it is not due to myocardial ischemia.

Musculoskeletal pain is very common in young individuals who increase their exercise abruptly (including the patient who acutely hyperventilates as part of an anxiety state—see Chapter 12). A history of unusual exertion with increased breathing plus tenderness of intercostal muscles usually suffices to make this diagnosis.

Pain caused by tracheitis or tracheobronchitis is a distinctive substernal burning sensation that is precipitated by coughing and is most often associated with viral respiratory infections. This is in contrast to the sharp, stabbing pleuritic chest pain that is experienced with pneumonia. The latter is clearly localized to the chest wall and arises from stretching the inflamed parietal pleura during breathing or coughing.

Other causes of chest pain include costochondritis (Tietze's syndrome), which is an anterior localized pain associated with tenderness over one or more costochondral junctions; herpes zoster which commonly causes unilateral aching and/or itching, limited to one dermatome, which may precede by several days the eruption of vesicles; rib fracture or bone metastases which are more chronic and pleuritic in nature; and cervical spine disease with referred pain to the chest. Acute stabbing chest pain can occur with a spontaneous pneumothorax, which occurs primarily in young men or in older patients with obstructive pulmonary disease. Frequently, a small (< 20%) pneumothorax is not accompanied by significant dyspnea in otherwise healthy individuals. Pleuritic chest pain associated with pulmonary emboli results from infarction of parenchymal lung tissue with irritation of the parietal pleura and almost always is associated with dyspnea; and in most patients, the chest roentgenogram will show an infiltrate. On the other hand, the pain associated with pulmonary hypertension is heavy and aching and often similar to that of cardiac ischemia (see Chapter 54). Gastrointestinal disorders, such as reflux esophagitis or gastric or duodenal ulcer are major sources of referred chest pain. They are usually distinguished from cardiopulmonary chest pain by their association with eating, and by their relief by antacids (Chapters 31 and 33).

Evaluation

Many of the common causes of noncardiac chest pain can be diagnosed by a thorough history and physical examination. Since discrete anatomic structures must be involved in order to cause noncardiac chest pain, the physical examination is more useful in the diagnosis of chest pain than it is in the diagnosis of dyspnea and hemoptysis. Inspection of the chest wall may reveal the characteristic unilateral eruption of herpes zoster along a dermatome. Light palpation over the chest wall will elicit pain and crepitus from fractured ribs. Mild pressure over the costochondral junctions anteriorly will reproduce the pain of the Tietze's syndrome. (In general, cardiac pain is not worsened by pressure over the chest wall.) In pneumonia or pulmonary infarction a distinct friction rub can be heard directly over the specific area of chest pain. With pericardial involvement a friction rub that varies with respiration or with the cardiac cycle is usually present. A thorough abdominal examination is important because diseases involving the abdominal visceral organs can cause referred chest pain that is indistinguishable from that produced by involvement of the thoracic structures. Often laboratory studies and a chest roentgenogram will not be necessary for the diagnosis of these common causes of chest pain.

Therapy

The treatment of chest pain requires therapy of the underlying disease process, as well as analgesic drugs for the pain itself. Nonspecific chest pain found in normal people requires reassurance; however, angina-like pain in smokers ideally requires first diagnostic testing to exclude ischemic heart disease followed by discontinuing cigarette smoking for both diagnosis and therapy. Tracheal irritation is limited to the duration of the viral illness but can be treated by cough suppression and bronchodilators (see under "Cough"). Tietze's syndrome is treated with standard anti-inflammatory agents and heat. While the pain of herpes zoster is often severe, it may be controlled with mild narcotics such as codeine 30 to 60 mg every 4 to 6 hours. Unfortunately, chest pain experienced in pulmonary hypertension does not respond to treatment with non-narcotic analgesics, and narcotics in sedative doses are required if the hypertension does not improve with treatment and if the pain is severe.

Pleuritic pain found in patients with pneumonia or pulmonary embolus responds to specific therapy of the inflammatory process. Nevertheless, narcotics may be needed to reduce splinting of the chest wall and thereby to prevent atelectasis. Codeine (60 mg) is usually adequate therapy but the physician should bear in mind the undesired cough suppressant action of this drug in inflammatory lung disease. In situations where pain is extreme an intercostal block is necessary. This is performed by local infiltration of the inferior surface of the rib near the spine with 5 to 10 ml of Lidocaine (1 to 2%). Although this therapy only lasts from 4 to 6 hours, local block in combination with the administration of narcotics often provides more long term control of pleuritic chest pain.

References

General

Burki, NK: Dyspnea. *Clin Chest Med 1:* 47, 1980.
  A good discussion of the mechanisms of dyspnea.
Fishman, AP: *Pulmonary Diseases and Disorders,* Vols. 1 and 2. McGraw-Hill, New York, 1980.
  The standard text of pulmonary medicine.
Hinshaw, HC and Murray MF: *Diseases of the Chest.* W. B. Saunders, Philadelphia, 1980.
  A practical approach to pulmonary medicine
Jones, NL, Campbell, EJ and Moran, WF: *Clinical Exercise Testing.* W. B. Saunders, Philadelphia, 1975.
  The standard text on this subject.
Ziment, I: *Respiratory Pharmacology and Therapeutics.* W. B. Saunders, Philadelphia, 1978.
  An exhaustive review of this subject.

Specific

1. Bell, WR, Simon, TL and DeMets, DL: The clinical features of submassive and massive pulmonary emboli. *Am J Med 62:* 355, 1977.
2. Biello, DR, Mattar, AG, McKnight, RC and Siegel, BA: Ventilation-perfusion studies in suspected pulmonary embolism. *AJR 133:* 1033, 1979.
3. Dalen, JE, Banas, JS, Jr, Brooks, HL, Evans, GL, Paraskos, JA and Dexter, L: Resolution rate of acute pulmonary embolism in man. *N Engl J Med 280:* 1194, 1969.
4. Friedman, GD, Siegelaub, AB and Doles, LG: Cigarette smoking and chest pain. *Ann Intern Med 83:* 7, 1975.
5. Irwin, RS, Rosen MJ and Braman, SS: Cough: a comprehensive review. *Arch Intern Med 137:* 1186, 1977.
6. Kaplan, J and Johns, CJ: Mycetomas in pulmonary sarcoidosis: non-surgical management. *Johns Hopkins Med J 145:* 157, 1979.
7. Kravitz, H, Gomberg, RM, Burnstine, RC, Hagler, S and Korach, A: Psychogenic cough tic in children and adolescents. *Clin Pediatr 8:* 580, 1969.
8. Lyons, HA: Differential diagnosis of hemoptysis and its treatment. Basics of RD published by The American Lung Association, 1976.
9. McNeil, BJ, Hessel, SJ, Branch, WT, Bjork, L and Adelstein, SJ: Measures of clinical efficacy. III. The value of the lung scan in the evaluation of young patients with pleuritic chest pain. *Nucl Med 17:* 163, 1976.
10. Rogers, RM, *et al.*: The management of massive hemoptysis in a patient with pulmonary tuberculosis. *Chest 70:* 518, 1976.
11. Snider, GL: When not to use the bronchoscopy for hemoptysis. *Chest 76:* 1, 1979.
12. Szucs, MM, Jr, Brooks, HL, Grossman, W, Banas, JS, Jr, Meister, SG, Dexter, L and Dalen, JE: Diagnostic sensitivity of laboratory findings in acute pulmonary embolism. *Ann Intern Med 74:* 161, 1971.
13. Terry, PB, Barth, KH, Kaufman, SL and White, RI, Jr: Balloon embolization for treatment of pulmonary arteriovenous fistulas. *N Engl J Med 302:* 1189, 1980.
14. Wynder, EL, Kaufman, PL and Lesser, RL: A short-term follow-up study on ex-cigarette smokers. *Am Rev Respir Dis 96:* 645, 1967.
15. Wynder, EL, Lemon, FR and Mantel, N: Epidemiology of persistent cough. *Am Rev Respir Dis 91:* 679, 1965.
16. Zavala, DC: Diagnostic fiberoptic bronchoscopy: techniques and results of biopsy in 600 patients. *Chest 68:* 12, 1975.

CHAPTER FIFTY-ONE

The Abnormal Chest Roentgenogram

PHILIP L. SMITH, M.D., and EUGENE R. BLEECKER, M.D.

The general physician will often, in the course of evaluation of a patient, be faced with the interpretation of an abnormal chest roentgenogram. Many physicians have the capability of taking chest roentgenograms in their office; others use the facilities of consultant radiologists. A knowledge of the significance of chest roentgenographic findings will allow the physician to plan further radiographic and diagnostic procedures.

It is essential that a chest roentgenogram always be compared with any previous available roentgenogram since a film only represents a single point on a spectrum. Often the most appropriate plan is observation of a specific lesion with serial chest roentgenograms.

SPECIFIC PATTERNS INDICATIVE OF AN ABNORMAL CHEST ROENTGENOGRAM

This section will review common abnormalities that indicate the presence of pulmonary disease that requires further evaluation.

Air Bronchogram (Fig. 51.1)

Normally, bronchi beyond the mainstem division cannot be seen; however, when lung tissue surrounding a bronchus is devoid of air due to either collapse or consolidation, an air bronchogram can be seen. The presence of an air bronchogram distinguishes a collapsed or consolidated part of the lung from an extrapulmonary density such as a pleural effusion. However, an air bronchogram is not present in every collapsed or consolidated lung because bronchi may fill with secretions or exudate. Therefore, its absence is less significant than its presence.

Silhouette Sign (Fig. 51.2)

The obliteration on a chest roentgenogram of a normally opaque structure in the chest by an abnormal pulmonary density is called the silhouette sign. If the physician has knowledge of thoracic anatomy and of spatial relations, he can use the silhouette sign to localize abnormalities within the lung parenchyma. Outlines of organs that are in contact with parenchymal infiltrates will be obliterated because the normal air interface is eliminated. On the other hand, intrathoracic lesions that are not anatomically contiguous will not interfere with the outlines of other nearby structures. For example, obliteration of the cardiac border localizes an abnormality to the right middle lobe or the lingular segment of the left upper lobe (Fig. 51.2). In contrast, an infiltrate that overlaps but does not obliterate the cardiac border is posterior and often represents a lower lobe lesion. Lower lobe abnormalities obliterate diaphragmatic borders while obliteration of the left border of the aortic knob, a posterior structure, occurs with lesions of the apical posterior segment of the left upper lobe.

Collapse (Fig. 51.3)

The collapse or diminution in volume of the whole lung, a lobe, or a segment of one of the lobes can be an important clue to the presence of asymptomatic pulmonary disease, such as bronchial carcinoma, or it may be the cause of symptoms, such as dyspnea in an asthmatic patient with mucous plugging. The primary mechanisms that cause pulmonary collapse are (a) bronchial obstruction either due to an intrinsic bronchial mass or to an extrinsic or intrinsic stenosis of the bronchus, (b) compression of the lungs from a large pleural effusion or from a pneumothorax, (c) peripheral bronchial plugging with subsequent pulmonary collapse, and (d) contraction of the lung secondary to chronic inflammatory disease. The signs of collapse are related to anatomic landmarks within the lung and are manifest by displacement of the septa in the lung, loss of aeration within the pulmonary parenchyma, and crowding of the vascular and bronchial lung markings. Other signs that are suggestive of collapse reflect the secondary effects of loss of lung volume such as elevation of the diaphragm, shift of the mediastinal structures toward the collapsed area, diminution in the size of a hemithorax, compensatory hyperinflation, hilar displacement, and tracheal deviation. These latter signs are much more difficult to interpret in patients with underlying lung disease in whom many of these signs may exist in the absence of collapse.

Pleural Effusion (Fig. 51.4)

Small amounts of free fluid within the pleural space will obliterate the costophrenic or costocardiac angles. Because the density of pleural fluid is greater than the density of the lung, a subpulmonic collection will displace laterally the crest of the diaphragm. An increased density between the stomach gas bubble and pulmonary tissue may also indicate the presence of fluid within the pleural space. The diagnosis of a large pleural effusion is not difficult because fluid within the pleural space on an upright chest roentgenogram will form a concave density across the chest cavity; decubitus roentgenograms will demonstrate free pleural fluid in the dependent hemithorax. If the patient is recumbent, as is often the case in emergency rooms, the pleural fluid will layer over the entire hemithorax, causing the lung to appear opaque.

Pneumothorax (Fig. 51.5)

A small collection of air is difficult to see within the pleural space. This diagnosis is aided by an expiratory chest roentgenogram that accentuates the amount of air within the pleural space by reducing the volume of air in the lung.

Abnormal Pulmonary Paranchymal Patterns

SEPTAL

Normally lung markings reflect vascular patterns within the pulmonary parenchyma and are rarely due to the bronchi or the lymphatics. There are three

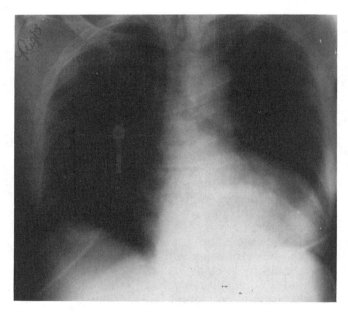

Figure 51.1 Air bronchogram. Patient presented with fever and sputum production: the initial roentgenogram demonstrates a branching air bronchogram seen behind the heart on the left which is consistent with a lower lobe infiltrate.

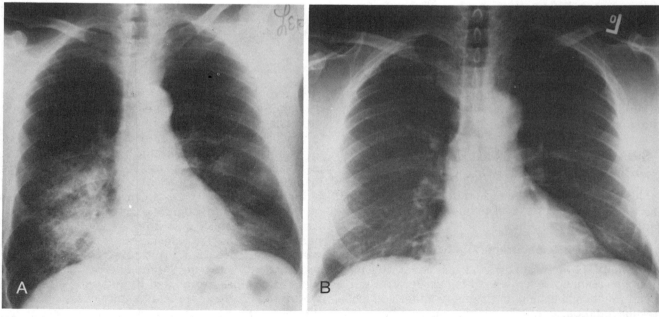

Figure 51.2 Silhouette sign. In this figure, a right middle lobe infiltrate obscures the border of the heart (A). A previous X-ray is shown for comparison (B).

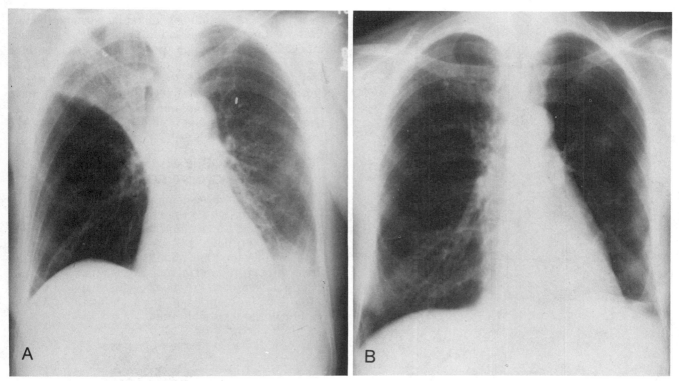

Figure 51.3 Collapse. This demonstrates collapse of the right upper lobe and partial collapse of left lower lobe in a patient complaining of cough and increased sputum (*A*). The right middle lobe fissure is displaced upwards and there is blunting of the left hemidiaphragm. Note there is no air bronchogram in either collapsed segment. Aggressive physical therapy was initiated and within 24 hours there is resolution of the collapse on the right and almost complete resolution on the left (*B*).

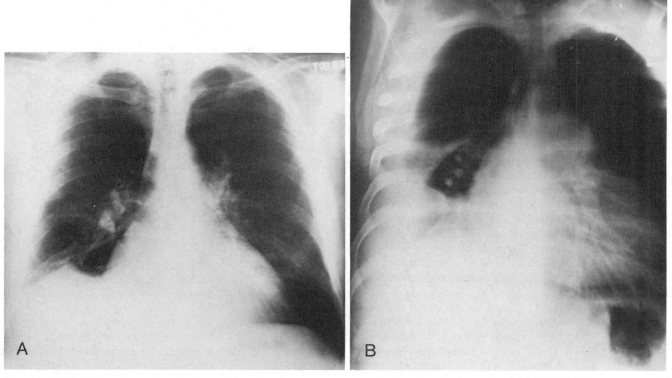

Figure 51.4 Subpulmonic effusion. The diaphragm appears to be elevated on the right (*A*). This represents subpulmonic fluid; when the patient is placed in the right lateral decubitis position (*B*), fluid layers on the right and tracks in the minor fissure and along the apex and diaphragm.

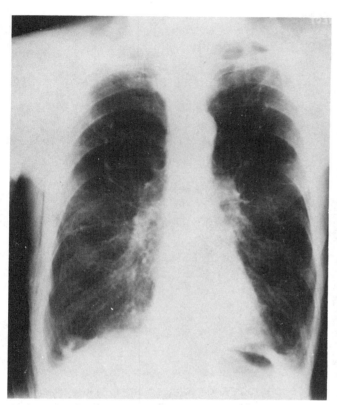

Figure 51.5 Pneumothorax. If the roentgenogram is not carefully examined, the pneumothorax in the right lower lung can be easily missed. Note the widespread bullae throughout the lung.

types of linear shadows that represent septal markings within the lung: Kerley A lines, thin nonbranching lines several inches long radiating from the hilum; Kerley B lines (Fig. 51.6), up to 1 inch in length found at the lateral lung bases, radiating from the pleura; and Kerley C lines, fine interlacing structures throughout the lung parenchyma that produce a spiderweb appearance. The most common cause of these lines is interstitial edema due to congestive heart failure.

DIFFUSE

Diffuse lung disease takes on two general patterns: diffuse interstitial disease and diffuse alveolar disease. *Alveolar infiltrates* (Fig. 51.7A) can be recognized by their fluffy margins, their coalescence into "rosette" formations, their occasional "butterfly" configuration, evolving hilar and central lung zones, and the presence of air bronchograms or air alveolograms.

An *interstitial pattern* may be primarily linear or reticular, and often consists of multiple discrete non-coalescent round nodules, 1 to 5 mm in diameter (Fig. 51.7B). Although there can be a summation effect, these small nodular densities retain a distinct identity as compared to the larger fluffier infiltrates characteristic of alveolar disease. In certain disease proc-

esses such as tuberculosis, histoplasmosis, or healed viral pneumonia, these nodules may calcify and thus appear more dense. The presence of honeycombing is pathognomonic of interstitial disease and pulmonary fibrosis. It can be identified on chest roentgenogram as round or oval, irregular air spaces that have a reasonably uniform diameter of 1 to 10 mm and are arranged in grape-like bunches, thus giving the impression of a bee hive.

COMMON PROBLEMS IN PATIENTS WITH ABNORMAL CHEST ROENTGENOGRAMS

In this section three general disease categories will be discussed in which the chest roentgenogram provides the basis for diagnosis and further evaluation. A general approach will be outlined including the initial evaluation that should be completed by the physician before referral to a pulmonary specialist or a thoracic surgeon. Frequently, this diagnostic evaluation can be completed in an ambulatory setting, with or without consultation.

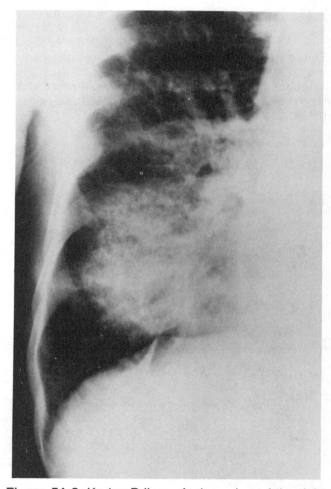

Figure 51.6 Kerley B lines. A close view of the right lower lung in a patient with congestive heart failure demonstrates horizontal linear lines that run to the edge of the lung.

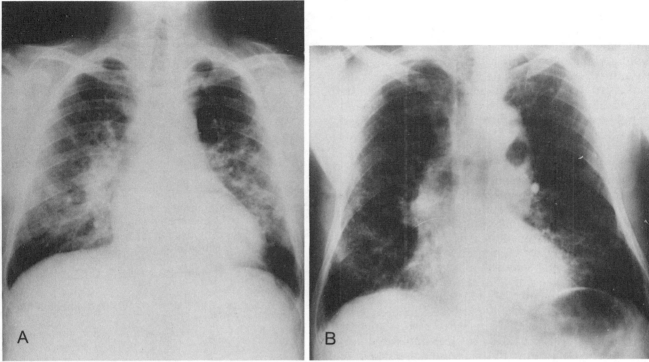

Figure 51.7 *A*, Alveolar patterns. This patient has progressive dyspnea after inhaling fumes from an automobile accident. Compared to *B*, little air is visible in the infiltrate because fluid is filling the alveoli. *B*, Interstitial pattern. This demonstrates bilateral interstitial infiltrates in a patient with progressive dyspnea and with fibrosis on biopsy. Compared to *A*, there is a lacy reticular appearance with accentuation of the air spaces by the fibrosis.

Recurrent or Slowly Resolving Bacterial Pneumonias

Obstructing pulmonary carcinoma must be considered in any patient who has a slowly resolving pneumonia. Most patients with bacterial pneumonia rapidly respond to antibiotic therapy, and their chest roentgenogram will return to normal over 3 to 6 weeks (see Chapter 27). Patients with chronic obstructive lung disease (Chapter 52) who have difficulty mobilizing their bronchial secretions and patients with superimposed congestive heart failure or with necrotizing pneumonia may have significant pulmonary infiltrates that persist for 8 to 12 weeks (1). If the patient shows symptomatic improvement with a decrease in both the amount and purulence of sputum, a decrease in fever, and slow but progressive roentgenographic clearing, further evaluation during this period is usually not warranted. If roentgenographic abnormalities persist and if there is other evidence of poor response to therapy or if the pneumonic infiltrate is found in an asymptomatic individual, further evaluation to exclude pulmonary carcinoma is warranted (see Chapter 53).

Patients with recurrent pneumonias (3) also must be evaluated for the possibility of lung cancer. More frequently, these patients have associated chronic diseases such as underlying airways disease, congestive heart failure, diabetes mellitus, or bronchiectasis. In evaluating patients with recurrent pneumonia, it is vital to review all previous chest roentgenograms to document the anatomic location and characteristics of the recurrent pneumonic infiltrate. In general, if a pneumonia recurs in multiple lobes, or in pulmonary segments that are unrelated anatomically, the likelihood of bronchogenic carcinoma is small. For example, a recurrent pneumonia that initially involves the right upper lobe and subsequently the lower lobe is unlikely to be the result of a single obstructive carcinoma. On the other hand, an infiltrate that occurs first in the right lower lobe and subsequently in the right middle lobe could be caused by a single mass lesion that occludes the bronchus intermedius. In addition to the anatomical location, it is important to consider the time during which recurrent pneumonias have occurred. If the interval is more than 3 years, the possibility of an underlying obstructing lung cancer is unlikely. However, chronic benign processes, such as a benign tumor or a congenital bronchial abnormality are still possible.

Apical Infiltrates

Frequently roentgenographic patterns that range from increased pulmonary markings or minor scarring to cystic or cavitary disease in the upper lobes will be interpreted by a radiologist as showing old granulomatous lung disease with possible active tuberculous infection. The evaluation of these patients includes questioning about previous tuberculous lung disease (including the type and duration of antituberculous therapy) and an assessment of the reactivity of the tuberculin skin test. Comparison with old chest roentgenograms is mandatory because the activity of an old granulomatous infection of the lung cannot be determined from an isolated chest roentgenogram. Frequently, old chest roentgenograms demonstrate that no change has occurred. The evaluation and treatment of patients with tuberculosis is discussed in Chapter 28.

Pleural Effusion

In general, when a pleural effusion is seen on a chest roentgenogram, examination of the fluid is imperative. The major exception to this rule is the patient who develops acute pulmonary edema associated with a rapidly developing pleural effusion that resolves with therapy for congestive heart failure (see Chapter 58). The physician should be able to perform a thoracentesis in order to investigate rationally the etiology of the effusion (Table 51.1). Some of the fluid should be collected in a heparinized tube so that cytologic examination can be performed, if necessary. Most pleural effusions are clear and straw-colored, and deviation from this is useful diagnostically. For example, a bloody effusion suggests pulmonary infarction or tumor, a lime-green effusion suggests tuberculosis, and viscous fluid with feculent odor strongly suggest an anaerobic empyema.

Pleural fluids can either be classified as transudates or exudates (2). An exudate is characterized by a pleural fluid protein concentration that is greater than 50% of the concentration of serum protein. Because of their high protein content, exudative pleural effusions usually have a specific gravity of more than 1.015, or protein concentration of greater than 3 g per 100 ml. A cell count and pleural fluid cytology should be performed since polymorphonuclear leukocytes in pleural fluid suggest acute inflammation and infection, while a predominance of lymphocytes suggests tuberculosis or malignancy. The presence of more than 5% pleural mesothelial cells usually excludes the diagnosis of tuberculosis. Low pleural fluid glucose concentrations occur in infections as well as in rheumatoid arthritis. If pleural effusion is bloody or appears infected, the patient should be hospitalized for further diagnostic studies and for therapy (pleural fluid pH, pleural biopsy, etc.)

Pneumothorax

There are three major types of pneumothorax: (a) spontaneous, (b) iatrogenic, and (c) traumatic. Of these, the internist is most commonly faced with a spontaneous pneumothorax either in a young healthy individual, or in the older patient with underlying pulmonary disease. In the former, a subpleural apical bleb ruptures into the pleural space causing varying amounts of air to collect. This is most commonly seen in 20- to 30-year-old males and is usually unrelated

Table 51.1
Causes of Pleural Effusion

Effusion	Common	Uncommon
Vascular	Congestive heart failure[a] Pulmonary infarction	
Metabolic		Hypoproteinemia[a] Cirrhosis[a] Nephrotic syndrome[a] Glomerulonephritis[a]
Malignancy	Metastatic disease	Mesothelioma
Infection	Bacterial (parapneumonic and empyema) Tuberculous	Mycoplasma (and other atypical pneumonias) Fungal Viral
Trauma	Hemothorax	Chylothorax
Gastrointestinal		Pancreatitis Esophageal rupture Subphrenic abscess
Collagen vascular disease		Systemic lupus erythematosus Rheumatoid arthritis
Miscellaneous		Asbestos exposure Drug hypersensitivity Postmyocardial infarction syndrome Meig's syndrome[a] Lymphoma and lymphatic abnormalities

[a] Usually transudative pleural effusion.

to activity, although 20% may admit to severe coughing at the time. In the older patient, emphysema with concomitant bullous disease is frequently associated with pneumothoraces. Pleuritic chest pain is a major manifestation of small pneumothoraces (10 to 20%) while dyspnea predominates in patients with larger collections of air.

After the diagnosis of pneumothorax is made, the generalist must decide whether the patient needs observation (ambulatory or inpatient) or consultation with a thoracic surgeon for insertion of a chest tube. Needle aspiration to expand the lung is discouraged since further laceration can occur. In general, patients with underlying lung disease must be hospitalized and must have a chest tube inserted since the leak seldom seals spontaneously. On the other hand, a young patient who is not in distress may be followed in the physician's office with a daily roentgenogram as long as the pneumothorax does not enlarge. There should be obvious shrinking of the space within 3–5

Table 51.2
Causes of Diffuse Alveolar Pulmonary Disease

Disorder	Common	Uncommon
Infection (pus)	Pneumonia	
Edema (fluid)	Cardiac and noncardiac pulmonary edema	
Hemorrhage (blood)		Anticoagulation
		Trauma
		Hemoptysis with aspiration
		Goodpasture's syndrome
		Idiopathic pulmonary siderosis
Cells	Sarcoidosis	Bronchoalveolar cell cancer
		"Eosinophilic" infiltrative disorders
Foreign material		Lipoid pneumonia
		Contrast media
		Alveolar proteinosis

Table 51.3
Causes of Diffuse Interstitial Pulmonary Disease

Disorder	Common	Uncommon
KNOWN CAUSES		
Infection		Miliary tuberculosis
		Fungal
		Viral and atypical pneumonia
		Pneumocystis infection
Collagen vascular disease	Scleroderma	
	Rheumatoid arthritis	
	Systemic lupus erythematosus	
Occupational (pneumoconiosis)	Asbestosis	
	Silicosis	
	Coal miner's pneumoconiosis	
Hypersensitivity and drug reactions	Extrinsic allergic alveolitis	Nitrofurantoin
		Cytotoxic drugs
Physical agents		Radiation
Vascular	Early heart failure	
Neoplastic		Lymphoma
		Lymphatic metastasis
UNKNOWN CAUSES		
Idiopathic pulmonary fibrosis	Sarcoidosis	Eosinophilic granuloma

days and eventually the lung should totally re-expand.

Diffuse Pulmonary Disease

While there are numerous causes of diffuse interstitial pulmonary disease, there are few causes of diffuse alveolar lung disease. Therefore, the distinction between an alveolar and an interstitial process is important. Unfortunately, it is not always possible to distinguish between the two entities and there may be a mixture of both. Moreover, a disorder that begins as an interstitial process can often merge into an alveolar process, such as early congestive heart failure progressing to severe pulmonary edema.

The causes of diffuse *alveolar* filling disease of the lung are shown in Table 51.2. The three most frequent causes are infection, edema, and hemorrhage and are characterized by rapid progression and regression. In contrast, diffuse interstitial lung disease develops more slowly. Therefore, the time course for the development of pulmonary symptoms and roentgenographic abnormalities is an important aspect in the differential diagnosis of diffuse lung disease.

While *interstitial* lung disease (Table 51.3) can be idiopathic, the primary goal in the evaluation is to determine whether a treatable disease is present. The initial medical history, physical examination, and laboratory testing should be oriented toward evaluating the patient for the presence of a pneumoconiosis secondary to occupational exposure, pulmonary involvement associated with collagen vascular disease, sarcoidosis, and granulomatous (tuberculous) infections of the lung. Once the more common causes of interstitial lung disease are excluded, the less common causes must be considered before the diagnosis of idiopathic pulmonary fibrosis is made. Often this process will require consultation with a pulmonary subspecialist who will guide this evaluation. Specialized pulmonary function testing including lung volume determination, diffusion capacities and cardiopulmonary exercise testing (see Chapter 54) are necessary in addition to routine spirometry. In many of these patients transbronchial biopsy using a fiberoptic bronchoscope may be recommended. The findings in lung biopsy are often useful in guiding therapy in patients with collagen vascular pulmonary diseases, sarcoidosis, idiopathic pulmonary fibrosis, and infectious disease. If the tissue obtained with transbronchial biopsy is inadequate for diagnosis, consultation with a thoracic surgeon for open thoracotomy and pulmonary biopsy may be indicated.

References

General

Felson, B: The chest roentgenologic workup—what and why? Convenient methods. Published by the American Thoracic Society. Basics of RD 8(5), 1980.
   A concise selective review.
Felson, B: Chest Roentgenology. W. B. Saunders, Philadelphia, 1973.
   An extensive basic approach to chest roentgenology.
Proto, AV: The chest radiologic workup—special studies. The American Thoracic Society. Basics of RD 9(1), 1980.
   A concise review of special roentgenographic studies of the chest.

Specific

1. Jay, SJ, Johanson, WG, Jr and Pierce, AK: The radiologic resolution of streptococcus pneumoniae pneumonia. N Engl J Med 293: 798, 1975.

2. Light, RW, MacGregor, I, Luchsinger, PC and Ball, WF: Pleural effusions: the diagnostic separation of transudates and exudates. *Ann Intern Med* 77: 507, 1972.

3. Winterbauer, RH, Bedon, GA and Ball, WC, Jr: Recurrent pneumonia. Predisposing illness and clinical patterns in 158 patients. *Ann Intern Med* 70: 689, 1969.

CHAPTER FIFTY-TWO

Obstructive Airways Disease

EUGENE R. BLEECKER, M.D., and PHILIP L. SMITH, M.D.

Obstructive diseases of the airways are the most common forms of pulmonary disease encountered in ambulatory practice. They include asthma (intermittent episodic bronchospasm), chronic obstructive bronchitis (bronchitis complicated by progressive airways obstruction), and emphysema (destruction of pulmonary structural elements causing obstructive lung disease). Although these diseases may differ in their clinical presentation, etiology, and prognosis, they all share the common feature of reduced expiratory airflow. Usually, patients with obstructive lung disease present with acute intermittent dyspnea at rest or with the insidious onset of progressive dyspnea during exercise. On the other hand, the diagnosis of early obstructive airways disease can only be made in asymptomatic patients by a decrease in forced expiration objectively measured with a spirometer (Fig. 52.1) (27). Furthermore, since the severity of airways obstruction often does not correlate with clinical symptoms such as wheezing and dyspnea, objective tests of pulmonary function are needed both to establish the initial diagnosis as well as to follow the clinical course of the disease (Table 52.1). To understand the pathophysiologic disturbances found in these patients and to assess the severity and prognosis in an individual patient, a review of some basic principles of airway mechanics is important.

PATHOPHYSIOLOGICAL ABNORMALITIES IN OBSTRUCTIVE LUNG DISEASE

To quantitate the amount of air leaving the lungs over a period of time, a forced expiration is performed into a spirometer which records the volume and speed of expiration. The factors that determine the speed and volume of a forced expiration are schematically represented in Figure 52.2. The lung is an elastic structure enclosed by the rigid chest wall with a potential cavity, the pleural space, located between. During normal respiration, the inspiratory

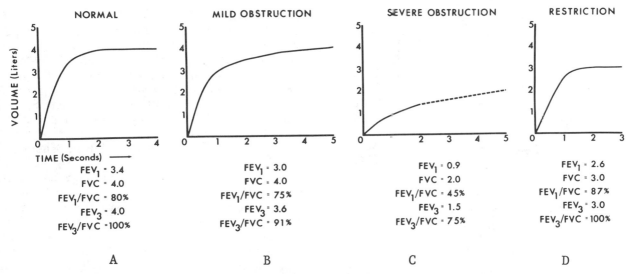

Figure 52.1 Spirographic tracings of forced expiration. Exhaled volume is plotted against time. The forced vital capacity (FVC) is represented by the total volume expired. One-second forced expiratory volume (FEV_1) is the volume of air expired during the first second. Three-second forced expiratory volume (FEV_3) is the volume of air expired during 3 sec. (*A*) Normal spirogram. (*B*) Spirogram from a patient with mild obstructive airways disease. The curve does not form a normal plateau and FEV_3/FVC % is reduced. (*C*) Spirogram from a patient with severe obstructive defect. If the spirogram were incorrectly terminated after 2 sec, the FVC would be artificially reduced (see text). When it is performed correctly (*dotted lines*) it is obvious that there is airway obstruction and that there is no restrictive disease. (*D*) Spirogram showing restrictive pulmonary disease (FEV_1/FVC is normal but FVC is reduced).

Table 52.1
Indications for Pulmonary Function Testing in Obstructive Airways Disease

To establish the presence and severity of airway obstruction
To evaluate objectively the reversibility of airways obstruction and the results of therapy
To assist in the differentiation between emphysema and other forms of airways obstruction
To serve as a basis to predict the course and prognosis of chronic obstructive disease
To evaluate work potential (see Chapter 3) or operative risks (see Chapter 83)

muscles contract, and both pleural and alveolar pressures become negative causing air to flow into the lungs. With expiration, air leaves the lungs as a result of their tendency to deflate when the respiratory muscles relax. Normally, as expiratory effort is increased, pleural pressure which surrounds the intrathoracic airways rises and compresses them (Fig. 52.2). This tendency for airways to collapse is opposed by the elastic properties of the lung that stabilize the bronchi and keep the airways open. Although slight airway compression occurs in normal subjects during a maximal expiratory effort, there is a marked tendency for airways to collapse in patients with emphysema in whom the structural components of the lung are destroyed.

Figure 52.3 diagrammatically illustrates bronchial morphology and the supporting elastic structures in the lung and illustrates how asthma, chronic bronchitis, and emphysema produce decreased expiratory air flow. In these diseases, forced expiration is limited by several factors (Table 52.2). In asthma, there is initial bronchospasm often followed by mucosal edema and retained secretions. During an acute asthmatic attack, bronchial smooth muscle may narrow and even close the airways causing air trapping and subsequent hyperinflation. In bronchitis, the onset of airflow obstruction may be insidious with initial mucous gland hyperplasia and retained bronchial secretions, especially in the peripheral airways (<2 mm). In addition, the presence of bronchial infection may lead to airway hyper-responsiveness to various inhaled agents (6) causing further smooth muscle bronchospasm. Finally, in emphysema, airways may collapse during normal tidal breathing because the structural elements of the lungs are destroyed.

PULMONARY FUNCTION TESTING IN OBSTRUCTIVE AIRWAYS DISEASE

Spirometry

Spirometry (Fig. 52.1) is the most useful pulmonary function test to assess airflow limitation in asthma and obstructive pulmonary disease. It is readily available in all pulmonary testing facilities and relatively inexpensive spirometers are also easily obtained (1,

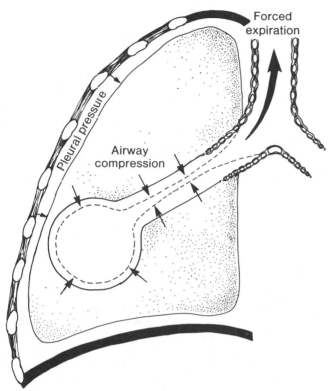

Figure 52.2 A schematic representation of the lungs and chest wall during a forced expiration. With maximal forced expiration, pleural pressure increases and becomes positive. At the point where pleural pressure exceeds intraluminal airway pressure, the airways are compressed. The structural components of the lung stabilize the airways, hold them open and oppose their tendency to collapse during expiration (see text).

16). Physicians who treat a significant number of patients with chronic obstructive airways disease should have a spirometer in their offices. Ideally, a spirometer should provide a graphic record of the patient's forced expiration, which should be maintained for at least 4 to 5 sec in order to measure both forced expiratory volume during the first second (FEV_1), and the forced vital capacity (FVC, the total volume that can be exhaled after a maximal inspiration). An electrical spirometer is less desirable, but if one is used, a graphic record is still necessary to evaluate the quality and reproducibility of the patient's effort and to calibrate accurately the speed and volume of the tracing (16). The American Thoracic Society has published guidelines for the use of spirometers (1). Three reproducible tracings should be made and the FEV_1 or another measurement of expiratory flow (maximal or midmaximal expiratory flow rates) should be calculated. Airway obstruction can be quantitated in three ways: measurement of absolute FEV_1; the FEV_1 as a percent of predicted, using readily available nomograms; and the ratio of FEV_1/FVC. Severe obstruction is usually present when the FEV_1 is less than 1.0 liter, 25% predicted, or

25–40% of the FVC. The ratio of the FEV_1/FVC is used to evaluate airways obstruction since pure restrictive ventilatory defects cause an equal reduction in the FEV_1 and the vital capacity; and the FEV_1/FVC ratio, therefore, will be normal (Fig. 52.1D). To confirm the diagnosis of airways obstruction the FEV_1/FVC should be reduced below 75 percent. Since patients with obstructive lung disease empty air from their lungs slowly (Fig. 52.1, B and C), their spirograms do not show a normal plateau. Therefore, if expiration is not prolonged, the forced vital capacity will be artifically reduced and the diagnosis of airway obstruction may be overlooked. For example, if a patient with obstructive airways disease exhales for only 2 sec, then the spirogram (Fig. 52.1C) will be artificially truncated. If it were stopped at 2 sec, the FVC would be recorded as 1.1 liters, the FEV_1 as 0.9 liter and the FEV_1/FVC as 78%. When it is correctly performed and expiration is prolonged (Fig. 52.1C, *dotted line*) the actual FVC becomes 2.0 liters and the FEV_1/FVC ratio (0.9/2.0) is 45%. Therefore, if the spirogram were not examined, an erroneous diagnosis of restrictive, rather than severe obstructive, lung disease would be made.

Patient Experience. There is little discomfort associated with spirometry in normal individuals or in patients with mild to moderate obstructive airways disease. After a nose clip is applied, the patient is instructed to take a deep inspiration, immediately followed by a forceful expiration that should continue for at least 4 sec. Forced expiration can result in coughing and, very rarely, cyanosis and hypoxemia in patients with severe airways disease and resting hypoxemia.

The peak expiratory flow rate can be measured in patients with asthma by use of inexpensive peak flow meters, which do not provide a printed record or a measurement of vital capacity. This peak flow meter can be used by a patient at home to monitor lung function serially during therapy (see below).

Complete Pulmonary Function Tests

Other pulmonary function tests that are useful in the detailed assessment of obstructive airways disease include the measurement of lung volumes, diffusion capacity, and arterial blood gases both at rest and during exercise (see Chapter 50, the section on dyspnea). The measurement of *lung volumes* quantitates the degree of hyperinflation that may be found either in patients with long-standing airway obstruction or in patients with acute asthma. Occasionally, initial clinical and symptomatic improvement in airways obstruction during recovery from an asthmatic attack will be reflected by a decrease in the degree of hyperinflation (46). The *single breath diffusion capacity* for carbon monoxide reflects the amount of functional alveolar capillary surface area available for gas exchange. The findings of expiratory airflow

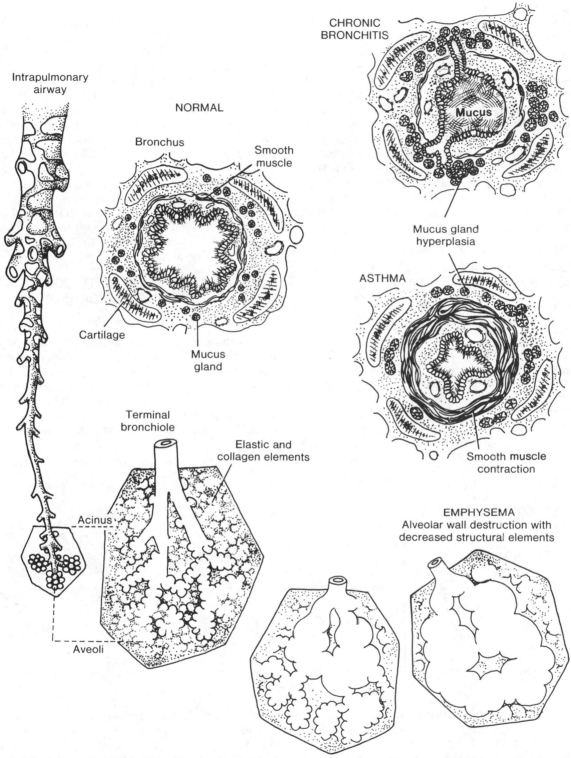

Figure 52.3 Schematic representation of the morphology of normal airways and lung parenchyma and the changes produced in these structures by asthma, chronic bronchitis, and emphysema (see text).

limitation, hyperinflation, and a reduced diffusion capacity often correlate with the presence of anatomic emphysema (17) (Fig. 52.8). There is no discomfort or risk during the measurement of lung volumes, but it is necessary that a patient be able to remain seated for 6 to 8 min, breathing a mixture of air and helium. Severely obstructed patients whose vital capacity is less than 1 liter cannot perform a single breath diffusion capacity since they must hold at least a 1-liter inspiratory volume for 10 sec.

Other pulmonary function tests such as the measurement of pulmonary compliance or airway resistance using a body plethysmograph are sophisticated tests that are not usually helpful in the routine management of patients with obstructive airways disease. Flow volume curves provide similar information to routine spirometry; however, the apparatus for this test is more complicated, is difficult to calibrate accurately, and is expensive. Nevertheless, many testing facilities use flow volume curves rather than spirometry. Flow volume curves are useful in the evaluation of extrathoracic airway obstruction and some examples of these curves in upper and lower airway obstruction are shown in Fig. 52.4 (18).

Early Detection of Airways Disease

The early diagnosis of chronic obstructive lung disease depends on sensitive pulmonary function

Table 52.2
Mechanisms of Airway Obstruction

Smooth muscle spasm
Mucosal edema
Mucous gland hyperplasia
Increased bronchial secretions
Airways collapse
Airways hyperreactivity to inhaled substances
(cigarette smoke, dust, histamine)

tests that correlate with the presence of peripheral airway obstruction (< 2 mm). Anatomically, these airways lack significant cartilage, have a smooth muscle wall that contains large numbers of mucus-secreting goblet cells, and rely entirely on the surrounding lung parenchyma for structural support. Correlations of the pathologic findings in the lungs of patients with early bronchitis and emphysema (17, 42) show abnormalities in these peripheral airways. Early peripheral airways disease may be predicted by a spirogram in which the FEV_1 is relatively normal (80% of predicted and the FEV_1/FVC ratio is 75%) but the FVC does not reach a plateau normally within 4 sec, thereby indicating slowly emptying parts of the lungs (21). This can be further quantitated by measuring the forced expiratory volume after 3 sec, the FEV_3, which is normally 98 to 100% of the FVC (FEV_3/FVC ratio: Fig. 52.1).

ASTHMA (INTERMITTENT OBSTRUCTIVE AIRWAYS DISEASE)

Definition

Asthma is difficult to define; for many physicians it simply implies wheezing from any cause. More specifically, asthma is a heterogeneous clinical syndrome that is characterized by intermittent dyspnea and wheezing resulting from widespread narrowing of the intrapulmonary airways. Unlike other causes of airflow obstruction, the key features in asthma are

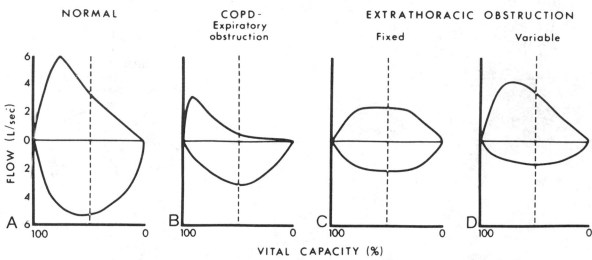

Figure 52.4 Flow volume curves (loops) of maximal forced expiration (*upper*) and maximal inspiration (*lower*). Expiratory and inspiratory flow is plotted against lung volume expressed as a percent of vital capacity. The *dotted line* can be used to compare flow rates at 50% of the vital capacity where inspiratory flow rates normally exceed expiratory flow rates. (*A*) Normal flow volume curves. (*B*) Flow volume curves illustrating expiratory airflow obstruction showing decreased flow rates at all points in lung volume throughout maximal expiration. (*C*) Fixed extrathoracic airway obstruction (cancer or fracture of the larynx) produces a pattern where there is a decrease and flattening of both inspiratory and expiratory flow volume curves. Inspiratory flow rate at 50% of the vital capacity is equal to similar expiratory flow rate. (*D*) Variable extrathoracic obstruction (vocal cord paralysis) produces a pattern where there is a decrease and flattening of maximal inspiratory flow volume curves. Inspiratory flow rates at 50% of the vital capacity are less than similar expiratory flow. (Modified from Hyatt and Black (18)).

reversibility of airway obstruction with relatively symptom-free periods between attacks and increased responsiveness of the airways to a wide variety of inhaled stimuli. The prevalence of asthma in the United States is estimated to be 3% of the population or almost 9 million people.

Types of Asthma

The above definition of asthma describes only the clinical characteristics of this heterogeneous disease. Asthma can also be classified according to precipitating factors, namely, the presence or absence of an allergic etiology. On the basis of clinical findings, more than half of an asthmatic population can be assigned to one of the five types that are listed in Table 52.3, although even these as well as the rest of the asthmatic population show considerable overlap in the clinical features of their disease.

NONALLERGIC INTRINSIC ASTHMA

The most common type of asthma is not due to allergy, but to poorly defined intrinsic factors. These asthmatics have persistent hyperreactivity of the airways to multiple nonallergic stimuli (see below). Although some intrinsic asthmatics have allergies that occasionally trigger an acute asthmatic attack, the usual clinical course of their disease does not correlate with their allergic hypersensitivities. Instead, asthmatic attacks may be related to infection, exercise, inhaled irritants, or psychologic stimuli. Although intrinsic asthmatics have significant eosinophilia in their blood and sputum, unlike patients with allergic asthma (see below), their serum IgE levels are normal. Asthmatic symptoms may begin at any age, but often start during adulthood. Commonly, patients may date the onset of asthma to an acute upper respiratory tract infection. Although intrinsic asthmatics may improve with appropriate therapy after their first attack, they subsequently develop chronic symptomatic asthma. Frequently the clinical manifestations of their disease are severe and have a tendency to persist throughout the year, showing variations in severity rather than complete symptomatic remissions. Some of these patients have chronic bronchitis that either complicates or precipitates asthmatic attacks (see below).

Asthma and Airways Hyperactivity. A characteristic feature found in all asthmatics is airways hyperreactivity, an exaggerated degree of bronchospasm induced by various inhaled agents (6). These agents include immunologic mediators, such as histamine and some prostaglandins; cholinergic agents, such as methacholine; and various irritants, such as dust, cigarette smoke, and cold air (exercise-induced asthma). Nonspecific airways reactivity is thought to correlate with asthmatic symptoms such as coughing and intermittent wheezing. Some patients with chronic obstructive lung disease also show increased airways reactivity. Neural reflex mechanisms may be partially responsible for bronchospasm induced by these inhaled irritants. These substances activate irritant receptors whose afferent pathways travel in the vagus nerves. Subsequent reflex bronchoconstriction is caused by activation of efferent vagal pathways. These same parasympathetic mechanisms mediate the cough reflex and control bronchial secretions. Some patients have symptoms only of airways irritability such as persistent coughing (see Chapter 50, section on cough). They have airways hyperreactivity to inhaled agents (methacholine) and their symptoms improve after treatment with bronchodilators (28). These patients probably have mild intrinsic asthma.

ALLERGIC EXTRINSIC ASTHMA

In 5–10% of asthmatics, clinical asthma is primarily caused by specific allergic factors. These stimuli include seasonal exposure to the pollens of grasses, ragweed, and trees, or to other specific allergens such as animal dander, dust, or some occupational agents. Allergic asthmatics frequently note the onset of recognizable symptoms early in life and relate a family or personal history of asthma or of other allergic diseases (allergic rhinitis, eczema, and urticaria). Many allergic extrinsic asthmatics also have attacks triggered by multiple nonallergic causes.

In these allergic patients, the intradermal injection of a specific allergen causes a wheal and flare reaction; inhalation of this same antigen causes airways obstruction. When a susceptible individual is exposed to an allergen, specific IgE or reaginic antibody is produced. This antibody sensitizes mast cells and basophils (2) and re-exposure to that allergen initiates a sequence of biochemical reactions within these sensitized target cells (Type I immunologic reaction) (see Chapter 22, Fig. 22.1). These reactions cause the formation, release, and synthesis of histamine, and other vasoactive substances which cause contraction of bronchial smooth muscle, alter vascular permeability, and attract inflammatory cells to the reaction site. In addition, these substances cause the pathophysiologic changes found in an allergic asthmatic attack (2).

The release of these mediators is inhibited by increases in cellular cyclic AMP (adenosine 3′:5′-monophosphate) and facilitated by increases in cyclic GMP (guanosine 3′:5′-monophosphate). β-Sympathomimetic agonists (such as isoproterenol) directly increase cyclic AMP and theophylline preparations (such as aminophylline) inhibit the activity of phos-

Table 52.3
Types of Asthma

Nonallergic intrinsic asthma
Allergic extrinsic asthma
Nonallergic extrinsic asthma
Asthma associated with chronic obstructive
   lung disease
Exercise-induced asthma

phodiesterase an enzyme that catalyzes the breakdown of cyclic AMP, thereby suppressing mediator release. Cholinergic stimulation, on the other hand, may enhance the release of mediators by increasing levels of cyclic GMP. These interactions are the basis for the pharmacologic treatment of allergic asthma.

NONALLERGIC EXTRINSIC ASTHMA DUE TO SPECIFIC AGENTS

In some patients, exposure to inhaled or ingested agents causes asthma that does not seem to be caused by the irritant effects of the inhaled substances nor is it mediated by classic immunologic reactions. However, recent studies have shown that some of these substances (toluene-2,4-diisocyanate (TDI) or phthalic acid anhydride) may cause their effects through immunologic mechanisms. They may act as haptens and combine with serum albumin to form a complete antigen that provokes an IgE-mediated asthma attack (24). When the exposure to these agents occurs in industrial settings, the reversible bronchospasm they produce is called "occupational asthma." Examples of these agents include metal fumes and salts (chromium, nickel, ammonium), wood (oak and western red cedar), vegetable, grain, and coffee bean dusts (flour—baker's asthma), industrial chemicals used in manufacturing processes of plastics, polyurethane foams (TDI, phthalic acid anhydride, epoxy resins, soldering fluxes), pyrolysis products of plastics (meat wrapper's asthma), enzymes (*Bacillus subtilis* detergents), as well as exposures during the manufacture of pharmaceutical agents (penicillin, pancreatic enzymes) (8) (see Chapter 7).

Aspirin and Other Drug Sensitivity. Other agents such as aspirin, nonsteroidal anti-inflammatory drugs (indomethacin and phenylbutazone), and tartrazine (yellow dye No. 5), a common coloring agent used in many foods and drugs, precipitate bronchospasm in 5 to 10% of all asthmatics (40) and urticaria in susceptible individuals (Chapter 22). While the precise mechanisms through which these ingested substances trigger asthma are unknown, it is felt that they are probably not initiated through classic IgE-mediated immunologic reactions. Asthmatics with aspirin sensitivity tend to be female and have associated nasal polyps and sinusitis. Bronchospasm occurs within 2 hours of the aspirin ingestion and severe reactions may be accompanied by vascular shock and, rarely, death. Therefore, asthmatics should avoid taking these substances, and challenges with these agents should be performed with extreme care. Table 22.12, Chapter 22, lists both prescription and nonprescription compounds that contain aspirin.

ASTHMA ASSOCIATED WITH CHRONIC OBSTRUCTIVE LUNG DISEASE

There are patients with chronic obstructive airways disease (chronic obstructive bronchitis or emphysema), whose disease is characterized by intermittent "asthmatic" attacks. A small number of these patients give a history of typical childhood asthma or of other allergic diseases. The importance of this somewhat artificial grouping is to emphasize that although the prognosis in these patients is determined by their chronic obstructive lung disease (see below), the pathophysiology and treatment of an acute exacerbation of bronchospasm is similar to that of typical asthma.

EXERCISE-INDUCED ASTHMA (COLD AIR)

Most asthmatics, regardless of etiology, develop wheezing and dyspnea after moderate to severe exercise, especially in cold environments. Some forms of exercise, such as running or bicycle riding, are more asthmogenic than others, such as swimming, where ambient air is usually warm and humid. Although the mechanism of exercise-induced asthma is still not completely understood, recently it has been shown that the production of postexertional asthma is directly related to increased heat loss from the pulmonary airways during exercise-induced hyperventilation. Thus, in experimental situations, exercise-induced bronchospasm can be prevented by having an asthmatic breathe air that is humidified and heated to body temperature (30). The response to exercise or cold air represents another example of airways hyperactivity in asthma. In some mild asthmatics, attacks of exercise-induced bronchospasm represent the primary clinical manifestation of their disease. Also, an elderly intrinsic asthmatic complaining of dyspnea on exertion outdoors on a cold winter day may actually be experiencing exercise-induced asthma rather than cardiac or pulmonary decompensation.

Clinical Presentation of Asthma

Usually asthmatic attacks are episodic, lasting hours to several days, separated by symptom-free periods during which airflow obstruction is absent or mild. Although the patient notes wheezing and coughing productive of white mucoid sputum during a mild asthmatic attack, he can perform ordinary tasks without difficulty. During more severe asthmatic attacks, however, he will experience exertional dyspnea that persists even at rest. Frequent coughing reflects airway hyperirritability. *Status asthmaticus* refers to a very severe and persistent asthmatic state that does not substantially improve despite intensive therapy.

Evaluation of Mild or Asymptomatic Asthma

HISTORY

A complete medical history is essential in the initial evaluation of patients with bronchial asthma to determine the overall severity, the specific factors which precipitate or aggravate symptoms, and the therapeutic modalities that are effective in an individual patient. The medical history should also establish the frequency and severity of asthmatic attacks as well as a description of exercise tolerance during symptom-free periods. If the asthmatic attacks are associated with bronchitis, the frequency, quantity, and duration of sputum production should be documented. The occurrence of seasonal exacerbations should alert the physician to the possibility of environmental factors such as ragweed or grass allergy (see Chapter 22, Fig. 22.3). A history of cough and wheezing precipitated by exposure to environmental cigarette smoke suggests the presence of nonspecific airways reactivity. On the other hand, a personal history of cigarette smoking is so unusual in asthma that it is more likely that such a patient actually has chronic obstructive pulmonary disease. The severity of exercise-induced bronchospasm should be elicited, especially in adolescents and young adults, in whom exercise asthma may interfere with normal social and physical development.

PHYSICAL EXAMINATION

Tachypnea, tachycardia, and a pulsus paradoxus (a drop in systolic blood pressure of greater than 15 mm Hg with inspiration) should be looked for. The upper airways should be examined for the presence of sinusitis, nasal polyps, or evidence of allergic rhinitis (boggy pale nasal mucosa, conjunctivitis). During the rest of the physical examination particular emphasis should be placed on breathing pattern, the use of accessory muscles of ventilation and the presence of rhonchi and rales during auscultation of the chest. If wheezing is not heard during quiet breathing, a maximal timed forced expiratory maneuver should be performed by asking the patient to blow out all the air in his lungs as fast as possible after a maximal inspiration. This will frequently induce wheezing not present during quiet breathing; and by timing the forced expiration, a simple index of airways obstruction is obtained. Normal subjects are able to perform a forced expiratory time in less than 4 sec, but with airflow obstruction the duration of expiration is greater than 5 or 6 sec.

LABORATORY TESTING

In mild asthmatics spirometry is useful to document baseline normal pulmonary function during a symptom-free period. In those patients with more severe asthma, spirometry provides an objective measure of severity and serves as a guide for therapy. For a transient time after the initial improvement from an acute attack, significant residual abnormalities in airways function often persist (27). Depending on the individual asthmatic, these residual abnormalities in airways function either resolve or persist with varying severity. This subclinical airways obstruction can serve as a focus for future recurrent asthmatic attacks. In asthmatics without superimposed chronic obstructive airways disease, blood gas analysis is indicated only to assess severe asthmatic episodes (see below). In older patients (> 40 years), especially

those with evidence of persistent airways obstruction or associated cardiovascular disease, baseline spirometry, an electrocardiogram, and a chest roentgenogram should always be obtained.

A complete blood count (CBC) with differential and sputum examination should be performed in asthmatics who have clinical findings of an acute infectious process. Eosinophils can make sputum appear grossly purulent; therefore, microscopic examination of the sputum in an asthmatic is necessary in order to avoid inappropriate use of antibiotics. Besides eosinophils, sputum may also contain Charcot-Leyden crystals (pointed elongated eosinophilic crystals) and Curschmann's spirals (mucous casts of small bronchioles) (13). If parenchymal pulmonary infection is suspected because of the presence of fever, purulent sputum, and physical findings such as rales and consolidation, a chest roentgenogram and sputum culture are indicated.

Skin testing (Chapter 22) is indicated to confirm the clinical suspicion of allergy. Common allergens that cause allergic asthma include ragweed pollens, various grasses, extracts of trees, molds indigenous to specific localities, and animal danders (cat, dog). Skin testing is most easily obtained by referral to an allergist. Total serum IgE is usually only moderately elevated in patients with allergic asthma and its measurement is not indicated in the routine clinical management of this disease. Specific serum IgE, measured by the radioallergosorbent test (RAST), provides information similar to that provided by allergy skin testing. Therefore, the RAST is helpful only when skin testing cannot be performed.

BRONCHIAL CHALLENGE PROCEDURES

Diagnostic testing with *exercise* or *inhalation challenge* with pharmacologic agents is occasionally useful to confirm the presence of hyperreactive airways in patients with questionable symptoms. These tests involve inhaling gradually increasing concentrations of either histamine or methacholine and observing spirometric changes in airflow obstruction (6). Similarly, an exercise challenge can be performed and pulmonary function can be quantitated during the first 30 min after maximal exercise. When positive, these tests can cause some mild to moderate distress in an asymptomatic asthmatic since a 20 to 30% reduction in FEV_1 is used as an endpoint for the diagnosis of hyperreactive airways. For example, an exercise challenge might help to confirm the diagnostic impression of exercise asthma in a young patient who complains of excessive coughing and dyspnea after physical exertion. These challenges require referral to a pulmonary function laboratory which is able to perform provocative testing. Inhalation challenge with specific antigen is almost never indicated since it does not distinguish allergic nonasthmatic patients (grass and ragweed hay fever) from asthmatics with these specific allergies (6). An exception is inhalation challenge in suspected occupational exposure when it may be important to establish the relationship between symptoms and a specific incriminating substance.

Acute Asthma

In order to understand fully the basis for the symptoms, signs, and laboratory findings that correlate with severe asthma, a review of the pathophysiology of acute bronchospasm is indicated.

PATHOPHYSIOLOGY OF ACUTE ASTHMA

Obstruction to expiratory airflow in acute asthma is initially caused by bronchial smooth muscle spasm that is followed, as the attack persists, by bronchial wall edema, inflammatory cell infiltration, and mucous plugging of the airways. With progressively more severe asthma ($FEV_1 < 1.5$ liters), the asthmatic is forced to compensate for bronchoconstriction in order to permit gas exchange to take place. He does this by breathing at high lung volumes since, as the lungs enlarge to total lung capacity, the airways are mechanically opened. Unfortunately, breathing in a hyperinflated state requires a marked increase in the inspiratory muscle forces, and results in varying degrees of dyspnea and fatigue. A reduction in vital capacity correlates with the degree of hyperinflation and, in very severe attacks, the vital capacity may be only slightly larger than the asthmatic's tidal volume. Therefore, the severity of the asthmatic attack is highly correlated with the two simple measures of forced expiration, the forced expiratory volume in 1 sec (FEV_1), and the forced vital capacity (FVC) (Fig. 52.1) (27, 36).

Another major physiologic change that occurs during a severe asthmatic attack is the development of pulmonary hypertension due to the direct effects of hypoxia and the mechanical effects of hyperinflation on the pulmonary vasculature. These changes are manifested by electrocardiographic abnormalities such as acute right axis deviation, "p" pulmonale, and right ventricular strain. In addition, the marked swings in pleural pressure during breathing in acute asthma affect left ventricular function and account for the development of pulsus paradoxus. A summary

Table 52.4
Pathophysiologic Changes in Acute Bronchial Asthma

Expiratory airflow obstruction (FEV_1 and expiratory airflow are reduced)

Breathing at high lung volumes to prevent airway closure at resting lung volumes (vital capacity is reduced)

Pulmonary hypertension (P pulmonale and right ventricular strain on ECG)

Large fluctuations in pleural pressure with respiration (pulsus paradoxus)

Ventilation-perfusion imbalance (arterial blood gases show hypoxemia always, hypocapnea (low $PaCO_2$) usually, and hypercapnea (high $PaCO_2$) only in very severe asthma)

Table 52.5
Objective Evaluation of Acute Asthma

Vital signs: tachycardia and pulsus paradoxus

Physical examination: use of accessory muscles of respiration with sternocleidomastoid contractions

Spirometry: reduced FEV_1 and increase in FEV_1 after administration of a bronchodilator

Chest x-ray: hyperinflation

ECG: acute cor pulmonale

Arterial blood gases (low PaO_2, low or high $PaCO_2$)

Sputum smear and culture: eosinophils

Table 52.6
Indications of Severe Asthma Necessitating Immediate Hospitalization (Acute Respiratory Failure)

$FEV_1 < 0.7$, FVC < 1.2 (absent bronchodilator response)

$PaO_2 < 50$ mm Hg, $PaCO_2 > 40$ mm Hg

Disturbances of consciousness, obvious exhaustion

Silent chest

Pulsus paradoxus > 15 mm

Pneumothorax or pneumomediastinum

of these pathophysiologic changes is listed in Table 52.4.

EVALUATION OF AN ACUTE ASTHMATIC ATTACK

Unfortunately, subjective symptoms such as dyspnea and wheezing do not correlate with severity of asthma (27) and the physician must rely on objective physical findings and laboratory tests to evaluate the acute asthmatic attack (Table 52.5). During the physical examination, the findings of a pulsus paradoxus and the use of accessory muscles of ventilation with sternocleidomastoid contractions correlate with the development of severe airflow obstruction, hyperinflation, and a marked reduction in FEV_1 ($< 40\%$ predicted or 1.25 liters) (27, 36).

When physical findings are present that suggest severe asthma, objective pulmonary function measurements should be performed in every asthmatic who is old enough to cooperate. An FEV_1 less than 1 liter or 25% predicted correlates with severe hypoxemia ($PaO_2 < 60$ mm Hg) (25). Spirometry should then be used to monitor the course of the asthmatic attack as well as the response to bronchodilator treatment. An absent bronchodilator response suggests status asthmaticus. If these physical findings and objective tests do not improve with therapy, then the patient should be sent to the Emergency Room for treatment. The findings listed in Table 52.6 indicate severe respiratory failure in status asthmaticus and require immediate hospitalization.

A chest roentgenogram is indicated in those patients with acute asthma who do not improve readily with initial treatment or those in whom pulmonary infection is suspected. The chest roentgenogram should be inspected for atelectasis due to mucous plugging of the airways, for pulmonary infiltrates due to infectious processes that could precipitate or complicate an asthmatic attack, and for a pneumothorax, or a pneumomediastinum. Furthermore, the presence of acute hyperinflation on a chest roentgenogram indicates a severe asthmatic attack (Fig. 52.5). The significance of electrocardiographic abnormalities consistent with acute cor pulmonale and pulmonary hypertension has been discussed. The measurement of arterial blood gases should be performed when physical findings and spirometry (FEV_1 < 1.25 liters or 40% predicted) suggest a severe asthmatic attack. Arterial hypoxemia develops during acute episodes of bronchial asthma (25), and in the very severe attack (FEV_1 < 0.7 liter or 10–15% predicted) hypoxemia can be life-threatening. Usually in mild to moderately severe asthmatic attacks alveolar hyperventilation is maintained and arterial CO_2 tensions are reduced. In asthma an arterial CO_2 tension that rises into the normal range or becomes elevated predicts imminent respiratory failure.

Differential Diagnosis

Because of its characteristic clinical presentation, acute bronchial asthma is easily differentiated from the other cardiopulmonary diseases that present with cough, wheezing, and dyspnea. In middle aged and elderly patients one must consider acute left ventricular failure with "cardiac asthma", pulmonary em-

bolism, or an infectious exacerbation of chronic obstructive pulmonary disease. Occasionally patients only complain of persistent coughing and deny wheezing or dyspnea. These patients often have pulmonary function tests which reveal mild obstruction, have bronchial hyperreactivity, and improve with bronchodilator treatment (27).

Airflow limitation produced by obstruction in the upper airways (larynx, trachea) caused by a foreign body, tumor, secretions, edema, inflammation, or tracheal malacia can sometimes be confused with lower airway obstruction. In upper airway obstruction, there may be a history of goiter, hoarseness, or prior endotracheal intubation. Physical examination usually reveals inspiratory stridor (wheezing during inspiration). Inspiratory flow volume curves (18), performed in a pulmonary function laboratory, show a reduction in inspiratory flows and a specific diagnostic pattern (Fig. 52.4). Direct or indirect laryngoscopy may visualize an anatomical abnormality.

Treatment of Asthma

Since asthma has multiple etiologies, its management requires a combined therapeutic approach that should attempt to maintain pulmonary function in a near normal state as well as to prevent recurrent asthmatic attacks (Table 52.7) Precipitating factors in an individual asthmatic must be identified and avoided. Clinical manifestations including broncho-

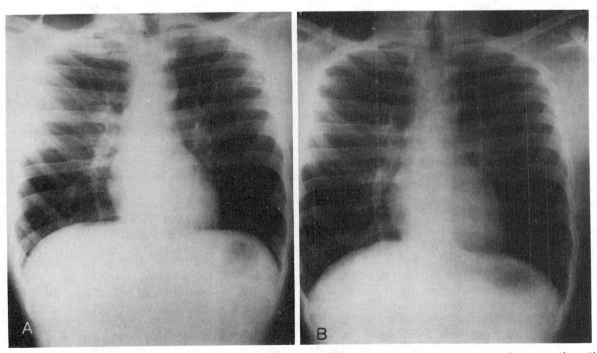

Figure 52.5 Acute hyperinflation in severe asthma. (*A*) Normal chest roentgenogram is an asthmatic. (*B*) Acute hyperinflation (lowered flattened diaphragms and widened intercostal spaces) in the same patient during a severe asthmatic attack. Pulmonary function tests showed a marked reduction in FEV_1 (0.8 liter, 18% predicted) and FVC (2.1 liters, 38% predicted) and an elevated total lung capacity (7.3 liters, 112% predicted).

Table 52.7
Treatment of Asthma

GENERAL MEASURES
    Control of environmental factors:
        Cigarette smoke, air pollutants
        Occupational exposures
        Control of environmental temperature and humidity
    Control of allergy to specific inhaled or ingested agents
    Control of emotional and psychologic factors
    Control of respiratory infections
SPECIFIC TREATMENT
    Pharmacologic
        Smooth muscle spasm—bronchodilators: local/systemic
        Inflammation (corticosteroids)
    Mechanical airways obstruction—mucus:
        Hydration—local/systemic
        Physical therapy
        Mucolytic agents: to be avoided
    Infection: appropriate antibiotics
    Hypoxemia: humidified oxygen
    Sedation: to be avoided

spasm and pulmonary infections must be effectively treated, while medical complications should be prevented.

AVOIDANCE OF PRECIPITATING FACTORS

As indicated above, numerous, often apparently unrelated factors, precipitate or worsen clinical asthma. Some of these stimuli are easily defined and controlled, while in other asthmatics the exact etiologies of an attack are difficult to determine with certainty. Knowledge of the triggers of asthma is of prime importance in its evaluation and treatment.

Environment. Asthmatics should avoid exposure to irritating dusts, sprays or aerosols, either at home or at work. For example, passive exposure of asthmatics to cigarette smoke, especially in enclosed spaces such as cars, airplanes, or poorly ventilated rooms, will cause worsening of airway function. The exact role of air pollutants in provoking asthma is still not completely known. However, it is known that ozone, sulfur dioxide, and nitrogen dioxide exposure can increase nonspecific airways reactivity in normal subjects and can cause symptoms and bronchospasm in asthmatics (6). Often occupational factors are not immediately obvious since asthmatic symptoms may occur several hours after leaving the work place (coughing and dyspnea awakening the patient from sleep). Since direct challenge with suspected provoking agents is not always practical and often dangerous, the etiology of an asthmatic's symptoms may be indirectly ascertained by systematically avoiding specific, potentially provoking factors. At home, the control of environmental temperature and humidity is accomplished with an air conditioner that will also help to filter pollens and air pollutants. The filter should be changed regularly to avoid the accumulation of sensitizing airborne molds and fungi.

In rare circumstances, removal to a more favorable climate may be indicated to control chronic asthma (see p. 458).

Allergy. Desensitization consists of injections of increasing concentrations of an antigen to which the asthmatic is sensitive, thereby inducing blocking antibody (IgG antibody that interferes with the antigen-antibody reaction). It is indicated when there are a limited number of allergens, demonstrated by skin testing, that appear to be etiologically related to an individual's asthma (20). Desensitization therapy is expensive, time-consuming, and not always effective. Therefore, before it is started, every attempt should be made to eliminate or reduce specific allergen exposure. At times, only a reduction in exposure to a known allergen can be effected. For example, if it is not possible to remove a household pet from the home of an allergic asthmatic patient, the pet should be excluded from the patient's bedroom. Down-filled pillows and shag rugs that accumulate dust should not be used.

Emotion. Asthmatic attacks can be produced and reversed in some patients by appropriate verbal suggestion (26). For example, less bronchodilation is produced by isoproterenol if the asthmatic is told he is being treated with a bronchoconstrictor rather than a bronchodilator. Therefore, the expectations of the asthmatic patient as well as of those treating him have a significant influence on the therapeutic efficacy of any given therapeutic regimen. Despite these considerations, all asthmatic patients must receive adequate medical treatment and symptoms should not be ignored because of possible psychogenic etiologies.

In some asthmatics, emotional factors play a much greater role in modulating the course of their disease and often cause difficult therapeutic problems. In addition, asthma can be a chronic, debilitating disease that in itself will stress the asthmatic and his family. Usually supportive measures initiated by a sympathetic physician, as well as by the patient's family members and friends, will avoid the need for psychiatric care. Occasionally, supportive psychotherapy will be useful, especially when counseling is available from a professional who is experienced in treating psychosomatic illnesses. In selected patients, mild sedatives (see Chapter 12) may be an adjunct to the total treatment regimen, but preferably other means should be used to help a patient cope with the anxiety caused by his disease. He should be assured of the concern of those around him, as well as the constant availability of adequate emergency care. Sedation is specifically contraindicated in severe (Table 52.6) asthmatic attacks since sedating a severely ill, exhausted asthmatic can result in acute respiratory failure (25) and even death.

An important adjunct to the psychosocial management of childhood asthma is the encouragement of a general exercise program. Asthma should not be an automatic excuse preventing participation in physical education and sports. With appropriate premedication asthmatics can participate in most activities. Some activities may be less asthmogenic than others (see exercise asthma). It is important not to isolate the asthmatic from his peers by unnecessary restrictive measures.

Infections. Upper respiratory tract infections can cause transient increases in nonspecific airways reactivity with persistent coughing, and occasional bronchospasm in nonasthmatics (Chapter 27, "Respiratory Infections," and Chapter 50, the section on cough). In fact, these reactions may be so severe and persistent that these "nonasthmatics" require treatment with bronchodilators. Therefore, it is not surprising that most asthmatics have attacks triggered by respiratory infections.

If there is clinical evidence of an acute bacterial respiratory infection associated with an asthmatic attack, antibiotic therapy should be initiated. Usually, the initial drug of choice is either tetracycline or ampicillin, administered for 7 to 10 days, unless the sputum smear or culture dictate the use of a different antibiotic regimen.

PHARMACOLOGIC TREATMENT

Pharmacologic therapy is the primary therapeutic modality used to treat reversible bronchospasm in asthma and in chronic obstructive lung disease (43). The five drug categories generally available include (a) sympathomimetics, (b) theophylline preparations, (c) antiallergic drugs, (d) anticholinergics, and (e) corticosteroids. Detailed knowledge of the mechanism of action and side effects of these drugs is important for every physician who takes care of patients with reversible airways disease. The selection of an appropriate drug regimen is complicated by the many preparations available for most of these agents. Specific combinations, dosage, and route of

delivery will often be determined by whether these drugs are used for preventive therapy in stable asthmatics or for the emergency treatment of acute asthma.

Sympathomimetic Agents. This group of drugs may be functionally divided into agents that have α- and β-sympathomimetic activities. More recently, β agonists have been further divided into those with β_1 and β_2 selective actions (Table 52.8). The undesirable side effects of β agonists are due to their β_1 actions which stimulate the cardiovascular system, causing tachycardia and arrhythmias. The β_2 actions of these drugs increase cyclic AMP levels in mast cells and bronchial smooth muscle, thereby inhibiting mediator release and directly dilating the airways smooth muscle.

Epinephrine has both α- and β-adrenergic effects, while *isoproterenol* has equal β_1- and β_2-sympathomimetic activity. Besides lack of specificity, these older sympathomimetics have a shorter duration of action because they are rapidly metabolized by catechol-ortho-methyltransferase (COMT), an enzyme present in high concentrations in the gut. Therefore, these drugs can only be administered by an aerosol or parenteral route and their duration of action is only approximately 30 min. Newer β_2-sympathomimetic agonists are not metabolized by COMT and thus have a longer duration of action than isoproterenol. These agents have progressively greater β_2 selectivity as shown in Table 52.8. Unfortunately, they still retain some β_1 cardiac side effects and furthermore, when administered systemically all cause skeletal muscle tremor, a specific β_2 side effect. This annoying side effect may occur even when oral treatment with terbutaline or metaproterenol is begun at reduced doses, but it frequently improves with continued therapy (2 weeks). *Ephedrine* is widely used because it is well absorbed orally, but its side effects include stimulation of the cardiac and central nervous systems, thereby limiting its usefulness. The

Table 52.8
β-Sympathomimetic Agonists

Generic Name	Trade Name	β_2 Selectivity	Inhalation Peak Effect (min)	Duration of Effect (hr)	Dosage Form
Isoproterenol	Isuprel Mistometer	$\beta_2 = \beta_1$	5–15	1½–1	Metered dose inhaler, 125 μg/puff Nebulized solution, 1:200
Isoetharine	Bronkosol Bronkosol Unit Dose Bronkometer	$\beta_2 > \beta_1$	5–15	3–4	Metered dose inhaler: 340 μg/puff Nebulized solution, 1%
Metaproterenol	Alupent	$\beta_2 >> \beta_1$	30–60	3–5	Metered dose inhaler, 0.65 μg/puff Nebulized solution, 5% Tablets, 10 and 20 mg
Terbutaline	Brethine Bricanyl	$\beta_2 >>> \beta_1$	30	4	Injection, 1 μg/ml Tablets, 2.5 and 5 mg
Albuterol	Proventyl, Ventolin	$\beta_2 >>> \beta_1$	60–90	4–6	Metered dose inhaler, 90 μg/puff
Fenoterol[a]	Berotec	$\beta_2 >>> \beta_1$	60	6–8	Metered dose inhaler, 200 μg/puff

[a] Pending release in the United States.

need to counteract these side effects has led to fixed dose combination tablets which contain ephedrine, a sedative, and a theophylline preparation. These drug combinations, although convenient and popular, do not meet the specific needs of an individual and usually do not deliver an adequate therapeutic dose of any of its components. Since newer β_2 agonists (metaproterenol and terbutaline) are well absorbed orally, they should replace ephedrine.

For the ambulatory treatment of asthma, the new β_2-sympathomimetic agonists can be used as aerosols to prevent asthmatic attacks caused by known trigger factors such as exercise, cold air exposure, or inhaled irritants. When therapy with an inhaled agent is begun, all patients should be shown how to use a metered dose inhaler, and thereafter, their technique should be checked periodically. Illustrations showing the correct technique are usually included in the package insert. This process should be performed as follows. At the end of a normal exhalation or at functional residual capacity, the inhaler should be held up to the open mouth and triggered at the beginning of a slow gradual inspiration to total lung capacity; slow, not rapid, inspiration should be particularly emphasized to the patient. A second inhalation of the drug can be taken immediately, or preferably the patient should wait 15 min before the second dose. This allows for deeper penetration of the aerosol into the lung since the first breath should dilate the airways. In patients who require continuous treatment for either short periods during an exacerbation or chronically because of persistent bronchospasm, two inhalations are taken every 6 to 8 hours. Recently, some physicians have been prescribing the use of inhaled sympathomimetics at more frequent intervals (every 3 to 4 hours). Although they find that this treatment is usually safe, it should not be used in patients with cardiac disease (31).

Often acute asthmatic attacks are initially treated in the physician's office, but when they are severe (Tables 52.5 and 52.6), treatment should be started in the office and the patient should then be sent to an Emergency Room. In an acute asthmatic attack, subcutaneous epinephrine (0.01–0.03 ml of 1:1000) or inhaled isoproterenol (two inhalations of 125 μg/metered dose/breath) are effective therapeutic regimens (31, 38), These medications can be repeated 3 times at 30-min intervals in young patients without heart disease. However, since both of these drugs have significant cardiac side effects, there is a trend to replace them with specific β_2 sympathomimetic agonists. *Isoetharine, metaproterenol,* and *albuterol* are available for aerosol administration and *terbutaline* and *fenoterol* will soon be released for aerosol administration (Table 52.8). Terbutaline is currently available for parenteral administration and is preferred to parenteral epinephrine because of its sustained action. However, repeat administration of parenteral terbutaline should be performed cautiously since this drug has a long duration of action (1 to 2 hours) and in high doses still produces unwanted cardiac side effects.

Theophylline Preparations. Numerous theophylline preparations are available for the treatment of reversible airways disease. The physician should become familiar with two of these compounds, choosing an inexpensive short acting agent (such as generic aminophylline) and a long acting preparation (such as Theo-Dur, Theovent, Somophyllin-CRT) (34). The toxic side effects of theophylline include stimulation of the central nervous system, nausea, vomiting, and inotropic and chronotropic cardiac actions. Toxic levels of these drugs cause grand mal seizures, cardiac arrhythmias, and even death (44). For the most part, gastrointestinal side effects are related to serum levels of theophylline and not to the direct effects of oral theophylline on the gut mucosa. Absorption from the gastrointestinal tract and metabolism of theophylline in the liver vary and may require adjustment of dosage in different individuals. The dose of theophylline should be reduced in patients with liver disease, congestive heart failure, or a history of seizures. Adolescents and heavy smokers often metabolize this drug more rapidly and may require increased doses. Ideally, peak plasma theophylline levels should be maintained between 10 and 20 μg per ml. At higher plasma levels, there is an increase in serious side effects, such as central nervous system irritability and cardiac tachyarrhythmias. In most ambulatory patients, the measurement of serum theophylline levels is usually not indicated, especially when there is a good therapeutic response and no evidence of side effects. However, in patients with altered theophylline clearance (liver or cardiac disease) or in those in whom high doses are required to achieve therapeutic effects, monitoring serum theophylline level is important. Blood should be sampled 1 to 2 hours after a drug dose to establish the peak serum level.

Initial therapy with oral aminophylline should start with 200 mg administered 3 or 4 times per day; however, some patients may require ultimately as much as 1200 to 1600 mg daily. The dose can be increased every 2 to 5 days while the patient is observed for therapeutic and toxic effects. The new, long acting theophylline preparations are very useful because patient compliance may be improved since they are only taken twice a day. Frequently, therapeutic levels are achieved with lower doses. Treatment with these preparations should begin with 200 mg twice a day and the dose should be increased by 100 mg increments every 2½ days. Many patients complain of nervousness, mild gastric distress, and headache when any of the theophylline preparations are started. These distressing side effects usually resolve during continued therapy (2 to 4 weeks).

Antiallergic Drugs. Cromolyn is a drug that does not act as a bronchodilator and, although its exact mechanism of action is unknown, it may stabilize mast cells preventing immunologic release of mediators (5) or improving nonspecific airways reactivity. It is administered as an inhaled dry powder, usually 3 to 4 times a day, which causes coughing and bronchospasm in some asthmatics. Because of these irritant properties, it is contraindicated in acute asthmatic attacks and it may be necessary to administer a nebulized sympathomimetic bronchodilator before cromolyn during routine use. However, a nebulized cromolyn solution without irritant properties will soon be commercially available.

Cromolyn is an effective prophylactic agent in some allergic and nonallergic asthmatic patients and is specifically useful in patients with significant exercise-induced asthma. Acute administration of one inhalation before exercise may prevent exercise-induced bronchospasm. It is usually used chronically in allergic asthmatics with known factors that specifically trigger asthma such as animal dander. Its effectiveness in patients with other forms of reversible obstructive airways disease is difficult to predict, but when effective, some severe asthmatics may be able to reduce systemic steroid requirements (see below). Some physicians are using cromolyn for the initial therapy of chronic allergic asthma. Initially it should be administered for a trial period of 2 to 4 weeks. Symptoms and objective pulmonary function tests (spirometry) should be used to assess its efficacy. Patients for whom cromolyn is prescribed should understand that its effect is to prevent but not to treat an asthma attack. This is important because many patients associate the use of inhaled medications with the symptomatic treatment of acute asthma.

Pretreatment with *antihistamines* does not prevent or reduce bronchospasm produced by inhaled specific antigen. Therefore, antihistamines should not be used to treat airways obstruction in allergic asthmatics. However, these drugs can be used to control allergic or vasomotor rhinitis (Chapter 22) in patients who also have asthma.

Anticholinergic Agents. One of the first forms of treatment for asthma was inhalation of anticholinergic agents. One rationale for the use of these drugs is that airway tone is maintained by the parasympathetic nervous system; inhaled anticholinergic agents block postganglionic efferent vagal neural control of airway tone and cause bronchodilation. Another reason is that anticholinergic agents also block reflex bronchospasm (see "Airways Hyperreactivity," p. 437). Use of these agents was abandoned until recently because of unwanted side effects such as drying of respiratory secretions, reduced bronchial mucociliary transport, blurred vision, urinary retention, and cardiac and central nervous system stimulation. Atropine is the most potent anticholinergic agent, but when inhaled some of it is absorbed systemically. Although atropine is frequently used to treat bronchospasm, it is not officially approved for use as a bronchodilator by the Federal Drug Administration. When atropine is used, a total dose of 1 to 2 mg (atropine sulfate parenteral solution) is inhaled from a hand nebulizer (DeVilbiss) every 4 to 8 hours. Some asthmatics as well as some patients with chronic obstructive bronchitis improve airways function with atropine treatment and it may be tried as an alternative to inhaled sympathomimetic agents (23). Recently, a new compound ipratropium (Sch 1000 or Atrovent), a quaternary ammonium compound, has become available for experimental use. It will soon be released commercially and is available at present from Boehringer-Ingelheim Ltd. for individual patients whose bronchospasm is improved only by inhaled atropine. Its major advantage is that it is not absorbed systemically during inhalation therapy (41). The exact role of these agents in the treatment of obstructive airways disease will be determined only after they are widely available.

Corticosteroids. Corticosteroids are effective agents for treating reversible obstructive airways disease, but their exact mechanism of action is unknown. They do cause bronchodilation, reduction in bronchial inflammation, and improve the response to β-sympathomimetic agents. The onset of their therapeutic effects is delayed and does not begin for 6 to 12 hours (29). Steroids may be administered as "burst" therapy for periods of 7 to 10 days in which high doses (40 to 80 mg of prednisone) are started and tapered rapidly (10 to 20 mg a day) over a 7- to 10-day period. "Burst" therapy is used to treat severe asthma attacks or acute severe exacerbations of bronchospasm in patients with reversible chronic obstructive lung disease. The major side effects from "burst" therapy are steroid-induced abnormalities in glucose metabolism. However, when corticosteroids are used to treat severe obstructive airways disease for *prolonged periods*, they may produce many other unwanted systemic side effects (Cushing's syndrome, adrenal pituitary supression, osteoporosis, etc). In addition, the patient's ability to deal normally with infectious processes is impaired. Since reactivation of tuberculosis can occur during chronic corticosteroid treatment, any patient with a positive PPD should receive simultaneous INH (isoniazid) prophylaxis. Acute adrenal insufficiency may occur during stressful medical or surgical illnesses (chapter 71). Whenever chronic steroid therapy is begun in an ambulatory setting, objective pulmonary function tests are required to evaluate its therapeutic effectiveness since some patients will feel better due to the euphoria produced by steroids, but have unchanged pulmonary function. The lowest effective dose should be employed and, if possible, alternate-day steroid therapy should be attempted. This should be done by decreasing the dose of prednisone by 5 mg every 2 to 3 days and measuring the FEV_1 periodically (weekly). When symptoms of bronchospasm worsen, the tapering process should be slowed. If bronchospasm improves after prolonged treatment, then further reduction or elimination of prednisone therapy may be possible. Aerosolized steroids (see below) or cromolyn may be useful to help reduce or even eliminate the need for systemic steroids in some patients.

Nonabsorbable corticosteroid aerosols (beclomethasone: Vanceril) are available. The technique for inhaler use described on page 444 should be reviewed with the patient who is beginning to use an aerosolized steroid. The use of these agents often permits a reduction or, if the patient is taking 20 mg of prednisone or less a day, even the elimination of oral steroid therapy. Treatment may also be initiated with these inhaled agents. Side effects from aerosolized steroid preparations are negligible, but include the development of oral candidiasis that is prevented by rinsing the mouth with water immediately after inhaling the steroids or treated by gargling with small doses of an antifungal agent (Nystatin). The usual dose of beclomethasone is 100 to 200 μg (2 breaths) inhaled 4 times a day. Whenever inhaled steroid therapy is started, the dose of oral steroids should be decreased slowly (5 to 10 mg weekly) in patients who have been treated with systemic corticosteroids for long periods of time. If patients being treated with beclomethasone have an acute exacerbation of asthma, treatment with oral prednisone should be reinstituted.

General Approach to Pharmacologic Therapy of Reversible Airways Disease

The purpose of this section is to integrate some of the principles of the pharmacologic treatment of bronchospasm that have been discussed separately under specific drug categories (43).

OCCASIONAL SYMPTOMATIC USE OF BRONCHODILATORS

During remission or in patients with very mild asthma (FEV$_1$ > 70% predicted), the occasional symptomatic use of aerosolized specific β_2-sympathomimetic agonists usually controls intermittent episodes of bronchospasm (Fig. 52.6). Alternatives to aerosol therapy are the use of theophylline derivatives or oral preparations of β_2-sympathomimetic agonists (metaproterenol, terbutaline). Such occasional use of bronchodilators can control intermittent episodes of bronchospasm and prevent bronchospasm from specific known stimuli (exercise, cold air, irritants). Also, cromolyn can be used intermittently to treat exercise-induced asthma.

CHRONIC BRONCHODILATOR THERAPY

There are two choices for initial continuous therapy in patient with reversible obstructive airways disease who cannot be managed with occasional intermittent bronchodilators. One choice is to treat these patients with aerosolized β_2-sympathomimetic agents. Ordinarily these drugs are effective and have fewer systemic side effects than theophylline preparations (31, 38). However, many physicians use theophylline as the drug of choice for chronic bronchodilator therapy. Those patients whose bronchospasm

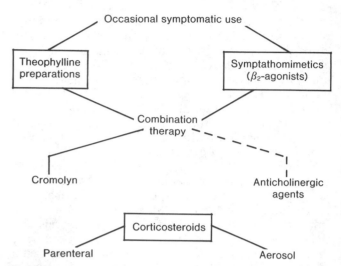

Figure 52.6 Approach to the pharmacologic treatment of reversible airways disease (see text).

is not controlled with a single bronchodilator require combination therapy. In these situations, oral theophylline preparations should be combined with inhaled specific β_2-sympathomimetics. There is experimental and clinical evidence suggesting that these agents have additive effects and combinations of these two classes of drugs produce greater bronchodilation than either drug does alone (45). Some patients will require both an oral theophylline and a sympathomimetic agent as well as aerosolized sympathomimetic agonists (see technique for use of inhalers on p. 444). The role of anticholinergic agents still needs to be determined. There are patients with chronic obstructive bronchitis who respond poorly to aerosolized β-sympathomimetics but show significant bronchodilation with inhaled atropine (23). Cromolyn provides effective prophylactic treatment for allergic and exercise-induced asthma. In allergic patients, this drug must be used continuously. Systemic corticosteroids should be reserved for status asthmaticus and for severe chronic asthma that does not respond to conventional therapy.

ACUTE ASTHMATIC ATTACKS

Less severe acute asthmatic attacks can be treated either with aerosolized β_2-sympathomimetics or oral theophylline preparations. If there are objective signs of severity (Tables 52.5 and 52.6), traditional regimens such as subcutaneous injections of epinephrine or inhaled isoproterenol are effective (38). More recently, systemic therapy with subcutaneous injections of terbutaline is being substituted for epinephrine. Also, the new selective β_2-sympathomimetic agents may be preferable to inhaled isoproterenol.

Depending on individual reliability, patients with reversible airways obstruction should be instructed what medications (usually a sympathomimetic aerosol or an oral theophylline compound) they can use for self-treatment before they must contact the physician (22). For example, an intelligent young adult asthmatic should know that he can use an inhaled β-sympathomimetic agonist more frequently (every 2 to 4 hours) and take an extra dose of aminophylline to self-treat a mild asthma attack. If he does not improve after a 4-hour period, then he should call his physician.

Other Specific Therapeutic Measures in Asthma

RESPIRATORY THERAPY

During acute asthmatic attacks, there is increased water loss from the respiratory tract and a tendency, especially in young children, to become dehydrated. Usually oral hydration is adequate. During the winter months when ambient room air is dry, a home humidifier will effectively increase the water content of the air. Care should be taken to clean these humidifiers to prevent the accumulation of molds or fungi. Rarely dehydration is so severe that parenteral or nebulized humidification becomes necessary. Both fine water particles and inhaled mucolytic substances from ultranebulizers irritate the airways and produce bronchospasm and coughing. Therefore, these forms of respiratory therapy should be avoided. Finally, there is no scientific basis for the use of intermittent positive pressure (IPPB) breathing ventilators either as a form of respiratory therapy or as a means of delivering bronchodilators (32).

OXYGEN

In rare cases when asthmatics with objective evidence of severe asthma (Tables 52.5 and 52.6) are treated in the physician's office, the administration of humidified oxygen may be indicated. If the patient does not improve, he should be sent to the Emergency Room. In the usual uncomplicated young asthmatic without chronic hypoventilation and CO_2 retention, there is little risk of causing respiratory failure by blunting the hypoxic ventilatory control. Only enough oxygen (28 to 35% venturi mask or 2 liters/min nasal cannula) should be administered to improve arterial PO_2 into a normal range (65 to 80 mm Hg).

Medical Complications of Reversible Airways Disease

There are a number of medical complications of asthma that may impair the patient's response to the usual therapeutic regimens (Table 52.9). In general, these complications should be sought if there is not an appropriate therapeutic response.

COMPLICATIONS OF PHARMACOLOGIC TREATMENT

In severe asthma, bronchodilators may cause a paradoxical fall in arterial oxygenation by altering the pulmonary homeostatic mechanisms that match ventilation and perfusion in the lungs. These falls in arterial oxygenation are small (5 to 10 mm Hg) and

Table 52.9
Medical Complications of Reversible Airways Disease

COMPLICATIONS OF BRONCHODILATORS
Paradoxical fall in arterial oxygenation
Paradoxical bronchospasm
Cardiac Arrhythmias
ATELECTASIS
PULMONARY INFECTIONS
Bronchitis
Pneumonia
AIR IN EXTRAPULMONARY SPACES
Penumothorax (tension)
Pneumomediastinum
ALLERGIC BRONCHOPULMONARY ASPERGILLOSIS

are easily treated with supplemental oxygen. Although this paradoxical hypoxemia is an indication for oxygen administration, it is not an indication to withdraw bronchodilator therapy.

Very rarely, the propellants used to aerosolize sympathomimetic and corticosteroid agents may provoke paradoxical bronchospasm. If an asthmatic complains of coughing and wheezing after using one of these aerosols, a different preparation should be employed.

Sympathomimetics and theophylline preparations stimulate cardiac activity and may cause arrhythmias, especially when used in therapeutic doses, in the presence of moderate hypoxemia or in elderly patients with pre-existing cardiac disease. However, arrhythmias can also be triggered by bronchospasm and hypoxemia during acute airways obstruction. In these situations, reversal of bronchospasm and improvement in gas exchange often improve the arrhythmias.

MECHANICAL AIRWAYS OBSTRUCTION

Mucus impaction in the airways may lead to microatelectasis or to the collapse of a pulmonary segment or of an entire lobe of the lung. Patients with major lobar collapse should be hospitalized. Frequently, the symptoms and physical signs of atelectasis are obscured during acute asthmatic attacks by wheezing and dyspnea. Therefore, atelectasis is best diagnosed with a chest roentgenogram (see Chapter 51). Usually, atelectasis will improve after treatment of bronchospasm, hydration and physical therapy (coughing, chest percussion, and postural drainage). Bronchoscopy to remove an obstructing mucus plug is rarely needed. In fact, in a patient with reactive airways disease and acute bronchospasm, it may even worsen bronchospasm and provide only temporary improvement of atelectasis.

INFECTION

While pulmonary infections often precipitate asthmatic attacks, bronchitis and pneumonia (see Chapter 27) frequently develop as a complication of asthma. Development of purulent sputum during the course of a prolonged or persistent asthmatic attack requires re-evaluation for superimposed infection, with a sputum smear and then appropriate antibiotic therapy.

EXTRAPULMONARY AIR

Rarely, air can accumulate abnormally in the extrapulmonary spaces. The presence of a pneumomediastinum is best detected by a chest roentgenogram, but it is frequently associated with subcutaneous air in the neck, thorax, and groin (palpable crepitus). Although no specific therapy is indicated, the patient should be hospitalized for careful observation because air may dissect into the pleural space. A pneumothorax can only be detected effectively by a chest roentgenogram and if a pneumothorax develops during an acute attack, regardless of its size, the patient should be hospitalized since the subsequent development of a tension pneumothorax can be life-threatening.

ALLERGIC BRONCHOPULMONARY ASPERGILLOSIS

Rarely, allergic bronchopulmonary aspergillosis complicates chronic asthma (39). These patients have airways obstruction that does not improve with usual therapeutic measures; they have febrile episodes associated with a cough productive of purulent sputum containing dark brown plugs, and a chest roentgenogram that shows focal bronchiectasis and mucus impaction. They often have pulmonary infiltrates that change location during serial roentgenographic studies. These patients usually have blood eosinophilia and serum precipitins as well as immediate and delayed skin reactions to aspergillus antigen. Early treatment with corticosteroids may improve bronchospasm and prevents progression to irreversible bronchiectasis. If this diagnosis is suspected, consultation with a pulmonologist or allergist is advisable.

Course and Prognosis of Asthma

The course and prognosis of pure bronchial asthma is not well understood. Traditionally, it is thought that uncomplicated asthma developing during childhood or early adult life is not a risk factor for progressive fixed obstructive pulmonary disease. However, there is also evidence that airways hyperreactivity and allergy are found more frequently in patients with severe obstructive pulmonary disease, so that these factors may be risks for the development of chronic airways obstruction. Further epidemiologic studies are necessary to define these relationships (4, 7, 21).

In general, when bronchial asthma begins at an early age, it usually improves, although the estimation of the rate of remission from childhood asthma varies in different studies from 30 to 70% (19). After a spontaneous remission, some childhood asthmatics will experience a recurrence of symptomatic asthma during adulthood. These latter patients, as well as patients with adult onset intrinsic asthma, often have asthma that is persistent and severe. Other patients who had a history of bronchial asthma during childhood, which seemed to resolve spontaneously, developed chronic progressive airways obstruction later in life. Additional risk factors such as chronic cigarette smoking and exposure to urban and industrial air pollution complicate their disease (see p. 451). Furthermore, it is unknown whether their history of bronchial asthma and associated airways hyperirritability are additional risk factors for the development of fixed obstructive lung disease.

Although death from asthma, or one of its complications, is rare, it does occur with a recorded incidence in the United States of 1 in 100,000 or approximately 2,000 deaths during the course of a year. Deaths in young asthmatics are usually preventable since they are caused by one of the medical or therapeutic complications that have been discussed. For example, in England in the early 1970s, increased mortality from bronchial asthma coincided with the marketing of high dose isoproterenol inhalers. It was postulated that these patients developed cardiovascular toxicity and arrhythmias from isoproterenol overdosage by the repeated use of these inhalers (11). Often acute respiratory failure and death in status asthmaticus are attributable to sedation of seemingly anxious patients whose respiratory drive is easily depressed because of their exhaustion. Asthmatics who manifest the objective signs of severe asthma (Tables 52.5 and 52.6) should receive rapid emergency treatment and should be hospitalized if they do not improve rapidly. Asthma can worsen as quickly as it can improve with appropriate therapy.

CHRONIC AIRWAYS OBSTRUCTION: CHRONIC OBSTRUCTIVE BRONCHITIS AND EMPHYSEMA

Patients with advanced chronic airways obstruction have a clinical course characterized by progressive loss of pulmonary function that eventually leads to respiratory failure and death. Usually management of these patients focuses upon the treatment of exacerbations of airways obstruction and pulmonary infection, basically providing palliative support for the complications of this disease. However, before the development of irreversible progressive airflow obstruction, there is a period when functional impairment and pathologic abnormalities are potentially reversible. Therefore, this discussion will emphasize not only the therapy of symptomatic obstructive lung disease, but also the identification of susceptible individuals at a time when the development of irreversible airways disease is preventable.

Chronic progressive airways obstruction is most commonly caused by chronic obstructive bronchitis and emphysema. Chronic bronchitis is defined in clinical terms but has certain pathologic correlates. In contrast, emphysema, a specific morphologic diagnosis, has associated clinical correlates, pulmonary function abnormalities, and characteristic roentgenographic patterns. In their pure forms, these two diseases represent distinct processes with different pathologic features and clinical manifestations. However, clinically they usually coexist (42).

It is very difficult to estimate the prevalence of chronic bronchitis and emphysema in the United States since there is often an insidious onset of respiratory symptoms and many patients are not diagnosed until relatively late. However, as much as 15 to 25% of the adult population has a history compatible with chronic bronchitis. How many of these have clinical airways obstruction is unknown. Autopsy series show that approximately 60% of adult men and 15% of adult women have evidence of emphysema.

Definitions
CHRONIC BRONCHITIS

Chronic bronchitis is defined as a clinical syndrome characterized by cough and sputum production that occurs on most days for at least a 3-month period during 2 consecutive years. Most often these symptoms are due to chronic bronchial irritation by agents such as cigarette smoke and air pollution which results in hyperplasia of goblet cells and mucus-secreting glands and in chronic mucus hypersecretion. By definition this excessive production of mucus is not due to specific diseases such as bronchiectasis, tuberculosis, or heart disease. Morphologic changes that correlate with the clinical diagnosis of chronic bronchitis are initially found in small airways (< 2 mm) and later progress to involve other parts of the tracheal bronchial tree (Fig. 52.3). The hypertrophied mucus glands occupy a greater proportion of the bronchial wall, which is inflamed, edematous, and eventually fibrotic. The lumina of peripheral airways are frequently filled with excess mucus (42).

Simple Chronic Bronchitis. A large proportion of patients who smoke develop chronic bronchitis. Most of these patients cough up a small quantity of mucoid sputum each morning. They either ignore this chronic cough or willingly accept it as a minor complication of cigarette smoking. Some of these patients will have intermittent episodes of purulent sputum production and occasional mild wheezing associated with upper respiratory tract infections. Many of these patients do not have a demonstrable impairment of expiratory airflow or an increased rate of decline in pulmonary function.

Chronic Obstructive Bronchitis. At the other end of the spectrum is a disease characterized by progressive air flow obstruction and chronic mucopurulent sputum production. The bronchi, normally sterile, are chronically infected. The factors that protect certain individuals and place others at risk for

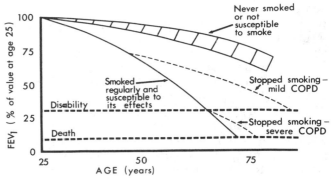

Figure 52.7 Effect of risk factors from smoking on the loss of lung function (FEV$_1$). The *upper curves* are derived from subjects who do not smoke or are not susceptible to the effects of smoking. They lose lung function gradually throughout adult life (15 to 30 ml/year). *Lower curves* show accelerated loss of lung function in subjects who are susceptible to the effects of cigarette smoke. At age 65 there is respiratory disability since FEV$_1$ has decreased to 25 to 30% of predicted (1 to 1.2 liters) and further functional deterioration will eventually cause death due to pneumonia, cor pulmonale, or respiratory insufficiency. If that subject stops smoking, life may be prolonged but a respiratory death will still eventually result. If intervention is initiated earlier in life (40 to 50 years) when there is mild COPD, accelerated loss of lung function is reversible and a respiratory death will be avoided. Although this figure illustrates theoretical loss of FEV$_1$ for an adult cigarette smoker, susceptible smokers will lose lung function at different rates thereby becoming disabled at different ages. (Modified from Fletcher and Peto (14).)

the development of air flow obstruction are not completely understood (see below). It is known that those who are susceptible to the effects of cigarette smoking and chronic bronchopulmonary infection have a progressive course, with accelerated loss of lung function that leads to pulmonary disability and eventual respiratory failure (Fig. 52.7).

EMPHYSEMA

Pulmonary emphysema is defined in anatomic terms and is a diagnosis that is made with certainty only by a pathologist. It is morphologically defined as permanent abnormal dilation and destruction of the alveolar ducts and air spaces distal to the terminal bronchioles. Each component of this definition is important. The enlargement must be permanent; therefore the temporary overdistension of the lung that occurs in asthma cannot be regarded as being emphysema. The enlargement must be abnormal; thus the changes that occur with normal aging cannot be considered to be true emphysema. Perhaps the most important concept is that there should be accompanying disruption of alveolar walls. Since the pathologic definition of emphysema is nonspecific, it is necessary to classify emphysema into anatomic subtypes. The most important, clinically, are centrilobular and panlobular emphysema (42).

Centrilobular Emphysema. This form is generally considered to represent the commonest type of emphysema. In centrilobular emphysema there is mainly destruction of the respiratory bronchioles and alveolar ducts which become confluent to form emphysematous spaces. Deposits of carbonaceous material are found in these areas. The distal alveolar sacs are often spared. The emphysematous lesions are located in the proximal acinar space at the center of the lobules between the conducting airways and the alveolar sacs. The major clinical association of centrilobular emphysema is chronic obstructive bronchitis due to cigarette smoking where pathologic abnormalities in the peripheral airways are the rule. Early disease with patchy pulmonary involvement does not cause roentgenographic abnormalities. But when it is far advanced, pathologic and roentgenographic examination shows that centrilobular emphysema is primarily located in the upper lung fields.

Panlobular Emphysema. This less common form of emphysema is characterized by uniform involvement of the pulmonary lobule with morphologic destruction of the distal structures and alveolar capillary membrane. Panlobular emphysema is less commonly associated with chronic bronchitis and cigarette smoking, tends to occur in the lower lung fields, is more frequently associated with the formation of cysts and bullae, and is found in patients with hereditary α_1-antitrypsin deficiency (see below) and with bronchiolar obliteration. Frequently the two major forms of emphysema occur in combination, with centrilobular emphysema in the upper lung zones and panlobular in the lower. However, pathologic distinction is difficult to make when severe disease exists.

Other forms of emphysema include paraseptal emphysema, which is associated with spontaneous pneumothorax, and irregular emphysema, which is found in patients with diffuse pulmonary fibrosis.

Etiology

There are many risk factors and proposed etiologies associated with the development of chronic obstructive airways disease. They are listed in order of relative importance in Table 52.10. Detailed knowledge of these factors is important in understanding those measures that may alter the progression and thus prevent the development of irreversible chronic airways obstruction.

AGE

The average nonsmoking adult shows a yearly decline of 15 to 30 ml in FEV_1 with increasing age. Thus an FEV_1 of 4 liters in a 25-year-old would be

Table 52.10
Risk Factors and Airways Obstruction (Approximate Order of Relative Importance)

AGE
INHALED IRRITANT AND NOXIOUS AGENTS
Smoking
Urban and industrial air pollution
HEREDITY
Familial incidence
α_1-Antitrypsin deficiency
SEX (MALE > FEMALE)
SOCIOECONOMIC STATUS
AIRWAYS HYPERREACTIVITY

expected to fall to almost 3 liters by age 65 (Fig. 52.7) (14). However, this normal loss of lung function is not associated with pulmonary disease. Additional risk factors add to the effects of this loss of pulmonary function and act synergistically to cause clinical airways obstruction (10, 21).

INHALED IRRITANT AND NOXIOUS AGENTS

The common factor that exists in the great majority of patients with chronic airways obstruction is exposure to inhaled irritant and noxious agents.

Cigarette Smoking. Cigarette smoke represents the most obvious and widespread pulmonary contaminant. Since 1940 when cigarette consumption in the United States increased to present high levels (10 lb of cigarettes per capita), there has been a progressive rise in the incidence and death rate from obstructive pulmonary disease and lung cancer. Various studies have shown that there is pathologic evidence of either chronic bronchitis or emphysema in patients with more than a 40-pack year history of smoking (defined as number of years smoking X packs of cigarettes per day). Furthermore, the risk of dying from chronic lung disease is from 3 to 14 times greater in smokers than in nonsmokers.

The deleterious effects of cigarette smoke may be specific or may be due to nonspecific effects of inhaled irritants on the tracheal bronchial tree. For example, stimulation of mucus secretion causes loss of normal mucociliary clearance mechanisms. Since infection often develops, inflammatory cells release proteolytic enzymes that may cause destruction of the pulmonary parenchyma by overwhelming the lungs' protective defences. Moreover, smoking also depresses the phagocytic function of the alveolar macrophage, increasing the tendency for respiratory infections (3).

Specifically, cigarette smoking seems to have a significant effect on loss of lung function and patients who smoke heavily decrease their FEV_1 by an average of 40 to 60 ml per year. A patient whose FEV_1 was 4 liters at age 25 would have an FEV_1 of 2 liters by the age of 65 (Fig. 52.7) (14). Unfortunately, some smokers lose lung function even more rapidly and approach a loss in FEV_1 of 60 to 80 ml per year. Nevertheless, patients who stop smoking appear to resume the normal 30 ml per year rate of decline within 1 year after the cessation of cigarette smoking. In some patients who continue to smoke, the rapid decline in lung function causes clinical obstructive pulmonary disease (Fig. 52.7) (10, 21).

Urban and Industrial Air Pollution. The effects of air pollution from exposure to urban or industrial environments on the development of chronic obstructive airways disease are unknown. Photochemical oxidant air pollutants include ozone and nitrogen dioxides which are formed by the effect of solar radiation on automobile and truck emissions. Low concentrations of sulfur dioxide and other particulate matter from the burning of fossil fuels are also present in an urban environment where there are also trace amounts of miscellaneous substances (arsenic, asbestos, cadmium, hydrogen sulfide, lead, and mercury). Periods of atmospheric inversions with increased environmental levels of air pollutants have been associated with exacerbations and even death in patients with cardiopulmonary disease. The sequelae of high exposures to these agents are airway inflammation, pulmonary parenchymal damage, and obstructive pulmonary disease. Furthermore, recent studies of low level exposures to all three of these agents demonstrate that they cause transient airways hyperreactivity in normal subjects and an exacerbation of respiratory symptoms in asthmatics (6). Therefore, it is probable that air pollution and cigarette smoking act synergistically to trigger symptomatic exacerbations and pulmonary function abnormalities in patients with chronic obstructive pulmonary disease. However, it is not known to what extent exposure to low levels of urban and industrial air pollutants contributes to the etiology and progression of pulmonary disease.

HEREDITY

Familial Incidence. First degree relatives of patients with chronic obstructive airways disease have abnormal lung function and an increased rate of decline of their FEV_1. This relationship holds even when other risk factors such as smoking are controlled. The relationship of this finding to the well-known familial aggregation of asthma, allergy, and airways hyperreactivity is poorly understood (see below) (21).

α_1-*Antitrypsin Deficiency.* While diseases such as cystic fibrosis are obvious inherited causes of obstructive lung disease that begin in childhood, α_1-antitrypsin deficiency is a rare genetic abnormality that causes liver disease in children and panlobular emphysema in adults. α_1-Antitrypsin deficiency should be suspected when emphysema develops without a history of chronic bronchitis or smoking in patients below the age of 45 or when multiple family members develop obstructive lung disease at an early age. Serum antiproteolytic activity is determined by

the Pi (inhibitor) phenotype. Normal individuals have two M genes and are considered MM phenotypes, whereas patients with α_1-antitrypsin deficiency have two Z genes or a ZZ phenotype. Homozygous α_1-antitrypsin deficiency is found in only 1 in 4000 people, but at least 60% of ZZ phenotypes will develop severe emphysema during adulthood. It is postulated that a deficiency of α_1-antitrypsin activity makes the lung vulnerable to damage by the endogenous proteolytic enzymes released by inflammatory cells. Inheritance is codominant so that the heterozygote, MZ, as well as several other mixed genotypes have intermediate levels of circulating antitrypsin. Recent evidence suggests that partial deficiency may also be a risk for the development of obstructive lung disease when other factors such as smoking are present. The diagnosis of this condition is discussed below (p. 454).

SEX

Male sex seems to be an important predisposing factor for the development of obstructive airways disease. Even in nonsmoking young males, there is still accelerated loss of lung function compared to nonsmoking premenopausal females. After menopause, women appear to have a more rapid decline in FEV_1 than similarly age-matched male controls (10, 21). In addition, the acute and chronic physiologic effects of cigarette smoking are different in men. In young men, cigarette smoking causes changes in peripheral airways function, while similar changes are not produced by cigarettes in premenopausal women. This is especially interesting since the earliest pathologic abnormalities of chronic bronchitis are in the peripheral airways. The reasons for these sex differences are unknown, but they may relate either to the protective effects of female sex hormones or to the deleterious effects of androgens.

SOCIOECONOMIC STATUS

People from lower socioeconomic groups seem to decrease FEV_1 at a faster rate than those from higher economic groups. While the risk factor is still found after controlling the effects of smoking, sex, and age, it may well relate to increased exposure of the respiratory tract to airborne pollutants in urban environments or to industrial exposures to noxious agents (10).

AIRWAYS HYPERREACTIVITY

Recent studies of first degree relatives of patients with obstructive lung disease show that those with hyperirritable airways lose lung function at accelerated rates (7). Also, patients with significant chronic airways obstruction who are hyperreactive to inhaled agents (methacholine) decrease their FEV_1 more rapidly (4). It is not known whether this airways hyperirritability develops as a consequence of obstructive lung disease or is a risk factor *per se*. Allergy may serve as a link between airways hyperirritability and hereditary factors since allergic factors are inherited, associated with hyperreactivity, and have been found with increased frequency in patients with far advanced obstructive lung diseases (21).

Clinical Presentation

HISTORY

Usually, patients with emphysema present with dyspnea and those with chronic obstructive bronchitis, with cough and sputum production. These two diseases are so interrelated that most patients have manifestations of both. It is useful, however, to recognize the characteristic features of these syndromes. These are summarized in Table 52.11. Although these clinical types represent extremes of a clinical spectrum, occasional patients are seen who qualify as having relatively pure emphysema (Type A) or bronchitis (Type B).

The usual patient with chronic airways obstruction has a long history of a chronic cough with mucopurulent sputum production. The onset of dyspnea is insidious but progressive. Frequently, these patients attribute their poor exercise tolerance to the effects of age or sedentary life-style and their chronic cough to the effects of smoking. Often they develop clinically apparent airflow obstruction (wheezing) during upper respiratory tract infections and the recovery period from these respiratory infections is prolonged. Eventually, dyspnea becomes so severe that it interferes with routine activities and medical attention is sought. In other patients, a respiratory tract infection triggers acute respiratory failure. Milder forms of obstructive airway diseases are often diagnosed as incidental findings during a routine physical exami-

Table 52.11
Clinical Findings in Emphysematous and Bronchitic Varieties of Chronic Airways Obstruction

Findings	Type A (Emphysema)	Type B (Bronchitis)
CLINICAL PRESENTATION:		
Dyspnea	Early onset, severe progressive	Insidious, onset, intermittent during infection
Cough	Onset after dyspnea	Precedes onset of dyspnea
Sputum	Scant and mucoid	Copious and purulent
Respiratory infection	Rare	Frequent
Body weight	Thin, weight loss	Normal or overweight
Respiratory insufficiency	Late manifestation	Frequent episodes
PHYSICAL EXAMINATION:		
Cyanosis	Absent	Often present
Plethora	Present	Absent
Chest percussion	Hyperresonant	Normal
Chest auscultation	Distant breath sounds, end expiratory wheezing	Rales, rhonchi, wheezes
Cor pulmonale	Often terminal	Common
LABORATORY EVALUATION:		
Hematocrit value	Normal	Occasional erythrocytosis
Chest roentgenogram	Hyperinflation with increased anteroposterior diameter and flat diaphragms. Attenuated vascular markings, bullous changes, small vertical heart	Increased bronchovascular markings with normal to enlarged heart and evidence of old inflammatory disease
PHYSIOLOGIC EVALUATION:		
Spirometry	Irreversible expiratory obstruction, airway closure	Expiratory obstruction, reversible component
Total lung capacity and residual volume	Marked increase	Mild increase
Lung elastic recoil	Marked reduction	Near normal
Diffusion capacity	Marked decrease	Normal or slight reduction
PaO_2		
Rest	Slightly decreased (65–75 mm Hg)	Marked decrease (45–65 mm Hg)
Exercise	Often falls	Variable (decrease to increase)
$PaCO_2$	Normal or low (35–40 mm Hg)	Normal or elevated (40–60 mm Hg)
Pulmonary hypertension	None to mild, worsens during exercise	Moderate to severe variable exercise response
PATHOLOGY	Widespread emphysema, may be panlobular	Chronic bronchitis with or without mild centrilobular emphysema

nation, a preoperative evaluation, or a medical evaluation for an unrelated disease. Occasionally, patients with chronic airways obstruction (emphysematous type) will be seen because of progressive weight loss that may initially suggest the presence of an occult malignancy.

When the diagnosis of advanced obstructive airways is well established, its course is relentlessly progressive. In patients with bronchitis, daily cough and sputum production usually increase, becoming more purulent and tenacious during infectious exacerbations. Some patients have difficulty clearing respiratory secretions during attacks of airflow obstruction. In these patients, the production of scant, viscous, purulent sputum may precede the development of respiratory failure. Wheezing and dyspnea are often persistent features of severe disease. Chronic hypoxemia causes cor pulmonale and the patient will note peripheral edema and weight gain. Some patients will experience asthmatic episodes that periodically worsen their baseline airways obstruction. Usually, these are associated with respiratory infections, but they may be triggered by any of the stimuli that precipitate an acute asthmatic attack.

PHYSICAL EXAMINATION

In individual patients, physical findings depend on the severity and type of chronic obstructive airways disease (Table 52.11). Vital signs may be normal or show tachypnea and a pulsus paradoxus (see p. 440) during severe bronchospasm. In milder forms of obstructive lung disease (FEV$_1$ > 1.2 liters), auscultation of the chest may be unremarkable or may reveal either rhonchi due to mucus within the airways or wheezing if bronchospasm is prominent. Breath sounds may be distant in patients with severe emphysema. Frequently, the diagnosis of airways obstruction is best made during the physical examination by performing a timed forced vital capacity. After inflating the lung to total capacity, the patient should perform a complete maximal expiration through an open mouth. This maneuver usually produces audible wheezing in patients with chronic obstructive airways disease while in patients with severe emphysema whose airways collapse, faint wheezing may be all that is heard. In everyone with significant expiratory airflow obstruction, the timed forced vital capacity will be prolonged beyond 4 to 5 sec. Many other respiratory findings occur with progressively severe disease and primarily reflect pulmonary hyperinflation. These include an increased anteroposterior diameter of the chest, widened intercostal spaces, hyperresonance, a decreased area of cardiac dullness, and low diaphragms. The same signs of severity found in patients with asthma, such as use of accessory muscles of respiration, occur in chronic airways obstruction during acute attacks of bronchospasm (Tables 52.5 and 52.6).

When cor pulmonale develops there is often cyanosis, a right ventricular heave, a holosystolic murmur along the left sternal border, an S$_3$ gallop, and varying degrees of hepatomegaly and peripheral edema. Neck veins will be distended and a large V wave with a Y descent is visible as pulmonary hypertension worsens, causing tricuspid valve dilation and insufficiency.

LABORATORY TESTING

Pulmonary Function Testing. The most characteristic functional defect in patients with chronic obstructive bronchitis and emphysema is decreased forced expiratory flow. This obstructive defect is best measured with a spirogram, which should be employed in the diagnosis and assessment of severity in chronic obstructive airways disease as well as for the evaluation of specific therapeutic regimens (see p. 434 for the patient experience during this procedure). It is also useful in predicting the prognosis, course, operative risk (see Chapter 83), and work potential (Table 52.1) (9, 12). In general, it is unusual for patients with an FEV$_1$ of 2 liters, or 50% of predicted, to experience significant dyspnea during normal physical activities. On the other hand, reduction of the FEV$_1$ below 1.2 liters is associated with dyspnea on mild exertion and significant disability. The severity of hyperinflation will be reflected by a reduction in vital capacity as well as by increases in lung volumes (46). Residual volume is usually elevated and, in emphysematous patients, total lung capacity is increased. When emphysema is present, the diffusion capacity of the lung is reduced, reflecting the loss of functional alveolar capillary membrane available for gas exchange. The presence of significant airways obstruction, hyperinflation, and a reduced diffusion capacity for carbon monoxide correlates with the pathologic finding of emphysema (Fig. 52.8) (17, 42).

Arterial Blood Gas Analysis. In evaluating and treating patients with significant chronic obstructive airways disease (FEV$_1$ < 1.2 liters), baseline arterial blood gas analysis is necessary to measure the level of oxygenation and adequacy of alveolar ventilation. When the FEV$_1$ is greater than 1.2 liters, resting arterial blood gases are usually relatively normal or show only mild hypoxemia. With more severe airways obstruction (FEV$_1$ <1.0 liter), the degree of hypoxemia and hypercapnea will depend on the ventilation perfusion abnormalities and pulmonary homeostatic mechanisms. Since hypoxemia correlates only roughly with the severity of airways obstruction as reflected by spirometry, arterial blood gases must be measured to evaluate the degree of resting hypoxemia in order to guide the treatment of cor pulmonale (see below). In addition to hypoxemia, it is important to know whether the patient has a chronically elevated arterial PaCO$_2$ indicating alveolar hypoventilation. The diagnosis of acute respiratory failure in patients with severe obstructive lung disease is usually made by finding either an acute fall in arterial oxygenation (absolute PaO$_2$ < 50 mm Hg) and/or an acute increase in PaCO$_2$ tension of more than 10 mm

Hg with associated acute respiratory acidosis. Such acute changes usually require hospitalization and intensive treatment.

Other Laboratory Tests. Normally, the mucopurulent sputum produced by patients with chronic obstructive bronchitis is infected with a mixed bacterial flora including *Streptococcus pneumoniae* and *Haemophilus influenzae.* Other pathogens may be present, depending on the frequency and type of broad spectrum antibiotic treatment. Sputum culture is usually indicated only when there is parenchymal pulmonary infection (pneumonia) and specific treatment will depend on the predominant organism seen on Gram stain and cultured from the sputum. A complete blood count will document erythrocytosis, which indicates significant hypoxemia, and eosinophilia, which may suggest allergic or asthmatic etiologies. A white blood count and differential count are helpful in the evaluation of pulmonary infection. An electrocardiogram may show arrhythmias, atrial hypertrophy (P pulmonale), and evidence of pulmonary hypertension (persistent S waves in the lateral precordial leads).

Patients who develop emphysema at an early age (45 or younger) without a history of cigarette smoking or chronic bronchitis, give a familial history of emphysema, or have roentgenographic evidence of panlobular emphysema should be screened with serum protein electrophoresis during symptom-free periods. If the α_1-peak is absent, then an α_1-antitrypsin level should be measured (available from a commercial laboratory). α_1-Antitrypsin is an acute phase reactant and should not be measured during periods of infection. If both the α_1-peak and antitrypsin level are low, then genetic phenotyping should be obtained if possible. This is important (21) for prognosis and genetic counseling. However, phenotyping is only done in a few medical centers in this country.

ROENTGENOGRAPHIC FINDINGS

As many as 50% of patients with significant chronic airways obstruction will have normal or near normal chest roentgenograms. In the others, there will be a variety of findings which are relatively nonspecific. Despite this, a chest roentgenographic examination is important both in the diagnosis and in the overall management of patients with airways obstruction. Specifically it is useful to exclude other associated pulmonary diseases such as pneumonia, atelectasis, or a pneumothorax.

Bronchitis. In patients with chronic obstructive bronchitis, there may be increased tubular markings, especially at the lung bases, that suggest thickening and disease of the bronchi. These patients may have increased vascular markings, evidence of pulmonary hypertension and right heart enlargement, but their roentgenograms usually do not show marked hyperinflation or cystic or bullous changes.

Emphysema. The diagnosis of emphysema can of-

ten be made from a chest roentgenogram when severe morphologic changes in the lung result in obvious roentgenographic findings (Fig. 52.8). In milder cases of emphysema, it is difficult to make a specific diagnosis. Many of the findings that are associated with emphysema only reflect hyperinflation which occurs in asthma or during a bronchospastic exacerbation in chronic obstructive bronchitis. The changes characteristic of hyperinflation include an increased radiolucency of the lungs, an increase in the anteroposterior diameter of the thorax, an enlarged retrosternal air space, and a low and flat diaphragm which makes a greater than 90° angle with the sternum on the lateral views (Fig. 52.8). Changes in vascular markings in the lung fields are often subtle and difficult to detect, especially when there is congestion of the pulmonary veins or parenchymal infection. Regional or generalized loss of vascularity in the peripheral lung fields with rapid tapering of the proximal branches of the pulmonary artery occurs more frequently in panlobular emphysema, especially in the lower lung fields. Centrilobular disease tends to show increased bronchovascular markings, especially in the lung bases. The pulmonary parenchyma needs to be examined carefully for the presence of cysts or bullae, although frequently these structures cannot be distinguished from the hyperlucent lung fields. Occasionally, an upper lobe bullus will be mistaken for a pneumothorax and a chest tube will be inserted inappropriately. Therefore, it is necessary to obtain a good quality baseline chest roentgenogram of every patient with moderate to severe obstructive airways disease. Although not indicated in the routine diagnosis of bullous disease, both chest tomography and computerized axial tomography (CT) scanning of the lung will visualize cystic spaces in the pulmonary parenchyma.

Cardiac Evaluation. The heart frequently appears small and is located in a vertical position. In the diagnosis of ventricular failure, the usual radiologic criteria for cardiac enlargement are not valid. Often one must look for subtle findings of a change in cardiac size by reviewing serial chest roentgenograms. More recently, new noninvasive diagnostic tests which include biplane echocardiography and gated heart pool scanning have become available to evaluate the function of both the left and the right ventricles (See Chapter 57).

MANAGEMENT OF THE AMBULATORY PATIENT

General Measures

The primary goal in managing the ambulatory patient with obstructive airways disease is to prevent progression of the disease. When the progression of irreversible airflow obstruction cannot be slowed, therapeutic goals include improving symptoms and decreasing pulmonary disability by treating the re-

A

	Actual	Predicted	% Predicted	Post BD[a]	Post/Pre BD[a]
SPIROMETRY					
FVC	2.32 liters (L)	3.99 L	58	2.50	107
FEV_1	0.98 L	3.17 L	30	1.15	117
FEV_1/FVC %	42	79.4		46	
LUNG VOLUMES					
(He dilution)					
TLC	7.82 L	6.29 L	124		
VC	2.86 L	3.99 L	71.7		
FRC	5.64 L	3.72 L	152		
RV	4.96 L	2.30 L	215		
DIFFUSING CAPACITY					
(single breath)					
DLCO[c] ml	11.6	24.4	47.5		
ARTERIAL BLOOD GASSES[b]					
PaO_2	56 mm Hg				
$PaCO_2$	48 mm Hg				
PH units	7.38				

[a] Bronchodilator.
[b] At rest, sitting, breathing room air.
[c] Diffusion capacity for carbon monoxide.

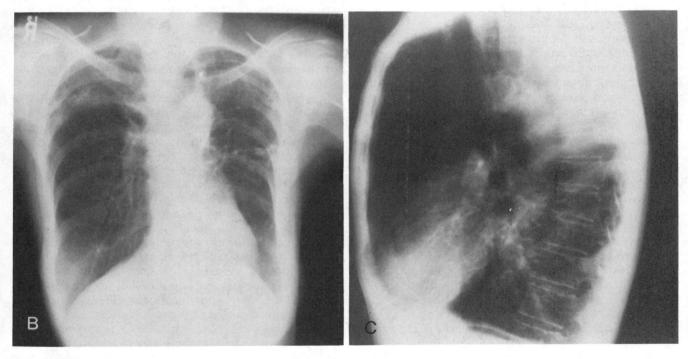

Figure 52.8   (*A*) Typical pulmonary function test results in a patient (male, 60 years old, 161 lb, 69 inches tall) with severe chronic obstructive pulmonary disease and probable emphysema. Forced expiration demonstrates a severe obstructive ventilatory defect with an immediate response to aerosolized bronchodilators. Spirograms do not reach a plateau, indicating slowly emptying areas of lungs. Lung volumes show an elevated total lung capacity (TLC) and residual volume (RV) indicating hyperinflation consistent with obstruction, suggesting early airway closure. Single breath CO diffusion capacity is reduced, indicating loss of effective alveolar capillary surface area for gas exchange. Reduced diffusion capacity and airway obstruction are consistent with the presence of emphysema. Arterial blood gases show an elevated carbon dioxide tension indicating hypoventilation, a mild compensated respiratory acidosis, and low oxygen tension with desaturation. This patient with chronic airflow obstruction is hyperinflated, has a reduced diffusion capacity suggesting emphysema and has hypoxemia associated with chronic CO_2 retention. His chest roentgenogram (*B* and *C*) is compatible with emphysema and shows hyperinflation and bullous changes with loss of vascular lung markings (see text).

versible components of bronchospasm, heart failure, and infection. It is clear that prevention and prompt treatment of exacerbations in chronic airways obstruction will improve the quality and duration of life.

The successful management of this chronic disease requires a comprehensive approach either by the physician or by a medical team that includes a therapist, vocational counselor, and visiting respiratory nurse clinicians as well as active participation by the physician. Studies have shown that patients consider their physician to be very influential. Whatever preventive and therapeutic measures are selected, they will be more effective if the physician actively coordinates and supports them. For example, it seems that physicians advise their patients to stop smoking only when there are findings consistent with overt lung disease such as objective evidence of abnormal chest roentgenograms, pulmonary function tests, or evidence of respiratory infection. Furthermore, in smoking cessation programs only 25% of participants said their physician actively participated and on further questioning most indicated that their physician would have been influential in affecting the outcome of the program (see Chapter 19).

If possible, the nurse, respiratory therapist, and physician should work together as a team, instructing the patient and his spouse. Ideally, general instruction should include information about pulmonary anatomy and physiology as well as basic information about the etiology and prognosis of chronic airways obstruction. This instruction can be given in individual as well as in group sessions and should be supplemented with visual aids and booklets which are published by the American Thoracic Society and available for distribution through the local (state) and national lung associations.

Even if therapeutic interventions do not markedly improve respiratory function, appropriate adaptation of a patient's life-style and recreational activities are worthwhile. For example, while exercise programs do not improve pulmonary function, they physically condition sedentary patients, making them able to participate in a wider range of activities (see below). In patients with severe disease resulting in curtailment of their usual recreational activities, counseling on alternative hobbies and activities may help prevent depression and maintain useful family interactions. Although sexual dysfunction is extremely common in these patients, this important aspect is rarely discussed with the physician. Sexual activity is often made easier by the use of supplemental oxygen or pretreatment with a bronchodilator. Alternatives include making the nondyspneic person the more active partner or the use of different positions (see Petty in "General References"). If the patient's disease precludes ambulation, then follow-up patient care is often best performed by home visits. The respiratory nurse clinician with the aid of the pa-

tient's spouse can facilitate this type of care. When the disease becomes terminal, the nurse and the physician can counsel the patient and his family about the possibility of dying at home (See Chapter 18). The physician should allay the patient's fears of suffocation and struggling since death is often peaceful, with the patient eventually dying in a coma secondary to CO_2 retention. Furthermore, one needs to discuss with the patient and his family whether resuscitative attempts such as intubation and prolonged mechanical ventilation in an Intensive Care Unit are appropriate and desirable. During this period, support from the physician, family, and clergy is vital. The patient may often be made comfortable with therapeutic modalities that include fluids, oxygen (see below), and sedation, if necessary.

Preventive Management

The *early diagnosis* of very mild peripheral airways disease is made with sophisticated pulmonary function testing that is not generally available. Furthermore, it is questionable whether physicians can motivate patients with subclinical asymptomatic disease to modify their life-style. However, there is a period when mild to moderate airways obstruction is easily diagnosed using a spirogram (Fig. 52.1) and modification of the patient's habits and treatment with bronchodilators, if indicated, may prevent the development of irreversible obstructive lung disease (Fig. 52.7). The routine screening with spirometry of patients at risk (greater than 35 years of age who have a significant smoking history or chronic bronchitis) will identify many patients with significant obstructive lung disease. For example, in our laboratory, approximately 35% of healthy Baltimore firemen between the ages of 25 and 45 who had screening spirometry as part of a physical examination exhibited at least mild degrees of airways obstruction. Prevention of the development of irreversible airways obstruction may well depend on behavior modification in such patients. Smoking cessation and the avoidance of industrial irritants will be better accepted by the patient when he knows the results of objective testing and the prognostic significance of these abnormalities. It is probable that the course of obstructive lung disease can be favorably altered by a systematic program (smoking cessation and bronchodilator therapy) in patients under 50 years of age with an FEV_1 more than 2 liters (21).

Important to any preventive regimen is complete *cessation of cigarette smoking*. This is especially true in any patient with homozygous PiZZ (α_1-antitrypsin deficiency). There are many smoking cessation programs and regimens that have been used with varying success rates. In evaluating the results of these programs, objective methods to assess their efficacy must be used (blood carboxyhemoglobin levels, sputum thiocyanate levels). Furthermore, the follow-up period must be long enough to judge that their effectiveness was not transient. At present, objective evaluation of these programs shows that only approximately 15 to 20% of subjects are able to abstain from smoking for 1 year. Strategies and methods for the physician to utilize in programs for smoking cessation are discussed in Chapter 19.

While *pulmonary infections* cannot be specifically linked to the progression of obstructive airways disease, the effective treatment of bacterial exacerbations is important since acute respiratory failure can be precipitated if exacerbations are not promptly treated. Furthermore, vaccination with anti-influenza and antipneumococcal vaccines may be useful in preventing pneumonia which can be devastating in patients with severe obstructive lung disease (see Chapter 30).

Reduction of Secretions

REMOVAL OF SECRETIONS

In patients with chronic airways obstruction and mucus hypersecretion, therapeutic interventions are aimed at the reduction and removal of respiratory secretions. Pulmonary secretions are normally cleared from the lung by mucociliary clearance and coughing. In obstructive airways disease, both of these mechanisms are impaired (see Chapter 50, section on cough). Often coughing is not effective because of airway collapse during forced expiration. Postural drainage and chest percussion can remove mucus secretions from the airways and these measures should be used by the ambulatory patient whenever there is persistent hypersecretion. Patient instruction in postural drainage and chest percussion can be obtained by referral to a Respiratory Therapy Department or the physician can learn these principles by referring to the literature such as given in "General References", (Respiratory Therapy). In addition, the mobilization of secretions is aided by pretreatment with two breaths of an aerosolized bronchodilator (β_2-sympathomimetic, see p. 443). Often the best times for this type of respiratory therapy are before retiring at night and after arising in the morning. Thus the patient may be able to sleep more restfully and also may be aided in clearing secretions that have accumulated during the night. If significant pulmonary hypersecretion is not present, these measures are not indicated (15).

AVOIDANCE OF IRRITANTS

Respiratory secretions will be stimulated both directly and reflexly by inhaled irritants. Furthermore, these substances cause bronchospasm which prevents mobilization of secretions. Therefore, smoking, urban and industrial pollutants, and other irritating inhaled substances must be avoided. This includes avoiding "passive smoking" by inhaling ambient air that is contaminated with tobacco smoke since this has been shown to increase airways obstruction in asthmatics.

ALTERATION OF SPUTUM CHARACTER

It has never been effectively proven that oral hydration will thin respiratory secretions and improve pulmonary function in obstructive lung disease (see "General References" (Conference on Scientific Basis of Respiratory Therapy)). Nevertheless, most physicians still recommend that patients without significant heart failure should drink approximately 1 liter of fluid daily.

Mucolytic agents are irritating substances that cause direct and reflex bronchospasm. Furthermore, liquefication of bronchial secretions in patients who are unable to mobilize them adequately with effective coughing may be deleterious.

Even if bronchial secretions are thick and viscous, treatment with a bland aerosol (normal saline) has not been shown to be effective. For example, patients with cystic fibrosis with thick bronchial secretions do not show improvement in clinical status after bland aerosol treatment (37).

TREATMENT OF INFECTION

Most patients with chronic bronchitis have a course that is characterized by intermittent infection with mucopurulent sputum. Treatment of these acute infectious exacerbations with a broad spectrum antibiotic that is active against *S. pneumoniae*, *H. influenzae*, and other common pathogens is indicated. Usually, a 7 to 10-day course of either ampicillin, tetracycline, or sulfamethoxazole is administered. In intelligent cooperative patients, antibiotic therapy may be initiated by the patient when he notes a change in sputum character or color. In general, continuous antibiotic therapy should be avoided unless there is evidence of persistent chronic infection or bronchiectasis.

Physical Therapy and Rehabilitation

INTERMITTENT POSITIVE PRESSURE BREATHING (IPPB)

Historically, IPPB machines have been used for both physical therapy and the delivery of bronchodilators. However, there is no scientific basis for the use of IPPB machines. In fact, IPPB may induce transient pulmonary overdistension that is harmful in these patients who are already hyperinflated (15, 32). IPPB may be useful in the delivery of medications to patients who are so severely obstructed that they are unable to take a deep breath from a freon-powered metered dose inhaler or hand bulb nebulizer (DeVilbiss). This circumstance is rare in ambulatory practice. Many patients who already have IPPB machines at home are so psychologically dependent on this form of physical therapy that the physician may decide that the use of such a machine should be continued. The administration of oxygen through any IPPB machine is contraindicated, because the oxygen mixture setting which supposedly delivers 40% oxygen usually administers much higher concentrations.

BREATHING EXERCISES

There is scientific evidence that pursed lip breathing may help an emphysematous patient maintain airways stability during expiration (see Petty, "General References"). Diaphragmatic exercises may give the patient a sense of well-being and may improve diaphragmatic muscle function. These breathing exercises are usually taught by a respiratory therapist. Specific details about them are available in the medical literature (15).

EXERCISE REHABILITATION

Exercise retraining programs do not improve pulmonary function, but they do seem to improve exercise tolerance and skeletal muscle function. Probably this is due to the nonspecific effects of training in sedentary poorly conditioned patients. Furthermore, after exercise training the patient may be able to perform a given level of exercise at a lower oxygen consumption and a lower minute ventilation. Community-based exercise training programs are more frequently available for cardiac rehabilitation (see Chapter 55). Occasionally, these may be adapted to the needs of patients with chronic obstructive pulmonary disease. If no organized programs are available, the physician should consider instructing his patients in an informal program of graded increases in physical activity (see (15) and "General References").

CHANGE IN ENVIRONMENT

In selected circumstances environmental change may be important therapeutically. Some patients seem to improve when they move from cold winter climates to either warm humid or warm dry climates. There is no evidence that the course of obstructive lung disease is altered by such environmental changes. Perhaps some of these patients improve by escaping from urban industrialized areas with air pollution. When such a move is contemplated, its social and economic effects must be carefully weighed by the patient and his family. Environmental changes are more important in patients with hypoxemia who live at high altitudes above 4000 feet where ambient oxygen is less than 120 mm Hg compared to 150 mm Hg at sea level. A move to a low altitude usually improves hypoxemia and decreases pulmonary hypertension. Since the adverse psychologic consequences of such a move may outweigh its medical benefits, those patients may do just as well remaining at high altitude by using treatment with low-flow oxygen (see below). Travel in an airplane or vacationing in high altitude areas may be contraindicated in patients with severe hypoxemia. Since airplane cabins are maintained at pressure equivalent to 5000 to 8000 feet, low-flow supplemental oxygen should be administered throughout flight to patients with arterial PaO_2 under 55. Also, vacations in high altitude locations (above 4000 feet) should be avoided in patients with severe chronic hypoxemia (PaO_2 less than 55 mm of Hg).

Treatment of Bronchospasm

Initial and maintenance therapy of bronchospasm is outlined in detail in the discussion of asthma in this chapter. In patients with chronic reversible airways disease, the principles of pharmacologic treatment are similar to those used in asthma; however, the response of patients to bronchodilators is usually not as marked. Some patients (Fig. 52.8) increase their FEV_1 only by 10 or 15% but the response of only a few hundred milliliters may provide significant improvement in exercise tolerance. A poor response to inhaled bronchodilators during laboratory testing does not preclude improvement after chronic therapy with pharmacologic agents. Such patients should have a repeat assessment of their lung function after a period of 1 to 2 months. If there is still no response to high doses of bronchodilators, patients with severe bronchospasm ($FEV_1 < 1.2$ liters) should be given a therapeutic trial with corticosteroids (see below). When there is no objective or symptomatic improvement, bronchodilators may be discontinued, although some physicians recommend continued maintenance therapy to prevent bronchospastic exacerbations. There is some evidence that patients who do not respond to inhaled β-sympathomimetic agonists may improve airways function with inhaled anticholinergic agents (see p. 445) (23). Very rarely, patients with a history of allergy or childhood asthma may improve with cromolyn (5).

If exercise tolerance is severely impaired by dyspnea, or if there is a poor or absent response to standard bronchodilators, a trial with *corticosteroids* is indicated (see p. 445). A favorable response to steroids occurs more frequently in patients with reversible airways disease when there is blood or sputum eosinophilia or when there is a previous history of allergy or asthma. Usually, a trial of systemic steroids such as prednisone (40 mg per day) is maintained for 3 to 6 weeks. Before, during, and after therapy, objective evaluation of lung function with spirometry is mandatory. Usually, systemic steroids are used in these trials because they are more effective than aerosolized preparations. If there is improvement, the steroid dose should be reduced while the patient is monitored with serial spirometry. Aerosolized corticosteroid agents can be used to supplement standard bronchodilators, can be used with systemic steroid therapy, or can even be substituted if the effective dose of oral prednisone is less than 20 mg per day. Prednisone doses less than 5 mg per day are not therapeutic and should be discontinued or aerosolized steroid agents should be substituted.

Treatment of Heart Failure

COR PULMONALE

In severe chronic airways obstruction ($FEV_1 < 1.0$ liter) pulmonary hypertension and cor pulmonale (Table 52.12) are caused by chronic hypoxemia ($PaO_2 < 50$ mm Hg). This severe hypoxemia also causes erythrocytosis, renal function abnormalities, impaired cognitive function, emotional instability, and dyspnea at rest and during exercise. Chronic low-flow oxygen therapy is indicated when severe oxygen desaturation persists despite appropriate treatment (Table 52.13) (15, 33). Other supplementary measures include the use of diuretics, salt restriction, and phlebotomy when the hematocrit value exceeds 60. When oxygen therapy is effective, erythrocytosis and peripheral edema usually improve. Since chronic therapy with oxygen is costly (approximately $3000 to $4000 per year for 2 liters of O_2 for 24 hours), it should be used judiciously. Furthermore, when high concentrations of oxygen are administered to severely hypoxemic patients with elevated levels of arterial $PaCO_2$, there may be depression of the respiratory drive, causing acute hypercapneic respiratory failure. Only enough oxygen to raise the resting arterial PaO_2 above 60 to 65 mm Hg is required.

The source of oxygen will be determined by the duration of daily therapy, the flow of oxygen required, and the mobility of the individual patient. For example, oxygen from a large compressed air tank or from an oxygen generator can be delivered to a sedentary patient who does not leave home. If tanks are used, one can be placed in the bedroom and the other in the area of the living quarters where the patient spends most of the day. The use of a costly portable oxygen apparatus is not indicated for a sedentary patient. On the other hand, a patient with exercise-induced hypoxemia who wants to continue to remain active may require a portable oxygen apparatus. Oxygen may be administered through a nasal cannula or through a Venturi mask. While the mask will deliver a complete range of specific oxygen concentrations (24 to 35%), nasal cannulas are usually preferred because they can be used during meals and do not interfere with coughing. A 1-liter flow rate through a nasal cannula delivers approximately 24 to

Table 52.12
Treatment of Heart Failure

COR PULMONALE
Oxygen
Salt restriction, diuretics, KCl
Phlebotomy
PULMONARY VASCULAR CONGESTION (LEFT VENTRICULAR FAILURE)
Salt restriction, diuretics, KCl
Digitalis (?) (increased sensitivity to digitalis in cor pulmonale)

Table 52.13
Low-Flow Oxygen Therapy in Obstructive Airways Disease

INDICATIONS
Pulmonary hypertension and cor pulmonale
Erythrocytosis
Neuropsychologic status
Exercise intolerance
COMPLICATIONS
Cost
Respiratory depression
METHODS OF DELIVERY
Source of oxygen (compressed air tank, O_2 generator, portable O_2 source)
Nasal cannula/Venturi mask
DURATION OF THERAPY
Intermittent—low-flow oxygen when resting $PaO_2 > 50$ mm Hg with:
Exercise-induced dyspnea and hypoxia; relieved by oxygen. Documentation by exercise testing
Nocturnal dyspnea restlessness, or insomnia: documented and relieved by oxygen
Continuous—$PaO_2 < 50$ mm Hg after treatment
Cor pulmonale and congestive heart failure
Diminished cognitive function
Persistent erythrocytosis

26% inspired oxygen concentrations while a 2-liter flow rate delivers approximately 28 to 30%.

The duration of oxygen therapy must be individualized for each patient. If the resting arterial PaO_2 is between 50 and 55 mm Hg, intermittent oxygen therapy should be considered for exercise-induced dyspnea or during nocturnal periods when there is evidence of restlessness or insomnia. In these situations, the effect of exercise (see Chapter 50, the section on dyspnea) or sleep (see Chapter 82, "Sleep Disorders") on arterial oxygenation must be documented. One cannot predict whether these moderate degrees of resting hypoxemia will worsen, stay the same, or improve during exercise. The clinical implications of arterial oxygen desaturation during sleep are not fully understood. Many patients with obstructive lung disease and moderate hypoxemia ($PaO_2 < 50$ to 60 mm Hg) have worse hypoxemia during sleep. If these changes are documented, low-flow oxygen should be employed to prevent the development of cor pulmonale. Continuous therapy with low-flow oxygen is indicated when the arterial PaO_2 is less than 50 mm Hg. In these situations, oxygen administration for at least 12 to 15 hours a day improves cognitive function and reverses pulmonary hypertension (15). Usually erythrocytosis will improve and repeated phlebotomies are not necessary.

LEFT HEART FAILURE

The diagnosis of left ventricular failure in patients with severe chronic obstructive lung disease is often difficult. Noninvasive cardiac testing may help to diagnose the presence of left ventricular dysfunction (see laboratory evaluation above). The treatment of left heart failure should begin with diuretics and salt restriction. Frequently slight pulmonary vascular congestion is sufficient to cause respiratory decompensation in these patients. The role of digitalis is very controversial and it should be used as a last resort (see Chapter 57). Many patients with endstage cor pulmonale have cardiac arrhythmias, especially multifocal atrial tachycardia, which are worsened by digitalis. Therefore, throughout the course of digitalis treatment, careful evaluation for toxic side effects is necessary.

Course and Prognosis of Chronic Airways Obstruction

It has been emphasized that lung function deteriorates with advancing age and risk factors, especially cigarette smoking, accelerate this loss of pulmonary function (Fig. 52.7) (14). Some subjects are more susceptible to these risk factors and lose lung function more rapidly. When the FEV_1 falls below 50% of predicted, its decline seems to be accelerated and unless progression is prevented, irreversible obstructive lung disease results. Pulmonary disability occurs when the FEV_1 is between 1 and 1.6 liters or about 25% of predicted (see Chapter 3).

Once obstructive airways disease is established, there is a tendency for the disease to worsen. In a general way, the prognosis of patients with airways obstruction can be estimated from their FEV_1 (9, 12). In moderate obstructive airways disease when the FEV_1 is more than 1.25 liters, the 5-year survival is similar to that determined by the patient's age and sex. If the FEV_1 remains above 1.25 liters, these patients continue to have near normal expected survival (9, 12). If there is evidence of cardiac disease, resting tachycardia, or if the FEV_1 is between 0.75 and 1.25 liters, 5-year survival decreases to approximately 66% of normal. This figure is further reduced to 33% if the FEV_1 is less than 0.75 liter or there is evidence of cardiac disease, tachycardia at rest, hypercapnea, or a very low pulmonary diffusion capacity for carbon monoxide (emphysema). There are obvious exceptions to these general estimates of prognosis (35) since the short and long term response to bronchodilator therapy may alter the progression of airways obstruction. However, it is very useful for the physician to have a general understanding of the prognosis of different levels of airways obstruction based on objective measurement of pulmonary function.

The progressive course of obstructive pulmonary disease should not justify withholding treatment from these patients. There is little doubt that symptoms as well as the quality of life can be markedly improved and life can be prolonged. Figure 52.9 illustrates the response to treatment and subsequent loss of pulmonary function in two patients with severe

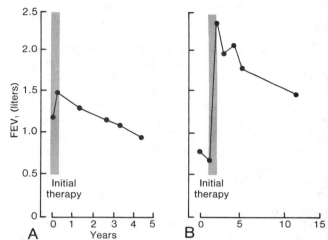

Figure 52.9 Response to treatment and subsequent loss of pulmonary function in two patients with severe chronic airways obstruction. (*A*) In this patient, initial therapy increased FEV_1 by 300 ml. However, from this improved FEV_1, there is still progressive deterioration of pulmonary function leading to an eventual respiratory death. (*B*) This patient was lost to follow-up for 1 year and FEV_1 deteriorated during this period. He had a better therapeutic response with marked improvement in pulmonary function. Although there was still progressive loss of lung function, from the new baseline FEV_1, respiratory disability was prevented during the 15-year follow up period. (modified from B. Burrows: *Lung Biology in Health and Disease*, *Vol. 9*, T. L. Petty (Ed.), Marcel Dekker, Inc., New York, 1978.

obstructive airways disease. In patient A, initial therapy increased FEV_1 (300 ml) but after this response, lung function deteriorated progressively leading to eventual respiratory failure and death. The second patient was lost to follow-up for 1 year and his FEV_1 deteriorated during this period. However, with therapy, there was marked improvement in pulmonary function. Although after treatment there was still progressive loss of lung function, respiratory disability was prevented during a 15-year follow-up period.

Expiratory airflow obstruction seems to be the major cause of disability and increased mortality in patients with chronic obstructive bronchitis and emphysema. There is considerable evidence that early changes in lung function can be detected and diagnosed with a spirogram (Fig. 52.1B). Serial measurements, perhaps at yearly intervals, in subjects who are at high risk for the development of chronic obstructive lung disease (cigarette smoking, chronic bronchitis, α_1-antrypsin deficiency, air pollution, etc.) would objectively demonstrate an abnormal rate of deterioration and provide the physician with essential diagnostic information. The effectiveness of preventive treatment of early obstructive lung disease would obviously depend on the physician's ability to modify those factors that are important in the etiology of airways disease in an individual patient. Therefore, a screening spirogram with measurements of FEV_1, FEV_3, and FVC is an important initial step in preventing the development of progressive irreversible airways obstruction.

General References

Normal and Abnormal Physiology

Murray, JF: *The Normal Lung.* W. B. Saunders, Philadelphia, 1976.
   This very readable text book provides a more extensive discussion of pulmonary mechanics, circulatory physiology, and acid-base balance.

West, JB: *Respiratory Physiology: The Essentials.* Williams & Wilkins, Baltimore, 1974.

West, JB: *Pulmonary Pathophysiology: The Essentials.* The Williams & Wilkins Company/Baltimore 1977.
   These two concise handbooks are excellent reviews of the essentials of pulmonary physiology and pathophysiology.

General textbooks of pulmonary disease

Fishman, AP: *Pulmonary Diseases and Disorders.* McGraw-Hill, New York, 1980.

Hinshaw, HC and Murray JF: *Diseases of the Chest.* W. B. Saunders, Philadelphia, 1980.
   These two general textbooks of pulmonary disease provide excellent extensive discussion of obstructive pulmonary disease.

Asthma

Patterson, R (Chairman) and Sogn, DD (Executive Secretary) (eds.): *Asthma and the Other Allergic Diseases—NIAID Task Force Report.* NIH Publication No. 79-387, May 1979.
   This extensive task force report by the National Institute of Allergy and Infectious Diseases provides an extensive discussion of asthma and allergic diseases. It is available for purchase from the Government Printing Office.

Weiss, EB and Segal, MS (eds.): *Bronchial Asthma: Mechanisms and Therapeutics.* Little, Brown, Boston, 1976
   Comprehensive multiauthored review of all aspects of bronchial asthma.

Chronic Obstructive Airways Disease

Hugh-Jones, P and Whimster, W: The etiology and management of disabling emphysema. *Am Rev Respir Dis* 117: 343, 1978.
   State-of-the-art review about the etiology and management of emphysema.

Petty, TL (ed.): Chronic obstructive pulmonary disease. In *Lung Biology in Health and Disease, Vol. 9.* Marcel Dekker, New York, 1978.
   This textbook is a comprehensive multiauthored review of all aspects of the diagnosis and the management (including respiratory therapy) of obstructive pulmonary diseases.

Epidemiology and Course of Chronic Obstructive Airway Disease

Macklem, PT and Permutt, S: The lung in the transition between health and disease. In *Lung Biology in Health and Disease, Vol. 12.* Marcel Dekker, New York, 1979.
   Extensive theoretical and practical multiauthored review of the epidemiology, etiology, and course of chronic obstructive lung disease.

Task Force Report: *Epidemiology and Respiratory Diseases.* NIH Publication No. 81-2019 October 1980.
   National Institute of Health publication that reviews the epidemiology and etiology of chronic respiratory diseases.

Respiratory Therapy and Pharmacologic Treatment

Lertzman, MM and Cherniack, RM: Rehabilitation of patients with chronic obstructive pulmonary disease. In *Lung Disease—State of the Art 1976–1977*, pp. 399–419. American Lung Association, 1978.
   State-of-the-art review discussing respiratory therapy and rehabilitation.

Proceedings of the Conference on the Scientific Basis of Respiratory Therapy, Temple University Conference Center at Sugarloaf. Philadelphia, May 2–4, 1974. *Am Rev Respir Dis* 110: 193, 1974.
   Excellent critical review of the scientific basis of oxygen, aerosol, physical, and IPPB therapy.

Shapiro, BA, Harrison, RA and Trout, CA: *Clinical Application of Respiratory Care*, Ed. 2. Year Book Medical Publishers, Chicago, 1979.
   Textbook with discussion of specific modes of respiratory therapy.

Ziment, I.: *Respiratory Pharmacology and Therapeutics.* W. B. Saunders, Philadelphia, 1978.
   Extensive review of pharmacologic treatment of obstructive lung diseases.

Specific References

1. ATS Statement: Snowbird Workshop on Standardization of Spirometry. American Thoracic Society, Medical Section of the American Lung Association. *Am Rev Respir Dis* 119: 831, 1979.
2. Austen, KF and Orange, RP: Bronchial asthma: the possible role of the chemical mediators of immediate hypersensitivity in the pathogenesis of subacute chronic disease. *Am Rev Respir Dis* 122: 423, 1975.
3. Ayres, SM: Cigarette Smoking and Lung Diseases: An Update. Basics of RD. Vol. 3, No. 5. American Thoracic Society, 1975.
4. Barter, CE and Campbell, AH: Relationship of constitutional factors and cigarette smoking to decrease in 1-second forced expiratory volume. *Am Rev Respir Dis* 113: 305, 1976.
5. Bernstein, IL, Johnson, CL and Ted, CS: Therapy with cromolyn sodium. *Ann Intern Med* 89: 228, 1978.
6. Boushey, HA, Holtzman, MJ, Sheller, JR and Nadel, JA: Bronchial hyperreactivity. *Am Rev Respir Dis* 121: 389, 1980.
7. Britt, EV, Cohen, B, Menkes, H, Bleecker, E, Permutt, S, Rosenthal, R and Norman, P: Airways reactivity and functional deterioration in relatives of COPD patients. *Chest* 77: 260, 1980.
8. Brooks, SM: Bronchial asthma of occupational origin. A review. *Scan J Work Environ Health* 3: 53, 1977.
9. Burrows, B and Earle, RH: Course and prognosis of chronic obstructive lung disease: a prospective study of 200 patients. *N Engl J Med* 280: 396, 1969.
10. Cohen, BH, Menkes, HA, Bias, WB, Chase, GA, Diamond, EL, Graves, CG, Levy, DA, Meyer, MB, Permutt, S and Tockman, MS: Multiple factors in airways obstruction. *Chest* 77: 257, 1980.
11. Conolly, ME, George CF, Davies, DS and Dollery, CT: Acquired resistance to beta stimulants: a possible explanation for the rise in the asthma death rate in Britain. *Chest* 63: 16, 1973.
12. Diener, CF and Burrows, B: Further observations on the course and prognosis of chronic obstructive lung disease. *Am Rev Respir Dis* 111: 719, 1975.
13. Epstein, RL: Constituents of sputum: a simple method. *Ann Intern Med* 77: 259, 1972.
14. Fletcher, C and Peto, R: The natural history of chronic airflow obstruction. *Br Med J* 1: 1645, 1977.
15. Fox, MJ and Snider, GL: Respiratory therapy: current practice in ambulatory patients with chronic airflow obstruction. *JAMA* 241: 937, 1979.
16. Gardner, RM, Hankinson, JL and West, BJ: Evaluating commercially available spirometers. *Am Rev Respir Dis* 121: 73, 1980.
17. Gelb, AF, Gold, WM, Wright, RR, Bruch, HR and Nadel JA: Physiologic diagnosis of subclinical emphysema. *Am Rev Respir Dis* 107: 50, 1973.
18. Hyatt, RE and Black, LF: The flow-volume curve: a current perspective. *Am Rev Respir Dis* 107: 191, 1973.
19. Johnstone, DE: A study of the natural history of bronchial asthma in children. *Am J Dis Child* 115: 212, 1968.

20. Lichtenstein, LM: An evaluation of the role of immunotherapy in asthma. *Am Rev Respir Dis* 117: 191, 1978.
21. Macklem, PT and Permutt, S: *The Lung in the Transition between Health and Disease.* Marcel Dekker, New York, 1979.
22. Maiman, LA, Green, LW, Gibson, G and MacKenzie, EJ: Education for self-treatment by adult asthmatics. *JAMA 241:* 1919, 1979.
23. Marini, JJ and Lakshminarayan, S: The effect of atropine inhalation in "irreversible" chronic bronchitis. *Chest 77:* 591, 1980.
24. Maccia, CA, Bernstein, IL, Emmett, EA and Brooks, SM: In vitro demonstration of specific IgE in phthalic anhydride hypersensitivity. *Am Rev Respir Dis 113:* 701, 1976.
25. McFadden, ER and Lyons, HA: Arterial-blood gas tension in asthma. *N Engl J Med 278:* 1027, 1968.
26. McFadden, ER, Luparello, T, Lyons, HA and Bleecker, ER: The mechanism of action of suggestion in the induction of acute asthma attacks. *Psychosom Med 31:* 134, 1969.
27. McFadden, ER, Kiser, R and DeGroot, WJ: Acute bronchial asthma: relations between clinical and physiologic manifestations. *N Engl J Med 288:* 221, 1973.
28. McFadden, ER: Exertional dyspnea and cough as preludes to acute attacks of bronchial asthma. *N Engl J Med 292:* 555, 1975.
29. McFadden, ER, Kiser, R, deGroot, WJ, Holmes, B, Kiker, R and Viser G: A controlled study of the effects of single doses of hydrocortisone on the resolution of acute attacks of asthma. *Am J Med 60:* 52, 1976.
30. McFadden, ER and Ingram, RH: Exercise-induced asthma. Observations on the initiating stimulus. Seminars in Medicine of the Beth Israel Hospital, Boston. *N Engl J Med 301:* 763, 1979.
31. McFadden, ER: Aerosolized bronchodilators and steroids in the treatment of airway obstruction in adults. *Am Rev Respir Dis 122:* 89, 1980.
32. Murray, JF: Review of the state of the art in intermittent positive pressure breathing therapy. *Am Rev Respir Dis 110:* 193, 1974.
33. Nocturnal Oxygen Therapy Trial Group: Continuous or nocturnal oxygen therapy in hypoxemic chronic obstructive lung disease. A clinical trial. *Ann Intern Med 93:* 391, 1980.
34. Piafsky, KM and Ogilvie, RI: Dosage of theophylline in bronchial asthma. *N Engl J Med 292:* 1218, 1975.
35. Postma, DS, Burema J, Gimeno, F, May, JF, Smit, JM, Steenhius, EJ, Weele, LTVD and Sluiter, HJ: Prognosis in severe chronic obstructive pulmonary disease. *Am Rev Respir Dis 119:* 357, 1979.
36. Rebuck, AS and Read, J: Assessment and management of severe asthma. *Am J Med 51:* 788, 1971.
37. Rosenbluth, M and Chernick, V: Influence of mist tent therapy on sputum viscosity and water content in cystic fibrosis. *Arch Dis Child 49:* 606, 1974.
38. Rossing, TH, Fanta, CH, Goldstein, DH, Snapper, JR and McFadden, ER: Emergency therapy of asthma: comparison of the acute effects of parenteral and inhaled sympathomimetics and infused aminophylline. *Am Rev Respir Dis 122:* 365, 1980.
39. Safirstein, BH, D'Souza, MF, Simon, G, Tai, EH-C and Pepys, J: Five-year follow-up of allergic bronchopulmonary aspergillosis. *Am Rev Respir Dis 108:* 450, 1973.
40. Samter, M and Beers, RF: Intolerance to aspirin. *Ann Intern Med 68:* 975, 1968.
41. Storms, WW, Dopico, GA and Reed, CE: Aerosol Sch 1000: An anticholinergic bronchodilator. *Am Rev Respir Dis 111:* 419, 1975.
42. Thurlbeck, WM: Aspects of chronic airflow obstruction. *Chest 72:* 341, 1977.
43. Webb-Johnson, DC and Andrews, JL: Bronchodilator therapy (two parts). *N Engl J Med 297:* 476, 1977.
44. Weinberger, M, Hendeles, L. and Bighley, L: The relation of product formulation to absorption of oral theophylline. *N Engl J Med 299:* 852, 1978.
45. Wolfe, JD, Tashkin, P, Calvarese, B and Simmons, M: Bronchodilator effects of terbutaline and aminophylline alone and in combination in asthmatic patients. *N Engl J Med 298:* 363, 1978.
46. Woolcock, A and Read, J: Lung volumes in exacerbations of asthma. *Am J Med 41:* 259, 1966.

CHAPTER FIFTY-THREE

Lung Cancer

PHILIP L. SMITH, M.D., and EUGENE R. BLEECKER, M.D.

EPIDEMIOLOGY

Lung cancer represents one of the most common malignant diseases facing Americans, especially with the increase in the elderly population and the increase in environmental pollutants. The death rate of this disease now approaches 117,000 per year in the United States with even higher rates elsewhere in the world (6). Although there is a predominant male to female ratio, recent statistics demonstrate a distinct rise in the incidence of lung cancer in women commensurate with their increased consumption of cigarettes (Fig. 53.1).

Cigarette smoking (see Chapter 19) still remains the

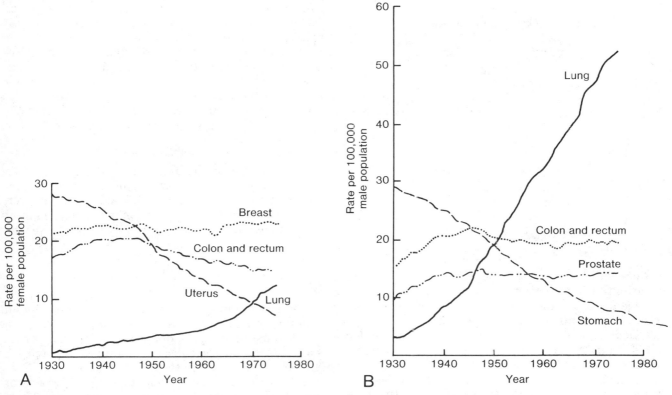

Figure 53.1 Age-adjusted cancer death rates from the four most common primary sources in United States women (*A*) and men (*B*), 1930 to 1975. Lung cancer in women will be the most common cause of death from malignancy by the 1990s if the present rate continues (Data from the U.S. National Center for Health Statistics and the U.S. Bureau of the Census. Adapted from H. C. Hinshaw and J. F. Murray: *Diseases of the Chest*, W. B. Saunders, Philadelphia, 1980.)

most important cause of lung cancer. The risk of developing cancer increases proportionately with the amount of smoking as is reflected by (a) the number of cigarettes smoked, (b) the number of years smoking, (c) the degree of inhalation, and (d) the "tar" and nicotine content of cigarettes smoked. Smoking of filter cigarettes or cigarettes with lower amounts of tar reduces lung cancer mortality rates, but these rates are still significantly higher than those of nonsmokers (16). In addition, exposure to various carcinogens such as asbestos, radioactivity, and the pollutants in the urban environment have led to an increased incidence of bronchogenic and pleural tumors (mesothelioma). Furthermore, smoking in combination with substances such as asbestos appears to act synergistically, probably due to the chronic effects of multiple irritants on the bronchial epithelium (7).

Although lung cancer has been classified into different cell types (Table 53.1), squamous cell cancer has offered the best opportunity to study the evolution of the disease. In both animals and humans the initial change is basal cell hyperplasia, followed by a change in cell shape which leads to cells that become atypical in appearance and, eventually, ends in localized cancer cells (carcinoma *in situ*). If the irrita-

tion stops at any point, it is postulated that these cellular changes may either arrest or revert to a normal state if the basement membrane has not been involved. This hypothesis is supported clinically by both a decrease in the death rate and in the amount of carcinoma *in situ* seen in exsmokers (2, 8).

SCREENING PROGRAMS

Since lung cancer is presumed to originate as described above and to take years before it advances to a clinically detectable stage, it would seem plausible that screening programs could detect nascent cancer. Since 1950 there have been several clinical trials designed to evaluate the early detection of lung cancer by sputum cytology and chest roentgenology (6), but none of these studies has shown a statistically significant reduction in the overall mortality from the disease. On the other hand, there is early evidence from more recent unpublished studies that annual screening with chest roentgenology and sputum cytology improves detection of lung cancer, increases the chances that the tumor can be resected, and increases 5-year survival of high risk patients (men who are heavy smokers and over age 45). Therefore, at present, it seems reasonable to screen with an annual chest roentgenogram and sputum cytology

Table 53.1
Histologic Classification of Lung Cancer

Class	Percentage of Cases
I. Squamous cell (epidermoid) carcinoma	30–35
II. Adenocarcinoma	30–35
III. Small cell anaplastic carcinoma (oat-cell carcinoma)	20
IV. Large cell undifferentiated carcinoma	15

only high risk patients who are concerned about the risk of developing lung cancer.

DIAGNOSTIC PROCESS

Symptoms

Most clinicians will evaluate patients for lung cancer after they have become symptomatic and/or have roentgenographic evidence of carcinoma. The most common presenting symptom is cough, followed by dyspnea, hemoptysis, and chest pain (see Chapter 50) (3). Hemoptysis is more commonly seen in patients with carcinomas that arise centrally in large airways and that either erode through the bronchus or become friable and bleed. Hemoptysis associated with a negative chest roentgenogram will occur in approximately 10 to 15% of patients with lung cancer (19). Dyspnea usually occurs when there is a large mass, associated pneumonia, or pleural effusion. Pain is most frequent when there is extension of the tumor beyond the lung parenchyma either into the adjacent mediastinum or thorax. In general, patients who are symptomatic at presentation have a poorer prognosis, and those who present with pain have the worst prognosis. Nevertheless, patients who are symptomatic for a longer time before their clinical presentation have a better prognosis than those who present with rapid onset of local and systemic symptoms, regardless of tumor type (5). Pain from a superior sulcus tumor (Pancoast tumor) unfortunately is often misdiagnosed as arthritis, and as a result, the patient may complain of shoulder pain for months before the correct diagnosis is made. Tumors that have metastasized outside the lung parenchyma can present with a multitude of symptoms depending on the organ involved. For example, the *superior vena cava syndrome* (facial swelling, distention of the veins of the neck, conjunctival injection, headache, convulsions) is occasionally seen in patients with tumors that involve the venous drainage to the right heart; or a *Horner's syndrome* (miosis, ptosis, enophthalmos, and reduced sweating) is seen in patients with tumors that invade the sympathetic nerve chain. Dysphagia, bone pain, or seizures may be seen when there is involvement of the esophagus, skeleton, or nervous system, respectively.

As opposed to these common clinical manifestations approximately 1 to 5% of patients with lung cancer present with various paraneoplastic signs or syndromes (Table 53.2). In general, neurologic manifestations are seen in more advanced lung cancer while connective tissue manifestations, such as hypertrophic osteoarthropathy, may antedate the diagnosis of tumor by as much as 2 years. Virtually any tumor may be associated with extrapulmonary symptomatology, although small cell and squamous carcinoma are most commonly responsible.

Physical Examination

The physical examination of the lungs is often unrevealing in patients with lung cancer unless obstruction of a major bronchus has occurred. However, the general physical examination may detect signs of extrapulmonary metastasis or of a paraneoplastic syndrome.

Laboratory

CHEST ROENTGENOGRAM

The laboratory diagnosis of cancer begins with an examination of the chest roentgenogram. While a roentgenogram does not diagnose the lesion, it serves as a focal point for subsequent procedures and for the sequence in which they will be performed. Centrally located lesions associated with atelectasis or pneumonia are most commonly squamous cell carcinomas. Adenocarcinomas and large cell carcinomas tend to arise as peripheral nodules and, therefore, are not associated with atelectasis or pneumonia. On the other hand, small cell tumors most commonly present with hilar adenopathy, often with no primary tumor visible on roentgenogram. Squamous cell carcinoma is the most frequently cavitating tumor, but even with this tumor, cavitation is uncommon. Cavitation represents either tumor necrosis that usually occurs in lesions larger than 2 cm or infection that develops into a lung abscess distal to the tumor. The solitary pulmonary nodule is discussed in detail below (pp. 466–468).

Approximately 15% of patients with lung cancer

Table 53.2
Paraneoplastic Syndromes

NEUROMUSCULAR SYNDROMES
  Encephalopathy
  Myelopathy
  Neuropathy—sensory, sensory motor
  Myopathy—myasthenia, Eaton-Lambert
CONNECTIVE TISSUE
  Hypertrophic pulmonary osteoarthropathy
  Scleroderma
ENDOCRINE-METABOLIC
  Cushing's syndrome
  Carcinoid syndrome
  Inappropriate antidiuretic hormone (ADH) syndrome
VASCULAR/HEMATOLOGIC
  Thrombophlebitis
  Purpura/Anemia

will present with a negative chest roentgenogram (19). This will occur predominantly in patients with hemoptysis from squamous cell carcinoma that arises proximally but is obscured by mediastinal tissues. Therefore, patients with their first episode of hemoptysis and a negative chest roentgenogram should be referred to a chest physician for further evaluation and possible bronchoscopy (see Chapter 50).

CYTOLOGY

The diagnosis of symptomatic lung cancer is made in approximately 80% of patients from the cytology submitted from spontaneously expectorated sputum or from bronchoscopy. Squamous cell tumors shed cells early into the airways and will have positive cytologies approximately 80% of the time whereas adenocarcinoma presenting as a peripheral lesion will have positive cytologies less than half the time. Peripheral lesions less than 2 cm in diameter will have positive sputum cytology infrequently. Screening sputum cytologies should be done before hospital admission. However, the completion of the diagnostic evaluation during hospitalization should not be delayed in situations where sputum cytologic examination is not readily available. In general, spontaneously expectorated sputum is the material most often submitted for cytologic exam. Patients should be instructed to produce a deep sputum sample by inhaling to total lung capacity in order to produce a forceful cough. Three to five early morning specimens should be collected in a tight fitting container, and if they cannot be submitted daily to the laboratory within 2 to 3 hours of collection, a fixative should be added so the specimens can be pooled and submitted together. Saccomanno's, containing 50% alcohol and approximately 7% carbowax, is one of the best fixatives; it can be prepared by the laboratory (11) and stored by the physician. More than five samples does not increase the incidence of a positive diagnosis of cancer. If the patient is not producing sputum, sputum induction by the inhalation of an aerosolized solution of saline can be helpful. The patient inhales, for 15 to 30 min, normal saline or a balanced salt solution (Hanks BSS) that is aerosolized by an ultrasonic nebulizer (DeVilbiss 3583). In general, sputum induction is not a routine office procedure and should be done by experienced personnel. In addition to the sputum collected immediately after induction, there is good material produced on the following morning. The addition of chest vibration or percussion does not improve the yield from sputum cytology. In cases where there is obstruction of the bronchus as evidenced by the physical examination or chest roentgenogram, it is reasonable to start collecting sputum after therapy, including antibiotics and perhaps bronchodilators, which may re-establish airway patency and allow sputum to be produced.

BRONCHOSCOPY

Bronchoscopy will generally be necessary either to diagnose patients suspected of having cancer or to determine resectability in those patients with positive sputum. Patients deemed inoperable may not need bronchoscopy. The fiberoptic bronchoscope has greatly aided in the diagnosis of lung cancer since smaller lesions can now be approached even though the lesion may not be visualized through the bronchoscope. Those lesions seen at bronchoscopy yield a diagnosis by biopsy or brushing in greater than 90% of cases. Fluoroscopy will be necessary to guide the biopsy forceps and brush in those cancers presenting as peripheral nodules beyond the vision of the bronchoscope. Depending on the experience of the operator and the size and location of the tumor, a positive diagnosis will be made on 30 to 70% of peripheral lesions. Tumors located near the apex of the lung or near the pleura most often do not yield a positive diagnosis, and these lesions are better approached by needle biopsy.

Patient Experience. In order to reduce patient expense, bronchoscopy may be performed on an ambulatory basis by a pulmonologist or a thoracic surgeon. The patient is told that he will have to fast (including liquids) 12 hours prior to bronchoscopy and that he will not be able to eat for approximately 4 hours after its completion when topical anesthesia wears off. The only discomfort the patient will experience is coughing caused by irritation of the trachea and main bronchi. There is usually no pain associated with this procedure. Risks include bleeding and pneumothorax in 5 to 15% of patients in whom transbronchial biopsy is attempted. However, most studies have shown that death is rare and almost always associated with a transbronchial biopsy which has caused significant bleeding.

NEEDLE BIOPSY

If a diagnosis of a lesion still has not been made, transpulmonary needle biopsy of the lung can be performed. This technique is most useful when a mass or nodule is located peripherally near the pleura or in the apex of the lung. It is especially useful in those lesions that are thought to represent metastatic disease since these tumors are difficult to diagnose by bronchoscopy, particularly when they are less than 2 cm in size. Needle biopsy is frequently the procedure of choice for superior sulcus tumors. The technique and experience of the operator are of paramount importance, and it is necessary that an individual at a given institution establish his own record for sensitivity and specificity for this procedure. In our own institution, the chance of making a positive diagnosis of cancer in a patient with proven tumor is 90%. When the pathology report indicates nonspecific inflammatory changes on two separate attempts, there is less than 5% chance of malignancy and under these circumstances we will consider following certain types of lesions by chest roentgenograms every few months and not doing further diagnostic procedures unless the lesions enlarge or cavitate. Needle biopsy generally requires hospitalization although in certain circumstances it can be performed in ambulatory patients.

Patient Experience. The patient should be informed that he will feel a mild pressure with the introduction of the needle. Otherwise, there is no significant pain associated with needle biopsy. Bleeding and pneumothorax occur in 30% of patients biopsied but only 10% of them require insertion of a chest tube. Contraindications to the procedure include large blebs that are in the direct path of the needle, a patient with an uncontrollable cough, in which case general anesthesia may be necessary, and contralateral pneumonectomy, in which case the production of a pneumothorax would be devastating. In addition, there is a relative contraindication to needle biopsy in patients with pulmonary hypertension since they have an increased risk of bleeding. However, patients with emphysema, although they have a greater risk of pneumothorax, can be biopsied.

MEDIASTINOSCOPY

Rarely, mediastinoscopy will be necessary to make the diagnosis of lung cancer. More commonly, the procedure is performed to "stage" the tumor (see below). In either case, the patient must be hospitalized. An anterior cervical or parasternal incision is made under general anesthesia, and biopsies are taken of any palpable lymph nodes. There is less than a 1% mortality and approximately a 5 to 10% complication rate that includes infection, pneumothorax, and bleeding.

EXTRAPULMONARY METASTASIS

At the time of initial diagnosis, approximately 30% of patients will have evidence of metastatic disease (3). In that event workup of the primary lesion ceases since metastatic cancer is a contraindication to any type of surgery. Approximately 60% of patients die as a result of bone, brain, or liver metastasis depending on the cell type (4). Adenocarcinoma and small cell carcinoma tend to metastasize earlier in their course than does epidermoid cancer. Except for small cell carcinoma, extensive evaluations for metastatic liver, brain, and bone disease are discouraged unless the following conditions exist: (a) if more than one of the liver function tests are abnormal, a liver scan should be performed; and if positive, a needle biopsy is indicated; (b) if bone pain is present, a bone scan will be the most sensitive test for detecting an abnormality. In addition, a skeletal roentgenographic survey can be ordered but is much less sensitive; (c) if the neurologic examination is abnormal, further evaluation is necessary and either a computerized axial tomography (CT) scan or brain scan should be obtained depending on which is available. In the case of small cell carcinoma, an extensive metastatic evaluation is always prudent, even in the absence of symptoms, since this type of tumor metastasizes early and is only responsive to chemotherapy or irradiation.

STAGING

Regardless of the diagnostic sequence chosen for an individual patient, the process should lead to an accurate histologic diagnosis and to accurate clinical staging. This information is essential for planning treatment and for understanding the prognosis, as discussed below. Table 53.1 lists the four histologic types of lung cancer. Tables 53.3 and 53.4 summarize the criteria for the clinical stages proposed by the American Joint Committee for Cancer Staging (14).

SOLITARY NODULES

Clinical

As opposed to patients with mass lesions on chest roentgenogram, those who present with solitary nodules are relatively asymptomatic. Solitary pulmonary nodules or "coin" lesions have been variously described as circumscribed densities ranging in size to 6 cm. Since lesions of 6 cm can hardly be classified as coin lesions, the term solitary pulmonary nodule is more appropriate to denote a lesion less than 6 cm in diameter. Until recently, most small pulmonary nodules were resected. Predictably, many benign lesions were removed; therefore, major efforts have been made to improve preoperative diagnostic accuracy.

Table 53.3
Tumor-Node-Metastases (TNM) System for Lung Cancer

T— Primary tumor
　T0: No evidence of primary tumor
　TX: Malignant cells in secretions but no radiographic or bronchoscopic evidence of tumor
　T1: Tumor less than 3.0 cm in greatest diameter, located beyond a lobar bronchus.
　T2: Tumor larger than 3.0 cm in diameter or any size with extension to hilum. At bronchoscopy tumor is at least 2.0 cm from the carina. No pleural effusion. Atelectasis or obstructive pneumonia, if present, involves less than an entire lung
　T3: Tumor of any size extending to chest wall, diaphragm, mediastinum, within less than 2.0 cm of carina (bronchoscopy) or with effusion or atelectasis of entire lung
N— Regional lymph nodes
　N0: None involved
　N1: Metastasis to ipsilateral hilar region
　N2: Mediastinal nodes involved
M— Distant metastases
　M0: None
　M1: Any metastases to distant sites

Table 53.4
Stages of Lung Cancer [a]

Occult carcinoma: TX, N0, M0
Invasive carcinoma
　Stage 1: T1, N0, M0; T1, N1,M0; T2, N0, M0
　Stage 2: T2, N1, M0
　Stage 3: T3 with any N or M; N2 with any T or M; M1 with any T or N

[a] See Table 53.3 for explanation of notations.

Laboratory

CHEST ROENTGENOGRAM

When evaluating an asymptomatic patient with a solitary pulmonary nodule, one should begin with a careful examination of the chest roentgenogram. The obvious first question facing the clinician is whether the nodule is benign or malignant since the diagnosis of a benign lesion will allow the physician to avoid unnecessary and extensive evaluations. There are specific roentgenographic features that will permit the physician to follow the patient with a reasonable assurance that a lesion is benign.

Growth. The first consideration is the growth characteristics of the mass. In the past, when old chest roentgenograms were available and a lesion had not changed in size for 2 years, it was considered benign; and this led to a "watch and wait" approach. However, some lesions that appear stable for 3 to 4 years are malignant; therefore, only lesions that have shown no growth for 5 years need no further evaluation. A prior film of similar quality must be used for comparison since reports of previous roentgenograms are not sufficient. If old films are available and growth of the nodule has occurred, a less specific technique is to quantify the volume change to determine whether the mass is malignant (15). A doubling time (double in volume) between 10 and 500 days suggests that the lesion is malignant, while doubling times of longer than 18 months are associated with benign lesions. This type of measurement is not simple, and when no old films are available, waiting for a lesion to grow may result in spread of the tumor. Therefore, observing a new lesion for growth is not recommended.

Calcification. Calcification represents one of the most reliable signs that a nodule is benign. The following patterns of calcification indicate a benign lesion: (a) a central dense calcified nidus, (b) a diffuse or irregular nodular deposit (*i.e.,* the popcorn-type calcification that occurs in hamartomas), (c) calcifications scattered throughout the lesion, and (d) a laminated pattern of calcium deposited in concentric layers throughout the lesion, a pattern that is found in granulomas. Finally, a few specks of calcium are not a reliable sign that a lesion is benign. Small amounts of eccentrically placed calcium visualized in a nodule can occur with scar carcinoma.

The roentgenographic diagnosis of calcification is often arbitrary and depends on interpretation. Siegelman *et al.* (17) have reported the use of the CT scanner to assess density and to distinguish benign from malignant lesions by grading the density of the nodule. More dense tissue has higher absorption and, therefore, higher CT density attenuation. Thus, while calcium diffusely spread throughout a lesion may go undetected on a standard chest roentgenogram, it results in a CT scan with a high attenuation number that allows separation of benign from malignant lesions. This method may prove useful in the ambulatory assessment of the solitary pulmonary nodule.

Shape/Size. The shape and configuration of a lesion do not provide help in deciding whether the nodule is benign or malignant. While malignant lesions tend to have poorly defined, fuzzy borders, are often lobulated, and sometimes notched, none of these signs is diagnostic of a malignant growth. For that matter, a discretely circumscribed, round, sharply defined nodule is not always benign. Although size itself offers little aid in deciding whether a lesion is benign or malignant, larger nodules are more frequently malignant and offer a poor prognosis (see Table 53.5). Until recently, most nodules less than 1 cm were felt to have such a small chance of being malignant that surgery was frequently thought unnecessary. However, this is not true as can be seen in Table 53.5. This is partly due to case selection, but also due to more sensitive radiographic techniques that allow visualization of smaller, less dense lesions.

Age. Although malignant solitary nodules can occur at any age, they are almost never seen (0.5%) in patients less than 30 years of age; therefore, lesions in this age group can simply be observed. However, a semiannual chest roentgenogram should be obtained for at least the first 2 years of follow-up.

METASTASIS TO LUNG

Approximately 7% of solitary pulmonary nodules represent metastatic disease (1, 12). Those patients presenting with a solitary pulmonary nodule due to metastatic disease will almost always have a prior history of cancer. Only 20% of metastatic nodules occur in patients with occult disease. Furthermore, there is no evidence that extensive metastatic workups will uncover these occult tumors. This means that of 100 solitary pulmonary nodules, 7 will be of metastatic origin, but only 1 or 2 will represent occult malignancies. Based on these statistics, it is unwise

Table 53.5
Comparison of Nodule Size and Malignancy

Centimeters	No. of Tumors		% Malignant
	Benign	Malignant	
Study A[a]			
>4	0	5	100
3–4	0	6	100
2–3	4	13	70
1–2	18	28	50
0–1	11	6	47
Study B[b]			
>4	9	56	87
3–4	20	59	75
2–3	91	105	50
1–2	225	78	34
0–1	104	8	5

[a] Adapted from Siegelman et al. (17), 1980.
[b] Adapted from Steele (18), 1963.

to look for an extrapulmonary primary tumor before precise diagnosis of the solitary nodule is undertaken. A complete medical history, physical examination, and laboratory evaluation, including urinalysis, liver function tests, and screening for occult blood from the gastrointestinal and genitourinary tract will be adequate to uncover most metastatic disease to the lung. If any of these tests are positive, the possibility of an extrapulmonary neoplasm should be investigated further.

STAGING

The actual sequence in evaluating a solitary pulmonary nodule is similar to that already outlined for bronchogenic carcinoma. Cytology will be positive in less than 20 to 30% of patients who present with peripheral nodules. Bronchoscopy will increase the yield if the lesion is greater than 1 cm. At some institutions needle biopsy is being used more frequently in the evaluation of the solitary pulmonary nodule in an effort to obtain tissue prior to thoracotomy. In situations where reliable needle biopsy is not available, physicians will need to proceed directly to thoracotomy for diagnosis. The staging of a solitary pulmonary nodule is not as complicated if the lesion is peripheral and less than 2 cm. These patients are usually asymptomatic, and if initial screening is negative and the tissue type is not small cell undifferentiated carcinoma, then curative resection can be attempted. If the lesion is located centrally or is greater than 2 cm, mediastinoscopy should be performed to exclude an inoperable tumor.

COURSE/MANAGEMENT

Prognosis

Even with treatment, the prognosis and course of lung cancer are dismal. The present overall 5-year survival for treated and untreated cancer of the lung is 5 to 10%. This is mostly due to delay in diagnosis since approximately 75% of tumors are unresectable based on clinical evidence of far advanced disease at the time of presentation. Furthermore, less than 50% of those considered clinically resectable (see below) can have their tumor removed when staging procedures are completed. Thus, of 100 patients with lung cancer, only 25 will undergo complete staging. Of these, 11 will be resectable and only 8 to 10 will be alive in 5 years. In general, if the tumor is unresectable, the median survival is 2 to 3 months. However, even in patients with unresectable cancer, the 2-year survival is 4% for cancer limited to one hemithorax (10). As with other cancers, survival is correlated with the histologic type of tumor and the stage at the time of presentation (Table 53.6). Squamous cell carcinoma and adenocarcinoma are associated with the best prognosis, while small cell carcinoma is associated with the poorest. Within the respective cellular groupings, those with more undifferentiated cell

Table 53.6
Two-Year Survival Rates (% Alive) Bronchogenic Carcinoma[a]

Cell Type	Stage		
	1	2	3
Squamous	46	39	11
Adenocarcinoma	45	14	7
Large	42	12	12
Small	6	5	3

[a] Adapted from the American Joint Committee for Cancer Staging and End Results (1974) (14). See Table 53.4 for definition of stages. This represents 2155 cases of histologically proved cancer. The staging was based on (a) physical examination, (b) chest roentgenogram, or (c) surgical procedures—bronchoscopy, mediastinoscopy, thoracentesis, biopsies.

types tend to have the worst prognosis. Tumor type becomes relatively unimportant if the carcinoma presents as a small nodule less than 1 cm. Frequently tumors contain more than one cellular element, and depending on the amount of tissue available and the number of specimens examined histologically, disagreement among pathologists frequently occurs. In addition, even the same pathologist, after reviewing different microscopic slides from the same tumor, may reclassify the tumor.

Treatment

Surgical resection remains the only proven therapy for non-small cell carcinoma. Attempts at "curative" radiation of any solitary pulmonary nodule are currently unacceptable. Irradiation of larger tumors is considered appropriate for the palliation of atelectasis associated with bronchial obstruction and for relief of symptoms associated with paraneoplastic syndromes. In certain instances irradiation is recommended to patients who have stage I or II disease, but who are considered inoperable (see below). Chemotherapy for small cell carcinomas often improves the quality and duration of life (13). Patients with such tumors should be referred to an oncologist for definitive therapy (see Chapter 8).

OPERABILITY AND RESECTABILITY

Before proceeding to lung resection, two questions facing the clinician are: first, operability: is the patient able to withstand an operation and resection? and second, resectability: can the tumor be resected? The determination of resectability should be made in consultation with a pulmonary physician and a thoracic surgeon. Whether a tumor can be removed is determined from information derived from bronchoscopy, mediastinoscopy, and, finally, visualization of the tumor at thoracotomy. Unfortunately, only a small number of tumors are resectable at the time of presentation although a higher percentage of patients will be alive at 5 years.

The determination of whether a patient is operable should begin as soon as the patient is suspected of having cancer since an inoperable patient can be spared an extensive workup that includes staging procedures. Factors such as age, coexistent medical conditions, and nutritional status are discussed in detail elsewhere (Chapter 8). While there are relatively few absolute criteria that preclude resection of the lung, patients with an FEV_1 less than 1 liter and a pCO_2 greater than 50 are poor candidates for any kind of resection. By using both the ventilation/perfusion lung scan and the spirogram, one can predict the amount of functional lung remaining after pneumonectomy, although this prediction is more difficult in patients undergoing lobectomy or segmentectomy. If the predicted postoperative FEV_1 is greater than 800 ml, resection can be performed on patients who otherwise might not have been considered operable candidates. It is important to remember that a normal blood gas does not exclude significant pulmonary disease since patients with emphysema and advanced obstructive lung disease can maintain relatively normal arterial blood gases (see Chapter 52). This underscores the need for obtaining the FEV_1 early in the evaluation, but a word of caution is necessary. Frequently, the initial evaluation reveals pulmonary function that precludes operation; however, after aggressive therapy, including bronchodilators for bronchospasm, antibiotics for infection, percussion and drainage for excessive secretions, and discontinuation of cigarette smoking, a marked improvement may be achieved so that a resection can be attempted.

OPERABLE PATIENTS

The course of lung carcinoma after curative resection is variable depending on the functional lung remaining. Often immediately postoperatively there is a significant amount of unsuspected bronchospasm which with conventional treatment improves promptly. Most patients with postoperative bronchospasm have underlying bronchitis with preoperative evidence of bronchospasm on spirogram; therefore, routine spirometry, before lung resection, is recommended. In addition spirometry postoperatively will aid in assessing whether there has been worsening of bronchoconstriction. After resection there appears to be some chronic compensatory hyperinflation of any remaining lung parenchyma; therefore, in time, pulmonary function can improve 20 to 30% over the immediate postoperative function, resulting in improved exercise capability. Normal activities can be resumed within several weeks of surgery, depending mostly on pulmonary reserve (see Chapter 83). Routine follow-up at least every 3 to 4 months for the first 2 years after resection is advised in order to detect metastasis, local recurrence, or a second primary. Sputum cytology and chest X-ray are recommended at least twice a year, especially in patients who continue to smoke.

INOPERABLE PATIENTS

If the patient is inoperable or the tumor is unresectable, and significant tumor remains or recurs, ambulatory treatment is directed at symptomatic relief. Dyspnea resulting from recurring pleural effusions can be effectively relieved in an ambulatory setting by repeated thoracentesis; chest tube drainage and sclerosing of the pleura can be employed (on referral to an oncologist or pulmonary physician) for more chronic resolution. Bone pain from metastasis often responds to local irradiation better than it does to narcotic sedation. Chest wall pain is the most difficult symptom to treat, but local intercostal blocks add to the analgesic effects of narcotics. Pneumonia often occurs when bronchogenic tumors obstruct major bronchi, and therapy with antibiotics alone is usually insufficient. In this situation, palliative irradiation may reduce the tumor size and temporarily allow drainage of the bronchus. Hemoptysis and the superior vena cava syndrome also may respond to radiotherapy. Consultation with an oncologist is useful for the primary physician when patients have residual tumor and are difficult to manage. Additional discussion of the care of the patient with incurable cancer is found in Chapter 8.

References

General

Baker, ER, Stitik, FP and Summer, WR: Preoperative evaluation of patients with suspected bronchogenic carcinoma. *Curr Prob Surg* Year Book Publishers, Chicago, 1974.
> *A good general review including more details about the surgical approach to cancer.*

Mittman, C and Bruderman, I: Lung cancer: to operate or not? *Am Rev Respir Dis* 116: 477, 1977.
> *A general review of the preoperative evaluation of the patient with lung cancer.*

Siegelman, SS, Stitik, FP and Summer, WR: *Pulmonary System: Practical Approaches to Pulmonary Diagnosis.* Grune & Stratton, New York, 1979.
> *To date, the most complete book on the procedures used to diagnose pulmonary disease. Includes useful, detailed clinical information on all procedures.*

Specific

1. Adkins, PC, Wesselhoeft, CW, Jr, Newman, W and Blades, B: Thoracotomy on the patient with previous malignancy: metastasis or new primary? *J Thorac Cardiovasc Surg* 56: 351, 1968.
2. Auerbach, O, Stout, AP, Hammond, EC and Garfinkel, L: Bronchial epithelium in former smokers. *N Engl J Med* 267: 119, 1962.
3. Boucot, KR, Cooper, DA, Weiss, W and Carnahan, WJ: The natural history of lung cancer. *Am Rev Respir Dis* 89: 519, 1964.
4. Cox, JD and Yesner, RA: Adenocarcinoma of the lung: recent results from the Veterans Administration lung group. *Am Rev Respir Dis* 120: 1025, 1979.
5. Feinstein, AR: Symptomatic patterns, biologic behavior, and prognosis in cancer of the lung. *Ann Intern Med* 61: 27, 1964.
6. Guidelines for the Cancer Related Checkup: *CA* 30: 1980.
7. Hammond, EC and Selikoff, IJ: Relations of cigarette smoking to risk of death of asbestos-associated disease among insulation workers in the United States (Biological Effects of Asbestos, Lyons, France). *IARC Sci Publ* 8: 312, 1973.

8. Hammond, EC: Evidence of the effects of giving up cigarette smoking. *Am J Public Health 55:* 682, 1965.
9. Hinshaw, HC and Murray, JF: *Diseases of the Chest,* pp. 463–523. W. B. Saunders, Philadelphia, 1980.
10. Hyde, L, Wolf, J, McCracken, S and Yesner, R: Natural course of inoperable lung cancer. *Chest 64:* 309, 1973.
11. Koss, LG: *Diagnosic Cytology and Its Histopathologic Bases, Vol. II,* Ed. 2. Lippincott/Harper, Philadelphia, 1979.
12. Lawhorne, TW, Jr, Baker, RR and Carter, D: Adenocarcinoma of the lung presenting as a solitary pulmonary nodule. *Johns Hopkins Med J 133:* 82, 1973.
13. Livingston, RE: Small cell carcinoma of the lung. *Blood 56:* 575, 1980.
14. Mountain, CF, Carr, DT and Anderson, WA: A system for the clinical staging of lung cancer. *AJR 120:* 130, 1974.
15. Nathan, H: Management of solitary pulmonary nodules. An organized approach based on growth rate and statistics. *JAMA 227:* 1141, 1974.
16. *Smoking and Health:* A report of the Surgeon General. U.S. Department of Health, Education, and Welfare, Washington, D.C., 1979.
17. Seigelman, SS, Zerhouni, EA, Leo, FP, Khouri, NG and Stitik, FP: CT of the solitary pulmonary nodule. *AJR 135:* 1, 1980.
18. Steele, JD: The solitary pulmonary nodule. Report of a cooperative study of resected asymptomatic solitary pulmonary nodules in males. *J Thorac Cardiovasc Surg 46:* 21, 1963.
19. Zavala, DC: Diagnostic fiberoptic bronchoscopy. *Chest 68:* 12, 1975.

SECTION 8

Cardiovascular Problems

CHAPTER FIFTY-FOUR

Angina Pectoris

GUSTAV C. VOIGT, M.D., and PHILIP D. ZIEVE, M.D.

Chest pain is one of the most frequent complaints of patients to physicians in an ambulatory practice (see Tables 1.3 and 1.4, Chapter 1). The major early objective in the diagnosis of such patients is the separation of noncardiac from cardiac pain. Chapter 50 describes the various causes of noncardiac pain and their distinguishing characteristics. This chapter describes the diagnosis and treatment of the commonest cause of cardiac pain, transient myocardial ischemia.

Ischemic heart disease due to atherosclerosis is one of the most prevalent ailments in the Western world; in the United States, it is the leading nontraumatic cause of disability and death. Most people recognize that chest pain may be an important symptom of ischemic heart disease and may be a prodrome of myocardial infarction (a "heart attack") and of sudden death. They know that it is important to see a physician as soon as possible when they experience chest pain. It is essential that physicians know how to respond to these people in order to make appropriate diagnostic and therapeutic decisions.

In the approach to the patient with chest pain, a detailed history and physical examination must not be replaced by sophisticated noninvasive or invasive cardiovascular procedures. Otherwise, unnecessary, sometimes painful, risky, and expensive procedures are overutilized; and the physician becomes less able to arrive at reasonable conclusions without such studies. Furthermore, a detailed history and physical examination permit the physician to tailor studies to meet more specifically the needs of the patient, thereby increasing the efficiency and yield of such procedures.

PATHOPHYSIOLOGY

Normally, the myocardium produces most of its energy by means of aerobic metabolism. When totally deprived of oxygen, the heart stops beating within a few minutes. Oxygen demands (Table 54.1) are a function of the amount of work that cardiac muscle is called upon to perform. That work, in turn, is a function of the heart rate, of the tension of the walls of the left ventricle, and of the contractility of the myocardium (25). Tension (T), described by the Laplace relationship ($T = P \cdot r/2h$), is directly proportionate to the ventricular blood pressure (P) and volume (r = radius of the ventricular cavity), and is inversely proportionate to the thickness (h) of the ventricular wall. Contractility essentially is the amount of work that the myocardium can do under a given load, and, in the normal heart, is influenced primarily by tone generated by the sympathetic nervous system and by catecholamines stored in cardiac muscle. These interrelationships which affect the heart's ability to do work also are important in the pathophysiology of heart failure (see Chapter 58).

In practical terms these concepts reveal why the heart is more prone to ischemia when its rate is increased (e.g., by exertion or emotional stress), when left ventricular tension is increased (e.g., by increased blood pressure or by ventricular dilation) or when myocardial contractility is increased (e.g., by a sympathetic discharge that accompanies exertion or emotional stress).

Oxygen supply (Table 54.1) is dependent on the oxygen content of the blood and on the volume of blood flowing through the coronary arteries per unit of time. Normally, the myocardium extracts from coronary blood as much oxygen as it can; this is reflected in the wide arteriovenous difference in oxygen concentration across the coronary circulation (coronary sinus blood has a very low oxygen saturation). Therefore, an increased demand for myocardial

oxygen can only be met by an increase in coronary blood flow. This flow is dependent on two major factors: aortic diastolic pressure (during systole the coronary arteries are squeezed and deliver much less blood to the myocardium) and coronary vascular resistance. Coronary vascular resistance is determined by the patency of the coronary blood vessels; when the vessels are narrowed by spasm or by an atherosclerotic plaque, oxygen demands may not be satisfied.

If the myocardium receives insufficient oxygen to satisfy its metabolic demands, the ischemia usually results in pain. Transient myocardial ischemia causes transient chest pain—*angina pectoris*; prolonged ischemia causes more prolonged chest pain because of *myocardial infarction.* The character of the pain (see below) is the same in both situations. When ischemic, the heart is much more susceptible to unstable electrical activity. The treatment of ischemia is directed at reducing myocardial demand for oxygen and at increasing the flow of coronary blood to the myocardium.

Table 54.1
Some Factors That Influence Myocardial Metabolism

Oxygen Demand	Oxygen Supply
1. Heart rate	1. Oxygen content of the blood

2. Tension (*T*) of the wall of the left ventricle[a]
  a. Ventricular blood pressure (*P*)
  b. Radius (*r*) of the ventricular cavity
  c. Thickness (*h*) of the wall
	2. Volume of blood flowing through the coronary arteries per unit of time

3. Contractility of the myocardium	

[a] $T = P \cdot r / 2h$ (see text).

RISK FACTORS

Both genetic and environmental factors influence the development of atherosclerotic heart disease. Recognition of these factors is especially important in so far as they may be modified to prevent disease. A pamphlet entitled "Risk Factors and Coronary Disease. A Statement for Physicians" is available from the American Heart Association (1); it summarizes the various risk factors that have been identified and makes recommendations for dealing with them (Tables 54.2 and 54.3).

Table 54.2
Risk Factors for Coronary Artery Disease

Factor	Comment	Documentation
Blood pressure (Chapter 59)	Risk is directly proportionate to increase of systolic or diastolic blood pressure	Excellent
Blood lipids (Chapter 72)	Risk is directly proportionate to increase in concentration of total cholesterol and of low density lipoprotein (LDL) and inversely proportionate to concentration of high density lipoprotein (HDL)	Excellent
Diabetes mellitus (Chapter 69)	Risk is 2 times control in diabetic men, 3 times control in diabetic women	Excellent
Cigarette smoking (Chapter 19)	Proportionate to number of cigarettes smoked per day (3 times control at a pack or more per day)	Excellent
Oral contraceptives (Chapter 90)	Risk is much greater in women over age 35	Excellent
Personality type	A competitive, driving person (so-called type A personality) is more prone to coronary artery disease	Good
Sedentary living (Chapter 55)	Individuals who do not exercise regularly may have a greater risk of myocardial infarction than do individuals who exercise regularly	Poor
Diet[a] (Chapter 72)	High lipid content of diet may potentiate coronary artery disease	Poor in humans Excellent in animals

[a] Obesity, alcohol, and caffeine—though claimed by some in the past to be risk factors—have not been established to be so.

Table 54.3
Primary Prevention of Coronary Artery Disease: Recommended Actions[a]

DEMONSTRATED RISK FACTORS THAT CAN BE MODIFIED
  Discontinue cigarette smoking
  Control hypertension
  Control blood lipids
  Monitor use of oral contraceptives
DEMONSTRATED RISK FACTORS THAT CANNOT OR PROBABLY CANNOT BE MODIFIED
  Identify ECG abnormalities
  Identify type A behavior
  Identify diabetes and gout
FACTORS THAT ARE NOT ESTABLISHED RISKS
  Encourage regular physical activity
  Monitor intake of alcohol and coffee

[a] Modified from AHA Committee Report (see text), *Circulation 62:* 449A, 1980.

It is difficult to assign a specific risk to a particular factor because often the risk is proportionate to the degree of exposure (e.g., the number of cigarettes smoked a day or the concentration of cholesterol in the blood) and because the various factors interact in a complicated way to compound the risk of disease in a given patient. However, the general physician should attempt to attenuate the risk associated with any of those factors that can be modified. Table 54.3 lists the proposals of the American Heart Association in this regard and indicates also those which are most likely to be effective in the primary prevention of coronary artery disease.

Although it is not a risk factor *per se,* recent myocardial infarction is a powerful predictor of new angina; almost half of those persons with no prior history of angina develop typical angina during the first year after a myocardial infarction (see Chapter 55 for additional discussion).

DIAGNOSIS

History

ONSET OF ISCHEMIC PAIN

Many patients with ischemic cardiac pain can document the circumstances and sometimes the date and time of their first pain. This is not so true in patients with pain of neuromuscular or gastrointestinal origin unless trauma or some catastrophe such as a bowel perforation has occurred. The ability of the patient to describe the first experience with chest pain is useful, therefore, in differential diagnosis.

CHARACTER AND LOCATION OF THE ISCHEMIC PAIN

The discomfort of myocardial ischemia is described differently by different people; some describe it as squeezing, crushing, burning, or smothering, whereas others describe it as a shortness of breath, or simply a feeling of heaviness. A sharp pain is unlikely to be of cardiac origin, but the patient should be asked to characterize it further, if he can, since "sharp" to some patients means "severe" rather than knifelike or piercing.

Typically, the discomfort is midline and substernal; it often radiates to the shoulder, arm, hand, or fingers—usually to the left. Radiation down the inside of the arm into the fingers supplied by the ulnar nerve is classic. Pain may radiate also into the neck, the lower jaw, or the intrascapular region. Occasionally, the patient may have pain only in a referred location and experience no chest discomfort at all. A patient may actually consult his dentist because he ascribes pain in the lower jaw, which is due to myocardial iscemia, to a toothache. The pain of myocardial ischemia is diffuse: rarely is the patient able to point with one finger to the location of the pain; when pain can be localized in that way, it is likely to be noncardiac in origin (see Chapter 50).

INITIATION OF ISCHEMIC PAIN

The most important diagnostic feature of the discomfort of myocardial ischemia is its relationship to exertion, to emotional stress, or to other situations which may either increase cardiac oxygen demand or decrease myocardial oxygen supply. The cause of atypical pain, pain in an unusual location or of an unusual character, may be clarified by this relationship. Pain that is experienced at rest, if it is due to cardiac ischemia, suggests unstable angina (see below, p. 486), variant angina (see below, p. 486), or myocardial infarction.

Anxiety is an important and often overlooked provoking factor in many patients. Myocardial oxygen demand may be increased by anxiety to an extent and duration greater than that produced by exercise, resulting in prolonged pain. This is important in understanding environmental factors in a patient with angina. The common cycle of anxiety producing chest pain and the pain in turn producing more anxiety should be recognized as an important mechanism of prolonged pain.

Angina is more likely to occur during cold or windy weather because of increased myocardial work and increased peripheral vascular resistance and perhaps because of cold-activated reflexes producing a decrease in coronary flow. Curiously, angina may occur only with an early daily activity or working period, such as an early morning shower or a walk from a car to a place of work. It is important to recognize this pattern because it has useful therapeutic implications (see below). Sometimes ischemic discomfort will follow a heavy meal, perhaps because of the shunting of blood to abdominal viscera and because of increased sympathetic tone. Nocturnal angina may be a consequence of left ventricular failure and often responds to digitalis or to diuretics (see below, p. 485). Similarly, patients who describe breathlessness and chest pain with exertion may have angina as a consequence of transient left ventricular failure (28).

Sometimes a patient will develop typical angina pectoris with work that involves the hands, arms, and shoulders, whereas the same patient may be able to walk at a brisk pace indefinitely without pain. It has been postulated that this phenomenon is due to the fact that smaller muscles use relatively more oxygen and that the use of smaller muscles in the upper extremities often involves *isometric activity* (increase in muscle tone with little shortening of muscle fibers), which increases peripheral arterial resistance. This increase in afterload (the resistance to ejection of blood from the heart) increases left ventricular ejection pressure, left ventricular work, and myocardial oxygen demand. In contrast, walking or the use of large leg muscles is not isometric; and the increased blood flow to the legs is accomplished in a setting of arterial dilation, decreasing peripheral resistance and allowing the heart to increase cardiac output at a lesser workload. It is important to establish these relationships for diagnosis and therapy.

Increase in *carboxyhemoglobin* level is an important cause of angina in some persons. The commonest ways in which this may occur are through exposure to high carbon monoxide (CO) levels in heavy traffic and through inhalation of CO in tobacco smoke. These two situations, both with implications for patient management, can be identified by careful history-taking.

RELIEF OF ISCHEMIC PAIN

Since angina is due to a discrepancy between oxygen supply and demand, relief of pain is achieved by increasing coronary blood flow or by decreasing oxygen demand. Cessation of effort or relief of anxiety decrease oxygen demand, and angina begins to disappear within minutes thereafter. So called "walk through angina" is uncommon. Most people must stop or at least slow the activity responsible for precipitating the pain before it is relieved. A history of relief of pain by sublingual nitroglycerin is also useful. However, the patient must be told that the use of nitroglycerin in this way is a diagnostic trial and that the prescription of nitroglycerin does not necessarily mean coronary artery disease. The physician and the patient both need to know also that the relief of chest pain by nitroglycerin is not specific for myocardial ischemia. For example, the pain of esophageal spasm is commonly relieved by nitroglycerin (see Chapter 31). A placebo effect may relieve chest discomfort due to other causes as well.

DURATION OF ISCHEMIC PAIN

Angina pectoris responds promptly to measures directed at reducing myocardial oxygen demand (cessation of effort usually) or at increasing coronary blood flow (e.g., administration of sublingual nitroglycerin). Pain is usually relieved within 5 min; if it persists beyond that time, it may not be due to myocardial ischemia (Chapter 50), but the possibility of myocardial infarction must be considered. If typical ischemic pain persists beyond 20 min, a myocardial infarction is likely and the patient should be hospitalized (see below, p. 486).

Physical Examination

The examination of a patient who complains of possible ischemic cardiac pain should be done with particular attention to uncovering circumstantial evidence that would support a diagnosis of cardiovascular disease: high blood pressure, evidence of abnormal lipid metabolism such as xanthomas (see Chapter 72), fundoscopic changes reflecting long-standing hypertension or diabetes, or evidence of peripheral vascular disease (Chapter 84).

Several physical findings suggest ischemic heart disease. A systolic bulge may be felt at the apex of the heart, especially when the patient lies in the left lateral decubitus position. A third or fourth heart sound (S-3 or S-4) may be heard. There may be a paradoxic split of the second heart sound caused by a delay in aortic valve closure because of a decrease in contractility of the left ventricle.

The opportunity to examine a patient during an episode of chest pain should not be missed. The examination should be done promptly while someone else sets up the electrocardiograph machine since it often takes several minutes to connect the machine, by which time the pain may have disappeared. Physical findings (e.g., S-4, paradoxical splitting of S-2) may be present transiently during an episode of chest pain; in such instances, they provide stronger evidence of ischemic heart disease than they do if they are found incidentally, when the patient is asymptomatic. The blood pressure should also be recorded if the patient is examined while he is experiencing chest pain; transient hypertension during an ischemic attack is seen commonly. In exercise stress testing (see below), hypertension is documented often before symptomatic or electrocardiographic evidence of ischemia. These observations emphasize the importance of blood pressure control in patients with ischemic heart disease (Chapter 59). Hypotension detected during myocardial ischemia may be a clue to global ischemia produced by left main coronary disease or its equivalent. This is important to recognize because early arteriography (see below) and bypass surgery should be considered in such patients.

Electrocardiogram

A 12-lead standard electrocardiogram (ECG) should be obtained in any patient with suspected ischemic cardiac pain.

The most reliable ECG sign of chronic ischemic heart disease is a Q wave (6), recorded by those leads of the ECG which are measuring electrical activity of a part of the myocardium that has been infarcted

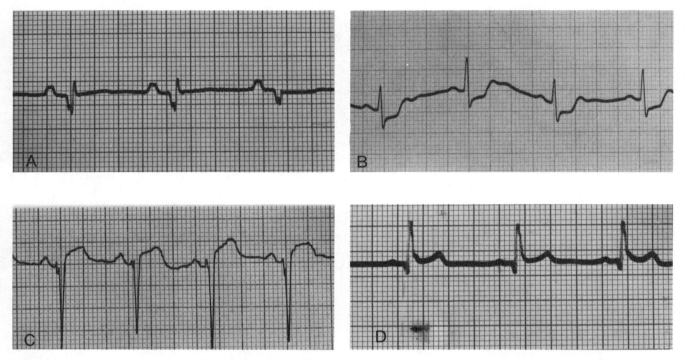

Figure 54.1 Electrocardiographic strips of patients with suspected ischemic heart disease. *A*, Q waves suggestive of chronic myocardial disease; *B*, ST depression developing after exertion; *C*, ST elevation during coronary artery spasm (variant angina); and *D*, early repolarization (a normal variant).

(Fig. 54.1*A*). Nonspecific ST-T wave changes, abnormalities of conduction (except for left bundle branch block—see below), and arrhythmias do not help to establish the diagnosis of myocardial ischemia. ST depression with a flat or down sloping ST segment indicative of subendocardial ischemia (Fig. 54.1*B*), is seen relatively rarely in the ECGs of patients with ischemic heart disease unless they are experiencing angina at the time the tracing is being recorded. On the other hand, these "ischemic" changes are seen commonly when a patient with ischemic heart disease is exercised to a point where he develops chest pain (see below). ST elevation at rest (Fig. 54.1*C*) suggests variant angina (see below) or myocardial infarction. T wave inversion in an ECG taken at rest is a nonspecific finding unless it is seen only when a patient is experiencing angina. Some important general guidelines concerning the ECG in evaluating chest pain are enumerated below, with the caution that some exceptions exist.

1. A patient who has not had a previous myocardial infarction and who has had *angina pectoris for less than a year* will usually have a normal ECG, if the ECG is done at a time when the patient is not experiencing chest pain. The finding of a normal resting ECG in such a patient is not good evidence against the diagnosis of coronary artery disease. Fifty percent of *all* patients with known coronary artery disease will have a normal resting ECG (17).

2. A patient with a normal resting ECG will usually have ischemic ECG changes *during an episode of*

angina. The absence of changes in such circumstances suggests that the pain is not cardiac. Also such patients will usually have a positive exercise stress test (see below).

3. Patients with *long-standing angina pectoris* usually have abnormal resting ECGs. They have evidence of previous myocardial infarction, left ventricular hypertrophy, conduction abnormalities, or nonspecific ST-T changes. A patient who has had chest pain for 5 years or more and who has a normal resting ECG probably has noncardiac chest pain.

4. A patient with a baseline abnormal resting ECG, due to *previous infarction, left ventricular hypertrophy, bundle branch block,* etc., may have no new ECG changes during an attack of angina. Such patients also can have an acute myocardial infarction with no new changes in their ECG.

5 *An abnormal resting ECG in the absence of other evidence* does not justify a diagnosis of ischemia or coronary artery disease. Although there is a high degree of statistical correlation between an abnormal ECG and coronary artery disease, the vast majority of people in whom this correlation exists have other evidence of coronary artery disease such as clinically documented infarction, typical angina pectoris, heart failure, cardiac enlargement, or arteriographically proven disease. When one sees a patient with a negative cardiac history, a normal cardiovascular examination, and an abnormal ECG, it is likely that the ECG abnormalities are due to some form of cardiac pathology other than coronary artery disease or that

there is no cardiac disease. The QRS abnormalities of infarction are conduction abnormalities which may have many causes (11), although the most common is infarction. Thus, a pattern suggesting old infarction can be seen in patients without coronary artery disease and may be due to healed myocarditis, to an infiltrative disease such as amyloidosis or sarcoid, or to Wolff-Parkinson-White syndrome (see Chapter 56). Similarly ST segment elevation suggesting acute infarction may be seen in the resting ECG of healthy persons with so-called "early repolarization." This pattern (see Fig. 54.1D) is found most often in young adult males, usually in the midleft chest leads but also in right chest leads and in limb leads. The ST elevation may reach 4 mm but there is no ST depression in reciprocal leads and the ST elevation usually normalizes during exercise. The presence of nonspecific ST-T abnormalities in an otherwise well person should not be regarded as evidence of heart disease in the absence of other confirmatory findings. Nonspecific ST-T abnormalities per se are rarely diagnostic of anything and that is why they are called "nonspecific."

6. There is a high degree of correlation between left bundle branch block and organic heart disease, especially coronary artery disease. Right bundle branch block, on the other hand, is seen commonly in the absence of other cardiac abnormalities. It is presumed that right bundle branch block in the absence of other evidence of cardiac disease is congenital; in many instances it is a totally benign finding.

7. Although there is a relationship between arrhythmias and cardiac disease, particularly coronary artery disease, most of the people in studies establishing these correlations have other evidence of heart disease and/or multiple risk factors. One is not justified in making a diagnosis of heart disease becaue of an arrhythmia in a patient who appears otherwise healthy. This should not be interpreted to justify a cavalier attitude toward arrhythmias. However, there are some people with life-long arrhythmias such as atrial fibrillation, complete heart block, ventricular premature beats, and paroxysmal ventricular tachycardia, who have no other evidence of disease and whose life expectancy is not obviously shortened. (Arrhythmias are dealt with in more detail in Chapter 56.)

Exercise Stress Tests

The role and the value of exercise stress testing are misunderstood by many health care providers. The exercise stress test is relatively safe and relatively inexpensive; when used in the context of the total clinical picture, it contributes valuable information about the patient with chest pain and/or with other cardiac symptoms.

The rationale behind exercise stress testing is simple. By increasing the work performed by the patient,

cardiac work is increased. This increase in work requires an increase in myocardial oxygen utilization which demands an increase in coronary blood flow. If narrowed or obstructed coronary arteries prevent the required increase in coronary blood flow, ischemia may occur and produce chest pain and/or ECG changes.

A variety of stress test techniques are available, but the most frequently used and best standardized require the patient to walk on a treadmill or an escalator, while permitting a controlled increase in workload by increasing rate and inclination of the device. Exercise on a bicycle ergometer is also commonly used. A bicycle ergometer may also permit a patient to exercise with his arms instead of his legs. This is particularly useful in patients who cannot use the treadmill, because of claudication, arthritis, or amputation, for example, and also in the evaluation of patients who have chest pain predominantly or exclusively with work that involves the arms and shoulders.

The stress test should be performed in a facility which permits monitoring during exercise, has a direct writing instrument to record and document the ECGs, and has equipment and staff trained to deal with arrhythmias and other cardiac emergencies. With properly selected patients and with an appropriately equipped laboratory and a trained staff, an exercise stress test is a safe procedure with reported mortality rates in the range of 0.01 % (24).

It is important to recognize that the exercise stress test is not just a technical procedure. Both the safety of the procedure and the information obtained are greatly enhanced when the team performing the study has sufficient clinical information to understand questions posed and to appreciate what limitations are necessary as far as the amount of work is concerned.

Ordinarily a patient exercises until a predetermined heart rate is attained. This is usually 80 to 90% of the maximum heart rate predicted on the basis of the patient's age (see Table 55.6, Chapter 55). This goal can be modified according to the pre-exercise evaluation of the patient and the needs of the patient and of his physician. In a young person in whom there is a low probability of ischemic heart disease, for example, attempting to reach the maximum heart rate or exercising the patient to the point of exhaustion is reasonable and adds to the sensitivity of the study. A negative study under such circumstances is yet stronger evidence against myocardial ischemia. On the other hand there is no obligation to reach a rapid heart rate or a high workload in an older patient in whom a negative study, no chest pain and no ischemic ECG changes, is clinically meaningful at a lesser workload. For example, the physician might decide that if the patient does not have angina and/or ischemic ECG changes at a workload approximating that patient's daily activity, further exercise stress testing is clinically meaningless. The physician is content that angina or ischemia does not occur during a patient's daily activity and he does not require more information about the patient's cardiovascular physiology for appropriate management.

CRITERIA

Criteria for a positive stress test vary among laboratories. Referring physicians must understand these criteria and the purpose for which they are being utilized. Depression of the ST segment with a flat or horizontal or down sloping ST segment is the typical ischemic change sought as "positive" electrocardiographic evidence of ischemia (Fig. 54.1B). If 0.5-mm ST depression is used as a criterion of positivity, the laboratory will produce results which are more sensitive but less specific—that is, there will be a higher proportion of false positive results. Conversely, if 2.0-mm ST depression is the criterion, the results will be more specific but less sensitive—that is, there will be a higher proportion of false negative studies. Most laboratories use 1.0-mm ST depression as a criterion of positivity, a compromise which provides a reasonable degree of specificity while avoiding a level of sensitivity which results in an overdiagnosis of ischemic heart disease. On the average, this common criterion results in false positive tests about 10% of the time (i.e, specificity is 90%) and false negative tests about 30% of the time (i.e., sensitivity is 70%).

In evaluating the results of exercise stress testing it is important to keep in mind Bayes' theorem: the *predictive accuracy* (number of subjects with true positive tests divided by the number of positive tests) of any diagnostic test is directly related to the sensitivity of the test (the percent of patients with the disease in whom the test is positive), the specificity of the test (the percent of patients without the disease in whom the test is negative), and the prevalence of the disease in the population studied. This relationship exists whenever the specificity of any test is less than 100%. In populations which have a high prevalence of disease the predictive accuracy will be very high even when sensitivity and specificity are low. Conversely, the predictive accuracy will be very low in groups of patients with a low prevalence of disease even when the procedure has high specificity and high sensitivity. Therefore, the predictive accuracy of an exercise stress test is dependent upon the characteristics of the population studied. In men with classic angina pectoris or previous myocardial infarction a positive exercise stress test will accurately predict the presence of occlusive coronary artery disease about 85% of the time (29). On the other hand, in asymptomatic patients with positive ST segment responses to exercise stress testing, the predictive accuracy is much lower. About 60% or more of these patients may have false positive tests (29); that is, arteriographic studies will not demonstrate significant coronary artery disease.

INDICATIONS FOR EXERCISE STRESS TESTING

There are at least seven indications for stress testing:

1. To *clarify the cause of chest pain*. This is probably the most common reason for recommending an exercise stress test in an ambulatory population. In some practices exercise stress tests will be recommended for many patients in order to provide reassurance that chest pain is not due to cardiac ischemia. The factors influencing sensitivity and specificity of the test (see above) must be kept in mind.

2. To *assess prognosis* in patients with known ischemic heart disease (see below).

3. To *decide whether a patient should have coronary arteriography*. The referring physician might decide, for example, that a patient with good exercise tolerance who has chest pain associated with 1 mm of ST depression in leads II, III, and AVF after maximum exercise will be treated medically, whereas the patient who has chest pain associated with several millimeters of ST depression in many leads after relatively minimal exercise should undergo coronary arteriography.

4. To *evaluate functional capacity* of patients in order to recommend appropriate activities. It may be helpful for the physician to know how much activity is necessary to produce evidence of ischemia in a given patient so that he can advise the patient about limitations in his activities. The physician should first ask the patient whether he has already done "stress tests" on himself—i.e., trials of various valued activities to determine which produce angina (most patients have done this). Often this testing is more useful than a formal stress test in deciding what to recommend to the patient. Some physicians feel that an exercise stress test is appropriate in an apparently healthy middle aged person who wishes to undertake a new physically stressful activity. For example, a preliminary exercise stress test is considered an appropriate part of the evaluation of a person who wishes to begin mountain climbing or serious running, especially if that person has previously led a largely sedentary life-style; the caveats regarding predictive accuracy (see above) should be recalled when interpreting stress tests in such persons.

Table 55.4 in Chapter 55 lists the metabolic equivalents (METS) of a number of common activities. Stress test data reported in terms of METS achieved before symptoms are useful for the physician in counseling his patient.

5. To *evaluate patients after myocardial infarction or coronary artery surgery* in order to determine appropriate exercise prescriptions. This is discussed in more detail in Chapter 55.

6. To *ascertain the effects of medical or surgical management of coronary artery disease*, particularly when baseline studies have been performed. The exercise stress test documents objectively whether or

not a patient has improved, and, if he has, to what extent. The documentation of improvements with a stress test is often reassuring to the patient.

7. To document the response of a *patient with a cardiac arrhythmia* to exercise and to document the response of the arrhythmia to therapy (see Chapter 56).

CONTRAINDICATIONS TO EXERCISE STRESS TESTING

There are a number of contraindications to stress testing:

1. *The recent onset of unstable angina* pectoris (see below) or *recent myocardial infarction* is a relative contraindication to exercise stress testing. Most of these patients should not be subjected to maximal exercise stress tests. However, *modified stress tests* can be done with a reasonable degree of safety in selected patients. The information obtained may be exceedingly helpful in making recommendations concerning activity and such studies may select a group of patients in whom coronary arteriography should be done earlier with an eye towards possible surgical intervention (see additional discussion in Chapter 55).

2. *Uncontrolled hypertension* is a relative contraindication and depends upon the level of blood pressure and upon the degree of end-organ impairment.

3. Exercise stress testing should not be performed in patients with severe *uncontrolled congestive heart failure* because of the risk of acute pulmonary edema, of hypotension due to low cardiac output, and of serious arrhythmias.

4. Signficiant *ventricular arrhythmias* are a relative contraindication to exercise stress testing. However, it may be difficult to know before the test whether a given ventricular arrhythmia is significant. For example, a patient with frequent multifocal premature ventricular contractions may show a decrease or an increase in ectopic activity when stressed; if ventricular ectopy increases with exercise, the test should be terminated.

5. Suspected *severe valvular disease*, particularly obstructive valvular disease such as mitral stenosis, aortic stenosis, or subvalvular aortic outflow obstruction, may impose serious risks to patients who are exercised. This is because the heart may be unable to increase cardiac output in response to an increased demand. With aortic stenosis, the demand for an increase in cardiac output may not be met, while at the same time peripheral vasodilation decreases peripheral vascular resistance, resulting in a marked fall in perfusion. Again, however, modified stress tests can probably be performed with a reasonable degree of safety in appropriately selected patients.

6. Exericise stress testing should be performed with caution in a *variety of conditions.* Exercise testing is contraindicated in patients with myocarditis, acute pericarditis, severe pulmonary hypertension, recent pulmonary embolism, intercurrent acute systemic illness, or significant infection. Patients with a high degree of atrioventricular block should be exercised cautiously since they may not be able to increase their heart rate appropriately. Patients taking medications such as reserpine and propranolol, particularly when these have been instituted recently, may be at some risk because these drugs limit heart rate or blood pressure response to exercise. Patients with severe chronic pulmonary disease may have difficulty when exercised, such as increased bronchospasm, increased hypoxemia, and cardiac arrhythmias. However, exercise stress tests in such patients, with concomitant pulmonary function studies and blood gas analyses, can provide useful information (see Chapter 52).

7. *Neurologic or orthopaedic disease* may make it difficult for the patient to engage in an exercise stress test. Modifications of stress testing, by use of a bicycle ergometer, for example, can sometimes circumvent these problems.

Patient Experience. The patient will be told that he will spend a total of 1 to $1\frac{1}{2}$ hours at the stress test laboratory; that he should not eat for at least 2 hours before the test; that the preceding meal should be light and should not contain butter, cream, coffee, tea or alcohol; and that he should wear clothes and shoes which are comfortable to walk in. He will also be told which of his regular medicines he should take on the day of the test (if he has not been told at the time the appointment was made, he should be instructed to telephone the stress test laboratory to inquire about his medication several days in advance). Before testing, ECG leads are applied to the chest and a blood pressure cuff is applied to one arm. The test consists of walking on a treadmill; the speed and the slope of the treadmill will be increased during the test. Alternatively, the test may consist of pedaling on a bicycle ergometer. The patient should be told that he will be asked to exercise to a point where he finds it uncomfortable; but that if he experiences chest pain, severe shortness of breath, claudication, or severe light-headedness, the test will be terminated. He should be told that he will not be asked to exercise to a degree inconsistent with his age and physical condition. The duration of the test will be determined by the time it takes to reach a maximum heart rate (usually no more than 10 to 15 min).

If radioactive scanning is included in the stress test (see below), the patient will receive an injection containing thallium-201 at the time of maximum exercise and will have cardiac scanning immediately after exercising and again 3 hours later.

OFFICE STRESS TESTING (MASTER'S TEST)

The use of submaximal office stress testing has decreased greatly in recent years. Popularized by Master and modified by many others, such studies have been replaced by maximal and near-maximal stress testing in specially equipped and staffed laboratories as described above. The utility and safety of doing any sort of exercise stress test in the office setting are questionable. The Master's two-step exercise test is much less sensitive than a treadmill exercise test; it will often be negative in patients with clinically evident ischemic heart diseases simply because the workload is insufficient to increase myocardial work significantly in many patients.

Radioisotopic Imaging (12)

Thallium-201 is the isotope most used for clinically assessing myocardial regional blood flow. Healthy myocardial cells rapidly extract thallium-201 shortly after it is injected intravenously; uptake is proportional to regional perfusion. Gamma emissions of low energy permit recording of the pattern of radioactivity. Areas of infarcted myocardium will show diminished or absent activity, so-called "cold spots." Perfusion defects are also seen in transiently ischemic muscles, and these defects disappear after the ischemic episode has passed.

Thallium-201 scans are commonly performed as part of an exercise stress test. Thallium is injected at the time of peak exercise, and images obtained shortly thereafter demonstrate the regional perfusion at the time of the stress. Images taken later will show redistribution of isotope if an abnormality revealed by the early images is due to transient ischemia; the abnormality will persist, however, or there will be only partial redistribution, if it is due to infarction.

Thallium scanning with exercise stress testing is more sensitive and more specific for detection of occlusive coronary artery disease than exercise stress testing alone (23). It is not reasonable, however, to recommend that all patients undergoing exercise testing should incur the additional expense of a thallium scan. The use of thallium with exercise stress testing is of particular value in those conditions which render ECG interpretation difficult or impossible—for example, left bundle branch block, Wolff-Parkinson-White syndrome, and patients who are more likely to have "false-positive" results of exercise stress tests, such as young patients (usually women) and patients with mitral valve prolapse or patients taking digitalis.

Besides its value in testing selected patients for exercise-related ischemia, thallium-201 scanning is useful in detecting evidence of a recent or remote myocardial infarction (e.g., in patients whose ECG shows nonspecific changes and whose event was too remote to be evaluated by measurement of cardiac enzymes). A resting defect on a thallium-201 scan is more sensitive than an ECG Q wave for identifying an old infarction.

Coronary Arteriography

Figure 54.2 shows diagrammatically the coronary arteries and their branches as they appear in angiogram images. Coronary arteriography provides direct information about the presence of coronary artery disease and about the distribution and severity of obstructing lesions. This procedure has greatly expanded our understanding of the prognosis of coronary artery disease (see below) and it has become a major tool for decision-making in the individual patient.

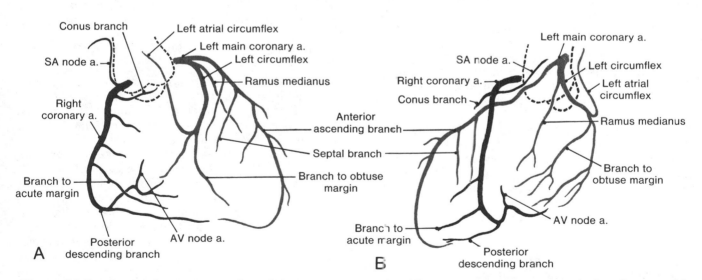

Figure 54.2 Anatomic representation of the coronary arteries. These vessels are represented as they would be seen on the angiogram. No attempt to convey the third dimension has been made. Careful study of the changes in position of the various branches with rotation of the heart is essential to intelligent interpretation of arteriograms. (*A*) Anteroposterior and (*B*) lateral. (Reprinted with permission from H. L. Abrams and D. F. Adams: The coronary arteriogram. First of two parts. Structural and functional aspects, *New England Journal of Medicine, 281:* 1276, 1969.)

INDICATIONS

Because of increasing experience and knowledge, a changing spectrum of indications for its use, and a variation in surgical aggressiveness concerning coronary artery disease, it is difficult to publish firm guidelines for the use of coronary arteriography. There are certain indications for coronary arteriography that are accepted generally. However, at the extremes are those who believe that coronary arteriography should be done as a last resort and those who believe that all (or almost all) patients with angina or myocardial infarction are suitable candidates for arteriographic study.

It is essential that a referring physician not abdicate his responsibility to a patient through the process of referral for catheterization and arteriography. The morbidity and mortality of the procedure in the chosen laboratory should be known. Ideally, each laboratory should systematically and periodically analyze its performance so that its results and risks are known to referring physicians.

The principal indications for arteriography are:

1. *To determine the operability* of patients who have failed maximal medical therapy (see below, p. 486). In such patients who have good left ventricular function there is about an 80% chance of operability. This indication is clear-cut since surgery offers an excellent chance for clinical improvement (see below, p. 486).

2. To permit *decisions concerning management in young patients with* coronary artery disease who desire to continue an active or stressful life-style; recommendations can best be made with knowledge of the anatomy of the disease and its prognosis (see below). This is particularly true if exercise stress testing or radioisotopic imaging suggests that there is a large amount of myocardium at risk of infarction.

3. To *detect left main or severe three-vessel coronary artery disease.* Patients with these lesions have a relatively higher mortality (see below, p. 481). Demonstration of the lesions is an indication for earlier surgery (see below).

4. To *evaluate patients who are being considered for noncoronary artery surgery* such as replacement of an aortic valve and who may benefit from preoperative assessment of the anatomy of the coronary arteries. In this way surgeons may elect to bypass some lesions or at least will know what lesions need to be bypassed if there are problems with left ventricular function during or immediately following cardiac surgery.

5. *To evaluate left ventricular performance.* If large segments of myocardium contract poorly or if overall ventricular performance is poor (as judged by measurement of ejection fraction or of left ventricular end-diastolic volume, see below), the risk of cardiac surgery is extremely high (18).

Technique and Patient Experience. Usually the patient is hospitalized the night before the catheterization. One hour before the procedure he is given a sedative, usually diazepam (Valium), 10 mg orally. What happens next depends upon the technique that is used.

By the Sones technique, an incision is made, under local anesthesia, over the right brachial artery, and the catheter is threaded through a small incision into the artery and then via the subclavian and brachiocephalic arteries into the aorta near the coronary sinuses. By the Judkins technique, a special catheter is inserted percutaneously into a femoral artery and then threaded up the aorta to the coronary sinuses. The tip of the catheter is moved into either the right or left sinus; contrast medium is injected; and then, under direct fluoroscopic visualization, the orifices of the right and left coronary arteries are injected sequentially with contrast medium. The patient is asked to hold his breath during the few seconds of the injection. The catheter used in the Judkins technique is designed to enter easily either the right or left artery, so that after one arterial system is visualized adequately, the catheter must be withdrawn and the complementary catheter must be inserted.

After the coronary circulation has been visualized, dye is injected directly into the left ventricular cavity to observe ventricular contraction and to look for aneurysms, mitral regurgitation, etc. (Another special catheter is introduced in the Judkins procedure for this phase of the study.) Ejection fraction (the ratio of stroke volume to end-diastolic volume) is measured, then the catheter is withdrawn, and (if the Sones technique has been used) the incisions are sutured.

During this procedure the patient feels slightly woozy from the sedation; there is no pain except for occasional mild midsternal burning when the dye is injected; he is usually discharged from the hospital the following day. (See also "Heart Catheterization," an illustrated brochure published for patients by the American Heart Association.)

COMPLICATIONS OF CORONARY ARTERIOGRAPHY

The major complications of coronary arteriography are death, myocardial infarction, and stroke. The minor complications include false aneurysms, arterial thrombosis, bleeding, allergy to contrast material (see Chapter 22), arrhythmias, and hypotension.

The risks of complications of coronary arteriography are related to the experience of the laboratory performing the studies and to the types of patients being studied. Risks will tend to be lower in young, otherwise healthy patients and higher in older patients with poor left ventricular function, particularly those with associated peripheral vascular disease. Risks are lower in those laboratories doing a large number of procedures and the low risk is related to the experience and proficiency of the team performing the study. In laboratories doing six or more procedures a week the overall mortality should be of the order of 0.1 (%). The risks of myocardial infarction and stroke should be comparable. Another way of evaluating the skill and proficiency of a laboratory is to look at the incidence of studies that had to be repeated because of inconclusive results with the original study. It should not be necessary to repeat more than 1–2% of studies. A newly established facility may take some time to reach a critical volume of coronary arteriographic studies before which there may be a higher risk of major and minor complications as well as an increased incidence of repeated studies.

INTERPRETATION OF CORONARY ARTERIOGRAPHY

There is often considerable variation among observers in the interpretation of coronary arteriograms. If there is 70% or more obstruction of a coronary artery, a significant impairment of coronary blood flow, even at rest, may be expected. A 50% narrowing may produce no significant decrease in flow at rest, but may produce serious physiologic impairment when there is an increase in myocardial oxygen demand. Sometimes the consulting cardiologist will utilize the combined results of stress testing and arteriography to decide whether a given coronary lesion may be important enough to consider bypassing. For example, marked ST depression with an exercise stress test associated with chest pain may indicate that there is a severe decrease in flow through a left anterior descending coronary artery even when the arteriogram demonstrates a lesion that is 50% or less obstructive.

PROGNOSIS

Mortality

The crude annual mortality rate after the onset of angina in persons without known infarction is about 5% (15). One-year survivors of an acute myocardial infarction have a similar long term prognosis. In contrast, the crude first-year mortality rate ranges between 5% and 10% for patients with unstable angina, for patients surviving 30 days after myocardial infarction, and for patients with stable angina of 2½ years' duration (2, 15, 20).

Stress testing (see above) helps to detect those patients with angina who have relatively good or relatively poor prognoses. Patients with typical symptoms of ischemia who have positive exercise stress tests have an annual incidence of subsequent events and mortality which is higher than patients who have negative stress tests (9). Symptomatic patients with equivocal tests will have intermediate risks. The prognosis is worse when ST depression is more down sloping, when the ST depression occurs earlier during exercise, when the degree to which the ST segments are depressed increases and when the ST depression persists longer after termination of exercise. This information may be helpful in selecting patients for further studies such as coronary arteriography.

Coronary arteriography (see above) identifies with considerable precision those subsets of patients with

relatively poor or relatively good prognoses, regardless of clinical manifestations of their coronary artery disease. The same anatomic spectrum of disease is found in patients with angina of various degrees, in patients with myocardial infarction without angina, and in patients with myocardial infarction plus angina of various degrees (21), i.e., these people have similar distributions of significant lesions in the left main (about 10%), left anterior descending (about 80%), left circumflex (about 65%), and right coronary (about 70%) arteries. However, longitudinal studies of patients who have had arteriograms have disclosed that the distribution of disease correlates with the risk of dying of the disease (14). In the first year after diagnosis, there is about a 30% mortality in patients with left main coronary artery disease and about a 15% mortality in patients with three-vessel disease (left anterior descending plus left circumflex plus right coronary). The first-year mortality is about 10% for patients with two-vessel disease, 8% with one-vessel disease when that vessel is the left anterior descending coronary artery, and about 5% when single vessel disease involves the circumflex or right coronary artery (3). Longer term studies show an annual mortality of about 10% in patients with three-vessel disease, about 7% in patients with two-vessel disease, and about 2% in patients with single vessel disease (3). The higher first year mortality is probably related to the events which prompted arteriographic studies in the first place.

Chapter 55 provides additional information about prognosis for subsets of patients with unstable angina or recent myocardial infarction.

Morbidity

Although angina may spontaneously remit after it has been present for a long interval (15) (either as a consequence of myocardial infarction or of collateral circulation), the *usual course* is one of periodic symptoms and, for many patients, progressive disease (gradually worsening angina, unstable angina, myocardial infarction, congestive heart failure, arrhythmias, or sudden death). Within 5 years of the onset of angina, about 1 in 4 men and 1 in 8 women will have a myocardial infarction (15).

The impact of angina upon a *patient's functional capacity* depends upon the nature of his usual activities and upon the status of his disease. As described below, pharmacologic and nonpharmacologic measures can make an important impact upon the limitation of activity created by angina, even though such measures usually make no impact upon the mortality risk. Overall, many patients with angina can continue to engage in most or all of their usual activities.

TREATMENT OF ANGINA PECTORIS

Medical Treatment

The basic objective in treating patients with angina pectoris is to relieve or prevent pain by improving

Table 54.4
Selected Drugs Used in the Treatment of Angina[a]

Class	Brand Name	Available Strengths	Usual Starting Dose	Usual Maximum Dose	Onset	Duration
NITRATES						
Nitroglycerin	Nitrostat and others	0.15-, 0.30-, 0.40-, 0.60-mg tablets, sublingual	1 tablet (0.4 mg) at time of, or in anticipation of, pain	2–3 tablets at time of pain	30 sec	3–5 min
Erythrityl tetranitrate	Cardilate	5-, 10-, 15-mg tablets, oral or sublingual; 10-mg tablets, chewable	5 mg sublingually in anticipation of pain or 10 mg oral or chewed 3 times a day	100 mg a day in divided doses	5 min (sublingual and chewed), 30 min (oral)	4 hr
Isosorbide dinitrate	Isordil, Sorbitrate and others	5-, 10-, 20-mg tablets, oral; 40-mg tablets or capsules, oral	10 mg every 4–6 hr	60–80 mg every 4 hr	15–30 min	4–6 hr
Nitroglycerin topical[b]	Nitro-Bid, Nitrol	2% ointment	½ inch every 4–6 hr as needed	4–5 inches every 3–4 hr	30–60 min	3–6 hr
Pentaerythritol tetranitrate	Peritrate and others	10-, 20-, 40-mg tablets, oral	10–20 mg 3 or 4 times a day	40 mg 4 times a day	30 min	4–6 hr
β-ADRENERGIC BLOCKERS						
Propranolol	Inderal	10-, 20-, 40-, 80-mg tablets, oral	10–20 mg 3 or 4 times a day	320 mg a day in divided doses	1–1.5 hr	4–6 hr
Nadolol	Corgard	40-, 80-, 120-mg tablets, oral	40 mg once a day	240 mg	1–2 hr	24 hr

[a] Other drugs, other doses of the drugs listed, and combinations of different drugs are marketed. The drugs and dosages shown are the ones most often used.
[b] A transdermal preparation has recently been released (see text).

the relationship between myocardial oxygen demand and supply (see above). This objective can be attained by increasing coronary blood flow and/or by decreasing myocardial oxygen demand. Angina occurring with exercise is due usually to an increase in myocardial oxygen demand which cannot be met because of fixed arterial obstruction. A decrease in or cessation of the work that produced angina usually results in a prompt reduction in myocardial oxygen demand. Thus, rest or a decrease in the level of activity may relieve angina in 1–2 min. When anxiety is a contributing or provoking factor, it may take longer for myocardial work to decrease and the episode of angina may be prolonged.

The major advance in the medical management of angina in recent years has been the demonstration that long acting nitrates and β-blocking agents can decrease the frequency of anginal attacks and can increase the exercise tolerance and work capacity of many angina sufferers. In general, the duration or intensity of exercise before angina is doubled when these drugs are used optimally.

Table 54.4 lists practical information about the drugs used most often in the treatment of angina.

NITRATES

Traditionally, nitroglycerin and related compounds have been the mainstay of the treatment of patients with angina pectoris. Initially these agents were thought to increase coronary blood flow by producing coronary artery dilation. Although nitrates may increase coronary blood flow in patients with spasm (see "Variant Angina" below) or may increase collateral flow to obstructed vessels, evidence suggests strongly that the mechanism of action of nitrates in most patients is not due to an increase in blood flow but to a decrease in myocardial oxygen demand. Thus, the beneficial effect of nitrates in patients with angina is due primarily to their effects on peripheral vessels. These compounds produce dilation of the venous circulation which in turn reduces venous return and decreases ventricular volume. The decrease in ventricular volume improves the efficiency of the heart and decreases wall tension. These effects reduce myocardial oxygen demand. Nitrates also produce, to a lesser degree, arterial dilation, thereby reducing the resistance to ventricular ejection, and these effects also produce a decrease in myocardial oxygen demand since they reduce left ventricular work.

Sublingual nitroglycerin is still the drug of choice for the relief and the prevention of discrete episodes of angina pectoris in most patients. In many patients with mild or infrequent angina, nitroglycerin is often the only medication required for the prevention or relief of pain. The initial dose should be small (0.4

mg) in order to minimize its unpleasant side effects (e.g., flushing, headache, light-headedness) in those patients in whom higher doses may be unnecessary.

Patients should be taught that it is important that their pain be relieved as soon as possible. Since many patients experience some premonitory symptoms before the development of chest pain, they should be instructed to take the nitroglycerin whenever they feel such symptoms. Use of nitroglycerin in this way may do more than simply prevent ischemic pain. Angina produces some anxiety which may increase heart rate and left ventricular contractility, increasing myocardial oxygen demand further. In turn, ischemia may be increased and the duration and severity of the pain may both be increased. Additionally, some patients, during periods of ischemia, develop serious arrhythmias, hypotension, or incipient heart failure which prompt administration of nitroglycerin may prevent. If pain is not relieved by 2 to 3 tablets of nitroglycerin or if tablets must be taken more often than every 30 to 60 min, the patient should be instructed to call his physician *immediately*, because of the danger of impending myocardial infarction (see "Unstable Angina" below). Since nitroglycerin may lose potency on storage, the physician should advise patients not to keep tablets longer then 3 to 4 months after opening the bottle; and that if pain is not relieved (especially if the side effects the patient usually notes are also absent) the problem may be due to a change in the drug rather than to a change in cardiac status. Prophylactic use of nitroglycerin is of particular value in patients who have mild or moderate angina in response to specific and reproducible stresses. For example, the patient who develops angina after walking from a car to a place of work can be taught to take nitroglycerin after the car is parked, wait a few minutes, and then walk to work, thereby preventing pain altogether. The use of prophylactic nitroglycerin before sexual intercourse may also prevent angina and alleviate the anxiety that is naturally associated with sexual activity when angina is anticipated.

It is important to teach the patient to use sublingual nitroglycerin correctly. The patient should take it while he is sitting to maximize the vasodilating effect (reduced in the supine position) and to avoid possible untoward effects of hypotension (increased in the standing position). When initiating treatment with sublingual nitroglycerin, it is advisable to administer the first dose in the office so that the patient can experience the side effects and receive reassurance from a physician or nurse that this is an expected response. Patients who start taking nitroglycerin at home may otherwise become so frightened by side effects that they may delay taking it or may avoid its use altogether. The most common side effects are flushing and headache; both may diminish with increasing usage of the drug.

Long Acting Nitrates. In recent years, it has been shown that long acting nitrates have a very important role in the control of angina. As shown in Table 54.4, long acting nitrates are available in a variety of preparations.

Careful studies of small numbers of patients have confirmed the clinical efficacy of two preparations— nitroglycerin ointment and isosorbide tablets (8, 22). Both of these preparations produce about a 50% increase in the exercise time before symptoms appear. These effects last from 4 to 6 hours after drug administration. Patients restudied on an average of 6 months after beginning isosorbide tablets maintained the same increase in exercise tolerance (8). The dose of nitrate needed to improve symptoms may be relatively high; fortunately, available preparations permit a great deal of flexibility in dose adjustment, as shown in Table 54.4.

In selecting among available preparations, the major considerations should be the known efficacy and convenience of a particular nitrate for the patient. Using these criteria, isosorbide is probably the best choice for ambulatory patients. The disadvantages of nitroglycerin ointment are that it is messy to apply, that it is difficult to apply similar amounts evenly each time, and that skin irritation may occur after prolonged use. Its major advantage is that it can be removed promptly if a patient develops a significant side effect (e.g., severe hypotension) shortly after it is applied. Many patients are treated in the hospital with nitroglycerin ointments; if its disadvantages become apparent after discharge, substitution of isosorbide is the best plan. (A recently released preparation of nitroglycerin (e.g., Transderm-Nitro) may obviate the disadvantages of the paste. It provides controlled release of 5 or 10 mg/day of nitroglycerin through a semipermeable membrane applied to the skin by means of an adhesive tape.)

The side effects of long acting nitrates are similar to those produced by sublingual nitrates. Many patients will have already experienced the headache produced by sublingual nitroglycerin before being treated with a long acting preparation. Because of persistent headache, some patients are unable to take long acting nitrates, although in most patients this is not a problem. Because long acting nitrates can produce orthostatic hypotension, and occasionally syncope, it is very important to check a patient's orthostatic blood pressure response before and after initiating or increasing a long acting nitrate. The two relative contraindications to long acting nitrates are a history of migraine or cluster headache and demonstrated orthostatic hypotension before initiating treatment.

β-BLOCKING AGENTS

β-Blockade by drugs such as propranolol (Inderal) effectively reduces the frequency and/or severity of angina in many patients.

In many respects β-blockade is an ideal approach

to the treatment of angina. It decreases heart rate, decreases contractility, and in many patients decreases systemic blood pressure. Any of these effects alone or in combination reduces myocardial oxygen consumption.

Since β-blocking agents decrease myocardial contractility and may increse left ventricular volume, they must be used with care in patients with cardiomegaly. In patients without failure or cardiac enlargement the beneficial effects on heart rate, contractility, and systemic blood pressure usually override the potential disadvantages of the side effects.

An added benefit for patients with ischemic heart disease is that β-blockade often effectively prevents arrhythmias. It may decrease or eliminate premature ventricular contractions (PVCs), and the ventricular rate in patients with atrial fibrillation may be decreased also. Decreasing PVCs is beneficial to patients with ischemic heart disease because such patients are at increased risk of ventricular tachycardia or ventricular fibrillation (5), particularly during an episode of ischemia. Furthermore, when PVCs are frequent, the number of hemodynamically effective beats is diminished, thus decreasing coronary as well as peripheral perfusion. In patients who are in atrial fibrillation, decreasing the ventricular response improves left ventricular dynamics by decreasing heart rate, increasing the diastolic filling period, and decreasing myocardial oxygen consumption.

The dose of propranolol or other β-blockers can be increased weekly until the desired effect is obtained. The heart rate is the best guide to maximal treatment; sinus bradycardia at a rate between 50 and 60 beats per min is a reasonable goal. It should be recognized that the doses necessary to produce bradycardia and to relieve angina pectoris vary considerably (see Table 54.4).

One of the most serious side effects of propranolol is increasing heart failure, which may be expressed first as decreased exercise tolerance. Reducing the dose and/or adding digitalis (7) may improve cardiac compensation and at the same time reduce the severity or frequency of anginal attacks. Propranolol is contraindicated in patients with intrinsic asthma. A history of allergic asthma or of bronchospasm during pulmonary infections should therefore be sought in all patients for whom propranolol is being considered. Furthermore, patients with chronic obstructive lung disease may develop increased bronchospasm from propranolol even if they have no history of allergic or intrinsic asthma; therefore, the drug should be used with caution, if at all, in these patients. Other relative contraindications for propranolol are insulin use (propranolol may block symptoms and signs of hypoglycemia) and peripheral arterial disease, particularly Raynaud's disease. Other side effects of propranolol include rash, fever, impotence, abdominal pain, nausea, gastric dilatation, depression, bad dreams, lethargy, and fatigue. The lethargy and fatigue may diminish with time without a reduction in dosage.

Other β-Blocking Agents. Because of the very extensive experience to date with propranolol, it remains the beta blocker of choice for patients with angina. Nadolol (Corgard) is the only other β-blocker which has been approved (in 1982) by the FDA for use in angina. Its unique advantage is its long half-life which permits administration once daily; because it is excreted entirely by the kidneys, the interval between doses should be increased in patients with renal insufficiency. In comparison studies it has been shown to be equivalent to propranolol in controlling angina. Metoprolol (Lopressor) and atenolol were still being reviewed for use in angina in 1982.

INITIATING AND ADJUSTING LONG ACTING DRUGS FOR ANGINA

Either a nitrate preparation or propranolol can be tried initially. If the patient fails to improve at the usual starting dose (see Table 54.4), the dose can be increased weekly until a response is achieved. If the type of treatment selected initially fails to help at a maximally tolerated dose, the other type can be added or substituted. Since the nitrates and beta blockers decrease myocardial oxygen demand by different mechanisms, the continued use of the two types of therapy is quite reasonable.

A number of relative contraindications to either long acting nitrates or β-blockers have been mentioned above; these contraindications are important in selecting the initial type of treatment in some patients.

Because of the known risk of precipitating worsening angina when a β-blocker is abruptly discontinued and because of indirect evidence for a similar problem when long acting nitrates are abruptly discontinued, these should always be tapered over 1 to 2 weeks when they are being stopped. Clearly, it is very important to warn all patients of the problems so that they do not casually stop and start these drugs; a corollary to this is the importance of explaining that these drugs are being prescribed chiefly to prevent symptoms, so that patients whose symptoms remit do not conclude that they can try stopping medication themselves.

A good argument can be made for administering propranolol to all patients with angina unless there is a specific contraindication. In patients who have infrequent or mild episodes of angina relieved promptly by rest or nitroglycerin, however, propranolol may add little or no benefit. In patients with more frequent or more severe episodes of angina, it is reasonable to initiate treatment with propranolol and to prescribe nitroglycerin for the relief of discrete episodes of pain. If propranolol is effective in reducing or eliminating angina pectoris, additional preparations may be unnecessary. In patients with maximal effects from β-blockade who continue to have pain, addition of a long acting nitrate preparation may bring symptoms under better control.

Since patients who fail to improve after *maximal medical management* for angina pectoris are considered candidates for coronary arteriography and possible surgery, it is important to define what maximal medical therapy constitutes. In practical terms, administration of propranolol in increasing doses, until bradycardia or side effects militate against further increase, in conjunction with a dose of long acting nitrates increased to the point where side effects begin to become intolerable, would be considered to constitute maximal medical management in most patients.

NEWER DRUGS

A new class of drugs that block the uptake of calcium ions by cell membranes has been developed recently. The most promising drug of this class is nifedipine. It is ordinarily prescribed in dosages of 10 to 30 mg every 6 hours. It appears to be as effective as nitroglycerin and propranolol in the treatment of stable angina pectoris and perhaps more effective in the treatment of coronary spasm (see below) (26). Because of limited experience with this drug, it would be prudent for the practitioner to prescribe it only after consultation with a cardiologist.

OTHER THERAPEUTIC CONSIDERATIONS

There are a number of other important considerations in the treatment of patients with angina.

Physical conditioning can improve the exercise tolerance of patients with stable angina (16). For interested patients, referral to a physician-supervised exercise program is the best plan. In recent years, most large communities have developed such programs for patients with coronary artery disease. Chapter 55 describes the physiologic basis of physical conditioning and describes a supervised exercise program for cardiac patients. The booklet entitled "Exercise Testing and Training of Individuals with Heart Disease or at High Risk for its Development: A Handbook for Physicians," available from the American Heart Association, provides additional information on this subject.

In addition to recommending exercise programs for selected patients, the physician should counsel patients with angina about physical activities which may increase their symptoms and should always ask them to raise any matters of concern about their regular activities. The energy requirements for a broad range of activities are summarized in Table 55.4 of the following chapter.

Hypertension is often present in patients with angina. There is a linear relationship between left ventricular work and myocardial oxygen demand (see above), and left ventricular ejection pressure increases in response to an increase in peripheral vascular resistance. Both systolic and diastolic hyperten-

sion can affect myocardial oxygen demand in this way. The physician should always attempt to reduce resting blood pressure to normal in patients with chronic hypertension, including those with isolated systolic hypertension. A reduction in blood pressure from 160/100 mm Hg to 130/85 mm Hg may achieve a reduction of 15% or 20% in myocardial oxygen demand. This can be of crucial importance in reducing the frequency and severity of angina pectoris in the hypertensive patient. Although any sympatholytic antihypertensive agent is reasonable in the hypertensive patient with angina (see Chapter 59), since propranolol has other antianginal properties and may control hypertension without diuretics in some patients, it is an excellent choice.

It is important to achieve a maximal level of pulmonary compensation in patients with angina and coexisting *lung disease* (see Chapter 52). Chronic hypoxemia and acidosis and the increased work of breathing in patients with pulmonary disease increase myocardial oxygen demand, or decrease myocardial oxygen delivery, or both. Abstinence from cigarettes, avoidance of environmental pollutants, and the judicious use of bronchodilators are also important in the overall management of such patients. In heavy smokers without clinical lung disease, a decrease in smoking may also decrease susceptibility to angina by eliminating the inhalation of carbon monoxide in tobacco smoke. Carbon monoxide exposure in heavy traffic should also be avoided in patients whose angina is precipitated in this setting.

The physician should never overlook the possibility of *hyperthyroidism* (Chapter 70) in patients with angina, particularly in those with increasing angina. Often, particularly in the older patient, other obvious signs of hyperthyroidism may not be present. For example, hyperthyroidism may be manifest only by an increased frequency or severity of angina, an increase in heart rate in people with atrial fibrillation, or by increasing heart failure.

Anemia also requires serious consideration, particularly when the hemoglobin concentration falls below 7 g/dl. This is the point at which cardiac output must increase to maintain peripheral oxygen delivery at rest.

Heart failure (Chapter 58) in patients with angina should always be treated. The real possibility that latent heart failure exists in patients with angina decubitus or nocturnal angina should be considered. Diuretics or the use of digitalis may be effective in such patients and may reduce the frequency and severity of angina or eliminate angina altogether.

Surgical Management of Angina Pectoris

Coronary artery bypass surgery is one of the most common surgical procedures performed in this country today. Our knowledge concerning the indications for the surgery and the effects of revascularization procedures on the coronary circulation and on morbidity and mortality is still developing. It is accepted generally that patients with incapacitating angina pectoris who have good left ventricular function and who have failed maximal medical therapy should be considered as candidates for coronary arteriography (see above) and subsequent surgery. It has been demonstrated that patients with left main coronary disease or its equivalent benefit symptomatically and have increased longevity following procedures designed to increase coronary blood flow (27). Recommendations regarding surgery for patients with lesions other than left main coronary lesions depend upon the consultant cardiologists' overall assessment of the patient.

The two surgical methods used today consist of saphenous vein bypass graft or implantation of an internal mammary artery into the native coronary artery circulation. The procedure that is used is often based on the surgeon's preference or experience. A well illustrated brochure, "Coronary Artery Bypass Surgery," which explains the procedure and the patient's experience, is available from the American Heart Association.

About 60% of *properly selected patients* will have complete (or nearly complete) relief of angina pectoris, and another 20% will have a significant decrease in angina (19). There will be a demonstrable increase in exercise tolerance following surgery in about 60 to 80% of such patients.

Patients with good left ventricular function have a 1 to 2% mortality rate from surgery. In addition, about 10% of patients will develop evidence of myocardial infarction during the perioperative period. The risk of complications from myocardial infarction in these patients, however, is small. The infarct occurs at a time when myocardial oxygen need is diminished because the patient is on cardiopulmonary bypass, and the infarct occurs in a setting where complications such as arrhythmias are recognized and treated promptly. Nevertheless, it does represent a risk as well as loss of functioning myocardium. Perioperative infarction is more likely to occur in patients with severe disease distal to a proximal obstruction.

Whether bypass surgery prolongs survival in patients without left main coronary artery disease or its equivalent is not entirely clear (4). The published studies do not provide a definitive answer in this regard. Until additional data are available, surgery should be recommended in this population primarily to improve the quality of life in patients who have failed a medical regimen and who have good ventricular function.

UNSTABLE ANGINA

Unstable angina is a term used to describe pain due to cardiac ischemia which is becoming more intense, is occurring more frequently—often provoked by diminishing effort (perhaps even at rest—

see below) and is being relieved less readily by nitroglycerin. The syndrome has also been called *crescendo angina* and *preinfarction angina*. Sometimes unstable angina will develop in a patient with previously stable, reasonably controlled angina; at other times, it will develop in a patient with recent onset of ischemic symptoms. During the episode, the ECG shows ST elevation or depression and/or T wave inversion which revert to normal when the pain has abated. Because of the increased risks of myocardial infarction and of sudden death and because of the need for aggressive medical therapy, patients with unstable angina should be hospitalized. Coronary arteriography is indicated in patients whose pain is not controlled by medical therapy to determine their suitability for coronary bypass surgery.

The prognosis and the medical management of these patients after hospital discharge is described in Chapter 55.

VARIANT ANGINA

Variant angina (*Prinzmetal's angina*) is, in a sense, unstable in that it occurs usually at rest but, unlike typical angina, does not occur on exertion or in response to emotional stress. Attacks of pain are experienced often at the same time each day, frequently awakening the patient early in the morning. During the attacks, there is ST segment elevation which reverts to baseline when the attack is over; there are also, in about a third of the patients, transient atrioventricular blocks and/or arrhythmias (including ventricular tachycardia or fibrillation). Unlike unstable angina, pain is usually promptly relieved by sublingual nitroglycerin.

It is now clear that *coronary artery spasm* (13) often plays a major role in the pathogenesis of variant angina. Two groups of patients have been identified. By far the larger group (85% of patients) have fixed, often proximal, obstruction of a major coronary artery; angina in this group frequently is associated with spasm of the artery near the site of obstruction. The variant syndrome in this group of patients commonly follows months or years of stable typical angina pectoris or follows a myocardial infarction. The ST elevation during the attack is likely to reflect anterolateral ischemia.

The smaller group with variant angina (15% of patients) have normal coronary arteries, but have spasm of one of the arteries that reduces blood supply to the myocardium, resulting in ischemic pain. These patients are usually younger than patients in the larger group and are predominantly women. There is usually no history of typical angina or of myocardial infarction. The ST elevation during the attack is confirmed by arteriography, either by the spontaneous occurrence of an attack during the procedure or by induction of an attack by the administration of ergonovine. Arteriography is important because patients with normal coronary arteries are obviously not candidates for bypass surgery and even patients with obstruction as well as spasm respond indifferently as a group.

β-Blocking agents such as propranolol are *contraindicated* in patients with variant angina. These drugs may potentiate coronary artery spasm because they allow α-adrenergic vasoconstriction to proceed unopposed by β-adrenergic activity. Therefore, nitroglycerin is the principal drug available for treatment of the condition. The recently released calcium channel blocking agent, nifedipine, appears to be effective in preventing spasm. Patients not controlled by nitrates may be prescribed this drug in dosages of 10 to 30 mg every 6 hours, but it would be prudent, since there is not yet widespread experience with it, to consult a cardiologist first.

References

General

Cohn, PF and Braunwald, E: Chronic coronary artery disease. In *Heart Disease, Vol. 2*, edited by E. Braunwald. W.B. Saunders, Philadelphia, 1980.
   A complete current discussion of the diagnosis and management of angina pectoris
Diamond, GA and Forrester, JS: Analysis of probability as an aid in the clinical diagnosis of coronary-artery disease. *N Engl. J Med 300:* 1350, 1979.
   A review of the application of Bayes' theorem to this problem.
Heberden, W: Commentaries on the history and cure of diseases. Available from the New York Academy of Science, Hofner Publishing Co., New York, 1962.
   The original, accurate, description of angina pectoris.

Specific

1. American Heart Association: Risk factors and coronary disease: A statement for physicians. *Circulation 62:* 449A, 1980.
2. Block, WJ, Jr, Grumpacher, EL, Dry, TJ and Gage, RP: Prognosis of angina pectoris. *JAMA 150:* 259, 1952.
3. Bruschke, AVG, Proudfit, WL and Sones, FM, Jr: Progress study of 590 consecutive nonsurgical cases of coronary disease followed 5–9 years; I. Arteriographic correlations. *Circulation 47:* 1147, 1973.
4. Chalmers, TC, Proudfit, WL, Feinstein, AR and DiBona, GF: Symposium: the scientific uses and abuses of the clinical trial: treatment of chronic stable angina with saphenous vein bypass grafting. Randomized Veterans Administration Cooperative Study. *Clin Res 26:* 229, 1978.
5. Chiang, BN, Perlman, LV and Ostrander, LD: Relationship of premature systoles to coronary heart disease and sudden death in the Tecumseh epidemiologic study. *Ann Intern Med 70:* 1159, 1969.
6. Cohn, PF, Gorlin, R, Vokonas, PS, Williams, RA and Herman, MV: A quantitative clinical index for the diagnosis of symptomatic coronary-artery disease. *N Engl J Med 286:* 901, 1972.
7. Crawford, MH, LeWinter, MM, O'Rourke, RA, Karliner, JS and Ross, Jr, J: Combined propranolol and digoxin therapy in angina pectoris. *Ann Intern Med 83:* 449, 1975.
8. Danahy, DT and Aronow, WS: Hemodynamics and antianginal effects of high dose oral isosorbide dinitrate after chronic use. *Circulation 56:* 205, 1977.
9. Ellstad, MH and Wan, MKC: Predictive implications of stress

testing: follow-up of 2700 subjects after maximum treadmill stress testing. *Circulation 51:* 363, 1975.
10. Gazes, PC Mobley, EM, Jr, Faris, HM, Jr, Duncan, R and Humphries, GB: Preinfarction (unstable) angina—a prospective study Ten years followup. Prognostic significance of electrocardiographic changes. *Circulation 48:* 331, 1973.
11. Goldberger, AL: Recognition of ECG pseudo-infarct patterns. *Mod. Concepts of Cardiovasc Dis 49:* 13 (March), 1980.
12. Hamilton, GW: Myocardial imaging with Thallium-201: the controversy over its clinical usefulness in ischemic heart disease. *J Nucl Med 20:* 1201, 1979.
13. Hilles, LD and Braunwald, E: Coronary-artery spasm. *N Engl J Med 299:* 695, 1978.
14. Humphries, JO, Kuller, L, Ross, RS, Friesinger, GC and Page, EE: Natural history of ischemic heart disease in relation to arteriographic findings. A twelve year study of 224 patients. *Circulation 49:* 489, 1974.
15. Kannel, WB and Feinleib, M: Natural history of angina pectoris in the Framingham study: prognosis and survival. *Am J Cardiol 29:* 154, 1972.
16. Kennedy, CC, Spiekerman, RE, Lindsay, Jr, MI, Mankin, HT, Frye, RL and McCallister, BD: One-year graduated exercise program for men with angina pectoris. *Mayo Clin Proc 51:* 231, 1976.
17. Mattingly, TW, Robb, GP and Marks, HH: Stress tests in the detection of coronary disease. *Postgrad Med 24:* 4, 1958.
18. Mitchel, BF, Alivizatos, PA, Adam, M, Guster, GF, Thiele, JP and Lambert, CJ: Myocardial revascularization in patients with poor ventricular function. *J Thorac Cardiovasc Surg 69:* 52, 1975.
19. Mundth, ED and Austen, WG: Surgical measures for coronary heart disease. *New Eng J Med 293:* 13, 75 and 124, 1975.
20. Norris, RM, Caughey, DE, Mercer, CJ and Scott, PJ: Prognosis after myocardial infarction. Six-year follow-up. *Br Heart J 36:* 786, 1974.
21. Proudfit, WL, Shirley, EK and Sones, FM, Jr: Distribution of arterial lesions demonstrated by selective coronary arteriography. *Circulation 36:* 54, 1967.
22. Reichek, N, Goldstein, RE, Redwood, DR and Epstein, ST: Sustained effects of nitroglycerin ointment in patients with angina pectoris. *Circulation 50:* 348, 1974.
23. Ritchie, JL, Zaret, BL, Strauss, HW, Pitt, B, Berman, DS, Schelbert, HR, Ashburn, WL, Berger, HJ and Hamilton, GW: Myocardial imaging with thallium-201: a multicenter study in patients with angina pectoris or acute myocardial infarction. *Am J Cardiol 42:* 345, 1978.
24. Rochmis, P and Blackburn, H: Exercise tests: a survey of procedures, safety, and litigation experience in approximately 170,000 tests. *JAMA 217:* 1061, 1971.
25. Sonnenblick, EH and Strobeck, JE: Derived indexes of ventricular and myocardial function. *N Engl J Med 296:* 978, 1977.
26. Stone, PH, Antman, EM, Muller, JE and Braunwald, E: Calcium channel blocking agents in the treatment of cardiovascular disorders; II. Hemodynamic effects and clinical applications. *Ann Intern Med 93:* 886, 1980.
27. Takaro, T, Hultgren, HW, Lipton, MJ, Detre, KM, and participants in the study group: The V.A. cooperative randomized study of surgery for coronary arterial occlusive disease; II. Subgroup with significant left main lesions. *Circulation 54 (suppl) III:* 107, 1976.
28. Taylor, SSH: Reversible left-ventricular failure in angina pectoris. *Lancet 2:* 902, 1970.
29. Weiner, DA, Ryan TJ, McCabe, CH, Kennedy, JW, Schloss, M, Tristani, F, Chaitman, BR and Fisher, LD: Exercise stress testing. Correlations among history of angina, ST-segment response and prevalence of coronary-artery disease in the coronary surgery study (CASS). *N Engl J Med 301:* 230, 1979.

CHAPTER FIFTY-FIVE

Rehabilitation after Myocardial Infarction

MAHMUD A. THAMER, M.D., and L. RANDOL BARKER, M.D.

EPIDEMIOLOGY

Care of the patient who has survived a myocardial infarction (MI) is a common problem in ambulatory practice. There are roughly seven million survivors of myocardial infarction in the United States at any time. Each year, there is an addition of approximately one million persons to this group, and about one million die (3). About two-thirds of survivors have had uncomplicated MIs and therefore have relatively good long term prognoses.

The majority of persons who have MIs are under the age of 60. It is estimated that in the United States 1 man in 5 will have an MI before the age of 60 and that 1 out of 10 to 15 men in this age group will die of atherosclerotic heart disease. These risks are 2 to 3 times lower in women (28).

Two epidemiologic observations underscore the importance of ambulatory care in reducing mortality due to coronary artery disease (CAD):

1. About three-quarters of all deaths from CAD occur outside the hospital.

2. In the past decade, the number of people dying of CAD in the United States has decreased about 17% (29); this decrease seems to be largely due to changes which have occurred outside the hospital (i.e., reduction in CAD risk factors and pre-hospital and post-discharge mangement of acute MI).

PROGNOSIS

Patients discharged following hospitalization in coronary care units (CCU) may be divided into three broad categories: those who have had a confirmed MI; those who have had unstable angina; and those who have had cardiac arrest without a confirmed MI. The different prognoses for patients in these three categories have been delineated in the past decade.

Survivors of Myocardial Infarction

MORTALITY

The overall first year mortality for hospital survivors of an MI is about 5 to 10%. Thereafter, the annual mortality remains between 3 and 5% for the next 15 years. These figures are the same for patients surviving transmural or subendocardial MIs (Fig. 55.1). Most of the deaths in the first year occur during the 3 months following discharge, and they occur chiefly in patients with one or more of the high risk characteristics listed in Table 55.1.

The classification of acute MI according to the presence and severity of congestive heart failure (CHF) on admission to the CCU developed by Killip is one of the most useful prognostic indices. Class I patients have no evidence of congestive failure on admission; class II patients have mild CHF; class III patients present with pulmonary edema; and class IV patients present with shock. Figure 55.2 shows the strikingly different survival rates among persons in these four classes, ranging from a 2-year survival rate

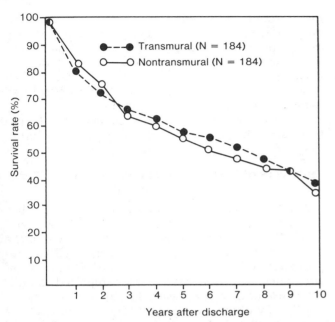

Figure 55.1 Survival rates in matched samples of transmural and nontransmural myocardial infarction patients discharged alive in metropolitan Baltimore, 7/1/66 to 6/30/67 and 1/1/71 to 12/31/71. (*Source:* M. Szklo *et al.*: Nontransmural MI: Prognostic implications, *Primary Cardiology, 6:* 76, 1980.)

Table 55.1
Characteristics Associated with Increase in Mortality following Discharge of Patients Who Have Had Myocardial Infarction (MI)[a]

ADMISSION CHARACTERISTICS:
  Congestive heart failure (chest X-ray or Killip classification) (2, 21)
  History of hypertension (32)
  Extent of left ventricular ischemia (radionuclide scintigraphy, cardiac enzymes) (7, 27)
CHARACTERISTICS AT DISCHARGE:
  History of a previous MI (32)
  Early (within 10 days) post-MI angina, with transient ST-T changes (25)[b]
  Ejection fraction ≤40% (radionuclide ventriculography, arteriography) (24, 32)
  Complex ventricular arrhythmia[c] (Holter monitor) (24)
  Proximal left or three-vessel coronary artery occlusive disease (arteriography) (32)
CHARACTERISTICS FOLLOWING DISCHARGE:
  Positive submaximal ECG stress test 2–3 weeks after MI (30)
  ECG abnormalities, especially S-T segment depression, ≥3 months after MI (33)
  Cigarette smoking (37)

[a] Numbers in parentheses are references.
[b] Mortality risk highest when ECG shows "ischemia at a distance," i.e., transient ischemic S-T changes in a myocardial location which is different from the location of the patient's MI.
[c] Multifocal premature ventricular contractions (PVCs), runs of two or more sequential ectopic ventricular beats, or PVCs with R on T pattern.

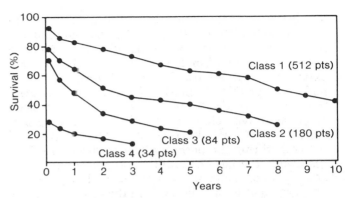

Figure 55.2 Survival after acute myocardial infarction based upon Killip classification (810 patients admitted to the Duke Medical Center Coronary Care Unit from 1967 to 1978). (*Source:* R. A. Rosati and P. J. Harris: *Prognosis: Contemporary Outcomes of Disease,* edited by J. Fries and G. E. Ehrlich, The Charles Press Publishers, Bowie, Md., 1981.)

of about 80% in Class I to less than 20% in class IV (21).

Of the other characteristics listed in Table 55.1, the most powerful predictors of mortality during the first year following an MI are a history of a previous MI; the development of early (within 10 days) post-MI angina accompanied by transient ST-segment or T-wave changes; an ejection fraction of 40% or less, complex ventricular arrhythmia, or the combination of these two (worst prognosis) at the time of discharge from the hospital; left main or three-vessel coronary artery occlusive disease; and a positive submaximal stress test within the first month following an MI.

MORBIDITY

Postinfarction angina occurs during the year following an MI in approximately 75% of persons who had angina before their MI, and it develops for the first time in about half of those who did not have it before their MI (36). In patients who are free of angina or other cardiac symptoms in the hospital, submaximal electrocardiogram (ECG) stress testing before discharge increases the ability to predict whether or not a patient will have angina after an MI. Angina after an MI occurs in 86% of patients with positive stress tests (96% of patients with both a positive stress test and a previous history of angina) and in 36% of those with negative stress tests (only in 20% of patients with both a negative stress test and no previous history of angina) (36).

Other medical complications include congestive heart failure, life-threatening arrhythmias, systemic emboli, and post-MI syndrome. The incidence of each of these problems is relatively low.

The *psychologic and social sequelae* during the year following an MI depend both upon the severity of the patient's MI and upon his psychosocial situation before the MI. Of survivors of MIs, 10 to 20% are never able to return to their former occupational and recreational activities, while the other 80 to 90% are able to do so within 2 to 6 months. Based upon extensive observations, Cassem has developed a hypothetical profile of emotional and behavioral reactions to an MI (Fig. 55.3); in this scheme, depression or maladaptive behavior related to pre-existing personality traits will be present in 10% or more of patients during the period following discharge from the hospital. It has been found that persistent denial, anxiety, depression, and dependency after an MI are all associated with a decrease in the rate of return to work and usual social activities, regardless of the patient's physiologic status (31).

Patients with Unstable Angina (see Definition, Chapter 54)

Patients discharged from the CCU with the diagnosis of unstable angina (or acute coronary insufficiency—MI ruled out) have a prognosis which is, in general, similar to that of patients with a completed MI (5 to 10% crude 1-year mortality). Patients with unstable angina also have an 8% 6-month risk and a 12% 1-year risk of developing myocardial infarction, which is essentially similar to the chance of recurrent MI for patients discharged with the diagnosis of completed MI (23).

In an individual patient with unstable angina, a more precise prognosis can be given when the distribution of coronary artery disease is known. Coronary arteriography has shown that left main coronary artery disease is more common in patients discharged with the diagnosis of unstable angina than in those discharged with the diagnosis of completed MI (15% versus 5%, respectively) (18). Another 10% have dif-

fuse coronary artery disease, 10% have normal coronary arteries (and are presumed to have coronary artery spasm as an etiology of their chest pain), and the remaining 65% are more or less equally divided between single, double, and triple coronary vessel disease. The prognoses associated with each of these patterns are described in Chapter 54.

The management of unstable angina after the patient is discharged from hospital is described on p. 499.

Survivors of Cardiac Arrests Who Have Not Had a Myocardial Infarction

The first year mortality of all survivors of cardiac arrest who have not had an MI is about 25%, with about three-quarters of deaths occurring within the first 6 months after hospital discharge. This is approximately 3 times the mortality rate of survivors of completed MIs. Two studies have reported the difference in prognosis in resuscitated patients, comparing those without and with an MI . In a study of 234 survivors of *out-of-hospital cardiac arrest*, followed for over 4 years, the rate of recurrence of ventricular fibrillation or sudden death in patients without an acute MI was 31% compared with 5% for patients admitted with electrocardiographic changes of acute MI. The median time to recurrent circulatory arrest was 20 weeks. More than 70% of the episodes of ventricular fibrillation were unexpected, occurring during sleep or during the usual activities of daily living (22). In a similar study of 230 patients discharged and followed for 3 years after *in-hospital cardiac arrest*, patients with and without MIs had similar mortality rates, i.e., about 30% by the end of the first year, 45% by the end of the second year, and 50% by the end of the third year (11).

The post-hospital management of patients who have survived idiopathic ventricular fibrillation must be highly individualized, based upon a thorough evaluation by a consulting cardiologist. Recent work suggests improved mortality rate in survivors of out-of-hospital cardiac arrest, when serum levels of antiarrhythmics are maintained in the therapeutic range (14).

REHABILITATION AND MANAGEMENT

The majority of patients discharged after MI can expect to return to most of their usual activities within 2 to 6 months. For a smaller number of patients, complications of their MI make this outcome impossible. In either situation, an organized plan for care should be followed, as summarized in Table 55.2. This plan should include the education of the patient so that he can participate in the rehabilitation process and should assure optimal monitoring and treatment of the patient by the physician; i.e., it can be divided into (a) education of the patient and his family and (b) management for the medical complications of MI.

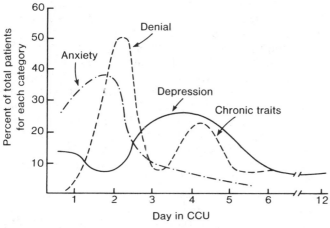

Figure 55.3 Hypothetical patterns and frequencies of emotional and behavioral reactions of coronary care unit (CCU) patients. (Adapted from: N. H. Cassem and T. P. Hackett: Psychiatric consultation in a coronary care unit, *Annals of Internal Medicine, 75:* 9, 1971, copyright American Medical Association.)

Table 55.2
Plan of Care for Survivors of Myocardial Infarction following Hospital Discharge

PATIENT EDUCATION (OBJECTIVES FOR ALL PATIENTS)[a]
    Understands disease process (damage to the heart which heals in a few months, leaves a scar)
    Understands likely prognosis
    Understands and follows progressive activity schedule[b]
    Understands approximate timetable for return to work
    Understands importance of controlling major risk factors (smoking, hypercholesterolemia, hypertension) and takes action to control them
    Knows how to recognize principal cardiac symptoms (angina, tachycardia, heart failure, hypotension) and understands how to use sublingual nitroglycerine
    Participates in group classes following discharge[c]
MEDICAL MANAGEMENT
    All patients:
        Review in-hospital course for prognostic characteristics (see Table 55.1) and for medications prescribed at discharge
        Assess and reinforce above patient education
        Check periodically for complications of infarction (see Table 55.5)
        Check for behavioral-psychiatric complications
        Check ECG 2–3 months following discharge
    Selected patients:
        β-Blocker treatment (when not contraindicated)
        Consider referral for physical conditioning[c]

[a] Essential to *include the patient's spouse* in all aspects of education.
[b] Serial exercise stress tests may be utilized to plan progressive activity (see text).
[c] If programs available in the community (see details on p. 497).

Although, to date, only smoking cessation (37) and β-blockade (3) have been shown convincingly to be associated with an improved prognosis after an MI, the comprehensive approach to care summarized in Table 55.2 is appropriate for most patients. It is likely that the efficacy of other aspects of care will be confirmed in the future (34). For example, a preliminary study has shown that the treatment of hypertension and hypercholesterolemia combined with physical conditioning probably reduces the chance of sudden death during the first 3 years following an MI (9); and studies which are in progress will soon indicate whether coronary artery bypass graft improves the prognosis in various subsets of MI survivors.

Physician-Patient Encounters

In general, each patient who has had an MI should be encouraged to telephone his physician at least once during the first week at home to discuss any questions which have arisen, and an office visit should be scheduled within 2 to 3 weeks of discharge. Before this visit, the physician should review the patient's hospital summary to determine whether adverse prognostic features were present (Table 55.1)

and to identify the medications prescribed at discharge. The visit should be divided between an assessment of the patient's progress in his rehabilitation (physical activity level, diet and smoking modifications, emotional status, understanding of the overall plan of care, expectation about return to work) and an assessment of his medical status (manifestations of ischemia and heart failure, blood pressure status, and review of current medications).

Because of the high frequency of *postinfarction angina* (see above), it is especially important at the first follow-up visit to describe this symptom to patients who have never had it and to point out to all patients that it may occur with the increased activity recommended for the coming weeks. Every patient should have a supply of sublingual nitroglycerin, and the correct use of this drug should be reviewed with him (see Chapter 54).

It is also very important to encourage the patient (or his spouse) to ask any questions which have arisen, however trivial. *Questions about specific activities* can be answered by referring to the information in Tables 55.3 and 55.4 (see "Activity Schedule," below).

Two or more additional office visits, similar to the first visit, should be scheduled during the 3 months following an MI and the patient should be encouraged to telephone at any time about symptoms or questions. At about 3 months, an ECG should be obtained which not only may provide helpful prognostic information (33), but will constitute the patient's new "baseline" ECG against which future ECGs should be compared.

Patient Education

Above all, the patient and his spouse need to be well informed about the following: the nature of his disease; cardiac symptoms; resumption of day-to-day physical activities; modification of major risk factors (smoking, hypertension, and hypercholesterolemia); and about the likely schedule for return to work. Nowadays, much of this information is provided before discharge, either by the CCU physician or by a cardiac rehabilitation nurse. Because patients may not retain the information they hear in the hospital, it is important to provide this information in writing and to assess and reinforce their understanding of it after discharge. The patient education booklet "After a Heart Attack" (available from the American Heart Association) gives a useful general account of the disease process, prognosis, CAD risk factors, and the rehabilitation process. Information about the patient's role in modifying cardiac risk factors is found in Chapter 19 (practical approaches to smoking cessation), Chapter 59 (treatment of hypertension), and Chapter 72 (low cholesterol diet).

Many community hospitals have developed *group classes* for survivors of MIs and their spouses, and evidence from one study indicates that this type of intervention is beneficial (19). Typically, patients and their spouses are invited to participate in a number of weekly meetings during the first or second month after discharge. Sessions are usully led by a nurse, a social worker, or a cardiologist with the objective of having participants raise questions about the recovery period so that they provide mutual support by sharing experiences with each other. Additional resources available in many communities are patient-run "heart clubs" and physician-supervised physical conditioning programs (see "Physical Conditioning" below). There are also several nationally distributed newsletters for patients with coronary artery disease.*

Activity Schedule

Table 55.3 contains a practical summary (for use by the patient) of symptom recognition and of a schedule of progressive physical activities for the first 3 months after an MI. For each month, the energy requirements of recommended activities are stated, in metabolic equivalents, METS† (1 to 3 METS for the first and second months, 3 to 5 METS for the third month); plans for a specific daily exercise (walking on a level surface) are stated; and a variety of useful hints are provided. Table 55.4 lists a broad array of activities corresponding to the recommended energy levels for the recuperation period and thereafter. Resumption of activities with different energy requirements should be gradual; in particular, the duration of certain activities should be short at first, with gradual increase, according to how the individual patient feels. The schedule in Table 55.3 can be given to most patients. A more aggressive plan can be developed for the individual patient if early physical conditioning, guided by serial stress testing, is available and is agreed to by the patient and his physician. Similar stress test-guided conditioning can also be planned for patients after the first 3 months of convalescence from an MI. These important aspects of rehabilitation are discussed in detail below (see "Physical Conditioning" p. 497).

Return to Work

Since the majority of patients have their first MI during their active working years, they are commonly concerned about returning to work. A tentative timetable for return to work should be discussed with the patient early after discharge. A number of factors should be taken into consideration. Generally, failure to return to work following an MI is due to psychologic rather than physical limitations (see "Psychologic Problems," below); telling the patient, soon after discharge, that he should *expect* to return to work will help to prevent disability due to psychologic

factors. Obviously the type of work is always an important consideration. Patients with occupations which involve mental stress and hectic schedules should be advised to return to work on a part time basis at first, leaving plenty of time for rest and relaxation. For patients whose work involves significant physical exertion, the timing of return to work can be based upon the information contained in Tables 55.3 and 55.4. From Table 55.4, it is evident that most occupations require an energy level of 6 METS or less. Occupational activities classified as heavy work, such as digging ditches, require energy expenditure of 7 or more METS. Certain activities may produce an increased work load on the heart because of psychologic stress (e.g., driving a vehicle) or because they entail significant isometric exercise (e.g., carpentry, plumbing, shoveling, operating pneumatic tools, or carrying objects heavier than 30 lb).

In order to evaluate objectively the impact of the patient's expected physical exertion upon his heart, ECG stress testing (see "Patient Experience," Chapter 54) and Holter monitoring, during simulated or actual occupational activities, can be obtained after the first 2 or 3 months of convalescence.

Patients with myocardial infarctions complicated by angina that is difficult to control, CHF, or arrhythmias should be evaluated in conjunction with a consulting cardiologist (see "Medical Complications" below) before a plan for return to work and other activities is recommended. Some of these patients will qualify for permanent medical disability (see criteria for disability due to coronary artery disease, Chapter 3, Table 3.1) or for job-retraining through vocational rehabilitation (see Chapter 3).

Sexual Activity

It is safe for patients who are symptom-free during usual activities of daily living to resume sexual intercourse within 4 to 6 weeks of their MI. Available data suggest that the energy requirement approximates 3 METS during foreplay and afterplay and 5 METS at climax (8). These are equivalent to the oxygen demands of a brisk walk around the block or of climbing one flight of stairs. In a study of patients after MI, coitus accounted for less than 1% of sudden deaths. These usually occurred during extramarital affairs in which the men were considerably older than their companions, and frequently were inebriated at the time of intercourse (35).

When counseling patients about resumption of sexual activity, the physician should give specific advice and should also encourage questions. Frequency of sexual intercourse can be similar to the frequency before the patient's MI. Sexual foreplay without completion of intercourse can be recommended to patients who wish to resume sex cautiously. In general, sex can be resumed in the position which was most gratifying before the MI; however, the patient should avoid positions in which he supports his weight on

---

* Example: *The Coronary Care Bulletin* (address: 3659 Green Road, Cleveland, OH 44122).
† One MET is the energy requirement at rest: 3.5 ml O_2/kg/min.

Table 55.3
Activity Schedule and Symptom Recognition for Patients Convalescing from Myocardial Infarction

GENERAL POINTS

All activities, including sitting and lying down, require energy. The amount of energy required to perform a specific activity is expressed as METS. One MET is your resting energy requirement. As activities become more strenuous, the amount of energy required (METS) also increases as does the workload imposed on your heart.

The schedule recommended in this program is based on the number of METS needed for various activities. Some specific recommendations are given for each of the first 3 months following your return to home. Table 55.4 gives the energy requirements for a wide variety of additional activities. If the table omits your favorite activities, ask your doctor about them.

Warnings: generally, the following activities impose an added strain on your heart and should be avoided, especially during the first 3 months after a heart attack:

1. Taking very hot or cold showers or baths.
2. Holding your breath while exercising, lifting, or straining.
3. Working in a bent or stooped position or with arms held above your head.
4. Work that requires continuous tensing of your muscles.
5. Working or exercising during very hot, cold, humid, or windy weather (in bad weather, plan your regular exercise at a nearby shopping mall).
6. Working or exercising during the first hour after a meal or after consuming alcohol.
7. Consuming excessive amounts of alcohol (*e.g.,* more than 1–2 ounces of whiskey, 2–3 beers, 1–2 glasses of wine).
8. Walking or exercising on a hill or an inclined surface.
9. Any activity which creates emotional stress or worry for you.

A RECOMMENDED ACTIVITY SCHEDULE

First Month (1–3 METS)

From Discharge to 1 Week

Regular exercise: walk 5 min at a leisurely pace once per day, on a level surface.

Some specific advice: this week, primarily get used to being at home. Occupy yourself with sit-down activities such as watching television, playing cards, sewing, painting, sketching, etc. Avoid lifting objects heavier than 5 lb or doing activities which require reaching above your head. You may go up and down the stairs. However, take your time and limit the number of times you need to climb them. Do all the things you were doing in the hospital. Get up and get dressed each day. You may be surprised at how tired and weak you feel. This is natural. Be sure to take rest periods when you need them, particularly after meals, before you exercise or climb the stairs.

Week 2

Regular exercise: walk 5 minutes at a leisurely pace twice per day

Some specific advice: continue all your previous activities, and add others such as taking rides in the car (however, no driving yet), cooking a meal, washing clothes in a machine (have someone else remove them), making your bed, attending a relaxing movie, going out to dinner, going shopping with your family (let others lift things from the shelves to the basket and carry the groceries), shooting pool, playing shuffle board, throwing a softball underhand, playing a piano or organ.

Weeks 3 and 4

Regular exercise: advance gradually to walking 10 minutes at a leisurely pace twice per day during these 2 weeks.

Some specific advice: continue your previous activities and others such as going to church, sweeping floors, polishing furniture, driving the car (beginning with short drives, avoiding heavy traffic).

Second Month (1–3 METS)

Regular physical exercise: progressively increase leisurely walking from 15 min once a day at a slightly faster pace to 20 min once or twice a day.

Some specific advice: the attached table of activities lists the approximate energy requirements of each. You may gradually increase your activities, by adding additional activities and spending more time at them; consult the attached table for activities requiring 3 METS or less.

Third Month (1–5 METS)

Regular exercise: increase gradually to walks at a faster pace, 15–30 min 1–2 times per day or more if you feel up to it.

Some specific advice: your doctor may permit you to return to your work on a part time basis, if the energy cost of your work does not exceed 5 METS. You should gradually expand the range and duration of physical activities that you engage in, selecting activities which require 5 METS or less.

RECOGNIZING HEART SYMPTOMS

Your heart will give you warning signs if it is not ready for increased activity. Here are some guidelines to use:

Pulse: Locate your pulse and count the number of times it beats for 15 sec and multiply that number by 4. This is your heart rate for 1 min. Take your pulse before you begin your walk or any new activity and at the end of the activity. Contact your doctor before resuming exercise if:

1. There is an increase of 20 heart beats or more per min in postexercise pulse over pre-exercise pulse.
2. If your heart rate exceeds 120 per min.
3. If you detect abnormal heart action: pulse becoming irregular, fluttering or jumping in chest or throat, very slow pulse rate, sudden burst of rapid heartbeats.

Chest Pain: Contact your doctor before resuming exercise if you experience pain or pressure in the chest, arm, or throat precipitated by exercise or following exercise. Remember to take your nitroglycerine and rest if you do experience pain.

Dizziness: Contact your doctor before resuming exercise if you become dizzy, light headed, or faint during exercise.

Breathing Difficulty: Contact your doctor before resuming exercise if you become short of breath during or after a new exercise; or if you awaken from sleep short of breath.

Table 55.4
Energy Requirements of Certain Activities[a]

Activity Level	Self-Care or Home	Occupational	Recreational	Physical Conditioning
Very light (3 METs or less)	Washing, shaving, dressing Desk work, writing, washing dishes Driving auto[b]	Sitting (clerical, assembling) Standing (store clerk, bartender) Driving truck[b] Crane operator[b]	Shuffleboard Horseshoes Bait casting Billiards Archery[b] Golf (cart)	Walking (level at 2 mph) Stationary bike (very low resistance) Very light calisthenics
Light to moderate (3–5 METS)	Clean windows Raking leaves Weeding Power lawn mowing Waxing floors (slowly) Painting Carrying objects 15–30 lb[c]	Stocking shelves (light objects)[c] Light welding Light carpentry[c] Machine assembly Auto repair Paper hanging[c]	Dancing Golf (walking) Sailing Horseback riding Volleyball Tennis (doubles) Sexual Intercourse[b] (see details in text)	Walking (3–4 mph) Level bicycling (6–8 mph) Light calisthenics
Moderate (5–7 METs)	Easy digging in garden Level hand lawn mowing Climbing stairs (slowly) Carrying objects 30–60 lb[c]	Carpentry (exterior home building)[c] Shoveling dirt[c] Pneumatic tools[c]	Badminton (competitive) Tennis (singles) Snow skiing (downhill) Light backpacking Basketball Football Skating (ice and roller) Horseback riding (gallop)	Swimming (breast stroke)
Heavy (7–9 METs)	Sawing wood[c] Heavy shoveling[c] Climbing stairs (moderate speed) Carrying objects 60–90 lb[c]	Tending furnace[c] Digging ditches[c] Pick and shovel[c]	Canoeing[c] Mountain climbing[c] Fencing Paddleball Touch football	Jog (5 mph) Swim (crawl stroke) Rowing machine Heavy calisthenics Bicycling (12 mph)
Very heavy (9 METs)	Carrying loads upstairs[c] Carrying objects 90 lb or more Climbing stairs quickly Shoveling heavy snow[c] Shoveling 10/min (16 lb)	Lumber jack[c] Heavy laborer[c]	Handball Squash Ski touring over hills[c] Vigorous basketball	Running (6 mph) Bicycle (13 mph or steep hill) Rope jumping

[a] *Source:* W. L. Haskell: Design and implementation of cardiac conditioning programs. In *Rehabilitation of the Coronary Patient*, p. 203, H. K. Hellerstein (ed.) John Wiley & Sons, New York, 1978.
[b] May cause added psychologic stress that will increase load on the heart.
[c] May produce disproportionate myocardial demands because of use of arms or isometric exercise.

his arms, as this type of work is isometric (see "Physical Conditioning" below) and may put extra stress on the heart. Sexual activity should be engaged in when both partners are relaxed, and extremes of ambient temperatures should be avoided. It is best to wait 2 or 3 hours after eating a large meal since this temporarily increases the work of the heart.

Inability to return to a previous pattern of sexual activity may be due to angina precipitated by intercourse, to new medications, or to psychologic stress associated with the recent MI. If an otherwise stable patient develops angina during intercourse, he should be advised to take sublingual nitroglycerin just before having sex. The evaluation and management of drug-induced and psychologic sexual dysfunction is discussed in Chapter 17.

Psychologic Problems

It is normal for patients to experience anxiety and temporary symptoms of depression during the first few weeks after discharge from the CCU. Most patients do well when encouraged to ventilate their concerns, when reassured that their response is normal, and when given a small supply of a minor tranquilizer (see Chapter 12) to be used if needed at bedtime and other times. As noted earlier ("Patient Education"), participation in group classes can also help patients adjust to changes in their lives following myocardial infarction.

Some patients have relatively severe psychologic and behavioral problems after MI which may interfere with their rehabilitation. The most common problem is *persistent depression*, which may have characteristics of a major or minor depressive illnesss or may resemble a grief reaction. The diagnosis and management of these problems are discussed in Chapter 14 (affective disorders) and 18 (grief reaction). Another common problem is *denial of illness* persisting beyond the first few days in hospital. The behavior associated with persistent denial may create substantial risks. This is especially true of patients who are extremely competitive and are used to controlling most of the circumstances of their lives. These patients typically attempt to resume their hectic living style immediately after returning home. When such patients are given ample and specific roles in observing and managing their heart disease (monitoring pulse rate, measuring blood pressure, keeping a diary of symptoms, etc.) and in drawing up plans for the resumption of activities, many of them will comply quite well with a plan of gradual rehabilitation (1). The consultation of a physician or psychologist skilled in behavior modification may be helpful in managing these patients.

Medical Prophylaxis

Cholesterol-lowering agents, β-adrenergic blocking agents, and anticoagulants and platelet inhibitors have all been tested as prophylactic agents in patients who have had an MI. Only β-blocking drugs have been shown convincingly to improve the prognosis in these patients (27a). Treatment with the β-blockers, metaprolol (Lopressor), propranolol (Inderal), and timolol (Blocadren) is associated with a significant reduction in mortality (all three drugs) and in the reinfarction rate (timolol only). The effectiveness of these drugs depends upon initiation of treatment within several days of the MI, i.e., while the patient is still in the hospital. The optimal duration of β-blocker prophylaxis has not been established, but patients should probably continue treatment for at least 1 year following discharge. Precautions regarding contraindications, side effects, and discontuation of β-blockers are described in Chapter 59.

Medical Complications

Table 55.5 lists the principal medical complications of MI, the procedures which may be useful in diagnosing or evaluating them, and potential therapies. In general, the use of sophisticated and costly procedures to evaluate these complications should be coordinated by a consulting cardiologist.

POSTINFARCTION ANGINA

As pointed out in the discussion of prognosis above, this is a very common problem in survivors of MIs. The medical management of angina is described in detail in Chapter 54. Because protection of the heart from transient ischemia may be especially important during recovery from an MI, the prescription of long acting nitrates and/or β-blockers to prevent angina is advisable in most patients who develop angina within the first 3 months following MI. After a patient has been angina-free for a number of months on these drugs, the drugs can be tapered and often discontinued if symptoms do not recur. Because of the very poor prognosis associated with angina occurring very early after an MI (25), patients with this problem should be referred to a cardiologist for consideration of coronary artery bypass surgery.

Table 55.5
Medical Complications of Myocardial Infarction

Complications	Diagnostic Procedures for Selected Patients[a]	Management Approaches
Angina or other evidence of reversible ischemia	ECG stress testing; radionuclide stress testing; coronary arteriography	Standard antianginal therapy (see Chapter 54). Coronary artery bypass for selected patients. Physical conditioning
Congestive heart failure	Radionuclide ventriculography and/or echocardiography (ejection fraction, segmental dysfunction, rupture, ventricular aneurysm)	Standard therapy for heart failure (see Chapter 58). Surgery in few selected patients
Arrhythmias	Holter monitor; ECG stress testing	Standard antiarrhythmic therapy (see Chapter 56)
Post myocardial infarction syndrome (Dressler's)	Echocardiography (pericardial effusion)	Aspirin or other antiinflammatory agents
Systemic emboli	Echocardiography (intracardiac thrombus)	Anticoagulant therapy (see Chapter 48). Surgery in selected patients

[a] Should be coordinated and interpreted by consulting cardiologist.

POSTINFARCTION CONGESTIVE HEART FAILURE

A small but significant proportion of patients develops chronic CHF after MI. This complication usually develops before discharge from the hospital. Nowadays, many patients have their left ventricular ejection fraction measured as part of their evaluation before discharge, so that those at increased risk of developing new CHF after discharge are known. The regimens described in Chapter 58 should be utilized in treating the CHF of patients after MI. In patients whose CHF is difficult to control, the combination of "preload" reduction with long acting nitrates and "afterload" reduction with hydralazine, in doses titrated for the individual patient, is often helpful. A small proportion of patients with persistent CHF may have segmental or global left ventricular dysfunction, which may improve significantly after coronary artery bypass surgery (10).

POST INFARCTION ARRHYTHMIAS

A substantial number of survivors of MIs are found to have complex ventricular arrhythmias on 24-hour ambulatory ECG monitoring, which is performed routinely after the first week of hospitalization in many hospitals. It has never been shown convincingly that antiarrhythmic therapy improves the prognosis of such patients; however, because of the poor prognosis associated with ventricular arrhythmias, it is current practice to attempt to control them medically and to confirm control by holter monitoring before or shortly after discharge. The drugs utilized to control arrhythmias are discussed in detail in Chapter 56. Once medical control of arrhythmias has been established, the patient should be treated for 3 to 6 months. If ECG monitoring shows no arrhythmia after this period, antiarrhythmic treatment can be stopped and the patient can be checked 1 week later for recurrent arrhythmia.

Studies are now in progress of the usefulness of membrane-active antiarrhythmic agents in the management of patients with the combination of complex ventricular arrhythmias and low ejection fractions at the end of their stay in the hospital. These studies may eventually provide clearer information about the optimal medical management of patients with this combination of high risk characteristics.

POST MYOCARDIAL INFARCTION (DRESSLER'S) SYNDROME (6)

It is estimated that 3 to 4% of patients develop this complication, usually within 1 to 6 weeks after a myocardial infarction. The syndrome is characterized by the pain of pericarditis (substernal pain, relieved by leaning forward and increased with inpiration); presence of a friction rub; fever; a pericardial effusion (which can best be demonstrated by echocardiography) and often a unilateral or bilateral pleural effusion.

The principal considerations in the differential diagnosis are pulmonary embolism and recurrence or extension of the recent MI.

When a patient develops the symptoms of Dressler's syndrome, he should be hospitalized immediately, and serial ECGs, cardiac enzymes, and a lung scan should be obtained. If these tests do not show pulmonary embolism, a new MI, or another explanation of the symptoms, the clinical diagnosis of Dressler's syndrome can be made. Echocardiographic evidence of a pericardial effusion and an elevated erythrocyte sedimentation rate provide additional evidence, although these findings are not essential for making the diagnosis.

Dressler's syndrome usually responds to salicylates or to indomethacin; in patients who do not respond to these drugs, prednisone gives prompt relief of symptoms. Once the diagnosis is secure and symptoms are controlled, the patient can be discharged. The anti-inflammatory drug chosen in hospital should be administered for 1 to 2 months. Prednisone should be withdrawn according to the schedule described in Chapter 71. Patients who have recurrent symptoms when anti-inflammatory treatment is discontinued should resume treatment for another month or longer.

SHOULDER-HAND SYNDROME

This syndrome, characterized by pain and stiffness of the shoulder and pain and swelling of the hand, may occur during the first 1 to 2 months following an MI. It usually affects the left side. This syndrome rarely occurs when patients are mobilized early after an MI. Management of the shoulder-hand syndrome is described in Chapter 80.

REFERRAL FOR CARDIOLOGIC CONSULTATION

Selected patients who have had an MI, especially relatively young persons, and patients with uncontrolled angina refractory to medical therapy, ventricular aneurysm with CHF refractory to medical therapy, evidence for "ischemia at a distance" (see footnote on Table 55.1 for definition), or mechanical complications such as ventricular septal defect (suggested by holosystolic murmur and thrill at the left sternal border) or papillary muscle rupture (suggested by refractory CHF and holosystolic apical murmur) may benefit from cardiac surgery, either by having their symptoms reduced or their prognosis improved (10).

In general, cardiac surgery should be postponed, if at all possible, for at least a few weeks following an MI. Patients with these complications should, however, be referred promptly to a cardiologist, to assure optimal medical therapy and to obtain an opinion about the advisability and the timing of cardiac surgery. The initial evaluative procedure chosen by the consultant may be one or more of the noninvasive procedures listed in Table 55.5 or coronary arteriography. The distribution of coronary occlusive disease associated with the best surgical results in patients after M.I. is the same as that described for patients with angina (see Chapter 54).

In the future, evaluation for coronary artery bypass surgery may be recommended for a broader group of patients, particularly in light of the poorer prognosis associated with an abnormal ECG stress test after MI, even in asymptomatic patients.

NONCARDIAC SURGERY

Noncardiac surgery carries a very high risk during the first 3 to 6 months following an MI (see Chapter 83 for details).

Physical Conditioning

Regular exercise, with the goal of attaining the physiologic adaptation known as the conditioning effect, is safe and beneficial for many patients after MI, just as it is for healthy persons. The activity schedule summarized in Table 55.3 is based largely on principles which underlie physical conditioning. Therefore, understanding of these principles is important in managing all patients who have had an MI regardless of whether or not they eventually undertake a formal conditioning program.

GENERAL PRINCIPLES

Dynamic versus Static Activity. Dynamic (isotonic, aerobic) activities entail rhythmic repetitive movements of large muscle groups against relatively small resistance. Such activities are of low intensity but can be performed for a long time. They include walking, jogging, running, cycling, swimming, rowing, rope jumping, skating, and cross country skiing. They decrease peripheral vascular resistance and increase cardiac output, the capacity of exercising muscles to extract oxygen, and total oxygen uptake by the body. It is the latter feature which earns them the appellation "aerobic" activities.

Static (isometric) activities, on the other hand, entail sustained, slow movement against resistance. They frequently involve the relatively small muscle groups of the upper extremities. Usually there is sustained contraction of the exercising muscle to a degree greater than 20% of maximal voluntary contraction. Examples are weight lifting, wrestling, push-ups, sit-ups, carrying packages or luggage, activities requiring lifting and straining such as shoveling, and the sustained use of hand grips. In such exercises there is increased peripheral vascular resistance with subsequent increase in diastolic pressure but relatively little increase in heart rate or cardiac output. Such exercises do not bring about enhancement in oxygen extraction by the exercising muscles or a significant increase in total oxygen uptake. Hence they are not aerobic.

The principal *hemodynamic* adaptation to aerobic

exercise in patients with heart disease is a decrease in peripheral arterial resistance. In normal people who practice aerobic exercise there are also changes in the heart itself, including increase in diastolic volume, increase in ejection fraction at rest and to a greater extent during exercise, and enhancement of contractility. There seems to be little, if any, of this central effect in patients with coronary artery disease, although recent data suggest that myocardial contractility may be enhanced (17). In particular, improvement in coronary collateral circulation or myocardial perfusion does not seem to occur as a result of physical conditioning in patients with heart disease (16).

Hormonal and Metabolic Effects of Training. In addition to the effect of training on the muscular and cardiovascular system, aerobic exercise is associated with beneficial changes in a number of other systems. There is increased vagal tone, lowering of catecholamines, decrease in serum triglycerides, increase in the ratio of high density to low density lipoprotein, reduction in adipose tissue, and augmentation in plasma fibrinolytic activity.

PHYSICAL CONDITIONING IN HEALTHY PERSONS

Healthy individuals can develop their own physical conditioning programs, utilizing the self-instruction programs described by Cooper (4) or others. The objective of conditioning programs is to reach an exercise level at which the body is achieving about 70% of maximal predicted oxygen uptake, a level which is attained when the heart rate reaches approximately 80% of the maximum predicted rate. Optimal physical conditioning is attained when a person engages in an aerobic activity in which this "target" heart rate is sustained for 20 min, at least 3 times per week. Table 55.6 lists target heart rates for healthy persons in various age groups. Lower levels of aerobic exercise also produce a partial conditioning effect.

When beginning a conditioning program, an un-

Table 55.6
Target Heart Rates for Healthy Persons, by Age (Approximately 80% Maximum Predicted Heart Rate) [a]

Age	Heart Rate
20–29	170
30–39	160
40–49	150
50–59	140
60–69	130

[a] *Source:* J. F. Parmley, Jr., S. Blair, P. C. Gazes, W. K. Giese, C. P. Summerall, and D. E. Saunders (eds.): Proceedings of the National Workshop on Exercise in the Prevention, Evaluation, and Treatment of Heart Disease. *Journal of the South Carolina Medical Association, 65* (suppl. 1): December, 1969.

conditioned person should follow a progressive schedule such as those recommended by Cooper (4). In addition, selected individuals should consult their physicians before beginning a program. In general, persons over the age of 35 and those at any age with risk factors for atherosclerosis should have a physical examination and a resting ECG. Exercise stress tests are recommended for individuals in a number of categories (12), as summarized in Table 55.7

PHYSICAL CONDITIONING IN PATIENTS FOLLOWING MYOCARDIAL INFARCTION

Benefits of Conditioning. Patients who have had an MI and have then attained the conditioning effect show favorable changes in psychometric tests, better control of angina, enhancement of work capacity, and, possibly, prolonged survival.

Psychometric testing has confirmed that exercise conditioning is associated with improvement in self-image and with a lightening of mood. Patients also show less anxiety, denial, and dependency; they appear to be better able to deal with day-to-day stresses; and they feel healthier and participate more actively in leisure time activities.

Because of the peripheral cardiovascular adaptation described above, angina pectoris occurs at higher exercise levels. Associated with the increase in the exercise threshold for angina and the increase in total oxygen uptake, there is an increase in work capacity; and at any level of work, the subject feels more comfortable and has greater stamina and endurance than he had before conditioning. Physically trained patients do continue to experience angina, but the level of cardiac work associated with angina is now reached at a higher external work load (20).

The effect of exercise training on longevity in patients after MI has not been established definitively. However, in the National Exercise and Heart Disease Project (NEHDP), the 3-year mortality for control and exercise groups was 7.3% and 4.6%, respectively, and the 3-year rate for recurrent MI for control and exercise groups was 7.0 and 5.3%, respectively (26). The number of participants (651) was not large enough to make these results statistically significant.

Risks of Conditioning. With proper selection, supervision, and precautions, physical conditioning for cardiac patients has proven to be remarkably safe.

Table 55.7
Recommendation for Stress Testing in Preventive and Rehabilitative Exercise Programs[a]

Status	Test or Training Mode
Healthy, under 35	No special test
Healthy, over 35	Stress test
Coronary prone, all ages	Stress test
Coronary stricken, all ages	Stress test

[a] Adapted from C. Long (ed.): *Prevention and Rehabilitation in Ischemic Heart Disease*, Williams & Wilkins, Baltimore, 1980 (12).

Table 55.8
Effect of Various Classes of Medications on Hemodynamic Status during Exercise[a, b]

Drug	Peak Heart Rate	Peak Systolic Blood Pressure
ANTIHYPERTENSIVES		
Hydralazine	↑	↓
Minoxidil	↑	↓
Clonidine	↓	↓
Guanethidine	↓	↓↓
Methyldopa	↓	↓
Prazosin	↑	↓
NITRATES	↑	↓
ANTIARRHYTHMICS	=	↓
β-BLOCKERS	↓	↓
DIGITALIS[c]	=	↑

[a] Adapted from A. C. P. Powles: The effect of drugs on the cardiovascular response to exercise, *Medicine and Science in Sports and Exercise*, 13: 252, 1981.
[b] ↓, decreased; ↑, increased; =, no discernible effect.
[c] Patients with congestive heart failure.

Cumulative data from over 1.5 million man-hours of exercise show that the risks of ventricular fibrillation, acute myocardial infarction, and death are 1/10,000-1/32,000, 1/253,000, and 1/116,000-1/212,000 man-hours of exercise, respectively (5).

Cardiovascular Medications and Conditioning. Many patients who have had an MI who are candidates for physical conditioning are taking one or more medications. Patients enrolled in a conditioning program should always be stress-tested (see below) while taking their regular medications; and the effects of their drugs upon the response to exercise should be considered in interpeting these tests. For example, because beta-blockers attenuate the response of the heart rate to exercise, heart rate is less useful as an endpoint for stress testing or as a function for the patient to monitor, and symptoms and ECG changes must be utilized to guide exercise intensity. Table 55.8 summarizes the effects of a number of commonly prescribed drugs on hemodynamic status. Persons taking a variety of drugs have been evaluated and have participated safely in physical conditioning programs. In fact, the majority of the patients in the NEHDP were taking one or more medications during the project. The most common drugs were nitrates, diuretics, and tranquilizers; but over 10% of subjects were taking β-blockers, antiarrhythmics, digitalis, or antihypertensives (15).

Referral for Conditioning. The decision to refer a patient for physical conditioning after an MI depends upon the patient's clinical status and motivation and upon the availability of a program designed for such patients. During the first 3 months following an MI, an activity schedule similar to that summarized in Table 55.3 is appropriate for most patients. After this, if the patient is interested and there are no contraindications, he should be offered the chance to join a physical conditioning program. If there is no supervised program in the community, patients who have had an uncomplicated MI can be advised to increase their exercise level gradually, utilizing the results of an ECG stress test to establish target heart rates, as described below.

Before beginning a conditioning program, the patient will have an ECG stress test (see Chapter 54 for description of the patient's experience), the results of which are utilized in planning his exercise program. In general, the conditioning heart rate is 70 to 85% of the maximum heart rate safely achieved on stress testing.

At many medical centers, physical conditioning is initiated routinely during the 3 months following the MI. In these early rehabilitation programs, serial stress tests guide the progress of the conditioning program. Figure 55.4 shows the results of such a stress test, performed 3 weeks after an MI in a patient who was preparing to begin a supervised exercise program

Contraindications. Contraindications to physical conditioning are poorly controlled angina, severe dyspnea at low workloads, moderate to severe uncontrolled hypertension (diastolic $\geq$ 110 mm Hg), complex arrhythmias, atrial fibrillation, second or third degree heart block, significant valvular or congenital heart disease, significant orthopedic or pulmonary limitations, chronic alcoholism, or recent acute physical or mental illness.

Training Sessions. Exercise sessions are supervised by personnel trained in exercise physiology and cardiopulmonary resuscitation, with immediate availability of monitoring and of resuscitative equipment. During the initial sessions, subjects usually have continuous ECG monitoring.

Sessions are usually held 3 times a week on nonconsecutive days. The total duration of an average session is about 45 min (5 to 10 min of warm-up, 30 min of exercise, and 5 to 10 min of cool-down calisthenics). The calisthenics involve stretching and range of motion exercises, which help to prevent musculoskeletal injuries and provide gradual and smooth acceleration or deceleration of the heart.‡ Aerobic exercise should last for about 30 min, at an intensity ranging between 70 and 85% of the maximum heart rate safely achieved on the recent ECG stress test. Exercise at 70 to 85% of maximal heart rate (or 50 to 68% of maximal oxygen uptake) is of sufficient intensity and safe enough for most patients to attain a good level of physical conditioning with a minimal risk of complications.

Training of a group of muscles by dynamic exercise is specific for that group, and there is little , if any, transfer of the training effect to other muscle groups. Therefore training of selected muscle groups, such as arm muscles, should be planned if work or leisure

activities require active use of these muscles. Aerobic training of upper extremities can be achieved by the use of shoulder wheels, rowing machines, and other devices. Bicycling, walking, jogging, aerobic dancing, and combinations of these exercises may be utilized for conditioning of the lower extremities. Swimming conditions the muscles of both upper and lower extremities.

Termination of Supervised Training. Criteria for terminating supervised exercise training and transfer to nonsupervised maintenance programs are not firmly established. However, clinical stability and demonstration of a peak functional performance capacity above 7 or 8 METs (see Table 55.4) are generally accepted exit criteria (5).

After a few months of supervised exercise, repeat stress testing is indicated to measure the change in work capacity and to assess more accurately the exercise intensity needed for optimal improvement. Continuation of exercise of appropriate duration, frequency, and intensity is necessary to maintain a state of physical fitness. Measurable deterioration in the conditioning effect occurs after missing only a few exercise sessions. The time required to retrieve lost ground seems to be directly related to the duration of time without exercise and to the degree of physical fitness achieved before cessation of exercise.

HOME CARE FOR ACUTE MYOCARDIAL INFARCTION

A controlled trial in Great Britain has shown that for patients with uncomplicated acute MIs the outcome is similar whether the patient is cared for in the home or in an intensive care unit (13). The authors concluded that home care was ethically acceptable for such patients. Because hospital care is the norm for an acute MI in the United States, it is unlikely that home care will gain significant acceptance here. However, for an occasional older person or for a person who consults his physician several days following an infarct, initial management at home may be appropriate. The scheme for rehabilitation after MI described in this chapter can be adapted to this situation.

MANAGEMENT OF UNSTABLE ANGINA AFTER DISCHARGE FROM HOSPITAL (18)

Of patients admitted to a hospital with unstable angina, 15 to 30% will continue to have pain despite vigorous medical management. Patients in this subgroup have a 25 to 45% 1-year mortality rate; therefore, most are evaluated for and referred for emergency coronary artery bypass surgery, an intervention which relieves or eliminates symptoms in the majority and improves the prognosis for those with left main coronary artery disease.

For the 70 to 85% of patients whose unstable angina

---

‡ See Chapter 64 for details regarding prevention and management of exercise-related musculoskeletal injuries.

EXERCISE STRESS TEST — CARDIAC REHABILITATION — BALTIMORE CITY HOSPITALS

Age __34__ Sex __M__

Occupation __Machinist, Beth Steel__

Last CCU Adm. __5/12-5/22/81__

  Dx. Inferior posterior lateral MI

  CPK 1322

  Complications:

  1) 10 beat ventricular tachycardia initially, controlled with lidocaine

  2) Angina

Symptoms since D/C __None__

_____

_____

Other Hx of CAD _____

  __Negative stress test 1972, 1975__

Medications: Last Taken

1) __Paste, ½ inch q4h__ __6/5/81 @ 4:00 p.m.__

2) _____   (D/C for test)

3) _____

Pt. _____

Hist.# _____ Date __June 6, 1981__

P.E. Supine BP __114/78__ HR __62__

  No murmurs, rubs or gallops

  Lungs clear

Resting EKG: Q and T waves decreased II, III, aVF, I, aVL, V5-6; ST elevated ½ mm. with R-R' I, aVL Tall R with peaked T wave V1-2

Risk Factors:

Smoking __2 ppd__	F.H. __Father died of MI (age 50)__	
HBP __No__	D.M. __No__	
Type A __No__	Obesity __No__	
Lipids __Normal__		

Target Rate: 130

POST EXERCISE

MIN	Speed/Slope*	METS	BP	HR	ST Changes	Arrhy	Comments	MIN	BP	HR	ST	Arrhy	Comments
0	– / –	–	120/92	84	Baseline	None	no Sx	0	145/95	132	Baseline	No	legs tired
2	1 / 0	1.2	140/100	87	"	"	"	2	114/85	94	"	"	
4	2 / 0	2	145/105	92	"	"	"	4	112/80	88	"	"	
6	2 / 3.5	3	140/115	98	"	"	"	6	112/84	75	"	"	
8	2 / 7	4	140/110	108	"	"	"	3	–	78	"	"	
10	2 / 10.5	5	150/120	112	"	"	legs tired	10	110/82	84	"	"	
12	2 / 14	6	150/120	128	"	"	"						
14	3 / 10	1 min 7	145/95	132	"	"	"						
16													
18													

* miles per hr /percent elevation

SUMMARY

Exercise Tolerance:

  speed __3__   H.R. __132__

  elevation __10__ Time __14 min. 30 sec.__

Workload Achieved:

  METS __7__

  O2 consumption __24__ (ml/kg/min)

N.Y.H.A. Class __I__

HR x BP __132 x 150 = 19,800__

IMPRESSIONS: 1) Adequate, negative early post MI submaximal stress test. 2) NYHA Class I

RECOMMENDATIONS:

1) May start monitored exercises in BCH program. Conditioning heart rate is to be about 105.

2) May gradually increase daily walking to 30 min. at 2 mph.

3) May return to work in 5 weeks (i.e., 2 months post myocardial infarction)

Figure 55.4 Example of a formal report of an electrocardiogram stress test, useful for planning the patient's rehabilitation.

responds to medical therapy, elective coronary arteriography should be planned within 1 to 2 months of discharge (see "Patient Experience", Chapter 54). For the approximately 10 to 15% of these patients who have significant left main coronary artery disease, coronary artery bypass surgery is recommended, as this seems to improve the patient's longevity. Bypass surgery probably also increases longevity in double and triple vessel disease. For the others, medical management is reasonable if symptoms are controlled adequately for the patient to return to his usual activities.

To date, the rehabilitation of the medically managed patient with unstable angina has not been studied as systematically as the rehabilitation of the patient after MI. These patients should receive education similar to that recommended for patients after MI regarding the nature of coronary artery disease, the recognition of symptoms, and the control of risk factors (see p. 491). Because these patients do not have an ischemic injury which takes 2 or more months to heal, they can usually be permitted to return to their usual activities more rapidly than patients who have had an MI. This is true particularly if their angina is well controlled and an ECG stress test shows minimal or no changes due to ischemia.

References

General

Long, C (ed): *Prevention and Rehabilitation in Ischemic Heart Disease*. Williams & Wilkins, Baltimore, 1980.
   Reviews in depth all aspects of prevention and rehabilitation of the patient with coronary artery disease.

Specific

1. Baile, WF and Engel, BT: A behavioral strategy for promoting treatment compliance following myocardial infarction. *Psychosomatic Med* 40: 413, 1978.
2. Battler, A, Karliner, JS, Higgins, CB, Slutsky, R, Gilpin, EA, Froelicher, VF and Ross, Jr, J: The initial chest x-ray in acute myocardial infarction, a prediction of early and late mortality and survival. *Circulation* 61: 1004, 1980.
3. Braunwald, E: Treatment of the patient after myocardial infarction. *N Engl J Med* 302: 290, 1980.
4. Cooper, KH (ed): *The New Aerobics*. Bantam Books, New York, 1970.
5. Council on Scientific Affairs, American Medical Association: Physician-supervised exercise programs in rehabilitation of patients with coronary heart disease. *JAMA* 1463, 1981.
6. Dressler, W: The post-myocardial-infarction syndrome. *Arch Intern Med* 103: 28, 1959.
7. Geltman, EM, Ehsani, AA, Campbell, MK, Schechtman, K, Roberts, R and Sobel, BE: The influence of location and extent of myocardial infarction on long-term ventricular dysrhythmia and mortality. *Circulation* 60: 805, 1979.
8. Hellerstein, HK and Friedman, EH: Sexual activity in the post coronary patient. *Arch Intern Med* 125: 987, 1970.
9. Kallio, V, Hamalainen, H, Hakkila, J and Luurila, OJ: Reduction in sudden deaths by a multifactorial intervention programme after acute myocardial infarction. *Lancet* 2: 8152, 1979.
10. Kent, KM, Borer, JS, Green, MV, Bacharach, SL, McIntosh, CL, Conkle, DM and Epstein, SE: Effects of coronary-artery bypass on global and regional left ventricular function during exercise. *N Engl J Med* 298: 1434, 1978.
11. Lemire, JG and Johnson, AL: Is cardiac resuscitation worthwhile? A decade of experience. *N Engl J Med* 286: 970, 1972.
12. Long, C: Exercise in the prevention and rehabilitation of ischemic heart disease. In *Prevention and Rehabilitation in Ischemic Heart Disease*, C. Long (ed). Williams & Wilkins, Baltimore, 1980.
13. Mather, HG, Pearson, NG, Read, KLQ, Shaw, DB, Steed, GR, Thorne, MG, Jones, S. Guerrier, CJ, Eraut, CD, McHugh, PM, Chowdhury, NR, Jafary, MH and Wallace, TJ: Acute myocardial infarction: home and hospital treatment. *Br Med J* pp. 334, 1971.
14. Myerburg, RJ, Conde, C, Sheps DS, Appel, RA, Kiem, I, Sung, RJ and Castellanos, A: Antiarrhythmic drug therapy in survivors of prehospital cardiac arrest: comparison of effects on chronic ventricular arrhythmias and recurrent cardiac arrest. *Circulation* 59: 855, 1979.
15. Naughton, JP: Pharmacological considerations in cardiac rehabilitation. In *Prevention and Rehabilitation in Ischemic Heart Disease*. C. Long (ed). Williams & Wilkins, Baltimore, 1980.
16. Nolewajka, AJ, Kostuk, WJ, Rechnitzer, PA and Cunningham, DA: Exercise and human collaterization: an angiographic and scintigraphic assessment. *Circulation* 60: 114, 1979.
17. Paterson, DH, Shephard, RJ, Cunningham, D, Jones, NL and Andrew G: Effect of physical training on cardiovascular function following myocardial infarction. *J Appl Physiol* 47: 482, 1979.
18. Plotnick, GD: Approach to the management of unstable angina. *Am Heart J* 98: 243, 1979.
19. Rahe, RH, Ward, HW and Hayes, V: Brief group therapy in myocardial infarction rehabilitation: three- to four-year follow-up of a controlled trial. *Psychosom. Med* 41: 229, 1979.
20. Redwood, DR, Rosing, DR and Epstein, SE: Circulatory and symptomatic effects of physical training in patients with coronary artery disease and angina pectoris. *N Engl J Med* 286: 959, 1972.
21. Rosati, RA and Harris PJ: Acute myocardial infarction. In *Prognosis Contemporary Outcomes of Disease*, J F. Fries and G. E. Ehrlich (ed). The Charles Press Publishers, Bowie, Md., 1981.
22. Schaffer, WA and Cobb, LA: Recurrent ventricular fibrillation and modes of death in survivors of out-of-hospital ventricular fibrillation. *N Engl J Med* 293: 259, 1975.
23. Schroeder, JS: Rule out myocardial infarction. In *Prognosis Contemporary Outcomes of Disease*, J. F. Fries and G. E. Ehrlich (eds). The Charles Press Publishers, 1981.
24. Schulze, RA, Strauss, HW and Pitt, B: Sudden death in the year following myocardial infarction. *Am J Cardiol* 62: 192, 1977
25. Schuster EH and Bulkley, B: Early post-infarction angina, ischemia at a distance and ischemia in the infarct zone. *N Engl J Med* 305: 1101, 1981.
26. Shaw, LW: Effects of a prescribed supervised exercise program on mortality and cardiovascular morbidity in patients after a myocardial infarction. *Am J Cardiol* 48: 39, 1981.
27. Silverman, KJ, Becker, LC, Bulkley, BH, Burow, RD, Mellits, ED, Kallman, CH and Weisfeldt, ML: Value of early thallium 201 scintigraphy for predicting mortality in patients with acute myocardial infarction. *Circulation* 61: 996, 1980.
27a. Sleight, P: Beta-adrenergic blockade after myocardial infarction *N Engl J Med* 304: 837, 1981.
28. Stamler, J: Acute myocardial infarction—progress in primary prevention. *Br Heart J* 33: 145, 1971.
29. Stamler, J: Primary prevention of coronary heart disease: the last twenty years. *Am J Cardiol* 47: 722, 1981.
30. Starling, MR, Crawford, MH, Kennedy, GT and O'Rourke, RA: Exercise testing early after myocardial infarction: predictive value for subsequent unstable angina and death. *Am J Cardiol* 46: 909, 1980.
31. Stern, MJ, Pascale, L and Ackerman, A: Life adjustment post-myocardial infarction. *Arch Intern Med* 137: 1680, 1977.
32. Taylor, GJ, Humphries, JO, Mellits, ED, Pitt, B, Schulze, RA, Griffith, LSC and Achuff, SC: Predictors of clinical course,

coronary anatomy and left ventricular function after recovery from acute myocardial infarction. *Circulation* 62: 960, 1980.

33. The Coronary Drug Project Research Group: The prognostic importance of the electrocardiogram after myocardial infarction. *Ann Intern Med* 77: 677, 1972.

34. Tristani, FE: National intervention trials and their descendants. In *Prevention and Rehabilitation in Ischemic Heart Disease*, C. Long (ed.), Williams & Wilkins, Baltimore, 1980.

35. Ueno, M: The so-called coition death. *Jpn J Legal Med* 17: 330, 1963.

36. Waters, DD, Theroux, P, Halphen, C and Mizgala, HF: Clinical predictors of angina following myocardial infarction. *Am J Med* 66: 991, 1979.

37. Wilhelmsson, C, Vedin, JA, Elmfeldt, D, Tibblin, G and Wilhelmsen, L: Smoking and myocardial infarction. *Lancet 1*: 415, 1975.

CHAPTER FIFTY-SIX

Arrhythmias

SHELDON H. GOTTLIEB, M.D., PHILIP D. ZIEVE, M.D., and GUSTAV C. VOIGT, M.D.

Contraction of the heart is normally the result of a well orchestrated electromechanical system. The orderly function of the system is maintained by the domination of the heart rate by a single pulse generator known as the *pacemaker*, by the relatively fast and uniform conduction of the electrical signal via specialized *conduction pathways*, and by the relatively long and uniform duration of the electrical signal relative to its velocity of conduction through these pathways, thereby assuring uniform electrical excitation and contraction of the heart. An *arrhythmia* is any disturbance in the normal sequence of impulse generation and conduction in the heart.

Arrhythmias may occur in the absence of heart disease, or may be symptoms of severe disease. They must be evaluated in the context of the clinical situation in which they occur. A precise etiologic diagnosis and an understanding of the pharmacology of the medications used are necessary to treat arrhythmias effectively.

PHYSIOLOGY OF IMPULSE GENERATION AND CONDUCTION

The Action Potential

Muscle contraction is stimulated by an electrical impulse, the action potential. In skeletal muscle, the action potential is transient, and the electrical activity is essentially dissipated before the beginning of contraction. In cardiac muscle, however, the action potential is sustained and lasts almost as long as the contraction itself (Fig. 56.1). In this way, the action potential not only stimulates contraction of the heart but also determines the duration and intensity of contraction. Furthermore, as long as the action potential is maintained, the heart cannot be stimulated to contract again.

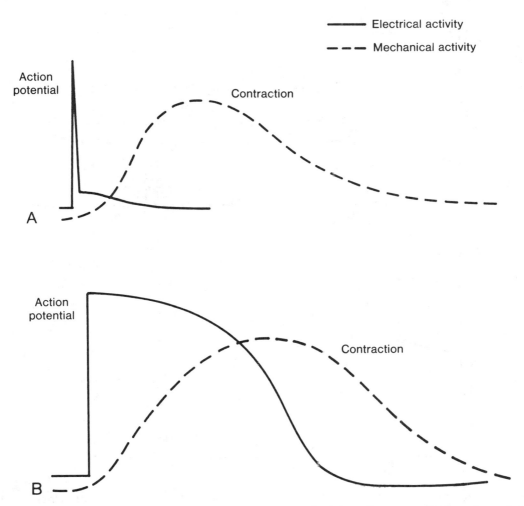

Figure 56.1 Comparison between relative time scales of electrical (*continuous curve*) and mechanical (*interrupted curve*) activity in skeletal (*A*) and cardiac (*B*) muscle. (*Source:* D. Noble: *The Initiation of the Heart Beat*, Clarendon Press, Oxford, 1975 (20).)

The action potential is generated by depolarization and repolarization of the muscle cell (Fig. 56.2). In the resting state the intracellular concentration of potassium is high and that of sodium low compared to the extracellular fluid. These gradients are maintained by metabolic activity within the cell membrane. The resting membrane potential is strongly negative (i.e., there is an electrochemical gradient across the membrane so that the inside of the membrane is negatively charged compared to the outside of the membrane). If an electrical stimulus is applied, the membrane becomes very permeable to sodium ions, which rapidly leak into the cell (phase 0). The membrane is thus depolarized (loses its negative charge) and, in fact, is transiently positively charged (overshoot). Repolarization occurs relatively slowly as first chloride (phase 1) and then, after a plateau (phase 2), potassium ions (phase 3) move back into the cell to restore the resting potential (phase 4).

RELATIONSHIP TO THE EKG

In the heart the phases of rapid depolarization and overshoot correspond to the QRS complex of the electrocardiogram; phase 2 corresponds to the ST segment; and phase 3, to the T wave (Fig. 56.2). During phase 2 the membrane is absolutely and, in phase 3, relatively, refractory to propagation of another electrical impulse.

FAST AND SLOW CURRENTS

Although in most cardiac tissue, excitation is propagated by the rapidly depolarizing sodium current (so that the action potential is conducted rapidly), excitation of the sinoatrial node and the proximal part of the atrioventricular node is propagated by a slowly depolarizing current generated by the influx of calcium ions into the cell. Also, in diseased cardiac muscle, the sodium current may be inhibited and depolarization may occur almost entirely via the slow calcium current; therefore the action potential may be conducted very slowly. This difference in conduction velocity between cells depolarized by the sodium versus the calcium current has important implications in both the generation and the treatment of arrhythmias (see below).

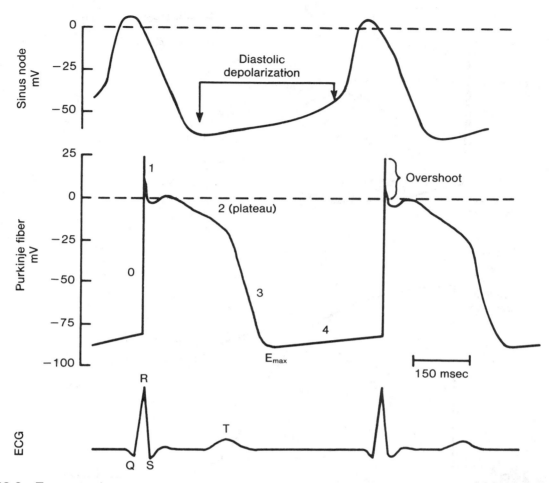

Figure 56.2 Transmembrane potentials from the sinus node and a Purkinje fiber. Note the spontaneous diastolic depolarization in the upper panel, characteristic of pacemaker fibers. The numbers in the middle panel are explained in the text. The lower panel shows the correlation of the time sequence of changes in the action potential and that of the surface electrocardiogram. Alterations in depolarization will be reflected in changes in the QRS duration of the surface record; those in repolarization will be associated with alterations in the Q-T interval. (*Source:* B. N. Singh, J. T. Collett, and C. Y. C. Chew: *Progress in Cardiovascular disease, 22:* 243, 1980 (23).)

PACEMAKER GENERATION

In most cells, the action potential will not be generated again until another electrical stimulus is applied. In pacemaker cells, slow spontaneous depolarization occurs until a threshold is reached whereupon phase 0 rapidly ensues (Fig. 56.2); this process is called *automaticity*. In the absence of heart block, the heart rate will be controlled by the pacemaker cells that depolarize most rapidly, because then the action potential is conducted rapidly throughout the heart and initiates rapid depolarization of other cells, even if they already have begun spontaneous slow depolarization. Automaticity is affected by the rate of slow spontaneous depolarization and by the threshold potential. Automaticity is enhanced by increased sympathetic tone, decreased vagal tone, increased catecholamine concentration in the blood, thyroid hormone, and by digitalis. It is suppressed by

decreased sympathetic tone, increased vagal tone, decreased thyroid hormone concentration, and by various drugs (e.g., the drugs used in the treatment of arrhythmias).

Impulse Generation and Conduction (Fig. 56.3)

SINOAURICULAR NODE

The sinoauricular (SA) node is composed of pacemaker cells located at the junction of the right atrium and the superior vena cava. The cells of the SA node spontaneously depolarize more rapidly than any other cells within the heart and the SA node therefore controls the heart rate.

ATRIAL FIBERS

The action potential generated by the SA node traverses the atrium rapidly along discrete bundles of specialized conduction tissue known as *internodal*

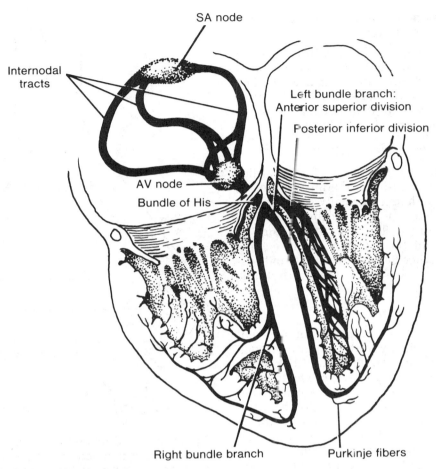

Figure 56.3 Anatomy of impulse conduction. (SA, sinoatrial, and AV, artrioventricular, nodes, respectively.) (*Source:* H. L. Greene and J. O. Humphries: In *Principles and Practice of Medicine*, Appleton-Century-Crofts, New York, 1980 (12).)

fibers. A specialized bundle of tissue connects the right and left atrium and the contractions of the atria are therefore nearly synchronous.

ATRIOVENTRICULAR NODE

The internodal fibers terminate in the atrioventricular (AV) node cells which lie at the junction of the right atrium and the interventricular septum just above the tricuspid valve and through which the action potential is conducted slowly. Electrical delay in the AV node allows the mechanical activity of the atria (which is slower than their electrical activity) to be synchronized with the mechanical activity of the ventricles. The AV node serves as a protective "gate" and will not respond to extremely rapid impulses generated in the atria, thereby protecting the ventricles from too rapid stimulation. The AV node may function as a subsidiary pacemaker if the SA node fails to pace.

BUNDLE OF HIS

When the action potential leaves the AV node, it enters the specialized conducting fibers known as the

bundle of His. The main bundle of His divides into three branches: the right bundle branch which runs along the right ventricular surface of the septum, the anterior superior branch which runs along the left ventricular surface of the septum, and the posterior inferior branch which runs along the posterior wall of the left ventricle. The action potential is conducted through the bundle branches into a widespread network of smaller fibers known as *Purkinje fibers* into the myocardium.

MECHANISM OF CARDIAC ARRHYTHMIAS

There are three basic causes of a disturbance in the rhythm of the heart: suppression of initiation or propagation of the action potential, ectopic pacemaker activity, and re-entry of the action potential into a pathway through which it has already passed. More than one of these mechanisms may be operative in producing a particular arrhythmia: e.g., ectopic supraventricular tachycardia in a patient with sinus node dysfunction.

Suppression of Initiation or Propagation of Action Potential

A disease process that interferes with pacemaker activity within the SA node or with the movement of the electrical impulse through the normal conduction pathways of the heart results either in abnormal slowing of the heart rate (bradyarrhythmia) and/or in one of the various forms of heart block.

Ectopic Pacemaker Activity

Enhanced automaticity of a part of the cardiac conduction system may result in the initiation of an impulse more rapidly than is normally generated by the SA node. If that happens episodically, occasional premature contractions will occur, the nature of which will depend on the location of the ectopic pacemaker. On the other hand, if there is rapid sustained firing of the ectopic focus, a tachyarrhythmia will be produced.

Re-entry

Alterations in the refractory period of adjacent pathways and of the velocity of the impulse through them may allow retrograde conduction of the action potential through one of the pathways. The forward (antegrade) conduction of the impulse is usually delayed or blocked in the pathway through which retrograde conduction occurs. The retrograde impulse then re-enters an adjacent pathway and is conducted forward again (Fig. 56.4). Sustained re-entry implies either unusual pathways for conduction of the action potential or poorly functioning and hence slowly conducting myocardium. Slow calcium currents (see above) may play an important role in sustained re-entry. Most premature contractions and most tachyarrhythmias are re-entrant rhythms.

DIAGNOSIS OF ARRHYTHMIAS: GENERAL CONSIDERATIONS

History

Arrhythmias may or may not cause symptoms. Symptoms, when they do occur, are due to an appreciation of the irregular rhythm (palpitations) or to a reduction in cardiac output (dizziness, light-headedness, syncope or chest pain). It is important to establish whether there are any factors that seem to trigger symptoms (e.g., drinking coffee, smoking, exercise, emotional stress) and whether there are symptoms of an underlying disease that may be associated with arrhythmia (e.g., heart failure, ischemic heart disease, thyrotoxicosis). The patient should be questioned specifically about the taking of stimulant drugs either illicitly (see Chapter 21) or as an ill-conceived attempt to lose weight (see Chapter 73).

Palpitations are heart beats that are sensed—usually because the beats are fast or irregular. However, they do not necessarily imply a significant arrhythmia and they may represent only sinus tachycardia

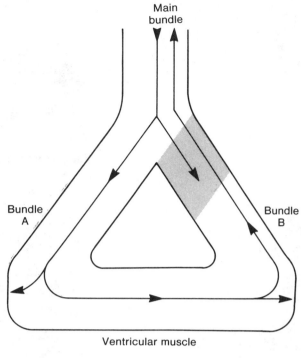

Figure 56.4 Sequence of activation of a loop of Purkinje fiber bundles (A and B) and ventricular muscle (VM) during re-entry. A region of unidirectional conduction block is indicated by the darkly shaded area in branch B. Conduction cannot occur through this area in the antegrade direction (from B to VM), but only in the retrograde direction (from VM to B). Slow conduction is present through the loop. The bottom of the figure shows a possible electrocardiographic pattern which may result from this type of re-entry. (*Source:* A. L. Wit, M. R. Rosen, and B. F. Hoffman: *American Heart Journal, 88:* 664, 1974 (26).)

in an otherwise healthy individual. Palpitations are usually described by patients as sensations of beating, flip-flopping, or as a throbbing in the chest. They are often localized to the area of the apex beat but rapid supraventricular tachycardias are commonly felt substernally or in the neck. Some people seem to sense the compensatory pause (see below) following an extra heart beat but some may sense the extra beat itself. Often the contraction following an extra beat is more powerful than a normal beat (so-called post-extrasystolic potentiation) and this stronger beat may be the one that is felt. Supraventricular beats are more commonly sensed as palpitations than are ventricular beats; and in fact potentially dangerous runs of ventricular tachycardia are commonly asymptomatic.

Light-headedness, dizziness, or syncope are common symptoms of significant arrhythmias. These symptoms and the conditions associated with them are discussed in detail in Chapter 78.

Physical Examination

An arrhythmia is best revealed on physical examination by inspection of the jugular pulse, palpation of the arterial pulse, and by auscultation of the heart.

Conditions associated with arrhythmia—e.g., heart failure (Chapter 58), chronic obstructive lung disease (Chapter 52), or valvular heart disease (Chapter 57)—can often be recognized by characteristic physical findings.

Inspection of the jugular venous pulse reveals atrial activity. If there is atrioventricular dissociation or complete heart block, so-called cannon waves may be seen intermittently in the jugular veins; they are due to ejection of blood back into the veins when the right atrium contracts against a closed tricuspid valve. Cannon waves that coincide with the arterial pulse may reflect supraventricular tachycardia. If there is atrial fibrillation, there are no atrial waves visible in the jugular pulse.

Palpation of the arterial pulse establishes the ventricular rate—at least of conducted beats—and rhythm. In conjunction with the jugular pulse, it may provide more specific information as well about the nature of an arrythmia.

Auscultation of the heart also establishes the ventricular rate and rhythm and the intensity of S-1, the most useful heart sound in the evaluation of arrhythmia. For example, variation in the intensity of S-1 during a regular tachycardia suggests AV dissociation; variation during a regular bradycardia suggests 2nd or 3rd degree heart block.

Use of the Electrocardiogram

It is essential to obtain an ECG when evaluating a patient who has an arrhythmia. Without it, with few exceptions, a specific diagnosis is impossible. Usually a surface resting ECG is all that is needed. Occasionally, ambulatory (Holter) monitoring or an exercise ECG is indicated to detect a sporadic arrhythmia or an arrhythmia that is induced by stress. Even less commonly, a complex arrhythmia cannot be diagnosed accurately by standard ECG, and an intracavity (His bundle) ECG must be obtained by catheterization in order to make a precise diagnosis.

SURFACE RESTING ECG

There are a number of features of the standard ECG which must be assessed:

Atrial Activity. Atrial activity is best assessed in leads 2, 3, aVf, and in V-1. The presence of P waves must be identified. If P waves are present, their configuration and their relationship to QRS complexes must be established. Normally the P-R interval is between 0.12 and 0.20 sec and each QRS complex is preceded by a P wave. If P waves are not present,

other evidence of atrial activity (fibrillation or flutter waves) should be sought.

Ventricular Activity. The duration of the QRS complexes (normally less than 0.10 sec) should be measured and the regularity of ventricular activity should be assessed. A basically regular rhythm may be interrupted by so-called premature beats—contractions that appear before the next regular beat is expected. If premature beats are present, it should be noted whether or not they have a fixed relationship to the preceding normal beat and whether or not their configuration is the same as the regularly occurring complexes.

AMBULATORY ECG (16)

The ambulatory (Holter) ECG records on magnetic tape the electrical activity of the heart—usually for a 24-hour period, although some newer models record for 48 hours. The recording device is small and does not interfere with virtually any of the patient's activities (except bathing and swimming). The technique is useful in the following circumstances:

1. Assessing whether suspicious symptoms—e.g., dizziness, light-headedness, palpitations, or syncope—in a patient with a normal resting ECG are due to an episodic arrhythmia.

2. Assessing whether episodic, but potentially life-threatening, arrhythmias are occurring in a patient with known heart disease (e.g., mitral valve prolapse or ischemic heart disease).

3. Assessing the efficacy of antiarrhythmic therapy or the function of a cardiac pacemaker.

The great majority of episodic arrhythmias are detected during 24 hours of Holter monitoring. If symptoms are very infrequent, however, and ambulatory ECG is unrevealing, it may be necessary to repeat the study periodically. It is important to ask the patient to keep a record of symptoms during the time that he is being monitored in order to determine whether those symptoms are, in fact, attributable to arrhythmia.

EXERCISE ECG

This technique is described in detail in Chapter 54. It is a useful test in the evaluation of patients who have symptoms suggestive of an arrhythmia during or after exercise or those with premature ventricular contractions—to determine if they become more or less frequent during or after exercise (see below, p. 518).

GENERAL PRINCIPLES IN MANAGEMENT OF ARRHYTHMIA

Once it has been established that a patient has a particular arrhythmia, the physician must decide whether treatment is necessary. That decision will be influenced by the effect of the arrhythmia on cardiac output, the potential for thromboembolic complications, the potential for degeneration of the arrhythmia into a more dangerous rhythm, and the relative risk of the treatment versus the relative risk of the arrhythmia to the patient's well-being and survival. It must also be determined whether the arrhythmia is constant or intermittent and whether it is secondary to a noncardiac process (e.g., hypoxia, electrolyte imbalance, fever) or a cardiac process (e.g., heart failure, pericarditis, digitalis intoxication), the correction of which will restore a normal cardiac rhythm.

If the physician determines that specific therapy is indicated, he must decide which of the various possible regimens is appropriate: one or more of the various antiarrhythmic drugs, a cardiac pacemaker, electrical conversion of the arrhythmia, or a combination of these.

Pharmacology of Antiarrhythmic Drugs

There are three major classes of antiarrhythmic drugs. *Membrane-active antiarrhythmic drugs* affect cell membrane properties such as rate of depolarization, conduction velocity, action potential duration, and refractory period. *β-Adrenergic blocking drugs* affect sympathetically mediated excitability and *calcium channel blocking drugs* affect calcium-mediated slow channel currents in the myocardium.

Table 56.1 shows some of the characteristics of the antiarrhythmic drugs that can be conveniently used to treat an ambulatory patient. Because lidocaine (Xylocaine) can only be administered parenterally and has a short half-life, it is limited to hospital use and is not included in the table. All of the drugs that are included can also be given parenterally (usually intravenously) but, again, this route of administration is limited almost exclusively to hospital use.

Most antiarrhythmic drugs have a low toxic:therapeutic ratio and some are exceedingly toxic (Table 56.2). The safe and effective use of antiarrhythmic drugs depends on a careful assessment of the etiology and physiology of an arrhythmia, and a knowledge of the pharmacology of the drugs that are used.

Digitalis, the other major drug used in the treatment of arrhythmias, acts indirectly as an antiarrhythmic agent by increasing vagal activity, thereby increasing the refractory period of the specialized conduction tissue of the atria and slowing the velocity of the action potential through the AV node. General considerations in the use of digitalis including dosages, choice of a preparation, and recognition and treatment of toxicity are discussed in Chapter 58.

MEMBRANE ACTIVE DRUGS

Quinidine

In addition to its direct effects on the heart, quinidine blocks parasympathetic stimulation by the vagus nerve and may enhance AV conduction (and the ventricular rate) in some patients. For this reason, patients with supraventricular tachyarrhythmias should be digitalized to suppress AV conduction before they are given quinidine. Quinidine also is a moderately potent inhibitor of α-adrenergic activity.

Several preparations of quinidine are available; quinidine sulfate is the recommended preparation on the basis of cost, but a prolonged release preparation containing gluconate (Quinaglute, Duraquin) may be preferred in some patients because it is less likely to cause gastrointestinal symptoms and can be given every 8 to 12 hours.

Table 56.1 shows the time necessary to reach a steady state after administration of usual doses of quinidine. If a faster effect is desired, loading doses may be given (e.g., 300 mg every 3 hours for 3 doses); in this circumstance hospitalization is advisable, both to monitor the effect of the drug and because the arrhythmia presumably is more dangerous.

Quinidine is used most often to prevent recurrence of supraventricular and ventricular tachyarrhythmias. It is also moderately effective, but is no longer the first approach, in the conversion of atrial flutter or fibrillation to normal sinus rhythm. The uses of the drug in specific situations are discussed below.

Toxicity. There are a number of possible toxic effects of quinidine. The most common are gastroin-

Table 56.1
Characteristics of Antiarrhythmic Drugs

Drug	Common Brand Name	Effects on ECG	Half-life (hr)	Time to Steady State (day)	Usual Oral Dose	Maximum Daily Dose (mg)	Therapeutic Plasma Levels
Quinidine	Generic	Prolongs QRS, QT, and (±) PR	6	1–2	200–600 mg q.6–8 h.	2400	3–7 µg/ml
Procainamide	Pronestyl	Prolongs QRS, QT, and (±) PR	3–4	1	500–1000 mg q.3–4 h.	8000	3–8 µg/ml[a]
Disopyramide	Norpace	Prolongs QRS, QT, and (±) PR	6–9	1–2	150 mg q.i.d.	1200	2–4 µg/ml
Propranolol	Inderal	Prolongs (±) PR, shortens QT	6	1	10–40 mg q.6h.	640	50–100 ng/ml
Phenytoin (diphenylhydantoin)	Dilantin	Shortens QT	24–36	3–5	300–400 mg a day	800	10–20 µg/ml

[a] It may also be important to measure, especially in patients in cardiac or renal failure, the level of the active metabolite of procainamide, N-acetylprocainamide (NAPA).

Table 56.2
Adverse Effects of Antiarrhythmic Drugs

Drug	Cardiac		Noncardiac	
	Common	Uncommon	Common	Uncommon
Quinidine	Decreased digoxin excretion (may precipitate digitoxicity)	Ventricular arrhythmias, myocardial depression, hypotension	Nausea, diarrhea, tinnitus, vertigo, rash, fever	Hepatic dysfunction, thrombocytopenia, hemolytic anemia
Procainamide	None	Myocardial depression	Nausea, vomiting	Agranulocytosis, lupus-like syndrome
Disopyramide	Myocardial depression, (should be used with caution in patients with severe or poorly compensated congestive heart failure)	Severe hypotension in absence of known heart disease	Anticholinergic effects— especially urinary retention, dry mouth, blurred vision, constipation, aggravation of narrow angle glaucoma	Acute psychoses, cholestasis
Propranolol[a]	Bradycardia, myocardial depression	Anginal syndrome may worsen if drug suddenly discontinued	Fatigue, nausea, vomiting, depression, impotence, potentiates bronchospasm in patients with asthma	Peripheral vascular insufficiency, hyperglycemia, alopecia
Phenytoin (Diphenylhydantoin)	None	Heart block	Cerebellar-vestibular effects, especially ataxia, nystagmus, vertigo; nausea, lethargy, seizures, rashes	Pseudolymphoma, megalobastic anemia, peripheral neuropathy

[a] Other β-blocking agents (metoprolol and nadalol) have the same adverse effects although bronchospasm and peripheral vascular insufficiency may be less likely with use of metoprolol.

testinal, especially diarrhea, and occur often within hours of administering the drug. Cinchonism (tinnitus, headache, visual disturbances) occurs occasionally. Hypersensitivity reactions (e.g., rash, arthralgias, immune thrombocytopenia, or hemolytic anemia) are rare. These reactions often necessitate substitution of another antiarrhythmic drug.

. Cardiac toxicity is usually dose-related, often signalled by a prolongation of the QT interval; QT prolongation of 50% or more beyond baseline is an indication for reduction of the dose of quinidine. Serious toxicity is manifest by a high degree of AV block, ventricular tachycardia or fibrillation—all emergency situations that may require cardiorespiratory support and warrant immediate hospitalization. Occasionally, patients taking quinidine die suddenly, sometimes with relatively low plasma levels of the drug. Patients with prolonged QT intervals before institution of therapy with quinidine may be more prone to sudden death and therefore probably should not be given the drug.

If patients taking quinidine are asymptomatic, ECGs need be recorded no more frequently than once a year; if they are symptomatic (e.g., complain of exertional chest pain, light-headedness, shortness of breath, etc.), more frequent tracings should be obtained (perhaps every 3 or 4 months, although no firm guidelines can be recommended).

Drug Interactions. Since patients prescribed quinidine are commonly being treated with digitalis as well, it is especially important to recognize that digoxin levels may increase significantly in patients given quinidine. The precise mechanism is unclear, but quinidine appears to decrease the excretion of digoxin by the kidneys, and therefore it is important to monitor serum digoxin concentrations when quinidine is first prescribed and to alter the dose of digoxin to prevent digitoxicity.

Quinidine is an α-adrenergic blocker and, if it is prescribed with vasodilators (e.g., nitrates, hydralazine, prazosin) or with potent diuretics (e.g., furosemide), may cause symptomatic (especially postural) hypotension.

Drugs that are metabolized by hepatic microsomal enzymes may alter the pharmacokinetics of quinidine; and conversely, quinidine may alter the kinetics of one of these drugs. For example, phenytoin may accelerate the metabolism of quinidine, shortening its effect; and quinidine may inhibit the metabolism of warfarin, prolonging its effect.

Procainamide

The suppressive effects of procainamide on the electrical activity of the heart are the same as those of quinidine; but, unlike quinidine, procainamide has very little effect on vagal or on α-adrenergic activity.

The drug has been thought to be most useful in preventing recurrence of ventricular arrhythmias, although in somewhat higher doses (4 to 8 g/day instead of the more usual 2 to 6 g/day) it is as effective as quinidine in preventing the recurrence of atrial arrhythmias and in converting atrial flutter or fibrillation to normal sinus rhythm.

Toxicity. The noncardiac toxicity of procainamide is different from that of quinidine. Gastrointestinal symptoms occur less often; and when they do, nausea and vomiting are more common than is diarrhea. Fever or granulocytopenia occurs occasionally.

Fifty percent of people taking procainamide develop antinuclear antibodies (ANA) within 3 months and 90% within 12 months (5, 17). Twenty to thirty percent of patients with ANA develop a lupus-like syndrome characterized by serositis (pleuritis, pericarditis, synovitis), fever, hepatomegaly and a positive LE preparation. Unlike classical systemic lupus erythematosus, vasculitis is not a manifestation of drug-induced lupus so that renal disease, for example, does not occur; and, most important, the syndrome abates, usually within months, when the drug is discontinued. The major threat of the syndrome is hemorrhagic pericarditis, and signs and symptoms of pericardial tamponade must be watched for.

Disopyramide

Disopyramide has direct membrane effects very much like quinidine and, like quinidine, blocks parasympathetic activity. It is licensed currently only for the treatment of specific ventricular arrhythmias: unifocal or multifocal premature ventricular contractions and ventricular tachycardia. Disopyramide is used in ambulatory practice primarily for patients with one of these ventricular arrhythmias who cannot tolerate quinidine or procainamide.

The noncardiac toxicity of disopyramide is due mainly to its anticholinergic effects; these include dry mouth, blurred vision, urinary hesitancy, and constipation. Nausea, vomiting, and diarrhea are less common than they are after administration of quinidine or procainamide. The cardiac toxicity of the drug is, in part, similar to that of quindine in that it can prolong the QT interval and produce ventricular tachycardia. Disopyramide may also cause or intensify heart failure or cause profound hypotension in patients who have compromised left ventricular function; it should be administered cautiously to such patients and stopped immediately if adverse reactions occur.

Phenytoin

Phenytoin decreases automaticity and the duration of the action potential in the Purkinje fibers of the myocardium. Its use is limited in the treatment of arrhythmias: its primary value is in the treatment of complex arrhythmias associated with digitoxicity, and therefore it is seldom prescribed as an antiarrhythmic agent in ambulatory practice. Occasionally, patients will be discharged from hospital and will be taking phenytoin for control of a ventricular arrhythmia that has proved resistant to other drugs (or that

has only been controlled by lidocaine, a drug that cannot be used on an ambulatory basis). Such patients are best followed in conjunction with a cardiologist.

Phenytoin toxicity is discussed in detail in Chapter 77.

SYMPATHETIC BLOCKING AGENTS

These drugs block the effects of catecholamines (which may potentiate the development of arrhythmias) and slow conduction in the atria, AV node, and myocardium.

β-Blockers are used primarily to lower the ventricular response in patients with atrial tachyarrhythmia; occasionally, in the process, they will convert paroxysmal atrial tachycardia, atrial flutter or fibrillation to normal sinus rhythm. In addition, ventricular arrhythmias initiated by exercise or ischemia (see Chapter 56) or associated with the prolonged QT syndrome (see below) may be prevented by these drugs. β-Blockers appear to be synergistic with digoxin, and relatively low doses of propranolol and digoxin, for example, may be very effective in controlling heart rate in patients with atrial fibrillation, or in maintaining normal sinus rhythm in patients who have been cardioverted.

Toxicity. β-Blockers sometimes, by blocking sympathetic tone, precipitate heart failure in patients with poor ventricular function (an effect that can be overcome by digitalis), and they are contraindicated in patients with bronchial asthma.

The four currently available β-blocking agents are propranolol, metoprolol, nadalol and atenolol. Propranolol is the preparation prescribed most commonly. Metroprolol (Lopressor) has less of an effect on bronchial smooth muscle than does propranolol and is safer to prescribe to patients with a history of bronchospasm (although considerable caution still must be exercised). Nadalol (Corgard) is long acting and may be useful in less compliant patients. Atenolol is also long acting and is relatively cardioselective. However, the drug has only recently been made available and experience with it is limited.

CALCIUM CHANNEL BLOCKERS: VERAPAMIL (1, 24)

At the time of this writing oral calcium channel blocking agents (see above, p. 503) are about to be approved for clinical use. Verapamil is the agent that has been studied most intensively as an antiarrhythmic drug. Its primary use appears to be in the control of supraventricular tachycardia. How effective the drug will be when administered orally (much of the work has been done by use of intravenous verapamil) to ambulatory patients is not yet clear nor is its long term toxicity.

Pacemaker Therapy

Implantable electrical pulse generators are the treatment of choice for patients with symptomatic bradyarrhythmias and heart block. In addition, specialized types of pacemakers may be used to terminate tachyarrhythmias by generating a current pulse which interferes with re-entrant tachycardias (socalled *overdrive pacing*). Modern pacemakers are less than 1 cm thick, weigh less than 70 g, and may function for 10 to 15 years. Pacemaker leads are easily implantable via a percutaneous transvenous technique and rarely become dislodged even during vigorous activity. Symptoms are relieved in a majority of patients who are symptomatic due to bradyarrhythmias and conduction block (see below).

Patient Experience. The units are implanted subcutaneously under local anesthesia in the pectoral area and the pacemaker lead is inserted via the cephalic vein or directly with the use of a special introducer into the subclavian vein and lodged in the apex of the right ventricle. The procedure takes about 1 1/2 hours; the patient experiences some discomfort when the anesthetic is injected and, often, an unpleasant sensation when the tissues are manipulated to create a pocket for the pacemaker unit.

After the procedure, patients, depending on their age and condition, are discharged from the hospital within 3 to 7 days. Patients with sedentary jobs may return to work approximately 2 weeks after pacemaker insertion, but patients with more active jobs should be kept off work for approximately 6 weeks to allow the wound to heal completely. After that, there is little or no discomfort and the unit feels like part of the chest wall. Patients may exercise if they wish, but should avoid extreme exertion (for example, doubles tennis rather than singles; jogging rather than hard running).

Patients with implanted pacemakers require careful, longterm follow-up. They must be seen approximately every 3 months and the function of the pacemaker must be assessed with a 12-lead ECG and a rhythm strip. The ECG documents that the complexes have not changed, implying that the pacemaker lead has not shifted position; and the sensing and pacing functions of the pacemaker are determined with the rhythm strip. Longterm follow-up is usually done in conjunction with a cardiologist.

It is important that the make of the pacemaker, its registration number, and its rate be entered into the patient's record and that the patient keep the registration card for the pacemaker on his person in the event of malfunction of the instrument or of an emergency intercurrent problem.

Cardioversion

The electrical conversion of atrial or ventricular tachyarrhythmias is done by the application of a short burst of direct current to the chest wall. The shock is synchronized with the QRS complex of the ECG to avoid applying it during the vulnerable period of the cardiac cycle when ventricular tachycardia or fibrillation might be induced.

Cardioversion is a more reliable technique for the conversion of tachyarrhythmias than is the administration of antiarrhythmic drugs. It may be required on an emergency basis if a patient has developed severe heart failure, hypotension or ischemia as a result of an arrhythmia. Otherwise the procedure should be planned with the cardiologist who will attempt the conversion.

Digitalis should be withheld for 1 day before the procedure to ensure that an excess amount of drug is not circulating, and quinidine, 400 mg every 6 hours, should be given for 1 day before the procedure to minimize the development of arrhythmia at the time of the conversion. (Some patients will convert to sinus rhythm after administration of quinidine.) It is not clear whether or not patients to be subjected to cardioversion should be treated with anticoagulants. It seems reasonable, however, to give anticoagulants to patients in chronic heart failure, who have a history of prior embolism, or who have mitral stenosis. Anticoagulation (see Chapter 48) in these circumstances should be maintained for 2 weeks before and 2 weeks after the procedure; many cardiologists maintain anticoagulation indefinitely in these patients.

Patient Experience. Cardioversion is done in a hospital with an anesthesiologist in attendance and with resuscitation equipment available. The patient is sedated, usually with 5 or 10 mg of intravenous diazepam or with intravenous Surital (thiamylal, a very short acting barbiturate), given to effect. Normally the patient cannot recall afterward the details of the procedure. For atrial fibrillation, cardioversion is attempted at 100 watt-seconds; the energy level is doubled repetitively and other shocks are administered until there is conversion or until a level of 400 watt-seconds is reached, after which the procedure must be terminated. Complications—embolism or a new arrhythmia—are unusual. After cardioversion, the patient is observed for a day or two and his rhythm is monitored, and then he is discharged. Quinidine is usually administered chronically in an attempt to prevent recurrence of the arrhythmia.

SPECIFIC ARRHYTHMIAS

Sinus Tachycardia

DEFINITION AND ETIOLOGY

In adults the normal sinus rate is 60 to 100 beats per min. Sinus tachycardia, a sinus rhythm at a rate greater than 100 beats/min, is usually a physiologic rhythm in that the rate is ordinarily appropriate to the physiologic state of the patient—a state that requires an increased cardiac output to meet increased metabolic demands. The maximum sinus heart rate that can be attained varies with age, but usually does not exceed 140 beats/min unless demands are excessive (vigorous exercise, for example). The common factors that stimulate an increase in the rate of sinus rhythm, other than exercise, are fever (an increase of approximately 10 beats/min for each Fahrenheit degree rise in body temperature), emotional stress, heart failure, and a variety of drugs that affect the autonomic nervous system (e.g., caffeine, aminophylline, amphetamines, alcohol, antidepressants, phenothiazines, etc.).

PHYSICAL FINDINGS

A regular rapid pulse and heart rate are detected although there may be a slight variation in rate—so-called sinus arrhythmia. S-1 is normal and the jugular pulsations are normal.

ELECTROCARDIOGRAM

A P wave precedes each QRS complex; the PR interval is normal for the rate (0.16 to 0.17 at rates over 130/min); and the P wave vector is normal (upright P waves in II, III, and aVf).

TREATMENT

In most cases persistent sinus tachycardia need not be treated; it is the underlying condition that requires therapy. Digitalis, especially, should not be used to treat a patient with sinus tachycardia unless he is in heart failure.

In the occasional patient with an unexplained sinus tachycardia in whom a thorough evaluation fails to reveal an underlying cause, and in whom tachycardia is symptomatic, the use of small doses of propranolol may be justified. Treatment should be initiated with 10 mg, 2 or 3 times a day. Recent experience has documented that low dose propranolol may also be helpful in treating the anxiety and tachycardia associated with anticipated stressful situations. Used only as necessary, doses of 20 to 40 mg of propranolol an hour before a public speaking engagement, for example, may help to relieve the associated anxiety and tachycardia experienced by some people.

Sinus Bradycardia

DEFINITION AND ETIOLOGY

Sinus bradycardia is a heart rate below 60 beats per min. Impulse generation in the sinus node is often slow in well conditioned people (e.g., long distance runners, heavy laborers). Inappropriately low sinus rates are commonly due to increased vagal tone such as is seen in association with pain, vomiting, or vasovagal syncope. A hypersensitive carotid sinus, more common in elderly people, may also result in marked bradycardia when the sinus is compressed by a tight collar or by the patient's tensing his neck. Parasympathomimetic drugs such as neostigmine, tranquilizers, phenothiazines, and digitalis and sympatholytic drugs such as reserpine or methyldopa also may produce sinus bradycardia. Vagally induced bradycardia may be severe and result in asystole (and loss of consciousness) when the stimulus is marked or prolonged or occurs in a hypoxic patient.

PHYSICAL FINDINGS

A regular slow pulse and heart rate are detected. S-1 is normal and the jugular pulsations are normal.

ELECTROCARDIOGRAM

A P wave precedes each QRS complex; the PR interval is normal for the rate (0.20 to 0.21) and the P wave vector is normal (upright P waves in II, III, and aVf).

TREATMENT

Asymptomatic sinus bradycardia discovered as an incidental finding does not require treatment. However, patients who present with symptoms of light-headedness or syncope and are found to have sinus bradycardia may have underlying sinus node disease or may be subject to paroxysms of tachycardia and bradycardia, the so-called "sick sinus syndrome" (see below). Patients with sinus bradycardia and symptoms should be evaluated with an ambulatory ECG to determine whether they are suffering from this condition. In any case, patients with symptomatic sinus bradycardia, not due to a drug, are best treated with permanent pacemaker implantation.

Sick Sinus Syndrome

DEFINITION AND ETIOLOGY

The term sick sinus syndrome refers to a heterogeneous group of arrhythmias involving defective impulse generation by the sinus node and/or abnormal impulse conduction in the atria. The syndrome is characterized by periods of inappropriate sinus bradycardia (often severe with rates between 25 and 40/min) which may precede or follow supraventricular tachyarrhythmias and by varying degrees of sinoatrial block including, sometimes, sinus arrest. The rubrics "bradycardia-tachycardia syndrome" or "tachycardia-bradycardia syndrome" are sometimes used, depending upon whether bradycardia precedes or follows a tachyarrhythmia.

The sick sinus syndrome is caused by degenerative fibrotic changes within the sinus node. It is often associated with similar abnormalities in other parts of the cardiac conduction system that result in varying degrees of atrioventricular and intraventricular block. These pathologic changes are much more common in patients over the age of 60; although their precise cause is unknown, they are often associated with hypertensive or ischemic heart disease.

SYMPTOMS AND SIGNS

Many patients are asymptomatic. When symptoms do occur, they are produced either by spontaneous sinus arrest or by the tachyarrhythmia itself (palpitations). If there is coexistent left ventricular dysfunction or coronary artery disease, symptoms of heart failure or of ischemia may occur.

The physical examination is often normal unless the patient is examined during an episode of brady-

or tachyarrhythmia in which case the findings will depend on the type of arrhythmia that is present (see below). Sometimes light carotid sinus massage will produce a symptomatic bradyarrhythmia in a patient with sick sinus syndrome who is in normal sinus rhythm.

ELECTROCARDIOGRAM

The ECG may be normal or may simply reveal sinus bradycardia. Often, there are varying degrees of sinoatrial block, characterized by varying P-P intervals on the ECG. Sometimes sinus arrest occurs, manifest by absent P waves and associated, usually, with a junctional escape rhythm. Some patients have slow atrial fibrillation reflecting a concomitant AV conduction abnormality (see above). The ECG changes of the various atrial tachyarrhythmias are described below in the discussions of these entities.

If there is a history of unexplained syncope or of palpitations and the resting ECG is normal, ambulatory ECG monitoring is indicated (see above, p. 507).

TREATMENT AND COURSE

The treatment of choice for patients with the sick sinus syndrome who are symptomatic from bradyarrhythmias is permanent pacemaker implantation (see above, p. 510). Otherwise symptoms are often progressive. Actually, even patients with relatively minor symptoms (e.g., light-headedness or dizziness) often will find that they feel significantly better after pacemaker therapy. Vagolytic drugs (atropine, for example) or β-adrenergic agonists (e.g., isoproterenol) are only of transient benefit.

Tachyarrhythmias associated with the syndrome are often not prevented by electrical pacing. However, pacing does allow the use of drugs such as digitalis and propranolol which depress the sinus node and increase the likelihood of sinus arrest or asystole. It is reasonable, after a pacemaker is implanted, to administer propranolol, 10 mg 4 times a day, and to increase the dose to 40 mg 4 times a day in an attempt to prevent tachyarrhythmias. If propranolol is not effective, digoxin should be administered as well. If tachyarrhythmias continue, consideration should be given, in conjunction with the consulting cardiologist, to the use of an antiarrhythmic drug (see above).

Patients with sick sinus syndrome have an incidence, unaffected by pacemaker therapy, of arterial embolization of approximately 10% per year (9). However there is no evidence yet to support the use of anticoagulant or antiplatelet drugs (aspirin or persantine) in this condition.

A high mortality rate is associated with the sick sinus syndrome in elderly people, usually because of coexistent atherosclerotic vascular disease (2, 27). Nearly half of patients over the age of 60 die within 2 years of pacemaker implantation (27).

Premature Atrial and Junctional Contractions

DEFINITION AND ETIOLOGY

Premature atrial and junctional contractions (PACs and PJCs) are commonly seen in patients who are otherwise well. They often are induced by the same stimuli that produce sinus tachycardia, especially caffeine or nicotine. However, in patients with congestive heart failure or chronic pulmonary disease PACs or PJCs may progress to atrial fibrillation or flutter.

SYMPTOMS AND SIGNS

Usually patients are unaware of premature atrial or junctional contractions. Occasionally they will note the PAC or PJC as a palpitation; and the physician, on listening to the heart or palpating the arterial pulse, will be aware of a slight irregularity in the cardiac rhythm.

ELECTROCARDIOGRAM

Premature atrial contractions are reflected in the ECG by a premature morphologically abnormal P wave followed by a premature morphologically normal QRS complex. Often these impulses are not conducted (Fig. 56.5) in which case, if the P wave is buried in the preceding T wave, a false diagnosis of sinus arrest may be made. At other times the premature impulse may be aberrantly conducted, the result of relative refractoriness of one of the bundle branches (usually a right bundle branch pattern is seen following the premature atrial beat).

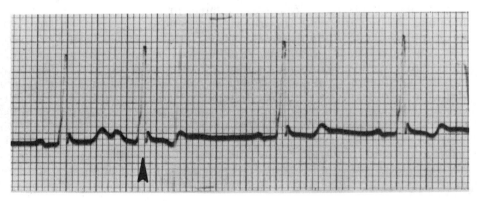

Figure 56.5 A premature atrial contraction (*arrow*). Note the normal configuration of the premature QRS complex.

Premature junctional contractions are reflected in the ECG by a retrograde P wave (negatively deflected in leads II, III, and aVf) which may follow, be hidden in, or precede a morphologically normal but premature QRS complex.

TREATMENT

Patients with premature contractions who are otherwise well do not require treatment.

Rarely, it may be necessary to prescribe digoxin or propranolol to reduce the frequency of PACs or to prevent their conduction to the ventricles in patients who have annoyingly frequent palpitations. In patients with underlying cardiac or pulmonary disease digitalization may prevent the progression of PACs to atrial fibrillation. Quinidine or procainamide is effective also in the control of PACs but the risk associated with the use of these drugs usually is not warranted (see above, p. 508).

Paroxysmal Supraventricular Tachycardia

DEFINITION AND ETIOLOGY

Supraventricular tachycardias (SVTs) are rapid heart rates (120 to 220 beats/min) triggered by a premature impulse generated anywhere between the sinus node and the AV junction. Most of these arrhythmias are due to re-entry (see p. 506)—usually in the AV node, occasionally through an accessory pathway or in the atria. Less often they are initiated by an ectopic atrial pacemaker.

About half the time, patients with SVTs have an otherwise normal heart (14). The common forms of heart disease associated with SVT are the pre-excitation syndrome (see below, p. 524), mitral valve prolapse (see Chapter 57), and atrial septal defect (see Chapter 57). Nonparoxysmal atrial tachycardia with block (due to gradually accelerated automaticity of an ectopic atrial focus) is a common manifestation of digitalis toxicity.

SYMPTOMS AND SIGNS

Patients are almost always aware of a suddenly rapid heart rate; usually there are no other symptoms but, if there is coexistent heart disease, patients may complain of shortness of breath or of ischemic chest pain. Often the patient will be able to terminate the arrhythmia abruptly by a Valsalva maneuver or by coughing. Frequently, polyuria will be experienced for as long as the arrhythmia lasts.

Attacks often occur spontaneously but may be precipitated by physical or emotional stress, caffeine, or nicotine. They may be as short as a few seconds and as long as several weeks. The frequency of the attacks is also quite variable; some people have attacks every day; some, only a few times during their entire life.

On examination, the physician will note a rapid regular arterial pulse and heart rate—often faster than that measured in patients with sinus tachycardia and usually not associated with the same stimuli. When the atria and ventricles contract simultaneously, cannon waves will be seen in the jugular veins.

ELECTROCARDIOGRAM

Paroxysmal SVT is characterized by a rapid regular heart rate. There is a fixed relationship of the P wave to the QRS complex. If the impulse is generated in the AV node, the P wave may be buried in the QRS complex but the process can be identified by the normal appearance of the QRS complex and by the regularity of the rate. When the P wave is visible, it may follow the QRS complex (some nodal re-entry rhythms, all accessory pathway re-entry rhythms) and will be inverted in leads II, III, and aVf. It may also precede the QRS complex and may appear morphologically normal (atrial re-entry or ectopic rhythm), in which case the diagnosis can only be made (by ECG) if the rate is high enough to make sinus tachycardia unlikely. The P wave also may be hidden in the T wave; but, again, the regularity of the rate and the usually normal duration of the QRS complex establishes the diagnosis.

If SVT occurs in association with an AV conduction abnormality, the ventricular rate will be slower than the atrial rate. The arrhythmia can be diagnosed by the rapid regular atrial rate. Various degrees of block may occur (see below)—for example, 2:1 AV block in which the atrial rate is twice the ventricular rate (Fig. 56.6).

Sometimes in patients with SVT there are coexistent bundle branch or intraventricular conduction abnormalities, and prolonged abnormal QRS complexes may occur. If P waves are not visible, the only way to distinguish this arrhythmia from ventricular tachycardia is by comparison with an ECG taken when the rate was slow (in which the abnormal QRS complexes will still be seen) and by the regularity and rate (ventricular rates greater than 160 beats/min are unlikely to represent ventricular tachycardia). If SVT occurs in a patient with an accessory AV conduction pathway (see below), conduction may be aberrant and it may not be possible with a surface ECG to distinguish the arrhythmia from ventricular tachycardia. If there is any question about which of these diagnoses is correct, urgent consultation with a cardiologist is in order.

TREATMENT AND COURSE

Therapy of paroxysmal SVT always starts with attempts to increase vagal tone. As mentioned above (see "Symptoms and Signs") the patient often has learned to do this himself. If the arrhythmia persists despite the patient's efforts, the physician should first apply carotid sinus massage. This must be done after auscultation of the carotid arteries to ensure that there are no bruits; if there are, carotid sinus massage is contraindicated. The carotid sinus is at the point of maximum impulse of the carotid artery in the neck. The right sinus should be massaged first

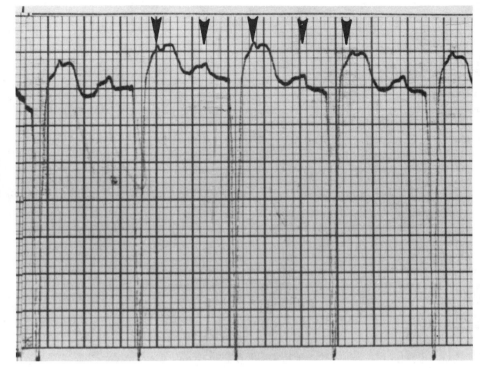

Figure 56.6 Supraventricular tachycardia with 2:1 AV block: The *arrows* point to consecutive P waves.

for up to 20 sec; if that has no effect, the left sinus should be massaged; the two sinuses should never be massaged simultaneously. During massage, the patient's ECG should be monitored continuously, and resuscitation equipment should be available.

If carotid sinus massage fails, pharmacologic therapy is indicated. This is best done in an emergency room or in a similar facility. If that is not logistically possible, the drug of choice is edrophonium (Tensilon), 5 to 10 mg intravenously; it usually converts the arrhythmia to normal sinus rhythm within 5 min. If, after administration of Tensilon, SVT persists, propranolol (1 mg intravenously every 5 min until conversion occurs or until 0.1 mg/kg has been given), digoxin (0.5 mg intravenously), phenylephrine (0.5 to 1.5 mg intravenously), or verapamil (10 mg intravenously followed, if necessary, by 10 mg 30 min later) should be given. One of these drugs is almost certain to be successful; rarely cardioversion is necessary.

Chronic administration of digoxin is indicated for prevention of recurrent attacks of SVT in patients with frequent symptomatic episodes. If the attacks recur despite digitalization, cardiology consultation is again indicated for advice about the use of antiarrhythmic agents and for possible diagnostic electrical pacing with intracardiac ECG to determine the precise nature of the arrhythmia and the regimen most likely to prevent it.

The *course* of patients with SVT is dependent on its cause. If the arrhythmia occurs in patients who are otherwise healthy, there is no morbidity between attacks and essentially no effect on survival. If it occurs in patients with underlying cardiac or pul-

monary disease, there is a real but undefined risk of heart failure, myocardial ischemia, or sudden death during an episode. Otherwise, survival is dependent on the nature and severity of the underlying disease.

If SVT occurs in association with an AV conduction abnormality (commonly 2:1 block), and the patient is taking digitalis, the drug should be withheld and serum potassium concentration should be measured. If the patient is hypokalemic, potassium repletion is, of course, in order; usually this can be accomplished by administration of oral potassium salts (i.e., 20 meq 3 times a day—see Chapter 42). Patients with refractory digitoxic arrhythmias with block should be hospitalized for more aggressive treatment. If SVT with atrioventricular block is not due to digitoxicity, it should be treated in the same way as SVT without block.

Multifocal Atrial Tachycardia

Multifocal atrial tachycardia is a chaotic supraventricular arrhythmia characterized electrocardiographically by varying morphology of the P waves, varying P-R intervals, and a rapid heart rate, usually 100–200 beats/minute; QRS morphology is normal and every QRS complex is preceded by a P wave (Fig. 56.7). The arrhythmia is usually seen in patients with serious underlying disease, especially decompensated chronic obstructive pulmonary disease, and is better treated by, for example, improving ventilatory function than by attempting directly to suppress the rhythm. Digitalis will not alter this arrhythmia (which is usually well tolerated) and therefore should not be administered.

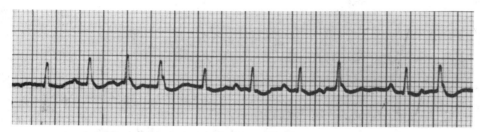

Figure 56.7 Multifocal atrial tachycardia. Note the variation in the morphology of the P waves and in the duration of the P-R intervals.

Atrial Fibrillation

DEFINITION AND ETIOLOGY

Atrial fibrillation is defined electrophysiologically as rapid uncoordinated generation of electrical impulses by the atria. It is usually triggered by a premature atrial contraction (see above) which, by reentry, generates multifocal impulses at a rate of 300 to 500/min. These impulses enter the AV node randomly; and, because of the slower rate of conduction of the AV node, not all of them are conducted. Therefore, the ventricular rate is slower than the atrial rate and is irregular. In untreated patients with normal AV conduction the ventricular rate is between 150 and 200 beats/min.

Atrial fibrillation may occur paroxysmally in people, even in young adults, who have no other evidence of heart disease. In such cases it often is associated with the same stimuli that produce other atrial arrhythmias (sinus tachycardia, premature atrial contractions, paroxysmal supraventricular tachycardia): physical or emotional stress, alcohol, nicotine, or caffeine. The major noncardiac illness associated with atrial fibrillation is hyperthyroidism; and in the presence of a fast ventricular response refractory to digitalis, atrial fibrillation may be the first clue to the diagnosis.

There are many forms of heart disease that predispose to the development of atrial fibrillation; the commonest are hypertensive, atherosclerotic, and rheumatic (especially when it involves the mitral valve), but almost every kind of myocardial disorder has been associated with it. Also, the tachyarrhythmic component of the sick sinus syndrome (see above) may be atrial fibrillation.

SYMPTOMS AND SIGNS

The only common symptom of atrial fibrillation is palpitations. If the ventricular response is fast (as it often is at onset of the arrhythmia), patients often complain of feeling "strange," weak, or faint as well. Since atrial contraction normally provides 20% of the total cardiac output, patients with incipient heart failure, ischemic heart disease, or valvular heart disease may develop symptoms (and signs) of those disorders (especially on exertion) when cardiac output is reduced as the result of atrial fibrillation.

Atrial fibrillation is characterized by an irregularly irregular heart beat and pulse with variation in intensity of the sounds (including murmurs) on both auscultation and palpation. It is prudent to look for signs of diseases known to be associated with atrial fibrillation (e.g., hypertension, mitral stenosis, and hyperthyroidism)—especially since those signs may be subtle or altered by the arrhythmia.

ELECTROCARDIOGRAM

The ECG shows rapid irregular fibrillatory atrial activity at rates between 300 and 500/min; no P waves are present. The ventricular rhythm is irregularly irregular, at rates which at onset are usually between 150 and 200/min—unless there is coexistent disease in the AV node in which case slower rates are likely (Fig. 56.8).

The QRS complex is usually morphologically normal. Occasionally there is aberrant conduction of an impulse in the ventricles, following a beat that has been preceded by a long pause. The aberrant beat usually has a right bundle branch block configuration. This so-called Ashman phenomenon is due to prolonged refractoriness of the (usually) right bundle branch after the long pause. It is important to distinguish these aberrant beats from ventricular premature beats. Apart from their typical relationship to a preceding long R-R interval, aberrant beats are often triphasic (RSR') and their initial vector is the same as that of the normally conducted beats; neither of these features is characteristic of ventricular premature beats.

TREATMENT AND COURSE

The approach to the treatment of atrial fibrillation should always include a search for underlying or precipitating factors. Treatment of the arrhythmia has two objectives: to slow the ventricular rate if it is fast and to convert the patient to sinus rhythm if possible.

Paroxysmal atrial fibrillation in a patient who does not have underlying heart disease often will revert to normal sinus rhythm once precipitating factors (e.g., stress, alcohol, nicotine) are removed. Specific treatment is indicated in the following circumstances: a rapid ventricular response associated with symptoms (e.g., extreme fatigue, syncope, angina, or shortness of breath); the presence of known underlying severe heart disease (e.g., aortic stenosis, severe mitral stenosis, ischemic heart disease, chronic congestive failure)—these patients are unlikely to revert to normal sinus rhythm spontaneously; persistent atrial fibrillation—especially if the resting ventricular rate is

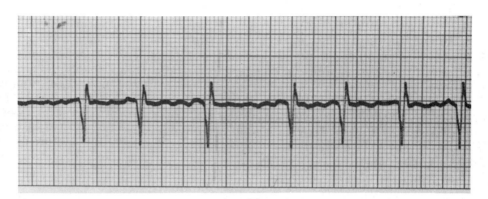

Figure 56.8 Atrial fibrillation. The ventricular rate is 90–100 beats/minute, indicative (since digitalis had not been administered) of an associated disorder of atrioventricular conduction.

greater than 110 beats/min or if the rate after moderate exercise (climbing a flight of stairs, for example) is greater than 150 beats/min.

Symptomatic patients and patients with underlying severe heart disease are best admitted immediately after onset of the arrhythmia to the hospital for cardioversion or for pharmacotherapy. Patients with persistent atrial fibrillation of less than 6 months' duration, particularly if there is no left atrial enlargement, should be hospitalized for elective cardioversion. Patients with atrial fibrillation that has lasted longer than 6 months or patients with large left atria are likely to be refractory to cardioversion. In general, cardioversion restores normal sinus rhythm in approximately 90% of patients but the relapse rate is high—50% in 1 year and 90% in 3 years (13)—unless the underlying disorder can be corrected or atrial fibrillation has been of short duration.

Asymptomatic or mildly symptomatic patients who have a rapid ventricular response should be treated with digitalis with a goal of a resting ventricular rate between 60 and 90 beats/min and a rate after modest exercise of below 150 beats/min. A loading dose by mouth of 0.75 to 1.0 mg of digoxin followed by 0.25 mg a day is ordinarily sufficient. If rapid digitalization is desired, it is best to hospitalize the patient and to administer intravenous digoxin. Approximately 20% of patients will convert to normal sinus rhythm after receiving digitalis.

If digitalization slows the rate, but the ventricular response is still too high, small doses of propranolol (10 to 20 mg 4 times a day) will often lower the rate further (see above, p. 510 for a general discussion of the use of this drug).

Patients who cannot or will not be cardioverted should receive an antiarrhythmic drug after they are digitalized (quinidine is ordinarily the first choice and will cause a return to normal sinus rhythm in about one-third of patients).

If the ventricular response is slow in untreated patients, there is an associated disorder of AV conduction. Such patients do not require specific therapy for the arrhythmia unless they are hemodynamically compromised (*i.e.*, in refractory heart failure) and their heart rate is under 60 to 70 beats/min, in which case, implantation of a pacemaker may be indicated.

Patients with atrial fibrillation are at increased risk of arterial embolization, especially if they have mitral stenosis and/or large left atria. For example, the Framingham study reported that, over a 24-year period, patients with chronic atrial fibrillation with and without rheumatic heart disease had a 17- and 5-fold increase, respectively, in the incidence of stroke (28). Overall the incidence of arterial embolization in patients with chronic atrial fibrillation is about 10% a year (9). It is the practice to give all patients the anticoagulant warfarin before elective cardioversion (see above, p. 511) and, although there are no good studies to support it, many physicians routinely treat with anticoagulants any patient with chronic atrial fibrillation if there are no contraindications. It seems reasonable to recommend anticoagulation for all patients who have had even one episode of arterial embolization as well as for patients with mitral stenosis or those who have paroxysmal atrial fibrillation as part of the sick sinus syndrome (see above, p. 512).

Apart from the morbidity and mortality associated with atrial embolization, the *prognosis* of patients with atrial fibrillation depends very much on whether there is underlying heart disease and, if there is, what the nature of it is.

Atrial Flutter

DEFINITION AND ETIOLOGY

Atrial flutter is a relatively coordinated rapid atrial activity due to re-entry of premature atrial impulses. Atrial beats are generated at about 300/min. Usually there is a 2:1 AV conduction block so that the ventricular response is about 150/min and, unlike atrial fibrillation, both atrial and ventricular responses are regular. Atrial flutter is almost always seen in patients who have underlying disease: ischemic heart disease, rheumatic heart disease, congestive cardiomyopathy, atrial septal defect, mitral valve disease, chronic obstructive pulmonary disease, and thyrotoxicosis—the same diseases often associated with atrial fibrillation. In contrast to atrial fibrillation, however, atrial flutter is not often seen in patients who are otherwise healthy.

SYMPTOMS AND SIGNS

Patients are usually aware of a rapid heart rate; whether or not other symptoms develop depends on the severity and nature of the underlying heart disease.

A regular rapid heart rate and atrial pulse are detected. Sometimes the flutter waves are visible in the jugular pulse. An S-4 is occasionally audible (in distinction to atrial fibrillation).

ELECTROCARDIOGRAM

The ECG shows rapid regular sawtooth flutter waves at about 300/min (Fig. 56.9); P waves are absent. The ventricular response is regular, usually at about 150/min and the QRS complex is ordinarily morphologically normal. If the AV node is diseased, higher degrees of AV block may be seen—usually a multiple of 2 (4:1, 8:1, etc). Aberrant conduction (see "Atrial Fibrillation") is unusual.

If the diagnosis is unclear, carotid sinus massage may help distinguish atrial flutter from other paroxysmal supraventricular tachyarrhythmias. It usually causes an abrupt temporary slowing of the rate and flutter waves, which may have been difficult to detect at a higher rate, will be visible in the electrocardiogram, most commonly in leads II, III, aVf and V1.

TREATMENT AND COURSE

Atrial flutter is an unstable rhythm and usually converts spontaneously to normal sinus rhythm or to atrial fibrillation. Because the rhythm is unstable and because patients usually have underlying heart disease, they are best hospitalized for observation and treatment. Unlike the situation in patients with atrial fibrillation, it is often difficult to lower the ventricular rate with digitalis in patients with atrial flutter. Nevertheless, digitalization is reasonable—especially if hospitalization must be delayed—since some patients will convert to normal sinus rhythm by administration of digoxin alone.

If there is no contraindication, however, electrical cardioversion is the treatment of choice if atrial flutter persists. Almost every patient can be converted to normal sinus rhythm, usually after application of a much lower current than is necessary to convert atrial fibrillation.

Digitalis (i.e., digoxin 0.25 mg a day) should be administered to prevent recurrences of atrial flutter. If digitalis is not effective alone, propranolol 20 to 40 mg every 6 hours or quinidine 200 to 300 mg every 6 hours should also be prescribed. All of these drugs are much more effective in preventing recurrence of flutter than they are in converting it to normal sinus rhythm.

Ventricular Premature Beats

DEFINITION AND ETIOLOGY

Ventricular premature beats (VPBs) are impulses generated in the ventricles, usually as the result of re-entry of an impulse conducted down from the atria through the AV node, but sometimes as the result of the firing of an ectopic (parasystolic) focus.

Occasional VPBs occur in many healthy people sporadically during their life, more frequently in older people. However, often VPBs are associated with underlying organic heart disease: e.g., ischemic heart disease, cardiomyopathy, or mitral valve prolapse. The frequency of VPBs may be increased in people both with and without heart disease by caffeine, alcohol, sympathomimetic drugs, tricyclic antidepressants, phenothiazines, hypokalemia, hypoxia, and excitement. VPBs are a common manifestation of digitoxicity. Exercise usually abolishes ventricular premature activity in normal people; if there is underlying heart disease, the effect of exercise is unpredictable, but an increase in the number of VPBs after exertion is highly suggestive of underlying disease.

SYMPTOMS AND SIGNS

Patients may not be aware that they have had a VPB, but often they experience a palpitation—either sensing the premature beat itself or the more forceful normal beat that follows it after a compensatory pause.

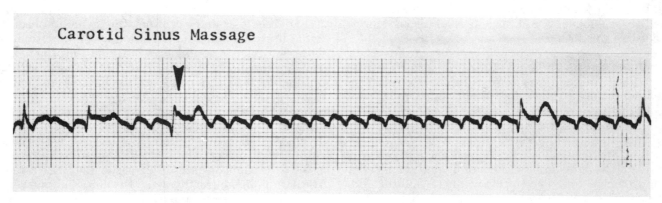

Figure 56.9 Atrial flutter. The flutter waves are clearly revealed after carotid sinus massage (*arrow*).

ELECTROCARDIOGRAM

The ECG shows a premature ventricular response with a morphologically abnormal, often bizarre, wide QRS complex. No P wave precedes a VPB but, by retrograde conduction, a P wave sometimes follows it. The ST segment and the T wave have an opposite vector from the QRS complex. Typically, a VPB is followed by a compensatory pause, i.e., the R-R interval between two normal beats separated by a VPB is the same as that between two normal beats separated by another normal beat (Fig. 56.10).

When VPBs are due to re-entry, they have a fixed temporal ("coupled") relationship to the preceding normal beats. When they are due to the firing of an ectopic (parasystolic) focus, they have no fixed relationship to the preceding normal beats but do have a regular pattern (i.e., the ectopic intervals are constant or are multiples of a constant). Ectopic beats may occasionally fuse with normal beats, producing a complex that is intermediate between the two (Fig. 56.11).

TREATMENT AND COURSE

Ventricular premature beats in patients with otherwise normal hearts are not harmful. However, there is an increased incidence of sudden death and of myocardial infarction in patients with VPBs who have underlying ischemic heart disease (15). It has not been demonstrated that suppression of VPBs in these latter patients alters their course (25). Since all antiarrhythmic agents have potentially serious side effects (see above, p. 508), the physician must consider for each patient the relative risks of treating or not treating VPBs. The following generalizations may be useful:

1. Apparently healthy young people with asymptomatic ventricular premature beats probably do not need treatment.

2. Apparently healthy young people with ventricular premature beats causing symptomatic palpitations also probably do not need to be treated. If symptoms interfere with normal life-style in spite of reassurance, a trial of low dose propranolol beginning with 10 mg, 4 times a day, and increasing if needed to 40 to 80 mg, 4 times a day, may abolish VPBs and relieve symptoms. Propranolol commonly produces a sensation of sluggishness in young people and often they will not continue the medication. In that case, nadalol (Corgard)—a long acting β-blocker—40 mg every morning, will often give symptomatic relief with good compliance.

3. Patients with known ischemic heart disease and symptomatic ventricular arrhythmias, especially symptomatic multiformed premature ventricular beats, should be treated. A history of recurrent ventricular tachycardia or ventricular fibrillation is always an indication for chronic antiarrhythmic therapy. Quinidine remains the drug of choice in initial doses of 200 mg 4 times a day. The dose should be titrated to serum levels of 3 to 7 μg/ml just before the next dose (the level should be measured every 3 or 4 days until the desired concentration is attained). In patients who do not tolerate quinidine, disopyramide, 100 to 150 mg every 6 hours, should be tried. The efficacy of the antiarrhythmic therapy should be assessed by an ambulatory ECG (see above, p. 507).

4. When ventricular arrhythmias occur in the setting of congestive heart failure, an attempt should be made to achieve a maximal state of cardiac compensation before instituting antiarrhythmic therapy.

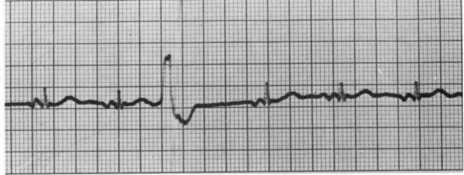

Figure 56.10 Premature ventricular beat. Note that the R-R interval between the two normal beats separated by the PVB is the same as that between two normal beats separated by another normal beat.

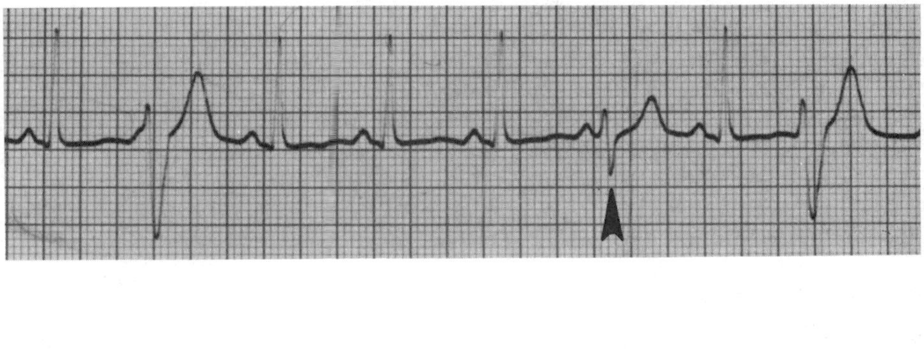

Figure 56.11 Premature ventricular beats due to the firing of an ectopic focus. The *arrow* points to a fusion beat.

Hemodynamic compensation may decrease or elimi-nate ventricular premature beats so that specific an-tiarrhythmic therapy is not needed. Disopyramide is a myocardial depressant and is specifically contrain-dicated in patients with marked cardiac enlargement and reduced contractility. Furthermore, patients in severe chronic heart failure are more likely to expe-rience problems such as hypokalemia, alkalosis, hy-poxemia, and digitalis toxicity, thus increasing the risk of serious side effects from antiarrhythmic agents.

5. Patients with recurrent symptomatic VPBs, re-current ventricular tachycardia, or ventricular fibril-lation may be best managed with a drug regimen which is selected using intracardiac electrophysio-logic techniques to assess the response to the drugs. This approach requires hospitalization and consul-tation with a cardiologist.

6. If VPBs have been suppressed for a year and if patients are asymptomatic, it is reasonable to discon-tinue antiarrhythmic therapy and to obtain an am-bulatory ECG 1 week later. If the arrhythmia does not recur the therapy need not be reinstituted.

Heart Block

Heart block, a delay or failure of conduction of the cardiac impulse, is categorized electrocardiographi-cally.

RIGHT BUNDLE BRANCH BLOCK (RBBB) (Fig. 56.12)

A delay or block of conduction through the right bundle branch causes a modest prolongation of the QRS complex (> 0.12 sec). The initial QRS vector is unaffected since this is accounted for largely by left ventricular depolarization. The right ventricle is ac-tivated by a spread of the action potential from the left ventricle, which is seen best in leads I and V6 where the S waves are wide and slurred and in V-1 where there is a double peak (R-R') of the R wave. RBBB is sometimes seen in the ECGs of patients who have otherwise normal hearts. More often it is asso-ciated with an underlying congenital or acquired disorder: e.g., cor pulmonale, interatrial septal defect, and hypertensive or ischemic heart disease. Patients with RBBB have an increased risk of cardiovascular morbidity and death from cardiovascular disease (21).

LEFT BUNDLE BRANCH BLOCK (LBBB) (Fig. 56.13)

A delay or block of conduction through the left bundle branch causes a marked prolongation of the QRS complex (0.14 to 0.16 sec). The entire sequence of ventricular depolarization is affected so that the QRS complex is widened and the QRS axis is directed to the left and posteriorly. Abnormal repolarization is reflected in the T wave, which is always in the opposite direction of the QRS complex.

LBBB always signifies heart disease—usually de-generative disease or ischemia.

HEMIBLOCKS

Left Anterior Hemiblock (LAH). When there is delay or block of the cardiac impulse in the anterior-

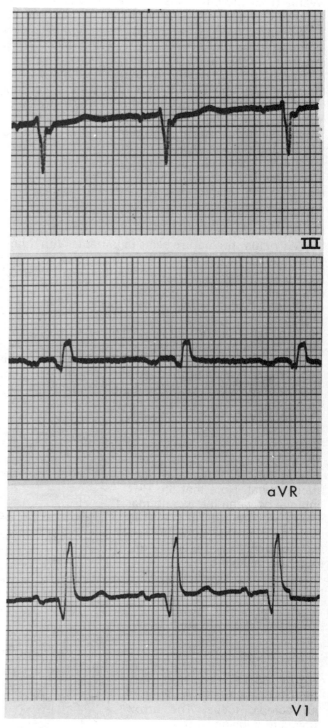

Figure 56.12 Right bundle branch block and left anterior hemiblock (bifascicular block).

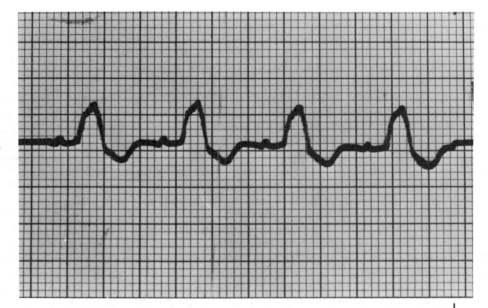

Figure 56.13 Left bundle branch block.

superior portion of the left bundle branch, the anterior-superior wall of the left ventricle is activated late, resulting in marked left axis deviation on the ECG (Fig. 56.12). The duration of the QRS complex is usually normal or slightly prolonged (<0.10 sec). The causes of left anterior hemiblock are the same as those of LBBB. LAH is occasionally seen in patients with no discernible heart disease. Whatever the cause, LAH is not in itself a poor prognostic sign and, at least in an ambulatory setting, requires no specific therapy (in hospital, some physicians would pace temporarily patients who developed LAH after a myocardial infarction).

Left Posterior Hemiblock (LPH). When there is delay or block of the cardiac impulse in the posterior portion of the left bundle branch, the posterior wall of the left ventricle is activated late. The ECG pattern of LPH is characterized by marked right axis deviation (> + 110°). The causes of LPH are the same as those of LAH and LBBB. Because the posterior portion of the left bundle branch is larger and better perfused than is the anterior-superior portion, LPH is less common than is LAH and usually indicates more extensive left ventricular disease.

BIFASCICULAR BLOCK

Right bundle branch block with left anterior hemiblock (manifest by RBBB pattern and left axis deviation— Fig. 56.12) or RBBB with LPH (manifest by a RBBB pattern and right axis deviation) indicates that only one pathway remains to maintain passage of the cardiac impulse from the atria to the ventricles. If bifascicular block is detected in an ambulatory setting, especially if there is a history of syncope or of light-headedness, a cardiologist should be asked to advise whether an intracardiac His bundle ECG (p. 507) is indicated. If the His-ventricle conduction time is prolonged, many cardiologists will recommend

pacemaker implantation to prevent morbidity or sudden death should complete heart block develop. The risk that unselected patients with bifascicular block will develop complete heart block is 5 to 6% a year (19). There is conflicting evidence, however, about the course of patients, generally, with bifascicular block; some report no increased morbidity (18); others, a considerably shortened survival (7, 8). Although there is not a consensus about how to deal with the problem, the prognosis seems to be related to the extent of the underlying disease.

FIRST DEGREE HEART BLOCK

Definition and etiology. The P-R interval normally varies with heart rate, but should not exceed 0.21 sec in people in normal sinus rhythm. First degree AV block is defined as a prolonged PR interval. The block may be due to a prolongation of conduction in any of the structures between the SA node and the bundle of His. Most commonly, when the QRS duration is normal, a long PR interval is due to a delay in conduction in the AV node. When first degree block coincides with left bundle branch block, it is likely that there is a delay in conduction in the His bundle. A prolonged PR interval with right bundle branch block may be due to a block in the AV node or in the bundle of His.

A prolongation of the PR interval is usually due to degenerative, ischemic, or inflammatory changes in the AV conduction systems. It is commonly seen in older people without other evidence of heart disease, in patients who have had an inferior wall myocardial infarction, or in association with myocarditis (including acute rheumatic fever). Drugs, such as digitalis, which affect vagal activity also may produce a first degree AV block.

Symptoms and Signs. First degree AV block in itself does not produce symptoms or abnormal physical findings except a first heart sound that is reduced in intensity (see Chapter 57).

Treatment and Course. Patients with first degree AV block who are asymptomatic and who have no other evidence of heart disease need not be treated. If patients with first degree block complain of light-headedness or dizziness, an ambulatory ECG should be obtained (see above, p. 507) since some of these patients may have episodic higher degrees of block.

SECOND DEGREE AV BLOCK

Definition and Etiology. Second degree AV block is present when some but not all P waves are followed by QRS complexes. Second degree AV block is due to conduction delay or block either in the AV node or in the conduction system below the AV node. The site of the block has important therapeutic implications (see below).

Mobitz-I or Wenckebach Second Degree AV Block (Fig. 56.14). Second degree AV block within the AV node results in the Wenckebach phenomenon, characterized by progressive lengthening of the PR interval for several cycles until the P wave is blocked completely; and the sequence begins again, often with a normal PR interval in the beat that follows the blocked P wave. In the absence of disease elsewhere in the conducting system, the QRS complex is normal. The "degree of Wenckebach" is characterized by the ratio of the number of P waves to the number of QRS complexes in each cycle of block. In other words, if block occurs after every third P wave, it is called 3:2 Wenckebach.

Since the conduction system below the AV node is usually intact, an AV junctional escape rhythm may be seen in patients with Wenckebach-type block. This rhythm is characterized by a regular rate of 40 to 60 beats per minute with normal QRS complexes and retrograde P waves that either closely precede, coincide with, or follow these complexes.

Since conduction through the AV node is influenced by vagal tone, Type I—second degree AV block may be precipitated by anything that increases vagal tone. It therefore is sometimes seen as a transient phenomenon in people with no other evidence of

heart disease. Otherwise, it is produced by the same processes that are associated with first degree AV block.

Mobitz-II Second Degree AV Block (Fig. 56.15). Mobitz-II block is defined as intermittent failure to conduct a P wave due to block below the level of the AV node. The PR interval of the conducted beat prior to a blocked P wave is usually normal. The block may be intermittent or may occur in a fixed 2:1 or 3:1 ratio. Coexistent bundle branch block is commonly seen. Progression to higher degrees of block or to asystole may occur rapidly.

Vagal influences have little effect on conduction below the AV node so that changes in vagal tone do not influence Mobitz-II block. However, the block may be precipitated by medications such as propranolol, which decrease conduction through the bundle of His. The common causes of Mobitz-II block are degenerative or ischemic changes within the His-Purkinje system.

Symptoms and Signs. Mobitz-I Second Degree AV Block: Patients are often asymptomatic but if vagal tone is increased (e.g., by digitalis or propranolol), profound bradycardia may ensue, sometimes with rates below 30/minutes. Such patients may complain of light-headedness, syncope, or extreme fatigue.

Physical findings are subtle; irregularity of the heart rhythm and arterial pulse may be noted when a beat is dropped. The first heart sound of the last beat before the dropped beat will be softer than that of the first beat after the pause (because of the variation in P-R interval—see Chapter 57).

Mobitz-II Second Degree AV Block: Symptoms and physical findings are similar to those of patients with Mobitz-I block except that they are not influenced by changes in vagal activity and the intensity of the first heart sound is constant.

Treatment and Course. Mobitz-I Second Degree AV Block: Asymptomatic patients need not be treated since the risk of rapid progression of the block and of asystole is slight. Symptomatic patients usually have pronounced bradycardia. If so, medications such as digitalis or propranolol, which may be increasing the block should be discontinued. If such

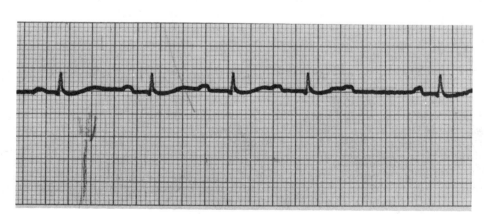

Figure 56.14 Mobitz-I or Wenckebach second degree atrioventricular block.

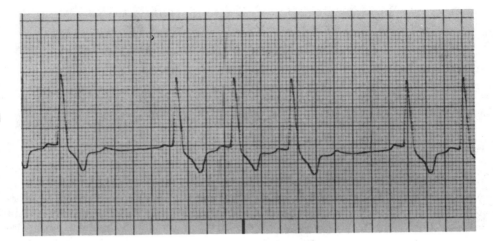

Figure 56.15 Mobitz-II second degree atrioventricular block.

medications are essential to the patient's management, a cardiac pacemaker should be implanted (see p. 510).

Mobitz-II Second Degree AV Block: Because of the risk of rapid progression of the block and of asystole, all patients, even if asymptomatic, should be treated with a permanent cardiac pacemaker.

Patients with a history of light-headedness or dizziness who have new bundle branch block should be suspected of having had Mobitz-II block. This suspicion often can be confirmed with the use of an ambulatory ECG (p. 507). An intracardiac ECG (p. 507), if necessary, may also show prolonged conduction through the His bundle. Patients with a known history of coronary artery disease and with new or increased bundle branch blocks who have a clear-cut history of syncope must be thought to have had Mobitz-II block or complete heart block until proven otherwise.

THIRD DEGREE (COMPLETE) HEART BLOCK

Definition and Etiology. Complete heart block occurs when there is total failure of conduction of impulses from the atria through the AV junction to the bundle of His (or, more rarely, if all three fascicles below the His bundle are diseased). The life of the patient then depends upon the escape of a ventricular pacemaker. A rhythm generated in the upper portion of the His bundle may have a QRS configuration nearly identical to that of normally conducted impulses and will have a rate between 40 and 60 beats/min (Fig. 56.16). It is more likely to be a stable rhythm than is a rhythm generated by a lower pacemaker. If the pacemaker is located more distally in the conducting system, the ventricular rate decreases; the QRS morphology becomes wider and more bizarre; and the risk of asystole increases. In children or young adults, complete heart block may occur due to congenital defects in development of the AV cushion or of the conduction system itself; escape rhythms are, in such cases, usually generated relatively high in the bundle of His. In older people complete heart block is most commonly due to degenerative and fibrotic changes in the conduction system (6). It is also seen sometimes in association with infiltrative disease of the myocardium (e.g., sarcoid or amyloid), inflammatory processes (e.g., rheumatoid arthritis), and myocardial infections (tuberculosis, syphilis, etc.) or ischemic heart disease. Occasionally digitalis toxicity may produce complete heart block.

Symptoms and Signs. A major symptom of complete heart block is sudden loss of consciousness (a Stokes-Adams attack), the result of asystole or of tachyarrhythmia (ventricular tachycardia or fibrillation). The asystole is due to failure of the ventricular pacemaker; the tachyarrhythmia, to escape of another focus when the idioventricular rate falls too low (a variant of the bradycardia-tachycardia syndrome—see p. 512). If the heart begins to pump effectively again within seconds—as it usually does—the patient promptly regains consciousness and is alert and oriented. If perfusion of vital organs is delayed, seizure-like activity (ordinarily not generalized) and even death may ensue. If they are unconscious for more than a few minutes, patients may not become fully alert for some hours.

Complete heart block in patients with underlying myocardial disease may cause symptoms of heart failure (see Chapter 58) primarily because of further reduction in cardiac output as the result of bradycardia.

Physical findings of heart block are all attributable to the dissociation between atrial and ventricular contraction: variation in the intensity of the first heart sound, variation in systolic blood pressure, variation in the intensity of heart murmurs and of 3rd and 4th heart sounds, and the appearance of cannon waves in the jugular pulse. The heart rate, of course, is slow.

Treatment and Course. The treatment of complete heart block is permanent pacemaker implantation. The life expectancy of treated patients with complete heart block who have no other evidence of cardiac or systemic disease is excellent and approaches that of

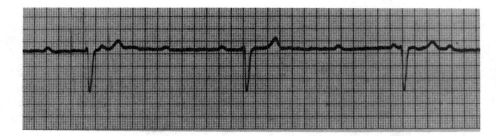

Figure 56.16 Third degree heart block.

their age-matched cohort. Patients with complete heart block due to coronary disease have a prognosis which is determined by the extent of their underlying coronary artery disease, and by their myocardial function.

Pre-excitation Syndrome

DEFINITION AND ETIOLOGY

The atria and ventricles are electrically isolated from each other by the AV groove and the electrical signal from the atria is conducted to the ventricle via the AV node and conducting system. If the AV groove is short-circuited by muscle fibers, if muscle fibers from the atria enter the His bundle below the AV node, or if muscle fibers from the His bundle bypass the bundle branches, a variable portion of the right or left ventricle will be depolarized early. These short-circuiting fibers are known as accessory atrioventricular, atrionodal, or nodoventricular fibers, depending on their location (Fig. 56.17).

The classic example of pre-excitation is the *Wolff-Parkinson-White (WPW) syndrome* which is due to accessory atrioventricular connections. This syndrome is characterized electrocardiographically by a short PR interval followed by a wide QRS complex, which is a fusion beat between the area of the ventricle which is preexcited and the area of the ventricle excited via normal conduction pathways (Fig. 56.18). The portion of the complex due to pre-excitation is called the delta wave because of its resemblance to the Greek capital letter Δ. If the accessory bundle connects the atria with the left ventricle, the electrocardiographic pattern resembles right bundle branch block (Type A WPW). If, on the other hand, the connection is with the right ventricle, the pattern resembles left bundle branch block (Type B WPW); the negative delta wave in lead II in this situation may be taken for a Q wave and the mistaken diagnosis of remote myocardial infarction may be made.

If the atrial fibers insert into the bundle of His and short-circuit the AV node, the PR interval is short, but no delta wave is seen since below the AV node conduction occurs along the usual pathways. This syndrome is known as the *Lown-Ganong-Levine (LGL) syndrome*. A number of other variants of pre-excitation have been described but are much rarer than these two relatively common disorders (11).

The ECG manifestations of pre-excitation may vary from time to time within a given individual since, if conduction occurs through the normal anatomic pathways, rather than through accessory fibers, no pre-excitation will be seen on the ECG. When pre-excitation is facilitated because of disease in the AV node or because of drugs that suppress conduction through the AV node (e.g., digitalis or propranolol) abnormalities on the ECG will be seen.

Re-entrant supraventricular arrhythmias are common in patients with pre-excitation syndromes (estimates vary from 13% (3) to 60% (4))—usually paroxysmal supraventricular tachycardia, but atrial fibrillation and flutter also occur. The morphology of the QRS complex during the tachyarrhythmia will depend on the direction in which the re-entrant tachycardia occurs. If re-entry occurs antegrade through the AV conducting system and retrograde through an accessory pathway, then the QRS duration during the tachyarrhythmia may be normal since the ventricle is depolarized in a normal direction through its normal specialized conducting tissue. If the circuit is established in the opposite direction, the QRS complex will be wide, with a bundle branch block pattern, because most or all of the ventricle will be depolarized by way of the accessory pathway, and easily can be confused with ventricular tachycardia.

SYMPTOMS AND SIGNS

The pre-excitation syndrome may be an incidental finding on an ECG or it may come to the attention of the physician because of symptoms. Other symptoms of tachyarrhythmia will depend on the nature of the arrhythmia and on the presence or absence of underlying heart disease.

There are no physical findings due to pre-excitation other than occasionally a loud S-1, except during periods of tachyarrhythmia; and then the findings depend on the type of arrhythmia that is present.

PREVALENCE

Pre-excitation syndromes are not rare. The prevalence of pre-excitation is between 1 and 30 per 1000 people (11). Accurate prevalence rates are difficult to obtain since short PR intervals with normal QRS durations are commonly seen in people without arrhythmias so that no studies are done to determine whether a bypass tract exists.

Pre-excitation syndromes occasionally may be associated with certain forms of congenital heart dis-

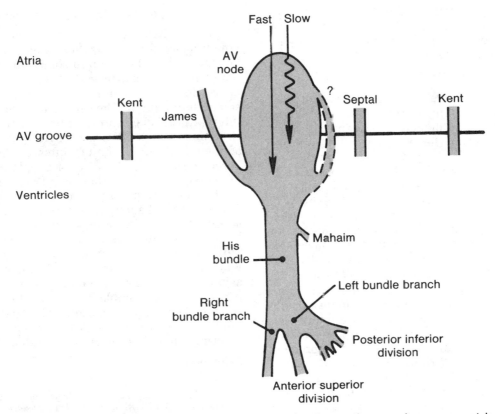

Figure 56.17 Schematic diagram of possible accessory conduction pathways. Accessory atrioventricular (AV) muscle bundles (Kent) are located in either the right or left AV groove or in the septum close to the AV node. Dual AV node pathways are represented by the fast and slow symbols. Accessory nodoventricular muscle bundles or accessory fasciculoventricular bundles (Mahaim) originate in the lower AV node, His bundle or bundle branches. Atrio Hisian or atriofascicular bundles (James) insert into the AV node, often the lower AV node. The pathway labeled ''?'' is a hypothetical intranodal bypass which could explain some short PR syndromes. (*Source:* H. L. Greene: *Johns Hopkins Medical Journal, 139:* 13, 1976 (11).)

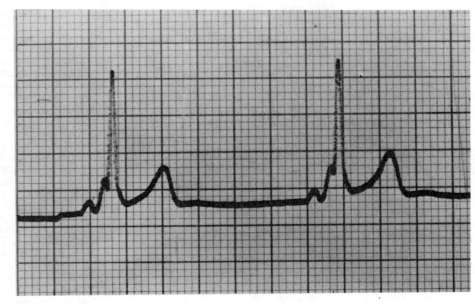

Figure 56.18 The Wolff-Parkinson-White syndrome.

ease. Pre-excitation of the WPW type is associated with the Ebstein's anomaly of the tricuspid valve, corrected transposition of the great vessels, and with hypertrophic cardiomyopathies.

TREATMENT AND COURSE

Asymptomatic patients need not be treated; their survival is the same as that of the normal population.

Patients with symptomatic supraventricular arrhythmias who, during the arrhythmia, have normal QRS complexes—indicating conduction over the normal pathways—are best treated with propranolol, 10 to 40 mg 4 times a day. If that approach fails, digitalis is a reasonable alternative (0.25 mg digoxin/day). Occasionally it will be necessary to administer quinidine or procainamide. Verapamil also may prove useful, but there is insufficient information at this point about the long term use of the drug orally. The use of these drugs is discussed on pp. 508–510.

Patients with symptomatic arrhythmias who, during the arrhythmia have wide QRS complexes, indicating conduction over the accessory pathways, should be hospitalized if possible for treatment with intravenous lidocaine or with quinidine or procainamide. Suppression of arrhythmic attacks thereafter should be attempted first with quinidine and then, if necessary, with procainamide or propranolol. *It is important that the physician be aware that digitalis is contraindicated in this situation:* by increasing the refractoriness of the AV junction, it may enhance conduction through the accessory pathway and induce a dangerously rapid ventricular response.

Patients with frequent arrhythmias, refractory to treatment and to suppression, may be candidates for an operation to transect the accessory pathway—identified during surgery by epicardial mapping. It has been reported that 90% of such operations are successful in preventing further arrhythmia (10), but currently few centers are able to do them.

The *course* of patients with pre-excitation syndromes is unpredictable—some have no or very infrequent arrhythmic attacks; others, despite therapy, have them frequently. Some patients have minimal symptoms during attacks, and others are incapacitated.

The long term survival of patients with pre-excitation who are subject to arrhythmic attacks is related to the severity of the arrhythmia. Patients with occasional palpitations or with easily controlled bouts of paroxysmal ventricular tachycardia are at low risk. Patients with bouts of atrial flutter or fibrillation and a rapid ventricular response are at considerable risk of ventricular fibrillation and of sudden death.

It is important that asymptomatic patients with pre-excitation who wish to engage in strenuous work have stress electrocardiography (Chapter 54 describes the technique and the patient's experience with it). Patients who develop tachyarrhythmias on exercise or have a documented history of tachyarrhythmias should not undertake strenuous exertion.

Long QT Interval Syndrome

An inherited syndrome has been described in which delayed repolarization is expressed as a long QT interval (> 0.45 sec). In some families the inheritance is autosomal recessive and is associated with nerve deafness; in others, the inheritance is autosomal dominant and hearing is normal. The long QT interval predisposes to re-entry ventricular tachyarrhythmias which often cause syncope and may cause sudden death (22). The QT interval should be measured routinely in the ECG of people who complain of syncope for which there is no explantion.

The most effective treatment of symptomatic patients is β-blockade with propranolol; if this does not suppress arrhythmic attacks, excision of the left stellate ganglion may be curative by interrupting sympathetic innervation of the heart. It is not known whether patients with long QT intervals who are asymptomatic benefit from propranolol, but certainly treatment is reasonable if there is a family history of sudden death. An exercise ECG is indicated in patients with negative personal and family histories to determine if arrhythmias can be induced by exertion.

References

General

Bigger, JT, Jr: Mechanisms and diagnosis of arrhythmias, and Management of arrhythmias. In *Heart Disease. A Textbook of Cardiovascular Medicine*, pp. 630 and 691. E. Braunwald (ed.). W. B. Saunders, Philadelphia, 1980.
   A comprehensive description, exhaustively referenced.
Schamroth, L: How to approach an arrhythmia. *Circulation* 47: 420, 1973.
   A practical approach to the analysis of arrhythmias.
Treatment of cardiac arrhythmias: *Med Lett* 16: 101, 1974.
   A brief synopsis of the treatment of the most common arrhythmias.

Specific

1. Antman, EM, Stone, PH, Muller, JE and Braunwald, E: Calcium channel blocking agents in the treatment of cardiovascular disorders; I. Basic and clinical electrophysiologic effects. *Ann Intern Med* 93: 875, 1980.
2. Aroestz, JM, Cohen, SI and Markin, E: Bradycardia-tachycardia syndrome: results in twenty-eight patients treated by combined pharmacologic therapy and pacemaker implantation. *Chest* 66: 257, 1974.
3. Berkman, NL and Lamb, LE: The Wolff-Parkinson-White electrocardiogram: a follow-up study of five to twenty-eight years. *N Engl J Med* 278: 492, 1968.
4. Bigger, JT: Mechanisms and diagnosis of arrhythmia. In *Heart Disease. A Textbook of Cardiovascular Medicine*, E. Braunwald (ed.). W. B. Saunders, Philadelphia, 1980.
5. Blomgren, SE, Condemi, JJ, Bignall, MC and Vaughn, JH: Antinuclear antibody induced by procainamide. A prospective study. *N Engl J Med* 281: 64, 1969.
6. Davies, M and Harris, A: Pathological basis of primary heart block. *Br Heart J* 31: 219, 1969.
7. Denes, P, Dhingra, RC, Wu, D, Wyndhan, CR, Amat-y-Leon, F and Rosen, KM: Sudden death in patients with chronic bifascicular block. *Arch Intern Med* 137: 1005, 1977.
8. Dhingra, RC, Denes, P, Wu, D, Wyndham, CR, Amat-y-Leon, F, Towne, WD and Rosen, KM: Prospective observations in patients with chronic bundle branch block and marked H-V prolongation. *Circulation* 53: 600, 1976.
9. Fairfax, AJ, Lambert, CD and Leatham, A: Systemic embolism in chronic sinoatrial disorder. *N Engl J Med* 295: 190, 1976.

10. Gallagher, JJ, Pritchett, ELC and Sealy, WC: The preexcitation syndromes. *Prog Cardiovasc Dis 20:* 285, 1978.
11. Greene, HL: Accessory atrioventricular conduction syndromes: a review. *Johns Hopkins Med J 139:* 13, 1976.
12. Greene, HL and Humphries, JO: Cardiac arrhythmias. in *The Principles and Practice of Medicine,* A. M. Harvey, R. J. Johns, V. A. McKusick, A. H. Owens, and R. S. Ross (eds.). Appleton-Century-Crofts, New York, 1980.
13. Jensen, JB, Humphries, JO, Kouwenhoven, WB and Jude, JR: Electroshock for atrial flutter and atrial fibrillation: follow-up studies on 50 patients. *JAMA 194:* 1181, 1965.
14. Josephson, ME and Kastor, JA: Supraventricular tachycardia: mechanisms and management. *Ann Intern Med 87:* 346, 1977.
15. Kannel, WB, Boylé, JT, McNamara, P, Quickenton, P and Gordon, T: Precursors of sudden coronary death: factors related to the incidence of sudden death. *Circulation 51:* 606, 1975.
16. Kennedy, HL and Caralis, DG: Ambulatory electrocardiography. *Ann Intern Med 87:* 729, 1977.
17. Kosowsky, BD, Taylor, J, Lown, B and Ritchie, RF: Long-term use of procaine amide following acute myocardial infarction. *Circulation 47:* 1204, 1973.
18. Kulbertus, HE, deLeval-Rutten, F, Duboir, M, *et al.:* Prognostic significance of left anterior hemiblock with right bundle branch block in mass screening. *Am J Cardiol 41:* 385, 1978.
19. Lister, JW, Kline, RS and Lesser, ME: Chronic bilateral bundle branch block: long-term observations in ambulatory patients. *Br Heart J 39:* 203, 1977.
20. Noble, D: *The Initiation of the Heart Beat,* p. 9. Clarendon Press, Oxford, 1975.
21. Schneider, JF, Thomas, HE, Kreger, BE, McNamara, PM, Sorlie, P and Karnel, WB: Newly acquired right bundle branch block. The Framingham study. *Ann Intern Med 92:* 37, 1980.
22. Schwartz, PJ, Periti, M, and Malliani, A: The long Q-T syndrome. *Am Heart J 89:* 378, 1975.
23. Singh, BN, Collett, JT and Chew, CYC: New perspectives in the pharmacologic therapy of cardiac arrhythmias. *Prog Cardiovasc Dis 22:* 243, 1980.
24. Stone, PH, Antman, EM, Muller, JE and Braunwald, E: Calcium channel blocking agents in the treatment of cardiovascular disorders; II. Hemodynamic effects and clinical applications. *Ann Intern Med 93:* 886, 1980.
25. Winkle, RA: Measuring antiarrhythmic drug efficacy by suppression of asymptomatic ventricular arrhythmias. *Ann Intern Med 91:* 480, 1979.
26. Wit, AL Rosen, MR and Hoffman, BF: Electrophysiology and pharmacology of cardiac arrhythmias; II. Relationship of normal and abnormal electrical activity of cardiac fibers to the genesis of arrhythmias. B. Re-entry, Section I. *Am Heart J 88:* 664, 1974.
27. Wohl, AJ, Laborde, NJ, Atkins, JM, Blomquist, CG and Mullins, CB: Prognosis of patients permanently paced for sick sinus syndrome. *Arch Intern Med 136:* 406, 1976.
28. Wolf, FA, Dawber, TR, Thomas, HE and Kannel, WB: Epidemiologic assessment of chronic atrial fibrillation and risk of stroke: the Framingham study. *Neurology 28:* 973, 1978.

CHAPTER FIFTY-SEVEN

Common Cardiac Disorders Revealed by Auscultation of the Heart

BARBARA B. BELL, M.D., and PHILIP D. ZIEVE, M.D.

HEART SOUNDS

First Heart Sound (S-1)

The first heart sound is a high frequency ("clicky") sound produced by closure of the atrioventricular (AV) valves, *i.e.,* M-1 (mitral valve closure) followed by T-1 (tricuspid valve closure). Mitral valve closure is louder than tricuspid valve closure.

Abnormally wide splitting of the first heart sound is produced by delays in closure of the tricuspid valve as in patients with right bundle branch block, ventricular ectopic beats, idioventricular rhythm, or with left ventricular pacing. In mitral stenosis, mitral valve closure may be so delayed that tricuspid valve closure may actually precede mitral valve closure.

A loud first heart sound indicates a mobile valve. *Increased intensity of the first heart sound* is associated with a rapid ventricular upstroke, which occurs when the ventricles are presented with an increased volume (e.g., ventricular septal defect and atrial septal defect) or with a wide open AV valve at the end of diastole, which occurs when there is shortening of the AV filling time (e.g., atrial tachycardia and conditions associated with a short PR interval) and when AV filling time is prolonged (e.g., mitral stenosis).

Reduced intensity of the first heart sound may indicate an immobile valve (e.g., severe mitral regurgitation or stenosis) or a long PR interval.

Second Heart Sound (S-2)

The second heart sound is produced by closure of the semilunar valves, i.e., A-2 (aortic valve closure) followed by P-2 (pulmonic valve closure). Normal splitting of the second heart sound occurs at the height of inspiration, when the splitting may be as wide as 0.10 sec, and is due to the increase in stroke volume in the right heart with the increase in venous return with inspiration. The two components of the second heart sound are synchronous and virtually single during expiration.

Abnormally wide splitting of S-2 without change in expiration is characteristic of an atrial septal defect or of anomalous pulmonary venous return. S-2 is widely split but variable in patients with pulmonary stenosis. In the presence of severe aortic stenosis, A-2 is delayed beyond P-2 resulting in wide splitting during expiration with no splitting during inspiration (reversed or paradoxical splitting). Paradoxical splitting of the second heart sound also occurs in the presence of a left bundle branch block, severe hypertension, or severe left ventricular failure.

Increased intensity of A-2 and P-2 are features of aortic and pulmonary hypertension, respectively. *A-2 or P-2 is of reduced intensity* when the aortic or pulmonic valve is immobile or severely thickened.

Gallops

The identification of a gallop sound affords valuable information concerning diagnosis, prognosis, and treatment. Gallops are diastolic sounds and appear to be related to the two periods of filling of the ventricles: the rapid filling phase (the S-3 or ventricular diastolic gallop) and the presystolic filling phase related to atrial systole (S-4 or atrial gallop).

The *atrial gallop sound or S-4* is a low frequency presystolic sound and is found in patients with primary myocardial disease, coronary artery disease, systemic or pulmonary hypertension, or severe aortic or pulmonic stenosis. The atrial gallop is an indication of severity of the underlying disorder and, as the patient's condition improves, the sound may become fainter or disappear. With ventricular hypertrophy an S-4 is a fixed finding of no prognostic significance.

The *ventricular gallop sound or S-3* is a low frequency sound. It occurs with the same timing as the normal physiologic third sound, approximately 0.14 to 0.16 sec after the second heart sound. The third sound is a normal finding in children and young adults up to the age of 30. An S-3 gallop is a feature of severe cardiac decompensation, whatever the un-

derlying cause (hypertension, coronary artery disease, rheumatic heart disease, etc.) and is an indication of a relatively poor prognosis.

Ejection Sounds ("Clicks")

Ejection sounds are produced at the time of ejection of blood from the left ventricle into the aorta or from the right ventricle into the pulmonary artery. The sound may originate in a thickened valve or in a dilated great vessel. The *aortic ejection sound* is located in the area of aortic auscultation—namely, from the second right intercostal space in a straight line to the cardiac apex, and occurs 0.05 sec after M-1. It is a high frequency sound, often called a "click." In the presence of systemic hypertension, the aortic ejection sound is an indication of severity. It disappears as hypertension improves. Aortic ejection clicks may also be heard in patients with aortic stenosis, aneurysm of the ascending aorta, and aortic insufficiency.

Pulmonic ejection sounds (or clicks) are frequently localized to the second left intercostal space and may increase in intensity with expiration. They occur immediately after M-1. Pulmonic clicks are a feature of valvular pulmonic stenosis and also of pulmonary hypertension.

A *midsystolic clicking sound*, with or without a late systolic murmur, may indicate mitral valve prolapse (see below).

Opening Snaps

An opening snap occurs because of a stenotic, but still mobile, mitral or tricuspid valve. The mitral opening snap is best heard between the pulmonic area and the cardiac apex. It occurs 0.04 to 0.12 sec after S-2 in early diastole. It is heard in patients with a thickened mitral valve. The earlier the snap, the more severe the stenosis. The tricuspid opening snap is best heard at the lower left or right sternal border and occurs immediately after S-2 in early diastole.

Murmurs

Evaluation of a heart murmur is one of the most common tasks which confronts a physician conducting a physical examination. Virtually all normal people have a systolic murmur during some period of their lives. On the other hand, a murmur may be a sign of serious underlying cardiac or noncardiac disease. It is important that the physician be able to distinguish the innocent murmur from those that reflect an underlying disorder and that he be able to select appropriately the tests, when necessary, that will lead to the precise diagnosis and to the proper management.

GENERAL CHARACTERISTICS OF MURMURS

A murmur is a series of audible vibrations produced by turbulence in the circulation. These vibrations can be characterized by intensity, pitch, shape, quality, and timing in the cardiac cycle, precordial location of maximal intensity, and radiation.

The *intensity or loudness of a murmur* is, by convention, graded on a scale of 1 to 6. A grade 1 murmur is audible only after concentrated auscultation. A grade 2 murmur is faint but readily audible. A grade 3 murmur is prominent but not loud. Grade 4 murmurs are loud and are frequently, but not always, associated with a palpable thrill. A grade 5 murmur is very loud. A grade 6 murmur is heard with the stethoscope held 1 cm above, but not actually touching, the chest wall.

The *pitch of a murmur* refers to the frequency of the sound—from high to low. High frequency murmurs usually reflect high velocity and/or high pressure.

The *shape of a murmur* refers to the change in intensity throughout the duration of the sound: for example, crescendo (increasing in intensity), decrescendo (decreasing in intensity), or constant.

The *quality of a murmur* refers to the nature of the sound: harsh, blowing, musical, cooing, rumbling, etc. Although these terms are not precise, they are useful in identifying various benign and significant conditions, as will be seen below.

The *timing of a murmur* is particularly important in establishing the cause of the sound—first, whether the murmur is systolic, diastolic, or continuous and second, whether it is heard in early, middle, or late systole or diastole. Murmurs that last throughout systole are called holosystolic. Late diastolic murmurs are sometimes called presystolic.

The *location of a murmur* refers to that site on the chest wall where the sound is loudest. The *direction of radiation* refers to the other sites where the murmur, though less intense, can still be heard; those sites may be outside the chest (the back or neck, for example). Aortic murmurs may be heard anywhere in a straight line from the second right interspace to the apex. Pulmonic murmurs are heard best at the second left intercostal space; tricuspid murmurs, at the lower left sternal border; and mitral murmurs, at the cardiac apex radiating into the axilla.

There are two kinds of systolic murmurs—ejection and regurgitant murmurs. The ejection systolic murmur may be an innocent flow murmur or it may reflect organic heart disease. The regurgitant murmur may be due to dilation of the annulus of the valve in an otherwise normal heart or may represent organic heart disease.

The *ejection murmur* is a crescendo/decrescendo (or "diamond-shaped") murmur caused by the turbulence of blood flowing through either the aortic or pulmonic valve. The murmur is most commonly midsystolic and ends before the second or closing sound (S-2) of the valve from which the murmur was generated; that is, aortic ejection murmurs end before A-2 and pulmonic ejection murmurs end before P-2. The loudness of the murmur depends in part on the pressure gradient across the valve and in part on

other factors, such as thickness of the chest, the cardiac output, etc.; the shape, on the acceleration and deceleration of blood flow across the valve as systole proceeds. When diastole is prolonged, for example, by premature ventricular contraction or by atrial fibrillation, ejection murmurs become louder because of the passage of a large volume of blood through the valve. In general, the larger the cardiac output, the louder the murmur. Increases in cardiac output due to hypermetabolic states such as anemia, fever, or thyrotoxicosis will increase the loudness of the murmur. Decreases in cardiac output such as congestive heart failure will decrease the loudness of the murmur.

Regurgitant murmurs are murmurs produced by backward flow of blood from a high pressure chamber to a compartment of lower pressure. Intensity may be constant as in mitral regurgitation, tricuspid regurgitation, or ventricular septal defect or may be decrescendo as in aortic and pulmonary regurgitation.

INNOCENT MURMURS

Innocent murmurs are a series of vibrations that are produced in the absence of significant abnormalities of cardiac anatomy or function (Table 57.1).

The innocent murmur can usually be distinguished from significant murmurs by the absence of other physical, radiologic, or electrocardiographic evidence of disease. Also, innocent murmurs are usually in early or midsystole, are grade 1 or 2 in intensity, and vary with respiration and/or position. Occasionally, echocardiography (see below) is done to clarify the etiology of a murmur, but more elaborate studies, such as stress tests, radionuclide studies, and cardiac catheterization, are employed only after it has been decided that a murmur is not innocent and that a more precise diagnosis is necessary.

The most common innocent systolic murmur of childhood and young adulthood that is clearly recognizable as benign based on the characteristics of the murmur alone, is the musical or *vibratory midsystolic murmur* (best heard at the lower left sternal border) that is caused by the vibration of the leaflets of the pulmonary valve.

The *venous hum* is a continuous murmur, loudest in the neck, caused by altered flow through the jugular veins. It can be eliminated by turning the patient's head, compression of the internal jugular vein on the side where the murmur is heard, or placing the patient in the supine position.

Table 57.1
Benign or Innocent Systolic Murmurs

Vibratory ejection systolic murmur
Continuous murmur of venous hum
Pulmonic ejection systolic murmur
Aortic ejection systolic murmur
Murmur associated with pregnancy

The *pulmonic ejection systolic murmur* is a systolic crescendo/decrescendo murmur generated by the flow of blood through the pulmonary valve. It is loudest in the left second intercostal space or at the midleft sternal border.

Similarly, the *aortic ejection systolic murmur* is an early systolic murmur generated by the flow of blood through the aortic valve. It is loudest in the right second intercostal space or at the apex of the heart. This innocent or flow murmur is the most common benign systolic murmur in the middle-aged or elderly patient and may have a cooing quality. ECG and echocardiogram may be necessary to rule out left ventricular hypertrophy and aortic stenosis.

Benign flow murmurs commonly are heard in *pregnant women*. Because of the normally increased stroke volume at 28 to 30 weeks of gestation, diastolic filling sounds and systolic ejection murmurs of turbulent flow are common. In pregnant patients also, an S-3 may be prominent enough to be confused with the mid-diastolic murmur of mitral stenosis. The S-3 of pregnancy may be distinguished from the murmur of mitral stenosis, however, by the absence of an opening snap and by the accompanying hyperdynamic apical movement. An echocardiogram is indicated in some patients to make a precise diagnosis.

In the pregnant patient it is critical to compare the femoral and brachial pulses and the blood pressures in the presence of a heart murmur, since coarctation of the aorta may present with a soft heart murmur and, if left undiagnosed, rarely may result in aortic dissection or rupture.

Clinical Applications of Echocardiography (19)

Echocardiography is a valuable adjunct to the clinical assessment in patients suspected of cardiovascular disease. This technique utilizes high frequency pulsed sound waves to record echoes of cardiac structures as they move within a beam of sound directed into the chest. Sometimes the cardiologist will use phonocardiography in combination with echocardiography to time the various normal and abnormal heart sounds more precisely.

A piezoelectric crystal is used to transmit a short pulse of ultrahigh frequency sound (1 to 8 kHz) into the tissues of the chest. The pulse transducer is placed at one point on the chest wall and rocked to inscribe an arc that will encompass several areas of the heart sequentially. It serves as a source of the sound beam and as a receiver of the echoes. It is of no discomfort to the patient; however, the patient must be able to lie flat for 20 min for performance of the test.

Echo spikes arise from the chest wall, right ventricular wall, interventricular septum, mitral leaflets, posterior left ventricular wall, aorta, and left atrium (Fig. 57.1). The size and function of these structures are analyzed and patterns of specific diseases may be recognized.

Two-dimensional echocardiography provides a sequential view of these structures and reveals, therefore, their function more precisely than does one-dimensional echocardiography. Instruments for two-dimensional echocardiography are not universally available, but where possible, both modes should be used for optimal visualization of the heart (19). Two-dimensional echocardiography is particularly helpful in assessing left ventricular function in patients with ischemic heart disease where regional structure and function are most important.

The echocardiogram is diagnostic in cases of idiopathic subaortic stenosis, mitral valve stenosis or

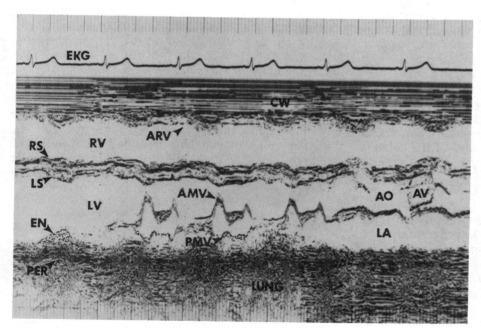

Figure 57.1 Normal one-dimensional echocardiogram. The tracing was taken as the transducer was scanned from the apex to the base of the heart. Ao, aorta; *AMV* anterior leaflet of the mitral valve. ARV, anterior wall of the right ventricle; *AV*, aortic valve opening; *CW*, chest wall; *EN*, posterior left ventricular endocardium; *LA*, left atrium; *LS*, left ventricular septum; *LV*, left ventricle; *PER*, pericardium. *PMV*, posterior mitral valve leaflet; *RS*, right ventricular septum; and *RV*, right ventricle.

prolapse, aortic regurgitation, and Ebstein's Anomaly of the tricuspid valve. The technique is helpful, but not diagnostic, in cases of aortic stenosis and atrial septal defect and other forms of congenital heart disease such as ventricular septal defect, tetralogy of Fallot, and bicuspid aortic valve.

SELECTED DISORDERS ASSOCIATED WITH ABNORMAL HEART SOUNDS

Aortic Stenosis

Stenosis of the aortic valve obstructs the flow of blood into the aorta and therefore raises the left ventricular pressure above the aortic pressure. The pressure gradient across the valve reflects the severity of the stenosis. The elevated pressure results in a concentric hypertrophy of the left ventricle. Symptoms develop when the left ventricle can no longer compensate for the pressure load; the heart fails and the cardiac output declines.

Aortic stenosis may occur at any one of several levels. The most common obstruction (75% of patients) is at the aortic valve, although subvalvular and supravalvular aortic stenosis may present with symptoms and signs of severity similar to those of valvular disease. It is particularly important to differentiate true aortic outflow obstruction from idiopathic hypertrophic disease which is a functional disorder (see Table 57.2 and below).

ETIOLOGY AND EPIDEMIOLOGY (21)

In patients below the age of 30, aortic stenosis is most likely to be due to a congenitally stenotic unicuspid valve. Between the ages of 30 and 65, a bicuspid aortic valve, which has become calcified and gradually more rigid over the years, is the most common cause of aortic stenosis. (One or two percent of the general population have a bicuspid aortic valve and 50% of these valves have calcified by age 50.) Rheumatic valvular disease accounts for only 6 to 27% of cases of isolated aortic stenosis in patients between the ages of 30 and 70 years. Over the age of 65, degeneration and sclerosis of the valve account for most cases of aortic stenosis. Except in the elderly, in whom the prevalence is the same in both sexes, isolated aortic stenosis is three to four times more common in men.

NATURAL HISTORY AND SYMPTOMS

Patients with aortic stenosis are usually asymptomatic until relatively late in the course of their disease. Mild to moderate obstruction does not compromise left ventricular function greatly, and even patients with severe stenosis may compensate for years before they develop symptoms. Symptoms ordinarily develop late in the sixth decade after which, if the lesion is not corrected, the average patient dies in about 4 years.

The earliest symptoms are easy fatiguability and excessive dyspnea after unusual exercise. Syncope or near-syncope with effort (see Chapter 78), angina (see Chapter 54), and dyspnea on unusual exercise (see Chapter 50) are indicative of severe valvular obstruction. Patients with heart failure survive less long (2 years) as a rule than do patients with syncope (3 years) or with angina (5 years) (22). Sudden death occurs in about 15% of symptomatic patients but, particularly worrisome, in about 5% of asymptomatic patients (22).

PHYSICAL FINDINGS

Patients with aortic stenosis usually have a loud (grade 3 to 4) systolic ejection murmur. The maximum intensity of the murmur is at the second right intercostal space and/or at the cardiac apex. At the apex the murmur often has a musical cooing quality. There is usually a thrill in the suprasternal notch or in the second right intercostal space. However, the loudness of the murmur may not correlate with the severity of stenosis. Also, if cardiac output is reduced, as in

Table 57.2
Comparison of Valvular Aortic Stenosis and Hypertrophic Cardiomyopathy

	Valvular Aortic Stenosis	Hypertrophic Cardiomyopathy
Symptoms	Dyspnea, angina, syncope or near-syncope	Dyspnea, angina, syncope or near-syncope
Signs	Systolic ejection murmur loudest at aortic area or at apex; louder if patient squats	Systolic ejection murmur loudest at left lower sternal border; louder if patient stands or performs a Valsalva maneuver
	A-2 may not be audible	A-2 usually audible
	S-4 common	S-4 very common
	Ejection sounds are common	Ejection sounds are uncommon
	Carotid upstroke is delayed	Carotid upstroke is brisk
ECG	Left ventricular hypertrophy (LVH) and strain pattern	LVH and strain pattern. Q waves in inferior and lateral leads are common
Chest X-ray	LVH is a late sign	LVH may occur but unpredictably
	Aortic valve is always calcified (may be seen only on fluoroscopy)	Aortic valve is not calcified
	Ascending aorta may be dilated	Ascending aorta is not dilated
Echocardiogram	Characteristic echos of valvular calcification and of valvular stenosis	Dysproportionate septal hypertrophy, systolic anterior displacement of mitral valve

congestive heart failure, or if the diameter of the chest is increased, the intensity of the murmur may be less than it otherwise would be. A late peak to the murmur does suggest severe obstruction, but this is difficult to appreciate with a stethoscope, and absence of the peak does not mean that obstruction is not severe. Augmentation of the murmur when the patient squats and diminution of the murmur when the patient stands or performs a Valsalva maneuver are characteristic of aortic stenosis.

The systolic murmur is an invariable sign of aortic stenosis; other cardiac sounds are dependent on the nature of the stenotic lesion. An early systolic ejection click is commonly heard when the valve is still mobile. The second aortic sound (A-2) is often not audible when the valve is rigid so that S-2 has only one component (P-2). Paradoxical splitting of the second heart sound, in the absence of left bundle branch block, is a sign of severity. A small pulse pressure (<30 mm Hg) also indicates severe obstruction (in elderly people, the pulse pressure may be normal despite severe stenosis). A slowly rising pulse—best assessed by palpation of a carotid artery—is characteristic. Under the age of 40, an S-4 is another sign of severe obstruction; over the age of 40, S-4 is common because of the high prevalence of hypertensive and ischemic heart disease and does not correlate with severity of stenosis.

The regurgitant early diastolic murmur of aortic insufficiency is heard in 30 to 40% of patients with aortic valve stenosis.

LABORATORY EVALUATION

An ECG, a chest X-ray, and an echocardiogram should be obtained routinely in a patient suspected of having aortic stenosis.

Electrocardiogram. The ECG is usually normal until stenosis becomes severe, at which point left ventricular hypertrophy (Fig. 57.2 and Table 57.3) and nonspecific ST depression and T wave inversion are common—but not invariable. In older patients particularly, an abnormal ECG cannot be relied upon to reflect severity since there are often other reasons why it might be abnormal.

Chest X-ray. Calcification of the aortic valve is always present in patients with aortic stenosis who are older than 35 to 40; but often fluoroscopy is necessary to reveal it. Poststenotic dilation of the ascending aorta is also commonly seen. The heart size and configuration are usually normal until the disease is far advanced.

Echocardiogram. Echocardiography reveals multiple diastolic echoes of aortic valve leaflets, due to valvular calcification, and, sometimes, an eccentric diastolic closure line. An increase in ventricular wall thickness on echocardiography implies severe obstruction, if there is no other cause for hypertrophy.

MANAGEMENT

Asymptomatic patients should be reassessed every 12 months so that signs of progressive disease can be detected promptly. Reassessment should include in-

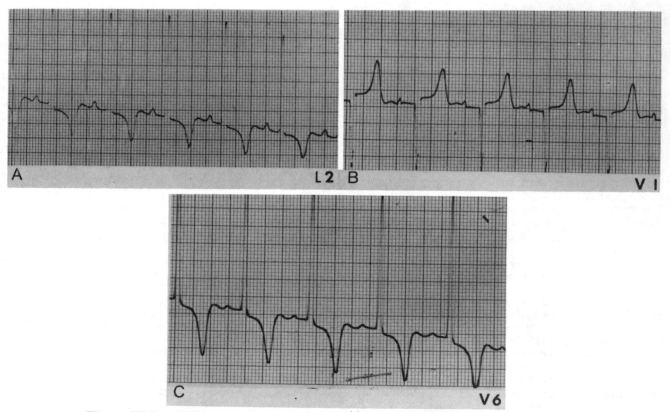

Figure 57.2   ECG of a patient with left ventricular hypertrophy (see Table 57.3).

Table 57.3
Principal Electrocardiographic Features of Left Ventricular Hypertrophy [a]

Electrocardiographic Criteria	Point System for Diagnosis [b]
Negative components of P in V$_1$ $\geq$ 1 mm and $\geq$ 0.4 sec	3 points
QRS	
Largest limb lead R or S $\geq$ 20 mm or largest chest lead S before transition or R after transition $\geq$ 30 mm	3 points
OR	
Largest S before transition plus largest R after transition = 45 mm:	
Frontal plane axis $\geq$ $-30°$	2 points
Duration in extremity lead $\geq$ 0.09 sec	1 point
Intrinsicoid deflection $\geq$ 0.05 sec	1 point
ST-T	
In general, opposite QRS:	
Without digitalis	3 points
With digitalis	1 point

[a] Modified from L. G. Horan and N. C. Flowers: *A Textbook of Cardiovascular Medicine*, edited by E. Braunwald, W. B. Saunders, Philadelphia, 1980, p. 229 (12).
[b] Interpretation of point score: 6 points, left ventricular hypertrophy; 5 points, probable left ventricular hypertrophy; and 4 points, possible left ventricular hypertrophy. If only voltage criteria are met, ECG may be designated as borderline, and the statement should be made that "left ventricular hypertrophy is suggested only by voltage and should be excluded by other clinical means."

terval history, pertinent physical examination, ECG, chest X-ray, and echocardiogram.

Patients should be cautioned to avoid undue exertion since acute heart failure, arrhythmia, and sudden death are more likely under such circumstances.

The risk of subacute bacterial endocarditis is increased in patients with aortic stenosis, and is unrelated to the severity of the stenosis (the risk is unchanged after aortic valve surgery—see below) (17). Therefore, antibiotic prophylaxis (see Chapter 83) is necessary before dental and surgical procedures.

Atrial arrhythmias are uncommon; if they occur, they must be treated aggressively (see Chapter 56) because they are more likely to cause angina, heart failure, or syncope than in a patient without aortic stenosis. β-Blocking agents are probably best avoided because they may compromise left ventricular function further. If heart failure develops, it should be treated with digitalis and diuretics (see Chapter 58), but great care must be taken to avoid volume depletion which may reduce cardiac output to a point where serious underperfusion of vital organs occurs.

Table 57.4 lists the indications for referral of a patient with aortic stenosis to a cardiologist. In general, referral is indicated if the diagnosis is unclear, if the patient is symptomatic, or if an asymptomatic

Table 57.4
Indications for Referral of Patients with Aortic Stenosis

If there is a question about the diagnosis
If the patient is symptomatic
If the asymptomatic patient has signs of severe obstruction:
  Physical signs:
    Small pulse pressure (<30 mm Hg)
    Late peak to systolic murmur
    Diminished A-2
    Paradoxical splitting of A-2
  ECG:
    Left ventricular hypertrophy
    ST depression, T wave inversion
  Chest X-ray: Concentric left ventricular hypertrophy
  Echocardiogram:
    Concentric left ventricular hypertrophy
    Calcification of aortic valve in patients under 60

patient has evidence of severe obstruction. Cardiac catheterization (see Chapter 54) is the definitive technique for assessing the severity and site of aortic stenosis. It should be performed in all symptomatic patients and in asymptomatic patients who have signs of severe disease. Hemodynamically significant stenosis is usually associated with a gradient of 50 mm Hg or greater (unless cardiac output is reduced, in which case the gradient may be much lower even if there is severe stenosis). The effective aortic valve orifice in patients with severe obstruction is usually less than 0.5 cm/m^2 body surface area (compared to 1.6 to 2.6 cm in normal people). At the time of catheterization, angiography is also done to assess left ventricular function, the patency of the coronary arteries and the degree, if any, of aortic regurgitation.

The cardiologist is likely to recommend replacement of the stenotic aortic valve with a prosthesis in all symptomatic patients and in asymptomatic patients with signs of severe obstruction who are found to have a large gradient or evidence, on angiography, of left ventricular dysfunction.

Operative mortality in patients without left ventricular failure is 5 to 10%; in patients with left ventricular failure, 10 to 25%. The patient's postoperative health and long term survival are dependent on a number of factors (age, general health, left ventricular function, etc) but overall the 5-year survival is approximately 80 to 85%, and the 10-year survival, approximately 70 to 75%. Most patients experience a considerable improvement in their sense of well-being and in their exercise tolerance (17). When patients die, however, their death is usually due to a cardiac complication (heart failure, myocardial infarction, or sudden death).

The surgeon has the choice of replacement of the diseased aortic valve with either a prosthetic device or with a porcine heterograft. The advantage of the porcine valve is the low rate of thromboembolism associated with it without anticoagulation (1 to 2% a year) compared to the rate associated with any one of the several prosthetic valves available despite anticoagulation (2 to 7% a year) (4). Patients with aortic stenosis are not at major risk of systemic thromboembolism, before or after cardiac surgery, unless they are in atrial fibrillation and/or have associated mitral valve disease. Therefore, the porcine valve may be a reasonable choice for them if technical considerations permit it. Ultimately, the surgeon must be the final judge of the type of artificial valve to use.

Hypertrophic Cardiomyopathy

Hypertrophic cardiomyopathy is a disease of cardiac muscle in which the ventricular septum is thickened disproportionately compared to the free wall of the left ventricle (asymmetric septal hypertrophy). The left ventricle is hypercontractile and during systole ejects essentially all of its blood, leaving a "clenched fist" with very high wall stress. The assymetric hypertrophy distinguishes this condition from those, such as hypertension and aortic stenosis, that cause secondary hypertrophy of the heart muscle (Table 57.2). A common, but not invariable, feature of the disease is obstruction to the left ventricular outflow tract.

ETIOLOGY AND EPIDEMIOLOGY

The etiology of hypertrophic cardiomyopathy is unknown, although there is evidence that it is usually inherited. Some patients become symptomatic when they are young adults, but the diagnosis is sometimes not made until much later in life. Men and women are equally likely to be affected. Most people with the disease are asymptomatic and the proportion of affected people who have become symptomatic is unknown.

NATURAL HISTORY AND SYMPTOMS

The most common symptom of hypertrophic cardiomyopathy is dyspnea, but patients also complain frequently of angina and of syncope or near-syncope. These symptoms are much more likely to be induced by exertion than to occur spontaneously.

Most symptomatic patients have a relatively stable, protracted course, but once marked symptoms develop, some patients become rapidly worse, with progressive heart failure, angina, or arrhythmias. Over a 5-year period in one study, most surviving patients (83%) were either stable or improved (25). The most troublesome feature of the illness is its propensity to cause sudden death. The incidence of sudden death is about 3 to 4% per year in patients with hypertrophic cardiomyopathy, but some families have a particularly high incidence. Unfortunately, there is no way to identify in any given patient an increased risk of sudden death; in fact, death may be the first manifestation of the disease.

PHYSICAL FINDINGS

The characteristic signs of the disease are a sustained left ventricular apical impulse, a loud S-4, and a harsh systolic ejection murmur, loudest at the left lower border of the sternum and often accompanied by a thrill. The location of the murmur helps distinguish the condition from valvular aortic stenosis. Other distinguishing features are as follows: the second heart sound (A-2) is usually audible; a diastolic murmur is rare; the pulse pressure is normal; ejection sounds are uncommon; and, most important, the upstroke of the carotid pulse is brisk. In addition, the murmur of hypertrophic cardiomyopathy is augmented when the patient stands or performs a Valsalva maneuver and is diminished when the patient squats—the opposite of the findings in patients with aortic stenosis.

LABORATORY EVALUATION

An ECG, chest X-ray, and echocardiogram should be obtained routinely in patients suspected of having hypertrophic cardiomyopathy.

Electrocardiogram. The ECG is abnormal in the majority of patients and is always abnormal in patients with obstruction. Typically, there is evidence of left ventricular hypertrophy (Fig. 57.2 and Table 57.3) and there is nonspecific ST depression and T wave inversion. Q waves are often seen in the inferior and lateral leads, reflecting septal hypertrophy.

Chest X-Ray. The left ventricle is sometimes enlarged, but unpredictably so. In contrast to aortic valvular stenosis, the aortic valve is not calcified and the ascending aorta is not dilated.

Echocardiogram. Echocardiography is diagnostic; it demonstrates a thickened ventricular septum, hypertrophied out of proportion to the posterior wall of the left ventricle. Also, the mitral valve apparatus is displaced anteriorly during systole.

MANAGEMENT

The goal of therapy is to reduce the hypercontractile state of the left ventricle. Currently this is best done by means of β-adrenergic blockade with propranolol (usual dose 10 to 40 mg, 4 times a day; if more than 320 to 400 mg a day are required, consultation with a cardiologist is warranted). Angina, especially, is often relieved in this way; but dyspnea also may be decreased as a result of a slower heart rate and of more time for the ventricle to fill. Although it is not clear that the risk of sudden death is reduced by β-blockade, most patients are symptomatically improved or at least stabilized by treatment.

Verapamil, a calcium channel blocking agent, reduces the hypercontractile state and may, when more widely used, change the natural history of this disease substantially (see Chapters 54 and 56).

Drugs which increase ventricular contractility or decrease ventricular volume are best avoided if possible—digitalis, vasodilators, β-adrenergic stimulants, and diuretics. Patients, even if asymptomatic, should avoid undue exertion (*e.g.,* running).

There is an increased risk of endocarditis in patients with hypertrophic cardiomyopathy and they should therefore receive antibiotic prophylaxis before dental and surgical procedures (see Chapter 83).

Surgical removal of a portion of the hypertrophied septum should be considered in severely symptomatic patients. Such a decision should be made in consultation with a cardiologist and a cardiac surgeon. Although the operative mortality is relatively high (5 to 10%), symptoms are usually relieved in patients who survive. In one series the incidence of sudden death appeared to be reduced after operation (25).

Atrial Septal Defect

Atrial septal defect of the ostium secundum type (in the midportion of the septum) is one of the most common congenital cardiac diseases that is diagnosed in adults. It causes, until late in the course (see below), a left to right atrial shunt with a volume overload of the right ventricle and overperfusion of the lungs.

ETIOLOGY AND EPIDEMIOLOGY

The defect is more common in females; the reported female to male ratio ranges from 1.5 to 3.5:1. Occasionally the defect is associated with other cardiac abnormalities. For example, 10 to 20% of patients with an atrial septal defect have mitral valve prolapse (13).

NATURAL HISTORY AND SYMPTOMS

Patients with atrial septal defect are usually asymptomatic until their third or fourth decade. Thereafter, symptoms invariably develop—usually dyspnea on exertion, fatigue, and palpitations—the result of heart failure and of supraventricular arrhythmias. Less commonly, symptoms of pulmonary embolism (Chapter 50) or paradoxical embolism (e.g., a stroke) occur. Virtually all patients are symptomatic by age 60. In fact, three-quarters of untreated patients are dead by age 50; and 90% by age 60. Increased pulmonary blood flow eventually produces pulmonary vascular disease and, consequently, pulmonary hypertension in about 15% of patients (5). When this happens, the left to right shunt first decreases and then reverses; it is at that point that cyanosis develops. Coexistent atherosclerotic or hypertensive cardiovascular disease may complicate the course of older patients with atrial septal defect and may make diagnosis and treatment more difficult.

PHYSICAL FINDINGS

Atrial septal defect usually causes a wide fixed split of the second heart sound, the result of late closure of the pulmonic valve, and a soft blowing systolic pulmonic ejection murmur. A low-medium frequency mid-diastolic flow rumble across the tricuspid valve is common. The precordium may be hyperdynamic with a palpable S-3. If pulmonary hypertension has developed (see below), clubbing and cyanosis may be observed, and P-2 will be ac-

centuated. Signs of right ventricular failure (edema, distended neck veins, hepatomegaly) are common late in the disease.

LABORATORY EVALUATION

An ECG, a chest X-ray, and an echocardiogram should be obtained routinely in a patient suspected of having an atrial septal defect.

Electrocardiogram. The ECG displays an incomplete right bundle branch block or rSR-1 in lead V_1 90 to 95% of the time with a vertical frontal plane axis or right axis deviation. Atrial fibrillation occurs commonly in symptomatic patients; atrial flutter and paroxysmal atrial tachycardia, less often.

Chest X-ray (Fig. 57.3). The chest X-ray in this disease is almost invariably abnormal and shows increased pulmonary vascularity with a prominent main pulmonary artery and increased heart size. The right pulmonary artery is usually more prominent than the left because of differential flow due to the jet effect.

Echocardiogram. The echocardiogram demonstrates paradoxical motion of the ventricular septum with respect to the posterior wall of the left ventricle. This is a nonspecific echo finding seen with volume overload of the right ventricle.

MANAGEMENT

If a patient is suspected of having an atrial septal defect, he should be referred to a cardiologist for

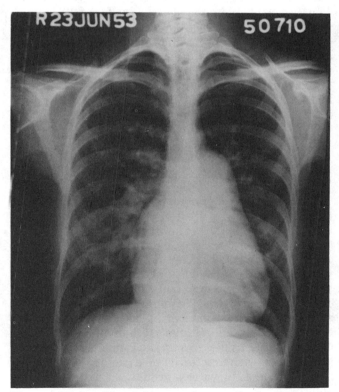

Figure 57.3 Chest X-ray of a patient with atrial septal defect (see text).

definitive diagnosis. The cardiologist will usually perform cardiac catheterization (see Chapter 54 for a description of the patient experience). All patients, even if they are asymptomatic, should have their defect repaired if pulmonary blood flow is more than 1½ times systemic blood flow. The operative mortality is less than 2%, although some degree of persistent right or left ventricular dysfunction is common in adults. If severe pulmonary hypertension has developed (pulmonary pressure equal to or greater than the systemic pressure), corrective surgery is contraindicated, but patients with lesser degrees of pulmonary hypertension may still benefit from repair of the defect. Survival after corrective surgery is influenced by the age of the patient and the degree of persistent cardiac dysfunction. Patients with otherwise normal hearts have normal survival rates after successful repair of the atrial defect and usually can resume normal activity.

Endocarditis prophylaxis is unnecessary for patients with atrial septal defect.

Mitral Regurgitation (3)

Mitral regurgitation may develop because of an abnormality of any part of the mitral valve apparatus: the valve leaflets, the chordae tendineae, the papillary muscles, or the annulus. Such abnormality may result in either acute or chronic signs and symptoms, depending on the nature of the lesion.

An incompetent mitral valve allows regurgitation into the left atrium of blood from the left ventricle. The reduced load on the ventricle reduces the tension in the ventricular muscle and allows it to utilize more energy in contraction. Therefore, in patients with chronic mitral regurgitation, cardiac output remains normal for years until, because of age or intercurrent disease, the ventricle no longer can compensate, and heart failure ensues. In patients with acute mitral regurgitation, ventricular compensation is inadequate and heart failure develops abruptly.

Chronic Mitral Regurgitation

ETIOLOGY AND EPIDEMIOLOGY

Chronic mitral incompetency in adults may occur in association with a great variety of disorders. Rheumatic fever, despite the marked decline in its incidence in recent years, still is the cause of 25% of cases—usually in association with some degree of mitral stenosis. Otherwise, chronic mitral regurgitation is most often due to congenital maldevelopment of the mitral apparatus, to an inherited (e.g., Marfan's syndrome or mitral prolapse—see below) or an acquired (e.g., systemic lupus erythematosus) disorder of connective tissue, to papillary muscle necrosis—the result of ischemic heart disease, or to idiopathic calcification of the valve—primarily a disorder of the elderly.

NATURAL HISTORY AND SYMPTOMS

Patients with chronic mitral regurgitation may remain asymptomatic for many years—even, if the regurgitation is not severe, for their entire lives. Characteristically, when symptoms do develop, they appear gradually over years as the left ventricle slowly loses its ability to compensate for the loss of more than half of its stroke volume back into the left atrium. Dyspnea and fatigue are the usual symptoms of left ventricular failure. Supraventricular arrhythmias, especially atrial fibrillation, are likely to develop if left atrial enlargement becomes marked, compromising somewhat the heart's ability to compensate. Acute pulmonary edema occasionally occurs but is uncommon. Sometimes severe pulmonary hypertension develops without much enlargement of the left atrium. Early surgical correction of the lesion in patients with pulmonary hypertension and signs of right ventricular hypertrophy is important.

In a series of unselected patients with mitral regurgitation, 80% treated medically survived 5 years; and 60% survived 10 years (20). Moderately to severely symptomatic patients do less well: in one report 46% of patients with chronic rheumatic mitral insufficiency survived 5 years (17).

PHYSICAL FINDINGS

A high pitched holosystolic murmur, loudest at the apex, is characteristic of chronic mitral regurgitation (patients with mild regurgitation may have only a late systolic murmur). The holosystolic murmur is constant in intensity and radiates always to the axilla and sometimes to the back and to the base of the heart. The murmur is intensified when the patient stands or performs a Valsalva maneuver and is diminished when he squats. If regurgitation is severe, the precordium is usually hyperdynamic and there is an S-3 gallop. S-1 is soft. If pulmonary hypertension has developed, an S-4 gallop, a loud P-2, and a right ventricular heave may be appreciated. Signs of right ventricular failure—edema, hepatomegaly, distended neck veins, hepatojugular reflux—may also be seen late in the course of this disease.

LABORATORY EVALUATION

An ECG, chest X-ray, and echocardiogram should be obtained routinely if a patient is suspected of having mitral regurgitation.

Electrocardiogram. The ECG shows evidence of left atrial enlargement (Fig. 57.4 and Table 57.5) and, if present, of atrial fibrillation. The pattern of left ventricular hypertrophy (Fig. 57.2 and Table 57.3) is often seen as well, primarily in patients with severe disease. A pattern of right ventricular hypertrophy (Table 57.6) indicating pulmonary hypertension is less common and, when seen, is cause for great concern.

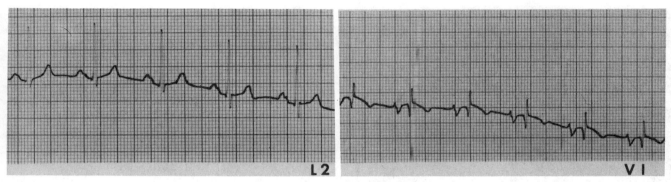

Figure 57.4 ECG of a patient with left atrial hypertrophy (see Table 57.5).

Table 57.5
Principal Electrocardiographic Features of Left Atrial Hypertrophy[a]

P wave:	
Axis	+45° to −30°
Amplitude (II, III, aV$_f$) duration Component (V$_1$)	> 0.11 sec (broad)
Early	Positive but inside normal
Late	Negative, ≥0.04 area units[b]

[a] Modified from L. G. Horan and N. C. Flowers: *A Textbook of Cardiovascular Medicine*, edited by E. Braunwald, W. B. Saunders, Philadelphia, 1980, p. 223 (12).
[b] Area units = mm-sec. One small block on standard ECG paper = 0.04 mm-sec.

Chest X-ray. Left ventricular and left atrial enlargement are common. On a posteroanterior (PA) film, elevation of the left bronchus and prominence of the left atrial appendage are the earliest signs of left atrial enlargement; a double density posteriorly is seen when the left atrium is grossly enlarged (Fig. 57.5).

Echocardiogram. Echocardiography demonstrates left atrial and left ventricular enlargement. Two-dimensional echocardiography may show that the valve does not close completely.

MANAGEMENT

Patients who do not have severe disease can be managed medically. Antibiotic prophylaxis against bacterial endocarditis should be administered before all dental and surgical procedures (Chapter 83). If atrial fibrillation is present, restoration of sinus rhythm should be attempted unless the left atrium is greatly enlarged or unless mitral regurgitation has been present for many years. (A detailed discussion of the treatment of atrial fibrillation is to be found in Chapter 56.) If heart failure develops, it should be treated by use of the measures described in Chapter 58; afterload reduction by use of an arteriolar vasodilator may be particularly useful in this condition: by lowering peripheral resistance, ejection of blood

Table 57.6
Electrocardiographic Criteria of Right Ventricular Hypertrophy in Adults without Conduction Defects Known NOT to Have Infarction[a]

Sign	Points[b]
Ratio reversal (R/S V$_5$:R/S V$_1$ ≤ 0.4)	5
qR in V$_1$	5
R/S ratio in V$_1$ > 1	4
S in V$_1$ < 2 mm	4
R in V$_1$ + S in V$_5$ or V$_6$ > 10.5 mm	4
Right axis deviation > 110°	4
S in V$_5$ or V$_6$ ≥ 7 mm and each ≥ 2 mm	3
R/S in V$_5$ or V$_6$ ≤ 1	3
R in V$_1$ ≥ 7 mm	3
S$_1$, S$_2$, and S$_3$ each ≥ 1 mm	2
S$_1$ and Q$_3$ each ≥ 1 mm	2
R′ in V$_1$ earlier than 0.08 sec and ≥ 2 mm	2
R peak in V$_1$ or V$_2$ between 0.04 and 0.07 sec	1
S in V$_5$ or V$_6$ ≥ 2 mm but < 7 mm	1
Reduction in V lead R/S ratio between V$_1$ and V$_4$	1
R in V$_5$ or V$_6$ < 5 mm	1

[a] Modified from L. G. Horan and N. C. Flowers: *A Textbook of Cardiovascular Medicine*, edited by E. Braunwald, W. B. Saunders, Philadelphia, 1980, p. 226 (12).
[b] Interpretation of point score: 10 points, right ventricular hypertrophy; 7 to 9 points, probable right ventricular hypertrophy or hemodynamic overload; and 5 to 6 points, possible right ventricular hypertrophy or hemodynamic overload. These criteria do not take into account serial ECG comparisons. Such additional data may alter the interpreter's impression of the likelihood of fixed enlargement or dynamic overload.

into the aorta, rather than back into the left atrium, is favored.

When patients become more than mildly symptomatic or if the diagnosis is unclear, referral to a cardiologist is indicated (Table 57.7). It is likely that cardiac catheterization and angiography (see Chapter 54) will be done to confirm the diagnosis, to establish the severity of the lesion, to evaluate the function of the left ventricle and, often, the patency of the coronary arteries. At this point a decision will be made about the value of operative repair of the lesion.

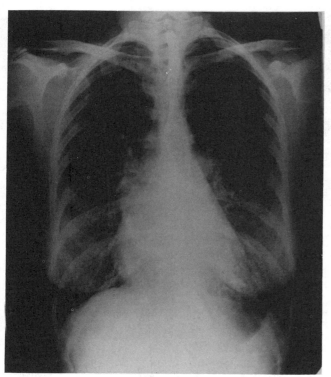

Figure 57.5   Chest X-ray of a patient with left atrial enlargement. Note the straight left heart border and the calcification of the wall of the left atrium.

Table 57.7
Indications for Referral of Patients with Mitral Regurgitation

Progressive dyspnea or fatigue
Development of supraventricular arrhythmia
A mildly symptomatic patient with progressive cardiac enlargement
Uncertainty about the diagnosis
Acute mitral regurgitation
Patients with mitral valve prolapse who have symptomatic arrhythmias or symptomatic mitral regurgitation

Unless the patient has severe noncardiac disease or unless left ventricular function is so severely reduced that the patient would not tolerate an operation, replacement of the defective valve with a prosthesis is very likely to be recommended. The operative mortality reported from various centers is 3 to 10%.

The health and survival of patients who have undergone successful valve replacement depends on a number of factors. Advanced age (over 60), the presence of concomitant mitral stenosis, poor left ventricular function (ejection fraction under 50%), and severity of symptoms preoperatively (New York Heart Association Class III or IV—see Chapter 58) are adverse factors which reduce long term postoperative survival. In general, patients with mitral regurgitation on the basis of ischemic heart disease do less well than do patients with rheumatic heart disease. Nevertheless, even patients with one or more adverse risk factors live longer, on the average, with a prosthetic valve than they would without one (10) and most patients are able to be more active than they were before surgery. The overall 10-year survival for patients who have undergone successful mitral surgery is approximately 70% (10). Postoperatively, anticoagulation with warfarin is used routinely to prevent thromboembolic complications (see Chapter 48).

Acute Mitral Regurgitation

ETIOLOGY AND EPIDEMIOLOGY

Acute mitral incompetence is most often due to rupture of the chordae tendineae, the cords that connect the valve cusps to the papillary muscles of the left ventricle. Most of the time the cause of the rupture is unknown, although occasionally rheumatic fever or acute left ventricular dilation can be incriminated. Much less commonly, acute mitral regurgitation will be caused by papillary muscle rupture (a rare complication of myocardial infarction) or by perforation of a mitral cusp as the result of bacterial endocarditis. The disorder is primarily encountered in middle-aged and elderly patients.

NATURAL HISTORY AND SYMPTOMS

Because the left atrium is suddenly presented with a volume load to which it cannot rapidly accommodate, acute pulmonary edema is much more common in patients with acute, compared to chronic, mitral regurgitation. The primary symptom of pulmonary edema is severe dyspnea at rest.

PHYSICAL FINDINGS

A harsh holosystolic murmur of constant intensity, loudest at the apex, is characteristic; if a posterior cord has ruptured, the murmur may radiate to the base of the heart, and may mimic the murmur of aortic stenosis. Sometimes an early or midsystolic, or even a crescendo-decrescendo, murmur is heard. An S-3 gallop is almost always heard and an S-4 gallop is common. Unlike the situation in patients with chronic mitral regurgitation, S-1 is normal or even loud. Signs of left sided heart failure (rales) and of right sided failure (edema, distended neck veins, etc) are also common.

LABORATORY FINDINGS

Chest X-ray. The chest X-ray shows marked pulmonary congestion. The left atrium and the left ventricle are minimally enlarged. These findings are the opposite of those found in patients with chronic mitral regurgitation.

Echocardiogram. Chamber enlargement is usually not seen; but increased systolic motion of the valve is common; and if the chordae have ruptured, the flailing chordae may be visualized.

MANAGEMENT

Patients suspected of having suffered acute mitral regurgitation should be hospitalized immediately for diagnosis, for treatment of acute heart failure, and for consideration for early operative repair.

Mitral Valve Prolapse (7)

ETIOLOGY AND EPIDEMIOLOGY

Systolic prolapse of a leaflet of the mitral valve into the left atrium has proved to be a very common phenomenon, affecting over 5% of the population (6, 14). Women are more likely to be affected than are men although the reported sex ratios vary considerably. The exact nature of this abnormality is not entirely clear; but in most cases the condition appears to be an inherited developmental abnormality (autosomal dominant), often in association with skeletal defects such as scoliosis or pectus excavatum. Myxomatous degeneration of these valve leaflets is common; a similar degenerative process is sometimes associated with a disorder of connective tissue (e.g., Marfan's syndrome or Ehlers-Danlos syndrome). Other patients have other cardiac abnormalities such as ischemic heart disease, hypertrophic or congestive cardiomyopathy, rheumatic valvulitis, or atrial septal defect.

NATURAL HISTORY AND SYMPTOMS

Most patients are asymptomatic and the condition is identified during a routine physical examination. Less often, patients complain of palpitations, chest pain, or dyspnea. The palpitations reflect arrhythmias (see below), the most common symptomatic cardiac abnormalities associated with the syndrome. The chest pain sometimes mimics angina (or, in fact, is angina if there is concomitant ischemic heart disease), but more often is sharp lancinating pain in the left chest, unrelated to exertion, and the cause of it is unknown. In about 15% of patients (16) symptomatic mitral regurgitation occurs, and patients complain of dyspnea, due to left ventricular failure.

It is now recognized that patients with mitral valve prolapse are at risk for embolic strokes. In a recent study 40% of patients under 45 who had had a stroke had mitral valve prolapse compared to 6.8% of matched controls (1).

The most feared complication of mitral valve prolapse, sudden death, is quite rare. The risk is higher in patients with a family history of sudden death.

PHYSICAL FINDINGS

The characteristic finding in patients with mitral prolapse is a midsystolic click, best heard at the lower left sternal border, due to sudden tensing of the prolapsed valve. It occurs later than the systolic ejection sound heard commonly in association with systemic hypertension (see p. 528). Very often the click is followed immediately by a crescendo late systolic murmur which continues until A-2.

The physical findings may vary from time to time in any given patient and may also vary with the position of the patient. In those relatively rare instances where chronic mitral regurgitation has developed, the typical physical findings—including the holosystolic murmur—of this condition will be encountered (see above).

LABORATORY FINDINGS

Electrocardiogram. The ECG is usually normal, especially in asymptomatic patients. Symptomatic patients may show nonspecific ST-T wave changes, usually in the inferior leads.

A variety of arrhythmias may occur in patients with mitral valve prolapse. The commonest are premature ventricular contractions (PVCs), and paroxysmal supraventricular tachycardia. When patients are exercised, it has been reported that many of them develop frequent PVCs and that up to 40% develop atrial arrhythmias (9).

Echocardiogram. The echocardiogram is diagnostic in this condition. It shows late systolic or holosystolic prolapse of one or both leaflets of the mitral valve. Often, however, the echocardiogram shows no abnormalities despite the typical cardiac findings. These patients probably have minor degrees of prolapse.

MANAGEMENT

Asymptomatic patients need no treatment, but should be reassessed by interval history, physical examination, and echocardiogram every few years. Those patients who have a systolic murmur should receive prophylaxis against bacterial endocarditis before dental or surgical procedures (see Chapter 83). (Patients who have only a click probably do not need prophylaxis.)

Patients with palpitations should have ambulatory electrocardiographic monitoring to determine the severity of their arrhythmia, and therapy should be prescribed on the basis of the type of arrhythmia that is present (see Chapter 56). Propranolol is often a drug of choice in the treatment of these patients and also in those with mitral prolapse who complain of chest pain (usual dose 10–40 mg, 4 times a day; if more than 320 to 400 mg a day are ineffective, a cardiology consultation is warranted). The mechanism of action of the drug in the relief of pain is unknown.

Patients with symptomatic mitral regurgitation should be treated as described above (p. 537).

Referral to a cardiologist is recommended at any time patients become symptomatic from arrhythmia or from chronic mitral regurgitation.

Mitral Stenosis

Stenosis of the mitral valve obstructs the flow of blood out of the left atrium and therefore raises the left atrial pressure above the left ventricular diastolic pressure. The pressure gradient across the valve is a measure of the severity of the stenosis. Because of the increase in left atrial pressure, there is an increase in pressure in the pulmonary blood vessels. The pulmonary congestion accounts for most of the symptoms of the disease.

ETIOLOGY AND EPIDEMIOLOGY

By far the most common cause of mitral stenosis in adults is rheumatic fever (although a history of rheumatic fever can be elicited in only 50% of patients with pure mitral stenosis). Pure mitral stenosis occurs in 40% of all patients with rheumatic heart disease. The rest of the time there is associated mitral regurgitation, aortic valve disease, and, uncommonly, tricuspid valve disease. Two-thirds of patients with rheumatic mitral stenosis are women.

NATURAL HISTORY AND SYMPTOMS

On the average, there is a latent period of nearly 20 years between an attack of acute rheumatic fever and the development of symptomatic mitral stenosis (24). Thus, symptoms usually do not develop before the fourth decade. The severity of symptoms is quite variable: some people in fact are never symptomatic; some are mildly symptomatic indefinitely; and some develop progressively severe cardiopulmonary decompensation. Of the patients with progressive disease, it has been estimated that an average of 7 years elapses between the onset of symptoms and the development of total disability (Class IV cardiac status—see Chapter 58). In one series the 5-year survival from that point in patients treated medically was only 15% (18).

Pulmonary congestion causes many of the symptoms of mitral stenosis: dyspnea, orthopnea, and paroxysmal nocturnal dyspnea. If left atrial pressure rises acutely because of a sudden stress, frank pulmonary edema may occur. Hemoptysis due to rupture of small bronchial veins or to pulmonary edema is not unusual.

As the disease progresses, pulmonary hypertension develops followed by symptoms of right heart failure: edema, distended neck veins, a tender liver, and ascites. At this point, the flow of blood into the left heart is limited, and the pulmonary arterioles hypertrophy, diminishing the risk of pulmonary edema. Low cardiac output is responsible for the fatigue which is a common complaint of patients at this stage.

Atrial fibrillation (Chapter 56) complicates the course of 40 to 50% of patients with mitral stenosis. The 20% reduction in blood flow across the mitral valve by the loss of left atrial contraction may intensify symptoms of heart failure and of fatigue.

At some time in their course, 20% of patients with mitral stenosis experience symptomatic thromboembolism—most often to the brain; 80% of these patients are in atrial fibrillation.

PHYSICAL FINDINGS

A mid-diastolic rumbling murmur with presystolic accentuation is characteristic of mitral stenosis. It is best heard, and is often limited to, the cardiac apex. To hear it, it may be necessary to turn the patient to the left lateral position and to have him expire fully.

Sometimes the patient must be exercised before the murmur is audible. The murmur is best heard with the bell of the stethoscope pressed lightly against the chest. A loud first heart sound (S-1) and opening snap (see above, p. 528) usually accompany the murmur when the valve is mobile.

Late in the course, signs of pulmonary hypertension (a loud P-2 and a right ventricular heave) and of right heart failure may be found.

LABORATORY FINDINGS

Electrocardiogram. The ECG shows left atrial enlargement (Fig. 57.4 and Table 57.5) in 90% of patients who are in sinus rhythm. With the development of pulmonary hypertension, signs of right ventricular hypertrophy appear (Table 57.6).

Chest X-ray. Left atrial enlargement (see p. 537 and Fig. 57.5) is seen in virtually all patients with symptomatic mitral stenosis, but the size of the left atrium does not correlate with the severity of stenosis. Late in the course right ventricular and right atrial hypertrophy will be seen as well. Symptomatic patients are also likely to show radiologic signs of pulmonary congestion—the severity of which will determine the findings that are seen (Chapter 58).

Calcification of the mitral valve is not unusual in patients with longstanding mitral stenosis, but this is better visualized by fluoroscopy than by a plain X-ray.

Echocardiogram. Mitral stenosis can be diagnosed by echocardiography, but its severity cannot be assessed. Mitral valve thickening can be seen; there is reduced excursion of the anterior leaflet of the valve and abnormal anterior motion of the posterior leaflet during diastole (it normally moves posteriorly).

MANAGEMENT

Asymptomatic patients need no treatment except prophylaxis for bacterial endocarditis when they are to undergo dental or surgical procedures (Chapter 83). Adult patients with rheumatic mitral stenosis do not ordinarily require prophylaxis for β-hemolytic streptococcal infection unless they have had an attack of rheumatic fever within the last 5 to 10 years or are in a population where β-hemolytic streptococcal infection is more prevalent (e.g., military personnel or hospital workers). When prophylaxis is necessary, the best regimen is 1 to 2 million units of benzathine penicillin G intramuscularly once a month.

Mildly symptomatic patients should be treated with diuretics and sodium restriction (see Chapter 58 for a detailed discussion of the treatment of heart failure). Digitalis, since it does not affect the hemodynamic abnormality, is not useful in this situation unless rapid atrial fibrillation develops. The treatment of atrial fibrillation is discussed in detail in Chapter 56, but it should be recognized that there is a 1 to 2% incidence of systemic thromboembolism at the time of conversion of atrial fibrillation to normal sinus rhythm in patients with mitral stenosis. The conversion, whether pharmacologic or electrical, should be done in the hospital. Patients with persistent sinus tachycardia who are not in heart failure may safely be treated with propranolol (10 to 40 mg, 4 times a day) to lower their heart rate.

Warfarin anticoagulants should be administered to patients with mitral stenosis who have had one or more episodes of systemic or pulmonary thromboembolism (see Chapter 48) or who are in atrial fibrillation.

Table 57.8 lists the reasons to refer patients with mitral stenosis to a cardiologist. In general referral is indicated to confirm the diagnosis, to assess the severity of the process, and to consider whether or not to recommend operative repair or replacement of the mitral valve. The cardiologist is likely to perform a cardiac catheterization to measure the size of the mitral orifice and to decide whether to recommend surgery for a patient with moderate or severe stenosis. However, the age of the patient, the presence of severe noncardiac disease, and the presence of other cardiac lesions (e.g., severe ischemic heart disease) will influence the recommendation. Patients with pulmonary hypertension or evidence of right ventricular hypertrophy should be referred even if asymptomatic.

The relatively poor prognosis of medically treated patients with progressive disease (see "Natural History and Symptoms" above) dictates that such patients, unless there are specific contraindications, should be offered surgery. The preferred procedure will depend on the anatomy of the valve at the time of operation. If possible a *mitral commissurotomy* will be performed. The operative mortality of this procedure is low (1 to 3%), and the long term results are excellent for a number of years. However, after commissurotomy, 10% of patients within 5 years and 60% within 10 years require reoperation because of restenosis or because of the development of symp-

Table 57.8
Indications for Referral of Patients with Mitral Stenosis[a]

Progressive dyspnea or recurrent attacks of pulmonary edema
Symptomatic disease of the aortic and/or tricuspid valve
Women, whether symptomatic or not, who wish to become pregnant
Patients whose symptoms have developed recently who have no history of rheumatic fever (to rule out an atrial myxoma)
Patients with chronic obstructive lung disease
Patients with angina pectoris
Patients with evidence of pulmonary hypertension (including right ventricular hypertrophy)

[a] Modified from R. O. Brandenburg et al.: Practical Cardiology, 5: 50, 1979 (2).

tomatic mitral regurgitation or of symptomatic aortic stenosis (11). If a prosthetic valve is implanted, the operative mortality is 3 to 10%; the course of patients who survive surgery depends on a number of factors (see p. 538), but certainly is better than that of symptomatic patients treated medically.

Aortic Regurgitation (8)

An incompetent aortic valve allows regurgitation into the left ventricle of blood ejected into the aorta. In order to compensate for the increased volume load, the left ventricle dilates and hypertrophies so that the effective stroke volume may for a long time be normal. Eventually, however, the left ventricle cannot maintain the work load and clinical signs and symptoms of heart failure ensue.

ETIOLOGY AND EPIDEMIOLOGY

Aortic regurgitation may be due to disease of the aortic valve cusps and/or to dilation of the aortic root.

Rheumatic fever is still the most common cause of chronic aortic valvular incompetence, although it now accounts for many fewer cases than it did 20 to 30 years ago. Bacterial endocarditis is the most common cause of acute aortic valvular incompetence. Congenital aortic valvular incompetence or traumatic rupture of a cusp of the aortic valve is relatively uncommon.

Chronic aortic regurgitation due to dilation of the aortic root is most commonly due to syphilitic aortitis (see Chapter 29) although, again, the incidence has dropped considerably. Other, relatively rare, causes include rheumatoid arthritis, ankylosing spondylitis, Reiter's syndrome, and congenital disorders of connective tissue (Marfan's syndrome, Ehlers-Danlos syndrome, and osteogenesis imperfecta). Acute aortic regurgitation due to dilation of the aortic root is most commonly due to a dissecting aneurysm—usually associated with medial necrosis of the aorta. Dissection is associated with systemic hypertension in approximately 50% of cases. Occasionally a primary disorder of connective tissue, such as Marfan's syndrome, can be incriminated.

Aortic regurgitation in general is more common in men than women, but there are specific exceptions (rheumatoid arthritis, for example).

NATURAL HISTORY AND SYMPTOMS

Patients with *chronic aortic regurgitation* remain asymptomatic sometimes for up to 20 years or have only mild dyspnea on exertion. When symptoms do develop (progressively more severe dyspnea, orthopnea, paroxysmal nocturnal dyspnea and, less often, angina), they reflect an ominous deterioration in the condition.

Patients with *acute aortic regurgitation* develop fulminant pulmonary edema because of the inability of the left ventricle to compensate for the sudden volume load and for the abrupt rise in left ventricular end-diastolic pressure. Marked dyspnea and weakness may be experienced virtually overnight and in most cases within 2 or 3 months. Other symptoms depend on the underlying cause: fever, for example, if it is endocarditis; severe pain in the chest or back, if it is a dissecting aneurysm.

PHYSICAL FINDINGS

Patients with *chronic aortic regurgitation* have a characteristic high frequency early diastolic decrescendo murmur, best heard at the aortic area and at the left sternal border. The duration (but not the intensity) of the murmur correlates with the severity of the lesion so that the murmur is holodiastolic in patients with severe aortic regurgitation. Often there is an accompanying harsh systolic ejection murmur as well, heard at the base of the heart. Severe aortic regurgitation may also cause a loud apical diastolic murmur (the Austin Flint murmur), simulating the murmur of mitral stenosis. Unlike the situation in true mitral stenosis, however, S-1 in patients with aortic regurgitation is often soft, the result of premature closure of the mitral valve, and there is no opening snap. If aortic regurgitation is moderate or severe, the pulse pressure is ordinarily wide, reflecting peripheral vasodilation. The combination of an increased systolic pressure and a reduced diastolic pressure (sometimes as low as 30 mm Hg) produces characteristic changes in the peripheral pulse (waterhammer pulse, "pistol-shot" sounds heard over the femoral artery, etc) and a typical bobbing of the head with each heart beat.

Patients with *acute aortic regurgitation* often show signs of left and right sided heart failure. The regurgitant diastolic murmur is lower pitched and shorter than it is in patients with chronic aortic incompetence; S-1 is often absent and S-3, uncommon with chronic regurgitation, is usually present. The pulse pressure is normal—the result of intense peripheral vasoconstriction.

LABORATORY FINDINGS

Electrocardiogram. The ECG also reflects the severity and duration of aortic regurgitation. Patients with chronic disease show the ECG pattern of left ventricular hypertrophy (Fig. 57.2 and Table 57.3), whereas patients with acute disease do not (although they commonly do show nonspecific ST-T wave changes).

Chest X-ray. The size of the heart in patients with aortic regurgitation depends on the duration and severity of the disease. Patients with chronic severe disease have very large left ventricles, but patients with acute regurgitation may have no cardiac enlargement at all.

Echocardiogram. Echocardiography is useful in the assessment of left ventricular function, the degree of hypertrophy of the left ventricle, and of the degree of dilation of the aortic root. Fluttering of the anterior

Table 57.9
Indications for Referral of Patients with Aortic Regurgitation[a]

Uncertainty about the diagnosis
Symptomatic chronic aortic incompetence (dyspnea, fatigue, angina)
Acute aortic imcompetence
Asymptomatic patients with evidence of severe chronic aortic incompetence: widened pulse pressure, holodiastolic murmur, progressive left ventricular hypertrophy

[a] Modified from R. O. Brandenburg *et al.: Practical Cardiology,* 5: 50, 1979 (2).

leaflet of the mitral valve during diastole is characteristic of moderate to severe aortic regurgitation and also indicates mobility of the mitral valve (a useful sign in ruling out significant mitral stenosis). Premature mitral valve closure is helpful in confirming very severe aortic regurgitation.

MANAGEMENT

Asymptomatic patients need not be treated, but should be assessed once or twice a year by interval history, physical examination, and chest X-ray. Yearly ECGs and echocardiograms should also be obtained. Prophylaxis for bacterial endocarditis is indicated when patients are to undergo dental or surgical procedures (Chapter 83).

If symptoms of heart failure develop, digitalis and diuretics should be prescribed. Also afterload reducing agents may be effective in otherwise unresponsive patients (see Chapter 58).

Table 57.9 lists the reasons to refer patients with aortic regurgitation to a cardiologist. In general, referral is indicated in patients with chronic disease to confirm the diagnosis and to consider whether or not to recommend aortic valve replacement for symptomatic patients and for asymptomatic patients with physical findings of severe disease (widened pulse pressure, holodiastolic murmur, increasing left ventricular enlargement). All patients with suspected acute aortic regurgitation should be seen by a cardiologist as soon as possible. The cardiologist is likely to perform cardiac catheterization (see Chapter 54) to assess the severity of the lesion, the presence of other valvular disease, and the function of the left ventricle. Recently radionuclide angiography has provided the cardiologist with a convenient noninvasive technique for making these measurements easily (see Chapter 58).

Patients with chronic aortic regurgitation do well until they become symptomatic. Thereafter, 50% of patients are dead within 2 years (15). Thus, valve replacement is warranted in all symptomatic patients, preferably before severe left ventricular dysfunction develops. The operative mortality is 5 to 10%, but of the patients who survive surgery, 50% live 10 years or more (23) and their quality of life is usually significantly improved.

References

General

Braunwald, E (Ed.): *Heart Disease. A Textbook of Cardiovascular Medicine.* W. B. Saunders, Philadelphia, 1980.
Encyclopedic review of cardiac physical examination, heart sounds, and cardiac graphic techniques.
Constant, J.: *Bedside Cardiology.* Little Brown, Waltham, Mass., 1976.
The best teaching text for understanding the physiologic basis of heart sounds and how to hear and describe them.
Tavel, M.E: The systolic murmur—innocent or guilty? *Am J Cardiol 39:* 757, 1977.
Concise characterization of the most commonly heard murmur in an ambulatory practice.

Specific

1. Barnett, JHM, Boughner, DR, Taylor, DW, Cooper, PE, Kostuk WJ and Nickol, PM: Further evidence relating mitral valve prolapse to cerebral ischemic events. *N Engl J Med 302:* 139, 1980.
2. Brandenburg, RO, Fuster, V and Guiliani, ER: Valvular heart disease. When should the patient be referred? *Practical Cardiol 5:* 50, 1979.
3. Braunwald, E: Mitral regurgitation: physiologic, clinical, and surgical considerations. *N Engl J Med 281:* 425, 1969.
4. Cohn, LH, Koster, GK, Mee, RBB and Collins, JJ, Jr.: Long term followup of the Hancock Bioprosthetic Heart Valve. A six-year review. *Circulation 60 (Suppl. 2):* 93, 1979.
5. Craig, RJ and Selzer, A: Natural history and prognosis of atrial septal defect. *Circulation 37:* 805, 1968.
6. Darsee, JR, Miklovich, JR, Nicoloff, NB and Lamb LE: Prevalence of mitral valve prolapse in presumably healthy young men. *Circulation 59:* 619, 1979.
7. Devereux, RB, Perloff, JK, Reichels, N and Josephson, ME: Mitral valve prolapse. *Circulation 54:* 3, 1976.
8. Goldschlager, N, Pfeifer, J, Cohn, K, Popper, R and Selzer, A: The natural history of aortic regurgitation. A clinical and hemodynamic study. *Am J Med 54:* 577, 1973.
9. Gooch, AS, Vicencio, F, Markanlov, V and Goldberg H: Arrhythmias and left ventricular asynergy in the prolapsing mitral leaflet syndrome. *Am J Cardiol 29:* 611, 1972.
10. Hammermeister, KE, Fisher, L, Kennedy, JW, Samuels, S and Dodge, HT: Prediction of late survival in patients with mitral valve disease from clinical, hemodynamic, and quantitative angiographic variables. *Circulation 57:* 341, 1978.
11. Heger, JJ, Wann, LS, Weyman, AE, Dillon, JC and Felgenbaum, H: Long-term changes in mitral valve area after successful mitral commissurotomy. *Circulation 59:* 443, 1979.
12. Horan, LG and Flowers, NC: Electrocardiography and vectorcardiography. In: *Heart Disease. A Textbook of Cardiovascular Medicine,* edited by E Braunwald, W. B. Saunders, Philadelphia, 1980.
13. Leachman RD, Cokkinos, DV and Cooley, DA: Association of ostium secundum atrial septal defects with mitral valve prolapse. *Am J Cardiol 38:* 167, 1976.
14. Markiewicz, W, Stoner, J, London, E, Hunt, SA and Popp, RL: Mitral valve prolapse in one hundred presumably healthy young men. *Circulation 53:* 464, 1976.
15. Massell, BF, Ameccua, FJ and Czohiczer, G: Prognosis of patients with pure or predominant aortic regurgitation in the absence of surgery. *Circulation 34 (Suppl 2):* 164, 1966.
16. Mills, P, Rose, J, Hollingsworth, J, Amara, I and Craige, E: Long-term prognosis of mitral-valve prolapse. *N Engl J Med 297:* 13, 1977.
17. Munoz, S, Gallardo, J, Diaz-Gorrin, JR and Medina, O: Influence of surgery on the natural history of rheumatic mitral and aortic valve disease. *Am J Cardiol 35:* 234, 1975.
18. Oleson, KH: The natural history of 271 patients with mitral stenosis under medical treatment. *Br Heart J 24:* 349, 1962.
19. Popp, RL, Rubenson, DS, Tucker, LR and French JW: Echocardiography: M mode and two-dimensional methods. *Ann Intern Med 93:* 344, 1980.
20. Rapaport, E: Natural history of aortic and mitral valve disease. *Am J Cardiol 35:* 221, 1981.
21. Roberts, WC: Anatomically isolated aortic valve disease: a case against its being of rheumatic etiology. *Am J Med 49:* 151, 1970.
22. Ross, J, Jr and Braunwald, E: Aortic stenosis. *Circulation 38 (Suppl. 5):* 61, 1968.
23. Samuels, DA, Curfman, GD, Friedlich, AL, Buckley, MJ and Austen, WG: Valve replacement for aortic regurgitation: long-term follow-up with factors influencing the results. *Circulation 60:* 647, 1979.
24. Selzer, A and Cohn, K: Natural history of mitral stenosis: a review. *Circulation 45:* 878, 1972.
25. Shah, FM, Adelman, AG, Wigle, ED, Gobel, FL, Burchell, HB, Hardarson, T, Curill, R, de la Calzada, C, Oakley, CM and Goodwin JF: The natural (and unnatural) history of hypertrophic obstructive cardiomyopathy. *Circ Res 34 (Suppl. 2):* 179, 1974.

CHAPTER FIFTY-EIGHT

Heart Failure

SHELDON H. GOTTLIEB, M.D.

DEFINITION

The amount of blood which the heart pumps per minute (the *cardiac output*) is normally precisely adjusted to the metabolic needs of the body. The cardiac output may increase by 2 or 3 times as an individual goes from sleep to exercise. An increase in cardiac output may occur within the space of one heart beat by a sudden decrease in vagal tone which causes an increase in *heart rate*. After several seconds of exercise, sympathetic tone increases which causes a further increase in cardiac output by increasing the heart rate and the amount of blood pumped per heart beat (the *stroke volume*). The increased cardiac output soon brings about an increase in the amount of blood returning to the right side of the heart (the *venous return*); also the heart further increases its output in response to the stretch in the heart muscle resulting from the increased volume of venous return (the *Frank-Starling* principle). If the heart is not able to pump enough blood to meet the metabolic needs of the body, compensatory mechanisms are brought into play by the heart, kidney,

lung, and peripheral vascular system. These adjustments cause symptoms and signs recognized as the syndrome of *heart failure*. *Acute heart failure*, manifest usually by pulmonary edema (recognized by the abrupt onset of extreme breathlessness) and evidence of alveolar edema by physical and radiological examination, warrants immediate hospitalization for diagnosis of the underlying and/or precipitating cause and for treatment. However, *chronic heart failure* is usually a problem that can be managed in an ambulatory setting.

EPIDEMIOLOGY OF HEART FAILURE

The *incidence* of heart failure is approximately 0.3 per 1000 per year below age 45, remains constant at approximately 3 per 1000 per year in the middle-age groups, and increases to 8 per 1000 in patients above the age of 70 (12). The incidence among men is approximately twice that among women (12).

The *prevalence* of heart failure increases greatly in patients above 60 years old (Fig. 58.1). Above the age of 70, women with congestive heart failure outnumber men. This is true in spite of the higher incidence in men and probably reflects the earlier mortality among men from coronary artery disease. Estimates of the prevalence rate for heart failure in patients above the age of 65 vary from approximately 20 to 65 per 1000 (7).

PHYSIOLOGY OF HEART FAILURE

The Heart as a Pump

LENGTH/TENSION RELATION: FRANK-STARLING MECHANISM AND PRELOAD

As heart muscle is stretched, it develops increased tension. The relationship of length to tension defines the *compliance* of heart muscle; the inverse of compliance is *stiffness*. If the ventricle is distended with blood, pressure is developed within the cavity. A higher pressure is needed to distend the ventricle to a given volume in a less compliant or stiffer ventricle. The pressure needed to stretch the ventricle to a given end-diastolic volume is called the *preload*, or left ventricular end-diastolic pressure (LVEDP). The relationship between the volume of the ventricle just prior to contraction and the force developed during contraction defines the *Frank-Starling law of the heart*. If the LVEDP is plotted against *stroke work*

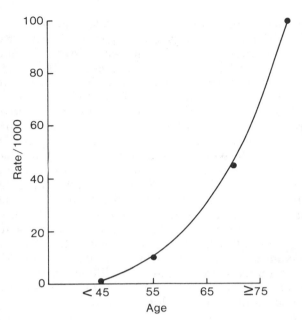

Figure 58.1 The prevalence of heart failure reported from physician's offices as a function of patient age. Note the marked increase in the 6th and 7th decades. Between 10% and 20% of patients older than age 60 followed regularly by a physician will have a history of heart failure. (From P. McKee *et al.: New England Journal of Medicine*, *285:* 1441, 1971 (12).)

(the stroke volume times the mean blood pressure), a *ventricular function curve* is defined (Fig. 58.2). It can be seen from this relationship that the normal ventricle is compliant and will develop an adequate amount of force during contraction with a relatively low preload. However, the failing ventricle requires a high preload in order to increase its stroke work (Fig. 58.2). The implications of this relationship are discussed below.

AFTERLOAD

Afterload is the dynamic resistance against which the heart contracts. It determines the degree of stress within the myocardium. Systolic blood pressure closely approximates and is clinically the most useful indicator of afterload. Afterload determines the ease or speed of ventricular contraction and hence the *ejection fraction* (that portion of the ventricular volume that is ejected with each beat) (Fig. 58.3).

CONTRACTILITY AND INOTROPIC STATE

The relationship of preload to stroke work defines the *functional state* of cardiac muscle (see above). The relative position of the curve defines the *inotropic state* of the muscle (see Fig. 58.2). For example, infusing the heart with an inotropic substance such as digitalis causes the ventricular function curve to shift to the left, to perform a higher stroke work at a given preload. In other words, the *contractility* of the heart is increased.

INTERRELATIONSHIP BETWEEN PRELOAD, AFTERLOAD, AND INOTROPIC STATE

The interrelationship between the preload, afterload, and inotropic state is summarized in Figure 58.3. If preload is kept constant, an increase in afterload will cause a depression in ventricular function. Thus, if afterload or blood pressure increases, ventricular function or ejection fraction decreases and the function of the ventricle may be restored to baseline by increasing the preload. A further increase in afterload leads to a further depression in ventricular function which again may be restored by increasing preload, or in clinical terms by increasing venous return or left ventricular end-diastolic pressure. Eventually, a limit is reached beyond which preload cannot be increased, as noted on the figure. This is the left ventricular filling pressure, the *preload reserve*, above which the pulmonary capillary oncotic pressure is exceeded, fluid passes into the aveoli, and pulmonary congestion occurs. Any increase in afterload which occurs when the preload reserve is reached will cause a decrease in ventricular function. The preload reserve varies with the compliance of the ventricle. If heart muscle is made stiffer or less compliant by a chronic disease process such as hypertension or aortic stenosis, or by an acute process such as ischemia, a higher filling pressure will be

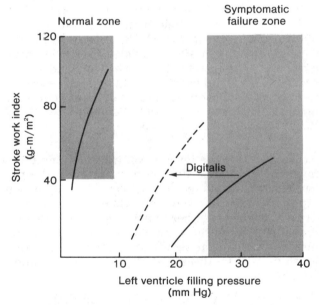

Figure 58.2 Ventricular function curves showing the relationship between left ventricular filling pressures and stroke work. The relative position of the curve defines the *inotropic state* of the heart. Note that for a given curve, *i.e.*, a given inotropic state, the *function* of the heart, or the amount of work the heart is capable of performing, varies with the left ventricular filling pressure. (Adapted from M. L. Weisfeldt: *The Principles and Practice of Medicine*, edited by A. M. Harvey *et al.*, Appleton-Century-Crofts, New York, 1980 (16).)

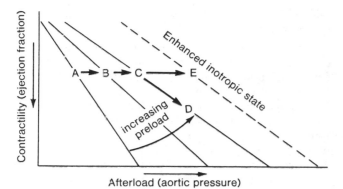

Figure 58.3 The interrelationship between preload, afterload, and inotropic state. The three *solid lines* are a family of curves at different levels of preload but with inotropic state kept constant. Taken together, they represent *ventricular function* as a function of both *preload* and *afterload*. Note that if preload is kept constant, an increase in afterload will cause a decrease in *contractility* as measured by the *ejection fraction*, but that when afterload is decreased to 0, the curves converge, because the *inotropic state* of the muscle is unchanged. As afterload increases, contractility may be maintained by increasing preload (shifting from *point A* to *B* to *C*). When preload reaches the point (*C*) at which an increase will cause pulmonary congestion, (the *preload reserve*) any further increase in afterload will decrease contractility (*point C* to *D*). Contractility may then be increased only by measures, such as digitalization, which enhance the inotropic state (*point D* to *E*). Patients are most sensitive to changes in afterload when their filling pressures are at the preload reserve. (Adapted from J Ross, Jr.: Afterload mismatch and preload reserve: a conceptual framework for the analysis of ventricular function. *Progress in Cardiovascular Disease, 18:* 255, 1976.)

necessary to set the level of ventricular function by means of the Frank-Starling principle; and the preload reserve will be reached sooner. The only way to improve ventricular function when the preload reserve is reached is either to decrease the afterload or to change the inotropic state, or contractility, of the muscle. The clinical significance of these interrelationships will be discussed at greater length under "Management."

BIOCHEMICAL BASIS FOR DECREASED CONTRACTILITY IN FAILING HEART

The contractile unit of heart muscle is the sarcomere, which consists of fibers of protein called *actin* and *myosin*. Actin and myosin interact with each other by interlocking protein cross bridges called *troponin*. The interlocking mechanism is facilitated by adenosine triphosphate (ATP) and magnesium. An inhibitory protein, *tropomyosin*, is present on the myosin fibers. Tropomyosin inhibits the interaction

between actin and myosin and allows the muscle to relax. Calcium inhibits the tropomyosin complex, frees the troponin cross bridges, and allows actin and myosin to interact and to develop tension. Calcium is therefore necessary for myocardial contraction to take place. Large amounts of calcium are stored within the heart in the capacious network of *sarcoplasmic reticulum* which is distinctive to heart muscle. *Excitation contraction coupling* takes place in heart muscle when an action potential, via mechanisms not yet understood, causes a release of calcium from the sarcoplasmic reticulum, thereby initiating contraction. In heart failure, there appears to be decreased energy available for cardiac contraction and slow transport of calcium into the sarcoplasmic reticulum following contraction, leading to a delay in relaxation of cardiac muscle. Clinically this is noted as an increase in resistance to filling or, in other words, a decrease in the *diastolic compliance* of the myocardium in heart failure.

Compensatory Mechanisms in Heart Failure
HEART RATE

If stroke volume remains constant, an increase in heart rate will cause a proportionate increase in cardiac output in patients in heart failure.

HYPERTROPHY AND DILATION

Left ventricular hypertrophy and dilation may allow compensation to be achieved for many years. The stress in the wall of the heart varies with the radius of the ventricular cavity. If the heart is subjected to a volume load, the heart dilates in order to accommodate the load and to increase its ability to eject the load (the Frank-Starling principle—see above). However, ventricular dilation causes an increase in ventricular wall stress which serves as a stimulus to ventricular hypertrophy. The hypertrophy is *eccentric*, so-called because it causes the left heart border to move laterally. Eventually the heart becomes both dilated and hypertrophied and the ratio of wall thickness to cavity size returns to normal, which returns wall stress to normal; therefore a state of compensated ventricular dilation is achieved. The response to a pressure overload is different. An increase in wall stress in the absence of volume overload leads to *concentric* hypertrophy; wall stress per unit area returns to normal but the cavity size is unchanged.

REDISTRIBUTION OF CARDIAC OUTPUT IN HEART FAILURE

There is a marked increase in peripheral vascular resistance and redistribution of cardiac output in heart failure. In less severe failure, where the resting cardiac output is normal, redistribution occurs only during exercise. In severe heart failure, where the resting cardiac output is significantly decreased, redistribution occurs at rest. The decrease in blood flow is most marked in the kidneys and the skin. Decreased renal blood flow causes a release of *renin* from the juxtaglomerular apparatus and therefore leads to an increase in plasma *angiotensin* activity. Angiotensin is a potent vasoconstrictor and acts both directly on smooth muscle and, indirectly, by increasing release of norepinephrine from vascular nerve endings. The increase in angiotensin activity leads to an increase in aldosterone production, which causes an increase in sodium reabsorption from the distal tubule of the nephron, thereby increasing plasma volume. The renal reabsorption of sodium is also facilitated by the decrease in cardiac output and in glomerular filtration rate, which causes an increase in the fraction of sodium reabsorbed in the proximal tubule of the nephron.

DIAGNOSTIC PROCESS

There is no one symptom, sign, or laboratory test which is pathognomonic of heart failure. Diagnosis must therefore be based on a process of clinical inference. The significance of symptoms and signs must be evaluated with regard to the patient's overall condition and to where the patient appears to be in the natural history of his disease. In ambulatory practice, a patient will often present to a new physician with the diagnosis of "heart failure" and will be taking medicine for this condition. In this situation, the physician should satisfy himself that the diagnosis of heart failure is correct before accepting it and maintaining treatment.

Diagnostic Classification of Heart Failure

ETIOLOGY OF HEART FAILURE

When the diagnosis of heart failure is made, it is essential to decide upon the most likely etiology, since the prognosis and the treatment of heart failure vary greatly depending upon its cause.

Heart failure is due to one of three basic mechanisms: an increased work load to which the heart cannot accommodate; a disorder of the myocardium so that it is unable to accommodate normal work loads; or a restriction of ventricular filling so that an adequate stroke volume cannot be achieved. Table 58.1 lists selected examples of these conditions. In this country systemic hypertension is the most common condition associated with heart failure (75% of cases), followed by ischemic heart disease, with or without hypertension (40% of cases) (7).

The most common precipitating causes of heart failure (Table 58.2) are noncompliance with medication or diet in a patient with previously compensated heart failure, acute myocardial infarction, and uncontrolled hypertension. In patients for whom the precipitating cause is not obvious, it is important to consider arrhythmia (Chapter 56) and pulmonary embolism (Chapter 50). In addition, it is important to

Table 58.1
Causes of Heart Failure[a]

INCREASED WORK LOAD TO WHICH HEART CANNOT ACCOMMODATE
  High output states:
    Hyperthyroidism[b]
    Anemia[a]
    Systemic arteriovenous fistulas[b]
    Certain dermatologic disorders (*e.g.*, psoriasis, erythroderma)
  Valvular regurgitation or left to right shunts[b]
  Increased impedance to ejection:
    Systemic hypertension[b]
    Pulmonary hypertension
    Pulmonic or aortic stenosis[b]
DISORDER OF MYOCARDIUM SO THAT IT IS UNABLE TO ACCOMMODATE NORMAL WORK LOADS
  Cardiomyopathies
  Myocardial infarction
RESTRICTION OF VENTRICULAR FILLING
  Pericardial constriction or effusion[b]
  Mitral and tricuspid valvular stenosis[b]
  Increased ventricular stiffness:
    Infiltrative myocardial disease (*e.g.*, amyloid)
    Ventricular hypertrophy
    Hypertrophic cardiomyopathy

[a] Adapted from M. L. Weisenfeldt (16).
[b] Indicates causes of heart failure which are potentially treatable by surgery or by specific therapy.

Table 58.2
Precipitating Causes of Heart Failure

FACTORS DECREASING MYOCARDIAL EFFICIENCY
  Myocardial infarction
  Ischemia
  Arrhythmia
  Hypoxia
  Alcohol and other toxic substances
  Recent initiation of a β-blocking drug
  Discontinuation of a cardiac glycoside
  Myocardial depressant drugs (*e.g.*, disopyramide, Adriamycin)
  Pericardial tamponade
  Myocardial infections (*e.g.*, bacterial endocarditis, myocarditis, parasitic infection)
  Vasculitis
FACTORS INCREASING CARDIAC LOAD
  Uncontrolled systemic hypertension
  Noncompliance with low salt diet
  Psychological stress
  Exercise, especially in extremes of heat or humidity
  Discontinuing diuretics, antihypertensive drugs, or afterload reducing agents
  Drugs which retain or contain sodium
  Infection
  Anemia
  Pulmonary embolism
  Thyrotoxicosis
  Acute valvular dysfunction

inquire about psychosocial stress, which has been shown to precede the onset of symptoms in as many as 50% of patients hospitalized for heart failure (14).

FUNCTIONAL CLASSIFICATION OF HEART FAILURE

The amount of exercise which a patient can perform without symptoms of heart failure determines his *functional class*. The functional classification scheme of the New York Heart Association is useful in categorizing patients (Table 58.3). Correctable disease may be present despite severe symptoms so that the functional classification provides useful prognostic information only within selected subsets of patients. Functional class is best determined by questioning the patient regarding his performance during daily activities. For example, a patient may be asked how many stairs he can climb before he has to stop and rest; or how heavy a load he can carry, and what work activities have had to be modified.

History

The most common symptom of heart failure is *dyspnea*. Dyspnea means uncomfortable breathing. It is not the shortness of breath experienced by normal people when they exercise or by anxious people when they hyperventilate (see also Chapter 50). Dyspnea in heart failure is a symptom of increased LVEDP leading to pulmonary venous and capillary congestion. The increase in pulmonary congestion causes an increased stiffness of the lungs and a decrease in the vital capacity. The work of breathing increases and breathing becomes rapid, shallow, and forced.

Orthopnea is dyspnea in the recumbent position. It is frequently experienced by patients with heart failure, although it may also be a symptom of patients with obstructive lung disease or with obesity. Blood normally pools in the lower extremities when a person is upright. When the patient who is in heart failure lies down, there is an increase in venous return to the heart which leads to an increase in pulmonary congestion because of the inability of the compromised left ventricle to accept and to pump the increased load. The severity of orthopnea is assessed by the number of pillows the patient must use to be able to breath comfortably.

Patients in heart failure with dyspnea and orthopnea often have a dry hacking *cough*; at times this is the patient's most troublesome symptom. The cough usually improves concomitantly with improvement in other symptoms.

Paroxysmal nocturnal dyspnea is characteristic of poorly compensated chronic heart failure. Patients commonly complain of paroxysmal dyspnea approximately 2 hours after falling asleep. It is often associated with bad dreams or nightmares and is relieved by sitting up or by getting out of bed and sitting in a chair. Because the dyspnea often is associated with wheezing, it must be distinguished from the nocturnal shortness of breath sometimes experienced by people with obstructive lung disease (see Chapter 52).

Fatigue is a common complaint of patients in heart failure. It is frequently described as a general sense of weakness or of lassitude. Some patients may complain of fatigue rather than dyspnea. In this setting fatigue is a symptom of low cardiac output, often due to overdiuresis following the aggressive use of potent diuretics.

A history of *edema* and or *weight gain* (from retention of salt and water) is often elicited from patients in heart failure. Many will also give a history of having taken digitalis in the past for a "heart problem."

Chest pain due to myocardial ischemia is common in patients in heart failure (see Chapter 54). Patients with preexisting poor left ventricular function may rapidly develop marked left ventricular dysfunction when their hearts become ischemic, or they may develop paroxysmal mitral regurgitation due to acute papillary muscle dysfunction. This may happen in association with exercise in patients with stable ischemic heart disease or may occur paroxysmally and at rest in patients with unstable ischemic heart disease or in patients who may be experiencing spasm of the coronary arteries (see Chapter 54). Paroxysmal dyspnea associated with exercise-induced ischemia is sometimes referred to as an "anginal equivalent." The symptomatic response to nitroglycerin does not by itself differentiate between dyspnea due to ischemia and dyspnea due to chronic congestive heart failure; sublingual nitroglycerin rapidly relieves congestion due to both conditions (see below).

Nocturia, a common symptom of heart failure, often occurs early in the illness. It is due to the redistribution in cardiac output that occurs in the recumbent position, restoring in part blood flow to the kidney which, in the upright position, has been diverted to other organs (see above).

Table 58.3
New York Heart Association (NYHA) Functional Classification of Cardiac Patients

Class I: No limitation. Ordinary physical activity does not cause undue fatigue, dyspnea, palpitation, or angina. Prognosis good

Class II: Slight limitation of physical activity. Such patients will be comfortable at rest. Ordinary physical activity will result in fatigue, palpitation, dyspnea, or angina. Prognosis good with therapy

Class III: Marked limitation of physical activity. Less than ordinary activity will lead to symptoms. Patients are comfortable at rest. Prognosis fair with therapy

Class IV: Inability to carry on any physical activity without discomfort. Symptoms of congestive failure or angina will be present even at rest. With any physical activity, increased discomfort is experienced. Prognosis guarded despite therapy

Decreased cardiac output by itself or in association with cerebrovascular disease may lead to *impairment in mental* function, ranging from mild confusion to overt psychosis. The most common neuropsychiatric complaints, however, are mild chronic anxiety and depression; these may be the presenting complaints, especially in elderly patients with previously undiagnosed heart failure.

Symptoms of congestion of the gastrointestinal system are common in patients with chronic, poorly compensated heart failure. Chronically increased right heart pressures cause passive congestion of the liver with swelling and discomfort in the right upper quadrant of the abdomen. In extreme cases there will be marked anorexia and weight loss due to gastrointestinal congestion. These symptoms are often compounded by the somewhat unpalatable low salt diet to which many of these patients must adhere.

Physical Findings in Heart Failure

The physical findings in heart failure depend upon which compensatory mechanisms are utilized to adjust the cardiac output to the metabolic needs of the body. Findings vary depending upon whether the heart failure is *compensated* or *uncompensated*.

UNCOMPENSATED HEART FAILURE

In chronic uncompensated or poorly compensated heart failure there will be signs of an attempt at cardiac compensation (increased heart size and heart rate) and signs of increased renin, angiotensin, and aldosterone activity (vascular redistribution and evidence of cardiac, pulmonary and peripheral congestion). Congestion is manifest by a ventricular gallop sound (S-3), rales, jugular venous distention, hepatojugular reflux, and by peripheral pitting edema.

Increased heart size may be recognized by inspection, palpation, and percussion of the precordium. The precordium should be palpated with the patient in the supine and in the left lateral position. The location, quality, and size of the point of maximal impulse (PMI) should be noted. The PMI of an eccentrically enlarged heart is displaced laterally and caudally and is heaving and diffuse. The PMI of a concentrically enlarged heart is not displaced but may be thrusting or sustained. The heart border should be percussed and its position relative to the PMI should be noted.

Sinus tachycardia, defined as a resting heart rate in an adult greater than 100 beats per minute, is a relatively sensitive but nonspecific sign of heart failure; it is a compensatory mechanism to increase cardiac output (see below). *Pulsus alternans*, a regular rhythm in which contractions are successively strong and weak, is most common in patients with increased resistance to left ventricular ejection (e.g., systemic hypertension) and is due to repetitive changes in stroke volume because of incomplete recovery of contractility by the failing heart.

The second pulmonic sound (P-2) is often accentuated in patients in left ventricular failure, because of increased pulmonary artery pressure. Paradoxic splitting of the second heart sound, an indication of prolonged left ventricular ejection time, may be heard in patients with chronic heart failure and is often associated with a left bundle branch block.

The *ventricular or S-3 gallop sound* is the most sensitive and specific sign of heart failure (8). The S-3 gallop sound is heard approximately 0.16 to 0.19 sec after the second heart sound (S-2) and is due to sudden restriction of filling in a relatively noncompliant left ventricle. It is usually heard directly over the PMI and may be audible only when the patient is in the left lateral position. The sound is low pitched and often may be sensed by the cadence of the heart's sounds rather than specifically heard. The cadence closely approximates the word "Kentucky," pronounced KYN-TUC'-KY. The middle syllable is accentuated to represent the loud second heart sound due to increased pulmonary artery pressure in patients in heart failure. The timing of the last syllable closely approximates the timing of the third heart sound when the word is repeated 100 times per minute.

Rales are high pitched sounds (similar to the sound of a clump of hair rubbed between the fingers) produced by the sudden filling with air of fluid-filled alveoli. They are a sign of moderately to severely decompensated left heart failure.

Neck vein distention and *hepatojugular reflux* are relatively insensitive but specific findings of heart failure. In chronic heart failure, right ventricular filling pressures will usually increase as the LVEDP increases. With time the right ventricle becomes increasingly more stiff and unable to accept a sudden volume load.

Neck vein distention is assessed while the patient is semirecumbent with the head turned slightly away from the examiner. Ideally the internal, rather than the external, jugular vein is inspected since the latter contains valves and may not reflect accurately the right heart pressure. Internal jugular venous distention is seen as a broad based filling in the anterior cervical triangle. However, since the external jugular venous system is often more easily identified, it may be used as an index of the pressure in the superior vena cava if the physician examines the neck properly. If the external jugular is compressed in the supraclavicular fossa, and the examining finger then strips the vein cephalad, blood will rise in the more proximal portion of the vein and the height of this volume of blood reflects the central venous pressure. The physician may choose an arbitrary reference point (such as 10 cm anterior to the posterior axillary line at the sternal angle—this approximates in many the level of the right atrium) and measure the column of blood above this point without regard for the angle of elevation of the thorax. The value of this observation is that accurate serial assessments are possible, permitting the physician to confirm worsening failure (increasing jugular venous pressure) or to recognize a too vigorous diuretic response (abnormally low jugular venous pressure).

Hepatojugular reflux is elicited by having the patient lie supine and semirecumbent at 45°. The patient is asked to breathe normally and is warned that the examiner will apply pressure over the right upper quadrant of the abdomen. Patients so warned will comply and will not hold their breath or perform a Valsalva maneuver which will make the sign impossible to elicit. The sudden increase in venous return causes right ventricular end-diastolic pressure and right atrial pressure to rise; and this will be seen as jugular venous distention.

Peripheral pitting edema is a relatively common, although not a specific, sign of heart failure. It occurs in the dependent portions of the body which in ambulatory patients means the feet and lower legs. Edema in heart failure is due to increased reabsorption of salt and water by the kidney. Because pitting edema in the lower extremities becomes detectable only when the leg volume increases by about 10%, an increase in weight may precede pitting edema as an early objective manifestation of decompensated heart failure in ambulatory patients.

Because of low cardiac output and vascular redistribution patients may have a slightly cyanotic cast to their skin and a drawn colorless look to their face. Their extremities may be cool and their nailbeds may be cyanotic.

COMPENSATED HEART FAILURE

In contrast to the findings in patients with acute or chronic uncompensated heart failure there may be few or no specific physical findings in compensated patients other than signs of increased heart size. A presystolic gallop or fourth heart sound (S-4) can be heard in most patients with longstanding high blood pressure or ischemic heart disease who are in normal sinus rhythm. The fourth heart sound is thought to be due to atrial contraction into a stiff ventricle. A soft systolic murmur, approximately grade 2, is commonly heard at the PMI in patients with chronic compensated heart failure. This murmur usually represents minor degrees of mitral insufficiency. The mitral regurgitation is not usually clinically significant but if the murmur is loud or if the patient complains of frequent episodes of paroxysmal dyspnea, a marked increase in mitral regurgitation during ischemia should be suspected and an attempt should be made to listen to the murmur while the patient is symptomatic.

Laboratory Diagnosis

CHEST X-RAY IN HEART FAILURE

The chest X-ray is the most useful diagnostic procedure for the evaluation of suspected heart failure

(8). The radiologic signs of heart failure are cardiac enlargement and pulmonary congestion.

There are a number of factors that influence heart size on the chest X-ray. These include body build, the depth of inspiration when the film is taken, and the chambers that are enlarged. Nevertheless, determination of the ratio of the transverse diameter of the heart to the greatest diameter of the chest, the *cardiothoracic ratio*, is a reliable and valid measurement of heart size and should be part of the data base of every patient who is thought to have or to have had heart failure. The normal cardiothoracic ratio is less than 0.5.

The pulmonary vasculature should be examined and signs of vascular redistribution caused by pulmonary venous hypertension and of enlarged hilar vessels caused by acute or chronic pulmonary hypertension should be noted.

Normally, the lower lobes of the lungs are better perfused than the upper lobes. The earliest radiologic sign of pulmonary congestion is reduction of blood flow to the lower lobes due to compression of vessels by extravascular fluid which has gravitated to the lung bases. In early heart failure, there is simply an equalization of the size of the vessels to the upper and lower lobes; but as congestion increases, the vessels to the upper lobes become more prominent, the so-called "cephalization" of flow. More severe failure is manifest by signs of interstitial edema and ultimately by alveolar edema and pleural effusion (Chapter 51).

ELECTROCARDIOGRAM

There are no ECG changes that are diagnostic of heart failure. The ECG may, however, reflect an underlying disease (e.g., left ventricular hypertrophy due to hypertension; Q waves or ST-T wave changes due to infarction) or the presence of an unstable rhythm (such as rapid atrial fibrillation) that has caused heart failure.

Patients with well compensated concentric or eccentric hypertrophy of the heart may show only relatively minor nonspecific ST-T wave changes. Grossly abnormal changes are seen in patients who have both dilation and hypertrophy of the left ventricle. The most common manifestations of left ventricular hypertrophy are increased voltage and ST-T wave changes. Although there are numerous ECG criteria for left ventricular hypertrophy (LVH), a clinically useful criterion is the index of Lewis: net positivity in lead 1 and net negativity in lead 3 = 1.7 mV or more (see also Table 57.3, Chapter 57). However, LVH should never be diagnosed on the basis of voltage changes alone; ST-T wave changes must be present in order to make the diagnosis.

Conduction abnormalities are common in patients in heart failure, especially left bundle branch block. Left bundle branch block may be an early sign of congestive cardiomyopathy, especially when it occurs in young patients. It is nearly always a sign of organic heart disease.

Left atrial enlargement is diagnosed by the presence of a negative P wave with an area of greater than 1 mm^2 in lead V_1. It commonly is seen in the ECG of patients with acute heart failure and disappears as the patient is treated.

Right ventricular hypertrophy is most reliably diagnosed in adults by a shift of the QRS axis towards the right greater than 90° (see also Table 57.6, Chapter 57). The QRS axis normally shifts toward the left with age.

Persistently upward coving of the ST segments in the precordial leads in the absence of left bundle branch block or significant intraventricular conduction delay is a reliable marker for the presence of a left ventricular aneurysm.

ECHOCARDIOGRAM

The echocardiogram, either one- or two-dimensional, is a reliable technique for determining ventricular size and thickness, the presence of valvular and other structural abnormalities, and the presence or absence of pericardial effusion. In one study, echocardiography supplied a specific diagnosis in 31% of patients who presented with cardiomegaly and/or heart failure of unclear etiology (11). The physician should consider echocardiography, therefore, for patients with suspected valvular or pericardial disease or for patients in whom the cause of heart failure is unclear. (The use of echocardiography in the diagnosis of valvular heart disease is discussed more fully in Chapter 57.)

Ejection fraction can be obtained by echocardiography by estimating end systolic and end diastolic volumes by measurement of the minor axis of the left ventricle; however, the technique is not reliable in patients with ischemic heart disease in whom there may be nonuniform contraction of the left ventricle.

RADIONUCLIDE ANGIOGRAPHY

Radionuclide angiography, sometimes called the "gated blood pool scan" is a technique for visualizing the cardiac chambers throughout the cardiac cycle. As most commonly performed, the patient's red blood cells are labeled *in vitro* with technetium-99m and are then injected intravenously. The intracardiac blood pool is scanned in multiple images with a scintillation camera which is synchronized (gated) with the ECG. A computer interfaces with the image from the scintillation camera, divides the cardiac cycle commonly into 16 equal segments, and displays on a television screen the images obtained sequentially in a continuous loop so that a moving image of the heart is seen. The technique is painless and exposes the patient to approximately the same amount of radiation as three plain films of the chest. The cost of radionuclide angiography is approximately 10 times that of an ECG.

The test, while expensive, has several advantages over any other method currently available for determining cardiac function. It is safe, essentially painless, and requires no special preparation of the patient. Studies have demonstrated excellent correlation of the images obtained with radionuclide angiography compared with ventricular contrast angiography (13).

Radionuclide angiography is an effective tool to differentiate between dyspnea due to cardiac and pulmonary causes, to evaluate left ventricular wall motion abnormalities including ventricular aneurysm, to evaluate left ventricular function reflected in the ejection fraction, to confirm the clinical diagnosis of cardiomyopathy, to evaluate left ventricular function after mitral valve replacement, and to detect hypertrophic cardiomyopathy and atrial myxoma. Radionuclide angiography is especially useful in establishing the prognosis of patients after myocardial infarction. Patients with an ejection fraction of less than 30% are particularly prone to increased morbidity and mortality (13).

The general physician will not ordinarily consider radionuclide angiography without the advice of a cardiologist. However, the technique may become more popular as an accurate way to complement the clinical assessment of the course of a patient with heart disease.

CARDIAC CATHETERIZATION

Cardiac catheterization (see Chapter 54) should be considered in any patient in chronic heart failure in whom an etiologic and anatomic diagnosis has not been made by noninvasive techniques. In a recent study in patients with chronic congestive heart failure in whom the etiology of the disease was not apparent, 28% were found to have coronary artery disease. Many of these patients had diabetes mellitus (2). Cardiac catheterization also may be the only way to diagnose occult valvular or pericardial disease or septal defects (see Chapter 57).

EXERCISE TESTING

It is often difficult to determine the functional status of patients claiming social security disability or workmen's compensation and functional limitation is frequently over- or underestimated. Recent studies have shown that the most precise determination of functional classification is given by exercise testing (5). The test should be obtained in consultation with a cardiologist and only if functional classification cannot be satisfactorily determined by clinical means.

MANAGEMENT

The goal of therapy is not merely to control symptoms but to treat specifically the underlying causes of heart failure if possible (see Table 58.1). If the underlying disease cannot be effectively treated, an attempt should be made to increase the capacity of the heart to do work and/or to decrease the amount of work that the heart has to do. Table 58.4 shows the various measures that can be utilized to accomplish these goals in ambulatory patients. These measures are discussed in detail below.

General Principles

LIFE-STYLE

It is not always possible to improve the function of the failing heart, but it usually is possible to decrease the metabolic needs of the body by encouraging a patient to stop smoking, to avoid emotionally stressful situations and people, and to get an adequate amount of rest. The physician must have a thorough understanding of the patient's work environment and the relationship of the patient to his spouse and family. The patient is more likely to change his life-style and priorities if the practitioner discusses the recommended therapy with both the patient and his family. The ambulatory patient should be encouraged to exercise, but to take care to avoid exertion to the point of causing further symptomatic cardiac decompensation. Sometimes this simply means performing the same activities more slowly.

There is a decreased stimulus to renin, angiotensin, and aldosterone production during supine rest, and even severely disabled patients may be able to lead socially useful and satisfying lives if they take a nap in the afternoon and in the early evening or before social or business engagements. Strict bedrest is rarely necessary.

It is important that the temperature and humidity of the patient's home and work environment be controlled as much as possible. Patients should be encouraged to have air conditioners for the summer months to reduce the extra demand placed on the heart by hot humid weather.

DIET

There is little evidence that a severely salt-restricted diet is of benefit in the long term in controlling heart failure in patients who respond well to moderate doses of diuretics. It is a common experience, however, that sudden increases in salt intake may precipitate acute heart failure in patients who have moderately well compensated but relatively severe heart failure. Holiday seasons are particularly dangerous in this regard, probably also because of the increased activity and emotional stress during these times. The physician must be aware of the various types of food which the patient is likely to eat. Most ethnic groups have certain foods which are prepared during festive occasions and many of these foods have a high salt content. Examples include "down-home cooking" among black people which is characterized by use of fatback or salt pork, and many foods prepared by traditional Jewish, Italian, or Polish cooks. Many patients attempt to substitute condiments in place of salt and are not aware that ketchup, hot sauce, etc., have high salt concentrations. A no-added-salt diet, which contains approximately 2 to 4 g of sodium, will suffice for most patients in compensated heart failure. Guidelines for planning this diet and a list of foods to be avoided by patients being treated for heart failure is given in Table 59.9 of Chapter 59.

Patients with heart failure may wish to know if they can continue to drink *alcoholic beverages.* In any patient with a cardiomyopathy apparently related to prolonged heavy alcohol use, total abstinence from alcohol may be essential to the management of heart failure. In other patients moderate alcohol use (e.g., wine with meals or a cocktail before dinner) is reasonable.

DRUGS WHICH PROMOTE POSITIVE SODIUM BALANCE

A number of drugs can promote a positive sodium balance: (a) renal sodium retention may be caused by corticosteroids, estrogens, and nonsteroidal anti-inflammatory agents other than aspirin and (b) some antacid preparations contain a significant amount of sodium (see Table 33.3, Chapter 33). Patients with heart failure should not receive these drugs, or, if the drugs are necessary, the patients should be monitored for and treated for increased symptoms of heart failure.

Drug Therapy (Table 58.5)

Heart failure is the result of mismatch between preload, afterload, and inotropic state; each of these factors may be adjusted by use of appropriate measures. Preload may be adjusted by the use of diuretic therapy, salt restriction, and venodilator therapy. Afterload may be adjusted by the control of hypertension and by the use of arteriolar dilating drugs. The inotropic state of the heart may be adjusted by the use of digitalis.

DIURETIC DRUGS

Diuretic drugs are used when it is not possible to treat the underlying cause of heart failure or when

Table 58.4
Measures Used in Ambulatory Treatment of Heart Failure

INCREASING CAPACITY OF HEART TO DO WORK
 Digitalis
 Antiarrhythmic drugs (Chapter 56)
 Pacemaker (Chapter 56)
DECREASING AMOUNT OF WORK THAT HEART HAS TO
  DO
 Rest
 Low sodium diet
 Diuretics
 Vasodilator drugs
 Home oxygen

Table 58.5
Characteristics of Selected Diuretic Drugs[a]

Generic Name	Brand Name	Preparation	Usual Daily Dose (mg)	Frequency of Dose per Day	Onset of Effect	Peak Effect	Duration
Chlorothiazide	Diuril	500-mg tablet	500–1000	1–2	1 hr	4 hr	6–12 hr
Hydrochlorothiazide	Generic, Hydro-Diuril, Esidrix	25/50/100-mg tablet	25–100	1–2	2 hr	4 hr	12 hr or more
Chlorthalidone	Generic, Hygroton	50/100-mg tablet	50–100	1	2 hr	6 hr	24 hr
Furosemide	Lasix	20/40/80-mg tablet	20–160	1–2	1 hr	1–2 hr	6 hr
Ethacrynic acid	Edecrin	50-mg tablet	50–100	1–2	30 min	2 hr	6–8 hr
Triamterene	Dyrenium	100-mg capsule	100–300	1–2	2 hr	6–8 hr	12–16 hr
Spironolactone	Aldactone	25-mg tablet	50–400	1–2	Gradual onset	2–3 days after initiation of therapy	2–3 days after cessation of therapy

[a] Modified from H. Frazier and H. Yager: *New England Journal of Medicine, 288:* 246, 455, 1973 (6).

signs and symptoms of heart failure persist despite treatment of the underlying condition. Diuretics reduce preload by increasing sodium and water excretion. However, if the contractility of the heart is depressed, reducing preload also reduces ventricular function (Fig. 58.2). Thus, diuretic drugs relieve symptoms of heart failure at a cost of reduced ventricular function. However, if the heart has dilated because of fluid overload, the decrease in ventricular wall stress and the improvement in ventricular contraction patterns brought about by a decrease in heart size following diuresis often lead to a prompt restoration of ventricular function.

There are three classes of diuretics in common use: thiazides, the so-called loop diuretics (ethacrynic acid and furosemide), and the potassium-sparing diuretics (spironolactone and triamterene) (Table 58.5) (see also Chapter 42).

The thiazides act on the distal convoluted tubule of the nephron; although their mechanism of action is unknown, they are thought to inhibit sodium transport and they cause a moderate increase in the excretion of sodium, chloride, and water. Potassium and hydrogen losses are accentuated because of the increased delivery of solute to the even more distal portion of the nephron where potassium secretion occurs and is modulated by aldosterone.

The loop diuretics inhibit tubular reabsorption of chloride and sodium in the thick ascending limb of the loop of Henle. These diuretics are potent and result in a substantial increase in the excretion of sodium, chloride, and water. Like thiazides, the loop diuretics increase the delivery of solute to the more distal portion of the nephron where potassium and hydrogen secretion is accentuated.

Potassium-sparing diuretics by themselves are only weak diuretics. However, they may be especially useful in combination with a thiazide or loop diuretic in preventing hypokalemia or when a patient becomes refractory to these more potent diuretics. The effect of thiazides and loop diuretics may be dampened by the reabsorption of sodium in the distal segment since they act proximal to the portion of the distal nephron where aldosterone influences sodium reabsorption. Spironolactone is structurally similar to aldosterone and competitively inhibits aldosterone binding to cellular receptors. Triamterene blocks sodium reabsorption and potassium excretion and does not compete with aldosterone or even depend on its presence to be effective. Both spironolactone and triamterene may cause life-threatening increases in the serum potassium level. Patients must not receive potassium supplementation while taking either of these drugs. Also, patients with renal failure are at increased risk for developing hyperkalemia if given these diuretics. In any patient serum potassium must be monitored carefully when these agents are used.

Use of Diuretic Drugs

Diuretic therapy should start with the lowest effective dose of a thiazide compound. Generic hydrochlorothiazide is the drug of choice. It is inexpensive, effective, and the tablet is small and easy to swallow. Many patients with mild heart failure may effectively control symptoms by use of the drug every other day or three times a week. Patients with progressive disease may become gradually resistant to the effect of thiazides and may require doses of 100 mg of hydrochlorothiazide a day for control of edema and dyspnea. Patients become resistant to thiazides when there is significant renal failure (such as when the serum creatinine is >2 to 4 mg/dl) or when renal blood flow is decreased markedly, as it may be in severe heart failure. There is no evidence that if one thiazide has failed, another will be effective.

When a patient becomes resistant to thiazide or has complications of thiazide therapy (see below), the loop diuretics—furosemide or ethacrynic acid—

should be prescribed. These drugs are often effective in relatively low doses. Furosemide is the more popular of the two drugs because gastrointestinal side effects are more common with ethacrynic acid, especially in higher doses. Furosemide should be started at a dose of 20 mg daily and increased as necessary for control of symptoms. A single dose should be administered each day, usually in the morning, although patients in severe failure may sleep better at night if the dose is given in the late afternoon.

Doses of furosemide as high as 1000 mg a day may be necessary in patients with severe heart failure associated with severe renal failure. At the point when more than 120 to 160 mg a day are required, however, the physician should reconsider whether or not the etiology of heart failure has been accurately determined and whether correctable causes of heart failure have been dealt with. If so, it is at this point (if not previously prescribed for potassium control) that a potassium-sparing diuretic—spironolactone or triamterene—should be added to the drug regimen. Triamterene is probably the drug of choice since it has a more rapid onset of action and may be less expensive than spironolactone when more than three tablets per day of spironolactone are required. Since these medications will ordinarily be used in patients who have received potassium supplementation, and who may have renal failure, the patient's electrolytes must be carefully monitored when these medications are started or when the dose is adjusted. Potassium supplementation should be stopped when the drugs are prescribed, and serum potassium again measured 1 week later. The usual dose of triamterene is 100 mg, 1 to 3 times a day; and of spironolactone, 25 to 100 mg, once or twice daily.

Side Effects of Diuretics

Hypokalemia (see Chapter 42). The thiazide and loop diuretics have marked kaliuretic effects and, especially in edematous patients (Chapter 42), hypokalemia is a common complication of the use of diuretic therapy. Hypokalemia may lead to fatigue and depression and frequently precipitates digitalis toxicity. The indication for and use of potassium salts in patients taking diuretics is fully discussed in Chapter 42.

Contraction of the Extracellular Volume. Diuretics are therapeutically effective by causing a net loss of sodium, chloride, and water. If the response is excessive, depletion of the extracellular fluid compartment (the maintenance of which depends on sodium and chloride) will occur. This may have catastrophic consequences such as hypotension (or postural hypotension) with precipitation of ischemia due to changes in cerebral, coronary, or renal blood flow. This complication is especially common when loop diuretics are used, but may occur following the use of thiazides or of combination diuretics. The physician should monitor carefully the patient, therefore, for evidence of excessive contraction of extracellular volume by assessment of his weight, the presence or absence of edema, the degree of fullness of the neck veins, and by assessment of the blood pressure and pulse. Not infrequently a dose of a diuretic which initiated diuresis will need to be reduced once cardiac compensation has improved.

Acid-Base Disturbance. By their different actions on the nephron, diuretics have an effect on acid-base balance. The thiazides and the loop diuretics are often associated with the generation and maintenance of a metabolic alkalosis. This usually requires no therapy. To correct the alkalosis, the associated volume and potassium deficiency would have to be corrected. If the volume were replenished, the effect of the diuretic would be negated. Therefore usually only potassium chloride supplements are given (see Chapter 42). If the alkalosis is thought to be detrimental, for example in patients with respiratory failure then either the diuretic should be discontinued or acetazolamide (Diamox) should be added to the regimen to diminish hydrogen ion excretion. The addition of acetazolamide will increase potassium excretion even more, so that special attention should be paid to potassium supplementation. The infrequency and complexity of this situation are such that a telephone consultation with a nephrologist before initiation of therapy with acetazolamide is appropriate.

Potassium-sparing diuretics may be associated with diminished hydrogen ion excretion and therefore with a mild metabolic acidosis. This is usually of no consequence and requires no treatment. If there is a question of treatment because of the severity of the acidosis, consultation with a nephrologist should be obtained.

Hyponatremia. The loop diuretics and the thiazides may be occasionally associated with hyponatremia by impairing free water clearance and therefore caution is especially appropriate in patients who tend to consume relatively large quantities of fluid. These diuretics also may be associated with hyponatremia where the extracellular volume has become contracted (a potent stimulus to the release of antidiuretic hormone) when fluid intake has not been restricted. In both of these instances, water restriction is mandatory. Usually this hyponatremia may be corrected by water restriction of less than 1 liter/day, but occasionally more severe restriction is necessary. Finally, the thiazides may be rarely associated with hyponatremia in euvolemic patients who also are severely potassium-depleted. This situation resembles clinically the syndrome of inappropriate secretion of antidiuretic hormone, although the exact mechanism of this complication is not fully known. The drug must be withdrawn should this complication develop.

Hyperuricemia. Thiazides, loop diuretics, and triamterene commonly elevate the concentration of serum urate by blocking urate secretion by the proximal renal tubules and/or by enhancing reabsorption through contraction of extracellular volume. Symptomatic gout, however, is not usual nor is the elevation of uric acid likely to cause renal injury or stone formation. Therefore, treatment, unless gout does occur, is not necessary.

Hyperglycemia. Thiazides and, less commonly, loop diuretics may cause glucose intolerance. Hypoglycemic therapy may be required (or changed, in diabetics already receiving a hypoglycemic agent) if the diuretic is to be continued (see Chapter 69).

Ototoxicity. Loop diuretics may impair hearing, usually reversibly, especially if large doses are taken or if the patient has renal insufficiency.

Other Effects. Thiazides are occasionally associated with a hypersensitivity-induced small vessel vasculitis (Chapter 47), with thrombocytopenia (Chapter 47), and with hypercalcemia (Chapter 71). Furosemide in high doses has been associated with the development of interstitial nephritis and renal failure, especially in patients with marked proteinuria. Spironolactone, a weak androgen antagonist, commonly causes gynecomastia and may reduce libido or even cause impotence; these side effects resolve within a few months of discontinuing the drug.

When diuretics have not adequately controlled the signs and symptoms of congestive heart failure, the physician should consider additional medication.

DIGITALIS

Inotropic drugs may help restore cardiac compensation by increasing the inotropic state, or contractility of cardiac muscle, thereby increasing the ejection fraction at a given preload and afterload, as described above (see p. 545). The only inotropic drugs currently available for oral use are the digitalis glycosides.

The digitalis drugs appear to improve contractility by increasing the delivery of calcium to the contractile apparatus of the heart. Digitalis inhibits sodium-potassium ATPase and it is postulated that this results in increase of influx of both calcium and sodium into the myocardial cell.

Indications for the Use of Digitalis Drugs. Despite more than 200 years of clinical experience with digitalis preparations, the indications for digitalis therapy remain controversial and there are conflicting reports regarding the utility of digitalis preparations in acute and chronic heart failure. Digitalis preparations may improve ventricular performance by moderating the heart rate of patients in atrial fibrillation or atrial flutter and by increasing ventricular contractility in some patients who are in heart failure. However, the degree to which digitalis preparations increase ventricular contractility is modest; the toxic : therapeutic ratio is small, and the drug must be pushed to near toxic limits in many cases before significant clinical effect is seen. Furthermore, the indiscriminate use of digitalis as a first-line medication for control of heart failure has led to its use in many patients in whom

heart failure is not due primarily to a decrease in the inotropic state of myocardial muscle. These include patients whose heart failure is due to valvular heart disease or to systemic hypertension, patients in whom heart failure is due to restrictions to ventricular filling (e.g., hypertrophic cardiomyopathy or pericardial tamponade), and patients in whom symptoms of fatigue are due to a decreased cardiac output induced by excessive diuresis.

Recommendations for Use of Digitalis Compounds.
1. Digitalis glycosides should be prescribed only for patients in congestive heart failure with dilated hearts (a cardiothoracic ratio > 0.5 suggests dilation; echocardiography however is the most precise way of demonstrating cardiac chamber size and thickness) and in whom the symptoms of heart failure appear to be due to a decreased inotropic state of heart muscle. It is also a useful drug for certain types of arrhythmias (see Chapter 56).

2. The practitioner should become familiar with the purified glycoside, digoxin, and should use it exclusively. It is well absorbed, can be used parenterally if necessary, and has an intermediate duration of action (half-life of 36 to 48 hours). The Burroughs Wellcome preparation of digoxin, Lanoxin, is the preferred digoxin preparation, because of variable absorption of many other brands.

3. The effect of digitalis on the patient's condition should be monitored and reassessed periodically. If there is no objective decrease in heart size within 1 or 2 months or increase in exercise capacity after a trial of digitalis therapy, the drug should probably be discontinued. Digitalis should be used cautiously in older patients and in any patient known to have impaired renal function. There is no evidence that elderly patients are intrinsically more sensitive to digitalis compounds, but they have a smaller body mass, often have impaired renal excretion of the drug, and have higher serum levels for a given oral dose of the drug.

4. The average dose of digoxin is 0.25 mg per day. In patients older than 65 years or in patients with known impairments of renal function, doses of 0.125 mg per day should be prescribed. Digitalization is best accomplished in the ambulatory patient by daily administration of the drug at the maintenance dosage. Within four or five half-lives of the drug (approximately 7 days) full digitalization is ordinarily achieved.

5. Digitalis may interact with other medications. It has recently been shown that the administration of quinidine causes a decrease in excretion of digoxin which may lead to digitalis toxicity (10). The use of thiazide and especially the loop diuretics may cause a decrease in renal blood flow and hypokalemia and therefore lead to digitalis toxicity. Cholestyramine and neomycin and some antacids impair digoxin absorption and may result in a subtherapeutic effect.

Recognition and Treatment of Digitalis Toxicity. Digitalis toxicity commonly is caused by administration of too much digitalis or by overdiuresis (often with associated hypokalemia), by intercurrent development of renal insufficiency, or by administration of drugs which interfere with digitalis excretion. Digitalis toxicity is especially common in older patients in an ambulatory practice. Approximately 10% of patients in the seventh and eighth decade being seen regularly by a physician will be taking digitalis (9).

The manifestations of digitalis toxicity are protean and may be difficult to recognize in older patients and in patients whose normal baseline level of function is not familiar to the practitioner. They include changes in the cardiovascular system, the gastrointestinal tract, and the central nervous system. The most frequent cardiac manifestations of digitalis toxicity are progressive slowing and regularization of the heart rate (i.e., development of a nodal rhythm) of patients in atrial fibrillation, and frequent premature ventricular contractions (PVC). Digitalis toxicity should be suspected in any older patient who is taking digitalis and has PVCs or any patient in atrial fibrillation whose heart rate falls below approximately 60 and becomes regular. Since digitalis both increases automaticity and decreases conduction through the AV node, paroxysmal atrial tachycardia (PAT) with block may be seen. The peripheral pulse in PAT with block is usually 100 to 120 beats per min (see Chapter 56). Cardiac toxicity may occur in the absence of other signs or symptoms of digitalis overdose.

Gastrointestinal side effects are common manifestations of digitoxicity. They include anorexia, mild nausea, and occasionally vomiting and diarrhea.

Digitalis may cause changes in the sensorium ranging from mild confusional states to frank delirium and psychosis. In an older patient it may be difficult to determine, without stopping the drug, whether these symptoms are due to primary cerebral disease or to digitalis excess.

The diagnosis of digitalis toxicity is based on clinical and laboratory findings. If symptoms compatible with digitalis toxicity are present, especially in an elderly patient who is also taking a diuretic, the drug should be stopped immediately. The patient should be examined in approximately 3 days and the symptoms should be reassessed. If symptoms have abated, a presumptive diagnosis of digitoxicity is warranted.

At the time of presentation, it is reasonable to measure the serum digoxin concentration. That is done in many commercial and hospital laboratories by use of a radioimmunoassay. It is important that the quality control of the laboratory be known, to ensure reliability of the procedure. On the average, a digitalized nontoxic patient will have a serum digoxin concentration of approximately 1.4 ng/ml; most toxic patients have concentrations 1.5 to 3 times this value. However, if a patient has symptoms compatible with digitalis toxicity and his serum digoxin level is within the normal range, toxicity has not been ruled out

since at therapeutic levels, hypokalemic (or hypercalcemic) patients may become digitoxic. Most patients with digitoxicity can be managed by temporary withdrawal of the medication and by reinstitution of it at a lower dose. Often, diuretic therapy must also be modified and/or potassium supplements administered. However, patients with symptomatic arrhythmias are best hospitalized for a few days so that they can be monitored closely.

Any patient who has become digitalis-toxic should have the indications for digitalis therapy carefully reviewed. In many cases the drug may be stopped without any apparent change in the patient's condition.

VASODILATOR THERAPY

A major advance in the treatment of heart failure in the past 10 years has been the introduction into clinical practice of vasodilator therapy. In ambulatory practice, these drugs should be considered for patients whose heart failure cannot be controlled by diuretics and digitalis. Three classes of vasodilators are available: drugs that act primarily on the venous system to reduce preload, drugs that act primarily on arterioles and thereby reduce afterload, and drugs that act as both veno- and arteriodilators (see Table 58.6).

Venodilators. Nitroglycerin in various dosage preparations is an effective venodilator. The hemodynamic effect of venodilators and diuretics is essentially the same. Both classes of drugs cause a decrease in preload, thereby relieving symptoms of vascular congestion (see Fig. 58.2). However, venodilators do so without inducing excessive potassium or fluid losses and a properly informed patient may use these drugs skillfully to reduce or eliminate disabling symptoms of pulmonary vascular congestion. Venodilators are most useful in patients with severe heart failure in whom the preload reserve is exceeded during exercise, resulting in excessive increases in LVEDP and resultant pulmonary vascular congestion. This may occur in association with ischemia in patients with ischemic heart disease or in association with advanced disease in patients with cardiomyopathy or end stage mitral or aortic regurgitation. These drugs are specifically contraindicated in patients whose failure is due to restrictions to ventricular filling such as hypertrophic cardiomyopathy or per-

Table 58.6
Vasodilators Useful in Treating Heart Failure

Principal Mechanism	Drugs
Venodilation	Nitroglycerine preparations
Arteriolar dilation	Hydralazine
Both mechanisms	Prazosin Hydralazine plus long acting nitrate

icardial tamponade and should be used with great caution in patients with aortic stenosis in whom a reduction in high preload levels may lead to a marked decrease in cardiac output.

The practitioner should be familiar with the use of nitrates in three forms (see also Chapter 54): a short acting sublingual nitrate, long acting nitrates taken orally, and nitroglycerin in a petrolatum base (Nitrol Paste). Sublingual nitroglycerin is generally used in a dose of 0.4 mg. The medication is sensitive to body heat, light, and moisture and must be kept in a carefully sealed brown glass container. Patients should be encouraged to purchase new sublingual nitroglycerin every 6 months to be sure that the medication is active. Sublingual nitroglycerin may be used liberally to control symptoms of pulmonary congestion during normal physical activity such as walking up stairs, shopping, and so forth. The use of oral forms of long acting nitroglycerin has been controversial because of reports of variable blood levels resulting from hepatic metabolism of nitrates in the portal circulation. However, it has recently been shown that high doses of oral nitrates will overwhelm the hepatic enzyme systems and that high and sustained blood levels of nitrates will be obtained (1). An effective medication is isosorbide dinitrate (generic, Isordil, Sokate) in doses of at least 20 mg orally, 4 times a day. If symptoms have not improved within a few days, the dosage should be increased. Doses as high as 40 to 60 mg orally, 4 times per day, may be used safely depending upon the patient's blood pressure response. Before and after each increase in the dose, the patient should be checked for orthostasis. If there is a drop of more than 10 to 15 mm systolic blood pressure, the dosage should be decreased slightly. Nitroglycerin, 2% in a petrolatum base, gives effective long acting venodilation but is messy and may be difficult for some patients to apply. It is best used under an occlusive polyethylene wrapping. The usual dose is 1 to 3 or 4 inches, 4 times daily. Again, titration of the dose depends on whether or not heart failure is improved and on whether orthostasis develops.

The most common side effects of nitrate therapy are headache, nausea, and skin irritation from the use of nitrol paste. Headaches can usually be controlled by aspirin and usually abate after 1 to 2 weeks of nitrate therapy. Gastrointestinal side effects can occasionally be eliminated by switching to a different preparation of long acting nitroglycerin or switching to nitroglycerin paste. Orthostatic hypotension requires a reduction in the dose or discontinuation of the drug.

Arteriolar Vasodilators. These drugs increase cardiac output by decreasing afterload, thereby decreasing the ventricular wall stress during contraction and allowing myocardial fibers to shorten more efficiently. The important influence of afterload on cardiac output has been discussed on page 545. A major component of afterload is peripheral vascular resistance. In recent years it has become recognized that the syndrome of heart failure is not due entirely to defects in left ventricular contraction. Activation of the renin-angiotensin-aldosterone system causes an inappropriate peripheral vasoconstriction and thereby a marked increase in afterload. The effects of arteriolar vasodilators may be seen by referring to Figure 58.3 in which the ejection fraction is plotted against the outflow resistance or afterload. These medications are most effective in patients with severe peripheral and pulmonary congestion, with decreased cardiac output often associated with decreased blood pressure, and with signs of peripheral hypoperfusion such as cool hands and peripheral cyanosis.

The most frequently used arteriolar vasodilator currently is hydralazine, but other medications also have been used in patients with heart failure (3). In properly selected patients and when used in effective doses, hydralazine may increase the cardiac output by as much as twofold. Careful studies performed on small numbers of patients weeks to months after initiation of hydralazine therapy have shown that this improved cardiac output may persist chronically in patients who respond initially (3).

Hydralazine for afterload reduction must be used cautiously in ambulatory patients. Doses of hydralazine less than 200 mg per day are rarely effective. If the patient's preload is not near maximum, hydralazine may cause a marked fall in blood pressure. In an ambulatory setting it is safest to start hydralazine in a dose of 10 mg and to observe the patient in the office for approximately 2 hours for signs of orthostasis. The patient can then be given a dose of 25 mg every 6 hours and observed the following day. If orthostatic hypotension or tachycardia is not observed, then the dose is increased to 50 mg every 6 hours. At an effective dose the patient's handshake, previously cool, becomes warm and firm; and the patient experiences a general sense of increased well-being and of decreased fatigue. The increased cardiac output may lead to an increase in renal blood flow, and diuretics often become more effective. If signs of peripheral vasodilation are not achieved, the dose of hydralazine should be increased to as high as 100 mg, 4 times a day. The major complication of hydralazine is a lupus-like syndrome. However, this syndrome usually does not become apparent until 18 to 24 months of treatment with hydralazine in doses above 200 mg per day. Because of the severity of their heart disease, most patients who require such large doses of hydralazine for afterload treatment of congestive heart failure will not live long enough to develop a lupus-like syndrome. Additional information about the properties of hydralazine and other vasodilators is provided in Chapter 59.

Mixed Veno- and Arteriodilators. In severe heart failure it is desirable to achieve both venous and arteriolar dilation simultaneously. Currently, this is best done by use of hydralazine and a long acting nitrate such as isosorbide dinitrate. *Prazosin* (Minipress), an oral antihypertensive drug, has both veno- and arteriodilatory actions and may therefore be useful as a single agent, but long term experience with the drug is not as extensive as it is with the hydralazine-long acting nitrate combination. The usual dose of prazosin is 2 to 5 mg every 6 hours, although some patients may require larger doses for effective afterload reduction. The effect of prazosin is often not noted at rest and some patients may develop tachyphylaxis to the drug. Additional information about prazosin is found in Chapter 59.

Captopril (4) blocks the action of angiotensin and causes a prompt sustained vasodilation in patients in severe heart failure. In addition, it blocks the production of aldosterone and thereby interferes with sodium reabsorption that commonly occurs in these patients. It may be an effective drug for patients with severe heart failure. The usual starting dose is 12.5 mg, 3 times a day, but doses as high as 100 mg, 3 times a day, may be necessary. Common side effects include skin rash and proteinuria. (See also Chapter 59.)

β-BLOCKER THERAPY

β-Blockade may be useful in the treatment of heart failure due to the following conditions: thyrotoxicosis, severe hypertension responsive to betablockade therapy, hypertrophic cardiomyopathy, and in patients with failure due to recurrent ischemia. The combination of betablockade therapy with nitrate therapy may be effective in patients with ischemic cardiomyopathy and chest pain. In all cases, β-blockade therapy is given until the resting heart rate falls below 70 beats per min and does not show a significant increase with mild to moderate exercise. This usually requires doses of propranolol of 160 mg daily in divided doses. Lower doses may be effective in patients with depressed hepatic blood flow or function due to congestive heart failure. *β-Blockade therapy should not be used in patients with uncompensated or poorly compensated heart failure.* It should be used with caution if at all in patients with bronchospasm. Metoprolol (Lopressor), a relatively selective betablocker, may be useful in patients with bronchospasm.

IMPORTANCE OF CONTROL OF HYPERTENSION IN PATIENTS IN HEART FAILURE

Hypertension increases ventricular wall stress, and therefore the afterload on the heart, and reduces the cardiac output, especially as the heart begins to fail. It is essential, therefore, that hypertension be controlled in patients in heart failure. This subject is discussed in detail in Chapter 59.

HOME OXYGEN THERAPY

Patients with severe end stage heart failure and marked arterial oxygen desaturation at rest due to low cardiac output or to concomitant pulmonary disease may often feel more comfortable with the use of home oxygen. Patients who require home oxygen therapy because of congestive heart failure rarely survive for more than 6 months to a year. The most efficient way to administer oxygen therapy at home is by means of tanks delivered to the house. This form of therapy is paid for in part, by Medicare, Medicaid, and by most private insurance plans. The physician should obtain an arterial blood gas determination to confirm the hypoxia before oxygen is prescribed.

ANTICOAGULATION THERAPY

Patients in severe chronic congestive heart failure are at great risk for pulmonary and peripheral emboli. The incidence of peripheral arterial embolization in these patients may be as high as 10% per year. A patient with a markedly dilated left ventricular cavity or a patient with a left ventricular aneurysm especially if in atrial fibrillation, should be considered for treatment with coumarin anticoagulants (see Chapter 48). Coumadin therapy may be hazardous in patients in severe heart failure who have wide swings in prothrombin time due to liver dysfunction.

Electrophysiologic Control of Heart Failure

Patients with persistent bradycardia due to sick sinus syndrome or complete heart block and patients with persistent tachyarrhythmias may develop heart failure. The treatment of these problems is discussed in Chapter 56.

Operative Correction of Mechanical Problems Causing Heart Failure

Any patient who is in heart failure because of a mechanical derangement of myocardial function should be considered for operative correction and consultation with a cardiologist should be obtained. The most commonly encountered correctable problems in patients with chronic congestive failure include valvular heart disease and atrial septal defect (Chapter 57) and ventricular aneurysm.

The possibility of a ventricular aneurysm should be considered in any patient with known ischemic heart disease and heart failure. Patients with known ventricular aneurysm who are uncomfortable performing their usual daily tasks should be referred for cardiologic consultation and consideration of aneurysmectomy. As noted above, radionuclide angiography and two-dimensional echocardiography are the best methods currently available for the noninvasive detection of ventricular aneurysms.

Coronary Artery Bypass Graft Surgery and Congestive Heart Failure

Patients with chronic congestive heart failure and angina pectoris (Chapter 54) should be sent for cardiologic consultation. Some of these patients will benefit by coronary artery bypass graft surgery, an aneurysmectomy, or an infarctectomy.

Community Health Services

Many community health services are available to help the physician deal with the patient and the patient deal with his illness.

HOME VISITS

In two situations, home visits by the patient's physician or by a visiting nurse should be considered in the management of a patient in heart failure: (a) when the patient has repeatedly returned to the office with heart failure due to dietary neglect or to failure to use his medications correctly and (b) when the home-bound patient's symptoms are so severe (NYHA class IV, Table 58.3) that he is unable to make an office visit without becoming exhausted.

INFORMATION BOOKLETS

The American Heart Association has useful booklets explaining low salt diets and other booklets explaining the management of congestive heart failure to the patient and his family.

Exercise Programs (Chapter 55)

Graduated regular exercise may benefit some patients with mild chronic heart failure and may be psychologically beneficial. However, there is no evidence that myocardial function can be improved by exercise. Isometric exercise is contraindicated in any patient in heart failure because of the extra work this demands of the heart. Exercise may be contraindicated entirely in left heart failure due to valvular heart disease and in most patients with functional Class III or Class IV congestive heart failure.

PROGNOSIS

The prognosis in heart failure is related to the etiology of the heart failure, the functional status of the patient, the initial response to treatment, the compliance of the patient, and the patient's age. Most patients in chronic congestive heart failure die suddenly, presumably from ventricular arrhythmia or from complications of cerebral and peripheral emboli.

In the Framingham Study, which included heart failure from all causes, the probability of dying within 5 years of onset of heart failure was 62% for men and 42% for women. The etiology of heart failure in most of these patients was hypertension and ischemic heart disease. The mortality from ischemic heart disease complicated by congestive heart failure is related to ventricular function; patients with an ejection fraction of less than 30% have a particularly poor prognosis and may have a mortality rate of 10 to 20% per year (15). Patients with heart failure due to regurgitant valvular lesions have a mortality in the same range. Heart failure complicating uncorrected aortic stenosis is a particularly ominous sign and the majority of these patients die also within 3 years (Chapter 57).

In general, prognosis is related to the age of the patient and to his functional class (p. 548), although there are few studies available in which functional class was accurately determined and prognosis was calculated on a stratified sample. Patients who are functional class II have an annual mortality of approximately 8%. Patients who are functional class III have a slightly higher annual mortality. Patients who are functional class IV rarely live longer than 18 months to 2 years. It is important that the practitioner not venture a prognosis to the patient and family until an optimal level of response to therapy has been achieved.

The mortality from congestive heart failure does not seem to have decreased in the last several years with newer forms of therapy although these enable patients with chronic heart failure to be more comfortable in their final years of life.

References

General

Braunwald, E (Ed.) Heart Disease. A Textbook of Cardiovascular Medicine. W. B. Saunders, Philadelphia, 1980.
    The current standard text. Exhaustively referenced.
Cohn, J and Franciosa, J: Vasodilator therapy of cardiac failure. N Engl J Med 297: 27, 254, 1977.
    Excellent review of newer concepts of therapy of heart failure.
Franciosa, J: Hypertensive left heart failure: pathogenesis and therapy. Hosp Pract 77, (Feb) 1981.
    Excellent account of the pathogenesis and treatment of the most frequently encountered form of heart failure.
Perloff, J, Lindgren, K, and Groves, B: Uncommon or commonly unrecognized causes of heart failure. Prog Cardiovasc Dis 12: 409, 1970.
    Exhaustive but readable review of commonly unrecognized causes of heart failure.

Specific

1. Abrams, J: Nitroglycerin and long-acting nitrates. N Engl J Med 302: 1234, 1979.
2. Boucher, C, Fallon, J, Johnson, R and Yurchak, P: Cardiomyopathic syndrome caused by coronary artery disease; III. Prospective clinicopathological study of its prevalence among patients with clinically unexplained chronic heart failure. Br Heart J 41: 613, 1979.
3. Cohn, J: Progress in vasodilator therapy for heart failure. N Engl J Med 302: 1414, 1980.
4. Davis, R, Ribner, H, Keung, E, Sonnenblick, E and LeJemtel, T: Treatment of chronic congestive heart failure with captopril, an oral inhibitor of angiotensin-converting enzyme. N Engl J Med 301: 117, 1979.
5. Franciosa, J: Functional capacity of patients with chronic left ventricular failure. Am J Med 67: 460, 1979.
6. Frazier, H and Yager, H: The clinical use of diuretics. N Engl J Med 288: 246, 455, 1973.
7. Gibson, T, White, K and Klainer, L: The prevalence of congestive heart failure in two rural communities. J Chron Dis 19: 141, 1966.
8. Harlan, W, Oberman, A, Grimm, R and Rosati, R: Chronic congestive heart failure in coronary artery disease: clinical criteria. Ann Intern Med 86: 133, 1977.
9. Klainer, L, Gibson, T and White, K: The epidemiology of cardiac failure. J Chron Dis 18: 797, 1965.
10. Leahey, E, Reiffel, J, Giardina, E and Bigger, T: The effect of quinidine and other oral antiarrhythmic drugs on serum digoxin. Ann Intern Med 92: 605, 1980.
11. Markiewica, W, Peled, B, Hammerman, H, Greif, Z, Hir, J and

Riss, E: Contribution of m-mode echocardiography to cardiac diagnosis. *Am J Med 65:* 802, 1978.

12. McKee, P, Castelli, W, McNamara, P and Kannel, W: The natural history of congestive heart failure: the Framingham study. *N Engl J Med 285:* 1441, 1971.

13. Nichols, A, McKusick, K, Strauss, H, Dinsmore, R, Block, P and Pohost, G: Clinical utility of gated cardiac blood pool imaging in congestive left heart failure. *Am J Med 65:* 785, 1978.

14. Perlman, L, Ferguson, S, Bergum, K, Isenberg, E and Hammarsten, J: Precipitation of congestive heart failure: Social and emotional factors. *Ann Intern Med 75:* 1, 1971.

15. Schulze, RA, Jr, Strauss, HW and Pitt, B: Sudden death in the year following myocardial infarction: relation to ventricular premature contractions in the late hospital phase and left ventricular ejection fraction. *Am J Med 62:* 192, 1977.

16. Weisfeldt, ML: Congestive heart failure: pathophysiology and the evaluation of ventricular function. In: *The Principles and Practice of Medicine,* edited by AM Harvey, RJ Johns, VA McKusick, AH Owens and RS Ross. Appelton-Century-Crofts, New York, 1980.

CHAPTER FIFTY-NINE

Hypertension

L. RANDOL BARKER, M.D.

In the National Ambulatory Medical Care Survey, management of hypertension was named as the principal reason for approximately 10% of office visits to internists (see Chapter 1, Table 1.3) and approximately 6% of visits to general and family practitioners (Table 1.4). The ambulatory care of this important condition is a longitudinal process requiring skill in enlisting the patient's cooperation and skill in selecting, monitoring, and adjusting treatment. This chapter focuses upon the distribution of hypertension in the population, the size of the risk of cardiovascular morbidity, and the value of treatment; upon the pathophysiologic characteristics of hypertension which elucidate both the morbidity produced by hypertension and the mechanism of action of antihypertensive drugs; and, principally, upon the longitudinal care of the patient.

EPIDEMIOLOGY

Each hypertensive patient seen in ambulatory practice comes from a universe of patients which has been studied extensively by epidemiologists and clinicians in recent years. The findings from these studies provide the rationale for the care of the individual patient. Because the patient with high blood pressure is usually asymptomatic, an understanding of the risks attending this condition and of the benefits of treatment is uniquely important.

Prevalence

As shown in the data from the Health and Nutritional Examination Survey (Fig. 59.1), the prevalence of hypertension, defined as a systolic blood pressure of ≥160 or a distolic blood pressure of ≥95, increases sharply with age and is more common in black subjects at all ages. These crude data, based on blood pressure measurement on a single occasion, overestimate the prevalence of sustained hypertension. On repeat examination, from 10 to 30% of patients presumed to be hypertensive will be found to have a *normal* blood pressure, defined as <140 over <90, and another 10 to 30% will be found to have *borderline* hypertension, defined as a pressure between 140/90 and 160/95 (5).

For clinical purposes, hypertension is usually defined as sustained diastolic blood pressure of ≥90. Of those individuals with sustained diastolic hypertension, approximately 70% have *mild* hypertension (diastolic 90 to 104), 20% have *moderate* hypertension (diastolic 105 to 114), and only 10% have *severe* hypertension (diastolic ≥115) (14).

These prevalence data indicate that the practicing physician will have to make decisions much more often for patients with mild hypertension than for those with moderate or severe hypertension. The data also explain why the absolute number of morbid events attributable to hypertension in any community is greatest in the population of patients with mild hypertension, although the risk of morbid events is much lower in this group than in the other two groups.

Risks

For the patient and the physician, the single most important concept in approaching hypertension is that high blood pressure increases the risk of symptomatic cardiovascular disease during the patient's entire life.

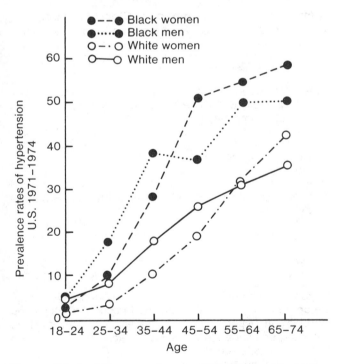

Figure 59.1 The prevalence of hypertension in the United States, defined as a systolic blood pressure of at least 160 mm Hg or a diastolic blood pressure of at least 95 mm Hg. Data from the Health and Nutrition Examination Survey, 1971 to 1974. (Source: Advance Data, Vital and Health Statistics of the National Center for Health Statistics, No. 1, October 18, 1976.)

Table 59.1
Risk of Cardiovascular Events According to Blood Pressure Status, Men and Women, 45 to 74 (Framingham Study: 18-Year Follow-up)[a]

Age	Average Annual Incidence per 1000 Population					
	Men			Women		
	Normal[b]	BHBP[c]	HBP[d]	Normal[b]	BHBP[c]	HBP[d]
45–54	8.3	14.6	23.4	2.4	5.0	8.9
55–64	15.5	29.3	44.4	6.2	14.2	22.7
65–74	16.4	31.9	52.3	8.3	24.9	33.2
45–74[e]	12.4	21.1	35.3	5.7	10.4	18.8

[a] Adapted from W. B. Kannel: Hypertension in Framingham. In *Epidemiology and Control of Hypertension*, edited by O. Paul. Symposia Specialists, Miami, 1975.
[b] Normal, ≤ 140/90.
[c] Borderline, 141/91 to 159/94.
[d] High, ≥ 160/95.
[e] Age-adjusted rates.

This concept has been elucidated by the longitudinal observations on subjects in the *Framingham study* (see Table 59.1 and Fig. 59.2). Adult subjects ranging in age from 45 to 74 years entered the study in 1951 through 1953 and were followed for 18 years. For practical purposes, the Framingham subjects (at entry) can be likened to patients making their first office visit to a physician at ages ranging from 45 to 74. Based on the average of blood pressures taken on three separate visits, these subjects were subgrouped into normal blood pressure, borderline hypertension, and hypertension, using the same criteria as the Health and Nutrition Evaluation Survey stated above. During 18 years of follow-up, each new cardiovascular event (meaning myocardial infarction, congestive heart failure, or cerebrovascular accident) was detected. The published analyses provide the practicing physician with a valuable profile of the long term risks associated with high blood pressure.

One table (Table 59.1) and one figure (Fig. 59.2) from the Framingham study have been selected to emphasize the following messages for the physician and his patient:

1. Risks rise progressively with each increase of both systolic and diastolic blood pressure.
2. In any interval of follow-up after initial evaluation, the annual risk of major cardiovascular events is much higher for older patients, as a function of both age and blood pressure at entry.
3. At all ages and blood pressures, the annual incidence of events is somewhat higher for men than for women, although the gradient of risk according to blood pressure is identical for both sexes at all ages.

By consulting the Framingham data, a physician can appreciate the degree of risk for an individual patient. For example, for a man 55 to 64 years old with a blood pressure ≥160/95, the risk of a stroke, myocardial infarction, or congestive heart failure during the ensuing 18 years is approximately 80%.

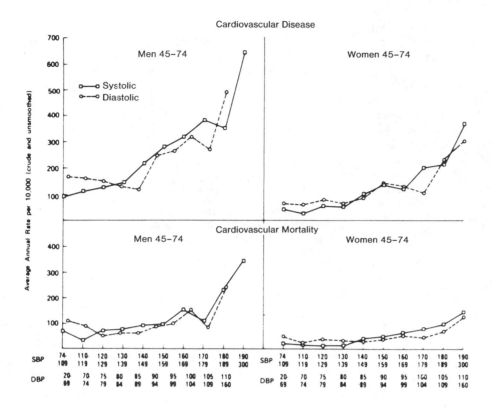

Figure 59.2 The incidence of cardiovascular morbidity (*top*) and mortality (*bottom*) during 18 years follow-up of the Framingham cohort, plotted according to systolic and diastolic blood pressure at the time of entry for men and women ages 45 to 74. (From W. B. Kannel and P. Sorlie: Hypertension in Framingham. In: *Epidemiology and Control of Hypertension*, edited by O. Paul. Symposia Specialists, Miami, 1975.)

Findings in the placebo-treated subjects in the *Veterans Administration Therapeutic Trial* (30) have added to the Framingham findings a more precise estimate of the risks attending diastolic hypertension. In this study, male subjects with sustained diastolic hypertension in the range 90 to 114 were treated with antihypertensive drugs or placebo tablets. Both groups were followed longitudinally for 3 years, and the 3-year morbidity rate was reported for the two groups and for a number of subgroups of interest to the practicing physician. Table 59.2 summarizes the attack rates in placebo-treated patients with entry diastolic pressures in two ranges (90 to 104 and 105 to 114) and shows the impact of two associated characteristics (age and presence/absence of established cardiovascular and renal morbidity at entry) upon these risks. Based on these data, the 3-year risk of morbidity in a male patient with left ventricular hypertrophy on electrocardiogram and a sustained diastolic blood pressure of 100 would be approximately 35%.

Risk Reduction

The results of several longitudinal studies indicate that control of hypertension reduces significantly the risk or morbidity and mortality attributable to hypertension.

VETERANS ADMINISTRATION TRIAL (Fig. 59.3)

This study was briefly described above. Treatment of hypertension reduced by 50% or more the expected

Table 59.2
Placebo-treated Subjects, Veteran's Administration Trial: Impact of Blood Pressure, Age, and Cardiovascular Abnormalities on Attack Rate[a]

Risk Factor at Entry	Number Randomized	Attack Rate[b]
CARDIOVASCULAR AND RENAL ABNORMALITIES[c] AND DIASTOLIC BLOOD PRESSURE (mm Hg):		
Without abnormality		
90–104	36	0.145
105–114	51	0.173
With abnormality		
90–104	48	0.352
105–114	50	0.426
AGE AND DIASTOLIC BLOOD PRESSURE (mm Hg):		
<50 years		
90–104	43	0.121
105–114	56	0.413
50+ years		
90–104	41	0.413
104–114	54	0.459

[a] Adapted from Veterans' Administration Cooperative Study Group on Antihypertensive Agents: Effects of treatment on morbidity in hypertension; III. Influence of age, diastolic pressure, and prior cardiovascular disease; further analysis of side effects. *Circulation*, 45: 991, 1972.
[b] Rate observed during 3 years.
[c] Criteria for abnormalities at entry: grade 2 or greater hypertensive retinopathy, cardiomegaly on chest X-ray, left ventricular hypertrophy on ECG, evidence of renal damage, myocardial infarction, congestive heart failure, cerebrovascular accident.

morbidity in the entire subgroup with diastolic blood pressures ≥105 and in those subgroups with diastolic 90 to 104 either who were over 50 or had one or more cardiovascular-renal abnormalities at entry to the study. Specifically, the risk of congestive heart failure, cerebrovascular accident, and progressive renal insufficiency was almost entirely eliminated, while there was no significant reduction in the risk of myocardial infarction. Treatment of the subgroup with diastolic pressure 90 to 104 who were under 50 years of age and had no cardiovascular abnormalities at entry reduced morbidity by less than 30%.

HYPERTENSION DETECTION AND FOLLOW-UP STUDY (HDFP)

In this study, reported in 1979 (14), systematic treatment and follow-up ("stepped care") were compared with usual care for hypertension in the community ("referred care"). There were approximately 10,000 participants, all having sustained diastolic pressures ≥90, recruited from probability samples in 14 communities. Death was the principal end point. After 5 years, analysis showed a statistically significant reduction in mortality for the group receiving stepped care compared with the group receiving referred care. This benefit was most pronounced in the subgroup with mild hypertension at entry (diastolic 90 to 104) and seemed to be related to the consistently better blood pressure control in the stepped care subjects (see Table 59.3). When demographic subgroups were analyzed, the statistically significant decrease in mortality was found for white men, black

men, and black women but not for white women; however, the difference in blood pressure control was least for participants in this demographic subgroup (white women).

Both the total incidence of events and the difference in incidence between stepped care and referred care in HDFP (Fig. 59.4) were far smaller than those

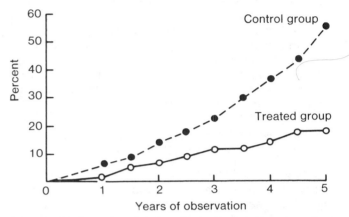

Figure 59.3 Life table analysis comparing percentage of incidence of cardiovascular complications over a 5-year period in control versus treated patients with initial diastolic blood pressure in the range of 90 through 114 mm Hg. (Source: Veterans Administration Cooperative Study Group on Antihypertensive Agents: II. Effects of treatment on morbidity in hypertension. *Journal of the American Medical Association*, 213: 1143, 1970, copyright, American Medical Association.)

Table 59.3
Percent of Stepped Care and Referred Care Participants at or Below Hypertensive Detection and Follow-up Program (HDFP) Goal Diastolic Blood Pressure (DBP) by DBP Stratum and Year of Follow-up[a]

Year	HDFP Goal Status[c]	Stepped Care DBP Stratum,[c] mm Hg				Referred Care DBP Stratum,[b] mm Hg			
		I (90–104)	II (105–114)	III (115+)	Total	I (90–104)	II (105–114)	III (115+)	Total
1	At or below goal	51.9	56.6	41.6	51.8	30.4	29.5	22.1	29.4
	Not at goal	42.1	37.0	52.9	42.2	61.8	61.8	69.6	62.6
	Unknown	6.0	6.4	5.5	6.0	7.8	8.7	8.3	8.0
2	At or below goal	57.2	59.4	47.6	56.7	34.9	31.8	28.5	33.7
	Not at goal	38.2	35.3	47.5	38.6	58.2	62.2	63.5	59.4
	Unknown	4.6	5.3	4.9	4.7	6.9	6.0	8.0	6.9
4	At or below goal	61.6	63.9	57.7	61.7	40.7	43.0	36.1	40.7
	Not at goal	31.5	28.6	36.1	31.3	47.3	45.0	51.4	47.2
	Unknown	6.9	7.5	6.2	7.0	12.0	11.9	12.5	12.1
5	At or below goal	63.8	69.6	63.6	64.9	43.0	48.3	39.1	43.6
	Not at goal	30.9	25.8	31.3	29.9	48.2	43.0	51.5	47.5
	Unknown	5.3	4.6	5.1	5.2	8.8	8.7	9.4	8.9

[a] From Hypertension Detection and Follow-up Program Cooperative Group: Five-year findings of the hypertension detection and follow-up program; I. Reduction in mortality of persons with high blood pressure, including mild hypertension. *Journal of the American Medical Association*, 242: 2562, 1979, copyright American Medical Association.
[b] At entry.
[c] HDFP defined goal DBP as 90 mm Hg for those entering with DBP equal to or greater than 100 mm Hg or receiving antihypertensive therapy, and a 10-mm Hg decrease for those entering with DBP of 90 to 99 mm Hg.

observed in the placebo trial of the Veterans Administration (Fig. 59.3); moreover, the finding of statistically significant differences depended upon the very large number of subjects in HDFP.

HDFP has provided additional evidence for the benefit of blood pressure control in the subset (diastolic 90 to 104) containing approximately 70% of hypertensive persons. The recently published results of an Australian trial comparing placebo and treatment in men and women with mild hypertension (diastolic 95 to 104) also demonstrated a modest benefit from treatment (26). Further evidence for or against active treatment of mild hypertension will be available when the results are known from a similar large scale British study (20).

PATHOPHYSIOLOGY OF ESSENTIAL HYPERTENSION

It is estimated that 95 to 99% of hypertensives do not have an identifiable anatomic or endocrinologic basis for their hypertension, and their problem has therefore been designated "essential hypertension." Nevertheless, a number of abnormal physiologic characteristics have been demonstrated in essential hypertension; these provide a conceptual basis for understanding the clinical consequences of hypertension and the mechanisms of action of antihypertensive drugs.

As indicated in Figure 59.5, the patient with established essential hypertension has an *increase in peripheral arterial resistance*; this is hypothesized to be the final consequence of either or both of two mechanisms illustrated in Figure 59.6; *i.e.*, inappropriate renal retention of salt and water or increased endog-

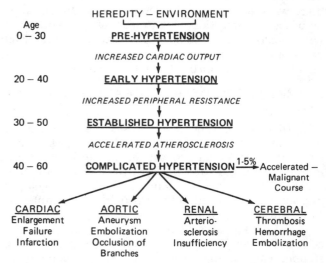

Figure 59.5 A representation of the natural history of untreated essential hypertension. (Source: N. Kaplan: *Clinical Hypertension*, Williams & Wilkins, Baltimore, 1978.)

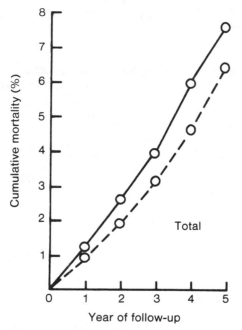

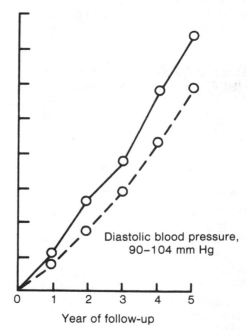

Figure 59.4 Hypertension Detection and Follow-up Program cumulative life table of all causes death rates, total and stratum 1 (diastolic blood pressure, 90 to 104 mm Hg). *Dashed line* indicates stepped care; *solid line*, referred care. (Source: Hypertension Detection and Follow-up Program Cooperative Group: Five-year findings of the hypertension detection and follow-up program; I. Reduction in mortality of persons with high blood pressure, including mild hypertension. *Journal of the American Medical Association*, 242: 2562, 1979, copyright, American Medical Association.)

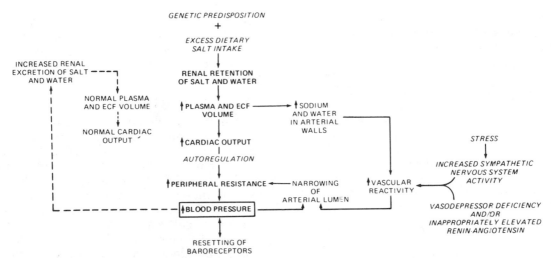

Figure 59.6 An overall scheme for the possible pathogenesis cf essential hypertension. The elevated blood pressure is shown by the *dotted lines* to increase renal excretion of salt and water, thereby returning plasma volume and cardiac output to normal. *ECF*, extracellular fluid. (Source: N. Kaplan: *Clinical Hypertension.* Williams & Wilkins, Baltimore, 1978.)

enous pressor activity. Possible antecedents for these mechanisms may be discovered in the history of a patient with established hypertension—e.g., a family history of hypertension and/or a personal history of excess salt ingestion for the first mechanism and evidence for chronic psychologic stress for the second. *Serial studies* on small numbers of subjects have suggested that a stage of increased cardiac output may precede the stage of increased peripheral resistance (Fig. 59.5). Clinically, this earlier stage may be manifest in some young hypertensives as a high resting pulse rate. In general, however, the evaluation of the individual patient will not yield much information about the dominant mechanism contributing to that individual's hypertension.

The major *complications* of untreated hypertension are named in Figure 59.5. These complications can be seen as the clinical manifestations of two pathophysiologic processes which are operating during the many "silent years" of increased peripheral resistance: first, chronic transmural trauma to the vessels in the arterial circulation, leading to accelerated atherosclerosis in large vessels and to obliterative changes in the small vessels; and second, chronic increase in the work load of the heart, leading to congestive heart failure and/or angina pectoris.

As noted in the discussion of epidemiology, blood pressure reduction markedly diminishes the risk of cardiovascular complications of hypertension. The mechanisms by which drug, dietary, or behavioral treatment operate may be appreciated in Figure 59.6. *Diuretics* decrease total body sodium, potentially reversing both of the processes underlying established hypertension (increased cardiac output and increased vascular reactivity). *Most sympatholytic drugs* are thought to decrease vascular reactivity, either by

diminishing α-adrenergic activity affecting arteriolar tone or by suppressing the activity of the renin-angiotensin system. The hypotensive response to β-adrenergic blocking agents may be related chiefly to decreased cardiac output, however. *Vasodilators* act chiefly on the arteriolar smooth muscle, decreasing tone and thereby decreasing peripheral resistance.

EVALUATION OF THE PATIENT

In this discussion, hypertension is defined as a diastolic pressure of 90 mm Hg or greater and the approaches recommended are based upon the general guidelines of the 1980 Report of the Joint National Committee on Detection, Evaluation, and Treatment of High Blood Pressure (see Table 59.4 and "General References").

Taking the Blood Pressure

In obtaining blood pressures, the physician should follow a number of standard practices, *i.e.*:

1. *Cuff selection*: Ideally, the rubber bladder in the cuff should be about 20% wider than the diameter of the arm and should encircle the arm without a significant gap or overlap.
2. Take the initial blood pressure when the *patient is relaxed*, usually in a sitting position. Check *both arms*. If there is a significant difference between arms, take all subsequent blood pressures in the arm with the higher pressure.
3. Use the *fifth Korotkoff sound* (disappearance) for diastolic pressure.
4. Before initiating antihypertensive treatment, take the blood pressure when the patient is *standing* in order to detect significant baseline orthostatic hypotension.

Table 59.4
Actions Recommended for the Evaluation and Treatment of Hypertension[a]

Diastolic Pressure (mm Hg)	Recommended Actions
PATIENT WITH AN INITIAL BLOOD PRESSURE ELEVATION:	
≥115	Immediate referral for remeasurement
95–114	Remeasure within 1 month
90–95	Remeasure within 3 months
PATIENT WITH CONFIRMED HYPERTENSION:	
≥115 (severe)	Treat promptly
105–114 (moderate)	Treat promptly
90–104 (mild)	Individualize treatment[b] (pharmacologic or non-pharmacologic)

[a] Adapted from Special Report: The 1980 Report of The Joint National Committee on Detection, Evaluation, and Treatment of High Blood Pressure. *Archives of Internal Medicine, 140:* 1280, 1980.
[b] The following coexisting factors support the decision to initiate pharmacologic treatment: presence of target organ damage, smoking, family history of premature cardiovascular complications, elevated systolic pressure, diabetes, and elevated cholesterol level.

5. *After starting or increasing antihypertensive drugs,* again check the blood pressure with the patient resting and with the patient standing, preferably after a standard exercise (e.g., 10 steps on a foot stool) as the orthostatic effect of drugs is usually most pronounced after exercise.

6. *Record* position, arm, blood pressure, pulse, and cuff size (therefore assuring that these conditions are duplicated when blood pressures are obtained at subsequent visits).

Clinical Classification

Evaluating hypertension for an individual patient consists of deciding which of four stages of hypertension is present (labile, chronic, accelerated, or emergency hypertension) and, for the patient with sustained hypertension, completing a baseline evaluation (see below). The classification of the patient should be accomplished carefully, for it provides the patient with a specific label (and notions) which will have a significant effect on his and his physician's future behavior. Two findings underline this point. First, almost half of those people who have been told they are hypertensive do not have sustained hypertension (5). Second, being labeled hypertensive may have significant "side effects" such as increased sick days, increased life insurance premiums, or certain employment restrictions (13).

On their initial visits, many patients will state that they have hypertension. For some of these, recorded blood pressures from other sources will be available. Some will be taking antihypertensive drugs, presum-

ably for sustained hypertension. Based upon this information and upon blood pressure recordings made at the initial and follow-up visits, the physician should decide independently which stage of hypertension is present.

LABILE HYPERTENSION

By definition, labile hypertension is present in any individual who has a recorded diastolic blood pressure of 90 or above, but has a usual diastolic pressure of less than 90. A labile rise in blood pressure can be produced in almost anyone by stressful events which provoke increased sympathetic nervous system activity. Therefore, it is no surprise that a high prevalence of labile hypertension has been found in community studies of hypertension. The best example is the Charlottesville community study (5) in which all adults having an elevated initial blood pressure were re-examined. Re-examination showed that the majority of adolescents and young adults (15 to 44 years old), half of those 45 to 55 years old, and a minority of those 55 or older had labile hypertension.

In practice, blood pressures should be measured on two or more separate occasions within 1 to 2 months to determine whether a patient with a high diastolic pressure has labile or sustained (*i.e.*, chronic) hypertension. If the diastolic pressure at the first visit is relatively high (e.g., ≥115), the repeat blood pressures should be obtained within 1 week.

It is estimated that 10 to 25% of labile hypertension progresses to chronic hypertension. Therefore, labile hypertensives should have their blood pressure checked carefully once each year. The physician should assure that such patients understand that they do not have sustained hypertension. In addition, they should be advised not to eat excess salt (see below, p. 579).

CHRONIC HYPERTENSION

By definition, hypertension is chronic if the diastolic pressure is consistently ≥90. In some patients, especially those with high initial pressures, electrocardiographic or X-ray evidence of left ventricular hypertrophy is adequate to confirm the suspicion of chronic hypertension at the first visit. Eye ground findings indicative of arteriosclerosis (grade 1, narrowing of arteriolar lumen; grade 2, arteriovenous nicking) are less reliable and less specific as indicators of chronic hypertension and should not be substituted for serial blood pressure measurements on separate occasions.

The prognosis in untreated chronic hypertension can be appreciated best in the data from the Framingham study, the Veterans Administration trial, and the HFDP trial summarized above.

ACCELERATED HYPERTENSION

By definition, hypertension is in the accelerated or malignant stage if the diastolic pressure is relatively high (e.g., ≥120) and there is clinical evidence of severe arteriolosclerosis, meaning either grade 3 or 4 hypertensive retinopathy (grade 3, hemorrhages and/or fresh exudates; grade 4, papilledema) or renal insufficiency for which there is no apparent cause except the hypertension.

The prognosis in untreated accelerated hypertension is extremely poor: approximately 95% of subjects will die of cardiac, renal, or central nervous system complications within 5 years of initial evaluation. Control of blood pressure and dialysis have dramatically improved the prognosis in these individuals.

HYPERTENSIVE EMERGENCY

By definition, a hypertensive emergency exists when severe elevation of the blood pressure will cause a catastrophic outcome within hours or days. Patients with two types of hypertensive emergency (hypertensive encephalopathy and dissecting aneurysm) may present initially in an ambulatory practice.

Hypertensive encephalopathy is the result of cerebral edema which develops gradually over 1 or more days in a patient with severe diastolic hypertension. In such a patient, global cerebral symptoms such as headache, confusion, and irritability have usually been present and progressive for hours or days. Papilledema is usually present.

Hypertensive encephalopathy is a clinical diagnosis which should be made only when intracerebral hemorrhage, which may also present with hypertension, has been excluded.

Thoracic aortic dissection results from an expanding hematoma in the wall of the aorta; in the patient who is dissecting, hypertension may promote perforation of the intima overlying the softened wall of the aorta. The patient with acute dissection will usually have a history of known hypertension and will present with a story of sudden "ripping" pain in the back.

Computerized tomography (CT scan) and contrast aortography are both very sensitive and specific diagnostic tests for dissection. By definition, a proximal dissection involves the aorta between the aortic root and the left subclavian artery and a distal dissection involves only that part of the aorta distal to the left subclavian artery.

Baseline Evaluation

The baseline evaluation of the patient with sustained hypertension should accomplish five objectives, *i.e.*:
1. Indicate the status of end organs affected by hypertension.
2. Identify clues to the presence of secondary hypertension.
3. Guide the selection of initial treatment.
4. Establish the pretreatment status of parameters commonly affected by antihypertensive drugs.

5. Detect the presence of additional cardiovascular risk factors.

Table 59.5 lists by source the information which should be obtained in the baseline evaluation to accomplish these five objectives.

END ORGAN STATUS

At baseline evaluation, most patients with chronic hypertension and many of those with accelerated hypertension have no symptoms attributable to their hypertension. In the past, it was thought that headache, tinnitus, epistaxis, and dizziness were symptoms of chronic hypertension, but community-based studies have demonstrated that these symptoms are not more prevalent in hypertensives than in normotensives. A minority of patients do have genuine hypertensive headaches, occipital in location, worse in the morning, and resolving with lowering of the blood pressure.

Heart

A history of congestive heart failure or of symptoms of coronary artery disease will occasionally be obtained at baseline evaluation. Auscultation of the heart commonly reveals accentuation of the aortic second sound and a systolic ejection murmur. Infrequent findings include a systolic ejection sound at the base of the heart, paradoxical splitting of the second heart sound, or a short high pitched diastolic murmur at the base. Objective evidence of cardiac hypertrophy is frequently found at baseline evaluation, either on physical examination (left ventricular heave or fourth heart sound) or on the electrocardiogram or chest X-ray. The 1962 National Health Survey showed that electrocardiographic and/or radiographic evidence of cardiac hypertrophy was present in approximately one-third of hypertensives under 44 years of age and over half of hypertensives 45 years and older (10). Electrocardiographic criteria for left ventricular hypertrophy are summarized elsewhere (Table 57.3, Chapter 57).

Eye

Traditionally, examination of the retina has been emphasized in the evaluation of hypertensive patients because it offers direct inspection of the vessels most affected by hypertension. Ophthalmic symptoms attributed to hypertension (decreased acuity due to retinal hemorrhages or retinal detachment) are very uncommon, however. Most patients with chronic hypertension have evidence of arteriolosclerosis (grades 1 and 2 hypertensive retinopathy), but these findings have little practical value as they are not specific for hypertension, and there is significant inter-observor and intra-observer variability in detecting them. On the other hand, grades 3 or 4 retinopathy should be sought in any patient with a high diastolic pressure, for these changes increase the importance of adequate blood pressure control within

Table 59.5
Baseline Evaluation of the Patient with Sustained Hypertension

Sources of Information	Objective Accomplished				
	End organ status	Etiology screening	Selection of initial treatment (see also Table 59.7)	Baseline status of parameter affected by treatment	Associated cardiovascular risk factor
PRIOR RECORDS:					
Prior BPs etc.	√	√	√	√	√
INTERVIEW:					
Prior HBP treatment			√		
Headache	√			√	
Sx[a] CHF	√		√	√	
Sx Angina	√		√	√	
Sx TIA/CVA	√		√		
Sx Claudication	√		√		
Age		√	√		
Oral contraceptives		√			√
Periodic Sx SNS[b]		√			
H/O[c] GU Sx	√	√			
Diet (salt intake)			√		
Cigarettes					√
Life-style			√		√
Understanding of HBP			√	√	
H/O Mood disturbance			√		
H/O Gout			√		
H/O Diabetes			√		√
PHYSICAL:					
Weight			√	√	√
BP both arms, resting and with exercise	√			√	
PR resting and with exercise	√	√	√	√	
Eye grounds	√				
Peripheral pulses	√				
Heart	√				
Lungs			√		
ABD (mass, bruit)		√			
LABORATORY:					
BUN	√	√	√	√	
K		√	√	√	
Na				√	
FBS				√	√
Uric Acid				√	
CBC				√	
Urinalysis	√	√			
ECG	√			√	
Chest X-ray	√	√		√	
Cholesterol				√	√

[a] Sx = symptoms.
[b] SNS = sympathetic nervous system.
[c] H/O = history of.

a short time (see discussion of accelerated hypertension above).

Kidney

Simple tests of kidney status (urinalysis and blood urea nitrogen or creatinine) are normal in the majority of hypertensives at baseline. In the patient with a high diastolic pressure, either an elevated blood urea nitrogen, or creatinine, proteinuria, or microscopic hematuria may be found as evidence for accelerated hypertension. Other forms of renal disease should be excluded in such patients before these findings are attributed to hypertension.

Central Nervous System

A history of established stroke or transient ischemic attacks or an asymptomatic carotid bruit may occasionally be present at baseline evaluation, but the majority of patients will have no evidence of cerebral vascular disease when first evaluated.

EVALUATION FOR SECONDARY HYPERTENSION

A few clues in the baseline evaluation identify those occasional patients who should be evaluated for hypertension secondary to a treatable primary condition. The rarity of these conditions is indicated by the reports from referral centers in which only 1 to 3% of patients have had a surgically correctable form of hypertension (8, 27).

These conditions and the clues to them are:

Current Use of an Oral Contraceptive. Clue: Patient currently using an oral contraceptive hormone. To confirm this etiology, there should be evidence for a normal blood pressure before oral contraceptive use; and the patient's blood pressure should become normal within 6 months of discontinuing oral contraceptives. (See additional details, p. 587.)

Renovascular Hypertension (RVH). Clues: The presence of an abdominal bruit radiating to the flank (with both systolic and diastolic components); a recent change from normal blood pressure to moderate or severe hypertension; a very high diastolic pressure (e.g., ≥120 mm Hg) in a person under 30 years of age; or evidence of accelerated hypertension.

If a patient has one or more of these findings and is a candidate for surgery, the physician may choose to order screening laboratory tests or to hospitalize the patient directly for renal arteriography. Alternatively, medical therapy, which is effective in most patients with RVH, may be selected initially. The usefulness of three screening tests, stimulated plasma renin activity (PRA), hypertensive intravenous pyelogram (IVP), and auscultation for an abdominal bruit, is summarized in Table 59.6.

Patient Experience. The patient can expect the following experience when undergoing radiologic evaluation for RVH. *Hypertensive IVP:* the patient takes nothing by mouth (NPO) for at least 12 hours and takes a laxative the night before. Contrast material is injected as rapidly as possible by the radiologist. Mild nausea is common during injection. The patient lies supine on the X-ray table for 15 min while X-rays are taken at 1, 2, 3, 4, 5, 10, and 15 min after dye injection. Total time in the radiology suite is 20 to 30 min. *Renal arteriography and renal vein renin sampling:* the patient is hospitalized, kept NPO, and given a laxative the evening before these studies. After local anesthesia, catheter-containing needles are inserted percutaneously into a femoral vein and a femoral artery. Substantial time is devoted to positioning of catheters, under fluoroscopic guidance. When dye is injected, the patient feels intense warmth in the abdomen for a few seconds. The patient is supine throughout the procedure. Total time in the radiology suite is usually 1½ to 2 hours.

Chronic Renal Disease. Clues: A history of hematuria, stones, or recurrent pyelonephritis; palpation of polycystic kidneys; microscopic urinalysis suggesting acute or chronic glomerulonephritis (red cell casts).

Primary Hyperaldosteronism. Clues: A baseline potassium level significantly below normal, with or without symptoms. Such patients should be asked about excess consumption of licorice which contains glycyrrhizinic acid, a moiety with mineralocorticoid-like acvtivity. The ambulatory evaluation of the patient with suspected primary hyperaldosteronism is discussed in detail in Chapter 42.

Pheochromocytoma (9). Clues: History of a hypermetabolic state (which may resemble hyperthyroidism) and of periodic clusters of symptoms of sympathetic nervous system hyperactivity (tachycardia, diaphoresis, palpitations, and orthostatic hypotension), especially when these are not provoked by psychologic stress and when there is no evidence for

Table 59.6
Usefulness of Screening Tests for Renovascular Hypertension (Singly and in Combination)[a]

Test	Sensitivity and Specificity[b]		Predictive Value[b]					
			Prevalence 1%		Prevalence 5%		Prevalence 10%	
	Sensitivity	Specificity	Positive test	Negative test	Positive test	Negative test	Positive test	Negative test
Intravenous pyelogram (IVP)	78	98	6.7	99.8	68.0	98.7	81[c]	97.6[c]
Plasma renin activity (PRA) >30[d]	27	95	5.2	99.2	22.1	96.1	37.5[c]	92.1[c]
Upper abdominal bruit[e]	39	99	28.3	99.4	67.0	96.8	81[c]	93.4[c]
All 3 done, 1 positive	93	92	11.6	99.9	38.0	99.6	57.8	99.2

[a] Adapted with permission from C. E. Grim: Sensitivity and specificity of screening tests for renal vascular hypertension. *Annals of Internal Medicine, 91:* 617, 1979. All values are percentages.
[b] See Chapter 1 for definitions.
[c] Calculated, not in original publication (courtesy of the author).
[d] Above 95th percentile for group of patients with essential hypertension, using peripheral venous plasma sample after 2 hours upright.
[e] Bruit with both systolic and diastolic components.

reactive hypoglycemia (see Chapter 71). Additional indications for screening a patient for pheochromocytoma are (a) a marked changed in blood pressure or heart rate in response to a minor injury, parturition, or general anesthesia, (b) a neurocutaneous syndrome (von Recklinghausen's or von Hippel-Landau syndrome), (c) a blood relative with a pheochromocytoma, (d) multiple endocrine neoplasia, Type II (medullary carcinoma of the thyroid or parathyroid adenoma, or both, with pheochromocytoma).

To screen patients for pheochromocytoma either total catecholamines, total vanillylmandelic acid (VMA), or total metanephrines should be measured in a single 24-hour urine specimen. Values for all three of these are elevated in the majority of patients with pheochromocytoma. With modern assay techniques, no foodstuffs and only a small number of drugs may interfere with test results (catecholamines, increased by methyldopa and L-dopa; metanephrines, increased by monoamine oxidase inhibitors; VMA, decreased by monoamine oxidase inhibitors and clofibrate, increased by nalidixic acid). Elevated VMA is virtually 100% specific and 97% sensitive for pheochromocytoma. Elevated metanephrines are virtually 100% sensitive, but there are some false positives. In the rare patient who has a normal blood pressure between paroxysms of hypertension, the urine specimen should be taken when the patient *is* hypertensive. Patients with positive screening tests should be hospitalized for radiologic localization of the tumor. For patients with suspected pheochromocytoma and normal screening tests, hospital admissions for provocative tests (histamine, glucagon, tyramine) or for the recently described clonidine suppression test (the plasma norepinephrine level is not suppressed by clonidine in patients with pheochromocytoma) (3a) should be considered, in consultation with an endocrinologist.

Coarctation of the Aorta. Clues: A relatively young patient (most will be recognized in the pediatric age group); decreased blood pressure in the lower extremities, suggested by diminished or absent femoral pulses and corroborated by blood pressures auscultated over the popliteal artery, using a large cuff; and evidence of collateral arterial vessels either on inspection of the trunk or on the plain chest X-ray. In a minority of patients, the coarctation occurs proximal to the left subclavian artery, and the blood pressure will be high only in the right arm. To confirm the presence of a coarctation, the patient must be hospitalized for aortography.

TREATMENT

Goals of Treatment

When sustained hypertension has been diagnosed, the initial goal of treatment is a normal blood pressure, defined as a diastolic pressure ≤90 mm Hg. An appropriate long term goal is the lowest diastolic pressure which can be attained safely (for practical purposes 70 mm Hg should be the lower limit). Partial reduction of blood pressure is an acceptable goal for patients in whom it is impossible to achieve a diastolic pressure of ≤90 mm Hg (25).

In most patients, satisfactory blood pressure control can be achieved within 2 to 3 months. In deciding whether treatment has altered the patient's blood pressure, it should be remembered that *a reduction of less than 10 mm Hg diastolic is not meaningful* (29). This is particularly important in deciding whether there has been a real response in the patient with mild hypertension. For example, evidence of a significant response in a patient with an average diastolic pressure of 95 mm Hg before treatment is a diastolic pressure of 85 mm Hg or less after treatment.

Promoting Compliance with Treatment

Compliance with treatment as a generic feature of ambulatory care is discussed in detail in Chapter 4. Because poor compliance is so common in hypertensive patients, the problem has been studied extensively in recent years; a number of strategies in patient care have been shown to improve compliance with antihypertensive treatment (16, 21). Some of these adherence-promoting strategies should be used routinely. Other, more intensive strategies should be used for those patients who prove to be especially noncompliant.

The following strategies should be used *routinely* from the outset of treatment:

1. Assuring that the patient knows several critical facts about hypertension: that it increases the risk of grave illness later in life; that it is usually asymptomatic when initially found; that treatment reduces the risk of grave illness; and that treatment is continuous for life. This information is covered well in patient-information pamphlets available from the American Heart Association and a number of drug companies. One of these should be given to each hypertensive patient *as an adjunct* to a verbal summary of this information by the physician or nurse.
2. Assuring that adherence to prescribed treatment is facilitated and is assessed carefully at each visit. This includes: adjusting the medication schedule to the patient's usual daily activities; inviting questions from the patient about the medication; and having the patient demonstrate that he knows the regimen.
3. Assuring that supervision is provided frequently enough. During the first year of treatment, this should be at least every 2 to 3 months, as scheduled visits.
4. Assuring that the practice is planned to maximize convenience for the patient, meaning that waiting time is brief, that telephone access to the practice is easy, that appointment changes are accommodated, and that prescription refills are easily obtainable.

For patients who do not comply regularly with

treatment, additional strategies have been shown to help:

1. Having the adult with whom the patient has the most contact (usually the spouse) become an active participant in promoting compliance. This other adult should know in detail the treatment regimen and should be asked to provide specific reinforcement for medication taking.
2. Arranging for periodic supervision in the patient's home by a visiting nurse, including blood pressure measurement, assessment of compliance with medications, and reinforcement of compliance.
3. Having the patient take and record his own blood pressure daily, using a sphygmomanometer designed for self-recording.
4. Having the patient participate in scheduled small group meetings which are coordinated by someone skilled in promoting group-support mechanisms.

In addition, several other important facts have been noted in studies of compliance in hypertension, *i.e.:*

1. Compliance-promoting strategies are additive.
2. Compliance decays in many patients who initially do well and in those noncompliers who improve after short term intensive interventions such as home visits. Because of the problem of compliance decay, it is important to maintain most routine compliance-promoting strategies continuously in the long term care of hypertensive patients.

3. The cost of drugs and side effects from drugs do not explain a large proportion of noncompliance in the treatment of hypertension.

Pharmacologic Treatment by the Stepped Method

For most patients, antihypertensive drugs will be selected as initial treatment. In some circumstances, an initial trial of nonpharmacologic management of hypertension is appropriate, as discussed below (pp. 579–580).

In the future, physicians may employ simple methods routinely to select the most appropriate drugs for individual patients with essential hypertension. For example, methods under investigation include measuring plasma renin activity and identifying a hyperkinetic circulation or angiotensin-dependent hypertension. At the present time, drug treatment for most patients should be initiated and modified according to the *stepped-treatment method* outlined in Figure 59.7.

With this method, diuretic therapy is always the *first step.* From 25 to 50% of patients respond satisfactorily to diuretics alone. The *second step* (adding a sympatholytic drug to the diuretic) and *third step* (adding to the diuretic a combinatin of the vasodilator hydralazine and a sympatholytic drug or one of the combinations of two sympatholytic drugs listed in Fig. 59.7) are reserved for patients who do not re-

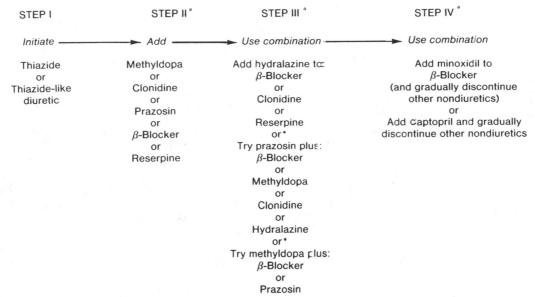

Figure 59.7 Stepped treatment. Asterisk (*) indicates combinations not mentioned in the stepped care regimens published in the 1980 report of the Joint National Committee on the Detection, Evaluation, and Treatment of Hypertension (see "General References"). They are included because they have been shown to be effective and thus they add greatly to flexibility in treatment when a Step III combination is indicated. Details regarding the use of each of these drugs are found on pp. 573–579.

a For patients in whom excess total body sodium is suspected, a loop diuretic should be tried instead of larger doses of Step II–IV drug(s).

Table 59.7
Factors Affecting Selection and Monitoring of Individual Antihypertensive Drugs[a]

Patient Factors	DIURETICS			NON-DIURETIC ANTIHYPERTENSIVE DRUGS											
	Thiazides	Loop	Potassium-conserving	Atenolol	Captopril	Clonidine	Guanethidine	Hydralazine	Metaprolol	Methyldopa	Minoxidil	Nadolol	Prazosin	Propranolol	Reserpine
Asthma or chronic obstructive pulmonary disease				W					W			W		W	
Angina								W			W				
Bradycardia				W			W		W			W		W	
Congestive heart failure				W			W		W			W		W	
Orthostatic ↓ BP baseline	W	W	W	W	W	W	W	W	W	W	W	W	W	W	W
Bifascicular/Trifascicular heart block				W					W			W		W	
Peripheral arterial insufficiency				W					W			W		W	
Digitalis use	Tox	Tox													
Diabetes	W	W	↑K												
Insulin use				IR					IR			IR		IR	
Irritable bowel							W			W					
Allergic rhinitis															W
Peptic ulcer															W
Vascular headache (migraine or cluster)								W			W				
Sexually active male			Imp	Imp		Imp	Imp		Imp	Imp		Imp		Imp	Imp
Depression				W		W			W	W		W		W	W
Baseline hyperkalemia				W	W										
Gout	W	W													
Chronic renal disease	D↑	D↑	↑K	D↓	D↓		D↓	D↓	D↓			D↓			D↓
Chronic liver disease						D↓	D↓		D↓	W	D↓		D↓	D↓	
Generic available	Yes							Yes							Yes
Monthly cost to patient															
Usually <$5.00	Yes														Yes
Often > $20.00		Yes	Yes	Yes	Yes	Yes	Yes	Yes	Yes	Yes	Yes	Yes	Yes	Yes	

[a] W, condition may be made worse by drug; Tox, digitalis toxicity risk increased (hypokalemia); Imp, sexual impotence may occur (includes spironolactone but not other potassium-conserving diuretics); D↑, dose may have to be increased to obtain desired effect; D↓, dose may have to be decreased and/or interval between doses increased, as excretion of drug may be impaired; and IR (insulin reaction), may block sympathetic nervous system manifestations of hypoglycemia, ↑K Increased risk of hyperkalemia.

spond adequately to diuretics alone. Each of the second step drugs is effective in 50 to 80% of patients who require more than diuretic treatment; almost all patients will respond to one of the second step drugs or to one of the combinations in Step III. The *fourth step* is recommended for the occasional patient with severe hypertension who fails to respond to or to tolerate the drugs in Steps I through III. Two potent (and costly) new drugs, minoxidil and captopril, are recommended instead of guanethidine, which was previously recommended as the fourth step drug; the reasons for this modification are summarized in the discussion of the individual drugs, below.

The *baseline evaluation often discloses information useful in selecting drugs* for an individual patient.

A frequently overlooked guideline is the patient's previous experience with specific antihypertensive drugs. Clearly, whenever there is a history of significant side effects or documentation of failure to respond, the drug(s) in question should not be selected. For each drug listed in Figure 59.7, there are one or more factors which may influence selection or dosage of the drug (Table 59.7).

The *blood pressure before treatment* is not a reliable predictor of the amount or kind of drug that an individual patient will need. In general, it is reasonable to initiate diuretic treatment alone and, if needed, to increase this to the maximum recommended dose. For those few patients with baseline diastolic pressures of 120 mm Hg or greater, it is reasonable to begin with a starting dose of a second step drug together with the diuretic. Such patients should be seen frequently until an effective regimen has been found; the response to all second step drugs (except diuretics and reserpine) will be apparent within 1 day of initiation or dose increase, meaning that daily evaluation and dosage adjustments can be utilized in treating patients with extremely high blood pressures.

In stepped-treatment, *diuretic therapy should always be maintained*, even in the patient whose blood pressure shows little or no response to a maximum dose of diuretic alone. This is because Step II to IV drugs promote renal sodium retention as a response to blood pressure lowering, attenuating the antihypertensive effect of the drug. This problem is overcome by maintaining sufficient diuretic treatment to prevent sodium retention; large doses of loop diuretics and/or the addition of diuretics which act on the distal tubule (potassium-conserving diuretics) may be needed to accomplish this in some patients as discussed below.

Clinical studies have confirmed the *efficacy of each of the combinations* of drugs shown in the third step in Figure 59.7. As noted in the figure, vasodilators (hydralazine and minoxidil) should always be added *after* the patient is taking a sympatholytic drug, in order to prevent vasodilator-induced symptoms (headache, tachycardia, angina). A specific combination may be more effective and better tolerated than the maximum dose of one of the second step drugs. Because all the drugs listed in Step III are effective when taken once or twice daily, these combinations do not create more complex schedules for the patient. Thus, a trial of one of the combinations should be considered whenever second step treatment fails.

Two or more of some antihypertensive drugs are available in *fixed-dose combination tablets* and more will probably be available in the future. The appropriate combination may provide additional convenience at no additional cost.

Characteristics of Individual Drugs

This section summarizes for each currently available antihypertensive drug six types of information:
1. *Mechanism* of action.
2. *Daily dose range* which is generally recommended; available tablet sizes; for some drugs, comments on maximum daily dose.
3. *Schedule(s) recommended*, with comments on the simplest schedules which are efficacious.
4. *Onset/resolution* time of the major antihypertensive action.
5. *Common side effects* (occurring in 5% or more of patients). The reported frequency of specific side effects varies greatly from study to study. The reasons: few studies have been designed specifically to detect side effects, methods of

detection are not standardized, and the patient groups reported are small, dissimilar, and not representative of the general population. In the few studies designed to detect the true incidence, it has been found that most patients notice and tolerate minor side effects when they begin taking antihypertensive drugs. An exhaustive and fully referenced account of reported side effects is found in McMahon's monograph, published in 1978 (see "General References"). Conditions which may increase the chance of some side effects for specific drugs are listed in Table 59.7.
6. *Combinations* with other antihypertensive drugs which have been shown to enhance the hypotensive effect.

DIURETICS USED FOR TREATING HYPERTENSION*

(General use began in 1962.)

Mechanism. Diuretics probably lower blood pressure by decreasing modestly the circulating volume and by decreasing peripheral resistance. A chronic increase in plasma renin activity has been demonstrated in diuretic-treated patients; this provides indirect evidence that the decrease in circulating volume persists as long as the patient is taking the diuretic. The potassium-conserving diuretics have only a mild antihypertensive effect. They are useful chiefly in combination with the thiazide and loop diuretics (see below).

Daily Dose Range. Ranges for the commonly prescribed diuretics are:

Thiazide and thiazide-like:
   Hydrochlorothiazide (Esidrix, HydroDIURIL, etc.) 25–100 mg (tablet sizes: 25, 50, 100 mg)
   Chlorothiazide (Diuril, etc.) 250–1000 mg (tablet sizes: 250 and 500 mg)
   Metolazone (Zaroxolyn) 2.5–10 mg (tablet sizes: 2.5, 5, 10 mg)
   Chlorthalidone (Hygroton) 25–100 mg (tablet sizes: 25, 50, 100 mg)
Loop diuretics:
   Furosemide (Lasix) 40 mg—no upper limit (tablet sizes: 20, 40, 80 mg)
   Ethacrynic acid (Edecrin) 50 mg—no upper limit (tablet size: 50 mg)
Potassium-conserving:
   Amiloride (Midamor) 5–20 mg (tablet size: 5 mg)
   Spironolactone (Aldactone) 25–100 mg (tablet size: 25 mg)
   Triamterene (Dyrenium) 100–300 mg (capsule size: 100 mg)
Combinations:
   Aldactazide (tablets containing spironolactone 25 mg, hydrochlorothiazide 25 mg)

---

* See Table 59.7 for factors affecting selection of these drugs.

Dyazide (capsules containing triamterene 50 mg and hydrochlorothiazide 25 mg)

Moduretic (tablets containing amiloride 5 mg and hydrochlorothiazide 50 mg)

For the first three drugs, the maximum diuretic and
hypotensive effect is seen at the maximum dose
listed. For chlorthalidone, the smallest dose, 25 mg, is
almost as effective as higher doses and there is less
disturbance of potassium balance at this dose. For
furosemide and ethacrynic acid, higher doses may
yield additional diuretic and hypotensive effects;
these two diuretics (particularly furosemide) are useful in patients with renal insufficiency and others
who do not respond to less potent diuretics.

Schedule. One to two times daily. The duration of
diuretic activity varies from several hours (furosemide) to 24 hours (chlorthalidone and metolazone),
but there is no evidence that using either a longer
acting diuretic or a divided schedule for short acting
diuretics is needed to control hypertension. When a
loop diuretic is prescribed in high dose to promote
excretion of excess sodium, it is most effective when
taken as a single large dose.

Onset/Resolution. The major antihypertensive response is seen within 1 to 2 weeks of initiating or
increasing a diuretic. Full resolution of antihypertensive effects occurs about 1 week after discontinuing
the drug.

Side Effects (Thiazide and Loop Diuretics). Mild
side effects such as increased urination and transient
orthostatic symptoms are very common when diuretics are initiated. Of the other side effects those seen
most commonly are: hypokalemia, gout related to
diuretic-provoked hyperuricemia, impaired glucose
tolerance, and increased cholesterol and triglyceride
levels (thiazides and chlorthalidone). Each of these
may require adjunctive therapy or, at times, discontinuation of diuretics. These problems are discussed
at greater length in Chapters 42 (hypokalemia), 66
(gout), 69 (diabetes), and 72 (hyperlipidemia). If diabetes is found at the baseline evaluation or if symptomatic diabetes is provoked in the course of long
term diuretic therapy, the physician should consider
substituting calorie and sodium restriction for diuretic therapy, utilizing second step drugs as needed.
Diuretic-induced increase in plasma lipid levels can
be prevented by adherence to a low cholesterol diet
(see Table 72.9); therefore, it is prudent to recommend
this to all patients when thiazide diuretic treatment
is started (11). Apart from allergy, there are no absolute contraindications for diuretics in hypertension.

USE OF POTASSIUM-CONSERVING DIURETICS

The potassium-conserving diuretics (amiloride, spironolactone, and triamterene) have a modest antihypertensive effect when used alone in some patients
with essential hypertension. Their principal value is
in combination with other diuretics when they func-

tion as adjuncts to avoid hypokalemia (see Chapter
42) or to enhance diuretic action. The latter indication
is occasionally seen in a patient who retains sodium
while taking diuretics and large amounts of second,
third, or forth step drugs; in such patients blood
pressure control may improve dramatically when
potassium-conserving drugs are added.

To avoid iatrogenic hyperkalemia, potassium-conserving diuretics should not be given concurrently
with potassium supplements or with captopril (see
below, p. 578) and should be used with caution in
diabetic patients because diabetics have an increased
risk of developing hyperkalemia when they take
these diuretics. Spironolactone has a number of undesirable endocrine side effects (especially gynecomastia and, occasionally, impotence). Therefore,
amiloride or triamterene are preferable to spironolactone in male subjects.

SYMPATHOLYTIC DRUGS (in alphabetic order)

β-Blocking Drugs*

The β-blocking drugs (in alphabetical order) are:
1. *Atenolol* (general use began 1981, trade name:
   Tenormin).
2. *Metaprolol* (general use began 1978, trade name:
   Lopressor).
3. *Nadolol* (general use began 1980, trade name:
   Corgard).
4. *Propranolol* (general use began 1976, trade
   name: Inderal).

Mechanism. One or more of the following mechanisms probably accounts for the major antihypertensive effect in patients who respond to β-blocking
agents: blockade of cardiac β-receptors with a resultant decrease in cardiac output, blockade of renal β-
receptors with inhibition of renin release, blockade
of central nervous system β-receptors with a decreased sympathetic outflow, or blockade of presynaptic β-receptors with decreased release of catecholamines. Evidence of some cardiac β-receptor blockade (heart rate of 64 beats or less per min at rest and
less than 80 per min after brief exercise in the office)
is present in most patients showing a decrease in
blood pressure. However, there is no clinically useful
way to determine which blocking mechanism is dominant in responders. Propranolol and nadolol are
nonselective β-blockers while metaprolol and atenolol are *cardioselective*. The major advantage of a
cardioselective β-blocker is the relative lack of β_2-
receptor blockade. β_2-Receptors mediate bronchodilation, dilation of resistance vessels, and the sympathetic response to hypoglycemia (tachycardia, sweating).

Daily Dose Range. Dose range is as follows:

Atenolol, 50–100 mg (tablet sizes 50, 100 mg)

---

* See Table 59.7 for factors affecting selection of these drugs.

Metaprolol, 100–500 mg (tablet sizes 50, 100 mg)
Nadolol, 40–320 mg (tablet sizes 40, 80, 120 mg)
Propranolol, 40–320 mg (tablet sizes 10, 20, 40, 80 mg)

Propranolol has a continuous dose-response curve and can be used in daily amounts greater than 320 mg to control hypertension. In contrast, atenolol produces little or no additional blood pressure reduction when the daily dose exceeds 100 mg.

Schedule. Propranolol and metaprolol: twice daily. Atenolol and nadolol: once daily. In small numbers of patients metaprolol has been shown to be as effective as atenolol when given only once a day.

Onset/Resolution. For all of the β-blocking drugs, the principal blood pressure response occurs within 2 to 4 hours of taking a prescribed dose, but the full antihypertensive effect may not be seen until the patient has taken the drug for 1 week. The principal antihypertensive effect of these drugs resolves within 1 to 2 days of discontinuing the drug. Whenever a β-blocking agent is being discontinued after prolonged use, it should be tapered over 1 to 2 weeks rather than abruptly stopped, because of the possibility of provoking angina, acute rebound to pretreatment blood pressure levels, or a number of other problems (e.g., anxiety, tachycardia, palpitations, tremor, perspiration, or increase in headaches in patients with migraine).

When switching a patient from one β-blocker to another, the following information should be used: equivalent daily nadolol doses are about 40 mg lower than propranolol doses and about 80% of metaprolol doses; β-blocking doses of metaprolol and propranolol are generally similar; and most patients exhibit β-blockade at a single dose, 50 mg, of atenolol.

Side Effects. The most common side effects are nausea, mild sedation, and fatigue. Sexual impotence has been reported occasionally. Of note is the fact that hypertensive athletes tolerate β-blocking agents well. With certain coexisting conditions, the β-blocking properties of these drugs may cause serious side effects. Absolute contraindications to the use of β-blockers are: severe bradycardia, low cardiac output, high degree heart block, severe asthma or chronic obstructive pulmonary disease, and severe peripheral vascular disease (e.g., gangrene, skin necrosis, severe or worsening claudication). For patients with mild asthma or chronic obstructive pulmonary disease, stable peripheral vascular disease, or stable insulin-requiring diabetes, low doses of the cardioselective agents, metaprolol and atenolol, may be safe and effective. It is recommended that a selective β_2-bronchodilator (see Chapter 52) be used concurrently whenever a β-blocking agent is prescribed for a patient with asthma or obstructive pulmonary disease.

Combination with Other Antihypertensive Drugs. The addition of the vasodilators hydralazine and minoxidil to β-blocking agents is often very effective. The combination of propranolol (and presumably other β-blockers) with prazosin or with methyldopa is also effective when there is only a partial response to either drug.

Clonidine (general use began 1975, trade name: Catapres)*

Mechanism. Evidence suggests that clonidine acts as an α-adrenergic stimulator which decreases sympathetic activity in the medulla oblongata, thereby diminishing sympathetic outflow to the peripheral vasculature. Clonidine suppresses renin release, but a relationship between this property and its antihypertensive effect has not been established.

Daily Dose Range. Range is 0.2 to 2.4 mg (tablet sizes: 0.1, 0.2, 0.3 mg).

Schedule. Twice daily. In contrast to methyldopa, the hypotensive effect of clonidine does not last 24 hours in patients given their total dose once daily.

Onset/Resolution. The major antihypertensive response occurs within 1 hour and remits after 8 to 16 hours. Because of the rapid onset of action, oral clonidine can be given hourly in doses of 0.1 or 0.2 mg in order to determine rapidly the dose needed to treat an individual patient. This property may be of value in the symptom-free patient with a very high pressure if blood pressure-lowering within a few hours is desired; however, apart from hypertensive emergencies, requiring hospitalization and parenteral treatment (see p. 567 above), there are no absolute indications for such rapid lowering of the blood pressure.

In a minority of patients, rapid *rebound to pretreatment blood pressure* with accompanying symptoms of increased sympathetic nervous system activity (tachycardia, perspiration, headache, palpitations) follows abrupt discontinuation of clonidine. Treatment for this problem is reinstitution of the drug. As there is no way to predict the few patients in danger of this severe reaction, all patients must be regarded as "at risk." In selecting antihypertensive drugs, patients known to be erratic in medication-taking should not receive clonidine, and all patients initiating clonidine therapy should be warned explicitly of the risk of discontinuing the drug.

Side Effects. The most common side effects are sedation, dry mouth, constipation, and orthostatic symptoms. Impotence has been reported. There are no absolute contraindications to the use of clonidine.

Combination with Other Antihypertensive Drugs: In a small number of reported patients, clonidine has been used with hydralazine to prevent the reflex sympathetic response to hydralazine (see p. 578). This combination is useful in patients needing Step III drugs who cannot take the more widely studied combination of β-blocking drugs and hydralazine,

---

* See Table 59.7 for factors affecting selection of this drug.

such as patients with a history of bronchospasm. Synergy between clonidine and prazosin has also been demonstrated.

Guanethidine (general use began 1959, trade name: Ismelin)*

Mechanism. Guanethidine depletes the stores of norepinephrine in peripheral tissues, but not in the central nervous system. Its hypotensive action is ascribed to the loss of sympathetic regulation of vessel tone in the venules and arterioles of the peripheral vascular system. Because its hypotensive property depends predominantly upon impaired venous tone, the effects of guanethidine are always more pronounced when patients are standing, particularly after exercise.

Daily Dose Range. Range is 10 to 200 mg (tablet sizes: 10, 25 mg). Guanethidine has a continuous dose-response curve and no established upper dose limit.

Schedule. Once daily.

Onset/Resolution. The major antihypertensive effect occurs within 3 to 5 days and remits within 1 to 2 weeks of discontinuing the drug.

Side Effects. Orthostatic exaggeration of the hypotensive response severely limits the usefulness of guanethidine. As shown in Table 59.8, many guanethidine-treated patients show one of two unsatisfactory patterns: a high resting pressure and an unacceptably low pressure after exercise or an unacceptably high resting pressure and a normal pressure after exercise. In addition, sexual dysfunction in male patients (impairment of ejaculation and/or erection) and diarrhea are very common.

Because of the risk associated with orthostatic hypotension and the availability of two new Step IV drugs, minoxidil and captopril, the initiation of guanethidine can almost always be avoided in the management of hypertension. Patients who currently take guanethidine should be monitored carefully, and an alternative drug should be considered whenever there is any suggestion that the exaggerated orthostasis is producing symptoms.

Combination with Other Antihypertensive Drugs. Guanethidine has been used effectively as a sympatholytic drug in conjunction with hydralazine. Because of its undesirable side effects, it provides no advantage over the other sympatholytic drugs which have been tested with hydralazine (β-blockers, clonidine, reserpine).

Methyldopa (general use began 1962, trade name: Aldomet)*

Mechanism. Recent evidence indicates that the derivative of methyldopa, methylnorepinephrine, displaces norepinephrine in the central nervous system and that the hypotensive effect of methyldopa is related to this process. Methyldopa suppresses renin

---

* See Table 59.7 for factors affecting selection of this drug.

Table 59.8
Blood Pressures of 16 Consecutive Patients Receiving Guanethidine, at Their Most Recent Visit[a]

Patient	Resting	Standing	Standing after Exercise	Guanethidine Dose[b] (mg)
1	190/120	140/114	124/94	50
2	210/132	134/100	100/84	50
3	170/120	170s/100	130/80	50
4	160/100	150/100	130/84	10
5	208/110	126/90	100/70	50
6	142/100	120/90	114/84	50
7	190/108	160/110	160/104	75
8	180/92	120/80	110/60	100
9	156/108	160/108	150/96	75
10	164/100	154/94	150/82	75
11	240/100	220/88	170/70	60
12	150/110	140/105	140/100	50
13	140/100	130/96	125/85	37.5
14	170/105	140/110	130/100	25
15	170/120	140/110	150/100	20
16	194/120	168/116	144/112	150

[a] From L. R. Barker: Guanethidine, exercise, and hypotension. *Lancet, 2:* 1297, 1976.
[b] All patients also on a diuretic.

release, but a relationship of this property to its antihypertensive action has not been clearly established.

Daily Dose Range. Range is 250 to 3000 mg (tablet sizes: 250, 500 mg). Although this dose range is publicized frequently, additional hypotensive response is rarely attained with doses greater than 2000 mg. Over long intervals of continuous treatment (*i.e.*, 10 years), most patients require a gradual increase in their daily dose of methyldopa to maintain satisfactory blood pressure control.

Schedule. Twice daily. In studies of small numbers of patients, the antihypertensive effect has persisted for 24 hours regardless of whether the daily dose was given on a 4 times daily, 3 times daily, twice daily, or once daily (at bed time) schedule. For patients who comply poorly or who experience side effects after daytime doses of methyldopa, a trial of a single daily dose at bed time is worthwhile.

Onset/Resolution. The major antihypertensive effect occurs within 4 to 6 hours of oral administration, and the hypotensive response remits within 1 to 2 days. Rapid rebound to pretreatment pressures, with or without symptoms, has been reported in a few patients after abrupt discontinuation of methyldopa.

Side Effects. The most common side effects are orthostatic symptoms, mood alteration, impotence (erectile dysfunction), and diarrhea (soft stools, 2 to 4 times daily). There are no absolute contraindications to the use of methyldopa.

Combination with Other Antihypertensive Drugs. The combination of methyldopa and propranolol is more effective than either drug alone. In patients who show a partial response to one of these drugs, adding a small amount of the other may at times be more practical than starting a different drug. This is especially true in the patient who may have failed to respond to two or more Step II drugs. Synergy between methyldopa and prazosin has also been demonstrated.

Prazosin (general use began 1976, trade name: Minipress)*

Mechanism. Prazosin blocks postsynaptic α-receptors in arterioles and venules, presumably decreasing blood pressure by impairing sympathetic tone at both sites. Prazosin does not block presynaptic α-receptors. This may explain why prazosin does not cause tachycardia and renin release, as both of these adaptive responses to blood pressure lowering are inhibited by activation of the presynaptic α-receptors.

Daily Dose Range. Range is 2 to 20 mg (capsule size: 1, 2, 5 mg). Although 20 mg is the recommended upper limit for hypertension, an additional antihypertensive effect may be attained at higher doses (up to 80 mg daily); in the patient with hypertension refractory to other drugs, a trial of high dose prazosin is therefore worthwhile.

Schedule. Twice daily. In a few carefully studied subjects, the antihypertensive effect has been shown to persist for 24 hours when the entire daily dose is taken at one time; this unconventional schedule can be tried in responders who comply poorly with a twice daily schedule.

Onset/Resolution. The major antihypertensive response occurs within 2 hours and remits after 24 hours.

Side Effects. The most common side effects are postural hypotension, headache, drowsiness, dry mouth, and palpitations. Sexual impotence is very uncommon.

Postural hypotension, usually without tachycardia and at times asymptomatic, occurs as a transient problem in up to half of patients during the first few days on prazosin. *Syncope* occurring within ½ hour after the initial dose of prazosin is a very rare, but severe, side effect. It may occur after taking a 1-mg dose. Clearly, warning and reassurance about postural symptoms (for the first few days) is important whenever this drug is prescribed. In addition, patients should either take their initial dose in the office (and be observed for about 1 hour) or they should be instructed to take it at bedtime, so that they will be recumbent during the initial adjustment to the drug. There are no absolute contraindications to the use of prazosin.

Combination with Other Antihypertensive Drugs. The combination of prazosin and a β-blocker is frequently effective in patients with severe hyperten-

sion which does not respond to either drug alone. Synergism has also been reported with clonidine, methyldopa and hydralazine.

The use of prazosin in the ambulatory management of congestive heart failure is discussed in Chapter 58.

Reserpine (general use began 1952)*

Mechanism. Chronic administration of reserpine depletes the stores of catecholamines in many tissues, probably by impairing the uptake of essential precursors. The antihypertensive effect is attributed to impaired uptake centrally and peripherally of dopamine, a precursor for the intracellular synthesis of norepinephrine.

Daily Dose Range. Range is 0.1 to 0.5 mg (tablet sizes: 0.1, 0.25 mg, generic available). Doses larger than 0.50 mg may further lower the blood pressure, but such doses produce excessive drowsiness in most patients and frank depression in a few.

Schedule. Once daily.

Onset/Resolution. The major antihypertensive effect occurs within 1 to 2 weeks and remits within 1 to 2 weeks of stopping the drug.

Side Effects. Frank depression occurs in some patients, and decrease in mental alertness is common. Both are dose-related. Nasal and gastric hypersecretion occurs at therapeutic doses and may produce nasal stuffiness or dyspepsia. An association between reserpine and breast carcinoma, reported in 1974, was not confirmed by carefully controlled observations. Because of the significant incidence of side effects and the availability of less offensive second step drugs, reserpine has not been recommended prominently in recent years. Two definite contraindications are history of peptic ulcer or depression.

Combination with Other Antihypertensive Drugs. In the Veterans Administration controlled trial (see above, p. 562), the combination of reserpine, hydralazine, and hydrochlorothiazide was shown to be highly effective. These three drugs are available in a fixed-dose combination tablet (Ser-Ap-Es) which contains 0.10 mg of reserpine, 25 mg of hydralazine, and 15 mg of hydrochlorothiazide.

VASODILATORS

Hydralazine (general use began 1951, trade name: Apresoline)*

Mechanism. Hydralazine directly relaxes smooth muscle in resistance vessels (arterioles and small arteries); it has a similar but lesser effect on capacitance vessels (venules and small veins). Secondary effects are a stimulation of renin release and a reflex increase in activity of the sympathetic nervous system (tachycardia, palpitations, headache, increased angina). Because of this property, hydralazine is recommended as a Step III drug to be added to a regimen containing a sympathetic inhibitor.

Daily Dose Range. Range is 20 to 400 mg (tablet

---

* See Table 59.7 for factors affecting selection of this drug.

sizes: 10, 25, 50, 100 mg, generic available). An upper limit of 200 mg is sometimes recommended because the risk of hydralazine-induced lupus increases at higher doses. However, 400 mg or more may be effective and appropriate in patients with severe hypertension who are difficult to control.

Schedule. Twice daily. If there is evidence that an individual patient's response does not persist for 12 hours, a 3 times daily schedule may be required. Hydralazine should be taken with meals, as absorption is maximal with food and blood pressure response may be erratic if the drug is taken irregularly with respect to eating.

Onset/Resolution. The major antihypertensive response occurs within 2 to 4 hours and remits within 12 to 24 hours.

Side Effects. The most common side effects (headache, palpitations, tachycardia) are seen when hydralazine is given without a sympathetic inhibitor. The uncommon but widely publicized lupus-like hydralazine syndrome has the following features in most affected subjects: occurs after 6 or more months of exposure to 200 mg or more daily, begins as new arthritis or arthralgia, rarely affects the kidneys, stimulates the production of antinuclear antibodies, and remits entirely within 6 months of discontinuing hydralazine. There are a number of other uncommon toxic reactions to hydralazine; but when used as a Step III drug, hydralazine is generally very well tolerated. There are no absolute contraindications to hydralazine when used in combination with a sympatholytic drug.

Combination with Other Antihypertensive Drugs. When hydralazine is added to any sympatholytic drug, the hypertension responds well in the majority of patients who are not controlled with the sympatholytic drug alone. The addition of hydralazine to one of the sympatholytic β-blocking agents is widely practiced, both because of the effectiveness of this combination and the predictable protection against reflex sympatholytic activity which the β-blockers provide. Synergism between hydralazine and prazosin has also been documented.

Minoxidil (general use began 1980, trade name: Loniten)*

Mechanism. Minoxidil relaxes arteriolar smooth muscle and is thus a peripheral vasodilator. Like hydralazine, it stimulates renin release and induces reflex hyperactivity of the sympathetic nervous system. Therefore, the patient should always be on an adequate dose of a sympatholytic drug (usually a β-blocker) before minoxidil is initiated.

Daily Dose Range. Range is 5 to 40 mg (tablet size: 2.5, 10 mg). Daily doses greater than 40 mg (up to 100 mg) may be effective. Because of its extraordinary potency, minoxidil should be initiated at a trial dose

of 2.5 mg; dose increases can be made daily until a response occurs.

Schedule. Once or twice daily. When minoxidil is being substituted for another drug (hydralazine for example), this drug should be continued until a response to minoxidil occurs; then the other drug should be gradually discontinued while the minoxidil dose is increased.

Onset/Resolution. The major antihypertensive effect occurs within 1 to 3 hours and remits within 1 to 2 days.

Side Effects. Fluid retention, often marked, occurs as a consequence of the hypotensive action of the drug; furosemide should be given in a dose adequate to eliminate the problem. Most patients develop hirsutism within 1 month of starting minoxidil, limiting greatly its usefulness in women. There are no other common side effects. Because the drug is relatively new, it is possible that additional problems will appear after more extensive use.

Combination with Other Antihypertensive Drugs. Like hydralazine, minoxidil should always be used in conjunction with a sympatholytic drug. All minoxidil studies to date have utilized β-blockers. Presumably the other sympatholytics which are effective with hydralazine (clonidine and reserpine) are also effective with minoxidil.

ANGIOTENSIN CONVERTING ENZYME INHIBITOR*

Captopril (general use began 1981, trade name: Capoten)

Captopril was approved for use in the United States in 1981. Because of the limited general experience with this drug and because of the risk of serious adverse effects, this drug should be utilized only in patients who do not respond to or cannot tolerate drugs in Steps I to III (see Fig. 59.7). Captopril offers an important advantage in the treatment of women refractory to Step III drugs, for whom minoxidil is usually unacceptable because of hirsuitism.

Mechanism. The blood pressure-lowering effect of captopril is attributed to the diminution of the concentration of the endogenous pressor, angiotensin II. Captopril inhibits the enzymatic conversion of angiotensin I to angiotensin II. The drug does not cross the blood-brain barrier, and its antihypertensive action is therefore strictly a peripheral effect.

Daily Dose Range. Range is 75 to 450 mg (tablet size: 25, 50, 100 mg). The drug should be initiated in a trial dose of 25 mg, 3 times daily. When it is being substituted for other drugs, these should either be discontinued or gradually tapered while captopril is being introduced. The dose of captopril may be increased daily in a patient with severe hypertension.

Schedule. Three times daily, at least 1 hour before meals (absorption is imparied when the drug is taken with meals).

Onset/Resolution. The major antihypertensive ef-

---

* See Table 59.7 for factors affecting selection of this drug.

fect occurs within a few hours of a dose and remits within 1 day. The full impact of a dose is seen after 1 to 2 weeks at that dose.

Side Effects. The commonest side effects of captopril are maculopapular rash and alteration of taste (decrease, total loss, or unpleasant taste). Both effects occur in 5 to 10% of persons within the first 1 to 2 months of use; both remit with either a temporary decrease in dose or discontinuation of the drug. The most serious adverse reactions are proteinuria and neutropenia. Proteinuria (equal or greater than 1 g per 24 hours) occurs in 1 to 2% of patients during the first year of treatment. In most cases, proteinuria subsides or resolves within 6 months even if captopril is continued. Patients should be monitored for proteinuria before treatment and monthly for the first year of treatment; if it develops, the risks and benefits of continuing treatment must be considered in the individual patient. Neutropenia occurs in less than 1% of patients, within 12 weeks of starting the drug; it remits promptly with discontinuation. The neutropenia develops gradually; therefore, it is prudent to obtain a white blood cell count every 2 weeks for the first 3 months of treatment. Patients should be warned to report any signs of infection during this period.

Combination with Other Antihypertensive Drugs. Like other antihypertensive drugs, the action of captopril is enhanced by concurrent use of a diuretic. Captopril prevents secondary hyperaldosteronism, which is dependent upon angiotensin II. This property has two important implications regarding diuretics: First, potassium-conserving diuretics should not be utilized in conjunction with captopril, as this combination increases the risk of hyperkalemia; and second, the development of hypokalemia is less likely during concurrent treatment with thiazide or loop diuretics, and potassium supplements should be given only for well-documented hypokalemia, with careful monitoring to avoid hyperkalemia. In general, captopril should not be used with agents affecting sympathetic activity as the sympathetic nervous system may be especially important in supporting the blood pressure in the event of acute hypotension. Theoretically, captopril may add to the antihypertensive effect of vasodilators (hydralazine and minoxidil), and this combination would be reasonable for a patient with very resistant hypertension.

Nonpharmacologic Aspects of Treatment

Four nonpharmacologic modalities may promote lowering of blood pressure: sodium restriction, weight reduction, physical exercise (sufficient to achieve the conditioning effect—see Chapter 55), and various techniques combining psychologic and physical relaxation (3, 17, 19, 22). All four have been shown to enhance the blood pressure lowering effect of antihypertensive drugs. Only weight reduction in obese subjects (19) and marked sodium restriction (meaning less than 1 g of sodium daily) (17) have been shown to control chronic hypertension. Because each of these four modalities requires significant changes in life-style, it is generally more difficult to achieve long term adherence to them than to drug treatment. Nevertheless, in initiating care for the individual patient, one or more of these modalities should be recommended as an adjunct to drug treatment. For highly motivated patients with mild or moderate hypertension, one or more of these can be tried as primary treatment.

WEIGHT REDUCTION AND SODIUM RESTRICTION

In 1979, the National High Blood Pressure Coordinating Committee published the following practical recommendations for weight reduction and sodium restriction in the care of and prevention of hypertension:

Weight Reduction:
1. Weight reduction should be considered routinely in the treatment of overweight borderline hypertensives, both for its potential in lowering blood pressure and for its general health benefits.
2. Practitioners should encourage weight reduction for the obese hypertensive patient, and if blood pressure is reduced to and maintained at normal levels, it should be used as definitive therapy.
3. For overweight patients who experience significant side effects from drugs, weight reduction should be considered as adjunctive therapy to help reduce drug dosages.
4. Persons with a family history of hypertension should avoid excessive weight gain and should reduce if overweight.
5. Prevention or control of obesity in the young should be regarded as having positive health benefits and as a possible preventive step for hypertension.

Chapter 73 contains a full discussion of obesity and its treatment.

Sodium Restriction:
1. Moderate sodium restriction (2 to 4 g daily) should be routinely prescribed and if blood pressure is reduced to and maintained at normal levels, it should be used as definitive therapy.
2. For patients who experience significant side effects from drugs, sodium restriction should be considered as adjunctive therapy to help reduce drug dosages or increase drug efficacy.
3. Persons with a family history of hypertension should be encouraged to restrict sodium intake even though they may not be hypertensive.
4. Practitioners recommending sodium restriction should indicate specific diets appropriate to each patient's condition and life-style and should ensure that the diet is explained satisfactorily.

Table 59.9 summarizes what the patient should know in order to follow a low salt (2- to 4-g sodium—"no-added-salt") diet.

EXERCISE AND RELAXATION

Similar guidelines have not been promulgated for physical exercise and relaxation techniques. Inexpensive books explaining how to engage in conditioning, or aerobic, exercise are readily available for the layperson; the physiologic basis for the conditioning effect is described in Chapter 55. The essential components of relaxation techniques are described in Chapter 12.

Although physicians may choose to try one of these as initial treatment for selected patients, they should inform all patients of the *implications of hypertension and antihypertensive drug therapy for ordinary physical activity*. Studies have shown that subjects with untreated hypertension have the same patterns of blood pressure fluctuation as normotensive subjects, only at higher pressures: with vigorous exercise, the systolic pressure rises (as much as 60 mm Hg) while the diastolic pressure does not change significantly; during sleep, systolic and diastolic pressure fall; and during an average day the blood pressure fluctuates over a systolic range of 20 to 40 mm Hg and a diastolic range of 10 to 20 mg Hg (12). Similar patterns have been found in patients being treated for hypertension with β-blocking drugs (31) and the combination of β-blockers and hydralazine (15); patterns have not yet been reported in patients taking other types of antihypertensive drugs. The impact of antihypertensives and other cardiovascular drugs on blood pressure during exercise is summarized in Chapter 55, Table 55.8. Overall, it is reasonable for the physician to inform his patient that hypertension does not make a person "different" and to reassure each patient that he can engage in all of his usual activities after beginning treatment for hypertension.

Table 59.9
Example of Information Given to Patients for Whom a Salt-Restricted Diet Is Recommended

You have been asked to regulate the salt in your diet. This is necessary to help control high blood pressure and/or to decrease excess body fluid which can result from many causes.

Years ago we had no medicines to decrease excess body fluid. It was necessary to restrict severely salt intake for this purpose. This strict diet was tasteless and expensive for the patient. Today we have medicines to help. It is no longer necessary for you to change all your eating habits.

It is important that you eat *less* salt than the average person, and that you eat essentially the *same amount of salt each day*. You will need to do the following things:

1. Do not add salt to your food at the table and use little salt in cooking. For most people, it is acceptable to use a salt substitute, but you should ask to be sure it is alright for you.
2. Do not eat foods that taste salty, such as pretzels and potato chips.
3. Know which foods are high in salt and avoid eating them or eat them only on special occasions, in small amounts. The following list should be of help:

MEATS:	*CONDIMENTS:*
Any meat smoked, cured or preserved in brine bacon	Meat tenderizer
Bacon	MSG "Accent"
Cold cuts	Celery salt
Cured beef	Garlic salt
Dried or chipped beef	Onion salt
Ham	Ketchup
Frankfurter	Mustard
Kidney	Pickles and relishes
Salt pork	Soy sauce and other commercial sauces
FISH:	*SNACK FOODS:*
Any canned, frozen, smoked, or cured fish	Potato chips
Anchovies	Pretzels
Sardines	Salted nuts
Salted cod fish	Olives
Smoked salmon, Herring, etc.	Salted peanut butter
	MISCELLANEOUS:
	Bicarbonate of soda
	Buttermilk
	Sauerkraut
	Tomato juice
	Cheese, except unsalted cottage cheese
	Seaweed

Most "fast foods" have added salt.

The following may have added salt (read the label):
Diet gelatin, sugar substitutes, canned vegetables.
Diet sodas have higher salt than regular sodas.

Remember: It is better to eat the same amount of salt each day rather than eat very little salt 1 day and several high salt foods the next.

Problems in the Course of Treatment

There are three problems which will occur during the long term treatment of most patients with hypertension: the need for adjustment of the antihypertensive regimen, instability in blood pressure control, and intercurrent or concurrent morbidity.

MEDICATION ADJUSTMENT

Within 2 to 3 months of initiating treatment, the average patient will have satisfactory blood pressure control. In the ensuing months and years, minor or major changes in the medical regimen will be needed for most patients. Each medication change requires the patient to learn a new habit and contains the potential for medication error. Therefore, whenever a medication adjustment is contemplated, the reason should be well-established. If the reason is loss of blood pressure control, this should be confirmed at two or more visits; if the reason is a possible drug side effect, this should also be confirmed at serial visits in some instances. When the adjustment involves a drug the patient is already taking, it is critical to *write down the change* for the patient, to avoid confusion with instructions on the current medication bottle.

INSTABILITY IN BLOOD PRESSURE CONTROL

Most patients have inadequate blood pressure control at an occasional visit during long term follow-up.

At those visits, the physician can usually identify the probable cause and design a plan to restore blood pressure control. A prompt follow-up visit should always be part of this plan. The differential diagnosis for instability in blood pressure control is summarized in Table 59.10, divided into common and uncommon causes.

Noncompliance. Noncompliance can be identified by review of medication taking. An effective way to approach this is illustrated in the discussion of interviewing skills in Chapter 1, pp. 12 and 13.

At certain times, the patient will simply omit the medication on the day of the visit. On the other hand, the patient may be taking medication faithfully but incorrectly. Because this may be due to an error in dispensing of medication, the physician should routinely check the patient's medication bottle.

History-taking is obviously important. If the patient has deliberately discontinued a medication, he will often explain his reasons.

If the patient denies noncompliance, this can be checked by having the patient take his medicine under supervision in the office and then measuring his blood pressure response for several hours.

Increased Salt Consumption. A significant increase in salt consumption may lead to a positive sodium balance, which can blunt the effects of antihypertensive drugs. This problem is not uncommon in the summer months. It should be expected whenever loss of blood pressure control is associated with a weight gain of 1 kg or more, with or without edema. Brief review of the patient's current diet will often substantiate this hypothesis. Management consists of having the patient resume moderate sodium restriction or substituting more potent diuretic treatment. Temporary use of furosemide (40 to 80 mg daily for 1 or more weeks) to eliminate excess sodium is often useful in this situation.

For patients in whom sodium overload is a recurrent problem, furosemide in doses adjusted to maintain a stable weight is very effective.

Psychologic Stress. In the patient who is adhering faithfully to treatment, psychologic stress may explain his failure to respond as usual to antihypertensive drugs. This is probably because increase in sympathetic nervous system activity is associated with psychologic stress.

Stress may be associated only with visits to a physician's office and the rise in blood pressure may be strictly transient. This problem can be minimized by assuring that the patient is at ease before taking the blood pressure and by repeating the measurement later in the visit if the initial pressure is high. When stress is suspected to result in erratic office blood pressures, blood pressure measurements taken at home by the patient or another responsible person provide better information for judging the effectiveness of treatment, and may spare patients from inappropriate increases in antihypertensive drugs and the associated side effects.

Psychologic stress may also be due to serious job- or family-related crisis. Brief inquiry may reveal additional stress-related symptoms, such as headache, dyspepsia, sleeplessness, irritability, etc. In such patients, management consists of supportive counseling and, at times, short term prescription of minor tranquilizers (see Chapter 12). This is the one situation in which minor tranquilizers may contribute to blood pressure control.

Concurrent Medications. A number of commonly prescribed and over-the-counter medications (Table 59.11) may attenuate the response to antihypertensive drugs. Therefore, inquiry about concurrent medications is always important in assessing unstable blood pressure control. Hypertensive patients should be told which common drugs are contraindicated, and that chronic use of drugs such as nonsteroidal anti-inflammatory agents and over-the-counter decongestants requires careful supervision of blood pressure.

Tolerance. With the possible exception of methyldopa, the development of tolerance to antihypertensive drugs has not been demonstrated. Therefore, whenever a patient appears to become "tolerant" to a drug which worked well initially, other causes of unstable blood pressure control should be sought.

After a number of years of taking methyldopa, many patients require larger amounts of the drug to maintain adequate blood pressure control. This find-

Table 59.10
Differential Diagnosis of Instability in Blood Pressure Control

COMMON CAUSES:
 Noncompliance
 Increased salt consumption
 Psychologic stress
UNCOMMON CAUSES:
 Concurrent medications
 Tolerance
 Refractory hypertension

Table 59.11
Medications Which May Attenuate Response to Antihypertensive Drugs

PROMOTES POSITIVE SODIUM BALANCE:
 Nonsteroidal anti-inflammatory drugs
 Corticosteroids
 Estrogens
 Sodium-containing antacids
SYMPATHOMIMETIC:
 Decongestants (oral)
 Amphetamines
 Bronchodilators
MECHANISM NOT ESTABLISHED:
 Tricyclic antidepressants
 Phenothiazines
 Monoamine oxidase inhibitors
 Oral contraceptives

ing may signify the development of true tolerance, or it may signify progressive hypertension. If the latter explanation is correct, a similar need for higher doses may be found with the other Step II drugs after they have been in general use for 10 or more years.

Refractory Hypertension. Rarely, a patient's blood pressure may become refractory to previously effective drugs, and none of the above causes will be found. In such patients, two questions must be answered:

1. *Is the hypertension really refractory to the patient's usual medication?* This question can be answered best by a brief hospital admission to ensure that the patient receives his medications correctly; because of the blood pressure lowering effect of bed rest, patients should be encouraged to remain active while in the hospital. Alternatively, supervision of medication-taking and blood pressure response in the office or at home by a nurse may suffice. It is usually found that these patients were failing to take their medication correctly, and that, under supervision, they respond appropriately.

2. *What is the reason?* (For the occasional patient whose refractory hypertension is confirmed.) Confirmed refractory hypertension in a previously responding patient strongly suggests that one of the causes of secondary hypertension is present. Evaluation for these will disclose a surgical cause (especially renovascular hypertension) for some patients. For those without surgically treatable hypertension, an effective drug regimen can almost always be found.

Occasionally, a newly diagnosed patient treated by the stepped method fails to respond to a variety of drugs and doses. This apparent primary refractoriness to antihypertensive drugs should also be evaluated by hospital or home supervision. For those patients found to be refractory to a variety of Step II or Step III regimens, one of the following three strategies usually works:

1. Use of a Step IV drug, minoxidil or captopril.
2. Use of high dose furosemide in conjunction with a Step II or Step III regimen.
3. Use of high dose prazosin.

CO-MORBIDITY

During long term treatment, most hypertensive patients will have acute or chronic conditions which require judicious adjustment of their antihypertensive drugs. For patients with selected chronic conditions, one or more antihypertensive drugs may be inappropriate, as summarized in Table 59.7. In this section we review those conditions which require extra caution with *any* antihypertensive drug regimen.

Acute Illness

From time to time, each patient with hypertension will have an intercurrent acute illness. The following

factors which increase a person's sensitivity to antihypertensive drugs may accompany some of those intercurrent illnesses:

1. Daily intake of all food, including salt, may be temporarily decreased.
2. The patient may be at bed rest for several days to several weeks. In previously healthy individuals, it has been demonstrated that bed rest for more than a few days produces a modest reduction in recumbent blood pressures and a marked reduction in standing blood pressure.
3. In patients with recurrent vomiting or diarrhea, fluid and electrolyte deficits may occur.
4. Hypotension, presumably due to vasodilation, may occur during febrile illnesses.

Short term decrease or withholding of antihypertensive drugs will protect such patients from the additional morbidity brought by hypotension or electrolyte depletion. Resumption of the full antihypertensive regimen should await return of the patient's hypertension. In some situations, for example following major surgery, the previous regimen may not be needed for 1 or more months.

Concurrent Chronic Illness

Cerebrovascular Disease. Hypertensive patients with suspected or known cerebral atherosclerosis should have their blood pressure lowered carefully to avoid hypoperfusion of an already compromised vascular network. Patients who develop typical orthostatic symptoms despite standing blood pressures in the "normal" range should have a trial of lower dose treatment or no treatment to determine whether positional cerebral ischemia is present.

In patients with completed strokes, controlled studies of antihypertensive treatment have shown both a reduction or no reduction in the occurrence of second strokes; these studies have not reported the incidence of other hypertensive morbidity in poststroke patients, particularly congestive heart failure, which should be reduced by antihypertensive treatment. Therefore, patients who remain hypertensive after their neurologic status has stabilized should be treated.

Coronary Artery Disease. In the hypertensive patient with angina pectoris, management of the angina always includes adequate blood pressure control.

The hypertensive patient who has a myocardial infarction may have a normal blood pressure or less severe hypertension during convalescence. Because this may be transient, the blood pressure should be evaluated at least monthly in the first 3 to 4 months after discharge.

Diabetes. In the patient with coexisting diabetes, consistent control of hyperglycemia will prevent erratic responses to antihypertensive drugs; the diabetic patient who periodically develops volume deficits from osmotic diuresis risks symptomatic hypotension. In the sizable subgroup of diabetics who have postural hypotension due to diabetic neuropathy, the risk of exaggerated hypotension accompanies any antihypertensive regimen; the orthostatic pressure and not the recumbent pressure should be monitored to determine the response to therapy in these and other patients with baseline orthostasis.

Asthma. In the hypertensive patient with coexisting asthma, blood pressure elevation may accompany episodes of increased bronchospasm. This may occur in untreated hypertensives as well as in those whose blood pressures are usually controlled on antihypertensive drugs. In treated patients, restoration of blood pressure control depends upon improvement in the asthma and not upon increased antihypertensive medications. As noted in Table 59.7, hypertensive patients with a history of bronchospasm should not receive β-adrenergic blocking agents.

PREPLANNED SURGERY (see Chapter 83)

HYPERTENSION IN ADOLESCENTS AND YOUNG ADULTS

Adolescents and young adults have not been included in the major studies of the epidemiology and treatment of hypertension. In recent years, preliminary findings about the natural history of hypertension in this age group and recommendations for management have been published. (See symposium on high blood pressure in the young (Kotchen and Havlik) in "General References.")

Epidemiology

A single longitudinal study, in Evans County, Georgia, has provided information about the prevalence of hypertension and the incidence of new hypertension in adolescents and young adults (28). The study utilized a probability sample of the population between the ages of 15 and 24 at entry. Hypertension was defined as an average of three diastolic blood pressure readings of 90 mm Hg or greater. At entry in 1960, the overall *prevalence of hypertension* was 14.6% (3.0% for subjects 15 through 19 years of age and 20.6% for subjects 20 through 24 years of age). The follow-up study in 1976, when all subjects were in their third or fourth decade, showed an overall prevalence of hypertension of 26.4%; during 16 years there was a 26% *incidence of new hypertension* for those 15 to 19 years old at entry and a 12% incidence for those 20 to 24 years old at entry. Overweight status and the development of obesity correlated highly with prevalence and incidence of hypertension, respectively. A small percentage of those hypertensive at entry had a normal blood pressure at follow-up; presumably they had labile hypertension when first examined.

In addition to prevalence and incidence rates, this study has yielded preliminary data on *long term morbidity* in the young adult with hypertension. During the first 10 years of follow-up (before the publication of the Veterans Administration study results), none of the hypertensive subjects was treated. An interim study in 1968 disclosed that a number of those hypertensive at entry had developed cardiovascular events attributable to hypertension. The 16-year follow-up in 1976 disclosed a much higher incidence of electrocardiographic abnormalities in those hypertensive at entry compared to those normotensive at entry.

Other epidemiologic studies of hypertension in young adults have indicated that labile hypertension may be more common than sustained hypertension in teenagers; that there is a striking incidence of sustained new hypertension between the ages of 15 and 25; and that most young adults with sustained hypertension have essential hypertension. The guidelines for baseline evaluation and for suspecting secondary hypertension are therefore the same as those summarized earlier (pp. 569–570). Oral contraceptive treatment is a particularly important etiology to consider in the baseline evaluation of all young women with hypertension (see below, p. 587).

Recommendations

In 1977, the National High Blood Pressure Coordinating Committee made the following recommendations for managing adolescent hypertension:

All adolescents with blood pressure levels above the 95th percentile (see Fig. 59.8) and a diastolic pressure of less than 100 mm Hg should receive the following surveillance and counseling:

1. Periodic blood pressure determination.
2. Advice on weight reduction, if needed.
3. Avoidance of salt abuse (placement on a moderate salt-restricted diet—5 g per day for teenagers, less for younger children).
4. Encouragement to be physically active.
5. Encouragement to discontinue smoking cigarettes (nonsmokers should be discouraged from starting the habit).
6. Examination for other risk factors (i.e., serum lipids, glucose, etc.).

All patients with sustained diastolic pressures of 100 mm Hg or greater should receive drug treatment by the stepped method. Methyldopa and β-blocking agents are recommended as Step II drugs.

For those patients whose diastolic pressure remains in the range 90 to 100 mm Hg after 1 year of nonpharmacologic management, drug treatment should be strongly considered.

Because of the psychologic and social stresses associated with adolescence, the care of a chronic condition such as hypertension requires special considerations in this age group (see Chapter 5).

HYPERTENSION IN OLDER PATIENTS

Physicians frequently find sustained hypertension in their older patients. This is not surprising in light of the data summarized above in Figure 59.1. In 1979, the National High Blood Pressure Coordinating Com-

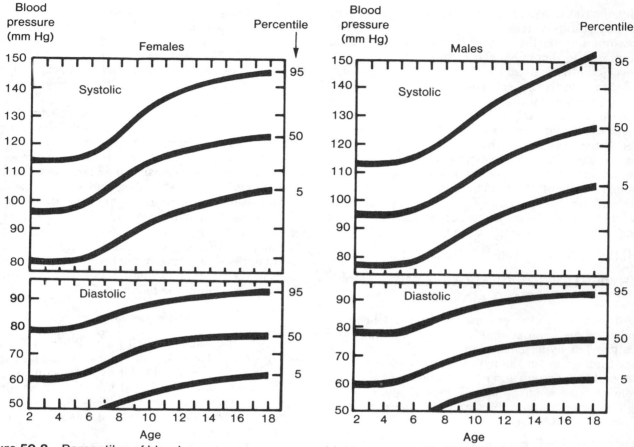

Figure 59.8   Percentiles of blood pressure measurement (right arm, seated). (Source: Report of the Task Force on Blood Pressure Control in Children. *Pediatrics, 59* (Supplement): 803, 1977.)

mittee announced its recommendations for the treatment of two subgroups of older patients with hypertension: those with systolic-diastolic hypertension; and those with isolated systolic hypertension (considered in the following section).

Recommendations

For older individuals with sustained diastolic pressures of 105 mm Hg or greater, stepped treatment to a goal pressure of 90 mm Hg or less is recommended. This recommendation is supported by the results of treatment in the subgroup of men with diastolic pressures of 90 to 114 mm Hg who were 60 years of age and older at entry to the Veterans Administration study (see Table 59.12). A similar placebo trial designed specifically to assess the effectiveness of treatment in older hypertensives was initiated in Europe in 1973. When completed, this study will provide information on both male and female subjects who were considerably older (mean age at entry 71 years) than the Veterans Administration subjects. An interim report from this study in 1978 indicated that both systolic and diastolic pressures can be reduced effectively and safely by the drugs used in the study: hydrochlorothiazide, triamterene, and methyldopa (2).

Caveats

Several special characteristics of older patients should be considered in deciding how to treat their hypertension.

Orthostatic hypotension unrelated to drugs is common in elderly subjects. Approximately one-fourth of those living at home have a 20 mm Hg or greater fall in systolic pressure upon standing (4). A combination of increase in sedentary activity and blunting of autonomic reflexes probably explains this. Thus it is particularly important to obtain baseline and follow-up standing blood pressures (including standing after walking) in older patients taking antihypertensive drugs.

Other characteristics of older subjects which increase the risk of chronic antihypertensive drugs include:

1. Salt and fluid intake may vary significantly from week to week.
2. Concomitant large vessel atherosclerosis (kidneys, brain, heart) may increase the risk of ischemic damage resulting from accidental drug-induced hypotension.
3. Medication-taking errors may be increased.
4. Drug excretion rates are generally reduced as a function of aging.

Table 59.12
Veterans Administration Trial Results in Patients 60 Years Old and Older [a]

	Placebo	Treated
NUMBER OF SUBJECTS	43	38
INCIDENCE OF MORBID EVENTS (%)	62.8	28.9
TYPE OF MORBID EVENT (No.):		
Cerebrovascular accident	10	3
Congestive heart failure	9	0
Accelerated hypertension	0	0
Coronary artery disease	5	5
Atrial fibrillation	2	0
Dissecting aneurysm	1	0
Other	0	3
Diastolic > 124 mm Hg	2	0
TOTAL	29	11

[a] Adapted from Veterans Administration Cooperative Study Group on Antihypertensive Agents: Effects of treatment on morbidity in hypertension; III. Influence of age, diastolic pressure, and prior cardiovascular disease; further analysis of side effects. *Circulation, 45:* 991, 1972.

Three precautions will minimize the risks of antihypertensive drugs in older patients: using the smallest recommended dose and increasing the dose very slowly; keeping the drug schedule simple; and promptly decreasing or discontinuing drugs if there are signs or symptoms of significant orthostatic hypotension or annoying side effects.

ISOLATED SYSTOLIC HYPERTENSION

Sustained isolated systolic hypertension (defined as a blood pressure ≥160/<90 mm Hg) is quite common in older patients and may be seen in any age group. The Framingham data and other studies have confirmed that systolic hypertension is an independent and powerful risk factor for cardiovascular morbidity. To date, there has been no formal study of the health impact of treatment for isolated systolic hypertension. However, in 1981 a multicenter controlled trial of treatment of isolated systolic hypertension in patients over 60 *was* initiated in the United States. In recent years, the physiologic basis for isolated systolic hypertension has been studied and practical recommendations for long term management have been published.

Pathophysiology (1, 23)

Isolated systolic hypertension may be found in patients at any age who have conditions associated with an increased cardiac output (arteriovenous fistula, patent ductus arteriosus, severe anemia, erythroderma, thyrotoxicosis, Paget's disease of the bone, etc.). However, in individuals without one of these conditions, the mechanisms for isolated systolic hypertension appear to be different in young and old

subjects. In younger subjects, there is a usually hyperkinetic circulation (increased heart rate, increased left ventricular ejection rate and cardiac indices, and normal peripheral resistance) and the hypertension responds to β-blocking agents. Older subjects usually have a normal heart rate, decreased left ventricular ejection rate and cardiac indices, and increased peripheral resistance; and the hypertension responds to vasodilator treatment.

Recommendations

In its 1979 statement on hypertension in the elderly, the National High Blood Pressure Coordinating Committee gave no definitive recommendations for isolated systolic hypertension, but stated that for the individual patient the goal should be an acceptable range (140 to 160 mm Hg) rather than a normal blood pressure (<140 mm Hg).

Treatment of isolated systolic hypertension should be strongly recommended for the following patients: those with left ventricular failure, those with poorly controlled angina, and those with consistently very high systolic pressure (*i.e.,* ≥200 mm Hg).

In each of these situations, reduction of the actual or potential increase in cardiac work due to systolic hypertension is the rationale for treatment. The stepped method for drug selection discussed earlier is appropriate.

HYPERTENSION IN PREGNANCY

Normally, the blood pressure falls slightly during the first and second trimesters of pregnancy and reverts to prepregnancy level in the third trimester. The fall in blood pressure is probably due to the general vasodilation which accompanies pregnancy. An increase in renin and aldosterone levels also occurs in normal pregnancy.

Based on previous records or history from the patient, it should be possible at the first prepartum visit to decide for most women whether they are usually normotensive or have chronic hypertension. This decision is very helpful in managing the several patterns of hypertension that may be associated with pregnancy. These are: pregnancy-induced hypertension (pre-eclampsia and eclampsia), chronic hypertension, and new postpartum hypertension. Management of the last-mentioned form of hypertension will usually be the task of the patient's primary physician, while management of the first two is the province of the physician supervising the pregnancy.

Depending upon the population and the criteria for hypertension, the reported incidence of hypertension during pregnancy varies from 5 to 30%. The hypertension is pregnancy-induced in about 75% of patients and chronic in the remaining 25%.

Pregnancy-induced Hypertension

Pregnancy-induced hypertension (PIH), or pre-eclampsia, is a syndrome in which the clinical data must be carefully considered before making the diagnosis, in particular to distinguish it from pre-existing chronic hypertension. Untreated PIH is associated with a high incidence of fetal mortality and maternal morbidity. The major pathophysiologic derangements are placental hypoperfusion, generalized vasospasm, and decreased glomerular filtration rate. The clinical manifestations which permit the firm diagnosis of PIH are:

1. *New* development of hypertension during the last trimester. The definition for hypertension in this instance is an absolute blood pressure exceeding 140/90 (on two occasions at least 6 hours apart) or a rise, between visits, of 30 mm Hg systolic or 15 mm Hg diastolic.
2. The development of *new* proteinuria during the last trimester.
3. The development of *new*, generalized edema during the last trimester (dependent edema alone is not a predictor of pre-eclampsia; it is seen in approximately one-third of pregnant women whose blood pressure remains normal).

In the patient who lacks the full clinical triad of findings, the following considerations may help to decide whether to treat her as if she is pre-eclamptic:

1. Does she have one of the known risk factors for PIH? The majority of affected women are primigravidas at the extremes of the child-bearing age range. A primigravida whose mother or a sister had eclampsia is at particularly high risk. These and other risk factors are summarized in Table 59.13.
2. Was the same degree of hypertension in fact present before the 20th week of gestation (i.e., chronic hypertension)?

Fortunately most PIH develops late in the third trimester when the fetus is mature and delivery can be planned promptly. The management for PIH which develops before the fetus is mature is hospital admission, modified bed rest, frequent monitoring of maternal blood pressure and fetal status, and antihypertensive drugs when the diastolic pressure exceeds 100. These measures are effective in resolving the manifestations of pre-eclampsia and ensuring a successful outcome of the pregnancy in almost all patients.

PIH resolves within 6 weeks of delivery. About 25% of primigravidas with PIH will develop PIH during a future pregnancy. Epidemiologic studies have shown, however, that women with a history of PIH do not have an increased risk of developing chronic hypertension (6). This finding is consistent with the concept that PIH is a specific and self-limited complication of pregnancy.

Chronic Hypertension in Pregnancy

Chronic hypertension will be seen more commonly in pregnant women who are in their 30s, as the prevalence of hypertension increases with age (Fig. 59.1). Because of the fall in blood pressure which occurs during the first two trimesters, a sustained blood pressure of 130/80 or above is the generally accepted criterion for chronic hypertension during these trimesters, and 140/90 is regarded as hypertension in the last trimester.

There are two important questions to consider in patients with chronic hypertension:

1. *Should a woman with chronic hypertension avoid pregnancy?* In the woman with mild to moderate hypertension, there is little or no increased risk to the mother or the infant. However, in a woman with evidence for major end-organ damage (significant cardiomegaly, renal impairment, or eye ground changes of accelerated hypertension), infant mortality is greatly increased. Such women should be advised to avoid pregnancy.
2. *How should chronic hypertension be treated during pregnancy?* In general, a patient who becomes pregnant while taking antihypertensive medication should remain on her usual medication unless she becomes hypotensive during the pregnancy. In these patients, it is important to confirm that chronic hypertension was documented adequately before drug treatment. For patients not taking antihypertensives whose chronic hypertension is discovered during the first or second trimester, the hypertension should be treated. This recommendation is based on the finding of improved fetal survival in a controlled trial of methyldopa treatment (without diuretics) for women with chronic hypertension, defined as a blood pressure exceeding 140/90 on at least three separate occasions (18).

New Postpartum Hypertension

New hypertension is detected occasionally at the 6th week postpartum visit. Within 1 year, some of these patients remain hypertensive, while most revert to a normal blood pressure (24). When the hypertension is first detected at the 6th-week visit, a urinalysis is critical in order to exclude the rare syndrome of postpartum nephrosclerosis. Women with diastolic blood pressures repeatedly above 100 mm Hg should be treated according to the stepped care strategy

Table 59.13
Risk Factors for Pregnancy-Induced Hypertension

Primagravida
Familial history of pre-eclampsia/eclampsia
Diabetes
Multiple gestation
Exremes of age
Pre-existing hypertensive vascular or renal disease
Hydatidiform mole
Fetal hydrops, but not isoimmunization *per se*
Previous history of pre-eclampsia/eclampsia

discussed earlier (p. 571). For women with mild hypertension (diastolic 100 mm Hg or less) and a normal urinalysis, conservative follow-up without drug treatment is appropriate for the first 6 months to 1 year. A small proportion of these women remain hypertensive after this interval, and they should be treated for chronic hypertension.

ORAL CONTRACEPTIVES AND HYPERTENSION

Longitudinal studies of women taking oral contraceptive pills (OCP) have shown the following:
1. A *mild increase in blood pressure* (systolic 5 to 6 mm Hg and diastolic 1 to 2 mm Hg) occurs shortly after initiating OCP in most women (32).
2. During the first 5 years of OCP use, there is a progressive rise in the blood pressure (mean 14 mm Hg systolic and 8 mm Hg diastolic) (32).
3. The reported incidence of *new hypertension* has varied from 3 to 6 per 1000 OCP users after 3 years of use. These rates were 2 to 3 times higher than the rates in comparable nonusers (7).

Population studies in recent years have shown that the OCP use does increase the risk of death from cerebrovascular and cardiovascular diseases. The absolute number of women affected is very small, but physicians must be aware of the potential hazards of this form of contraception.

The physiologic basis for the modest increase in blood pressure accompanying OCP use may be volume expansion. After 3 weeks, it has been found that most individuals show a 100 to 200 mEq increase in total body sodium. In addition, increased renin and aldosterone activity are found. There is no difference in the degree of these changes between those women who remain normotensive and those who develop hypertension. A history of pregnancy-induced hypertension does not increase the risk of OCP-induced hypertension and is not a contraindication to OCP use. Furthermore, there are no contraindications to OCP use in the patient with well-controlled chronic hypertension who may wish to use this kind of contraception.

Approach to the Patient

The use of oral contraceptives has played a major role in the reduction of unwanted pregnancy during the past 20 years (see Chapter 90). Most physicians will find that a substantial proportion of women in the child-bearing age range are OCP users or will select OCP prophylaxis. Therefore, it is important to have an approach to the occasional woman who may develop hypertension while on oral contraceptives. The following approach is recommended:
1. Assure that a baseline blood pressure is obtained before OCP use.
2. Dispense no more than a 6-month supply at one time.

3. Measure the blood pressure at least every 6 months. If the patient develops hypertension or if the blood pressure rises significantly (though remaining below 140/90), the patient should be advised to select another form of contraception, and when this has been done OCP should be discontinued.
4. Approximately one-half of women developing hypertension during OCP use will revert to normal blood pressure within 3 months of discontinuation of OCP use. If the blood pressure does not revert to normal, the patient should be managed for chronic hypertension as described earlier in this chapter.
5. In the OCP user who develops hypertension and must continue OCP use, treatment for sustained hypertension as outlined earlier is appropriate.

References

General

Chesley, LC: *Hypertensive Disorders in Pregnancy.* Appleton-Century-Crofts, New York, 1978.
  Monograph covering many aspects of hypertension in pregnancy.
Kaplan, NM: *Clinical Hypertension.* Williams & Wilkins, Baltimore, 1978 (new edition scheduled 1982).
  Monograph covering in detail what the clinician needs to know about essential and secondary hypertension.
Kotchen, T and Havlik, R (editors): High blood pressure in the young. *Hypertension* 2: I-1 to I-133, 1980.
  Entire issue devoted to papers presented at a 1979 symposium.
McMahon, FG: *Management of Essential Hypertension.* Futura Publishing New York, 1978.
  Monograph providing a systematic account of each available antihypertensive drug, particularly useful for compilation of reported side effects. Extensive referencing is provided.
Paul, O: *Epidemiology and Control of Hypertension.* Stratton Intercontinental Medical Book Corp., New York, 1975.
  Multicontributor symposium covering all significant information about epidemiology of hypertension prior to 1975.
Perry, HM and Smith, WM: *Mild Hypertension: To Treat or Not to Treat.* The New York Academy of Sciences, New York, 1978.
  Mult author symposium covering critically the many unanswered questions about mild hypertension.
The 1980 Report of the Joint National Committee on Detection, Evaluation, and Treatment of High Blood Pressure. *Arch Intern Med* 140: 1280, 1980.
  Specific recommendations based on the consensus of a national panel of experts.

Specific

1. Adamopoulos, PN, Chrysanthakopoulis, SG and Frohlich, ED: Systolic hypertension: nonhomogeneous diseases. *J Cardiol* 36: 697, 1975.
2. Amery, A, Berthaux, P and Birkenhäger, W, *et al.:* Controlled trial: antihypertensive therapy in patients above age 60. *Acta Cardiol* 33: 113, 1978.
3. Boyer, JL and Kasch, FW: Exercise therapy in hypertensive men. *JAMA* 211: 1668, 1970.
3a. Bravo, EL, Tarazi, RC, Fouad, FM, Vidt, DG and Gifford, RW: Clonidine-suppression test; a useful aid in the diagnosis of pheochromocytoma. *N Engl J Med* 305: 623, 1981.
4. Caird, FI, Andrews, GR and Kennedy, RD: Effect of posture on blood pressure in the elderly. *Br Heart J* 35: 527, 1973.
5. Carey, RM, Reid, RA, Ayers, CR, Lynch, SS, McLain, WL and Vaughan, ED, Jr: The Charlottesville blood-pressure survey. Value of repeated blood-pressure measurements. *JAMA* 236: 847, 1976.

6. Chesley, LC, Annitto, JE and Cosgrove, RA: The remote prognosis of eclamptic women: sixth periodic report. *Obstetrics 124:* 446, 1976.

7. Fisch, IR and Frank, J: Oral contraceptives and blood pressure. *JAMA 237:* 2499, 1977.

8. Gifford, RW, Jr: Evaluation of the hypertensive patient. *Chest 64:* 336, 1973.

9. Gitlow, SE, Mendlowitz, M and Bertani, LM: The biochemical techniques for detecting and establishing the presence of a pheochromocytoma. *Am J Cardiol 26:* 270, 1970.

10. Gordon, T and Waterhous, AM: Hypertension and hypertensive heart disease. *J Chronic Dis 19:* 1089, 1966.

11. Grimm, RH, Leon, AS, Hunninhake, DB, Lenz, K, Hannan, P and Blackburn, H: Effects of thiazide diuretics on plasma lipids and lipoproteins in mildly hypertensive patients. *Ann Intern Med 94:* 7, 1981.

12. Hamer, J, Fleming, J and Shinebourne, E: Effect of walking on blood pressure in systemic hypertension. *Lancet 2:* 114, 1967.

13. Haynes, RB, Sackett, DL, Taylor, DW, Gibson, ES and Johnson, AL: Increased absenteeism from work after detection and labeling of hypertensive patients. *N Engl J Med 299:* 741, 1978.

14. Hypertension Detection and Follow-up Program Cooperative Group: Five-year findings of the hypertension detection and follow-up program; I. Reduction in mortality of persons with high blood pressure, including mild hypertension. *JAMA 242:* 2562, 1979.

15. Koch, G: Haemodynamic adaptation at rest and during exercise to long-term antihypertensive treatment with combination of β-receptor blocking and vasodilator agent. *Br Heart J 38:* 1240, 1976.

16. Levine, DM, Green, LW, Deeds, SG, Chwalow, J, Russell, RP and Finlay, J: Health education for hypertensive patients. *JAMA 241:* 1700, 1979.

17. Morgan, T, Gillies, A, Morgan, G, Adam, W, Wilson, M and Carney, S: Hypertension treated by salt restriction. *Lancet 1:* 227, 1978.

18. Redman, CWG, Beilin, LJ, Bonnar, J and Ounsted, MK: Fetal outcome in trial of antihypertensive treatment in pregnancy. *Lancet 2:* 753, 1976.

19. Reisin, E, Abel, R, Modan, M, Silverberg, DS, Eliahou, HE and Modan, B: Effect of weight loss without salt restriction on the reduction of blood pressure in overweight hypertensive pa-

tients. *N Engl J Med 298:* 1, 1978.

20. Report of Medical Research Council Working Party of Mild to Moderate Hypertension: Randomised controlled trial of treatment for mild hypertension: design and pilot trial. *Br Med J 1:* 1437, 1977.

21. Sackett, DL: The hypertensive patient; 5. Compliance with therapy (editorial). *Can Med Assoc J 121:* 259, 1979.

22. Shapiro, AP, Schwartz, GE, Ferguson, DCE, Redmond, DP and Weiss, SM: Behavioral approaches to the treatment of hypertension: review of the clinical status. *Ann Intern Med 86:* 626, 1977.

23. Simon, AC, Safar, MA, Levenson, JA, Kheder, AM and Levy, BI: Systolic hypertension: hemodynamic mechanism and choice of antihypertensive treatment. *Am J Cardiol 44:* 505, 1979.

24. Stout, ML: Hypertension six weeks postpartum in apparently normal patients. *Am J Obstet Gynecol 27:* 730, 1934.

25. Taguchi, J and Freis, ED: Partial reduction of blood pressure and prevention of complications in hypertension. *N Engl J Med 291:* 329, 1974.

26. The Australian therapeutic trial in mild hypertension (editorial). *Lancet 1:* 1261, 1980.

27. Tucker, RM and Labarthe, DR: Frequency of surgical treatment for hypertension in adults at the Mayo Clinic from 1973 through 1975. *Mayo Clin Proc 52:* 549, 1977.

28. Tyroler, HA, Heyden, S, Sneiderman, C, Heiss, G and Hames, C: A 16-year follow-up of blood pressure in young adult residents of Evans County. Medical Horizon Symposium: Hypertension in Childhood and Adolescents, Pittsburgh, September 1976.

29. Varady, PD and Maxwell, MH: Assessment of statistically significant changes in diastolic blood pressures. *JAMA 221:* 365, 1972.

30. Veterans Administration Cooperative Study Group on Antihypertensive Agents: II. Effects of treatment on morbidity in hypertension. *JAMA 213:* 1143, 1970.

31. Watson, RDS, Stallard, TJ and Littler, WA: Influence of once-daily administration of β-adrenoceptor antagonists on arterial pressure and its variability. *Lancet 1:* 1210, 1979.

32. Weir, RJ, Briggs, E, Mack, A, Naismith, L, Taylor, L and Wilson, E: Blood pressure in women taking oral contraceptives. *Br Med J 1:* 533, 1974.

SECTION 9

Musculoskeletal Problems

CHAPTER SIXTY

Shoulder Pain

NOBLE M. HANSEN, M.D.

Shoulder pain is a common complaint in ambulatory practice. Most often the general physician can establish the correct diagnosis and can direct therapy without an orthopaedic or rheumatogic consultation. This chapter will review the major causes of shoulder pain and provide a basis for treatment of these conditions.

REFERRED PAIN (Table 60.1)

When a patient complains of shoulder pain, the physician should consider first that the pain might be referred from another region of the body. Unlike a primary disorder of the shoulder, referred pain is not made worse when the patient actively moves his shoulders.

Shoulder Pain Referred from Cervical Spine or Thoracic Outlet

Problems arising in the *cervical spine* (see Chapter 61) often produce shoulder pain as a major manifestation; but on closer questioning, the patient usually will have some pain in the neck as well. In addition, the pain will be exacerbated by motion of the neck. It is important to evaluate this possibility by having the patient extend, flex, and rotate his neck. This will increase or elicit pain due to cervical disc disease, degenerative joint disease, or other cervical problems.

Table 60.1
Causes of Referred Shoulder Pain

CERVICAL SPINE DISEASE AND THORACIC OUTLET
  SYNDROME
DISORDERS IN OTHER PARTS OF THE BODY:
  Heart or pericardial disease
  Pleural disease—*e.g.*, carcinoma of the superior parts of
    the lung
  Diaphragmatic irritation—*e.g.*, subphrenic abscess
  Gallbladder disease

Further, pain arising from a problem within the cervical spine will often extend beyond the shoulder to below the elbow.

The *thoracic outlet syndrome* is a less common cause of shoulder pain and results from compression of vascular and neural structures between the 1st rib and the clavicle or between the anterior and middle scalene muscles. The thoracic outlet syndrome may be caused by a variety of structural disorders such as an unusual insertion of the anterior scalene muscle or the presence of a cervical rib (usually arising from the 7th cervical vertebra). Most often the symptoms are weakness, numbness, and pain throughout the entire arm in the distribution of the ulnar nerve. These symptoms can often be exacerbated by asking the patient to assume an exaggerated military position with the shoulders held backward and downward. The symptoms may also be elicited and the radial pulse may weaken or disappear when the patient compresses the neurovascular bundle by extending the neck and rotating it toward the examined side just after a deep inspiration.

Shoulder Pain Referred from Other Regions of the Body

Diseases of various viscera may cause pain to be referred to the shoulder, sometimes without any other evidence that a problem exists. Ischemic heart disease, pericarditis, carcinoma of the lung, and gallbladder disease are especially common processes that should be considered when the clinical presentation suggests that shoulder pain is referred.

ANATOMY, FUNCTION, AND PATHOPHYSIOLOGY OF THE SHOULDER

For the physician properly to diagnose and treat disorders of the shoulder he should understand several aspects of shoulder anatomy (Fig. 60.1). At the superior aspect of the shoulder, just lateral to the acromion, are the supraspinatus and infraspinatus tendons which comprise what is called the *rotator cuff*. These tendons function to initiate elevation of the arm through the first 20° of abduction. The *biceps tendon* runs anteriorly across the head of the humerus into the glenoid portion of the shoulder joint. It functions to aid movement of the arm directly forward from the body. This tendon runs in a bony groove in the head of the humerus. Problems of the tendinous portions of the shoulder will account for the vast majority of complaints of shoulder pain seen in an ambulatory practice.

The rotator cuff tendons arise from the lateral aspect of the head of the humerus and sweep underneath the rigid arch formed by the acromion and the acromiocoracoid ligament. As the shoulder is abducted actively, the rotator cuff tendons become impinged against the bony arch and the humeral head (Fig. 60.1). During this impingement, the blood flow

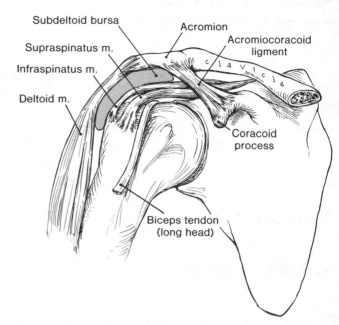

Figure 60.1 Coronal section of shoulder anatomy. Note the relationship of the subdeltoid bursa lying next to the supraspinatus tendon, but being separate from the shoulder joint. Note the acromion which is in a position to impinge the supraspinatus tendon on abduction of the arm.

through the rotator cuff tendons is markedly decreased and may be totally obliterated as the arm is abducted (4). In this region of intermittently decreased blood flow, progressive degenerative changes occur frequently after the age of 30. Inflammation in the rotator cuff tendons and/or the biceps tendon may accompany this degenerative process; and pain is characteristically brought on as the inflamed tendon is compressed or impinged against the rigid acromial arch (1). The unique anatomy and pathophysiology explain two important clinical observations. First, the patient usually gives a history of recurrent exacerbations of symptoms from the underlying degenerative process. Second, the symptoms are related to activity. Therefore, it is extremely important to consider recreational or occupational demands on the shoulder joint when managing these patients.

PRIMARY DISORDERS OF THE SHOULDER

A history of trauma is most important in the assessment of primary shoulder problems. Significant trauma indicates the need for an X-ray of the shoulder joint to rule out the possibility of a nondisplaced fracture or of dislocation. However, the majority of patients with shoulder pain will have a problem located in the tendinous portion of the shoulder joint. The three major problems are: acute tendinitis, chronic tendinitis, and adhesive capsulitis. An X-ray of the shoulder is not needed when these problems are suspected; it should be obtained, however, if pain persists or worsens in spite of conservative therapy (see below). For this reason the physician will want to ensure follow-up in 1 to 2 weeks either by telephone or an office visit. This encounter will also permit the physician to educate the patient about exercises and activities which may help prevent recurrences (see below).

Acute Tendinitis

DIAGNOSIS

Acute tendinitis of the shoulder is a dramatic illness. The rapid onset of severe pain is characteristic, and the pain can be incapacitating. The patient complains of pain over the anterior or lateral aspect of the shoulder resulting in the characteristic "deltoid ache." The pain frequently will radiate down to the elbow, but should not involve the forearm or neck, as referred pain sometimes does (see above). Motion of the shoulder, especially arm abduction (compression of the rotator cuff), is very painful. The most characteristic physical finding is localized tenderness over one of the rotator cuff tendons or the biceps tendon. Tenderness directly at the superior aspect of the shoulder just lateral to the acromion is in the region of the supraspinatus tendon and tenderness just posterior to this is in the region of the infraspinatus tendon. If the arm is externally rotated and the anterior aspect of the humeral head is palpated, the biceps tendon in its groove can be felt; commonly tenderness will be localized at this point. When the biceps tendon is inflamed, active external rotation and then elevation of the arm will give maximum discomfort. While an X-ray of the shoulder is not necessary for the diagnosis of tendinitis, if obtained, it may show calcium within the rotator cuff just superior and lateral to the humeral head. Deposits of calcium begin within the rotator cuff tendon itself but occasionally extend into the subdeltoid bursa. These deposits can form within 24 to 48 hours, and they frequently resolve as the symptoms subside. Occasionally, the calcium may persist long after symptoms have disappeared and in this case its presence is of no concern. It is important to understand that the primary inflammatory process is occurring within the rotator cuff tendon itself and that the subdeltoid bursa becomes inflamed secondarily. The terms subacromial bursitis, subdeltoid bursitis, or "bursitis" of the shoulder are commonly used interchangeably and have led to the erroneous idea that the primary inflammatory response is within the bursa.

TREATMENT

In considering treatment, it should be emphasized that tendinitis is generally a self-limited illness lasting up to 2 weeks. The most important complication, in those who do not initially respond, is adhesive capsulitis (see below).

The initial aim of treatment of acute tendinitis is to relieve pain. In mild cases, the shoulder should be rested in a sling and the patient should be given an oral anti-inflammatory agent such as aspirin, 600 to 900 mg 4 times a day. The patient should understand that he is not taking aspirin as an analgesic but as an anti-inflammatory agent; and, therefore, it must be taken regularly. If aspirin does not provide relief, a 5-day course of phenylbutazone, 100 mg, 3 to 4 times a day is usually very helpful. The long term use of phenylbutazone is contraindicated because of the increased risk of bone marrow toxicity. If the patient is having very severe pain, an analgesic such as codeine, 30 to 60 mg, every 4 to 6 hours, for several days may be helpful. Also, the application of moist or dry heat for 20 to 30 min 2 or 3 times/day may provide comfort and muscle relaxation.

If the response to this treatment after 2 weeks is not adequate, local injections of a glucocorticoid preparation into the region of maximum tenderness may give immediate dramatic relief. This procedure may be performed by the general physician using a 22 gauge needle; the steroid is injected in a dose of 1 ml of Aristospan, Celestone, or Kenalog combined with 3 ml of 1% Xylocaine. An occasional patient will not respond to initial treatment, and an X-ray may show a significant calcium deposit in the tendon; aspiration of the calcium with a 16 gauge needle, usually by an orthopaedist or rheumatologist, may provide immediate relief to such patients.

As the pain of acute tendinitis subsides following initial treatment, the patient should begin gentle range of motion exercises (Fig. 60.2), to prevent the development of adhesive capsulitis (see below). The physician may teach the exercise to the patient. It is best that the patient perform circumduction exercises by bending forward 90° at the waist and dangling the arm straight down and then swinging the elbow in a circular fashion. This will allow the shoulder to move without the patient actively using the rotator cuff tendons to elevate the arm. Another home exercise is to have the patient stand facing a wall and to flex the shoulders forward until the fingers touch the wall; then the fingers are "walked" up the wall, carrying the arm and shoulder into full forward flexion. Either or both of these exercises can be done for 10 min twice a day.

Quite often attacks of acute tendinitis are recurrent; thus, a change in recreational or occupational activity may be necessary. If the patient is not able to regain full range of motion of the shoulder within 2 to 4 weeks, a physical therapy consultation should be requested. The therapist can supervise the exercises and encourage the patient to do them. If there is still a poor response or continuing pain after a period of 2 weeks, a consultation by an orthopaedist or rheumatologist is appropriate. However, there is, in general, no place for surgery in the treatment of acute tendinitis of the shoulder.

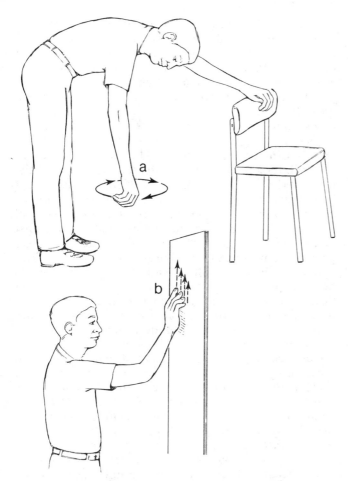

Figure 60.2 Range of motion exercises of the shoulder. (*a*) Circumduction exercises of the shoulder and (*b*) the wall-climbing exercises for the shoulder as described in the text.

Chronic Tendinitis

DIAGNOSIS

Chronic tendinitis of the shoulder has the same basic etiology as acute tendinitis. It is, however, a milder but more persistent problem. The patient most often develops activity-related pain over the lateral or anterior aspect of the shoulder and upper arm. The patient often recognizes a particular motion or activity which makes the pain worse. Active elevation of the arm almost always causes the pain to worsen because of impingement of the tendons; however, passive range of motion is normal. There is mild tenderness over the rotator cuff or biceps tendon.

TREATMENT

Treatment consists of the application of dry or moist heat, gentle circumduction exercises, and anti-inflammatory agents such as aspirin, 600 to 900 mg 3 to 4 times a day. Other nonsteroidal anti-inflammatory agents (for example indomethacin, 25 to 50 mg 4 times/day) may be tried if aspirin is not effective.

Usually the patient's discomfort is not so severe that phenylbutazone is required. If the tenderness is particularly severe and localized, injection of a glucocorticoid preparation as described above can give significant relief; this is especially effective when the biceps tendon is involved. The patient should be instructed to avoid any aggravating activities.

If the patient does not respond to conservative therapy in several months or if there are repeated episodes of protracted pain, an orthopaedic consultation is indicated. The consultant should obtain or review an X-ray of the shoulder and should search for *aggravating mechanical factors*, such as spur formation along the acromion which has led to increased impingement. There are several surgical procedures designed to remove parts of the coracoacromial arch to decrease impingement of the inflamed rotator cuff, but these all require hospitalization and general anesthesia (2). In addition if there is biceps tendinitis, this tendon may be removed from its groove in the humeral head and attached more distally to the shaft of the humerus.

Finally, in the patient with chronic pain not helped by conservative therapy the consultant will need to consider the less common complication of a tear of the rotator cuff tendons (3). This diagnosis should be considered when the physical examination reveals weakness in elevation of the arm and atrophy of the deltoid, supraspinatus, and infraspinatus muscles. Occasionally, there is a palpable cleft in the rotator cuff tendon. In suspected cases the consultant will suggest an *arthogram of the shoulder*. This requires an injection into the shoulder joint of approximately 15 ml of Renograffin mixed with air, followed by X-rays to see if the dye remains within the joint or flows through a tear of the rotator cuff into the subdeltoid bursa as shown in Figure 60.3. Ordinarily, the subdeltoid bursa does not connect with the shoulder joint. In individuals who are over the age of 40, the rotator cuff usually tears because of attrition. In these patients there are no sudden symptoms, and often surgical repair of the tear is quite difficult. Frequently, the best result that can be obtained from surgery of a tear of a rotator cuff in patients in this group is some decrease in the pain, but residual loss of motion persists. In some older individuals rotator cuff tears are associated with hydroxyapatite crystal deposition (see "Milwaukee Shoulder," in Chapter 66). In younger individuals, there is more often an acute episode leading to sudden tear of the rotator cuff, and in this instance early surgical repair may give much better results.

Adhesive Capsulitis ("Frozen Shoulder")

DIAGNOSIS

This problem is characteristically seen in patients who are between the ages of 40 and 70 years. It is more common in women and is usually preceded by a period of inactivity of the shoulder (for example,

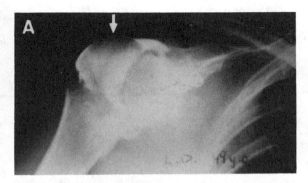

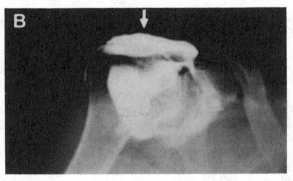

Figure 60.3 (A) Normal shoulder arthrogram. The superior aspect of the joint should be smooth with a fine layer of contrast material. (B) Rotator cuff tear. Note extravasation of the dye from the glenohumeral joint into the subdeltoid bursa, indicating a large tear of the rotator cuff tendon.

following a stroke, a shoulder injury, or an exacerbation of chronic tendinitis). The patient presents with slowly progressive stiffness of the shoulder that is usually painless or is associated with mild discomfort in the anterior and lateral aspect of the shoulder. The patient may also complain that he is unable to bring his hand to his mouth when he eats or that he has difficulty in combing his hair. On physical examination marked reduced passive range of motion of the glenohumeral joint will be demonstrated; but the shoulder is usually not tender. The examiner should put a hand on the top of the shoulder to prevent elevation of the scapula (which could mask loss of glenohumeral motion) and should then passively abduct the arm. The maximum angle between the humerus and the side of the chest with the scapula fixed is a measure of motion between the glenoid and humerus; normally the angle is at least 90°

NATURAL HISTORY

Adhesive capsulitis may last as long as 1 to 2 years. Generally, the patient's range of motion slowly improves, although a complete return to full range of motion is very unlikely. Most often a satisfactory range of motion is achieved which permits the patient to raise his hand to the back of the head, the mouth, and the low back.

PREVENTION

Adhesive capsulitis is a potential complication whenever a patient's shoulder is immobilized, and eventually it may represent a greater disability than the primary reason for immobilization. This complication can be prevented if range of motion exercises of the shoulder are initiated as soon as acute pain subsides.

TREATMENT

The primary aim of treatment of adhesive capsulitis is gradually to increase the activity of the shoulder. A specific exercise program in passive and active motion of the shoulder should include forward flexion and abduction and rotation of the shoulder and should be performed at a minimum of 10 min twice daily. Circumduction exercises and wall-climbing exercises—Figure 60.2—are excellent. It is important that the patient understand (a) that improvement is expected over the course of months, not days or weeks, and (b) that the range of motion achieved may not be entirely normal but, it is to be hoped, will permit him to reach his hand to his head, mouth, and back. Long term use of anti-inflammatory medications usually has no place in the treatment of adhesive capsulitis; but a 2-week course of an anti-inflammatory medication during the initiation of treatment may be helpful if pain is exacerbated. Occasionally injection of a glucocorticoid (see above) into the region of the shoulder joint at the initiation of therapy is useful if discomfort prevents adequate exercising. Prescribing an analgesic medication to allow physical therapy is important. Most patients are adequately treated by the primary physician after an initial physical therapy consultation which will aid the patient in understanding the exercise program. If the patient fails to improve the range of motion of his shoulder after several months of therapy, consultation with an orthopaedic surgeon is indicated. Very occasionally, manipulation of the shoulder under general anesthesia and simultaneous glucocorticoid injection into the shoulder joint may improve the patient's range of motion which then can be maintained by further physical therapy.

References

General

Bateman, JE: *The Shoulder and Neck*, Ed. 2. W.B. Saunders, Philadelphia, 1978.
    Complete book on the shoulder containing a complete differential diagnosis. Excellent discussion of anatomy and biomechanics of the shoulder joint.
Kozin, F: *Painful Shoulder and the Reflex Sympathetic Dystrophy Syndrome in Arthritis and Allied Conditions*, Ed. 9, edited by DJ McCarty. Lea & Febiger, Philadelphia, 1979.
    Excellent detailed review of shoulder pain from the rheumatologist's perspective.

Specific

1. Linge, B, van and Mulder, JD: Function of the supraspinatus muscle and its relation to the supraspinatus syndrome. *J Bone Joint Surg* 45B: 750, 1963.

2. Neer, CS, II: Anterior acromioplasty for the chronic impingement syndrome in the shoulder. *J Bone Joint Surg 54A:* 41, 1972.
3. Neviaser, JS: Ruptures of the rotator cuff of the shoulder. New concepts in the diagnosis and operative treatment of chronic ruptures. *Arch Surg 102:* 483, 1971.
4. Rathbun, JB and Macnab, I: The microvascular pattern of the rotator cuff. *J Bone Joint Surg 52B:* 540, 1970.

CHAPTER SIXTY-ONE

Neck Pain

NOBLE M. HANSEN, M.D.

Neck pain is a common problem. Nearly 50% of individuals over 50 years of age experience neck pain at some time. Since there are many structures in the neck that, when diseased, may cause pain, as well as multiple sources of referred pain, the physician must systematically evaluate patients who complain of neck pain. This chapter provides a review of the skeletal structures of the neck; the method of evaluation for complaints of neck pain; a description of common problems and their treatment; and guidance for referral of selected patients with neck pain.

ANATOMY AND SOURCES OF PAIN (Fig. 61.1)

The cervical spine consists of seven vertebral bodies connected by an *anterior and a posterior longitudinal ligament*. These ligaments provide stability when the neck is flexed and extended. The vertebral bodies are joined by *intervertebral discs* composed of a gel-like material (the *nucleus pulposus*) which absorbs increased pressure applied to the spine. The nucleus pulposus is contained within an *annulus fibrosus*, a fibrous structure ringing the outer margin of the disc. During the 4th decade of life, both the nucleus pulposus and the annulus fibrosus undergo progressive degeneration, seen microscopically as a loss of the fibrous pattern and of the collagen alignment. As a result, the ability of the disc to absorb shocks is reduced. There are *facet joints* found between vertebral elements posteriorly, one on each side of the spine; they are apophyseal (projecting) joints with a synovial lined capsule. It is within these small joints in the posterior spine that true osteoarthritis can occur—osteoarthritis being a breakdown of the articular cartilage within the joints. The *neural foramina*, located laterally on either side of the vertebral bodies, are the canals through which the individual nerve roots emerge from the spinal canal. The spinal canal and the foramina can be encroached upon by a bulging intervertebral disc or an osseous proliferation (bony spur) originating in a vertebral body, a facet joint, or from the bony margin of a

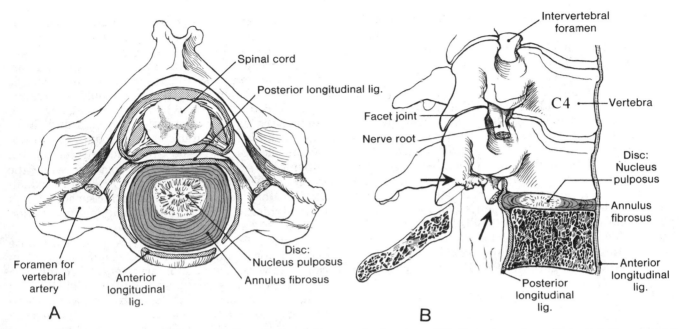

Figure 61.1 Anatomy of disc and ligaments of the cervical spine. (*A*) Superior view. Note relationship of anterior and posterior longitudinal ligament to the intervertebral disc. (*B*) Lateral view. Note relationship of intervertebral foramen to the intervertebral disc and facet joint. Bulging of the intervertebral disc or bone spurs forming from the facet joint may cause compression of the nerve root within the intervertebral foramen (*arrows*).

neural foramina (Fig. 61.1). When the encroachment involves a nerve root, pain in the distribution of that root (radicular pain) may occur. The facet joint capsules and the intervertebral disc are innervated by fine unmyelinated nerves (called C-fibers) which have simple nerve endings. When these nerve endings are stimulated by degenerative disease within the disc or joint capsules, the patient may experience pain which is referred to the posterior aspect of the neck at any level. The pain felt in the neck may not be at the cervical level from which the nerve is arising. In addition, C-fiber stimulation can cause pain to be referred to the interscapular area, superiorly and laterally over the shoulders, and in the lower arm and the hand. C-fiber stimulation occasionally causes a decrease in sensation in the lower arm and in the hand. Spasm of any of the many muscles of the neck region is also a common source of pain.

EVALUATION OF THE PATIENT

History

The date of onset of the patient's symptoms and of any associated trauma should be ascertained. A history of trauma is an indication for a complete set of cervical spine X-rays (see below). Often, knowledge of the specific activity the patient was performing at the onset of pain will be quite helpful in establishing the cause of the pain. Prolonged extension of the neck, such as occurs in people doing overhead work, is a common occupational situation which can give rise to pain in the cervical region. It is quite common

that a patient sustains a minor twisting injury or trauma to the neck and does not experience neck pain within the first 24 hours. The patient's first pain may then begin to appear and may progress. Reproduction or increase of pain by neck motion is very helpful in localizing the problem to the cervical spine rather than to a referred source (Table 61.1). It is also important to know if the pain is felt outside the neck as well, such as in the head, posteriorly between the scapulae, about the shoulder, down the arm, or in the hand. The patient should be asked about decreased sensation in his hands and, if he is able, to say specifically which fingers are involved. If the pain and numbness are felt in a dermatome distribution, this indicates nerve compression (Table 61.2). Pain associated with motion of the shoulder is not characteristic of cervical spine disease and should make the physician consider the problem to be within the shoulder joint (see Chapter 60). Symptoms such as dizziness, visual changes, and ataxia are not usually associated with cervical problems arising from simple nerve root compression or degenerative disc disease, but may be found when bony spurs encroach on the vertebral foramina (Fig. 61.1) and compress the vertebral arteries. These relatively rare symptoms usually occur when the neck is in a certain position, and are usually of short duration.

Physical Examination

In the physical examination of the patient, the physician should first determine the range of motion of the neck, including flexion, extension, rotation, and lateral bending. Normally, the chin can be placed easily upon the anterior chest and the neck can be extended so that the patient is looking directly above. Normally, there is almost 90° of rotation of the neck to both sides. Simple hyperextension of the neck commonly exacerbates the pain caused by cervical disc degeneration. The patient should be asked to extend his neck and maintain this position for a period of 30 sec to see if the pain is made worse. Putting direct compression on top of the head also may produce pain in the patient with degenerative disc disease. This pain is often exacerbated by compressing the head while the neck is extended. The posterior neck muscles are palpated for muscle spasm, which may be asymmetric and may give the patient the appearance of torticollis (wry neck). Next, the shoulder should be subjected to a range of motion to see if this elicits pain within the shoulder itself.

Selected neurologic tests (see Fig. 75.2 and Table 81.6) are important in the evaluation of the patient with neck pain, including: reflex testing of the upper and lower extremities; muscle strength testing of the upper extremities; and sensory testing of the upper extremities. The reflex testing should include the biceps, triceps, brachioradialis, quadriceps and gastrocnemius tendons, and the Babinski test. Muscle strength in the upper extremities should include the biceps (flexion of elbow), triceps (extension of elbow), wrist extensors and flexors, hand and finger flexors and intrinsic muscles of the hand. The intrinsic muscles of the hand are tested by having the patient hold the fingers tightly together while the examiner tries to separate them. A sensory examination is then performed. An objective sensory deficit is one which conforms to a dermatome distribution (see Fig. 75.2 and Table 81.6).

Occasionally, cervical spine problems can cause cervical myelopathy when a bone spur forms posteriorly at the margin of an intervertebral disc and then impinges on the spinal cord producing signs of cord compression: increased reflexes in the lower extremities with a positive Babinski sign. A spinal cord tumor at this level could give similar findings.

Laboratory Assessment

If the history reveals an episode of recent trauma or if the neurologic examination reveals abnormalities, a complete set of cervical spine X-rays should be obtained. These films should include an assessment of levels C1 through C7 with oblique and open-mouth odontoid views. These X-rays will help the physician rule out fracture or metastatic disease. There is not, however, a good correlation between clinical symptoms or signs and degenerative abnormalities on X-ray. In fact in asymptomatic individuals after the age of 40, cervical degenerative changes (spondylosis) are common and after the age of 50 are evident in over 90% of individuals (1). On the other hand, there may be serious cervical disease with minimal or no changes on X-ray. If there is no history

Table 61.1
Sources of Referred Pain the Neck

DISORDERS OF THE HEAD:

Migraine or tension headache—pain anterior or posterior

Sinus infection—most often the pain is anterior but occasionally posterior, especially when muscle spasm is present.

Temporal-mandibular joint problem—usually pain is anterolateral

DISTANT LESIONS:

Irritation of the surface of the diaphragm innervated by the phrenic nerve (C3, 4, and 5)—frequently shoulder as well as low neck pain, but more medial diaphragmatic lesion may be associated with just neck pain. An example is gastric ulcer

The clue to referred pain is the absence of any tenderness in the neck or of exacerbation of symptoms with manipulation of the neck

Table 61.2
Characteristic Findings at Individual Cervical Nerve Root Levels

Nerve Root	Disc Level	History	Examination[a]
C3	(C2–3)	Pain into the back of the neck and around the mastoid process	No reflex changes. Electromyographic changes only
C4	(C3–4)	Pain into the back of the neck to the levator scapulae to anterior chest	No reflex changes. Electromyographic changes only
C5	(C4–5)	Pain into side of neck to the superior lateral shoulder, numbness over the deltoid muscle	Deltoid muscle atrophy and weakness of shoulder abduction
C6	(C5–6)	Pain to the lateral aspects of the arm and forearm and into the thumb and index finger with numbness of thumb and dorsum of hand	Weak biceps and brachioradialis muscles and decreased biceps and brachioradialis tendon reflexes
C7	(C6–7)	Pain into the mid-forearm to middle and ring finger	Triceps muscle weakness with decreased triceps muscle reflex
C8	(C7–T1)	Pain to the medial aspect of the forearm into the ring and small finger with numbness of the ulnar border and small finger	Triceps weakness with weakness of intrinsic muscles of the hand

[a] Sensory testing will usually show abnormalities in dermatome of the affected nerve root (see Fig. 75.2).

of trauma, initial X-rays are not necessary, but should be obtained if there is an inadequate response after 1 or 2 weeks of therapy.

Computerized tomography is also useful in the evaluation of problems of the upper cervical spine (2), especially after significant trauma when X-ray studies reveal no abnormality or if the positioning necessary for regular X-rays is difficult. Bone scans using radionuclides may be helpful when neoplastic disease is suspected; however, arthritis or positioning artifacts may confuse interpretation (6).

SELECTED SYNDROMES ASSOCIATED WITH NECK PAIN

Many problems of the neck may result in neck pain (Table 61.3). Because the most common problems—cervical disc disease and cervical spondylosis (degenerative changes)—may have similar manifestations, they are discussed together based on the presence or absence of neurologic findings (see below); and two other common problems, stiff neck and whiplash injury are discussed separately.

Pain with Nerve Root Compression

DIAGNOSIS

The objective signs of nerve root compression are muscle weakness, a decreased reflex, and decreased sensation in a dermatome distribution.

Patients with nerve root compression present with the acute or gradual onset of posterior neck pain which radiates to the shoulder and down one arm into the lower arm and often into the hand itself. The pain will occasionally radiate into a finger which corresponds to the dermatome of the nerve root involved. The pain is made worse by movement of the neck and by extreme neck positions. The patient may, in addition, complain of decreased sensation in the arm and of paresthesia in the hand. The physician should bear in mind that a patient may have nerve root compression from the cervical spine, but have little or no neck and arm pain; and instead have arm weakness and loss of sensation. Nerve root compression can be caused by impingement of the nerve by a cervical disc—most common in younger individuals, or by osseous proliferation which can impinge upon the nerve as it exits through its foramen—most common in patients over 50 (5).

MANAGEMENT

Patients with neurologic findings are probably best referred to an orthopaedist or to a neurosurgeon for more complete examination and followup. If muscle weakness and sensory impairment are of such a degree that they would be unacceptable if permanent,

Table 61.3
Selected Problems of the Neck Which May Result in Neck Pain

Problem	Comment
Arthritis	Especially rheumatoid (see Chapter 67) and degenerative joint disease (see text and Chapter 65)
Disc Disease	See text
Fibrositis	See Chapter 63
Infection	Osteomyelitis or soft tissue infection—look for point tenderness
Neoplasia	Myeloma or metastatic disease is associated with point tenderness and X-ray abnormalities
Neuritis	Any nerve may be involved. A relatively common one is the spinal accessory nerve. Look for tenderness over the nerve—lateral aspect of upper 1/3 of sternomastoid muscle
Platybasia	A congenital disorder which may not manifest symptoms before age 40 or from Paget's disease, X-rays show characteristic changes (i.e., invagination of the base of the skull)
Sprain	Whiplash (see text)
Structures in neck	Any organ or structure located in the neck may become a source of neck pain. Careful examination will detect abnormalities such as thyroiditis, lymphadenitis, or tender carotid artery (carotodynia)
Tendinitis	Any tendon may be involved but occipital and sternomastoid are particularly common. Local tenderness is a clue
Torticollis (wry neck)	Diagnosis is usually obvious by observation. An underlying structural problem could produce reflex muscle spasm; and therefore, with an initial episode an underlying problem (such as tumor or infection) should be considered
Trauma	Because of the danger of cord injury, trauma associated with neck pain should be carefully evaluated
Vascular	Arteritis or dissection may cause neck pain

immediate surgical decompression should be considered. The orthopaedist or neurosurgeon will evaluate these patients further with computerized tomography or myelography.

In mild cases of nerve root compression, treatment consists first of immobilization of the neck by use of a *soft cervical collar* which should allow slight flexion of the neck. If the collar forces the neck into some extension, it may exacerbate the symptoms. A soft cervical collar, made of foam rubber and stockinette and fastened behind the neck, serves more as a reminder to a patient to restrict his neck motion, as it will actually only restrict approximately 25% of flexion-extension and approximately 20 and 10% of rotational or lateral motion, respectively (3). These collars are well tolerated, inexpensive, and easily accessible (made in the office or available in pharmacies). Cervical collars that more fully restrict neck movements (such as the Philadelphia collar, Somibrace, four-poster brace, or cervicothoracic brace) are difficult to use, more expensive, and should be recommended only after consultation with an orthopaedist or neurosurgeon.

If the pain is severe, *bed rest* may be necessary. It is helpful to place a small pillow under the nape of the neck to provide proper positioning. If muscle spasm is present, moist or dry *heat* applied to the neck may give symptomatic relief. *Analgesia* using aspirin, 300 to 600 mg every 4 to 6 hours may help. If a stronger analgesic becomes necessary, the addition of codeine, 30 to 60 mg orally 3 or 4 times daily may be used. While not a first line agent, a muscle relaxant may be helpful (see Chapter 62) if symptoms persist after 3 or 4 days.

The acute phase usually lasts only 1 or 2 weeks. When symptoms have been recurrent, intermittent *cervical traction* can provide excellent relief and should be used after the exacerbation subsides. This is performed initially by a physical therapist. For a period of 30 min, 15 to 20 lb of chin halter traction is applied to the neck. The neck must be positioned in slight flexion; extension, which could worsen symptoms, must be avoided. After several sessions, the patient can be instructed in the use of a home cervical traction unit which then can be applied for 30 min at a time, up to 3 times/day for several months. Should the acute symptom not subside or if new signs develop, referral to an orthopaedist or a neurosurgeon is necessary for confirmation of the diagnosis, and for consideration of the use of a complex brace and possible surgery.

Even when symptoms and signs subside there is, unfortunately, a relatively high rate of recurrence of symptoms. It is therefore important for the physician to educate the patient in activities or positions which should be avoided and in exercises which may help relieve muscle spasm (Figs. 61.2 and 61.3).

Pain without Nerve Root Compression

DIAGNOSIS

The majority of patients who present with neck pain have no objective neurologic findings. Changes in sensation in the lower arm or hand can occur from C-fiber irritation from degenerative disc disease or from degeneration of the facet joints within the neck and, therefore, may be present without true nerve root compression. The patient may present either with an *acute onset* of pain (most of the time a disc herniation) or with a *slowly progressive* discomfort (most often from degenerative joint disease) which has been building over several months. In the acute disc herniation syndrome, the patient presents with the rather sudden onset of neck pain which is associated with decreased range of motion of the cervical

spine, bilateral muscle spasm, or occasionally asymmetric muscle spasm which produces torticollis (wry neck). The patient may have pain in the shoulder or arm, but have no objective weakness or sensory findings on examination. X-rays of the cervical spine may be entirely normal.

TREATMENT

Initial treatment is basically the same as that outlined above for patients with nerve root compression. The neck is "immobilized" with a soft cervical collar; local heat and analgesics also may give symptomatic relief. Muscle relaxants (see Chapter 62) may be tried if symptoms persist after 3 or 4 days of initial treatment. When the pain has subsided, the patient may benefit from intermittent cervical traction. In patients who have a chronic, more insidious onset of pain, it is helpful to examine the patient's occupational situation more closely to see if there are exacerbating circumstances. Any activity that creates prolonged extension of the neck, such as overhead work (e.g., painting) may aggravate a pre-existing problem. If after initial treatment pain lasts more than 2 or 3 weeks, X-rays of the cervical spine should be obtained to look for a possible vertebral collapse, metastatic disease, or foraminal encroachment by bone. The treatment is based on the severity of the symptoms. In milder cases, anti-inflammatory medication, such as aspirin, 600 to 900 mg, 3 or 4 times/day, may be adequate, or one of the nonsteroidal anti-inflammatories, such as ibuprofen (Motrin) 400 mg, 4 times/day, may be tried over a course of 2 or 3 weeks. The patient should be informed that his symptoms often may be chronic or recurrent and he should be advised about how to avoid recurrences (Fig. 61.2).

If an acute severe episode of neck pain in this situation does not respond to treatment within the first week or two, the patient should be referred. When the symptoms are more mild and chronic, a trial of treatment for several months would be reasonable before referral. Further evaluation by an orthopaedic surgeon or a neurosurgeon will include a complete cervical spine X-ray and a computerized cervical tomogram or myelogram to identify the problem and its location. If a herniated disc is identified, consideration can be given to its removal with anterior interbody fusion. This operation can give excellent relief of pain if the correct level of involvement has been identified (7,8).

Stiff Neck

Stiff neck is very common and is not a diagnosis, but rather a description of a symptom. Strain of the muscles or ligaments, of the neck, cold-induced muscular spasm, fibrositis, or neuritis are all possible causes. The problem is characterized by posterior cervical muscular spasm on one or both sides. The spasm usually lasts only 1 to 4 days, and is relieved by the application of heat and by mild analgesics such as aspirin, 600 mg 4 times/day or acetamino-

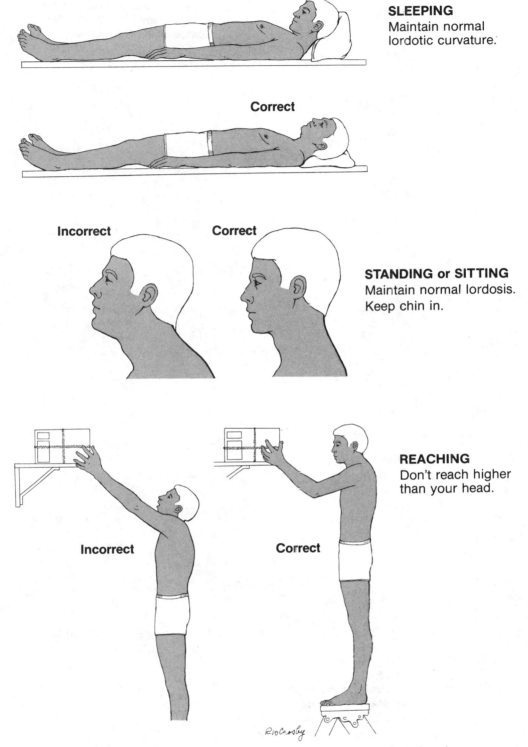

SLEEPING
Maintain normal
lordotic curvature.

STANDING or SITTING
Maintain normal lordosis.
Keep chin in.

REACHING
Don't reach higher
than your head.

Figure 61.2 Position to prevent recurrence of neck pain.

phen (Tylenol), 300–600 mg four times/day. The patient should receive advice about relieving muscle spasm and preventing recurrences (Figs. 61.2 and 61.3). Should the discomfort last beyond a week, an underlying disorder should be considered (e.g., disc disease), and an evaluation should be initiated.

Whiplash (4)

MECHANISM

Whiplash is a term given to acute injuries of the neck caused by sudden extension of the cervical spine. In this country, the most common cause is a

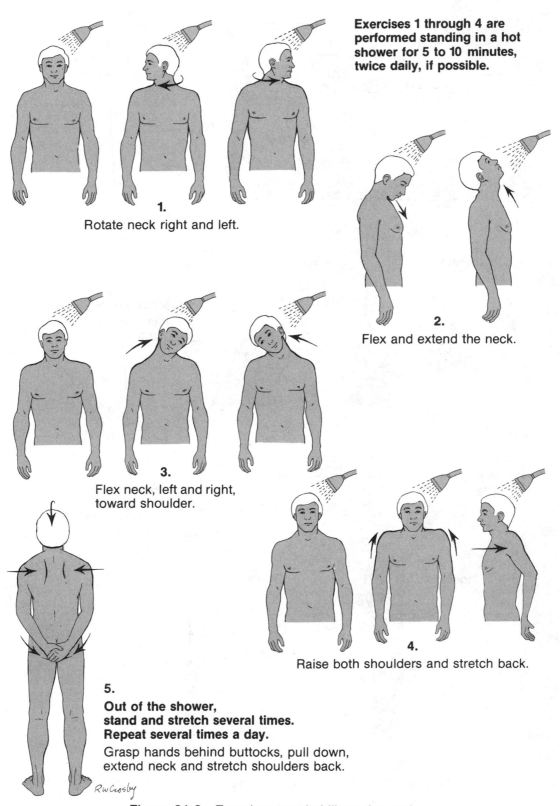

Exercises 1 through 4 are performed standing in a hot shower for 5 to 10 minutes, twice daily, if possible.

1.
Rotate neck right and left.

2.
Flex and extend the neck.

3.
Flex neck, left and right, toward shoulder.

4.
Raise both shoulders and stretch back.

5.

Out of the shower, stand and stretch several times. Repeat several times a day.

Grasp hands behind buttocks, pull down, extend neck and stretch shoulders back.

RwCrosby

Figure 61.3 Exercises to rehabilitate the neck.

rear-end automobile collision. It has been shown experimentally in cadaver studies that when the neck is suddenly and forcefully hyperextended, the muscles of the anterior neck are torn, including the sternomastoid and longest coli muscles. A retropharyngeal hematoma can result; the anterior longitudinal ligament of the cervical spine may tear; and separation of the disc from the vertebral body can occur.

Patients with whiplash are frequently involved in litigation and compensation situations, which makes physicians skeptical of their complaints; it is, however, well documented experimentally that significant injury can occur by this mechanism.

DIAGNOSIS

It is not uncommon for the patient to be without discomfort initially. Pain usually begins several hours to 1 or 2 days after the injury. The patient experiences pain in the posterior and/or anterior region of the neck. It commonly radiates to the occipital aspect of the head and it may radiate to the shoulders and down the upper lateral aspect of the arms. Occipital headaches can occur. Disc herniation and nerve root compression rarely occur from whiplash injury. X-rays following whiplash injuries are usually normal. There may be, however, some loss of the normal cervical lordosis which is an indication of muscle spasm and of splinting of the neck.

TREATMENT

If muscle spasm or limitation of motion is present, the patient should be placed in a soft cervical collar (see above). Analgesics, in adequate doses, should be given. The patient should be warned that extension of the neck will exacerbate his pain. Heat applied to the cervical spine, either moist or dry, may give symptomatic relief, but does not speed healing. The patient should be encouraged to do his daily work and activities as much as possible. If the patient has severe pain and muscle spasm at the initial injury, his clinical course will probably last 4 to 6 weeks. When the patient's pain subsides and he has full range of motion without muscle spasm, the soft collar can be gradually discontinued, and the patient should also be advised of the methods of relieving muscle spasm and preventing recurrent symptoms (Figs. 61.2 and 61.3). If there are no symptoms of nerve root compression, the patient should be treated for a long period of time, perhaps a year, before consideration of further workup.

All patients with whiplash injury, especially those with nerve root signs, are probably best seen at least once by an orthopaedist or neurosurgeon for confirmation of the diagnosis and for follow-up should the symptoms not resolve in a reasonable time.

References

General

Bland, JH and Nakano, KK: Neck pain. in *Textbook of Rheumatology*, edited by WN Kelly, ED Harris, S Ruddy, and CB Sledge. W.B. Saunders, Philadelphia, 1981.
   An excellent discussion of the anatomy and biomechanisms and of the diagnosis, treatment, and differential diagnosis of common cervical spine problems.
Disease of the Intervertebral Disc: *Orthop Clin North Am* 2(No. 2): 1971.
   Excellent coverage of anatomy, histology, and pathophysiology of degenerative disc disease.
Rothman, RH and Simeone, FA: The Spine. W.B. Saunders, Philadelphia 1975.
   An exhaustive textbook with excellent chapters covering anatomy, differential diagnosis, cervical disc disease, and arthritis of the spine.

Specific

1. Elias, F: Roentgen findings in the asymptomatic cervical spine. *NY J Med* 58: 3300, 1958.
2. Gehr, RB, Rothman, SL and Kier, EL: The role of computed tomography in the evaluation of upper cervical spine pathology. *Comput Tomogr* 2: 79, 1978.
3. Johnson, RM, Hart, DL, Simmons, EF, Ransby, GR and Southwick, EF: Cervical orthoses. *J Bone Joint Surg* 59: 332, 1977.
4. Macnab, I: "The whiplash syndrome." *Orthop Clin North Am* 2: 389, 1971.
5. Odom, GG, Finney, W and Woodhall, B: Cervical disc lesions. *JAMA* 166: 23, 1958.
6. Oppenheim, BE and Cantez, S: What causes lower neck uptake in bone scans? *Radiology* 124: 749, 1977.
7. Robinson, RA, Walker, AE, Ferlic, DC and Wiecking, DK: The results of anterior interbody fusion of the cervical spine. *J Bone Joint Surg* 44A: 1569, 1962.
8. Scovill, WB: Types of cervical disc lesions and their surgical approaches. *JAMA* 196: 479, 1966.

CHAPTER SIXTY-TWO

Low Back Pain

ANDREW F. BROOKER, M.D., and JOHN R. BURTON, M.D.

As many as 65% of the population experience low back pain at some time in their lives, and this problem is a major cause of time lost from work (7). While perhaps as many as one-third of these patients do not seek the advice of a physician (11), the remainder do so; and, therefore, most physicians often will need to evaluate patients with this problem. This chapter reviews the patterns of back pain most frequently described by patients and the process of evaluating these patients and outlines acute and intercritical treatment.

Symptoms of low back pain most often begin in the 3rd and 4th decade of life, and approximately 60 to 65% are not associated with trauma, lifting or strain (10). The back is a complex anatomic and functional region which is not easily analyzed. Therefore, it is often very difficult to diagnose precisely patients complaining of back pain. Physicians must use considerable judgment in deciding how best to evaluate and manage these patients. Most important, serial observation is a critical component in the care of patients with low back pain.

ANATOMY AND BIOMECHANICS OF THE LUMBAR AREA

Figure 62.1 emphasizes the anatomic complexity of the lumbar region and illustrates the important structures in the region.

The lumbar vertebrae are exposed to tremendous forces. This is due principally to the magnification of stresses which result from the lever effect of the arm in lifting and to vertical forces associated with man's upright position. Figure 62.2 demonstrates how lifting an object away from the body introduces the lever magnification phenomenon resulting in a marked increase in forces on the vertebral body and discs. Because each intervertebral disc is a fluid system, there is a hydraulic pressure created whenever a load is placed on the axial skeleton. This hydraulic pressure magnifies 3 to 5 times the force that occurs on the annulus fibrosus. This force is akin to the hoop stress which occurs in a barrel when pressure is applied to its liquid content. The ability of the annulus fibrosus to withstand stress decreases significantly with age, and by 60 years many individuals have only 50% the strength in these fibers that they had at age 30.

The lumbar spine, however, is not just an isolated structure. Much support is obtained by the muscles and ligaments and by the muscles of the thoracic and abdominal cavities. These latter structures act as a sort of muscular cylinder which helps to decrease the load on the axial skeleton by as much as 30% in the lumbar area and 50% in the thoracic spine (13).

ASSESSMENT OF PATIENTS WITH LOW BACK PAIN

Important information will always be obtained from the history and physical examination in the patient with low back pain.

History

The history may provide a clue that the cause of low back pain may not be a regional problem. The patient's *age* is the first important fact. Older individuals, especially those over 60 years of age who are seen with new back pain, are more likely to have referred pain or a less common cause of back pain than are younger individuals. Further, any history of *systemic illness*—such as fever, weight loss, gastrointestinal or genitourinary symptoms or arthritis—should suggest a less common cause of the back pain (see below).

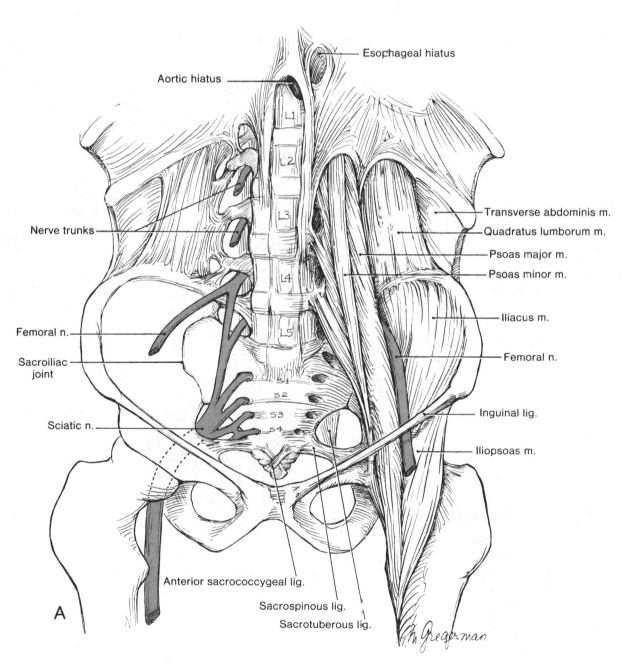

Figure 62.1   Normal anatomy: (*A*) anterior and (*B*) posterior views (p. 604).

The *occupational* and *recreational history* will provide information about predisposing factors, as well as about features of the patient's life which may need to be modified should the problem become chronic.

A thorough assessment of the *chronological development* of the pain and of the factors which *aggravate* and *alleviate* the pain will guide the physician in directing the evaluation and management of the patient. The *pain should be characterized* with respect to its severity, quality, localization, and duration to aid determination of the etiology as well as the anatomic localization of the problem. Historical evidence of motor or sensory *nerve root irritation* or of *sphincter dysfunction* (bladder or bowel incontinence) should be sought.

Physical Examination

The examination of the back should receive special emphasis, but a general physical examination should also be done in those patients in whom referred pain or a less common cause of back pain is suspected.

EXAMINATION OF THE BACK AND ASSOCIATED MUSCULOSKELETAL AREAS

The patient should wear only a gown which opens in the back and should be barefoot.

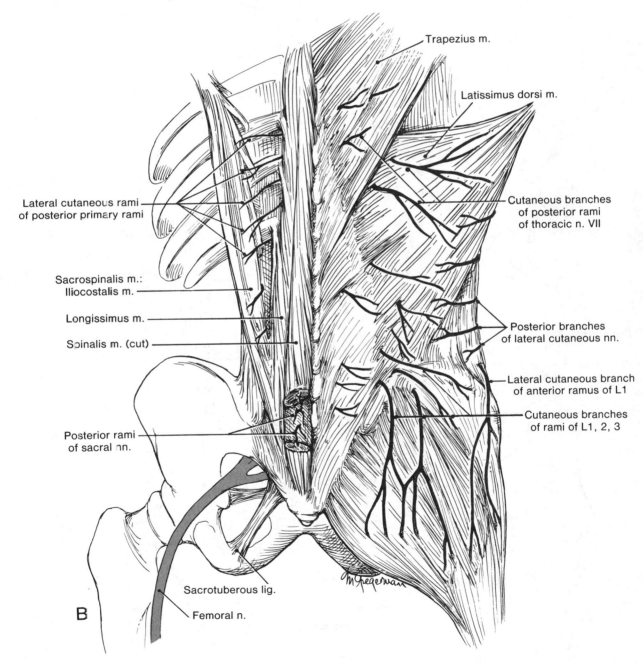

Trapezius m.

Latissimus dorsi m.

Cutaneous branches of posterior rami of thoracic n. VII

Lateral cutaneous rami of posterior primary rami

Sacrospinalis m.: Iliocostalis m.

Longissimus m.

Spinalis m. (cut)

Posterior branches of lateral cutaneous nn.

Lateral cutaneous branch of anterior ramus of L1

Cutaneous branches of rami of L1, 2, 3

Posterior rami of sacral nn.

Sacrotuberous lig.

Femoral n.

B

Fig 62.1B

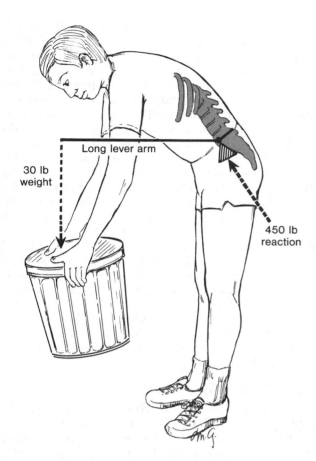

Figure 62.2   Forces in the lumbar area.

First, the patient should be examined while he is *standing*. The spinal column should be checked for scoliosis, kyphosis, or lordosis. Firm palpation of the paravertebral muscles and of each vertebral spine should be performed. Isolated tenderness of one or two spinous processes suggests a local problem such as compression fracture, abscess, or tumor.

Mobility of the spine should then be assessed. The patient should bend forward to attempt to touch his toes. During this process there should be a normally smooth rhythm down and up. If the rhythm is interrupted or is hesitant, a problem with a facet joint or significant lower back muscle spasm may be present. Similarly, lateral flexion and extension should be assessed. Lateral flexion is usually preserved in disc disease but may be absent, for example, in patients with ankylosing spondylitis.

The patient should be examined *sitting with his legs dangling* over the edge of the examining table. The deep tendon reflexes of the knees and ankles should be tested. They assess the reflex arcs involving the nerve roots, L4, and S1, respectively. An absent reflex may signify nerve root irritation due to a herniated intravertebral disc. While the patient remains seated, the physician should perform a *straight leg examination* by straightening the patient's knee Flexion of the hip and extension of the knee stretches

the lumbar nerve roots; and if radicular pain (down the leg and not limited to the back) is produced by this maneuver, nerve root irritation is present. The irritation can be confirmed by lowering the leg just to the point where the pain disappears and then dorsiflexing the foot which again stretches the nerves and reproduces pain. This sign, if positive, suggests a herniated disc or, less commonly, bony impingement of a nerve root caused by degenerative disease of a facet joint, lumbar stenosis, or rarely, a tumor of the cord or surrounding structures. The absence of radicular pain, especially in an individual over age 30 years, does not rule out a herniated disc which may be too small or in the wrong location to irritate the nerve roots. This variant method of straight leg testing serves as a check on the standard method.

Next, the patient assumes the *supine* position, so that a *standard straight leg raising test* can be performed. This is done by extending the knee of the side expected to be involved and then slowly flexing the hip. Normally the hip can be flexed to 80° without pain, except perhaps for some tightness in the hamstring muscles and behind the knee. A positive test is manifested by pain or paresthesia in the sciatic distribution (i.e., posterior aspect of the thigh, leg, and the foot) on the affected side or on both. It is an indication of nerve root irritation. Following this test the unaffected or well leg should be raised, thus performing the *crossed straight leg raising test*. This procedure causes tension and stretch of the nerve roots of the opposite (affected) side and results in pain in the affected lower extremity. When this test is positive, there is a very high (6, 8, 17) but not absolute (16) correlation with disc herniation.

Next, *sensory assessment* of the buttock, perineum, and lower extremities can be accomplished. Figure 75.2 shows the relevant sensory dermatomes which can be evaluated by pinprick and touch. Abnormalities will help localize a lesion and when present will help the physician decide on the need and urgency of an orthopaedic or neurosurgical consultation. An important component of the sensory assessment is the search for signs which would suggest the presence of a *cauda equina syndrome* (compression of the lower portion of the spinal cord and its nerve roots). This syndrome, if present, is an indication for immediate hospitalization and neurosurgical or orthopaedic consultation. The signs of compression of the lower end of the spinal cord are saddle anesthesia, loss of anal sphincter tone (assessed by rectal examination) and cremasteric reflexes, as well as historical evidence of bowel and bladder dysfunction.

A *detailed assessment of motor function* in the legs will also help to localize a lesion in the patient in whom neurologic involvement is suspected (see also Table 81.7). This assessment should include, while the patient is sitting, the knee extensors (L2–4), the dorsiflexors of the foot (L4–5, 51), and the plantar flexor of the foot (S1–2). In order to demonstrate subtle weakness, the patient should stand and walk normally as well as on heel (gastrocnemius muscle group—S1–2) and toe (tibialis anterior muscle—L4–5). The symmetry of the buttock also can be assessed at this time (gluteus maximus—L4–5, S1–2).

Finally, an assessment of the *hip, sacroiliac, and knee joints* should be done, as abnormalities in these joints may cause back or leg pain and mislead the physician into assuming that a primary lumbar problem is present. The hip and knee joints should be assessed by moving these joints through a normal range of motion; this is done with the patient supine in order to exclude nonarticular discomfort which may be generated by active movement. The sacroiliac joint is best assessed when the patient is supine with the knee flexed and the ankle placed on the opposite straight leg at the knee. The physician places his hands on the flexed knee and the ipsilateral anterior superior iliac spine and, by pressing down, the sacroiliac joint on that side is stressed. When the patient is not supine, firm pressure over the sacroiliac joints will also elicit discomfort when sacroiliitis is present.

EXAMINATION OF OTHER REGIONS

Because pain may be referred to the back or may be due to changes in the back that are part of a systemic process, a selective general examination is important in some patients, particularly if (a) the patient is over 50 years of age, (b) there is fever, (c) historical clues suggest a systemic process, (d) the assessment of the back is normal, or (e) the back discomfort persists or progresses in spite of conservative therapy.

Metastatic cancer of the spine is especially common from primary tumors of the breast, lung, prostate, thyroid, and rectum. These regions should therefore be examined carefully. Further, an abdominal examination and, in women, a pelvic examination are necessary. Referred pain from cancer may also be felt in the back. For example, pancreatic lesions may cause pain to be referred to the high lumbar or low thoracic vertebral region. Bowel or urinary tract lesions may cause pain to be referred to the mid or low lumbar region, and disease located in the pelvis may cause lower lumbar or sacral pain. Particular attention to the lymph nodes may provide a clue to the presence of an intra-abdominal lymphoma.

Important also is the assessment of the adequacy of the arteries emanating from the lower aorta. Abnormalities here may cause pain due to ischemia in the back, buttock, or lower extremities during exertion. In addition to diminished pulses and bruits over arteries, cutaneous signs of ischemia (ulcers, loss of hair or nails) should be sought in the legs or feet (see also Chapter 84).

Laboratory Evaluation

X-RAY EVALUATION

It is usually not necessary to obtain an X-ray of the lumbar spine when patients with back pain are first evaluated. The study is important in checking for the less common causes of back pain rather than in diagnosing the more common problems of acute or subacute lumbar disc disease or of muscular strain in which the X-ray will be normal or nonspecific. By age 50, 67% of normal individuals show evidence of "disc disease" characterized by narrowing of one or more disc space and disc calcification; and an additional 20% of individuals are found to have lumbar osteophyte formations alone and only 13% of individuals at this age have normal lumbar X-rays. On the other hand, abnormal X-rays are seen in less than 5% of individuals who are less than 20 years of age (9). Two-thirds of patients with evidence on X-ray of lumbar degenerative disc disease are asymptomatic. Also, there is no correlation between the presence of facet joint osteoarthritis and symptoms (12). Lumbar X-rays should be obtained whenever there is a suspicion back pain has a less common cause and especially if the patient does not respond within 3 weeks to conservative therapy. In this setting less common causes of low back pain such as a collapsed vertebra, or osteoblastic or an osteolytic lesions may be detected by the X-ray.

OTHER LABORATORY TESTS

These tests should be performed when back pain is suspected to be due to a less common cause. While the evaluation may be quite varied, several screening tests are particularly helpful: urinalysis (renal disease), stool occult blood (intestinal cancer), complete blood count and differential and erythrocyte sedimentation rate (inflammatory or neoplastic disease), serum calcium and alkaline phosphatase (diffuse bone disease) and, in males, acid phosphatase (metastatic prostatic cancer). Other tests may be indicated based on the suspicion of the diagnostic possibilities.

Serial Observation

It is most important for the physician, when first evaluating a patient with back pain, to establish rapport and to ensure follow-up of the patient either by telephone or by a subsequent office visit, since an absolute diagnosis of the specific cause of back pain is often impossible at the initial visit. Even when there is a history of trauma, the diagnosis is not certain since, for example, 10% of patients with neoplasia as a cause of back pain give a history of trauma (7). Even when there is no initial clue in the history or in the physical examination, a serious or less common disorder is not ruled out.

If on reassessment there are symptoms or signs of progression or if there is an incomplete response to treatment, re-evaluation with an eye to an alternative diagnosis is necessary. After conservative management for an episode of back pain, 40% of patients will be symptom-free in 1 week and symptoms will have remitted in 75% by 3 weeks (5). Regardless of the initial problem formulation, follow-up contact with the patient within 3 weeks is mandatory. By following this approach routinely, considerable initial laboratory testing can be avoided and clues to the presence of an underlying less common and potentially serious disorder will not be missed. This follow-up also provides an opportunity for education regarding recurrent symptoms (very common) and for advice regarding prophylactic measures (see below).

COMMON REGIONAL (NONSYSTEMIC) BACK SYNDROMES

Three problems account for the majority of complaints of low back pain: acute and subacute lumbar disc disease and muscle strain (facet joint) syndrome.

Acute Lumbar Disc Disease

The annulus fibrosus degenerates with time, which predisposes to disc rupture and to herniation of the nucleus pulposus (Fig. 62.3), resulting in the acute lumbar disc syndrome. There may be mild transient episodes of low back pain associated with this degenerative process, but it is herniation that produces the sudden severe discomfort. A sudden increase in the pressure in the lumbar spine which might occur with a flexion injury, lifting with the arms extended away from the body (the lever magnification of stresses), a sudden lurch or even a sneeze or cough can precipitate the rupture. However, many patients who have a ruptured disc will not give a history of injury or of a sudden increase in pressure. Lumbar disc disease is most common at the L4–5 level and at the L5–S1 level and is less common between the other vertebral bodies. Acute lumbar disc disease is less common than subacute disc disease or muscular strain syndrome (see below).

DIAGNOSIS

Patients with this problem describe severe back, buttock and/or leg pain which is either unilateral or bilateral. The pain may be so severe that the patient resists examination and splints the back in an awkward position of lateral lumbar flexion and hip flexion. The patient is still or else moves very slowly. Any suggestion of restlessness or pain worsened by quiet rest in bed suggests the dangerous cauda equina syndrome (see above). The diagnosis of acute lumbar disc herniation is most likely when examination (see above) reveals signs of nerve root irritation with either a loss of motor function, loss of deep tendon reflexes, and/or a localized sensory deficit.

MANAGEMENT

The patient will often be so uncomfortable that immediate hospitalization and urgent orthopaedic or neurosurgical consultation is necessary. After hospital admission a decision must be made about further confirmation of a neurologic deficit (occasionally necessary by electromyography, which may show denervation of leg muscles) or about myelography or computerized axial tomography (CT) of the lumbar region. These latter techniques will show a defect in the spinal canal, usually from a herniated disc or rarely from another lesion (e.g., neural tumor). Because there is less morbidity, many consultants prefer CT for initial confirmation of a herniated disc (3); although neither CT or myelography are completely free from false negative results. Depending on the patient's response to initial treatment and on the above studies, surgery may be considered. Most patients, however, will respond to conservative therapy. When followed for several years, patients treated surgically or conservatively have the same fitness for work. Also, approximately 60% of those who had surgery and approximately 40% who were treated conservatively will be symptom-free when studied 8 years posthospitalization (14). Those with conservative therapy, however, may have, more symptoms in the earlier posthospitalization period.

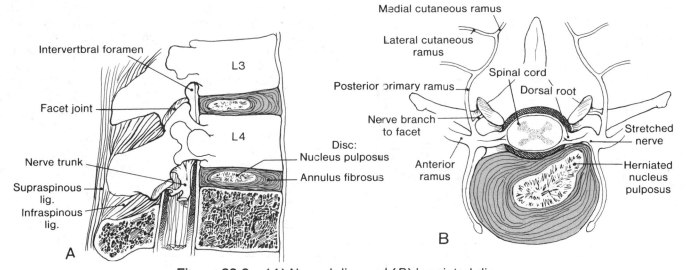

Figure 62.3   (A) Normal disc and (B) herniated disc.

Should the patient not be hospitalized initially, very close surveillance is necessary with immediate hospitalization should signs progress or should the pain not promptly remit. The conservative management of patients with this problem is discussed in the section on subacute lumbar disc disease as patients with this latter syndrome are more frequently managed at home (see below).

Subacute Lumbar "Disc" Disease

This problem is similar to acute lumbar disc disease, but is not sudden or totally incapacitating. Frequently, the history is of several weeks' or even years' duration. The disease is caused either by a herniated disc or by a bony spur impinging on a nerve root.

DIAGNOSIS

The patient with this problem describes back, buttock, or lower extremity pain (usually radiating below the knee) that is most commonly unilateral. Examination usually reveals evidence of irritation of a specific nerve root resulting in loss of a localized motor or sensory neurologic function or of an absent deep tendon reflex (L5–S1 disc, ankle; or L3–4 or L4–5 disc, knee). The straight (or crossed straight) leg raising test is often positive. In this situation, conservative management at home is most appropriate. However, re-evaluation and/or consultation is mandatory should neurological symptoms or signs progress or if a prompt remission of symptoms does not occur.

MANAGEMENT

Recumbency is the natural position associated with the lowest intradiscal pressure. The patient should therefore be advised to adhere to *strict bedrest* for a minimum of 3 to 4 days. To minimize back motion, he should either have a bed-board placed under his mattress or have the mattress moved to the floor. He should position a small pillow beneath his head and knees, as shown in Figure 62.4. This relaxes the muscles and relieves stretch on the nerve roots. An equally comfortable position is the semifetal position. The patient should be out of bed only for bathroom use. The application of *heat* by a heating pad for 20 to 30 min several times a day (on low or medium

setting with a protective towel between skin and pad to prevent burns) will often relieve muscular spasm and thereby provide comfort. Occasionally a patient will feel that heat worsens symptoms, in which case heat application should be discontinued. Application of moist heat is not practical when the patient is supine in bed; but it may be used (and is preferred by some patients) for symptomatic relief once the patient is out of bed. Moist heat may be accomplished by using hot towels, a shower, a tub bath, or a heat pack which produces sustained heat for up to ½ hour (available at pharmacies). Analgesics such as codeine, 30 to 60 mg in combination with aspirin or acetaminophen (Tylenol) every 4 to 6 hours, may be necessary for the first several days. Subsequently, acetaminophen or aspirin alone is usually sufficient to control pain. An *anti-inflammatory agent* such as aspirin, 600 mg 4 times a day, is an important adjuvant to rest. The patient should understand that aspirin is being prescribed for its anti-inflammatory qualities and that it should be taken regularly during the period of significant symptoms. If the patient cannot tolerate aspirin, a nonsteroidal anti-inflammatory agent such as indomethacin (Indocin) 25 to 50 mg 3 or 4 times a day, may be prescribed. The nonsteroidal anti-inflammatory agents, however, have not been shown to be more effective than aspirin. *Muscle relaxants* are not first line therapeutic agents, but they may be used in the occasional patient who has not responded in a day or two to the above treatments. Carisoprodol (Soma), 350 mg 4 times a day, has been found in controlled studies to be more effective than placebo in relieving discomfort in patients with low back pain (1). Cyclobenzaprine (Flexeril), 10 to 20 mg 3 times a day, has also been shown more efficacious than placebo in the treatment of intractable pain syndromes with muscle spasm, but is associated frequently with a dry mouth, drowsiness, and dizziness (2). Diazepam (Valium), highly touted as a muscle relaxant, has been variably shown to be no more effective to slightly more effective than placebo (14). Its sedating properties, however, may be useful in the patient who finds adherence to bedrest difficult. Only a 3- to 7-day supply should be given because of its potential for abuse.

When improvement occurs after 3 or 4 days, the

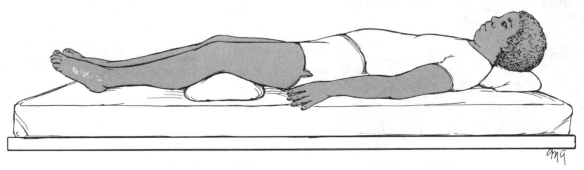

Figure 62.4   Recumbent position.

patient may be permitted out of bed for short leisurely walks. Sitting should be avoided as it will tend to increase intradiscal pressure and may cause a recurrence of pain. Over a period of 1 to 2 weeks, ambulation is increased with a gradual decrease of the dose of analgesic until the patient can return to his usual activities without medication. During this recovery period it is especially important to advise the patient to avoid activities which greatly increase the forces applied to the lower spine (e.g., lifting, pushing, force on outstretched upper extremity as in making beds or vacuuming, lurching, or bending). Should the patient fail to respond or should a recurrence occur, he should be re-examined and a orthopaedic or neurosurgical consultation should be con-

sidered. For the patient who is recovering satisfactorily, a variety of exercise programs have been advocated, but simple isometric flexion exercises are the most effective. These exercises (Fig. 62.5) should be recommended as soon as pain subsides. Additional exercises that stretch the lumbar sacral muscles (Fig. 62.6) also may provide comfort. Exercises which are designed to strengthen the abdominal musculature, such as sit-ups with the knees flexed or straight leg raising, have been shown to magnify markedly the lower lumbar intradiscal forces, could exacerbate symptoms, and are not recommended.

With continued healing the discomfort should resolve entirely, and the patient then can be advised about prophylactic measures (see below).

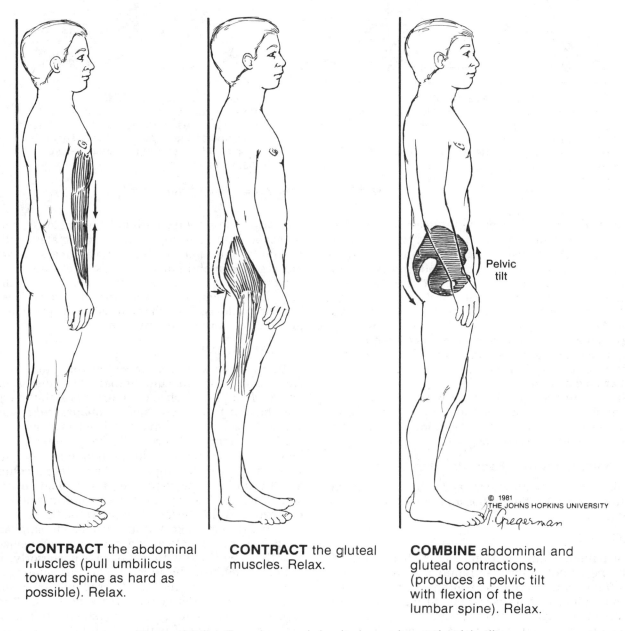

© 1981
THE JOHNS HOPKINS UNIVERSITY

CONTRACT the abdominal muscles (pull umbilicus toward spine as hard as possible). Relax.

CONTRACT the gluteal muscles. Relax.

COMBINE abdominal and gluteal contractions, (produces a pelvic tilt with flexion of the lumbar spine). Relax.

Figure 62.5   Exercises—abdominal muscles and pelvic tilt.

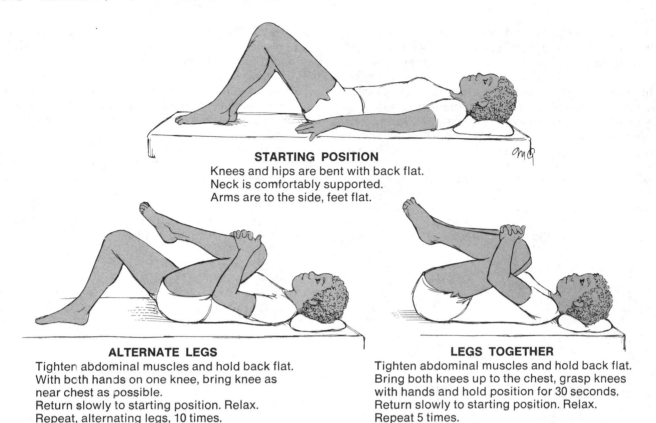

STARTING POSITION
Knees and hips are bent with back flat.
Neck is comfortably supported.
Arms are to the side, feet flat.

ALTERNATE LEGS
Tighten abdominal muscles and hold back flat.
With both hands on one knee, bring knee as
near chest as possible.
Return slowly to starting position. Relax.
Repeat, alternating legs, 10 times.

LEGS TOGETHER
Tighten abdominal muscles and hold back flat.
Bring both knees up to the chest, grasp knees
with hands and hold position for 30 seconds.
Return slowly to starting position. Relax.
Repeat 5 times.

Figure 62.6 Knee-chest exercises.

Physical therapy is usually not necessary in managing these patients; and, in particular, active exercise programs may intensify symptoms and should be avoided. Therapy such as ultrasound, shortwave, diathermy, heat or cold packs may provide short term relief, but there is no evidence that there is any effect on the disc lesion or any long term effect on symptoms. Also, such therapy is often quite inconvenient for patients and therefore may detract from overall compliance. Lumbar traction has not been shown to be more effective than bed rest in the treatment of lumbar disc disease.

There is an occasional patient with this syndrome that may benefit from a *lumbosacral support*. However, these devices are more commonly used in muscle strain syndromes (see below).

Muscular Strain (Facet Joint) Syndrome

This common syndrome is caused by an exertional or stress injury to the lumbosacral muscles or to the facet joints.

DIAGNOSIS

The patient complains of pain in the back, buttock, or in one or both lower extremities. Usually symptoms follow a recent increase in physical activity for that individual such as gardening, lifting, or an infrequently played sport. Usually the patient experiences no (or only minimal) discomfort during or immedi-

ately after the activity. Within the next 12 to 36 hours, however, pain develops and is associated with a feeling of muscular stiffness. Over hours to days, increased pain and musuclar spasm develop.

Examination of the back (see above) may show nonspecific signs of muscle spasm and of loss of lumbar lordosis; but characteristically there is no evidence of nerve root irritation.

MANAGEMENT

The treatment for this large group of patients is the same as it is for subacute lumbar "disc" disease (see above). In addition, once the patient is ambulating he may benefit from the use of a *lumbosacral support*. While these devices have not been evaluated in a controlled study, theoretically they could provide benefit by increasing intra-abdominal pressure, which will provide support to the vertebral column; and by limiting (or reminding the patient to limit) spinal motion (clearly the spine is not immobilized, however). A lumbosacral support is fitted by an orthotist (brace maker) at an orthopaedic appliance shop. The most practical and most common device is a cloth corset fitted with metal stays posteriorly. The patient should use the support when ambulating and then, as healing occurs, should gradually be weaned from the use of the corset over a period of 2 to 3 weeks until usual activities are resumed. It is important for this group of patients to *return gradually* to full activity as an abrupt return would likely cause a recurrence of low back pain. As in the other syndromes associated with back pain, the physician should establish rapport at the first visit and ensure follow-up since a less common cause of back pain could present with the symptoms and signs of muscle strain. Prompt re-evaluation is necessary should the symptoms not improve or should progressive symptoms or signs develop.

When patients are completely free of symptoms and are performing at a moderate level of activity, an exercise program can be initiated (see below).

LESS COMMON SYNDROMES

There are other regional and systemic disorders which are manifest by complaints of low back pain.

Lumbar Stenosis

Some people have a congenitally narrow spinal canal. Frequently, however, symptoms do not begin until after the age of 35 or 40. Characteristically irritation of multiple nerve roots at different levels on both sides is found, and this is the clue to the diagnosis. When lumbar stenosis is considered, orthopaedic or neurosurgical consultation is appropriate. Laminectomy gives very satisfying results; whereas conservative therapy may be associated with progressive neurologic dysfunction in the lower extremities.

Sacroiliitis

Pain from an inflammatory process of the sacroiliac joint is not uncommon. Frequently the process is manifest as leg or buttock pain rather than as back pain. It may be the first symptom of ankylosing spondylitis when it is identified in a young man. Sacroiliitis may also be seen in older men and women because of a nonspecific inflammatory process in this joint. A clue to the presence of sacroiliitis is tenderness when the joint is stressed while the patient is in the prone or in the supine position (see p. 606). Conditions affecting the sacroiliac joint are discussed in Chapter 68.

Vertebral Fractures

Vertebral compression fractures are common and usually the result of a flexion injury when the spine is abruptly and violently flexed as it is, for example, during jumping. The force needed to compress a vertebral body in healthy bone is considerable. However, when the bone is diseased, as, for example, in osteoporosis, multiple myeloma, metastatic cancer, or hyperparathyroidism, the injury may be relatively insignificant. Pain is usually localized and immediate, although it may be delayed for several days following the fracture. Often tenderness over the vertebra indicates the presence of this problem, but an X-ray is necessary to confirm the diagnosis. With lumbar or thoracic vertebral compression fractures, management includes rest, adequate analgesia, and gradual ambulation when the patient is pain-free. A lumbosacral support or, for the patient with a thoracic vertebral fracture, a chair-back brace may be helpful in alleviating pain. It is important in the evaluation to consider a process (such as multiple myeloma) that may have weakened the bone and predisposed it to fracture.

Other Causes

Many other regional or systemic problems may cause patients to come to physicians with complaints of back pain. The more usual of these are listed in Table 62.1.

MANAGEMENT OF INTERCRITICAL PERIOD

While most patients with low back pain have a complete remission of symptoms within 3 weeks (5), many patients will experience a recurrence. For this reason the physician should discuss with the patient ways to prevent recurrence. The important subjects of posture, weight control, exercise, and activities will need to be discussed.

Figure 62.7 shows some correct and incorrect *postures* and practical advice which may be useful to provide patients who have had low back pain. *Weight reduction* is desirable in the obese patient, as excessive weight directly increases the load on the lower vertebral column and its supporting structures. *Exercises* designed to strengthen the muscles of support

Table 62.1
Some Less Common Causes of Low Back Pain[a]

REFERRED PAIN
(A clue that the pain is referred is the absence of any tenderness, limitation of motion, or aggravation of pain or spasm during the physical examination of the back.)
  Sacral pain—from a pelvic problem
  Lower lumbar pain—from a lower abdominal disease process
  Lower thoracic and upper lumbar pain—upper abdominal disease process
SYSTEMIC OR REGIONAL DISEASES SOMETIMES ASSOCIATED WITH BACK PAIN
  Infections—tuberculosis, osteomyelitis, spinal or epidural abscess
  Neoplastic disease—primary myeloma, lymphoma, retroperitoneal sarcoma or neural tumor—metastatic disease
  Metabolic disease—osteoporosis (see Chapter 71), osteomalacia, Paget's disease
  Postural back pain (increased lordosis as, *e.g.*, with high heel use)
  Psychiatric cause of back pain, *e.g.*, depression (see Chapter 14)

---

[a] These causes should be considered when the patient fails to respond to conservative treatment or if there is suspicion on initial evaluation.

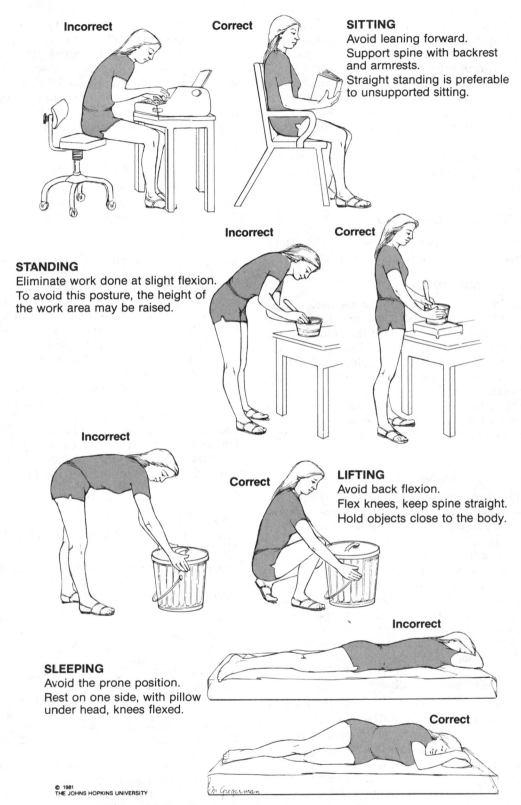

SITTING
Avoid leaning forward.
Support spine with backrest and armrests.
Straight standing is preferable to unsupported sitting.

STANDING
Eliminate work done at slight flexion. To avoid this posture, the height of the work area may be raised.

LIFTING
Avoid back flexion.
Flex knees, keep spine straight.
Hold objects close to the body.

SLEEPING
Avoid the prone position.
Rest on one side, with pillow under head, knees flexed.

© 1981
THE JOHNS HOPKINS UNIVERSITY

Figure 62.7   Postural attitudes—correct/incorrect.

are frequently prescribed although they have not been shown to be preventive. However, weakness of muscles regularly occurs with bedrest and with mod-ified activity that is part of the treatment of patients with acute back pain syndromes. Also, it has been demonstrated that sudden loading of the spine when the back is flexed and when the knees are straight markedly increases lumbar forces compared to when the knees are bent and the back is straight. Exercises which strengthen the quadriceps (extend knees) are theoretically sound, and include swimming, cycling, or jogging on a flat surface. In addition, because the abdominal musculature is important in supporting the spine when a weight is brought to bear on it (see above) exercises that strengthen the abdominal musculature (Fig. 62.5) are important. More complex exercise programs are likely to be followed by only an occasional patient and therefore are not recommended.

Work or athletic *activities may need to be modified*, although there is no convincing support for the concept that heavy labor or lifting predisposes to the development of low back pain (15). Several points are, however, worth emphasis: (a) improper technique in lifting produces backache, (b) there is a high incidence of low back pain in those people who either sit for prolonged periods or who are unable to sit at all during the work day, (c) sudden maximal physical activity results in a high incidence of back pain. Further, there is evidence that back pain occurs more frequently in individuals who consider their occupation to be physically hard and in those who feel that the work that they perform is particularly stressful to the spine (4). These observations are important for the physician to bear in mind as he educates the patient about recurrences of back pain after the acute episode has resolved.

References

General

Heljet, AJ and Gruebel Lee, DM: *Disorders of the Lumbar Spine.* J. B. Lippincott, Philadelphia, 1978.
   A readable well illustrated monograph on low back pain problems.

Macnab, I: *Backache.* Williams & Wilkins Co., Baltimore, 1977.
   A very well organized, practical text with many helpful schematic illustrations covering all aspects of low back pain.

Specific

1. Baratta, RR: A double-blind comparative study of Carisoprodol, Propoxyphene, and placebo in the management of low back syndrome. *Curr Ther Res 20:* 233, 1976.
2. Brown, BR, Jr and Womble, J: Cyclobenzaprine in intractable pain syndromes with muscle spasm. *JAMA 240:* 1151, 1978.
3. Carrera, GF, Williams, AL and Houghton, VM: Computed tomography in sciatica. *Radiology 137:* 433, 1980.
4. Dehlin, O, Hedenrud, B and Horal, J: Back symptoms in nursing aides in a geriatric hospital. *Scand J Rehabil Med 8:* 47, 1976.
5. Dillane, B, Fry, J and Kalton, G: Acute back syndrome—a study from general practice. *Br Med J 3:* 82, 1966.
6. Hakelius, A and Hindmarsh, J: The significance of neurological signs and myelographic findings in the diagnosis of lumbar root compression. *Acta Orthop Scand 43:* 239, 1972.
7. Horal, J: The clinical appearance of low back disorders in the city of Gothenburg, Sweden *Acta Orthop Scand* Suppl. 118: 1, 1969.
8. Hudgins, WR: The predictive value of myelography in the diagnosis of ruptured lumbar discs. *J Neurosurg 32:* 152, 1970.
9. Hult, L: The lumbar insufficiency-lumbago-sciatica syndrome. *Acta Orthop Scand* Suppl 16: 32, 1954.
10. Hult, L: Cervical, dorsal and lumbar spinal syndromes. *Acta Orthop Scand* Suppl. 17: 1, 1954.
11. Kane, EL, Leymaster, C, Olsen, D, Woolley FR and Fisher, FD: Manipulating the patient. A comparison of the effectiveness of physician and chiropractor care. *Lancet 1:* 1333, 1974.
12. Lawrence, JS, Bremner, JM and Bier, F: Osteo-arthrosis. Prevalence in the population and relationship between symptoms and x-ray changes. *Ann Rheum Dis 25:* 1, 1966.
13. Morris, JM, Lucas, DB and Bresler, B: Role of the trunk in stability of the spine. *J Bone Joint Surg 43A:* 327, 1961.
14. Quinet, RJ, and Hadler, NM: Diagnosis and treatment of backache. *Semin Arthritis Rheum 8:* 261, 1979.
15. Rowe, ML: Low back pain in industry. *J Occup Med 11:* 161, 1969.
16. Vaz, M, Wadia, RS and Gokhale, SD: Another cause of a positive crossed-straight-leg-raising test. *N Engl J Med 299:* 779, 1978.
17. Woodhall, B and Hayes, GJ: The well-leg raising test of Fajersztajn in the diagnosis of ruptured lumbar intervertebral disc. *J Bone Joint Surg 32A:* 786, 1950.

CHAPTER SIXTY-THREE

Bursitis, Tenosynovitis, and Fibrositis

GREGORY B. KELLY, M.D.

BURSITIS

General Considerations

DEFINITION

Bursitis, the inflammation of a bursal sac, is a very common problem. Bursal sacs are subcutaneous structures lined with synovial membrane which secretes and absorbs fluid. The bursae provide, thereby, a lubricating mechanism between structures such as bones, ligaments, tendons, muscles, and skin. Although usually isolated, occasionally they are in communication with a joint space. There are over 150 such structures in the body, but the number is not fixed and a new bursa may appear wherever there is friction between structures (1).

Most instances of bursitis can be diagnosed properly and treated in the office by the general physician; however, occasionally, because of the location of the bursa, the uncertainty of the diagnosis, or frequent recurrences of the problem, referral to an orthopaedist or rheumatologist may be necessary.

ETIOLOGY

The most common cause of bursitis is trauma; less often, a systemic process such as rheumatoid arthritis or gout causes the inflammation. Septic bursitis is especially a concern in patients with superficial bursitis (such as olecranon or prepatellar bursitis) (4).

MANIFESTATIONS

Bursitis is particularly common in middle-aged and older individuals of either sex, but the reason for this age distribution is not known. Patients with acute bursitis usually describe the abrupt onset of localized pain and discomfort which is worsened by any movement of the structures adjacent to the bursa. Frequently, there is a history of trauma or of repetitively performed activity. Fever is occasionally present.

When the inflamed bursa is superficial, an obvious swelling may be present which is often erythematous and tender. On the other hand, inflammation in deep bursae may be manifest only by regional tenderness and by some limitation of motion.

ASPIRATION OF BURSAE

When there is identifiable swelling that is fluctuant, especially accompanied by fever or evidence of surrounding cellulitis, it is important to aspirate fluid from the bursa. This may be easily accomplished by the general physician when the bursa is superficial (Table 63.1). The appearance of the fluid varies, depending on the cause. It should be analyzed routinely (Table 63.1) in order to establish the diagnosis (Table 63.2).

THERAPY

If a septic bursitis is identified, the patient should be hospitalized to receive parenteral antibiotics and repeated aspiration of the bursa. Gout, pseudogout,

Table 63.1
Technique of Aspiration of Superficial Bursae (or Joints) and of Analysis of Bursal (or Synovial) Fluid

1. Determine by palpation the area of maximum tenderness and/or fluctuance and outline with indelible pen
2. Determine and outline with an indelible pen any structures to be avoided
3. Clean the skin with iodine solution such as povidone (Betadine)
4. Anesthetize the skin with Xylocaine in the area of planned aspiration
5. An 18 gauge needle should be used to aspirate
6. The fluid should be grossly inspected by the physician and analyzed for the following:
   (a) Cell count and differential—fluid needs to be in a tube containing anticoagulant
   (b) Glucose and total protein—fluid needs to be placed in a tube without anticoagulant
   (c) Type of crystals (see Chapter 66)
   (d) Gram stain and culture using transport media (even in the absence of a high white cell count)
   (e) Mucin clot analysis
      (1) Add 1 to 2 drops of bursal fluid to 1 ml of 2–5% acetic acid in a test tube
      (2) Shake the mixture a few moments and observe the clot (good, if clot remains intact and this is normal or a noninflammatory state; poor, if clot disintegrates and this represents inflammatory disease states (see Table 63.2)

or rheumatoid arthritis should be treated with anti-inflammatory agents (see Chapter 66).

Usually traumatic bursitis will heal spontaneously if the area of the inflammation is rested. The spontaneous healing, however, requires several weeks and therapy shortens this period considerably. Therefore, if sepsis and crystalline disease are ruled out, the treatment outlined in Table 63.3 is indicated.

If there is no initial response to treatment, then the patient should be treated by an *injection* into the inflamed bursa of a mixture of Xylocaine and depo-steroid (Table 63.4).

Usually, injection of an inflamed bursa with Xylocaine results in an immediate and dramatic relief of pain and this response indicates that the proper site has been injected. The anti-inflammatory effect of the steroid injection is seen in approximately 72 hours. If a satisfactory response has not occurred, the bursa may be reinjected in approximately 2 weeks. Waiting for 2 weeks before reinjection provides ample time to rule out iatrogenic sepsis which occasionally occurs after a steroid injection. If a bursitis does not respond to two steroid injections, orthopaedic consultation is necessary, as rarely definitive treatment by *surgical excision* of the bursa may be necessary.

Specific Forms

Several forms of bursitis are particularly common; their unique aspects are described here.

Table 63.2
Patterns of Bursal (or Joint) Fluid Findings in Common Problems

	Trauma	Sepsis	Inflammation Rheumatoid Arthritis	Inflammation Microcrystalline
Color of fluid	Bloody, xanthochromic	Yellow to cloudy	Clear yellow to cloudy	Clear yellow to cloudy
WBC/RBC	<1200/many	10,000–200,000/few	1000–20,000[a]/few	1000–20,000[a]/few
Protein	Normal	Slightly decreased	Slightly increased	Slightly increased
Glucose	Normal	Decreased	Slightly decreased	Slightly decreased
Crystals	–	–	–	+[b]
Mucin clot	Good to intermediate	Poor	Poor	Poor
Culture	–	+	–	–

[a] Cell count in noninfected inflammatory fluid may sometimes be as high as it is with sepsis; thus the need for culture.
[b] Gout: negatively birefringent sodium urate (see Chapter 66). Pseudogout: positively birefringent sodium pyrophosphate (see Chapter 66).

Table 63.3
Treatment of Bursitis

1. Splint where feasible
2. Application of heat for 20–30 min several times a day; i.e., heating pad at low heat and wrapped in a towel to prevent burning
3. Anti-inflammatory agents: aspirin, 600 mg, 4 times a day (emphasize to patient that regular doses are required for sustained anti-inflammatory effect). If aspirin is not tolerated, a newer nonsteroidal anti-inflammatory agent such as indometacin (Indocin), 25–50 mg, 3–4 times a day (other nonsteroidal anti-inflammatory agents may be used and are discussed in Chapter 67)
4. Improvement is usual in several days but the anti-inflammatory agent should be continued an additional 4–5 days to prevent recurrence
5. If no significant response is noted in 5–7 days and if sepsis has been ruled out, the bursa may be injected with Xylocaine and/or a steroid preparation (see Table 63.4).

Table 63.4
Methods of Injection of Bursae or Joints with Xylocaine and/or Depo-glucocorticoid Preparations[a]

1. Be certain sepsis has been ruled out (Tables 63.1 and 63.2)
2. Outline both area of injection and surrounding structures that should be avoided by use of an indelible pen
3. Prepare the skin carefully with an iodine-containing solution such as povodine (Betadine)
4. Anesthetize the skin with intradermal Xylocaine
5. Mix 2–3 ml of 1–2% Xylocaine with 20–40 mg of a depo-glucocorticoid (such as Aristocort or Kenalog) being sure the steroid is well suspended and inject the bursa with some of this mixture using a 20–22 gauge needle

[a] Notes of caution: (a) injection into the skin will cause atrophy and thus should be avoided; the patient should understand that there is a possibility of this complication; and (b) injection into tendons may cause degeneration and, in time, rupture and these structures should be avoided.

OLECRANON BURSITIS

This very common form of bursitis—also called student's or miner's elbow—is easily recognized by its location just behind the olecranon process of the ulna. Its special features are: (a) it is frequently associated with systemic disease, such as rheumatoid arthritis of gout; (b) symptoms frequently are chronic, in that they have been present for 2 or 3 weeks before a patient sees a physician; and (c) it is a common site for septic bursitis following trauma and may be associated with surrounding cellulitis (3, 4). If rheumatoid arthritis or gout is present, it is important to realize that sepsis sometimes coexists. Traumatic olecranon bursitis is usually hemorrhagic, although xanthochromic fluid may be present.

Swelling in the area of the olecranon bursa should always be aspirated (see Table 63.1 and 63.2) and a culture should always be obtained.

Therapy. Therapy depends on the characteristics of the fluid. If gout is present, specific therapy is indicated (see Chapter 66). Traumatic bursitis responds to simple removal of fluid; but if the fluid reaccumulates a steroid injection (Table 63.4) should

be given. If sepsis is identified, the patient should be hospitalized for parenteral antimicrobials and frequent aspiration and an X-ray of the elbow should be obtained to rule out osteomyelitis.

PREPATELLAR BURSITIS

Prepatellar bursitis (housemaid's or carpenter's knee) is a very common form of bursitis, easily recognized by its location in front of the patella. It is most often caused by trauma from kneeling, but it may also be a site of sepsis and the bursa, for this reason, should always be aspirated, even if it feels dry (5).

ANSERINE BURSITIS

The anserine bursa is fan-shaped and lies between the confluence of tendons and the tibia bone at the anterior medial aspect of the knee just below the joint space. Anserine bursitis is most often seen in individuals with arthritis, such as degenerative joint disease, and is recognized by its location; the pain is typically produced when the knee is flexed.

If there is surrounding erythema or if the patient is

febrile, aspiration should be attempted because sepsis, although uncommon, may be present. Therapy depends on the findings (see Tables 63.2 and 63.3). When injection therapy is used, the solution should be injected in a fan-shaped pattern so that the entire bursa is treated.

ISCHIAL BURSITIS (7)

The ischial bursa is located over the ischial tuberosity close to the sciatic nerve. When a person is sitting, the ischial bursae are covered only with subcutanous tissue and skin; when a person is erect, the gluteus maximus also covers the bursa.

The most common reason for inflammation of this bursa is trauma, such as may occur in bicycling. It also may be a site of hemorrhage after minor trauma, especially in patients who have been taking anticoagulants. It is rarely a site of sepsis.

Usually the inflammation results in an abrupt onset of pain, but occasionally the onset is more insidious. Because of the close proximity of the sciatic nerve to the bursa, there may be an associated neuritis resulting from pressure on the nerve which causes pain to radiate into the leg. Motion of the hip will result in intensification of pain so that frequently a patient will limit his stride on the affected side. Moreover, the patient often sits on one buttock to relieve pressure on the bursa. Direct pressure over the ischial tuberosity will cause sharp pain. In addition, the pain is intensified when the patient is supine and his hip is passively flexed. The pain may also be elicited by the *Patrick test*. This is performed with the patient in the supine position with the knee flexed and with the heel of the involved extremity resting on the contralateral knee; the application of pressure in a posterior direction to the flexed knee causes pain in the inflamed bursa. A rectal examination also may reveal tenderness and induration over the ischial tuberosity.

The differential diagnosis of ischial bursitis includes lumbar spine disease and thrombophlebitis. Localization of the pain over the ischial tuberosity and the finding of induration near the ischial tuberosity on rectal examination establishes the diagnosis of ischial bursitis. In the absence of these findings, a positive Patrick test is still diagnostic. However, on occasion, the patient may need further evaluation for a back problem (see Chapter 62) or for thrombophlebitis (see Chapter 48).

Aspiration of the bursa, even when it is inflamed, is not recommended because it is often difficult to localize and the surrounding structures, especially the sciatic nerve, may be injured. If aspiration is indicated because there is associated fever and, therefore, the possibility of septic bursitis, the patient should be referred to a rheumatologist or an orthopaedist for immediate evaluation.

Standard therapy (Table 63.3) usually provides dramatic improvement within 2 to 3 days; but if there has been associated leg pain or weakness from sciatic nerve inflammation, those symptoms may persist for several months.

Ultrasound, administered by a physical therapist, is effective, especially when symptoms are chronic, and it should be considered if initial therapy has not relieved the symptoms within several days.

If the diagnosis is unclear, if there is a question of sepsis, and if the patient does not respond within a week to therapy, consultation with a rheumatologist or orthopaedist is recommended. If the diagnosis is confirmed, the consultant may aspirate the bursa and, if sepsis is ruled out, inject it with Xylocaine and depo-corticosteroids, which often results in dramatic improvement.

SEMIMEMBRANOSUS-GASTROCNEMIUS BURSITIS (BAKER'S CYST) (2)

The semimembranosus-gastrocnemius bursa—commonly called a cyst—lies in the posterior medial aspect of the knee behind the femoral condyle and in 50% of individuals is continuous with the knee joint. Inflammation of this bursa is most commonly associated with other knee problems such as rheumatoid arthritis or degenerative arthritis. The bursa is rarely traumatized or infected. When the bursa is inflamed, pain is the major manifestation, especially during activities that require movement of the knee. Contraction of the quadriceps (knee extension) compresses the suprapatellar bursa (which communicates often with the knee joint) causing fluid in the knee joint to flow directly into the semimembranosus-gastrocnemius bursa, thereby causing pain. A Baker's cyst can also be associated with calf swelling and tightness (the bursa descending several centimeters into the leg). Tenderness is present over the bursa and often the patient complains of pain when the gastrocnemius muscle group is stretched—a positive Homans' sign. The location of the swelling often leads to confusion with thrombophlebitis or with a popliteal aneurysm. For this reason, careful examination, including palpation of the venous and arterial systems, is necessary. When there is any doubt about the diagnosis, special diagnostic studies and appropriate consultation as outlined in Chapter 67 and 84, respectively, may be indicated.

The condition is often refractory to medical therapy. If there is no response to treatment in several days, referral to an orthopaedist or rheumatologist is indicated. Because of the important structures in the popliteal fossa (artery, nerve, and vein), aspiration of the bursa by the general physician is not recommended. Unlike other types of bursitis, steroid injections are only palliative so that surgery, which provides definitive therapy, should be considered.

ILIOPECTINEAL BURSITIS

The iliopectineal bursa lies anterior to hip joint with which it communicates in approximately 15% of individuals. It lies between the inguinal ligament and the iliopsoas muscle just lateral to the femoral artery. Pain is the most frequent manifestation of iliopectineal bursitis; swelling may result in a bulge resembling a femoral hernia (see Chapter 88) below the inguinal ligament. Extension of the hip (for example, during walking) intensifies the pain so that the patient often limits the stride of the affected side. The anterior crural nerve (the largest branch of the lumbar plexus) lies just below the bursa and it may be irritated from bursal inflammation; resulting neuritis causes pain in the thigh which often is also intensified by walking and there may also be weakness of anterior muscles of the thigh. When a bursa is quite enlarged it may compress the femoral vein resulting in edema in the affected leg.

If a hernia can be ruled out (see Chapter 88), the bursa should be aspirated, provided the femoral artery can be distinguished, medial to the site of aspiration. If there is doubt about the diagnosis, referral to an orthopaedist or a rheumatologist is indicated. Aspiration and injection with Xylocaine results in lasting improvement. Injections should be administered only by someone familiar with the anatomy of the area and with experience in injecting it.

TROCHANTERIC BURSITIS (6)

The trochanteric bursa lies in the lateral aspect of the thigh over the greater trochanter of the femur and is closely associated with tendons of the glutei muscles. The problem primarily affects older individuals. Most cases are of unknown etiology although many are thought to result from osteoarthritis. Trauma accounts for approximately 20% of cases and sepsis is rare. The onset of abrupt pain, frequently with radiation to the knee or even to the groin, is most common. Discomfort is intensified by movement from the sitting to the standing position.

On examination there is tenderness over the bursa. An X-ray of this area is indicated, as frequently calcium is identified and its presence supports the diagnosis. The hip joint can be evaluated by X-ray and so that problems resulting in referred pain which may simulate trochanteric bursitis can be ruled out.

Therapy, as outlined in Table 63.3, is usually quite effective. If calcium has been identified on X-ray, it is usually in the area of the inflammatory process and, for this reason steroid injection should be aimed at the calcium.

TENOSYNOVITIS

Inflammation of a sheath of a tendon is a relatively common problem. For the most part, only long tendons have sheaths. Tenosynovitis most often occurs from exercise, especially when a tendon has been used repetitively when the individual is not properly conditioned (see Chapter 64). Tenosynovitis also may be part of a generalized inflammatory process such as systemic lupus, dermatomyositis, rheumatic fever, gout, or gonorrhea. Sometimes, tenosynovitis is the first manifestion of one of these diseases.

Tenosynovitis often affects the tendons of the hand. It is manifest most commonly by pain which is intensified with movement of the inflamed part. Frequently, there is localized tenderness and heat. Occasionally, a friction rub is felt and/or heard when the appropriate muscle is contracted.

When tenosynovitis is identified in the absence of trauma, a systemic disease should be suspected and, if present therapy of that disease is obviously important. Gonorrhea, especially, should be suspected in sexually active individuals, if inflammation involves the tendons of the ankle or wrist. Using Transgrow media, culture of the endocervical canal and rectum in women and of the urethra in men is indicated (see Chapters 26 and 45).

If the tenosynovitis has developed because of trauma, such as exercise or because of unknown reasons, nonspecific therapy, as for bursitis (Table 63.3), is appropriate. If the fingers are splinted, they should be in the position of function (see Chapter 64). If symptoms persist after 3 or 4 days of conservative therapy, the peritenon (loose tissue surrounding the tendon) should be injected with Xylocaine and a corticosteroid (such as Aristocort or Kenalog) after the tendon is outlined with an indelible pen (Table 63.4). Occasionally, symptoms are recurrent in which case referral to a rheumatologist or orthopaedist is indicated.

STENOSING TENOSYNOVITIS (DE QUERVAIN'S DISEASE)

Stenosing tenosynovitis is not a complication of tenosynovitis; rather, it occurs primarily when trauma is severe and localized. In stenosing tenosynovitis either a nodule forms on a tendon or an actual stenosis of a tendon sheath of a long tendon develops. This results in the affected part "sticking" in a position. The patient is unable to flex a digit fully or else, once it is flexed, the digit locks and literally must be straightened by external force until it suddenly snaps free. When stenosing tenosynovitis is present in a long tendon of the hand, it is called trigger finger or thumb. Stenosing tenosynovitis is caused by repeated trauma, but it is occasionally seen in association with rheumatoid arthritis, amyloidosis, pregnancy, and myxedema.

The treatment is identical to that of bursitis as outlined in Tables 63.3 and 63.4. If the patient resists several weeks of conservative therapy, surgical release may be necessary. When a nodule is palpated, it should be injected with a small amount of corticosteroid (such as 10 to 20 mg of Aristocort or Kenalog) with a small amount of Xylocaine and, frequently, it will resolve in several weeks (8).

FIBROSITIS (5)

Fibrositis is a misleading term; since it is not associated with inflammation and since no pathologic change in the tissues has been identified. Rather, it is a *pain amplification disorder* and, in part, is related to a disorder of non-REM (rapid eye movement) sleep (see Chapter 82). It is common and it affects men and women, middle-aged and older.

Symptoms

Patients with this problem complain of profound pain, stiffness, and exhaustion that are increasingly intolerable and unremitting. Often the symptoms are more profound in the winter and frequently they are exacerbated by exposure to bright lights or loud noises. Stiffness is usually profound, usually occurs daily and lasts for several hours or even, occasionally, throughout the entire day. The stiffness is diffuse, affecting many different muscles and joints. Typically, a sleep disturbance is present, with nocturnal restlessness and early morning fatigue.

The *examination* may be diagnostic and shows exquisitely tender areas of skin. These areas are constant and are particularly likely to occur in some of 14 of the more common trigger sites (Fig. 63.1). Frequently, the patient senses an area of swelling, although examination usually does not confirm this.

Almost always, this syndrome is associated with other problems, especially rheumatoid arthritis (Table 63.5); however, it does not parallel the activity of these diseases.

A *definitive diagnosis* of fibrositis requires the presence of all of the following criteria: (a) diffuse aching of at least 3 months duration, (b) disturbed sleep pattern, (c) tenderness in 12 of the 14 trigger sites (Fig. 63.1), and (d) skin-fold tenderness over the scapula (demonstrated by pinching a fold of skin in that region).

Therapy is directed at correction of the sleep disorder by use of a tricyclic antidepressant amitriptyline (Elavil), or doxepin (Sinequan), each 25 mg, 4 to 6 hours before bedtime. The doses of these agents must be increased every several days (to maximum doses) until restful sleep occurs. (Excessive dosage results in increased morning drowsiness; if this occurs the dose should be decreased.) The exact mechanism of action of these two antidepressant agents is not known, although it is suspected that they specifically affect a phase of disturbed sleep by increasing serotonin levels in the brain (these increased levels are known to be associated with sleep). Occasionally, the patient taking these mediations will notice the onset of frightening dreams; these will generally pass within several days or weeks and improved compliance can result if the physician explains this complication to the patient. Additional details about the use of tricyclic antidepressants are contained in Chapter 14. The patient should not be given a benzodiazepine such as Valium, as this may intensify the problem.

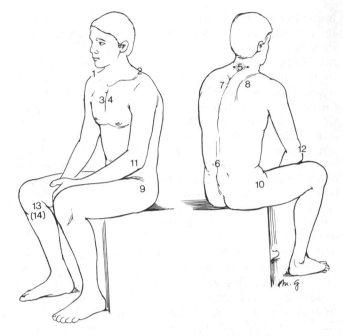

Figure 63.1 The more common trigger sites of fibrositis. *1, 2,* midpoint of upper fold of trapezius muscle; *3, 4,* second costochondral junction most often on the superior surface (occasionally there is also tenderness of more inferior costochondral junctions); *5,* area immediately anterior to the trapezius muscle, on the right and left sides; *6,* along the L4–S1 interspinous ligaments; *7, 8,* at the origin of the supraspinatus muscle near the medial border of the scapula; *9, 10,* in the upper and outer quadrant of the buttocks; *11, 12,* the tennis elbow site at the lateral epicondyle just distal to the radial head; *13, 14,* over the medial collateral ligament of the knee, proximal to the joint line and anterior to the semimembranosus and semitendinosus tendons; the medial fat pad.

The physician should note: (a) it is important to apply deep firm pressure when examining these trigger sites; (b) these areas, except site 6, are often somewhat tender to deep firm pressure in normal individuals; the discomfort is extreme in patients with fibrositis; and (c) the areas of tenderness are reproducible and very defined; pressure applied 1 or 2 cm away, except at site 5, does not produce discomfort. (Adapted from: H. A. Smythe and H. Moldofsky: *Bulletin on Rheumatic Diseases, 28:* 938, 1977 (5).)

Nonspecific therapy such as the application of heat for 15 to 20 min several times a day to the most symptomatic sites may be helpful. Although injection of a local anesthetic (such as Xylocaine) into an area of extreme tenderness may provide dramatic relief, it is of no lasting benefit and, therefore, should be avoided. Furthermore, anti-inflammatory agents are usually not helpful in treating fibrositis, although they may aid in controlling an underlying problem such as rheumatoid arthritis. Occasionally, if there is

Table 63.5
Causes of Secondary Fibrositis[a]

CONNECTIVE TISSUE DISEASE
  Any may be associated with this syndrome but it is more common with rheumatoid arthritis
SKIN DISEASE
  Erythema nodosum, psoriasis
INFECTION
  Syphilis, tuberculosis, brucellosis, streptococcal infections, bacterial endocarditis, gonorrhea, rubella, and viral hepatitis
ENDOCRINE
  Hypothyroidism, hyperparathyroidism
MALIGNANT DISEASE
DRUG REACTION
  Hypersensitivity vasculitis and drug-induced lupus
INFLAMMATORY BOWEL DISEASE
SARCOIDOSIS

[a] Adapted from W.P. Beetham: Diagnosis and management of fibrositis syndrome and psychogenic rheumatism. *Medical Clinics of North America*, 63: 422, 1979.

no response to therapy, the patient may need to be referred to a rheumatologist for confirmation of the diagnosis and to help support the primary physician in his treatment of a patient with this often therapeutically frustrating problem.

References

General

Pinals, RS: Traumatic arthritis and allied conditions. In: *Arthritis and Allied Conditions*, Ed. 9, edited by DJ McCarthy. Lea & Febiger, Philadelphia, 1979.

Smythe, HA: Nonarticular rheumatism and psychogenic musculoskeletal syndromes. In: *Arthritis and Allied Conditions*, Ed. 9, edited by DJ McCarty. Lea & Febiger, Philadelphia, 1979.
    These chapters provide a reference resource on fibrositis, bursitis, and tendinitis.

Specific

1. Bywaters, EGL: Bursae of the body. *Ann Rheum Dis 24*: 215, 1965.
2. Doppman, JL: Baker's cyst and normal gastrocnemius-semimembranosus bursa. *AJR 94*: 646, 1965.
3. Ho, G, Tice, AD and Kaplan, SR: Septic bursitis. *Ann Intern Med 89*: 21, 1978.
4. Simonelli, C, Zoschke, D, Bakhurst, A and Messner, R: Septic bursitis *Ann Intern Med 98*: 975, 1978.
5. Smythe, HA and Moldofsky, H: Two contributions to understanding of the fibrositis syndrome. *Bull Rheum Dis 28*: 298, 1977.
6. Spear, IM and Lipscomb, PR: Non-infectious trochanteric bursitis and peritendinitis. *Surg Clin North Am 32*: 1217, 1952.
7. Swarbout, R and Compere, E: Ischiogluteal bursitis—the pain in the arse. *JAMA 227*: 551, 1974.
8. Younghusland, DZ and Black, JD: De Quervain disease. *Can Med Assoc J 89*: 508, 1963.

CHAPTER SIXTY-FOUR

Exercise-related Musculoskeletal Syndromes

RONALD P. BYANK, M.D.

Sports such as jogging, marathon running, golf, tennis, softball, bowling, and many others are an integral part of the lives of millions of Americans.* Consequently, physicians are contacted frequently by patients with exercise-related syndromes. This chapter describes for a number of common exercise-related syndromes the mechanism of injury, the usual signs and symptoms, the treatment, the indications for referral, and the methods of preventing recurrences of the problem.

PROBLEMS OF THE KNEE (Fig. 64.1)

Meniscal Injury

DEFINITION AND MECHANISM OF INJURY

Tears of the medial or lateral meniscus (a disc-shaped fibrous cartilage) of the knee are common.

* See Chapter 55 for a discussion of physical conditioning from the standpoint of the cardiovascular system.

SUPERIOR VIEW

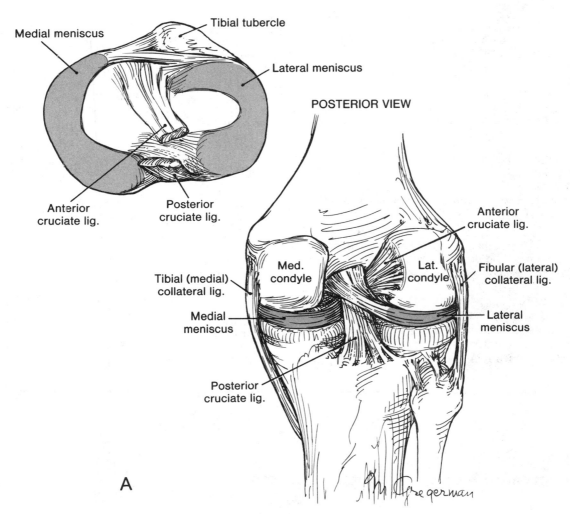

Figure 64.1 (*A*) Important structures of the knee.

When a rotary force is applied to the flexed knee joint, the meniscus is trapped between the femur and the tibia; then when the knee is extended, the cartilage may be torn (4). Tears of the medial meniscus are about 10 times as common as those of the lateral meniscus. This problem is encountered, especially, in individuals who play football and basketball, as well as in persons who are bowlers, golfers, or baseball players.

SYMPTOMS AND SIGNS

The patient who sustains a twisting flexion injury of the knee develops a sudden onset of pain, an inability to flex the knee fully, or to bear weight. Examination reveals the presence of knee joint effusion and tenderness over the joint line, either medially (medial meniscus injury) or laterally (lateral meniscus injury). Sometimes the onset is insidious and the patient notes episodes of knee effusion or of clicking or locking of the knee (which may last for

several minutes or several hours). Examination of patients who suffer from this more chronic condition often reveals only minimal joint line tenderness; certain maneuvers are helpful in the diagnosis of meniscal injury; they are, however, more likely to be diagnostic in patients with acute symptoms.

The *McMurray test* is performed with the patient lying supine with the hip and knee fully flexed and the foot rotated outward to its full capacity to test the medial meniscus and inward to test the lateral meniscus—Figure 64.2*A*. The knee is extended with the foot at first rotated out and again with it rotated in and a painful click in the knee indicates a positive test. Not all meniscal tears will result in a positive test. The *Apley* or grinding test is performed by flexing the knee 90° when the patient is in the prone position, and then rotating the tibia internally and externally on the femur while compressing the leg against the femur, and then repeating the rotation while pulling the leg in a direction from the femur—Figure 64.2*B*. Pain during compression may be due to

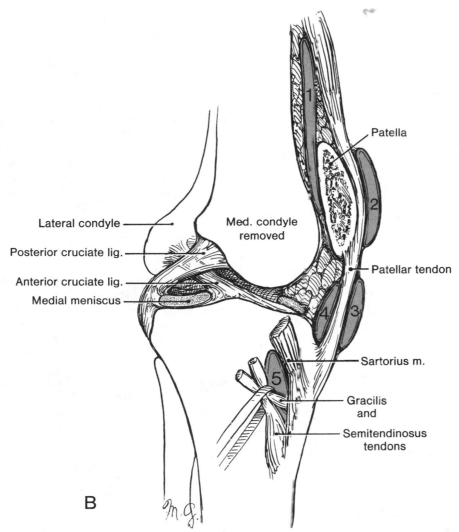

Lateral condyle

Posterior cruciate lig.

Anterior cruciate lig.

Medial meniscus

Med. condyle removed

Patella

Patellar tendon

Sartorius m.

Gracilis and

Semitendinosus tendons

B

Figure 64.1 (B) Five bursae of the knee: 1, suprapatellar; 2, prepatellar; 3, superficial patellar tendon; 4, retropatellar tendon; 5, pes anserinus.

a meniscal tear and pain while pulling the leg is likely from a ligamentous injury.

Examination of the knee joint should always include, in addition to these maneuvers, an evaluation for ligament instability (excess motion on rotating and moving the flexed knee anteriorly, laterally, medially, and posteriorly on the femur). The injured knee should always be compared to the normal knee, which should be examined first. The laxity of ligaments varies tremendously between individuals and, therefore, assessment of the normal knee is a useful guide to evaluation of the injured knee. If there is any evidence of ligament instability, referral to an orthopaedist should be accomplished urgently.

ADDITIONAL EVALUATION

X-rays of the knee should always be obtained to rule out other problems such as loose bodies within the knee, osteochrondritis dissecans, fractures, or arthritis. If a large effusion is present, it should be aspirated for two reasons: first, removal of the fluid will result in relief of discomfort; and second, if a hemarthrosis is present, it may indicate a serious injury and the patient should be referred to an orthopaedist. If referral cannot be accomplished for several days, the knee should be splinted with a knee immobilizer (see below). Aspiration of the knee joint is easily accomplished after preparing the skin with an iodine-containing solution (such as Betadine) and anesthetizing it with Xylocaine. The easiest approach to aspiration is generally medially at the patellofemoral joint.

DIFFERENTIAL DIAGNOSIS

The various diagnostic possibilities (see above) are best ruled out by evaluation of the X-ray of the knee, as clinical examination is not precise for this purpose.

TREATMENT AND PROGNOSIS

Initial treatment consists of immobilization of the injured knee with a knee immobilizer (a rigid support

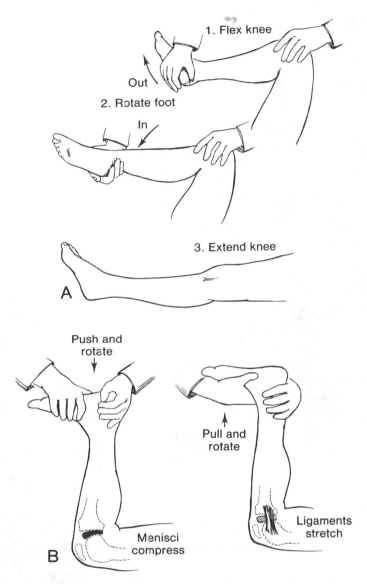

1. Flex knee

Out

2. Rotate foot

In

3. Extend knee

A

Push and rotate

Pull and rotate

Menisci compress

Ligaments stretch

B

Figure 64.2   (*A*) McMurray test and (*B*) Apley test.

available from large pharmacies or orthopaedic appliance stores). An Ace bandage is not sufficient to provide stability, although it may help to diminish effusion. The patient should use crutches to keep his weight off the knee and should elevate the injured extremity when he lies down. Ice packs should be applied to the knee for 15 min several times a day to reduce swelling.

Most often symptoms subside within 14 days; if symptoms resolve, the prognosis is variable. In the instance of a small tear, complete healing may occur without subsequent symptoms. On the other hand, a larger tear may result in recurrent symptoms after initial improvement. Therefore if symptoms persist beyond 2 weeks with conservative treatment or if they recur following return to normal activity, an orthopaedic referral is indicated for consideration of an arthrogram and/or arthroscopy to establish the

diagnosis. An *arthrogram* is an X-ray of the joint and requires the injection of iodinated contrast material and air into the joint space. This is done by a radiologist or orthopaedist after administration of local anesthesia. After the procedure, which generally is well tolerated, crutches should be used for 1 to 2 days during which time only mild analgesics are usually needed. *Arthroscopy* which may be accomplished in 15 to 30 min by the orthopaedist using local or general anaesthesia, involves the insertion of the arthroscope (a 2- to 4-mm diameter instrument) through a stab wound in the anterior lateral aspect of the knee. The patient usually requires crutches for 2 to 3 days and mild analgesics. If the diagnosis is confirmed, surgical excision of the torn portion of the meniscus or of the entire meniscus may be necessary and may be performed either by arthroscopic surgery or through arthrotomy.

Following surgery for a torn meniscus, the patient is often able to return to light sports activity within 6 to 8 weeks, but it may be 3 months or longer before he can resume activities such as running or tennis. A proper postoperative conditioning period of supervised physical therapy is important and will consist of strengthening the quadriceps muscles and of range-of-motion exercises to ensure normal mobility of the knee. Joint space narrowing and arthritic change almost always follow meniscectomy, but may not limit a patient's activity significantly.

PREVENTION

This injury occurs by chance when a rotational force is applied to the knee when it is in the flexed position; it cannot be prevented by conditioning.

Patellofemoral Arthralgia (Chondromalacia (1, 2))

DEFINITION AND MECHANISM OF INJURY

Patellofemoral arthralgia refers to pain originating from the patellofemoral joint associated with changes in the articular cartilage of the patella. The patellar cartilage shows softening, which is caused by lateral subluxation or hypermobility of the patella, usually due to an increased angle (Q-angle) between the quadriceps and patellar tendon, and by patella alta. The normal *Q-angle* is up to 20°; if it is greater than this, increased lateral displacement of the patella results (Fig. 64.3). An abnormal Q-angle is sometimes associated with excessive pronation of the feet (flat feet). *Patella alta* is an anatomical variant in which the patella rides more proximally than usual, so that it becomes hypermobile. Patella alta can be identified on X-ray when the patellar tendon length exceeds the maximum length of the patella by more than 1 cm (Fig. 64.4). Normally, the lengths of these two structures are equal. Patients with a variation in hip joint anatomy that results in compensatory external tibial torsion (external rotation of lower leg in axial plane, slew-foot) will also have lateral displacement

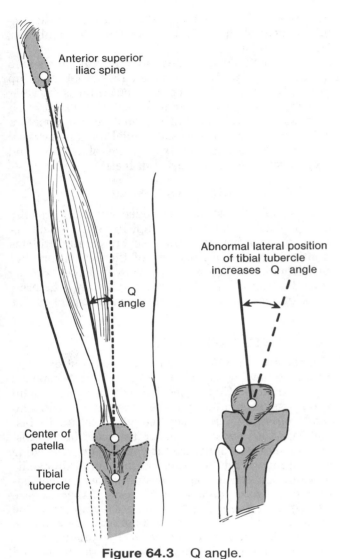

Figure 64.3   Q angle.

Figure 64.4   Patella alta. *P*, patella; *PT*, patellar tendon.

of the patella and excess wear of the patellofemoral joint.

Chondromalacia is a very common disorder especially in inexperienced adolescent and young adult runners who do not properly condition themselves, but accelerate their activities too rapidly.

SYMPTOMS AND SIGNS

Pain, usually described as a soreness or aching around or under the patella, is the hallmark of this problem. The discomfort is aggravated by running up hills, climbing stairs, kneeling, or hyperflexing the knee. Pain frequently disappears during activity only to recur just at the end of or after activity. The patient may also complain of the knee "locking"; however, upon careful questioning, this locking is found to be only very transient and is not the true locking that is experienced in tears of the meniscus (see above).

Physical examination reveals any or all of the anatomical abnormalities described above. Patella alta and hypermobility of the patella are very frequent. Pain and/or crepitus with patellofemoral manipulation or palpation of the articular surface of the patella is usually present. Attempts to push the patella laterally may cause pain and involuntary contracture of the quadriceps, the so-called *apprehension sign*. If the patient extends his knee from 30° of flexion to full extension against resistance, pain will result. A knee effusion is frequently present.

ADDITIONAL EVALUATION

X-rays of the knees should be obtained routinely and should include a tangential or sunrise view to look for lateral subluxation of the patella, often with a hypoplastic lateral trochlear facet of the femoral sulcus.

DIFFERENTIAL DIAGNOSIS

Other problems which occasionally may be confused with chondromalacia are prepatellar bursitis (Fig. 64.1*B*) (localized to the prepatellar bursa, see Chapter 63), retropatellar (also called infrapatellar) tendon bursitis (Fig. 64.1*B*) (localized to the area below the patella and behind the tendon), pes anserinus bursitis (Fig. 64.1*B*) (inflammation in the bursa that lies deep to the combined insertion of the sartorius, gracilis, and semitendinosus tendons into the proximal medial tibial metaphysis), fat pad syndrome (trauma-related inflammation of the infrapatellar fat pad) (Fig. 64.1*B*), meniscal injury (see above), ligamentous instability of the knee, arthritis, and osteochondritis dissecans. Hip or pelvic disease are associated with referred pain from sciatic nerve root irritation. These problems can be differentiated by careful physical and radiological examination; if there is any doubt, referral to an orthopaedic surgeon is appropriate.

TREATMENT AND PROGNOSIS

Therapy is initiated as soon as possible after the appearance of symptoms. The use of crutches for up to 7 days to rest the knee is important; and the application of ice to the knee for approximately 15 min several times a day will help to decrease swelling. In addition, anti-inflammatory medications should be prescribed, such as aspirin, 600 mg 4 times a day or, if aspirin is not tolerated, other nonsteroidal anti-inflammatory agents such as indomethacin (Indocin), 25 to 50 mg 3 to 4 times a day.

After the initial 24 hours, the application of ice may be discontinued and moist heat may be applied for 15 to 20 min several times a day. The patient should avoid vigorous sports activities until symptoms subside, which often takes several weeks. Progressive resistance exercises of the quadriceps should be supervised by a physical therapist to maximize quadriceps strength and stability. The course of patients with this problem is unpredictable. Orthopaedic referral is usually necessary if the patient has been forced to abandon his major sport for more than a few weeks, or if the problem recurs. Intra-articular steroid injections by the orthopaedist may alleviate symptoms, but this treatment must be restricted, as it will increase cartilage deterioration if done to excess. Correction of the tracking problem in the patellofemoral joint may require the use of an orthotic to correct excess pronation of the foot (see Chapter 99), or the use of a cartilage knee brace (a heavy elastic brace containing a horseshoe-shaped pad to stabilize the patella—available from large pharmcies or orthopaedic appliance stores). Occasionally, surgical treatment of chondromalacia is necessary if conservative treatment fails. Surgery is designed to prevent subluxation of the patella. Results are variable depending on the extent of the problem and the type of surgery but, occasionally, the patient may not be able to return to sports which place stress on the knee.

PREVENTION

Prevention of chondromalacia requires the use of proper foot gear (see Chapter 99), often including the use of orthotics, and "proper conditioning" of the athlete by gradually increasing his level of activity and by the performance of stretching exercises (see below).

PROBLEMS OF THE LEG

Shin Splints (3)

DEFINITION AND MECHANISM OF INJURY

Shin splints are the occurrence of pain over the anteriomedial aspect of the mid to distal portion of the lower leg—Figure 64.5 (site A). They are caused by overuse of the muscles of this region as may occur with running, jogging, or sustained walking. The pain is thought to result from tendinitis of the posterior tibial tendon and by periostitis from the pulling of this muscle from its bony attachment along the medial aspect of the tibia, the interosseous membrane, and the fibula.

Shin splints develop most often in individuals who (a) are not properly conditioned, (b) do not warm-up properly, (c) run on hard or uneven surfaces, (d) wear improper foot gear, or (e) have anatomical abnormalities such as variation in the anatomy of their hip joint with resultant excessive tibial torsion (external rotation of tibia in the axial plane, slew-feet), and hyperpronation of the feet (flat feet).

SYMPTOMS AND SIGNS

Shin splints are characterized by pain, usually gradual but occasionally abrupt in onset, which occurs during or just after exercise. Frequently, athletes continue to exercise in spite of the discomfort; but occasionally the pain is so severe that the exercise must be stopped. Examination reveals only the presence of tenderness along the medial aspect of the tibia.

DIFFERENTIAL DIAGNOSIS

If the area of tenderness is localized, a stress fracture may have occurred, although it is quite unusual in the tibia or fibula (see below). A compartment syndrome is similar but the location of pain and tenderness is different (see below). Occasionally fascial hernias, tenosynovitis, or tears of the interosseous membrane may produce symptoms suggesting shin splints; and, for this reason, an orthopaedic consultation should be requested if there is persistence of the symptoms after 3 weeks of therapy (see below) or if there is recurrence of symptoms. The orthopaedist will confirm the diagnosis and will look for anatomical abnormalities which predispose to this condition (see below). Also, an X-ray (indicated when symptoms are prolonged or recurrent) of the leg in the case of shin splints, will occasionally show irregular bone formation of the tibia or fibula as a result of periostitis. A radionuclide bone scan is more sensitive than an X-ray and may be necessary if the diagnosis is uncertain. A positive bone scan shows increased uptake of radionuclide by the tibia, fibula, or interosseous membrane.

TREATMENT AND PROGNOSIS

Ice packs should be applied several times a day for 15 min at a time in order to reduce swelling and inflammation. The patient should avoid, for several weeks, the exercise which has precipitated the problem. The use of an elastic wrap on the lower leg provides some comfort and the prescription of anti-inflammatory agents such as aspirin, 600 mg 4 times a day, will help control the inflammatory process.

Acute shin splints should resolve in 3 weeks; and, after this, conditioning is necessary before the patient can return to his sport. The syndrome rarely recurs if conditioning has been correct.

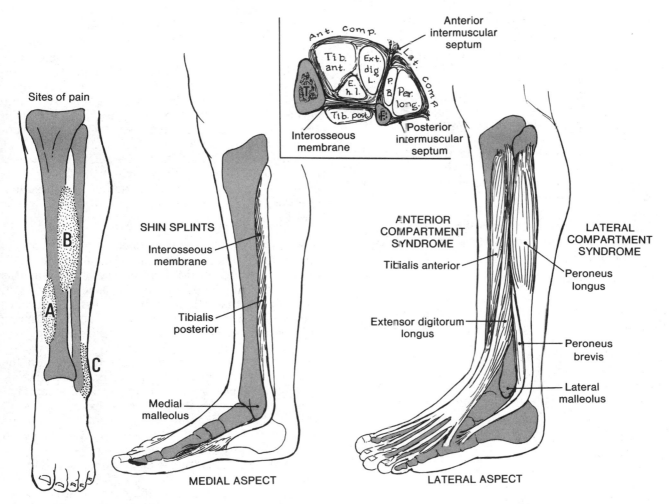

Figure 64.5 Sites of pain and relevant anatomy of (*A*) shin splints, (*B*) anterior compartment syndrome, and (*C*) lateral compartment syndrome.

PREVENTION

Prevention of this problem requires stretching exercises before physical activity (see below), running or walking on soft level surfaces, and use of proper shoes (Chapter 99). An orthotic device may also be prescribed by an orthopaedist or podiatrist if hyperpronation of the feet or excessive tibial rotation is present. These also will be helpful in preventing recurrences.

Compartment Syndromes

DEFINITION AND MECHANISM OF INJURY

There are two compartments in the leg which are prone to injury and subsequent swelling: the anterior (tibial) compartment and the lateral (peroneal) compartment. The anterior compartment syndrome is also called lateral shin splints and occurs when an athlete runs to excess on his toes or on a hill, or runs with shoes that have a sole which is too flexible.

Compartment syndromes are usually seen in competitive runners and they are much less common than shin splints.

SYMPTOMS AND SIGNS

Anterior Compartment Syndrome. The patient notices pain in the extensor muscles of the leg and in the lower leg, ankle, and foot. Discomfort usually occurs during or just after exercise. Examination reveals tenderness and often swelling of the anterior compartment, which is located over the midlateral aspect of the lower leg—Figure 64.5 (site *B*).

Lateral Compartment Syndrome. In this situation the pain is located in the posterolateral aspect of the ankle above and behind the lateral malleolus—Figure 64.5 (site *C*); this is the area where the peroneal tendons are located. Frequently the patient feels as if his ankle has "given out." This syndrome is caused by excessive pronation of the foot (flat foot) and ankle (eversion) in runners with hypermobile ankles (weak ankles).

TREATMENT AND PROGNOSIS

Initially, ice should be applied for 15 min several times a day, and the patient must rest from exercise for 3 to 4 weeks. Anti-inflammatory agents, such as aspirin, 600 mg 4 times a day, are very helpful in controlling the inflammatory response. Once symptoms subside, the patient should condition himself before returning to full exercise. This conditioning requires pre-exercise stretching (see below), especially of the muscles that are involved, and then gradual return to running. The patient should have well designed running shoes (see Chapter 99), should avoid toe running, and should always run on a level surface.

In the management of the lateral compartment syndrome an orthopaedist or podiatrist should be consulted to evaluate the use of an orthotic device or heel wedge to prevent hyperpronation, which predisposes to recurrence of the problem.

The prognosis for patients with either of these compartment syndromes is excellent provided the patient is properly conditioned.

DIFFERENTIAL DIAGNOSIS

Should symptoms not respond within a 7- to 10-day period, an X-ray of the area should be obtained to rule out other causes, such as a stress fracture or osteoid osteoma. A compartment syndrome also can be confused initially with thrombophlebitis, cellulitis, or vascular insufficiency and these should all be investigated by means of serial observations and appropriate specific tests when indicated.

PREVENTION

Prevention of compartment syndromes requires stretching exercises (see below) before running, especially of the musculature involved in each of the compartments, and the use of good quality running gear, often including orthotics.

PROBLEMS OF THE ANKLE AND THE FOOT

Achilles Tendinitis

DEFINITION AND MECHANISM OF INJURY

Achilles tendinitis is inflammation of the heel tendon and surrounding tissue and is due to overuse. The problem is most often caused by repetitive stretching of the tendon when the athlete is not properly conditioned. However, even with good conditioning it occurs in athletes who run on hills or who wear shoes with rigid soles. Furthermore, structural abnormalities such as tibia vara (bow-legged deformity), tight hamstring and calf muscles, a cavus foot (high arched foot often with claw toes), and a varus (inverted) heel deformity predispose to Achilles tendinitis. Initially, the peritenon (loose soft connective tissue surrounding the tendon) is inflamed, but in chronic cases the tendon itself undergoes mucoid degeneration with the formation of longitudinal fissures and often nodule formation in the degenerate tendon.

This problem is commonly seen in recreational athletes, as well as in more serious runners.

SYMPTOMS AND SIGNS

The athlete with this problem notices a burning sensation in the heel, usually early during a run, which then lessens or disappears completely as running progresses. The discomfort often recurs upon completion of the run, in which case it is often more severe. Occasionally, a runner may note heel pain soon after awakening from sleep, which then subsides with daily activities.

On examination there is local or diffuse tenderness in the Achilles tendon; and, when the condition is chronic, there may be a tender nodule in the tendon, crepitus, and swelling.

TREATMENT AND PROGNOSIS

The application of an ice pack to the area for 15 min several times a day will provide comfort and reduce swelling. Anti-inflammatory agents such as aspirin, 600 mg 4 times a day for several days, will help control the inflammatory process. The runner should rest for several days, then reduce his running mileage and avoid hills until symptoms have been absent for 10 to 14 days. Exercises which gently stretch the tendon are important to condition the runner (see below) and to prevent recurrences. If symptoms persist, a rest from exercise for a period of 3 to 4 weeks or longer may be necessary to permit healing. Local injection of corticosteroids into the Achilles tendon should be avoided as this can weaken the tendon and cause a rupture.

In resistant cases, physical therapy, especially ultrasound, is helpful. In addition, when the syndrome is severe, splinting or casting of the ankle joint and the use of crutches are necessary to immobilize the Achilles tendon. In mild cases, with initial treatment and then proper conditioning, the prognosis is excellent. If the condition does not respond to therapy within 1 to 2 weeks, an orthopaedic consultation should be obtained since occasionally surgery is necessary. If surgery must be performed, it is unlikely that the athlete will be able to return to running, although other exercises such as swimming or cycling may be readily performed.

PREVENTION

Prevention of this problem requires the use of good running shoes (see Chapter 99) with flexible soles, a well molded Achilles pad, and a rigid heel counter. If the runner has a cavus foot (see above) an orthopaedist or a podiatrist should be consulted about the use of an orthotic device.

Plantar Fasciitis (Heel Spur)

Plantar fasciitis or heel spur syndrome is the most common cause of heel pain; it occurs most often in people who hike or run, but it may also occur in individuals who are not athletic. This problem is fully discussed in Chapter 99.

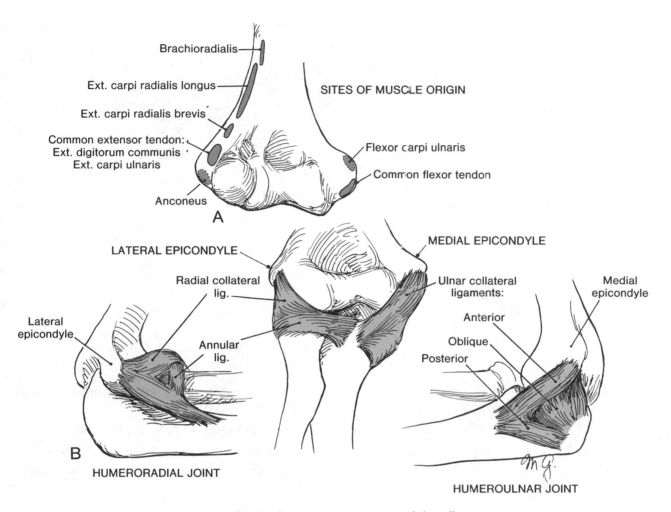

SITES OF MUSCLE ORIGIN

Brachioradialis

Ext. carpi radialis longus

Ext. carpi radialis brevis

Common extensor tendon:
Ext. digitorum communis
Ext. carpi ulnaris

Flexor carpi ulnaris

Common flexor tendon

Anconeus

A

LATERAL EPICONDYLE

MEDIAL EPICONDYLE

Radial collateral lig.

Lateral epicondyle

Annular lig.

Ulnar collateral ligaments:

Anterior

Oblique

Posterior

Medial epicondyle

B

HUMERORADIAL JOINT

HUMEROULNAR JOINT

Figure 64.6   Important structures of the elbow.

PROBLEMS OF THE ELBOW (Fig. 64.6)

Tennis Elbow

DEFINITION AND MECHANISM OF INJURY

The term "tennis elbow" refers to inflammation in the region of the lateral epicondyle of the humerus at the origin of the common extensor muscles; it is a common exercise-related syndrome. It is caused by activities that combine excessive pronation and supination of the forearm with an extended wrist. Although the mechanism by which tennis elbow is produced is not known, the actual cause of pain may be due to radiohumeral synovitis or bursitis, tendinitis of the common extensor origin, traumatic epicondylitis or periostitis of the lateral epicondyle, or entrapment by scarring of a branch of the radial nerve in this region.

This problem is quite common in individuals performing activities such as tennis, badminton, and bowling, as well as with many non-sports-related activities such as using a screwdriver or a wrench.

SYMPTOMS AND SIGNS

The onset of symptoms is usually gradual. Physical examination reveals tenderness over the lateral epicondyle or over the radiohumeral joint. The proximal common extensor muscle is often tender to palpation and, on occasion, there is swelling in this area. The elbow usually has a normal flexion and extension, although the latter may sometimes be temporarily painful. Supination and, especially, pronation may be painful if they are performed against resistance. Pain can be elicited by stretching the wrist extensors by holding the elbow fully extended with the forearm pronated and the wrist maximally palmar flexed—Figure 64.7.

ADDITIONAL EVALUATION

The history and physical examination are diagnostic and further studies are not indicated unless symptoms fail to improve with treatment. In that case, an X-ray of the elbow should be obtained; on occasion, there may be calcium deposits noted at the lateral epicondyle of the humerus.

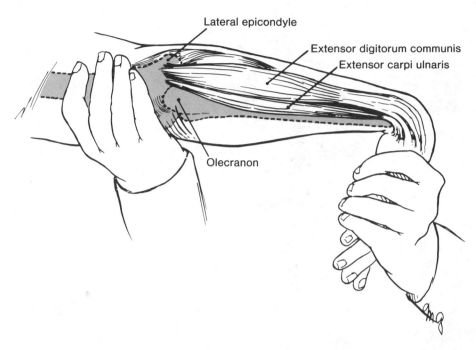

Figure 64.7 Tennis elbow.

TREATMENT AND PROGNOSIS

The painful arm should initially be immobilized in a sling or, if symptoms are severe, immobilized in a long arm splint with the wrist held in dorsiflexion to rest the extensor tendons. Aspirin or other anti-inflammatory agents such as indomethacin (Indocin), 25–50 mg 3 to 4 times a day will help diminish the inflammation. The injection of the area at the point of tenderness with a mixture of 3 ml of 1 to 2% Xylocaine and 1 ml of glucocorticoid suspension (such as Aristocort or Kenalog) followed by the use of a sling for 1 or 2 weeks often provides dramatic relief of pain. A second injection may be repeated in approximately 3 weeks if symptoms fail to improve or if they recur during this period.

The prognosis is quite variable and depends to a large extent on the patient's activities; but it may recur even in patients who are conscientious about their activity. If symptoms recur or if they fail to respond promptly to treatment, an orthopaedic consultation is indicated. Surgery may occasionally be required. The type of surgery depends on the problem and occasionally a return to the vigorous activity that precipitated the problem may not be possible.

PREVENTION

Prevention of this problem requires conditioning of the muscle groups in the forearm and wrist through an exercise program. This program often needs to be specialized, and a physical therapist should be consulted. Often the use of a tennis elbow strap (available at sports stores) in the area of the muscle mass of the proximal portion of the forearm is helpful since it decreases strain of the common extensor origin at the lateral epicondyle.

Medial Epicondylitis (Golfers's Elbow)

DEFINITION AND MECHANISM OF INJURY

Medial epicondylitis of the elbow is due to inflammation of the tissues in the area of the medial epicondyle where the muscles that flex and pronate the wrist originate. It is caused by overuse of these muscles.

This problem is less common than tennis elbow and is seen in individuals performing repetitive pronation exercises such as occur in golf.

SYMPTOMS AND SIGNS

The manifestations of this problem are very similar to those of tennis elbow except that the location is in the area of the medial, rather than the lateral, epicondyle.

TREATMENT, PROGNOSIS, AND PREVENTION

These aspects are similar to those of tennis elbow.

SPRAINS AND AVULSION FRACTURES

Definition and Mechanism of Injury

A sprain is defined as a partial or complete rupture of the fibers of a ligament, as well as a stress injury to the joint capsule. When the ligament is strong, it does not rupture, but a chip of bone may be avulsed from the insertion of the ligament. These injuries are most common around the ankle, knee, elbow, and fingers. Violent muscle action in athletes, especially adolescents, may avulse a traction epiphysis (apophysis), usually at one of three sites on the pelvis: (a) anterior superior iliac spine from sartorius avulsion, (b) anterior inferior iliac spine from rectus femoris avulsion, and (c) ischial tuberosity from avulsion of the hamstring (Fig. 64.8). Also, injuries to the joint capsules and ligaments of the fingers are particularly common.

Sprains and avulsion fractures result from sudden forceful muscle contraction and are very common in athletes.

SYMPTOMS AND SIGNS

The hallmark of a sprain or an avulsion fracture is pain in the area of the injury. Physical examination reveals swelling and stiffness of the involved joint with increased pain as the patient attempts to use it. The joint may be unstable if the ligament rupture is complete. Maximal swelling and tenderness are usually localized at the area of the sprain or fracture, especially if it is superficial as in the ankle, knee, or finger.

ADDITIONAL EVALUATION

X-rays of an injured area must be done to establish the diagnosis of an avulsion fracture.

If joint instability is found on examination, a consultation from an orthopaedic surgeon should be requested. Also, stress X-rays, especially of the ankle, knee, and finger are often done by the orthopaedic surgeon either under local or general anesthesia to evaluate the degree of instability of the joints.

Surgical intervention by the orthopaedic surgeon to repair joint instability is occasionally necessary, especially in injuries in the area of the ankle and knee; even after surgery, an athlete will often not be able to return to the activity which resulted in the injury.

TREATMENT AND PROGNOSIS

The initial treatment of sprains and/or avulsion fractures consists of immobilization of the area with

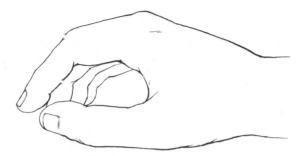

Figure 64.9   Position of function of fingers.

a splint, elevation, and application of ice for approximately 15 min several times a day to decrease swelling, and the prescription of analgesics such as aspirin or acetaminophen (Tylenol) alone or in combination with codeine, 30 to 60 mg, every 4 to 6 hours. If the injury is in the area of the ankle or knee, the patient must keep his weight off the injured joint by the use of crutches. If it can be applied, a compression dressing using an Ace bandage is useful to help decrease swelling As the initial edema begins to subside, which occurs usually in 1 or 2 days, the ice packs may be discontinued and warm soaks or hot packs may be applied for approximately 15 min several times a day. Occasionally, heat makes the condition worse in which case it should obviously be discontinued. Immobilization of the sprained or fractured part must be continued until satisfactory healing has occurred, at which time progressive mobilization of the joint is instituted. It is important to immobilize a finger for no more than 3 weeks and then only in the *position of function*, in order to avoid permanent stiffness of the joint (Fig. 64.9). Ankle sprains usually must be immobilized for 3 to 6 weeks and, on occasion, may take 3 months to heal. Immobilization is best accomplished by the use of an ankle splint (a rigid device available from large pharmacies or orthopaedic appliance stores) or by the means of a posterior plaster splint.

The prognosis is quite variable and depends to a large extent on the location of the injury; but with proper treatment and with subsequent conditioning of the patient the prognosis is generally good.

PREVENTION

The prevention of sprains and avulsion fractures requires proper conditioning, especially by the performance of stretching exercises (see below) before exertion, and the use of proper foot gear and protective equipment.

STRESS FRACTURES

Definition and Mechanism of Injury

A stress fracture is a crack, which is sometimes minute, that can occur in almost any bone that has been repetitively subjected to impact. The most common sites of stress fractures are the metatarsal shafts,

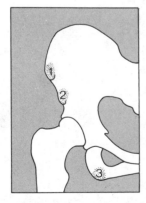

Figure 64.8   Common sites of avulsion fracture: (*1*) anterior superior iliac spine, (*2*) anterior inferior iliac spine, and (*3*) ischial tuberosity.

especially the second and third metatarsals, the distal fibula, the proximal tibia, and the symphysis pubis. Stress fractures may, however, occur in other bones such as the lumbar vertebrae, the sacroiliac joint, the distal femur, the distal aspect of the tibia, and the lateral malleolus.

Stress fractures occur most commonly from walking or running, usually when an athlete has tried to do too much too fast, has used improper shoes, or has exercised on hard surfaces. Stress fractures occur in both poorly conditioned individuals and in highly conditioned athletes.

SYMPTOMS AND SIGNS

A patient who has sustained a stress fracture notices the gradual onset of aching of the affected bone during or just after exercising. Examination reveals localized tenderness and occasional swelling.

ADDITIONAL EVALUATION

The diagnosis depends on the symptoms and signs since X-rays of the affected area are usually normal at first; only after 2 to 4 weeks (sometimes longer) they may show bone resorption at the fracture site

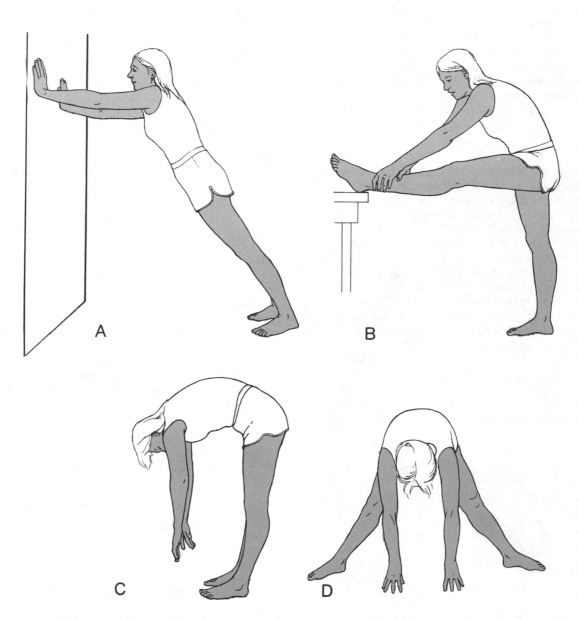

Figure 64.10   (*A*) Stretch the Achilles tendon by leaning forward with the feet flat and placed at least four feet from the wall. (*B*) Stretch the hamstring and gastrocnemius muscle groups by elevating the leg and bending forward as far as possible. (*C*) Stretch the hamstring and back muscles by touching the toes slowly; bouncing should be avoided. (*D*) Stretch the adductor muscle by gradually spreading the legs as far apart as possible; place the fingers on the floor for support.

and/or the formation of callus (new bone). A radionuclide bone scan is positive, however, before the fracture can be identified on X-ray, and the scan may remain positive for up to 2 years after the injury. Therefore, a bone scan is indicated if symptoms persist more than a few weeks and X-rays are negative.

DIFFERENTIAL DIAGNOSIS

Tibial stress fractures may be confused with pes anserinus bursitis, shin splints, and bone tumors, especially osteoid osteoma. If there is uncertainty about the correct diagnosis, the general physican should request a consultation from an orthopaedist.

TREATMENT AND PROGNOSIS

The treatment of stress fractures involves complete immobilization of the injured part in a splint. If the injury is in a lower extremity, the patient should not bear weight on it. The injured part should also be elevated, and ice should be applied initially for approximately 15 min several times a day until the swelling subsides, which usually occurs in 24 to 36 hours. After the swelling has subsided, heat may be applied for 15 min several times a day; but this should be discontinued if the discomfort is made more severe, which occasionally occurs. Pain should be controlled with aspirin or acetaminophen (Tylenol) alone or combined with codeine, 30 to 60 mg every 4 to 6 hours as needed.

Metatarsal stress fractures should be treated initially with a cast which should be left on 4 to 8 weeks. (If the physician is unfamiliar with the application of a short leg cast, referral to an orthopaedist is indicated.) Stress fractures of the tibia and fibula require more prolonged periods of immobilization and may require a cast for up to 12 weeks or longer. All patients with suspected stress fractures of the tibia or fibula should be seen by an orthopaedist.

With proper treatment and then appropriate conditioning, the prognosis is excellent and most patients will be able to return to normal sports activities.

PREVENTION

Prevention of stress fractures requires proper conditioning with pre-exercise stretching exercises, proper footwear, and avoidance of hard surfaces and of too rapid an acceleration of physical activity.

STRETCHING EXERCISES

It has been pointed out that the occurrence (and recurrence) of some of the problems described in this chapter can be prevented by several measures—that is, selecting good shoes (see Chapter 99 for a description and illustration), not increasing the amount of stress on the musculoskeletal system too rapidly, and stretching the major muscle groups of the lower extremity before participating in sports. The four stretching exercises which should be practiced routinely are illustrated in Figure 64.10. Each exercise should be done for both sides for 15 to 30 sec at a time for a total of 10 to 15 min before engaging in sports activities.

References

General

Brody, DM: Running injuries. *Ciba Clinical Symposia*, 32, Nov. 4, 1980.
   An excellent review of running injuries, including superb anatomical illustrations and a description of specific stretching exercises.
Turek, SL: Orthopaedics. Principles and Their Application, Ed. 3. W. B. Saunders, Philadelphia, 1977.
   A very comprehensive orthopaedic textbook.
Mirkin, G and Hoffman, M: *The Sports Medicine Book*. Little, Brown, Boston, 1978.
   An excellent general reference book for sports medicine containing descriptions of stretching exercises.

Specific

1. Ficat, RP and Hungerford, DS: *Disorders of the Patello-femoral Joint.* Williams & Wilkins, Baltimore, 1977.
2. Insall, J: Chondromalacia patellae. *J Bone Joint Surg* 58A: 1, 1976.
3. Slocum, DB: The shin splint syndrome—medical aspects and differential diagnosis. *Am J Surg* 114: 875, 1967.
4. Slocum, DB and Larson, RL: Rotatory instability of the knee. *J Bone Joint Surg* 50A: 211, 1968.

CHAPTER SIXTY-FIVE

Degenerative Joint Disease

ALEXANDER S. TOWNES, M.D.

The common occurrence, the chronic and often benign course, and the lack of definitive treatment of degenerative joint disease or osteoarthritis have generated a general apathy and disinterest on the part of many physicians about this disease. A common attitude also among patients is that this form of arthritis is an inevitable consequence of aging and must be accepted as such. Advances in understanding of the pathophysiology of degenerative joint disease, especially in the past decade, have accomplished a great deal in dispelling these undeserved attitudes. As a result a better perspective of the multiple etiologic factors potentially involved in this disease, and a better understanding of the clinical problems presented by patients with this disorder have developed.

Degenerative joint disease is particularly important to the general physician who sees ambulatory adult patients. Estimates indicate that approximately half of all visits to physicians for joint disease are for this diagnosis. Degenerative joint disease is the most common arthritis diagnosed in a general practice (7).

PREVALENCE

Prevalence of degenerative joint disease increases with advancing age, beginning perhaps as early as the third decade of life and being almost ubiquitous as detected by radiography or by biochemical changes in articular cartilage in the seventh and eighth decades and beyond. It is fortunate and important, however, that clinical symptoms are not necessarily associated with structural changes, so that estimates of prevalence based on these findings exceed the magnitude of the clinical problem. Thus, symptoms and clinical findings of degenerative joint disease are not an inevitable accompaniment of aging. However, symptoms and findings are uncommon below age 35 and are more frequent above age 65, with perhaps as much as 30 to 40% of the population age 65 and above having some symptoms related to this diagnosis.

PATHOPHYSIOLOGY

The pathogenesis of degenerative joint disease is probably multifactorial; however, the final common pathway is believed to be *injury to articular cartilage*, which then undergoes a sequence of changes resulting eventually in loss of its proteoglycan matrix, cellular proliferation in attempted repair, release of enzymes with more destruction of all cartilage elements, and proliferation of subchondral bone. Changes are most severe in or may be confined entirely to areas of maximal stress on the articular cartilage, most striking in weight-bearing areas of the large joints. Although one hypothesis suggests a primary synovial lesion (2), most observers have concluded that the chronic synovitis which is found in more advanced cases of degenerative joint disease is probably secondary to cartilage degeneration with reaction to detritus shed into the joint cavity from this process. An important role of crystalline deposits of calcium pyrophosphate or hydroxyapatite in the synovial inflammatory response in certain patients, especially those with more advanced osteoarthritis, has been demonstrated (5). Remodeling and microfractures of subchondral bone with hardening and loss of ability to absorb stress as primary mechanisms in production of osteoarthritis have also been suggested (9).

Since there are no nerve fibers in articular cartilage, there are no symptoms due to early changes in the joints. There are multiple sources of pain, however, as the disease progresses. Periosteal irritation as a result of proliferating bone, denuded bone, microfractures of subchondral bone, stress on ligaments as a result of loss of cartilage and joint incongruity, low grade synovitis, effusion, and spasm of surrounding muscles are all potential sources of pain in osteoarthritis.

ETIOLOGY AND PREDISPOSING FACTORS

The cause of degenerative joint disease is not known. It is quite likely that there are multiple causes and many factors which may influence disease expression, some of which are listed in Table 65.1.

Because of multiple etiologic mechanisms in the pathogenesis of osteoarthritis, the history should seek to determine specific factors which may be implicated in each patient. Heredity may be important, especially in development of Heberden's nodes (12) (see below). A family history may also draw attention of the patient to the benign occurrence of these bony enlargements in elderly family members and serve to reassure them regarding their course.

Obesity is perhaps an obvious factor, but its extent and duration are important in assessing potential damage to weight-bearing joints, especially the knees. Preceding trauma may be important in subsequent development of degenerative arthritis in a joint damaged by ligamentous instability, meniscal tear in the

Table 65.1
Factors Contributing to Development of Osteoarthritis

AGING
  Diminished proteoglycan aggregation
  Diminished resistance of cartilage to fatigue fracture
    (? defective collagen network)
  Decreased resiliency of soft tissues
  Loss of normal anatomical relationship (hip)
HEREDITY
  Heberden's nodes
  Primary generalized osteoarthritis
  Postural or developmental defects (e.g., scoliosis, slipped
    capital femoral epiphyses or Legg-Calvé-Perthes disease.
  Metabolic defects (ochronosis, Wilson's disease)
ABNORMAL DISTRIBUTION OF MECHANICAL STRESS
  Postural or developmental defects
  Joint instability or hypermobility
  Local incongruity of joint surfaces post-traumatic, after
    meniscectomy, prolonged immobilization
  Obesity (abnormal stress on knees due to thigh adiposity)
EXCESSIVE REPETITIVE STRESS
  Occupational
  Sports-related
  Associated with neuropathy
CRYSTALLINE DEPOSIT DISEASE
  Calcium pyrophosphate
  Hydroxyapatite
PREVIOUS INFLAMMATORY JOINT DISEASE
METABOLIC ABNORMALITIES
  Ochronosis
  Wilson's disease
  Acromegaly
  ? Diabetes mellitus

knee joint, etc. Traumatic episodes with sufficient damage to induce these abnormalities are likely to be severe enough to be recalled, for example, as severe "sprains" with swelling lasting several days or longer following a sports-related or other injury. Prior joint surgery with removal of a torn meniscus in the knee is also a predisposing factor to osteoarthritis of the knee. Repetitive stress of minor trauma may also predispose to development of osteoarthritis (for example, in knees of basketball players) and may account for osteoarthritis in joints not commonly affected (e.g., elbows of baseball pitchers and elbows as well as shoulders of air hammer operators). Lifelong postural or mechanical defects also predispose to degenerative changes as the result of abnormal distribution of stress to the joint when force is applied. Since abnormalities such as varus or valgus deformities of the knees may also occur as a result of osteoarthritic damage to the joint, the history is important in determining which came first.

Degenerative joint disease may also be associated with other disease states: preceding inflammatory arthritis; metabolic diseases, such as ochronosis, with deposition of metabolites in cartilage; diseases predisposing to chondrocalcinosis such as hemochromatosis and hyperparathyroidism; and acromegaly. Diabetes mellitus may also predispose to osteoarthritis, although this association is less well documented.

GENERAL CLINICAL FEATURES

History

Characteristically there is involvement of only one or a few joints in osteoarthritis. Joints commonly affected and those usually spared are shown in Table 65.2. Since the presentations of patients may differ, depending upon the pattern of joints involved and predisposing factors, some of these presenting symptoms will be highlighted separately after a general discussion of the symptoms and findings in this disease.

Degenerative joint disease usually begins insidiously and progresses slowly. Aching discomfort early in the course characteristically increases in severity with use of the joint; therefore it tends to reach a peak after the day's activity and is relieved by rest. Pain is often aching in character and may be difficult for the patient to localize precisely. It is usually felt in the areas surrounding the involved joint. However, it is important to remember that hip pain may be referred to the medial aspect of the thigh, the lateral portion of the buttock, or to the knee. Morning stiffness and stiffness after rest may be absent, or if present, lasts only 15 to 20 min or less, in contrast to a longer duration in inflammatory joint disease such as rheumatoid arthritis. However, in advanced disease stiffness may be more profound, and pain may occur at rest. When joint destruction is marked, the patient may be kept awake at night by the pain.

As the disease progresses, large pieces of degener-

Table 65.2
Distribution of Joint Involvement in Osteoarthritis

COMMONLY AFFECTED
  Hands:
    Distal interphalangeal (Heberden's nodes)
    Proximal interphalangeal (Bouchard's nodes)
    Carpal-metacarpal of the thumb (joints between 1st
      metacarpal and greater multangular and between
      greater multangular and navicular)
  Knees
  Hips
  Spine:
    Cervical
    Lumbar
    Thoracic
  Feet:
    Metatarsophalangeal (especially 1st)
USUALLY SPARED
  Hands:
    Metacarpophalangeal
    Carpal-metacarpal (except 1st)
  Wrists
  Elbows
  Shoulders

ated cartilage may shed into the joint, producing loose bodies which may cause locking or giving away of the joint in addition to pain.

There are no systemic symptoms in osteoarthritis. This is an important negative feature of the history which helps to differentiate this disease from other forms of arthritis.

Physical Findings

Early in the disease there may be no physical findings. Most patients who present with symptoms will have some pain on passive motion of the involved joints or on motion against resistance. This is frequently a sense of crackling or crepitus as the joint is moved, probably due to joint surface incongruities and irregularities of opposing cartilaginous surfaces. Crepitus may be exaggerated by movement with weight-bearing or by manual compression of the joint during movement (for example, compression of the patella against the condyle of the femur when patellofemoral arthritis is present). In more advanced disease, joint motion may be limited and gross deformities may develop. Tenderness along the joint line is common, but may be mild or absent. In contrast to most inflammatory joint diseases, soft tissue swelling is usually absent or minimal in osteoarthritis except in its most advanced stages. Bony enlargement and irregularity is common, especially in the hands at the distal interphalangeal joints (Heberden's nodes) and less commonly in the proximal interphalangeal joints (Bouchard's nodes). Joint effusions are relatively infrequent compared to more inflammatory forms of joint disease. However, they may occur, especially in the knees. There is usually no detectable heat or redness over involved joints, although some warmth

may be present as the disease progresses and chronic synovitis develops.

Physical examination of the patient with osteoarthritis should always include a careful evaluation of the neurological system and peripheral vascular system since disease in these systems may produce pain or limited motion in an extremity which may be erroneously attributed to degenerative joint disease (see under "Differential Diagnosis").

Laboratory Findings

Degenerative joint disease is characterized by normal laboratory tests unless it is associated with some other disease process. In particular the erythrocyte sedimentation rate (ESR) is characteristically normal, in contrast to the inflammatory arthritides. Mild and transient elevation of ESR may occasionally be associated with the acute inflammatory events described below, or may be due to intercurrent disease elsewhere.

Examination of synovial fluid is helpful when effusion is present in a large joint. Synovial fluid in osteoarthritis is usually of the noninflammatory type, i.e., with good viscosity, white blood cells < 2000 per mm^3, protein content < 4 g/d, glucose approximately equal to a simultaneous serum glucose, and a good mucin clot when mixed with acetic acid (see Tables 63.1 and 63.2). When crystals of calcium pyrophosphate or hydroxyapatite are present (see Figure 66.1 and Table 66.1) the white cell count of the fluid may be elevated and protein content increased.

X-ray Findings

Radiographic findings are important in the diagnosis and differential diagnosis of degenerative joint disease since certain abnormalities are characteristic of this disorder. Therefore X-ray examination of the affected joints is indicated in the evaluation of most patients to confirm the diagnosis and to determine the extent of abnormalities present. However, it is important to point out that in early disease X-rays may be normal, and even with characteristic findings of joint narrowing and proliferation of subchondral bone with spur formation, symptoms may be absent. Hence, the importance of relating radiographic findings to the history and physical examination cannot be overemphasized. In general the more severe the radiographic changes, the more likely the patient is to have symptoms and findings of osteoarthritis. Radiographic findings from the earliest to the most advanced changes are listed in Table 65.3 and examples of X-rays are shown in Figure 65.1.

For evaluation of *hands* a single anteroposterior (AP) view of both hands is sufficient in most cases. Both *hips* can be visualized on a single AP film of the pelvis; more specific films may be required if an abnormality is detected or if findings do not correlate with the clinical picture. AP and lateral films are required for adequate evaluation of the *knee* joint.

Table 65.3
X-Ray Findings in Osteoarthritis

EARLIEST:
  No abnormality
EARLY:
  Slight loss of articular cartilage thickness (narrowing of
    radiologic joint space)
MODERATE:
  Marginal osteophyte formation
LATE:
  Loss of cartilage space (often focal in weight-bearing
    joints)
  Sclerosis of subchondral bone
  Subchondral cyst formation
  Loose bodies
  Subluxation or deformity

Special views of the patella ("skyline" view) may also be required to demonstrate the extent of patellofemoral arthritis. In evaluating the *spine*, AP, lateral, and oblique views are needed, the latter to visualize the neural foramina and the localization of nerve root compression by bony spurs.

CLINICAL PATTERNS OF OSTEOARTHRITIS

Heberden's Nodes

These bony enlargements of the distal interphalangeal joints are more frequent in women and commonly begin to appear in the fifth or sixth decade of life. They are often asymptomatic but a source of concern on the part of many patients who may view them as an outward sign of aging or as the beginning of a more serious and disabling arthritic disorder. Thus the physician must be aware of and prepared to deal with the emotional investment of the patient which may focus concerns about declining functions (including menopause) upon an obvious change in physical appearance such as Heberden's nodes. With a curt dismissal, no explanation of the true significance of this abnormality, and no opportunity for the patient to ventilate her concerns the physician will miss an important therapeutic opportunity.

Primary Generalized Osteoarthritis

This term was applied by Kellgren and Moore (6) to a group of patients whom they characterized as having osteoarthritis involving the distal and proximal interphalangeal joints and the carpometacarpal joint of the thumb in addition to involvement of multiple other joints (hips, knees, metatarsophalangeal, and spine). This pattern of osteoarthritis is uncommon; it affects mostly middle-aged women who have a positive family history of a similar disorder. Occasionally in early phases they will have had some inflammatory symptoms with an elevated ESR and an episodic course. It is suggested that these patients constitute a subgroup of patients with a heritable form of osteoarthritis which involves multiple joints and which perhaps has some distinctive radiologic features. However, the nature of the proposed heritable factor and whether these patients are clearly different from others with primary osteoarthritis have not been determined. It is important to recognize the syndrome clinically, primarily in order to differentiate it from rheumatoid arthritis and other polyarticular diseases.

Erosive Osteoarthritis of Hands

This term has been applied to patients with severe osteoarthritis of the hands (distal interphalangeal (DIP) and proximal interphalangeal (PIP) joints) in which extensive erosion of subchondral bone occurs with eventual deformity and significant limitation of motion of the finger joints (8). These patients also may have episodes of acute inflammation in these joints and their surrounding tissues. X-rays reveal the extensive bony erosion and subchondral cyst formation which may be interpreted incorrectly as rheumatoid or gouty erosions. The distribution of involvement in DIP and 1st carpometacarpal joints, sparing the metacarpophalangeal and wrists, should easily establish the true nature of the process. From the clinical point of view this syndrome is important because of the severity of symptoms and physical findings which are not common in milder forms of osteoarthritis of the hands.

Hip

Hip involvement is potentially the most painful and disabling joint abnormality in osteoarthritis. It is more often unilateral. Developmental defects in the structure of the hip including congenital hip dysplasia, slipped capital femoral epiphysis, or unrecognized avascular necrosis may have gone undetected but have predisposed the patient to develop osteoarthritis; with age, disturbance of the normal anatomical relationship between femoral head and acetabulum may also predispose to osteoarthritis. In contrast to osteoarthritis of the knee, obesity is not a major causal factor in osteoarthritis of the hip.

Pain, which early in the disease is associated with weight-bearing and movement, may become severe even at rest, and night pain is common in advanced disease. Patients may walk with a limp or with an abnormal gait. Pain and limitation of motion during internal rotation and extension are early physical signs and subsequently all motions may be painful and restricted. Clear identification of pain on motion of the hip is important in differentiating hip disease from other causes of pelvic pain. Flexion and adduction contracture and shortening may occur as disability progresses. Most patients who are symptomatic will have characteristic changes of osteoarthritis on X-rays of the hip. Progression of disease is variable but perhaps more likely to occur rapidly in the hip than in other joints.

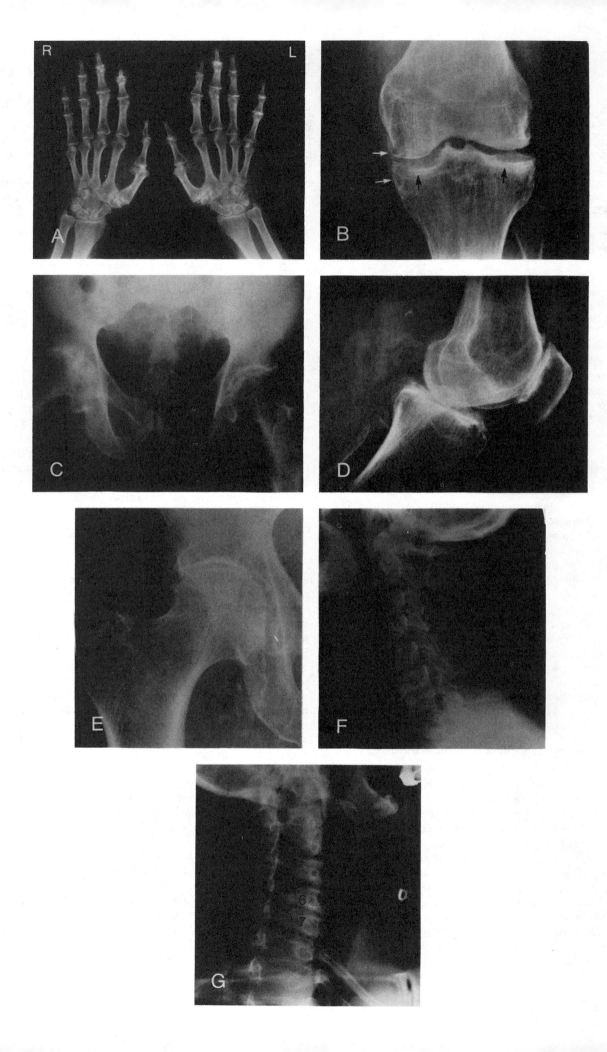

Knee

The knee is the most common symptomatic joint in osteoarthritis. There is a definite relationship to obesity, and the weight-bearing areas of the medial compartment are most often involved. Patellofemoral joint involvement is also common.

Chondromalacia patellae (see also Chapter 64) is a syndrome occurring usually in younger individuals (2nd, 3rd, and 4th decades) probably resulting from trauma and shearing forces against the patella as it contacts the femur in midflexion. Knee effusion is frequently associated with this syndrome. In younger patients with knee effusion who do not respond to rest, arthroscopy may be indicated and will show characteristic changes. In this instance, surgery may be indicated (see below). The relationship of this rather common syndrome to osteoarthritis is not entirely clear, although a distinct etiologic mechanism and pathology have been suggested.

Spinal Syndromes

Degenerative joint disease can result in neck or back pain which may be acute or chronic (see Chapters 61 and 62). Particularly in cervical spine involvement, symptoms may be more related to referred pain than to neck pain. These syndromes can also result in pain without obvious nerve root compression or neurologic abnormalities. Low cervical spine involvement can cause pain which is usually aching or burning in quality referred to the upper anterior chest, to the lower border of the scapula, and radiating down the arm to the elbow. Confusion with anginal pain may occur, but the history is usually clear that pain is localized to one side and occurs at rest, particularly during the night or in the early morning after sleep (probably due to positioning of head during sleep). Although it may also be exacerbated by activity during the day, pain related to cervical arthritis does not subside rapidly with rest and is not related to specific exertion. Physical examination usually can reproduce the pain on extremes of movement of the neck or with manual compression of the cervical segments in hyperextension rotation or lateral flexion. Degenerative arthritis of the thoracic spine can also cause radicular pain in the thoracic area, but this is surprisingly uncommon in contrast to frequent radiologic findings of spur formation in the thoracic spine, probably because of the anterior position of most of these bony abnormalities.

Another spinal syndrome, the relationship of which to osteoarthritis is not clear, is diffuse idiopathic skeletal hyperostosis (DISH). Table 65.4 lists the radiologic criteria for this diagnosis (10). Despite extensive hyperostosis and bony bridging between

Table 65.4
X-Ray Abnormalities in Diffuse Idiopathic Skeletal Hyperostosis[a]

SPINAL

Laminated calcification and ossification along the anterior lateral aspect of the vertebral bodies continuing across the disc spaces and varying in thickness from 1 to 20 mm (see Fig. 65.2A, arrow)

Bumpy spinal contour appearance from increased bone deposition located at the anterior disc space margins (see Fig. 65.2A)

Radiolucent disc extension (i.e., L-, F- or Y-shaped lucencies within the bone deposition along the anterior disc margin) (see Fig. 65.2B, arrow)

Radiolucency beneath deposited bone linearly located between the anteriolateral calcification and the vertebral bodies (see Fig. 65.2A, arrow)

EXTRASPINAL

(Frequent and distinctive features which permit a diagnosis even without spinal X-rays)

Bony proliferation

Ligament calcification, ossification

Para-articular osteophytes

(These changes are always present in the pelvis and in approximately 75% of cases in the heel and foot and less commonly in the elbows, knees, shoulders, humerus, wrist, and hands)

[a]Adapted from D. Resnick et al.: *Seminars in Arthritis and Rheumatism, 7:* 153, 1978 (10).

Figure 65.1 (A) Hands of patient with degenerative joint disease. Note the following characteristics: soft tissue enlargement on right over the second distal interphalangeal joint (Heberden's node); the loss of joint space and bony proliferation of all distal interphalangeal joints especially 2 and 3 in the right hand and 3 in the left hand; involvement of carpal metacarpal joint of both thumbs with narrowing and increased density of subchondral bone; and normal metacarpal phalangeal joints and wrist joints. (B) X-ray of knee showing degenerative joint disease with loss of joint space (cartilage) especially in medial compartment, sclerotic subchondral bone, subchondral cysts, and early marginal spurs especially on lateral side. (C) Pelvic film of a patient with advanced degenerative joint disease in the right hip. Notice the joint space narrowing and proliferation of subchondral bone. The left hip shows the minimal change of marginal sclerosis. (D) Lateral X-ray of same knee (in B) illustrating involvement of patellofemoral joint with narrowing and spur formation superiorly. (E) X-ray of a hip showing relatively early degenerative joint disease. Notice the narrowed joint space and spur formation of femoral head at upper margin of acetabulum. (F) X-ray of the lateral cervical spine showing degenerative joint disease. Note narrowing of C5-6, and especially C6-7 interspace with anterior lipping and spur formation. (G) Oblique X-ray view of cervical spine of same patient (F) showing osteophytes encroaching on neural foramina C5-6, C6-7.

the vertebral bodies, motion and function are usually maintained since the apophyseal joints are usually spared. This syndrome is chiefly important because of its impressive radiographic appearance (Fig. 65.2), the diffuse bony changes with hyperostosis, and the importance of distinguishing it from ankylosing spondylitis.

"Acute" Exacerbations of Osteoarthritis

Patients with degenerative joint disease may present occasionally with acute or subacute painful episodes with swelling of the affected joint. These episodes are usually superimposed upon more typical preceding symptoms and signs of osteoarthritis, but may be the event precipitating an initial visit to the physician. In these patients there may be evidence of inflammation with pain, swelling, warmth, and some erythema on occasion. When the knee is involved there may be a joint effusion. The episodes, which may be precipitated by minor trauma, probably are caused by sudden release into the joint of large amounts of cartilaginous debris and/or microcrystalline deposits contained therein, and very rarely by complicating sepsis. In a study by Huskisson et al. (5) either calcium pyrophosphate, or hydroxyapatite crystals, or both were found in a high proportion of knee effusions of patients with such episodes, but, in addition, in a significant proportion of unselected patients with osteoarthritis of the knee with effusion. Thus the concurrence of crystalline deposit disease and osteoarthritis seems to be well established, although the relationship of cause and effect is not yet clear. From the clinical point of view, however, this interrelationship provides a better understanding of these acute inflammatory episodes which punctuate the course of otherwise typical osteoarthritis (see also Chapter 66). Sepsis may occasionally complicate an osteoarthritic joint, but it is a much less common event than occurs in a rheumatoid arthritic joint.

For these reasons a patient with established osteoarthritis who develops an acutely swollen, painful, hot joint should have the joint aspirated and the fluid analyzed (see Tables 63.1 and 63.2) because of the possibility of there being either a complicating microcrystalline induced or a septic arthritis.

DIAGNOSIS AND DIFFERENTIAL DIAGNOSIS

The diagnosis of degenerative joint disease is based upon the history and physical findings related to the joints, the absence of systemic signs, and typical radiologic findings. Differentiation from other forms of arthritis is usually not difficult, with the possible exception of some of the more unusual diffuse or inflammatory patterns of involvement described above. Consideration of the age of the patient, the

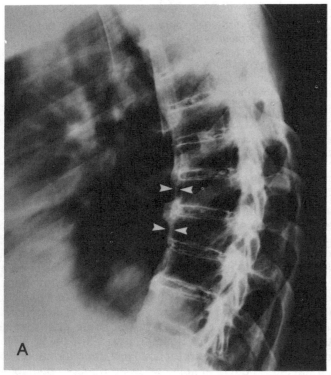
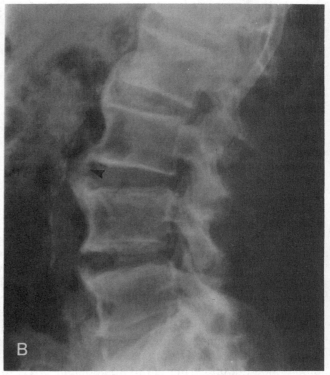

Figure 65.2 (A) Lateral X-ray of thoracic spine of patient with diffuse idiopathic skeletal hyperostosis. (B) Lateral X-ray of lumbar spine of patient with diffuse idiopathic skeletal hyperostosis. Prominent bony fusion and lipping anteriorly are seen.

distribution of the joints involved, and the radiologic findings will usually lead to the correct diagnosis.

The most common errors in differential diagnosis occur in attributing symptoms of pain or restricted movement to degenerative joint disease when the problem is not the joints. Since X-rays may demonstrate changes of degenerative joint disease in asymptomatic or mildly symptomatic patients, the physician must rely upon a careful history and physical examination to localize the disease to the joints. Table 65.5 lists other disorders, also common in older age groups, which often give rise to pain, and painful or restricted movement, and which may be erroneously attributed to degenerative "arthritis" unless a careful examination is done.

MANAGEMENT

There is no cure for degenerative joint disease and no therapy which can be directed toward the specific pathophysiology of cartilage degeneration. However, much can be done to relieve symptoms, minimize disability, and perhaps to delay progression of the disease. Certainly a nihilistic approach to therapy, e.g., "go home, take aspirin, and accept the fact you are getting older" which has been common advice in the past, is not justified. The criteria for the determination of medical disability under Social Security are listed in Table 3.5 on page 28.

General Measures

PATIENT EDUCATION

Explaining to the patient the nature of the disease, that other joints are not likely to be involved, that progression of disease is slow, and that preservation of function is likely will reassure most patients. For

Table 65.5
Differential Diagnosis of Osteoarthritis: Extra-articular Causes of Pain or Restricted Movement

BONE DISEASE
    Osteopenia or osteoporosis (see Chapter 71)
    Malignancy: myeloma, metastatic
    Paget's disease
PERIARTICULAR SOFT TISSUE ABNORMALITIES
    Soft tissue contractures (Dupuytren's, post cerebrovascular accident, or debilitating disease with disuse)
    Tendinitis or bursitis (see Chapter 63)
    Reflex dystrophy
NEUROMUSCULAR DISEASES
    Neuropathy (diabetic, alcoholism, B_{12} deficiency) (see Chapter 81)
    Parkinsonism (see Chapter 79)
    Tardive dyskinesias (see Chapter 79)
    Senile dementia with rigidity (see Chapters 16 and 79)
VASCULAR DISEASES (see Chapter 84)
    Atherosclerotic
    Diabetic
    Vasculitic

the patient with Heberden's nodes or mild disease in other joints, this reassurance and understanding will be the most important therapeutic step in management.

REST

Pain and discomfort of degenerative joint disease are frequently exacerbated by use, especially continuous use or weight-bearing. Further, excessive use of joints already damaged by osteoarthritis may accelerate cartilage degeneration. Therefore, rest is an important modality of treatment for osteoarthritis. Short periods of rest through the day are usually more effective than less frequent longer periods. With weight-bearing joints, rest is particularly important. Many patients, especially elderly ones, have the notion that use of a joint becomes limited if rested too much, so that needless overuse is common. When an understanding of the value of rest and reassurance about function is given, they will often quickly learn to live within their own limitations without undue restrictions of activity and with improvement in symptoms.

USE OF CANES, CRUTCHES, AND WALKERS

In more severe disease, rest from weight-bearing and stability when walking may be partially achieved by the use of a crutch, a cane, or a walker. The patient's attitude about the use of such assistive devices is an important consideration here since some will interpret their cane as a sign of infirmity and fail to use it, while others may carry it proudly as a badge of dependency even when it is not needed. Instruction in proper use of a cane, a crutch, or a walker should be given by the physician or a physical therapist. It should be remembered that the object is to take weight off the affected limb; thus a cane or a crutch should always be used on the opposite side and used simultaneously with the affected limb for weight bearing. A walker does not provide this type of unilateral support, but it may be needed in patients with bilateral knee pain or in patients whose instability requires more support than that provided by a cane or a crutch.

CORRECTION OF POSTURAL OR MECHANICAL STRAIN

This is an important consideration in patients with poor body mechanics. Thus the patient with pronated feet (see Chapter 99) will have excessive stress on the knees and low back. Genu varus or valgum will stress the lateral or medial compartment excessively. Instruction in proper lifting and avoidance of unnecessary strain on certain joints or muscles by occupational or other activities may also need attention—for example, use of a cervical pillow in the patient with neck involvement (see also Chapters 61 and 62).

PHYSICAL THERAPY

Simple measures can be prescribed for home use without the need for referral to a physical therapist in patients with mild disease. However, the physician must be sure that the patient understands directions. Reinforcement on subsequent visits is also important to ensure compliance. Patients with more advanced disease should be referred to a physical or occupational therapist for more extensive instruction in an exercise program, joint protection maneuvers, use of assistive devices, gait training, and the like.

Heat. Application of heat often provides symptomatic relief of pain, reduces muscle spasm, and facilitates subsequent performance of an exercise program. Most patients prefer moist heat, which can be applied for 15 to 20 min via bathtub, hot towels, or commercially manufactured packs. Electric heating pads may also be used. Paraffin wax baths may be useful in patients with extensive hand involvement. With all modalities of heat therapy, temperatures above 110°F (43°C) and prolonged or uninterrupted use should be avoided, to prevent skin damage. Use of diathermy, ultrasound, heat cabinets, and the like offers little advantage in most cases and requires a physical therapist.

Exercise. Goals of an exercise program are to maintain or improve function by preserving range of motion and improving muscle strength. The latter is important to help stabilize the joint and, by maintaining soft tissue cushioning of stress, to reduce the stress applied to the joint. Gradual conditioning is important so that muscle pain and soreness are not aggravated. Maintenance of quadriceps strength is particularly important in osteoarthritis of the knee. This can be accomplished by beginning with slow full extension of the knee against gravity, and then, as symptoms and progress allow, by extension with progressively increasing weight attached to the lower leg (an old pocketbook or bag with a strap to which are added canned goods of specific weight from the pantry shelf will suffice). In patients whose pain prevents active quadriceps strengthening, isometric exercises are useful. With the knee extended the patient is instructed to tighten the quadriceps maximally so that the patella becomes fixed, to hold for 10 to 15 sec by count, release, and repeat. Exercise should be graded according to the ability of the individual patient and carried out at least three times per day for optimal effect. In general, if muscle soreness or joint pain is worse after exercise, the intensity of the exercise should be reduced or progression halted until symptoms subside. Swimming is also a valuable means of exercise which does not involve weight-bearing stress. Bicycling also provides exercise with less weight-bearing stress than walking.

Other measures. For cervical spine disease gentle overhead traction may improve symptoms. This can be accomplished at home with a halter device and pulley and may be combined with the use of a soft cervical collar (see Chapter 61).

Many patients report remission of stiffness and pain and a sense of joint protection through the use of elastic supports around the joint. Such devices used at the knee, however, often obstruct venous circulation in the leg and cause edema, so that their use is not generally recommended. Wearing nylon stretch gloves may provide relief for some patients with extensive hand involvement (1).

DIET

Control of obesity (Chapter 73) is important in osteoarthritis of the knees, hips, and metatarsophalangeal joints. Otherwise there is no dietary imperative either to omit or to eat any specific foods, vitamins, or nutrients. Patients should be cautioned against food fads and unwarranted claims of relationship of diet and osteoarthritis.

Drug Therapy

NONSTEROIDAL ANTI-INFLAMMATORY DRUGS

Nonsteroidal anti-inflammatory (NSAID) and analgesic agents are the mainstay of drug treatment of osteoarthritis. For patients with mild disease, pain is usually related to mechanical factors rather than to inflammation. Thus, analgesic doses are all that is required. Aspirin is an effective analgesic and usually is well tolerated in divided doses of 1.2 to 2.4 g/day. Acetaminophen may be equally effective as an analgesic in patients unable to take aspirin.

Although mild by comparison to that of rheumatoid arthritis, the inflammatory component of osteoarthritis becomes more evident as the disease progresses and may warrant the use of anti-inflammatory doses of salicylates or other NSAID. The average dose of aspirin required may vary from 3.6 to 4.8 g/day for anti-inflammatory effect. At this dose gastrointestinal side effects of aspirin including gastric ulceration and increased blood loss in the stool are common. This may be largely obviated by the use of enteric coated aspirin, but erratic absorption in some patients requires a measure of blood salicylate level after several days of therapy to ensure an optimum level of 15–25 mg/dl. Other salicylate preparations such as choline salicylate (Arthropan liquid 870 mg/5 ml, available without prescription), chlorine magnesium salicylate (Trilisate 1500 mg), and salicylsalicylic acid (Disalcid 500 mg) both requiring a prescription, are also effective and have better gastrointestinal tolerance than aspirin, but are also significantly more expensive, about equal in cost to other nonsteroidal anti-inflammatory drugs.

A large number of NSAID (11) in addition to salicylates are now available and more are being developed. It is probable that the efficacy and side effects of aspirin and the nonsteroidal anti-inflammatory agents are mediated largely through the ubiquitous prostaglandin system by inhibition of cyclooxygenase enzymes which are involved in the synthesis of prostaglandins from fatty acids of the cell membrane, principally arachidonic acid. The anti-inflammatory potency, duration of action, and the side effects of each agent are somewhat variable because of the differences in tissue distribution and metabolism of the various drugs. For example indomethacin (Indocin) is a potent NSAID which penetrates most tissues including the central nervous system. Tolmetin (Tolectin) has a somewhat similar molecular structure and efficacy, but because it is largely excluded by the blood brain barrier, has fewer central nervous system side effects such as headache and psychic disturbances. Sulindac (Clinoril) is converted to an active metabolite after absorption so that it bypasses and does not inhibit the local gastroprotective effect of prostaglandins in the gastric mucosa. Naproxen (Naprosyn) differs from other propanoic acid derivatives in its longer half-life in the plasma, so that intervals between doses can be increased. Aspirin irreversibly acetylates platelet cyclooxygenase for the life of the platelet, whereas other compounds reversibly inhibit platelet thromboxane production. In controlled clinical trials none of the NSAID has been shown to differ significantly from aspirin in efficacy in the treatment of osteoarthritis or other forms of arthritis, although the frequency of side effects has been lower with some of these drugs than with regular aspirin. Also, any one agent may be unaccountably more effective than another, so that a trial and error approach is often warranted.

Some of the factors in choice of a NSAID include cost (11), frequency of administration required (a major factor in compliance), and side effects, which may be variably tolerated by different patients (see Table 67.5 for list of side effects and dosage). Aspirin is clearly the cheapest and generally the drug of first choice in treatment of osteoarthritis.

CORTICOSTEROIDS

Intra-articular injection of suspensions of corticosteroids (see Table 63.4) has been shown to be useful in the management of osteoarthritis, when associated with effusions in large joints such as the knee (4). If prolonged relief lasting several months is not achieved with one or two injections, this therapy should not be continued. The risk of serious side effects including enhanced destruction of the joint and infection may follow repeated injections, which should therefore be avoided.

There is absolutely no indication for systemic administration of corticosteroids in the management of osteoarthritis.

Orthopaedic Surgery

The orthopaedist should be consulted in management of patients with osteoarthritis who have a problem of malalignment or major instability in weight-bearing joints, for symptoms or findings of loose bodies in the joint, and for intractable pain with advanced disease of the hips or knees. Osteotomy may correct malalignment. Arthroplasty to improve instability and remove loose bodies, meniscal fragments, and perhaps large spurs may be useful in some patients. Joint replacement offers excellent results in patients with osteoarthritis of the hip (3). Joint replacement is less successful in the knee, but is advantageous in some patients with advanced disease. Arthrodesis (i.e., surgical fusion of the joint) is still useful in patients with unilateral, intractable, and severe knee involvement.

Recurrent symptoms of chondromalacia patellae may also be an indication for orthopaedic referral. Arthroscopy can confirm the diagnosis, and surgery may be indicated in some patients, although there is not uniform agreement on the procedure or its outcome.

PREVENTION

Since the etiology of degenerative joint disease is uncertain, so is its prevention. However, recognition of predisposing factors and elucidation of normal physiology of articular cartilage suggest certain prudent steps which can be recommended.

Immobilization with avoidance of joint stress gives rise to biochemical changes in cartilage similar to early lesions in osteoarthritis. Thus normal stress and functioning of joints is important in maintenance of normal cartilage physiology. Perhaps one can abstract from this that a sedentary and inactive life is not good for the integrity of articular cartilage. Further, since strong periarticular muscles lend stability and help absorb stress applied to joints and since obesity adds stress to weight-bearing joints, it seems logical to conclude that physical conditioning to maintain muscle strength, and a lean habitus may be important in prevention of degenerative joint disease. Soft tissues tend to lose mobility with advancing age and such changes have been shown to increase impact stress of joints. Physical conditioning may retard this loss of mobility and therefore should be encouraged in aging individuals.

At the same time it is evident that repetitive stress, especially when abnormally applied, is a strong predisposing factor to osteoarthritis. Thus correction of abnormal mechanical forces from developmental or postural defects, avoidance of unusual occupational stress, and avoidance of traumatic injury to joints are important in prevention of osteoarthritis.

References

General

Brandt, KD: Pathogenesis of osteoarthritis. In *Textbook of Rheumatology, Vol. II*, edited by WN Kelley, CD Harris, S. Ruddy and CB Sledge. W. B. Saunders, Philadelphia, 1981.

Blanc, JH and Stalberg, SD: Osteoarthritis: pathology and clinical patterns. In *Textbook of Rheumatology, Vol. II*, edited by WN Kelley, CD Harris, S Ruddy and CB Sledge. W. B. Saunders, Philadelphia, 1981.

Robertson, WD: Management of degenerative disease. In *Textbook of Rheumatology, Vol. II*, edited by WN Kelley, CD Harris, S Ruddy and CB Sledge. W. B. Saunders Philadelphia, 1981.

These three chapters provide an in-depth review of all aspects of osteoarthritis.

Specific

1. Ehrlich, GE and DiPiero, AM: Stretch gloves: nocturnal use to ameliorate morning stiffness in arthritic hands. *Arch Phys Med Rehabil 52:* 479, 1971.
2. Glynn, LE: Primary lesion in osteoarthritis. *Lancet 1:* 574, 1977.
3. Harris, WH: Total joint replacement. *N Engl J Med 297:* 650, 1977.
4. Hollander, JL: Treatment of osteoarthritis of the knees. *Arthritis Rheum 3:* 564, 1960.
5. Huskisson, EC, Dieppe, PA, Tucker, AK and Channel, LB: Another look at osteoarthritis. *Ann Rheum Dis 38:* 423, 1979.
6. Kellgren, JH and Moore, R: Generalized osteoarthritis and Heberden's nodes. *Br Med J 1:* 181, 1952.
7. Marsland, DW, Wood, M and Mayo, F: Content of family practice; I. Routine order of diagnosis by frequency, and II. Diagnosis by disease category and age/sex distribution. *J Fam Pract 8:* 37, 1976.
8. Peter, JB, Pearson, CM and Marmnor, L: Erosive osteoarthritis of the hands. *Arthritis Rheum 9:* 365, 1966.
9. Radin, EL, Parker, HG, Pugh, JW, Steinberg, RS, Paul, IL and Rose, RM: Response of joints to impact loading; III. Relationship between trabecular microfractures and cartilage degeneration. *J Biomech 6:* 51, 1973.
10. Resnick, D, Shapiro, RF, Wiesner, KB, Niwayama, E, Utsinger, PD and Shaul, SR: Diffuse idiopathic skeletal hyperostosis (DISH) [ankylosing hyperosteosis of Forestier and Rotes-Querol]. *Semin Arthritis Rheum 7:* 153, 1978.
11. Simon, LS and Mills, JA: Non-steroidal anti-inflammatory drugs. *N Engl J Med 302:* 1179 and 1237, 1980.
12. Stecker, RM: Heberden's nodes, heredity in hypertrophic arthritis of the finger joints. *Am J Med Sci 201:* 801, 1941.

CHAPTER SIXTY-SIX

Crystal-induced Arthritis

ALEXANDER S. TOWNES, M.D.

INTRODUCTION

Gout was the first form of arthritis that was recognized to be caused by the deposition of (urate) crystals in the joints and periarticular tissues. It is now known that other crystalline substances—most commonly calcium pyrophosphate dihydrate and hydroxyapatite—also are implicated in the pathogenesis of certain kinds of arthritic disease. Although disorders associated with these various crystals differ in etiology and in specific characteristics, they have in common the deposition of crystals in and around joints, the propensity to episodes of acute inflammatory arthritis, and sometimes the development of a destructive arthropathy. It is therefore appropriate to consider these varied clinical disorders together under the unifying concept of crystal-induced arthritis.

Mechanisms of Crystal-induced Arthritis

The inflammatory properties of crystals such as sodium urate and calcium pyrophosphate dihydrate when injected into joints or soft tissues depend upon the interaction of the crystals with plasma proteins and the phagocytosis of the crystals by polymorphonuclear leukocytes (PMN). Leukocytes which have phagocytized crystals generate and release a potent low molecular weight chemotactic factor, a glycopeptide, which attracts more neutrophils and amplifies the response. During the process of phagocytosis, leukocytes also release into the surrounding tissue lysosomal enzymes which further activate mediators of inflammation. Urate crystals, by the nature of their electrostatic surface charge, also interact with other plasma proteins to activate the complement system and the kinin system, contributing further to the inflammatory response.

Although the events which trigger acute inflammation are not entirely clear, it seems likely that there is, in association with rapid changes in serum urate concentration, a sudden release of a sufficient volume of crystalline material from tissue sites into joint spaces to begin the cycle of phagocytosis and inflammation (8, 9).

The invariable association between phagocytosis of crystals and the acute inflammatory response is important clinically since demonstration of crystals within leukocytes from synovial fluid constitutes a convenient method of making a definitive diagnosis in patients with acute inflammatory crystal-induced arthritis.

Although gouty arthritis and other crystal-induced diseases are usually characterized by symptoms and signs of acute inflammation, sometimes destructive arthropathy occurs with little evidence of inflammation.

Crystal Identification

The identification of crystals in synovial fluid or in periarticular tissue is fundamental to the diagnosis and management of patients with crystal-induced arthritis. Crystals of monosodium urate are best identified by placing a drop of aspirated tissue fluid directly on a glass slide and by examining the wet preparation through a microscope under polarized light (15); the crystals are difficult to see under non-polarized light. Although specialized equipment is ideal, crystals can be demonstrated adequately in the physician's office by placing a plastic polarizing lens (made from an old pair of sunglasses, for example) between the light source and the microscopic stage, and by placing another lens in the body or in the eyepiece of the microscope. When one lens is rotated so that the field becomes dark, the negatively bire-fringent urate crystals (i.e., crystals capable of bending light rays in two planes; the notation of negativity is an arbitrary term used by physicists to describe the direction of bend), dimly seen in ordinary light, stand out brightly and can be identified within the cytoplasm of polymorphonuclear leukocytes. If a red plate compensator is used (one can be fabricated by wrapping a glass slide longitudinally with two layers of transparent (cellophane) tape (occasionally more layers of tape are required)) (2), the crystals are even more easily identified since the field turns red and crystals parallel to the axis of the compensator will appear yellow, while those perpendicular to the axis will appear blue. Monosodium urate crystals are usually needle- or rod-shaped. The size varies but some large crystals equal to or larger than the diameter of the leukocyte are usually seen. A slide prepared in this manner may be kept for several hours at room temperature; however, once the cells die and lyse, evaluation is less valid. In the event the aspirated fluid cannot be examined immediately, it may be preserved overnight by refrigeration in a plain test tube.

Monosodium urate crystals (which are usually present in abundance) are pathognomonic of gout (see Table 66.1 and Fig. 66.1). Absence of crystals is strong evidence against the diagnosis, and especially if leukocytosis is significant, infection or another diagnosis should be considered.

Monosodium urate is usually easily distinguished from calcium pyrophosphate dihydrate (CPPD) on the basis of morphology and of characteristics of the crystals under polarized light (see Table 66.1 and Fig. 66.1). CPPD crystals vary much more in size and shape from rod-like to rhomboid and irregular forms, are usually much shorter, and are never needle-like. They are usually refractile without polarized light and do not increase appreciably in brilliance when the light is polarized. They are weakly positively birefringent and change color in the opposite direction to urate when the red plate compensator is used (i.e., blue when parallel to the axis and yellow when perpendicular).

Because CPPD crystals are small and do not stand out in polarized light, they are overlooked more frequently by the occasional observer. Routine reports from unspecialized clinical laboratories are often falsely negative.

Other crystalline materials which may be seen include those from previously injected corticosteroids (which appear as crystals of varying and unusual configuration), and occasionally cholesterol crystals

Table 66.1
Identification of Crystals in Synovial Fluid

MONOSODIUM URATE
  Morphology:
    Rod- or needle-shaped
    Length usually approaches diameter of polymorphonuclear leukocyte (PMN)
  Polarized light:
    Stand out brightly when field is dark
    Strongly negatively birefringent
  Red plate compensator:
    Yellow crystals parallel and blue crystals perpendicular to axis
CALCIUM PYROPHOSPHATE DIHYDRATE
  Morphology:
    Rhomboid, rod, or irregular rhomboid shape
    Length variable, often smaller than one lobe of a PMN nucleus
  Polarized light:
    No increase in refractile appearance when field is dark
    Weakly positively birefringent
  Red plate compensator:
    Blue crystals parallel and yellow crystals perpendicular to axis
HYDROXYAPATITE
  Not usually seen with ordinary or polarized light microscopy
  Microspheroid clusters with alizarin red (available in histology laboratories)
  Usually requires electron microscopy or radioactive carbon label binding for demonstration

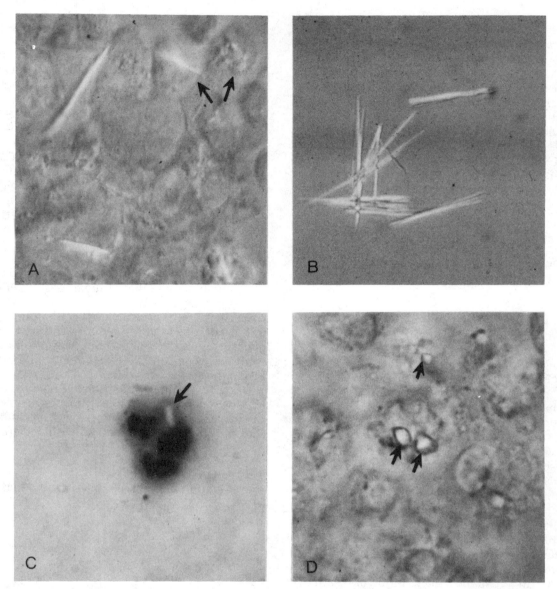

Figure 66.1 (*A*) Urate crystals in synovial fluid examined by polarized light microscopy. Note the needle shape and variable size but many have a larger diameter than white blood cells (oil immersion). (*B*) Urate crystals from tophus examined by polarized light with red plate compensator (oil immersion). (*C*) Calcium pyrophosphate dihydrate (CPPD) crystal in white blood cell found on gram stain (oil immersion). Note the shape and size relative to nucleus and cytoplasm. Gram stain is not the usual method of demonstration, but is occasionally useful. (*D*) Wet preparation of synovial fluid demonstrating varied size and shape of CPPD crystal phagocytized by white blood cell (oil immersion lens, polarized light). Size and shape varies from squat rhomboid to rod-shaped. Note several crystals in some cells.

which are easily distinguished from all of the above (resembling a folded envelope). Contaminating crystalline or refractile substances such as EDTA anticoagulant, talc, etc. can be avoided by use of careful technique.

GOUT

Gout is a syndrome that is caused by an alteration in purine metabolism, the end-product of which is uric acid. This alteration results in hyperuricemia and in the deposition of urate crystals in various tissues. Periodic attacks of acute inflammatory arthritis, characteristic of gout, are due to the deposition of urate crystals in and about joints. *Primary gout* is caused by an inborn error in the production or excretion of uric acid. *Secondary gout* is caused by an increased breakdown of nucleic acids in association with one of a variety of acquired diseases or by impaired excretion of urate as a consequence of acquired renal disease (Table 66.2).

Most patients with gout (approximately 85%) have,

Table 66.2
Causes of Hyperuricemia[a]

With Increased Urinary Uric Acid	With Normal or Low Urinary Uric Acid
10–25% of primary gout (defect unknown)	75–90% of primary gout (defect unknown)
Specific enzyme defects with primary gout	
Secondary causes:	Secondary causes:
Myeloproliferative disease	Renal insufficiency
Lymphoproliferative disease	Lead intoxication
Hemolytic anemias	Drugs:
Obesity	Salicylates (low dose *i.e.* <2.4 g/day)
Glycogen storage disease	Diuretics
Exercise	Pyrazinamide
Psoriasis	Ethambutol
	Nicotinic acid
	Alcohol
	Others
	Obesity
	Sarcoidosis
	Starvation

[a] Modified from J. B. Wyngaarden and W. N. Kelley: *Gout and Hyperuricemia*. Grune & Stratton, New York, 1976.

usually for unknown reasons, an elevated renal threshold for the excretion of uric acid. The rest (approximately 15%) overproduce uric acid, although precise enzymatic defects in purine catabolism only rarely have been identified. Production and excretion of uric acid are best assessed by measurement of urate in a 24-hour sample of urine; normally less than 600 mg/day are excreted if the diet for 5 days has been free of foods that are rich in purines (fish, meat, and poultry; especially the solid organs of these food sources); while there is considerable dietary variation, an excretion of more than approximately 750 to 800 mg/day while eating a nonrestricted diet may be considered indicative of overproduction in the absence of purine gluttony (4).

Normal levels of serum urate vary widely in the population, with a range of 3 to 8 mg/dl; also, there may be spontaneous variation within individuals. The upper limit of normal for serum urate measured by the uricase method usually is considered to be 7.0 mg/dl for adult males and 6.0 mg/dl for females. Ranges may be higher by 1 mg/dl or more if automated colorimetric methods, commonly used in multiphasic screening tests, are employed.

Serum "uric acid" concentration is primarily a measurement of urate. The concentration of urate and uric acid are related to pH: at normal blood and interstitial fluid pH of 7.40, the ratio of urate to uric acid is approximately 45 to 1; as the pH falls—e.g., in the urinary tubule—the relative concentration of uric acid rises (e.g., at a pH of 4.50 the urate to uric acid ratio is approximately 0.06 to 1).

Prevalence

Gout is estimated to occur at a lifetime frequency of 3 per 1000 population in the United States. It is 10 times more common in males in all its forms and is rare in premenopausal females. Gout is infrequent below age 30 and increases in frequency to a plateau at about age 60. Age at onset is probably related to the duration and severity of preceding hyperuricemia. Gout is more common in obese or in hypertensive people, although the relationships are complex. The frequency of gout in hypertensive subjects, for example, is magnified if they are treated with thiazide diuretics (see also p. 650). Gout is also more common in patients with a chronically high alcohol intake, especially if they also are obese or have mildly impaired renal function. Associations of gout with hyperlipidemia and with atherosclerotic coronary disease have also been reported, but these relationships need further clarification.

Clinical Features (Table 66.3)

ACUTE ARTHRITIC ATTACK

The acute arthritic attack is the hallmark of gout. It is characterized by the onset of pain, swelling, and discomfort which progress rapidly to a peak level of intensity within 24 to 36 hours after onset. The pain is often severe enough to prevent use of the affected joint or even for the patient to bear the weight of bed clothing. The metatarsophalangeal joint of the great toe is the most commonly affected joint, followed by the forefoot, heel, ankle, knee, wrist, fingers, and elbow. The great toe is affected at some time during the course of perhaps 90% of gouty subjects. Usually a single joint is involved early in the course of the disease but pauciarticular arthritis (two or three joints) may occur; polyarticular (more than three joints) onset is rare. Polyarticular gout is more common in late disease associated with soft tissue tophi. Recurrent acute arthritis is more common in previously affected joints.

There are several events which may trigger an acute attack of gout: trauma, an acute illness such as an acute myocardial infarction, dietary indiscretion, overuse of alcohol, starvation, and recent administration of drugs which lower serum urate concentration.

Table 66.3
Clinical Features of Gout

EPIDEMIOLOGY
    Sex: Males 10 to 1; Rare in premenopausal women
    Age: Usually middle age or older (peak age 60)
ACUTE GOUT
    History:
        Acute attacks, recurrent, with disease-free intervals
        Rapid progression to peak severity within 24 hours
    Physical findings:
        Usually monoarticular with swelling, tenderness, erythema, and intense inflammation
        Big toe metatarsophalangeal joint commonly involved (podagra)
        Forefeet, heels, ankles, knees, wrists, fingers, elbows, and other joints may be affected
        Occasionally polyarticular
        Fever may occur
    Laboratory: Joint aspiration with leukocytosis and identification of urate crystals is diagnostic
INTERCRITICAL GOUT
    No symptoms or findings except hyperuricemia
    Toe aspiration may reveal urate crystals
CHRONIC GOUT
    Often polyarticular
    Symptoms may persist between attacks
    Tophi are common (approximately 90–95%)
    Deformities may develop

Most of these events are associated with rapid changes in serum urate concentration, and it has been postulated that such changes cause dissolution of tissue deposits with discharge of crystalline material locally to induce the acute attack.

A family history of gout should be sought in patients with primary gout, and especially in those patients who excrete excess amounts of uric acid in whom a specific enzyme defect may be suspected. However, a positive family history is obtained in less than half of gouty subjects so that a negative history is of no differential diagnostic value.

On physical examination of the patient with acute gouty arthritis there is frequently erythema overlying or adjacent to the affected joints, especially when small joints are involved. The erythema often involves only a localized area rather than the entire joint. The intensity of the inflammatory reaction frequently results in a mistaken diagnosis of cellulitis, a diagnosis which may appear to be supported by a fever which may reach 101°F (38°C) or higher. Joint swelling usually is marked and joint effusion is also common. Tenderness on palpation or motion of the affected part also usually is marked.

The intensity and severity of these classical acute signs and symptoms may vary from one attack to another, and may be less evident when a large joint such as the knee is involved, especially in elderly patients and in patients with polyarticular gout. However, the history will almost always indicate rapid progression to a peak intensity within 24 to 36 hours, an important feature in differential diagnosis.

Laboratory findings may include a mild leukocytosis and an elevated erythrocyte sedimentation rate. Serum uric acid almost always is elevated but is of limited diagnostic value because of the frequency of hyperuricemia in the absence of gout, and because the acute attack, which is related principally to the concentration of tissue urate, may occur at a time when the serum urate may be normal as a result of previous drug administration (such as high dose aspirin (> 3.5 g/day) or another uricosuric agent) or of spontaneous variation. Examination of the synovial fluid provides diagnostic findings in almost all instances in which it can be obtained. There is a brisk leukocytosis with polymorphonuclear leukocytes which, when examined under polarized light, can be seen to contain phagocytized urate crystals (see section on crystal identification).

The acute attack is self-limited and even without treatment will subside in several days to weeks. Once the acute attack subsides or is treated, there are no residual joint symptoms—another important point in differential diagnosis.

Recurrent acute attacks are usual: approximately 75% of patients will have a second gouty attack within 2 years of their first and most of these will have occurred within the first year; occasionally 10 years or more may elapse between attacks (20).

INTERCRITICAL GOUT

Between acute attacks of gout, patients will be totally asymptomatic with no abnormal physical findings unless tophi are present or unless the disease has progressed to the chronic phase. If the patient's first visit to the physician is at this stage, a presumptive diagnosis can be made on the basis of a history of a typical prior attack, especially if there have been multiple attacks, and on the basis of hyperuricemia. A definitive diagnosis of gout can be established even in intercritical gout by aspiration of the flexed great toe joint with a 22 gauge needle under local anesthesia, using a dorsolateral approach perpendicular to the plantar surface—a procedure which is usually well tolerated. In a recent study urate crystals were identified in 14 of 15 patients, including some who had not had symptomatic involvement of their toe (18). This approach may be taken if confirmation of the diagnosis is important in deciding about management (e.g., to rule out gout if another diagnosis seems possible).

CHRONIC GOUT

This form of the disease is infrequent, especially since the advent of effective therapy to control hyperuricemia. Patients with chronic gout frequently have some persistent symptoms (such as morning stiffness) and manifest signs of synovial tissue thickening and some joint deformity. Acute exacerbations are still frequent and are often polyarticular. Tophi (soft tissue deposits of sodium urate) are present in 90 to 95% of patients. The rate of formation of tophi seems to be a direct function of the level and duration of hyperuricemia. Tophi are chalky or pinkish, gritty, usually superficial deposits which are felt in joints or tendons, over pressure points, or in the pinnae of the ears. Large tophi may look like bulbous swellings of the joints or, when they are located over the extensor surface of the forearm or in the ulnar bursa, may be mistaken for rheumatoid nodules. In such circumstances, aspiration or biopsy of tophi with demonstration of urate crystals will confirm the diagnosis of chronic gout. The actual concurrence of gout and rheumatoid arthritis is extremely rare.

EXTRA-ARTICULAR MANIFESTATIONS

It has long been known that primary gout may be associated with renal disease in three forms: *chronic gouty nephropathy, nephrolithiasis,* and *acute uric acid nephropathy.*

Chronic gouty nephropathy develops after many years of hyperuricemia and results from the deposition in the interstitial medullary tissue of sodium urate crystals which cause, ultimately, an interstitial nephritis. The frequency of this complication, until recently, had been assumed to be high. Recent controlled studies, however, indicate that the incidence of renal insufficiency solely from gout and hyperuricemia is low and that renal dysfunction is usually mild; most often renal failure in patients with gout can be attributed to age, vascular disease, or primary renal disease (1, 3). Renal failure from primary gout and hyperuricemia is usually silent and suspected only because of the identification of a mild abnormality of the concentration of blood urea nitrogen or of serum creatinine. Some patients will have slight proteinuria; only a few will be found to have peripheral tophi. It is not known whether secondary gout is associated with the development of chronic gouty nephropathy. The evaluation and management of patients who have renal failure is discussed in Chapter 44.

Uric acid nephrolithiasis accounts for only a small number of patients who have urinary calculi (see Chapter 43). However, approximately 20% of patients with gout develop calculi although the stones may antedate acute gouty arthritis by years. From a different perspective, about 25% of patients with uric acid calculi have an abnormal serum urate concentration. The prevalence of uric acid calculi increases proportionate to the concentration of serum urate or to the excretion of uric acid whether or not gout is present. In one study, in men, serum levels of urate of 7 to 8 mg/dl, 8 to 9 mg/dl, and >9 mg/dl were associated with renal stones in 12.7%, 22%, and 40%, respectively (5). Also in gouty patients, urinary excretion rates of <300, 300 to 700, 700 to 1,100, and >1100 mg/24 hours of uric acid were associated with a prevalence of renal stones of 11, 21, 35, and 50%, respectively (21). The development of uric acid calculi is related not only to uric acid excretion but also to urinary pH and concentration. This subject is more fully discussed in Chapter 43.

Acute uric acid nephropathy is associated with a sudden increase in urate production and a marked rise in uric acid excretion, resulting in the formation of microcrystals in the renal tubules. This most often occurs in patients with lympho-or myeloproliferative disorders especially during treatment. Acute uric acid nephropathy is rarely encountered in ambulatory practice.

Differential Diagnosis

During the acute attack gout must be differentiated principally from acute infectious arthritis and from other forms of crystal-induced arthritis. It is important therefore to aspirate joint fluid for smear and culture as well as for crystal identification. Infectious arthritis is associated with a very low synovial fluid glucose not found in gouty fluids.

X-rays (Fig. 66.2)

In the early course of gout, X-rays are normal except for acute soft tissue swelling. As the disease

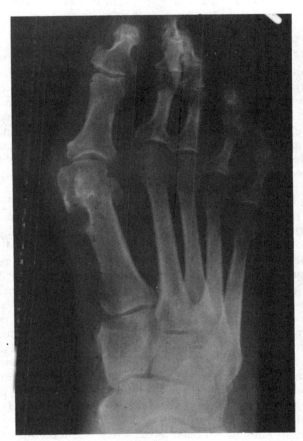

Figure 66.2   X-ray of foot in patient with gout showing soft tissue swelling over first metatarsophalangeal joint and typical gouty erosion: away from joint margin, punched out with overhanging edge and no osteoporosis.

progresses, lucent areas of urate deposits may be seen in bone adjacent to the joints. These lesions may be mistaken for the erosions that are seen in rheumatoid or other arthritides but may be distinguished from them in that osteoporosis and bony sclerosis, which are common in other erosive diseases, are not present. Overhanging margins of bone are said to be characteristic of gouty erosions, but are not frequently found.

X-rays of gouty joints are thus indicated mainly to evaluate the extent of possible tophaceous deposits in patients with gout of long duration, and only occasionally are indicated as an aid to diagnosis or differential diagnosis.

Management

If the diagnosis of gout can be established with certainty by the demonstration of urate crystals, the treatment is relatively simple and straightforward. Hospitalization is seldom required unless the diagnosis is in doubt; even the most severe case can be effectively managed on an ambulatory basis. The key elements in management are control of the acute attack and compliance with therapy administered to reduce serum urate and to prevent recurrent attacks and progression to chronic tophaceous gout.

MANAGEMENT OF THE ACUTE ATTACK

If the diagnosis of acute gout is established or if gout has been diagnosed previously by the identification of urate crystals in the affected joints, rapid relief can be obtained in almost all cases by the administration of nonsteroidal anti-inflammatory drugs in appropriate doses. Indomethacin (Indocin) 50 mg (i.e., two 25-mg capsules) every 6 hours for 6 to 8 doses is dramatically effective. There are few side effects if the dose is then quickly reduced to 25 mg every 6 hours after the initial response and maintained until the attack is completely resolved, usually no more than 5 to 7 days. Alternatively other nonsteroidal anti-inflammatory drugs may be used; see Table 67.5 in Chapter 67. Phenylbutazone (Butazolidine), a potent anti-inflammatory agent, has been largely replaced by better tolerated drugs.

Colchicine is the time-honored drug for treatment of acute gout; but its efficacy is limited by side effects which are almost invariable if an adequate dose is administered orally. The usual regimen is 0.6 mg every 2 hours up to 16 doses until relief is obtained or until side effects, usually diarrhea, nausea, or vomiting, develop. It is no longer necessary to subject a patient to severe diarrhea when he already has a very painful joint, so that oral colchicine has largely been replaced by nonsteroidal anti-inflammatory agents. They are at least as effective and have fewer side effects. The exception is in the well instructed patient who immediately after recognizing the onset of an acute attack of gout can institute oral colchicine and in doing so can abate the attack with a few doses and with minimal side effects.

Intravenous administration of colchicine rapidly provides a therapeutic plasma level of the drug and does not cause gastrointestinal side effects. It is particularly useful in treatment of acute gout when the patient cannot take medication by mouth and in the patient with peptic ulcer disease, or with another contraindication to the use of nonsteroidal agents. Two milligrams of colchicine (available in ampoules containing 1 mg in 2 ml) diluted with isotonic saline to 20 ml and given slowly (i.e., over 10 min) intravenously usually provide relief within 6 to 8 hours and, if necessary, may be followed by 1 or 2 doses of 1 mg in 20 ml of isotonic saline intravenously in 12 to 24 hours, not to exceed 4 mg in 24 hours. Reduced dosage is necessary in patients with impaired renal function. Care must be used to prevent extravasation of colchicine into the soft tissues since it may cause necrosis.

A diagnostic therapeutic trial of colchicine has limited value (except with podagra, see below) since acute gout of several days duration may not respond to colchicine and since pseudogout due to calcium pyrophosphate dihydrate-induced arthritis often shows a dramatic response as well.

Drugs administered to lower serum urate have no place in the treatment of the acute gouty attack. In fact, these agents may cause exacerbation of acute attacks by the associated changes in plasma urate levels (see above).

Acute Podagra. Podagra is an acute inflammatory arthritis of the first metatarsophalangeal joint and is a characteristic manifestation of gout. Other acute arthritides are much less likely to involve the great toe. It is quite difficult to aspirate the first metatarsophalangeal joint when it is acutely inflamed (it is much easier to aspirate during an intercritical period, see above); in fact an inexperienced physician may cause marked discomfort for the patient. For this reason, if the physician is inexperienced he should make a presumptive diagnosis on clinical grounds, supported by the demonstration of an elevated serum urate concentration, although this finding is not always present. In this situation, the diagnosis will be further strengthened by the resolution or marked improvement of the problem within 6 to 8 hours after the administration of intravenous colchicine by the physician in his office. A response of early podagra to colchicine is more specific for gout than is a response to a nonsteroidal anti-inflammatory agent and is suggested when a patient is first seen and the diagnosis has not been definitively established.

INTERCRITICAL GOUT

The efficacy of colchicine in doses of 0.6 mg 1, 2, or 3 times daily (dose frequency depends on control; most require two doses a day) in reducing the frequency of acute attacks of gout has been well established (20). Thus, prophylactic colchicine should be given to all patients who have had more than one episode of acute gout to prevent recurrent attacks or to reduce the frequency of those attacks. In patients without tophi (nontophaceous gout), with infrequent acute attacks and with mild hyperuricemia (i.e., <9 to 10 mg/dl), this therapy may be all that is required. Some patients who have nontophaceous gout with infrequent attacks of arthritis (e.g., <1 or 2 a year) and who have relatively mild hyperuricemia (i.e., < 9 to 10 mg/dl) may as an option elect not to take regular colchicine prophylaxis; in this instance, the episodic use of a nonsteroidal anti-inflammatory drug such as indomethacin (Indocin) (see above) is appropriate to control acute attacks. However, in most patients with persistent hyperuricemia of 10 mg/dl or higher, the serum urate concentration should be reduced to prevent recurrent gout and to reverse the accumulation of urate in the tissues. In this instance, colchicine prophylaxis should be continued until the patient has been free of attacks for at least 3 to 6 months after the concentration of serum urate has returned to normal.

Two classes of drugs that lower serum urate concentration are available: *uricosuric agents* promote urinary excretion of urate by blocking tubular urate reabsorption, and *allopurinol* (Xyloprim) decreases production of urate through inhibition of purine metabolism. Indications for the use of allopurinol are a history of urinary calculi or the presence of renal insufficiency, of chronic tophaceous gout, of excessive basal urinary uric acid excretion (i.e., >750 to 800 mg/24 hours), or of high levels of serum urate associated with secondary gout. Uricosuric agents are most effective in patients with nontophaceous gout with normal renal function and normal uric acid excretion (i.e., <750 to 800 mg/24 hours). Evaluation of *urinary uric acid excretion* is thus important not only as a clue to the mechanism of hyperuricemia (Table 66.2) but in the choice of therapy.

Probenecid (Benemid) is the uricosuric agent of choice because of its well established safety and its relatively long duration of effect. An initial dose of 0.5 g twice daily should be increased to 1.5 g daily or to a maximum of 2 g/day (in 2 or 3 divided doses) to achieve a serum urate concentration consistently below 6.5 mg/dl, the level required to produce a urate gradient from tissue to plasma and to prevent further deposition of urate. In order to minimize the chance of precipitating a recurrent arthritic attack, the uricosuric agent should not be initiated until at least a week after an acute attack of gout has subsided and only after colchicine prophylaxis (see above) has been initiated for 3 or 4 days. The principal side effect of probenecid is gastrointestinal distress, but there is a risk of the formation of uric acid calculi in the renal tubules in the first week (the period of negative uric acid balance) of therapy, especially when there is a large basal uric acid excretion (i.e., 600 to 800 mg/day); this risk can be eliminated if the patient drinks 2 to 3 liters of fluid/day and takes an alkalizing agent such as sodium bicarbonate or citrate salt (Polycitrate) 0.5 to 1 mEq/kg body weight in 5 or 6 doses a day to keep the urine pH above 6.0 to 6.5 for the first week of uricosuric therapy. Small doses of aspirin (2.4 g/day) block the effect of probenecid on renal excretion of urate and should be avoided.

Sulfinpyrazone (Anturane) is a more potent uricosuric agent but must be given every 4 to 6 hours (400 to 600 mg/day) for maximum effect. This agent, which is an analog of phenylbutazone, may cause gastric ulceration and platelet dysfunction. For these reasons, it should be used only when probenecid or allopurinol (see below) is not tolerated.

Allopurinol (Xyloprim) is a potent agent which reduces the concentration of serum urate. Since it blocks urate production, it is particularly useful in patients with renal dysfunction or with uric acid calculi. Serious side effects of rash, fever, leukopenia, hepatitis, and/or occasionally a generalized vasculitis occur in less than 2% of patients. These symptoms are most likely to occur within the first 2 months after initiation of therapy so that patients should be kept under close surveillance during this period. Toxicity seems to be enhanced when the drug is administered concomitantly with thiazide diuretics. Allopurinol (Xyloprim, available in 100 and 300 mg tablets) should be started at a dose of 200 mg daily and increased gradually (i.e., over 2 or 3 weeks) until the serum urate is consistently below 6.5 mg/dl; no more than 300 mg should be administered as a single dose. Prolonged use of doses in excess of 300 mg twice a day increases the risk of toxicity.

Concomitant use of allopurinol and probenecid has been advocated (17). These agents seem to have an additive effect in lowering serum uric acid. However, use of a single agent is preferable if possible.

Compliance is the major factor in the effective therapy of intercritical gout. Patients feel well between attacks, and continued compliance with medications requires reinforcement in patient education and in follow-up visits to ensure maintenance of normal serum levels of urate.

CHRONIC GOUT

Compliance with appropriate therapy should eliminate this phase of gout except for a few patients with severe disease who are intolerant of one or more drugs used in treatment. Prolonged use of nonsteroidal anti-inflammatory agents (including aspirin in doses greater than 3.5 g/day—a uricosuric dose) may be required in some of these patients for adequate control of inflammation and chronic symptoms. Effective reduction in serum urate for months or years will result in dissolution of tophi and in general improvement. However, very large tophi may require surgical removal.

TREATMENT OF ASYMPTOMATIC HYPERURICEMIA

Asymptomatic hyperuricemia (>7 mg/dl in males and >6 mg/dl in females) should be evaluated first by assessment of urine uric acid excretion. If urinary uric acid is significantly elevated (>600 mg/day on low purine diet or >750 to 800 mg/day in the absence of purine gluttony), a careful search for causes of hyperuricemia (see Table 66.2) should be made and consideration should be given to allopurinol therapy in order to prevent urinary stones and chronic renal insufficiency from interstitial deposition of urate. However, in the majority of such patients urine uric acid will be normal or reduced despite hyperuricemia. In this situation, some of these patients may subsequently develop gouty arthritis, but the risk of urinary stones or renal disease is much less than if the urine uric acid excretion were elevated. Fessel *et al.* (3) have suggested that azotemia attributed to hyperuricemia is of no clinical significance until serum uric acid levels reach 13 mg/dl in men and 10 mg/dl in women. The expense and potential toxicity of therapy to lower serum urate, therefore, is probably not warranted since therapy can be successfully initiated if gout develops (7); this issue is controversial, however, and some would initiate therapy when serum levels are consistently >9 mg/dl in the hope of preventing potential renal damage and acute gout (19).

HYPERURICEMIA SECONDARY TO DIURETICS

The renal tubular handling of uric acid is complex: there is complete glomerular filtration followed by tubular resorption, tubular secretion, and further tubular reabsorption. The reabsorption of uric acid is in part modulated by the volume of extracellular fluid (expansion increases excretion and contraction decreases excretion). Diuretics modify the renal handling of uric acid by their effect on volume and also some diuretics may directly affect urate transport. Thiazides regularly cause a dose-related rise of the serum urate level. This elevation is reversed upon withdrawal of the agent. The increase in concentration averages 1 to 2 mg/dl but occasionally may be 4 to 5 mg/dl. Furosemide also is frequently associated with a rise in concentration of serum urate; less commonly ethacrynic acid, acetazolamide, and rarely triamterene are associated with hyperuricemia. Spironolactone *per se* is not associated with hyperuricemia.

The incidence of gout after the initiation of a diuretic is a complex issue. Other factors which affect the incidence of gout—such as hypertension or obesity—are often present in diuretic-treated patients. Approximately 1 to 10% of hypertensive patients with hyperuricemia secondary to diuretic therapy actually develop gout. This risk increases in patients with known gout and those patients with diseases associated with elevation of serum urate, such as myeloproliferative disorders or psoriasis. Also in association with diuretic therapy uric acid excretion is diminished and there is no increase in the incidence of urinary calculi. The risk of developing urate nephropathy is unknown (see above). For these reasons expectant management of patients with asympto-

matic hyperuricemia secondary to diuretics is appropriate.

Should acute gout develop, treatment as described above may be initiated. Intercritical gout is managed similarly to primary gout and uricosuria therapy with probenecid (if there is no renal failure) or therapy with allopurinol to decrease production of urate may be used. Stopping the diuretic is usually associated with a slight fall in the plasma urate concentration but many patients will continue to have attacks of gout. Therefore, if a patient develops gout while taking diuretics, and the need for the diuretic continues, it is best to treat the gout as discussed above and continue the use of the diuretic.

CALCIUM PYROPHOSPHATE DIHYDRATE (CPPD)-INDUCED ARTHRITIS

Pseudogout is a syndrome caused by the deposition of calcium pyrophosphate dihydrate in fibrocartilage and joint tissue and in ligaments and tendons with an occasional resulting inflammatory response. It most often is idiopathic but may be associated with certain other diseases (see below).

Inorganic pyrophosphate is an important metabolite in many biosynthetic reactions where it is removed from macromolecules through the action of pyrophosphatases. It is adsorbed to hydroxyapatite and is probably involved in the regulation of mineralization, both in the accretion from amorphous calcium phosphate and in the dissolution of crystalline hydroxyapatite.

Prevalence

Chondrocalcinosis increases in frequency with age; it is present in about 5% of the adult population at the time of death and in 20 to 30% of people above age 80. The exact prevalence of CPPD disease is not known. In one series of consecutive patients with newly diagnosed crystal-induced arthritis, CPPD disease accounted for about one-third of the cases (10). Males are probably affected more than females with a ratio of males to females of 1.5:1 in the largest reported series (10).

Etiology

Familial cases with an autosomal dominant inheritance have been described (16) in which chondrocalcinosis appears at an earlier age. These families are uncommon and many of these patients will remain asymptomatic for many years; the metabolic defect has not been identified, however. Most cases of CPPD disease are sporadic and idiopathic; a few are associated with one of a variety of metabolic diseases. Many of the diseases associated with deposits of CPPD involve metabolic abnormalities in connective tissues, but the precise mechanisms of CPPD crystallization are unknown. A list of these associated diseases is presented in Table 66.4.

Table 66.4
Diseases Associated with Calcium Pyrophosphate Dihydrate (CPPD) Deposition Disease

Gout
Hemochromatosis—hemosiderosis
Hyperparathyroidism
Hypomagnesemia
Hypophosphatasia
Hypothyroidism
Neurogenic arthropathy

Clinical Features (Table 66.5)

Patients are usually middle aged to elderly at the time of onset of arthritic symptoms. There are several possible patterns of presentation: about one-quarter present with *self-limited acute gout-like attacks (pseudogout)* predominantly affecting the knees and wrists, but occasionally involving other joints, including rarely the first metatarsophalangeal joint. Monoarticular attacks are the rule, but involvement of symmetrical joints and polyarthritis may occur rarely. Symptoms are often less intense than they are in gout, but the presentation is variable and some attacks may be quite severe. Systemic symptoms, including fever to 101°F (38°C) or more, may occur as in gout, and patients are frequently misdiagnosed as having infection. Attacks are often exacerbated by trauma and by acute illness. Long intervals (sometimes years) between attacks are common.

In about half the patients, and especially in women, the presentation *resembles osteoarthritis* with bilateral involvement, especially of the knees. The wrists, the metacarpophalangeal (MCP) joints, hips, shoulders, elbows, or ankles also may be affected. Acute exacerbations occur in about half of these patients with features that resemble osteoarthritis except that the disease is more progressive and destructive. Varus or valgus knee deformities are common and extensive calcification around the patella may be seen on X-ray. Flexion contractures may occur also. The relationship to ordinary osteoarthritis is still unclear, except that the involvement of joints not usually affected in osteoarthritis (MCPs, wrists, shoulders, elbows) suggests a different pathogenesis (see also Chapter 65).

In a few patients persistent subacute inflammation with fatigue, morning stiffness, and synovial swelling in multiple joints lasting weeks or months *resembles rheumatoid arthritis.*

A few patients also have been reported with severely *destructive arthritis* resembling the Charcot joints of neuropathic arthropathy but associated with a normal neurological examination (13). CPPD disease may also be associated with a true neuropathic arthritis due to tabes dorsalis.

Laboratory Findings

Patients may have peripheral leukocytosis and an elevated erythrocyte sedimentation rate in associa-

Table 66.5
Clinical Features of Calcium Pyrophosphate Dihydrate (CPPD) Deposit Disease

EPIDEMIOLOGY
  Age: Middle aged or elderly
SITE
  Knee and wrist most common joints involved
  Metacarpophalangeal joints, hips, shoulders, elbows, ankles may be affected
  Arthritis usually monoarticular
PATTERN
  Acute gout-like attacks with symptom-free intervals in 25%
  Osteoarthritis-like disease in 50%, with superimposed acute attacks in half of these patients
  Rheumatoid-like polyarthritis in 5%
  Neuropathic-like arthritis without neurological damage
  Asymptomatic chondrocalcinosis in 20%
LABORATORY
  Synovial fluid shows leukocytosis and characteristic CPPD crystals

tion with acute or subacute attacks of arthritis. The synovial fluid will show polymorphonuclear leukocytosis which may exceed 50,000/cu mm in acute pseudogout, but is more commonly in the range of 15,000 to 25,000. Crystal identification is the key to diagnosis (see above). In the absence of acute or subacute inflammation, leukocyte counts may be low (<2000 per cu mm) and crystals may be largely extracellular.

Because of the occasional association with other disorders (Table 66.4), the patient's serum calcium, phosphorus, alkaline phosphatase, and uric acid should be measured, although they will usually be normal (12). Because pseudogout may be the presenting manifestation of hemochromatosis and because of the importance of early diagnosis in this disorder, measurement of serum ferritin is also indicated if there is any suspicion of this diagnosis.

X-ray Findings

The typical X-ray findings of CPPD deposit disease are punctate and linear calcifications (chondrocalcinosis) seen most frequently in the fibrocartilage of the menisci of the knee, usually bilaterally (Fig. 66.3). Other fibrocartilages may show similar changes including the disc in the distal radioulnar joint, the symphysis pubis, the lip of the acetabulum or the glenoid fossa or intervetebral discs. Hyaline cartilage may also be involved with similar punctate linear calcifications which may be identified as a dense line parallel to the subchondral bone. Calcification in the soft tissues of the joint capsule and occasionally in ligaments and tendons may also be seen but is less characteristic. In patients with the type of CPPD disease that resembles osteoarthritis, subchondral cyst formation with bony collapse may be prominent. Osteophyte formation is variable and inconsistent.

These radiographic findings may be helpful in suggesting or confirming the diagnosis of CPPD disease.

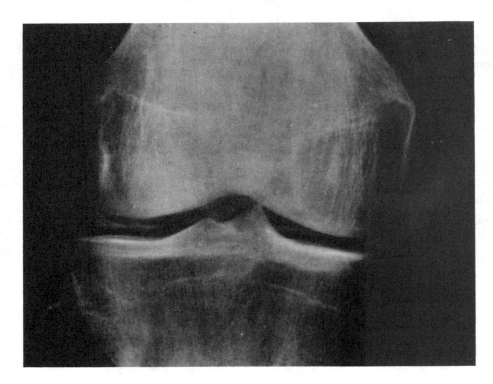

Figure 66.3   X-ray of knee of a patient with chondrocalcinosis. Stippled calcification of the medial and lateral menisci is easily identified.

However, it may not be possible to visualize the extent of deposits radiographically, and their absence does not exclude the diagnosis if typical crystals can be demonstrated in synovial fluid or in biopsy material.

Management

There is no therapy which influences the deposition or resolution of tissue deposits of CPPD. In the acute episode diagnostic aspiration of synovial fluid with removal of crystals and leukocytes may provide significant clinical improvement. Local injection of depo-corticosteroid is often effective and avoids potential side effects of systemic drug therapy (see Chapter 63, for technique). Efficacy of colchicine has been debated, and although it is sometimes effective, especially if given intravenously, the use of indomethacin (Indocin) or other nonsteroidal anti-inflammatory agents is generally preferred as described above for acute gout (see above). Since many of these patients are elderly (and may therefore have an impaired glomerular filtration rate), caution regarding renal toxicity of these agents should be exercised (see Chapter 44, Table 44.5). In patients with only recurrent acute attacks no therapy is indicated between attacks, but early administration of anti-inflammatory agents on exacerbation may minimize or abort attacks. Therapy for patients with more subacute inflammation or for those with osteoarthritis-like disease is similar to that described for osteoarthritis (see Chapter 65), except that anti-inflammatory levels of drugs may be required for optimal symptomatic control.

HYDROXYAPATITE-INDUCED ARTHRITIS

The capacity of hydroxyapatite crystals to induce an inflammatory response was first appreciated in some patients with acute tendinitis (14). More recently hydroxyapatite crystals have been identified in patients with osteoarthritis, especially in association with acute inflammatory episodes (6), and in patients with destructive arthropathy of the shoulder joint (11). The latter, termed *Milwaukee shoulder*, is associated with painful limited shoulder motion, complete disruption of the rotator cuff, and extensive degenerative changes in the bone. Further definition of the role of hydroxyapatite in crystal-induced arthritis and of the spectrum of its clinical manifestations will be forthcoming as identification of crystals is applied more widely. At this time the physician need only be aware of the potential inflammatory properties of this crystalline material and consider its implication in the above clinical situations.

References

General

Howell, DS: Diseases due to the deposition of calcium pyrophosphate and hydroxyapatite. In *Textbook of Rheumatology*, edited by WN Kelley, ED Harris, Jr, S Ruddy and CB Sledge: W. B. Saunders, Philadelphia, 1981.

WN Kelley: Gout and related disorders of purine metabolism. In *Textbook of Rheumatology*, edited by WN Kelley, ED Harris, Jr, S Ruddy and CB Sledge. W. B. Saunders, Philadelphia, 1981.

These chapters in this comprehensive textbook provide an up-to-date review of all aspects of crystal-induced arthritis.
Steinbroker, O and Neustadt, PH: Aspiration and injection therapy. In *Arthritis and Musculoskeletal Disorders*. Harper & Row, Hagerstown, MD, 1972.

This is a very practical manual to aid the physician in the techniques of joint aspiration.

Specific

1. Berger, L and Yu, TF: Renal function in gout. *Am J Med 59:* 605, 1975.
2. Fagan, TJ and Ludsky, MD: Compensated polarized light microscopy using cellophane adhesive tape. *Arthritis Rheum 17:* 256, 1974.
3. Fessel, WJ, Siegelaub, AB and Johnson, ES: Correlates and consequences of asymptomatic hyperuricemia. *Arch Intern Med 132:* 44, 1973.
4. Gutman, AB and Yu, TF: Uric acid nephrolithiasis. *Am J Med 45:* 756, 1968.
5. Hall, AP, Barry, PE, Dawber, TR and McNamara, PM: Epidemiology of gout and hyperuricemia. *Am J Med 42:* 27, 1967.
6. Huskisson, EC, Dreppe, PA, Tucker, AK and Cannell, LB: Another look at osteoarthritis. *Ann Rheum Dis 38:* 423, 1979.
7. Liang, MH and Fries, JF: Asymptomatic hyperuricemia: the case for conservative management. *Ann Intern Med 88:* 666, 1978.
8. Malawista, SW: Gouty inflammation. *Arthritis Rheum 20:* 5241, 1977.
9. McCarty, DJ: The gouty toe—a multifactorial condition. *Ann Intern Med 86:* 234, 1977.
10. McCarty, DJ: Pseudogout and pyrophosphate metabolism. *Adv Intern Med 25:* 363, 1980.
11. McCarty, DJ, Halverson, PB, Carrera, GF, Brewer, BJ and Kozen, F: "Milwaukee shoulder"—association of microspheroids containing hydroxyapatite crystals, active collagenase and neutral protease with rotator cuff defects; I. Clinical aspects. *Arthritis Rheum 24:* 464, 1981.
12. McCarty, DJ, Silcox, DC, Coe, F, Jacobelli, S, Reiss, E, Genant, H and Elliman, M: Diseases associated with calcium pyrophosphate dehydrate crystal deposition. A controlled study. *Am J Med 56:* 704, 1974.
13. Menkes, CJ, Simon, F, Delrieu, F, Forest, M and Delbarre, F: Destructive arthropathy in chondrocalcinosis articulosis. *Arthritis Rheum (Suppl) 19:* 329, 1976.
14. Pinals, RS and Short, CL: Calcific periarthritis involving multiple sites. *Arthritis Rheum 7:* 359, 1964.
15. Phelps, P, Steele, AD and McCarty, DJ, Jr: Compensated polarized light microscopy. *JAMA 203:* 508, 1968.
16. Reginato, A, Valenzuela, F, Martinez, V, Passaro, G and Daza, KS: Polyarticular and familial chondrocalcinosis. *Arthritis Rheum 13:* 197, 1970.
17. Rundles, RW, Metz, EN and Silberman, JR: Allopurinol in the treatment of gout. *Ann Intern Med 64:* 229, 1966.
18. Weinberger, A, Schumacher, HR and Agudelo, CA: Urate crystals in asymptomatic metatarsophalangeal joints. *Ann Intern Med 91:* 56, 1979.
19. Wyngaarden, JB and Kelley, WN: *Gout and Hyperuricemia.* Grune & Stratton, New York, 1976.
20. Yu, TF and Gutman, AB: Efficacy of colchicine prophylaxis in gout. Prevention of recurrent gouty arthritis over a mean period of five years in 208 gouty subjects. *Ann Intern Med 55:* 179, 1961.
21. Yu, TF and Gutman, HB: Uric acid nephrolithiasis in gout. Predisposing factors. *Ann Intern Med 67:* 1133, 1967.

CHAPTER SIXTY-SEVEN

Rheumatoid Arthritis

ROBERT L. MARCUS, M.D., and PHILIP D. ZIEVE, M.D.

DEFINITION

Rheumatoid arthritis is a chronic inflammatory systemic disease of unknown etiology. Patients with the disease ordinarily come to the physician because of involvement of their joints in the inflammatory process. During the course of the illness, the majority of the patients' complaints and the primary therapeutic efforts of the physician continue to focus on arthritis.

The symptoms and signs of rheumatoid arthritis and the changes that it produces in affected tissues are not specific to this illness. Therefore, the diagnosis is usually made clinically after the accumulation of sufficient data from the history, physical examination, and laboratory studies. The persistence of many of these findings is important in this regard.

EPIDEMIOLOGY

There appears to be considerable variation in the prevalence of rheumatoid arthritis both in this country and around the world. In part the prevalence of the disease depends on the criteria used in establishing the diagnosis. In the United States somewhere between 0.5% and 3.8% of women and 0.1% and 1.3% of men (4) are afflicted by the disease. It is likely that the application of relatively strict criteria in the diagnosis of rheumatoid arthritis excludes some patients with more mild disease.

Although rheumatoid arthritis may present at any age, it most commonly affects patients between the third and sixth decade, with a peak incidence between the ages of 35 and 45. Women are afflicted approximately 2 to 3 times as often as men.

HISTOPATHOLOGY

Early in its course, tissues affected by rheumatoid disease show nonspecific inflammatory changes. In more advanced disease, synovia are infiltrated by granulation tissue (pannus) that is characteristic but not pathognomonic of the disorder. The proliferation of the pannus may result ultimately in the erosion of cartilage, bone, and supporting tendons that produces the deformities of end-stage disease (see below, p. 656).

HISTORY

The presentation of the disease (Table 67.1) varies from situations in which the diagnosis is obvious to ones in which the presentation is so atypical that it suggests other conditions. Diagnosis may be complicated further by the occasional coexistence or emergence of rheumatoid arthritis in the setting of another disease (such as gout or pseudogout, see Chapter 66; fibrositis, see Chapter 63; or deep vein thrombosis, see Chapter 48) which may cause similar signs and symptoms.

The typical case of rheumatoid arthritis begins insidiously with the slowly progressive development of symptoms and signs over a period of weeks to months. Occasionally, however, patients will experience an acute onset, usually polyarticular, within 24 to 48 hours; sometimes an acute presentation appears to be associated with either emotional or physical stress (for example, loss of a loved one or a recent injury).

Nonspecific systemic symptoms, primarily fatigue, malaise, and depression, are common (approximately 75% of patients) but not invariable, and may precede other symptoms of the disease by weeks to months. Usually the patient does not feel tired upon awakening but complains of rather severe fatigue 4 to 6 hours later. Fever occurs in perhaps 20% of patients; and then is almost always low grade (37–38°C; 99–100°F); a higher fever suggests another illness, such as infection.

Arthritic symptoms (and signs) provide the definitive clues by which a specific diagnosis is made. Often the patient first notices stiffness (see below) in one or more joints, usually accompanied by pain on movement and by tenderness in the joint. The number of joints that are involved is highly variable, but almost always the process is eventually polyarticular. The American Rheumatism Association, in its criteria for the diagnosis of rheumatoid arthritis (6), has emphasized the importance of persistent swelling of the joints for greater than 6 months, stating that soft tissue swelling of (or increased fluid in) a joint, followed by swelling of another joint within 3 months, as well as simultaneous swelling of symmetrical joints, are characteristic features of the disease. Any joints may be involved; but the ones involved most often are the proximal interphalangeal (PIP) and metacarpophalangeal (MCP) joints of the hands, the wrists (particularly at the ulnar-styloid articulation), knees, elbows, temporomandibular joints, hips, ankles, and metatarsophalangeal joints. Some patients have involvement of only one joint; and others develop arthritis of virtually all of their peripheral joints. Most patients (approximately 90%) are somewhere between these extremes.

Morning stiffness may be a feature of any inflammatory arthritis but is especially characteristic of rheumatoid arthritis (almost all patients complain of

Table 67.1
Symptoms and Signs of Rheumatoid Arthritis

Symptoms		Signs	
Extra-articular	Articular[a]	Extra-articular	Articular
Fatigue	Morning stiffness	Rheumatoid nodules	Pain on passive motion
Depression	Pain and tenderness	Lymphadenopathy	Tenderness
Malaise	Swelling	Splenomegaly	Swelling
Anorexia		Ocular disease	Heat
		Entrapment neuropathies	Typical deformity

[a] Persistence (6 months or more) and symmetrical nature of signs and symptoms are important, but not invariable, diagnostic features.

it) and, in fact, is a useful gauge to measure the activity of the disease. The symptom is defined as stiffness in affected joints which persists at least for several hours (the average is 3 to 4 hours), thus distinguishing it from the transient gelation phenomenon of degenerative arthritis which lasts but a few minutes (see Chapter 65). Similar stiffness may of course occur after any prolonged period of inactivity. A number of hypotheses have been proposed to explain this symptom, but a definitive explanation has yet to be given.

It is typical of patients with rheumatoid arthritis that their symptoms wax and wane, especially at the beginning of the illness. Because of this and because objective signs may not be present at first, it is not unusual that the diagnosis is delayed for months or even years. During this time the physician can best serve the patient by reassurance, careful interval history and periodic physical examination (see below), and, if appropriate, selected screening tests (p. 657). Symptomatic treatment with anti-inflammatory drugs may be instituted during this period (p. 663).

PHYSICAL EXAMINATION

A complete physical examination initially, and then a limited examination every 3 to 6 months, is important in patients with suspected rheumatoid arthritis, not only to make the diagnosis but to establish a baseline against which to assess the possible later development of both articular and extra-articular disease.

However, the primary focus of examinations in the physician's office will be the joints—repeated examinations and careful records of the status of affected joints, determined by history and previous examinations. The presence and status of rheumatoid nodules should be assessed repeatedly as well (see below).

Joints

Swelling is the most measurable change that occurs in a joint that is affected by rheumatoid arthritis. The physician should attempt to quantitate serially the degree of swelling by the use of a tape measure and, in the case of small joints, by the use of a jewellers tape, if possible (3). The first change in involved joints is usually synovial thickening, appreciable as slight swelling; eventually, soft tissue swelling beyond the synovium and increased amounts of fluid within the joint space produce more readily recognizable (and, often, persistent) changes. In the hands, where the disease is often first manifest, typical fusiform swelling of the PIP joints commonly occurs (Fig. 67.1); the distal interphalangeal joints are less often involved. The metacarpophalangeal joints and the wrists are swollen even more often than are the PIP joints. The elbows, knees, ankles, and MTP joints are other common sites of disease where swelling may be readily apparent. Swelling of symmetrical

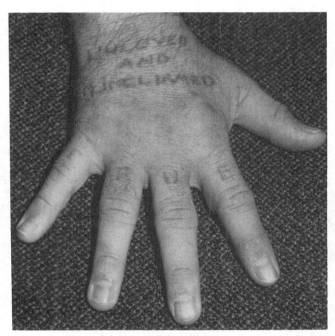

Figure 67.1   Typical fusiform swelling of the PIP joints.

joints, although not invariable, is characteristic of rheumatoid arthritis (see above, p. 654).

In contrast to gout (see Chapter 66) or to septic arthritis redness of affected joints is not a prominent feature of rheumatoid arthritis.

Tenderness and pain on passive motion, although not specific for rheumatoid arthritis, are the most sensitive indices of inflammation of a joint. If patients do not complain of these symptoms during an examination, it is unlikely that they have active inflammatory disease. It is important for the physician to apply gentle but firm pressure when examining a joint so that tenderness due to inflammation will be elicited, but not so much pressure that a normal joint will be inappropriately symptomatic. Inflamed joints are also usually warmer than normal joints; the examiner may assess this best by feeling with the back of his fingers.

The *range of motion* of the joint is not a very reliable measure of rheumatoid activity. The restricted movement of the badly deformed joint *is* obviously a reliable finding; but with respect to joints that are less flagrantly involved, it is more difficult for the physician to be entirely certain about the meaning of a limited range of motion.

Weakness is a common feature of patients with rheumatoid arthritis; but, like range of motion, it is not easy to assess. The fatigue produced by the illness (see above) may contribute to an overall sense of weakness; but weakness of one or more limbs or parts of limbs may be caused by muscle atrophy, a result of joint deformity and of disuse. However, weakness may only seem to be present at times when, because of pain, the patient is unwilling to apply his full strength.

Permanent deformity may be an endstage of the inflammatory process that is first apparent as joint swelling. Persistent tenosynovitis and synovitis may lead to the formation of synovial cysts, which sometimes rupture (see below), to displaced tendons, and to compression by synovial fluid of the normal supporting structures of the joint (leading, for example, to muscle atrophy). These anatomic changes result in *flexion contractures*, *subluxation* (incomplete dislocation) of articulating bones, and to bony *ankylosis*. Typical visible changes include ulnar deviation of the fingers at the MCP joints (Fig. 67.2), hyperextension or hyperflexion of the joints of the fingers (Fig. 67.3), and ankylosis of the carpal and tarsal joints. Ankylosis of other joints is rare and may be a distinguishing feature when comparing rheumatoid arthritis to diseases that mimic it. Displaced toes (upward) with hallux valgus formation are also common.

Synovial cysts are common in patients with rheumatoid arthritis and can be readily seen and palpated overlying the joints with which they communicate. Synovial cysts of the popliteal space (Baker's cysts) may develop in patients with a variety of disorders of the knee, but seem to be especially prevalent in patients with rheumatoid disease. If popliteal cysts rupture, the signs and symptoms resemble closely those of acute thrombophlebitis (calf swelling and tenderness—even a positive Homan's sign). Proper therapy depends on the physician's ability to make the right diagnosis. An arthrogram (performed by injection of a radio-opaque dye into the joint, followed by an X-ray of the knee) often will show the cyst and its connection with the joint space (Fig. 67.4). Decompression of the cyst by aspiration of synovial fluid from either the joint or the cyst and injection of a corticosteroid into the joint usually effectively relieve the symptoms of the condition.

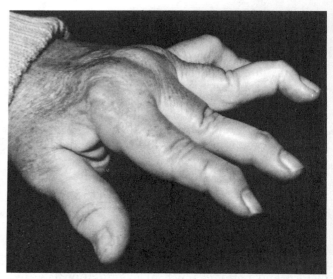

Figure 67.3 Hyperextension and hyperflexion of joints of the fingers.

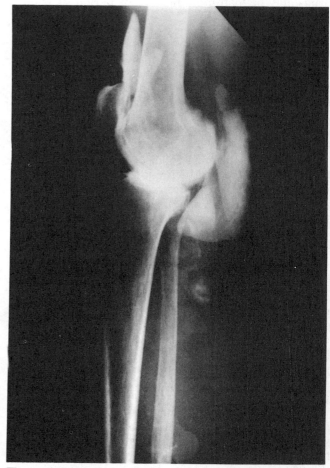

Figure 67.4 Arthrogram of a synovial cyst with dissection into the calf. (Courtesy of Jack Bowerman, M.D.)

Rheumatoid Nodules

Although not specific for rheumatoid arthritis (they also may be seen in patients with systemic lupus

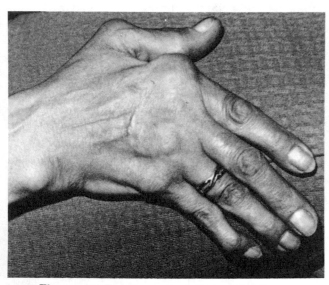

Figure 67.2 Ulnar deviation of the fingers.

erythematosus and with rheumatic fever), rheumatoid nodules, when present, do constitute a major criterion for diagnosis of the disease. Nodules occur in 20 to 30% of patients with rheumatoid arthritis and are found most commonly subcutaneously at pressure sites such as the extensor surface of the elbows and of the forearm and hand, the ischial tuberosities, the back of the head, and the base of the spine. Rarely nodules may arise in visceral organs such as the lungs or heart (p. 661). The subcutaneous nodules vary in size from a few millimeters to several centimeters and may either be fixed to surrounding connective tissue or be freely movable beneath the skin. Occasionally, nodules may erode into a contiguous structure or ulcerate through the surface of the skin; but most often they produce no symptoms; and the patient is only aware of them, if at all, if they produce an unwanted cosmetic effect.

Lymphoid Hyperplasia

Lymphadenopathy, either local or generalized, occurs in 25% or more of patients with rheumatoid arthritis; and is probably more common than that in seropositive patients. The nodes are nontender, firm, and freely movable; and, although the diagnosis of lymphoma sometimes is considered, the process almost always proves to be benign. When biopsied, the nodes show a proliferation of normal plasma cells, consistent with the immunologic reactivity of the disease. *Splenomegaly* occurs more rarely (5 to 10% of patients), occasinally in association with *Felty's syndrome* (see p. 661).

LABORATORY TESTS

Baseline laboratory information in patients with suspected rheumatoid arthritis should include an hematocrit value, white blood cell count and differential count, an erythrocyte sedimentation rate, and a rheumatoid factor titer. In selected patients, synovial fluid analysis, additional serologic studies, appropriate X-rays, and biopsies may also be important (see below).

Hematology

A mild *anemia* with hematocrit values in the range of 30 to 34% occurs in approximately 25 to 35% of patients with rheumatoid arthritis. In most cases the reduced red cell mass is due to the so-called anemia of chronic disease (see Chapter 46) and is a normocytic-normochromic process characterized by low serum iron, low serum iron-binding capacity, and a normal or increased serum ferritin concentration. However, occasionally true iron deficiency anemia develops because of intercurrent stress ulceration and/or because of the irritative effects of aspirin (see below, p. 663) on the gastric mucosa.

The *white count* is usually normal in patients with rheumatoid arthritis, but occasionally is elevated in patients with a great deal of inflammatory disease and rarely is depressed (especially in association with Felty's syndrome, see p. 661). Similarly the platelet count is usually normal but also may be elevated in association with the inflammatory process and may be reduced in patients with Felty's syndrome.

The *erythrocyte sedimentation rate* (ESR), most reliably measured by the Westergren method, is usually elevated in patients with rheumatoid arthritis and is an excellent way to follow the activity of the disease (see below).

Serology

RHEUMATOID FACTORS

These are antibodies that react with the Fc fragment (a part of the molecule that can be produced in the laboratory by enzymatic cleavage of immunoglobulin G (IgG)). Although they may belong to any of the three major classes of immunoglobulins—IgG, IgM, and IgA—rheumatoid factors, as measured for clinical purposes, are IgM antibodies. The antibodies are by no means pathognomonic of rheumatoid arthritis, nor do they seem to be involved in its pathogenesis, but they *are* detectable in the serum of 70 to 80% of patients with the disease (5). A significant titer of rheumatoid factor is one of 1:80 or greater. The titer does not correlate with the activity of disease but it does appear that patients with very severe erosive arthritis or with extensive extra-articular disease are likely to have relatively high titers.

Rheumatoid factor is also detectable in the serum of many patients without rheumatoid arthritis; most of these patients have had demonstrated or presumed chronic antigenic stimulation such as prolonged infection (bacterial endocarditis, tuberculosis, viral hepatitis), collagen vascular disease, chronic lung disease (pulmonary fibrosis, asthma), and dysproteinemia (myeloma, macroglobulinemia, mixed cryoglobulinemia). Also, transient appearance of rheumatoid factor may occur in patients who have been recently vaccinated or who have had a self-limited viral infection. Finally, rheumatoid factor may be detected in the serum of apparently normal people, especially people over the age of 50, where its prevalence is anywhere from 10 to 25%, depending on the assay.

All of the clinical tests for rheumatoid factor depend on the agglutination, by serum which contains it, of particles (sheep red cells, latex, bentonite) coated with aggregated human or animal IgG. There is some variation in sensitivity of detection of rheumatoid factor according to which technique is used, so that the clinician should be familiar with the procedure used by his reference laboratory.

ANTINUCLEAR ANTIBODIES

Antinuclear antibodies, as usually measured, are present in approximately 20 to 30% of patients with rheumatoid arthritis; although, as in the case of rheumatoid factor, these antibodies can be detected more often in these patients if more sensitive tests are utilized. In comparison to systemic lupus erythematosus (SLE) the titer of antinuclear antibodies is ordinarily low in patients with rheumatoid disease. LE-cell preparations also are positive in 10 to 20% of

Table 67.2
Synovial Fluid[a]

	Normal	Rheumatoid (Inflammatory) Arthritis	Noninflammatory Arthritis
Color	Clear	Yellow-white	Clear to pale yellow
Clarity	Transparent	Turbid	Transparent
Viscosity	Very high	Low	High
Mucin clot	Good	Fair to poor	Fair to good
Spontaneous clot	None	Often	Often
White cells (per cumm)	<150	3000–50000	<3000
Polymorphonuclear leukocytes (%)	<25	>70	<25
Serum-synovial fluid glucose difference	0	≥30	≤5
C'H5O: Protein	>2.5	<2.5[b]	>2.5

[a] Modified from D. J. McCarty: Synovial fluid. In *Arthritis and Allied Conditions*, Ed. 9, p. 51, edited by D. J. McCarty. Lea & Febiger, Philadelphia, 1979.

[b] This ratio is low in the synovial fluid of patients with inflammatory arthritis associated with immune complex formation (rheumatoid arthritis, systemic lupus); it is normal or high in the synovial fluid of patients with other inflammatory arthritis (infection, gout, Reiter's syndrome).

patients with rheumatoid arthritis; the distinction between SLE and rheumatoid arthritis therefore depends primarily on the total clinical presentation rather than on the serologic tests.

SERUM COMPLEMENT

Serum hemolytic complement (C'H50) is generally normal or increased in patients with rheumatoid arthritis, although rarely patients with longstanding seropositive disease will show a slight decrease in serum complement. The test is most useful in helping to distinguish the patient with early rheumatoid arthritis from patients with early SLE in whom it is often markedly decreased.

Synovial Fluid

Synovial fluid should be analyzed when there is some doubt about the cause of effusion in a patient with monoarticular or polyarticular arthritis. If the primary physician is not familiar with the technique of arthrocentesis or if he does not feel comfortable about tapping the joint in which there is an effusion, the patient should be referred to a rheumatologist or to an orthopedic surgeon. The patient should be told that the overlying skin will be anesthetized before the aspiration, that he will experience minimal discomfort, and that his ability to use the joint will not be affected.

Early in the course of rheumatoid arthritis joint fluid may not show the characteristic inflammatory changes that ultimately develop (Table 67.2). Thereafter, however, the normally clear fluid becomes yellowish white and turbid and, because of the degradation of hyaluronic acid by lysosomal enzymes, the viscosity of the fluid falls considerably and the so-called mucin clot becomes poor. (A simple method of testing the mucin clot is to add 1 ml of joint fluid to 4 ml of 2% acetic acid (Fig. 67.5)). Fluid aspirated from an inflamed joint also often clots spontaneously,

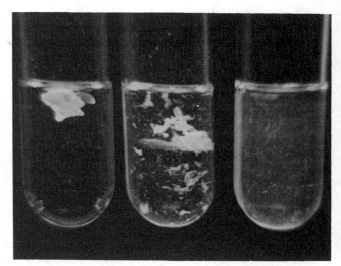

Figure 67.5 Mucin clot test demonstrating (*left to right*) good, intermediate, and poor mucin clots.

another feature distinguishing it from normal. There is considerable variation in the total white cell count and the neutrophil count in synovial fluid of rheumatoid joints, but in general many more leukocytes (predominantly neutrophils) are present than are seen in the fluid of either normal joints or joints that are arthritic but are not acutely inflamed. If the physician is familiar with the use of a counting chamber, cell counts can be done in the office with normal saline as a diluent. At the same time, a smear can be made and stained for differential counting of white cells. If the physician is unable to perform these counts, the fluid should be transported to an appropriate laboratory, in which case the fluid should be added to a tube containing EDTA to prevent clot formation. The cells will not lyse even if 4 to 6 hours pass before they are counted. However, rapid transport to the laboratory is essential so that an accurate glucose measurement can be made. The difference between the concentration of glucose in the serum and that in the fluid of inflamed joints is much greater than the difference between the serum glucose level and that in fluid of uninflamed joints. However, only rarely is the synovial fluid glucose less than half the serum level (in contrast to septic arthritis).

A reduction in total hemolytic complement (C'H50) in synovial fluid can be of diagnostic significance when the patient with rheumatoid arthritis has an atypical presentation. It need not be measured routinely, especially in patients in whom the diagnosis is known, unless there is concern about possible complicating articular infection (see Table 67.2). If measured, C'H50 in serum should be measured simultaneously. It is also important to remember that, if the protein concentration is low in synovial fluid, complement activity will be proportionately low as well; therefore it is necessary to measure protein concentration in the joint fluid any time that complement activity is to be assessed. For complement determination the joint fluid and serum should be packed in ice and transported to the laboratory within hours of its collection. If that is not possible, the specimens may be stored at −20°C (the usual temperature of a freezer in a refrigerator) for up to 1 week.

Radiology (Fig. 67.6)

Roentgenograms are rarely necessary in the diagnosis of rheumatoid arthritis, but are useful in following the progression of the erosive process. Furthermore, X-ray changes lag behind and require sufficient time (months) to evolve in a characteristic manner, impairing their usefulness early in the course of the disease.

Radiologic findings vary in rheumatoid arthritis depending on the duration and severity of the illness. Early in the disease X-rays may show nothing other than soft tissue swelling. Thereafter periarticular osteoporosis may develop; and it is usually most noticeable in the small joints of the hands, wrists, and feet. With progression of the disease, narrowing of the joint space occurs due to loss of cartilage, and juxta-articular erosions appear, generally at the point of attachment of the joint capsule. In end-stage disease, large cystic erosions of bone may be seen; bony proliferation may occur because of degenerative changes that follow inflammation; and the marked deformities that are visible to the naked eye (see above p. 656) are also visible radiologically.

Biopsies

Because the histology of rheumatoid arthritis is characteristic only in far advanced cases (see above, p. 654), synovial biopsy is rarely helpful in the management of the condition, even if diagnosis is in doubt. On the other hand, biopsy of a rheumatoid nodule will almost always permit a specific diagnosis of rheumatoid arthritis to be made (see above, p. 656). However biopsy of a nodule is only indicated if the diagnosis is unclear, in which case, consultation should first be requested from a rheumatologist; if he concurs, the patient should be referred to a surgeon for the procedure.

EXTRA-ARTICULAR DISEASE

Rheumatoid arthritis is potentially a chronic inflammatory *systemic* disease. Although the joints are almost always the principal focus of the illness, other organ systems may also be involved, either because of rheumatoid granuloma formation or because of a generalized vasculitis. Usually (but not invariably) extra-articular manifestations of rheumatoid arthritis occur in patients with relatively more severe disease.

Ocular Disease

Ocular manifestations of rheumatoid arthritis occur in up to 15% of patients, most commonly in association with *Sjögren's syndrome* (a condition characterized by salivary gland enlargement and impaired formation of saliva and of tears, resulting in a dry mouth and dry eyes). Episcleritis and scleritis are less common; they are manifest either by discomfort or by actual pain in the affected eye. The physician may be able to see the lesions on the surface of the eye (erythema and nodularity); but in any case, because of the very rare possibility of scleral perforation, he should refer these patients to an ophthalmologist; unfortunately, neither medical nor surgical therapy is very effective in healing these lesions.

Neurologic Disease

Entrapment neuropathies (for example, the carpal tunnel syndrome) sometimes occur in patients with rheumatoid arthritis because of compression of a peripheral nerve by inflamed edematous tissue. This problem is discussed in Chapter 81. *Cervical myelopathy*, secondary to arthritis of the cervical spine, is a particularly worrisome complication; if caused by *atlantoaxial subluxation*, permanent—even fatal—neurologic damage may ensue. Neurosurgical consultation should be sought at the first sign of cord compression (radicular pain, difficulty voiding, focal weakness). Atlantoaxial subluxation can be diagnosed before any sign of neurologic dysfunction if lateral films of the cervical spine are obtained while the patient's neck is flexed. Such a study is appropriate in all patients with rheumatoid arthritis who complain of neck pain.

Pleuropulmonary Disease

Pleural and pulmonary manifestations of rheumatoid arthritis occur more often in men, usually in association with seropositivity (see below). Pleural

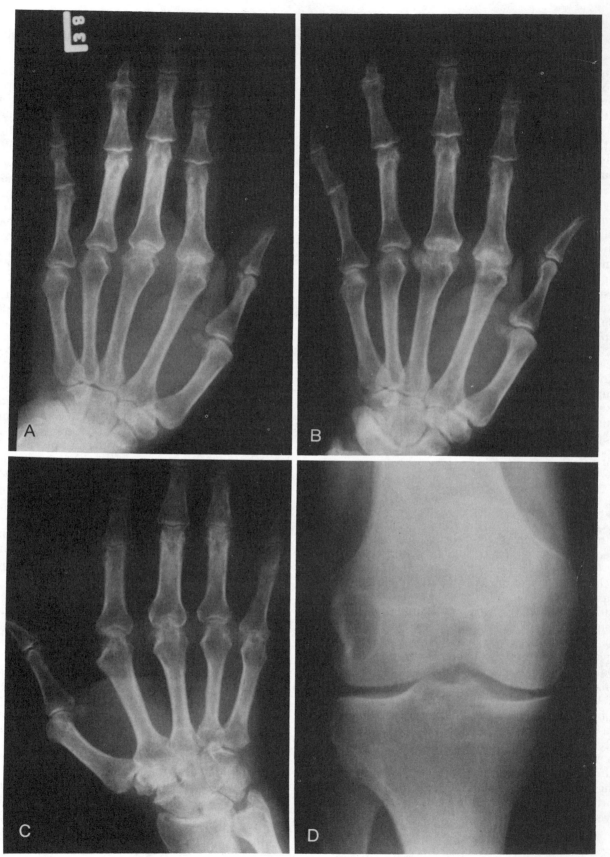

Figure 67.6 Radiologic changes in rheumatoid arthritis. (*A*) Early joint space narrowing in 2nd and 3rd metacarpophalangeal joints. (*B*) Cystic changes, erosions, and further bony proliferation in 2nd and 3rd metacarpophalangeal joints. (*C*) Periarticular osteoporosis, most noticeable in the interphalangeal joints, and numerous marginal erosions and cysts in the carpal bones and metacarpal heads. (*D*) Joint space narrowing in a knee; there is a large cyst in the lateral femoral condyle.

thickening and asymptomatic small pleural effusions are the most frequent signs of pulmonary involvement, but rarely large effusions occur that limit breathing and require drainage. The effusions may be either transudates or exudates; however, over 70% of the time the glucose concentration of the fluid is low (less than 30 mg/100 ml) (2). The effusions appear to be caused by a nonspecific pleuritis, but sometimes they are associated with subpleural rheumatoid nodules. Rarely parenchymal nodules are seen as well and are usually asymptomatic; but cavitation simulating cancer or tuberculosis may occur. The physician must always make certain through careful evaluation of each patient that a pleural or pulmonary lesion is, in fact, rheumatoid in origin and not due to a complicating, intercurrent process.

The most troublesome manifestation of rheumatoid lung disease is diffuse interstitial fibrosis with progressive respiratory insufficiency; however, a cause and effect relationship between this process and rheumatoid arthritis is not clearly established. Patients with symptomatic pleuropulmonary manifestations of rheumatoid arthritis should be followed in consultation with a rheumatologist and/or a pulmonologist.

Cardiac Disease

Cardiac manifestations of rheumatoid arthritis, especially pericardial thickening and small pericardial effusions, are relatively common at autopsy (1), but are quite unusual clinically. Symptomatic pericarditis occurs rarely (and equally as often in men and women); heart disease and cardiac conduction abnormalities occur even more rarely. Patients with symptomatic pericarditis may respond to 30 to 40 mg of prednisone a day, administered for 1–2 weeks, but that decision should be made in consultation with a rheumatologist.

Felty's Syndrome

Felty's syndrome is characterized by rheumatoid arthritis, splenomegaly, and leukopenia—predominantly granulocytopenia. Patients with the syndrome usually are older, have a high titer of rheumatoid factor, and have arthritic deformities. Recurrent bacterial infections and chronic refractory leg ulcers are the major complications, and splenectomy may benefit patients whose infections are severe.

Rheumatoid Vasculitis

Vascular inflammation is found in 10 to 25% of patients with rheumatoid arthritis who are autopsied. Its role in the pathogenesis of the disease is unclear. In a very small proportion of patients (less than 1%) a syndrome of accelerated vasculitis (7) is seen, characterized by distal cutaneous ulcerations (Fig. 67.7) and gangrene, peripheral polyneuropathy, and visceral (intestinal, renal, cardiac, cerebral) ischemia. There seems to be a positive correlation between the long term administration of corticosteroids and the

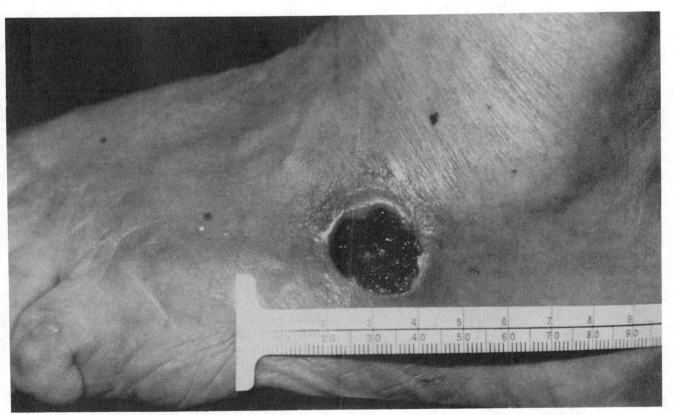

Figure 67.7   Vasculitic ulcer on the foot of a patient with rheumatoid arthritis.

severity of this process. The syndrome ordinarily emerges after years of seropositive, persistently active, rheumatoid arthritis. Immediate consultation with a rheumatologist and, usually, hospitalization are indicated.

COURSE

Rheumatoid arthritis is a variable illness, and its course cannot be predicted precisely in a given patient. The disease develops slowly, but progressively, over months or years in most patients and remains persistently symptomatic. Degree of disability is probably directly proportionate to the severity and the duration of the inflammatory process. Although treatment certainly can alter the course of the illness, complete remission is unlikely in people who have had symptomatic rheumatoid arthritis for a year or more. In this situation, seropositivity correlates to some extent with sustained disease. There is no clear-cut way to predict which patients will develop significant deformities (subluxation, ankylosis, etc., see above, p. 656); most will not; on the other hand, a recent study has shown that 60% of patients with rheumatoid arthritis are unable to work 10 years after onset of their illness (9). A minority of patients (approximately 25%) will have a course characterized by remissions and exacerbations—often with months or even years during which they are asymptomatic; a few have permanent remissions. Such patients often have an abrupt onset of their disease, which paradoxically may herald a better prognosis. Some patients who at first have episodic attacks of arthritis ultimately develop a more typical sustained progressive course.

MANAGEMENT

General Principles

Rheumatoid arthritis is not a disease that can be cured, but it usually can be controlled by proper therapy. It is important that the patient understands the illness, its variability and chronicity, and that it is probably a problem that he must deal with for the rest of his life. Thus he must maintain contact on a regular basis with his primary physician; the frequency of visits will depend on the severity of the inflammatory process and on the nature of any extra-articular disease. The physician should maintain a chart, documenting serial measurements which reflect the course of the illness (Table 67.3). Furthermore, it is essential to remember that intercurrent problems can mimic a flare in the rheumatoid process i.e., a septic joint, tuberculosis, pleurisy, drug-induced leukopenia, tumor, etc.). Careful re-evaluation of the patient with a flare-up is critical, especially when it is unsuspected or appears atypical.

Rest is an important feature of the management of rheumatoid arthritis. Although the value of complete bedrest, even in the actively symptomatic patient, is questionable, 8 to 9 hours sleep at night and a 2-hour

Table 67.3

Measurements to Be Made Serially in Patients with Rheumatoid Arthritis[a]

Duration of morning stiffness
Time of onset of fatigue
Aspirin need/day
Grip strength
Number of joints that are tender or are painful on passive motion
Degree of swelling of affected joints
Erythrocyte sedimentation rate (Westergren)

[a] Adapted from D. J. McCarty: Clinical assessment of arthritis. In *Arthritis and Allied Conditions*, Ed. 9, edited by D. J. McCarty. Lea & Febiger, Philadelphia, 1979.

rest period in the middle of the day are reasonable goals for everyone with active disease. Also, vigorous activity (heavy work, brisk exercise) probably should be avoided because of the danger of intensifying joint inflammation. On the other hand, patients should be urged to maintain a modest level of activity, both at work and at home.

Physical therapy should be instituted as soon as possible after the diagnosis of rheumatoid arthritis is made and should be maintained on a daily basis indefinitely. Passive range of motion exercises (moving the joints through a full range of motion) are important in preventing contractures and muscle atrophy and should be taught by the primary physician. Sometimes the help of another family member or of a friend is necessary for the patient to be able to accomplish these exercises. If necessary, advice about specific active exercises and about splinting of acutely symptomatic joints should be sought from a physiatrist, a rheumatologist, or a orthopaedist—depending on the availability and expertise of these specialists.

The application of *heat* for 20 to 30 min to painful joints often relieves pain temporarily and relaxes tight muscles. Heat may be especially useful just before physical therapy. Patients often prefer moist heat, but dry heat is equally effective.

During periods when the inflammatory process is particularly intense, especially if they occur at the onset of the illness, *hospitalization* is helpful in removing the patient from the stresses of his everyday life, in beginning a structured rehabilitation program, and in evaluating the effect of drugs (see below) on the illness.

There is increased susceptibility of the rheumatoid joint to infection, usually by Gram-positive organisms. Whenever a single joint flares up or is accompanied by increased body temperature or follows a recent procedure (*e.g.*, dental), infection should be ruled out by means of synovial fluid examination (see p. 658).

Drug Treatment: A Stepped Method

Drugs are used in rheumatoid arthritis for their anti-inflammatory effects. They are always used in conjunction with the general measures of heat, physical therapy, etc. discussed above. Although there is no question that drugs reduce the signs and symptoms of the disease, it is still not known whether they alter its ultimate course (see below for a discussion of the characteristics of specific drugs).

A stepped method of treating patients with rheumatoid arthritis, similar to that used in the treatment of hypertension (see Chapter 59) is a reasonable approach (Table 67.4). With this method, aspirin is always the first step. Approximately 75% of patients will show some response to this drug. If aspirin cannot be tolerated or if inflammation is not adequately controlled within 2 to 4 weeks, another nonsteroidal anti-inflammatory drug (NSAID—see details below) is prescribed as a second step (8). Unless aspirin toxicity has developed, there is no compelling reason why it cannot be administered together with an NSAID. However, there is no good evidence that the combination of any two NSAIDs are better than one. It is also true that any one NSAID may be unaccountably more effective than another, so that a trial and error approach is often warranted.

If arthritis appears to progress despite aspirin or NSAID, a third step is indicated. Some rheumatologists use a gold compound at this point while others use an antimalarial agent first. In general, antimalarials are probably better utilized in patients with relatively mild, although persistent, disease; and gold, in patients with relatively more active disease. The consulting rheumatologist should play a major role, at least by telephone, in these often difficult therapeutic decisions. Fifty to seventy percent of patients improve after 2 to 4 months of chrysotherapy. If no response has occurred within 6 months, or if toxicity is observed (see below), the drug is discontinued. If there is a good response, gold is given in a reduced dosage indefinitely. The response to antimalarials is also delayed, with increasing improvement noted up to 6 months; in patients who do respond, continued use of the drugs dictates that the patient be examined by an ophthalmologist every 6 months so that early signs of ocular toxicity, the major side effect, can be detected (see below).

Table 67.4
Stepped Method of Treatment of Patients with Rheumatoid Arthritis

Step	Drug(s)[a]
1	Aspirin
2	Another nonsteroidal anti-inflammatory drug (NSAID)
3[b]	Gold or Antimalarial
4	D-Penicillamine
5	A cytotoxic drug

[a] Corticosteroids are adjuncts in this program.
[b] Steps 3 and 4 may be taken in consultation (at least by telephone) with a rheumatologist; Step 5 *must* be taken in consultation with a rheumatologist.

If there is an inadequate or toxic response to gold and/or antimalarial drugs, the fourth step in the treatment of rheumatoid arthritis is the use of D-penicillamine. Approximately 80% of patients will respond to this drug after it is given for 3 or 4 months. The use of D-penicillamine is often limited by its toxic effects (see below); and again, it should not be given without the advice, at least by telephone, of a rheumatologist. In patients who respond favorably, the drug can be administered indefinitely at a relatively low maintenance dose (see below). Since penicillamine chelates heavy metals, gold must be discontinued before initiation of penicillamine therapy.

The fifth step in the treatment of rheumatoid arthritis, the use of cytotoxic drugs, should be reserved for the occasional patient with rapidly progressive, otherwise uncontrollable, life-threatening disease—especially patients with severe extra-articular manifestations of the illness. These drugs should be prescribed only by a rheumatologist and then only after the patient understands fully the possible long term toxicity (see below).

Corticosteroids should be used as adjuncts, either systemically or intra-articularly, during the stepped program for patients who need briefly a more potent anti-inflammatory effect. An acutely inflamed, very painful joint will often respond dramatically to an intra-articular injection of hydrocortisone. The injection should be administered by a rheumatologist or an orthopaedist unless the primary physician is experienced with the technique. Patients with severely painful flare-ups of polyarthritis may require limited courses (1 to 3 weeks) of oral prednisone, 10 to 15 mg per day. Maintenance steroids should not exceed 10 mg per day, because of the danger of steroid dependence and harmful side effects. Many patients may receive major benefit from an alternate day schedule of 10 to 15 mg prednisone. In rheumatoid arthritis, low dose therapy is the rule.

Purely analgesic drugs (acetaminophen, narcotics) should not be prescribed chronically to patients with rheumatoid arthritis, because of the danger of masking signs and symptoms of inflammation without suppressing the inflammation itself. In that setting, progressive joint destruction might occur without the physician's being aware of it. Furthermore, drug dependency is a hazard in patients who have a chronic disease that causes persistent pain indefinitely.

Characteristics of Individual Drugs

FIRST STEP DRUGS: ASPIRIN

Mechanism. Aspirin inhibits the synthesis of prostaglandins, cyclic fatty acids which mediate a wide variety of physiologic reactions through their effect on cellular cyclic adenosine monophosphate production. Whether this inhibition accounts for the anti-inflammatory effects of aspirin is not known.

Dosage. The starting dose of aspirin is 900 mg (3 tablets) 4 times a day. The drug should be taken during meals and with a bedtime snack to minimize gastrointestinal side effects (see below). Salicylate levels should be monitored every few weeks at first to ensure that an adequate dose is being administered; a therapeutic level is 20 to 25 mg/100 ml. If such a level is not achieved with the starting dose, one or more tablets a day are prescribed until the desired level is attained or until mild tinnitus or mild deafness is experienced. If the patient does develop tinnitus or deafness, he should stop taking aspirin until the symptom disappears; and then the total daily dose should be reduced by one tablet until a dose is reached that does not produce symptoms. Most patients, however, will not develop tinnitus or deafness below serum salicylate levels of 30 mg/100 ml. After each change of dosage, it may take a week for a new steady state to be achieved.

Usual Time to Maximal Effect. The maximum anti-inflammatory effect of aspirin is achieved within 10 to 14 days. The patient must be told of the importance of taking the medicine exactly as prescribed in order for the therapeutic effect to be achieved.

Side Effects. Tinnitus (see above) and dyspepsia (nausea, heartburn, anorexia) are common side effects of aspirin therapy; both can be controlled: tinnitus, by reducing the dosage; dyspepsia, by taking the aspirin with food. Enteric coated aspirin reduces the incidence of dyspeptic symptoms and, although absorption is somewhat reduced, an effective dosage can usually be achieved by appropriate monitoring of salicylate levels. Buffered aspirins are more expensive than, and have no clear-cut advantage over, the standard preparation.

The most troublesome side effects are gastrointestinal bleeding and peptic ulceration, due primarily to the irritative effect of the drug on the gastric mucosa. These problems occur in less than 5% of patients, and

are reasons to substitute a second step drug. Because of the inhibition of platelet function by aspirin (see Chapter 48), it should never be prescribed to a patient with an underlying bleeding tendency (including patients taking anticoagulant drugs).

SECOND STEP DRUGS: NSAID (Table 67.5)

Mechanism. The mechanism of action whereby these drugs inhibit inflammation is unknown. Many of them, like aspirin, inhibit prostaglandin synthesis, but the relationship between this effect and their clinical effect is not established.

Dosage. See Table 67.5. Whichever NSAID is selected, a relatively low dose should be initiated, maintained for 2 weeks, and then gradually increased at 2-week intervals until a maximum therapeutic effect is achieved or until mild toxicity has been observed (exceptions are phenylbutazone and oxyphenbutazone—see below). If a particular preparation is not tolerated or is ineffective, a trial with another NSAID may be initiated. As noted above, there is no proof that the administration of more than one NSAID is better than the administration of any one single agent. Assays of these various drugs are not widely available so that, unlike the situation with aspirin, the clinician must depend entirely on the patient's response to therapy to gauge dosage.

Usual Time to Maximal Effect. Ten to fourteen days.

Side Effects. All anti-inflammatory agents have the potential of producing dyspepsia and, to a lesser extent, peptic ulceration and gastrointestinal bleeding. Phenylbutazone (and oxyphenbutazone) imposes a special risk of (rarely) producing aplastic anemia and therefore should be given only for acute flareups of arthritis and should not be prescribed for

Table 67.5
Second Step Drugs For Rheumatoid Arthritis: Nonsteroidal Anti-inflammatory Drugs

Generic Name	Brand Name	Dosage Range (available strengths)	Side Effects[a]
Indomethacin	Indocin	25–50 mg q.i.d. (25- and 50-mg capsules)	Dyspepsia[1] → headache[2] → gastrointestinal (GI) bleeding,[4] peptic ulcer
Tolmetin	Tolectin	400–600 mg t.i.d. (200- and 400-mg capsules)	Dyspepsia[2] → GI bleeding,[4] peptic ulcer, rash
Ibuprofen	Motrin	400–600 mg q.i.d. (300- and 400-mg tablets)	Dyspepsia[2] → GI bleeding,[4] rash, headache
Naproxen	Naprosyn	250–325 mg b.i.d. (250-mg tablets)	Headache[3] → GI bleeding,[4] dyspepsia, rash
Fenoprofen	Nalfon	600–800 mg q.i.d. (300-mg capsules; 600-mg tablets)	Dyspepsia[2] → headache,[3] rash
Sulindac	Clinoril	150–200 mg b.i.d. (150- and 200-mg tablets)	Dyspepsia,[3] diarrhea, constipation, rash, headache → tinnitus,[4] edema
Phenylbutazone[b] (and oxyphenbutazone)	Butazolidine (and Tandearil)	200 mg b.i.d. (100-mg tablets) and 200 mg b.i.d. (200-mg tablets)	Edema,[3] dyspepsia → GI bleeding,[4] peptic ulcer, rash, aplastic anemia

[a] In decreasing incidence: [1]over 25%, [2]10–25%, [3]5–10%, and [4]under 5%.
[b] Should not be used for more than a short course (4 days or less) because of the risk of aplastic anemia..

more than 4 to 5 days. In contrast to aspirin, each of these drugs is relatively expensive, the monthly cost averaging over 20 dollars.

THIRD STEP DRUGS: GOLD AND ANTIMALARIALS

Mechanism. a. *Gold*—a number of mechanisms have been postulated but none has been proved to explain the effect of gold in patients with rheumatoid arthritis.

b. *Antimalarials*—similarly, the mechanism of action of antimalarials in patients with rheumatoid arthritis is unknown.

Dosage. a. *Gold* (gold sodium thiomalate (Myochrysine) or gold thioglucose (Solganol)) therapy should be initiated at 10 mg (1 ml) intramuscularly; if this is tolerated, 25 mg intramuscularly should be given the second week; and if that is tolerated, 50 mg intramuscularly should be given weekly until a response has occurred or until a total of 1 g has been given. If there *is* a favorable response, therapy should be maintained with 50 mg intramuscularly each month. Gold is best injected into the gluteal muscles while the patient is lying down; he should remain lying for about 10 min after the injection.

b. *Antimalarials* (hydroxychloroquine, 200 mg tablets; chloroquine is no longer recommended because of its greater ocular toxicity). Hydroxychloroquine is given in a dose of 200 mg a day.

Usual Time to Maximal Effect: a. Gold—4 to 6 months.

b. *Antimalarials:* 3 to 6 months.

Side Effects. a. *Gold*—a pruritic rash occurs in one-third or more of patients and is the major reason why the drug is not tolerated. Sometimes the rash will disappear if treatment is withheld for a week and then reinstituted at a lower dose (25 mg). Proteinuria occurs commonly (10% of patients); nephrotic syndrome, rarely. Bone marrow depression and isolated immune thrombocytopenia are also rare complications. Side effects ordinarily abate if treatment is stopped; occasionally a chelating agent (British anti-Lewisite—BAL) is required if severe toxicity occurs, in which case, hospitalization is indicated.

b. *Antimalarial*—the major side effect is irreversible retinopathy with visual impairment; at the dosages recommended, this complication is very rare, but still warrants baseline and periodic (6-monthly) ophthalmologic examinations (funduscopic exam, measurement of visual acuity and of visual fields). Dyspepsia and skin rash occur occasionally and respond to withdrawal of the drug.

FOURTH STEP DRUG: D-PENICILLAMINE

Mechanism. Penicillamine chelates metals, interferes with cross-linking of collagen fibrils, and disrupts sulfhydryl-disulfide bonds; but whether any of these actions explains the effects of the drug in patients with rheumatoid arthritis is unknown.

Dosage. Penicillamine (Cuprimine, Depen) is available in 125- and 250-mg capsules. Therapy is started at a daily dose of 250 mg and then increased at intervals of 3 months, as necessary, to 500, and then 750 mg per day. The drug should be given to patients 1 hour before they intend to eat, to effect maximum absorption.

Usual Time to Maximal Effect. Four to six months.

Side Effects. Pruritis, skin rash, and dyspepsia are the common adverse reactions to penicillamine (over 10% of patients); proteinuria occurs less often (approximately 5% of patients). These untoward responses are reversible if the drug is withdrawn. Nephrotic syndrome and bone marrow depression occur more rarely, but are less likely to be reversible.

FIFTH STEP DRUGS: CYTOTOXIC AGENTS

Mechanisms. These drugs interfere with the synthesis of nucleic acids, one of the consequences of which is suppression of the immune response. The explanation for the effect of cytotoxic agents in patients with rheumatoid arthritis is unknown, but presumably relates to these basic mechanisms.

Dosage. The drugs most commonly used are cyclophosphamide (Cytoxan) and azothioprine (Imuran). The dose schedules range from 1.5 to 2.5 mg per kg per day (100 to 200 mg). The drugs are available as 25- and 50-mg tablets.

Usual Time to Maximal Effect. Six to eight months.

Side Effects. Probably the most common side effect, in the first few months in this dose range, is a slowly falling blood cell count secondary to dose-related marrow depression; this effect is reversible if the drugs are withdrawn. The most serious side effect is the increased incidence, over a period of years, of malignant neoplasms (bladder cancer and lymphoproliferative and myeloproliferative neoplasms); it is this effect, more than any other, which limits the use of these agents for the treatment of rheumatoid arthritis. Thus, these agents (especially cyclophosphamide) should be strictly reserved for life-threatening complications of the rheumatoid process (e.g., vasculitis). Other less serious, but still important, complications of cytotoxic drugs are azoospermia and amenorrhea (cyclophosphamide), hemorrhagic cystitis (cyclophosphamide), increased susceptibility to infection, and dyspepsia.

Surgery

Surgery may be useful at various stages of the course of rheumatoid arthritis. Early synovectomy may sometimes be helpful in relieving extreme pain and in slowing joint destruction. Later, tendon repairs, arthroplastic procedures, and joint replacement may be necessary. The patient, the primary physician, the rheumatologist, and the orthopaedist should participate in the consideration of such operations.

Summary of Indications for Hospitalizations or for Referral to a Specialist

See Tables 67.6 and 67.7.

Table 67.6
Indications for Hospitalization of Patients with Rheumatoid Arthritis

Early in the course for assessment of the extent of the disease and for institution of a therapeutic regimen (p. 662)

At the time of acute painful flareups of arthritis

For assessment and treatment of severe manifestations of extra-articular disease (p. 659).

Table 67.7
Indications for Referral of Patients with Rheumatoid Arthritis for Consultation

TO A RHEUMATOLOGIST:
1. If there is any question about the validity of the diagnosis
2. If a synovial tap is indicated and the primary physician is not comfortable in performing the procedure (an orthopaedist can also do this procedure)
3. For advice about splinting (an orthopaedist can also provide this advice)
4. If the therapeutic regimen reaches the third step and at each step thereafter (see p. 662)—at least by telephone before Steps 3 and 4, in person, before Step 5
5. If there is any consideration of corrective surgery (an orthopaedist can also provide this advice)
6. If there are severe manifestations of extra-articular disease

TO AN ORTHOPAEDIST:
1. For advice about splinting
2. If there is any consideration of corrective surgery

TO A PHYSICAL THERAPIST:
1. Soon after diagnosis to advise and institute appropriate physical therapy.

References

General

Kelley, WN, Harris, ED, Jr, Ruddy, S, and Sledge, CB (eds): *Textbook of Rheumatology*. W. B. Saunders, Philadelphia, 1981.
   A comprehensive, extensively referenced, especially well illustrated text.
McCarty, DJ (ed): *Arthritis and Allied Conditions*, Ed. 9. Lea & Febiger, Philadelphia, 1979.
   A comprehensive extensively referenced text; the information about rheumatoid arthritis is scattered among a number of chapters.
Williams, RC: *Rheumatoid Arthritis as a Systemic Disease*. W. B. Saunders, Philadelphia, 1974.
   An easily read book, emphasizing extra-articular disease.

Specific

1. Lebowitz, WB: The heart in rheumatoid arthritis (rheumatoid disease). A clinical and pathological study of sixty-two cases. *Ann Intern Med* 58: 102, 1963.
2. Lillington, GA, Carr, DT and Mayne, JG: Rheumatoid pleurisy with an effusion. *Arch Intern Med* 128: 764, 1971.
3. McCarty, DJ: Clinical assessment of arthritis. In *Arthritis and Allied Conditions*, Ed. 19, p. 131, edited by DJ McCarty. Lea & Febiger, Philadelphia, 1979.
4. O'Sullivan, JB and Cathcart, ES: The prevalence of rheumatoid arthritis. Follow-up evaluation of the effect of criteria on rates in Sudbury, Massachusetts. *N Engl J Med* 76: 573, 1972.
5. Plotz, CM and Singer, JM: The latex fixation test; II. Results in rheumatoid arthritis. *Am J Med* 21: 893, 1956.
6. Ropes, MW, Bennett, GA, Cobb, S, Jocox, R and Jessas, RA: 1958 Revision of diagnostic criteria for rheumatoid arthritis. *Arthritis Rheum* 2: 16, 1959.
7. Schmid, FR, Cooper, NS, Ziff, M and McEwen, C: Arteritis in rheumatoid arthritis. *Am J Med* 30: 56, 1961.
8. *The Medical Letter on Drugs and Therapeutics*: Non-steroidal anti-inflammatory drugs for rheumatoid arthritis: 22: 29, 1980.
9. Yelin, E, Meenan, R, Nevitt, M and Epstein, W: Work disability in rheumatoid arthritis: effects of disease, social, and work factors. *Ann Intern Med* 93: 551, 1980.

CHAPTER SIXTY-EIGHT

Sacroiliitis: Ankylosing Spondylitis and Reiter's Syndrome

FRANK C. ARNETT, JR., M.D.

ANKYLOSING SPONDYLITIS

Definition

Chronic inflammation of the sacroiliac joints, sacroiliitis, may occur as an isolated clinical syndrome or as a component feature of several other chronic rheumatic disorders. Sacroiliitis is considered the *sine qua non* for early *primary ankylosing spondylitis*; however, this latter diagnosis should only be applied when symptoms or signs indicate ascension of inflammation into additional segments of the axial skeleton. *Secondary forms of sacroiliitis* or spondylitis may complicate the clinical course in 10% of patients with inflammatory bowel disease (ulcerative colitis and Crohn's disease), 5 to 10% of those with psoriatic arthritis, and nearly one-third of those with Reiter's syndrome. The dominant clinical problems which bring the patient with primary spondylitis to a physician and require careful management over many years relate to pain, limitation of motion, and deformity of the spine. In secondary spondylitis the same principles of diagnosis and management of the axial problem apply, but must be accompanied by attention to the cutaneous, gastrointestinal, genitourinary, and peripheral articular manifestations of the primary disorders.

The pathogenesis of axial inflammation is unknown; however, there is a strong hereditary component marked by the histocompatibility antigen, HLA-B27. This genetic marker is strongly associated with sacroiliitis and spondylitis regardless of clinical setting (Table 68.1). Approximately 90% of patients with primary ankylosing spondylitis have HLA-B27 Conversely, if "normal" individuals with HLA-B27 are carefully assessed, clinical and/or radiographic evidence of disease can be found in nearly 20% (3). In addition to this genetic predisposition, certain environmental agents appear to be associated with these diseases in the B27-positive host. There is increasing evidence that certain *Klebsiella* species in the gastrointestinal tract may be implicated in the pathogenesis of primary ankylosing spondylitis (4). A secondary spondylitis may occur in the setting of Reiter's syndrome which has been triggered by certain gastrointestinal or genitourinary infections (see Reiter's Syndrome).

Prevalence

The prevalence of spondylitis parallels the frequency of HLA-B27 in different populations in the United States and other regions of the globe. This tissue type occurs in 8 to 10% of caucasian Americans and the disease occurs in 1 to 2% of the white population (Table 68.1). Black Americans have a much lower frequency of both disease and the HLA-B27 antigen (13). On the other hand, there is a high frequency of spondylitic disease and of HLA-B27 in American Indians (7). In other parts of the world, ankylosing spondylitis is common in Europeans but is found rarely in African Blacks or Orientals, again reflecting the relative frequency of the B27 marker.

Histopathology

The spondylitic diseases are characterized by chronic inflammation involving *synovial joints*, especially those in the axial skeleton, *fibrous joints* such as sacroiliacs and symphysis pubis, and nonarticular bony areas where tendons and fascia have their *insertions* (*enthesopathy*). The chronic inflammatory infiltrates are nonspecific and histologically indistinguishable from those of rheumatoid arthritis. On the other hand, unlike the rheumatoid process where there is cartilaginous and bony destruction, this inflammatory process tends to promote new bone formation and fusion across previous articulations. This ossification and calcification of the articular and ligamentous structures of the spine results in eventual fusion, and gives rise to the characteristic radiographic findings.

History

The typical patient with sacroiliitis or ankylosing spondylitis is a young white man under the age of 40 years (Table 68.2). Women appear to be affected less often than men; however, this may be due to underrecognition of the disease in females. The initial symptoms of the disorder in women may be peripheral or cervical arthritis, and low back involvement

Table 68.1
Classification of Spondylitis and Frequency of HLA-B27[a]

Classification	
PRIMARY	
Sacroiliitis	90%
Ankylosing spondylitis	90%
SECONDARY	
Spondylitis of inflammatory bowel disease	50%
Psoriatic spondylitis	50%
Reiter's disease with spondylitis	90%
INFECTIOUS	
Sacroiliitis	Not increased
Discitis	Not increased
Osteomyelitis	Not increased

[a] Found in 8 to 10% normal white and 2 to 4% of black Americans.

Table 68.2
Clues to Early Ankylosing Spondylitis

A young man (or women)
Pain/stiffness in buttocks, low back, chest wall
　Worse with rest
　Better with exercise
Sciatic-like pains
Family history of spondylitis
History of iritis

may be absent or overshadowed by these complaints. Many are misdiagnosed and labeled seronegative rheumatoid arthritis (see Chapter 67). Therefore, the physician must be mindful of these differences between men and women and consider an emerging spondylitic process in young women presenting with a seronegative arthritis. Similarly, children are also more likely to develop a peripheral oligoarticular lower extremity arthropathy, and symptoms in the axial skeleton may not develop for many years, if ever. Their illness is often labeled juvenile rheumatoid arthritis (1).

The usual presenting symptoms of sacroiliitis or ankylosing spondylitis are those of pain and stiffness in the low back or buttocks. These symptoms begin insidiously, and the patient has usually noticed them for at least 3 months before seeking medical advice. Unlike mechanical low back syndromes, the pain and stiffness of inflammatory disease are characteristically worsened by rest and improved by exercise. The patient is unable to rest at night or sit for prolonged periods and must arise and walk in order to obtain relief. Like discogenic disease, however, symptoms of shooting pains into the buttocks and down the posterior or lateral thighs may mimic sciatica. These pains are usually transient and not associated with any demonstrable neurologic deficits. Frequently, patients will already have been evaluated myelographically and/or treated conservatively or surgically for presumed disc disease.

With time the disease progresses into the lumbar and thoracic regions. Chest wall pain occurs frequently and may mimic pleuritic or pericardial pain syndromes. Progressive limitation of spinal movements ensues, and patients may note more difficulty in bending forward, the development of a stooped posture, and actual loss of height. Finally, the disease process reaches the cervical spine, and if appropriate preventive measures are not taken, the neck may become fused in a kyphotic position. Although other peripheral joints are uncommonly affected, the root joints (hips and shoulders) eventually become involved in 50% of patients. Occasionally fusion of the back may be entirely asymptomatic, and the patient will develop complaints only when the disease reaches the cervical spine, hips, or shoulders (11).

Additional important historical facts should be sought in the assessment of the patient. The family history will be positive for a first-degree relative with spondylitis in 16% of patients (10). The past history should seek out prior episodes of peripheral arthritis, perhaps beginning in childhood, or even an episode of Reiter's syndrome. Acute anterior uveitis (iritis) may have been a harbinger of the articular syndrome, and at least 25% of patients will have iritis at sometime before or during their course of illness. The review of systems as well as the family history should seek out symptoms or diagnoses of psoriasis or inflammatory bowel disease in the patient or his family members. The patient with spondylitis may have

relatives with psoriasis or inflammatory bowel disease but never manifest these disorders himself (5).

Physical Examination

A complete physical examination initially and every 4 to 6 months is important in patients with suspected inflammatory back disease. This practice ensures the diagnosis and provides the baseline with which the physician can assess future articular or extra-articular complications or the superimposition of unrelated systemic or musculoskeletal disorders. It must be emphasized that ankylosing spondylitis is a disease where the patient requires management over decades, and each new complaint cannot necessarily be ascribed to the basic disease process. Thus, while the primary focus of examinations will be the musculoskeletal system, especially the axial skeleton, shoulders, hips, and peripheral joints, additional attention must be directed toward the eyes, heart, skin, and gastrointestinal tract.

ARTICULAR FEATURES (Table 68.3)

There are few measurable abnormalities in early spondylitis. In fact the patient with *sacroiliitis*, despite significant symptoms of pain and stiffness in the low back region, may have an entirely normal physical examination. At most, there may be tenderness on direct palpation of these joints in the buttocks or upon compression of the pelvis. Stressing the sacroiliac joint to elicit pain (see p. 606) may also be useful.

Those abnormalities which eventually appear in the patient who has progressive disease relate to loss of range of motion and deformity in mobile structures. After evaluation of the sacroiliac regions the physician should next direct his attention to the *lumbar spine*. The patient with lumbar involvement has often lost the normal lordosis, and there is flattening of that segment of the back. In addition, there is loss in range of motion when the patient attempts

Table 68.3
Physical Examination in Ankylosing Spondylitis

SACROILIAC JOINTS	THORACIC SPINE
Tenderness	Increased kyphosis
Pain with compression/ stress	Tenderness
LUMBAR SPINE	Pain with rib cage compression
Tenderness	Decreased chest expansion
Paravertebral muscle spasm	CERVICAL SPINE
Loss of lordosis	Tenderness
Decreased flexion:	Pain on motion
Schober test (<5cm) (see text)	Muscle spasm
Abnormal finger-floor	Decreased motion
Decreased lateral motion and extension	Kyphosis, decreased lordosis
HIPS, SHOULDERS	Occiput to wall movement (see text)
Pain on motion	
Decreased range	

to bend forward and touch his toes. It should be recalled that hip motion accounts for 90° of the flexion of trunk on the lower extremities and that the lumbar spine provides the remaining stretch by reversing its lordosis and becoming kyphotic. It is important to obtain serial measurements of the distance between the patient's fingertips and the floor with maximal forward bending. Another objective measurement of lumbar motion is the *Schober test*: With the patient standing erect, a horizontal line is drawn at the L5–S1 region and another line 10 cm above that. With forward flexion the distance between these two points should increase to 15 cm in the normal lumbar spine. This test is best applied and interpreted in the young patient since lumbar motion normally decreases with age. Lateral bending of the lumbar spine should also be assessed at the same time.

Involvement of the *thoracic spine* is determined subjectively by the patient's complaints of pain or stiffness in that region and by demonstrable tenderness along the vertebral column and paravertebral muscles. Compression of the rib cage laterally and over the sternum may also elicit pain. Objective determination of fusion of the costovertebral joints is obtained by measuring the chest expansion. A tape measure is placed around the patient's chest wall at the nipple line, and the change in circumference from full expiration to full inspiration is measured. Less than 3 cm is considered abnormal.

The range of motion of the cervical spine should be determined for extension, right and left rotation, lateral flexion, and forward flexion. Loss of extension is usually the earliest abnormality, and as the disease progresses there is a tendency for the patient to develop fixed deformity in the forward flexed position. Therefore, another rough estimate of developing cervical kyphosis is the occiput-to-wall measurement. This is obtained with the patient placing his heels against the base of the wall and attempting to extend his neck fully to touch the wall with the back of his head. This is normally readily accomplished.

Examination of the range of motion and elicitation of any pain on motion of both shoulders and hips is important since from one-third to one-half of patients will develop involvement of these root joints at some-time during the course of the disease. Less often, peripheral joints become inflamed, but usually only transiently. The joints most commonly involved are the knees, ankles, and wrists. Approximately 10% of patients with ankylosing spondylitis will complain of pain in the heels either at the Achilles tendon insertion or over the attachment of the plantar aponeurosis in the sole of the foot. Swelling is usually not apparent in these areas, but tenderness to direct palpation is found.

EXTRA-ARTICULAR FEATURES (Table 68.4)

Cardiac abnormalities occur in less than 5% of patients with ankylosing spondylitis. The most com-

Table 68.4
Extra-articular Manifestations and Complications of Ankylosing Spondylitis

CARDIAC	5%
First degree atrioventricular block	
Second and third degree atrioventricular block	
Aortic regurgitation	
OCULAR	25%
Acute iritis	
Chronic iritis	
NEUROLOGIC	Rare
Cauda equina syndrome	
Cord injury due to fractures	
AMYLOIDOSIS	4%
PULMONARY FIBROSIS	Rare

mon, first degree atrioventricular (AV) block, can be determined only electrocardiographically. A history of palpitations or syncope and the finding of a slow or irregular pulse on examination should alert the physician to higher degrees of AV block. At times a cardiac pacemaker is required for serious arrhythmias or complete AV dissociation. Aortic regurgitation due to inflammatory thickening of the aortic valve and root is another serious cardiac complication. Once the diastolic murmur becomes apparent there is usually cardiac decompensation requiring valve replacement in 1 to 2 years.

Iritis occurs in approximately 25% of patients with ankylosing spondylitis and does not necessarily parallel the course of the articular disease. Its onset is usually abrupt and unilateral with intense pain, redness, and photophobia as the cardinal symptoms. Immediate ophthalmologic attention is required to prevent serious damage to the anterior chamber of the eye. Local corticosteroids are usually successful in abating an acute episode; however, frequent slit lamp examinations determine the response and help dictate whether systemic steroids are required.

The *cauda equina syndrome* is a rare but serious neurologic complication of spondylitis (see also p. 605). It is believed to be related to entrapment of exiting lumbar and sacral nerves through the inflamed spinal column; however, compressive inflammatory lesions within the spinal column may be found in some cases and are surgically remediable. Patients with ankylosing spondylitis should be questioned regularly about parasthesias and pain or weakness in the legs, as well as symptoms of bladder and/ or bowel sphincter dysfunction. *Other neurologic sequelae* of the disorder include injuries to the spinal cord from fracture dislocation of a rigid and brittle spine. The neck is especially prone to fracture, and paraplegia or quadriplegia may result.

Secondary amyloidosis can be found in approximately 4% of patients with ankylosing spondylitis, usually after many decades of persistent inflammatory disease. Proteinuria and nephrotic syndrome indicate renal involvement, which is usually the most serious organ manifestation of amyloid.

Apical pulmonary fibrosis, sometimes with cavity formation, is rare and usually is of no clinical consequence. This radiographic abnormality may mimic tuberculosis, and *vice versa.*

Laboratory Tests

Radiographic evaluation of the sacroiliac joints provides the single most specific test for this disorder. Although a diagnosis of sacroiliitis/spondylitis can be suspected based on the history and physical examination, definitive diagnosis cannot be established without radiographic findings. A single anteroposterior view of the pelvis is usually adequate to define sacroiliitis; however, at times special views such as Ferguson's or oblique views are necessary to evaluate fully the integrity of the sacroiliac joints. The earliest radiographic change is usually bony sclerosis on both sides of the joint margins. Shortly thereafter bony erosions occur (Fig. 68.1). There is eventual fusion across the joint space with subsequent loss of the early sclerotic changes (Fig. 68.2). Sacroiliitis is not infrequently confused with the radiographic anomaly, *osteitis condensens ilii*, where there is symmetrical sclerosis on the iliac side of each sacroiliac joint without any erosions. This finding is most common in young women who have borne children.

If the inflammatory disease has progressed beyond the pelvis, an early radiographic finding on lateral lumbar spine films is "squaring" of the vertebral bodies. This phenomenon may also be seen in the thoracic and cervical regions. The apophyseal joints of the spine become fused and, presumably due to immobility, diffuse osteoporosis ensues. Calcification and ossification of the ligamentous structures between vertebral bodies results in the characteristic

syndesmophytes seen on X-ray, *i.e.*, the bamboo spine.

Radionuclide scanning (scintigraphy) of the sacroiliac joints has recently been advocated as a sensitive test in early disease, before radiographic changes are observed. Unfortunately, there are wide ranges of tracer uptake in normal sacroiliac joints, and there is a great deal of controversy regarding their specificity. They may be useful in detecting unilateral sacroiliitis and are probably of most value in localizing pyogenic infections in the sacroiliac joints and other spinal structures (8, 9).

Hematologic studies are usually normal. In patients with severe disease, however, there may be a mild normocytic-normochromic anemia reflective of chronic disease. The white blood cell count is usually

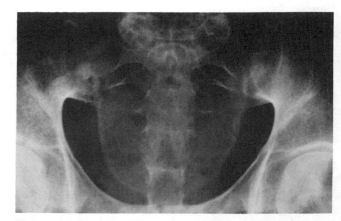

Figure 68.2 Late X-ray changes of sacroiliitis showing complete fusion of the joint space and loss of the early sclerotic change.

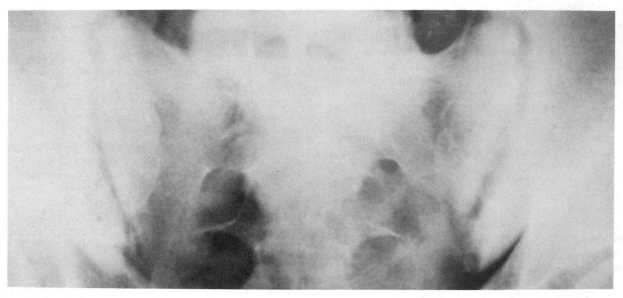

Figure 68.1 Relatively early X-ray changes of sacroiliitis showing bony sclerosis on both sides of the joint margins. Joint space erosions, a later manifestation of the disease, are present also.

normal as is the platelet count, although again those with highly inflammatory disease may demonstrate mild thrombocytosis. The erythrocyte sedimentation rate is usually elevated. *Serologic studies* are characteristically negative for rheumatoid factor and antinuclear antibodies, and serum complement levels are normal.

Tissue typing: HLA-B27 occurs in 90% of patients with sacroiliitis or spondylitis. This genetically determined tissue type occurs in approximately 8% of the normal white American population. Recently, HLA typing by many commercial laboratories has become available to practicing physicians and when properly used may be a helpful diagnostic aid in the assessment of a patient with low back symptoms or seronegative peripheral arthritis (12). It must be emphasized, however, that indiscriminate HLA typing cannot be substituted for a thorough clinical and radiographic evaluation of the patient. In fact, determination of B27 is rarely needed in making the diagnosis of spondylitis. There are unusual circumstances, however, where the patient gives a strong history suggestive of inflammatory back disease but in whom the radiographs are not yet diagnostic of sacroiliitis. It is in such situations that HLA typing may be helpful, most especially for children and women with early or atypical disease. Even then a positive B27 *does not confirm* a diagnosis of sacroiliitis, but provides supporting data for the diagnosis when the most specific finding (radiographic sacroiliitis) is not present.

Many patients will already know their tissue type or wish to have the test performed because of the hereditary impact of disease on their family. In these circumstances the physician must offer proper genetic counseling. The facts should be simply presented to the patient as they are currently known. It should be emphasized that spondylitis is not usually a life-threatening or crippling disorder and that symptoms can be controlled medically in the majority of patients. The likelihood that a family member will develop inflammatory back disease is low. Since HLA antigens, including B27, are inherited in a Mendelian dominant fashion, the risk of inheriting this tissue type would be 50% for each of a patient's children (this assumes that the opposite parent is negative for B27). Even if a child inherits this tissue type, his likelihood of developing arthritis is only 20% (see p. 667). Therefore, without any knowledge of HLA status, every child of a patient with B27-positive spondylitis has roughly a 10% (50% times 20%) chance of developing spondylitis.

The 90% probability of never developing this form of arthritis needs to be emphasized to patients concerned about this hereditary factor.

Course

It is impossible to predict the ultimate course of any patient presenting with sacroiliitis. The inflam-matory process may remain confined to these isolated joints or it may progressively ascend into the lumbar, thoracic, and cervical spinal segments. Likewise, the duration of time from onset of symptoms to fusion of higher spinal segments is highly variable. Thus, each patient should understand the nature of this illness and the need for *continued medical surveillance*, as well as the principles of physical and pharmacologic management of the disorder (Table 68.5).

Management

PHARMACOLOGIC

Anti-inflammatory drugs are used to relieve the pain and stiffness of the disease and to promote the patient's ability to perform the physical exercises so important to maintaining a good posture. It is unclear whether these drugs actually affect the natural history of the disease since no long term controlled studies are available. It seems likely, however, that they do alter and improve the overall functional capacity of the patient. Most often their use is required throughout the person's life; but, occasionally when symptoms completely remit, the anti-inflammatory agent may be tapered over several weeks and reinstituted if symptoms recur. Silent progress of the disease may occur; therefore, the physician should closely monitor these patients even when they are not on medication.

Salicylates (aspirin) may be tried as the initial anti-inflammatory drug. An initial dose of three tablets four times per day is usually sufficient to attain blood salicylate levels that are anti-inflammatory (15 to 25 mg/dl). Blood salicylate levels should be measured and the dosage adjusted to attain these levels. The majority of patients with ankylosing spondylitis will not have a dramatic response to salicylates; however, a trial of these inexpensive agents is often warranted before consideration is given to more potent and expensive nonsteroidal anti-inflammatory drugs.

Indomethacin (Indocin) is effective therapy in many patients in dosages up to 75 to 100 mg per day. Although hematologic reactions are far less common with this drug compared with phenylbutazone (see below), gastrointestinal intolerance and peptic ulcer disease as well as the central nervous system effects of severe morning frontal headache, vertigo, depression psychosis, hallucinations, and feelings of dis-

**Table 68.5
Principles of Management in Ankylosing Spondylitis**

Ensure patient understanding of disease process and objectives in management
Alleviation of pain and stiffness with anti-inflammatory drugs
Physical measures to maintain posture and range of motion in affected areas

sociation, may limit its usefulness. Additional *newer nonsteroidal anti-inflammatory agents* are now available including tolmetin (Tolectin), sulindac (Clinoril), naproxen (Naprosyn), and others which may prove more useful in individual patients or in those intolerant of indomethacin (see Chapter 67).

Phenylbutazone (Butazolidin, Azolid) appears to be the most effective agent in the majority of patients with spondylitic disease. Its long term use is indicated in patients with very active disease unresponsive to other anti-inflammatory agents; however, because of its potential serious side effects (see below), its prolonged use is not recommended without a thorough understanding by the patient of these risks (see below) and without consultation from a rheumatologist. The dosage varies from 200 to 400 mg per day with occasional patients requiring 600 mg for several days in order to suppress highly aggressive disease. Phenylbutazone has a long serum half-life (approximately 80 hours) and a single daily dose may be possible in some patients. The majority, however, will require divided doses usually 2 to 3 times per day. Lower doses should be used in older patients and in those with hepatic and renal disease. There are multiple interactions of this drug with other pharmacologic agents such as sulfa drugs (increased sulfonamide effect), anticoagulants (increased anticoagulation effect), oral hypoglycemics (increased sulfonylurea hypoglycemia), and phenytoin (increased phenytoin toxicity), and the physician should make himself aware of interactions between any other drug his patient is currently taking. The most serious potential side effect of phenylbutazone therapy relates to bone marrow suppression. Aplastic anemia, pancytopenia, granulocytopenia, or thrombocytopenia occur approximately 2 to 10 times for each one million prescriptions filled. Gastrointestinal effects include nausea, vomiting, peptic ulcer disease, and gastrointestinal bleeding. The drug should be used cautiously in patients with compromised cardiovascular status since fluid retention can result in congestive heart failure or pulmonary edema. Reduction of salt intake, especially in older patients, may reduce edema and the likelihood of fluid overload. Other side effects include skin rashes, hepatotoxicity, myocarditis, acute parotitis, vertigo, and anaphylaxis. Thus each patient should be informed of the potential side effects of phenylbutazone use, especially the hematologic ones, and consent to this avenue of therapy. Furthermore, complete blood counts should be obtained every 1 to 2 weeks during the first 3 months of therapy and every 4 to 6 weeks thereafter; however, once a fall in the blood count occurs from aplasia, stopping the drug usually will not reverse the process. If the patient is noncompliant or cannot obtain adequate hematologic follow-up, alternative agents should be used.

Radiation therapy to the spine was once an effective means of relieving pain. This form of treatment is no longer recommended because of the risk of subsequent leukemia.

PHYSICAL MEASURES

While anti-inflammatory agents relieve the pain and stiffness of spondylitis, an equally important function is their promotion of the patient's ability to perform the physical therapy program necessary to prevent spinal deformity and loss of motion in the joints. In fact, such a program can usually not be instituted until symptoms have been brought under control. The natural history of the disease should be explained so that the patient understands the rationale for the exercise program which he must follow (and which the physician will need to reinforce) over many years. An erect posture when sitting or standing should be encouraged. The patient's bed should be quite firm or should be supported by a bed board. Use of a pillow should be avoided or the smallest possible pillow should be used to prevent flexion of the neck. Sleeping in the prone position is most efficacious in promoting spinal extension, but the supine position is adequate if there is good support. The patient should refrain from sleeping on his side in a curled up posture.

An active exercise program to promote extension of the back, and range of motion of the axial and peripheral joints as well as breathing exercises to maintain chest expansion should be instituted and executed two to three times per day. Referral to a physical therapist to provide specific instructions and to determine that the patient is performing well is a good investment. Swimming is an excellent exercise for the patient with ankylosing spondylitis.

If spinal structures undergo complete ankylosis, the danger of spinal fracture after even minor trauma is increased. This is especially true in the neck, where whiplash types of injury occur. Thus, the spondylitic patient should take special precautions to prevent injury, including the use of a soft cervical collar when automobile riding or when walking on slippery surfaces.

Prognosis

The prognosis for ankylosing spondylitis is excellent. The majority of patients can be managed successfully by pharmacologic and physical means. Most continue to lead productive lives in their chosen professions, and change in vocational plans is usually not indicated. The morbidity from articular and extra-articular complications is low, and life-span is not reduced significantly, if at all. In many instances pain in an affected area of the spine disappears after that segment has fused and often disease halts at a particular segment and does not proceed to others. While these facts should be optimistically presented to the patient, they are not cause for laxity in following the postural and exercise program and maintaining close medical surveillance.

REITER'S SYNDROME

Definition

Unlike ankylosing spondylitis, Reiter's syndrome is primarily a peripheral arthritis. It shares with ankylosing spondylitis, however, a predisposition to affect young white men, and a tendency for sacroiliitis or spondylitis, inflammation of tendon and fascial attachments, uveitis, the same cardiac complications, and a strong association with HLA-B27 (75% positive). Although classically defined as the triad of nongonococcal urethritis, conjunctivitis, and arthritis, it has recently been found that the majority of patients do not express the classical triad, and that approximately 40% of patients will have arthritis as the only feature of the triad. This latter group has been termed "incomplete Reiter's syndrome," and diagnosis depends upon recognition of the typical pattern of arthritis, the presence of mucocutaneous lesions, and other features that are discriminating (2). Reiter's syndrome may, in fact, be the most common cause of arthritis in young men, even exceeding the prevalence of ankylosing spondylitis. Women are less often affected and comprise only 10 to 15% of most series. The diagnosis and management of the disease focus primarily on symptoms and signs referable to the joints and nonarticular musculoskeletal structures. The diagnosis is made on clinical grounds based upon a constellation of symptoms and signs. Typing for HLA-B27 may be a useful diagnostic aid in the incomplete or atypical case.

History and Examination

The principal clues to the diagnosis of Reiter's syndrome are summarized in Table 68.6. The patient presenting with Reiter's syndrome is usually a young white male between puberty and age 40. Blacks and Orientals are affected far less commonly, presumably due to the relatively low frequency of HLA-B27 in these groups. The reason for low female affectability is unclear.

The disorder occurs in two settings. First, the disease may follow an episode of diarrhea caused by *Shigella*, *Salmonella*, or *Yersinia* (see Chapter 25). This postdysenteric form constitutes approximately 15% of most series in the United States. Second, the endemic form is believed to result from venereal exposure to unknown pathogens. Much of the evidence supporting this notion is debatable and clearly there are a large number of patients with Reiter's disease where no antecedent diarrheal or venereal event can be ascertained.

In the classical form, urethritis with mild dysuria and a mucopurulent discharge is usually the first symptom, followed shortly by conjunctivitis. Arthritis is usually the last feature of the triad to appear, usually from several days up to 1 month following the onset of urethritis. The arthritis is typically in the lower extremities, involving only one to four joints, most commonly the knees, ankles, and small joints of the feet. The patient notes pain, swelling, heat, and erythema over the joints in the majority of cases of this highly inflammatory disease. In addition to frank arthritis, over 50% of patients will have nonarticular musculoskeletal pain. Heel pain due to inflammation of the plantar aponeurosis or Achilles tendon insertion is one of the most prominent symptoms of the disease and may be one of the most disabling. Diffuse swelling of digits (sausaging), especially the toes, also occurs in over 50% of patients and is indicative of involvement not only of the joints but of tendons and periosteal structures.

The mucocutaneous features of Reiter's syndrome are often asymptomatic and must be sought on physical examination. These include (a) painless shallow oral ulcers usually on the tongue and palate, (b) circinate balanitis manifested by shallow moist painless ulcers on the glans penis in uncircumcised men or a dry scaling eruption on the glans in the circumcised, (c) hyperkeratosis and crumbling of nails, and (d) keratoderma blennorrhagica, a papulosquamous skin eruption usually beginning on the palms and soles which closely resembles pustular psoriasis.

Additional features include fever in approximately one-third of patients, weight loss, and uveitis. The disease may begin abruptly and run a toxic course, or very insidiously and pursue an indolent one. Not infrequently heel pain is the first symptom, and this complaint in a young man should raise the question of emerging Reiter's syndrome.

Laboratory Tests

Hematologic studies will usually demonstrate a mild normocytic normochromic anemia characteristic of chronic disease. The hematocrit value rarely falls below 30%. A modest leukocytosis in the range of 10,000 to 15,000/cu mm with a mild shift to the left occurs frequently in those with an acute toxic presentation. Thrombocytosis with platelet counts in the range of 400,000 to 600,000/cu mm is found in approximately one-third. The erythrocyte sedimentation rate is usually elevated.

Serologic studies for rheumatoid factor and antinuclear antibodies are negative. Serum complement is typically normal or elevated as an acute phase reactant. *HLA typing* will reveal the B27 antigen in

Table 68.6
Clues to the Diagnosis of Reiter's Syndrome

A young man with arthritis
Preceding diarrhea, urethritis, or conjunctivitis
Lower extremity oligoarthritis (knee, ankle, foot)
Heel pain and/or sausaging of digits
Rash on soles, penis; painless oral ulcers; dystrophic nails
Fever, weight loss, leukocytosis

HLA-B27 antigen

75% of cases, but is rarely required in diagnosing the disease. *Radiographs* are typically normal early in the course of the disease; however, over time, periostitis may be seen involving the calcaneus or along the shafts of swollen digits. Should sacroiliitis appear, it is more likely to be unilateral in this disease than in ankylosing spondylitis. In severe disease cartilage may be lost in joint spaces and bony ankylosis may ensue.

Synovial fluid has the characteristics of a moderate inflammatory process with a poor mucin clot, white blood cell counts ranging from 5,000 to 50,000/cu mm, elevated protein, normal glucose, and a high complement (in contradistinction to the synovial fluid hypocomplementemia of rheumatoid arthritis). Culture shows that the synovial fluid is sterile. *Synovial biopsy* demonstrates an acute and chronic inflammatory process which is nonspecific and indistinguishable from that of many other inflammatory synovitides and therefore it is not usually necessary. Urethral stains and cultures are negative for gonococci in the majority, although the concurrence of gonococcal urethritis with Reiter's syndrome has been documented. Therefore, this culture should not be overlooked.

Course and Prognosis

Reiter's syndrome follows a self-limited course and completely resolves in 3 months to 1 year in approximately one-third of patients. Another 30 to 40% of patients will have relapses after months or years of quiescence. It has been estimated that a patient with this disease has a 15% chance of having another episode each year for as long as 30 years. Less commonly, a chronic progressive course ensues resulting in articular destruction and fusion of peripheral, and usually axial skeletal joints. Disability results primarily from severe heel pain, deformities of the feet, visual loss due to uveitis, and, less commonly, cardiac complications. Approximately 10% of patients will become permanently disabled and unable to work (6).

Management

Treatment is directed toward suppressing the inflammatory process in joints and tendon insertions and preventing deformity of the peripheral and axial skeleton. Likewise, uveal tract involvement requires close follow-up and treatment by an ophthalmologist in order to prevent permanent visual loss. Phenylbutazone and indomethacin have been found to be most effective in suppressing the articular inflammation in this disease. Salicylates are helpful in a minority of patients but may be worthy of trial. Dosage recommendations and adverse side effects are similar to those for ankylosing spondylitis. Systemic corticosteroids may be necessary to treat severe uveitis or inflamed joints which have been unresponsive to phenylbutazone or other nonsteroidal anti-inflammatory drugs, and in these instances consultation with a rheumatologist is suggested. At times, intra-articular corticosteroid injection (usually performed by a rheumatologist) may be useful when systemic therapy has not completely suppressed the inflammatory process. Only occasional patients with extensive cutaneous and articular disease will require more radical therapy (e.g., cytotoxic drugs) and consultation with a rheumatologist should be sought in these circumstances. Anti-inflammatory agents are generally continued for several months and then tapered in those whose symptoms are completely controlled. However, many patients will need continued, lifelong anti-inflammatory agents to suppress the inflammatory activity of the disease. Also, approximately 30 to 40% (see above) of those who have had symptomatic remissions will experience a relapse and require the reinstitution of anti-inflammatory medications. *Tetracycline or erythromycin* may be effective in treating the nongonococcal urethritis; however, it is unclear whether this therapy influences the subsequent emergence or course of the articular disease.

Physical measures are important adjuncts in the management of this disorder as in ankylosing spondylitis. There is a tendency for fusion of peripheral joints as well as axial ones. During acute inflammatory episodes, rest is important, and severely inflamed joints should be splinted to ensure comfort for the patient. As soon as inflammation can be brought under control with drugs, it is important that affected joints be exercised to maintain their ranges of motion. At first passive range of motion should be encouraged in all affected joints. Later, more active range of motion and strengthening exercises should be prescribed as the patient improves.

Painful feet, especially heels, may be helped by shoe inserts which shift weight-bearing to nonaffected areas (see also Chapter 99).

References

General

Bluestone, R: Ankylosing spondylitis. In *Arthritis and Allied Conditions*, Ed. 9, edited by DJ McCarty. Lea & Febiger, Philadelphia, 1979.

Sharp, JT: Reiter's syndrome. In *Arthritis and Allied Conditions*, Ed. 9, edited by DJ McCarty. Lea & Febiger, Philadelphia, 1979.

These two chapters provide comprehensive reviews of those two common forms of sacroiliitis.

Specific

1. Arnett, FC, Bias, WB and Stevens, MB: Juvenile-onset chronic arthritis: clinical and roentgenographic features of a unique HLA-B27 subset. *Am J Med 69:* 369, 1980.
2. Arnett, FC, McClusky, OE, Schacter, BZ and Lordon, RE: Incomplete Reiter's syndrome: discriminating features and HL-A W27 in diagnosis. *Ann Intern Med 84:* 8, 1976.
3. Calin, A and Fries, JF: Striking prevalence of ankylosing spondylitis in "healthy" W27 positive males and females. *N Engl J Med 293:* 835, 1975.
4. Edmonds, J, Macauley, D, Tyndall, A, Liew, M, Alexander, K,

Geczy, A and Bashir, H: Lymphocytotoxicity of anti-Klebsiella antisera in ankylosing spondylitis and related arthropathies. *Arthritis Rheum 24:* 1, 1981.

5. Enlow, RW, Bias, WB and Arnett, FC: The spondylitis of inflammatory bowel disease. *Arthritis Rheum 23:* 1359, 1980.
6. Fox, R, Calin, A, Gerber, RC and Gibson, D: The chronicity of symptoms and disability in Reiter's syndrome. *Ann Intern Med 91:* 190, 1979.
7. Gofton, JP, Chalmers, A, Price, GE and Reeve, CE: HL-A27 and ankylosing spondylitis in B.C. Indians. *J Rheumatol 2:* 314, 1975.
8. Gordon, G and Kabins, SA: Pyogenic sacroiliitis. *Am J Med 69:* 50, 1980.
9. Greyson, ND: Radionuclide bone and joint imaging in rheu-matology. *Bull Rheum Dis 30:* 1034, 1980.
10. Hochberg, MC, Bias, WB and Arnett, FC: Family studies in HLA-B27 associated arthritis. *Medicine (Baltimore) 57:* 463, 1978.
11. Hochberg, MC, Borenstein, DG and Arnett, FC: The absence of back pain in classical ankylosing spondylitis. *Johns Hopkins Med J 143:* 181, 1978.
12. Khan, MA: Clinical application of the HLA-B27 test in rheumatic disease. *Arch Intern Med 140:* 177, 1980.
13. Khan, MA, Braun, WE, Kushner, I, Grecek, DE, Angus Muir, W and Steinberg, AG: HLA-B27 in ankylosing spondylitis: differences in frequency and relative risk in American blacks and Caucasians. *J Rheumatol 3:* 39, 1977.

SECTION 10

Metabolic and Endocrinologic Problems

CHAPTER SIXTY-NINE

Diabetes Mellitus

ROBERT I. GREGERMAN, M.D.

DEFINITION AND CLASSIFICATION

Diabetes mellitus is a condition characterized by an abnormality of glucose utilization and associated with elevation of blood glucose concentration. Approximately 10 million people in the United States are diabetic by this definition. Diabetes mellitus is not a single distinct disease entity. The commonest varieties of diabetes mellitus are known to be associated with abnormalities of insulin secretion and concentration, with cellular resistance to insulin action, and with vascular abnormalities such as basement membrane thickening. Nonetheless, diagnosis is based on the finding of persistently abnormal blood glucose concentrations at some time in life.

Until recently there has been no general agreement on the classification of diabetes mellitus, based either on etiology or manifestations. A new terminology has recently been proposed by the National Diabetes Data Group of the National Institutes of Health (8). This classification is followed in this chapter; it has the endorsement of at least the majorities of the American Diabetes Association and of many diabetologists in both the United States, the United Kingdom, and elsewhere (Table 69.1).

Table 69.1
Classification of Diabetes Mellitus and Other States of Glucose Intolerance

Type of Diabetes	Former Terminology	Clinical Characteristics
INSULIN-DEPENDENT TYPE (IDDM, TYPE I)	Juvenile diabetes Juvenile onset-type diabetes Ketosis-prone diabetes Brittle diabetes	Onset usually in youth but occurs at any age. Insulin deficiency requires exogenous insulin to prevent ketosis-acidosis. Non-insulin-dependent phases may occur during natural history. 10–12% of all cases

NON-INSULIN-DEPENDENT TYPES (NIDDM, TYPE II):
  Nonobese NIDDM
  Obese NIDDM
	Adult onset diabetes, maturity onset diabetes (MOD), stable diabetes, nonketosis-prone diabetes; in young people was called maturity onset diabetes of youth (MODY)	Onset generally after age 40, but may occur in young; not insulin-dependent or ketosis-prone, but may need insulin for control of persistent hyperglycemia; periods of ketosis-acidosis may occur during stress of illness; weight control of obese subtype may ameliorate disease. 80% of all cases

OTHER TYPES:
  Diabetes mellitus associated with
    Pancreatic disease
    Hormone excess due to endocrine disease or hormone treatment (steroids of glucocorticoid type)
    Drug use
    Insulin receptor abnormalities
	Secondary diabetes	Diagnosis demands usual abnormalities of glucose handling and documentation of associated condition

Impaired glucose tolerance (IGT)
  Nonobese IGT
  Obese IGT
  IGT associated with certain conditions and syndromes
  Drug (chemical) induced
  Insulin receptor abnormalities
  Genetic syndromes
	Asymptomatic diabetes; chemical diabetes; subclinical diabetes; borderline diabetes; latent diabetes	Diabetes is based on abnormality of glucose handling: may represent a stage of development of diabetes, although most remain in this class for years or revert to normal glucose tolerance

Gestational diabetes mellitus (GDM)	Gestational diabetes	Glucose intolerance has *onset* during pregnancy; does not include diabetic who becomes pregnant: increased risk of perinatal complications and future diabetes

Non-insulin-dependent Diabetes Mellitus (NIDDM: Type II)

This is the commonest form of diabetes mellitus and accounts for about 80% of patients presenting with an abnormality of glucose metabolism. The majority of patients are obese. Patients with NIDDM are neither absolutely dependent on treatment with insulin nor ketosis-prone. Nonetheless, treatment with insulin may be necessary in order to control hyperglycemia which leads to symptoms through osmotic diuresis. Furthermore, such patients do sometimes develop insulin dependence as the result of stress (severe infections, trauma). NIDDM is very likely a heterogeneous disorder. Although most patients are over age 40 at the time of diagnosis, this type of disease is also seen in young persons, and it is for this reason that older terms such as "maturity onset type diabetes" should be abandoned.

NIDDM has a much more obvious familial pattern of expression than does insulin-dependent diabetes mellitus (IDDM, see below). Included in the group of NIDDM are patients who develop the disease before they reach adulthood (formerly known as "maturity onset diabetes of the young" or MODY). Behavioral and possibly environmental factors appear to be involved in the onset of NIDDM. Especially prominent is the role of excessive caloric intake and subsequent obesity in 60 to 90% of cases. In this type of diabetes, association with certain histocompatibility antigen (HLA) subtypes and antibodies to islet cells has not been found. Blood insulin levels are variable and may be normal, subnormal, or even supranormal; insulin resistance is common. However, measurement of insulin concentration has no diagnostic usefulness.

Insulin-dependent Diabetes Mellitus (IDDM: Type I)

This type of diabetes—which accounts for about 10% of cases—*generally* has its onset in childhood or in early adulthood, hence the former name "juvenile onset diabetes mellitus." However, that designation was misleading, since this type of diabetes can occur at any time of life. Moreover, its essential characteristic is that insulin dependence is absolute; without insulin therapy, ketosis-acidosis usually ensues rapidly. Although the disease is probably heterogeneous, genetic determinants are important in most of these patients (see below). Rare cases may have a viral basis, but even in these, genetic predisposition may be important. A minority of siblings of patients with IDDM develop diabetes; when tested initially, these individuals may show only impaired glucose tolerance but eventually develop overt IDDM. Increased or decreased frequency of certain histocompatibility antigens, abnormal immune responses and autoimmunity, and antibodies to islet cells have been demonstrated in IDDM. None of these findings is currently useful in a diagnostic sense.

Inheritance and Genetic Counseling

The genetics of IDDM (formerly juvenile) and NIDDM (formerly adult onset) are different; surprisingly, familial expression is greater in the latter group. The precise genetics, however, are not clear, and prediction of the occurrence of diabetes in offspring of diabetic parents is not possible; even statistical estimates are crude (6). The prevalence of overt diabetes in offspring of conjugal diabetic parents is remarkably low, ranging from 3 to 12% in most reports. Contributing to the difficulty of prediction are the criteria for detection of diabetes (overt diabetes vs. diabetes detected by glucose tolerance testing; see pp. 680–683) and age of onset.

The conclusion that hereditary factors are more important in NIDDM than in IDDM comes from studies of twins. If expression of diabetes were based entirely on genetic grounds, one would expect 100% concordance for diabetes in monozygotic twins; but this is not the case for patients diagnosed when young (before age 40). Only in twins in whom diagnosis is made later in life is 100% concordance approached. Thus, environmental factors must be important in younger diabetics.

Studies of ethnic groups show distinctive patterns of diabetes and superimposed geographic (environmental) effects upon these patterns. The most easily apparent determinant is obesity. Certain American Indian tribes show a remarkably high prevalence of diabetes (Pima; Navajo); obesity appears to be the major factor in expression of the disease in these people. In terms of the patterns of disease, in South Africa, black and Indian populations have similar environments and diets, but only the black diabetics are ketosis-prone. In contrast, the Indians have more frequent vascular disease. In non-Indian populations in the United States, no such distinctive ethnic or racial patterns have been recognized to date.

Parents who have produced an insulin-dependent diabetic offspring often wish to know the risk to future offspring. Prenatal HLA typing of fetal cells obtained at amniocentesis could be compared to that of the diabetic sibling; a fetus with the same HLA identity would increase the risk, but the accuracy of the prediction would still be only about 50%. The imprecise nature of this assessment is in contrast to the nearly 100% certainty of predicting Tay-Sachs disease or Down's syndrome. Thus, even with an accurate family history and pedigree, together with chemical assessment of diabetes (glucose tolerance testing), only crude predictions can be made for a couple who wish to know their own chances of developing diabetes and to know the risk for their offspring (6).

At this point, only a few generalities seem safe. Prospective parents should not be told to avoid procreation merely because one parent is diabetic. Even when both parents are diabetic, the risk seems relatively low. If avoidance of pregnancy is decided upon, a diabetic mother may be at increased risk from several commonly used contraceptive measures, although the evidence for this increased risk is not firm. Estrogen-based contraceptives may be unwise because of possibly increased risk in the diabetic of vascular thrombosis and hyperlipidemia. Intrauterine devices may possibly produce infection more often in a diabetic. Thus, mechanical means of contraception such as diaphragm or condom would seem to be the safest methods (see Chapter 90).

Other Types of Diabetes

Sometimes diabetes is associated with another condition or disease; usually the association is infrequent but more common than in the general population (Table 69.2). This heterogeneous group includes some disorders in which there is a clear relationship between the associated disease and the diabetes and others in which an association has been noted but is not well understood. For example, in pancreatic insufficiency due to pancreatitis, insufficient insulin may be produced and insulin-dependent diabetes mellitus ensues. At the opposite extreme, an associ-

Table 69.2
Diseases Associated with Diabetes Mellitus or Abnormal Glucose Tolerance

ENDOCRINE DISORDERS
  Acromegaly
  Aldosteronism
  Glucocorticoid excess (Cushing's syndrome; iatrogenic)
  Hyperthyroidism
  Pheochromocytoma
AUTOIMMUNE DISORDERS
  Adrenal insufficiency (Addison's disease)
  Hashimoto's disease
  Hypoparathyroidism
  Myasthenia gravis
  Pernicious anemia
  Polyglandular failure (adrenals/gonads/thyroid)
  Primary hypothyroidism
OTHER DISORDERS
  Chronic pancreatitis

ation between aldosterone excess in primary aldosteronism and diabetes mellitus has been observed, but the mechanism is not clear. Glucocorticoid excess, as in Cushing's syndrome or steroid therapy, may produce diabetes mellitus. Recently, rare cases of diabetes associated with antibodies to insulin receptors have been described.

Problems in Classification of Individual Patients

On occasion, classification may be difficult. For example, an adult presenting with ketosis-acidosis may be erroneously classified as IDDM when in fact the individual's diabetes is of the NIDDM type, with insulin dependence having been precipitated by the stress of infection. Similarly, the process of distinguishing between a patient with IDDM and a thin NIDDM patient for whom insulin has merely been prescribed may require discontinuation of the insulin therapy, a procedure which may be impractical. Diagnostic procedures necessary to exclude the possibility that the diabetes is one of the other types (e.g., Cushing's syndrome, hemochromatosis, etc.) may not have been performed. In addition, for those patients in whom diagnosis was based on an abnormality of glucose tolerance, diagnostic criteria may not have been met, or may have been equivocal (see p. 681). In these situations, classification should be considered tentative.

CLINICAL PRESENTATION

Most diagnoses of diabetes mellitus are now made at an asymptomatic stage of the disease as a result of routine blood tests which reveal elevation of blood glucose concentration. In some institutions where the diagnosis is actively sought, glucose tolerance tests reveal many cases. Of those patients who are symptomatic at time of diagnosis, most will complain of increased frequency of urination (polyuria), excessive thirst with increased fluid intake (polydipsia), and, if the disease is very severe, increased appetite and increased food consumption (polyphagia) associated with weight loss. All of these symptoms are manifestations of excessive blood sugar and of secondary glucosuria. Other symptomatic manifestations include blurred vision, vaginitis (usually due to monilial infection), and skin infections. Furuncles and carbuncles, once common, are now rarely seen, but intertriginous moniliasis is common in the obese. Oral moniliasis is uncommon.

Usually, these symptoms are present for weeks or months before medical attention is sought. The onset of symptoms is often insidious and may be attributed by the patient, or even by the physician, to emotional factors or to a common problem such as a urinary tract infection. Indeed, the diagnosis may be missed for a time because the physician "knows" that the patient is not a diabetic on the basis of previous evaluation.

Some patients present with absent or minimal di-abetic, i.e., glucosuria-related, symptoms but have already developed complications of the diabetic state such as neuropathy or, more commonly, vascular disease. However, only rarely will a patient be unaware of diabetes and yet present with severe complications of the disease such as diabetic ophthalmopathy or nephropathy.

DIAGNOSIS

Elevation of blood sugar concentration is the hallmark of diabetes mellitus. Glucosuria alone is not a diagnostic finding, however, since rare individuals may have a renal tubular glucose "leak" (renal glucosuria) at normal concentrations of blood sugar. Only infrequently will individuals show diagnostically elevated blood sugar levels before glucosuria develops ("elevated renal threshold").

New Criteria for Diagnosis of Diabetes Mellitus

New criteria have been suggested as follows (Tables 69.3 and 69.4) (8): (a) unequivocal elevation of plasma glucose (PG) concentrations associated with classic symptoms of diabetes mellitus, or (b) elevation of fasting plasma glucose (FPG) on more than one occasion, or (c) elevation of PG following an oral glucose challenge on more than one occasion. A single elevated FPG or a single oral glucose tolerance test never establishes the diagnosis.

In most modern laboratories glucose is determined in plasma or serum. Plasma and serum values are identical, but both are 5 to 15% higher than are obtained using whole blood. The physician should be aware of the laboratory's procedure, lest inappropriate diagnosis is made because of methodologic differences.

Impaired Glucose Tolerance (IGT) vs. Diabetes Mellitus

The standards promulgated in Tables 69.3 and 69.4 are not arbitrary, but have been derived from many studies and numerous considerations, including prospective studies conducted in the United States and Britain over the past 15 years. These standards, first published in 1979, supersede those in general use for many years. The older standards for the oral glucose tolerance test (OGTT) were clearly set at levels of blood sugar that were too low and reduced the specificity of the test (high number of false positive results). Perhaps most widely used in the past were the criteria of Fajans and Conn and standards promoted by the U.S. Public Health Service, World Health Organization, etc. In general, the upper limits of normal at 1 hour had been set at between 180 and 195 mg/dl; and for 2 hours, at 140 to 160 mg/dl.

Although some disagreement will inevitably exist on all standards, perhaps the most important point for the clinician to recall is that no single value of fasting glucose or combination of values in glucose tolerance tests sharply divides diabetics from nondi-

Table 69.3
Normal Plasma Glucose Concentrations [a]

Fasting state (10–16 hr postprandial)	
Venous plasma	<115 mg/dl
Venous whole blood	<100 mg/dl
Capillary whole blood	<100 mg/dl
2-Hour oral glucose tolerance test (OGTT)	
Venous plasma	<140 mg/dl
Venous whole blood	<120 mg/dl
Capillary whole blood	<140 mg/dl

Values between those which are diagnostic (see Table 69.4) and those which are normal should be considered *non*diagnostic. Impaired glucose tolerance (IGT) is considered present when three criteria are met: (a) fasting level is below diagnostic, (b) 2-hr value is intermediate, and (c) some other value (½, 1, 1½) must be elevated to:

Venous plasma	>200 mg/dl
Venous whole blood	>180 mg/dl
Capillary whole blood	>200 mg/dl

[a] To express values as millimoles/liter, multiply glucose in mg/dl × 0.056. Serum and plasma values are the same.

Table 69.4
Diagnosis of Diabetes: Diagnostic Concentrations of Glucose

Fasting state (10–16 hr postprandial)
  Venous plasma [a]   >140 mg/dl
  Venous whole blood >120 mg/dl
  Capillary whole blood >140 mg/dl
Oral glucose tolerance test (OGTT) *preparation*: fasting 10–16 hr during which no caffeine-containing drinks or smoking is permitted.
  75-g glucose (40 g/m^2)
    Use in nonpregnant adults: (1.75 g/kg for children. Up to 75 g maximum). Dosage form: flavored water, 25 g glucose/100 dl. Drink over 5 min. Obtain blood samples at 0, ½, 1, 1½, 2 hr
    Test positive for diabetes mellitus: *both* the 2-hour sample *and* at least one other sample must meet following criteria:
      Venous plasma   >200 mg/dl
      Venous whole blood >180 mg/dl
      Capillary whole blood >200 mg/dl
  100-g glucose
    Use only in pregnant adults: obtain blood samples at 0, 1, 2, 3 hr
    Test positive for diabetes mellitus: *two* or more of the following values must be met or exceeded:

	Venous plasma (mg/dl)	Venous Whole Blood (mg/dl)	Capillary Whole Blood (mg/dl)
Fasting	105 mg/dl	90	90
1 hr	190	170	170
2 hr	165	145	145
3 hr	145	125	125

[a] Serum and plasma values are the same.

abetics. Most populations exhibit a continuous unimodal distribution of values, usually skewed to the higher end. (An exception is the Pima Indian population in which bimodal distribution of both fasting and 2-hour post-glucose values is seen (10)). The Fajans and Conn criteria were simply statistically based, *i.e.*, individuals were deemed diabetic if their 1-, 1½-, and 2-hour values were greater than 2 standard deviations above the mean for a group of healthy adults who were less than 50 years old. In contrast, the new criteria are derived from prospective observations of the fate of individuals whose glucose concentrations fall within certain ranges. The conclusions from such studies are as follows:

1. Individuals whose plasma glucose levels during the OGTT fall between normal (1 hour < 160 mg/dl; 2 hours < 140 mg/dl) and diabetic should be clearly classified into a group (impaired glucose tolerance, IGT) separate from those with overt glucose intolerance.

2. In this IGT group, one can expect 1 to 5% per year to develop symptomatic diabetes mellitus or diagnostically abnormal glucose tolerance. On the other hand, many such individuals eventually show normalization of glucose tolerance while still others remain in the IGT range. The higher the blood sugar within the range of IGT, the greater the tendency for tolerance to deteriorate.

Perhaps the most convincing evidence on IGT progression has come from a long term study of Pima Indians (2, 8, 10). The risk of progression to overt diabetes in this group was clearly related to the level of glucose within the range of 160 to 200 mg at 2 hours (3 times that of persons with lower values). In this group, however, the rate of decompensation to overt diabetes was still only 3% per year.

3. Treatment of the IGT group with oral antidi-abetic (hypoglycemic) agents had no effect on the eventual development of diabetes.

4. Diabetic microvascular complications (retinopathy or nephropathy) do *not* develop in individuals with IGT. On the other hand, in the study of Pima Indians, values > 240 mg/dl were associated with such changes.

SIGNIFICANCE OF IMPAIRMENT OF GLUCOSE TOLERANCE FOR DEVELOPMENT OF CARDIOVASCULAR DISEASE

Although morbidity and mortality from cardiovascular disease is unequivocally increased in patients with clinical diabetes mellitus, the issue of the impact of IGT on such events is unsettled. The National Diabetes Data Group Study concluded that morbidty and mortality from arteriosclerotic disease appeared to be significantly increased in patients with IGT, although to a lesser degree than the 2- to 3-fold increase seen in overt diabetes (8). On the other hand, no such conclusion could be drawn from later studies in 15 populations of the impact of IGT on development of coronary artery disease (11). In some of these studies, a strong relationship was found between IGT and coronary heart disease death rates, but in others no such relationship was evident. No satisfactory explanation is available to explain these discrepancies. At this time, IGT cannot be designated as an established risk factor for coronary heart disease or other cardiovascular diseases.

Fasting Plasma Glucose (FPG)

Elevation of FPG should be followed up by several repeat measurements of the FPG on different days. Since over 90% of individuals with repeated elevations of FPG will have an abnormal glucose tolerance test (OGTT), little is gained by proceeding directly to such a test. FPG may be elevated by stress and illness, but is actually less subject to this change than is the OGTT. When an illness results in elevation of FPG (or an abnormal OGTT) only to revert to normal with recovery, the question which arises is whether a "diabetic" state has been unmasked or whether the transient elevation is simply the result of disturbed carbohydrate metabolism associated with the illness. Only long term follow-up may sometimes provide an answer. In the interim, the individual may be deemed to have IGT (see above). The terms subclinical, preclinical, chemical, latent, and borderline diabetes, etc., should be avoided, both because of their uncertain meaning and because of the psychologic trauma and economic penalties (e.g., insurance ratings, job qualifications) that are often needlessly created.

The 2-Hour Postprandial Blood Sugar as a Screening Test

This frequently used procedure should be abandoned. Only infrequently will a gross elevation of postprandial sugar be seen when the FPG is normal. Initially nondiagnostic but abnormal elevations (e.g., 140 to 200 mg/dl) are often not observed on follow-up testing with an OGTT. Even a normal glucose concentration 2 hours postprandially has no established value for predicting that an OGTT would be normal. The 2-hour postprandial blood sugar with glucose added to the meal is similarly to be avoided.

Use of the Oral Glucose Tolerance Test

Diagnostic criteria for the OGTT are listed in Tables 69.3 and 69.4; Table 69.4 also shows how the test is performed. The OGTT is not necessary if there is unequivocal elevation of plasma glucose in a patient who has classic symptoms of diabetes or if the fasting plasma glucose is elevated on more than one occasion (see p. 681). Indeed, in the absence of signs and symptoms of diabetes, relatively few clinical indications exist for attempted establishment of a diagnosis of diabetes mellitus solely by use of the OGTT.

INDICATIONS

The physician may wish to perform the test because of a positive family history. Occasionally, he may wish to prognosticate for a sibling of a diabetic. The OGTT does have a place in diagnosis during pregnancy (see below). The test is also sometimes performed in an individual who manifests premature atherosclerosis or has unexplained neuropathy or retinopathy. However, under such conditions a positive OGTT is ordinarily, at most, no more than suggestive of a cause of the disorder at hand. For example, premature atherosclerosis certainly occurs in nondiabetics and in the face of normal glucose tolerance. Perhaps a greater constraint on the use of the OGTT for early diagnosis is the realization that, given the limitations of currently available therapeutic measures, the physician does not—except in obese individuals—undertake therapy directed at improvement of an abnormal OGTT. In many patients, therefore, no immediate therapeutic benefit is likely to result from uncovering an abnormal OGTT. Moreover, the "labeling effect" associated with an abnormal OGTT may create unnecessary morbidity in a previously healthy person.

LIMITATIONS

A number of other considerations impose limitations on the usefulness of the OGTT. A variety of illnesses, both acute and chronic, produce abnormalities of the OGTT. Infection, trauma, drugs, and even physical inactivity may produce a "diabetic" OGTT (Table 69.4). Following myocardial infarction, many weeks may be required before normal glucose tolerance is again seen, and at least 2 weeks may be required after a febrile illness. Testing with OGTT should certainly be postponed under these circumstances. Reduced food intake with less than 150 g of carbohydrate/day can also produce an abnormal test within a few days as can fasting beyond 16 hours. Even performance of the test in the afternoon rather than in the morning may produce elevated levels of blood sugar. Smoking immediately before or during the test can produce an abnormal result, as may the ingestion of caffeine-containing drinks (coffee, tea) in the period of fasting. If nausea, vomiting, or diaphoresis occurs during the test, the results are invalid and the test should be terminated. A repeat test may not necessarily provoke these symptoms. Beyond all of these caveats, great variability in any patient's OGTT response is well established, so that a diagnosis of diabetes *cannot* be established on the basis of a single abnormal test.

Drug Effects on Glucose Tolerance

Table 69.5 gives a list of drugs and related substances which have been reported to be associated with decreased glucose tolerance and even with the development of symptomatic diabetes mellitus. The agents most often responsible are glucocorticoids (cortisone, prednisone, etc.) and the diuretics used in the long term therapy of hypertension. Potassium depletion—which can be present even when serum potassium is normal—is one mechanism by which diuretics can produce glucose intolerance. Other

Table 69.5
Drugs Associated with Abnormal Glucose Tolerance or Diabetes Mellitus

HORMONES AND RELATED AGENTS
  ACTH
  Catecholamines (epinephrine, isoproterenol, levodopa)
  Dextrothyroxine
  Estrogens (oral contraceptives)
  Glucocorticoids (cortisone and derivatives)
  Thyroxine and triiodothyronine (toxic doses)
DIURETICS AND ANTIHYPERTENSIVE DRUGS
  Chlorthalidone (Hygroton, Combipres, Regroton)
  Clonidine (Catapres, Combipres)
  Ethacrynic acid (Edecrin)
  Furosemide (Lasix)
  Thiazides (Diuril, Hydrodiuril, etc.)
PSYCHOACTIVE AGENTS
  Chlorprothixene (Taractan)
  Haloperidol (Haldol)
  Lithium (Lithane, Eskalith)
  Phenothiazines (Thorazine, Trilafon, Etrafon, Triavil, etc.)
  Tricyclic antidepressants
    Amitriptyline (Elavil, Endep, Triavil, etc.)
    Desipramine (Norpramin, Pertofrane)
    Doxepin (Adapin, Sinequan)
    Imipramine (Presamine, Tofranil)
    Nortriptyline (Aventyl)
MISCELLANEOUS
  Antineoplastic drugs (L-asparaginase, streptozotocin)
  Indomethacin
  Isoniazid (INH)
  Nicotinic acid

drugs also affect glucose tolerance, but do so much less often. Despite their tendency to decrease glucose tolerance, these drugs should not be withheld when medically indicated. A common error is to fail to use a diuretic in a diabetic hypertensive patient for fear of exacerbating glucose intolerance. Although blood pressure control may be attempted by using nondiuretic agents (see Chapter 59), failure to achieve satisfactory blood pressure control should prompt the physician to proceed with use of a diuretic. If glucose tolerance worsens, therapy with the usual modalities for control of blood sugar should then be instituted. If the patient is already receiving insulin, an increase of insulin dose may be all that is needed. Similar considerations pertain to the use of glucocorticoids. The course of diabetes provoked by the administration of corticosteroids or diuretics, once these agents have been discountinued, is variable.

Other Aspects of the Glucose Tolerance Test Including Effect of Age

Previous schemes for interpretation of the OGTT include summation of the fasting and 2-hour glucose levels, etc. These approaches are usually arbitrary and should be abandoned.

The effect of age on glucose tolerance is a special circumstance. Although age has no effect on fasting plasma glucose, the values in the OGTT tend to increase with age. One method for dealing with this

phenomenon was to report any given value as a percentile rank. Although this was a reasonable approach, the diagnostic criteria of the National Diabetes Data Group, as proposed above, takes into account this effect of age (8). By this approach, aging merely results in IGT and is associated with the corollaries of this state, viz., the possibility of higher risk for development of atherosclerotic disease and overt diabetes.

Gestational Diabetes

The term gestational diabetes (GDM) refers only to women who become overtly diabetic during pregnancy. Women who are known to have diabetes and become pregnant are not included. The majority of gestational diabetics return to a state of normal glucose tolerance postpartum. GDM occurs in some 1 to 2% of all pregnancies. Such patients are at increased risk (about 30%) for developing diabetes within 5 to 10 years after parturition.

Proper management of the patient with GDM is important, since the increased morbidity and mortality of poorly controlled diabetes can be greatly reduced. Indications for detection of such patients using the OGTT include recognition of glucosuria, family history of diabetes, a history of stillbirth or fetal malformations, spontaneous abortions, and an earlier heavy baby (see p. 705).

Previous (PrevAGT) and Potential (PotAGT) Abnormalities of Glucose Tolerance

Persons with a normal OGTT who previously showed either IGT or overt diabetic hyperglycemia should be classified as PrevAGT. These individuals are not to be considered diabetic and should not be labeled, as in the recent past, with the terms prediabetes or latent diabetes. The economic and psychosocial stigmata of such labels are not justified. Furthermore, if, following development of glucose intolerance during pregnancy or some other occasion, an individual reverts to normal OGTT, reclassification to PrevAGT is warranted. The stress associated with trauma, burns, surgery, and infection may also result in hyperglycemia or abnormalities of OGTT which revert to normal and warrant classification as PrevAGT.

The term potential abnormality of glucose tolerance (PotAGT) should never be used as a diagnostic label for any person. The term is useful only in research.

TREATMENT OF DIABETES MELLITUS

Education of the Patient

Of those chronic conditions which are common in ambulatory practice, diabetes stands apart because of the broad scope and the critical importance of patient education and long term management. For all diabetics, the following factors are important: the impact of diet on diabetes; the implications of diabetes for ordinary activities; recognition of the signs of worsening diabetes; the importance of proper care of the feet; and the clarification of misconceptions about diabetes. For patients receiving insulin, the following additional actors are important: correct administration of insulin, the unique constraints which insulin therapy places on dietary management and changes of activity, the recognition of the symptoms of hypoglycemia, and the adjustment of insulin dose during intercurrent illness.

The patient's response to being informed of a diagnosis of diabetes varies widely. Many patients have already suspected the diagnosis as the result of previous observations of similar symptoms in family members. These individuals are often also aware of the complications of the disease (loss of vision, amputations) and the use of "the needle" (insulin self-administration). Transient anxiety or depression occurs frequently and should be anticipated by the physician. Management of these minor mood disturbances is described in Chapter 12.

Many patients are reluctant to accept the need for self-injection of insulin, and many physicians are unwilling to press the issue. The result is poor control, inappropriate use of oral hypoglycemic drugs, or both. Reluctance of both patient and physician may stem from unfamiliarity with the techniques. In point of fact, insulin injection is simple and almost without discomfort. A firm attitude on the part of the physician will overcome patient reluctance in almost all cases. The use of disposable syringes has eliminated the inconvenience of sterilization while the modern thin, very sharp, plastic-hubbed or syringe-attached needles render the injections practically painless. Aspects of technique are described below (p. 690).

A substantial proportion of "new" diabetics will quickly reveal a noncompliant pattern of handling their particular chronic illness. These patterns are usually difficult to alter. Perhaps the best way to prevent the development of poor compliance is to educate the patient and other members of the patient's household from the outset (see Chapter 4 for a detailed discussion of compliance-promoting strategies).

EDUCATIONAL PROCESS

The educational process should be as frank and as authoritative as possible, since much misinformation is apt to deluge the patient. Misconceptions should be explained and countered. The physician is not often able to undertake and continue this process in the detail it deserves; therefore, a nurse or other trained individual should be available whenever possible to instruct the new diabetic and to continue the educational process as necessary. Excellent booklets are available from the American Diabetes Association and pharmaceutical manufacturers as adjuncts to personal instruction as are a variety of teaching films and newsletters dealing with all aspects of diabetic care (5). In all aspects of management the need for reinforcement and continuing patient education must be stressed. Even the most intelligent patient often needs reiteration of treatment principles and procedures.

The goal of such instruction is correct patient self-care. Even such procedures as altering the dose of insulin to conform to changing needs should, whenever possible, be taught. Successful management is never possible without such education. On the other hand, all patients will need assistance from time to time. Telephone contact with the physician should be available and encouraged. Many problems of adjustment of insulin dosage, etc., can and should be handled by telephone in order to avoid excessive use of office time and unnecessary expense and loss of work time for the patient. Finally, the need for education of key members of the patient's family should not be forgotten. Alterations of diet and of eating patterns are not often made easily and may not be made at all if a spouse is unaware, for example, that punctual meals are essential for the patient receiving insulin therapy.

Diet Therapy

Different diet strategies guide therapy for diabetes, depending on whether one is dealing with an obese, non-insulin-dependent (NIDDM) patient or an individual of appropriate weight who has insulin-dependent disease (Table 69.6). For the obese NIDDM diabetic, the immediate and long term goals are *weight reduction*, and almost any weight reduction scheme (diet plan) will suffice (see Chapter 73). Ideally, diet composition should approximate that shown in Table 69.7. Most such patients are not symptomatic and do not require therapy with insulin or oral hypoglycemic agents for control of symptoms. The latter, if used, have the advantage that they do not complicate a low calorie diet. Simultaneous institution of a weight reduction program and treatment with insulin, if prescribed, often lead to hypoglycemia and must be approached cautiously. The short term goal of insulin therapy under these conditions is the relief of symptoms due to hyperglycemia. No attempt at "tight" control should be made at this time; such efforts should be deferred until efforts at weight loss have ended.

The importance of weight reduction for the obese diabetic cannot be overstated. Population studies indicate that most diabetes is either made manifest by obesity in genetically predisposed persons or is actually caused by obesity. Hence, most overt diabetes in obese patients is potentially either preventable or "curable" by weight reduction provided that the diabetes has not been present for more than a few years. However, most patients are unable to achieve and/or maintain a weight that will reverse overt diabetes, even though they are made aware of the necessity for doing so. Chapter 73 on obesity and Chapter 4 on compliance deal with this problem in greater detail.

The second goal of diet therapy is prevention of atherosclerotic disease. The evidence that this major problem of the diabetic *may* be preventable is to a large degree based on comparisons of the prevalence of atherosclerotic disease in different populations with widely varying diets. A detailed discussion of the evidence bearing on this issue can be found elsewhere (13, 14). In any case, the diabetics in this country who have followed conventional diabetic diets—at least until about 1970—have had the highest rate of coronary disease seen anywhere in the world (3 times the rate of the general population). Because of this and the evidence from population studies, the American Diabetes Association recommended in 1971 that its old standard diabetic diets be abandoned. Unfortunately, the new diets, high in starch and low in saturated fats, have not been widely accepted by either physicians or patients, perhaps because of the long-held notion that carbohydrate is harmful to the diabetic (Table 69.7). In fact, the new relatively high carbohydrate diets do not result in higher blood glucose levels. Similarly, the notion that high carbohydrate diets increase hyperlipidemia is not corroborated by observations in diabetic patients. Another problem in instituting the new dietary approach is the lack of standardized diets to replace the old ones. The American Diabetes association has taken the view that diets should be individualized. Such individualization may be logical but seems to be beyond the capacity of all but the most sophisticated centers, even though in theory any dietitian could construct such a diet.

A guiding principle of individualization of diabetic diets should be the recognition that individual food preferences must be respected whenever possible. The dietitian should obtain the patient's *preferred* dietary history and then attempt to construct the diet around these preferences. Such an approach is demanding for the dietitian, but the issuance of a standardized "American" diet to a diabetic from an ethnic minority simply guarantees noncompliance.

DIET DURING INSULIN THERAPY

Any patient receiving insulin faces a special problem with diet, one that for the insulin-dependent patient is usually even more difficult than for the individual with NIDDM. Unlike patients who are not receiving insulin—who require no special timing of meals and whose total intake can vary from day to day—the pattern of food intake for the individual receiving insulin must be quite rigid. Total caloric intake must be distributed among the meals of the day, which usually include midafternoon and bedtime snacks as well, so that insulin dose can be adjusted according to the patient's needs. The reverse procedure, selection of an insulin dose and adjustment of total caloric intake to this dose, is unphysiologic and should never be used. Occasional patients strive to reduce insulin dosage by senseless starvation, incorrectly assuming that insulin dose has some relationship to "severity" of their disease. Needless to say, patients must be dissuaded from such practices.

The exact composition of the diet for the IDDM patient is less important—from the point of view of blood sugar control—than is the constancy of food intake from day to day. Insulin effect (duration, intensity), even for a particular type of insulin, varies from patient to patient. Accordingly, avoidance of extremes of blood sugar concentration (hypo- and hyperglycemia) requires some adjustment of food

Table 69.6
Dietary Strategies for Diabetics [a]

Strategy	Obese, Non-insulin-requiring [b]	Lean, Insulin-requiring
Reduce caloric intake	Yes	No
Improve pancreatic β cell function (disease reversal)	Weight reduction effective	Not possible
Day-to-day dietary constancy	Not critical	Yes—essential
Extra feedings	No	Yes
Consistent timing of meals	No	Yes—essential
Extra food for exercise	No	Usually
Frequent small feedings during intercurrent illness	No	Yes

[a] Modified from West (13).
[b] Includes patients on oral hypoglycemics.

Table 69.7
Distribution of Major Nutrients in Normal and Diabetic Diets (United States)

Diet	Nutrients (Percent of Total Calories)						
	Starch and other polysaccharides	Sugars and dextrins	Total carbohydrate	Fat		Protein	Alcohol
				Total	% Polyunsaturated		
"Typical" diet	25–35	20–30	45–50	35–45	30	12–20	0–10
Traditional diabetic diet	25–30	10–15	35–40	40–45	30	15–20	0
Newer diabetic diets	30–45	5–15	45–55 [a]	25–35	50	12–25	0–6

[a] Even higher levels of starch and lower levels of fat would be desirable, but are seldom possible in Western societies because they differ too much from the traditional diets of these cultures. Table modified from West (13).

apportionment for each individual. However, one should attempt to simulate as closely as possible the patient's usual pattern of food intake. The main modification is usually to add between-meal snacks. Once an acceptable food pattern has been established and insulin dose adjusted to that pattern, the patient must adhere to the program if extremes of blood sugar are to be avoided. Patients learn by trial and error how much latitude they can tolerate. Problems, not easily solved, are encountered in individuals who engage in strenuous sports or work which varies from day to day. Such persons may have to eat more on some days than others or make frequent adjustments of their insulin dose. Rigid control of blood sugar is not possible in such cases.

The major adaptive problem with diet in insulin-treated individuals is the need for most patients to eat "mechanically," i.e., by-the-clock. No longer can the individual wait for hunger to prompt a meal; nor can he approach dining out at a restaurant with indifference to the time the meal will be served. To do so is to court a major hypoglycemic episode. However, delay of a meal may be unavoidable. In order to prevent hypoglycemia in this circumstance, about 10 g of carbohydrate per half hour should be ingested. This can be provided by 6 oz (180 ml) of a sugar-containing soda ("soft drink"), a palatable pre-meal alternative to a candy bar.

ESTIMATION OF CALORIC NEEDS

Caloric requirements for maintenance of weight vary somewhat from individual to individual but are mainly determined by activity level. Required calories are *approximately* 40 kcal/kg or 20 kcal/lb for an adult with "normal" activity. Thus an individual of 70 kg may require 2800 kcal, although some lean men performing ordinary activities may require as much as 3000 to 3500 kcal/day. Individuals who perform manual labor may need 4000 or more kcal, while sedentary persons may need only 2000 kcal or less.

In prescribing diets caloric requirements are often underestimated. Physicians commonly prescribe an 1800-kcal diet for maintenance even if it is grossly inadequate for a particular patient's caloric needs. Prescription of such a diet leads to frustration and noncompliance. Overzealous decreases of calories for weight reduction may be equally defeating. When maintenance of weight is the goal, a careful dietary history by a skilled dietician may give a good starting point for establishment of an individual's needs; the prescribed diet may then become simply a modification of that patient's ordinary pattern.

OTHER ASPECTS OF DIET AND INSULIN THERAPY

After a dietician estimates the constituents that will be acceptable to a patient, joint discussion should be held with the spouse or other involved family members. Cooperation and participation of a spouse in the process may be essential for successful adaptation which, for practical reasons, may require that both partners participate in the diet modifications.

The intelligent use of diet exchange lists (food equivalents) is necessary for most IDDM patients. Such lists are available from the American Diabetes Association, the American Dietetic Association, and most hospital dietetic units. There is no necessity for such exchanges in NIDDM.

Special "diabetic" or "dietetic" foods are expensive and usually are unnecessary. Some such foods do contain less free sugar than is ordinarily the case, but the patient must read the labels carefully to avoid self-deception.

Exercise during Insulin Therapy. The patient must be instructed on dietary self-management in several situations. Modest exercise (walking briskly) requires about 10 g of extra carbohydrate/hour. Vigorous exercise (basketball playing) requires about an extra 20 to 30 g/hour (e.g., 360 ml of soda). To some extent the hypoglycemic effect of exercise may be greater if the insulin has been injected into an extremity being exercised. Most patients prefer to inject insulin into the thigh, but persons who engage in vigorous exercise (jogging, other sports, manual labor) may have to use abdominal or arm injection sites to avoid excessive insulin effect due to exercise-induced rapid absorption.

Effect of Anorexia. When a patient with IDDM develops anorexia because of short term common illness ("cold," "flu," gastroenteritis), insulin should not be discontinued, but a modest (one-third) reduction of the normal dose may be needed. Every effort should be made to ensure intake of 50 g of carbohydrate in every 8-hour period to avoid both ketosis and hypoglycemia.

Selection of Patients for Oral Hypoglycemic Drugs or Insulin Therapy

NON-INSULIN-DEPENDENT DIABETES

As previously noted, the initial approach to the obese non-insulin-dependent (NIDDM) patient is weight reduction. Such therapy—if followed—can be expected to reduce blood sugar within a few weeks. If fasting plasma glucose (FPG) is less than 200 to 300 mg/dl, glucosuria will not ordinarily produce enough symptoms to be troublesome during this period and no additional drug therapy (oral hypoglycemics or insulin) is needed. Even a FPG of 300 to 400 mg/dl is ordinarily well tolerated. These patients are not ketosis-prone; no urgency exists for instituting drug therapy. On the other hand, symptomatic glucosuria, persisting for weeks despite efforts at (or actual) weight loss, should not be ignored. In this case, drug therapy is indicated for symptomatic relief and can be discontinued if weight reduction is successful.

In the past, many NIDDM patients with symptomatic disease have been treated with oral hypoglycemic drugs (see p. 695). However, even asymptomatic patients have also been treated for only modest elevations of FPG or even for abnormal glucose tolerance. Such treatment may improve or normalize glucose tolerance. Extrapolation of results from patient surveys relating abnormalities of glucose tolerance to development of complications of diabetes would suggest that such treatment might be beneficial. However, no evidence exists to support this possibility. In fact, a study of long term use of tolbutamide—although controversial—suggests that the drug itself may increase the frequency of occurrence of cardiovascular problems. Thus, at present, drug therapy of modest elevations of FPG or OGTT abnormalities is not warranted.

The official recommendation of the American Diabetic Association, the AMA Council on Drugs, and the Food and Drug Administration is that sulfonylureas be limited to patients with symptomatic NIDDM who cannot be controlled by diet and in whom addition of insulin is impractical and/or unacceptable.

The indications for use of insulin in patients with *asymptomatic* NIDDM are unclear. Although evidence is accumulating that modest elevations of blood sugar do indeed relate to at least some of the complications of diabetes (2), no prospective studies are available to demonstrate that insulin therapy of patients with asymptomatic hyperglycemia (FPG or OGTT) are benefited. Insulin therapy is certainly indicated for control of *symptomatic* diabetes (see above, p. 680) in NIDDM that cannot be controlled with diet.

INSULIN-DEPENDENT DIABETES

The IDDM patient should be started on insulin therapy as soon as insulin need is apparent. Ordinarily these patients have been hospitalized for treatment of ketoacidosis and have been switched from short acting insulin, used in the treatment of the acute phase, to an intermediate or long acting preparation. The insulin dependence has been established by the occurrence of the acute episode. Unless this acute event was precipitated by stress in an otherwise NIDDM patient, insulin dependence is usually absolute and permanent. Occasionally in adults (more often in children), insulin requirement may decrease or even disappear over several months; relapse is the rule in such cases.

OTHER CIRCUMSTANCES REQUIRING INSULIN THERAPY

Some patients who are not, strictly speaking, insulin-dependent also need insulin therapy. Patients with NIDDM may develop grossly uncontrolled hyperglycemia during stress (trauma, infection, surgery). Whether or not ketosis ensues, the gross hyperglycemia may produce severe osmotic diuresis and its sequelae. Obviously, such patients require control of hyperglycemia with insulin therapy which may be discontinued as soon as the situation war-

rants. Most young people of normal weight who develop diabetes will require insulin, even though they are not ketosis-prone. The group of children or young adults recently described and termed MODY (maturity onset diabetes of youth) are also candidates for insulin, although many may be managed on diet alone.

Occasional adults, usually thin and not necessarily exhibiting much glucosuria, may exhibit unexplained weight loss and lack of well-being. Such patients may show dramatic improvement with insulin.

Some patients will be encountered who are receiving insulin therapy needlessly. Typically these are elderly individuals with NIDDM who have already developed an array of medical problems, usually cardiovascular. The degree of blood sugar control with large amounts of insulin (50 to 100 units) is poor. Although aggressive use of insulin will certainly normalize blood glucose, the development of hypoglycemia is risky in such persons. On the other hand, abrupt discontinuation of insulin in these patients often results in no worsening of diabetic control and reveals that, in fact, no significant insulin effect has been manifest. Adherence to a proper diet will usually suffice in such cases and will actually control hyperglycemia to a greater degree than does the use of insulin.

NORMOGLYCEMIA AS A GOAL OF INSULIN THERAPY

In view of the growing evidence that control of hypoglycemia may prevent development of the microvascular complications of diabetes (2), no one would argue that normalization of blood sugar with insulin is undesirable, but that is not achievable with present treatment schemes if unacceptable episodes of hypoglycemia are to be avoided. When should at least an effort be made to reach the goal of near-normal blood sugars? In which patients? Individuals with NIDDM tend to have relatively stable blood sugars and predictable responses to insulin. An attempt at therapy should be made in such patients. In most, at least the fasting plasma glucose can be normalized without great difficulty (see Table 69.3). Patients with IDDM are much more difficult to manage, and not even an approach to normalization is achievable in most. Many physicians nonetheless go through an agonizing trial with such patients, only to have the effort end in failure and frustration for all involved. Usually several types and mixtures of insulin are tried along with both single dose and multiple dose schedules. If one or two doses of NPH or Lente insulin a day are unsuccessful (see below), it is extremely unlikely that more elaborate schemes will succeed. Often at the end of a grand effort—which has failed—the patient is on a dose of insulin which reflects the effort if not the "tight control" that was sought (e.g., two doses a day of a mixture of short and intermediate acting insulin). At that point, defeat

Table 69.8
Characteristics of Commonly Used Insulin Preparations

Type	Physical State	Modifying Protein	Peak Action (hr)	Duration of Effect (hr)
SHORT ACTING (RAPID ONSET)				
Regular (CZI)	Clear solution	None	1–2	6–8
Semilente	Suspension (turbid)	None	2–4	8–14
INTERMEDIATE ACTING				
NPH	Suspension (turbid)	Protamine	3–8	18–36
Lente	Suspension (turbid)	None	3–8	18–36
LONG ACTING				
Protamine zinc (PZI)	Suspension (turbid)	Protamine	8–12	18–36
Ultralente	Suspension (turbid)	None	8–12	18–36

should be accepted and a simpler treatment scheme adopted.

Types of Insulin

Most of the preparations now in use are suspensions of insulin which have been chemically or physically modified to prolong their action following subcutaneous injection. The characteristics of these insulins are summarized below and in Table 69.8.

CRYSTALLINE ZINC INSULIN (CZI; REGULAR INSULIN)

This unmodified insulin is a completely dissolved ("clear") preparation the main use of which is for acute therapy of ketoacidosis in hospitalized patients. In the ordinary treatment of ambulatory patients, regular insulin is rarely used alone, but rather is mixed with other insulins. Although the duration of action of regular insulin injected subcutaneously is said to be about 6 to 8 hours with peak action at 2 to 4 hours, recent work shows that in most diabetics who have been receiving insulin for some time, the duration of action is actually quite prolonged. This phenomenon is presumably due to the attenuating effect of insulin-binding antibodies. In occasional patients receiving more than one dose of long acting insulin daily, regular insulin may be given as the second dose. Very rarely, regular insulin may be used 3 or 4 times daily as sole therapy for extremely unstable ("brittle") diabetics. This preparation is also now being used experimentally for continuous subcutaneous injection with portable infusion pumps.

PROTAMINE ZINC INSULIN (PZI)

This preparation, a loose chemical combination of insulin with the carrier protein, protamine, was the first long acting insulin. Until recently, PZI was amorphous material containing an excess of protamine which precluded addition of regular insulin. However, all PZI now available is crystalline, contains no excess protamine, and can be mixed with regular insulin. Indeed, the commonly used NPH insulin approximates such a mixture (see below). PZI has a duration of action exceeding 24 hours.

PZI is rarely used by itself. Exceptions include diabetics who are not eating because of intercurrent acute or chronic illness. Other patients who may benefit from PZI are those who experience unacceptably frequent episodes of insulin-induced hypoglycemia when the "intermediate" insulins are used. Such individuals are so-called "brittle" diabetics. When a long acting form is to be used as sole therapy, some authorities have preferred—because of its allegedly more predictable effect—Ultralente insulin to PZI.

NEUTRAL PROTAMINE HAGEDORN INSULIN (NPH; ISOPHANE INSULIN)

This preparation is a standardized crystalline suspension prepared from regular insulin and protamine. Often termed "intermediate acting," NPH in fact exhibits rather rapid onset of action and a duration of action usually over 24 hours. Ideally, with a single injection of NPH, the short acting component provides insulin effect during the day when meals are elevating the plasma glucose, while the long acting portion of PZI provides insulin effect through the night. For many patients the achieved ratio of insulin effects is satisfactory. However, if NPH is not satisfactory, other mixtures of insulins can be prepared as needed (see below). NPH insulin is always given subcutaneously in either one or two injections daily.

THE LENTE INSULIN SERIES

This group of insulins was devised at a time when PZI contained excess protamine, thus precluding the preparation of mixtures of short acting Regular with long acting PZI. Controlled addition of zinc was used to prepare a microcrystalline, rapidly absorbed and rapidly acting material (Semilente insulin) and another crystalline product with much slower absorption and longer action, Ultralente insulin. These insulins avoided the use of a foreign protein, protamine, and could be mixed in varying proportions. In some geographic areas, in both the United States and abroad, the Lente insulins are used almost exclusively.

Semilente Insulin. This preparation is similar to regular insulin in onset and duration of action, although its effects are somewhat slower in onset and more prolonged. Semilente is always given subcutaneously. The chief use of Semilente is in mixtures with Ultralente; otherwise indications are similar to those for regular insulin.

Ultralente Insulin. This preparation has a duration of action exceeding 24 hours and is indistinguishable from PZI. Ultralente may, like PZI, occasionally be used alone (see PZI). However, the main use of Ultralente is as the long acting component in the mixture that is known as Lente insulin.

Lente Insulin. This material is a 30:70 mixture of Semilente and Ultralente insulins. Duration of action and uses are essentially identical to that of NPH.

MIXTURES OF INSULINS

The usual goal of conventional insulin therapy is a single injection once daily. If this goal is to be reached, insulin effect must be prolonged sufficiently to produce normoglycemia in the morning and at the same time provide adequate daytime control of the increases of blood glucose that occur postprandially. While the use of NPH or Lente insulin is often successful, the patterns of effect that these insulins provide are not always satisfactory. Either one of two scenarios is observed. In the first, the excessive daytime hyperglycemia and glucosuria dictates the need for additional rapidly acting insulin. Thus, regular insulin is added to NPH or Lente; or Semilente is added to Lente. The second and opposite situation is seen when a single injection of NPH or Lente controls daytime hyperglycemia and glucosuria, but the total duration of action is inadequate, resulting in hyperglycemia at the beginning of the next day. Under these circumstances, additional long acting component is needed. Ultralente can be added to Lente, or a mixture of Semilente and Ultralente can be used with a ratio of 20:80 or 10:90. In this situation many diabetologists, rather than attempt to control fasting (overnight) hyperglycemia by addition of more long acting insulin to a single injection, prefer to give a second small dose of NPH or Lente Insulin. The a.m. dose may have to be reduced somewhat, resulting in a "split-dose" program (see below, "Insulin Therapy"). Such regimens seem especially useful in "brittle" diabetics, in some persons who have been receiving insulin for many years and in whom the duration of insulin effect seems to lessen, in persons requiring relatively large doses of insulin (greater than 60 units daily), and during pregnancy.

Commercial Insulin Preparations

NEW INSULIN PREPARATIONS OF INCREASED PURITY

Until the last few years, all available preparations regardless of type were of essentially the same purity. With the realization that the commercial products did contain small amounts of other related and unrelated proteins (proinsulin, insulin degradation

products, etc.) and that these impurities might possibly contribute to "insulin allergy," antibody formation, etc. further purification procedures were introduced. The ordinary insulins (Lilly, Squibb) now in greatest use are >98% pure. Beginning in 1972 these materials were unofficially designated "single peak" insulins, because they are pure enough to appear as such on gel chromatography. Still more highly purified material was introduced a few years ago into the U.S. market by several European manufacturers (Novo; Nordisk) and is unofficially termed "monocomponent" insulin. Similar preparations were made available by Lilly, the major U.S. manufacturer, and in 1980 the preparation became commercially available. The unofficial term for this was "single component" insulin. Henceforth, this material will be known simply as purified pork insulin (Iletin II, pork; Lilly).

Although the highly purified insulins are currently being aggressively marketed in the United States by their European manufacturers, no proof is available that they offer the patient or physician any advantage. They do offer a considerable (severalfold) increase in cost. Most of the problems encountered with insulin in the past disappeared with introduction of the relatively pure "single peak" insulins after 1972. Allergic reactions and lipoatrophy were the two most troublesome events; both do appear to have been related to impurities.

Allergy to insulin is most commonly a local reaction at the site of injection. Local redness, swelling, heat, and itching occur within minutes to an hour after injection and persist for a few hours to a day, often with formation of an area of induration. Such reactions, no longer common, would occur during the first few weeks of therapy and usually disappear as therapy was continued. Rarely, similar reactions develop many hours or up to a day after injection (delayed hypersensitivity).

Systemic allergic reactions, with or without a local reaction, are rare; they are manifest by urticaria, angioedema, and even anaphylactic shock (IgE-mediated; see Chapter 22). Such reactions seem to occur most often in persons who have previously received insulin and appear during reinstitution of therapy after a lapse of months or years. Local reactions may progress to systemic ones; if this seems to be occurring, one should treat the patient before anaphylaxis occurs. The first maneuver involves a trial of highly purified insulin. If this approach fails, drugs such as antihistamines and glucocorticoids are helpful, but persistent insulin allergy is best treated by desensitization. With the patient receiving no antihistamines or steroids and no insulin in the preceding 12 to 24 hours, the procedure involves injection of 0.1-ml volumes of insulin which has been diluted 1:100 in 0.1% human serum albumin to prevent adsorption losses or to glass. An initial dose (0.001 unit) is given intradermally. Subsequent doses of 0.1 ml contain doubling amounts (units). After several intradermal injections at 30-min intervals, the subcutaneous route is used. If a reaction occurs, epinephrine may be administered; the dose of insulin is reduced, but the process is continued. This procedure requires a series of solutions of insulin. These may be prepared by the physician or pharmacist, but are also available in kit form by telephone request to Dr. John Galloway, Eli Lilly Co., Indianapolis, Indiana. Special kits and instructions for desensitizing patients who have delayed hypersensitivity reactions are also available from the same source.

Insulin lipoatrophy is now an uncommon event. Harmless but disfiguring localized atrophy of subcutaneous fatty tissue occurs around the site of insulin injections and is sometimes seen simultaneously with insulin allergy. The process may be related to impurities in insulin preparations rather than to insulin itself, since newer preparations ("single peak") are much less likely to produce this problem. In addition, the injection of highly purified "monocomponent" or "single component" insulins into the atrophied areas has sometimes resulted in disappearance of the atrophy.

Insulin lipohypertrophy is even less common than insulin atrophy. This phenomenon is probably due to an intrinsic action of insulin and has not been improved by use of purer insulins. Repeated injections into the same area do appear to predispose to lipohypertrophy.

TRADE NAMES, UNIT DESIGNATIONS, AND SYRINGES

Lilly designates all of its insulin as Iletin. The newest, most highly purified material is Iletin II. Squibb uses no trade name, while foreign manufacturers have regrettably introduced a bewildering array of designations.

All insulin, regardless of type or source, is standardized at a specific concentration per ml. The symbol U refers to the insulin concentration in units/ml. Until 1973 when U-100 was introduced into use in the United States, the standard forms were U-80 and U-40. The shift to U-100 was made in the expectation of phasing out the old strengths and with the hope of reducing confusion by patients. By 1980 about 90% of the insulins in use were U-100, and U-80 was no longer being manufactured by Lilly. Within the next few years U-40 insulins will probably be withdrawn from the U.S. market.

Several sizes of syringe are available for use with U-100. A 1-ml syringe can be used for all doses up to 100 units, but most accurate dispensing of less than 30 units is made when syringes of 0.5-ml capacity are used. The bores of these syringes are smaller and the scales are consequently expanded. Occasional patients require more than 100 units per single injection. For such use 2-ml syringes (200-unit capacity) are manufactured, but these are in short supply and are difficult to obtain. The use of disposable plastic syringes with attached needles has greatly simplified use of insulin and is preferred by almost all patients (Becton-Dickinson: B-D, or equivalent). Reusable glass syringes requiring detachable needles are also available. Special syringes are available for use by patients with severe impairment of vision which prevents them from accurately measuring their insulin dose. However, a simple solution to this problem is often possible. Disposable syringes can be prefilled with ordinary sterile precautions by an able person (relative, friend) and safely stored in a refrigerator for at least a week.

INSULIN INJECTION TECHNIQUE

Following initial instruction the patient should be observed during self-administration of insulin to be certain that the correct volume is being drawn into the syringe and that the technique of injection is proper. Sterilization of the skin with an alcohol wipe is not necessary, although the injection site should be clean. If the injection is made through skin that is wet with alcohol, unnecessary burning discomfort will be produced.

For use in ambulatory patients insulin preparations should always be given subcutaneously. Most needles in present use are ½ inch in length. Unless the individual is very thin, the best technique involves insertion of the needle at 90° to the skin surface. If the patient is very thin, or the needle is ⅝ inch in length, or the site is covered by thin skin, the needle may be inserted at up to 45°. The objective is a subcutaneous rather than intradermal or intramuscular injection. Following injection, the area should not be massaged, since that may accelerate absorption.

The choice of injection site is of importance, since the rate of insulin absorption—and hence the duration and magnitude of insulin effect—varies considerably between anatomic locations. Absorption is slowest from the thigh, fastest from the anterior abdominal wall, and intermediate from the arm. In addition, absorption from an exercising extremity is accelerated (p. 686). The long used technique of rotation of sites is perhaps unwise and may contribute to erratic control. On the other hand, the repeated use of precisely the same spot within a site should be avoided.

BEEF VS. PORK INSULINS

All insulin sold in the United States is derived from beef or pork pancreas. Most ordinary preparations marketed by Lilly are a variable mixture of beef (bovine) and pork (porcine) insulins with the beef derived component predominating (about 70%), but the precise proportions varying with available supply. The products marketed by Squibb are derived entirely from beef. Lilly's most highly purified material (Iletin II) is exclusively prepared from pork sources. Porcine insulin differs from the human form by only a single amino acid, while the beef material has several additional amino acid substitutions. As a result, pork insulin is, in some persons, less allergenic than the beef material. Clinically, this is of significance in occasional cases of insulin allergy and may affect insulin requirements. Switching a patient from beef-pork or all-beef preparation to an all-pork material will double cost and may result in reduction of 30% in the number of units needed. Such a maneuver is hardly cost-effective. On the other hand, an inadvertent shift of preparations may result in loss of blood sugar control or hypoglycemia.

Human insulin is not currently available for general clinical use. Such material has, however, already been produced by bacterial recombinant DNA techniques and, together with partially synthetic human insulin, has undergone clinical testing in Europe. Whether such materials will offer any advantages over currently available insulins remains to be established.

Insulin Therapy

STRATEGIES OF INSULIN ADMINISTRATION: INITIATION OF THERAPY

The fundamental information which the patient should understand when insulin therapy is initiated is reviewed in Table 69.6. Institution of insulin therapy coincides with or follows the establishment of a diet (see above). As pointed out earlier, relative constancy of food intake is essential. If such dietary compliance cannot be assured, the goal of insulin therapy should be no more than the avoidance of symptomatic hyperglycemia and ketoacidosis. Otherwise, tighter control will unquestionably result in hypoglycemic episodes. In any case, insulin therapy cannot possibly achieve good control when diet is varying. The goal of insulin therapy—under optimal conditions—is the closest *practically achievable* approach to normalization of the blood sugar (see "Normoglycemia as a Goal of Insulin Therapy," p. 687).

First attempts at blood sugar control in almost all ambulatory patients should be done with an intermediate acting insulin (NPH or Lente). A safe initial dose for a non-insulin-dependent patient who has not received previous insulin therapy is 20 units for a nonobese individual and 30 units for an obese patient.

Previously treated patients often require higher initial doses. Insulin-dependent patients will ordinarily have been started on insulin therapy while in the hospital, but the scheme below can be used for further adjustment of dose for both types of patient.

The dose of insulin can be increased by 5 units every 3 days until satisfactory control is approached. Usually, such a program will bring the patient under control within a few weeks. Increments of 10 units every 3 days are also safe if the patient is markedly symptomatic or if no effect is apparent within a week. During this time the patient should be monitoring urine glucose (see "Monitoring Insulin Therapy"). A telephone call to the physician can be made every week or 10 days, but the patient should be encouraged to proceed with the adjustments of dose as planned and should not require or expect a physician's instructions at each dose increment. Unnecessary dependence is thus discouraged and the patient's involvement in management is enhanced.

When glucosuria begins to subside, almost always first apparent as decreased glucosuria or aglucosuria in the first a.m. specimen, the dose of insulin should be held constant until such time as fasting plasma glucose (FPG) can be obtained. Sometimes glucosuria first subsides during the day rather than in the a.m. If this pattern develops, the dose of insulin should be held constant until both FPG and the plasma glucose (PG) at the aglucosuric time are measured. At the time the PG is measured, a double voided urine sample should be obtained and glucosuria should be measured simultaneously. A few such determinations allow an estimate of the patient's renal threshold; thereafter the physician can approximate the PG for that particular individual from the glucosuria. From the point of development of aglucosuria during some portion of the day to eventual "control" requires continued adjustment of insulin dosage, almost always upward, and adjustment of the patient to the diet and the routine of monitoring. During this time the patient often needs reassurance that the period of close dependency on the physician will soon come to an end. Every effort must also be made to avoid rigidly scheduled visits to the physician's office or the clinical laboratory that interfere with the patient's livelihood or important personal affairs. Such intrusions will only discourage the patient and promote future noncompliance. On the other hand, achievement of reasonable control should not be prolonged and should be possible within a few weeks. When months pass and the patient's control remains irregular, seems to follow no pattern, or is marked by many hypoglycemic episodes, the problem is either noncompliance (see Chapter 4), usually dietary, or improper prescription of insulin. Noncompliance in the use of insulin can sometimes be ascertained by comparison of frequency of insulin purchase with the volume predicted by prescribed therapy. For example, a 10-ml vial of U-100 insulin contains 1000 units; if the patient receives 50 units daily, a vial should last 20 days (1000/50).

Many patients will not be controlled with a single dose of intermediate acting insulin (NPH or Lente; see "Mixtures of Insulin"). In these individuals hyperglycemia and glucosuria improve; the late a.m. or afternoon glucose measurements are the first to show a tendency to normalize. However, the long acting component of the insulin preparation is insufficient to ensure normoglycemia in the fasting state, i.e., in the early morning. Two maneuvers can be tried. Usually, the addition of a pre-dinner dose of the same

Table 69.9
Monitoring of Urine Glucose[a]

Diagnostic Method	Glucosuria (g/100 ml)						
	0	0.1	0.25	0.5	0.75	1	2
Clinitest	Blue		Blue-green trace	Green (+)	Green-brown (++)	Brown-orange (+++)	Orange (++++)
Testape	Yellow	Green-yellow (+)	Green (dark) (++l)	Green-blue (+++)			Black (++++)
Clinistix	Pink		Pink (+)	++	Purple (+++)	Nonquantitative	
Diastix	Aqua	Light green trace	Green (+)	Green-brown (++)		Yellow-brown (+++)	Brown (++++)

[a] Note that the colors in the different methods do not indicate comparable degrees of glucosuria. All colors should be matched against the chart supplied by the manufacturer. Clinitest will indicate up to 4–5% glucosuria, provided that 2 drops of urine rather than 5 drops are used. A number of products are available to test for ketones, including Acetest tablets and strips such as Ketostix. The cost of these materials varies widely. Materials that test for both glucose and ketones (e.g., Keto-Diastix) are much more expensive than those which test for glucose alone. Attention should be given to the shelf stability of these preparations. Storage under improper conditions of temperature and/or humidity will lead to inaccuracies of testing.

intermediate acting insulin can be made, sometimes requiring a concomitant reduction of the a.m. dose. For example, if such a patient is receiving 60 units daily, up to 15 units may be given in the evening—usually before the dinner meal—and the a.m. dose can be reduced to 50 units. Additional increments of 5 units may then be made to either dose, depending on whether the fasting or postprandial glucose needs lowering. Patients requiring a "split-dose" schedule, as this is sometimes called, usually are receiving 60 units or more daily. To avoid a two-dose schedule the alternate approach of increasing the long acting component can be instituted. In this case, the Lente insulins are best employed (see "Types of Insulin"). If the patient is already receiving NPH, a switch to the same dose of Lente is made. Ultralente insulin may then be mixed with Lente in daily increments of 5 to 10 units. Since Lente insulin is already a mixture of Semilente and Ultralente in a proportion of 30:70, addition of Ultralente merely alters this ratio in favor of the longer acting component, thus providing a greater likelihood that early a.m. PG will be controlled without producing midday hypoglycemia. To some extent, addition of more long acting component does, however, effect a lowering of glucose even during the day. In any case, some patients can be controlled on a single dose of insulin in this way. For the patient who does not want a second daily injection, this approach may be worthwhile.

Many patients given an intermediate acting insulin readily achieve normoglycemia in the fasting state, but have heavy glucosuria during the day, i.e., postprandially. In such individuals, addition of Semilente insulin to Lente provides short acting effect during the period when hyperglycemia needs control. For this purpose one may also add regular insulin to NPH or to Lente.

Much effort can be expended in such "fine tuning." Once the FPG is normalized, efforts to achieve "tight control" during the day can sometimes be made successfully, but often result in unacceptable hypoglycemic episodes. In the absence of evidence that "tight control," as currently achievable, is effective in preventing complications of diabetes, one may properly question the desirability of extreme machinations of this type in the ordinary case. This point is not in conflict with the evidence that hyperglycemia may be important as a cause of increased cardiovascular disease. The point is simply that "tight control" is usually unachievable in most diabetics, at least with current techniques.

MONITORING INSULIN THERAPY

Efficacy of treatment in the ambulatory patient should be monitored by measuring FPG and urine glucose. Normalization of FPG—more reproducible than postprandial sugars—represents the basic or "coarse" adjustment of insulin dose, while postprandial normalization can be viewed as the "fine" adjustment. No useful purpose is served by attempts to adjust postprandial PG before normalization of the FPG is achieved; only thereafter should PG be monitored at midafternoon or before the evening meal. Urine glucose monitoring before meals and before bed time is also important and too often neglected (Table 69.9). Double voiding technique should be used whenever possible, especially for the first morning specimen, if the patient has not voided during the night. While heavy daytime glucosuria is still present, no useful purpose is served by additional frequent monitoring of PG. On the other hand, when afternoon (before dinner) glucosuria has cleared, PG determination—like that of FPG—becomes essential to determine whether the PG has reached, or is approaching, hypoglycemic levels. The development of such episodes is, of course, an indication of need for adjustment of the treatment program, usually reduction in insulin dose.

In ketosis-prone patients, the urine should also be monitored for ketonuria. This can be accomplished using Acetest tablets, or one of the combination "stix" (Table 69.9). Ordinarily, monitoring for ketones is not necessary as a routine procedure.

The optimal frequency of monitoring of FPG and/ or of urinary glucose must be determined for each patient. During initiation of therapy, determination of glucosuria 4 times daily (first voided a.m. specimen, pre-lunch, pre-dinner and at bedtime) is essential if insulin is to be varied (increased) as described above. Typically, FPG must be determined every week or two while insulin dose is being adjusted, and thereafter less often—perhaps monthly or even every 2 to 3 months. The required frequency depends on the degree of control which is being sought. For most patients the *practical* goal will be avoidance of fasting and postprandial hyperglycemia and the prevention of heavy glucosuria. It is for such patients that the monitoring schedule has been described above. If "tight control" is the goal, a much more frequent schedule is necessary, especially if daytime glucosuria is to be eliminated. In the patient with NIDDM, complete absence of glucosuria can sometimes be achieved without the need for frequent determinations of FPG, but in patients with IDDM the monitoring of "tight control" is a very demanding process. For such patients home monitoring of blood glucose is now possible with the use of one of several devices (reflectance photometers) and capillary blood. With highly motivated patients who can afford the cost of the instrument (about $300), long term management by this means is possible, apparently with significant improvement or near normalization of blood sugar in many, although at least two doses of insulin a day are necessary. Whether this approach to control of blood sugar is effective in the long term prevention of the complications of diabetes mellitus remains to be established. The present experimental clinical use of "open-loop" insulin infusion pumps is also assisted by home monitoring of plasma glucose.

Long term monitoring of overall blood sugar control by measurement of one of the chronic *effects* of hyperglycemia has been advocated. Glucose reacts nonenzymatically in a concentration-dependent manner with the amino groups in proteins to produce glycosylated derivatives. One of several such proteins is hemoglobin A_{1C} (HbA$_{1C}$), a minor hemoglobin component of red cells. Normally HbA$_{1C}$ does not exceed 4% of total hemoglobin. A correlation has been established between the degree of hyperglycemia and HbA$_{1C}$. In poorly controlled diabetics, the content of this component may double. Although it can be used clinically, at present this type of monitoring is principally of research interest.

FACTORS AFFECTING INSULIN REQUIREMENT DURING CHRONIC THERAPY

Insulin Resistance. Classically, the term insulin resistance refers to a state in which the requirement for insulin exceeds 200 units daily. This type of insulin resistance is usually due to the development of antibodies to insulin (see below). Even in the absence of antibodies to insulin, however, a variety of observations have clearly shown that resistance to insulin contributes to the hyperglycemia of diabetes mellitus. This resistance—or decreased sensitivity to insulin—is most apparent in the diabetes that is associated with obesity and the state now termed non-insulin-dependent diabetes mellitus. Even nondiabetic obese individuals who maintain *normal* levels of blood sugar do so by secreting supranormal amounts of insulin.

Although obese diabetics are insulin-resistant in terms of their glucose homeostasis and certain aspects of lipoprotein metabolism, their metabolic state is not so deranged as to allow development of ketoacidosis. In the majority of insulin-resistant diabetics, weight reduction will reverse the insulin resistance. Glucose tolerance often improves to (or toward) normal and the need for insulin to control hyperglycemia may decrease or disappear. In contrast, some nonobese patients with NIDDM have lower than normal levels of plasma insulin. Such patients comprise a spectrum of combinations of insulin resistance and insulin deficiency.

Recent evidence suggests that sulfonylurea compounds, in addition to their action in facilitating insulin release, may act by returning insulin sensitivity toward normal, perhaps by increasing insulin receptors. The use of these drugs is dictated, however, by other considerations.

Increases of Insulin Requirement. The stress of infection or trauma may increase insulin requirements quickly. Usually the site of any infection that is severe enough to produce this effect is obvious, or at least there is good evidence of an infectious process (fever, leukocytosis). Only rarely will a search for a hidden focus provide an explanation for changing insulin requirements or even for the development of ketoacidosis. Most episodes of ketoacidosis that are not related to stress are not caused by an increased insulin requirement. Rather, such episodes are usually related to noncompliance, although this may be unintentional as when the patient mistakenly omits insulin because of intercurrent viral illness. In the past a common cause of an *apparent* increase in insulin requirement was use of the wrong insulin concentration (U-40 for U-80). Insulin requirement tends to increase after the end of the first trimester of pregnancy (see below).

A slow increase of insulin requirement (for the commonly used insulin of beef-pork origin) occurring over months may be related to development of insulin antibodies of the IgG type. Usually the patient may be stabilized at a new, higher, dose level. Under these circumstances, the duration of action of short acting insulin is often prolonged, while intermediate or long acting insulins may not carry a 24-hour effect. Insulin requirement may exceed 200 units per day and administration may become a problem. A switch to purified pork insulin may result in up to a 30% decrease in requirement. Occasionally, a short course of glucocorticoid therapy is necessary to effect a dose reduction. Prednisone (40 to 60 mg daily), rather than increase insulin requirement, will usually produce a dramatic fall in insulin requirement beginning at 7 to 10 days. Hospitalization should be considered after the first 5 days of such therapy in anticipation of rapid decrease of insulin requirement. When the decrease occurs, glucocorticoid therapy can be abruptly discontinued. Recurrence of the resistant state is infrequent and may not occur for months or years.

Still another type of insulin "resistance" has been recently recognized. It has long been appreciated that in most patients a modest proportion of the insulin injected subcutaneously undergoes local destruction by tissue proteinases. However, in some patients very large amounts may be destroyed in this way leading to massive *apparent* resistance. In these individuals, when insulin is injected subcutaneously together with a proteinase inhibitor, required insulin dose is greatly reduced. This phenomenon may explain the large difference frequently observed between insulin dose required by intravenous route and that given subcutaneously. At present no insulin additive is approved that obviates this problem, and one can only inject as much insulin as seems to be required.

Decreases of Insulin Requirement. Vigorous exercise reduces blood glucose and, in anticipation of such activity, the dose of insulin may need to be reduced (see p. 686).

During pregnancy, insulin requirement drops during the first trimester, rises and may double during the second and third trimesters, and falls suddenly at delivery (see below). Diabetics who develop nephropathy often show a decreased insulin requirement. A tendency to normoglycemia or even to hypoglycemia develops occasionally in patients previously requiring insulin who develop chronic congestive heart failure. Development of adrenal or pituitary insufficiency will also result in a decreased insulin requirement.

HYPOGLYCEMIA DURING INSULIN THERAPY: RECOGNITION, PREVENTION, AND TREATMENT

Hypoglycemia is, of course, an inevitable effect of an excessive insulin dose. Especially when severe, hypoglycemia causes central nervous system symptoms ranging from headache, confusion, and visual disturbances to personality change, seizures, unconsciousness, and transient hemiparesis. When hypoglycemia occurs during waking hours and is accompanied by the usual symptoms of epinephrine release (tremor, sweating, tachycardia, and palpitations), there is no problem in recognizing the condition. Even mild hypoglycemia (plasma glucose 40 to 50 mg/100 ml) can produce epinephrine release as a compensatory and corrective physiologic response. However, under certain circumstances, the occurrence of hypoglycemia cannot be easily identified.

By far the most frequent cause of hypoglycemia in the diabetic receiving insulin therapy is failure of the patient to eat at normal times. Despite repeated warnings many patients not only miss meals, but obfuscate the treatment program further by lying to the physician about food intake. The physician must be ever on guard but tactful in constantly considering this possibility.

Diabetics who develop autonomic neuropathy may lose their hypoglycemia-induced adrenergic symptoms. Such patients are at risk for major disaster. Other patients who are receiving β-adrenergic blocking drugs (such as propranolol) may also lose their warning symptoms and may, in addition, develop marked hypertension during an episode of hypoglycemia.

Excessive insulin action may occur during the night or early morning hours. The hypoglycemia-induced release of epinephrine and other counter-regulatory hormones (cortisol, growth hormone, glucagon) causes rebound hyperglycemia, glucosuria, and ketonuria (Somogyi effect). If the physician notes an elevated blood sugar at this point and prescribes still more insulin, the result is further hypoglycemia, perpetuation of the cycle, and possible serious consequences. The physician is obliged to question the patient carefully for clues to the presence of nocturnal hypoglycemia leading to this sequence such as nightmares, night sweats, and headache during the night or on arising. Often, but not always, the pattern of daytime glucosuria shows minimal spill. Reduction of insulin dose by 10% in IDDM and up to 30 to 40% in NIDDM will often identify and correct the situation. In the latter patients, such a brief and substantial reduction in insulin dose can be made with impunity.

The immediate therapy of hypoglycemia is ingestion of food, preferably sugar. Patients should carry a ready carbohydrate source such as candy and must realize that a tiny piece of such material will not suffice. If available, sweetened juice or a soft drink is most satisfactory. A tablespoon of sugar added to fruit juice or merely dissolved in a glass of water will produce relief in 10 to 20 min. Family members or friends should be instructed in the treatment of such an emergency and should not waste time in attempting to reach medical assistance before administering sugar. Although no objection exists to seeking emergency medical care after sugar is given, the problem is usually resolved by the time medical assistance can be obtained. If no obvious cause is apparent for the episode of hypoglycemia—such as a missed meal which is subsequently eaten—the patient should be on guard for recurrence over the next few hours, during which time repeated ingestion of sugar, at hourly intervals, may be advisable.

Most patients will never require emergency medical assistance for treatment of hypoglycemia. However, occasional individuals will be prone to this problem and sometimes cannot be treated by the simple means described. Either because of a hypoglycemia-related alteration of mental status or because of unconsciousness, such persons will not be able to take oral sugar. A safe and effective emergency therapy is administration of 1 mg of glucagon subcutaneously by a person instructed in this technique. Glucagon is readily available in single dose form (1 mg vial) and should be kept available during initiation of insulin therapy and in hypoglycemia-prone persons. About 10 to 15 min are required for an obvious effect on sensorium. As soon as possible, oral sugar should then be given. An effort should always be made to identify the cause of the hypoglycemic episode and to reduce dosage or take other appropriate action to prevent recurrence.

Oral Hypoglycemic Drugs (Sulfonylureas)

MECHANISM OF ACTION

Within a few years after their introduction 25 years ago, these drugs came into wide use for the treatment of NIDDM. The acute hypoglycemic effects of the sulfonylureas appear to be mediated through insulin release. However, in chronic administration, during which blood glucose has been lowered, no increase of plasma insulin is apparent. Recent studies on the mechanisms of action of these drugs show both an increase in the number of insulin receptors and a potentiation of insulin action. Numerous effects other than the desired hypoglycemic action of the sulfonylureas have been studied in connection with drug-drug interactions of these compounds (see below).

CURRENT PLACE IN THERAPY: UNIVERSITY GROUP DIABETES STUDY (UGDP)

Although sometimes used to good purpose for treatment of symptomatic hyperglycemia, oral hypoglycemic drugs were often administered to patients with NIDDM who could have been treated with diet (i.e., by weight reduction). Many patients with minimal fasting or postprandial hyperglycemia or other abnormalities of glucose tolerance were also given these drugs.

A multicenter long term cooperative study (University Group Diabetes Program, UGDP) attempted to assess the usefulness of these agents in asymptomatic diabetics by comparing tolbutamide with diet and insulin treatment. The study began a vitriolic controversy beginning in 1970 when it first reported that tolbutamide-treated patients fared no better than those given placebo and indeed had a higher cardiovascular (but not overall) death rate. Since that report, diabetologists have been divided concerning the usefulness (or dangers) of these agents. While the harmfulness of these agents seems now, on reanalysis of the data, to be open to serious question, the long term benefits in terms of prevention of complications of diabetes remain questionable. It is almost certain that the original UGDP study was too brief and too few patients were studied to have permitted answers to questions concerning prevention of complications. A number of other studies of this issue have now concluded that sulfonylureas do not result in harmful effects.

THERAPEUTIC EFFECTS VS. SIDE EFFECTS

No doubt exists that short term symptomatic relief of hyperglycemia and its sequelae can be obtained in most NIDDM patients treated with sulfonylureas. This result can be most gratifying in properly selected patients. For example, patients who may have difficulty in self-administering insulin because of visual or other physical handicaps may benefit symptomatically from use of sulfonylureas. On the other hand, the use of sulfonylureas is not harmless, because of their intrinsic pharmacologic action in lowering blood glucose and a number of toxic effects. Hypoglycemia can occur and may be both severe and protracted, especially in the elderly or in patients with decreased renal function. Administration of certain of these agents to elderly patients, especially to patients with impaired cardiovascular function, may produce water retention and a syndrome identical to that of inappropriate secretion of antidiuretic hormone (SIADH) with severe hyponatremia and symptoms as profound as coma (12). The volume expansion that occurs may precipitate or worsen congestive heart failure. Chlorpropamide (Diabinese) is the classic offender in this regard, although tolbutamide (Orinase) has been rarely involved as well.

CANDIDATES FOR THERAPY WITH SULFONYLUREAS

Obese NIDDM patients who have not responded to a weight reduction diet or who, having started on a diet, need interim symptomatic relief from hyperglycemia that is producing osmotic diuresis (polyuria, polydipsia) may benefit. Typically these individuals are over age 40 and are more likely to respond if their diabetes has been present for only a few years. Other candidates are those who are unwilling to accept insulin therapy or in whom the risks of hypoglycemia seem unacceptable. The latter might include persons with occupations involving hazardous conditions (vehicle or dangerous equipment operators). Still others include nonobese individuals in whom insulin therapy is unacceptable, but for whom persistent hyperglycemia is felt by the physician to constitute a long term risk factor for atherosclerotic and microvascular disease.

Although most physicians would currently be reluctant to change therapy to an oral agent for a patient who is managing well with insulin, such a change—if undertaken—is more likely to succeed if the diabetes has required less than about 40 units of insulin. Patients with a previous history of ketoacidosis are ordinarily not candidates for a transfer from insulin. A history of hyperosmolar nonketotic coma

Table 69.10
Characteristics of Hypoglycemic Drugs (Sulfonylureas)

Compound	Trade Name	Tablet Size (g)	Daily Dose Range (g)	Duration of action (hr)	Doses per Day	Route of Inactivation
Tolbutamide	Orinase	0.5	1–3	12	2–3	100% in liver
Chlorpropamide	Diabinese	0.1 0.25	0.1–0.5	36+	1	80% metabolized, unknown site(s); 20% excretion by kidney as intact drug; 100% excretion as intact drug *plus* metabolites, activities unknown
Acetohexamide	Dymelor	0.25 0.5	0.5–1.5	12–18	1–2	Partial liver metabolism; 100% kidney excretion as active metabolites plus unchanged drug
Tolazamide	Tolinase	0.1 0.25 0.5	0.25–1.0	12–18	1–2	Partial liver metabolism; partial excretion via kidney

does not preclude a successful change from insulin. Patients with no tendency to ketosis, but whose diabetes is so severe that it has produced weight loss, may not respond to sulfonylureas given as initial therapy but may respond after hyperglycemia has been controlled for a short time with insulin.

Oral agents should not be prescribed for certain patients: individuals with a history of ketoacidosis, unless the latter has developed in relation to stress; patients with a history of severe toxic reaction to a sulfonylurea; and patients with severe hepatic or renal disease, although correct choice of an agent may make such therapy possible (see Table 69.10).

Effectiveness. In optimally selected patients about one-half can be expected to experience normalization of fasting blood sugar while about one-third will not respond. In others, some drug effect will be evident, perhaps to a degree which permits symptomatic relief. Maximal drug effect can be expected within a few days to a week. Those who do not respond during initial therapy are considered to be "primary" sulfonylurea failures. In other cases, following a month or more of good response, the drug seems to become ineffective ("secondary" sulfonylurea failure). The frequency of this response has been estimated at 3 to 10%. Many secondary failures are due to noncompliance. Only occasionally in secondary failure will a switch from a maximal dose of one agent to another be successful.

Transfer from Insulin or from One Sulfonylurea to Another Sulfonylurea. An ineffective agent may be stopped abruptly and a new one started. NIDDM patients receiving insulin can also be abruptly switched, provided that they do not need more than 40 units of insulin. A need for maximal doses of sulfonylurea can usually be anticipated in such cases. If the patient has manifested ketosis in the past, as for example during stress, but is otherwise thought to be a candidate for a switch to an oral agent, the

dose of insulin may be cut in half as the drug is started. Subsequent monitoring over the next few days will show whether the oral agent can control hyperglycemia or must be abandoned.

Choice of Drug. Tolbutamide is the only sulfonylurea studied in the UGDP. Although the Food and Drug Administration's admonitions concerning other oral agents extrapolate from this study of tolbutamide, it may be useful to remember that the related available drugs might have fared better or worse. This caveat aside, there is little to lead one to choose between the available agents (Table 69.10) except that the longer acting drugs need not be taken as often. The frequency of toxicity with tolbutamide is very low, probably lower than with the other agents, even at maximal doses. Chlorpropamide should never be used at a dose greater than 500 mg per day (above which hepatic toxicity is frequent). Because of the unique ability of chlorpropamide among the sulfonylureas to produce a syndrome of drug-induced water intoxication (SIADH) (see above), this drug should be avoided in the elderly in whom this effect has been seen almost exclusively. Acetohexamide is the least used of all the agents, partly because it was introduced later than tolbutamide and chlorpropamide and partly because of lack of aggressive marketing. Tolazamide, the newest of the sulfonylureas available in this country, was introduced 15 years ago but has been marketed vigorously only within the past few years. Phenformin, a biguanide (not a sulfonylurea), was withdrawn from the market in 1977 as an "imminent hazard to the public health" after 18 years of general use. Fatal lactic acidosis, hypertension, and persistent tachycardia were associated with its use. The drug is available free of charge to any physician who files an application with the Food and Drug Administration, but for practical purposes use of phenformin has been abandoned by all but a few diabetologists.

For many years, "second generation" sulfonylureas have been in wide use outside the United States. These drugs are safe agents and, although up to 200 times more potent than the older sulfonylureas, do not offer clear advantages over the older drugs. No long term studies of the UGDP type are available with these agents. Glyburide (glibenclamide; Micronase) and glipizide (Glibenese; Minodiab) are the most likely candidates for introduction into the United States in the near future.

Comparative Cost. At present, the approximate monthly retail cost of therapy with these drugs is from $10 to $50 depending on the dose and the agent used. Two of the drugs, tolbutamide and chlorpropamide, are currently available in their generic forms at one-half to one-third the price of the trade name products. The cost of insulin therapy may be significantly less than that with the oral agents, depending on the doses required.

INSTRUCTION TO THE PATIENT ON USE OF SULFONYLUREAS

The obese patient must be made to realize that diet, *i.e.*, weight reduction, is the mainstay of therapy. In order to avoid unnecessary anxiety, the current status of the UGDP controversy should be discussed with the patient and the possible risks and goals of therapy clearly outlined. Although hypoglycemia is not common with the sulfonylureas, when it does occur, it is likely to be both severe and prolonged. The symptoms of hypoglycemia should be clearly described to the patient, family and/or friends, and corrective measures outlined (see "Insulin Therapy"). The possibility of drug-drug interactions (see below) should be mentioned lest another physician prescribe a drug which potentiates or decreases the effectiveness of the sulfonylureas. Loading doses of sulfonylureas may have a place in patients under observation in hospital but should not be used in ambulatory patients.

MONITORING THERAPY WITH SULFONYLUREAS

Since patients receiving sulfonylurea drugs are not ketosis-prone and have fairly stable diabetes, monitoring is relatively simple. Similar considerations apply to patients being treated with diet alone. Patients who have fasting plasma glucose (FPG) in or near the normal range exhibit little or no fasting glucosuria but may show glucosuria in the postprandial state. Such patients can check their overnight (early a.m.) urine samples for glucose as infrequently as once a week or even every 2 weeks. More important they should understand that appearance of glucosuria where none had been evident or the worsening of glucosuria is an indication for contact with a physician. Similarly, these patients must be taught that, should they develop symptoms and signs of uncontrolled hyperglycemia (heavy glucosuria, polyuria,

polydipsia), prompt advice from a physician is absolutely necessary. Testing for urinary acetone is not necessary unless the patient has glucosuria and at some earlier time had an episode of ketoacidosis, perhaps during stress.

FPG should be determined every few months in most patients and is the only useful means of monitoring sulfonylurea-treated patients who respond to treatment with normalization of blood sugar. Development of hypoglycemia—which may be detected before symptoms develop—is an indication for downward adjustment of drug dosage.

Some patients relentlessly monitor their urine at very frequent intervals—perhaps daily—even though years pass without glucosuria. Such practices are to be discouraged, but certain patients persist despite advice to the contrary, perhaps out of compulsiveness or because of their constant need for reassurance.

SPECIAL CONSIDERATIONS IN TREATMENT OF THE GERIATRIC PATIENT

Some elderly patients may best be treated with oral agents. These individuals may have special problems (e.g., poor vision or manipulative skills) which make self-administration of insulin more difficult than usual. Moreover, simple symptomatic therapy may be the foremost consideration in these individuals. On the other hand, many elderly persons can manage insulin therapy, especially of the type that is not excessively aggressive, and age alone should not deter the physician from appropriate institution of insulin therapy. As noted above (p. 690), insulin syringes can be prefilled and stored in the refrigerator for 1 to 2 weeks; this plan is useful for the older person who cannot accurately draw up the correct amount of insulin. The elderly are especially likely to suffer from multiple diseases and to use multiple drugs. The risk of drug-drug interactions in this group is therefore greater than in younger individuals (see below). The elderly are also especially prone to development of severe and prolonged hypoglycemia with use of the sulfonylureas, which may be related, in part, to the decrease of renal function that normally accompanies aging and that may be worse in the diabetic. Decreased renal function (glomerular filtration rate; creatinine clearance) is frequently present in the elderly even when the serum creatinine is normal, since creatinine production decreases with age as muscle mass decreases. Thus, sulfonylureas which are disposed of exclusively by excretion (acetohexamide) or in part by this route (chlorpropamide; tolazamide) are more likely to produce hypoglycemia when renal function decreases. Chlorpropamide is also uniquely capable of inducing enhanced endogenous antidiuretic hormone action and of inducing a water intoxication syndrome, a phenomenon seen almost exclusively in elderly diabetics (12). Tolbutamide and tolazamide are probably the safest of the sulfonylureas for use in the elderly; the initial dose should be low and increases should be made cautiously. Loading doses should not be used in the elderly.

DRUG-DRUG INTERACTIONS

A variety of drugs enhance the hypoglycemic action of sulfonylureas, while others decrease their effect. The magnitude of the effects varies with the different sulfonylureas. Several mechanisms are involved, some of which are known. Among the more commonly used drugs, salicylates, some sulfonamides, chloramphenicol, phenylbutazone and its derivatives, and bishydroxycoumarin all enhance the hypoglycemic action of the sulfonylureas either by displacement of binding to plasma proteins or by interfering with metabolic disposal. Propranolol (Inderal) and other blockers may mask the hypoglycemia-induced release of epinephrine and thus prolong and intensify the hypoglycemic reactions. Propranolol, by blocking insulin release, may also precipitate hyperosmolar coma. Clonidine (Catapres) may, like propranolol, mask the signs and symptoms of hypoglycemia. Acute ingestion of alcohol can enhance hypoglycemia; chronic alcohol use accelerates metabolic disposal of sulfonylureas and antagonizes their hypoglycemic action. Sulfonylureas, especially chlorpropamide, interfere with the metabolism of alcohol and may produce a disulfiram-like (Antabuse) effect (see Chapter 20). The thiazide diuretics, chlorthalidone, furosemide, and ethacrynic acid may produce hyperglycemia even in normal persons and antagonize the sulfonylureas. Another commonly used drug, the anticonvulsant, phenytoin (Dilantin), also has an antagonist action. Numerous other drugs may enhance or negate the effect of the sulfonylureas; equally important, the sulfonylureas themselves produce numerous alterations of drug action. These problems should not be overstated, but the physician should be aware of these possibilities and interactions.

Treatment of "Other Types" of Diabetes Mellitus (Secondary Diabetes)

Drug-induced diabetes (e.g., thiazides) and diabetes associated with the use of glucocorticoids are usually not ketosis-prone and ordinarily resemble that of NIDDM. Treatment with sulfonylureas may be tried, but insulin is often necessary. Withdrawal of the offending agent does not always ameliorate the diabetic state. The possibility of precipitating diabetes in patients with a strong family history should not deter the physician from the judicious use of diuretics or glucocorticoids when these agents are necessary. Similarly, a diabetic who is already receiving insulin should not be denied diuretic therapy (e.g., when hypertension develops) or glucocorticoids for fear of "aggravating" the diabetes. If such aggravation occurs, usually only an increase of insulin dose is necessary to reestablish the previous state of control.

Diabetes secondary to *chronic pancreatitis* or *pancreatectomy* should be treated with insulin. The insulin requirement is usually 20 to 40 units per day. The patients should be instructed to follow the dietary strategy outlined for insulin-dependent diabetes in Table 69.6. Alcoholic patients with this form of diabetes are particularly difficult to manage if they continue to drink heavily and eat erratically.

COMPLICATIONS OF DIABETES MELLITUS

Diabetes mellitus is the third leading cause of death in the United States today. Most of these deaths are due to the complications of the disease—primarily those complications associated with accelerated atherosclerosis and with chronic renal failure (Fig. 69.1). The risk of both atherosclerotic heart disease and of atherosclerotic peripheral vascular disease is increased approximately 3-fold in diabetics and is proportionate to the duration of disease (both in patients with NIDDM and with IDDM). Atherosclerotic disorders are discussed in Section 8 and in Chapters 80 and 84; chronic renal failure is discussed in Chapter 44.

Diabetic Neuropathy

(See Chapter 81 for a general discussion of peripheral neuropathy.)

The incidence of neurologic deficit in diabetes mellitus is not known, although it is clear that in most patients the occurrence and severity of involvement are related to duration of the disease (Fig. 69.1). The most commonly appreciated abnormality is that which afflicts peripheral sensory nerves. Several types of sensation are involved (pain, proprioception, vibration), and can lead to such uncommon but striking disorders as neuropathic arthropathy. Less well appreciated are the autonomic disorders which give rise to disturbances of cardiovascular function (postural hypotension; resting tachycardia), genitourinary function (impotence; bladder dysfunction), and gastrointestinal function (nocturnal diarrhea; fecal incontinence). Motor deficits are much less common but may occur with striking suddenness. Weakness is distal (neuropathic) rather than proximal (myopathic), although a specific type of myopathy also occurs in diabetics (see "Diabetic Myopathy" below).

PERIPHERAL SENSORY NEUROPATHY

Classically, the deficit is distal, with the lower extremities being first affected, followed by the upper extremities. The term "stocking-glove" distribution is appropriate. In more sophisticated terms, the disorder is a symmetric polyneuropathy with a proximal-distal gradient of dysfunction. In severe cases, even the sensory innervation of the trunk is involved; in this instance the most distal fibers are those of the anterior abdomen and low thorax. Rarely, even the distal

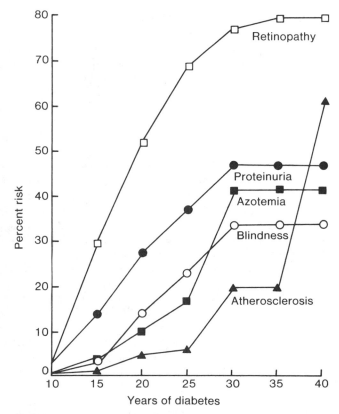

80

Figure 69.1 Complications of diabetes mellitus as a function of duration of the disease. (From M. B. Davidson: *Journal of Chronic Diseases*, *34:* 5, 1981 (2).)

portion of the cranial nerves are affected (e.g., the distal sensory portion of the trigeminal nerve). The patterns of loss are not specific for diabetes mellitus and can be seen in such diverse states as amyloid neuropathy and toxic (e.g., lead) neuropathies. Whether the process represents a "dying-back" of those nerves which are longest or is the cumulative result of randomly scattered lesions along the nerve trunks is not known.

The nerve damage may first produce hyperesthesia and dysesthesia, including tingling and burning sensations. Later, a variety of symptoms are experienced including sensations of numbness or heaviness. Patients often complain that their feet feel "dead" or that they have a sensation of walking on a soft or nonexistent surface. Loss of ability to perceive both temperature and firmness give rise to these complaints. Severe, spontaneous, short-lived leg pains and cramps are common.

On neurologic testing skin hypoesthesia is the commonest finding (pinprick, two-point discrimination, light touch). The hypoesthesia and loss of temperature perception lead to unappreciated skin trauma and predispose to infection. The sensory loss in the finger tips can prevent the blind diabetic from learning Braille letters.

PERIPHERAL MOTOR NEUROPATHY

Much less common and less well recognized are the motor function abnormalities that occur as part of diabetic neuropathy. The intrinsic muscles of the feet are those most commonly involved. Interosseus atrophy produces inability to separate toes, but more important, allows the foot to assume abnormal positions. When claw or hammer toe develops, new pressure points appear at the tips of the toes and along the dorsal aspects; hyperkeratosis, callus formation, and ulceration follow. The interosseous atrophy that may affect the hands does not lead to total loss of function, but does result in weakness of grip. Diffuse weakness of the legs and upper extremities may also occur.

NEUROPATHIC FOOT ULCERS

(See also Chapter 85.)

The combination of sensory loss and motor weakness with anatomic deformity leads to pressure points and to eventual ulceration. Typically, these ulcers occur on the sole of the foot. Remarkably, the ulcers may heal repeatedly only to recur in the same location, but recurrence is not inevitable.

THERAPY OF PERIPHERAL NEUROPATHIES

The therapy of ulceration is primarily one of local foot care. Since callus formation aggravates the tendency to increase local pressure and worsens ulceration, regular debridement is essential. Some patients can be taught debridement techniques, which may at least delay the intervals between visits for this purpose, but usually periodic professional assistance is essential. Such care is often best provided by podiatrists (see Chapter 99). Fitting of custom-made molded shoes is very helpful and is essential in some cases for prevention of ulceration.

Medical therapy is probably useless, except for analgesics as needed. Codeine or a similar agent is often necessary for relief of pain and it may be required chronically. A number of drugs (phenytoin, amitriptyline, carbamazine, and diphenhydramine) have been recommended for treatment of pain in peripheral neuropathy, but there have been no controlled trials to test their efficacy (see Chapter 81 for additional details). Vitamin therapy is also frequently given, but vitamins are almost certainly useless for this purpose. Prompt and vigorous antibiotic therapy of infection in ulcerated areas is essential.

MONONEUROPATHIES

Mononeuropathy (mononeuritis simplex and multiplex) may occur in *any* superficial nerve (simplex) or asymmetric simultaneous combination (multiplex). The lower extremities are more commonly involved (femoral, lateral femoral cutaneous, sciatic, peroneal) than the upper (ulnar, radial, etc.). Onset is usually sudden with intense, often cramping and lancinating pain (see Tables 81.6 and 81.7). Typically, the pain is worse at night and, when the lower extremities are involved, may be relieved by pacing about.

At onset, diagnosis can only be surmised, although tenderness along a nerve trunk is very suggestive. Herpes zoster may be suspected, especially when hyperesthesia occurs, but when no vesicles appear and muscle weakness and atrophy are eventually evident, the diagnosis becomes obvious. The prognosis is quite good, with complete recovery within a few months being the rule.

Cranial and Oculomotor Neuropathies. These mononeuropathies are distinguished from other mononeuropathies mainly by their location. Pain and headache may be present. The commonest nerves involved are III (palebral ptosis; pupillary function undisturbed), VI (inward deviation of eye; diplopia), IV (inward and upward deviations; diplopia). Recovery within 2 months is almost universal. When the facial nerve is involved, distinction from Bell's palsy is not possible (see Chapter 81), although the diabetic variety tends to be less severe and recovery is usually complete.

ABNORMAL SWEAT PRODUCTION

Almost always associated with other evidence of diabetic autonomic neuropathy, this complication in its typical form produces heat intolerance and increased sweating (hyperhydrosis) of the upper half of the body with decreased or absent sweating (anhydrosis) below the midtrunk. In other cases, anhydrosis is generalized and recognition of the complication may be difficult. In women the condition may be confused with menopausal sweats.

A consequence of impaired sweating includes failure to recognize hypoglycemia (see p. 694). This is a serious problem, since one of the warning signals of insulin reaction is lost. Many elderly patients, including those without diabetes mellitus, already have impaired sympathetic responses as a result of aging rather than of diabetes.

Diabetic Myopathy (Amytrophy)

This is a rare but devastating complication of diabetes mellitus which may be confused with diabetic neuropathy. Severe proximal muscle weakness and pain usually affect the pelvic girdle and thigh muscles, although upper truncal musculature can also be involved. The typical patient is an elderly, NIDDM patient with mild disease. Men are more frequently affected than are women. Onset may be fairly rapid, and low grade fever and elevated erythrocyte sedementation rate may be present. Cerebrospinal fluid protein may be very high. Muscle biopsy shows fiber degeneration. Prognosis for improvement is good, but significant residuals are common.

Cardiovascular Dysfunction

In addition to abnormalities of innervation that result in abnormal cardiovascular reflexes (see be-

low), diabetic cardiac denervation apparently accounts for the phenomenon of painless myocardial infarction, which is said to occur in more than 30% of diabetics who experience an acute event. Diagnosis is difficult unless acute electrocardiographic changes are apparent. Precipitation of unexplained ketoacidosis or myocardial failure may divert attention to these secondary events.

RESTING TACHYCARDIA

Heart rates of 90 to 100 beats/min are common in patients with autonomic neuropathy; occasionally even higher rates are observed. Parasympathetic damage is the apparent explanation; the sympathetics appear to be less affected. Propranolol is useful if therapy is needed. In severe cases, the tachycardia subsides over the years as denervation becomes more complete and the sympathetics are also lost.

Several noninvasive tests are available to assess the presence of autonomic cardiovascular dysfunction. These include the Valsalva maneuver, beat-to-beat heart rate variation, and the lying-to-standing heart rate response. Such assessments are more subtle indicators of the presence of autonomic dysfunction than is postural hypotension. These tests are rarely of use clinically, but do allow objective assessment. The consequences—or at least the associations—of these abnormal cardiovascular reflexes in diabetics are important. Once they have developed, there is a marked decrease of 5-year survival. Sudden death—not attributable to myocardial infarction—has been described in many such patients (4).

POSTURAL HYPOTENSION

The most readily recognized and a most troublesome cardiovascular abnormality is postural hypotension (see Chapter 81). The patient may complain merely of dizziness or faintness on standing, or the problem may be more severe, with visual disturbances and syncope. These symptoms may be confused with episodes of hypoglycemia. Remarkably, some patients with fairly marked postural hypotension are asymptomatic.

On initial examination, every diabetic patient should be checked for a postural decrease in blood pressure. In addition, a check for postural hypotension should be made whenever a potentially aggrevating condition occurs. The onset or aggravation of postural hypotension is often associated with the beginning of therapy with a variety of drugs often used in diabetics such as antihypertensive drugs, including diuretics, vasodilators/antispasmodics such as nitroglycerin (glyceryl trinitrate), antidepressants (tricyclic), and phenothiazines. Occasional diabetic patients may be unable to tolerate effective doses of these drugs because of this problem.

The mechanism of this disorder is thought to reside in the efferent limb of the baroreceptor arc secondary to damaged sympathetic vasoconstrictor fibers in the splanchnic bed, muscles, and skin. Diminished plasma renin responses to postural change have been noted in such patients, as have abnormalities of plasma norepinephrine, but the role of these defects is not clear.

A variety of mechanical maneuvers including the use of antigravity or "space suits" have been recommended but are not useful. Drug therapy with vasopressors such as phenylephrine or combinations of tyramine or amine-containing cheeses and monoamine oxidase inhibitors have had their advocates. For patients with severe postural hypotension, the most useful drug is the mineralocorticoid, fludrocortisone (Florinef). In doses of 0.1 to 1.0 mg/day, the drug is often helpful, but since one of its actions is to expand fluid volume, it can produce edema, precipitate cardiac failure, or produce severe hypertension in the recumbent state. Refractoriness may eventually occur. In mild cases, the simple advice that the patient assume upright positions slowly by sitting on the edge of the bed after recumbency may help avoid syncopal episodes, while continuing postural hypotension, though easily measured, may not be especially symptomatic (also see Chapter 81).

Digestive System Dysfunction

Most of the disorders of the gastrointestinal tract in diabetes are related to disturbances of motility. Esophageal motor dysfunction can be demonstrated on testing but is usually not a clinical problem.

Atony of the stomach (gastroparesis diabeticorum) is often asymptomatic, but may be troublesome. Diagnosis is apparent—sometimes as an incidental finding—on barium X-ray of the upper gastrointestinal tract. Occasionally a syndrome of vomiting is accompanied by gastric atony, but mere delay and unpredictable emptying of the stomach may produce irregular diabetic control in already difficult to manage patients with IDDM. Metoclopramide (Reglan) is said to be effective in this disorder (see Chapter 33).

Small bowel dysfunction is common and symptomatic leading to "diabetic diarrhea." Typically the diarrhea is nocturnal. Fecal incontinence may occur and is very distressing. The disorder tends to be episodic, with attacks lasting from a few days to weeks or rarely months. Watery brown diarrhea, usually without steatorrhea, is typical. On barium X-ray studies of the small bowel the findings are those of disturbed motility. Despite the distressing symptoms, the patient appears well; weight loss is uncommon. When steatorrhea occurs, pancreatic exocrine insufficiency and sprue syndrome, more common in diabetics than in the general population, enter the differential. Fully developed sprue is associated with gross evidence of malabsorption. A trial of antibiotic therapy (e.g., tetracycline, 250 mg 4 times a day for 2 weeks) may improve the diarrhea and the malabsorption if the latter is due to small bowel stasis and bacterial colonization. Symptomatic treatment with

antispasmodics (e.g. Lomotil) may be useful, especially when attacks of diarrhea are short-lived.

Large bowel complaints, especially of constipation, are common in the elderly. It does not appear that diabetics are especially prone to any additional problems in this regard.

Patients with poorly controlled diabetes may develop fatty changes of the liver. Hepatomegaly and/or elevations of liver enzymes may occur. Effective control of blood sugar results in disappearance of these abnormalities.

Bladder Dysfunction (Neurogenic Bladder)

The symptoms of bladder dysfunction in diabetics are often overlooked (1). Onset is insidious and occurs over many years. Most patients (80%) will have clinical evidence of neuropathy affecting other systems. The first clinical manifestation of bladder dysfunction is an increase in the interval between voidings until urine is passed only twice or even once daily. A need to strain, slow stream, dribbling, and sensation of incomplete voiding may be present. These symptoms should be routinely solicited from diabetics, especially when there are symptoms or signs of peripheral neuropathy.

Demonstration of residual urine is the hallmark of clinically symptomatic cystopathy, but many diabetic patients, when studied by cytometric techniques, have objective evidence of a neurogenic involvement and a grossly enlarged bladder well before clinical symptoms are evident (1). At this stage, residual urine is not present and other urinary tract abnormalities (recurrent infections) are not evident. The concept that residual urine invariably leads to bacteriuria and infection is widely held but has been challenged and attributed to associated, age-related disorders of bladder outlet (benign prostatic hypertrophy; descensus of the bladder and cystocele).

A variety of cystometric and other procedures are employed for diagnosis of cystopathy. In recent years gas as a filling medium has been introduced, along with sphincter electromyography, flow measurements (uroflowmetry), and urethral pressure profiles. These procedures are useful in distinguishing diabetic cystopathy from associated nondiabetic disorders and help determine treatment programs. A long, low pressure curve with lack of sensation until the bladder capacity is reached, together with increased bladder capacity, establishes the diagnosis. These studies require consultation with a urologist.

Therapy is either medical or surgical. When considerable bladder distention is present, a period of decompression, usually with an indwelling catheter, for about 2 weeks, is helpful in re-establishing bladder function. Many relatively early cases can thereafter be managed through use of suprapubic pressure (Credé maneuver) every 3 hours. If residual urine is reduced to 100 ml or less, no further therapy may be needed. Otherwise, parasympathetic drugs such as bethanechol (Urecholine) (10 to 20 mg, 3 to 4 times daily, or larger doses twice weekly) may be helpful. Intermittent self-catheterization is also useful. If these maneuvers are not effective, transurethral surgery (vesicle neck resection or limited electroincision) is highly effective in many cases. Urinary incontinence is only rarely a problem with this procedure. Vigorous antibiotic therapy is often necessary to prevent recurrent infections and their complications. Long term urologic follow-up is mandatory.

Sexual Dysfunction

The frequency of erectile impotence is high in diabetes, perhaps 50 to 60% overall, but it is, like many other complications of diabetes, related to duration of disease. The problem seems to be a type of autonomic neuropathy involving the pelvic parasympathetic nerves.

Impotence is a common problem in nondiabetic men, and the problems leading to such impotence must be included in the differential diagnosis in the diabetic. Psychogenic factors probably account for the large majority of nondiabetic cases. Although no evidence suggests that psychogenic problems are any more common in diabetics, neither are diabetics immune to psychogenic disturbances. The onset of diabetic impotence is usually slow (6 months to several years), often associated with retrograde ejaculation, and impotence eventually becomes complete. Despite this, libido is characteristically retained. While patients with psychogenic impotence often report nocturnal erections and emissions and may retain masturbatory activity, all of these are absent in diabetic impotence.

An important point on clinical examination is that testicular sensitivity to pressure sufficient to cause pain is retained in psychogenic cases, but is often greatly diminished or lost in the diabetic in whom accompanying sensory neuropathy is common.

The endocrinologic possibilities should be considered because they are potentially treatable, but it is rare to find an endocrine basis for impotence in the diabetic. Testosterone secretion, easily verified by plasma testosterone measurement, is invariably normal in diabetics; therefore, as one would expect, testosterone therapy is useless. Prolactin excess has been recently touted as a cause of impotence, but if that is the case, it must be extremely rare.

A variety of drugs, especially ones which are often used in diabetics, may cause impotence. The most common offenders are the nondiuretic antihypertensives (see Chapter 59).

Several studies report that, in contrast to the male, sexual function in diabetic women appears to be unaffected by the disease. Others have asserted that many diabetic women lose ability to achieve orgasm (3).

The differential diagnosis and therapy of impotence is discussed in detail in Chapter 17. In recent years, considerable success has been achieved in diabetics by use of penile implants, including inflatable prosthetic devices.

Neuropathic Arthropathy (Charcot's Joint; Diabetic Charcot's Foot)

This complication of diabetes is frequently unrecognized or misdiagnosed. The disorder is a progressive, degenerative change of the bony structure of the foot, most often involving the tarsal and tarsometatarsal joints (60%), but also the metatarsalphalangeal joints (30%) and the ankle (10%). The prevalence has been estimated at 1 in 680 cases, but the disorder is probably more common. The patient presents with a swollen foot, often attributed to or associated with recent trauma. The foot may be painful or may be remarkably free of pain, considering the appearance. Examination shows moderate to gross deformity of the foot with "rocker-bottom" subluxation of the midtarsal region or subluxation of the metatarsophalangeal joints. Usually the foot is erythematous and warm to the touch. An infected neuropathic ulcer may be present. More often than not, the pulses are intact. Physicians unfamiliar with this presentation are likely to diagnose some other type of inflammatory arthritis or osteomyelitis and their impression may be "verified" by the X-ray findings. In these early stages, the X-rays show severe osteoarthritis, but, as the disease progresses, there is complete destruction of the involved joints with resorption of the metatarsal heads and phalangeal diaphyses. A variety of other bony changes occurs including fractures, joint effusions, and subluxations. When these changes are at the maximal stage, i.e., when soft tissue involvement is most prominent, the diagnosis of osteomyelitis is frequently entertained, especially when there is an associated, often infected, ulcer. Synovial biopsy showing a thickened synovium containing osseous debris may provide the correct diagnosis and avoid the necessity of embarking on a prolonged and difficult course of antibiotic therapy for suspected osteomyelitis.

Diabetic Charcot's foot may also be confused with the changes associated with osteoarthritis, and gouty, rheumatoid, and psoriatic arthritis. Consultation by an orthopaedic surgeon, rheumatologist, or podiatrist to confirm the diagnosis and to assist with therapy is almost always indicated.

Treatment is based on the cessation of further trauma to the affected area, which is best accomplished by elimination of weight-bearing. Hospitalization may be necessary for this purpose. Reduction of edema and signs of inflammation may take several weeks. Immobilization with a cast may be helpful, but should not be undertaken in the acute stage and, if used, should be done with great care to ensure the integrity of the areas covered by the cast. Simpler bootlike devices may also be used. Crutches can be used at this point, followed eventually by a walking cast. Up to 4 months of treatment may be required.

Thereafter, molded or contoured shoes are essential to proper long term management. Surgical intervention is inadvisable, although occasionally a stabilization procedure may be required if conservative therapy fails. Amputation is not indicated unless osteomyelitis unequivocally coexists or the entire process fails to respond to prolonged conservative efforts. Despite the discouraging appearance of the foot at its worst stages, sufficient healing and stabilization to produce a useful foot can be anticipated.

Other Foot Problems in the Diabetic. A number of common foot problems (e.g., bunions, calluses, corns, fungal infections, and ingrown toenails) can lead to devastating complications in diabetic patients. Prevention through proper foot care and early recognition and treatment are important considerations in the long term care of every diabetic patient. These problems are discussed in detail in Chapter 99.

Diabetic Nephropathy

Progressive renal failure is another life-threatening complication of diabetes. The relationship between hyperglycemia (or insulin deficiency) and the development of microangiopathy with eventual nodular glomerulosclerosis (Kimmelstiel-Wilson disease) remains to be unequivocally established, but experimental evidence is accumulating in favor of such a relationship. Moreover, from observations in man, it now seems clear that the factor is either hyperglycemia, *per se*, or some other factor in the internal milieu of the diabetic that is responsible for the development of diabetic renal disease, since kidney transplants in diabetic patients often develop typical lesions of diabetes.

The clinical course of diabetic nephropathy and the impact of failing renal function on insulin requirement and the oral hypoglycemic drugs is discussed in Chapter 44.

Infections

Although it has never been unequivocally established that diabetics are more prone to infections than nondiabetics, most clinicians will encounter patients who have experienced repeated bacterial or fungal skin infections (carbuncles, furuncles, external otitis, moniliasis) or gastrointestinal moniliasis at sometime before the diagnosis of diabetes was made or in association with uncontrolled hyperglycemia. Most authorities seem to agree that—once established—infections in the diabetic are more difficult than usual to treat and patients are prone to develop complications. Experimentally, hyperglycemia inhibits the phagocytic activity of granulocytes, a factor which may contribute to lowered host resistance. Control of blood sugar, therefore, should be part of any treatment program for an infection.

Urinary tract infections are an especially troublesome problem in diabetics. Although infections are not clearly increased in incidence, a greater prevalence of complications is obvious. Half of all cases of papillary necrosis occurs in diabetics. Diabetic patients also seem prone to develop infections with unusual pathogens. However, no statistical case has been made for the desirability of suppression of asymptomatic bacteriuria in diabetics. Development of pyelonephritis is an indication for immediate hospitalization and vigorous antibiotic treatment; risk of renal carbuncle formation is a special hazard for the diabetic.

Diabetic Retinopathy

This complication of diabetes mellitus has become one of the leading causes of blindness in the United States. In IDDM patients retinopathy first begins to be evident after about 10 years. By the time diabetes has been present for 15 to 20 years, about one-third of patients have severe disease and another one-half have obvious but lesser degrees of progressive retinal involvement. Patients with NIDDM also develop retinopathy, apparently with less frequency (2), but when retinopathy does develop in this older group, the process seems to progress even more rapidly than it does in IDDM patients.

BLINDNESS IN DIABETIC RETINOPATHY

The visual loss in diabetic retinopathy is potentially even more severe than in blindness due to other causes. Many persons who are legally blind (defined as visual acuity less than 20/200 in both eyes) due to causes other than diabetes have slow onset of visual loss, thus allowing time for adaptation. In addition, they often retain reasonably full visual fields and visual acuity at or close to the legal limit. Such persons can see well enough to ambulate independently and can perform a variety of common activities (self-care, housework). With the aid of special devices they may be able even to read newsprint and can engage in some occupations. In contrast, the visual loss of diabetic retinopathy is often due to sudden hemorrhage or retinal detachment and frequently leaves the patient with only light perception. In addition, the diabetic frequently already has other complications of the disease when blindness develops.

Although total blindness afflicts only a minority of diabetic patients (2), a larger number suffer some degree of loss of visual acuity due to macular edema, the commonest cause of visual loss in diabetics.

TYPES OF RETINAL DISEASE IN DIABETES

A crude but convenient classification of diabetic retinal disease is nonproliferative (synonym, "background"), preproliferative, and proliferative retinopathy. The latter, more advanced stage, is the point at which sudden and massive visual loss becomes a problem.

Nonproliferative and Preproliferative Retinopathy. The earliest lesions—readily visible with an ordinary ophthalmoscope—are the region of the macula: microaneurysms, punctate retinal hemorrhages, hard exudates, soft exudates ("cotton wool"), and so-called intraretinal microvascular anomalies (IRMAs). Both microaneurysms and small intraretinal hemorrhages appear as red dots, and both tend to fade within months. Distinction can best be made by fluorescein angiograms in which only microaneurysms "light up." This procedure often identifies extensive intraretinal disease when only a few abnormalities are evident by ophthalmoscopy. Hard exudates, which are glistening yellow or white lipid deposits located in the outer retinal layers, surround areas of capillary obliteration. Soft exudates develop in infarcted areas within the inner retinal layers; they disappear within a few weeks. IRMAs are dilated, hypercellular vessels which are thought to represent either dilated capillaries or intraretinal vascular proliferation. These telangiectatic vessels are identifiable using the green filters of an ordinary ophthalmoscope but are best seen in the secondary phase of fluorescein angiograms during which they leak dye into the retina. IRMAs occur adjacent to areas of capillary closure.

Even the presence of only background retinopathy already indicates areas of intraretinal vascular occlusion with resulting nonperfusion. Decreased visual acuity at this stage requires an ophthalmologist's examination to determine with stereoscopic techniques whether *macular edema* is present. It is not generally appreciated by internists that even without proliferative disease, macular edema may result in visual loss as severe as the 20/200 level. Spontaneous improvement is not common but may occur. In the absence of accompanying proliferative disease, patients at this stage can usually ambulate freely and can engage in some occupations. Ability to read a newspaper except with a vision aid is unlikely and the patient will have to relinquish driving a vehicle because driver's license vision requirements will no longer be met.

Preproliferative disease is said to be present when venous beading occurs in the large retinal veins or when there are many soft exudates, extensive hemorrhages or many IRMAs.

Proliferative Retinopathy. Retinal ischemia is a stimulus to new vessel proliferation (neovascularization). The growth of new vessels into the vitreous causes contraction of the vitreous gel and traction on both new vessels and the retina, thus setting the conditions for retinal detachment and hemorrhage into the vitreous.

TREATMENT OF DIABETIC RETINOPATHY

Two forms of surgical therapy are now available for the treatment of proliferative retinopathy and its complications. Photocoagulation is of proven value in the prevention of visual loss due to proliferative disease, while vitrectomy restores and appears to stabilize vision after hemorrhage and/or retinal detachment.

Photocoagulation Therapy. Since the introduction of the xenonarc photocoagulator in 1959, the approach and rationale of therapy has changed markedly. While the xenonarc polychromatic light source has continued in use, monochromatic devices such as the argon laser have also been extensively used. Initially, therapy was directed at patches of proliferating vessels, but it became apparent that such treatment was not effective in stabilizing proliferative disease. It was noted, however, that in some patients destruction of a large portion of the peripheral retina seemed to arrest the proliferative process. Eventually this approach led to an interinstitutional study called the National Diabetic Retinopathy Study (DRS). Half the patients were treated with the xenonarc; the other half with the argon laser. Multiple (several hundred) burns were placed in the retinal periphery. Within a few years the efficacy of both light sources was established in treatment of nearly 2000 patients. A reduction of severe visual loss of nearly 60% was apparent in patients with proliferative or severe background disease (9).

At this time, the place of laser treatment of macular edema by a study such as the DRS has not been established. Some authorities feel that such therapy is ineffective and may actually decrease central vision, but the issue is not settled.

Patient Experience. Photocoagulation therapy is an outpatient procedure usually performed in several sessions. Ordinarily only topical (corneal) anesthesia is necessary. Occasionally, some discomfort may be experienced during the procedure, in which case a local anesthetic is injected into the retro-orbital tissues to allow a completed, pain-free procedure.

Vitrectomy for Proliferative Retinopathy. Hemorrhage into the vitreous is the usual indication for vitrectomy, a procedure which removes old blood and opaque vitreous and can be combined with cataract extraction. Retinal detachment resulting from traction bands which are formed in the vitreous is another indication for vitrectomy. Provided that the retina has not been torn by the proliferative disease, reattachment occurs within several weeks. Other repair procedures can be attempted. Recently, as an extension of vitrectomy, the removal of preretinal membranes has been introduced.

The results of vitrectomy are dramatic in restoring sight after vitreous hemorrhage. In addition, stabilization of vision can be expected when the traction process is encroaching on the macula. Remarkably, vitrectomy appears to cause actual regression of proliferative retinopathy and may be an effective alternative to photocoagulation in patients who retain good visual acuity. This issue is under active investigation in a newly initiated Diabetic Retinopathy Vitrectomy Study (DRVS).

INDICATIONS FOR REFERRAL TO AN OPHTHALMOLOGIST

All diabetic patients with evidence of background retinopathy or with decreasing visual acuity should be referred for follow-up to an ophthalmologist with expertise in retinal disease. In addition, frequent monitoring of intraocular pressure to detect glaucoma is mandatory in older diabetics (see Chapter 95). Prevention of blindness due to diabetes is now a reality. No longer is ophthalmologic referral a mere formality in these cases.

DIABETES DURING PREGNANCY

Fetal Mortality

Statistics vary widely on the effect of diabetes on survival of the fetus. In some studies the more severe the diabetic state, the worse the perinatal survival, but other studies fail to show a close relationship. Agreement is present only in the case of patients with diabetic nephropathy (White Class F) or proliferative retinopathy (Class R). In these individuals perinatal survival appears to be diminished. Overall, and without regard to the severity of the disease, conventional therapy has resulted in 75 to 90% fetal survival. Ketoacidosis occurs in 2 to 10% of diabetic pregnancies and is associated in these cases with fetal losses of 80 to 100%.

Maternal Mortality and Morbidity

Maternal mortality during pregnancy is definitely increased and at 0.5% is about 20 times that in nondiabetics. Most deaths are due to ketoacidosis or to hypoglycemia, the latter usually occurring in the first trimester or immediately postpartum, times at which insulin requirements often decrease. Obviously, optimal management could eliminate most or all of these deaths. Some deaths which may not be preventable include infections following cesarean section or hemorrhage following traumatic delivery of a large infant. Diabetics with overt heart disease (ischemic heart disease, congestive heart failure) have a very high mortality (75%) when allowed to go to term. Such patients should never become pregnant or should have an abortion if pregnancy occurs.

Maternal morbidity also increases during the diabetic pregnancy. Polyhydramnios occurs in 25% of pregnancies (10 times greater incidence than expected). Asymptomatic bacteriuria (20%) and frank pyelonephritis (7%) occur 3 times more often than in the general population. Pyelonephritis is said to occur in 25% of bacteriuric diabetics and is associated with a very high rate of fetal loss.

Implications of Minimal Diabetes for the Pregnancy

Concern over the problems of the overtly diabetic mother and the fetus has resulted in attempts to determine the effects of even minimal diabetes on the pregnant state and in screening for the presence of diabetes by glucose tolerance tests. Identification of such diabetics has led to studies which purport to show increased perinatal mortality up to 3 to 4 times expected for the general population while other studies have refuted such claims. The most extreme enthusiasts for identification of such individuals sometimes go on to treat with insulin in order to maintain postprandial blood sugar levels which are normal for pregnancy (lower than ordinary normal values; see Table 69.4). Claims have been made that these procedures can be followed in ambulatory patients without undue or unacceptable hypoglycemia. However, frequent and sometimes prolonged hospitalizations and multiple episodes of hypoglycemia almost invariably accompany such an approach. Moreover, no evidence has been presented that such therapeutic heroics significantly affect perinatal mortality. At present such therapy is experimental and cannot be considered to be established.

Diagnosis of Diabetes during Pregnancy

Diabetes developing *de novo* during pregnancy is termed gestational diabetes (p. 683). No diagnostic problem exists when gross hyperglycemia occurs along with glucosuria. However, diagnosis by glucose tolerance testing *during pregnancy* requires special consideration. Since the fasting plasma glucose (FPG) is normally 10 to 20 mg lower during pregnancy than in the nonpregnant state, special criteria for the diagnosis have been established (see Tables 69.3 and 69.4; note also that the dose of glucose is 100 g). Use of the oral glucose tolerance test (OGTT) for the diagnosis of diabetes is certainly dominant in nonpregnant individuals, but the intravenous glucose tolerance test (IVGTT) has a few strong supporters for pregnant patients. Unfortunately, no studies are available to indicate which test is better able to identify women at risk for diabetic complications of pregnancy.

Indications commonly used for testing include family history of diabetes, previous delivery of a large infant (>4000 g; 8.8 lb), previous delivery of an infant with a congenital anomaly, previous unexplained stillbirth, polyhydramnios, obesity, and glucosuria. However, the criteria for obesity are vague, and a minor degree of glucosuria is frequent in normal pregnancy and may be seen in 25% of pregnant women, if a sensitive method of testing is used in the postprandial state. Use of these criteria will result in screening 25 to 50% of pregnant women with an OGTT, while only about 3 to 6% of women so tested will be found to be diabetic. Since the figure for the entire population of pregnant women is about 3%, the commonly used screening criteria are obviously not very useful. Others have proposed a preliminary oral glucose load of 50 g combined with a single blood glucose at 1 hour. Only those individuals with a value greater than 130 mg/100 ml are screened by an OGTT.

This procedure correctly identifies 80 to 90% of diabetics but has 15 to 20% "false positives."

The rationale for labeling any individual whose OGTT meets the criteria in Table 69.4 as a diabetic is not clear. This approach makes no provision for a state of gestational glucose intolerance. Furthermore, in many studies the prognosis for the pregnant state and the perinatal morbidity of infants born of mothers with an abnormal OGTT but with essentially normal FPG does not differ from normal (see above). If one accepts the claim that perinatal mortality is increased in the infants of women with gestational diabetes discovered by OGTT, the question must then be asked whether therapy beyond that which is normally recommended to prevent excessive weight gain is warranted. The answer to this question receives no consensus. Some obstetricians tend to aggressive management while internists are often reluctant to embark on complicated treatment programs which many consider to be of unproven value.

Management of Overt Diabetes during Pregnancy

INSULIN THERAPY

Patients with overt diabetes receiving insulin therapy should be monitored to establish optimal control of blood sugar. Although many obstetricians favor hospitalization with frequent daytime blood sugar determinations ("glucose panel") as an aid to establishment of optimal control, the procedure is useless unless patient compliance can be foreseen after the hospitalization.

Several studies have reported that "tight control" is associated with reduction of fetal loss from 25% to 3 or 4%. On the basis of this information, the goal of insulin and diet therapy should be the closest approximation of normalization of blood sugar that is possible while avoiding therapeutic heroics, i.e., multiple and prolonged hospitalizations solely for the purpose of blood sugar control. Normal fasting blood sugar (not exceeding 85 mg/100 ml) and postprandial blood sugars which do not exceed 140 mg/100 ml would be considered "tight control" by most. However, some obstetricians strive for blood sugar levels averaging 100 mg/100 ml, a goal probably impossible to achieve without prolonged hospitalizations and excessively frequent hypoglycemia.

Most patients will require two doses of intermediate acting insulin or a mixture of intermediate and short acting insulin. A few NIDDM patients may have satisfactory control on a single dose of insulin. It should be kept in mind that insulin requirements often decrease in the first trimester only to rise progressively as pregnancy proceeds. Frequent monitoring of glucosuria and ketonuria is an invaluable guide to ambulatory management, as it is in the nonpregnant patient. While frequent blood sugar determinations are helpful, they do not replace urine monitoring. Minor ketonuria due to carbohydrate lack is common but can usually be distinguished by rough quantitation of the ketonuria and, if necessary, of the blood sugar measurement. Determination of plasma bicarbonate and plasma "ketones" should be made if any doubt still exists. The development of ketoacidosis is an indication for immediate hospitalization.

DIET THERAPY

Diet therapy is often modified slightly to include increased protein intake. Weight gain of about 25 lb (11.5 kg) is expected and acceptable in both normal and diabetic pregnancy. Severe weight control, previously advocated by some, has been abandoned.

TIMING OF DELIVERY

This issue has been argued for decades, since it was recognized that the incidence of stillbirths in diabetics increases beyond the 36th week. However, attempts to deliver infants early (before 40 weeks) has resulted in a high rate of cesarean section and a high rate of neonatal loss due to neonatal respiratory distress syndrome. Attempts have been made to determine fetal lung maturity by amniotic fluid phospholipid measurements (lecithin/sphingomyelin ratio). Other monitoring measurements include the urinary estradiol quantitation. These monitoring issues remain controversial and are largely determined by prevailing obstetrical dogma.

COUNSELING THE DIABETIC WOMAN—RISKS OF PREGNANCY

The issue of the complexity of diabetic management is not likely to deter pregnancy. On the other hand, the possibility of diabetes in the newborn or young child is often of great concern; this issue has already been discussed (see "Inheritance and Genetic Counseling"). Other questions concern maternal and fetal mortality. While the diabetic mother without overt complications suffers little or no increased risk, the fetal issues must be presented with candor. Of special importance beyond that of infant survival is the problem of an increased risk of congenital abnormalities and long term neurologic abnormalities in children of diabetic mothers (7). Whether complications of diabetes are accelerated by pregnancy is not clear. The long term survival of the diabetic with microvascular disease is already significantly compromised and an honest prognosis in this regard may deter pregnancy, not necessarily because of concern over acceleration of the diabetic complications, but out of concern for the future welfare of a child born to a mother whose state of health may be poor and whose survival is threatened.

References

General

Diabetes Care. A publication of the American Diabetes Association since 1979.
   This journal for the practitioner contains reviews and practical articles.

National Diabetes Data Group: Classification and diagnosis of diabetes mellitus and other categories of glucose intolerance. *Diabetes 28*: 1039, 1979.

The latest criteria for diagnosis; a milestone in our concepts of the problem. Many references. Reprints available from: Westwood Building, Room 607, National Institutes of Health, Bethesda, MD 20205.

Podolsky, S (ed): *Clinical Diabetes: Modern Management*. Appleton-Century-Crofts, New York, 1980.

A multiauthored text including some outstanding authorities. Many references, diet tables, photographs, etc. Especially good portions relevant to management of ambulatory patients.

Williams, RH (ed): *Textbook of Endocrinology*, Ed. 6. W. B. Saunders, Philadelphia, 1981.

The latest edition of this standard textbook contains good chapters relating to diabetes.

Specific

1. Bradley, WE: Diagnosis of urinary bladder dysfunction in diabetes mellitus. *Ann Intern Med 92* (Part 2): 323, 1980.
2. Davidson, MB: The continually changing "natural history" of diabetes mellitus. *J Chronic Dis 34*: 5, 1981.
3. Ellenberg, M: Sexual dysfunction in diabetic patients. *Ann Intern Med 92* (Part 2): 331, 1980.
4. Ewing, DJ, Campbell, IW and Clarke, BF: Assessment of cardiovascular effects in diabetic anatomic neuropathy and prognostic implications. *Ann Intern Med 92* (Part 2): 308, 1980.
5. FILMS: Millner, Fenwick, Inc.: Diabetic Teaching Films. 2125 Greenspring Dr., Timonium, MD 21093. NEWSLETTERS: *Diabetes in the News*. 233 East Erie St., Suite 712, Chicago, IL 60611 (no charge; junior high school level or above); *Forecast*. 600 5th Ave., New York, NY 10020 (about $15/year; high school level or above).
6. Goldstein, S and Podolsky, S: Inheritance of diabetes and genetic counseling. In *Clinical Diabetes: Modern Management*, Chap. 1, pp. 1–22, edited by S Podolsky. Appleton-Century-Crofts, New York, 1980.
7. Haworth, JC, McRae, KN and Dilling, LA: Prognosis of infants of diabetic mothers in relation to neonatal hypoglycemia. *Dev Med Child Neurol 18*: 471, 1976.
8. National Diabetes Group: Classification and diagnosis of diabetes mellitus and other categories of glucose tolerance. *Diabetes 28*: 1039, 1979.
9. Preliminary Report on Effects of Photocoagulation Therapy: *Am J Ophthalmol 81*: 383, 1976.
10. Rushforth, NB, Miller, M and Bennett, PH: Fasting and two-hour post-load glucose levels for the diagnosis of diabetes. *Diabetologia 16*: 373, 1979.
11. Stamler, R and Stamler, J (eds): Asymptomatic hyperglycemia and coronary heart disease. A series of papers by the International Collaborative Group, Based on Studies in Fifteen Populations. *J Chronic Dis 32*: 683, 1979.
12. Weissman, PN, Shenkman, L and Gregerman, RI: Chlorpropamide hyponatremia. Drug-induced inappropriate antidiuretic-hormone activity. *N Engl J Med 284*: 65, 1971.
13. West, KM: Diet therapy of diabetes: an analysis of failure. *Ann Intern Med 79*: 425, 1973.
14. West, KM: Diet and diabetes. *Postgrad Med 60*: 209, 1976.

CHAPTER SEVENTY

Thyroid Disorders*

ROBERT I. GREGERMAN, M.D.

* Substantial portions of this chapter were published in R. I. Gregerman: The thyroid gland. In *The Principles and Practice of Medicine*, Ed. 20, edited by A. M. Harvey *et al.* Appleton-Century-Crofts, New York, 1980.

INTRODUCTION

Disturbances of thyroid growth and function are among the most common endocrinologic disorders encountered in ambulatory practice. Excessive production of the thyroid hormones, thyroxine (T_4) and triiodothyronine (T_3) (Fig. 70.1) results in hyperthyroidism, or thyrotoxicosis; decreased hormone production, in hypothyroidism. Generalized enlargement of the thyroid, regardless of cause, is termed goiter. Focal enlargement of the thyroid is termed a "nodule" and is usually benign. Either goiter or focal enlargement may be associated with abnormal thyroid function. Goiter can produce anatomic changes ranging from the simply cosmetic to obstruction of contiguous structures such as the trachea and esophagus.

Thyroid Regulatory Mechanisms

The principal regulatory mechanism of the thyroid is the hypothalamic-pituitary-thyroid negative feedback control system. The hypothalamus secretes thyrotropin-releasing hormone (TRH), which travels via the hypophyseal portal system to the pituitary, where it stimulates release of thyroid-stimulating hormone (TSH). TSH stimulates many aspects of thyroid activity including hormone synthesis, thyroid growth, and the release of thyroid hormones. Secretion of TSH by the pituitary is inhibited by the thyroid hormone—thus the term "negative feedback loop."

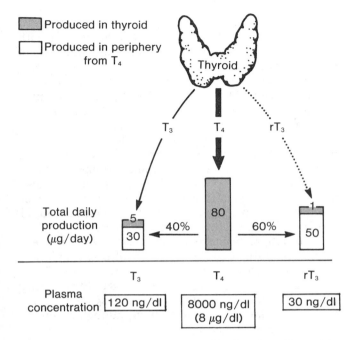

Figure 70.1 Production rates by the thyroid and in the periphery of thyroid hormones and their mean concentrations in the plasma.

Iodide from plasma is concentrated by an active process (iodide "pump") which can maintain a thyroid/plasma iodide ratio as high as 500 to 1. Iodide is thereafter converted through a series of enzymatic steps resulting in the formation of T_3 and T_4 bound within the thyroglobulin sequence. The iodide pump activity transports a number of anions other than iodide, a phenomenon which has been exploited diagnostically and therapeutically. For example, the pertechnetate anion, as the radioactive isotope ^{99m}Tc, has been widely used for thyroid imaging, although ^{123}I is now preferred.

The minimal daily requirement of iodide is only about 100 to 200 μg, an amount which is determined by obligatory loss, mainly through the kidney. The minimal daily requirement is enormously exceeded by dietary intake; for example, iodinated salt provides about 1000 μg in a normal 10-g daily intake. Thus, iodide deficiency, once common in the United States and elsewhere, is essentially unknown except in remote areas of the underdeveloped world.

Any chemical substance that interferes with thyroid hormone function or release may lower blood hormone concentration and induce compensatory hypertrophy of the gland (goiter) via stimulation of TSH secretion. Certain substances are known to prevent iodide accumulation by impairment of the iodide "pump." Other substances interfere with hormone synthesis or inhibit hormone release. Clinically useful agents which have been employed for therapeutic effects in states of excess hormone production (hyperthyroidism) are known to act at one or another of these points. Perchlorate, no longer commonly used

therapeutically, inhibits the iodide "pump." The thiocarbamide drugs interfere with hormone synthesis by blockade of incorporation of iodide into the tyrosines ("organification") and of the coupling reactions in iodothyronine formation, but have more effect on coupling than on organification. Lithium ion (currently in wide use for the treatment of depressive illness, Chapter 14), interferes with thyroglobulin proteolysis and hormone release and may result in goiter and, occasionally, hypothyroidism. Iodide itself in pharmacologic amounts interferes with hormone formation and release and in some individuals is a goitrogen.

Metabolic Effects of Thyroid Hormone

The thyroid hormones exert their actions through a variety of mechanisms. A classic thyroid hormone effect is on basal metabolic rate (BMR), the basis for the first laboratory method for clinical assessment of thyroid status. The numerous known actions of thyroid hormone range from specific stimulation of mitochondrial oxidative metabolism to the nuclear regulation of protein synthesis. Thyroid hormones also exert specific regulatory effects on membrane physiology, e.g., potentiation of catecholamine effects. This action of thyroid hormones explains the signs of exaggerated sympathetic activity in hyperthyroidism and the effectiveness of the therapy of this condition by β-adrenergic blockade.

Hormone Transport

The thyroid hormones in the blood are T_4 and a much smaller quantity of T_3. Both hormones are tightly but reversibly bound to several plasma proteins, mainly thyroid hormone binding globulin (TBG). In the normal person 65 to 70% of the thyroid hormones are bound to TBG, about 15% to the secondary carrier, thyroxine-binding prealbumin (TBPA), and about 15% to albumin. Variations of TBG occur in many clinical states and account for most of the changes in T_4 concentration in plasma that are seen in diseases other than hypo- and hyperthyroidism. Small quantities of T_4 (0.03%) and T_3 (0.3%) are not protein-bound but are unbound or "free" and in rapid equilibrium with the protein-bound fraction.

The concentrations of free T_4 and T_3 in plasma are thought to reflect the amount of hormone exerting an effect on tissues. Clinical status in a number of conditions correlates with free T_4 rather than with total hormone in plasma. A good example of this correlation is the normal pregnant state in which total T_4 is high, but in which there is no evidence of free thyroid hormone excess. The explanation is that plasma TBG is elevated, a consequence of the hyperestrogenism of pregnancy.

In some pathologic states that affect the quantity of TBG in plasma (Table 70.1), and hence the total T_4, the absolute concentration of free T_4 may not adjust to a normal value. During illness, factors other than the concentration of TBG and TBPA appear to determine the free hormone concentration, presumably by affecting the affinity of the TBG-T_4 interaction.

Metabolism and Interconversion of Thyroid Hormones

Practically all tissues metabolize and degrade the thyroid hormones, but the liver is quantitatively most important and is a site at which regulation of hormone degradation occurs. T_4 metabolism is the major source (80%) of circulating T_3 in the normal individual. The normal thyroid secretes mainly T_4 and only a small amount of T_3 (Fig. 70.1). Only in hyperthyroidism, iodine deficiency, and certain other pathologic circumstances is T_3 sometimes the predominantly secreted hormone.

Most of the T_4 secreted (about 85%) is ultimately deiodinated and further degraded. The physiologically most important pathway involves conversion of about 35% of the T_4 to metabolically active T_3, which is itself further deiodinated. About an equal amount of T_4 is converted to reverse T_3 (rT_3) (Fig. 70.1). Although not active in calorigenesis, rT_3 does antagonize a number of the effects of T_3 and thus may have some physiologic importance. In a variety of pathologic states the formation of T_3 is inhibited, whereas that of rT_3 is reciprocally enhanced. Measurement of rT_3 has some usefulness in the differential diagnosis of the "euthyroid sick syndrome" (see "Differential Diagnosis" under "Hypothyroidism").

LABORATORY TESTS OF THYROID FUNCTION AND OF THYROID DISEASE

Most thyroid "function" tests assess secretory activity of the thyroid gland only indirectly. Measure-

Table 70.1
Factors Affecting Thyroxine-Binding Globulin (TBG)

TBG INCREASED
    Estrogens:
        Oral contraceptives
        Pregnancy
    Hypothyroidism
    Acute hepatitis
    Cirrhosis
    Genetic TBG excess
    Acute intermittent porphyria
    Perphenazine (Trilafon)
TBG DECREASED
    Androgens
    Anabolic steroids
    Cirrhosis
    Glucocorticoids
    Nephrotic syndrome
    Severe chronic nonthyroidal illness
    Cushing's syndrome
    Genetic TBG deficiency

ments of blood hormone concentrations, the most commonly used tests, cannot be equated directly with the rate of hormone production, although they reflect that rate when plasma binding of hormones is normal. However, a variety of illnesses, drugs, and alterations of physiologic state affect plasma binding. Accordingly, proper interpretation of plasma hormone concentrations demands concomitant assessment of plasma binding. Thyroid gland function can be assessed somewhat more directly by measurement of thyroidal iodide accumulation ("uptake"; RaIU) using isotopes of iodide (^{131}I, ^{123}I). These tests also must be properly interpreted, since uptake of tracer is only an approximation of the accumulation of stable iodide and of hormone synthesis.

Other laboratory tests are useful in the assessment of thyroid status and the diagnosis of thyroid disease but are not, strictly speaking, tests of thyroid function. Such tests include measurements of the integrity of the physiologic feedback control system (TSH), thyroid autoantibodies, and the immunoglobulins related to Graves' disease.

Measurements of Plasma Hormone: Plasma T_4 and T_3

The commonly used and important tests of thyroid function are measurements of the levels of T_4 and T_3, as determined by radioimmunoassay or other specific methods. Unlike the case with older techniques, no chemical interference is produced by drugs or iodine-containing substances, but it must be kept in mind that such agents may affect the actual level of thyroid hormones in blood. rT_3 is occasionally also used in differential diagnosis, especially of ill patients. The value of T_4 is certainly the single most important measurement in clinical evaluation of thyroid disease. However, interpretation of a given value (concentration) must take into account whether T_4 binding to plasma proteins is normal. Accordingly, T_4 must be assessed in conjunction with determination of TBG (see below). Normal values of the common tests are given in Table 70.2.

"Free T_4": Measurement of Non-Protein-Bound Thyroid Hormone in Plasma

The "free T_4" of plasma is estimated by separate measurements of the non-protein-bound T_4 (equilibrium dialysis) and the total T_4; their arithmetic product equals the free T_4. The dialyzable (non-protein-bound) T_4 normally approximates only 0.03% of the total.

The free T_4 hypothesis (see p. 709) has been helpful as a physiologic concept. Determination of the free T_4 for clinical purposes is often useful, but the measurement has serious limitations. In some states, such as pregnancy or during estrogen therapy, both T_4 and TBG are elevated and thyroid status is accurately reflected by the free T_4. The dialyzable fraction is decreased, but since the T_4 is elevated, the free T_4 is

Table 70.2
Thyroid Function Tests[a]

	Plasma T$_4$ (μg/dl)	Plasma T$_3$ (ng/dl)	T$_3$ Resin Uptake (T$_3$U) (%)	T$_3$ Resin Uptake Ratio (T$_3$UR)	TSH (μU/ml)	Free T$_4$ (FT$_4$) (ng/dl)	Free T$_4$ Index (FTI)[b]
Normal mean	8	120	30	1	—	1.5	8.0
Normal range	5–12	80–160	25–35	0.85–1.15	0–6	1.0–2.0	5.8–10.6
Confidence limits	±1	±20	±2	±0.05	±2	±0.3	—

[a] See text for limitations of interpretation of normal ranges. Confidence limits (95%) of a single value are approximate and depend on both the laboratory and the level within the range.

[b] The FTI on any sample is calculated as T$_4$ × T$_3$UR, but the normal range for the FTI is determined empirically. The units of the FTI depend on whether the percentage T$_3$ resin uptake or the T$_3$ resin uptake ratio is multiplied times T$_4$.

normal. In hyperthyroidism, free T$_4$ reflects thyroid status better than total T$_4$, since the altered metabolic state itself lowers TBG; in some cases a normal or borderline elevation of T$_4$ is associated with an elevated free T$_4$. In hypothyroidism, TBG is often elevated and the free T$_4$ is decreased more than is the total T$_4$.

Problems of interpretation of the free T$_4$ arise in many seriously ill patients. A variety of nonthyroidal diseases ranging from acute infections to liver disease can result in elevation of the free T$_4$. In these situations, the patient is usually euthyroid with a normal T$_4$; the free T$_4$ is elevated only because the dialyzable fraction is increased. An explanation for this phenomenon is not readily available. Altered concentrations of neither TBG nor TBPA account for the increased free T$_4$. The appearance of a factor in plasma which interferes with protein binding of T$_4$ has been postulated. Thus, an elevated free T$_4$ is not a specific finding related solely to thyroid status.

Estimates of TBG: T$_3$ Resin Uptake and "Free T$_4$ Index" (FTI)

The T$_3$ uptake test (T$_3$U) is not to be confused with the concentration of T$_3$ in plasma. The T$_3$U is not a thyroid function test, but merely provides an indirect estimate of the concentration of plasma TBG. To some extent, T$_3$U is also influenced by the quantity of T$_4$ in plasma, i.e., by the degree of saturation of the T$_4$ (and T$_3$) binding sites on TBG. The T$_3$U may be replaced by direct quantitation of TBG. Technically the T$_3$U is measured by adding a tracer quantity of T$_3$ and a nonspecific T$_3$ binding absorbent resin to the sample of plasma to be tested. The tracer distributes itself between nonspecific binding sites on the absorbent and specific binding sites on TBG. Resin-bound tracer is therefore reciprocally related to the quantity of TBG in the plasma. The test result is expressed as a percent or as a ratio of the test sample to that of the laboratory's control plasma (T$_3$U ratio).

The usefulness of the T$_3$U is in interpreting a given level of T$_4$. A high (or low) T$_4$ can be interpreted as reflecting increased or decreased T$_4$ secretion only if the plasma binding of T$_4$ is normal, i.e., only if the TBG (T$_3$U) is normal. Otherwise, to reach a proper conclusion about thyroid function, disturbance of binding must be considered along with the high (or low) T$_4$. For convenience the T$_4$ and T$_3$U have been combined to give a so-called free T$_4$ index (FTI) by simply multiplying one number times the other. This procedure "compensates" for the high or low T$_4$ value which results from abnormality of TBG concentration. In most, but not all, cases, FTI closely parallels free T$_4$.

Tests of the Negative Feedback System

THYROID-STIMULATING HORMONE (TSH)

Plasma TSH is invariably elevated in primary hypothyroidism because of reduced feedback inhibition by the decreased concentrations of the thyroid hormones. The measurement of plasma TSH is important both in the diagnosis of primary hypothyroidism and in monitoring the adequacy of thyroid hormone replacement therapy (see below). Elevation of plasma TSH is the most sensitive indicator of hypothyroid status. Elevations of TSH are reliably measured by radioimmunoassay techniques currently available. However, by most assay methods plasma TSH of normal subjects is below the sensitivity of the method; many of the values reported to be within the normal range are nonspecific.

SUPPRESSION TESTS: USE OF T$_4$ AND T$_3$

In several thyroid diseases, gland function becomes independent of TSH, i.e., nonsuppressible by amounts of exogenous thyroid hormone that inhibit normal pituitary secretion of TSH. Nonsuppressibility is seen in hyperthyroidism due to any cause, in cases of hyperfunctioning adenoma ("hot nodule") with or without hyperthyroidism, and in some cases of nontoxic nodular goiter. About one-half of patients with Graves' ophthalmopathy without hyperthyroidism have nonsuppressible thyroid function. Return of suppressibility in the course of Graves' disease indicates clinical remission, and the test is therefore a useful guide to therapy as well as diagnosis. Testing for suppressibility is done with T$_3$ or T$_4$ with the use of a 50% decrease of radioiodide uptake as the endpoint. T$_4$ is given as a single 3-mg dose or 25 μg of T$_3$ are given every 8 hours. Radioiodide uptake is measured at 6 to 8 days (see p. 726).

THE TRH TEST

Parenterally administered TRH produces release of TSH from the pituitary. Response to TRH is abnormal in several clinical circumstances and is diagnostically useful. Confirmation of a diagnosis of primary hypothyroidism is possible when the plasma TSH elevation is borderline, since an exaggerated plasma TSH response will be seen. The *increment* of TSH following TRH does not normally exceed 30 μU/ml, but elevations several times this amount may be seen in cases of borderline hypothyroidism. The most common use of the tests is as an alternative to the T_3 suppression test in the diagnosis of hyperthyroidism. Hypersecretion of thyroid hormones producing even minimal elevation of blood hormone levels blunts or abolishes the normal response to TRH. The TRH test is also useful in the differential diagnosis of severely ill patients with low plasma T_4 (see "Euthyroid Sick Syndrome vs. Hypothyroidism"). The TRH test is of limited use in the elderly in whom lack of TRH response is normal.

The test is performed by injecting 500 μg of TRH intravenously. Plasma TSH is measured before injection and at 20 and 30 min. A significant response is an increase of more than 2 μU/ml. The general physician can easily perform the TRH test in his office. (The TRH (Thypinone) can be bought through any commercial pharmacy.)

Thyroidal Radioiodide Uptake (RaIU) Tests

The rate of tracer iodide accumulation (^{131}I, ^{123}I) in the thyroid can be measured by using times ranging from a few minutes to the plateau of accumulation (24 hours). These procedures, although still in wide use, have been rendered almost obsolete by the simpler and less expensive measurements of hormone concentrations in plasma. The diagnostic usefulness of the RaIU is also seriously limited by the "saturation" of Western diets with iodide. This has resulted in RaIU values that are too low to discriminate normal function from hypofunction, so that the test is now useless for the diagnosis of hypothyroidism. It is still of use in hyperthyroidism although, since results are "normal" in up to 50% of cases of hyperthyroidism, a normal RaIU does not exclude the diagnosis. One important use of the test is in patients with hyperthyroidism associated with thyroiditis. If this condition is suspected, an RaIU is important; a low value deters inappropriate therapy. The RaIU is also subject to interference by chemical agents and certain clinical states; both produce false positive and false negative results. The RaIU should no longer be used for the *routine* evaluation of thyroid function.

Immunologic Tests

Assay of antibodies to thyroidal antigens (thyroglobulin, microsomes), so-called thyroid autoantibodies, are useful in determining the presence of autoimmune thyroiditis (see below, p. 721, "Hashimoto's Disease"). Measurement of thyroid-stimulating immunoglobulin (TSI) (see "Graves' Disease") is not yet readily available. The long acting thyroid stimulation (LATS) test, still available in some laboratories, is useless. TSI measurements, when available, are useful in the pregnant patient, since high levels are associated with an increased likelihood of neonatal hyperthyroidism. A fall in TSI is a good indicator of remission in Graves' disease and will probably be useful for this purpose as the test becomes available.

Other Tests

A variety of *scintiscan* or *imaging techniques* are available to delineate the anatomy of the thyroid and to distinguish functional from nonfunctional tissue, a consideration in the differential diagnosis of thyroid neoplasms. Currently, ^{99m}Tc pertechnetate (TcO$_4^-$) is most widely used, but ^{123}I is the imaging agent of choice. (Some tumors will accumulate pertechnetate, thereby obscuring the diagnosis.)

Ultrasound imaging (sonography) is now a routine procedure for distinguishing cystic from solid nodules, an important point in differential diagnosis of these lesions. Moreover, ultrasound can accurately assess the *size* of nodules, providing an objective basis for evaluation of medical therapy.

Needle biopsy is rapidly assuming the status of a routine procedure in many centers. In proper hands, needle biopsy is a safe, outpatient procedure which gives a diagnosis in most cases. *Fine needle aspiration* with cytologic examination is not as reliable as needle aspiration biopsy. Although both procedures may fail to distinguish benign adenomas from well differentiated follicular carcinomas (7), an important limitation of the technique, the procedure undoubtedly helps avoid many operations and may provide much needed reassurance for the patient. Needle biopsy is performed ordinarily by an endocrinologist or a surgeon who has been trained in the technique. The procedure, performed under local (cutaneous) anesthesia, is ordinarily painless. The only significant complication is local hemorrhage, but this is uncommon and usually of minor degree.

Nonspecificity of Thyroid Function Tests in Nonthyroidal Illness

The clinician should realize that thyroid function tests may be non-specifically altered in many nonthyroidal diseases, *i.e.*, these tests are *not specific* when severe illness is present (Table 70.3). Moreover, a variety of drugs affect both thyroid function and the function tests (Tables 70.1 and 70.4). Some examples of these considerations are presented below; extensive discussions can be found elsewhere (3).

EFFECTS OF GONADAL AND ADRENAL HORMONES

Estrogens (pregnancy, contraceptives) raise, and androgens lower, T_4 by altering plasma TBG. Gluco-

Table 70.3
Nonthyroidal Illness: Effects on T₄, Free T₄, and TBG in Plasma [a]

	Effects on T$_4$	Free T$_4$	TBG
LIVER DISEASE			
Active hepatitis	↑	↔↑	↑
Cirrhosis	↑ ↓	↔↑	↑ ↓
Cholangitis	↑	↔↑	↑
RENAL DISEASE			
Nephrotic syndrome	↔↓	↔	↔↓
Uremia, chronic	↔↓	↔↓	↔↓
INFECTIONS	↓	↑	↔
MALNUTRITION	↓	↑	↔↓

[a] Most illnesses and even such minor alterations of physiologic state as decreased food intake will produce a decrease of plasma T$_3$.

Table 70.4
Drug and Hormone Effects on Plasma T₄ and TBG

Gonadal Hormones	Effect on T$_4$	Free T$_4$	Effect on TBG
ESTROGENS	↑	↔↓	↑
Oral contraceptives			
Pregnancy			
ANDROGENS	↓	↔	
Testosterone			↑
Anabolic steroids			
GLUCOCORTICOIDS	↓	↔	↓
Cushing's syndrome			
Pharmacologic uses			
PSYCHOTROPIC DRUGS			
Perphenazine (Trilafon)	↑	↔	↑
ANTICONVULSANTS			
Phenytoin (Dilantin)	↓	↔↓	↔
HEPARIN	↔	↑	↔
ADRENERGIC BLOCKERS			
Propranolol (Inderal)	↔ (↓ T$_3$)	↔	↔
GALLBLADDER DYES	↔ ↓ (↓ T$_3$)	↔↓	↔

corticoids inhibit thyroid activity acutely by interfering with TSH secretion and affect the pituitary's responsiveness to TRH. The plasma T$_4$ is lowered during chronic glucocorticoid therapy, due mainly to a decrease of TBG. When dexamethasone is given acutely, the plasma T$_4$ decreases slightly and T$_3$ falls sharply.

LIVER DISEASES

A variety of alterations of thyroid function tests are produced by liver diseases. Early in infectious hepatitis, the T$_4$ is elevated secondary to an increase of TBG. Chronic liver disease produces many abnormalities in an unpredictable fashion. T$_4$ may be increased or decreased in parallel with TBG and the T$_3$U. Free T$_4$ is often elevated with no obvious relationship to the TBG. T$_3$ is usually low. A frequent and unexplained abnormality is elevation of TSH, although the response to TRH is not exaggerated as it is in hypothyroidism. RaIU is often elevated in acute alcoholic hepatitis with or without cirrhosis and in some cases of cholangitis. These changes have been attributed both to iodide depletion and to acceleration of T$_4$ metabolism.

RENAL DISEASES

The nephrotic syndrome is often associated with depressed T$_4$, but the decrease is not always explained by a lowering of the TBG. In chronic renal disease, the *means* of T$_4$, TBG, and the FTI are not significantly different from normal, but the *range* is greater and values may exceed the usual normal limits. Some patients with severe chronic renal failure receiving long term dialysis show a progressive decrease of T$_4$. These patients and those with the nephrotic syndrome may represent examples of the recently recognized "euthyroid sick syndrome" (see "Hypothyroidism"). As one would expect in any chronic illness, the plasma T$_3$ is depressed.

INFECTIONS, MALNUTRITION, AND DRUGS

The T$_4$ may drop early in the course of acute infection and free T$_4$ may rise. Neither change is accounted for by an alteration of TBG. During starvation, plasma T$_3$ falls. Free T$_4$ is often increased without relation to the TBG. Plasma T$_3$ is often decreased in the elderly, a change which has been attributed to aging, but is in fact due to diminished food intake and nonspecific illness. Closely correlated alterations of T$_3$U and plasma TBG have been reported in protein-calorie malnutrition. Some pharmacologic agents affect the thyroid hormones of plasma (1). Phenytoin (Dilantin) lowers the T$_4$ and free T$_4$, often into the hypothyroid range. Although plasma TSH may be somewhat elevated, clinical hypothyroidism is not seen. Heparin acutely elevates the free T$_4$. The mechanisms of these changes are not known. Propranolol decreases plasma T$_3$ by inhibition of the normal T$_4$ deiodination route; rT$_3$ is increased. A similar effect is produced by some radiopaque contrast media used for visualization of the gallbladder.

Interpretation of Thyroid Function Tests: Statistical Considerations

No single numerical value divides normal from abnormal in any thyroid function test. The upper and lower limits of normal for plasma T$_4$, free T$_4$ index, and T$_3$ are set at ± 2 standard deviations from the mean. By definition, therefore, 2.5% of normal persons will have abnormal values at each end of the distribution. To complicate the issue, a small number of hyperthyroid or hypothyroid persons have values that fall within the normal range. In addition to the statistical overlap, one must recall that both biologic day-to-day variation and unavoidable analytic error further obscure the dividing line between normal and abnormal. For example, 95% confidence limits of a single T$_4$ test are ± 1 μg/dl at the upper and lower limits of the normal range. For all of these reasons, and because of the occasional instance of laboratory or reporting error, a single determination can neither establish nor exclude a diagnosis with anything more than reasonable statistical certainty. Therefore, all abnormal values should be confirmed before therapy is undertaken.

HYPERTHYROIDISM (THYROTOXICOSIS)

Hyperthyroidism, the clinical state resulting from an excess of thyroid hormone, is the most common functional disorder of the thyroid. Although essentially the same clinical picture results from any of several distinct pathologic processes (Table 70.5), selection of proper therapy demands that the correct diagnosis be established. The most common variety of hyperthyroidism is Graves' disease, an autoimmune process also known as diffuse toxic goiter. Only slightly less common is hyperthyroidism due to a hyperfunctioning nodular goiter (toxic nodular goiter). Occasionally hyperthyroidism is due to a solitary hyperfunctioning adenoma. Recently hyperthyroidism has been seen with increasing frequency as a transient phenomenon in the evolution of thyroiditis (4, 8, 11). The other causes of hyperthyroidism listed in Table 70.5 are so rare that they are not usually encountered in ordinary practice.

Graves' Disease

Graves' disease is a complex disorder comprising toxic goiter, ophthalmopathy, and occasionally dermopathy. At any given time during the course of the disease, one of these manifestations may be an isolated finding. Graves' ophthalmopathy and Graves' dermopathy can occur independently of thyroid hormone excess. Recently, the view has been expressed that ophthalmopathy and dermopathy are closely related but separate and overlapping immunologic disorders (10).

Table 70.5
Causes of Hyperthyroidism[a]

COMMON
    Graves' disease
    Toxic nodular goiter
        Multinodular
        Uninodular
    Hyperthyroidism in association with thyroiditis
RARE
    Thyrotoxicosis due to TSH or TSH-like stimulator
        Choriocarcinoma or hydatidiform mole
        Embryonal cell carcinoma of testis
        Pituitary tumor with TSH excess
        Idiopathic TSH excess
    Toxic thyroid carcinoma
    Hyperthyroidism due to exogenous thyroid hormone
        Factitia
        Medicamentosa (iatrogenic)
    Toxic struma ovarii

[a] Listed in approximate decreasing order of frequency.

A variety of abnormal immunoglobulins are found in the plasma of patients with Graves' disease. Some of these immunoglobulins have TSH-like activity, and are designated thyroid-stimulating immunoglobulins (TSI); they are antibodies to the normal receptor sites for TSH. The reasons for development of abnormal immunoglobulins in Graves' disease are not clearly understood. Recent thinking views Graves' disease as a failure of T-cell surveillance rather than as a response to thyroid antigens released from thyroid damaged by unknown causes (10).

The plasma of patients with Graves' ophthalmopathy contains a factor (exophthalmos-producing substance (EPS)), which produces exophthalmos and other abnormalities of orbital tissues in suitable test animals. In Graves' ophthalmopathy, the extraocular muscles show interstitial edema, increased connective tissue, fatty infiltration, and infiltration with lymphocytes. Eventually, gross degenerative changes such as fibrosis may occur (see "Ophthalmopathy of Graves' Disease," below).

Dermopathy, a unique, albeit unusual, finding in Graves' disease, consists of more or less circumscribed areas of mucopolysaccharide deposition, typically over the shins, hence the term "pretibial myxedema." This unfortunate designation unjustifiably suggests a relationship between the very different type of generalized mucopolysaccharide deposition in hypothyroidism and the localized deposition in Graves' disease. No relationship exists between these processes.

Clinical Presentation and Diagnosis of Hyperthyroidism

HISTORICAL FEATURES

The presentation of the patient with hyperthyroidism is highly variable (Table 70.6). The severity of the thyrotoxic aspect is determined not only by the degree of hormone excess but also by its rapidity of onset, its duration, and by the age of the patient. The "typical" patient presents with one or more of the following *spontaneous* complaints: "nervousness," weight loss, palpitations (which at first may be intermittent), enlarging neck mass (goiter), change in appearance of eyes (Graves' disease), or symptoms of heart failure.

As the disease progresses in severity, skeletal muscle wasting occurs, which tends to involve especially the limb girdle musculature, producing a proximal myopathy. This problem may result in weakness, expressed, for example, as great difficulty in climbing stairs or, on examination, in arising from a squatting position. Exertional dyspnea, without evidence of cardiac failure, is common and may be related to the myopathy.

The "nervousness" is typically irritability, inability to concentrate, restlessness, or overt emotional lability, but it is the tremor that most often leads the patient to express this complaint. Impairment of nor-

Table 70.6
Signs and Symptoms of Hyperthyroidism

Organ or System	Signs and Symptoms
ADRENERGIC MANIFESTATIONS	Excess sweating, heat intolerance, palpitations, tachycardia, tremor, lid lag, stare, nervousness, and excitability
HYPERMETABOLISM AND CATABOLISM	Increased appetite, weight loss
ONE SYSTEM PREDOMINANCE	
Eyes[a]	Periorbital edema, exophthalmos (proptosis), chemosis, ophthalmoplegia, papilledema
Cardiac	Arrhythmia, congestive heart failure
Muscle	Fatigue and weakness, muscle wasting, proximal myopathy, periodic paralysis
Gastrointestinal	Increased frequency of bowel movements, pernicious vomiting
Bone	Acropachy, osteoporosis, hypercalcemia
REPRODUCTIVE	Infertility, abortion, scanty menses, testicular atrophy, gynecomastia
MENTAL	Anxiety, irritability, psychosis, insomnia
SKIN	Onycholysis, ''pretibial'' myxedema, hyperpigmentation

[a] Graves' disease only.

mal sleep pattern with frequent wakenings is common.

The weight loss classically occurs in the face of increased appetite, although frequently no obvious change in appetite is noticed or there may actually be anorexia, especially in elderly patients. The only prominent gastrointestinal symptom is increased frequency of bowel movements but true diarrhea is not seen.

The "heat intolerance" of hyperthyroidism is often apparent only on questioning. Commonly the patient will admit to having reduced the number of covers used on the bed at night, or to the development of new and unusual habits such as sleeping in the nude or with feet extended from under the blankets. Sweating is increased but is not usually a spontaneous complaint.

Skin changes are hardly ever noticed by the patient and "silky skin" or hair is only rarely seen on examination. Hair loss is not infrequent, usually noticed as thinning of the scalp hair by women. Other skin changes include occasional cases in white persons of diffuse hyperpigmentation with darkening noted mostly over extensor surfaces of elbows, knees, and small joints. In black patients, darkening of skin is common.

PHYSICAL FINDINGS

The thyroid is palpably enlarged in 95% of patients with hyperthyroidism. Asymmetric enlargement is common, especially in patients with toxic nodular goiter. Extreme vascularity of the gland may result in palpable or audible blood flow, a bruit, usually heard over the enlarged lobes but occasionally best heard more rostrally over the superior thyroidal arteries. A bruit over the thyroid of a hyperthyroid patient is usually diagnostic of Graves' disease; this finding is not present in patients with toxic nodular goiter.

The cardiovascular findings include sinus tachycardia, systolic flow murmurs, and wide pulse pressure, commonly, and atrial fibrillation, occasionally. The apex impulse is often prominent and forceful. Cardiac failure may develop in severe cases of long duration, especially in elderly persons.

The *eye findings* can be separated into those that occur as a result of thyroid hormone excess and those that are part of the ophthalmopathy of Graves' disease. Excessive thyroid hormone enhances sympathetic tone. The innervation of the eyelids is partially under sympathetic control. Lid retraction with increased scleral visibility above and below the iris, along with infrequent blinking, leads to the "stare" so commonly seen. Failure of the lid to follow promptly movements of the globe ("lid lag") is another manifestation of the same process. When Graves' ophthalmopathy is present, there is forward protrusion of the globe. This process may be unilateral at first and is often asymmetrical. The protrusion represents true proptosis and contributes an additional component to the stare produced by increased sympathetic tone. Extraocular muscle weakness results in limitation of ability to converge and to perform extreme movements of gaze. Strabismus and diplopia are more severe manifestations. The most serious complications of Graves' ophthalmopathy are infiltrative (p. 719).

The *dermopathy* of Graves' disease occurs most commonly on the legs ("pretibial myxedema"), but also can be seen on the dorsum of the foot, or on the back, the hands, or even the face. The plaque usually has a sharp, raised margin and may have an orange peel-like appearance. The affected areas are often intensely pruritic.

Clubbing of the fingers and toes is rare (thyroid acropachy) and distinguishable radiographically from that seen in pulmonary disease. A common sign is separation of the distal portion of one or more fingernails from their nailbed (onycholysis).

DIAGNOSIS

Recognition of Graves' disease in a typical case is not difficult, but, because of its frequently insidious onset, an absence of eye findings or of an overtly enlarged thyroid, or because of involvement of one or relatively few organ systems, the diagnosis may be missed for months or years.

The usual thyroid function tests will substantiate the diagnosis in most cases. If the results of the T_4 and free T_4 index are borderline or normal, the plasma T_3 must be measured, since hyperthyroidism may be due to elevation of T_3 alone. "T_3-toxicosis" (see p. 720) however, occurs in less than 5% of cases. Occasionally, all the tests of thyroid hormone levels are borderline. If the clinical suspicion of thyrotoxicosis is strong, every effort should be made to obtain laboratory confirmation by measurement of RaIU, the T_3 suppression test, or the TRH test (see above). Clinical trials of antithyroid drugs should be avoided.

DIFFERENTIAL DIAGNOSIS

In some patients, particularly elderly ones, the clinical picture may not suggest hyperthyroidism and only an astute clinician will promptly consider the correct diagnosis. Such patients may present with only unexplained weight loss or weakness. Occult neoplasm may first be suspected and the diagnosis of hyperthyroidism may be missed entirely or considered only after extensive evaluation fails to yield a diagnosis. These are the patients often labeled "apathetic hyperthyroidism." The term implies lethargy—which is in fact not often present—but should rather be used to denote that group of individuals who for unclear reasons lack the signs of sympathetic hyperactivity and hence do not exhibit tachycardia, lid retraction, tremor, etc.

Congestive heart failure or atrial fibrillation may be the presenting manifestation. So-called thyrocardiac patients have been incorrectly thought to be resistant to ordinary doses of digitalis. This is occasionally true, but a normal response to conventional therapy for cardiac failure or an arrhythmia should not be considered incompatible with a diagnosis of hyperthyroidism.

Some patients with anxiety may present with tachycardia, tremor, irritability, and weakness simulating hyperthyroidism. The "anxiety" of thyrotoxicosis is more likely to appear as irritability and hyperkinesis than as an expressed feeling of anxiety. The typical anxiety state often exhibits features of depression which are usually absent in hyperthyroidism. In depression, weight loss is invariably accompanied by anorexia, a relatively unusual symptom of hyperthyroidism (see p. 715).

The characteristic ophthalmopathy of Graves' disease may offer the first clue to the diagnosis. However, ophthalmopathy may not be accompanied by hyperthyroidism and may be unilateral. The T_3 suppression test or TRH test will substantiate the diagnosis in most but not all cases of euthyroid Graves' ophthalmopathy. Without evidence of either thyroid hyperfunction, disturbance of the negative feedback system, or dermopathy, the diagnosis of Graves' ophthalmopathy cannot be made with absolute assurance. Indeed, other diseases of the orbit or retroorbital space must be considered. Computerized axial tomography of the skull and the orbital contents and high resolution sonography are useful diagnostic tools. These procedures can visualize the enlarged extraocular muscles of Graves' ophthalmopathy, although such enlargement is also seen in pseudotumor. In many cases of Graves' ophthalmopathy, without hyperthyroidism, other aspects of Graves' syndrome eventually become apparent.

When hyperthyroidism is found in a patient without goiter or exophthalmos, suspicions of factitious hyperthyroidism may be warranted. An RaIU test and scan will establish whether the thyroid is functional, and scintiscan will sometimes give evidence for enlargement that is not palpable. A very low uptake and a normal sized gland on scintiscan suggests ingestion of thyroid hormone or the presence of thyroiditis with hyperthyroidism (see below, p. 720).

Therapy

Hyperthyroidism due to Graves' disease is frequently a self-limited process that terminates within a year or two in about one-half of patients. This natural history strongly influences selection of therapy. Other therapeutic considerations relate to the age of the patient and the presence or absence of complications.

Since there are currently no means of controlling the underlying cause of the disease, presumably thyroid-stimulating immunoglobulin (TSI) production, therapy is designed to interfere with thyroid hormone synthesis by drugs or by ablation of thyroid tissue by radioiodide or surgery. Opinions differ on approaches, but the views expressed here probably closely approximate a consensus of conservative medical opinion. Each form of therapy has advantages and disadvantages; none provides a simple, definitive solution and none is truly curative. The objective of therapy is to assure minimal morbidity from both the therapy and the disease. The therapy of hyperthyroidism due to causes other than Graves' disease is discussed separately.

THIOCARBAMIDE ANTITHYROID DRUGS

These agents will predictably control excessive production of thyroid hormone in essentially all cases, although in only about one-half of cases will a permanent remission of the hyperthyroidism be seen. Of these latter cases, about one-half will become hypothyroid in the period about 15 to 20 years after successful treatment and onset of remission. Relapses may occur within 6 months to a year or even longer after apparent remission, but such relapses are uncommon except in postpartum patients.

Restoration of the clinically euthyroid state requires at least 4 to 8 weeks, although clinical improvement is usually seen much sooner. Antithyroid drugs are ordinarily the preferred *initial* treatment for children, some young adults without complications or other medical problems, and the pregnant patient. The antithyroid drugs are also routinely used as preliminary therapy in patients who are to be treated by surgery (see below, p. 719). The objective in these cases is to ensure euthyroid status at the time of operation. Patients who are to be treated with radioiodide (see below, p. 718) are also frequently treated with an antithyroid drug pre- and/or postablation.

Radioiodide is slow in producing its effect and may have to be given in multiple doses; use of an antithyroid drug before or after such therapy is therefore a temporary but useful adjunct.

In the United States, only two thiocarbamide drugs are available, propylthiouracil and methimazole (Tapazole). Propylthiouracil may have an advantage when speed in restoration of euthyroid status is an urgent consideration. Propylthiouracil, unlike methimazole, in addition to its effects in inhibiting thyroid hormone synthesis, also inhibits conversion of T_4 to T_3 in peripheral tissues. Methimazole, on the other hand, is longer acting than propylthiouracil and may be given on a less frequent dosage schedule, thus facilitating compliance. In most adults with hyperthyroidism, 100 to 150 mg of propylthiouracil every 8 hours or 20 to 30 mg of methimazole every 12 hours will usually suffice as initial therapy, whereas maintenance is often possible with 50 to 100 mg of propylthiouracil twice daily or 5 to 10 mg of methimazole once or twice daily. If at these relatively low maintenance doses of antithyroid drug, the plasma T_4 falls below normal, efforts to "titrate" the dose further are frequently tedious and unsuccessful, and should be avoided. A euthyroid state can be achieved under these circumstances by the *addition* of oral thyroxine, usually at somewhat less than full replacement dose.

Special Considerations in the Use of Antithyroid Drugs. Although the recommended dose will control the disease in the vast majority of cases, some individuals clearly need higher doses. If the patient is severely ill, larger doses should be given from the beginning. The risk of an adverse drug effect may be increased, but this is not established and should not be a consideration under such circumstances. In order to achieve total blockade of hormone synthesis, as much as 200 mg of propylthiouracil every 4 hours may be necessary. Since methimazole has a longer duration of action, it need not be given so often, but 30 to 40 mg, 3 times daily, may be needed in some cases.

Time-honored treatment schedules suggest that a period of 12 to 18 months of therapy be used before consideration is given to discontinuation of the drug. At that point, a few indicators are helpful in predicting success or failure of the outcome. Patients who have continued to require large doses of the drug are almost certain not to have achieved remission. On the other hand, reduction in thyroid mass during therapy is often predictive of lasting clinical remission. A test for restoration of the normal negative feedback system (thyroid suppressibility) is sometimes helpful as a guide in determining whether therapy can be discontinued. To perform the test, the antithyroid drug is discontinued. The patient is given 75 μg of T_3 (Cytomel) daily or a single 3-mg dose of T_4. RaIU is then determined after 1 week. Low postsuppression 24-hour uptake (<10%) predicts reasonably accurately that the patient will remain in remis-

sion. An uptake above the normal range almost invariably indicates continuation of active disease. Intermediate values are not useful. If continued disease activity seems to be present, discontinuation of therapy is inadvisable and will almost certainly result in clinical relapse and needless morbidity.

If a suppression test or clinical signs suggest that remission has been reached, antithyroid drug therapy is terminated and the patient is observed. If the status is indeterminate, antithyroid drug may be reduced to one-half the maintenance level for 3 to 6 months in the expectation that if recurrence occurs, it will be blunted. Prophylactic use of propranolol (see below) during withdrawal of antithyroid drugs is a useful maneuver that prevents emergence of symptoms of overt hyperthyroidism should relapse occur. Routine determination of plasma T_4 or T_3 every 3 to 4 weeks allows early recognition of return of thyroid overactivity.

If the hyperthyroid state recurs, treatment with antithyroid drug may be reinitiated for another course (*i.e.*, 1 year) or alternative therapy may be undertaken (^{131}I or surgery). A second course of antithyroid drug has a significant chance of inducing remission. In selected patients, prolonged or even indefinite drug therapy is reasonable, but with most patients such an approach is not desirable.

Minor side effects of drug therapy occur in about 10% of patients. Skin rashes, the most common side effect, are usually seen in the first months of therapy, and often disappear even if therapy is continued. Antihistamine drugs are useful in controlling urticaria and pruritus. Leukopenia is not uncommon, but is usually not severe and is dose-related. If the absolute number of polymorphonuclear leukocytes falls below 2000, the dose should be reduced or the drug discontinued. If the side effects are not tolerated, a switch to another agent will allow continuation of therapy in about half the cases. *Major complications* of drug therapy occur in less than 0.1% of cases. Agranulocytosis is the most dreaded complication. Unlike leukopenia, agranulocytosis from thiocarbamides is not dose-related and is of such sudden onset that routine blood counts are of no help in prevention. The patient should, however, be instructed to contact the physician promptly if severe sore mouth or sore throat and fever occur. Fortunately, most patients with agranulocytosis recover, albeit after a stormy course. Other toxic reactions include drug fever and arthralgias, both of which appear to be dose-related. Elevations of alkaline phosphatase activity are commonly seen in patients receiving propylthiouracil. If other liver enzymes are normal, the drug may be continued, but persistent laboratory evidence of hepatocellular damage is an indication for discontinuation of therapy. White blood count should be monitored after several weeks of therapy and following increases of drug dose. Liver enzymes should be measured every 3 to 6 months.

ADJUNCTIVE DRUG THERAPY

Iodide. Iodide in the treatment of hyperthyroidism should be reserved for patients with severe illness. Occasionally, iodide therapy produces severe dermatitis. Use of iodide may preclude for many weeks the use of radioactive iodide, the thyroid uptake of which will be greatly diminished.

Iodide is the best agent available for inhibiting hormone release and is useful in patients who need rapid correction of the hyperthyroid state. Iodide also has a time-honored place in preoperative preparation (see below, p. 719) for thyroidectomy, to reduce vascularity of the gland. When given following radioiodide therapy, iodide seems especially effective in accelerating restoration of euthyroid status.

The dose of iodide is one drop of a saturated solution (50 mg) of potassium iodide 2 times a day; larger doses are often given but are unnecessary. Lugol's solution is a pharmacologic concoction containing iodine and iodide which has no virtue over iodide alone.

Adrenergic Antagonists. The symptoms and signs of thyrotoxicosis that are related to sensitization of the sympathetic nervous system are in large measure abolished by β-adrenergic blocking drugs. The current agent of choice is propranolol. The indications for its use are *severe* tachycardia, tremor, sweating, and agitation. Propranolol is effective for relief of these manifestations of hyperthyroidism, but does not appreciably affect excessive metabolic rate or reverse the catabolic state of severe cases. Propranolol has occasional undesirable side effects and is relatively contraindicated in some individuals (e.g., those with asthma). Concern is often expressed that patients with heart disease may be thrown into congestive heart failure or that heart failure, if present, may worsen. On the other hand, some patients with congestive heart failure may respond well to the drug when excessive heart rate is a major contributing factor. Other uses for propranolol are in the prevention of symptoms during trial withdrawal of an antithyroid drug and while awaiting the effects of ^{131}I therapy. Most patients require propranolol in doses of at least 160 mg daily, but doses up to 720 mg may be necessary. The drug should be discontinued as soon as the patient is rendered euthyroid by other therapy.

RADIOACTIVE IODIDE THERAPY

Radioactive iodide (^{131}I) is uniformly effective therapy; it is simple to administer and inexpensive. It is the preferred form of therapy for most adults with Graves' disease and is much to be preferred over surgery.

The single disadvantage of radioactive iodide is that hypothyroidism is a frequent consequence. For many years, concern was expressed over the possibility of producing carcinoma of the thyroid, leukemia, or genetic damage in the future offspring of women in their childbearing years. All of these concerns have been shown to be groundless. Although low doses of external radiation do produce carcinoma of the thyroid, the higher doses used for treatment of hyperthyroidism do not. Long term follow-up of treated patients over the past 30 years has failed to substantiate any such risk or any increased risk of leukemia. The amounts of radiation to the ovaries from therapeutic doses of radioiodide used for therapy of hyperthyroidism are lower than those delivered by diagnostic X-ray procedures and can be expected to produce no genetic effects. Thus, radioiodide therapy for hyperthyroidism can be considered for any adult patient.

Hypothyroidism follows radioiodide therapy in the immediate few months after therapy in a more or less dose-related fashion. Large doses predictably eliminate hyperthyroidism with certainty but totally ablate the thyroid with great regularity. Small, single doses render the patient euthyroid with 50 to 70% likelihood but unavoidably still produce hypothyroidism within a year in about 10% of cases. Furthermore, of the patients rendered euthyroid, 3 to 4% per year develop hypothyroidism over the ensuing 20 years.

One may question whether the high frequency of post-treatment hypothyroidism constitutes a significant disadvantage of radioiodide therapy. The answer is that, for the majority of those who become hypothyroid, replacement therapy with thyroxine is a trivial inconvenience. For these patients, the advantages of radioiodide therapy far outweigh the one disadvantage. Unfortunately, a few patients, despite warnings to the contrary, discontinue their required lifelong replacement therapy, become lost to follow-up, and suffer all the consequences of long-standing hypothyroidism and myxedema.

Some physicians advocate the use of deliberately ablative doses of [131]I. This approach to therapy certainly greatly simplifies patient management and is reasonable in view of the high probability of post-therapy hypothyroidism regardless of dose. Nonetheless, most physicians do not advocate deliberate ablation unless the patient has experienced a major complication of hyperthyroidism (e.g., severe heart disease) or has complicating medical problems that demand prompt control. In young patients who are tolerating their disease reasonably well, most physicians prefer to use small doses of ^{131}I, repeated if necessary, until the patient is euthyroid. Such an approach does not, of course, guarantee that hypothyroidism will be avoided.

As discussed below (p. 720), larger (10 to 30 mCi) doses of [131]I *are* appropriate initially in the treatment of toxic nodular goiter.

In the past, elaborate schemes have been used to estimate the required dose of [131]I. Unfortunately, none of these has proven helpful, since the biologic sensitivity to radiation effect, the most important variable, is not measurable. Currently, in a typical "low dose" treatment scheme patients with small glands are given 2 to 3 mCi, while those with moderately enlarged to large glands are given 5 to 10 mCi. Ablative doses approximate 15 mCi. Because of the unpredictable response with nonablative doses, antithyroid drugs are often used initially to render the patient euthyroid. Antithyroid therapy is then interrupted for 48 hours before the ^{131}I is given and reinstituted 24 hours afterward. Alternatively, an antithyroid drug can be initiated 24 to 48 hours following therapy with ^{131}I. Similar approaches combining antithyroid drug and ^{131}I are almost routinely used in patients with severe or complicated hyperthyroidism, e.g., thyrocardiac disease.

Radioactive iodine can be administered only by an appropriately licensed physician—usually an endocrinologist or a nuclear medicine physician. Thereafter, no special precautions need be taken by the patient.

The undocumented notion has long persisted that radiation thyroiditis may produce excessive release of thyroid hormones 7 to 14 days after therapy, with the possibility of consequent worsening of the clinical state. This complication, if it occurs at all, must be rare. Nonetheless, prudence dictates a conservative approach in precarious patients, e.g., those in congestive heart failure, who are best brought to euthyroid status or are at least significantly improved by antithyroid drug therapy before ablation with ^{131}I. At 3 months following ^{131}I, when the short term radiation effect becomes maximal, the antithyroid drug can be discontinued or tapered, provided, of course, that the laboratory and clinical evidence indicates return to euthyroid status. Otherwise, another dose of ^{131}I may be required.

SURGICAL THERAPY

For many years surgical ablation of the thyroid, e.g., subtotal thyroidectomy, was the main therapy for hyperthyroidism. This procedure still has its advocates, especially for young adults and for children who cannot be successfully treated with antithyroid drugs. In the hands of experienced surgeons, subtotal thyroidectomy is certainly effective therapy attended by minimal morbidity. However, complications include the small but real risk of anesthesia/operative mortality, recurrent laryngeal nerve damage with vocal cord paralysis, permanent hypoparathyroidism, and most commonly, hypothyroidism. The latter two complications are, to a certain extent, unavoidable and are not merely the consequence of poor surgical technique. In addition to about a 10% occurrence of immediate postsurgical hypothyroidism, 2 to 3% of patients become hypothyroid each year following surgery, a figure only slightly lower than that following therapy with ^{131}I. A higher complication rate must be expected when the operation is performed by surgeons with limited experience in thyroid surgery. Surgery also is followed by a significant (5%) rate of recurrent hyperthyroidism, sometimes occurring many years later. In this case, even the most enthusiastic supporters of surgical treatment agree that recurrent hyperthyroidism should never be treated by a second operation, since the frequency of major complications rises to an unacceptable level.

TREATMENT OF HYPERTHYROIDISM DURING PREGNANCY

Hyperthyroidism during pregnancy, almost invariably due to Graves' disease, should be treated with an antithyroid drug. Surgery has been used successfully during pregnancy, but has no advantage and may be associated with increased fetal losses. Radioactive iodide is contraindicated. Therapy with antithyroid drugs during pregnancy is guided by two considerations. First, the antithyroid drugs freely cross the placenta and can, in large doses, produce goiter and hypothyroidism in the infant. Second, thyroid hormones do not cross the placenta from mother to fetus. The dose of antithyroid drugs should be the minimal amount adequate to control the hyperthyroidism. A dose of drug which totally blocks hormone synthesis along with a replacement amount of thyroxine is not appropriate during pregnancy. When ordinary doses of antithyroid drug are used, the fetus is usually born without goiter, but as a precaution the dose is often reduced, if possible, during the last month of pregnancy. Iodide should not be used during pregnancy, since the fetal thyroid is especially susceptible to the goitrogenic effect of iodide. Monitoring the plasma hormone level requires determination of free T_4 or the free T_4 index, since T_4 is normally elevated during pregnancy in association with the increased TBG.

TSI (see p. 714) of Graves' disease cross the placenta and enter the fetal circulation. Occasionally, the newborn infant is hyperthyroid as a result of this passive transfer of antibodies. The physician caring for the newborn should always be alerted to this possibility.

Ophthalmopathy of Graves' Disease

The exact frequency of ophthalmopathy in Graves' disease is not known, but most patients have either no obvious infiltrative eye involvement or show only minimal to moderate proptosis. Severe exophthalmos occurs in no more than a few percent of cases of Graves' disease. Proptosis becomes more than a cosmetic concern when the eyelids fail to close, setting the stage for corneal ulceration. Paresis of the extraocular muscles producing diplopia can also be troublesome and may require use of an eye patch or corrective surgery. The most disturbing and rarest eye involvement is chemosis or marked inflammation and edema of the conjunctivae and periorbital soft tissues. Ophthalmopathy of this severity is termed malignant or infiltrative exophthalmos. Rarely, optic neuritis leading to blindness occurs. The therapy of severe ophthalmopathy, which may include decompression of the orbit, is accomplished by an ophthalmologist (2).

Graves' ophthalmopathy follows a temporal course which may be totally dissociated from the hyperthyroidism, the treatment of which should be independent of and uninfluenced by the eye disease. Despite claims to the contrary, no form of treatment of hyperthyroidism has any advantage for control of the ophthalmopathy. The notion persists that induction of hypothyroidism may aggravate exophthalmos. Development of clinical hypothyroidism should therefore be avoided, especially when exophthalmos is present.

Hyperthyroidism Associated with Thyroiditis (Lymphocytic Thyroiditis with Spontaneously Resolving Hyperthyroidism; Postpartum Thyroiditis with Hyperthyroidism; Silent Thyroiditis)

Classical subacute thyroiditis (see below, p. 728) has long been known to be associated occasionally with short-lived, self-limited hyperthyroidism. The explanation for this phenomenon has been that the destructive inflammatory process causes release of preformed thyroid hormone. The hyperthyroidism invariably disappears within a few months.

In the past few years, another, apparently distinct variant of the thyroiditis-hyperthyroidism syndrome, has been recognized. These patients present with modest thyroid enlargement which is *nontender*. No prior history of viral illness can be obtained. The radioiodide uptake is very *low*, as it is in subacute thyroiditis, while the T_4 and T_3 are high. About one-half of cases have significant elevations of thyroid antibodies, and about one-half of these high titers subside within a few months. A propensity of the condition to occur in the postpartum period has been noted, sometimes in successive pregnancies, and sometimes followed by the development of hypothyroidism. On biopsy the changes seen differ from those of the peak phase of classical subacute thyroiditis, but the latter, in its late stages of evolution, may be indistinguishable from that of lymphocytic thyroiditis. Whether lymphocytic thyroiditis with spontaneously resulting hyperthyroidism (silent thyroiditis) is a new disease, as has been suggested by some, or is a newly recognized variant of subacute thyroiditis is a matter of debate (4, 8, 11).

It is important to obtain a radioiodide uptake measurement in all patients with hyperthyroidism who do not clearly have Graves' disease (*i.e.*, who do not have associated eye findings) or toxic nodular goiter. A very low radioiodide uptake will establish the diagnosis of hyperthyroidism associated with thyroiditis and allow the physician to avoid inappropriate therapy (radioiodide or surgery). Treatment with an antithyroid drug *may* be useful; propranolol (see above, p. 718) affords symptomatic relief and may be all the treatment that is necessary.

Hyperthyroidism Associated with Nodular Goiter (Toxic Nodular Goiter)

Toxic nodular goiter is usually seen in adults in midlife or in the elderly. While the typical patient with Graves' disease usually relates symptoms extending over a few months to a year, the history in toxic nodular goiter is often much longer. Many years may pass before diagnosis. Because of the patient's age and the duration of illness, severe cardiac or musculoskeletal involvement is common.

Toxic nodular goiter appears to arise in the pathologic evolution of some cases of nodular goiter. Most nodular goiters (see below, p. 724) are initially TSH-dependent, *i.e.*, suppressible with exogenous thyroid hormone. Eventually, some of these goiters develop autonomous areas with other regions of relatively decreased activity. Nodular goiters at this stage of evolution do not secrete enough hormone to produce clinical hyperthyroidism but show nonsuppressible function. A few of these autonomously functioning goiters evolve to a stage where excessive production of hormone and clinical hyperthyroidism ensue.

If the usual laboratory tests (T_4, free T_4 index) are borderline, special tests such as measurement of T_3, suppression with thyroid hormone, or TRH stimulation should be considered. The suppression test can be undertaken cautiously in the elderly patient without overt heart disease, but should not be used if heart disease is obvious. The test is more helpful in excluding the diagnosis than in establishing a state of hormone excess, since a significant number of cases of nontoxic nodular goiter are also not suppressible. The TRH test is of limited value in the elderly.

Therapy of toxic nodular goiter is best accomplished with ^{131}I. Rather large doses, in the range of 10 to 30 mCi, are usually necessary. Hypothyroidism occurs much less frequently following ^{131}I therapy for nodular goiter than for Graves' disease. If the clinical situation demands prompt relief of the hyperthyroidism, an antithyroid drug can be used following the therapeutic dose of ^{131}I, since the response to radioiodide is often slow and multiple doses may be needed. Otherwise ^{131}I given alone is simple therapy, without side effects, and easily monitored by measurements of plasma T_4. Other therapeutic considerations including the use of adjunctive therapy follow those outlined for the therapy of Graves' disease with one exception. In hyperthyroidism due to toxic nodular goiter, antithyroid drugs alone cannot be expected to produce a lasting remission.

Hyperthyroidism Due to Excessive Secretion of T_3; "T_3 Toxicosis"

In most cases of hyperthyroidism, the thyroid secretes excessive quantities of both T_4 and T_3. However, in perhaps 5% of cases, T_3 is the predominant hormone secreted. T_3 toxicosis may occur in hyperthyroidism due to Graves' disease, toxic multinodular goiter, or autonomous adenoma. The patient who appears clinically hyperthyroid but whose T_4 is normal should have plasma T_3 measured. T_3 toxicosis sometimes occurs early in the course of hyperthyroidism due to Graves' disease and can develop during therapy with an antithyroid drug. Continuing clinical findings of hyperthyroidism during such therapy—and despite a normal or low T_4—should raise the possibility that T_3 toxicosis is present and that more, rather than less, antithyroid drug is needed.

Thyroid Storm (Thyrotoxic Crisis)

This dreaded complication of hyperthyroidism is now only rarely encountered. When thyroid storm does occur, it is usually in the setting of a severe medical or surgical stress imposed on a patient with uncontrolled or unrecognized hyperthyroidism. Clinical features of full-blown thyroid storm include fever, sometimes to the level of extreme hyperpyrexia, marked tachycardia, great irritability, diarrhea, and hypotension. Thyroid storm often progresses rapidly to delirium and coma. Any such severe exacerbation of hyperthyroidism demands hospitalization and urgent consultation with an endocrinologist.

HYPOTHYROIDISM

Hypothyroidism, the metabolic state resulting from deficient thyroid hormones, is relatively common. Most cases can be diagnosed even when symptoms and signs are minimal, provided that the physician considers the diagnosis and seeks appropriate laboratory confirmation. The manifestations of hypothyroidism are varied and to a large measure age-dependent. Myxedema is a severe form of hypothyroidism which results in deposition of mucopolysaccharides in the skin and other tissues, producing a characteristic appearance and a constellation of physical findings. The term myxedema is commonly but incorrectly used interchangeably with hypothyroidism. *Primary hypothyroidism* is a term used to indicate that the hormone deficiency results from a disease or other process within the thyroid gland. *Secondary hypothyroidism*, much less common, results from lack of thyrotropin (TSH) secretion, a result of pituitary or, rarely, hypothalamic disease. The thyroid is usually smaller than normal and not palpable. Almost invariably the hypothyroidism is part of a generalized decrease in pituitary function that has resulted from postpartum necrosis, pituitary tumor, pituitary apoplexy, or, rarely, granulomatous disease.

Etiology

Currently, the commonest cause of hypothyroidism is iatrogenic, *i.e.*, the result of therapy of hyperthyroidism with radioiodide or by surgery. Spontaneous cases occur as an idiopathic process of thyroid atrophy or in association with Hashimoto's thyroid-

itis. Hypothyroidism from other causes is uncommon. A clinical classification is given in Table 70.7.

Idiopathic hypothyroidism may in most cases be the result of long-standing Hashimoto's thyroiditis. This conclusion is based mainly on the frequent occurrence of high titers of autoantibodies to thyroid antigens in both hypothyroidism and in Hashimoto's thyroiditis. In addition, both occur frequently in association with other autoimmune diseases such as pernicious anemia. As a clinically encountered thyroid abnormality, Hashimoto's thyroiditis is second in frequency only to nontoxic nodular goiter and is by far the most common cause of goitrous hypothyroidism.

DRUG-INDUCED HYPOTHYROIDISM

A *variety of drugs* can produce hypothyroidism that is invariably associated with goiter formation. Only a few in current use have such an effect. Lithium, currently in wide use for the treatment of manic-depressive illness (see Chapter 14), is one such agent. If goiter occurs, lithium need not be stopped; addition of thyroxine relieves the hypothyroidism and causes regression of the goiter. Overtreatment of hyperthyroidism with an antithyroid drug will, of course, produce hypothyroidism. Iodide in pharmacologic amounts is an antithyroid drug and will also occasionally produce goiter and hypothyroidism as in patients given long term iodide therapy for asthma or other chronic lung disease. However, most adults who are susceptible to the antithyroid action of iodide have an underlying thyroid abnormality, such as Hashimoto's thyroiditis (see below, p. 728) or radioiodide-treated Graves' disease.

Table 70.7
Clinical Classification of Hypothyroidism[a]

HYPOTHYROIDISM WITHOUT GOITER (DECREASE OF THYROID TISSUE MASS)
    Postablative for hyperthyroidism (radioiodide therapy or surgery)
    Idiopathic atrophy
    Developmental defect (congenital)
    Pituitary or hypothalamic disease
HYPOTHYROIDISM WITH GOITER
    Chronic thyroiditis (Hashimoto's disease, etc.)
    Drug-induced (antithyroid drugs, iodide, lithium, sulfonylureas, etc.
    Iodide deficiency (remote geographic areas)
    Genetic biosynthetic defects

[a] Hypothyroidism in the United States is now most commonly the consequence of therapy for hyperthyroidism. Hypothyroidism due to idiopathic atrophy of the thyroid is second in frequency. Developmental defects (*e.g.*, lingual thyroid) are rare. Hypothyroidism with goiter is nearly always due to Hashimoto's thyroiditis, rarely to a drug. Genetic biosynthetic defects are rare and usually become manifest in childhood.

Clinical Features

Hypothyroidism in the adult is highly variable in presentation. Usually, onset is insidious, often occurring over many years, with the result that the symptoms go unappreciated by patient and physician alike. The nonspecificity of the symptoms also contributes to the delayed diagnosis. No predictable progression of symptoms is apparent, but easy fatiguability, lethargy, increased sleep requirement, cold intolerance, muscle aching, and stiffness are perhaps the commonest early symptoms. The skin is dry and scaling. Hair loss is frequent. The eyebrows become sparse, the face "puffy," *i.e.*, full, with edema of the periorbital areas. The voice often becomes low pitched and rough. Constipation is common and may be severe enough to produce megacolon; sometimes the diagnosis is suggested by the radiologist from the results of a barium enema. Diminished hearing, especially in old persons, is easily overlooked or attributed to "aging." Ordinarily, the affected individual becomes abnormally placid, but agitation, frank psychosis, or dementia may occur. Paresthesias of the hands due to carpal tunnel syndrome are common. Diminished sexual function is the rule. Women often experience menorrhagia. Rarely, galactorrhea may be seen in women of childbearing age. Fertility is diminished, but pregnancy may occur and normal delivery is possible. The newborn is euthyroid, unless the mother's hypothyroidism is drug-related or the hypothyroidism is of the rare familial athyrotic variety.

SEVERE HYPOTHYROIDISM WITH MYXEDEMA

In spontaneous cases of hypothyroidism, only with severe, long-standing disease does extensive deposition of mucopolysaccharide occur, producing the clinical state of myxedema. Rarely, myxedema may develop rapidly after radioiodide or surgical ablation of the thyroid for hyperthyroidism.

In myxedema, a variety of manifestations can be appreciated on physical examination and, of course, they vary with the severity and duration of the disease. The skin, in addition to being dry and scaling, is typically cool. The scaling may be extensive so that large flakes are shed over the elbows and knees. The subcutaneous tissues may be infiltrated by mucopolysaccharides so that the skin appears to be "thickened" or "doughy." In the elderly, atrophy of the epidermis may occur simultaneously, producing a stiff, translucent, parchment-like appearance. Yellow-orange discoloration of the skin may be evident, especially in the palms. The presence of edema is not obvious, since pitting is not noted except in extreme cases complicated by hypoproteinemia. An exception is the collection around the eyes of "bags of water." This finding is not, however, specific for hypothyroidism. The tongue is sometimes enlarged. The heart rate is usually slow (sinus bradycardia). The heart may appear enlarged, due either to dilation of the myocardium or pericardial effusion. Pleural effusions and ascites may also be present, sometimes even in cases that are otherwise not clinically severe. Dilutional hyponatremia, clinically indistinguishable from the syndrome of inappropriate antidiuretic hormone excess, may be present. The deep tendon reflexes characteristically show a delay in their relaxation phase, the so-called "hung-up reflex." This is a highly suggestive finding but may be seen occasionally in other diseases. Mental functioning is slowed, as reflected in the characteristically slow speech. The reading speed may be greatly reduced. Hearing loss may be severe or of a degree apparent only on audiometric testing. Cerebellar dysfunction, if present, is usually evident only on extensive neurologic testing, but in rare cases is grossly apparent as ataxia.

Myxedema Coma

This severe, often fatal, event is an infrequent complication of long-standing disease and is typically seen in the elderly patient. Myxedema coma is often associated with or precipitated by pneumonia, peritonitis, or some other serious infection. Severe respiratory failure is a major feature and can be due to a variety of factors ranging from upper airway obstruction to impaired chest wall mechanics.

Since elderly patients often become hypothermic on exposure to cold or during sepsis, the diagnosis of myxedema coma is more frequently considered than actually confirmed. Any of these events demand hospitalization.

Laboratory Findings

In primary hypothyroidism, the combination of low plasma T_4, free T_4 index (or free T_4), and high TSH is diagnostic. Difficulties in diagnosis are encountered only in occasional cases. The plasma T_3 is usually low, but since T_3 decreases in a variety of nonthyroidal illnesses ranging from malnutrition to liver disease, its measurement is not useful for diagnosis of hypothyroidism. Furthermore, it is normal in many patients with mild hypothyroidism. In hypothyroidism due to pituitary or hypothalamic disease the TSH is low or "normal." The TRH test is ordinarily not necessary for diagnosis of primary hypothyroidism, but can be helpful when the T_4 and TSH are borderline. In this situation, an exaggerated response to TRH may be seen (TSH increment >30).

In addition to the definitive diagnostic tests, a variety of other laboratory abnormalities are encountered, although they serve no useful diagnostic purpose. A common laboratory finding is elevation of plasma enzymes which originate in skeletal muscle: creatine phosphokinase (CPK), serum glutamic oxaloacetic transaminase (SGOT), serum glutamic pyruvic transaminase (SGPT), and lactic dehydrogenase (LDH). Fractionation studies show that when these enzymes are elevated in hypothyroidism, they do not originate in cardiac muscle. Other abnormalities include electrocardiographic changes (such as flattened or inverted T waves, minor ST segment depressions, and low amplitude QRS complexes) and abnormalities of blood gas measurements due to hypoventilation. Anemia (see Chapter 46), usually normocytic and normochromic, may be present, as may macrocytic anemia of coexistent vitamin B_{12} deficiency (pernicious anemia). An abnormality of red cell shape (spiculation) also has been described in hypothyroidism.

Differential Diagnosis

The most difficult problem in diagnosis is the simple clinical appreciation of the possibility that the patient may be hypothyroid. Once suspected, the subsequent history, physical examination, and, particularly, laboratory findings will easily establish the diagnosis in all but a few cases. However, some special problems may be encountered. Any elderly patient who is sick, pale, and puffy faced becomes a suspect for the diagnosis, especially if an adequate history cannot be obtained. A patient with atypical chest pain, nonspecific electrocardiographic abnormalities, and elevated CPK or SGOT is not infrequently labeled as having ischemic heart disease and myocardial infarction; the proper diagnosis may be hypothyroidism. A patient with the nephrotic syndrome might be mistaken for one having hypothyroidism. However, although the plasma T_4 may be low (TBG is low in some nephrotic patients), the free T_4 index (or free T_4) is normal. More important, the patient with the nephrotic syndrome will have features characteristic of that disorder, *i.e.*, massive proteinuria and hypoalbuminemia (see Chapter 44).

"EUTHYROID SICK SYNDROME" *VS.* HYPOTHYROIDISM

The diagnosis of hypothyroidism in severely ill patients presents special problems (2). Patients with the simulating "euthyroid sick syndrome" are usually elderly, often have sepsis, and have a low T_4 and T_4 index but a normal TSH and a normal response to TRH. Plasma rT_3 is often elevated. It is not likely that one will encounter such patients often in an ambulatory practice.

Treatment

The best preparation for ordinary use is T_4 (levothyroxine; sodium L-thyroxine, Synthroid). T_3 (liothyronine, Cytomel) is also effective and sometime preferable for treatment of goiter, but has no special advantage for routine therapy of hypothyroidism and has the distinct disadvantage that one cannot monitor the plasma T_4 to determine adequacy of replacement. Combinations of T_4 and T_3 and desiccated thyroid should no longer be used.

Traditionally, initiation of thyroid hormone replacement therapy has been cautious and conservative and has utilized dosage schedules that ensure slow restoration of a normal metabolic state. While the principle is rational, the practice is often faulty. Therapy should be adjusted to the individual case, with several points in mind. If the patient is not elderly and has never had overt cardiac disease, overcautious initiation of therapy will result only in needless prolongation of the hypothyroid state with its attendant morbidity. If the patient has evidence of preexisting cardiac disease, therapy should be started slowly, but unnecessary delay should be avoided. Only rarely will serious heart disease, such as angina pectoris, prevent at least partial therapy sufficient to eliminate myxedema, if not full correction of hypothyroidism.

The usual hypothyroid patient, without complicating medical problems, may be started on full daily replacement dosage. Even with this therapeutic schedule, the clinical response will be very slow. One can expect several months to pass before restoration of the normal metabolic state.

The objective of therapy is to restore the euthyroid state. Enough thyroxine is given daily to maintain the plasma T_4 at the upper range of normal, or, ideally, to the point where the TSH is restored to normal. Most persons need about 0.15 mg per day; only rarely is as much as 0.2 mg necessary and more is hardly ever needed. Elderly patients often require only 0.1 mg daily. Recently, concern has been expressed over the bioavailability of hormone in certain generic preparations and even lack of standardization of certain brands of thyroxine. Determination of plasma T_3 during therapy with T_4 is unnecessary.

If the patient is elderly or has known cardiovascular disease, a daily dose of 0.025 to 0.05 mg of T_4 should be started, with 0.05-mg increases at 2-weekly intervals.

Hypothyroid patients who require surgery are poor risks until their thyroid status is at least partially corrected, a process that requires 3 to 4 weeks with ordinary oral therapy. Elective surgery is best delayed in such patients. In an urgent situation, an intravenous dose of T_4 is probably warranted to prepare the patient for surgery in a few days. The increased susceptibility of hypothyroid persons to respiratory depression by conventional doses of many CNS active drugs should be borne in mind. This increased drug sensitivity has been responsible for precipitation of myxedema coma.

GOITER

A goiter is an enlarged thyroid gland. The term implies nothing about the functional state of the gland. Goiter is the most common thyroid abnormality. *Diffuse goiter*, also called simple goiter, is a gland that is uniformly and symmetrically enlarged without apparent irregularities. (Some use the term *simple goiter* to denote any nontoxic or nonhyperfunctioning gland, regardless of its anatomy.)

In some areas of the world thyroid enlargement is so common as to be termed *endemic goiter*. Before the widespread introduction of iodized salt these areas were common, but this is no longer the case. Endemic goiter, for practical purposes synonymous with iodine deficiency goiter, is now found only in selected geographically isolated areas of the underdeveloped world. The term *sporadic goiter* refers to thyroid enlargement as now encountered in the United States and other developed areas. Sporadic goiter is seen in a few percent of the population and increases in frequency with age. The cause is unknown.

Causes

Any process that prevents the synthesis of normal quantities of thyroid hormones will produce goiter. If impairment of hormone synthesis is severe enough, goiter formation is associated with reduction of blood hormone levels, eventually to be followed by clinical hypothyroidism. The mechanism of the thyroid enlargement in this situation is increased pituitary TSH secretion via activation of the feedback system. The resulting increased thyroid mass is a compensatory mechanism which may allow sufficient hormone synthesis to occur so that the patient remains euthyroid. Drugs that interfere with thyroid hormone synthesis (thiocarbamides, lithium, iodides, etc.) can lead to goiter. Withdrawal of a goitrogenic drug results in regression of the goiter, as will administration of enough T_4 or T_3 to suppress endogenous TSH secretion.

Recognition

A mass in the base of the neck is the usual mode of presentation of goiter. Occasionally a scintiscan shows enlargement that cannot be readily appreciated on physical examination. Rarely, an enlarged thyroid is neither visible nor readily palpable but is incidentally found by X-ray of the chest or esophagus when either a retrosternal mass is noted or the trachea or esophagus is found to be deviated. Except in subacute thyroiditis, pain is not a usual symptom but can develop during cyst formation or hemorrhage, a fairly frequent event in multinodular goiter.

Obstruction of the trachea or esophagus can be produced, but dysphagia should not be readily attributed to minor degrees of thyroid enlargement. Hoarseness may occur due to involvement of the recurrent laryngeal nerve, but this is rare in benign enlargement, and its occurrence suggests thyroid neoplasm.

Differential Diagnosis

Clinical and laboratory assessment of thyroid function should be made in all cases of goiter. The clinician must recognize that the functional state may change with time, sometimes rather rapidly, and hence the precise diagnosis may not be possible on a single examination. Goiter in association with hyper-

thyroidism suggests Graves' disease, toxic nodular goiter, or a hyperfunctioning ("hot") nodule. Hypofunction in association with goiter is likely to represent Hashimoto's thyroiditis (see "Hypothyroidism"), but other possibilities such as drug ingestion may have to be excluded. Rarities such as an infiltrative process (amyloid disease, metastatic neoplasm) and the inherited defects of hormone synthesis (organification or coupling defects) have to be kept in mind (Table 70.7).

If the clinical and laboratory assessments indicate normal thyroid function, the diagnosis of euthyroid goiter is made. Multinodular enlargement almost always indicates a process of many years standing. Differentiation of diffuse enlargement from nodular enlargement may require scintiscanning, since small nodules may be missed on physical examination. When only small, nonpalpable nodules are present, an optimally performed scan may show irregular ("patchy") uptake of tracer, but even the best scintiscanning techniques can delineate nodules of only about 1 cm in size. A goiter composed of many such small nodules may appear to represent a non-nodular thyroid on both physical examination and scan. Thyroid autoantibodies are elevated in the blood of most patients with goiters due to Hashimoto's thyroiditis. A proper history will point to possible drug-related goiter. Rapidity of enlargement may help differentiate benign from malignant lesions, while the presence or absence of pain will help in identifying inflammatory thyroiditis (see below, p. 728).

Treatment

Although thyroid enlargement is idiopathic in sporadic goiter, the process is nevertheless dependent on the presence of TSH. Administration of a physiologic quantity of thyroid hormone results in suppression of TSH release. When TSH secretion is chronically suppressed in this manner, the enlarged thyroid eventually regresses or at least ceases to enlarge. This suppression therapy may be accomplished with thyroxine (T_4; sodium L-thyroxine; levothyroxine) or triiodothyronine (T_3; liothyronine; Cytomel). The dose should not be excessive. T_4 at a dose of 0.15 mg $\pm$ 0.05 mg daily is ample. T_3 is given at a dose of 50 to 75 μg daily. Some evidence suggests that T_3 may be effective in a greater proportion of cases.

Suppression therapy must be monitored. The physician must be certain that the gland is suppressible, since perhaps as many as 20% of nontoxic nodular goiters are autonomous. Other goiters may represent inapparent euthyroid Graves' disease. These patients may, if not monitored, develop iatrogenic hyperthyroidism due to the exogenous thyroid hormone. Monitoring of therapy also assures that an adequate amount of hormone is being given. Although regression of goiter is evidence of adequacy of therapy, the physician should be certain that the dose is adequate in those cases that do not show obvious regression.

Several laboratory methods can be used to monitor suppression therapy. Suppression of RaIU was once the standard method of assessing adequacy of dose and suppressibility, but is less useful now because of the low RaIU so often seen in normal persons. However, the RaIU is still the only currently available method to assess suppression in patients administered T₄.

Suppression therapy with T₃ has the advantage that the plasma T₄ falls to a level below normal if suppression is adequate, thus obviating the need for RaIU testing and assuring patient compliance. When T₄ is used for suppression therapy, a plasma T₄ which is not in excess of normal provides assurance that the dose is not excessive. Monitoring of suppression by RaIU should be done no sooner than 3 weeks after beginning suppression therapy with T₄ or 1 week with T₃. If plasma T₄ is monitored during therapy with T₃, a month should elapse.

If the treated gland is diffusely enlarged, obvious regression by 6 months is to be expected in about one-half of cases. Nodular glands are less likely to respond and any response that occurs is slower. Even if complete regression is not accomplished, prevention of further glandular enlargement can be expected.

Several years may be necessary to discern regression of a long-standing multinodular goiter, and during that time one or more nodules may become more easily palpable as the relatively normal portions of the gland regress. Some confusion may occur if the physician interprets this as a progression of the disease or as the appearance of a malignant area.

Suppression therapy is often properly performed for cosmetic reasons. Suppression therapy is also clearly indicated for individuals with many years of life expectancy during which time mechanical problems may develop. However, little is to be gained by treatment of patients whose glands are known not to have changed in size over many years and who are, therefore, unlikely to develop difficulties. A clear and unequivocal indication is found in the patient who has already had surgery for goiter. Recurrence of goiter is frequent in such persons but can predictably be prevented with suppression therapy.

Once started, suppression therapy is usually continued indefinitely but can be terminated or withdrawn if regression occurs. Some goiters do not recur; in those that do, therapy can be reinstituted. Suppression therapy does not lead to permanent loss of TSH secretion, even after decades of thyroid hormone administration, although rare individuals may manifest a brief period of hypothyroidism when prolonged therapy is withdrawn.

Goiter so large as to produce not merely a deviation but significant tracheal compression, as assessed by plain X-ray views of the trachea, or to interfere with swallowing is now a rarity. In these cases, surgery, although attended by significant morbidity, should be considered, since suppression therapy is unlikely to be effective in significantly reducing the size of such large goiters. Radioiodide therapy can be considered in these cases, especially in the elderly or in individuals with other serious medical problems. Multiple doses are usually required. While the response is slow, useful reduction in the size of the goiter may be achieved.

The frequency of carcinoma in multinodular goiter has been debated for years. Unwarranted concern has resulted in countless unnecessary operations (see p. 727).

THYROID NEOPLASMS

One of the most frequent abnormalities of the thyroid is a localized area of enlargement commonly known as a nodule. In evaluating a thyroid nodule, the possibility of malignancy is the main concern. About 90% are benign adenomas or cysts; the remaining ones are lesions of varying degrees of malignancy.

Benign Thyroid Neoplasms: The Solitary Nodule

Many solitary nodules are true adenomas and are encapsulated. While most benign adenomas are relatively hypofunctioning, follicular adenomas may exhibit normal or greater than normal function, i.e., they take up iodine and elaborate thyroid hormone. The growth of most benign adenomas, hypofunctional though they may be, is dependent on endogenous TSH. Adenomas whose function is independent of TSH are termed autonomous.

Benign thyroid nodules are present in at least 5% of the population, but clinically aggressive thyroid carcinoma is rare. In a group of over 200 patients with thyroid nodules identified in the Framingham Study (4% of 5000 patients examined, ages 30 to 60) and followed for 15 years, none developed clinically evident malignancy. In that population, new thyroid nodules continued to appear at a rate of about 1 per 1000 persons per year, about twice as frequently in women as in men (9).

CLINICAL APPROACH

The first point to be established is whether the patient really has only a single nodule. Palpation by an experienced examiner is essential. Frequently, the "solitary" nodule turns out to be one of several nodules in a nontoxic nodular goiter. A single nodule in a clearly enlarged thyroid has a similar connotation, since the enlarged gland is likely to be harboring many small, nondiscrete nodules. Although most patients with a nodule are euthyroid at presentation, T₄ index should be determined for confirmation. If any question about hyperthyroidism exists (see below), plasma T₃ should also be measured.

The next essential question is that of the functional state of the nodule relative to the remaining thyroid tissue, since the hyperfunctioning nodule is almost invariably benign. When scintiscanning is performed, accumulation of isotope in the nodule can approximate that of the surrounding gland ("warm" nodule), be greater ("hot" nodule) or less ("cold" nodule). A hot nodule can be considered benign (99.8% with ^{123}I). "Warm" nodules are far more likely to be benign than not, but the statistics are not so unequivocal as they are for the hot nodule.

The "Hot" Nodule. Management of the hot nodule depends on whether an excessive amount of thyroid hormone is being produced. The autonomous hot nodule, if it produces an amount of hormone equal to or greater than that of normal gland output, suppresses TSH; the remaining normal tissue then becomes relatively inactive and may not be visible, or may be only poorly visible, by scintiscan. In cases in which the nodule is hyperactive but has not clearly suppressed the remaining thyroid tissue, demonstration of autonomous function may depend on a scintiscan after a period of suppression (see p. 711) with administered thyroid hormone.

If the amount of hormone produced by the adenoma considerably exceeds normal, thyrotoxicosis should be clinically apparent. Usually T_4 and T_3 are produced in excess. However, hyperthyroidism due to T_3 alone (T_3 toxicosis) is fairly frequent with such hyperactive nodules.

The natural history of the hot nodule is variable. Over a 10-year interval about one-third will show little change, one-third will become frankly hyperactive, and the remainder will become "cold," sometimes with obvious hemorrhagic infarction and cystic degeneration. Treatment of the hot nodule that is producing hyperthyroidism can be satisfactorily accomplished with radioactive iodine or surgery. Prophylactic ablative therapy is not indicated. Suppression therapy with thyroid hormone is, of course, not effective and will lead to iatrogenic hyperthyroidism.

The "Cold" Nodule. In the evaluation of the cold nodule, it should be borne in mind that 90% of such lesions are benign; only 10% are malignant and almost all of these are very slow growing and of low grade malignancy.

Two additional procedures, now widely available, can provide a diagnosis and avoid unnecessary surgery. They should be performed sequentially, if possible. *Ultrasound* (sonography) examination accurately identifies about 10% of all "cold" nodules as cystic. Almost all (98%) predominantly cystic lesions represent benign adenomas; mixed cystic-solid lesions are less certainly benign. A large proportion of patients with "cold" nodules can be spared surgery by this simple, noninvasive technique. *Needle biopsy* may also be useful (see p. 712) (7).

A conservative approach to the cold nodule, involving a trial of suppression therapy, is recommended. Lesions less than 2.5 cm in diameter can be handled in this way with great safety. Regression (or stability) of the nodule over a 6-month period indi-

cates benign disease; such patients can be followed indefinitely with continued suppression therapy. An objective and accurate estimate of nodule size for follow-up purposes can be made with sonography.

Considering the probability that 90% of cases treated in this way represent benign disease in the first place and the low grade malignancy of almost all of the remaining cases, this approach is reasonable. However, close follow-up is necessary to ensure that appropriate therapy is instituted should the lesion enlarge further during suppression therapy or should lymph nodes become palpable.

Thyroid Carcinomas

GENERAL CONSIDERATIONS

About 95% of thyroid carcinomas are of the papillary or follicular variety; of these, 80 to 90% are papillary carcinomas. Anaplastic and medullary carcinomas probably account for no more than 5% of the total. The relative frequency of the various types of thyroid carcinomas is markedly age-dependent (see p. 727).

Occult thyroid carcinoma (defined as lesions with the histologic appearance of carcinoma, but less than 1.5 cm in diameter) is found in 5 to 10% of U.S. and European populations and 30% of Japanese samples at autopsy. Death from thyroid carcinoma is as rare in Japan as in the United States. Clearly, occult carcinoma behaves as a benign disease and does not warrant aggressive management.

In the United States, about 10,000 new cases of thyroid carcinoma are seen each year, but only about 1000 persons die. Most of these deaths result from the aggressive forms of the disease, *i.e.*, anaplastic lesions, the unusually aggressive follicular carcinomas, and a few from the very uncommon aggressive papillary lesions. Only rare deaths are attributable to medullary carcinoma.

THERAPEUTIC CONSIDERATIONS IN THYROID CARCINOMA

Papillary Carcinoma

Enough information is now available to provide support for a middle-of-the-road approach, one which falls between that which advocated thyroid hormone suppression therapy without surgery and that which has employed radical surgery alone. Long term observations have now also reasonably defined the role of radioiodide ablation therapy (6).

Surgery for Papillary Carcinoma. Follow-up at 10 years indicates a recurrence rate of about 20% for subtotal resection *vs.* 10% for total removal of the gland. Deaths due to carcinoma are 1.5 and 0.5%, respectively. The differences are statistically significant. However, the complication rate for total thyroidectomy (hypoparathyroidism, vocal cord paralysis) remains high. As a result, many surgeons have now adopted a modified or "near total" thyroidectomy. In this procedure the affected side is completely removed; most of the contralateral lobe is also removed but the posterior capsule is left, together with the tip of the upper pole. Visibly involved lymph nodes are always removed but radical neck dissection is not justified even in the presence of obviously involved nodes (6).

The presence of cervical node metastases at operation or the extent of lymphadenectomy does not seem to influence either recurrence or death rate. The death rate in lesions under 2.5 cm without local invasion and without evident distant metastases at the time of surgery is less than 1% in 10 years and 4 to 8% in the less favorable categories (6).

Postoperative Therapy: TSH Suppression and Ablation with Radioiodide. Postoperative therapy with full replacement doses of thyroxine will suppress endogenous TSH, reduce recurrence, and is routine in all cases. In addition, postsurgical ablative therapy with radioactive iodide has a role, although not all cases of localized disease need such therapy. The patient with a minimal papillary lesion needs no such therapy but the patient with a large, locally invasive lesion should receive ablative therapy with ^{131}I. In cases with an intermediate sized lesion, without invasion of the thyroid capsule and without lymph node metastases, the recurrence rate is greatly reduced by treatment with radioiodide, and deaths from recurrent disease may be completely abolished. The hesitation to use radioiodide routinely stems from the unwarranted fear of radiation-induced leukemia. Doses of ^{131}I smaller than those customarily recommended may be equally effective. In contrast to the constraints on radioiodide therapy of localized disease, known metastatic disease should always be treated vigorously.

Follicular Carcinoma

This tumor is somewhat more aggressive than papillary carcinoma, tends to be angioinvasive, and may metastasize to bones and lungs. The tumor may bypass regional lymph nodes, a marked difference from papillary disease. The most important prognostic feature is invasion, either through the tumor capsule or into blood vessels. Unlike papillary carcinoma, primary tumor size at presentation does not appear to influence prognosis (12).

The clinical presentation may be very different from that of papillary disease; the patient may present with metastatic disease involving lungs, bone, brain, or spinal cord. In these cases the primary tumor may be small and initially overlooked. Only rarely do the metastases produce sufficient thyroid hormones to cause thyrotoxicosis.

The surgical approach to follicular carcinoma should be that taken for papillary carcinoma. Suppression therapy with thyroid hormone replacement is routine. Postoperative ablative therapy with radioiodide appears warranted, especially for those pa-

tients with overtly invasive disease. However, the case for routine postoperative use of ^{131}I ablation therapy in the treatment of follicular carcinoma is not statistically established (12).

Anaplastic Carcinoma

This carcinoma is relatively uncommon; its frequency depends on the age of the population. Anaplastic carcinoma is very rare in children and in adults under the age of 35. By age 50, as many as 10% of cases of thyroid carcinoma are due to anaplastic disease and by age 80, by which time the incidence of thyroid carcinoma has fallen markedly, nearly half of the cases that do occur are of this variety. The disease is locally invasive in a highly aggressive fashion and quickly produces pain, dysphagia, hemoptysis, and hoarseness. Death usually occurs within 6 to 12 months. Surgically resectable disease without evidence of metastases, even if it has extended outside the thyroid capsule, can be associated with a long term survival (20 to 30%). It is important to distinguish the small cell type from lymphoma of the thyroid. This rare disease, unlike anaplastic carcinoma, is radiosensitive and amenable to chemotherapy.

Medullary Carcinoma

Medullary carcinoma accounts for 1 to 2% of all thyroid cancers. The tumors arise from the parafollicular or C-cells and produce thyrocalcitonin. Both sporadic and familial varieties are known. The sporadic case typically presents as a solitary nodule, while the familial variety is often multifocal and part of a multiple endocrine adenomatosis syndrome. Diarrhea occurs in some patients. Thyrocalcitonin in plasma is elevated in the basal state or after stimulation with calcium or pentagastrin infusion. When surgical excision is performed before regional nodes have become involved, 90% of patients survive for 10 years. Once the nodes are involved, only 40% survival can be expected. Medullary carcinoma does not appear to respond to suppression therapy with thyroid hormone.

THE QUESTION OF CARCINOMA IN THE MULTINODULAR THYROID

The risk of *clinically significant* carcinoma in a nontoxic nodular goiter is low. Occult carcinoma will be found in a significant proportion of such cases. However, the approach to such occult lesions is no different from that to occult carcinoma in the nonnodular gland. Demonstration of multinodularity by palpation or its suggestion by scan leads some physicians to a firm recommendation against surgical intervention. Suppression therapy is recommended, but only for prevention of further gland enlargement and not out of concern for malignancy. Others feel that large nonfunctioning nodules within multinodular goiters should be treated with suppression therapy for a period of 6 months. Failure to regress is considered an indication for surgical excision. However, since most large nodules in multinodular goiters do not regress within such a period of time, while a significant number may actually become more prominent as less abnormal tissue regresses, this approach is certain to result in unnecessary surgery. Serial sonographic estimates of nodule size may prove useful in such cases.

RADIATION-ASSOCIATED THYROID CARCINOMA

Low dose irradiation of the thyroid is a stimulus to thyroid carcinogenesis, with a latency period of one to several decades.

In recent years thyroid carcinomas have been reported to occur in increased incidence in patients who received radiation therapy some years earlier for enlarged tonsils, adenoids, or thymus; acne; cervical lymphadenopathy, etc. A distinction must be made between treatment with penetrating external radiation and local irradiation with point sources (radium rod and plaque treatment). Thyroid carcinoma has not been related to such limited exposure.

In the reports purporting to show a relationship between external radiation and the development of thyroid carcinoma, as many as one-third of irradiated individuals have been found to develop thyroid carcinoma. Papillary and follicular carcinomas have been seen in about the same ratio as in nonirradiated patients. A relationship between exposure to radiation and development of medullary and anaplastic carcinoma has not been observed. The biologic behavior of radiation-induced carcinomas appears to be similar to the behavior of those that appear spontaneously.

Almost as rapidly as this association between clinical radiation therapy to the head and neck and thyroid carcinoma has been noted, reports refuting this association have appeared (see (5) for references). Accordingly, the approach to the patient with a history of irradiation to the head and neck is not currently standardized. If no thyroid abnormality is palpable, re-examination of the patient at 2-year intervals should suffice. Routine scanning procedures for patients with nonpalpable lesions is not indicated. Although many nonpalpable lesions (0.5 to 1.0 cm) can be detected by optimal use of methods now available, and although the frequency of carcinomas in irradiated patients with abnormalities on scan alone is probably similar to that in patients with palpable disease, the issue at stake here is the natural history of such small lesions. Lesions too small to be palpable are clinically, if not pathologically, benign, and should be managed conservatively.

In the postirradiation patient with a palpable nodule, a conservative approach is presently warranted for the following reasons: (a) even those reports which suggest an association claim no more than an increase of carcinoma from 10% of nodules in nonirradiated persons to 30% of nodules in those radiated.

(b) Most nodules that are carcinomas behave in an extremely benign manner. (c) The entire association is in doubt (5). Clearly, prudence demands that these patients should receive the care recommended above for other patients with palpable nodules; but a widespread surgical assault on these cases is not warranted.

THYROIDITIS

Pyogenic (Suppurative) Thyroiditis

Pyogenic or suppurative thyroiditis, also known as acute thyroiditis, is very rare and most physicians will never encounter a case. The thyroid infection usually follows bacteremia, but can occur as an isolated, primary event. The gland shows typical signs of an acute inflammatory process.

Riedel's Thyroiditis

Riedel's thyroiditis is another rare but indolent and painless form of thyroiditis. The intense induration associated with this process makes the clinical differentiation from infiltrating neoplasm difficult.

Hashimoto's Thyroiditis

This entity is also common (see "Hypothyroidism"; "Goiter"; and Table 70.7). This process is painless and usually produces only modest enlargement of the thyroid. Nodularity is the rule. Distinction from nontoxic nodular goiter is made by the presence of high titers of thyroid autoantibodies in the serum of 80 to 90% of patients with Hashimoto's thyroiditis.

Subacute Thyroiditis

This entity, also known as granulomatous or de Quervain's thyroiditis, is common. Many mild cases are probably never diagnosed. The term subacute is often deceiving and sometimes inappropriate. Although the onset may be insidious, it is perhaps just as often acute over several days. Many patients give a history of recent antecedent upper respiratory tract infection.

The earliest symptoms may be referred pain, usually to the ear, but pain can appear to originate in the jaw or occiput. This phase may last a few hours or days before tenderness and discomfort in the thyroid area becomes apparent. Rarely, the patient is concerned only with the referred pain and unaware of thyroidal tenderness until examination makes it apparent. When the onset is acute, the symptoms and signs are more likely to be severe. Initially, pain and swelling of the thyroid are often unilateral, but the process usually does not remain localized for more than a few days. Systemic symptoms include fever, especially in acute cases, and a sensation of intense fatigue and malaise. The course may be protracted with symptoms persisting for months, although usually they subside within a week or two.

Erythrocyte sedimentation rate is elevated. Early in the disease, the thyroidal radioiodide uptake is depressed, while plasma T$_4$ is elevated. Mild cases have no or only borderline abnormalities of the tests. Significant titers of thyroid autoantibodies are not common but can be seen.

Clinical hyperthyroidism is occasionally seen with subacute thyroiditis (see above). Rarely hypothyroidism occurs and lasts several months. Permanent hypothyroidism is unusual.

THERAPY

Therapy for subacute thyroiditis is symptomatic. The patient should be strongly reassured concerning the benign, self-limited character of the disorder. Thyroid tenderness often responds within several days to aspirin in doses sufficient to maintain therapeutic (anti-inflammatory) blood levels. Codeine should be added if neck discomfort is severe. In less than 10% of cases the process may be severe enough to require glucocorticoid therapy (30 to 60 mg of prednisone daily or equivalent). Glucocorticoid produces prompt relief of pain and tenderness but, if the disease is severe enough to require its use, will usually be necessary for weeks to several months. Relapse is common when therapy is discontinued, and retreatment may be necessary.

Lymphocytic Thyroiditis (Silent Thyroiditis)

This newly recognized process occurs in association with hyperthyroidism and is discussed on p. 720.

References

General

DeGroot, LJ (ed): *Radiation-associated Thyroid Carcinoma. Grune & Stratton, New York, 1977.*
   An extensive discussion of the development of the subject with additional information on many aspects of thyroid carcinoma. For an update of the radiation-related aspects, see (5) for additional references.

Werner, SC and Ingbar, SH (eds): *The Thyroid, Ed. 4. Harper & Row, New York, 1978.*
   A comprehensive textbook on all aspects of the subject.
Williams, RH (ed): *Textbook of Endocrinology, Ed. 6. W. B. Saunders, Philadelphia, 1981.*
   The latest edition of this standard textbook contains an excellent chapter on the thyroid.

Specific

1. Anonymous: *Medical Letter 23:* 30, 1981. Effects of drugs on thyroid function tests.
2. Gregerman, RI: The thyroid gland. In *The Principles and Practice of Medicine,* Ed. 20, edited by AM Harvey, RJ Johns, VA McKusick, AH Owens and RS Ross. Appleton-Century-Crofts, New York, 1980.
3. Gregerman, RI and Davis, PJ: Effects of intrinsic and extrinsic variables on thyroid hormone economy. In *The Thyroid,* Ed. 4, edited by SC Werner and SH Ingbar. Harper & Row, New York, 1978.
4. Hamburger, JI: Pitfalls in the laboratory diagnosis of atypical hyperthyroidism. *Arch Intern Med 139:* 96, 1979.
5. Maxon, HR, Saenger, EL, Thomas, SR, Buncher, CR, Kereiakes JG, Shafer, ML and McLaughlin, CA: Clinically important radiation-associated thyroid disease. *JAMA 244:* 1802, 1980.
6. Mazzaferri, EL, Young, RL, Oertel, JE, Kemmerer, WT and Page, CP: Papillary thyroid carcinoma: the impact of therapy in 576 patients. *Medicine 56:* 171, 1977.
7. Miller, JM, Hamburger, MD and Kini, S: Diagnosis of thyroid nodules. Use of fine needle aspiration and needle biopsy. *JAMA 241:* 481, 1979.
8. Nicolai, TF, Brosseau, J, Kettrick, MA, Roberts, R and Beltaos, E: Lymphocytic thyroiditis with spontaneously resulting hyperthyroidism (silent thyroiditis). *Arch Intern Med 140:* 478, 1980.
9. Vander, JB, Gaston, EA and Dawber, TR: The significance of nontoxic thyroid nodules. Final report of a 15-year study of the incidence of thyroid malignancy. *Ann Intern Med 69:* 537, 1968.
10. Volpé, R: The role of autoimmunity in hypoendocrine and hyperendocrine function. With special emphasis on autoimmune thyroid disease. *Ann Intern Med 87:* 86, 1977.
11. Walfish, PG and Ginsberg, J: Letter. *Ann Intern Med 88:* 128, 1978.
12. Young, RL, Mazzaferri, EL, Rahe, AJ and Dorfman, SG: Pure follicular carcinoma: impact of therapy in 214 patients. *J Nucl Med 21:* 733, 1980.

CHAPTER SEVENTY-ONE

Selected Endocrine Problems: Disorders of Pituitary, Adrenal, and Parathyroid Glands; Pharmacologic Use of Steroids; Hypo- and Hypercalcemia; Water Metabolism; Hypoglycemia

ROBERT I. GREGERMAN, M.D.

PITUITARY DISEASES

Disorders of the pituitary gland are manifest by disturbance of function (hyper- or hyposecretion of trophic hormones), by anatomic encroachment on adjacent structures (enlargement of tumors), or by a combination of these processes. Many of the cases of hormone hypersecretion are due to benign tumors—often clinically inapparent microadenomas. Most commonly a small adenoma produces an excess of prolactin with resultant galactorrhea. Most cases of galactorrhea, however, are functional, in some cases idiopathic and in others due to drugs.

When a pituitary tumor is large enough to produce increased pressure within the sella turcica, enlargement and erosion of the bony walls of that structure either produce no symptoms or may cause headache.

Tumor enlargement superiorly—the direction of least resistance—leads to encroachment upon the adjacent optic chiasm and may produce visual field defects. Pituitary tumors large enough to be anatomically apparent are frequently associated with failure of hormone secretion (hypopituitarism), a process which results in end-organ failure (hypoadrenalism, hypogonadism, and/or hypothyroidism). The pituitary may also be affected by a wide variety of systemic illnesses, including granulomatous, infectious, vascular, and neoplastic processes, but all are extremely uncommon causes of hypopituitarism.

A related problem is that of craniopharyngioma. This developmental abnormality may simulate pituitary tumor. The lesion is usually outside the pituitary and presents as a suprasellar mass lesion readily evident on computerized tomography. Most cases are manifest during childhood.

Clinical Presentations

When a patient presents with evidence of *decreased endocrine function*, routine evaluation must include consideration of whether the process is due to pituitary disease—i.e., "secondary" gland failure, or is "primary"—i.e., in the end-organ. For example, in most patients with hypothyroidism thyroid-stimulating hormone (TSH) is elevated due to failure of normal inhibition of the negative feedback loop. However, if TSH is not elevated in the face of hypothyroidism, the possibility of hypopituitarism must then be further evaluated. Similarly, in patients with hypogonadism an easy differential diagnosis can be made, since determinations of follicle-stimulating hormone (FSH) and luteinizing hormone (LH) levels invariably will be elevated if there is primary end-organ failure. In patients with adrenal insufficiency, however, the plasma adrenocorticotropic hormone (ACTH) does not always clearly differentiate primary from secondary disease. In cases of *endocrine hyperfunction*, pituitary function may also be evaluated but not necessarily routinely (see "Hyperthyroidism", chapter 70, p. 714; and "Adrenocortical hyperfunction," p. 736).

Not infrequently, the issue of pituitary disease is raised inadvertently. The patient's complaints lead to radiologic examination of the skull because of headaches, suspected sinusitis, injury, or for some other reason. An enlarged or an abnormal sella turcica is noted. The issue then arises concerning further evaluation of what may be an incidental finding. Referral to an endocrinologist is appropriate at this point, but further evaluation by the nonspecialist is also possible.

Evaluation of an Abnormal Sella Turcica

The sella turcica as seen in ordinary X-rays of the skull may appear deceptively normal or may appear abnormal when it is not. Polytomograms are more useful in delineating the anatomy of this structure, but even this procedure is often deceptive. Asymmetry, a double contour, and erosions of the cortical bone forming the sellar outline and of the clinoid processes are all criteria for sellar abnormality. The volume of the sella can be calculated and compared to normal values. Sellar enlargement is probably the most reliable finding on tomography. If the sella is shown to be abnormal, computerized tomography (CT) should be undertaken. This procedure is essential in evaluation of the possibility of suprasellar extension of tumors. If a suprasellar mass is shown, the patient should be referred for ophthalmologic examination of the visual fields, preferably with a red dot, the most sensitive technique for detection of field defects produced by suprasellar masses. For the evaluation of intrasellar lesions, CT has not been especially useful until very recently. However, the most advanced CT scanners can show details of intrasellar contents and are probably superior to polytomography for evaluation of the sella itself.

Empty Sella Syndrome

An enlarged sella does not always mean that a pituitary tumor is present. Not infrequently extensive evaluation leads to demonstration of an empty sella turcica. Such patients are often discovered during evaluation of skull X-rays obtained for reasons other than suspected hypopituitarism—usually headache—and, indeed, usually have no clinical endocrine disease. The cause of the empty sella syndrome is not known, but open communication of cerebrospinal fluid through a defect in the diaphragma sellae and/or a ruptured cyst have been postulated. In most cases, a rim of normal pituitary tissue remains and pituitary function, which should be routinely evaluated, is normal; in some there is minimal hypopituitarism and/or a visual field defect for reasons which are not clear but could represent a previous cyst. The diagnosis can be suspected from CT which fails to show enhancement, but definitive diagnosis and differentiation from intrasellar tumor may not be possible without a pneumoencephalogram that demonstrates entry of air into the sella turcica. This procedure is not ordinarily warranted unless the issue is whether surgery or radiation therapy is required for suspected tumor as, for example, when headache is severe and intractable. In such cases, neurologic or neurosurgical consultation is indicated.

Chromophobe Adenomas

Chromophobe adenomas, the commonest of the pituitary tumors, account for about 85% of cases with most occurring between ages 30 and 60. Not infrequently chromophobe adenomas occur in association with parathyroid or pancreatic islet cell adenomas and are sometimes associated with the Zollinger-Ellison syndrome (see Chapter 33). These associations constitute the syndrome of multiple endocrine adenomatosis (MEA), Type I. When the pituitary is not involved, but pheochromocytoma, medullary thyroid carcinoma, and—occasionally—parathyroid adenomata occur together, the syndrome is termed MEA, Type II.

Chromophobe adenomas are usually noninvasive but may infiltrate local structures and on rare occasions even behave as locally malignant lesions. Long thought to be "functionless," many are now known to be prolactinomas. The term chromophobe adenoma belongs to the era in which pituitary tumors were classified by their histologic staining characteristics (chromophobe, eosinophile, and basophile). A more precise classification can now be constructed which is based on the secretory product of the tumor (e.g., somatotrope tumor, growth hormone-producing), but the old terms persist.

Pituitary function remains clinically normal until more than 75% of the normal pituitary has been destroyed by the adenoma. Hypogonadism is usually the earliest evidence of a hormone deficiency state (60 to 80% of cases) but hypothyroidism as an initial manifestation is almost as common. Adrenal insufficiency is usually the last problem to develop and is often inapparent except on laboratory testing. In about 10% of cases, diabetes insipidus develops.

Prolactin and Galactorrhea

Bilateral breast discharge may be the first clue to the presence of a prolactin-secreting chromophobe adenoma. In many cases discharge from the breast is minimal and may be apparent only on physical examination when a few drops of milk may be expressable. Breast enlargement may occur in the male, but prolactin excess is an uncommon cause of gynecomastia (Chapter 74). Prolactin secretion appears to inhibit the secretion of gonadotropins and hence may also be associated with evidence of hypogonadism including impotence and amenorrhea (Chapter 74).

Most cases of galactorrhea are not due to tumor but rather are due to a functional disturbance of prolactin secretion, which in turn is either spontaneous or related to the use of certain drugs. In either case, the hallmark of galactorrhea is an increase of the concentration of prolactin in plasma. Radioimmunoassays for prolactin are widely available and present no special problems of interpretation (see below). The drugs most commonly incriminated in the production of galactorrhea are reserpine, phenothiazines, tricyclic antidepressants, α-methyldopa (Aldomet), and estrogens (oral contraceptives). If no drugs are involved, a functional disorder is still likely, but some cases will be due to chromophobe adenoma. Rarely, galactorrhea occurs secondary to hypothyroidism.

The degree of prolactin elevation is strongly suggestive of the cause of the disorder. Levels of prolactin greater than 200 ng/ml are essentially diagnostic of tumor, even in the absence of changes in the sella. Low levels of prolactin (less than 50 ng/ml) are much more likely to be due to a functional disorder, but in many cases differentiation is not possible by this means. A significant proportion of the normal population harbors a nonsecreting microadenoma which is evident only at autopsy. Other normal persons may have minor abnormalities of the sella on polytomography (2). Hence, demonstration even of such a change does not prove the presence of a functional microadenoma.

Many cases of galactorrhea, with or without microadenoma, can be successfully treated with the drug bromocriptine (Parlodel) which may lower the prolactin, abolish the galactorrhea, and restore normal menses. Treatment with bromocriptine can be undertaken by the nonspecialist provided that tumor is not likely. If prolactin levels are very high or if radiographic evidence of tumor is present, an endocrinologist should be consulted.

The indications for surgical intervention should be anatomic. Small tumors confined to the sella, or even those with some degree of suprasellar extension and associated with limited visual loss, are best treated by transsphenoidal surgery (see "Acromegaly"). Microadenomas can often be successfully removed and normal pituitary function restored. With marked suprasellar extension, a transfrontal surgical approach may be needed. This is a much more formidable procedure. In many cases a large tumor cannot be completely removed; postoperative radiation therapy will prevent clinical recurrence in these instances.

Acromegaly

Pituitary tumors that produce an excess of growth hormone result in the clinical state termed acromegaly. If the growth hormone excess occurs before cessation of growth, gigantism occurs. When growth hormone excess begins in the adult, the most common clinical feature suggesting the presence of acromegaly is insidious alteration of facial appearance over many years. Old photographs may be useful in helping to identify such changes. The various physical findings include enlargement (lengthening) of the mandible, sometimes with separation of the teeth; coarsening of facial features due both to overgrowth of frontal, malar, and nasal bones and soft tissue overgrowth producing widening of the nose and protrusion of the lips; enlargement of the hands and feet, often noted by increasing glove and shoe size; and dermatologic changes which include skin thickening and sebaceous gland enlargement (hydradenitis). Very commonly, patients present with a nerve entrapment (carpal tunnel) syndrome. Osteoarthritis and diabetes mellitus, while frequently seen in this disorder, are too common to provide a clue to the presence of acromegaly. Tumors large enough to produce sellar enlargement may lead to headache; suprasellar extension may result in visual field defects.

The laboratory diagnosis is simple in overt cases but requires dynamic testing in mild cases. Elevation of serum growth hormone (GH) in the fasting, basal state to values consistently greater than 10 ng/ml is strongly suggestive of the diagnosis. However, stress and physical activity may also elevate the GH levels. Elevated values must therefore be confirmed with a test of the ability of glucose to suppress the GH. During a standard glucose tolerance test (Chapter 69), the GH—determined simultaneously with the glucose—should normally fall to a value less than 5 ng/ml. Most acromegalics show no fall of GH, while a few exhibit a "paradoxical" rise during the test. Laboratory evidence of elevated and nonsuppressible GH warrants referral to an endocrinologist, as does the presence of equivocal clinical or laboratory findings.

TREATMENT OF ACROMEGALY

Treatment should be directed by an endocrinologist. Irradiation of the pituitary, usually by external high voltage techniques, has been standard treatment for years. Such therapy is effective but is usually extremely slow in its effect and may take several years to produce maximal suppression of hormone production. Surgery is indicated when there is a need for rapid reduction of the elevated growth hormone (e.g., for cosmetic reasons in a young woman with early disease; visual field loss; or intractable headache). Transsphenoidal operation is now standard for most cases and should, if at all possible, include an attempt at selective removal of a microadenoma. The transsphenoidal operation involves minimal morbidity, a very low rate of complications, and essentially no mortality.

Cushing's Disease

When evidence is obtained for overproduction of glucocorticoids and testing suggests the presence of adrenal hyperplasia (see "Adrenal Diseases"), X-ray evaluation of the sella turcica is in order. Only rarely will an abnormality be evident, even on CT. Most cases of Cushing's disease with adrenal hyperplasia are, nonetheless, due to a basophilic microadenoma of the pituitary (see p. 737).

PITUITARY FAILURE (HYPOPITUITARISM)

Idiopathic Causes

Patients are occasionally encountered in whom pituitary failure occurs without evidence of pituitary tumor or of another anatomic defect demonstrable by current techniques. Some of these patients are eventually found to have infiltrative processes (sarcoidosis, histiocytosis, lymphoma). Hypopituitarism in these patients is diagnosed by the demonstration of end-organ failure occurring in the absence of the expected elevation of trophic hormone. Isolated deficiencies of trophic hormones also occur but are rare. Among these, the most likely to be encountered is hypogonadotropic hypogonadism in the male, sometimes associated with anosmia (Kallmann's syndrome) In these patients, no anatomic basis is apparent.

Sheehan's Syndrome (Postpartum Pituitary Failure)

Massive uterine hemorrhage occurring at delivery occasionally results in pituitary infarction and panhypopituitarism. In this syndrome, failure of postpartum lactation and absence of menses are attended by debility and other evidences of end-organ failure. Because of improvements in obstetrical care (prompt treatment of hemorrhage), such cases are now rare.

Pituitary Apoplexy

On rare occasions hemorrhagic infarction of a pituitary tumor may lead to severe headache and/or signs of a rapidly expanding intracranial abnormality. Skull films or tomograms of the sella turcica are abnormal. Another rare but recently recognized phenomenon is that of pituitary infarction ("apoplexy") occurring during the course of a febrile illness, presumably viral. Intense headache lasts for days and is usually but not always severe enough to require hospitalization. The acute febrile illness subsides with symptomatic therapy and without specific clinical or radiographic findings, only to be followed later by the development of hypopituitarism. Both men and women can be affected.

Hormone Replacement Therapy of Hypopituitarism

Pituitary insufficiency, regardless of the cause, is treated with thyroid hormone (thyroxine, see p. 723) adrenal glucocorticoid (cortisol, see p. 735) and gonadal hormone (testosterone, see p. 784; or an estrogen, see p. 795). At the present time, pituitary trophic hormones are not available for routine clinical use; furthermore, they are not necessary for maintenance of normal health and vigor. Occasionally, young women may be candidates for therapy with gonadotropins in order to produce ovulation and restore fertility. Such therapy is possible but available at only a few centers. In males, normal libido and sexual performance can be assured with testosterone therapy. Restoration of fertility in the male is also possible with the use of a combination of gonadotropins, but such therapy is not generally available.

Disturbances of Pituitary Function Due to Nonendocrine Disease

Perhaps more common than decreased pituitary function resulting from intrinsic pituitary disease is altered gonadotropin secretion on a functional basis. Many illnesses can affect the functional integrity of the hypothalamic-pituitary-end-organ axis. This phenomenon is most obvious as disturbance of menstruation in women (see Chapter 74). Any disease which results in malnutrition can produce decreased gonadotropins and (secondary) amenorrhea. Alcoholism is an outstanding example. Liver disease need not be present in alcoholism in order to produce amenorrhea, but a variety of liver diseases are themselves associated with loss of menses. The common factor seems to be malnutrition.

The classical example of nonendocrine illness that simulates an endocrine disturbance is anorexia nervosa (see Chapter 5). In this psychiatric disturbance, which results in severe malnutrition with resultant weight loss, the most marked disturbance of endocrine function is cessation of menses resulting from a decrease of gonadotropins. Other trophic hormones are not affected. Thyroid function is usually normal. Axillary and pubic hair are retained, giving important clinical evidence for the preservation of adrenal function. Although cortisol secretion is low (urinary steroid excretion is decreased), this results from slow metabolic disposal of cortisol rather than decreased ACTH secretion; plasma cortisol is normal. Growth hormone may be elevated, a consequence of starvation due to any cause. The diagnosis of anorexia nervosa should be based on the association of psychiatric abnormalities and obvious decrease in food intake. The tests described will serve merely to support the diagnosis.

Other diseases may also result in secondary amenorrhea due to failure of gonadotropin secretion. These include such diverse conditions as severe emotional disturbances, marked obesity, poorly controlled diabetes, and severe chronic infections.

ADRENAL DISEASES

Adrenocortical Insufficiency (Addison's Disease)

In ambulatory patients the clinical presentation of adrenocortical insufficiency is related to a number of chronic complaints which are nonspecific in character. Although a high index of suspicion will certainly result in far more tests than positive diagnoses, detection of this relatively rare problem demands such an approach. The alternative is needless morbidity culminating in acute hospitalization for full-blown disease, i.e., vascular collapse with Addisonian "crisis."

ETIOLOGY AND ASSOCIATION WITH OTHER AUTOIMMUNE DISEASES

Adrenocortical insufficiency is now most commonly due to "autoimmune" disease and is associated with the presence of antibodies to adrenal tissue. Most other cases are secondary to pituitary disease. Tuberculosis, once a common cause, now only rarely produces adrenocortical insufficiency, probably because of decreased frequency of tuberculosis and because of effective therapy. Many cases of autoimmune adrenocortical insufficiency are associated with autoimmune thyroiditis (Hashimoto's disease),

although the two problems may develop years apart. The simultaneous occurrence of autoimmune thyroid and adrenal disease is termed Schmidt's syndrome. Rarely, autoimmune adrenocortical insufficiency, autoimmune hypothyroidism, and autoimmune gonadal failure occur in the recently recognized syndrome of "polyglandular failure." There is also an association of autoimmune adrenocortical insufficiency with pernicious anemia and Sjögren's syndrome, and probably with systemic lupus erythematosus. Other rare causes of adrenocortical insufficiency include histoplasmosis and sarcoidosis.

CLINICAL PRESENTATION

Chronic symptoms include anorexia, weight loss, weakness, and decreased physical endurance. Vomiting may occur and abdominal pain, sometimes resembling that of peptic ulcer disease, can be a presenting feature. Other symptoms include mental sluggishness, irritability, and symptoms of either postural hypotension or of hypoglycemia. In primary adrenal insufficiency, increasing pigmentation (white patients) or further darkening of skin (black patients) may be noted. Loss of axillary and pubic hair—an important finding when present—may occur in females. Such hair loss is commonly overlooked on physical examination and is hardly ever volunteered as part of the history.

Physical examination often shows postural hypotension. Pigmentation is diffuse but in addition is especially evident in creases of the hands, the areolae, over pressure areas (knuckles, elbows), and in new scars. Pigmentation of buccal mucous membranes is a pathognomonic finding in white patients but is a normal finding in blacks. Lymphadenopathy is occasionally seen. When the adrenal insufficiency is secondary to pituitary disease, additional findings may relate to the manifestation of a pituitary tumor (headache, visual loss), to hypothyroidism (Chapter 70), and to hypogonadism (Chapter 74).

LABORATORY EVALUATION

Classically, hyponatremia associated with hyperkalemia and some degree of azotemia provided the clues to the diagnosis. These latter abnormalities are manifestations of severe disease and may be absent in the less severe cases that are likely to be encountered in an ambulatory practice. A variety of other nonspecific abnormalities occur, occasionally including anemia, lymphocytosis, and eosinophilia.

Laboratory diagnosis of adrenal insufficiency must be made or excluded by determination of plasma cortisol. Determinations of plasma cortisol made without prior adrenal stimulation by injected ACTH have many limitations. In this regard both the normal diurnal rhythm of cortisol and the high degree of variability of plasma cortisol in normal persons must be kept in mind. Plasma cortisol can be initially measured at any time of the day, and a normal value

(15 to 25 µg/dl) will exclude the diagnosis. However, afternoon determinations may be "low" simply because of the normal p.m. drop and even the fasting a.m. cortisol is highly variable. Values lower than 5 µg/dl at any time are highly likely to be due to adrenal insufficiency. Intermediate values (5 to 10 µg/dl) may be seen in less severe cases and may overlap those of normals. Thus, measurement of unstimulated plasma cortisol is useful, especially in excluding the diagnosis, but may fail to detect mild cases or may yield indeterminate values.

Plasma ACTH can be determined by radioimmunoassay. An elevated level will be seen in primary adrenal insufficiency because of lack of inhibition of the negative feedback system. However, the high cost and relative lack of reliability make measurement of plasma ACTH only an adjunct to diagnosis which has its major usefulness primarily in establishing a diagnosis of secondary (pituitary) adrenocortical insufficiency.

Evaluation of the significnce of low or borderline values of plasma cortisol should always be made by administering exogenous ACTH and then measuring plasma cortisol again—after the adrenal stimulation. The ease with which such testing is performed—and the frequent failure of unstimulated plasma cortisol values to give definitive information—provides a cogent argument for use of ACTH stimulation as the preferred screening procedure for adrenal insufficiency. Many variations of ACTH stimulation tests have been advocated. A simple and reliable procedure is the intravenous injection of 0.25 mg of synthetic ACTH (Cortrosyn) (see below). Plasma cortisol obtained 3 to 4 hours after injection will normally increase 2 to 4 times over baseline and will be above the normal baseline range. Patients with adrenocortical insufficiency do not show a response. If the test is positive (no response), confirmation should be made with an 8-hour intravenous infusion of ACTH and at least two plasma cortisols obtained between 6 and 8 hours. The dose of ACTH is the same. Expected increments of cortisol are somewhat greater in the latter test.

Synthetic ACTH is now readily available. This compound is preferred over the older preparations of natural material, since adverse reactions are not seen with the synthetic peptide. If the natural (aqueous) ACTH is used, it is given in a dose of 25 units in the manner described for the synthetic material. Rapid "1-hour" screening tests with either type of ACTH should be avoided, since the increment of cortisol is less than when a longer period is used. The 1-hour test is therefore more difficult to interpret and less reliable. ACTH gel should not be used in testing for adrenocortical insufficiency.

Tests of adrenal function based on urinary excretion of steroid metabolites (17-ketogenic (17-KGS)) or 17-hydroxysteroids (17-OHS)) should be avoided as initial tests for adrenal insufficiency. These tests offer no advantage over plasma cortisol measurements and often yield artifactually low values due to incomplete collection of urine. Following stimulation with ACTH, determination of urinary steroids can, however, provide useful confirmation of the plasma cortisol response. The adrenal response to ACTH is slow in secondary adrenal insufficiency and requires stimulation for up to 3 days. However, other tests of pituitary function are available and serve better to identify the presence of adrenal insufficiency resulting from pituitary disease (see "Pituitary Disease").

Although the adrenal mineralocorticoid, aldosterone, may be low in adrenal insufficiency, the hormone is secreted by the zona glomerulosa rather than the more central portion of the adrenal cortex and may be relatively unaffected by processes which destroy much of the adrenal. Therefore, measurements of plasma and urinary aldosterone have no place in routine diagnosis of adrenocortical insufficiency.

TREATMENT OF ADDISON'S DISEASE

The Addisonian patient should be made to realize the importance of taking hormone therapy regularly and of understanding self-care during situations of stress. Unless both patient and physician cooperate in this effort, the life of the Addisonian patient becomes a series of hospitalizations requiring emergency therapy for crises, most of which are avoidable.

Steroid Replacement Therapy. Under normal circumstances patients are given 20 to 30 mg of cortisol (or equivalent) daily. Recommended dosage schemes vary. The simplest and least expensive therapy is 12.5 mg (one-half of a 25-mg cortisone tablet) taken twice daily (morning and evening). In another scheme, 10 to 15 mg of cortisol (hydrocortisone) are used on the same schedule. Some authorities prefer to simulate the normal diurnal rhythm of cortisol secretion, although no evidence indicates that this scheme is of any benefit. In this approach, 15 to 20 mg of cortisol are given on arising and 5 to 10 mg in the evening. Equivalent doses of prednisone or another glucocorticoid (see Table 71.2) may be used but have no advantage. Their use may, indeed, dictate a requirement for additional mineralocorticoid therapy, since glucocorticoids such as prednisone, dexamethasone, etc., have much less mineralocorticoid activity than does cortisol (or cortisone). Overtreatment with glucocorticoids should be avoided. Frequent increases of dose for treatment of nonspecific complaints are a common practice but are to be deplored, since iatrogenic Cushing's syndrome is a real hazard to the long term well-being of patients with Addison's disease.

The requirement for glucocorticoids (cortisol) is, of course, increased during stress. In the ambulatory patient, minor stress can be handled by a properly instructed and motivated patient. Telephone contact with the physician is also useful—or even essential—

on many such occasions, especially in the early months of therapy before the patient's ability to deal with these episodes has been demonstrated. The commonest stress for the ambulatory patient is a nonspecific often viral, febrile illness. Ordinarily, a febrile response to 101°F (38°C) or thereabouts which is unaccompanied by vomiting or diarrhea can be handled by simply increasing the cortisol dose to 50 to 75 mg daily in divided doses. A more severe episode (e.g., bronchitis) may require 100 mg. The occurrence of vomiting or significant diarrhea requires contact with a physician and may demand the use of parenteral glucocorticoids.

The need for hospitalization during stress must be determined by the physician and depends on the circumstances. It is obviously prudent to be cautious, but in this long term, chronic illness frequent and precipitous hospitalizations should be avoided. Many minor events can be handled by judicious increase of steroid dosage. Preoperative management is described elsewhere (Chapter 83).

Although not all patients with fully developed adrenal insufficiency require mineralocorticoid therapy in addition to cortisol replacement, such therapy is usually started when the diagnosis is made. Initial dose is 0.1 mg of fludrocortisone daily (Florinef, 0.1 mg tablets). Aldosterone is not available for therapy of Addison's disease. Only rarely will patients require more than 0.1 mg of fludrocortisone. In the past doses as high as 0.2 mg daily were used, but hypertension and edema were common. Some individuals require as little as 0.05 mg every other day. Adequacy of therapy can be judged by determinations of serum sodium and potassium and clinical parameters, including normalization of blood pressure without postural hypotension. When, during stress, the dose of cortisol is increased beyond 50 to 75 mg daily, fludrocortisone therapy becomes unnecessary, since the mineralocorticoid activity of cortisol is sufficient to maintain self-balance when taken in greater than baseline physiologic amounts.

Patient Education. The patient and members of the patient's household should be educated about the symptoms of Addisonian crisis and how to respond in emergencies. In addition, the patient should carry an identification document or wear an inscribed bracelet identifying the Addisonian state and instructing therapy. Appropriate information in addition to name, address, and telephone number should read approximately as follows:

"I am a patient with adrenal insufficiency (Addison's disease). If I am seriously injured, found unconscious, or am vomiting, I should be given an injection of dexamethasone, as emergency treatment for Addisonian crisis. A filled syringe is with my belongings. Notify my physician [name, telephone number] or other medical authority immediately."

Syringes containing dexamethasone phosphate (4

mg in 1 ml of water) are available for patients and can be conveniently carried.

All patients with Addison's disease should eat a diet which contains a liberal quantity of sodium (100 to 150 mEq/day), regardless of whether mineralocorticoids are used. In event of intercurrent diarrhea or profuse sweating, additional salt should be consumed. Electrolytes should be checked periodically (every 3 to 4 months during the critical first year of therapy). Mineralocorticoid therapy should be cautiously reduced if edema, hypertension, or hypokalemia are noted and salt and/or mineralocorticoid increased if postural hypotension, hyponatremia, or hyperkalemia appear. Overtreatment with glucocorticoids should be carefully avoided. Over the long term, it should be borne in mind that, if the Addison's disease is idiopathic (*i.e.*, autoimmune), related diseases and their own manifestations may appear at any time (hypothyroidism, hypoparathyroidism, hypogonadism).

Adrenocortical Hyperfunction

The adrenals produce several steroid products: glucocorticoids (chiefly cortisol), mineralocorticoids (chiefly aldosterone), and so-called adrenal androgens (a group of steroids collectively termed 17-ketosteroids (17-KS)). Clinical disorders are known which affect predominantly the secretion of one or

Table 71.1
Adrenocortical Hyperfunction

GLUCOCORTICOID EXCESS PREDOMINATES
  Adrenal hyperplasia (60–70% of all cases):
    1. Pituitary microadenoma secreting ACTH (most cases of adrenal hyperplasia)
    2. Nonendocrine tumor secreting ACTH (rare)
  Adrenal neoplasm (30–40% of all cases):
    1. Adrenal adenoma ⎱
    2. Adrenal carcinoma ⎰(about equal in frequency)
ADRENAL ANDROGEN EXCESS PREDOMINATES (HIRSUTISM/VIRILISM)
  Some adrenal adenomas
  Some adrenal carcinomas
  Partial adrenogenital syndrome[a]
ALDOSTERONE EXCESS
  Primary aldosteronism:
    1. Adrenal adenoma
    2. Adrenal nodular hyperplasia
  Secondary aldosteronism:
    1. Salt and volume depletion, including diuretic use and various disease states causing increased production of renin
    2. Juxtaglomerular cell hyperplasia or tumor (rare)

[a] Complete enzymatic defects in steroid synthesis are rare and are invariably manifest early in life as adrenal insufficiency and abnormalities of genital development. In ambulatory adults, partial defects of synthesis of cortisol lead to compensatory adrenal hyperplasia with production of excessive quantities of adrenal steroids with weak androgenic activity. Hirsutism, with or without virilism, ensues (see Chapter 74).

other of these hormones. Table 71.1 lists these disorders of adrenal hyperfunction. Most are rather uncommon or rare, but some essentially functional disorders are frequently encountered. The approach presented here is predominantly oriented to the recognition—or exclusion—and initial evaluation of these diseases in ambulatory patients. Once the practitioner is reasonably certain that a problem exists, detailed evaluation often requires consultation with an endocrinologist and sometimes hospitalization for special procedures. However, many relatively simple tests to define the situation can and should be performed on an ambulatory basis. It must be appreciated that details of diagnostic workups vary widely even among specialists and are in constant evolution as new hormone assays and tests emerge.

CUSHING'S SYNDROME (GLUCOCORTICOID EXCESS)

Etiology

In this syndrome a supraphysiologic amount of glucocorticoid (cortisol) is secreted along with varying amounts of adrenal androgens. Most cases are due to hypersecretion of ACTH from the pituitary with resultant adrenal hyperplasia (Cushing's disease). In recent years it has become apparent that almost all of these cases are due to pituitary microadenomas that produce excessive amounts of ACTH (see "Pituitary Diseases"). A smaller number of these cases are due to adrenal adenoma or carcinoma. Cushing's syndrome may also occasionally be caused by ectopic production of ACTH by malignant tumors. Of these tumors, small cell carcinoma of the lung is most commonly involved. When a tumor causes Cushing's syndrome, the malignancy is usually obvious, although rarely a small neoplasm may be inapparent when the evidence of glucocorticoid excess first appears.

Clinical Presentation

The severity of the signs and symptoms depends on the magnitude of the steroid excess, the rapidity with which it develops, and the degree to which androgen production is increased. The signs and symptoms of glucocorticoid excess are familiar to all physicians who have seen the entire picture of this disease emerge as the result of long term treatment of patients with prednisone and similar drugs. Glucocorticoid excess produces increased deposition of subcutaneous fat in the face ("moon facies"), while deposition of fat in the upper body produces "buffalo hump" and truncal obesity. Skin changes include telangiectasia over the face, atrophy and thinning of the skin with easy or spontaneous bruising, ecchymoses, and development of purplish abdominal striae. Hyperpigmentation is sometimes seen. Muscle weakness results from so-called steroid myopathy and is especially prominent in the shoulder and pelvic girdle areas. The extremities become thin as muscle wasting occurs. Eventually bone mineral loss occurs producing osteoporosis with its resultant back pain. Crush fractures of the vertebrae are common and frequently spontaneous, while hip or wrist fractures may occur following minimal trauma. Hypertension and diabetes mellitus are common. Hypokalemia may occur. Probably less well recognized are the psychiatric disturbances which result from chronic glucocorticoid excess. Lability of mood, depression, mania, and frank psychoses may all be precipitated by glucocorticoid excess.

Androgenic effects occur from both the intrinsic properties of the glucocorticoids and the associated production of adrenal androgens. With glucocorticoid excess alone only mild signs are usually evident, i.e., hirsutism (facial, extremities, truncal) and acne. More profound androgen effects that include virilization suggest adrenal tumor. These signs include frontal baldness in women, oligomenorrhea, increase in muscle mass, and enlargement of the clitoris. Androgenic effects cannot, of course, be appreciated in men.

Differential Diagnosis

Obesity and Hirsuitism. In women obesity is frequently associated with hirsutism, hypertension, and/or diabetes. When weight gain is rapid, striae may appear. These findings often raise the possibility of Cushing's syndrome and provoke laboratory screening for this disorder. Very few of such patients will be found to have Cushing's syndrome.

One-half of obese persons have increased cortisol production which is a phenomenon resulting from the obese state. In these individuals the urinary excretion of steroid metabolites is increased and falls into the range of that seen in Cushing's syndrome. However, in distinction from Cushing's syndrome, such obese individuals have plasma cortisol concentrations which are normal rather than elevated. Furthermore, the suppressibility of the pituitary-adrenal axis in obesity is also normal (see "Laboratory Diagnosis" below). The obesity-related increase of urinary steroid metabolite excretion is one of several reasons why such measurements are to be avoided for screening purposes.

Psychiatric Illness. Psychiatric symptoms are common in Cushing's syndrome. However, in the past few years it has also been appreciated that depressive illness may be associated with markedly excessive production of glucocorticoids (13). These patients do not appear clinically to have full-blown Cushing's syndrome, but at least some clinical features suggest the diagnosis and lead to laboratory investigation. Differentiation from true Cushing's syndrome may be difficult at first, but the differential diagnosis eventually becomes clear, since remission of the psychiatric disturbance results in disappearance of the abnormal laboratory findings.

Laboratory Diagnosis

General. The tests of adrenal and pituitary function fall into two groups: (a) static measurements of blood or urine steroids or (b) dynamic testing of the pituitary-adrenal axis. Both procedures are useful and may be combined. With regard to the measurements themselves, in blood both plasma cortisol and ACTH can be assayed. In urine, assays are available for cortisol ("free cortisol"), two different groups of cortisol metabolites (17 hydroxycorticosteroids (17-OHCS) and 17-ketogenic steroids (17-KGS)), and the adrenal androgens (17-ketosteroids (17-KS)) which also include some cortisol metabolites.

Screening for Suspected Cushing's Syndrome. Many patients with Cushing's syndrome have mild disease. Steroid production in such individuals is not greatly increased and there is considerable overlap with normal values. Accordingly, determination of plasma cortisol or urinary steroid excretion is not likely to be helpful. Screening can best be performed with an abbreviated suppression test with use of dexamethasone. A single oral dose of 1 mg is given between 11 p.m. and midnight and the plasma cortisol is measured at 8 to 9 a.m. Normal patients will show suppression of cortisol to less than 5 μg/dl. If the test is abnormal, a more involved but more reliable suppression test is performed in which dexamethasone is given orally at a dose of 0.5 mg every 6 hours for 2 days. Plasma cortisol, urinary 17-OHCS, or both can be monitored by this test. The plasma cortisol at the end of the suppression period should be suppressed to less than 3 μg/dl. Urinary 17-OHCS during the second 24 hours should not exceed 2.5 mg. Suppression is normal in obesity but may be abnormal in patients with psychiatric illness.

Other Screening Procedures. An alternative screening procedure is measurment of the 24-hour urinary excretion of cortisol (free cortisol). This test is relatively sensitive. Minimal elevations of plasma cortisol tend to result in marked increases of urinary cortisol. The test is not affected by obesity, but may be altered in patients with psychiatric illness.

The normal diurnal rhythm of plasma cortisol tends to be obliterated in Cushing's syndrome. In normal individuals, the 4 p.m. cortisol is on an average 50% of that obtained in the early a.m. Although widely advocated for diagnosis, determination of this rhythm by measurement of a.m. and p.m. cortisol is not a reliable screening procedure.

Interpreting Tests and Additional Diagnostic Maneuvers

Unfortunately, both false positive and false negative screening tests are occasionally seen. If the tests are equivocal and the clinical features strongly suggestive, referral to an endocrinologist is appropriate. In expert hands, a variety of maneuvers can usually establish or exclude the diagnosis and differentiate among the causes of Cushing's syndrome, but familiarity with the specialized test procedures is essential. Often a degree of laboratory precision is required that is not always achieved by ordinary commercial laboratories. Useful tests likely to be employed in such consultations, in addition to those described, include multiple samplings of plasma cortisol throughout the day and night ("integrated blood levels"), determinations of urinary excretion of steroids on multiple occasions, variations of the dexamethasone suppression test with the use of different doses of the steroid, and plasma ACTH measurements by special techniques.

Until strong laboratory evidence is at hand to indicate that steroid production is abnormal, procedures such as X-rays of the skull, tomography of the sella turcica, and CT of the adrenal areas are not justified. These procedures are not useful in screening, although they are important in determining the locus and etiology of steroid excess once this phenomenon has been established.

Treatment of Cushing's Syndrome

Surgery remains the treatment of Cushing's syndrome due to an adrenal adenoma. Although surgical removal of the adrenals (bilateral adrenalectomy) has been accepted for years as the most effective therapy for Cushing's disease (adrenocortical hyperplasia), this treatment is being rapidly abandoned. Induction of permanent adrenal insufficiency, the risk of development of an enlarging pituitary adenoma accompanied by hyperpigmentation (Nelson's syndrome), and significant operative mortality and morbidity are drawbacks of adrenalectomy for this condition. However, it has been recently realized that most cases of Cushing's disease can be treated by transsphenoidal surgical removal of a pituitary microadenoma, and this approach has rapidly become the preferred therapy (17). Long term follow up studies are not yet available, but current enthusiasm seems justified. Medical therapy with the adrenolytic agent, mitotane (o,p-DDD), is also effective, either alone or preferably in combination with pituitary irradiation. The selection of the therapeutic approach for the individual patient should be made by an endocrinologist.

ADRENAL ANDROGEN EXCESS

If evidence of Cushing's syndrome coexists with signs of androgen excess, the 24-hour excretion of 17-KS should be measured along with 17-OHCS or 17-KGS. The 17-KS measurement is, however, of no use in *routine* screening for Cushing's syndrome. Elevated values do occur, but do so less frequently than do the other indices of cortisol production. However, an argument can be made for including a single, 24-hour determination of urinary 17-KS in the initial screening workup for Cushing's syndrome, provided there is clinical evidence of androgen excess. When adrenal tumor is present, measurement of urinary 17-KS may be the most abnormal test. Some adrenal tumors (benign adenomas or carcinomas) produce enormous amounts of 17-KS. In suspected cases of adrenal tumor, measurement of 17-KS is specifically indicated. Serum testosterone will also be elevated in such cases.

Hirsutism. Hirsutism without virilism is extremely common (see Chapter 74). The combination of hirsutism plus virilism, which is exceedingly rare, is invariably associated with elevated 17-KS. When such a patient is encountered, referral to an endocrinologist is the most appropriate course. In adults, most cases will prove to be caused by adrenal tumors. Other causes, e.g., entities such as congenital adrenal hyperplasia (female pseudohermaphroditism, isosexual precocity in males, hypertension, and salt loss) all become apparent in childhood. Only a few cases (due to 21-hydroxylase deficiency) have ever been seen in adults.

Other Adrenal Diseases

MINERALOCORTICOID EXCESS

The classical condition resulting from mineralocorticoid excess is primary aldosteronism due to a benign adrenocortical adenoma (Conn's syndrome). Clinical features include hypertension and the manifestations of hypokalemia. A significant number of cases are due to bilateral adrenocortical nodular hyperplasia. The evaluation of this condition is described in Chapter 42.

MINERALOCORTICOID DEFICIENCY

Aldosterone deficiency is part of classical adrenal insufficiency (Addison's disease) but may also occur as a selective, functional deficiency state in the syndrome of hyporeninemic hypoaldosteronism. The identifying feature is hyperkalemia. The syndrome is described in Chapter 44.

PHEOCHROMOCYTOMA

This rare catecholamine (epinephrine, norepinephrine) producing tumor is usually considered in relationship to the evaluation of hypertension and is described in Chapter 59.

PHARMACOLOGIC USES OF STEROIDS AS ANTI-INFLAMMATORY AND IMMUNOSUPPRESSIVE DRUGS

Most steroid (glucocorticoid) usage is related to treatment of diseases other than adrenal insufficiency. The doses used exceed those of physiologic output and are best termed "supraphysiologic" or, simply, pharmacologic. The anti-inflammatory and immunosuppressive properties of these drugs constitute an invaluable part of the modern therapeutic armamentarium, but such uses, at least when prolonged, are invariably associated with side effects. Short term uses are much safer, if not entirely innoc-

uous. Although the glucocorticoid and mineralocorticoid actions of steroids have been chemically dissociated, no such separation has been possible for desired vs. undesired effects. All available glucocorticoids share these properties to an equal degree, although potency (effectiveness per milligram) varies widely (Table 71.2). Despite this fact, certain glucocorticoid compounds have tended to become associated with the treatment of particular conditions, e.g., dexamethasone for treatment of cerebral edema. Often no secure pharmacologic base supports such practices. On the other hand, legitimate pharmacologic differences between available preparations do exist which include different rates of absorption, metabolic disposal, and solubility. Exploitation of such properties is seen in dermatologic use. Triamcinolone and fluocinolone acetonides appear to be much more effective than hydrocortisone for cutaneous use, a

Table 71.2
Commonly Used Glucocorticoids

Generic Name	Common Trade Name(s)	Equivalent Potency (mg)[a]	Sodium retention relative to cortisol
FOR ORAL USE			
Cortisol (hydrocortisone)	Cortef	20	—
Cortisone[b]	—	25	1
Prednisone	Deltasone Meticorten Delta-Cortef	5	0.1
Prednisolone	Meticortelone Sterane	4	0.1
Methylprednisolone	Medrol	4	0
Triamcinolone	Aristocort, Kenacort	4	0
Dexamethasone[c]	Decadron	0.75	0
Betamethasone[c]	Celestone	0.6	0
FOR PARENTERAL USE			
Cortisol	Solu-Cortef		
Methylprednisolone	Solu-Medrol		
Triamcinolone	Aristocort		
Dexamethasone	Decadron		
Betamethasone	Celestone		
FOR TOPICAL USE			
Triamcinolone	Aristocort, Kenalog		
Fluocinolone	Synalar		
Betamethasone	Valisone		
FOR INHALATION			
Beclomethasone	Vanceril		

[a] Also equivalent to daily physiologic replacement when given in divided doses.
[b] Cortisone acetate has long been given parenterally (intramuscular route) as well as orally; however, recent evidence indicates that this compound is unpredictably absorbed from injection sites and cannot be relied upon to produce adequate blood levels.
[c] This compound has a relatively long duration of action and should not be used for alternate-day glucocorticoid therapy.

Most of the compounds listed are available in generic forms. All are marketed as ester derivatives or salts of esters, e.g., cortisol sodium hemisuccinate (Solu-Cortef). For practical purposes, only cortisol and cortisone have significant salt-retaining (mineralocorticoid) action.

phenomenon apparently related to properties of absorption. Another example is the use of beclomethasone (Vanceril) as an aerosol in the treatment of asthma.

Adverse Effects

Untoward effects of glucocorticoids are listed in Table 71.3. These problems are related to dose and—

Table 71.3
Untoward Effects of Chronic Glucocorticoid Therapy

ACUTE
Fluid/Electrolyte disturbances
  Sodium retention
  Fluid retention
  Potassium depletion
  Hypokalemic alkalosis
Gastrointestinal
  Peptic ulcer (hemorrhage, perforation)
  Ulcerative esophagitis
Endocrine
  Precipitation of diabetes mellitus
Ophthalmic
  Glaucoma
Neurologic
  Mood swings
  Acute psychosis
  Convulsions
CHRONIC
Fluid/Electrolyte disturbances
  See above, plus hypertension
Musculoskeletal
  Muscle weakness
  Muscle atrophy
  Steroid myopathy
  Osteoporosis/pathologic fractures
  Aseptic necrosis of femoral or humeral heads
  Tendon rupture
Gastrointestinal
  Pancreatitis
Dermatologic
  Impaired wound healing
  Atrophy of skin (fragility)
  Ecchymoses
  Increased sweating
Neurologic
  Convulsions
  Increased intracranial pressure
  Insomnia
  Euphoria
  Depression
Endocrine
  Menstrual irregularities
  Carbohydrate intolerance/diabetes mellitus
  Adrenal atrophy/disruption of normal response to stress (iatrogenic Addison's disease)
Ophthalmic
  Cataracts
  Glaucoma
Hematologic
  Thromboembolism
Other
  Weight gain
  Increased susceptibility to infections

equally important—duration of therapy (7, 10). No contraindication ever exists to a single dose of glucocorticoid, regardless of the size of that dose. Thus, treatment of an allergic reaction with one or a few doses carries no risk. Chronic therapy, however, should be instituted only after consideration of the risk-benefit ratio. Therapy that is not intended as chronic may become so. For example, asthmatic patients may be so impressed by relief afforded by systemic steroids that other modalities are abandoned and the patient becomes totally dependent on glucocorticoids.

Side effects of steroids are closely related to desired effects. Anti-inflammatory effects are obviously desirable when treating a disease such as rheumatoid arthritis. However, many inflammatory responses are beneficial, as for example the inflammatory responses associated with bacterial infection. In this situation, glucocorticoids may inhibit a useful inflammatory response which otherwise would serve to localize the process. Thus, one ordinarily avoids pharmacologic doses of glucocorticoids when infection requiring an antibiotic is necessary. Not infrequently, however, patients receiving glucocorticoids develop an infection. Ordinarily, steroid therapy is not discontinued; rather, vigorous antibiotic therapy is instituted and the dose of steroid is kept at as low a level as the clinical situation allows, thus preventing clinical evidence of adrenal insufficiency and the development of nonspecific but serious symptoms (see "Steroid Withdrawal Syndrome," p. 741).

Adverse effects of steroids are related not only to duration of therapy but to dose used. Obviously, one should attempt to use a minimally effective dose. Nonetheless, some persons seem especially vulnerable to unwanted side effects. Poorly nourished, debilitated, and elderly patients are all more prone to the muscle-wasting effects of steroids. Postmenopausal women—already prone to develop osteoporosis—are especially vulnerable to the demineralization which accompanies steroid use. Genetically predisposed individuals may develop overt diabetes mellitus when given glucocorticoids. Peptic ulcer disease may be reactivated and complications such as bleeding or perforation may be precipitated. Tuberculosis, clinically inapparent except for a positive tuberculin test, may become active. The role of isoniazid prophylaxis in this situation is described elsewhere (Chapter 28).

Topical Therapy

Whenever steroids can be used locally, such use is preferred, especially when long term treatment is involved. Although absorption may be complete from a local site, the amount of steroid required is often far less when use is local. One thus avoids—to some extent—systemic effects, side effects, and pituitary-adrenal suppression. In addition to dermatologic use of topical steroids, treatment of some ophthalmologic conditions, allergic rhinitis, asthma, and of localized joint disease are examples of this principle.

Intermittent Therapy

Usually, severe disease requires initiation of steroid therapy given as multiple daily doses. When the disease intensity has waned (e.g., 1 to 2 weeks), conversion to alternate-day therapy can be made. Intermittent therapy of this type should always be considered whenever long term use is contemplated. Such therapy is to be preferred because pituitary-adrenal suppression is not likely and the adverse effects of glucocorticoids are minimized (7, 10). When initiating intermittent therapy the daily divided dose is given as a single morning dose. After this dose has been shown to be tolerated for several days, the single daily dose may be doubled and given as a single dose every other day. Thereafter, the dose given every other day can be reduced slowly, as clinically indicated. The "off" day, particularly when alternate-day therapy is first started, may result in the patient becoming symptomatic. To handle this situation small doses of glucocorticoid may be given on this day. Nonsteroidal anti-inflammatory agents may also be helpful in ameliorating symptoms at this time and in easing the transition.

Use of Adrenocorticotropic Hormone

The clinical indications for use of ACTH rather than a glucocorticoid are practically nonexistent. ACTH was available for clinical use even before cortisone. It is clear that in sufficient amounts (100 units) long acting preparations (gel or zinc suspensions) given once daily are capable of stimulating adrenal secretion of up to 300 mg of cortisol daily. However, disadvantages are multiple: the route is parenteral; magnitude of response is unpredictable; mineralocorticoid effects (salt and fluid retention, potassium wasting) are considerable; response in patients previously treated with glucocorticoids is slow and unpredictable. The only advantage is that adrenal responsiveness is maintained during therapy. Combined ACTH-glucocorticoid therapy has been advocated for this reason, as has the occasional injection of ACTH to prevent adrenal atrophy. The advantage of such an approach over that of intermittent glucocorticoid therapy is not clear. Moreover, when ACTH is used alone in high doses for a prolonged period, pituitary suppression occurs even though adrenal suppression does not. Another disadvantage of ACTH therapy is failure to produce more than the equivalent of 300 mg of cortisol (60 mg of prednisone) despite maximal stimulation of the adrenals. Such a dose, while considerable, may be insufficient to produce the desired anti-inflammatory effect. The only current, fairly widespread use of ACTH is in the treatment of multiple sclerosis. It is not clear that such use is supported by anything more than anecdote.

Withdrawal from Chronic Glucocorticoid Therapy

Treatment with glucocorticoids (cortisone, hydrocortisone, prednisone, etc.) produces suppression of the hypothalamus-pituitary-adrenal axis; the output of ACTH falls and there is subsequent adrenal atrophy and an inability to respond to stress with increased cortisol output. The time required for initial suppression is highly variable, but all patients receiving daily pharmacologic doses of glucocorticoids for more than 1 week should be presumed to have a suppressed response to stress. If stressed by surgery, trauma, or severe infection these patients should be treated with replacement glucocorticoids as if they had Addison's disease. On the other hand, glucocorticoids may be discontinued abruptly after 2 to 4 weeks of pharmacologic steroid therapy provided that the patient is not under stress, since baseline—as opposed to stress-related—adrenal function will almost always be adequate. Patients who have been treated with alternate-day steroid therapy are not at risk, since pituitary-adrenal function seems well preserved in these individuals (7, 10).

When it becomes desirable to terminate glucocorticoid therapy, the question arises of how to accomplish this goal while avoiding adrenal insufficiency. In the presence of active underlying disease, for which the glucocorticoids may have been given in the first place, a dilemma quickly becomes apparent. The nonspecific symptoms of adrenal insufficiency may be similar or identical to those of the disease that was under treatment. In addition, the occurrence of the "steroid withdrawal syndrome" (see below) may further compound the issue.

WITHDRAWAL SCHEDULE

No single scheme can solve this difficult clinical problem although many have been proposed (3). However, a few general points can be made. First, even after prolonged therapy, in the absence of active underlying systemic disease, symptoms of adrenal insufficiency should not be expected until the daily dose of glucocorticoid drops below physiologic replacement (30 mg of cortisol, 7.5 mg of prednisone, or equivalent; see Table 71.2). At this point most patients will tolerate a single 20- to 30-mg daily dose of cortisol (or 5 to 7.5 mg of prednisone). Continuation for 2 months at this level should ensure some degree of recovery of pituitary-adrenal function. Further withdrawal begins to re-establish the normal pituitary-adrenal relationship. Additional reductions of 5 mg of cortisol can be made every 2 to 3 weeks over the next 2 months or, alternatively, an every other day program can be tried over the same period; the glucocorticoid can then usually be stopped without producing symptoms. Assessment of the functional status of the patient's adrenals at this point is described elsewhere (see "Recovery from Pituitary-Adrenal Suppression" below).

STEROID WITHDRAWAL SYNDROME

Abrupt withdrawal of pharmacologic doses of glucocorticoids, even after months of therapy, does not always produce chemical evidence of adrenal insufficiency. Nonetheless, the patient may experience many of the symptoms of adrenal insufficiency, e.g., lethargy, malaise, anorexia, nausea, vomiting, myalgias, fever, and—in severe cases—desquamation of skin in a manner resembling exfoliative dermatitis. Such patients may be found to have normal or elevated levels of cortisol. This phenomenon is not simply adrenal insufficiency, but rather is a pharmacologic withdrawal syndrome. Symptoms subside promptly with reinstitution of glucocorticoid therapy (1).

RECOVERY FROM PITUITARY-ADRENAL SUPPRESSION

After long term glucocorticoid therapy (pharmacologic doses for a year or more), recovery of normal pituitary-adrenal responsiveness does not occur readily (8). At least several months must elapse, even if the patient receives no exogenous steroid therapy during that time. In the first month after withdrawal, both pituitary and adrenal function remain depressed (low plasma ACTH and low plasma cortisol). Over the following 4 months, pituitary function recovers (plasma ACTH is elevated), but adrenal function remains subnormal (plasma cortisol is lower than normal). Eventually, adrenal function recovers (plasma cortisol levels normalize) while elevated plasma ACTH falls and returns to normal. The entire process may require up to 9 months. During this interval the patient may fare well, provided there is no stress, but replacement therapy with glucocorticoids may become necessary at any time. Accordingly, no patient should be considered to have normal pituitary-adrenal function unless at least 1 year has elapsed after complete withdrawal of chronic glucocorticoid therapy. Occasional patients seem never to recover normal responsiveness. Ideally, therefore, all patients with a history of chronic steroid therapy should be tested for normal responsiveness 1 year after withdrawal.

Assessment of a glucocorticoid-treated patient's adrenal function under baseline conditions is not difficult. Both plasma cortisol measurements and urinary excretion of steroid metabolites give a reasonable estimate of such baseline function. However, predicting the response to stress is more difficult. Hypothalamic-pituitary function usually recovers first, followed by adrenal function. Accordingly, a normal response to exogenous ACTH usually indicates recovery of the entire axis (see p. 735 for details of testing with ACTH). A more complete assessment of the integrity of the axis can be made by induction of hypoglycemia with insulin (insulin tolerance testing). Hypoglycemia triggers ACTH release and the adrenal's cortisol secretory response. A normal insulin tolerance test assures that if the patient is subjected to stressful circumstances, replacement therapy with steroids will not be necessary. If neither an ACTH nor an insulin tolerance test has been done,

clinical assessment, including perhaps plasma cortisol determinations or empirical treatment with glucocorticoids becomes necessary. In the suppressed individual, testing with metyrapone (Metopirone), an adrenal 11-hydroxylase inhibitor sometimes used for evaluation of the integrity of the hypothalamic-pituitary-adrenal axis, may be misleadingly normal.

HYPOCALCEMIC STATES

Hypocalcemia is a relatively uncommon problem in ambulatory patients. The classic cause of hypocalcemia is idiopathic hypoparathyroidism, but most cases encountered are a consequence of inadvertent surgical ablation of the parathyroids during thyroidectomy or of a metabolic disturbance such as renal failure. The causes of hypocalcemia are listed in Table 71.4.

Clinical Manifestations of Hypocalcemia

The symptoms of hypocalcemia are primarily neuromuscular and are not usually evident until the serum calcium falls below about 8 mg/dl and often considerably lower. Mild symptoms are totally nonspecific and include psychologic manifestations (irritability; mood changes; depression), paresthesias, and muscle cramps. More severe symptoms are delirium, psychosis, tetany (including laryngeal stridor), and seizures. Neuromuscular irritability can often be demonstrated by the twitching which is induced by tapping over the facial nerve just anterior to the ear. A positive response is contraction of the facial muscles around the lip (Chvostek's sign). Another clinical maneuver is compression of the upper arm by a blood pressure cuff with the pressure elevated above the systolic pressure. A positive response is spasm of the hand induced within 3 min (Trousseau sign). Signs

Table 71.4
Causes of Hypocalcemia[a]

HYPOCALCEMIA WITH HIGH SERUM PHOSPHATE
Postablative hypoparathyroidism (post-thyroidectomy)
Idiopathic hypoparathyroidism
Pseudohypoparathyroidism
Renal failure
HYPOCALCEMIA WITH LOW OR NORMAL SERUM PHOSPHATE
Malabsorption (vitamin D deficiency)
Magnesium deficiency (alcoholism)
Renal rickets (renal tubular acidosis; phosphate diabetes; cystinosis; Fanconi syndrome; vitamin D-resistant rickets)
Medullary carcinoma of thyroid

[a] The serum alkaline phosphate is elevated whenever severe metabolic bone disease is present. Parathyroid hormone is depressed in idiopathic hypoparathyroidism and may be depressed in magnesium deficiency. Parathyroid hormone is regularly elevated in renal failure and in pseudohypoparathyroidism. Urine calcium is depressed in most hypocalcemic states, except when the rare renal tubular calcium-wasting syndromes are responsible for the hypocalcemia.

of chronic hypocalcemia include patchy hair loss, scaling of skin, atrophy and brittleness of fingernails, and cataract formation. Candidiasis is common. Calcification of the basal ganglia may be seen on X-ray examination of the skull. Either osteosclerosis or osteopenia may occur depending on the etiology of the hypocalcemia.

Laboratory Findings

Hypocalcemia can be said to be present when the serum calcium falls below 8.5 mg/dl. However, since almost half of serum calcium is protein-bound, reduction of serum protein by 1 g/dl lowers the serum calcium by about 0.8 mg/dl. The level of serum calcium must, therefore, always be evaluated in the context of the serum protein concentration; the serum magnesium concentration should also be evaluated at the same time (see below, "Other Causes of Hypocalcemia"). Plasma parathyroid hormone (PTH) is low or nondetectable in idiopathic or postablative hypoparathyroidism and in some cases of hypocalcemia due to magnesium deficiency, but is elevated in pseudohypoparathyroidism, renal failure, malabsorption, and vitamin D deficiency. The interpretation and indications for determination of PTH levels are discussed below.

Idiopathic Hypoparathyroidism

This condition is rare. Although most patients are diagnosed in childhood, some do not exhibit the disease until adult life. Occasionally familial, the idiopathic disease is autoimmune, frequently associated with high titers of antibodies to parathyroid tissue, and may be seen in association with other autoimmune endocrine diseases (adrenal insufficiency, Hashimoto's thyroiditis) and pernicious anemia.

Postthyroidectomy Hypoparathyroidism

Probably the most common cause of hypoparathyroidism, this condition is a complication of surgical thyroidectomy. The hypocalcemic state may become evident immediately after surgery, but often takes many years to develop, presumably due to slowly progressive interference with the blood supply to the parathyroids. Routine screening of serum calcium in patients who have had thyroidectomy will reveal many asymptomatic patients. Most of these individuals will seem to need no therapy, but in view of the subtle neuromuscular changes which can result from hypocalcemia, careful consideration should always be given to this issue. Hypoparathyroidism does not occur following radioiodide therapy of thyroid disease, even if hypothyroidism has been produced.

Pseudohypoparathyroidism

This is a rare disorder of genetic origin (X-linked dominant trait). In addition to hypocalcemia and its manifestations, there are associated skeletal developmental defects which result in short stature, shortening of metacarpals and metatarsals, and round face. Clinical manifestations attributable to hypocalcemia may not appear until adult life. The biochemical basis of the hypocalcemia is end-organ resistance to the action of PTH. The combination of hypocalcemia, elevated parathyroid hormone, and typical skeletal abnormalities is virtually diagnostic. In the absence of skeletal abnormalities, diagnosis depends on demonstration of resistance to administered PTH, a specialized procedure requiring referral to an endocrinologist.

Treatment of Hypoparathyroidism and Pseudohypoparathyroidism

The treatment of all forms of hypoparathyroidism is similar. A few patients with idiopathic or postablative PTH deficiency can be managed with calcium supplements alone. The dose is 1 to 2 g as calcium daily. Since calcium gluconate and lactate contain only about 10% calcium, one must administer 10 to 20 g of these salts; the carbonate contains 40% calcium. Numerous tablets must be taken; patient compliance is a common problem. Every effort should be made to work out an acceptable, palatable, and economic program with a consistently available preparation for what is invariably lifelong therapy.

The second mainstay of therapy is vitamin D. The most commonly used preparation in the past has been ergocalciferol (vitamin D_2; Calciferol), the dose is usually 50,000 or 100,000 units daily, although higher doses may be necessary. The compound is available in 50,000-unit (1.25 mg) capsules. The sole advantage of ergocalciferol is cost; it is by far the least expensive form of vitamin D therapy. The disadvantage of ergocalciferol is somewhat unpredictable toxicity with resultant hypercalcemia and all of its manifestations (see p. 744). Because vitamin D is fat-soluble, toxicity may last for many weeks or even months after discontinuation of therapy. Glucocorticoids are effective therapy for hypercalcemia due to vitamin D toxicity.

A possibly preferable vitamin D preparation is its synthetic analog, dihydrotachysterol (DHT; Hytakerol) The dose varies from 0.2 to 2 mg daily. The compound is available as tablets and as an oil. The advantage of therapy with DHT is more rapid onset of action than D_2 and more rapid reversibility of toxicity upon withdrawal of the drug. The only disadvantage of DHT is its relatively high cost. Yet another effective compound is 1,25 dihydroxy vitamin D_3 (calcitriol; Rocaltrol), the natural, active form of vitamin D. This compound is more rapid than DHT in onset and has a shorter duration of effect but has the disadvantage of even greater cost. The dose is 0.25 to 1.0 μg daily. Both 0.25- and 0.5-μg tablets are available.

The approach to chronic therapy of hypoparathyroidism is institution of a relatively fixed calcium intake at a total level of about 2 g, which is about 1 g over regular dietary intake. Thus, a patient whose normal daily calcium intake approximates 1 g needs an additional 1 g of calcium in the form of supplementary calcium salts (see above). Instruction of the patient by a dietician is essential. Vitamin D, in whatever form is selected, is given simultaneously, with adjustments of dose at weekly or biweekly intervals depending on the serum calcium level. The goal of therapy is a serum calcium of 8.5 to 9.5 mg/dl. Hypercalcemia is to be avoided. Once a stable level of serum calcium is reached (1 to 2 months), the patient can be monitored at monthly intervals and eventually every 3 to 4 months. The possibility of toxicity due to hypercalcemia is always to be kept in mind. Even mild hypercalcemia predisposes to nephrocalcinosis and nephrolithiasis in these patients.

Hypocalcemia Due to Other Causes

When hypocalcemia is related to malabsorption, efforts to correct that situation should be undertaken, but simultaneous treatment with vitamin D and calcium may be indicated.

One relatively common cause of hypocalcemia is alcoholism with resultant magnesium deficiency. Overt malnutrition need not be present. The mechanisms by which alcohol abuse produces magnesium depletion include decreased dietary intake and alcohol-facilitated renal excretion of magnesium. Magnesium depletion results in both impaired secretion of PTH and impaired PTH action. Intramuscular magnesium therapy normalizes the serum calcium within hours.

Other diseases associated with hypocalcemia include osteomalacia (vitamin D and/or calcium deficiency) and variants of the Fanconi syndrome (a spectrum of renal tubular abnormalities). The hypocalcemia associated with renal failure is described in Chapter 44.

HYPERCALCEMIC STATES

In recent years routine, automated blood analyses have come to include determinations of serum calcium. This development has led to the detection of many cases of hypercalcemia, most of them mild and asymptomatic. The demonstration of hypercalcemia always requires investigation.

Etiologies

In an ambulatory setting the most common cause of minimal, asymptomatic hypercalcemia is probably that associated with use of thiazide diuretics, an occurrence in perhaps 25% of cases treated with these drugs. The problem is fully reversible upon withdrawal of the drug. Once established as the cause of the hypercalcemia, thiazide therapy may be continued if otherwise clinically indicated and the hypercalcemia is minimal. In the rare case where the serum calcium exceeds 12 mg/dl, one may switch to an alternative, non-thiazide diuretic.

Another common cause of benign hypercalcemia in ambulatory patients is hyperparathyroidism. Small, indolent, probably harmless parathyroid adenomas produce hypercalcemia in 1 of 1000 patients screened (9). The approach to such patients is described below (see p. 745).

Some ambulatory patients who are found to have hypercalcemia will have weight loss, anorexia, etc. A calcium elevation in this setting is ominous. Since minimal elevations of calcium (less than 12.0 mg/dl) are ordinarily asymptomatic, the patient's symptoms of anorexia, weight loss, etc., are more likely attributable to the underlying disease, rather than to the incidental and associated but minimal hypercalcemia. The calcium elevation, however, is a finding which suggests a malignant process, e.g., carcinoma of the lung or breast, etc. These patients are usually promptly hospitalized for diagnostic procedures and therapy of the underlying disease.

In the event that malignancy is not apparent, the differential diagnosis includes primary hyperparathyroidism (see below). At this point, determination of PTH concentration is useful in elucidating the cause of the hypercalcemic state. However, one should not rely on only a PTH assay to determine the cause of the hypercalcemia. A normal PTH on repeated determinations excludes a diagnosis of hyperparathyroidism (see below), but an elevated PTH does not necessarily indicate its presence. PTH assays do not always reliably differentiate between hypercalcemia due to hyperparathyroidism and that due to PTH-producing tumor. Elevations of PTH are often due to ectopic PTH production by tumors. Although tumor-produced PTH is not identical to normal PTH, the antibodies used to quantitate PTH often fail to distinguish between these substances. Recent improvements in PTH assays with more specific antibodies have improved diagnostic accuracy, but absolute specificity is not yet possible (15). Results will vary with the laboratory and depend on the assay used. Information concerning specificity may not be available from a particular commercial laboratory.

A variety of other circumstances produce hypercalcemia. These are listed in Table 71.5.

Therapy of Hypercalcemia

The treatment of hypercalcemia due to hyperparathyroidism is discussed elsewhere (see "Primary Hyperparathyroidism").

Therapy to control hypercalcemia is not commonly initiated in ambulatory patients. Most often the hypercalcemia or its underlying cause will have required initial therapy in a hospital. However, when the acute symptoms of hypercalcemia have been controlled during hospitalization, long term palliative therapy may be needed for the ambulatory patient.

Table 71.5
Causes of Hypercalcemia

Condition	Comment
COMMON CAUSES	
Thiazide drugs	Mild elevation (not >12.5 mg/dl); requires 2 or more weeks to subside
Hyperparathyroidism	Frequently asymptomatic; commonly discovered on routine blood test
Malignancy	Commonest cause in hospitalized patients; may lead to initial encounter in ambulatory patients
Spurious	Inappropriate technique while drawing blood (venous stasis produces hemoconcentration)
RARE CAUSES	
Multiple myeloma	Severe disease is evident
Milk alkali syndrome	Requires use (abuse) of alkali ($NaHCO_3$) and large quantities of milk or calcium salts
Hypervitaminosis D	Usually 50,000 units or more daily
Thyrotoxicosis	Severe disease is evident
Paget's disease of bone	Immobilization necessary
Immobilization	Body cast in adolescent males; patients with Paget's disease of bone; quadriplegia
Sarcoidosis	Hyperglobulinemia usually present
Chronic renal failure	Very uncommon; may exacerbate after transplantation or during hemodialysis
Adrenal insufficiency	Hemoconcentration present
Idiopathic elevation	Mild elevation in postmenopausal women; may revert to normal with physiologic estrogen therapy

In malignancy, glucocorticoids (20 to 60 mg of prednisone daily) may control hypercalcemia, as may indomethacin (100 to 200 mg daily) in a small proportion of cases. Mithramycin is an effective agent for control of hypercalcemia of any cause, but this drug is ordinarily used only for the treatment of hypercalcemia due to tumor. Usually such therapy is given in a hospital, but ambulatory treatment is also feasible. The drug is given intravenously. At a dose of 25 μg/kg (15 μg/kg if hepatic disease is present or bone marrow function is impaired by disease or other drugs) side effects are not usually seen. Several days are often needed for a response to become apparent, but the effect often lasts for many days or even weeks. Calcitonin (Calcimar) is an effective calcium-lowering agent for many hypercalcemic states and can be self-administered. This hormone must be given subcutaneously on a daily or several times weekly schedule. The principal use of calcitonin is in the treatment of Paget's disease of bone. The major side effect is nausea and vomiting in a small percentage of cases. Glucocorticoids are often effective in lowering hypercalcemia due to sarcoidosis, vitamin D intoxication, and the milk-alkali syndrome. Mild hypercalcemia in elderly postmenopausal women may sometimes respond to physiologic amounts of estrogen (12). Treatment of hypercalcemia with phosphates administered orally is sometimes possible, especially in mild hyperparathyroidism (see below).

Often partial control of hypercalcemia is sufficient to relieve symptoms; complete normalization of calcium level is often neither desirable nor necessary.

Primary Hyperparathyroidism

The term primary hyperparathyroidism refers to autonomous hyperfunction of one or more parathyroid glands. Hypercalcemia is the hallmark of this disorder. Secondary hyperparathyroidism, on the other hand, is a physiologic or pathophysiologic homeostatic response to situations that lower blood calcium.

The most common cause of primary hyperparathyroidism is a solitary benign adenoma (85% of patients). In a small proportion of patients more than one adenoma is present, and in the remainder the cause is idiopathic hyperplasia. Carcinoma of the parathyroid is rare (less than 1% of patients). Hyperparathyroidism may be familial and may occur as part of the syndrome of multiple endocrine adenomatosis (MEA; p. 732).

DIAGNOSIS

Most patients are now detected by routine automated analysis of blood electrolytes. The symptoms or sequelae of hypercalcemia may also alert the physician to the diagnosis (Table 71.6). Once the diagnosis is suspected, it is most important to establish beyond any doubt the presence of hypercalcemia. Multiple determinations of serum calcium should be made in a laboratory where a high degree of precision is assured. Because of spontaneous fluctuations of the serum calcium and because of analytical error, values that are only minimally elevated (10.5 to 12.0 mg/dl) must be repeated many times. The resulting *mean* level should be used for diagnostic purposes, not the last—sometimes normal—value obtained.

Table 71.6
Symptoms and Signs of Hypercalcemia

SHORT TERM (READILY REVERSIBLE)
   General: weakness, anorexia, weight loss, fatigue
   Gastrointestinal: nausea, vomiting, constipation
   Genitourinary: polyuria, azotemia
   Musculoskeletal: bone aches
   Neurologic: lethargy, sleepiness, difficulty concentrating, confusion, psychosis
   Cardiovascular: bradycardia, electrocardiographic abnormalities (short Q-T, arrhythmias, digitalis toxicity)
   Ophthalmologic: difficulty focusing
   Dermatologic: pruritis
LONG TERM (IRREVERSIBLE OR SLOWLY REVERSIBLE)
   Gastrointestinal: peptic ulcer, pancreatitis
   Genitourinary: renal calculi (colic, hematuria); nephrocalcinosis; polyuria
   Skeletal: bone loss (osteopenia); subperiosteal resorption, bone cysts, pseudogout
   Neuromuscular: muscle atrophy
   Ophthalmologic: band keratopathy; conjunctival calcifications

Once hypercalcemia is established as being present (greater than 10.5 mg/dl on multiple determinations), the next (or simultaneous) step is to determine the likelihood of the presence of other causes of hypercalcemia (see Table 71.5). Finally, assay of PTH in blood should be performed (see below).

Other routine laboratory studies may include low serum phosphorus and, in severe cases with bone involvement, elevation of serum alkaline phosphatase. Other more elaborate indirect tests of PTH hyperfunction—none of which is useful for screening purposes—include the calculation of the tubular reabsorption of phosphate (TRP) and determination of urinary excretion of cyclic adenosine monophosphate (cyclic AMP). These tests, if they are to be used at all, are best performed by specialists. Other abnormalities in laboratory tests occur but are not useful for screening or in differential diagnosis, since they occur nonspecifically. Patients with hypercalcemia, regardless of cause, usually show hypercalciuria, but hypercalciuria may also occur without hypercalcemia. Increased excretion of hydroxyproline occurs, as it does in other bone diseases.

In severe cases of long duration, X-ray studies of various bones will reveal a variety of changes suggestive but not diagnostic of hyperparathyroidism. Demineralization (osteopenia) and subperiosteal resorption is most obvious in the clavicles and the hands, while the lamina dura of the teeth may be resorbed. Cystic changes occur in skull and long bones. None of these changes is likely to be seen in mild cases. X-ray studies are not useful for screening purposes.

Parathyroid Hormone Assays. These radioimmunoassays, now widely available from commercial laboratories, are quite useful but have several limitations. Specificity of the assay varies among laboratories, due to the use of different antibodies. Some laboratories offer several different PTH assays, each of which has its own advantages and limitations. The most commonly used procedure, the so-called "C-terminal" assay, measures a peptide fragment derived from PTH. This assay, as performed on peripheral venous blood (plasma or serum) is the most sensitive test for detecting hyperparathyroidism, but it is also elevated by impaired renal function, due in part to decreased peptide fragment excretion, and is frequently elevated in normal elderly persons, especially women over about age 65. The elevations seen in primary hyperparathyroidism are often only modest (e.g., 50% greater than the upper limits of normal). Accordingly, at least two or three assays should ordinarily be obtained. The assay also measures PTH-like materials produced by tumors.

Several other assays are also available; these measure "intact" hormone or N-terminal fragment(s). Interestingly, although these assays are more specific and less likely to be elevated in cases of ectopic (tumor) production of PTH, they are also less sensitive in detecting primary hyperparathyroidism, being

normal in nearly half of cases. In chronic renal failure, where secondary hyperparathyroidism is invariably present, the "intact hormone" assays are not artifactually raised by retention of PTH fragments, as are the C-terminal assays, and more or less reflect the degree of secondary hyperparathyroidism.

Steroid Suppression Test. Although most cases of hyperparathyroidism and of other hypercalcemic states can be diagnosed by the means described, the etiology of occasional cases of hypercalcemia remains in doubt. In these, a short course of prednisone therapy (30 to 40 mg daily for 10 to 14 days) may help diagnostically. The hypercalcemia of hyperparathyroidism does not respond to such therapy. While only about one-half of cases of hypercalcemia due to malignancy respond, hypercalcemia due to diseases that are not always apparent—such as sarcoidosis, vitamin D intoxication, and milk-alkali syndrome—respond consistently. Daily determinations of blood calcium should always be obtained during such a test.

Further Evaluation. Having established the presence of hypercalcemia and elevation of PTH, and having excluded by appropriate means malignancy, impaired renal function, and other conditions in Table 71.5, the diagnosis of hyperparathyroidism is reasonably well established. However, the urinary excretion of calcium should be determined at this point. Recently, benign familial hypercalcemia due to parathyroid hyperplasia has been described. These patients—for reasons which are not understood—do not have hypercalciuria or other complications of minimal hypercalcemia and do not need surgical intervention. In most cases of hyperparathyroidism referral to an endocrinologist should be made if the diagnosis is in doubt or if surgery is contemplated.

THERAPY

In diagnosed patients the main question is whether surgical intervention is warranted. The rate of development of complications (urolithiasis, emotional disorders, bone disease, decreased renal function, peptic ulcer, pancreatitis) in patients with asymptomatic hypercalcemia has been recently estimated and is quite low. However, the decision for or against surgery will obviously be based not only on the presence of such problems, but on such factors as patient age, associated medical illness, etc. (5, 9). In occasional patients, medical management of the hyperparathyroidism may be indicated (see below).

SURGICAL THERAPY

If a decision is made to treat the patient surgically, referral to a surgeon experienced in parathyroid/thyroid exploration is warranted. In such experienced hands, an adenoma, if present, will be located and easily removed in 90 to 95% of cases. Parathyroid hyperplasia, which accounts for 10% of cases of hyperparathyroidism, is usually easily identified. In such cases, the surgeon should be prepared to perform a near-total parathyroidectomy. Second neck explorations are technically difficult and may result in unnecessary morbidity (damage to the recurrent laryngeal nerve). Accordingly, any hyperplastic parathyroid tissue that is left behind should be identified with clips. As an alternative, many surgeons are now removing all parathyroid tissue from the neck and transplanting a portion of one hyperplastic gland to an accessible location, usually a sternocleidomastoid muscle or into the forearm.

Failure to identify an adenoma and absence of hyperplasia may require partial thyroidectomy—the adenoma may be imbedded in the thyroid—or exploration of the anterosuperior mediastinum. This procedure may be performed at the time of initial surgery or at some time later. Such "details" obviously involve the surgeon's preference and experience, but should be considered and discussed before surgery. If the neck has already been explored unsuccessfully, selective venous catheterization studies with sampling of PTH levels is a useful procedure for preoperative localization of the tumor. Only a few major medical centers can perform this procedure. Such localization studies are not indicated before initial surgery.

MEDICAL THERAPY

The medical therapy of hyperparathyroidism with phosphate is ordinarily limited to those patients in whom surgery is not desirable but who require therapy. Although intravenous phosphate therapy carries the risk of soft tissue calcium deposition, no such problem attends the use of phosphate given orally. Sodium-potassium phosphate salts given orally (K-Phos; Neutra-Phos) may produce diarrhea. Dosage should be titrated upward as tolerated. A sodium-free preparation is also available (Neutra-Phos-K) for use in patients whose sodium intake should be restricted. Asymptomatic patients with mild hypercalcemia should probably not be treated with phosphate.

DISORDERS OF WATER METABOLISM

The combination of excess thirst, increased intake of water, and increased output of urine is a common clinical presentation of a number of conditions (Table 71.7). In most of these, the symptoms are related to some event which results in excessive loss of fluid via the kidney. For example, hyperglycemia results in a large solute load (glucose) being presented to the renal tubules; an obligatory loss of water (osmotic diuresis) ensues. Hypercalcemia produces abnormalities of renal tubular function which results in impaired ability to concentrate urine. Lithium, widely used for treatment of bipolar affective disorders (manic-depressive illness), impairs the action of antidiuretic hormone and thereby produces water loss

Table 71.7
Causes of Polyuria[a]

Disorder	Mechanism
Glucosuria (diabetes mellitus)	Osmotic diuresis
Excessive intake of water	Psychogenic
Various drugs	Often due to anticholinergic effects producing dryness of mouth; possible central effects
Decreased antidiuretic hormone (ADH) effect	Deficiency of ADH secretion (idiopathic diabetes insipidus or due to pituitary-hypothalamic disease); nephrogenic diabetes insipidus
Renal disease, plus renal effects of potassium depletion, hypercalcemia, and lithium therapy	In all of these disorders, impairment of renal concentrating ability is present
Hyperthyroidism	Impairment of urinary concentrating ability; decreased salivary flow

[a] Disorders associated with increased urine volume.

Table 71.7 lists some of the conditions producing polyuria and their mechanisms.

Disorders of water metabolism are uncommon in ambulatory patients, but the commonest is probably that of psychogenic water drinking. In this disorder, the patient's psychiatric state alters normal behavior in such a way as to produce compulsive water drinking. Many of these patients have poorly defined psychiatric disorders. Occasional individuals begin excessive water intake on receiving "health advice" from a lay source, i.e., the notion that drinking large quantities of water is healthful. Regardless of the cause, once such behavior is started, a compulsive behavior pattern tends to persist and is reinforced by a pathophysiologic mechanism. Whatever the cause, large urine output, if it persists for a long time, produces a reversible impairment of urine-concentrating ability due to washout of renal medullary solutes. Thus, the behavior pattern, though basically of psychogenic origin, may become self-perpetuating. Attempts to have the patient restrict water intake when urinary concentrating ability is impaired under these conditions leads to continued water loss and the resulting hyperosmolality leads to intense thirst. "Weaning" from excessive water intake may be very difficult.

A rare disorder of water metabolism in ambulatory patients is diabetes insipidus, a deficiency of antidiuretic hormone (ADH, arginine vasopressin; AVP). This condition is either idiopathic—in which case it is unassociated with other evidence of pituitary-hypothalamic disease—or, more commonly, is secondary to pituitary disease (tumor) or other disease in the hypothalamic-pituitary stalk-pituitary area (craniopharyngioma; aneurysm). Other rare causes include a variety of infiltrative diseases (sarcoidosis, tuberculosis), head trauma—especially with basal skull fracture or neurosurgical procedures, and central nervous system infections. The most common illness mimicking diabetes insipidus is the drug-related disorder which results from use of lithium for bipolar affective illness. Another very rare condition resembling lack of ADH results from an inherited renal tubular resistance to antidiuretic hormone, nephrogenic diabetes insipidus.

Approach to the Patient with Polydipsia and Polyuria

The history should be corroborated by family or friends if possible. Important historical points are rapidity of onset of symptoms, a preference for use of iced water, and nocturnal drinking habits. Sudden onset and preference for iced water are classical for diabetes insipidus. Numerous spontaneous awakenings at night in order to drink and urinate also strongly suggest this diagnosis, while absence of such nocturnal events is in favor of functional disease. A careful psychiatric history is important. The use of drugs should be noted (6).

Initial laboratory workup should be simple. Urine glucose should be measured. An a.m. serum sodium and/or osmolality determination along with serum potassium, calcium, urea nitrogen, and creatinine should be made. The patient should collect all urine over one or more 24-hour periods. The sample should be examined to determine the volume, osmolality, and total creatinine excretion, the latter serving as a marker for completeness of the collection. Measurement of urine specific gravity is obsolete and should not be used.

These preliminaries will define the problem and provide an insight into the diagnosis. Unless considerable glucosuria is present, the patient's problem is not due to uncontrolled diabetes mellitus, even if blood glucose is incidentally elevated. The presence of a normal serum sodium and/or osmolality indicates only that the process is not severe enough to have overwhelmed the ability to excrete water or the homeostatic (thirst) mechanism. Elevated serum osmolality strongly suggests diabetes insipidus; the opposite finding indicates psychogenic water drinking. The presence of normal serum calcium and potassium excludes several metabolic problems, while abnormalities of calcium, potassium, or renal function will make it clear that the problem is not primarily one of water metabolism (see Table 71.7).

At this point most patients will have normal findings in serum but a large volume of urine with low osmolality. Normal urine volume ranges up to 2500 ml; urine osmolality is decidedly low when the value is well below that of serum, i.e., less than 300 mOsm/kg (the urine is maximally dilute at 50 to 70 mOsm/kg). In both diabetes insipidus and psychogenic water drinking urine volume will usually exceed 4 liters daily. Values less than 5 to 6 liters daily do not distinguish between these possibilities but do indicate less than complete diabetes insipidus, in which urine volumes approach 10 to 12 liters daily, as they may in cases of severe psychogenic water drinking. If the serum sodium/osmolality is low and the urine volume is large with low osmolality, a diagnosis of psychogenic water drinking is likely.

Diabetes Insipidus *vs.* Psychogenic Water Drinking

Having established the presence of a large urine volume of low osmolality together with normal serum electrolytes, additional testing is necessary to establish a diagnosis. Referral to an endocrinologist or nephrologist is appropriate at this juncture, although under optimal conditions further efforts to establish the diagnosis on the ambulatory patient may be undertaken before referral (see below). Hospitalization for testing under "metabolic" conditions is nearly always to be preferred in these cases; however, most *ordinary* hospital conditions are not appropriate for the gathering of definitive information on water handling.

The first additional test is that of water deprivation. Best performed during the day when monitoring is possible, the patient remains recumbent and refrains from fluid intake; all urine is collected in hourly batches for 6 hours. Volumes and osmolalities are determined on each sample. Body weight is determined hourly. When the urine volume and osmolality seem to have stabilized after several hours, antidiuretic hormone (ADH; Pitressin) is given (5 units, aqueous, subcutaneously). Urine osmolality and volume are then determined every 30 min for an additional 90 to 120 min. If at any point drop in body weight exceeds 3%, the ADH should be injected and the test terminated over the next 90 min.

In the normal individual, urine volume will fall and osmolality will rise over several hours. Urine osmolality will exceed 500 mOsm/kg. Administration of ADH produces an additional increase in urine osmolality, but the increase will be small if the level is already high. In the patient with partial diabetes insipidus, the plateau is at 300 mOsm/kg with an increase to at least 500 mOsm/kg after ADH; some patients will not respond maximally (osmolality 1000 mOsm/kg). Patients with nephrogenic diabetes insipidus will not respond to ADH. A prompt fall of urine volume and an increase of urine osmolality may not occur in some patients with psychogenic water drinking. These patients are often overhydrated and may not reach plateau levels for as long as 12 hours. If the diagnosis is still doubtful at this point, referral for consultation should be made. Further tests can be performed to provoke ADH release by infusion of hypertonic saline. Administration of intravenous ADH and other special maneuvers may be necessary. X-rays of the sella turcica and CT scans of the area of the sella, although usually negative, are important in cases of diabetes insipidus to rule out space-occupying lesions. Anterior pituitary function must be assessed when diabetes insipidus is diagnosed.

Treatment

The treatment of psychogenic water drinking involves psychiatric counseling. These patients are difficult to manage, especially if they become severely hyponatremic. "Weaning" such patients from water may also be a slow process not only because of the profound nature of their psychiatric disturbance, but because of their acquired inability to concentrate urine, a process which is only slowly reversible.

The treatment of diabetes insipidus involves use of ADH in some form. Until the last few years Pitressin Tannate in oil was the preferred agent. This material is given intramuscularly. Great care must be taken to suspend the insoluble hormone before injection. The usual dose is 5 U every 24 to 72 hours, depending on the duration of effect in a particular individual. Antidiuretic hormone may also be administered as a nasal spray. Two forms are available; lysine vasopressin, with an effect which lasts only 4 to 6 hours, has been largely replaced by the synthetic analog, desmopressin (DDAVP). This material acts for 12 hours or longer. DDAVP is a great advance in the therapy of diabetes insipidus. Nasal absorption may be impaired by rhinitis or respiratory tract infections, during which treatment with Pitressin Tannate may be necessary. Patients with partial diabetes insipidus can sometimes be managed with chlorpropamide (Diabinese; 250 to 500 mg daily), a drug which potentiates endogenous ADH. However, hypoglycemia is a significant hazard. Clofibrate (Atromid-S) is another drug which has been used to treat diabetes insipidus. Nephrogenic diabetes insipidus, both idiopathic and secondary to lithium, is partially responsive to thiazide diuretics (11).

Syndrome of Inappropriate Secretion of Antidiuretic Hormone (SIADH)

The clinical manifestations of this disorder are due to hyponatremia and the diagnosis is based on that finding. The causes are multiple. Classically, the disturbance was related to ectopic production of ADH by a neoplasm. The tumor most likely to produce this syndrome is a small cell (oat cell) carcinoma of the lung, but many other tumors have also been shown to produce the same syndrome. The presence of a tumor is usually obvious, but occasionally it may be clinically occult. In addition, a variety of acute and chronic diseases of the central nervous system can produce an identical syndrome. Drugs, acting centrally, may also produce ADH hypersecretion (morphine, barbiturates (11)). The best described drug-related SIADH which is likely to be encountered in an ambulatory patient is that due to chlorpropamide (Diabinese) during the therapy of diabetes mellitus (Chapter 69). In this case, the disturbance is due to potentiation of ADH action, although increased ADH release may also be involved (11).

TREATMENT

The treatment of SIADH is usually that which is related to the underlying disease or involves withdrawal of drug therapy (e.g., chlorpropamide; Diabinese: see Chapter 69). Water restriction is effective, but is difficult to maintain in an ambulatory setting. Lithium has been occasionally useful. Demeclocycline, a tetracycline analog, is an ADH antagonist and is effective in some cases. An ADH peptide analog which blocks ADH action has been recently developed and offers promise for therapy, but the agent is not yet available for clinical use.

HYPOGLYCEMIA

Since the symptoms of hypoglycemia are rather nonspecific, hypoglycemia is properly more often suspected than present. Chemical hypoglycemia, defined as a plasma sugar of less than 50 mg/dl, may not be symptomatic, although levels less than 30 mg/dl are nearly always associated with symptoms (see Chapter 69 for discussion of plasma versus blood glucose values).

Hypoglycemia produces symptoms by two mechanisms: (a) by triggering the release of epinephrine, one of several homeostatic responses which tend to normalize a low blood sugar and (b) by deprivation of the nervous system of its essential energy source.

The causes of hypoglycemia are numerous, but by far the most common is a benign functional disturbance of insulin secretion which is temporally associated with absorption of food from the gastrointestinal tract. Most other hypoglycemic events are seen in diabetics being treated with insulin. A few other conditions producing hypoglycemia are associated with insulin overproduction, the rarest of which is an insulinoma. In most situations hypoglycemia is due not to insulin excess but to disturbances of glucose production, as in ethanol ingestion, or rarely to glucose overutilization, as in the presence of certain extrapancreatic tumors. The causes of hypoglycemia are listed in Table 71.8.

Clinical Diagnosis

PRESENTATION OF THE PROBLEM

In some patients the history will suggest to the physician that the patient is experiencing periodic hypoglycemia. Other patients will themselves suggest to their physician that hypoglycemia accounts for the symptoms. Much has been written in the lay literature about hypoglycemia, and many books attribute the entire range of human miseries to this disorder. Needless to say, the case has been overstated. The physician encountering such a patient may find mere

Table 71.8
Causes of Hypoglycemia

POSTPRANDIAL STATE
    Reactive (idiopathic)
    Early diabetes mellitus
    Ethanol ingestion
    Postgastrectomy state
FASTING STATE
    Insulin excess:
      1. Insulin injection
      2. Sulfonylurea ingestion
      3. Insulinoma
    Alcohol ingestion
    Hormonal deficiencies:
      1. Adrenal insufficiency
      2. Pituitary insufficiency
    Prolonged fasting in normal women
    Liver disease
    Extrapancreatic tumors
    Renal failure (chronic end-stage)

reassurance ineffective, so convincing is some of the lay literature in this area and so obsessed are some patients. However, the physician inevitably embarks on a search, either to confirm or refute the suspected diagnosis. Unfortunately, failure to document the presence of hypoglycemia may not serve to dispose of the issue, while generation of dubious or equivocal laboratory results may merely serve to prolong the preoccupation, initiate useless diets, or even delay diagnosis of serious but unrelated disease.

"NON-HYPOGLYCEMIA"

The frequency with which self-diagnosis of hypoglycemia occurs depends on the population, but in one study from Los Angeles, the problem was very common. The condition has been termed "non-hypoglycemia" and extends the concept of "non-disease," as it originates from misattributes of the physician, such as misinterpretation of laboratory values, to misattributes of the patient (16). Identification of such individuals is important as is their re-education (4). The ready acceptance by patients of hypoglycemia as a diagnosis is perhaps related to its social acceptability, the comfort received from attributing vague symptoms (e.g., fatigue, mental "fogginess") to a "real" disease, the satisfaction of an escape into dietary rituals, and possibly relief from the anxiety that life-threatening or at least serious disease may be lurking.

The recognition of "non-hypoglycemia" requires a careful history which fails to demonstrate the legitimate symptoms of hypoglycemia as well as a clear demonstration that glucose metabolism is normal (see below). Exclusion of other organic disease is routine (Table 71.8). Finally, psychiatric disease must be considered, based on positive findings rather than merely on an exclusion of apparent organic illness.

If the evaluation fails to establish the presence of *bona fide* hypoglycemia, the physician is left with the issue of the therapy of "non-hypoglycemia." This difficult problem includes at least three steps which have been termed (a) disattribution, (b) explanation and ventilation, and (c) reattribution (16). Disattribution involves confrontation of the patient with the results of the test procedure. For some patients the mechanics or ritual of the procedure itself are impressive and therefore helpful. If the patient clings to the diagnosis of hypoglycemia despite strong evidence to the contrary, the physician should attempt to explore the reason for the patient's need to do so. During this process, an effort should be made to have the patient fully explain his notions about hypoglycemia and ventilate about what might happen if those notions are challenged. Finally, the physician must either provide an alternate explanation for the symptoms—reattribution—along with a treatment plan or be prepared to assist the patient in accepting an uncertain and ambiguous situation. Unless grossly apparent emotional problems become evident during this process, psychiatric referral should be made after considerable deliberation and only after an effort has been made by the internist to resolve the problem.

DEFINING HYPOGLYCEMIC SYMPTOMS

Because laboratory confirmation may be extremely difficult in some cases, an extraordinarily careful history is essential. The degree to which the history is convincing will determine the vigor with which a rather nebulous diagnosis is to be pursued. Two issues guide the process. First, what exactly are the symptoms? Second, do the symptoms occur postprandially or in the fasting state?

Adrenergic vs. Neuroglycopenic Symptoms. Two groups of symptoms and signs are associated with hypoglycemia. Many of the symptoms of hypoglycemia relate to stimulation by low blood glucose of the release of epinephrine. These comprise the first group and are termed *adrenergic* or sympathetic. Usually these symptoms are of rapid onset and more than one is ordinarily present. Ordinarily they last only 15 to 30 min, and include sweating, a sensation of hunger, and anxiety. Irritability and palpitations are often mentioned but are rarely spontaneous or prominent complaints.

The second group of symptoms is related to glucose deprivation of the central and, to a lesser extent, peripheral nervous systems. These symptoms may be termed *neuroglycopenic* and when severe mimic those of central nervous system hypoxia. Minimal symptoms are headache, mental dullness, and sudden fatigue. Confusion and visual disturbances (blurring, dimming of vision) are associated with moderate to severe hypoglycemia, while unconsciousness and seizures are indications of very severe hypoglycemia.

While adrenergic symptoms are mainly postprandial, neuroglycopenic symptoms, especially those of severe variety, are seen in association with fasting hypoglycemia. Minor neuroglycopenic symptoms may also be seen in the postabsorptive state, but symptoms severe enough to cause loss of consciousness are rare and should not be readily attributed to this cause. When severe symptoms do occur in the postprandial state, great difficulty in establishing a diagnosis may be encountered. The duration of this type of hypoglycemia is so short that, by the time the patient is seen by a physician and a blood sugar determination is obtained, the glucose has often returned to normal.

Postprandial vs. Fasting Hypoglycemia. An accurate history is essential in order to identify the hypoglycemia as either postprandial or fasting. The subsequent evaluation and the diagnostic possibilities segregate clearly once this distinction is made. If a distinction can be made based on the history, the alternate type of hypoglycemia should no longer be considered since the two types do not coexist.

Postprandial (Reactive) Hypoglycemia. In this situation the patient has no problem on arising and before breakfast. Similarly, no difficulty is experienced if the patient sleeps late. The symptoms usually develop 2 to 5 hours after a meal.

Inquiry concerning the patient's dietary habits may be revealing. Some patients restrict carbohydrate intake intermittently. When this is done and a large carbohydrate meal follows, hypoglycemia may be precipitated. A history of previous gastrointestinal surgery (gastrectomy) is also important. The amount of alcohol consumed should be noted, since ethanol ingestion may precipitate hypoglycemia, even in the nonfasting patient (see below). Often the patient may recall milder symptomatic episodes experienced over a long period, since the intensity of postprandial hypoglycemia tends to wax and wane over the years. A family history of diabetes should be sought. Postprandial hypoglycemia can be an early manifestation of diabetes mellitus of the non-insulin-dependent type (see Chapter 69). Although symptoms and signs of anxiety or depression may be present, they have no diagnostic usefulness.

General physical examination can be expected to be negative. Even when early diabetes mellitus is found by glucose tolerance testing to be the cause of the hypoglycemia, complications of diabetes that can be found on physical examination (retinopathy, neuropathy) will not be present.

Laboratory Evaluation

Although ordinary meals do not consist of carbohydrate alone, the only practical and standardized test for detection of postabsorptive hypoglycemia is the glucose tolerance test. For this purpose, the test as described for diagnosis of diabetes mellitus (Chapter 69) is modified to include more frequent sampling (30-min intervals) and a longer period (5 hours). The patient is observed during the entire test. Correlation of blood sugar values with clinical symptoms is essential. If the patient develops hypoglycemia associated with symptoms and signs which reproduce those ordinarily experienced, a diagnosis of postabsorptive hypoglycemia can be considered established. A more precise diagnosis depends on the type of curve observed (see below). If symptoms occur in the absence of hypoglycemia, the diagnosis is psychiatric. If hypoglycemia is seen but no symptoms occur, the hypoglycemic response may simply not have been severe enough to have triggered symptoms. The diagnosis then remains presumptive. A repeat test may succeed in reproducing the clinical situation.

CRITERIA FOR DIAGNOSIS OF HYPOGLYCEMIA

Plasma glucose values are greater than 50 mg/dl during glucose tolerance testing in 75% of *normal, asymptomatic* persons. However, some normal individuals show values which fall to 50 mg/dl or somewhat lower and may exhibit hypoglycemic symptoms during the test, even though they never have such symptoms spontaneously. Thus, even a finding of hypoglycemia during testing may not necessarily explain the observed symptoms. In addition, occasional normal individuals may reach levels below 35 mg/dl without any symptoms at all.

Plasma insulin determinations in connection with the glucose tolerance test are of no particular use in interpreting the results. Variability is very great and in no sense diagnostic.

TYPES OF HYPOGLYCEMIC RESPONSE DURING GLUCOSE TOLERANCE TESTING

Early Diabetes Mellitus. The fasting glucose is normal. In the first 2 hours, values diagnostic of diabetes mellitus are reached, although the highest values are usually between 200 and 250 mg/dl (Chapter 69). Thereafter, between 3 and 4 hours, the glucose falls to its lowest value and below 50 mg/dl.

Postgastrectomy State. Plasma glucose rises rapidly and may reach a peak over 300 mg/dl by 1 hour, following which a rapid decline occurs. The lowest value is seen at 2 to 3 hours.

Idiopathic. In this response the blood glucose values in the first 2 hours are normal, but at about 3 hours a fall to hypoglycemic levels occurs. Values usually return to baseline by 5 hours.

Management of Postprandial Hypoglycemia

EARLY DIABETES MELLITUS

If the patient is obese, weight reduction may normalize the glucose tolerance and abolish the hypoglycemic episodes. If the patient is not obese, dietary manipulation can be attempted, but no standardized approach is available. The diet most likely to succeed is one which simulates that now recommended for diabetes generally, *i.e.*, a diet which contains a high proportion of complex carbohydrates rather than simple sugars (Chapter 69). Also important is the distribution of food intake into small meals—often as many as six. Alcohol may be an aggravating factor in producing hypoglycemia and should be restricted, at least on a trial basis. Caffeine (coffee, tea) need not be restricted. Sulfonylurea drugs are not useful.

POSTGASTRECTOMY STATE

As many as 75% of asymptomatic patients who have had a gastrectomy will show reactive hypoglycemia during a glucose tolerance test. The therapy of symptomatic patients is similar to that described above: frequent small meals and restriction of simple sugars. The anticholinergic drug propantheline (Pro-Banthine), 7.5 mg taken 30 min before meals, may be helpful. This drug inhibits gut motility and delays gastric emptying. At this dose, side effects (blurred vision; dry mouth) are minimal. Propranolol (Inderal) often blocks symptoms but does little to affect hypoglycemia and therefore may be hazardous.

IDIOPATHIC

The course of this disorder is obscure. Some patients may present with anxiety and/or depression in association with onset of hypoglycemic symptoms. Although diet manipulation and/or propantheline therapy as described above may ameliorate the hypoglycemia, additional treatment may be needed for the psychologic aspects. Recent introduction of high protein, low carbohydrate diets for weight reduction has also led to difficulties in some persons. Carbohydrate restriction followed by carbohydrate ingestion leads to the hypoglycemia in these individuals. Ethanol (doses of 3 oz of gin or equivalent) may potentiate reactive hypoglycemia in normal subjects.

Fasting Hypoglycemia

The classical entity associated with fasting hypoglycemia is the insulinoma, but such insulin-secreting tumors are very rare and other causes of fasting hypoglycemia should be eliminated before embarking on the difficult task of establishing the presence of an insulinoma.

Fasting hypoglycemia in a well-nourished or obese individual suggests insulinoma, drug (sulfonylurea) ingestion, or insulin self-administration. Debilitation suggests hepatic disease (most often related to chronic alcohol abuse) or, rarely, extrapancreatic tumor. The history, physical examination, and routine laboratory studies will readily identify patients with chronic congestive heart failure or chronic renal disease, two other conditions occasionally associated with fasting hypoglycemia. Other aspects of these problems as well as endocrine deficiencies and alcohol abuse as causes of hypoglycemia are discussed below.

LABORATORY EVALUATION

When symptoms of hypoglycemia occur in the fasting state (usually overnight but in any case longer than 4 hours following a meal) a number of diagnostic possibilities more serious than those associated with postprandial hypoglycemia must be considered. However, the first step in evaluation of the problem is to establish the existence of hypoglycemia. Assuming that the symptoms are not so profound as to have caused coma, in which case hospitalization is mandatory, an overnight fast followed by determination of plasma glucose is the simplest screening procedure. This procedure may have to be repeated several times. If hypoglycemia cannot be documented in this way, the period of fasting may have to be extended to 24, 48, or even 72 hours. Hospitalization and close monitoring are necessary under these circumstances.

A sex difference in response to fasting is well-established. Normal males may fast for up to 72 hours and will not show fasting plasma glucose (FPG) below 50 mg/dl. In contrast, women often exhibit a progressive fall in the concentration of plasma glucose during prolonged fasting. At 72 hours the majority of women have a concentration of glucose less than 50 mg/dl and some as low as 25 mg/dl. Thus, prolonged fasting to establish the diagnosis of fasting hypoglycemia is not always useful since so many normal women will become hypoglycemic.

INSULINOMA

This tumor occurs with equal frequency in men and women and at any age. Symptoms of headache on arising, confusion before breakfast, or nocturnal or early a.m. seizures may be present for years before the diagnosis is suspected. Hyperinsulinism may produce abnormal hunger, weight gain, and obesity. Neuropsychiatric symptoms may lead to neurologic or psychiatric evaluations or to hospitalizations. In some of these cases, permanent neurologic deficits have been seen and are presumably related to long duration of symptomatic hypoglycemia before diagnosis.

Diagnosis. In addition to the demonstration of hypoglycemia, the determination of plasma insulin is important. During fasting in normal persons both glucose and insulin levels decline and the ratio of immunoreactive insulin (IRI) and glucose (G) is maintained at less than 0.3 (mU IRI/mg G/dl). In most patients with insulinoma an abnormally high ratio of IRI/G is apparent after even overnight fasting. These determinations should be made repeatedly, since fasting hypoglycemia and an abnormal ratio of IRI/G often occur only intermittently even in patients with subsequently proven insulinomas. In addition, a single abnormal ratio determination never establishes the diagnosis. The physician should be very cautious in accepting the accuracy of IRI values obtained from commercial laboratories. Proinsulin levels are elevated in patients with insulinoma and can be a useful adjunct. A variety of other useful procedures should, if necessary, be conducted by an endocrinologist. If fasting fails to provoke hypoglycemia (see above), the patient should exercise for 2 hours (bicycle exerciser), a procedure which raises glucose levels in normal persons, but lowers plasma concentration further in patients with insulinoma. Provocative tests of insulin secretion (tolbutamide, leucine, glucagon) can be utilized with appropriate caution. Suppression of endogenous insulin C-peptide is another useful procedure in difficult cases, but requires induction of hypoglycemia by infusion of insulin under controlled conditions, a procedure which must be performed by an endocrinologist in a hospital. Computerized axial tomography and sonography can localize tumors of 2 to 3-cm size. Selective angiography can sometimes identify even smaller tumors. These procedures must not be used as alternatives to the tests described above but should be performed after demonstration of abnormal secretion of insulin. The definitive treatment of an insulinoma is surgical.

INSULIN AND SULFONYLUREA SELF-ADMINISTRATION

Occasional nondiabetic patients, usually family members of diabetics or persons with medically related occupations (nurses, technicians), engage in surreptitious insulin administration. Physical examination may reveal needle marks. Other clues can be provided by the presence of antibodies to insulin, which are present only in persons given insulin of animal origin, or by the measurement of insulin C-peptide. In persons who are secreting insulin, C-peptide is also produced concomitantly, but C-peptide is not present in commercial insulin and will be very low or absent when hypoglycemia is induced by exogenous insulin.

Oral hypoglycemic drugs (sulfonylureas; see Chapter 69), like insulin, may occasionally be abused and cause fasting hypoglycemia. The drug can be detected by analysis of the blood, although only specialized laboratories perform these measurements.

ALCOHOL ABUSE

This problem probably produces hypoglycemia more commonly than any other single cause. As stated above, ingestion of ethanol can produce postprandial hypoglycemia in normal, well-nourished persons who engage in "social" drinking. However, fasting hypoglycemia related to ethanol ingestion occurs in chronic alcohol abusers and especially those who are malnourished. The situation most likely to provoke hypoglycemia is cessation of food intake and continued ingestion of ethanol over the ensuing 10 to 20 hours. Under these circumstances, ethanol intoxication, i.e., drunkenness, may mistakenly be thought to be responsible for the symptoms.

LIVER DISEASE AND CHRONIC CONGESTIVE HEART FAILURE

Although hypoglycemia can be seen in the course of severe, acute hepatitis or as a result of chronic passive congestion in long-standing congestive heart failure, liver disease does not usually produce hypoglycemia. Patients with severe cirrhosis may occasionally have fasting hypoglycemia, but the development of hypoglycemia in such a patient should suggest the presence of a hepatoma. In patients with well differentiated hepatoma, hypoglycemia may be an early symptom.

ENDOCRINE DISEASE

Glucocorticoids and growth hormone are important regulators of glucose metabolism. Thus, either pituitary insufficiency or adrenal insufficiency (primary or secondary to hypopituitarism) can result in hypoglycemia as a presenting manifestation. The diagnosis of these disorders is described elsewhere in this chapter.

References

General

DeGroot, LJ (ed): *Endocrinology, Vols. 1–3.* Grune & Stratton, New York, 1979.
   A comprehensive, multivolume textbook containing a great deal of information. Poorly indexed.
Felig, P, Baxter, JD, Broadus, AE and Frohman, LA (eds): *Endocrinology and Metabolism.* McGraw-Hill, New York, 1981.
   A new textbook of manageable proportions.
Hershman, JM (ed): *Management of Endocrine Disorders.* Lea & Febiger, Philadelphia, 1980.
   A short textbook.
Williams, RH (ed): *Textbook of Endocrinology, Ed. 6.* W. B. Saunders, Philadelphia, 1981.
   The latest edition of this standard textbook contains detailed coverage of most aspects of the topics considered in this chapter.

Specific

1. Amatruda, TT, Jr, Hurst, MM and D'esopo, ND: Certain endocrine and metabolic facets of the steroid withdrawal syndrome. *J Clin Endocrinol Metab 25:* 1207, 1965.
2. Burrow, GN, Wortzman, G, Rewcastle, NB, Holgate, RC and Kowacs, K: Microadenomas of the pituitary and abnormal sellar tomograms in an unselected autopsy series. *N Engl J Med 304:* 156, 1981.
3. Byyny, RL: Withdrawal from glucocorticoid therapy. *N Engl J Med 295:* 30, 1976.
4. Cahill, GF and Soeldner, JS: A non-editorial on non-hypoglycemia. *N Engl J Med 291:* 905–906, 1974.
5. Coe, FL and Favus, MJ: Does mild, asymptomatic hyperparathyroidism require surgery? *N Engl J Med 302:* 224, 1980 (editorial); and rebuttal (letters), Incidence of primary hyperparathyroidism. *N Engl J Med 302:* 1312, 1980.
6. Davis, FB and Davis, PJ: Water metabolism in diabetes mellitus. *Am J Med 70:* 210, 1981.
7. Fauci, AS, Dale, DC and Balow, JE: Glucocorticoid Therapy: mechanisms of action and clinical considerations. *Ann Intern Med 84:* 304, 1976.
8. Graber, AL, Ney, RL, Nicholson, WE, Island, DP and Liddle, GW: Natural history of pituitary-adrenal recovery following long-term suppression with corticosteroids. *J Clin Endocrinol Metab 25:* 11, 1965.
9. Heath, H, III, Hodgson, SF and Kennedy, MA: Primary hyperparathyroidism. Incidence, morbidity, and potential economic impact in a community. *N Engl J Med 302:* 189, 1980.
10. Melby, JC: Systemic corticosteroid therapy: pharmacology and endocrinologic considerations. *Ann Intern Med 81:* 505, 1974.
11. Miller, M and Moses, AM: Drug-induced states of impaired water excretion. *Kidney Int 10:* 96, 1976.
12. Roof, BS and Gordan, GS: Hyperparathyroid disease in the

aged. In *Geriatric Endocrinology, Vol. 5, Aging*, pp. 33–79, edited by RB Greenblatt. Raven Press, New York, 1978.

13. Sachar, EJ (ed): *Hormones, Behavior, and Psychopathology*. Raven Press, New York, 1976.

14. Spiegel, RJ, Vigersky, RA, Oliff, AI, Echelberger, CK, Bruton, J and Popkack, DG: Adrenal suppression after short-term corticosteroid therapy. *Lancet 1*: 630, 1979.

15. Stewart, AF, Horst, R, Deftos, LJ, Cadman, EC, Lang, R and Broadus, AE: Biochemical evaluation of patients with cancer-associated hypercalcemia. *N Engl J Med 303*: 1377, 1980.

16. Yager, J and Young, RT: Non-hypoglycemia is an epidemic condition. *N Engl J Med 291*: 907, 1974.

17. Zervas, NT and Martin, JB: Management of hormone-secreting pituitary adenomas. *N Engl J Med 302*: 210, 1980.

CHAPTER SEVENTY-TWO

Plasma Lipids and Hyperlipidemia

DAVID E. KERN, M.D., and MARC R. BLACKMAN, M.D.

Although abnormalities of plasma lipids are common among individuals in Western industrialized societies and have major prognostic significance, the general physician who attempts to diagnose and manage lipid disorders may feel confused and frustrated. This is so because of the proliferating, but still incomplete, knowledge about the metabolism of lipids and the pathophysiology and treatment of lipid disorders. This chapter reviews these subjects and attempts to put them into a context that is clinically useful to the practicing physician.

LIPID AND LIPOPROTEIN NOMENCLATURE AND COMPOSITION (Table 72.1)

Each of the major lipid classes—cholesterol, cholesterol esters, triglycerides, and phospholipids—enters and circulates in the blood in association with one or more specific proteins, termed *apoproteins*. The resulting *lipoproteins*, which confer miscibility upon otherwise insoluble lipids, are complex structures.

The major classes of lipoproteins can be separated from each other by differences in density (ultracentrifugation), net surface charge (electrophoresis), and by other properties. Ultracentrifugation, which provides the most useful means of classification, separates lipoproteins into five principal classes. From the least dense (and also the largest) to the most dense (and also the smallest), they are chylomicrons, very low density lipoproteins (VLDL), intermediate density lipoproteins (IDL), low density lipoproteins (LDL), and high density lipoproteins (HDL).

Each lipoprotein contains characteristic proportions of lipids and type-specific apoproteins such that, with increasing lipoprotein density, the relative amount of lipid decreases and that of apoprotein increases. Thus, triglycerides are the major component of chylomicrons (80 to 90%) and of VLDL (50 to 70%), while cholesterol (about two-thirds as cholesterol ester) is the major component of LDL (45 to 50%) and an important constituent of HDL (15 to 25%). Conversely, apoproteins make up 1 to 2% of chylomicrons and about 50% of HDL.

All known lipid disorders are associated with altered plasma levels of one or more lipoproteins.

LIPIDS AS RISK FACTORS FOR ATHEROSCLEROSIS

Hypercholesterolemia, cigarette smoking, and high blood pressure are currently acknowledged to be the

Table 72.1
Classification and Characteristics of Lipoproteins

Class (Based on Ultracentrifugation)	Migration on Paper Electrophoresis	Cholesterol Content (%)	Triglyceride Content (%)	If Elevated, Plasma Appearance[a]
Chylomicron (very, very low density lipoprotein)	Chylomicrons remain at origin	2–7	80–90	Floating creamy layer with clear infranatant
Very low density lipoprotein (VLDL)	Pre β	10–22	50–70	Turbid
Intermediate density lipoprotein (IDL)	Slow Pre β	30	40	Slightly turbid
Low density lipoprotein (LDL)	β	45–50	5–10	Clear
High density lipoprotein (HDL)	α	15–25	3–5	Clear

[a] After standing for 12 hours at 4°C.

three major risk factors for the development of atherosclerotic vascular disease. It has been estimated that men in the highest 10% of exposure for all three factors have about a 30-fold greater chance, over a period of 9 to 12 years, of demonstrating clinical manifestations of coronary heart disease (CHD) than those in the lowest 10% of exposure (15,17). When data from women are similarly compared, the risk is less, but still substantial (15).

It has been demonstrated in several large prospective studies among diverse populations that total (or LDL) cholesterol and HDL cholesterol are independent risk factors. While there is a strong positive correlation between the subsequent development of CHD and elevated plasma levels of total (or LDL) cholesterol, there is an inverse correlation between HDL cholesterol levels and risk of CHD that is at least as strong. Over the range of plasma total cholesterol or of HDL cholesterol levels found in an average American population, the risk of CHD can vary (roughly) 5-fold. Total serum cholesterol levels have less predictive value beyond the age of 50 or 60, although HDL cholesterol levels and the ratio of HDL cholesterol to LDL cholesterol remain useful predictors in this age group. Levels of plasma triglyceride and VLDL do not appear to be independent risk factors for CHD (6).

Current epidemiologic data are insufficient to define the risk of fasting chylomicronemia or of elevated levels of IDL. The available information, derived from retrospective reviews of small groups of patients or from case reports, suggests that fasting chylomicronemia is associated with recurrent episodes of abdominal pain and pancreatitis, but is not associated with CHD. On the other hand, there does appear to be an enhanced risk of premature ischemic cardiovascular disease in patients with dysbetalipoproteinemia—a disorder characterized by elevated levels of IDL and of an abnormal lipoprotein, β-VLDL, and by low HDL levels.

While the risk from lipid disorders is greatest for CHD, there is also a lesser, but still increased, risk of cerebrovascular disease (8) and of peripheral vascular

disease (13). Also, there is an inverse correlation between levels of HDL cholesterol and risk of cerebrovascular disease and of peripheral vascular disease.

PHYSIOLOGY OF LIPID AND LIPOPROTEIN TRANSPORT

Plasma chylomicrons contain exogenously (i.e., dietary) derived triglycerides, and are detectable normally in the postabsorptive, but not in the fasting state. In contrast, endogenous triglycerides are synthesized in the liver from fatty acids, the origins of which vary with the diet. Triglycerides are released from the liver as VLDL. Metabolism of chylomicrons and VLDL occurs initially at the capillary endothelial surfaces of extrahepatic tissues by the action of a specific enzyme, lipoprotein lipase, which removes triglycerides from both lipoproteins. Further catabolism of chylomicrons and of VLDL is effected by the combined actions of HDL and the enzyme lecithin cholesterol acyltransferase (LCAT), secreted by the liver. The coordinated actions of lipoprotein lipase and HDL and LCAT transform chylomicrons and VLDL to chylomicron remnants and LDL, respectively. Chylomicron remnants are removed and degraded by the liver, where fatty acids derived from their triglycerides serve as substrates for endogenous triglyceride synthesis. Plasma LDL serve as the major carrier for cholesterol.

Cholesterol is an integral structural component of plasma membranes, and is a synthetic precursor of steroid hormones and bile acids. The liver and intestine are the major sites of its production. Cholesterol is excreted only by the liver, which secretes cholesterol and bile acids into the biliary tract. Approximately 300 to 500 mg of cholesterol are absorbed daily from the usual American diet. Alterations in dietary cholesterol intake or in the enterohepatic circulation of cholesterol or bile acids (e.g., via cholestyramine or T-tube drainage) lead to reciprocal changes in hepatic cholesterol synthesis.

Since most (65 to 70%) plasma cholesterol exists in

LDL, there is a strong positive correlation between plasma measurements of LDL cholesterol and those of total cholesterol. Transport of LDL to extrahepatic tissues leads to degradation of this lipoprotein and utilization of its cholesterol. Approximately two-thirds of LDL is catabolized by an LDL receptor pathway, whereby LDL are bound to specific cell surface receptors, internalized, degraded by lysosomal enzymes, and the products are released into the extralysosomal cytoplasm. The resulting free cholesterol then regulates cellular cholesterol metabolism. Abnormalities of the LDL receptor pathway are now recognized as causes of several disorders of lipid transport (see "Pathophysiology"). The remaining one-third of LDL is catabolized by a receptor-independent scavenger mechanism, which is probably localized in the reticuloendothelial system. Unlike the LDL receptor pathway, the scavenger mechanism does not appear to be subject to feedback control.

Recently, attention has focused upon elucidating the structure and function of plasma HDL (4), but further research is necessary to determine what function(s) of HDL is (are) responsible for the known inverse relationship between plasma HDL levels and the prevalence of coronary heart disease.

THE LIPID HYPOTHESIS

The lipid hypothesis is a unifying theory set forth to explain the interrelationships among hereditary factors, environmental influences, lipid metabolism, plasma lipids, and disease (Fig. 72.1). According to this theory, environmental factors (such as diet, exercise, and smoking) and endogenous metabolic factors (which are genetically determined), either individually or conjointly, determine plasma lipid levels. Abnormal plasma lipid levels, in turn, may promote or cause clinical sequelae (such as coronary heart disease). While this theory is strongly supported by several lines of evidence, a major point of controversy has been the failure so far to demonstrate unequivocally whether maneuvers that favorably alter plasma lipid levels can decrease the risk of CHD in humans.

HYPERLIPIDEMIA

Definition

There are no generally agreed upon absolute levels of cholesterol and triglycerides above which a diagnosis of hyperlipidemia can be made. Since plasma lipid levels have a unimodal, near normal distribution in most populations, and since risk seems to increase continuously over a broad range of lipid values, there are no precise cutoff points that can be used to segregate individuals into normal and abnormal categories. Furthermore, in contrast to hypertension, for example, no therapeutic trials have identified specific plasma lipid levels above which therapy is indicated.

Although hyperlipidemia is often operationally diagnosed on the basis of total (or LDL) cholesterol or triglyceride levels above the 95th percentile, a percentile-based definition is of limited value because plasma lipid distributions vary between and within populations. For example, total cholesterol levels (and the prevalence of CHD) are much higher in North American and Northern European populations than they are in the Japanese population. A person diagnosed as hyperlipidemic in Japan would probably be classified as normal in the United States.

Finally, use of the term "hyperlipidemia" fails to account for the now well-established role of HDL cholesterol in the prediction and possibly in the pathogenesis of atherosclerosis. Low, rather than high, plasma levels of HDL cholesterol correlate with subsequent disease.

It is best to consider plasma lipids as risk factors which predict and may cause disease or which may be caused by disease (e.g., primary or secondary disorders of lipid metabolism), rather than to consider hyperlipidemia per se as disease. Despite these caveats, use of the term hyperlipidemia is common; and, therefore, it is used in this chapter to mean a plasma total (or LDL) cholesterol or plasma triglyceride level above the 95th percentile in a reference population.

The distributions of total cholesterol, total triglyceride, and HDL cholesterol values among North

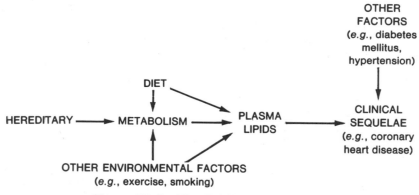

Figure 72.1 The lipid hypothesis.

American participants in the Lipid Research Clinics Prevalence Study are available for reference (10). While the participants in this study do not represent a random sample of the entire North American population, they do encompass a broad range of sociodemographic groups and certain important trends have been noted. Plasma levels of total (and LDL) cholesterol and triglycerides increased substantially with age until about 50 to 65 years, after which they tended to reach a plateau or fall. Triglyceride levels were higher in males than in females and in whites than in blacks. HDL cholesterol levels were higher in preadolescent boys than in girls. However, during adolescence HDL cholesterol levels fell in males and then remained relatively stable until age 50 to 60, when they started to rise again. In females, HDL cholesterol levels rose gradually with age, surpassing male levels in adolescence. HDL cholesterol levels were higher in blacks than in whites, particularly among men. These variations according to age, sex, and race must be considered when assigning a range of normal or a percentile to an individual's lipid level (Tables 72.2–72.4).

Classification

PRIMARY VS. SECONDARY

For clinical purposes hyperlipidemic states have been classified as either primary (endogenous disorders of lipid metabolism) or secondary. The latter are associated with an identifiable disease or condition and are reversible with control or eradication of that

Table 72.2
Plasma Total Cholesterol Distributions (mg/dl)[a, b]

	White							Black					
Age	Male			Female			Age	Male			Female		
	5th%	Mean	.95th%	5th%	Mean	95th%		5th%	Mean	95th%	5th%	Mean	95th%
15–19	113	150	197	120	158	203	10–19	120	160	205	124	165	211
20–24	124	167	218	125	172	228	20–29	—[c]	179	—	124	177	235
25–29	133	182	244	130	176	229	30–39	138	192	253	132	185	243
30–34	138	192	254	131	179	238	40–49	148	207	267	146	202	268
35–39	146	201	270	141	186	245	50–59	—	207	—	—	217	—
40–44	151	207	268	147	195	253	60+	—	221	—	—	234	—
45–49	158	212	276	152	205	268							
50–54	158	213	277	163	218	285							
55–59	156	214	276	169	226	294							
60–64	159	213	276	173	229	296							
65–69	158	213	274	171	230	297							
70+	151	207	270	167	226	228							

[a] Source: Adapted from reference 10.
[b] Levels determined by routine chemistry laboratories may be 30 mg/dl or more higher than those determined by a standardized research laboratory.
[c] Percentile not given if $N < 100$.

Table 72.3
Plasma HDL Cholesterol Distributions (mg/dl)

	White[a]							Black[b]	
Age	Male			Female			Age	Male	Female
	5th%	Mean	95th%	5th%	Mean	95th%		Mean ± S.D.	Mean ± S.D.
15–19	30	46	63	35	52	74	15–19	53 ± 11	54 ± 11
20–24	30	45	63	33	53	79	20–24	—	—
25–29	31	45	63	37	56	83	25–29	58 ± 15	57 ± 10
30–34	28	46	63	36	56	77	30–34	54 ± 13	60 ± 13
35–39	29	43	62	34	55	82	35–39	53 ± 16	59 ± 15
40–44	27	44	67	34	58	88	40–44	58 ± 20	62 ± 19
45–49	30	45	64	34	53	87			
50–54	28	44	63	37	62	92			
55–59	28	48	71	37	62	91			
60–64	30	52	74	38	64	92			
65–69	30	51	78	35	63	98			
70+	31	51	75	33	61	92			

[a] Source: Adapted from reference 10.
[b] Source: Adapted from reference 16. Values are mean ± standard deviation.

Table 72.4
Plasma Triglyceride Distributions (mg/dl)[a]

Age	White Male 5th%	White Male Mean	White Male 95th%	White Female 5th%	White Female Mean	White Female 95th%	Age	Black Male 5th%	Black Male Mean	Black Male 95th%	Black Female 5th%	Black Female Mean	Black Female 95th%
15–19	37	78	148	39	75	132	10–19	31	59	102	36	65	110
20–24	44	100	201	40	89	165	20–29	—[b]	81	—	38	77	137
25–29	46	116	249	40	89	172	30–39	42	107	224	38	80	150
30–34	50	128	266	41	89	176	40–49	52	126	294	43	99	188
35–39	54	145	321	41	94	194	50–59	—	142	—	—	104	—
40–44	55	151	320	47	105	209	60 +	—	109	—	—	120	—
45–49	58	152	327	47	112	228							
50–54	58	152	320	54	120	238							
55–59	58	141	286	56	126	257							
60–64	58	142	291	57	127	240							
65–69	57	137	267	60	131	241							
70 +	58	130	258	60	131	235							

[a] Source: Adapted from reference 10.
[b] Percentile not given if $N < 100$.

disease or condition. Some causes of secondary hyperlipidemia are listed in Table 72.5. These primary and secondary states may be associated with one or more hyperlipidemic patterns (Table 72.6).

PHENOTYPIC

Both primary and secondary hyperlipidemias can be classified phenotypically by their plasma lipid patterns (Table 72.7). Usually, all that is required is measurement of plasma levels of *total cholesterol* and *fasting triglycerides*, together with *observation of a fasting plasma sample* which has been left undisturbed overnight in a refrigerator at 4° C. Elevated levels of total (or LDL) cholesterol do not affect the appearance of plasma, whereas hypertriglyceridemia associated with increased levels of VLDL imparts a uniform turbidity to plasma, and hypertriglyceridemia associated with chylomicronemia is characterized by a creamy supernatant fraction which floats on top of the plasma (Fig. 72.3). The unusual type III phenotype, which may be suggested by clinical findings (see below), requires electrophoresis for identification of the abnormally migrating VLDL and IDL. Knowledge of the phenotypic classification is not necessary for appropriate management of hyperlipidemic patients. Table 72.7 is provided for reference, since this classification is widely used.

GENOTYPIC

Primary hyperlipidemias can also be classified genotypically (11) (Table 72.8). This classification derives from studies of plasma lipid distributions in relatives of hyperlipidemic patients. Although the monogenic disorders are clearly defined, they account for only a minority of patients whose lipid levels are above the 95th percentiles of values in the general population. However, the monogenic forms may be associated with a greater risk of disease (5).

Table 72.5
Causes of Secondary Hyperlipidemia

Exogenous:	Alcohol, oral contraceptives, estrogens, corticosteroids, diuretics (thiazides, chlorthalidone), obesity, nutritional (diet high in cholesterol/saturated fat)
Endocrine:	Diabetes mellitus, hypothyroidism, Cushing's disease, Addison's disease, acromegaly, hypopituitarism
Liver:	Obstructive or parenchymal disease, hepatoma
Renal:	Nephrotic syndrome, chronic renal failure, hemodialysis
Acute stress situations:	Acute myocardial infarction, sepsis, burns
Pregnancy	
Pancreatitis	
Dysgammaglobulinemias:	Multiple myeloma, macroglobulinemia, systemic lupus erythematosus
Gout	
Viral infections	
Other:	Glycogen storage disease, lipodystrophies, progeria, acute intermittent porphyria, anorexia nervosa, Klinefelter's syndrome

Although among a group of affected relatives a single genotype may present as more than one phenotype (Table 72.8), in any given individual the phenotype tends to be stable. The interrelationships among primary, secondary, phenotypic, and genotypic classification systems are illustrated in Table 72.6.

PREVALENCE

The prevalence of hyperlipidemia (as defined above) in the United States is 5%. Among hyperlipidemic individuals, the type II and type IV phenotypic patterns are by far the most common. Estimated gene frequencies for the monogenic disorders are included in Table 72.8.

Table 72.6
Interrelationships among Secondary, Phenotypic, and Genotypic Classification Systems[a]

Elevated Lipoprotein Class[b]	Phenotype[b]	Genotype	Secondary Disorders
Chylomicrons	I	Familial lipoprotein lipase deficiency, other	Dysglobulinemias, uncontrolled diabetes mellitus, hypothyroidism
LDL	IIa	Familial hypercholesterolemia, familial combined hyperlipidemia, polygenic hypercholesterolemia	Nephrotic syndrome, hypothyroidism, dysglobulinemias, Cushing's syndrome, exogenous steroids, diuretics, acute intermittent porphyria, excessive dietary cholesterol and saturated fat, hepatoma
LDL and VLDL	IIb	Familial combined hyperlipidemia, familial hypercholesterolemia	Nephrotic syndrome, dysglobulinemias, Cushing's syndrome, exogenous steroids, diuretics, stress-induced, excessive dietary cholesterol and saturated fat
βVLDL, IDL	III	Familial dysbetalipoproteinemia, unclassified	Hypothyroidism, dysglobulinemias, diabetic ketoacidosis
VLDL	IV	Familial hypertriglyceridemia, familial combined hyperlipidemia, sporadic hypertriglyceridemia, Tangier disease	Obesity, poorly controlled diabetes mellitus, dysglobulinemia, chronic renal failure, dialysis, contraceptive steroids, alcohol, exogenous steroids, diuretics, Cushing's syndrome, estrogen use, nephrotic syndrome, hypopituitarism, glycogen storage disease (type I)
VLDL and chylomicrons	V	Familial hypertriglyceridemia, familial lipoprotein lipase deficiency (during pregnancy)	Same as for Phenotype IV
Abnormal lamellar lipoproteins causing increased total cholesterol	—	Familial LCAT deficiency	Cholestasis (with lipoprotein X), hepatic failure (with lamellar HDL)

[a] Adapted from R. J. Havel et al.: Lipoproteins and lipid transport. In Metabolic Control and Disease, edited by P. K. Bondy and L. E. Rosenberg, W. B. Saunders, Philadelphia, 1980.
[b] Most common patterns.

PROBLEMS OF CLASSIFICATION

There are three major problems with the present classification systems:

1. They do not use HDL cholesterol level, which is a strong predictor of CHD.
2. They are not based upon an understanding of lipid metabolism or of its pathogenetic significance.
3. Their clinical usefulness is limited.

While it is important for therapy to be able to distinguish primary from secondary hyperlipidemia, it is *possible* to identify adequately and to manage most individuals with abnormal lipid patterns *without* typing them, either genotypically or phenotypically. Knowledge of the genotype, however, is essential for genetic counseling. Furthermore, an understanding of the phenotypic and genotypic classifications is a prerequisite for following therapeutic and other advances in the field, since this terminology is used in much of the clinical literature.

Pathophysiology

The pathophysiologic mechanisms underlying the various primary and secondary hyperlipidemias are as yet incompletely understood.

Familial hyperchylomicronemia (type I) is a rare autosomal recessive disorder in which persistent or recurrent hyperchylomicronemia (fasting and postabsorptive) results from a marked deficiency in activity of the enzyme lipoprotein lipase (LPL).

Derangements of LDL receptor or postreceptor function are responsible for certain hypercholesterolemic disorders. Fibroblasts (and other cell types) from patients with *familial monogenic homozygous hypercholesterolemia (type IIa)* have been studied *in vitro* and several LDL receptor abnormalities have been found (2). As a result of these abnormalities, LDL catabolism is severely impaired, and is dependent to variable extents on the receptor-independent scavenger mechanisms (see "Physiology of Lipid and Lipoprotein Transport"). LDL receptor function is decreased to a lesser extent in cells from patients or relatives heterozygous for this disorder.

Familial dysbetalipoproteinemia (type III) is associated with accumulation of an abnormal lipoprotein, β-VLDL (which is probably an abnormal VLDL remnant), the circulatory removal of which is impaired.

The pathogenesis of *primary endogenous hypertriglyceridemia (type IV)* is poorly understood. Many

Table 72.7
Hyperlipidemia Phenotypes and Associated Clinical Manifestations

Type	Prevalence	Cholesterol	Triglyceride	Plasma[a]	Ultracentrifugation	Electrophoresis	Age of Onset (Primary Form)	Xanthomas[b]	Other Clinical Manifestations
I	Rare	↑	↑↑	Clear plasma, creamy supernatant	↑↑ Chylomicrons	Chylomicrons	Infancy or childhood	Eruptive, tubero-eruptive	Recurrent abdominal pain, other GI symptoms, lipemia retinalis, hepatosplenomegaly
IIa	Common	↑↑	→	Clear	↑↑ LDL	↑↑ β	Childhood for homozygous FHC,[c] late childhood to middle age for heterozygous FHC, adulthood for others	Tendinous, xanthelasma, tuberous; planar (homozygous)	Premature CHD, arcus corneae, aortic stenosis (homozygous FHC), arthritic symptoms
IIb	Common	↑↑	↑	Clear	↑↑ LDL, ↑ VLDL	↑↑ β, ↑ pre β			
III	Rare to uncommon	↑	↑ or ↑↑	Slightly turbid	↑ VLDL, ↑ IDL, (↓ LDL) (↓ HDL)	Broad β	Adulthood (occasionally late adolescence)	Planar (especially palmar), tuberous, tendinous	Premature CHD and peripheral vascular disease, male > female, obesity, abnormal glucose tolerance, hyperuricemia, aggravated by hypothyroidism, good response to therapy
IV	Most common	– or ↑[d]	↑↑	Turbid	↑↑ VLDL	↑↑ pre β	Early to late adulthood	Usually none; rarely eruptive, or tuberoeruptive	CHD and peripheral vascular disease, obesity, abnormal glucose tolerance, hyperuricemia, arthritic symptoms, gall bladder disease
V	Uncommon	↑	↑↑	Turbid plasma, creamy supernatant	↑↑ Chylomicrons, ↑↑ VLDL	↑↑ Chylomicrons, ↑↑ pre β	Childhood to middle age, usually adulthood	Eruptive, tubero-eruptive	Recurrent abdominal pain, other gastrointestinal symptoms, lipemia retinalis, hepatosplenomegaly, peripheral paresthesias, abnormal glucose tolerance, hyperuricemia

[a] Plasma obtained after 12 hr of fasting, left undisturbed in refrigerator overnight.
[b] Seen only in a minority of patients, but the frequency increases as plasma lipid levels rise.
[c] FHC, familial hypercholesterolemia.
[d] Cholesterol normal if triglycerides < 400 mg/dl.

Table 72.8
Genotypic Classification

MONOGENIC
  Familial hypercholesterolemia—presents as IIa > IIb, autosomal dominant, 0.1–0.5% estimated gene frequency
  Familial hypertriglyceridemia—presents as IV (rarely V), autosomal dominant, 1% estimated gene frequency
  Familial combined hyperlipidemia (familial multiple lipoprotein type hyperlipidemia)—presents as IIa, IIb, or IV (rarely V), autosomal dominant, 1.5% estimated gene frequency
  Familial lipoprotein lipase deficiency—presents as I, autosomal recessive, rare
  Familial dysbetalipoproteinemia—presents as III > IV, genetics uncertain, rare
POLYGENIC
  Polygenic—presents as IIa > IIb or IV, more common than monogenic forms
SPORADIC
  Sporadic—presents as IV > IIa or IIb, no hereditary pattern demonstrated, more common than monogenic forms
UNCLASSIFIED

studies have failed to account for the effects of obesity *per se* on VLDL-triglyceride metabolism, or to distinguish among genetic and various nongenetic primary endogenous hypertriglyceridemias, or between endogenous and mixed hyperlipidemias. In most patients, hypertriglyceridemia results from increased hepatic production of VLDL and triglycerides, while in others, decreased extrahepatic VLDL-triglyceride catabolism is responsible.

In patients with *type V hyperlipoproteinemia*, the relative roles of derangements in VLDL production and catabolism, as well as of triglyceride metabolism, remain speculative. Although postheparin LPL activity (a standard test) has been shown to be normal in such patients, deficiency of an LPL cofactor has been demonstrated, suggesting that enzyme function may not be normal.

In patients with *insulin-dependent diabetes mellitus (IDDM)* and acute diabetic ketoacidosis, increased plasma triglyceride levels result primarily from enhanced hepatic production of VLDL and triglycerides. In patients with chronic, poorly controlled IDDM, hypertriglyceridemia results primarily from reduced extrahepatic lipolysis of triglyceride-rich lipoproteins, and from decreased fatty acid storage in adipose tissue.

Although clinically significant hypertriglyceridemia after *alcohol ingestion* occurs most often in patients with underlying primary hypertriglyceridemia, modest alcohol-related elevations of plasma triglycerides can occur transiently in any individual. Hyperlipidemia leads to pancreatitis in a substantial number of alcoholic patients, but it has not been established that the reverse sequence occurs. The mechanisms for, and significance of, increased plasma HDL levels after acute or chronic alcohol use are not known.

Exogenous estrogens increase hepatic production of VLDL and triglycerides and, to a lesser extent, their rate of removal by extrahepatic tissues. The result is elevation of plasma triglyceride levels by as much as 25% to 50%. HDL levels are also increased. These effects can be prevented somewhat by combining (e.g., in oral contraceptives) the estrogen with certain progestational agents.

Primary hypothyroidism is associated with several defects in lipoprotein catabolism, including impaired LDL-receptor function. As a result, total and LDL cholesterol levels are elevated, as are levels of IDL and β-VLDL. This latter anomaly can mimic that found in patients with familial dysbetalipoproteinemia.

In patients with *chronic renal failure*, including those on maintenance hemodialysis, VLDL levels are elevated, while LDL levels are normal, and HDL levels are low. Decreased LPL activity and insulin resistance are important factors promoting the VLDL abnormality. The relationship between altered VLDL and HDL levels and the accelerated atherogenesis that occurs in some of these patients is not understood.

Abnormal lipid/lipoprotein patterns that are found in patients with certain other forms of secondary hyperlipidemia are illustrated in Table 72.6.

Clinical Manifestations

Adverse clinical sequelae of hyperlipidemic states are manifest most often by disorders of the vascular, dermatologic, and gastrointestinal systems. The relationships between phenotypic classifications and clinical manifestations are outlined in Table 72.7.

VASCULAR
As discussed previously, elevated levels of plasma LDL cholesterol, manifest usually as hypercholesterolemia (i.e., elevated plasma total cholesterol), and subnormal levels of HDL cholesterol, are independent risk factors for the subsequent development of CHD. The earlier the onset of symptomatic CHD, the more likely it is that a lipid abnormality is present. In the most severe form of hypercholesterolemia, homozygous monogenic familial hypercholesterolemia, CHD usually develops in childhood and very few patients survive past age 30. In the heterozygous monogenic form, clinical cardiac disease usually develops any time from late childhood to middle age (average age: 40 years in men; 50 years in women). While hypertriglyceridemia and elevated VLDL do not independently predict the development of CHD, this lipid pattern is frequently seen in patients with CHD and peripheral vascular disease. The rare primary disorder, familial dysbetalipoproteinemia (type III), also seems to be associated with a high incidence of CHD and peripheral vascular disease, and may be especially amenable to therapy. Fasting chylomicronemia has not been shown to be associated with increased risk for the development of CHD.

DERMATOLOGIC

Xanthomas may occur in all the hyperlipidemias; however, they are present in a minority of hyperlipidemic individuals. They occur with increasing frequency as the plasma lipid levels rise. They are cutaneous and/or subcutaneous papules, plaques, or nodules characterized histopathologically by localized collections of lipid-laden histiocytes (foam cells). The presence or absence of xanthomas should always be noted. If present, their appearance (see below) can provide useful information about the nature of the underlying lipid disorder (Table 72.7). Unless tendons (especially the Achilles tendon) are palpated, tendon thickening characteristic of tendon xanthomas may be missed. Xanthomas are divided morphologically into several types:

1. *Tendinous* (Fig. 72.2A)—firm subcutaneous masses, which arise in tendons and occasionally in ligaments, fascia, or periosteum. They characteristically move in concert with the associated tendon, and can appear as diffuse thickenings of the tendon. They most often occur on the Achilles tendons and the extensor tendons of the hands, knees, and elbows. The overlying skin is normal in color.

2. *Tuberous* (Fig. 72.2, *B* and *C*)—soft cutaneous and subcutaneous nodules which may harden with age and increasing fibrosis. Occasionally, they occur as superficial extensions of tendon xanthomas. They can also form from the confluence of eruptive xanthomas, an intermediate stage being called *tuberoeruptive* xanthomas. They occur most often on extensor surfaces and areas subjected to trauma, such as the elbows, knees, dorsa of the hands, heels, and buttocks. The overlying epidermis can be normal in color or have a yellow or orange hue.

3. *Eruptive* (Fig. 72.2, *D* and *F*)—small (1 to 4 mm) cutaneous papules, which tend to appear in crops, often coincident with an abrupt rise in plasma triglyceride levels. Compared to the other types of xanthomas, they contain more inflammatory cells, free fatty acids, and triglycerides and fewer foam cells and cholesterol esters. They most often occur over pressure areas, such as the buttocks, parts of the trunk, elbows, and knees. They often have a yellow center and red halo.

4. *Planar* (Fig. 72.2, *E, G, H*)—flat, slightly elevated cutaneous lesions, which occur most often in skin folds and scars, but can be more widely distributed. When present on the eyelids, they are called *xanthelasma*. When located on the palms, they are called palmar xanthomas, and when confined to the palmar creases, *xanthoma striata palmaris*. They tend to be yellow or yellow-brown.

Hypercholesterolemia is associated with tendinous, planar, and tuberous xanthomas. Severe hypertriglyceridemia and chylomicronemia are associated with eruptive, and occasionally tuberoeruptive or tuberous xanthomas. Palmar xanthomas are char-acteristic of familial dysbetalipoproteinemia and florid obstructive liver disease. Planar xanthomas on the body or palms in the presence of a type II lipid profile suggest homozygous monogenic familial hypercholesterolemia. The presence of tendinous or tuberous xanthomas or premature xanthelasma with a type II lipid profile suggests either heterozygous or homozygous monogenic familial hypercholesterolemia, as opposed to the polygenic or nongenetic forms. Tendon xanthomas are found in one-third to one-half of heterozygotes. The usual relationships between phenotype and xanthoma type are outlined in Table 72.7.

Occasionally, xanthomas appear in the absence of a hyperlipidemic state. For example, xanthelasma occur commonly in normolipidemic older individuals and in nonwhites, whereas planar xanthomas can occur in patients with lymphoma, leukemia, or myeloma.

Differences exist in the responses to treatment of the various hyperlipidemia-associated xanthomas. Thus, tendon xanthomas are the most resistant to treatment and, in practice, seldom disappear. In contrast, eruptive and planar xanthomas can disappear within a few weeks after return of plasma lipid levels toward normal.

GASTROINTESTINAL

As many as 35% to 55% of patients with fasting chylomicronemia experience episodes of recurrent abdominal pain. Symptoms are ordinarily associated with marked elevations of plasma triglyceride levels (greater than 1000 to 2000 mg/dl). Abdominal pain may be so severe that it prompts unnecessary surgery, particularly if the lipid disorder is not suspected. The pain is often associated with pancreatitis, although the responsible pathogenetic mechanism is not well understood. It should be noted that routine serum amylase determinations are frequently subject to technical artifact when hyperlipidemia is present, due to the presence of an amylase-inhibiting factor which may or may not be triglyceride. In such cases, a more reliable estimate of the serum amylase value can be obtained by determining amylase levels on serial dilutions, until the value obtained no longer changes with further dilution. Another cause of abdominal pain may be rapid hepatic or splenic enlargement with capsular distension. Often the cause is unclear. Gastrointestinal symptoms other than abdominal pain, such as nausea, vomiting, borborygmi, and diarrhea also occur.

Other Clinical Associations

Other clinical concomitants of hyperlipidemia include the following: premature arcus corneae (grayish white corneal ring due to lipid droplets) in hypercholesterolemia (elevated LDL); aortic stenosis in homozygous monogenic familial hypercholesterolemia; achilles tendonitis in heterozygous monogenic

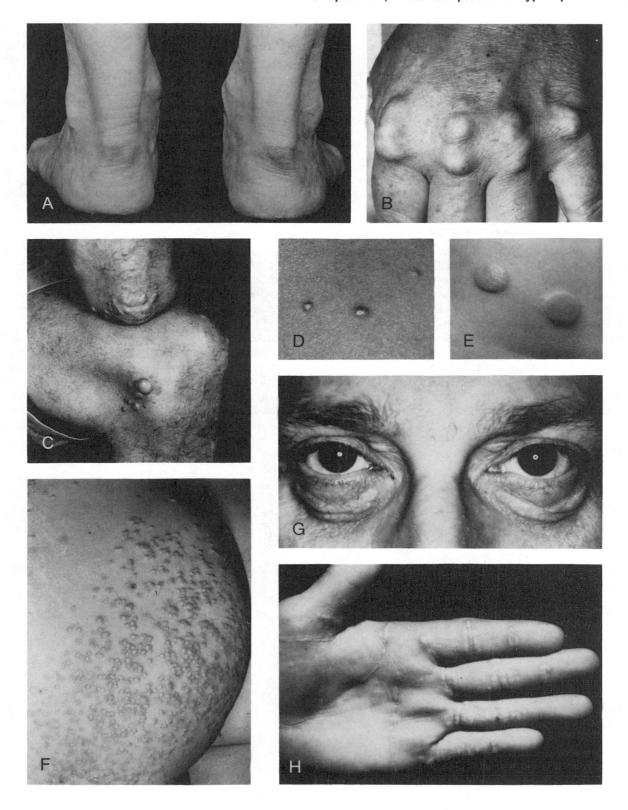

Figure 72.2   Dermatologic manifestations of lipid disorders. (*A*) tendinous xanthomas, (*B*) tuberous xanthomas, (*C*) tuberous xanthomas, (*D*) eruptive xanthomas, (*E*) planar xanthomas, (*F*) eruptive xanthomas, (*G*) planar xanthoma on eyelids (xanthelasma), and (*H*) planar xanthomas confined to palm creases (xanthoma striata palmaris).

familial hypercholesterolemia; obesity, glucose intolerance, hyperinsulinemia, hyperuricemia, and perhaps cholelithiasis in association with hypertriglyceridemia and elevated VLDL; recurrent polyarthralgias, arthritis, tenosynovitis, and sicca-like syndromes in hypertriglyceridemia (elevated VLDL) or hypercholesterolemia (elevated LDL); lipemia retinalis (cream colored retinal vessels) in chylomicronemia (evident when plasma triglycerides rise above 3,000 mg/dl, obvious when they exceed 10,000 mg/dl).

EVALUATION AND MANAGEMENT

Indications for Evaluation

Determination of plasma lipid levels is recommended in two situations: (a) For the development of a data base in young or middle-aged adults. It could be argued that this is not necessary until it has been unequivocally demonstrated that the correction of an identified abnormality improves the associated increased health risks. Nevertheless, a screening determination of plasma total (or LDL) cholesterol and, if a reliable laboratory is available, an HDL cholesterol is recommended because the physician will gain valuable prognostic information about the patient which will influence the general management of that individual. For example, interventions which are known to affect plasma lipid levels adversely (Table 72.5) might be avoided and the management of other clearly treatable CHD risk factors (such as cigarette smoking or hypertension) might be more aggressively pursued. (b) To provide a data base in patients at increased risk of having a lipid disorder: Thus, a personal or family history of atherosclerotic disease (especially if premature), a family history of hyperlipidemia, a nonreversible cause of secondary hyperlipidemia (Table 72.5), the chronic use of agents known to affect plasma lipid levels adversely (Table 72.5), or the observation of symptoms or physical findings associated with hyperlipidemic states (see above and Table 72.7) should all prompt further evaluation.

Laboratory Testing for Lipid Disorders

Determination of plasma levels of total and HDL cholesterol (not affected by recent dietary intake), triglycerides (requires a 12-hour fast), and observation of plasma which has been refrigerated overnight (requires a 12-hour fast) (Fig. 72.3) are suggested. Determinations should always be repeated once or twice to ensure reliability. This is especially true of plasma HDL levels, because there is a relatively narrow range of normal values making even small differences in levels prognostically important, and because HDL cholesterol is currently determined in

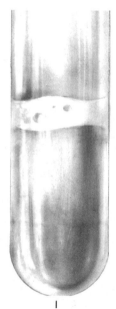 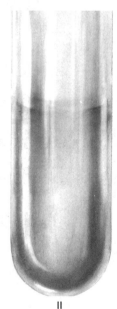 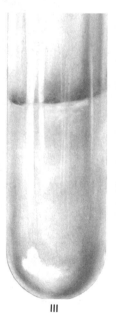 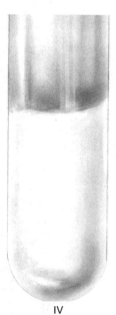 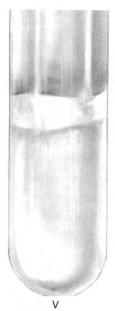

I	II	III	IV	V
Increased levels of triglycerides associated with ↑ chylomicrons (very VLDL)	Increased levels of total LDL cholesterol	Increased levels of cholesterol and triglyceride associated with abnormally migrating VLDL and IDL	Increased levels of triclycerides associated with ↑ VLDL	Increased levels of triglycerides associated with both ↑ VLDL and ↑ chylomicrons
Creamy Supernatant on top of clear plasma	Normal appearance clear plasma	Slight uniform turbidity	Uniform turbidity	Uniform turbidity and creamy supernatant

Figure 72.3 Appearance of plasma in various hyperlipidemia states. (Plasma obtained after 12 hours of fasting, left undisturbed in a refrigerator overnight.)

clinical laboratories by a method that is not entirely reliable. When triglyceride concentration is high (greater than 400 mg/dl), the plasma should be ultrafiltered to remove VLDL which interferes with the test; the physician should ask the laboratory about the preparation in such circumstances. The HDL cholesterol levels should always be measured before embarking upon specific hypocholesterolemic therapy; a mildly elevated plasma total cholesterol level due to a high plasma HDL cholesterol does not require treatment.

When chylomicronemia is suspected and plasma triglyceride levels exceed 400 mg/dl, but the standing plasma test is negative, lipoprotein electrophoresis provides a more sensitive means for detecting chylomicrons.

Evaluation of the plasma lipids should generally be delayed until 12 weeks after myocardial infarction, sepsis, or burns since lipid levels can be transiently altered by these acute events.

In patients with elevated fasting triglyceride levels and turbid plasma (elevated VLDL), baseline fasting glucose and uric acid levels may be useful because of the frequency of carbohydrate intolerance and hyperuricemia.

Therapy

When hyperlipidemia is diagnosed (plasma lipid levels above the 95th percentile for the appropriate sex, age, and race), secondary causes should be identified (Table 72.5) and treated. If the secondary hyperlipidemia is not reversible or primary hyperlipidemia exists, appropriate diet therapy should be instituted.

The aim of therapy is to achieve and maintain lipid levels in the normal range.

DIET (Table 72.9)

It is now well-established that plasma lipid levels can be altered by dietary manipulations. Under controlled conditions (such as in a metabolic unit), plasma levels of total (or LDL) cholesterol may be reduced by 30% or more and of triglyceride or VLDL by as much as 80% or more. Fasting chylomicronemia can also be eliminated. Under ambulatory conditions, where diets tend to be less restrictive and noncompliance more common, reductions in lipid levels are less dramatic. For example, among prospective studies of cholesterol lowering diets, the decrease in plasma cholesterol averaged 15.6% (range 8.5 to 22%).

Cholesterol Lowering Diets (Table 72.9). Diets designed to lower plasma cholesterol levels are characterized by a restriction of *dietary cholesterol* to 100 to 300 mg per day and a reduction of *saturated fat intake,* with or without a marked increase in dietary *polyunsaturated* fat. Restrictions in dietary cholesterol and saturated fats independently contribute to the reduction in plasma cholesterol levels. An increase in dietary polyunsaturated fat will result in

Table 72.9
Dietary Treatment of Hyperlipidemia[a]

HYPERCHOLESTEROLEMIA (↑ LDL CHOLESTEROL)
1. Cholesterol restriction (100–300 mg/day)
2. Reduction in saturated fat to <10% of total calories
3. Increase in polyunsaturated fats (see text)

The above objectives may be achieved by monitoring the following foods:

Foods to limit (partial list): meat, especially non-lean and organ meat; shellfish (high in cholesterol, low in fat); fat; egg yolk; cream; whole milk; butter; ice cream; most cheeses; artichoke; avocado; coconut; cocoa butter; palm oil

Foods allowed (partial list): fish; deskinned chicken; egg white and egg substitutes; skim milk, sherbet; cottage cheese; yogurt made from skim milk; vegetable oil (especially safflower and corn oil); vegetable margarines; vegetables other than those listed above

HYPERTRIGLYCERIDEMIA (↑ VLDL)
1. Loss of excess weight (total calories restricted)
2. Alcohol restriction, if needed
3. Low cholesterol, low saturated fat, increased polyunsaturated fat diet, if needed

CHYLOMICRONEMIA
1. Fat restriction (5–20% of total calories)
2. Medium chain triglycerides allowed (see text)
3. Vegetable fat (5 g) to supply essential fatty acids
4. Loss of excess weight and elimination of alcohol are indicated when plasma VLDL triglyceride elevations accompany the chylomicronemia (see text)

Note: Shellfish (high in cholesterol but low in fat) are allowed

---

[a] Practical booklets for both physicians and patients are available at no cost from the Lipid Metabolism Branch, National Institutes of Health (see "When to Obtain Consultation" (p. 768)). There is also much useful information in Rifkind and Levy (see "General References"). Since a fat restricted diet can be complex, consultation with a dietician is usually required.

further, though less marked, plasma cholesterol reduction. The influence of dietary fiber on plasma cholesterol levels is complex and controversial, so that no definitive recommendations can be made at present regarding optimal dietary fiber content in a hypocholesterolemic diet.

The typical North American diet has a polyunsaturated:saturated fat (P:S) ratio of 0.4. The diet recommended by the American Heart Association (1) as a preventive measure for the entire population would reduce cholesterol intake to less than 300 mg/day, decrease total fat intake from 40% to 30 to 35% of total calories, reduce saturated fats to less than 10%, and increase polyunsaturated fats to as high as 10% of total calories. The P:S ratio of such a diet would be about 1.0.

Little information exists on the effects of widespread or prolonged use of diets rich in polyunsaturated fats (e.g., P:S ratio ≥1.5). However, it appears that such diets can promote formation of lithogenic bile and actually can increase the incidence of symptomatic biliary tract disease. Although data from a single study suggested that such diets are associated with an increased risk of malignant disease (12), this finding was not supported when data from several trials were pooled (3). However, the relationship between cholesterol level and cancer risk remains an open question, as emphasized by the recent report of an adverse association between serum cholesterol level and incidence of colon cancer in men in the Framingham Study (18).

Maximal effect of a hypocholesterolemic diet usually occurs within 6 weeks. Clinical observations suggest that patients with monogenic familial hypercholesterolemia (especially the homozygotes) respond less well to dietary therapy than do patients with polygenic or nonhereditary forms of hypercholesterolemia.

The effect of cholesterol-lowering diets on HDL cholesterol levels is of great interest, but remains poorly understood. Interestingly, individuals who consume modest amounts of alcohol regularly have higher HDL cholesterol levels than those who do not. However, immoderate daily alcohol consumption should not be recommended because of its numerous well-known adverse effects, because it sometimes raises plasma triglyceride levels, and because of the lack of evidence demonstrating a role for it in the prevention of CHD. The benefits *versus* risks of modest regular alcohol consumption are unknown.

Triglyceride Lowering Diets. Diets designed to reduce plasma triglyceride and VLDL levels emphasize the loss of excess weight by total caloric restriction. Plasma triglyceride levels usually fall, often to normal, after a few days of caloric restriction. The reduction is maintained as long as weight loss continues at a rate of 1 to 2 lb (0.5 to 1 kg) per week. If normal weight is attained and maintained, further therapy may not be necessary. If hypertriglyceridemia persists or occurs in individuals of normal weight, a cholesterol-lowering diet, as outlined above, may be effective. Alcohol intake should be restricted since it can cause a striking rise in triglyceride levels in some patients with hypertriglyceridemia. Although extreme increases in the carbohydrate content of a diet can cause transient and, rarely, sustained hypertriglyceridemia, there is no firm evidence to suggest that total carbohydrate restriction is helpful in the treatment of hypertriglyceridemia. There is conflicting evidence regarding the effect on the plasma triglyceride level of excessive intake of sucrose (common sugar); its role, if any, in glucose-tolerant individuals is of much smaller magnitude than that of dietary fat. The rationale for dietary restriction of simple sugars is based mainly upon the need to avoid excess caloric intake (and to prevent dental caries) and not upon any direct effect of these substances on plasma lipids. Obesity is inversely correlated with HDL cholesterol levels; moreover, there is evidence to suggest that plasma HDL cholesterol levels rise during weight reduction.

Chylomicron Reduction. Treatment of fasting chylomicronemia (type I) involves the restriction of dietary fat intake to 5 to 20% of total calories (0.5 g of fat/kg body weight is a reasonable starting point). The fat deficit should be corrected predominantly by substitution of complex carbohydrates. Since medium chain triglycerides are transported directly from the intestine to the liver in the portal circulation without incorporation into chylomicrons, they (available as MCT oil) may be added to the diet to enhance its palatability. Five grams of vegetable fat rich in polyunsaturates should be included to prevent essential fatty acid deficiency.

Dietary fat is severely restricted until fasting chylomicronemia is eliminated and clinical symptoms prevented or reduced in frequency; dietary fat is then chronically restricted to whatever degree is necessary to prevent fasting chylomicronemia. The efficacy of fat restriction in preventing recurrent abdominal pain is supported by clinical observations of individual patients.

When fasting chylomicronemia is accompanied by elevation of VLDL triglyceride (type V), therapy is initiated with a triglyceride-lowering diet. Severe restriction of dietary fat is required only when hypertriglyceridemia is marked and abdominal symptoms are present. A modest reduction of fat intake to approximately 30% of total calories is all that is required in the asymptomatic patient. Elimination of alcohol is often very effective.

Efficacy of Diet Therapy in the Prevention of CHD. Although the clinical efficacy of cholesterol-lowering diets in the prevention and reversal of CHD has been clearly demonstrated in animals and suggested by epidemiologic observations in man (14), dietary trials in humans have given varied results, probably because of methodologic problems.

DRUGS

In general, drug treatment is recommended only after an initial 6-week to 3-month trial of diet therapy has proved unsuccessful. Moreover, diet therapy should be continued during drug treatment since the effects of each are often additive. Because of the need for chronic therapy, the risks of toxicity, and the uncertain benefits of drug treatment, careful deliberation is required before embarking upon the long term use of any hypolipidemic drug.

Although various pharmacologic agents have been reported to lower levels of total cholesterol and total triglycerides by as much as 40% and 80%, respectively, in most clinical trials the actual reductions in mean levels of these lipids were considerably less. The response to therapy varies with the lipid disorder being treated, patient compliance, the baseline level of plasma cholesterol or triglyceride (the higher the starting level, the greater the percentage reduction), and probably with other ill-defined factors. Patients with homozygous monogenic familial hypercholes-

Table 72.10
Lipid-Lowering Drugs

BILE ACID SEQUESTERING RESINS—(Cholestyramine, colestipol)
Mechanism: Anion exchange resins which bind bile acids, resulting in increased hepatic synthesis of cholesterol and bile acids, increased fecal excretion of cholesterol, and usually a net reduction of plasma cholesterol levels.
Efficacy: Decreases total and LDL cholesterol up to 25–40% (onset 4–7 days, maximal effect within 2 weeks).
Pharmacokinetics: Not absorbed, but may bind other drugs (*e.g.*, thiazides, digitalis preparations, anticoagulants, phenobarbital, thyroxine, phenylbutazone, iron)
Side effects: (a) *Common*—unpleasant sandy/gritty preparations, gastrointestinal (G.I.) (constipation, nausea, abdominal discomfort, flatulence, etc.), lowered serum folate levels; (b) *uncommon*—G.I. (steatorrhea), hyperchloremic acidosis (small patients on high doses), fat-soluble vitamin deficiency; (c) *possible*—(?)increased risk of cholelithiasis
Administration: (a) cholestyramine—12–32 g/day, given b.i.d. to q.i.d. before or during meals; supplied as Questran 9-g packets each containing 4 g of active drug; (b) colestipol—15–30 g/day, given b.i.d. to q.i.d. before or during meals; supplied as Colestid in 5-g packets or 500-g bottles
Preparations should be taken in water or juice. Other medicines should be taken 1 hr before or 4 hr after dosage. Monitor serum folate levels and consider supplemental multivitamins with folic acid
Clinical use: Drugs of first choice in the treatment of hypercholesterolemia, because of their relative safety and efficacy
CLOFIBRATE (Atromid-S, 500 mg)
Mechanism: Not well understood, seems to increase the rate of intravascular catabolism of VLDL and IDL to LDL, may increase lipoprotein lipase activity
Efficacy: Decreases triglycerides/VLDL within 2–5 days (mean reduction 22% in Coronary Drug Project, up to 80% reduction in some patients), may decrease or increase LDL cholesterol (mean decrease in total cholesterol of 6% in Coronary Drug Project), reduces IDL in type III
Pharmacokinetics: Completely absorbed; peak concentration within 4 hr; metabolized in liver and excreted in urine; elimination divided into two kinetic phases, the slower with a half-life of 12–

15 hr; may enhance the action of oral anticoagulants, phenytoin, oral hypoglycemic agents, and furosemide by displacing them from plasma albumin binding sites.
Side effects: (a) *Usually*—well tolerated; (b) *occasional*—2–3-fold increase in the incidence of cholelithiasis; other G.I. (nausea, diarrhea, weight gain); reduced libido, impotence; unusual flu-like syndrome; (c) *uncommon*—rash, alopecia, breast tenderness, reversible abnormality in liver function, hepatomegaly, etc.; (d) *unknown*—(?)thromboembolism, (?)intermittent claudication, (?)arrhythmia, (?)neoplasia
Administration: 2g/day, given in 2–3 divided doses
Clinical use: Drug of choice in the treatment of elevated VLDL triglyceride; of particular utility in Type III. Use with caution in the presence of hepatic or renal insufficiency
NICOTINIC ACID (such as Nicobid (time-released), 125, 250 or 500 mg, or Nicolar, 500 mg)
Mechanism: Diverse effects on lipid metabolism including: decreased hepatic synthesis of VLDL, increased synthesis of HDL, inhibition of lipolysis in adipose tissue, increase in lipase activity
Efficacy: Decreases VLDL triglycerides within 1–4 days (mean 26% in Coronary Drug Project, range up to 80% depending on pretreatment levels); decreases LDL cholesterol, onset 5–7 days, maximal effect 3–5 weeks (mean decrease 10% in Coronary Drug Project, range up to 30%)
Pharmacokinetics: Well absorbed p.o.; in the high doses used it is partially metabolized in liver and partially excreted unchanged in urine; plasma half-life is about 45 min
Side effects: (a) *Common*—cutaneous flushing and pruritis, which diminish after several weeks of therapy; G.I. (nausea, diarrhea, abdominal pain, abnormal liver function); (b) *less common*—dermatologic disorders (*e.g.*, increased pigmentation); activation of peptic ulcer; arrhythmia; gout; urinary frequency and dysuria; glucose intolerance, etc.
Administration: Gradual increase over 1–3 weeks from 300 mg/day to 2–9 g/day; given in t.i.d. dosage; give with meals to diminish side effects
Clinical use: Second-line drug (because of side effects) in the treatment of elevated LDL cholesterol or VLDL triglyceride

terolemia may respond less well to treatment with drugs or diet than do patients with heterozygous monogenic, polygenic, or nonhereditary hypercholesterolemia. A recent study has shown that the combination of colestipol and nicotinic acid holds therapeutic promise for normalizing LDL cholesterol levels in patients with heterozygous familial hypercholesterolemia (7).

Clinically useful information pertinent to the most commonly prescribed lipid-lowering drugs (cholestyramine, colestipol, clofibrate, and nicotinic acid) is provided in Table 72.10. The usefulness of these drugs in the treatment of the different types of hyperlipidemia is outlined in Table 72.11. The use of other drugs by the primary physician is not recommended, either because of a general lack of experience in their use and the potential for long term toxicity, or because of demonstrated toxicity.

Efficacy of Drug Therapy in the Prevention of CHD. The clinical trials of hypolipidemic drug therapy, on the whole, have been larger, better designed, and more recently executed than the diet trials, but again, the results have been promising, yet inconclusive.

Table 72.11
Drug Treatment of Hyperlipidemia

HYPERCHOLESTEROLEMIA (↑ LDL Cholesterol) (Types IIa, IIb)

First line:	Cholestyramine or colestipol
Second line:	Clofibrate, nicotinic acid
Third line[a]:	Probucol, neomycin, others

HYPERTRIGLYCERIDEMIA (↑ VLDL, ↑ IDL) (Type III, IV, V, IIb)

First line:	Clofibrate
Second line:	Nicotinic acid

CHYLOMICRONEMIA (↑ TG in Chylomicrons) (Type I)
No effective drug therapy

[a] These drugs should be used only in consultation with a medical specialist in lipid disorders.

Most of the methodologic problems of previous studies have been obviated by the design of the Lipid Research Clinics Coronary Primary Prevention Trial which is in progress (9).

EXERCISE

Evidence has accumulated over the past decade that regular isotonic exercise favorably affects plasma lipid levels. Most of the exercise programs which have been evaluated, including jogging, rapid walking, swimming, bicycling, cross-country skiing, and mountain climbing have involved 30 min or more of continued effort at 70 to 85% of maximal heart rate at least 3 times weekly. HDL cholesterol levels have fairly consistently been shown to rise (approximately 20%) and triglyceride levels to fall (approximately 25%) with exercise.

It is currently unknown whether regular exercise programs can prevent or retard the development of vascular disease.

SMOKING

HDL cholesterol levels have been found to be lower in people who smoke cigarettes than in nonsmokers or exsmokers. Moreover, an inverse relationship exists between the number of cigarettes smoked daily and the level of HDL cholesterol. Smoking cessation has been associated with a modest rise in plasma HDL level. It is not known what proportion of the increased risk of CHD associated with smoking is mediated through alteration in the plasma lipids or via other mechanisms. There is, however, substantial evidence that smoking cessation reduces CHD risk.

OTHER

Bolder forms of therapy (such as ileal bypass, portacaval shunt, plasma exchange, or extracorporeal hemoperfusion) exist for the severely hypercholesterolemic patient who is resistant or only partially responsive to diet, exercise, and lipid-lowering drugs. However, these therapies should be considered experimental and should be carried out only in consultation with a specialist in lipid disorders.

WHEN TO OBTAIN CONSULTATION

Consultations with a specialist in lipid disorders should be obtained when:

1. Lipid levels are *inadequately controlled* after treatment of secondary causes and after diet and initial drug therapy.

2. A *familial or monogenic form* of hyperlipidemia is suspected. The consultant can help with genetic screening, the use of third-line drugs, and the choice of more experimental forms of therapy when necessary. He may also be able to provide information on the reliability with which commercial laboratories in a given area measure plasma lipid levels.

The Lipid Metabolism Branch, National Heart, Lung and Blood Institute, National Institutes of Health, Bethesda, Maryland 20205, can provide the names of centers actively participating in the Lipid Research Clinics Program.

HEALTH MAINTENANCE ADVICE FOR INDIVIDUALS WITHOUT LIPID DISORDERS

Certain maneuvers that favorably alter plasma lipid levels and are safe can be recommended. *Smoking cessation*, which is of proven therapeutic efficacy in the prevention of lung cancer, chronic pulmonary disease, and CHD, and in the reduction of overall mortality, is associated with a modest rise in HDL cholesterol levels. *Regular isotonic exercise* raises HDL cholesterol levels and the HDL:LDL cholesterol ratio, and lowers plasma triglyceride levels. It also improves cardiovascular conditioning, serves an adjunctive role in weight control therapy, is inversely correlated with the frequency of CHD events, seems to increase the individual's sense of well-being, and may favorably affect resting blood pressure. *Avoidance of significant obesity* (i.e., greater than 20% to 30% above ideal body weight) by appropriate caloric intake and regular exercise should prevent hypertriglyceridemia, raise HDL cholesterol levels, and prevent or ameliorate numerous other complications as discussed elsewhere (see Chapter 73). General use of the *American Heart Association recommended diet* (1) (also available from regional American Heart Association offices), which consists of modest restrictions in cholesterol and saturated fat intake and a modest increase in polyunsaturated fat intake, should prove mildly hypocholesterolemic and could result in an overall reduction in the incidence and prevalence of CHD.

References

General

Ahrens, EH, Jr and Connor, WE (co-chairmen): Report of the task force on the evidence relating six dietary factors to the nation's health. *Am J Clin Nutr 32:* 2622, 1979.
   Comprehensive reviews of the role of dietary cholesterol, fat, carbohydrate, and alcohol in human disease.
Havel, RJ, Goldstein, JL and Brown, MS: Lipoproteins and lipid transport. In *Metabolic Control and Disease,* p. 393, edited by PK Bondy and LE Rosenberg. W. B. Saunders, Philadelphia, 1980.
   Comprehensive review of hyperlipidemic states, with major emphasis on lipid metabolism.
Kannel, WB, Castelli, WP and Gordon, T: Cholesterol in the prediction of atherosclerotic disease. New perspectives based on the Framingham Study. *Ann Intern Med 90:* 85, 1979.
   Review of the role of total, LDL and HDL cholesterol and triglyceride in the prediction of coronary heart disease.
Rifkind, BM and Levy, RI: *Hyperlipidemia, Diagnosis and Therapy.* Grune & Stratton, New York, 1977.
   Excellent, clinically oriented, well referenced text on hyperlipidemia.
Tyroler, HA (ed): Epidemiology of plasma high-density lipoprotein levels. The Lipid Research Clinics Prevalence Study. *Circulation 62*(suppl. IV): IV-1 to IV-136, 1980.
   Review of the role of HDL cholesterol as a predictor of atherosclerotic disease and of the environmental factors which affect HDL cholesterol levels. Includes data from the Lipid Research Clinics Prevalence Study.

Specific

1. AHA Committee Report: Diet and coronary heart disease. *Circulation 58:* 763, 1978.
2. Brown, MS and Goldstein, JL: Familial hypercholesterolemia: a genetic defect in the low-density lipoprotein receptor. *N Engl J Med 294:* 1386, 1976.
3. Ederer, F, Leren, P, Turpeinin, O and Frantz, ID, Jr: Cancer among men on cholesterol-lowering diets. *Lancet 2:* 203, 1971.

4. Glomset, JA: High density lipoproteins in human health and disease. *Adv Intern Med 25:* 91, 1980.
5. Goldstein, JL, Schrott, HG, Hazzard, WR, Bierman, EL and Motulsky, AG: Hyperlipidemia and coronary heart disease; II. Genetic analysis of lipid levels in 176 families and delineation of a new inherited disorder, combined hyperlipidemia. *J Clin Invest 52:* 1544, 1973.
6. Hulley, SB, Rosenman, RH, Bawol, RD and Brand, RJ: Epidemiology as a guide to clinical decisions. The association between triglyceride and coronary heart disease. *N Engl J Med 302:* 1383, 1980.
7. Kane, JP, Malloy, MJ, Tan, P, Phillips, NR, Freedman, DD, Williams, ML, Rowe, JS and Havel, RJ: Normalization of low-density-lipoprotein levels in heterozygous familial hypercholesterolemia with a combined drug regimen. *N Engl J Med 304:* 251, 1981.
8. Kannel, WB, Gordon, T and Dawber, TR: Role of lipids in the development of brain infarction: The Framingham Study. *Stroke 5:* 679, 1974.
9. Lipid Research Clinics Program: The coronary primary prevention trial: design and implementation. *J Chronic Dis 32:* 609, 1979.
10. Lipid Research Clinics Populations Studies Data Book: Volume I. The prevalence study. U.S. Department of Health and Human Services, Public Health Service, National Institutes of Health. NIH Publication No. 80-1527, 1980.
11. Motulsky, AG: The genetic hyperlipidemias. *N Engl J Med 294:* 823, 1976.
12. Pearce, ML and Dayton, S: Incidence of cancer in men on a diet high in polyunsaturated fat. *Lancet 1:* 464, 1971.
13. Shurtleff, D: Section 30. Some characteristics related to the incidence of cardiovascular disease and death. Framingham Study, 18-year follow-up. Part of WB Kannel and T Gordon: The Framingham Study: An Epidemiologic Investigation of Cardiovascular Disease. DHEW Publication No. (NIH) 74-599, 1974.
14. Stamler, J: Population studies. In *Nutrition, Lipids, and Coronary Heart Disease*, pp. 25–88, edited by R Levy, B Rifkind, B Dennis and N Ernst. Raven Press, New York, 1979.
15. Truett, J, Cornfield, J and Kannel, W: A multivariate analysis of the risk of coronary heart disease in Framingham. *J Chronic Dis 20:* 511, 1967.
16. Tyroler, HA, Glueck, CJ, Christensen, B and Kwiterovich, PO: Plasma high density lipoprotein cholesterol comparisons in black and white populations. *Circulation 62* (suppl. IV): IV-99, 1980.
17. Wilhelmsen, L, Wedel, H and Giosta, T: Multivariate analysis of risk factors for coronary heart disease. *Circulation 48:* 950, 1973.
18. Williams, RR, Sorlie, PD, Feinleib, M, McNamara, PM, Kannel, WB and Dawber, TR: Cancer incidence by levels of cholesterol. *JAMA 245:* 247, 1981.

CHAPTER SEVENTY-THREE

Obesity

MARC R. BLACKMAN, M.D.

Obesity, defined as an excess of total body fat, is one of the most prevalent chronic medical disorders in the world. Numerous complex, as yet ill-understood, interactions among predisposing genetic and environmental factors influence the initiation, development, and persistence of excess adiposity. Although mild obesity does not appear to increase mortality (1,16), in more obese patients, morbidity and mortality vary directly with the amount of excess body fat and the presence of certain associated medical and behavioral abnormalities. Evaluation and management should therefore be directed predominantly toward those individuals with persistent, symptomatic, significant obesity. Since the long term results of most treatment regimens have been poor, there is an urgent need to promote a variety of effective societal and individual approaches for prevention of excess adiposity.

DEFINITION

Obesity vs. Overweight

Obesity must be distinguished from overweight, which refers to an increase in body weight due to increased bone, muscle, or fat. Although the two terms are usually used synonymously, errors do occur in equating obesity with overweight, as for example in the muscular athlete with normal or decreased body fat. Since body composition and, in particular, body fat normally vary with age, sex, diet, physical activity, and population group, it is important to compare measurements of body fat in individual patients with those derived from appropriate control groups.

Methods for Quantifying Adiposity

Numerous methods exist for assessing and quantifying adiposity, but the simplest, most common, and most reliable clinical approaches involve either determination of relative weight or measurement of skin-fold thickness. In the former approach, a patient's weight is expressed as a percentage or ratio of ideal weight, such as that issued in the Metropolitan Life Insurance Company's Build and Blood Pressure Study of 1959 (17). Of the various indices of weight and height tested, the body mass index [weight/(height)^2] has the highest correlation with other measures of body fat (see Fig. 73.1). Although measurements of skin-fold thickness (using standardized calipers) are useful in assessing body fat in population studies, the technique is often less reliable in individual patients than are direct measurements of weight and height.

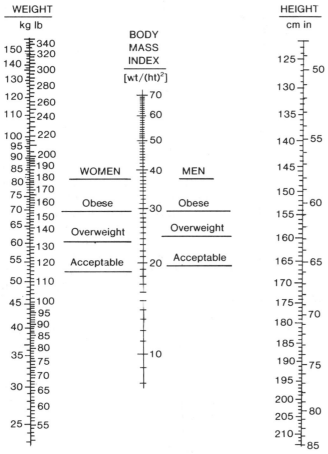

Figure 73.1   Nomogram for body mass index. (From G. A. Bray (ed): Obesity in America, DHEW Publication No. (NIH) 79–359, U.S. Government Printing Office, Washington, D.C., 1979.)

CLASSIFICATION

The heterogeneous nature and the many approaches to evaluation and management of the obesity syndromes have made classification schemes necessary but nonuniform. Categorization can be conveniently based upon anatomic/developmental and etiologic criteria.

Anatomic/Developmental

Patients with *youth-onset* (< 15 to 20 years old) obesity more often have generalized obesity with both hyperplasia and hypertrophy of their adipocytes. Patients with *adult-onset* (> 15 to 20 years old) obesity more often have a centripetal distribution of excess fat and adipocyte hypertrophy without an increase in the number of fat cells (2,11). Although there is a considerable overlap between the two groups, the classification is conceptually and practically useful.

Other, much less common types of obesity fall within the anatomic classification. The *lipodystrophies* are localized accumulations of excess fat, most commonly single or multiple lipomas. The latter are inherited as an autosomal dominant trait. *Dercum's disease* (adiposis dolorosa) and *Weber-Christian disease* are two rare illnesses of unknown etiology characterized by focal (occasionally painful) distributions of single or multiple nodules of histologically normal fat.

Etiologic

Various organic and environmental factors, none mutually exclusive, are included within the etiologic classification of obesity.

ORGANIC FACTORS

Hyperplastic (youth-onset) obesity appears to be inherited. However, even in patients with an apparent genetic predisposition to obesity, environmental influences seem to be important determinants of body weight (see below).

In both experimental animals and in man, certain *primary endocrine disorders* are important causes of obesity. These include hyperinsulinism, hypercortisolism, and deficiencies of growth hormone, thyroid hormone, or sex steroids.

Hyperinsulinemia can result from appropriate or surreptitious use of exogenous insulin, or from insulin hypersecretion by benign or malignant pancreatic neoplasms.

Hypercortisolism most often is iatrogenic, resulting from excess administration of exogenous glucocorticoids. Much less commonly, true Cushing's disease or syndrome is responsible.

Since *growth hormone* exerts an influence on conversion of fat stores into energy for body growth and protein deposition, its absence, either due to pituitary dysfunction or removal, leads to increased adiposity which is reversible by administration of the hormone.

Although *thyroid hormones* directly modulate the overall basal metabolic rate (BMR), hypothyroidism *per se* is most often associated with modest or no weight gain. Morbid obesity (defined below) due solely to hypothyroidism has not been documented, whereas moderate weight loss because of anorexia disproportionate to the decrease in BMR is occasionally seen.

The *polycystic ovary (Stein-Leventhal) syndrome,* a fairly common group of disorders in young women, is characterized by mild obesity, hirsutism, oligomenorrhea, and infertility in association with mild hypothalamic-pituitary-ovarian (and possibly adrenal) dysfunction. The obesity and the menstrual abnormalities are often ameliorated after ovarian wedge resection.

Hypothalamic obesity is a rare disorder associated most often with the presence of a craniopharyngioma or, less often, with other neoplastic or inflammatory diseases near the hypothalamic ventromedial nuclei, sites in the brain that appear to be involved in the control of normal feeding and satiety.

In addition to insulin and glucocorticoids, other *pharmacologic agents* induce increases in food intake and in body fat. The most commonly used are phenothiazines, oral contraceptives, and the antihistamine, cyproheptadine (Periactin). Weight gain associated with the latter drug probably results from its antiserotoninergic properties.

ENVIRONMENTAL FACTORS

In view of the obvious imbalance between energy input and expenditure in obese individuals, it is not surprising to find numerous clinical studies that document the importance of nutritional habits and patterns of physical activity in the development of excess adiposity. The adverse effects of an absolute or relative excess in total caloric intake, of a maldistribution of foodstuffs (especially too much fat or carbohydrate), and of the general increase in sedentary life-styles are particularly important.

In contemporary affluent societies, obesity is most frequently associated with behavioral and psychologic determinants that affect both the circumstances and substance of food intake. Although numerous studies have sought to identify the obese persona, it appears that no such diagnostic personality profile exists. Nonetheless, a major psychologic distinction between youth- and adult-onset type of obesity may reside in the distorted perception of body image that is frequently associated with obesity in childhood and adolescence. Thus, in the latter group, affected individuals often believe that their body habitus and weight are normal, a phenomenon rarely encountered in adult-onset obesity. Moreover, in contrast to certain commonly held notions, it appears that obese individuals are often depressed, are unhappy about being fat, and are relieved by successful and sustained weight loss.

Socioeconomic factors exert strong influences on the development and persistence of obesity in individuals as well as in population groups. In the United States obesity is more common in: (a) children and adults from the lower socioeconomic groups, (b) black vs. white women, (c) white vs. black men, and (d) first generation Americans vs. their descendants. Interestingly, when body weights of women of similar ages were compared, those women born later in this century were less heavy than women born in the early 1900s; the opposite trend appeared true for men (12). The reason for this is unclear, but may be related to the steadily increasing fashion consciousness and emphasis on exercise among American women, and to the generally more sedentary work habits and lifestyles of men.

Morbid Obesity

Morbid obesity defines a subset of patients who are 50 to 100%, or 100 lb (45.5 kg), above their ideal body weights. A predominantly genetic origin, with onset of disease in youth, a generally relentless progression through life, and a long term cure rate of less than 5% are characteristic. In contrast, the onset and progression of the usual forms of mild-to-moderate adult-onset obesity are influenced more by psychosocial factors. Whereas patients with youth-onset morbid obesity often suffer from distorted perceptions of body image, this has not been true of patients with adult-onset disease. The latter group, however, has been characterized as generally lacking in internal cues that control food intake, thus being more susceptible to external, environmental eating cues. This observation, confirmed in numerous psychologic studies, has exerted a major influence upon the philosophy and design of behavior modification programs.

PREVALENCE

Determination of the prevalence of obesity requires the application of standardized, accurate techniques for quantifying body fat to large scale epidemiologic surveys, both within and between various population groups. Most current information is derived from measurements of relative weight and/or skin-fold thickness(es) conducted by life insurance company actuaries, as part of National Health surveys, or in studies of the factors that predispose to cardiovascular disease or diabetes mellitus. As suggested by the previous discussion, the prevalence of obesity varies considerably with sex, age, socioeconomic, religious, ethnic, and other factors.

Results of a recent Health and Nutrition Examination Survey (HANES 1, 1971 to 1974) by the National Center for Health Statistics are depicted in Table 73.1. For persons in the 20 to 74 age range, a greater percentage of men than women were 10 to 19% overweight, 18.1% vs. 12.6%, respectively. In contrast, women were more commonly 20% or more overweight, 23.8% vs. 14.0%, respectively. Moreover,

Table 73.1
Prevalence of Overweight[a]

Age	Men		Women	
	10–19%	20% or more	10–19%	20% or more
20–74	18.1%	14.0%	12.6%	23.8%
20–24	11.1	7.4	9.8	9.6
25–34	16.7	13.6	8.1	17.1
35–44	22.1	17.0	12.3	24.3
45–54	19.9	15.8	15.1	27.8
55–64	18.9	15.1	15.5	34.7
65–74	19.1	13.4	17.5	31.5

[a] Percent population deviating by 10–19% and by 20% or more from desirable weight (estimated from regression equations of weight on height for men and women ages 20–29 years, obtained from HANES 1). United States, Health and Nutrition Examination Survey, 1971–1974. (From G. A. Bray (ed.): Obesity in America, DHEW Publication No. (NIH) 79-359, U.S. Government Printing Office, Washington, D.C., 1979.)

the percentage of men and women ages 25 to 74 who were 20% or more overweight was higher in the 1971 to 1974 study than in a similar 1961 to 1962 survey.

In the U.S. Public Health Service Ten State Nutrition Survey of 1968 to 1970 (10), the prevalence of obesity in adolescents was determined by measurement of triceps skin-fold thickness. With use of the criterion of skin-fold thickness greater than the 85th percentile of adult values (18.6 mm in men and 25.1 mm in women), obesity in adolescents was found to vary with age from 11 to 39% for white males, and from 9 to 19% for white females. White male adolescents were more obese than their black counterparts. In this study there were no consistent relationships between obesity and socioeconomic status. However, Stunkard et al. (20) have emphasized the importance of social factors in the prevalence of obesity or overweight in childhood. In one study (20) overweight children from lower socioeconomic groups were identified by age 6, whereas overweight children from upper socioeconomic groups could not be identified until age 8, and there were fewer at later ages in childhood.

In the much publicized longitudinal study of approximately 5000 individuals in Framingham, Mass. (12), about 15% of men and 20% of women had relative body weights greater than 30% above ideal. Moreover, 3% of men and 9% of women were more than 50% overweight. Within any age cohort, both men and women had a progressive increase up to age 45 to 49 years, after which weights stabilized or fell. In studies of changing body composition with age, it is clear that, even with stable weights, the proportion of body fat increases and that of lean body mass decreases with advancing years.

The Seven Country Study of Keys et al. (13) (Table 73.2) provided comparative data on obesity and overweight, utilizing criteria of skin-fold thickness and relative weight; by either criterion men from the

United States were among the most corpulent examined.

PATHOGENESIS

Energy Intake

In the United States the typical diet is composed of approximately 40 to 45% carbohydrate, 40% fat, and 15 to 20% protein. Energy intake that exceeds energy expenditure is the cardinal pathogenetic mechanism promoting an increase in body fat. Although there is evidence to support the idea that body weight is fairly closely regulated over long periods of time, body composition changes considerably with age, as noted previously. The numerous factors controlling normal food intake and distribution, storage, and expenditure of energy represent a complex, highly integrated series of events, as yet only partially understood.

Until recently, it was thought that normal control of hunger and satiety in man resided in certain nuclei of the lateral and medial hypothalamus, respectively, and that other neural, nutritional, endocrine-metabolic, gastrointestinal, and psychologic factors exerted their influences by impinging upon these sites. Current evidence favors a more diffuse localization of feeding and satiety "centers" involving not only the perihypothalamic area but portions of the limbic system and cerebral cortex as well.

Energy Expenditure

Even after adjustments for differences in age, sex, and body weight, energy expenditure varies considerably among normal adults. Under resting conditions, there are adaptations to the amount and type of food ingested that allow for increased or decreased utilization of nutrients and that maintain a stable weight in most people.

In our sedentary society physical exercise plays a

Table 73.2
Prevalence of Overweight and Obesity in Groups of Men from Seven Countries[a]

Country	Percent of Sample	
	Overweight[b]	Obese[c]
Japan	2	2
Greece	11	11
Finland	15	14
Yugoslavia	19	29
Italy	33	28
Netherlands	13	32
United States	32	63

[a] Data adapted from A. Keys (13), from G. A. Bray: The obese patient. In Major Problems in Internal Medicine, Vol. IX, edited by L. H. Smith. W. B. Saunders, Philadelphia, 1976

[b] Overweight = men 10% or more over standard weight.

[c] Obesity = men with sum of triceps and subscapular skin-fold >28 mm.

relatively minor role in energy expenditure. Short term vigorous exercise such as weight lifting, competitive contact sports, etc. often leads to increases in dietary intake, utilization of muscle glycogen stores, and muscle mass. In contrast, frequent, sustained, moderate aerobic exercise such as jogging, swimming, etc., mobilizes fat stores.

Despite the apparent long term control of general energy balance and body weight in normal persons, there is no conclusive evidence of an endogenous set-point (e.g., glucostatic, lipostatic, or thermostatic) that modulates adipose tissue mass.

The recent observations of altered indices of cellular sodium potassium ATPase activity in red blood cells (5) and in liver (4) from obese subjects, as compared to controls, suggest possible pathophysiologic mechanisms by which cellular thermogenesis, and therefore the efficiency of energy expenditure, might be perturbed in human obesity. The mechanisms by which external and cognitive controls exert their effects await elucidation.

NATURAL HISTORY

Much information has been adduced to show that obese infants and children become obese adults more often than do their lean counterparts. In addition, youth-onset obesity tends to be more severe and persistent, and more resistant to treatment, than are the usually milder forms of later onset. This may be due to the fact that weight loss and decrease in adiposity per se result predominantly from a decrease in adipocyte size and not number, so that adipose hyperplasia (usually youth-onset) (see p. 770) is ordinarily irreversible. In contrast, there is greater therapeutic promise for the more common, normocellular adult-onset obese population.

Metabolic Concomitants

Although the exact roles of all organic and environmental factors in the pathogenesis of obesity remain to be elucidated, certain metabolic concomitants of excess adiposity have been characterized. Numerous studies document the close association between obesity and diabetes mellitus and suggest that obesity per se is diabetogenic. Obesity leads to increased pancreatic insulin production and hyperinsulinemia, both basally and after stimulation by ingestion of glucose, amino acids, etc. Evidence exists that the hyperinsulinemia is due to insulin resistance at the tissue level (e.g., liver, adipose tissue, and skeletal muscle) (14), caused in some individuals by a decrease in the number of cell surface receptors for insulin, and in others by aberrant, insulin-dependent intracellular glucose metabolism. However, some investigators feel that hyperglycemia and hyperinsulinemia are due predominantly to excess caloric—principally carbohydrate—intake and not to insulin resistance. Finally, it has been proposed that chronic hyperinsulinemia leads to a further decrease in the number of cell surface insulin receptors (i.e., "down-regulation"), the latter serving as an adipocyte response to prevent episodes of hypoglycemia.

There is a significant association between obesity and the presence of hyperlipidemia, especially hypertriglyceridemia. This latter relationship probably results, at least in some patients, from the hyperinsulinemia-induced increase in hepatic triglyceride synthesis and formation of triglyceride-rich very low density lipoproteins (VLDL), although this hypothesis requires further confirmation. Hypercholesterolemia and increased endogenous cholesterol synthesis are also more frequent in obese patients, and may be responsible for their increased risk of cholesterol gallstones.

Many patients with adult-onset truncal obesity appear cushingoid. Simple obesity is associated with an increased cortisol production rate leading to increased hepatic steroid metabolism and increased urinary excretion of certain steroid conjugates. Such patients typically have increased urinary 17-hydroxycorticoids; however, plasma cortisol, urinary free cortisol, and overnight dexamethasone suppression tests are usually normal.

Salt and water retention is a common problem in obese patients, and is in part mediated by increases in aldosterone secretion induced by dietary carbohydrate and, to a lesser extent, protein intake.

Onset of normal menarche does not occur until a critical body weight is reached (usually 40 to 45 kg), a finding that explains the earlier menarche in women with youth-onset obesity. Menstrual abnormalities, such as dysfunctional uterine bleeding, amenorrhea, and infertility, are also more common in obese women, and are often associated with aberrant cyclical reproductive hormone function (subnormal levels of follicle-stimulating hormone (FSH) in the follicular phase, and of progesterone in the luteal phase.

Other important endocrine or metabolic sequelae of obesity, the mechanisms for which are unclear, are decreased growth hormone responses to provocative stimuli and hyperuricemia. The former, by decreasing the availability of a lipolytic hormone, permits excess fat accumulation, while the latter is responsible for the increased prevalence of gout in obese individuals.

Risks

A large body of research and anecdotal data has suggested that obesity and overweight exist as graded phenomena, and that there is strong positive correlation between the degree of excess adiposity and increased morbidity and mortality, the latter particularly from cardiovascular and cerebrovascular diseases. It now appears that this hypothesis must be somewhat modified.

Critical analysis of data derived from retrospective life insurance studies (16) suggested that there was no significant increase in mortality until body weight rose to values greater than 30% above ideal body weight. Data from a large number of prospective studies also suggest that severe to extreme, but not mild to moderate, obesity is associated with decreased longevity. Moreover, morbid obesity is not, *per se*, a risk factor for premature dying; rather, it exerts its deleterious effects by influencing known risk factors, such as hypertension, hyperlipidemia, and diabetes mellitus. Finally, in a recent analysis of several large scale community surveys, Andres (1) has also confirmed the apparent lack of increased mortality among aged individuals with mild-to-moderate obesity, and has suggested that more epidemiologic and clinical research be focused on possible beneficial effects of mild obesity. It seems likely that public health and other officials, as well as individual physicians, will become more cautious in their advice regarding evaluation and management of patients with mild to moderate obesity.

Medical Consequences

The major physiologic and medical concomitants of moderate to extreme obesity are depicted in Table 73.3. Although a direct pathophysiologic link between obesity and these conditions has not been unequivocally established, in each instance, the morbidity associated with the condition is proportional to the degree of excess adiposity, and is partially or totally

Table 73.3
Possible Medical Consequences of Obesity

ENDOCRINE-METABOLIC:
  Hyperglycemia, hyperinsulinemia, insulin resistance
  Hypertriglyceridemia, hypercholesterolemia ($\uparrow$VLDL $\uparrow$LDL $\downarrow$HDL)
  $\uparrow$ Cortisol production but normal plasma cortisol, diurnal rhythm, urine free cortisol and overnight dexamethasone suppression
  Early menarche, menstrual abnormalities, hirsutism
  $\downarrow$ Growth hormone, basally and after provocative stimuli
  Hyperuricemia, gout
CARDIOVASCULAR:
  Hypertension
  Coronary artery disease
  Congestive heart failure
  Varicose veins
  Cerebrovascular disease
PULMONARY:
  Hypoventilation (*e.g.*, Pickwickian) syndromes
  Chronic respiratory infections
GALLBLADDER:
  Cholelithiasis (cholesterol gallstones)
MUSCULOSKELETAL:
  Osteoarthritis
  Chronic orthopaedic problems
  $\downarrow$ Ambulation
RENAL:
  Nephrotic syndrome (normal or nonspecific biopsy)
ONCOLOGIC:
  Endometrial and (?) breast carcinoma
DERMATOLOGIC:
  Acanthosis nigricans
  Chronic skin infections
PSYCHOSOCIAL:
  Depression, loss of self-esteem
  $\downarrow$ Employability

reversed after successful weight loss. In addition, obesity, particularly when severe, frequently exacerbates or complicates the course of a variety of other illnesses, for example, by delaying surgical procedures, enhancing operative risks, prolonging convalescence from many illnesses, and exacerbating unstable behavioral patterns.

EVALUATION AND MANAGEMENT

Evaluation

The initial evaluation of the obese patient should include a medical and psychosocial history, physical examination, and appropriate laboratory and other studies. The history will usually indicate whether the patient has youth-onset or adult-onset obesity. It is particularly important to identify any medical or psychologic factors that may motivate the patient to lose weight or that militate for or against certain treatment plans.

Although secondary obesity is rare, its importance lies in its reversibility after identification and specific therapy of the underlying medical or pharmacologic disorder. Special emphasis should therefore be placed on screening an obese patient for any contributing endocrine-metabolic process and on obtaining a history of medication use.

Evidence of glucose intolerance should be sought by obtaining fasting blood glucose levels with the patient on a regular (or, preferably, high carbohydrate) diet, and comparing the results to those from age- and sex-matched controls. The oral glucose tolerance test is not ordinarily necessary to make the diagnosis of adult-onset diabetes mellitus. Hypercortisolemia should be suspected in any plethoric, hypertensive patient with centripetal obesity, hypokalemia, and glucose intolerance. A normal overnight dexamethasone suppression test (*i.e.*, 1.0 mg of oral dexamethasone at 11 p.m., followed by an 8 a.m. plasma cortisol <5 μg/dl) eliminates the diagnosis of endogenous hypercortisolemia with a high degree of certainty. Clinically significant hypothyroidism can usually be ruled out when the free thyroxine index (*i.e.*, serum T_4 $\times$ resin T_3 uptake) is normal. On occasion, hyperthyroid patients "outeat" their increased BMR and complain to the physician of weight gain. The finding of menstrual irregularities, mild hirsutism (but not virilization), and obesity in a young woman prompts suspicion of the polycystic ovarian syndrome, a diagnosis made more likely by the additional findings of a mildly elevated serum testosterone level (60 to 100 ng/dl), flat basal body temperature curve (*i.e.*, no ovulation), and palpable abnormalities on pelvic examination. Diseases of the hypothalamic-pituitary region should be considered in obese patients with otherwise unexplained neuroendocrine abnormalities. Certain rare syndromes, such as the Prader-Willi syndrome (obesity, short stature, hypogonadism, and mental retardation), are usually recognized in childhood by their characteristic clinical presentations.

In addition to the above, fasting blood samples should be sent for determinations of triglyceride, total cholesterol, and uric acid levels. Most patients with hyperlipidemia have acquired (*i.e.*, secondary), not genetic (*i.e.*, primary) hyperlipidemias, and will respond to appropriate diet regimens. Finally, in patients with clinically apparent or suspect hypoventilation syndromes, pulmonary function should be tested.

A useful algorithm for the outpatient evaluation of the obese patient has been published by Bray and coworkers (3).

Management of Mild to Moderate Obesity

Based upon the initial assessment of the patient, the physician should ascertain the type and degree of obesity, including the medical or psychologic urgency for weight loss, the patient's motivation and readiness for weight loss, and the most suitable treatment plan. Since the usual form of simple adult-onset, mild to moderate obesity appears not to carry an increased risk of morbidity or mortality (see pp. 773-774), it should be treated conservatively, if at all, by a combination of moderate diet, regular exercise, and patient-motivated nutritional education and behavioral relearning. There is no justification for the use of anorexigenic drugs in the treatment of the problem. If the patient asks for them, the physician should explain that they are minimally effective, are of no help in maintaining weight loss, and that many of them are dangerous (see below p. 777). Moreover,

the patient should be cautioned against the purchase of patent medicines. It is now clear that several lay organizations for weight reduction (e.g., Weight Watchers and Take Off Pounds Sensibly (TOPS)) are as capable as health professionals in effecting weight loss in this category of obese patient.

For most adults, a balanced diet containing 1500 to 1800 calories per day is necessary for maintenance of ideal body weight under conditions of basal activity. Thus, modest caloric restriction to 900 to 1200 calories/day for women and 1200 to 1500 calories/day for men is appropriate, with small increases proportionate to increases in levels of physical activity. It is often useful to advise patients who are motivated to diet to purchase one of the readily available, inexpensive calorie counters and to use the information to limit their daily diet to a specific number of calories. In general, daily modest exercise programs should be tailored to the individual patient's ability and enjoyment. Regular physical conditioning will facilitate weight loss, as well as decrease or abolish obesity-associated hyperinsulinemia and insulin resistance, hypertriglyceridemia, hyperuricemia, and systolic and diastolic hypertension and will improve cardiovascular, respiratory, and musculoskeletal problems. A goal of a loss of 1 or 2 lb (0.5 to 1 kg) a week is appropriate whenever a patient embarks on a weight reduction program.

Improved nutritional understanding often results from effective and practical dietary counseling. Diet sheets and booklets that set forth easy to understand and follow recommendations, particularly when attuned to the sociocultural and economic characteris-

---

**BALTIMORE CITY HOSPITALS
WEIGHT CONTROL PROGRAM**

Name: _____ Date: _____

Day: Mon.   Tues.   Wed.   Thurs.   Fri.   Sat.   Sun.   (circle one)

Exercise or activity: A. Type_____   Minutes_____   B. Type_____   Minutes_____

Time	Minutes	Food Type	Amount	Meal/ Snacks	Hunger Yes No	Body Position	Activity while Eating	Location of Eating	Eating (with Whom)	Feeling

Time: starting time for a meal or snack; Meal/snack: indicate type of eating by the appropriate letter—M (meal) or S (snack). Hunger: check yes or no.

Figure 73.2 Food diary for identification of abnormal behavioral patterns leading to excess food intake.

tics of the patient, are especially valuable. Improved patterns of eating behavior should be encouraged. Specific suggestions should include smaller, more frequent, or regular meals, eaten more slowly, in defined surroundings. Use of food diaries is especially helpful (Fig. 73.2), particularly in identifying abnormal behavioral patterns leading to excess food intake. For the patient who makes a significant effort, reinforcement of the improved eating behavior by his physician is important in maintenance of weight reduction. Usually formal consultation with a professional behavioral therapist is not required.

Management of Morbid Obesity

Morbid obesity (see p. 771) is associated with a measurably increased morbidity and mortality, as well as with a generally poor response to conventional methods of moderate caloric restriction. Although there are hazards associated with each of the more intensive forms of treatment, in many severely obese patients the risks and disadvantages of being overweight greatly exceed those of treatment. In some individuals, behavioral modification (see below) may offer a more effective, and safer, management option.

DIET

Significant weight loss (up to 5 to 6 kg/week) can be achieved by prolonged (4 to 8 weeks) *starvation* of motivated, hospitalized morbidly obese patients. Within 1 to 2 years following such treatment, however, fewer than 25% to 30% of these patients have maintained their initial weight loss, and in the long term, fewer than 5% attain their ideal body weight. A major hazard of such treatment is the excessive loss of lean body mass, and thus negative nitrogen balance, that occurs predictably within the first 1 or 2 weeks of starvation, and continues at a somewhat lower rate thereafter. Other complications of this technique include orthostatic hypotension, ketoacidosis, electrolyte and vitamin deficiencies, weakness, decreased libido and impotence, menstrual irregularities, hyperuricemia and acute gout, renal uric acid calculi, emotional disturbances, and, rarely, sudden death. Despite these potential disadvantages, the need for hospitalization and the high incidence of recidivism, total fasting appears to be a generally safe and efficacious technique for inducing significant short term (*e.g.*, presurgical) weight loss when supervised by physicians experienced in the technique.

Supplemented fasting is a technique that exploits in an ambulatory setting several of the advantages of total fasting, particularly those of significant short term weight loss and high patient adherence. In general, patients consume 1 to 1.5 g of protein/kg of desirable body weight, enough to prevent loss of lean body mass, in a hypocaloric (*e.g.*, 300 to 500 calories/day) diet supplemented by adequate hydration, potassium salts, and other vitamins and minerals. In one study of nearly 1200 patients who were followed

clinically and biochemically at frequent intervals, approximately 75% to 80% of the patients lost more than 40 lb (18 kg) (7). Moreover, hypertension and glucose intolerance, as well as the need for appropriate medications, disappeared or diminished in the majority of affected patients; other benefits, such as improved exercise tolerance, ambulation, pulmonary, psychosocial, and employment status also became evident. The disadvantages of the technique are similar to, but of lesser magnitude than, those described above for total fasting; there have been, in addition, several sudden cardiac deaths in patients without known preexisting heart disease. A major problem with supplemented fasting is that the initial success rate drops to about 25% on subsequent attempts at fasting after major weight regain.

A variant of the supplemented fast, the *"liquid protein"* diet, has been widely used in this country in recent years, and consists of a very poor quality protein, collagen hydrolysate, supplemented with tryptophan. Because of the ready commercial availability of this diet, many obese patients have consumed it without appropriate vitamin or mineral supplementation or medical supervision. In one report (21), more than 60 sudden cardiac deaths were documented during or shortly after discontinuation of this diet. Although electrocardiograms often showed prolonged QT intervals, decreased QRS voltages, and refractory ventricular dysrhythmias, electrolyte abnormalities such as hypokalemia and hypocalcemia were not invariably present. Some autopsy studies have revealed a nonspecific cardiac muscle atrophy similar to that seen in protein-calorie malnutrition states in man and experimental animals. More recently, transient, potentially life-threatening cardiac dysrhythmias were detected by 24-hour Holter monitoring, but not by standard 12-lead electrocardiograms, in 3 of 6 morbidly obese, hospitalized patients followed for 40 days on a commercially available liquid protein diet (15). In none of the 6 patients was there an antecedent history of cardiac disease, and in all the patients Holter monitoring was normal before and after the study diet. Except for mild hypokalemia in one of the affected patients, none of many routine chemical or metabolic parameters distinguished between patients with and without cardiac abnormalities. The Food and Drug Administration requires that warning labels be placed on all protein-supplemented diets, and has suggested restricting such diets to certain individuals, all of whom should be aware of the potential hazards and should be followed by physicians experienced in using such diets. However, in view of the latter study, it appears prudent to discontinue use of these diets until the mechanisms of their cardiac toxicity are elucidated.

There are numerous, palatable balanced and unbalanced low-calorie diets in common use. Many patients find it easier to follow regimens that limit caloric intake by eliminating entire food groups, such as carbohydrates, or by providing nutritionally adequate food homogenates. Perhaps the benefits of these approaches derive both from a perception that they are more "medicinal" and from diminution in external feeding cues.

Diets that are very low in calories (fewer than 800 calories/day) and carbohydrates are usually ketogenic. They are particularly popular because of the commonly held ideas that (a) nutritional ketosis exerts an anorexic effect, (b) greater weight loss ensues than after a balanced diet containing an equal number of calories, and (c) such diets spare body protein better than do balanced diets. There are no unequivocal data to support the first two notions. Although low carbohydrate, low caloric diets do generally cause a more profound early (1- to 2-week) diuresis of salt and water than do balanced diets, the rate of fat loss is no greater. Moreover, hypocaloric, low carbohydrate diets, like fasting and supplemented fasting, are associated with weakness, dehydration, postural hypotension, and occasional hyperuricemia and acute gout.

In conclusion, the safest diets are balanced and contain more than 800 calories daily. The numerous fad diets that are hypocaloric and unbalanced, particularly when medically unsupervised, should be avoided.

How effective are dietary attempts at long term weight loss? Although quantitation of successful weight loss has been defined differently by various investigators, numerous studies confirm that only 10% to 20% of obese patients who initially lose significant amounts of weight on diets maintain or increase that weight loss several years later. Although all factors that promote such success or failure remain unknown, it has been shown that ability to continue in a diet program (nearly 25% of patients drop out within the first few weeks) and emotional stability are important. The appearance of pathologic depression during or after dietary weight loss is well recognized, and is more common in juvenile-onset obese patients, in whom the baseline distortion of body image is often accompanied, paradoxically, by a perception of larger body size with progressive weight loss.

BEHAVIOR MODIFICATION

The basis for behavior modification therapy in the management of obesity rests upon the finding that many obese patients, particularly those of adult onset, respond predominantly to external, rather than internal, feeding cues. Both classical Pavlovian (aversive) conditioning and Skinnerian (operant) conditioning have been used successfully. The latter approach, which offers rewards or contracts, or modification of the environment, to change eating behavior, has been associated with greater patient satisfaction and, correspondingly, lower dropout rates. Weight loss resulting from behavior modification, unlike that produced by dietary, pharmacologic, or surgical therapy, has not been associated with serious

adverse side effects. Although these techniques offer great therapeutic promise, particularly when used in conjunction with diet and exercise programs, not all obese individuals will respond to this form of therapy, a fact which underscores the need for improved categorization and prognostication of obesity subtypes.

The short and long term efficacy of group therapy for obesity has also been examined, and appears similar to that of individual therapy, a finding that should prompt more effective use of trained therapists. Few data have been published by any of the lay, self-help groups that advertise success at weight reduction, such as Weight Watchers, TOPS, etc., but anecdotal impressions by experienced therapists suggest that these groups achieve short term results as good as, and long term results as poor as, those in medically supervised programs.

PHARMACOLOGIC THERAPY

There is no known pharmacologic agent for the treatment of obesity that is reliably effective, devoid of short and long term adverse side effects, and inexpensive and readily available. The anorexigenic derivatives of phenethylamine (Table 73.4), which include the amphetamines and fenfluramine, are the most commonly prescribed drugs. All possess certain pharmacologic properties like those of epinephrine and norepinephrine; however, their various chemical modifications have led, to differing extents, to decreased cardiovascular and central nervous system

Table 73.4
Anorectic Agents Currently Employed for the Treatment of Obesity in the United States[a]

Generic Name	Proprietary Name	DEA Schedule[b]
d,l-Amphetamine	Benzedrine and others	II
Methamphetamine	Desoxyn and others	II
Phenmetrazine	Preludin	II
Phendimetrazine	Plegine	III
Benzphetamine	Didrex	III
Chlorphentermine	Pre-Sate	III
Clortermine	Voranil	III
Mazindol	Sanorex	III
Fenfluramine	Pondimin	IV
Diethylpropion	Tenuate, Tepanil	IV
Phentermine	Fastin, Ionamin (resin)	IV

[a] From G. A. Bray (ed.): Obesity in America, DHEW Publication No. (NIH) 79-359, U.S. Government Printing Office, Washington, D.C., 1979.
[b] Drug Enforcement Administration: The schedules of the Controlled Substances Act are numbered in order of decreasing potential for abuse; drugs in Schedule II (amphetamine, methamphetamine and phenmetrazine) are the most restricted.

Table 73.5
Drugs of Unproved Efficacy or Safety in the Treatment of Obesity[a]

Human chorionic gonadotropin
Cholecystokinin
Glucagon
Indomethacin
Biguanides
Neomycin, cholestyramine
Diuretics, laxatives
Bulk fillers (methylcellulose)
L-Dopa
Hydroxycitrate
Amylase inhibitors
Thyroid hormones

[a] Adapted from G. A. Bray (editor): Obesity in America, DHEW Publication No. (NIH) 79-359, U.S. Government Printing Office, Washington, D.C., 1979.

toxicity and preservation of anorexigenic properties. In a detailed analysis of the safety and efficacy of this group of drugs, the Food and Drug Administration has examined clinical data from nearly 10,000 patients reported in a large number of double-blind and two-drug comparison studies. At the end of 20 weeks, patients on drug and placebo had equal drop-out rates, while patients taking drugs averaged about ½ lb (0.25 kg)/week greater weight loss. Moreover, there were no significant differences in weight loss when any drugs in this class were used. Intermittent therapy (2 to 4 weeks on, 1 to 2 weeks off), was often as effective as uninterrupted treatment, except with fenfluramine, which sometimes led to depression after the drug was stopped.

Although the most frequent side effects of the anorexigenic drugs are insomnia and dry mouth, and, for fenfluramine, depression and diarrhea, the major obstacle to their more widespread use is their potential for inducing physical and/or psychologic dependence.

Table 73.5 lists other drugs, purported to promote weight loss, which are also of unproved efficacy or safety in humans, and should not be used in the management of obesity.

SURGICAL THERAPY

Because of the increased morbidity and mortality associated with extreme degrees of obesity, and the generally unsatisfactory results produced by more conservative therapies, several surgical techniques have been devised to effect substantial weight loss in massively obese patients. In general, surgery should be reserved for psychologically stable, motivated patients with (a) massive obesity (usually 100 lb (45 kg) or more above ideal body weight) and repeated failures on strict diet and other therapies; (b) severe medical consequences of obesity (e.g., hypertension, diabetes mellitus, hyperlipidemia, orthopaedic problems) refractory to conventional therapy alone; and (c) unremitting, severe obesity-related despair and loss of self-esteem.

The most frequently used procedure, *jejunoileostomy*, is performed by anastomosing the distal jejunum to the terminal ileum either as an end-to-side or end-to-end procedure; in the latter approach, the defunctionalized bowel is drained with an ileocolonic anastomosis. The major benefits from successful surgery have been (a) permanent (if no reanastomosis) weight loss varying from 10 to 15 to 100 kg within 1 to 3 years postoperatively. This weight loss results primarily from a marked decrease in food intake (despite normal appetite), and only secondarily from an iatrogenic chronic malabsorption syndrome; (b) substantial improvement in blood pressure, hyperinsulinemia, and glucose intolerance, hyperlipidemia, etc.; and (c) dramatic improvement in sense of well-being and self-esteem (18).

Unfortunately, the list of adverse effects associated with the intra- or postoperative course of jejunoileostomy patients has grown progressively more formidable. Even in large medical centers with experienced personnel, the overall mortality rate following surgery varies from 3 to 5%. Serious perioperative complications include pulmonary embolus, renal failure, wound infection, gastrointestinal bleeding, and pancreatitis. Among the adverse long term effects are chronic diarrhea and flatulence, malabsorption with electrolyte and vitamin imbalance, cholelithiasis, urinary tract stones (calcium oxalate), hyperuricemia, polyarthralgias, intestinal bacterial overgrowth (pseudo-obstructive megacolon and bypass enteropathy), and progressive hepatic dysfunction leading to hepatic failure. In one large series (9) 58% of patients experienced potentially life-threatening complications or major reoperations; 17% of patients required surgical reversal of reanastomosis, usually because of severe hepatic cirrhosis and failure.

Gastric bypass surgery (8) induces significant weight loss by promoting decreased oral food intake while preserving normal gastrointestinal absorptive and digestive function. The proximal 10% of the stomach is fashioned into a 60- to 100-ml pouch by anastomosis to the jejunum through a 1.2-cm channel, thus producing rapid gastric filling, slow emptying, and prolonged satiety. One year postoperatively, weight loss in approximately 1500 reported patients averaged 30 to 35% of baseline weight, with one-third of patients losing 50 kg or more. Since carbohydrate and bile acids are absorbed normally after gastric bypass, diabetes mellitus and hypercholesterolemia are usually unchanged; however, liver function often improves, and malabsorption, electrolyte and vitamin imbalance, and kidney stones do not occur. By taking frequent small feedings of high caloric foods, it is possible for patients to "outeat" the bypass. The overall mortality rate has been reduced from 3 to 1%, but has been as high as 27% in patients over 50 years old. Complications of the procedure include channel ulcers or obstruction, bile reflux, and the dumping syndrome. A variant of the gastric bypass, the gastroplasty, involves creation of a 6- to 12-mm stoma separating a proximal 60- to 100-ml gastric pouch from the distal stomach.

Although more research is needed to determine the long term efficacy and safety of gastric bypass surgery and its variants, it appears that these procedures may be of benefit in the treatment of selected morbidly obese patients. In contrast, the striking complication rates associated with jejunoileal bypass procedures militate strongly against use of this technique in all but the most extreme instances.

PREVENTION OF OBESITY

As is evident from the preceding discussion, psychological and sociocultural factors play prominent roles in the development of nearly all types of obesity. Since the long term results of therapy for both mild-to-moderate and morbid obesity are so unsatisfactory, much more attention should be paid to prevention of excess body fatness.

The finding that behavior modification techniques can benefit not only individual obese patients, but also groups of such people, even in commercially run weight-reducing programs, is provocative, and suggests that this approach to weight reduction may have much wider application. The ability to modulate community awareness of, and responsivity to, the need for maintenance of optimal weight has been proved by results of the Stanford Heart Disease Prevention Program, which succeeded in a highly coordinated effort to decrease various of the risk factors of cardiovascular disease in three demographically matched communities (6).

Stunkard recently has suggested a variety of new, imaginative approaches to obesity prevention that could be initiated, singly or in combination (19). For example, organized industry, given the proper (financial) incentive, could: (a) increase the number and availability of quality, commercially run weight reduction programs, and provide data regarding their short and long term efficiacies; (b) develop new, more nutritious low calorie food products; (c) offer a wide variety of reasonably priced health foods throughout the general restaurant and food service (e.g., vending machines) industries; (d) increase, perhaps with aid from the sporting goods industry, the number of health and sports clubs; and (e) promote widespread improvement in general health habits by decreasing life insurance premiums for individuals who maintain normal body weight, blood pressure, etc. Analogous untapped potential for fostering good general health patterns, including the maintenance of optimal body weight, resides in other influential segments of our society, such as the media, education establishment, government, worksite, and various volunteer agencies.

References

General

Albrink, MJ (ed): Obesity. *Clin Endocrinol Metab* 5: No. 2, 1976.
    Excellent, in-depth reviews of clinical and basic research in obesity.

Anderson, AE and Margolis, S: Eating disorders: obesity and anorexia nervosa. In *The Principles and Practice of Medicine*, Ed. 20, edited by AM Harvey, RJ Johns VA McKusick, AH Owens, Jr and RS Ross. Appleton-Century-Crofts, New York, 1980.
    Concise, practical, clinical approach.

Bray, GA: The obese patient. In *Major Problems in Internal Medicine*, Vol. IX, edited by LH Smith. W. B. Saunders, Philadelphia, 1976.
    Major text, comprehensive and lucidly written.

Bray, GA (ed): Obesity in America, DHEW Publication No. (NIH) 79–359, U.S. Government Printing Office, Washington, D.C., 1979.
    Valuable resource, summary of recent NIH symposium.

Buchwald, H (ed): Morbid obesity. *Surg Clin North Am* 59: No. 6, 1979.
    Good account of a multidisciplinary approach to the extremely obese patient.

Specific

1. Ancres, R. Influence of obesity on longevity in the aged. In *Advances in Pathobiology*, No. 7, Aging, Cancer, and Cell Membranes, pp. 238–246, edited by C Borek, CM Fenoglio and DW King. Thieme-Stratton, New York, 1980.
2. Björntorp, P: Effects of age, sex, and clinical conditions on adipose tissue cellularity in man. *Metabolism* 23: 1091, 1974.
3. Bray, GA, Jordan, HA and Sims, EAH: Evaluation of the obese patient; 1. An Algorithm. *JAMA* 235: 1487, 1976.
4. Bray, GA, Kral, JG and Björntorp, P: Hepatic sodium-potassium-dependent ATPase in obesity. *N Engl J Med* 304: 1580, 1981.
5. DeLuise, M, Blackburn, GL and Flier, JS: Reduced activity of the red-cell sodium-potassium pump in human obesity. *N Engl J Med* 303: 1017, 1980.
6. Farquhar, JW, Maccoby, N, Wood, PD, et al.: Community education for cardiovascular health. *Lancet* 1: 1192, 1977.
7. Genuth, SM, Castro, JH and Vertes, V: Weight reduction in obesity by outpatient semistarvation. *JAMA* 230: 987, 1974.
8. Griffen, WO: Gastric bypass for morbid obesity. *Surg Clin North Am* 59: 1103. 1979.
9. Halverson, JD, Wise, L, Wazna, MF and Ballinger, WF: Jejunoileal bypass for morbid obesity. A critical appraisal. *Am J Med* 64: 461, 1978.
10. Health Services and Mental Health Administration: Ten State Nutrition Survey 1968–1970. DHEW Publication No. (HSM) 72–8130. Washington, DC. U.S. Government Printing Office, 1972.
11. Hirsch, J and Batchelor, B: Adipose tissue cellularity in human obesity. *Clin Endocrinol Metab* 5: 299, 1976.
12. Kannel, WB and Gordon, T: Obesity and cardiovascular disease. The Framingham Study. In: *Obesity. Proceedings of a Servier Research Institute Symposium on Obesity. Servier Institute Monograph*, edited by WL Burland, J Yudkin and P Samuel. Churchill Livingstone, Edinburgh, 1974.
13. Keys, A (ed): Coronary heart disease in seven countries. American Heart Association Monograph No. 29, 1970.
14. Kolterman, OG, Insel, J, Saekow, M and Olefsky, J: Mechanisms of insulin resistance in human obesity: evidence for receptor and postreceptor defects. *J Clin Invest* 65: 1272, 1980.
15. Lantigua, RA, Amatruda, JM, Biddle, TL, Forbes, GB and Lockwood, DH: Cardiac arrhythmias associated with a liquid protein diet for the treatment of obesity. *N Engl J Med* 303: 735, 1980.
16. Seltzer, CC: Some re-evaluations of the build and blood pressure study, 1959, as related to ponderal index, somatotype and mortality, *N Engl J Med* 274: 254, 1966.
17. Society of Actuaries: *Build and Blood Pressure Study, Vol. 1*. The Society, Chicago, 1959.
18. Solow, C, Silberfarb, PM and Swift, K: Psychosocial effects of intestinal bypass surgery for severe obesity. *N Engl J Med* 290: 300, 1974.
19. Stunkard, AJ: Obesity and the social environment: current status, future prospects. *Ann NY Acad Sci* 300: 298, 1977.
20. Stunkard, A, d'Aquili, E, Fox, S and Filion, RDL: Influence of social class on obesity and thinness in children. *JAMA* 221: 579, 1972.
21. Van Itallie, TB: Liquid protein mayhem. *JAMA* 240: 144, 1978.

CHAPTER SEVENTY-FOUR

Common Problems in Reproductive Endocrinology: Hypogonadism, Gynecomastia, Impotence, Hirsutism, Galactorrhea, Frigidity, Menopause, Menstrual Abnormalities

S. MITCHELL HARMAN, M.D., Ph.D., and J. COURTLAND ROBINSON, M.D.

Few general physicians feel comfortable or competent with sexual and reproductive medicine. This is in part because neither medical school nor postgraduate training has given sufficient emphasis to this subject to engender the confidence that comes with familiarity. Thus, most physicians view complaints involving the reproductive system as esoteric or rare, and hence the province of the specialist (*i.e.*, endocrinologist, urologist, or gynecologist). Also, the subject of sex, although more openly dealt with than in former years, still may produce feelings of embarrassment in both patient and physician.

In fact, sexual and reproductive dysfunction is not rare in the general population. Nearly 50% of men will experience one or more periods of impotence between the ages of 20 and 50 (7); as many as 10% of married couples will have difficulty with conception; and approximately 1 in 400 male births will have Klinefelter's (XXY) syndrome (6).

Furthermore, the new freedom with which sex and reproduction are discussed socially and treated in the popular media, and the advent of scientific investigation of human sexuality have altered the expectations of the patient population. "Normal" sexual function is now an objective of many men and women and dysfunction is legitimately viewed as a health problem. Such problems are now more likely to be brought openly to a physician than in former times, when reticence and modesty were the social norm. Thus it is important that the generalist be familiar with the major disorders of reproductive function and have adequate knowledge of the points of history, techniques of physical diagnosis, and modes of laboratory investigation to allow him to distinguish patients who require reassurance or can be treated simply in the office from those who need referral to a specialist for more complex testing and therapy.

SEXUAL AND REPRODUCTIVE PHYSIOLOGY

Levels of Sexual Differentiation

The sexual differentiation of individuals can be viewed as a continuum proceeding in time from conception to adulthood and in biologic "depth" from genetic to social and psychologic as follows: (a) *genetic sex* is determined at conception when the egg, bearing an X chromosome, is fertilized by a sperm bearing either a Y (XY = male) or X (XX = female) chromosome. The genetic sex determines (b) *gonadal sex*—the development of an ovary or testis from the undifferentiated primitive gonad. (c) *Primary sex*—the embryonic testis secretes testosterone, which in turn causes the development of a penis and scrotum. In the absence of a testis the embryo develops a uterus and fallopian tubes, and, without androgen, female external genitalia form, so that the primary sex is female. The primary sex characteristics identify the individual's sex at birth (d) *secondary sex* changes occur at puberty and are the result of greatly increased secretion by the gonads of sex steroid hormones. In males growth of body and pubic hair, beard growth, increase in muscle mass, deepening of voice, and onset of male libido with ejaculations and increased frequency of erections are characteristic effects of testosterone. In the female, rounding of body contours with breast growth and subcutaneous deposition of fat in the hips and buttocks, and also the onset of menses, are effects of cyclic estrogen secretion, while growth of pubic and axillary hair and probably libido are manifestations of adrenal androgen secretion. Both sexes experience a spurt of body growth at puberty, which is then followed by closure of epiphyses and cessation of growth of long bones. It is the hormone-dependent secondary sex characteristics which provide clues to adult sexual identity and which form the underpinning of (e) *tertiary sex* which is the way in which an individual identifies him or herself. There are few mammalian species whose level of sexual dimorphism is as extreme as that of humans. This is reflected by the fact that our identification as man or woman is crucial to balanced psychologic and social function and is a critical component of our self-image. The physician must bear in mind that any change which seems to alter a patient's masculinity or femininity is perceived as profoundly threatening and has power to harm well beyond its biologic manifestations.

Male Reproductive Physiology

Activity of the male reproductive system is regulated by the hypothalamus which produces, at irregular intervals of 40 to 120 min, surges of secretion of a decapeptide, luteinizing hormone releasing hormone (LHRH), into capillaries of the median eminence, which drain into the pituitary portal veins. LHRH induces pituitary gonadotropic cells to episodic secretion of two glycoprotein hormones, luteinizing hormone (LH) and follicle-stimulating hormone (FSH). FSH induces spermatogenesis in the seminiferous tubules while LH acts on the Leydig (interstitial) cells of the testis to stimulate testosterone secretion. Testosterone, the major circulating androgenic steroid, is partially bound in plasma to a protein, sex hormone binding globulin (SHBG), which decreases its clearance rate and also serves as a testosterone reservoir. In most target cells testosterone is reduced to 5α-dihydrotestosterone which binds to specific cytoplasmic hormone receptor proteins and is translocated to the cell nucleus. Once in the nucleus the testosterone-receptor complex activates particular genes which in turn leads to specific protein synthesis

and to altered cellular activity. In addition to its masculinizing activity, testosterone also acts in concert with FSH on the seminiferous tubules to induce growth, lumen formation, and spermatogenesis. Testosterone is needed for growth of and secretion by the prostate and seminal vesicles. More general body effects include positive nitrogen and calcium balance (with bone and muscle formation) and increased function of apocrine and sebaceous glands of the skin, which often results in comedones and acne. Another important effect of testosterone is to "feed back" to the hypothalamus and pituitary to inhibit secretion of gonadotropins. Thus, the reproductive hormones form a "closed loop" autoregulated system.

Female Reproductive Physiology

The hypothalamic pituitary relationship is similar to that of males, except that the complex modulation of hormone secretion in women normally results in a cyclic rather than tonic reproductive pattern. In women LH stimulates the interstitial-thecal tissue to make androgen and, to some extent, the estrogens estradiol and estrone. In concert with FSH these steroids produce growth of ovarian follicles by proliferation of granulosa cells. Granulosa cells convert thecal androgens to estradiol and a dominant follicle emerges as the major source of estradiol secretion, while adjacent follicles undergo atresia. Rising estrogen secretion in this follicular phase of the cycle induces proliferation of the uterine endometrium, and by a "positive feedback" effect, a sudden surge of LH secretion around day 14 of the cycle. This LH surge results in ovulation. LH then induces the follicle to become a functioning corpus luteum producing both estradiol and progesterone during the latter half, or luteal phase, of the cycle. Progesterone acts to produce a secretory endometrium, rich in glycogen and, in concert with estrogen, causes a negative feedback effect which gradually reduces the secretion of LH and FSH. With loss of gonadotropic support, the corpus luteum involutes, steroid secretion diminishes, the endometrium, left without estrogen and progesterone stimulation, sloughs off as the menstrual flow, and the stage is set for the next cycle. Ovarian estradiol is the major estrogen during the reproductive period and is primarily responsible for inducing and maintaining female secondary sex characteristics. Some estrogen, mainly estrone, is formed peripherally in fat, liver, kidney, and other tissues by conversion of adrenal and ovarian androgenic precursors. The secretion of these androgens also increases at puberty.

Male and Female Hormones and Libido

The reader is referred to Chapter 17 for a description of the stages of the sexual response which characterize sexual physiology in men and women. It is not clear in humans precisely to what extent sex hormones influence these events. There is no doubt that men completely deprived of testosterone (*i.e.*, chemical or physical castration) experience a gradual loss (over 1 to 2 years) of interest in sex, reporting an absence of sensations of arousal in response to sexual cues (*e.g.*, female nudity) and also loss of erections and ejaculation. Many also report heightened emotional sensitivity, weepiness, and loss of aggressive interest, ability to concentrate or drive toward career goals, etc. Experimental evidence suggests a direct effect of testosterone on the central nervous system (4). In women, there is no such obvious relationship between libido and sex hormones, but some data exist to suggest that women are more likely to initiate sexual contact during phases of the menstrual cycle when androgen activity is highest (1), and women with androgen-secreting tumors often report heightened sex drive with increased sexual content of dreams and fantasies. It has also become apparent in recent years that the pituitary hormone, prolactin, which in women is responsible for lactation, is probably an "antisexual" hormone which reduces libido and potency in both sexes (3). In women, estrogens are necessary to maintain the vagina and the external genitalia in their mature reproductive states. In the absence of adequate estrogen, genital atrophy may result in pain on intercourse, with resultant loss of interest in sexual activity (see below).

SEXUAL AND REPRODUCTIVE DYSFUNCTION IN THE MALE

Hypogonadism

ETIOLOGIES

Failure of the testicle to secrete adequate testosterone to develop or maintain male secondary sex characteristics and libido results in the syndrome of male hypogonadism. In order to investigate and diagnose these patients it is helpful to classify the failure as shown in Table 74.1.

Central. An example of *central, genetic, primary* hypogonadism is Kallmann's syndrome, which is characterized by hyposmia, and is due to a defect in hypothalamic LHRH secretion. *Acquired* hypothalamic failure may occur with diencephalic tumors. Pituitary hypogonadism is also *central* and usually *acquired.* Etiology may be infectious (*e.g.*, tuberculosis or mycosis), traumatic, vascular (as in infarction with pituitary apoplexy), or most commonly neoplastic (either chromophobe adenoma, or craniopharyngioma). *Central* hypogonadism may also be associated with functioning pituitary tumors, such as those which secrete prolactin (prolactinoma) or growth hormone (acromegaly). Occasionally pituitary hypogonadism is congenital and idiopathic.

Gonadal. Acquired causes of *gonadal* hypogonadism include trauma and infection (usually viral or granulomatous). Autoimmune damage to the testis may occur either alone or as part of a complex of multiple endocrine failure (Hashimoto's thyroiditis,

Table 74.1
Classification of Male Hypogonadism

Classification	Criteria
ACCORDING TO LOCATION OF LESION	
Central (hypothalamic or pituitary)	Gonadotropins ↓ or → Testosterone ↓
Gonadal (testis)	Gonadotropins ↑ Testosterone ↓
Peripheral (failure of end organ response)	Gonadotropins ↑ Testosterone ↑ or →
ACCORDING TO ETIOLOGY	
Genetic	History, (especially family history) Buccal smear, karyotype
Acquired	History, physical examination, radiology Evidence of infection, trauma, neoplasia, etc.
ACCORDING TO TIME OF ONSET	
Primary (failure of pubertal development)	History, physical examination
Secondary (loss of previously developed libido and secondary sex characteristics)	History, physical examination

idiopathic Addison's disease, adult-onset diabetes mellitus, hypoparathyroidism, or pernicious anemia). Occasionally a varicocele will produce partial hypogonadism. Whether these entities result in *secondary* or *primary* failure depends on the time of life at which the damage occurs.

The most common cause of *genetic gonadal* hypogonadism is Klinefelter's syndrome which is due to chromosomal nondisjunction producing XXY genetic sex. These patients have very small, firm testes and gynecomastia. They usually enter puberty, but fail to progress fully and present as phenotypic males with impotence, small phallus, and, often, gender confusion. *Genetic gonadal* hypogonadism may also occur if one or more critical enzymes in the steroid synthetic pathway leading to sex hormones is missing. Usually such defects are common to the adrenal and testis and produce female primary sex in XY individuals.

Peripheral. Peripheral hypogonadism is always genetic and causes a continuum from complete androgen insensitivity or "testicular feminization" in which the phenotype is female (with normal estrogenization at puberty but lacking a uterus, and hence menses) through varying degrees of partial sensitivity in which midline fusion of labioscrotal structures is highly variable (Reifenstein syndrome) producing gender confusion, and ending with minor defects such as hypospadias and cryptorchidism.

APPROACH TO THE PATIENT

The approach to the patient should be directed first at determining whether hypogonadism truly exists, then at its etiologic classification, and finally at providing appropriate therapy and/or referral for the specific condition diagnosed.

Patient Presentations. Patients are frequently brought to the attention of physicians by parents concerned with failure of pubertal onset or progression (see also Chapter 5). *Primary* hypogonadism may stem from almost any of the etiologies cited above and must be differentiated from so-called "constitutional delayed puberty" which is an idiopathic self-limited, familial condition. A strong family history of "late blooming" and beginning enlargement of the testicles is reassuring in this regard. A set of standards for pubertal development of adolescent boys is available (20) (see Chapter 5, Table 5.5). In general, any boy reaching 17 years of age without signs of pubertal onset, or who begins but does not proceed through puberty, or who has other associated signs or symptoms (e.g., severe headaches) of disease (e.g., a pituitary tumor) which produces hypogonadism deserves further investigation. Another presentation is genital intersexuality. A finding of hypospadias, cryptorchidism, or ambiguous genitalia in a patient with complaints suggesting hypogonadism should lead to further diagnostic procedures. The gradual loss of male secondary sex characteristics and libido is a third presentation of male hypogonadism. This may be so insidious as to be taken for "normal" by the patient, especially one progressing from middle toward old age, so that it is only noticed in association with the investigation of some related condition, such as hypothyroidism, adrenal failure, severe headaches, renal tuberculosis, etc. Finally, and probably most common, is the complaint of impotence which may be the earliest manifestation of hypogonadism, but is also seen in various other physical and psychologic conditions. Impotence is discussed more completely below and also in Chapter 17.

History. A proper history should include a chronicle of pubertal progression, with time of onset of pubic hair, beard growth, voice change, growth spurts, erections, and ejaculations recorded as accurately as recollection allows. Of critical interest are loss or diminishment of libido and erections or ejaculations, slowing of beard growth, thinning of body and pubic hair, changes in the breast (*i.e.,* swelling or tenderness), and loss of aggressive impulse or drive. The presence of headaches, double vision, or reduced peripheral vision may give clues to a pituitary tumor. Symptoms of hypothyroidism, adrenal failure, acromegaly, diabetes, anemia, pulmonary disease, and autoimmune disease should be sought. A history of urologic problems, cryptorchidism, hypospadias, or episodes of orchitis is important. Finally, a family history of delayed puberty or of other endocrine abnormalities may be revealing.

Physical Examination. The physician should first note the body habitus and facies. Does the patient look mature or babyish, masculine or feminine? A lower body segment (greater femoral trochanter to floor) longer than the upper segment and arm span greater than height comprises "eunuchoid" proportions and suggests pubertal or prepubertal hypogonadism. Good muscle mass and axillary hair militate against long-standing hypogonadism. Male pattern baldness is an androgen-dependent process. The presence of comedones, especially in the tragus of the ear (a very common location) is a good sign of androgen activity. Complexion should be noted, since increased pigmentation suggests primary adrenal failure, and dry flaky skin, hypothyroidism. Vital signs should be taken and the presence of hypertension or of postural hypotension should be noted as possible indicators of adrenal enzyme defects or of Addison's disease. Special attention should be paid to the eyes for limitation of extraocular movements, papilledema, or restriction of visual fields, all suggestive of an intracranial tumor. Examination of the male breast should include careful palpation for the subareolar thickening and nodularity which may be the only evidence of gynecomastia (see p. 785), and squeezing of the nipple to elicit galactorrhea, which, though rare in males, is pathognomonic of a prolactinoma. Careful attention should be paid to the genitals with observation of pubic hair pattern (which should extend up the linea alba to the umbilicus), penis size and location of urethral meatus, scrotal rugation and pigmentation, and size and turgor of the testicles. The normal adult testis should be no less than 15 ml in volume (approximately 4.0 × 3.0 cm) and have the resistance to palpation of a firm ripe plum. An "over-ripe" softer feeling strongly suggests testicular atrophy. Careful palpation of the left side of the scrotum while the patient performs a Valsalva maneuver may reveal the presence of a varicocele; significant varicoceles are always on the left and approximately 5% of them are associated with lower testosterone production from both testes (venous drainage from the left testis crosses over to the right). Rectal examination should assess prostate size, since the prostate shrinks with testosterone deficiency. Careful neurologic examination should include testing of the sense of smell to detect Kallman's syndrome.

DIFFERENTIAL DIAGNOSIS

The two basic hormone tests which give the most information about suspected male hypogonadism are the serum *testosterone* and *gonadotropin* measurements. These are readily available from most commercial laboratories and are generally accurate within 20%. Normal adult males will have morning serum testosterone levels not less than 300 (and usually 450 to 700) ng/dl in most laboratories. Borderline values between 250 and 350 ng/dl are suspicious. Abnormal or suspicious determinations should be repeated at least once for confirmation since there is considerable variability both in radioimmunoassay determination and from time to time within individuals. Serum LH usually is from 2 to 30 mIU/ml and

Table 74.2
Additional Investigations Useful in the Evaluation of Hypogonadism

Type of Failure	Radiologic Procedures	Hormone Measurements	Other Tests
Central	Skull film (sella) Polytomography CT scan with contrast Pneumoencephalogram (rarely) Cerebral angiogram (rarely)	Prolactin Thyroxine TSH Cortisol (a.m.)	Visual fields (formal) Clomiphene test LHRH test
Gonadal	Bone age (if primary)	Thyroxine Cortisol (a.m.)	Buccal smear Karyotyping Gonad biopsy
Peripheral	None	None	Receptor determination (research laboratory only)

FSH from 2 to 16 mIU/ml, but different assays will have different ranges of normal. Low or *normal* LH and FSH in the presence of subnormal testosterone defines central hypogonadism. Elevated gonadotropins indicate gonadal failure.

Further investigation of patients with proven hypogonadism should probably be undertaken by a specialist in endocrinology. Table 74.2 lists various investigative procedures and types of patients for whom they are pertinent.

Referral to a urologist for testicular biopsy may be helpful in diagnosing traumatic or infectious damage. Biopsy shows shrinkage and hyalinization of tubules in Klinefelter's syndrome. This procedure can often be done on an ambulatory basis under local anesthesia. However, it may cause hemorrhage and considerable pain and about a week is required for full recovery. Therefore, it usually should be undertaken only after at least a telephone consultation with an endocrinologist.

THERAPY

There are three basic aims of therapy in patients with central hypogonadism. The first is to suppress or remove any intracranial mass whose size or extent threatens vision or brain function. This may be accomplished by neurosurgery or radiation therapy depending on the type and size of the lesion. The second aim, to suppress abnormal hormone secretion, is applicable to prolactinomas too small to threaten vision or brain function. Treatment with bromocriptine (Parlodel), 2.5 mg, 3 times daily, with meals and continued indefinitely, has proven effective in lowering serum prolactin, increasing gonadotropins and testosterone, and in restoring libido (3). Interestingly, the mere replacement of testosterone by injection has not restored sexual competence so long as prolactin levels remained elevated. The third aim, which is to replace deficient androgen, may be necessary in either central or gonadal hypogonadism. This is best accomplished by intramuscular injection of 200 to 300 mg of testosterone enanthate in oil (such as Delatestryl) every 2 to 4 weeks. The dose may be started at 200 mg every 4 weeks, after which the dose and interval can be adjusted depending on duration of the symptomatic (libido, sexual potency) therapeutic effect. Oral androgen preparations are generally less effective. In *central* hypogonadism, 3 times weekly injections of 2,000 to 4,000 IU of human chorionic gonadotropin (hCG) (such as Pregnyl or Follutein) will normalize testosterone levels, generally within a month of initiation of therapy, and may also stimulate spermatogenesis. hCG is used because of its LH-like activity. Human LH is otherwise not available. Because of the requirement for more frequent injections as compared to testosterone, hCG should replace testosterone only in those patients with central hypogonadism who want to have children. Follow-up of treated patients should include questions about sexual function, assessment of habitus, beard growth, and depth of voice. Libido and potency usually return within a few weeks of initiating treatment, while secondary sex characteristics improve gradually over 6 months to a year. Determination should be made as to whether gynecomastia or prostate enlargement with symptoms of urethral obstruction are occurring as a side effect of therapy.

Gynecomastia

IMPORTANCE

Significant enlargement of the male breast is a phenomenon which requires a physician's attention so that those cases with a serious hormonal and/or neoplastic etiology can be distinguished from the common benign idiopathic form.

ETIOLOGIES

Increase in breast tissue is common as sex steroids rise in early adolescence (up to 65% of boys age 14), but it regresses spontaneously (to less than 15%) by age 17. The incidence increases again in the 20s, remains stable around 25%, and increases again to about 60% in the 50s. This idiopathic gynecomastia is nearly always less than 5 cm in diameter and causes no symptoms (24). Neoplastic hormone secretion is a rarer but important cause of breast enlargement. Noticeable gynecomastia of >5 cm in diameter may be the first clue to the presence of an adrenal or testicular neoplasm or to a prolactinoma. In the case of adrenal tumors there is usually, but not always, an associated Cushing's syndrome. Various malignant tumors may secrete chorionic gonadotropin, which can overstimulate testicular steroid production and thus lead, indirectly, to gynecomastia. Hypo- and hyperthyroidism have been associated with breast enlargement. The taking of exogenous estrogen either purposely (by individuals with gender confusion or with prostate carcinoma) or incidentally because of estrogenic activity of various medications (e.g., Valium, cimetidine, spironolactone, digitalis glycosides) should always be considered. Another iatrogenic cause is peripheral conversion to estrogens of excess androgens from testosterone or hCG therapy. Gynecomastia is common in liver failure. Finally, true gynecomastia must be differentiated from the "gynecoid" breast seen in obesity and/or old age, which contains increased fatty tissue, but not glandular breast tissue, and also from carcinoma of the male breast.

APPROACH TO THE PATIENT

History. The duration and age of onset of breast swelling is important. The presence of tenderness or discharge and the quality of the discharge (clear, turbid, bloody) should be noted. Any symptoms of hypogonadism (see above) should be elicited, as should symptoms of hypothyroidism (see Chapter 70) or Cushing's disease. Careful medication history and sexual history may reveal an exogenous etiology.

Physical Examination. In general the examination should be the same as for hypogonadism (see above) with the addition that signs of Cushing's disease and thyroid disease should be emphasized (see Chapter 70). Deep palpation of the upper abdomen may reveal an adrenal tumor or downward displacement of the kidney by such a tumor. Careful bimanual palpation of the testicles may detect a secretory tumor (androblastoma). Examination of the breast must be directed at differentiating between presence of breast tissue (firm, slightly lobulated, and symmetrically distributed from the nipple outward with a limited boundary); fat (softer, diffusely distributed, and with no clear separation from surrounding subcutaneous adipose); and tumor (hard, nodular, frequently tender, often fixed to skin or underlying muscle, asymmetric with regard to the nipple). Milky nipple discharge on firm squeezing suggests prolactinoma; clear or bloody discharge suggests breast cancer. Unilateral breast enlargement should increase the suspicion of neoplasia, but asymmetry is not uncommon (10 to 15%) in patients with idiopathic gynecomastia. The decision whether further investigation is required depends on the age of the patient, the rapidity of enlargement of the breast, and the degree of

such enlargement. Men between 18 and 45 years of age with recent onset of rapidly enlarging mammary glands, or glandular breast tissue diameter greater than 5 cm, or with symptoms or signs suggesting hypogonadism, hypothyroidism, or Cushing's disease should receive further attention.

DIAGNOSTIC PROCEDURES

Determinations of serum estrogens (estrone and estradiol) are seldom helpful. Serum *testosterone* and *gonadotropin* (LH and FSH) determinations are indicated as are serum *prolactin* and specific determination of *serum hCG*. Elevation of 24-hour urinary 17-ketosteroid indicates an adrenal etiology in which case adrenal hyperfunction should be investigated. Patients with firm, nodular, unilateral enlargement should be referred for surgical biopsy.

THERAPY

Drug-induced gynecomastia remits gradually (several months) if the drug can be discontinued. Treatment of primary endocrine disease (e.g., prolactinoma, adrenal tumor, hCG-secreting carcinoma, etc.) should usually be undertaken by an appropriate specialist once the diagnosis is clear. When "idiopathic" gynecomastia is a cosmetic problem, plastic surgical excision of breast tissue is usually the therapeutic method of choice.

Impotence

In this section, impotence and loss of libido will be considered only as they relate to physical disorders. For more general treatment of sexual dysfunction the reader is referred to Chapter 17. Briefly, impotence is the inability to achieve or maintain erection satisfactorily to effect penetration and ejaculation. Transient or occasional impotence is common and not evidence of a medical problem, but a pattern of repeated episodes over more than a month should be investigated. Impotence may or may not be accompanied by loss of sexual desire, depending on the etiology.

ETIOLOGIES

A disorder of any of the systems which maintain the sexual response and apparatus may lead to impotence: (a) psychologic (see Chapter 17); (b) vascular—diminished blood supply to the pelvic area (e.g., aortic atherosclerosis or peripheral vascular disease) may result in impotence with intact libido; (c) neuropathic—damage to the peripheral pelvic autonomic nerves (e.g., peripheral neuropathy due to diabetes mellitus or heavy metal poisoning) or damage to the central nervous system (e.g., spinal injury due to tumor, trauma, or multiple sclerosis, or brain damage from a variety of causes) may inhibit or obliterate the sexual response; (d) toxic—various drugs, especially alcohol and opiates can acutely and chronically diminish sexual ability (other medications affecting the autonomic and central nervous system, especially tranquilizers and all sympathicolytic antihypertensives may be associated with impotence); (e) debilitative—various severe and chronic medical illnesses (e.g., malignancy, renal failure) are commonly accompanied by loss of sex drive and/or impotence; and (f) endocrine—hypogonadism (see p. 782) and prolactinoma (see p. 782) have been discussed as causes of impotence. Other endocrine diseases frequently producing reduced sexual function are hyper- and hypothyroidism, Cushing's syndrome, and acromegaly. In one series of patients referred to a major diagnostic center for persistent symptoms without apparent psychiatric etiology, 35% were found to have endocrine disorders (28).

APPROACH TO THE PATIENT

History. The duration of symptoms, the frequency with which intercourse is attempted, and the percent of attempts ending in erectile failure should be recorded in order to determine whether the impotence is absolute or relative and if it is progressing. Impotence unaccompanied by loss of libido suggests a neurologic or vascular problem, whereas loss of interest in sexual activity is consistent with either hypogonadism or a psychologic etiology. Preservation of morning erections is evidence against vascular or neuropathic disease; however, in the cited series (28) 14% of patients with an endocrine etiology still had morning erections. A history of medication use and substance abuse should be diligently sought. The physician should also ask about symptoms of hypo- or hyperthyroidism, Cushing's disease, and diabetes, peripheral neuropathy (paresthesia, hyperesthesia, burning or shooting pains) or central nervous system disease, and vascular disease (claudication, angina, cold extremities, skin ulcers).

Physical Examination. The physical examination should pay particular attention to the manifestations of hypogonadism described above (p. 783), to signs of thyroid or adrenal disease (Chapter 70) and also signs of peripheral vascular disease (peripheral pulses, skin temperature, skin atrophy or hair loss) (Chapter 84) and central or peripheral neuropathy (Chapter 81).

DIAGNOSTIC PROCEDURES

Hormone determinations should be used to investigate for hypogonadism (p. 783), or prolactinoma (p. 782). If historical or physical findings lead to a suspicion of thyroid or adrenal disease, appropriate tests should be undertaken (Chapter 70). A fasting blood sugar should always be obtained. If peripheral neuropathy seems a likely etiology, this can often be confirmed by referral to a urologist for bladder manometrics and to a neurologist for nerve conduction velocity measurements (see also Chapter 81). Diagnosis of vascular causes may require Doppler estimation of penile blood flow and/or selective angiography.

THERAPY

Therapeutic efforts should be directed at the specific entity underlying the impotence, whenever one can be found. Psychologic impotence may respond to various therapeutic modalities depending on its severity and associated problems (see Chapter 17). Vascular causes may require revascularization by surgery or implantation of a penile prosthesis. Neuropathic impotence is occasionally reversible with removal of the inciting lesion (e.g., spinal cord tumor) but, if irreversible, may also be treated with an implantable penile prosthesis, though results will vary depending on whether the spinal ejaculatory center or afferent pathways are damaged. Drug-induced impotence will usually be reversed by discontinuation of the offending agent. Therapy of hypogonadism has been discussed (see p. 784). If sexual function does not improve within 6 weeks after specific therapy for an organic cause has been instituted, consideration should be given to the possibility that the experience and expectation of sexual failure are inhibiting the response even though the primary etiology is no longer present. Such "secondary" psychological impotence may respond to psychological or behavioral therapy (see Chapter 17).

Aging

A series of investigations conducted from 1966 to 1976 found that men's testosterone levels declined with age and protein binding of testosterone to SHBG increased with age, resulting in a profound decrease in mean free (bioavailable) testosterone. These changes were accompanied by an increase in circulating estrone and estradiol and in gonadotropins (9). More recent work, in which older men were carefully selected to match the younger men in terms of health, obesity, alcohol intake, social class, etc. revealed only an increase in gonadotropins and minimal increase in SHBG but no change in total or free sex steroids with age (10). Thus, there does not appear to be "male menopause" in healthy middle class American men. Despite the stability of serum testosterone and other sex steroids, these same men, and men in many other studies, have reported a steady decrease both in sexual appetite and ability with decreases in frequency of intercourse from an average of 2.6 events per week to less than 2 per month by age 70 to 75 (21). This decrease cannot be blamed on hypogonadism, but probably reflects changes in other (i.e., nervous and vascular) systems occurring with age. There are no satisfactory scientific data to support a beneficial effect of administration of androgens in aging men. Until and unless such data become available, this practice should be discouraged.

SEXUAL AND REPRODUCTIVE DYSFUNCTION IN WOMEN

Common Problems

HIRSUTISM AND VIRILIZATION

Growth of coarse dark hairs in various body areas depends on the action of androgens. The pattern of appearance of hair reflects the relative sensitivity of different skin zones to androgen effect. While pubic and axillary hair appear in both sexes, further hair growth diverges due to different androgen levels. Although male patterns vary, maximum expression of androgen effect includes hair development over the face, limbs, chest, linea alba, and back. In those carrying genes for "male pattern baldness," high levels of androgens are also associated with loss of scalp hair, first at the temporal hairline and later the crown.

Most women (80%) develop some dark hair growth over the legs and forearms without much facial hair, while about one-third have some hair over the chest or extending along the linea alba. Abnormal amounts of androgens result in the male distribution of hair growth, the state of "hirsutism." Very high levels of androgen production lead to virilization with increased muscle mass, clitoral enlargement (>2.0 cm), deepening of voice, male pattern baldness, development of acne, and malodorous perspiration.

Excess body hair without signs of virilization is termed "simple" hirsutism. Hirsutism with virilization is rare, almost always due to adrenal or ovarian tumor, congenital adrenal hyperplasia, or male pseudohermaphroditism, and therefore these patients should be referred to an endocrinologist.

Hirsutism without Virilization. Although simple hirsutism may rarely be an early manifestation of Cushing's syndrome or an adrenal or ovarian neoplasm, most cases will fall into a group termed "idiopathic" or "constitutional." This typically develops during the late teens, although slow progression may not produce troublesome amounts of hair for 10 years after onset of menses. In half to two-thirds of these patients somewhat excessive ovarian production of androgens (testosterone and/or androstenedione) is demonstrable, and is usually associated with oligomenorrhea and decreased fertility. Ovarian structure may show hyperthecosis or polycystic ovarian disease. The combination of hirsutism, obesity, acne, amenorrhea, and polycystic ovaries is known as the Stein-Leventhal syndrome. These individuals produce excessive quantities of estrogen precursors (testosterone and Δ^4-androstenedione) and normal quantities of estrogen.

In perhaps half of all cases of simple hirsutism, elevated serum testosterone is not demonstrable, but recently, about one-half of these cases have been shown to have increased plasma "free" (*i.e.*, non-protein-bound) testosterone due to reduced sex hor-

mone binding globulin. Increased hair follicle conversion of testosterone to the more potent dihydrotestosterone has been demonstrated in some of the remaining cases and other causes of increased sensitivity to androgens have been postulated.

Racial and ethnic factors are also important determinants of hair growth. Women of Asian ancestry and Caucasian women of northern European origins usually have relatively little facial or extremity hair. In contrast, Caucasian women of Mediterranean origins frequently develop mustache, beard, or sideburn hair. The immediate family history is also important (e.g. hirsutism in an individual of Mediterranean origins with a strong family history is most unlikely to require laboratory studies). The timing of onset is also important. Sudden development of hirsutism, many years after onset of menses, is likely to be due to tumor.

Transitory hirsutism may occur during pregnancy and occasionally during menopause. A number of pharmacologic agents can produce hirsutism including: glucocorticoids, phenytoin (Dilantin), minoxidil, diazoxide, and oral contraceptive agents. Rare causes include chronic local skin trauma and porphyria cutanea tarda.

Differential Diagnosis. A careful ethnic and family history are essential. The temporal evolution of the process should be noted, including the menstrual history. Physical signs of virilization should be sought. Cases with virilism need referral to an endocrinologist, while those with severe ovarian dysfunction require the attention of a gynecologist for therapy of abnormal menstruation or impaired fertility.

The decision to proceed with laboratory testing depends on the severity of the hirsutism. Laboratory studies can be performed sequentially, if financial considerations are dominant, or simultaneously. Plasma testosterone, which is of ovarian and rarely adrenal origin, is measured first. Normal serum testosterone suggests idiopathic hirsutism and excludes major ovarian disorders. Not excluded are mild cases of ovarian hyperthecosis with abnormal androstenedione production or decreased sex hormone binding globulin (increased "free" or bioavailable androgen). The uncovering of such borderline cases is usually not worthwhile since management would be unaffected.

If the testosterone is elevated to between 85 and 200 ng/dl, ovarian hyperthecosis or polycystic ovaries (Stein-Leventhal) is most likely. These patients should have determinations of serum follicle-stimulating hormone (FSH) and luteinizing hormone (LH). Normal values suggest ovarian hyperthecosis, while increased LH and low-normal or reduced FSH are highly suggestive of polycystic ovary disease.

Levels of testosterone greater than 200 ng/dl suggest a diagnosis of ovarian neoplasm, a very rare entity, and further diagnostic workup should be directed by specialists. This may include sonography, computerized axial tomography, and/or ovarian vein catheterization. In the absence of elevated serum testosterone, an adrenal origin must still be excluded. Elevated serum dehydroepiandrosterone-sulfate (DHEA-S) or 24-hour urinary excretion of 17-ketosteroids (17-KS) suggests adrenal neoplastic disease. Elevations of urinary pregnanetriol and/or plasma 17-α-hydroxyprogesterone suggests congenital adrenal hyperplasia (21-hydroxylase deficiency) which occasionally has its clinical onset in the teens or twenties. Finally, tumor is excluded by suppression with dexamethasone (see Chapter 71). Failure of suppression is indicative of adrenal neoplasm. Congenital adrenal hyperplasia is diagnosed when the levels of DHEA-S or 17-KS fall to 10–20% of baseline.

Therapy. The therapy of simple hirsutism is usually local and essentially cosmetic, even when there is a hormonal abnormality, because medical reduction of androgen excess does not rapidly affect the presence of existing hair and is often incomplete. Patients on medical therapy should be cautioned not to expect rapid results, since dedifferentiation of androgenized follicles may require 6 to 18 months even when androgen excess is totally eliminated. The major benefit to be expected is prevention of progress of the hirsutism, with variable degrees of reversal coming later as therapy is continued.

Local measures include bleaching, wax stripping, shaving, plucking (tweezing), the use of hair removal creams (depilatories), and electrolysis. Contrary to popular belief, such measures do not accelerate the growth rate of hair. Plucking may cause local infection. Wax applications or hair removal creams are effective but may be irritating and must be used with care. All of these procedures must be repeated at intervals. Electrolysis and thermolysis are effective procedures for permanent removal of hair, but are expensive and uncomfortable. Effectiveness and safety (avoidance of burns, scarring, and infection) are dependent on the technique of the operator. Referral of the patient requires that the physician be familiar with the electrologist's skill. Under the best of circumstances, electrolysis is generally successful in destroying about 50% of the follicles treated at one time. Thus, several repetitions are invariably required.

Medical therapy is directed toward the suppression of androgen production. Although such therapy appears more rational when androgen excess is demonstrable, idiopathic cases may also respond. Adrenal suppression, although introduced on the erroneous assumption that androgens of adrenal origin were responsible for most cases of hirsutism is, nonetheless, effective in about one-third of cases. This seems to be due to reduction of ovarian androgen production which is either directly dependent on ACTH or indirectly dependent on ovarian conversion of circulating adrenal steroids. Adrenal suppression is directly effective in cases of congenital adrenal hyperplasia.

This form of therapy is simple and usually free from side effects. Dexamethasone is given as a single dose of 0.5 or 0.75 mg orally at bedtime which reduces the morning peak of ACTH secretion. Signs of glucocorticoid excess are unlikely to occur nor is chronic adrenal suppression with adrenal insufficiency a problem. Normal adrenal responsiveness is restored within a few days of discontinuation. Insomnia and appetite stimulation may occur.

The alternative form of medical therapy, suppression of ovarian androgen production with a cyclically administered estrogen-progestin combination (oral contraceptive), is effective in about one-half of cases. Estrogens also increase concentration of plasma sex hormone binding globulin, reducing the circulating free androgens. Since progestins have some intrinsic androgen-like activity on hair follicles, a combination which minimizes the content of progestational agent may be the most appropriate. A combination of 80 μg mestranol and 1 mg norethindrone (Ortho-Novum, 1/80 or Norinyl 1+80) is satisfactory, as is ethinyl estradiol, 0.05 mg, and norgestrel, 0.5 mg (Ovral). Combinations containing 100 μg mestranol and 2 mg norethindrone (Ortho-Novum, 2 mg or Norinyl-2) are also satisfactory.

Disadvantages of oral contraceptives include their cardiovascular and other undesirable effects (see Chapter 90). The multiple disadvantages of administering these agents must be weighed when they are to be prescribed for an essentially benign problem. Suppression of ovarian androgen production by oral contraceptives precludes pregnancy. Thus therapy must be interrupted when fertility is desired and the drug withheld until pregnancy is terminated. Hirsutism may recur during this time.

Rarely, combined adrenal-ovarian suppression may be used if neither alone is effective. Several other agents have been used successfully for the medical therapy of hirsutism. Medroxyprogesterone acetate (Provera), 100 mg intramuscularly every 2 weeks, or 30 to 40 mg orally reduces testosterone production and interferes with testosterone action at the tissue level. A variety of side effects may be encountered. Spironolactone (Aldactone) at a generally well-tolerated dose of 25 mg twice daily, also appears to suppress ovarian androgen production (26). Cyproterone acetate is a competitive inhibitor of androgen action at the level of the hair follicle. None of these agents is currently approved in the United States for the treatment of hirsutism.

DYSMENORRHEA

Dysmenorrhea, painful menstruation, is a very common problem. It is considered *primary* when it appears within a year or two of the menarche, a problem therefore of teenagers, and *secondary* when the painful menstruation appears as a result of a specific pathologic process such as fibroids, endometriosis, pelvic inflammatory disease, or an intrauterine contraceptive device. This secondary form, therefore, usually occurs in women who are well past the menarche and when it occurs, the physician should seek an initiating cause, as the problem will not resolve without control of the inciting disorder.

Primary dysmenorrhea is the development within 1 or 2 days of the onset of menstruation of either crampy or sustained lower abdominal and pelvic pain which may radiate into the legs and which may be associated with nausea, vomiting, irritability, or abdominal distention. In a few patients, symptoms may be so severe that performance of their usual daily activities is not possible. Usually the discomfort is most severe during the initial several hours and then begins to fade and is usually gone within 2 or 3 days. The episodes become less severe with increasing age and often disappear spontaneously within 5 or 10 years after the menarche or after pregnancy.

The pathogenesis of primary dysmenorrhea is not completely understood, but it requires ovulation and it is felt to result from excessive myometrial contractions, possibly due to an excess formation of uterine prostaglandins.

Mild forms of dysmenorrhea require only mild analgesic therapy such as aspirin or acetaminophen and reassurance from the physician that the symptoms will resolve in time. There are a number of preparations available without prescription which are marketed for menstrual cramps. Most are combination tablets and none are proven to be more effective than aspirin or acetaminophen alone. Examples of these combination tablets are: Femcaps (aspirin, phenacetin, citrate, ephedrine, and atropine) or Midol (aspirin, caffeine, and cinnamedrine).

When symptoms are more severe or incapacitating, therapy with agents with antiprostaglandin activity greater than that of aspirin or acetaminophen may be effective. Nonsteroidal anti-inflammatory agents, all of which have antiprostaglandin activity, should be tried. Ibuprofen (Motrin, 400 mg, 4 times/day, for 5 to 6 days) and mefenamic (Ponstel, 250 mg, 4 times/day, for 5 to 6 days) have been approved by the FDA for use in dysmenorrhea. Other nonsteroidal anti-inflammatory agents such as indomethacin (Indocin, 25 mg, 4 times/day for 6 doses) and naproxen (Naprosyn, 500 mg, 4 times/day for 5 doses) have been shown to be effective in the treatment of dysmenorrhea, but have not been studied as extensively and have not yet been approved as analgesics by the FDA. These drugs are most effective if given just before menstrual flow begins and continued for 2 to 3 days thereafter. However, because of the uncertainty of the effects of these agents in early pregnancy, it is suggested that their use be delayed until the beginning of menstrual flow in those patients who are sexually active and who are not using effective means of birth control. The patient should use one agent as a trial for three cycles and then this should be discontinued if there has been an inadequate response in controlling the symptoms. It is currently unknown whether one nonsteroidal anti-inflammatory agent might be effective when another has failed.

Oral contraceptive agents suppress ovulation and thereby dramatically control dysmenorrhea; these agents may occasionally be necessary for management of this problem when it is severe. The use of oral contraceptive agents is fully discussed in Chapter 90.

The unusual patient who does not respond to these therapies should be seen by a gynecologist for evaluation for an undetected problem causing secondary amenorrhea or to provide more experienced guidance in the drug therapy of primary amenorrhea.

ABNORMAL VAGINAL BLEEDING BEFORE MENOPAUSE

During the 35 to 45 years of menstruation nearly all women will have occasional variations in bleeding pattern. In women approaching the menopause, irregularity of the menstrual cycle is typical, as described below. In younger women, most changes in bleeding pattern will be of the type called dysfunctional uterine bleeding (DUB), which is defined as abnormal bleeding for which no anatomic source can be found. Most DUB is related to anovulation, generally as a manifestation of alterations in pituitary-gonadal physiology described as "idiopathic hypothalamic oligo-amenorrhea" (see below). DUB may also be seen in the hirsutism-anovulation syndrome (e.g. Stein-Levinthal). A variety of physical and emotional stresses can precipitate DUB. In a few patients, abnormal vaginal bleeding will be related to unsuspected pregnancy or to anatomic problems.

Women will often describe abnormal bleeding first to their general physician, and will often be concerned about cancer. Therefore, it is important for the general physician to have a systematic approach to this problem. With careful history-taking and a limited evaluation, a working diagnosis and plan can usually be developed in the office.

Table 74.3 lists the various causes of abnormal vaginal bleeding in the premenopausal woman.

HISTORY. The patient should be asked how the abnormal bleeding differs from that which occurs during her normal cycle in terms of volume, timing, and quality, and when the normal pattern changed. *Menorrhagia* is present when menstruation occurs at the usual time but blood loss is greater than usual (e.g., the patient has to change pads more frequently, pads contain more blood than usual, or bleeding lasts several days longer than usual). This characteristic is consistent with DUB, leiomyomata uteri, endometrial polyps, or an underlying medical problem (e.g., hypothyroidism). *Metrorrhagia* is present when the patient has vaginal bleeding (usually spotting) between otherwise normally spaced periods. This characteristic may be found with leiomyomata, polyps, or local vulvar vaginal problems, but carcinoma of the endometrium or cervix and break-through bleeding related to oral contraceptives may also present this way.

Table 74.3
Causes of Abnormal Vaginal Bleeding in the Premenopausal Woman

1. Dysfunctional uterine bleeding (hypothalamic idiopathic anovulation)
2. Perineal causes: bladder pathology, hemorrhoids
3. Vulvar causes: infection, laceration, tumor
4. Vaginal causes: infection, laceration, tumor, foreign body
5. Cervical causes: infection, erosion, polyp, carcinoma
6. Uterine causes: infection, polyp, leiomyomata, carcinoma, intra-uterine device (IUD)
7. Ovarian causes: infection, polycystic ovary (Stein-Levinthal)
8. Pregnancy: threatened abortion, complete abortion, ectopic pregnancy
9. Oral contraceptive pills
10. Systemic medical conditions: bleeding diathesis (especially thrombocytopenia), thyroid disease, others

Menometrorrhagia indicates the presence of both menorrhagia and metrorrhagia. *Polymenorrhea* is present when menstruation occurs at intervals of less than 21 days. *Oligomenorrhea* is present when menstruation occurs at intervals of greater than 35 days. These two patterns are more commonly associated with alterations in hormone balance (*i.e.*, DUB) often precipitated by physical or emotional stress.

The history can also provide *evidence of ovulation*. This may be very helpful since most DUB is usually associated with failure to ovulate. Features associated with ovulation include 1) mittelschmerz (mild or moderate pain in one iliac fossa at mid-cycle, indicating rupture of an ovarian follicle), 2) increased mid-cycle mucus (due to the secretory effect of progesterone), 3) premenstrual molimina (abnormal fullness, headaches, and irritability immediately preceding the onset of bleeding), 4) dysmenorrhea, and, 5) a biphasic basal body temperature pattern (at time of ovulation, the temperature usually rises 1° Farenheit or ½° Centigrade and remains elevated until the onset of bleeding).

Sexually active women should be asked what type of contraception they are using and questioned regarding symptoms suggesting pregnancy. Breakthrough bleeding (metrorrhagia) is not uncommon in women using oral contraceptives, especially during the first year of use. Pregnancy-related bleeding is a problem in the first trimester, when it may be difficult to distinguish clinically whether the patient is pregnant. Almost always, the patient will have missed her period, and she may have morning sickness, frequent urination, and other early symptoms of pregnancy. Bleeding may be due to one of several conditions. *Threatened abortion* is characterized by bleeding before the loss of the fetus; this occurs in 10% of pregnancies and ultimately about half will have healthy babies. *Spontaneous abortion* is characterized by intense cramping and bleeding with passage of clots. The abortion may be complete (the uterus is empty and no further management may be needed) or incomplete (partial loss of uterine contents and need for prompt attention by a gynecologist). *Ectopic pregnancy* is characterized by a missed period followed by abnormal bleeding which may range from spotting to heavy bleeding. There may be associated unilateral pelvic pain.

The history should include inquiry about an *abnormal vaginal discharge* or other symptoms of pelvic infection or irritation (Chapter 91). A chronic pelvic infection may cause any of the abnormal bleeding patterns described above.

In patients with menorrhagia, polymenorrhea or oligomenorrhea, the history should include a brief inquiry about several medical conditions. Severe *thrombocytopenia* may cause menorrhagia, but coagulation abnormalities, including anticoagulant therapy, rarely cause abnormal vaginal bleeding. The patient with abnormal vaginal bleeding due to thrombocytopenia will usually have other manifestations of this problem (Chapter 47). *Hypothyroidism* may cause menorrhagia while hyperthyroidism tends to be associated with oligo-amenorrhea. The patient's history should therefore include a check for symptoms of thyroid disease (Chapter 70).

When *dysfunctional uterine bleeding* is suspected (absence of features of ovulation and lack of evidence for other causes), the patient should be asked about recent changes in her general health and in her daily activities. Among the factors which may precipitate DUB are diet change, weight gain or loss, emotional stress, jogging and other strenuous activities, sleep loss, mental strain, chronic medical conditions, and alcohol or illicit drug use.

PHYSICAL EXAMINATION. All patients complaining of abnormal vaginal bleeding should have a pelvic examination, to look for obvious anatomic causes of the bleeding. It is important not to defer the examination because of the bleeding. Hemorrhoids, vulvar conditions, vaginitis and cervicitis, cervical polyp or cervical erosion, and leiomyomata uteri are the principal anatomic problems which may be identified. Vulvovaginal and cervical sources of bleeding should be suspected especially in patients who describe metrorrhagia or post-coital bleeding.

The patient should also be checked for echymoses and petechiae, especially in the lower extremities, and for physical signs of thyroid disease.

LABORATORY TESTS. A hemoglobin concentration or a hematocrit value should always be obtained, and, in an actively bleeding patient, orthostatic blood pressure and heart rate should be checked. In addition, every woman with a change in her bleeding pattern should have a Pap smear evaluated (Chapter 92). Sexually active women should always have a pregnancy test.

If the history or physical examination suggests the possibility of a bleeding diathesis, a platelet count, bleeding time, prothrombin time, and partial thromboplastin time should be obtain (Chapter 47). Thyroid function tests should be obtained if thyroid disease is suspected on clinical grounds.

WORKING DIAGNOSIS AND MANAGEMENT. *Anatomic causes.* The general evaluation described above is sufficient to identify most of the anatomic causes for abnormal bleeding in the pre-menopausal woman. A history of typical ovulatory symptoms increases the likelihood that the bleeding is due to an anatomic problem or a chronic medical condition. Because uterine problems (*e.g.*, fibroid tumors, and, much less commonly, endometrial cancer) are more frequent in women over 35, these patients should be evaluated by a gynecologist if they develop *any* unexplained change in their bleeding pattern, especially if a change persists for more than two cycles. When definite pelvic pathology or pregnancy is detected or suspected, the patient should be referred promptly to a gynecologist, except in the case of vaginitis or cervicitis, which may be treated by the general physician (Chapter 91). The evaluation which a gynecologist will perform for possible gynecologic cancer is described in Chapter 92.

When a primary medical condition seems to explain the patient's problem, this condition should be managed appropriately (thrombocytopenia: see Chapter 47; thyroid disorders: see Chapter 70).

Dysfunctional Uterine Bleeding (DUB). For the large number of women in whom the working diagnosis is dysfunctional uterine bleeding, the general physician may elect to manage the problem himself or refer the patient to a gynecologist. The most common cause of DUB is anovulation. In this case no corpus luteum is formed so that a progesterone-primed endometrium is not produced. If levels of estrogen are fairly high, the endometrium will continue to proliferate, become hyperplastic, then break down irregularly and bleed.

When dysfunctional bleeding has been a problem for a brief period (three to four months), appropriate management consists of explaining the problem to the patient and having her modify obvious precipitating factors whenever this is possible. If her menorrhagia is particularly heavy and is interfering with her usual activities, the problem can be controlled promptly by prescribing a 21-day package of a combination oral contraceptive such as Ovral-21. She should be given the following written instructions: take the first three tablets immediately, then take one tablet twice daily for the next nine days. Within 24 hours, the current bleeding will be suppressed, and she will then have withdrawal bleeding at the end of the 9-day course. If the primary stress causing her DUB is not modified, the DUB will persist, and referral to a gynecologist is appropriate.

Patients with persistent DUB, especially those in whom there is a problem of infertility, should be referred to a gynecologist or reproductive endocrinologist. Two objective findings which help to confirm the absence of ovulation are the lack of a biphasic basal body temperature pattern described above and a failure of serum progesterone to rise during the patient's menstrual cycle. The two pieces of data should be obtained if possible before referral. DUB will occur in some women in whom these data indicate ovulation. The usual explanation is that there has not been adequate progesterone produced to promote proper shedding of the endometrium. An endometrial biopsy will often be performed by the consulting gynecologist. This biopsy can confirm either the absence of ovulation (the endometrium will be proliferative, indicating only an estrogen effect) or the presence of ovulation (the endometrium will be secretory, reflecting a progesterone effect, or it may show a mixture of proliferative and secretory changes). Depending upon these findings and additional investigations, the gynecologist will develop a management plan for the patient.

OLIGO-AMENORRHEA

Gonadal dysfunction in women nearly always presents as alteration of the menstrual pattern, either irregular and infrequent menses (oligomenorrhea) or cessation of menses (amenorrhea). Oligo-amenorrhea (the syndrome of few or no periods) may be classified as in Table 74.4. Classification will provide clues to the etiology and hence to prognosis and therapy.

Primary. *Primary central* amenorrhea *with maturational failure* suggests idiopathic or genetic gonadotropin deficiency of pituitary or hypothalamic origin. A patient with *primary gonadal* failure is likely to have Turner's syndrome (XO sex chromosomes and no ovaries). *Primary* amenorrhea *with normal maturation* may be due to *peripheral* causes as simple as imperforate hymen with obstruction of menses, or

Table 74.4
Classification of Female Hypogonadism (*i.e.* Oligo-amenorrhea)

Classification	Criteria
ACCORDING TO TIME OF ONSET	
Primary (no onset of menses)	History
Secondary (cessation of established menses)	
ACCORDING TO SOMATOTYPE	
Maturation failure (juvenile)	Physical examination
Feminized (normal secondary sex)	
Masculinized (hirsute, deep voice, increased muscle mass, clitoromegaly)	
ACCORDING TO LOCATION OF LESION	
Central (hypothalamic or pituitary):	Gonadotropins ↓ or →
a. Without galactorrhea	
b. With galactorrhea	
Gonadal (ovarian failure)	Gonadotropins ↑
Exogeneous (disruption of menses by drugs, stress, or illness of other than reproductive organs)	History, physical examination, various laboratory and radiologic tests
ACCORDING TO ETIOLOGY	
Genetic (chromosomal or familial)	History, buccal smear, karyotype
Acquired (infectious, neoplastic, traumatic, surgical, hemorrhage or infarction, autoimmune)	History, physical examination, radiology, other special procedures

as serious as congenital uterine agenesis. A special case of this latter kind is testicular feminization (see p. 782).

Secondary. Feminized patients with *central secondary* amenorrhea may have brain tumors or anorexia nervosa, but most commonly, have idiopathic hypothalamic amenorrhea. Pituitary amenorrhea is usually *acquired* and is frequently accompanied by deficiencies in other hormone axes (adrenal, thyroid). Etiologies are the same as in the male (see above).

Gonadal secondary amenorrhea can be due to infection (e.g., tuberculosis), neoplasm (Krukenberg tumor—metastasis of gastrointestinal neoplasm to ovary), trauma, surgery, or an autoimmune disorder. This latter category is often associated with a syndrome of polyglandular failures (see p. 782) and is the most common cause of "idiopathic premature menopause."

Exogenous. *Exogenous* amenorrhea may be caused by hyper- or hypothyroidism, starvation, liver failure, renal failure, or severe stress, as in grief or mental illness. Another form of exogenous interruption may come from consumption of substances of abuse (opiates, alcohol) or prescribed medications (major tranquilizers, estrogens).

GALACTORRHEA

Galactorrhea is the production of milk (confirmed by demonstrating fat after staining the fluid with Sudan stain) by a non-nursing individual who is not recently postpartum. *Secondary central* amenorrhea is frequently (15%) accompanied by galactorrhea. Galactorrheic amenorrhea is often (42%) due to the presence of a prolactin-secreting pituitary adenoma which may or may not be readily detectable (macro- *vs.* microadenoma) (15). Other causes of galactorrheic amenorrhea include medication (INH (isoniazid), phenothiazines), recent pregnancy, hypothyroidism, and idiopathic hypothalamic dysfunction. It is not uncommon for a woman who has nursed to have mild persistent galactorrhea (without amenorrhea) for up to 5 years after weaning. In these cases prolactin levels are normal (< 30 ng/ml).

Approach to Women with Reproductive Endocrine Dysfunction

The diagnostic approach to female reproductive disturbances is aimed at classifying the kind of disorder (see above), identifying or eliminating specific disease entities which require medical or surgical treatment, and, having done this, determining to what extent the remaining symptoms represent a problem to the patient and treating these problems appropriately.

HISTORY

The physician should determine whether the problem is primary or secondary. A chronicle of pubertal events should be recorded including earliest budding of breast tissue (thelarche), pubic hair darkening and lengthening (pubarche), onset of menstrual flow (menarche), and time of growth spurt and its cessation. A menstrual history includes the average interval between menses, their regularity and when irregularity developed, date of last period and previous period before that, the duration of flow and its magnitude, presence of ovulatory pain (mittelschmerz), premenstrual tension, and dysmenorrhea. The latter three findings suggest ovulatory cycles. A pregnancy and nursing history (mature and premature deliveries, abortions, success with and duration of lactation, and living children's ages) and history of gynecologic surgery (including dilation and curettage) are pertinent. A history of breast changes (swelling, tenderness, discharge) should be determined. The physician should ask whether the patient is troubled by growth of excessive hair, and if so, what is the duration of symptoms, the location and severity of the problem, and the treatment used, if any. Also of interest are symptoms of masculinization: increased libido with greater sexual appetite or increased sexual dreaming and fantasies, voice deepening, and frontal hair loss. Symptoms of estrogen deficiency (hot flashes, vaginal discharge with dyspareunia, and breast atrophy) are important. A careful history of medication and drug use, including oral contraceptive agents, may be helpful. A further general history should include weight gain or loss, dietary habits, symptoms of diabetes, adrenal or thyroid disease, and history of tuberculosis or liver, renal, or CNS problems. A family history should include ethnic origin and familial occurrence of reproductive and other endocrine dysfunctions (e.g., hirsutism, oligomenorrhea, hypothyroidism).

PHYSICAL EXAMINATION

On inspection the physician should note body habitus (obese or wasted, mature or childlike, masculine or feminine). The presence or absence of pubic and axillary hair, distribution of coarse dark hair on chest (periareolar, midsternal), abdomen, buttocks, and extremities, and the density of such hair must be noted. The quality of the patient's voice should be evaluted. Examination of breasts and pubic hair should include an estimate of their stage of maturity based on available standards (19) (see Chapter 5, Table 5.4) and nipples should be squeezed to look for galactorrhea. On pelvic examination it is important to look for clitoromegaly (> 2.0 cm in length), state of the vaginal mucosa (dry *vs.* moist, thick and rugated *vs.* thin and atrophic), discharge, presence or absence and size and consistency of cervix and uterus, and also to attempt to estimate whether ovaries are enlarged (cystic) or not. In primary amenorrhea without maturation, signs of Turner's syndrome (wide set eyes, shield chest, wide set nipples, "webbing" of neck, short 4th metacarpal, and signs of aortic coarctation) should be sought. The remainder of the general physical examination (eyes, abdomen, etc.) should be as described in the evaluation of male hypogonadism (see p. 783) stressing signs of an intracranial mass lesion and thyroid or adrenal disease.

DIAGNOSTIC PROCEDURES

All women with secondary amenorrhea should be considered pregnant until proven otherwise (even if sexual activity is not admitted, as, in adolescence, it may not be). Specific hCG assay is the most sensitive test for pregnancy (see Chapter 90). Further testing should be delayed until pregnancy is ruled out.

Serum estrogen determinations usually cannot distinguish low normal from deficiency, therefore, estrogen status should be assessed as follows. Cells for vaginal cytology should be obtained at the time of pelvic examination so that a maturational index can be estimated (see Chapter 91). A progesterone withdrawal test (7 days of 10 mg of medroxyprogesterone acetate (Provera) orally or a single 100-mg dose of progesterone in oil i.m.) will result in withdrawal bleeding within a few days (2 to 5 if oral and 7 to 10 if i.m.) after the drug administration if estrogen levels are adequate. If there is no bleeding, a 21-day course of estrogen (0.02 or 0.05 mg of ethinyl estradiol (Estinyl)/day) with 5 to 10 mg of medroxyprogesterone acetate (Provera) for the last 7 days should be administered. Absence of vaginal bleeding at this point indicates an absent or severely damaged endometrium, sometimes secondary to previous overvigorous dilation and curettage (Ashelman's syndrome).

Serum or urinary gonadotropins are used to classify hypogonadism as *gonadal* (elevated) or *central* (low or normal). The investigation of *central* hypogonadism should include a serum prolactin, especially if galactorrhea is present. Prolactin values between 30 and 100 ng/ml are elevated but may be consistent with prolactinoma or hypothalamic (idiopathic) galactorrhea. Values greater than 100 ng/ml nearly always mean that a prolactinoma is present (15). Further testing should be undertaken by appropriate specialists and is similar to that outlined for patients with male hypogonadism (Table 74.2). If hirsutism is present, the serum testosterone and urinary 17-ketosteroids should be measured (see p. 787).

Therapy in Women with the Oligo-amenorrhea Syndrome

ABSENCE OF MENSES

The mere fact of amenorrhea is disturbing to some women, but not to others. Women with idiopathic oligo-amenorrhea who desire regular periods can be treated with low dose estradiol plus progestin regimens in cyclic fashion as outlined below. Where fertility is an issue, appropriate referral should be made.

GALACTORRHEA

Women with hyperprolactinemia can be treated by transsphenoid removal of an adenoma (if present) or by suppression with bromocriptine (Parlodel) 2.5 mg, 2 or 3 times/day, which treatment frequently also restores libido (see "Frigidity and Female Endocrine Dysfunction," below), suppresses lactation, and restores menses and fertility.

INTRACRANIAL TUMOR

If vision or brain function is threatened, surgery or radiotherapy is indicated. If only a microadenoma is present, it may be legitimate simply to follow visual fields and X-rays at intervals of 6 months to 1 year and treat hormone deficiency appropriately.

ESTROGEN DEFICIENCY STATE

Estrogen deficiency is not a frequent occurrence in young women with central secondary amenorrhea, but may occur in some women, especially those with hyperprolactinemia (16). It may be defined by a failure to develop withdrawal bleeding after progestin administration, plasma estrogen less than 25 pg/ml, and/or failure to ovulate and menstruate after being given clomiphene citrate (clomid) 50 to 100 mg/day for 5 days. It is the rule in gonadal hypogonadism. Symptoms, complications, and therapy are discussed in the section on menopause (see below).

Frigidity and Female Endocrine Dysfunction

DEFINITION

As in the male, female hyposexuality can be divided into reduced sexual interest or appetite (inhibition of desire), failure of arousal (inhibition of excitement), and anorgasmia (for a more complete discussion, see Chapter 17). Discussion below will be limited to physical and especially endocrine etiologies.

ETIOLOGIES

Organic etiologies of female hyposexuality include diabetes mellitus with peripheral neuropathy, hyperprolactinemia, hypogonadism with estrogen deficiency, and organic disease of the vagina, uterus, fallopian tubes, or ovaries with resultant dyspareunia. Various endocrine (e.g., hyper- or hypothyroidism) and other systemic debilitating diseases can also cause loss of interest in sex.

HISTORY

Questions should be the same as those asked of the patient with female hypogonadism (see above). Additional questions should be asked about dyspareunia. If there is pain or discomfort on intercourse, it is important to know if it occurs with attempts at penetration (local vaginal or vulvar problems) or only after deep penetration (pelvic disease—e.g., leiomyoma, endometriosis, salpingitis). The physician should determine whether there was a previous history of satisfactory sexual activity, and if so, the time and circumstances of onset of its deterioration. Careful questioning should reveal to what extent the problem is one of loss of interest, excitation (lubrication and heightened pelvic blood flow), or orgasm.

A history of symptoms of diabetes or peripheral neuropathy and of thyroid, adrenal, or other serious systemic disorders should be obtained. Medication use (tranquilizers, oral contraceptives) and substance abuse (opiates, alcohol) are also pertinent.

PHYSICAL EXAMINATION

The physical examination should be conducted in the same way as for patients with female hypogonadism (see p. 792). Careful attention should be given to the genitalia, uterus, and adnexa for evidence of infection, atrophy, or neoplasia. Endometriosis is sometimes detected on rectovaginal examination by palpation of nodules in the space between the rectum and vagina (pouch of Douglas). Testing of peripheral sensation should be thorough.

DIAGNOSTIC PROCEDURES

If evidence of hypogonadism exists, appropriate tests should be made (see p. 793). Measurement of serum prolactin may be helpful even in patients without apparent galactorrhea or amenorrhea (see p. 793). Patients with pelvic disease should be referred to a gynecologist for further evaluation and therapy.

THERAPY

Therapeutic efforts should be directed at the specific organic etiology whenever possible. Estrogen deficiency should be replaced (see below) and hyperprolactinemia should be treated surgically or medically (see above). When no organic cause is evident after careful examination, consideration of various modes of psychological diagnosis and treatment is appropriate (see Section 2, "Psychiatric and Behavioral Problems").

Problems of Menopause

DEFINITION

Menopause is the irreversible cessation of the female reproductive cycle and menses which follows from a permanent loss of ovarian response to gonadotropins. This change generally occurs spontaneously between the ages of 45 and 55 in American women, with an average age of 50. Destruction or cessation of function of the ovary prior to age 40 is referred to as premature menopause. Hysterectomy terminates menstrual bleeding, but not ovarian function, and hence, does not constitute a true menopause. In any year between 1981 and 2000, there will be approximately 30 million women of postmenopausal age (roughly one-third of the female population in the United States). Thus, an understanding of the medical problems of the menopausal period is important for all general physicians.

PHYSIOLOGY

Although it has long been known that the menopausal ovary is nearly depleted of primary follicles, the hormonal events of the perimenopausal period have only recently been elucidated. The work of Sherman and Korenman (27) and others has shown that after age 35 to 40 there is a tendency for serum estradiol to decrease, probably reflecting a reduction in the responsive cohort of follicles at onset of a cycle. This results in less feedback inhibition which in turn raises FSH levels and leads to a shortened follicular phase of the cycle (earlier ovulation), so that women in their late 30s may go from a regular 28- or 29-day menstrual interval to one of 25 to 27 days. In the early 40s the luteal phase may also become inadequate with lower progesterone levels and early dissolution of the corpus luteum, resulting in further shortening of the cycle. Estradiol levels continue to decline. Next, anovulatory cycles and "missed" cycles, with long quiescent periods in which gonadotropins are high and estradiol very low, begin to occur. For a year or two menses are irregular and occur with reduced frequency, but occasional ovulatory cycles are seen. Finally cyclic bleeding ceases. FSH and LH levels become greatly elevated in serum and urine. Usually the FSH increase is greater. The ovary may still contain a few follicles, but these do not respond to gonadotropin. Estradiol levels become extremely low and adrenal estrone becomes the major estrogen.

PSYCHOLOGIC SYMPTOMS

Epidemiologic and clinical studies have shown that there is not an increase in mental illness attributable to menopause and that, in particular, women who develop depression during the menopausal years do not have a distinct syndrome, an absence of previous depression, or an absence of other life-stress precipitants (31). There are, however, many cultural misconceptions about this period (e.g., expectations of loss of sexual interest and ability and expectations of an increased incidence of mental illness), and often these misconceptions propagate feelings of inadequacy, somatic symptoms such as fatigue, and other complaints. The organic changes of the menopause may reinforce these symptoms, and many women have had their symptoms worsened even further by the comment from a physician that the phenomenon is "an expected part of aging."

In spite of the lack of evidence that psychologic symptoms accompanying menopause are due to estrogen deficiency, many women have been given estrogens for their psychologic complaints. Reported benefits are probably due to a placebo effect. The physician should try to educate each patient about the menopause and should evaluate her for any underlying psychologic disturbances. Women who develop significant psychologic problems during the menopause should be managed appropriately, as described in the chapters in Section 2 of this book.

ESTROGEN DEFICIENCY STATE

Ovarian estrogen production is minimal after the menopause. Ovarian interstitial and hilus cells still retain some secretory capacity, but produce mainly small amounts of testosterone and androstenedione. Most estrogen is therefore formed from peripheral conversion of androgen, 75% of which comes from the adrenal. There is evidence that this rate of conversion is greater in obese women, who therefore tend to have higher estrogen levels postmenopausally. Estrogen deficiency results in various symptomatic manifestations in approximately 70% of postmenopausal women.

Hot Flashes. Nearly 50% of menopausal women complain of a sudden sensation of flushing and extreme warmth, followed by profuse sweating and sometimes shaking or tremor. These episodes occur at irregular intervals of 30 to 120 min and may awaken the patient at night. In about 15% they are severe enough to limit normal daily activities. Recent investigations have shown that these episodes, objectively identifiable by altered skin and core temperature and skin resistance, are closely related temporally to episodic gonadotropin secretion by the pituitary gland. They precede LH and FSH secretory rises by just a few minutes (30). LH and FSH secretory episodes are generally increased in amplitude, but not frequency during the menopause, probably reflecting derepression of neurosecretory activity of the hypothalamus by loss of estrogen feedback. It is theorized that this exaggerated excitation of neurosecretory nuclei may spread to the adjacent thermoregulatory centers in the hypothalamus, setting off the "hot flash" (which is thus a sort of "hypothalamic seizure").

Genital and Breast Atrophy. The female reproductive organs undergo striking changes at the time of the menopause. Pubic hair becomes sparse and lank, and may turn gray. The labia majora lose their fullness as subcutaneous adipose is withdrawn from them and the mons veneris, thus exposing the labia minora. The skin and mucous membranes of the genitalia become thin and dry. The vaginal pH becomes more alkaline as glandular secretion of glycogen is lost. This change and the mucosal atrophy may result in a chronic vaginitis with itching, discharge, and local tenderness (see Chapter 91). Many women report decreased lubrication at intercourse and dyspareunia. The cervix, uterus, and fallopian tubes also shrink. Estrogen deprivation also is implicated in the relaxation of pelvic ligaments and muscles which may result in uterine or bladder prolapse and contributes to the disturbing symptom of stress incontinence. At the same time glandular breast tissue atrophies, the breasts lose adipose and become shrunken and pendulous. There is a decrease in the erectile response of the nipple.

Osteoporosis. Accelerated loss of calcium from bone, increasing from 0.5% to an average of 1% of bone mass per year, at the time of the menopause (or with any cause of severe estrogen deficiency), has been well documented in a number of studies (22,23). Besides estrogen deficiency, dietary calcium deficiency, relative calcium malabsorption (perhaps due to reduced levels of or response to 1,25-dihydroxyvitamin D_3 in the gut), increased parathyroid hormone, and reduced exercise have all been considered as contributing factors. Calcium loss is mainly from trabecular bone. The vertebrae, femoral head, and radius contain high proportions of trabecular bone. This loss results in 8 times as many fractures in postmenopausal women compared with age-matched men. The incidence of fractures is greater in white than in black women, probably reflecting greater initial bone mass in blacks. Early in the disease process, crush fractures of the vertebral bodies predominate, causing loss of height, stooped posture (Dowager's hump), and sometimes back pain. Later, hip and forearm fractures become common. It has been estimated that, if a white woman lives to be 90 years of age, she has a 20% chance of hip fracture. About 1 million bone fractures occur annually in women over 45 years of age of which 150,000 are hip fractures. The death rate within 3 months of hip fracture is a staggering 16%, usually from complications of surgery and/or prolonged hospitalization. Repeated fractures are all too likely in the survivors. With approximately 30 million women at risk in the United States in any year until 2000 A.D., postmenopausal osteoporosis is a public health problem of major magnitude.

ENDOMETRIAL HYPERPLASIA AND CARCINOMA

With loss of regular shedding of the endometrium the incidence of endometrial hyperplasia, due to the unopposed tonic effects of residual (adrenal) estrogen, begins to rise. This lesion is rarely seen in cyclic premenopausal women, but occurs more frequently in young women with a pattern of irregular anovulatory bleeding. Hyperplasia also appears to be more common in obese postmenopausal women, probably because of increased aromatization of androgens to estrone in fatty tissue. Endometrial hyperplasia, especially the atypical adenomatous pattern, characteristic of unopposed estrogens, appears to be a precursor of endometrial carcinoma. The latter lesion is also more common in young anovulatory and postmenopausal obese women (14).

The incidence of endometrial carcinoma begins to rise at age 45, reaches a peak at about 0.08% (80 per 100,000) at age 70, and falls off thereafter. It is usually detected because of postmenopausal vaginal bleeding, is invasive (into myometrium and vessels) in only about 10% of cases, and has a relatively good prognosis if treated promptly by hysterectomy. It results in very few deaths, being both relatively rare and frequently curable.

ESTROGEN REPLACEMENT THERAPY

Benefits. It is clear that use of estrogen is highly effective, compared with placebo, in suppressing the symptoms of the "hot flash" (17). Even low doses

(0.02 mg/day of ethinyl estradiol (Estinyl) or 0.625 mg/day of Premarin), which have no measurable effect on circulating serum gonadotropins, have been found effective. Such therapy is often given for 6 months to a year and then tapered; hot flashes recur in about 50% of cases, however. In this instance, a more prolonged course of low dose estrogens, cyclic, progestin-opposed estrogen therapy (see below), or clonidine (see below) may be useful. Genital atrophy, vaginitis, and dyspareunia are all relieved by estrogen therapy, which may be systemic or local (by means of estrogen-containing cream). This latter form of therapy is not necessarily advantageous in preventing systemic effects of estrogen, since estrogens are taken up through the vaginal mucosa in unpredictable but significant amounts (25). Finally, estrogen replacement has been shown to be effective in reducing calcium loss and decreased bone density (12) and also the actual number of fractures (2) in estrogen-deficient women. Thus, there is no doubt that estrogens are highly efficacious in reducing the major problems associated with menopausal estrogen deficiency.

Risks. The risk of estrogen therapy of greatest current concern to the practicing physician and patient population is endometrial carcinoma (see above). A number of recent studies have demonstrated that postmenopausal estrogen therapy, as commonly practiced in the United States, *i.e.*, 0.625 to 1.25 mg of oral conjugated estrogens (Premarin) given daily without interruption, is associated, after 2 or more years of therapy, with a 6- to 8-fold increase in incidence of endometrial carcinoma (18). Recently, however, Hulka has demonstrated that monthly interruption (see below) of therapy and/or use of nonconjugated estrogen reduces the relative risk of invasive carcinoma to about 1.3 (not statistically significant) (13). Furthermore, it is apparent from other studies that the use of an oral progestin for 7 to 10 days of the cycle to mature the endometrium does not produce any excess endometrial hyperplasia or endometrial carcinoma (8,29). It is also of interest that women treated for up to 10 years with cycles of combined estrogen-progestin for birth control have not shown increased endometrial carcinoma, despite the high doses of estrogen employed. Thus it appears that cyclic, progestin-opposed estrogen therapy is free of this risk. One objection to this mode of therapy is that many women will find continuation or resumption of monthly vaginal bleeding unacceptable. Another is that such bleeding will be confusing to the physician trained to assume that postmenopausal bleeding indicates disease. It can be pointed out, however, first, that continued menstruation may be a small price to pay for even partial protection from osteoporosis and its distressingly frequent complications, not to mention prevention of genital atrophy, etc., and, second, there is no reason why regular monthly bleeding should be any more confusing to the physician in a 70-year-old woman than in a 35-year-old. In either case, it is intermenstrual spotting or unexpectedly heavy flow which should alert the physician to the necessity for investigation. Furthermore, even if this mode of therapy should result in some slight increase in the risk of endometrial carcinoma, comparison of incidences of morbidity and mortality show that endometrial carcinoma is a relatively rare and infrequently fatal disease, while osteoporotic fractures are very common and often crippling or fatal.

Although data have been presented on both sides of the issue, the best current information supports the conclusion that neither estrogens contained in oral contraceptives nor estrogens used for postmenopausal replacement therapy (11) are associated with an increased incidence of breast cancer. The high doses of estrogen in oral contraceptives have been shown to have a number of pharmacologic side effects which are fully discussed in Chapter 90. Because orally administered estrogens reach the liver first in high concentration, there is no dose of oral estrogen which will provide precise physiologic replacement and also avoid the potential for harmful side effects. Even though only one of the known complications (gallbladder disease) has actually been found with estrogen replacement therapy, these effects which include increased risk of thromboembolic disease, hypertension, and atherosclerosis are a legitimate consideration. Development of a convenient method of administering systemic (rather than portal) estrogen in physiologic doses cyclically for 3 weeks at a time would probably minimize these risks, but as yet such a method is not available. The physician must therefore weigh the risks and benefits in his own mind. We believe the current evidence favors the use of estrogen replacement therapy continuously after the menopause, especially in women with premature loss of ovaries (under age 40) and in white women, especially those at high risk (*i.e.*, small stature and slender builds, and smokers). This therapy is contraindicated in known cases of breast cancer and probably in women with a high risk of breast cancer (see Chapter 86), and in women who have suffered from stroke, phlebitis, or pulmonary emboli. The use of progestin is not necessary in those women who have had a hysterectomy. A regimen of 21 days of 1 mg of micronized estradiol (Estrace) or 0.02 mg of ethinyl estradiol (Estinyl), with the addition of a suitable progestin (e.g., 5 to 10 mg of medroxyprogesterone acetate, Provera) for the last 10 days is recommended. This is followed by 7 days without therapy before resumption of the cycle. Current cost for such a regimen is approximately $4.50 per month. The use of androgens adds little or nothing to this form of therapy and is not justified. Until further evidence confirms the absence of risk of endometrial carcinoma, an endometrial biopsy should probably be done on such patients at the initiation of therapy and every 2 years thereafter or if intermenstrual bleeding occurs (see Chapter 92).

ALTERNATIVES TO ESTROGEN THERAPY

There is no good alternative to estrogen for genital atrophy. As noted above, local estrogen cream produces unpredictable systemic estrogen absorption and thus has only illusory advantages over systemic therapy. Clonidine (Catapres), 0.5 mg twice daily has been shown to be effective in reducing the "hot flash" symptom (5). Other modes of therapy for prevention of osteoporosis include regimens of increased exercise, supplementation of diet with approximately 1500 mg of calcium (one 8-oz glass of milk and one 600-mg tablet of calcium carbonate 3 times a day) and use of vitamin D (1000 U/day). In patients > 70 years old as much as 10,000 U/day of vitamin D may be required to restore calcium absorption to normal. None of these regimens has been proven as effective as estrogen replacement and they should probably be used in conjunction with, rather than instead of, estrogen therapy.

Postmenopausal Bleeding

Postmenopausal bleeding is defined as any vaginal bleeding which occurs in a woman who has had no menstrual periods for 1 year.

Postmenopausal bleeding must always be investigated because approximately 10% of women with such bleeding will be found to have a malignant process of some kind. The remainder have various problems such as endometrial hyperplasia, polyps, infections, traumatic lacerations, etc. It is important that patients be educated that any bleeding after 1 year of menopause is abnormal and needs to be reported to the physician.

HISTORY

The management of postmenopausal bleeding begins with a careful review of the history with respect to duration, frequency, and the characteristics of the bleeding in terms of color, amount, and flow. The presence or absence of hormone therapy is important. Even if cyclic hormones are being used, heavy bleeding or bleeding at unexpected times in the cycle should still be investigated.

PHYSICAL EXAMINATION

A careful physical examination should be undertaken. The abdomen must be evaluated for suprapubic masses and lower abdominal tenderness. The external genitalia must be inspected for neoplasia and/or atrophic changes. The vaginal mucosa should be inspected for atrophy or lacerations. The cervix must be visualized and a Pap smear obtained if needed. The size, shape, and position of the uterus must be noted and the adnexae evaluated for enlargement or tenderness. A rectal examination may reveal the presence of hemorrhoids and/or fissures. Samples of stool and of urine should be obtained for analysis for occult blood. These latter procedures may suggest the rectum or bladder rather than the uterus or genitals as the source of bleeding.

DIAGNOSTIC PROCEDURES

Patients with obvious lesions of the vulva, vagina, or cervix should have a direct biopsy taken for pathologic evaluation. Patients with significant adnexal disease should be further investigated by intravenous pyelogram, barium enema, flat plate of the abdomen, and sonography. Bleeding from nonmalignant causes such as atrophic vaginitis, or traumatic lacerations secondary to intercourse, should not postpone the next and most important step, namely referral of the patient to a gynecologist for dilation and curettage (if the uterus is present).

Cervical biopsies are indicated only if the Pap smear is borderline or abnormal. The physician should know that general anesthesia for a D and C may be recommended by the gynecologist for patients who are obese, who have a low tolerance for pain, or who are new to the physician. In those patients who have been seeing the physician for annual examinations and who have negative Pap and pelvic examinations over a number of years, a D and C under local anesthesia is usually a very satisfactory procedure and requires minimal hospital time.

References

General

Eskin, BA (ed): *The Menopause, Comprehensive Management.* Masson, New York, 1980.
    Excellent summary of pertinent clinical issues and menopausal physiology.
Gregerman, RI and Bierman, EL: Aging and hormones. In *Textbook of Endocrinology,* Ed. 6, edited by R. H. Williams. W. B. Saunders, Philadelphia, 1981.
    Thorough discussion of endocrine relationships involved in osteoporosis and of effects of aging on reproductive endocrinology.
Paulsen, CA: The testis. In *Textbook of Endocrinology,* Ed. 6, edited by RH Williams. W. B. Saunders, Philadelphia, 1981.
    Definitive chapter on pathophysiology of the male reproductive system.
Ross, GT and Vande Wiele, RL: The ovaries. In *Textbook of Endocrinology,* Ed. 6, edited by RH Williams. W. B. Saunders, Philadelphia, 1981.
    Detailed step-by-step instruction on diagnosis and management of disturbances of female reproductive endocrinology.

Specific

1. Adams, DB, Gold, AR and Burt, AD: Rise in female initiated sexual activity at ovulation and its suppression by oral contraceptives. *N Engl J Med* 299: 1145, 1978.
2. Aitken, JM, Hart, DM and Lindsay, R: Estrogen replacement therapy for the prevention of osteoporosis after oophorectomy. *Br Med J 3:* 515, 1973.
3. Carter, JN, Tyson, JE, Tolis, G, VanVliet, S, Faiman, C and Friesen, HG: Prolactin secreting tumors and hypogonadism in 22 men. *N Engl J Med* 299: 847, 1978.
4. Davidson, JM: Hormones and sexual behavior in the male. *Hosp Pract 10:* 126, 1975.
5. Edington, RF, Chagnon, JP and Steinberg, WM: Clonidine (Dixarit) for menopausal flushing. *Can Med Assoc J* 123: 1, 1980.
6. Federman, D: *Abnormal Sexual Development* p. 27. W. B. Saunders, Philadelphia, 1968.
7. Frank, E, Anderson, C and Rubinstein, D: Frequency of sexual dysfunction in normal couples. *N Engl J Med* 299: 111, 1978.
8. Gambrell, RD, Massey, FM, Castaneda, TA, Ugenas, AJ and

Ricci, CA: Reduced incidence of endometrial cancer among postmenopausal women treated with progestogens. *J Am Geriatr Soc 27:* 389, 1979.

9. Harman, SM: Clinical aspects of aging of the male reproductive system. In *The Aging Reproductive System*, p. 29, edited by E Schneider. Raven Press, New York, 1978.

10. Harman, SM and Tsitouras, PD: Reproductive hormones in aging men; I. Measurement of sex steroids basal luteinizing hormone and Leydig cell response to human chorionic gonadotropin. *J Clin Endocrinol Metab 51:* 35, 1980.

11. Hoover, R, Gray, IA, Cole, P and MacMahon, B: Menopausal estrogens and breast cancer. *N Engl J Med 295:* 401, 1976.

12. Horsman, A, Gallagher, JC, Simpson, M and Nordin, BEC: Prospective trial of estrogen and calcium in postmenopausal women. *Br Med J 2:* 789, 1977.

13. Hulka, B, Kaufman, DG, Fowler, WC, Grimson, RC and Greenberg, BG: Predominance of early endometrial cancers after long-term estrogen use. *JAMA 244:* 2419, 1980.

14. Judd, HL, Lucas, WE and Yen, SSC: Serum 17β-estradiol and estrone levels in postmenopausal women with and without endometrial cancer. *J Clin Endocrinol Metab 43:* 272, 1976.

15. Kleinberg, DL, Noel, GL and Frantz, AG: Galactorrhea: a study of 235 cases, including 48 with pituitary tumors. *N Engl J Med 296:* 589, 1977.

16. Klibanski, A, Neey, RM, Beitins, IZ, Ridgway, CE, Zervas, NT and McArthur, JW: Decreased bone density in hyperprolactinemic women. *N Engl J Med 303:* 1511, 1980.

17. Lauritzen, C and VanKeep, PA: Proven beneficial effects of estrogen substitution in the postmenopause: a review. *Front Horm Res 5:* 1, 1978.

18. Mack, TM, Pike, MC, Henderson, BE, Pfeiffer, RI, Gerkins, VR, Arthur, M and Brown, SE: Estrogen and endometrial cancer in a retirement community. *N Engl J Med 294:* 1262, 1976.

19. Marshal, WA and Tanner, JM: Variations in pattern of pubertal changes in girls. *Arch Dis Child 44:* 291, 1969.

20. Marshall, WA and Tanner, JM: Variations in pattern of pubertal changes in boys. *Arch Dis Child 45:* 13, 1970.

21. Martin, CE: Sexual activity in the aging male. In *Handbook of Sexology*, p. 813, edited by J Money and N Musaph. Elsevier-North Holland, New York, 1977.

22. Meema, S, Bunker, ML and Meema, HE: Preventive effect of estrogen on postmenopausal bone loss. *Arch Intern Med 135:* 1436, 1975.

23. Nordin, BEC, Gallager, JC, Aaron, JE and Horsman, A: Postmenopausal osteopenia and osteoporosis. *Front Horm Res 3:* 131, 1975.

24. Nutall, FQ: Gynecomastia as a physical finding in normal men. *J Clin Endocrinol Metab 48:* 338, 1979.

25. Schiff, I, Tulchinsky, D and Ryan, KJ: Vaginal absorption of estrone and 17β-estradiol. *Fertil Steril 28:* 1063, 1977.

26. Shapiro, G and Evron, S: A novel use of spironolactone: treatment of hirsutism. *J Clin Endocrinol Metab 51:* 479, 1980.

27. Sherman, BM and Korenman, SG: Hormonal characteristics of the human menstrual cycle throughout reproductive life. *J Clin Invest 55:* 699, 1975.

28. Spark, RF, White, RA and Connolly, PB: Impotence is not always psychogenic. Newer insights into hypothalamic-pituitary-gonadal dysfunction. *JAMA 243:* 750, 1980.

29. Sturdee, DW, Wade-Evans, T, Paterson, MEL, Thom, M and Studd, JWW: Relations between bleeding pattern, endometrial histology, and estrogen treatment in menopausal women. *Br Med J 1:* 1575, 1978.

30. Tataryn, IV, Meldrum, DR, Lu, KH, Frumar, AM and Judd, HL: LH, FSH, and skin temperature during the menopausal hot flash. *J Clin Endocrinol Metab 49:* 152, 1979.

31. Weissman, MM: The myth of involutional melancholia. *JAMA 242:* 742, 1979.

SECTION 11

Neurologic Problems

CHAPTER SEVENTY-FIVE

Evaluation of the Patient with Neurologic Symptoms

BARRY GORDON, M.D., Ph.D., and ALFRED C. SERVER, M.D., Ph.D.

This chapter describes approaches to history-taking, physical examination, and laboratory evaluation which are most useful in ambulatory patients with neurologic symptoms. One or more of these approaches is appropriate in patients with each of the neurologic problems discussed in subsequent chapters (headache, dizziness, vertigo, syncope, seizures, cerebrovascular disease, peripheral neuropathy, tremor, and Parkinson's disease).

NEUROLOGIC HISTORY AND PHYSICAL EXAMINATION

General Principles

Four types of information should be obtained (or inferred) whenever there is a new neurologic symptom: the temporal evolution of the symptom, any associated symptoms, the specific abnormality of neurologic functions, and the anatomic localization of the problem. Figures 75.1 and 75.2 summarize those facts which are most often needed for anatomic localization. Additional details regarding the anatomic relationships of peripheral nerves are shown in Chapter 81, Figures 81.1 and 81.2.

It is important to remember that most individual neurologic symptoms or signs are not specific for one functional or anatomic disturbance or for one etiology (e.g., loss of a reflex is not necessarily due to motor nerve damage, a hemiparesis is not necessarily due to cerebrovascular disease, and a resting tremor is not necessarily due to Parkinson's disease). The constellation of findings from the history and physical examination, however, is often quite specific. Therefore, a good history and physical examination are adequate for making a working diagnosis for most neurologic problems encountered in office practice.

An Example. A physically active patient with a history of recurrent low back pain for many years gives a 3-day history of increased back pain, numbness on the back of the right leg extending to the foot, and some clumsiness of

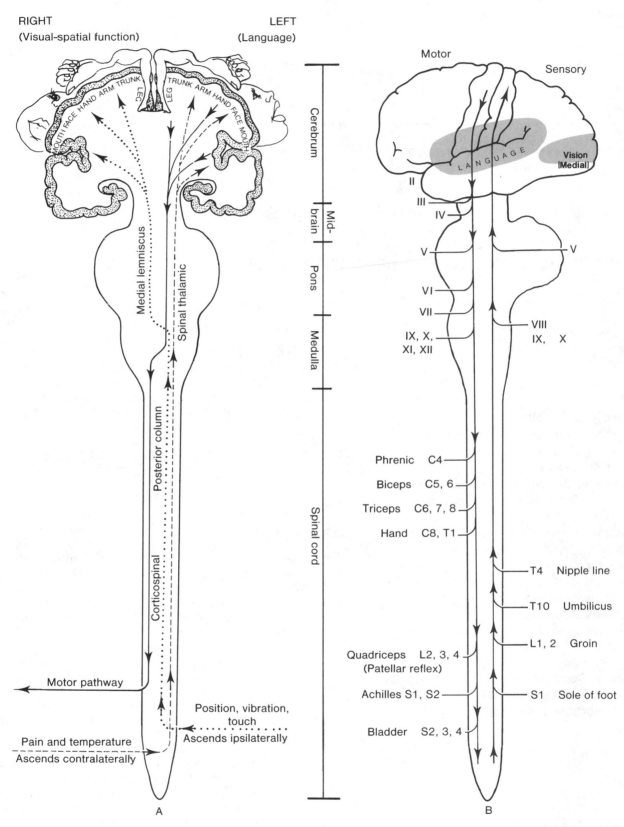

Figure 75.1   Schematic of neurologic localization. (A) Anterior and (B) lateral schematic of central nervous system localization. Upper motor neuron signs and nonradicular sensory signs can only define the *side* of the lesion (A); in general, they do not reveal the *level* of the lesion. Presence or absence of other neurologic signs or symptoms can help specify the level of a localized neurologic problem (B).

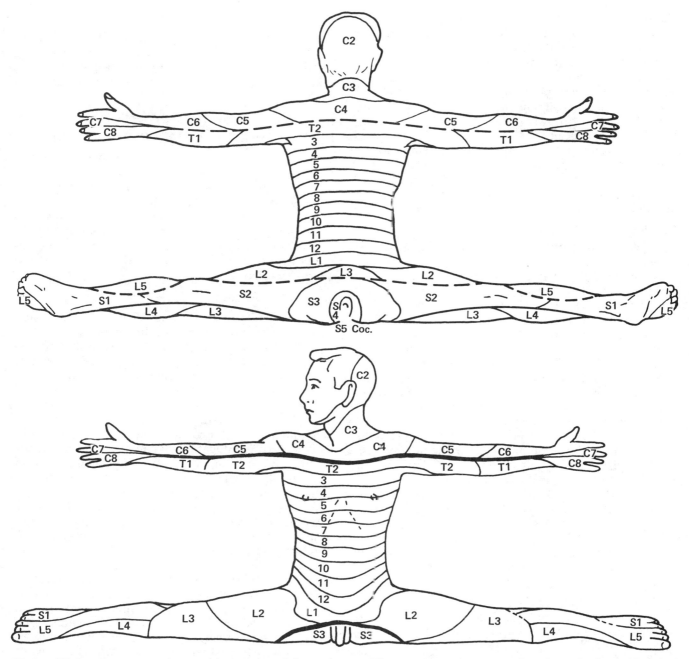

Figure 75.2   Cutaneous innervation areas of dermatomes. The numbers correspond to the spinal cord level of the dermatome. *C*, cervical; *T*, thoracic; *L*, lumbar; and *S*, sacral. (From W. Haymaker and B. Woodhall: *Peripheral Nerve Injuries*, Ed. 2. W. B. Saunders, Philadelpnia, 1962.)

the leg. Symptoms began about 1 day after he dug up his garden. Physical findings are consistent with lower motor neuron impairment at the level of S1. Working diagnosis: herniated disc at the L5–S1 level.

Depending on the circumstances, either a brief (but adequate) examination of each general neurologic function may be required or only selected areas of the nervous system may need evaluation.

Brief Neurologic History

HIGHER FUNCTIONS AND CONSCIOUSNESS

Handedness. Are you right-handed or left-handed?

Language. Have you had any problems with your thinking or with your speech? (Minor word-finding difficulty is very common in normal people, as are brief lapses of memory.)

Memory. How is your memory? What kind of

things do you forget? (To family: any problems with concentration, memory, or general abilities noted?)

Acute Cerebral Dysfunction. Have you ever fainted, lost consciousness, felt dizzy, or had a seizure (fit, convulsion)?

Mood. How are your spirits? Do you feel depressed? Are you worrying a great deal? How do you feel about the future? About yourself (confident, hopeless, helpless, guilty)?

Hallucinations/Delusions. Have you seen or heard things that are unusual or that you think are not there? Does your imagination seem to play tricks on you? What do you feel is wrong? Is there anything or anybody affecting you?

CRANIAL NERVES

Nerve I (Olfactory). Not tested in brief history and physical.

Nerve II (Optic Nerve and Vision). How is your vision? Do things seem blurred or are there patches where it is hard for you to see? Have you ever lost the vision in one eye or had trouble seeing out of one side or in one direction?

Nerve III, IV, and VI (Extraocular Motions). Have you ever had any double vision?

Nerve V (Trigeminal Nerve). Have you ever had any numbness over your face or difficulty chewing?

Nerve VII (Facial Nerve). Have you ever had any weakness in your face or paralysis of your face?

Nerve VIII (Auditory-Vestibular Nerves). How is your hearing? Have you had any ringing in your ears or difficulty hearing out of one side? Any loss of balance, spinning sensations, or dizziness?

Nerves IX, X, and XII (Glossopharyngeal, Vagal, and Hypoglossal). Any problems chewing or swallowing your food? Does it seem to get caught anywhere? Where? What kinds of foods do you have problems with? (Liquids are often the most difficult foods for patients with neurologic problems.)

MOTOR

Have you noted any weakness in your arms or legs? Is it there all the time or does it seem to come and go? Have you noted any twitching in your muscles? Where? How often? Any wasting of your muscles?

GAIT

Do you have any problems with walking? What kind? Where does it happen?—Climbing up stairs, walking certain distances, etc.? Do you feel unsteady on your feet? Do you get any cramps in your legs? Under what circumstances?

FINE MOTOR AND CEREBELLAR FUNCTION

Have you noticed any shaking or any difficulty in writing, drawing, buttoning, etc.?

SENSATION

Have you had any numbness, tingling, or pain in your arms, legs, or feet? Where? Does position change or any other factor seem to bring it on?

BLADDER/BOWEL

Any problems in starting to urinate or in urinating? Any difficulty with constipation or diarrhea? Any uncontrolled urination or stool evacuation? If so, was it associated with the urge to urinate/defecate or was it spontaneous?

Brief Neurologic Examination

HIGHER FUNCTIONS AND CONSCIOUSNESS

The questions suggested in the history plus observations made throughout the history and physical examination are usually sufficient for determining level of consciousness, language functioning, visual-spatial functioning, mood, and level of intelligence. Systematic mental status examinations appropriate for patients with psychiatric problems and for patients with dementia are described in Chapters 9 and 16, respectively.

CRANIAL NERVES

Nerve II (Optic Nerve and Vision). Check vision (make sure that patients wear their glasses, if needed) with the use of the Snellen chart or by having the patient read from a newspaper, each eye separately. Check fields by confrontation (each eye separately) using finger wiggle. Examine fundi.

Nerve III, IV, and VI (Extraocular Movement and Pupils). Make patient move eyes into all principal positions of gaze (horizontal, vertical, diagonal), observe for dysconjugate movements and ask, while testing, about diplopia. Look for nystagmus and lid lag also. Check pupils for size, symmetry, reaction to light. (Normal pupil size for young adults is 3 to 5 mm. In the elderly, normal pupils are often 2 to 3 mm. A slight degree of pupillary asymmetry, 1 mm or less, is present in about 5% of the normal population; it usually varies from hour to hour and day to day, and it decreases in bright light.)

Nerve V (Trigeminal Nerve). Corneal reflexes should be tested at corresponding points on the cornea of each eye, by having the subject look up and away from the testing swab. (There are wide variations in corneal sensitivity among normal individuals; some subjects, particularly those who have worn contact lenses, have virtually no response at all. Asymmetry is the most important clue to disease.)

Nerve VII (Facial Nerve). Inspect for asymmetry of the nasolabial folds when the face is not moving. Have the patient show teeth, close eyes, frown. (Intact persons may have a slight degree of resting asymmetry of the face; this is particularly common in edentulous persons. Normally both sides should move briskly together on showing teeth, smiling, etc. Lag on one side may be a sign of a slight seventh nerve palsy, central or peripheral.)

Nerves IX and X (Glossopharyngeal and Vagus). Inspect the uvula for position and for motion with "Ahh." Test the gag reflex on both sides of the pharynx, looking for asymmetry of response. (Some people have asymmetry of the resting uvula. Also, bilaterally hyperactive to bilaterally absent gag responses are within the normal range.)

Nerve XI (Accessory Nerve). Observe shoulder shrug; should be symmetric.

Nerve XII (Hypoglossal Nerve). Inspect the tongue at rest in the mouth; have the patient protrude it and move it to both sides. (The tongue normally has small twitches which are not pathologic fasciculations; it should protrude in the midline.)

MOTOR EXAMINATION

Adventitious Movements. Observe for tremor and other spontaneous movements. (See additional details in Chapter 79.)

Bulk. Examine for asymmetries of muscle mass. (Denervation will cause loss of muscle bulk, reaching a maximum by 4 months; disuse over months to years will also cause a decrease in muscle bulk, e.g., in the legs of patients who are permanently bedridden.)

Muscle Tone (Resistance to Passive Motion). Test tone by passively flexing and extending the upper and lower extremities. Normal tone is a slight firmness of muscles and slight resistance to passive motion. In *hypotonia*, the muscles are flaccid, without resistance to passive motion. This may mean lower motor neuron or cerebellar disease.

There are several subtypes of *hypertonia*:

Rigidity is increased resistance to passive motion throughout the whole range of motion around a joint.

In *spasticity*, the initial passive motion is easy, but then there is a tightening of the muscle ("spastic catch") possibly followed by a sudden release ("clasp-knife effect"). Spasticity usually affects only one set of muscles around a joint (in the upper extremities, the biceps, forearm pronators, and finger flexors; in the lower extremities, the quadriceps, hamstrings, plantar flexors).

In *gegenhalten or paratonia*, resistance is present in all directions, but varies with the examiner's force and speed. It often seems to be voluntary ("fighting back"). Gegenhalten is seen normally in infants, but appears pathologically in adults with dementias or frontal lobe disease.

Voluntary Strength. Voluntary strength should be sampled in several major muscle groups. Test elbow extension and flexion, hand and finger extension, grip strength (with two fingers), hip flexion (with patient sitting), knee flexion, knee extension, foot dorsiflexion. Also observe the patient's gait (see below).

If desired, the following rating scale can be used:

    0 = No movement
    1 = Flicker
    2 = Able to move with gravity eliminated (e.g., lateral
        motion of arm when recumbent)
    3 = Able to move against gravity
    4 = Able to move against resistance
    5 = Normal strength.

(In conversion reactions and malingering, strength on formal testing is usually jerky or "giving." With sudden passive motions in the opposite direction, the examiner may be able to demonstrate that the muscles can produce normal force. The examiner may note that the subject can do some voluntary activities, e.g., combing hair, reaching for objects, getting up or sitting down, etc., with muscles which the patient states are "too weak" to use for such motions on formal testing.)

REFLEXES

The most important reflexes to test are the biceps (C5–6), triceps (C6–8), patellar (L2–4), achilles tendon (S1–2), and plantar flexion ("Babinski"). (Activity of the reflexes varies widely among patients and can vary in the same individual depending upon his emotional status and upon his ability to relax his muscles. As in the rest of the examination, asymmetries between two sides generally carry more weight than symmetric reflex changes; comparison must be made with the muscles relaxed to a similar degree and with the two extremities in identical positions. A *decrease* in the reflex or reflexes is generally due to disruption of the sensory or motor nerves (or both) of the reflex loop itself. Sometimes decreased reflexes are seen immediately after a cerebrovascular accident, in which case interpretation does not depend on the reflexes alone. *Increased* reflexes mean upper motor neuron (UMN) disease located anywhere from just above the anterior horn cell to the cerebral cortex. A *Babinski response* is dorsiflexion of the big toe, which may be associated with dorsiflexion and spreading of the other toes and dorsiflexion of the foot. The classic Babinski response is slow and deliberate. Nonspecific withdrawal may resemble the Babinski reflex, but it is usually rapid and the patient usually complains of subjective distress; a reliable Babinski sign can and should occur in the absence of any patient discomfort from the stimulus. A Babinski sign may be found in the absence of other UMN signs, as an indicator of UMN disease.)

SENSATION

The patient should be tested for symmetry and for differences in proximal and distal perception, in all four extremities. Test sensitivity to pinprick (lateral spinothalamic tract) and test both proprioception and vibratory sense (posterior column). (There are normal differences in pinprick perception over different areas of the body—for example, it is decreased over the beard area—but patients generally ignore these differences. Patients who do not can give very confusing responses and must be told to ignore small subjective differences. Repeat testing is often important to determine the reliability of a patient's response. Vibration sense should be tested with a 128 cycles per second (cps) tuning fork. Loss of vibration sense is often the earliest detectable abnormality in peripheral neuropathy. Mild distal loss of pin and vibration sense is very common in otherwise normal elderly patients.)

FINE MOTOR AND CEREBELLAR

Have the patient touch his thumb sequentially to each of the fingers of each hand separately, observing for speed, effort, and rhythm. Test finger-to-nose-to-finger (subject has to touch examiner's moving finger, then touch his own nose, then touch the examiner's finger again, etc.) for speed, rhythm, intention tremor, and inaccuracy (dysmetria). Ask the subject to tap each foot separately; observe for differences in speed, ease, and rhythm. (In these tests, normal subjects show equal ability with either side or are slightly better on the side of their preferred hand. Slowness and subjective effort on repetitive movements, without a loss of rhythm, are characteristic of UMN lesions. Relatively preserved speed with erratic movements and loss of rhythm may be seen in cerebellar disease. Finger-nose-finger testing may be affected by tremor of various types as described in Chapter 79.)

STATION AND GAIT

Observe for any tendency to list or any need for support while sitting, standing, or walking. Observe regular walking. Have the patient walk heel-to-toe. Have the patient walk on his heels and toes (tests strength and balance). Perform Romberg test (feet together in young patients, slightly apart in older patients).

In *cerebellar disease*, there is a wide base (legs widely separated), unsteadiness, and lateral reeling (lateral reeling can be evaluated by having the patient walk around a chair in both directions; he will tend to walk into the chair when it is on the affected side and to veer away from the chair when it is on the unaffected side). Because of his fundamental abnormality of motor coordination, the patient with cerebellar disease affecting the lower extremities cannot participate in a Romberg test which requires standing with the two feet together; this is not an "abnormal Romberg test."

In *sensory ataxia* (loss of proprioception), there is uncertainty, slapping or stamping of the feet, and a "positive" Romberg test (means that the patient loses his balance with eyes closed but can avoid falling when his eyes are open because of visually mediated vestibular or cerebellar compensation).

In a *spastic gait* (in UMN disease), the leg does not flex, but circumducts and there is foot dragging (the toe of the sole of the patient's shoe becomes disproportionately worn); there is also loss of arm swinging on the spastic side.

In a *parkinsonian gait*, there is unilateral or bilateral loss of arm swinging; the patient is bent forward; and there is rigidity, shuffling, and festination (the upper part of the body advances ahead of the lower extremities; gait becomes faster as if to catch up).

In *lower motor neuron (LNM) paralysis* of the pretibial and peroneal muscles, there is drop-foot; hip flexion is preserved, and the patient lifts the foot very high, advances it by swinging it forward, then slaps it down.

In *frontal lobe disease*, gait may be wide-based, shuffling, and slow, and turning is very slow, but there is no weakness or loss of sensation.

Special Considerations in Evaluation of Neurologic Symptoms

The neurologic symptoms seen in ambulatory patients are often less florid than those of patients hospitalized for neurologic disease, and many of these symptoms are related to prior acute neurologic events. There are two important considerations in the evaluation of ambulatory patients with neurologic symptoms: the variability in patient performance over time; and the difference between the manifestations of upper motor neuron (UMN) and lower motor neuron (LMN) lesions.

VARIABILITY OVER TIME

In dealing with abnormalities of the peripheral nerves, spinal cord, and brainstem, the physician can expect symptoms and signs to remain about the same after the basic problem has stabilized; subsequently, alterations of the findings usually reflect a change in the patient's disease. On the other hand, the performance of patients with ostensibly stabilized cerebral disease may vary greatly from minute to minute, hour to hour, or day to day. The variability affects the psychomotor domain, *e.g.*, performance of everyday tasks, memory, speech and language, and mood.

Examples:

1. The patient may be able to dress, fix breakfast, and bring in the mail one morning; be incapable of these tasks the next morning; and perform them correctly on the third morning.

2. The patient may remember his wife's name in the morning but not in the evening of the same day.

3. The aphasic patient may be able to say something one minute and be unable to say it several minutes later.

4. The stroke survivor's affect may vary from depressed to euphoric from hour to hour and day to day.

As a result of this type of variability, members of the patient's family may become confused and, often, quite angry at the patient. They may frequently contact the physician to inquire whether a change in behavior means that the disease is getting worse; or they may conclude that the patient is capable of doing certain tasks but "just not trying" sometimes. When the pattern is clearly one of waxing and waning, the family should be reassured that, just as intact individuals have their "good days" and "bad days," brain-damaged subjects do also, but in exaggerated and different ways. The evaluation and management of behavior changes of patients with cerebral damage is discussed in more detail in Chapters 16 (dementia) and 80 (stroke).

DIFFERENCE BETWEEN UPPER AND LOWER MOTOR NEURON SYMPTOMS

The manifestations and the course of upper motor neuron (UMN) and lower motor neuron (LMN) damage differ fundamentally. UMN lesions affect the pathways bringing a command from the cortex to the anterior horn cell. UMN function depends upon integrity of the cortex and the corticospinal and corticobulbar tracts. LMN lesions affect the final common pathway for muscle movements. LMN function depends upon the integrity of the anterior horn cell in the spinal cord and its nerve fiber for carrying impulses to the muscle cell. A number of points are helpful in recognizing or distinguishing these common problems when they are less overt, which is often the situation in patients seen in office practice.

Upper Motor Neuron Lesion Syndrome. If a UMN lesion is total, paralysis of voluntary movements will be total. However, there may be preservation of involuntary movements, such as those associated with yawning, laughing, crying, or anger.

When there is weakness (paresis) rather than paralysis due to UMN damage, the following patterns of weakness are seen.

In the face, the lower muscles are usually involved. There is variable but often some involvement of the orbicularis occuli (producing a widened palpebral fissure and weakness of eye closure); but the forehead is completely spared. This is in contrast to LMN (peripheral) seventh nerve damage where usually both the upper and lower facial muscles are involved (although sometimes mild peripheral seventh nerve weakness—e.g., early Bell's palsy, an LMN lesion—can mimic this pattern). One additional differential point is that the LMN lesion will produce the same amount of weakness with both a voluntary and an involuntary movement (e.g., laughing). A UMN seventh nerve paresis (from a stroke, for example) may not be apparent when the patient is laughing or crying involuntarily but may only be present when the patient is asked to smile voluntarily.

In the arm and leg, distal muscles are affected by UMN lesions much more than proximal muscles. In addition, some specific motor functions are affected more than others: In the arm, shoulder abduction and external rotation; in the forearm, extension and supination; in the wrist and finger, extension; in the hip, flexion; in the knee, flexion; and in the foot and toe, dorsiflexion.

Whether or not the muscles are weak in an UMN lesion, voluntary movements are typically slowed and require greater effort than usual; and the affected limb's ability to make fine movements is lost. A patient with a very mild hemiparesis may be able to squeeze the examiner's hand with normal strength, but his movements are slower and clumsier than usual; he may be unable to easily use his fingers individually; also, when asked to extend both arms with his eyes closed, there may be downward and inward drift of the weak arm (pronator sign). In the lower extremity, a patient with such a mild defect may be able to dorsiflex his foot voluntarily. However, he may not be able to do this very rapidly (as revealed on attempted foot tapping); and the movement may not be automatically coordinated with walking, resulting in a "drop foot."

Typically (but not invariably),' UMN lesions are accompanied by spasticity and hyperreflexia.

Lower Motor Neuron Lesion Syndrome. Weakness resulting from a permanent LMN lesion is fixed and unchanging. Only those muscles served by the involved spinal cord segment or peripheral nerve are weak. There are none of the widespread effects characteristic of an UMN lesion. Atrophy is usually apparent within several weeks after an LMN lesion, in contrast to UMN lesions where atrophy is slight and late (many months). Pathologic fasciculations may be present in affected muscle groups, distinguishable from benign occasional muscle twitching by the fact that they are frequent and they occur only in the denervated muscles. Muscles are usually flaccid and hyporeflexic or areflexic. If a peripheral nerve has been involved, there may be associated hypesthesia or anesthesia.

Mixed UMN and LMN Lesions. In some situations, UMN and LMN lesions may occur together. For instance, *spinal cord injury* will typically give signs of a LMN lesion at the level of the injury, due to localized destruction of the anterior horn cells and their nerve roots; below the level of the injury, there may be a partial or complete UMN syndrome with spasticity, hyperreflexia, and preserved involuntary reflexes. Likewise, *amyotrophic lateral sclerosis,* an idiopathic degenerative disease, affects both pyramidal tract cells and anterior horn cells. Along with LMN-type weakness, fasciculations, and wasting (more pronounced in the upper extremities), these patients often have lower extremity hyperreflexia and Babinski signs.

Neurovascular Examination

This section describes a systematic approach to the neurovascular examination. This examination is especially important in patients in whom cerebrovascular disease or an increased risk of cerebrovascular disease is the problem (see Chapter 80). The examination includes an assessment of the heart and peripheral vasculature with emphasis on the vessels of the head and neck.

HEART AND PERIPHERAL VESSELS

The radial arteries should be simultaneously palpated at both wrists to determine any asymmetry in pulse amplitude or timing (pulse delay). The brachial arterial blood pressure should be measured in both arms with the patient supine, sitting, and standing. Unequal blood pressures in the two arms (≥ 20 mm Hg difference in systolic and diastolic pressure) is suggestive of a stenotic lesion of the subclavian artery on the side with the lower pressure. Orthostatic hypotension, defined as a fall in systolic pressure of greater than 15 mm Hg on moving from a supine to upright position, may be important in explaining symptoms in some patients.

A detailed cardiac examination can provide evidence of cardiomegaly, valvular disease, or an arrhythmia, each of which may predispose a patient to having a stroke. Finally, a complete assessment of the peripheral vasculature, for evidence of widespread atherosclerosis, should include palpation and auscultation of the femoral arteries and palpation of the arterial pulses in the feet.

VESSELS OF HEAD AND NECK

The evaluation of the vessels of the head and neck should follow the time-honored format of inspection, palpation, and auscultation.

Inspection. Prominence of the superficial *temporal artery* with erythema, and, occasionally, ulceration of the overlying skin, in a patient with persistent malaise is suggestive of giant cell arteritis, an inflammatory process which can lead to retinal and/or cerebral infarction (see Chapter 76).

Dilation of the *episcleral arteries* of an eye can result from occlusion of the ipsilateral internal carotid artery (in this instance, the hemisphere on the side of the occlusion is being supplied in a retrograde fashion by the external carotid artery through enlarged ophthalmic arteries). The *funduscopic examination* allows direct visualization of the retinal vessels, and changes resulting from atherosclerosis, hypertension, or diabetes can be detected. Moreover, the absence of an expected change can be informative, as in the case of the hypertensive patient with normal retinal vessels on the side of a severely stenosed carotid artery (in this instance, occlusive disease of the ipsilateral carotid artery protects the retina from the effects of chronic hypertension). A detailed funduscopic examination may also demonstrate emboli, seen as white or refractile elements in the retinal arterioles. These emboli may be composed of cholesterol, platelets and fibrin, or calcium and are suggestive of atherosclerotic carotid occlusive disease or cardiac valve disease.

Palpation. The value of palpation of the cervical vessels has been the subject of debate. Reports of embolic stroke following firm palpation of a diseased carotid artery have left many clinicians with a sense of trepidation regarding manipulation of this vessel. The current consensus, however, is that gentle palpation of the carotid artery can be performed with limited risk and will occasionally provide useful information as to the status of the vessel. Perhaps more valuable and certainly less dangerous is palpation of the superficial temporal and facial arteries which are branches of the external carotid artery. A weak or absent pulse in these arteries on one side of the head is suggestive of ipsilateral occlusive disease of the external or common carotid artery. In contrast, an increase in pulsation in these vessels may result from stenosis or occlusion of the ipsilateral internal carotid artery causing collateral flow through the external system. Finally, the finding of a tender superficial temporal artery with decreased pulsation may support other data consistent with the diagnosis of giant cell arteritis.

Auscultation. Following auscultation of the heart to rule out the possibility of a transmitted cardiac murmur, the examiner should proceed to the following sites: the clavicular regions over the subclavian arteries; the lateral and anterior aspects of the neck along the paths of the vertebral arteries (as they course through the cervical vertebrae) and of the carotid arteries up to their bifurcation at the angle of the jaw; the occipital, temporal, and parietal regions of the cranium; and the orbits. The finding of a cephalic bruit in an adult raises the possibility of an arteriovenous malformation, while a cervical bruit is suggestive, but not diagnostic, of atherosclerotic occlusive disease. In addition to its location, a bruit can be characterized on the basis of its duration, loudness, and pitch. These parameters can provide information on the degree of stenosis of the involved vessel (Fig. 75.3). Moreover, by following these parameters in subsequent examinations, a progression to greater stenosis over time can be detected.

USE OF DIAGNOSTIC PROCEDURES

The general physician may refer a patient for any of several diagnostic procedures in evaluating a neurologic problem. For several commonly ordered procedures, the following information is provided here: definition, principal indications, limitations, and what the patient experiences during the procedure.

Skull X-rays

DEFINITION OF PROCEDURE

"Routine skull X-rays" refers to a set of films which include three standard views: lateral, anteroposterior (AP), and inclined AP. Many other views are possible, and may be indicated in specific conditions (e.g., basal skull views for a patient with atypical trigeminal neuralgia).

PRINCIPAL INDICATIONS

1. Known or suspected significant head trauma.
2. Minimal or possible head trauma, for medicolegal reasons.
3. Suspected pituitary tumor.
4. Suspected problems involving the bones: e.g., metastatic tumor (osteoblastic or osteolytic), myeloma, or Paget's disease.

LIMITATIONS

The skull X-ray has very little value anymore as a general screening test for intracranial disease. Relatively few neurologic conditions are associated with

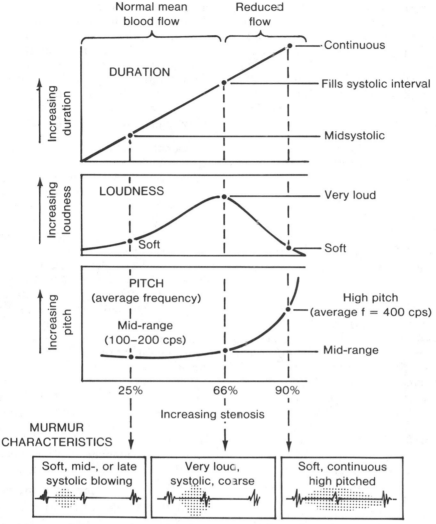

Figure 75.3   Effect of increasing stenosis on the duration, loudness, and pitch of a murmur. (Reproduced with permission from: J. F. Toole and A. N. Patel: *Cerebrovascular Disorders*, Ed. 2. McGraw-Hill, New York, 1974.)

bony changes; even when such changes are present, they can generally be evaluated better by procedures with greater sensitivity, specificity, and often nearly equivalent cost and risk, such as computerized tomography (see below).

Patient Experience. The patient should be informed that he will be asked to keep his head in several uncomfortable positions for short periods of time; accurate positioning might be impossible with patients who have neck problems or with the elderly.

Spine Films

DEFINITION OF PROCEDURE

Standard spine films are usually AP and lateral views; oblique and flexion/extension views usually must be ordered specifically.

PRINCIPAL INDICATIONS

1. Suspected cervical spondylitic radiculopathy— in this case, oblique films are necessary to examine the intervertebral foramina through which the roots pass.

2. Suspected cervical or lumbar stenosis or spondylolythesis.

3. Suspected vertebral fracture.

4. Suspected metastatic tumor.

5. To rule out other problems such as tumor, fracture, and infection in patients with suspected spondylosis or disc disease.

LIMITATIONS

Interpretation of "positive" findings: asymptomatic cervical spondylosis and interspace narrowing due to disc degeneration are so common after age 40 (see Chapter 61) that their presence has limited usefulness in the absence of more specific findings from the history and physical examination. Negative films provide good evidence against spondylosis as the cause of radicular symptoms.

X-rays are indirect studies; they do not show soft tissue or the actual status of the cord and nerve roots;

these must be inferred. In patients with herniated intervertebral discs, films are usually normal or show only nonspecific intervertebral narrowing. However, patients with congenitally small bony canals (cervical or lumbar stenosis) are at high risk for these soft tissue problems occurring secondary to degenerative changes in the discs and ligaments; the radiologist should be specifically asked about these possibilities if they are clinically relevant.

Patient Experience. The patient must cooperate for several views. Patients with neck problems or the elderly may be unable to position themselves for adequate cervical spine films.

Electroencephalography (EEG)

DEFINITION OF PROCEDURE

This is a record of the minute (1 to 50 microvolt) electrical rhythms and other electrical activity of the brain.

PRINCIPAL INDICATIONS

1. Known or suspected seizure disorders (see Chapter 77). (Recording during sleep or after sleep deprivation significantly increases the chances of a useful diagnostic examination; for complex partial seizures, nasopharyngeal leads record from the medial temporal regions where most of these seizures originate, and therefore can slightly increase the yield of the study.)

2. Confirmation of focal brain lesions in the absence of other evidence (e.g., to help localize a stroke).

3. Confirmation of diffuse brain disease, such as cerebral degeneration (e.g., Alzheimer's), delirium, cerebral vasculitis, drug effect or withdrawal. (Because the general criteria for normal are broad, serial EEGs on the same subject are most helpful in these situations to confirm/disprove pathology.)

4. Sleep disorders (see Chapter 82)—routine and special EEG recording techniques are often indicated.

LIMITATIONS

General. An EEG records only relatively gross waves of electrical activity. Only one-third of the cerebral cortex is accessible to standard surface EEG recording, and disturbances have to extend over a wide area of cortex before they can be recorded. Furthermore, many different etiologic processes produce the same kind of electrical disturbances.

Negative EEG. Since the EEG is not very sensitive, a single negative EEG is not convincing evidence for the absence of most diseases. For example, up to 20% of patients even with known epilepsy have normal interictal records. Serial or repeated negative EEGs may be far more significant.

"Mildly Abnormal" EEG. Depending upon the reader and classification scheme, many (5 to 30% or more) of normal adult EEGs can be classified as minimally or mildly but nonspecifically abnormal in some way. The relevance of these interpretations

must be judged in the context of the patients' problems, but should often not be given very much weight because of the broad range of normal. This is particularly true in infancy, childhood, adolescence, and old age. For instance, temporal slow activity (usually on the left, occasionally on the right or bilaterally) is a normal finding after the age of 40 in as many as 30 to 40% of subjects; it may be confused with the slowing produced by a focal brain lesion.

Patient Experience. Subjects are asked to lie down or recline while surface electrodes are attached with electrode paste (which tenaciously clings to hair, so that women should not get their hair done before coming for the study). The total procedure takes an average of about 40 to 60 min, with 20 to 30 min of actual recording time. For most of the actual recording, the patient will simply be asked to lie calmly with his eyes closed. Additional studies which most laboratories routinely perform include recording during hyperventilation (for 3 to 5 min) and photic simulation with a repetitive flash. (For many tracings, subjects will be encouraged to fall asleep if they can. Some laboratories induce sleep with oral chloral hydrate.)

The EEG is extremely sensitive to patient movement, sweating, or muscle tension; any of these may make a tracing uninterpretable.

For Sleep-Deprived EEGs. The patient is generally asked to stay up all night the night before, and the EEG is done in the laboratory first thing in the morning.

Nasopharyngeal leads are generally applied through the nostrils after local anesthesia of the nasopharynx by spray; they may be annoying and they may interfere with nasal breathing, but they should not hurt.

Carotid Dopplers

DEFINITION OF PROCEDURE

The carotid Doppler examination is an ultrasonic study of blood flow in the supraorbital artery, with and without superficial temporal artery compression. The supraorbital artery is a branch of the internal carotid, and it also has anastomotic connections with the superficial temporal artery. With a patent internal carotid, flow through the supraorbital artery should be unaffected by compression of the temporal artery (the direction of flow may transiently reverse as the internal carotid supply compensates). However, with significant compromise of the internal carotid circulation, supraorbital artery flow becomes totally dependent upon the superficial temporal artery supply and will be abolished by compressing it. It is this that the Doppler study assesses. This study is, therefore, dependent both upon a hemodynamically significant alteration of flow in the internal carotid (usually meaning a greater than 90% stenosis) and upon the "normal" pattern of vascular supply to the supraorbital artery.

PRINCIPAL INDICATIONS

Suspected significant internal carotid artery stenosis (carotid bifurcation): a Doppler study has approximately 90% sensitivity and specificity as an indicator of significant (greater than 90%) carotid bifurcation stenosis.

LIMITATIONS

This procedure is not useful for suspected verte-brobasilar disease. It often is normal if there is less than 90% occlusion. It does not reveal plaque ulceration or intracranial vascular disease in the carotid siphon or middle cerebral artery. A negative Doppler study does not completely rule out significant stenotic disease; 10% of even highly stenotic lesions will be missed by the Doppler because of collateral flow to the supraorbital artery. It is never a substitute for thorough investigation of suspected cerebrovascular disease if otherwise indicated.

Patient Experience. Subjects sit or recline with their eyes closed while an ultrasound-conducting gel is applied to the supraorbital region. An ultrasonic probe is then held over the artery for a few minutes while the temporal artery is being compressed and released. There is no appreciable discomfort or risk.

Isotope Brain Scanning

DEFINITION OF PROCEDURE

Normally, the blood-brain barrier is impervious to the carrier of the radioactive isotope used in brain scanning. Breakdown of the blood-brain barrier caused by infarct, tumor, or other disease permits migration of the isotope carrier into the brain and, if enough breakdown has occurred, the brain scan is positive in that region.

PRINCIPAL INDICATIONS

Isotope brain scan is not the procedure of choice for any suspected diagnosis except early brain abscess. For most other suspected intracranial disease, computerized tomography is preferable (and no more costly).

LIMITATIONS

The isotope scan has comparatively low sensitivity and spatial resolution (limited to lesions >2 cm). It has limited discriminating power, i.e., infarct, abscess, and tumor can give a similar appearance. Timing of the scan is important. For example, in a brain infarction, the isotope scan is usually not positive for the first 10 days to 2 weeks; it then becomes positive but reverts back to "normal" a few weeks later. It is not useful for intracerebral hematomas; it is unreliable for subdural hematoma (except when large); it gives poor visualization of the cerebellum; it gives no effective visualization of the brainstem; and it is not useful for hydrocephalus, atrophy, old infarction, or other quiescent structural damage. Finally, scalp and skull lesions (bruises, contusions, Paget's disease) can produce prominent artifacts.

Patient Experience. Patients may be given sodium per-chlorate orally shortly before the injection of isotope to block carrier uptake in the choroid plexus. Then the patient is required to lie still for the (variable) period of time it takes to accomplish each scan by overhead scintillation counters (usually a fairly massive piece of machinery which is moved over the patient's head). There are no appreciable risks.

Computerized Tomography (CT Scanning)

DEFINITION OF PROCEDURE

Computerized tomography uses narrow X-ray beams to exploit the differences in X-ray absorption between different kinds of intracranial tissues. Without contrast, the CT scanner can differentiate between the density of bone, calcified tissue, blood, grey matter, white matter, cerebrospinal fluid (CSF), and air. Its resolving power is proportional to how marked these density differences are: modern CT scanners can reveal hematomas only several millimeters wide, and infarcts of perhaps a centimeter to perhaps 1.5 cm wide. Although CT scan results are typically presented as horizontal slices through the brain, present technology allows slices to be reconstructed in the vertical plane, or any other, to give a better perspective on abnormal findings.

Intravenous injection of dye (usually Renograffin) is used to enhance the X-ray contrast of vascular lesions and will diffuse into an area of blood-brain barrier breakdown to increase the X-ray absorption density there.

CT scanning is highly sensitive and often diagnostic; as such, it has a place in both screening and specific investigation. When done without contrast injection, it is essentially free of risk. When done with contrast, the risk is that of the contrast material itself: frequently, a warm flush in the face, nausea, and sometimes vomiting. In approximately 1 case in 100,000 there is the possibility of death from the contrast injection. Many conditions can be screened for without the use of radiographic contrast; this should be strongly considered in patients where the most common abnormalities do not require contrast for visualization (e.g., dementia syndrome evaluation) and in the elderly where the risks are somewhat greater.

PRINCIPAL INDICATIONS

Evaluation of intracranial problems where structural alteration is known or suspected; e.g., tumor, ischemic cerebrovascular disease, hemorrhagic cerebrovascular disease, atrophic degenerative disease (Alzheimer's, Huntington's), hydrocephalus, or subdural hematoma.

LIMITATIONS

The clinician should be aware that CT scanning is neither infinitely sensitive nor infallible. A CT scan should not be performed unless there is a definite suspicion of its being positive. For instance, a CT scan after a transient ischemic attack (TIA) may be normal; this finding does not detract from the significance of the event and the need for further study. Furthermore, a negative CT scan does not exclude actual structural damage. The lesion site may not have been included in the slices done as part of a routine examination, or the damage may not have caused enough change in local absorption density to contrast with its surroundings. (This is not uncommon in cerebral infarction a week or so after the initial insult, when the original edema has cleared, and new vessel formation (and phagocytosis) have not yet begun to affect brain density.) A CT scan can also be negative because the damage is in an area of the brain which is poorly seen, such as the brainstem or spinal cord, or outside of the brain tissue itself.

Patient Experience. The patient is asked to lie down with his head inside what looks like a washing machine. In some scanners, a bag of water is pumped up around the head, but there is no direct contact. Straps will usually be applied over the forehead to prevent motion. (Patient motion will seriously impair the quality of the scanning and may make the scan uninterpretable.) Contrast material may be given intravenously, by single bolus, or by intravenous drip. The procedure takes 5 to 20 min, depending upon the scanner.

General References

Ackerman, RH: Noninvasive carotid evaluation. *Stroke 11:* 675, 1980.
  Brief up-to-date review of Doppler studies.
Baker, AB and Baker LH (eds): *Clinical Neurology* (3 volumes). Harper & Row, Hagerstown, Md., 1976 (with yearly updates).
  Although not the most comprehensive survey of neurologic diagnosis and practice, many of its chapters are well-recognized for their succinctness and clarity, and yearly updates of this loose-leaf book keep the information up to date. Some specific chapters of interest:
  DeJong, RN: Case taking and the neurologic examination.
  Peterson, HO and Keiffler, SA: Neuroradiology. *(A discussion of plain skull films, arteriography, pneumoencephalography, brain scanning.)*
  O'Leary, JL and Landau, WM: Electroencephalography and electromyography. *(Short introductions to EEG and EMG.)*
Weisburg, LA: Computer tomography in the diagnosis of intracranial disease. *Ann Intern Med 91:* 87, 1979.
  Good general review.

CHAPTER SEVENTY-SIX

Headaches and Facial Pain

BARRY GORDON, M.D., Ph.D., and L. RANDOL BARKER, M.D.

EPIDEMIOLOGY

While various epidemiologic surveys of headache are not always comparable or consistent with one another, all agree on the magnitude of the problem: 80 to 90% of the normal adult population reports recurrent headache, and in 30 to 50% of this population headaches were described as severe or disabling at times. Women clearly suffer disproportionately from headaches, both in terms of numbers affected and severity of headaches; the reported prevalence in women varies from slightly higher to as much as 3 times higher than in men (6, 13, 18).

Findings from the 1977 to 1978 National Ambulatory Care Survey (NACS) provide a profile of that subset of headache sufferers who go to a physician for headache. In this survey of office practice, headache was the seventh most frequent symptomatic reason for visits to all physicians; it accounted for approximately 2% of all visits to internists, general practitioners, and family practitioners. Table 76.1 adapted from the NACS, indicates the differences in visit rate for headache with respect to age group and sex of patients. Table 76.2 shows the distribution of headache duration reported by these patients; almost one-half of visits were for headache of less than 1 week's duration.

One aspect of the epidemiology of headache which deserves emphasis is the lower prevalence of recurrent headache in persons 65 and older. Fifty-seven percent of men and 43% of women in this age group report themselves as headache-free, and only 18 to 30% report disabling or severe headaches (17). On the other hand, as indicated in Table 76.1, the frequency of visits to physicians by those persons who do have headache increases with age.

Of all patients with headache, 80% or more will have what has been described as tension (muscle contraction) headache. Two to 7% will have migraine headaches, usually common migraine. In practice, physicians see a disproportionate number of patients with migraine, since these individuals are much more likely to seek medical attention than those with tension headache (13). In addition, the physician is likely to see a number of patients with nonmigrainous

Table 76.1
Average Annual Rate of Office Visits for Headache, According to Sex and Age of Patient: United States 1977–1978[a]

Sex and Age (yr)	Average Annual Visit Rate per 1,000 Persons
BOTH SEXES	
All ages	43.2
Under 15	17.6
15–24	31.4
25–44	53.8
45–64	60.2
65 and over	63.9
FEMALE	
All ages	55.4
Under 15	15.8
15–24	40.8
25–44	67.0
45–64	82.0
65 and over	81.8
MALE	
All ages	30.3
Under 15	19.4
15–24	21.7
25–44	39.7
45–64	36.3
65 and over	38.4

[a] Adapted from B. K. Cypress: Headache as the reason for office visits, National Ambulatory Medical Care Survey: United States, 1977–1978. Advance Data, Vital and Health Statistics of the National Center for Health Statistics. Number 67, January 7, 1981.

Table 76.2
Percent of Office Visits with Headache as a New Problem with Respect to Sex of Patient and Time Since Onset of Complaint: United States, 1977–1978[a]

Time Since Onset of Complaint	Female (%)	Male (%)
Less than 1 week	43.9	49.3
1–3 weeks	16.3	22.7
1–3 months	16.1	13.6
More than 3 months	20.5	13.7

[a] Adapted from B. K. Cypress: Headache as the reason for office visits, National Ambulatory Medical Care Survey: United States, 1977–1978. Advance Data, Vital and Health Statistics of the National Center for Health Statistics. Number 67, January 7, 1981.

vascular headaches due to systemic infections with fever (1). Likewise, the relatively uncommon organic syndromes associated with significant headache (such as cluster headache, exertional headache, temporal arteritis, and sinusitis) are likely to be overrepresented in a physician's office.

Life-threatening causes of headache are rare. In a study of a community hospital emergency department, 1% of patients complaining of acute headache had a subarachnoid hemorrhage or meningitis (1). In specialized headache clinics, which generally cater to preselected patients with more chronic problems, serious conditions (usually tumors, increased intracranial pressure, arteriovenous malformations, and the like) are found in about 5% of referrals. However, not surprisingly, such conditions (especially brain tumor) are often the major concerns of patients who come to a physician for evaluation of acute or chronic headaches.

GENERAL APPROACH TO THE PATIENT WITH HEADACHE
History
The history provides by far the most useful information for evaluating headache, particularly a careful account by the patient of the current or most recent episode. The following questions are especially helpful in the differential diagnosis of headache (the interpretation of the patient's answers to these questions is discussed in detail in the sections on specific headache syndromes):

1. *Associated factors*: Is there any warning of the attack (prodromal feeling, focal numbness or weakness, or visual symptoms including the fortification hallucinations of classic migraine)? Is the patient aware of any factors that can bring on these headaches (alcoholic ingestion, vasodilator use, psychosocial stresses, perimenstrual period, foods, drug use, position, sexual intercourse, exertion, tobacco)? What drugs is the patient taking for other conditions? To what does the patient attribute the headache?

2. *Temporal features*: How does the headache be-

gin—suddenly, or by building up slowly over a period of several hours or even days? When does the headache occur? Does it waken the patient from sleep or is it present on awakening? What is the frequency of headaches (have the patient recount the past month's and the past year's pattern)? How long do the headaches last (maximum, minimum, average)? Have there been intervals of weeks or months without the headache?

3. *Character and location of pain:* What kind of pain is the patient experiencing with the current headaches (bandlike, squeezing, pressure, pounding, or throbbing)? Where is the pain located (one side of the head, all over the head, in the eyes, radiating up the back of the neck, etc.)? Does the pain radiate anywhere or seem to spread during the course of attack? How severe can the headaches be (on a scale of 1 to 10)? How does the patient rate this headache pain to the pain of other headaches or other situations (e.g., is it the "worst ever" or "the worst pain in my life")?

4. *Aggravating and alleviating factors:* Does anything make the headache pain worse (bending, sneezing, straining, coughing)? What factors seem to help the headache (lying down, pressing on the temples, avoidance of work, simple analgesics, narcotics, or other medications)? How is the patient currently treating the headache?

5. *Associated neurologic symptoms:* Does the patient have associated symptoms during the headaches such as spots before the eyes (very common in both tension and migraine headaches); inability to tolerate light, sound, touch or movement; nausea and/or vomiting; focal numbness or weakness?

6. *Prior evaluation:* Has the patient been evaluated for the headaches and what has he been told as a result of this evaluation? It is important to request previous records for all patients who give a history of severe, disabling headache, irrespective of the reported duration of the present headache problem or the nature of the previous evaluation; sometimes even just requesting the records reminds the patient of a 10- to 20-year history of severe headache and multiple visits; sometimes the previous records confirm this despite a patient's poor recall. In either case, this information can be particularly valuable in evaluating a patient who describes recent onset of severe headaches.

7. *Functional impact:* How are the headaches currently affecting the patient (work and social relationships)?

8. *Family and household history:* Is there any history of headaches in the parents, siblings, children or in other people living in the patient's household? What type?

Physical and Laboratory Examination

As stated, information obtained in the history will usually suggest the probable basis for a patient's headache. The appropriate requirements for the physical examination and the laboratory examination are thus described under each type of headache below. The extent of the physical examination indicated may vary from no examination (e.g., in a patient with headache following vasodilator therapy), to an examination focused upon structures which may be the source of the headache (e.g., sinuses), to an extensive neurologic and laboratory examination (the patient with progressive focal neurologic signs).

Principles of Initial Treatment

Most patients with headache can be treated presumptively for tension or migraine headache, as described below. A fuller investigation should be carried out in patients who show either of the following situations after initial treatment: (a) Those patients who fail to respond to treatment of the presumed condition. Even in this situation, the extent of the evaluation should be tempered by the circumstances and the patient's expectations. For example, a middle-aged patient who fails a conservative treatment regimen for recent onset of what appear to be migraine headaches should have an earlier and more extensive evaluation than a middle-aged patient with 20 years of apparent tension headaches, and an unfailingly normal examination, who has not responded to the full spectrum of therapeutic options. (b) Those patients who show significant changes in complaints or physical findings which point to one of the less common causes of headache discussed below.

TREATMENT EXPECTATIONS

A recent study compared physicians' expectations in the management of headaches with the expectations of their patients (8). The majority of the physicians in this study expected that their patients would demand pain relief and not care very much about getting an explanation of their problems or medications. In contrast, only 31% of the patients themselves felt that pain relief itself was most important; 46% rated an explanation of their problem as their most important concern.

When treating the usual tension or migraine headache, the physician should neither expect always to achieve total relief of headache pain, nor should the patient be misled into thinking that this is always possible. The patient must be educated to understand realistically the limitations of drug therapy and the potential for drug side effects, which, in some cases, can be more distressing than the headaches. Selection of a treatment regimen is complicated by the high placebo response rates (20 to 40%) and by the variable natural history of headaches. Because of this variability, a detailed baseline history of the patient's headache problems is important for subsequent assessment of the patient's response to treatment.

SPECIFIC HEADACHE SYNDROMES

Tension (Muscle Contraction) Headache

In the absence of any rigorous criterion or physiologic markers, the term "tension headache" has been applied to what is probably a heterogeneous group of patients suffering from headache.

PATHOGENESIS

The symptoms of this type of headache are presumed to be caused by contraction of scalp and neck muscles. The muscle contraction is thought to be a somatic consequence of coexisting psychosocial stress in the patient's life, although the stress cannot always be identified. Neither increased muscle tension nor precipitating stress is specific for tension headaches; both are also common in migraine, which is the prototype of vascular headache (see below). Table 76.3 summarizes the data obtained by Friedman et al. in 1954 (2) on the frequency of several characteristics in a large number of patients and shows considerable overlap between tension and migraine headaches.

PRESENTATION

Tension headache is usually described as a squeezing, "bandlike" tightness or pressure sensation which is felt bilaterally and which may be generalized, occipital, frontal, or bitemporal. However, some patients with otherwise typical tension headaches complain in addition of throbbing pain (suggestive of vascular headache), or sharp shooting pain (suggestive of neuralgia); these may be the only manifestations of tension headache in occasional patients. Patients frequently complain of spots before their eyes when the pain is intense, but these are not the true fortification hallucinations of migraine (see below). The duration of the headache varies from minutes to hours to days. Some patients complain of continuous headaches which have been unremitting for years; this kind of headache is almost always due to tension. Moreover, a history of increased psychosocial stress will often be associated with headache episodes. Finally, the patients may report some relief of pain with massage of their scalp (as may patients with migraine headache).

Physical examination is unremarkable except for neck or scalp muscle tenderness, in some patients, and occasionally an exaggerated physiologic tremor (see Chapter 79) due to anxiety.

TREATMENT

Nonpharmacologic. It is usually helpful to explain to the patient the presumed pathogenesis of tension headache, i.e., scalp and neck muscle contraction or "tension." This information helps the patient to understand both the benign nature of his headache and its possible relationship to psychosocial stress. As explained elsewhere (Chapter 10), concerned listening to a patient's story often helps to reduce somatic symptoms due to stress. The physician can also help by encouraging any effort made by the patient to reduce the stressful situations. For nonpharmacologic relief of symptoms, massage of the scalp and neck muscles by another person should be recommended; in addition, any other procedure which the patient

Table 76.3
Characteristics of Migrainous and Tension Headaches[a]

	Migraine (%)	Tension (%)
Age at onset		
<20 years	55	30
>20 years	45	70
Premonitory symptoms	60	10
Frequency		
Daily	3	50
<Weekly	60	15
Duration		
Constant, daily	0	20
1–3 days	35	10
Throbbing pain	80	30
Location		
Unilateral	80	10
Bilateral	20	90
Vomiting with attacks	50	10
Family history of headache	65	40

[a] Adapted from N. H. Raskin and O. Appenzeller: *Headache.* W. B. Saunders, Philadelphia, 1980; as modified from A. P. Friedman et al.: *Neurology, 4:* 773, 1954.

may have found helpful should be encouraged by the physician (as long as he believes it to be harmless).

Pharmacologic. Symptomatic treatment with drugs is an important adjunct to the general measures just described; for selected patients, prophylactic drug treatment can also be tried. Most patients will have used headache remedies containing aspirin or acetaminophen before consulting their physician about treatment. For mild to moderate headaches, however, an additional trial of these mild analgesics should be recommended if they have not been taken at the usual effective dose (600 mg every 4 to 6 hours).

A number of drugs are widely prescribed for patients with moderately severe intermittent headaches unresponsive to aspirin or acetaminophen. These drugs include codeine sulfate; propoxyphene (Darvon); and two products which contain combinations of analgesics, sedatives, and caffeine: Fiorinal (butalbital, caffeine, aspirin, phenacetin); and Percodan (oxycodone, aspirin, phenacetin, caffeine). Each of these drugs can lead to habituation and dependency (see Chapter 21). Therefore, it is unwise to initiate treatment with these drugs unless it is clear the patient can use them appropriately for limited periods.

Prophylaxis can also be tried for the occasional patient whose tension headaches are very severe or very frequent. The best results (60% improved vs. 22% or placebo) have been obtained with the tricyclic antidepressant amitriptyline (Elavil), given in daily doses of 50 to 100 mg at bedtime (5). (A detailed discussion of the use of this drug is found in Chapter 14). Somewhat less benefit was obtained with prophylactic benzodiazepine anxiolytic drugs (diazepam, Valium; chlordiazapoxide, Librium) in the same study.

Migraine

Migraine headache is divided into two subgroups—*classic migraine* which denotes a syndrome of headache with associated characteristic premonitory sensory, motor, or visual disturbances; and *common migraine* which denotes a syndrome in which there is no neurologic disturbance preceding the headache.

PATHOGENESIS

The symptoms of a migraine headache are attributed to sequential changes affecting intracranial and extracranial arteries.

The initial change is *vasoconstriction*, which, when it produces brain ischemia, is responsible for the fortification hallucinations (see below), transient hemiparesis or hemiparesthesias, confusion, and vertigo that can be seen in classic migraine. While vasoconstriction presumably also occurs in common migraine, it seems to be below the threshold necessary to produce obvious symptoms and instead is perhaps responsible for the prodomal unease and warning that these patients may experience. Vasoconstriction is thought to last from ½ hour to several hours in a typical migraine attack.

The initial vasoconstriction is followed by *vasodilation* of the affected vessels, resulting in typical "vascular headache" pain—pain which throbs in unison with the pulse. Some patients even report noticing dilated, throbbing, aching vessels over one side of the scalp during an episode. Patients often report some relief during the attack by pressure on the temples, which presumably decreases blood flow to the dilated temporal arteries.

Usually the vasoconstrictive symptoms are resolving or have resolved by the time the headache (vasodilation symptoms) starts. In some patients, however, these symptom groups overlap, perhaps because some vessels remain vasoconstricted while others are becoming vasodilated.

EPIDEMIOLOGY AND NATURAL HISTORY

The lack of a simple, specific test for migraine headache and variations in the definition of migraine headache make it difficult to determine the prevalence and natural course of this condition. Nevertheless, some characteristics are clear.

From 20 to 50% of migraine headache sufferers have a positive family history for migraine, usually in one parent. This seems to be particularly true with patients who have classic migraine.

The onset of migraine is usually between the ages of 15 through 25, and the headaches are more common in women. While recurrence is usually a hallmark of migraine headache, some patients have only rare episodes, or even only a single typical episode in their lives. Migraine episodes usually become less frequent and less severe with age.

The perimenstrual period (particularly before the onset of bleeding, when levels of estradiol are falling), oral contraceptives (particularly off-days, presumably due to falling estrogen levels), and menopause are associated with migraine headaches. The following substances may initiate headaches in susceptible subjects: vasodilators (nitrates and antihypertensives); alcohol; chocolate; cheeses, wines, and other foods containing tyramine; and monosodium glutamate. Caffeine or ergotamine withdrawal can also cause headaches (presumably by rebound vasodilation). The patient should be asked about these associations and any others which he may have noted.

DIAGNOSIS AND DIFFERENTIAL DIAGNOSIS

The following are reasonably well established criteria for the working diagnosis of a migraine headache:

1. *Prodomal warning* of some kind, ranging from vague malaise to focal neurologic symptoms. So-called fortification hallucinations are almost specific for classic migraine; these are slowly enlarging scotomata which are surrounded by luminous angles and which slowly change shape and appear to move across the visual fields (see Fig. 76.1) (rarely occipital lobe tumors or arteriovenous malformations may produce the same effects).

2. *Unilateral head pain* during any one attack. The pain usually increases gradually, reaching a peak in several hours and lasting for several hours to a day in typical cases. Attacks lasting 2 to 3 days are not uncommon, and some migraine attacks last for 1 to 2 weeks. The pain is usually described as "pounding" or "throbbing." Although headaches are typically unilateral during a single attack, most patients will have attacks on both sides of the head. However, in

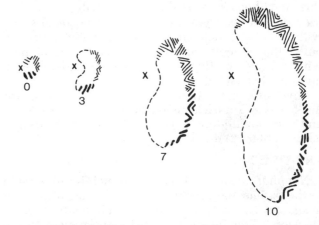

Figure 76.1 Lashley's maps of the progression of his own fortification spectra at varying time intervals after the onset of a migrainous attack. The *X* in each instance indicates the visual fixation point. The numbers represent minutes. (From N. H. Raskin and O. Appenzeller: *Headache.* W. B. Saunders, Philadelphia, 1980; as appeared in K. S. Lashley: *Archives of Neurology and Psychiatry, 46:* 331, 1941, copyright American Medical Association.)

20% of patients, headaches will always be on the same side.

Even these criteria are not broad enough to encompass all the manifestations of migraine headache. Other frequent symptoms include photophobia, sonophobia, nausea, vomiting, and generalized malaise. The headache itself is usually described as throbbing, but may also be described as aching or stabbing. Furthermore, scalp muscle contraction may occur, so it is not unusual for a patient with migraine to develop bilateral headache and scalp tenderness, features typical of tension headache. In this instance, the headache is referred to as "mixed headache" or "migraine/tension variant headache."

In the *differential diagnosis* of migraine, the most important considerations are transient ischemic attacks (TIAs) or other cerebrovascular events, particularly in middle-aged and older patients (see Chapter 80 for details). Migrainous ischemia usually occurs in patients with a prior history of similar attacks, often in young adulthood; the family history in these cases tends to be particularly strong. Symptoms of migrainous vasoconstriction typically last ½ hour to several hours; TIAs usually last less than 5 min (although a longer time course is possible). Headaches should be a prominent component of the migrainous ischemic event; while headache may occur in up to 25% of patients with transient ischemic events, it is usually relatively mild and transitory. Some patients with suspected migrainous ischemic events, particularly those with "migraine equivalents" (ischemic symptoms without headache) should be evaluated for TIA before their symptoms are attributed to migraine.

TREATMENT

The vast majority of migraine sufferers can be helped by treatment, principally pharmacologic treatment.

Nonpharmacologic. The most useful nonpharmacologic treatment is elimination or avoidance of known trigger factors, when this is possible. Common drugs which may trigger an attack are nitrates, vasodilators, indomethacin, and oral contraceptives. Another common trigger factor, often less tractable, is psychologic stress. Whenever possible such stress should be decreased, as discussed above under tension headache. Less common trigger factors which can be eliminated are excess coffee use, dental problems, and irregular sleep habits. There are no consistently implicated dietary trigger factors; however, each patient should be encouraged to try eliminating any dietary component or other trigger factor which he can identify.

During an established attack, a patient usually feels better reclining in a dark cool room. This is the only practice other than drug treatment which appears to be helpful.

Pharmacologic. Mild attacks: Patients with mild migraine attacks often obtain relief from aspirin or acetaminophen, used as described above under tension headache.

Moderate and severe attacks: At the start of an attack in a patient with moderate to severe migraine, ergotamine tartrate is the agent of choice. Because of its relative specificity, ergotamine may be administered at the onset of symptoms as a therapeutic trial to confirm a clinical suspicion of migraine headache. The action of ergotamine has traditionally been attributed to its vasoconstrictor property, but the reason for its effectiveness in aborting migraine symptoms is not understood clearly.

Ergotamine is available in preparations which permit administration by multiple routes (see Table 76.4). The ideal route is one which is convenient, leads to prompt absorption of the drug, and is not affected by vomiting. Both suppositories and sublingual preparations meet these criteria well. Ingested tablets may be vomited and are therefore less reliable. Recommended schedules for ergotamine administration are summarized in Table 76.5. The objective of these schedules is to attain a total dose which is effective, but which is below the dose that produces nausea and vomiting. Traditionally this has been accomplished by taking additional doses at 30 and 60 min if the first dose is ineffective.

Because of the variability of response to ergotamine doses, Raskin and Appenzeller (see "General References") recommend that each patient should be told how to determine the dose which produces nausea for him (the nauseating dose). This is done by following the traditional schedule on a headache-free day; the cumulative dose attained just prior to the nauseating dose would be the appropriate total therapeutic dose (the subnauseating dose) for that patient to take (all at once) at the onset of future attacks.

A number of points are important in instructing a patient about the use of ergotamine. Above all, the patient should understand that ergotamine is not a "pain killer," but that it is used to interrupt the vascular events causing migraine pain. He should understand that for maximum benefit he *must* take ergotamine at the onset of prodromal symptoms or headache (waiting for the headache to become well-established is a common problem in patients who report no benefit from ergotamine). In order to assure immediate access to his medicine, the patient should be advised to carry some with him at all times. The patient should be informed that taking more than the recommended maximum daily dose (see Table 76.5), carries the risk of peripheral vasoconstriction in addition to nausea and vomiting. Because ergotamine preparations have a short shelf-life, the patient should be instructed to obtain a new supply if he fails to obtain benefit from his medicine or if he has not used it for many months. Finally, patients should be warned not to use ergotamine more than twice in the same week.

Occasionally the patient has *side effects* from er-

Table 76.4
Ergot-containing Drugs[a]

Brand and Generic Names	Route[b]	Ergot Alkaloid	Caffeine	Belladonna	Other
Bellergal	p.o.	Ergotamine 0.3 mg		0.1 mg	Phenobarbital 20 mg
Bellergal-S	p.o.	Ergotamine 0.6 mg		0.2 mg	Phenobarbital 40 mg
Cafergot	p.o.	Ergotamine 1 mg	100 mg		
Cafergot	p.r.	Ergotamine 2 mg	100 mg		
Cafergot-PB	p.o.	Ergotamine 1 mg	100 mg	0.125 mg	Phenobarbital 30 mg
Cafergot-PB	p.r.	Ergotamine 2 mg	100 mg	0.25 mg	Phenobarbital 60 mg
D.H.E. 45	i.m./i.v.	Dihydroergotamine mesylate 1 mg/ml			
Ergomar	s.l.	Ergotamine 2 mg			
Ergonovine	p.o.	Ergonovine 0.2 mg			
Ergostat	s.l.	Ergotamine 2 mg			
Ergotamine	s.c./i.m.	0.25 mg/0.5 ml or 0.5 mg/l ml			
Ergotamine	Inhal.	0.36 mg/puff			
Ergotamine	p.o.	1 mg			
Ergotrate	p.o.	Ergonovine 0.2 mg			
Gynergen	p.o.	Ergotamine 1 mg			
Medihaler Ergotamine Aerosol	Inhal.	Ergotamine 0.36 mg/puff			
Migral	p.o.	Ergotamine 1 mg	50 mg		Cyclizine 25 mg
Wigraine	p.o.	Ergotamine 1 mg	100 mg	0.1 mg	Phenacetin 130 mg
Wigraine	p.r.	Ergotamine 1 mg	100 mg	0.1 mg	Phenacetin 130 mg

[a] Adapted from N. H. Raskin and O. Appenzeller: *Headache.* W. B. Saunders, Philadelphia, 1980.
[b] p.o., per os; p.r., per rectum; i.m., intramuscular; i.v., intravenous; s.l., sublingual; s.c., subcutaneous; Inhal., inhalation.

Table 76.5
Recommended Schedules of Ergotamine for Treating a Migraine Attack

Route	Strength per Dose	Initial Dose[a]
Sublingual (s.l.)	2 mg (tablet)	2 or 3 mg (1 or 1½ tablets)
Rectal (p.r.)	1 mg (suppository) 2 mg	1 or 2 mg
Oral (p.o.)	1 mg (tablet) 2 mg	1 or 2 mg
Aerosol (inhal.)	0.36 mg per puff (fine powder in cannister)	1 or 2 puffs

[a] Repeated at 30 and 60 min if necessary. This constitutes maximal total dose for 1 day.

gotamine even when taken at the subnauseating dose. These include abdominal cramps, muscle cramps, vertigo, diarrhea, and distal parenthesia; less commonly, syncope, tremor, angina pectoris, and claudication may occur. Most patients, however, tolerate the drug well.

The relative contraindications to ergotamine use are established angina and symptomatic peripheral arterial disease. Traditionally, hypertension has been named as a contraindication; Raskin and Appenzeller (see "General References") point out, however, that hypertensive patients can safely take the drug, citing early reports which showed no increase in blood pressure. Normotensive patients do show a transient 10 to 20 mg Hg increase in systolic and diastolic pressure. Whenever there is concern about the effect of ergotamine on the blood pressure of an individual patient, the blood pressure response to ergotamine should be measured in the physician's office, following the protocol for determining the subnauseating dose of ergotamine outlined above.

For an *established, severe migraine headache,* simple analgesics usually do not help. For this reason, reliable patients should be given small supplies of either codeine (60 mg) or meperidine hydrochloride (Demerol) (50 to 100 mg), to be taken as needed if ergotamine and other measures have failed to abort an attack. This measure may save a patient many unnecessary trips to the physician's office.

PROPHYLACTIC THERAPY

Prophylactic therapy for migraine should be considered when the patient has two or more attacks per week or when he has less frequent attacks which cannot be controlled with ergotamine and which disrupt employment or social life.

The decision regarding prophylaxis must be the patient's after the distinction between symptomatic and prophylactic therapy has been explained clearly. Even a patient who has not had adequate relief from routine measures may forego prophylactic treatment because of the inconvenience, expense, and possible side effects of continuous drug therapy. Furthermore, for each of the drugs used prophylactically for migraine, a relatively long trial period (up to several months) may be necessary to assess its effectiveness; and trials with a number of drugs may be necessary. These facts should also be explained to the patient. Finally, the patient should understand that during the trial of prophylaxis he can continue the usual measures for treating his migraine attacks.

Those drugs which have been effective in migraine prophylaxis together with dose ranges and common side effects are listed in Table 76.6.

The following general conclusions can be drawn about migraine prophylaxis (11):

1. Fifty percent or more of patients report some improvement in their migraine syndrome during the first year, compared with a reported improvement in 25% of "control patients" (patients who choose not to take prophylaxis); during the second year of prophylaxis, the response rate may be lower.

2. Most of the improvement consists of a decrease in frequency or severity of headaches—freedom from headaches occurs in only a minority of patients.

3. Each of the drugs which has been tried (Table 76.6) gives similar results; failure of one drug does not predict response to another, so that a sequential trial of different drugs is reasonable.

4. Those drugs which have the least toxicity and which are known best to the physician should be tried first (for the generalist, these are propranolol and amitriptyline).

Each patient who chooses prophylactic therapy should be asked to keep a log in which to record the frequency and severity of headaches and the nature of any associated factors. As stated, improvement may occur either as a decrease in frequency of attacks, or a decrease in the severity of the attacks, or both; the patient's log will determine whether any improvement has occurred.

THE PATIENT WITH INTRACTABLE MIGRAINE HEADACHES

A small number of migraine sufferers do not find relief from intractable and disabling headaches, even after prolonged and thorough attempts at therapy. For a complete assessment and an adequate trial of therapy, these patients should be referred to a neu-rologist. During particularly incapacitating episodes, hospital admission should be considered to provide adequate rest and treatment with potent analgesics.

Cluster Headache

Cluster headache is probably a variant of migraine (7). It has previously been designated by a number of names, e.g., Horton's headache, histamine headache (a misnomer), and migrainous cranial neuralgia. Episodes of pain occur in clusters extending over days to weeks, thus giving the syndrome its name. Most episodes last from 4 to 6 weeks and are followed by long pain-free intervals. The intervals between episodes range from 3 months to 5 years, occasionally longer; most patients, however, have one or two episodes per year. Eventually the problem ceases altogether.

Cluster headache is much less frequent than migraine in the population. It occcurs predominantly in middle-aged men. Onset usually occurs between the age of 20 and 50. There is no evidence for a familial basis for cluster headache.

MANIFESTATIONS

In a typical attack, there is sudden stabbing or burning pain in the eye, orbit, and cheek on one side. The pain is usually excruciating. Unlike patients with migraine, patients with cluster headache are usually agitated and they often pace the floor during the attack. Characteristically, the patient also describes ipsilateral lacrimation, rhinorrhea, and conjunctival injection. Ipsilateral ptosis and miosis may also occur; this is thought to be due to compression of the sympathetic plexus by the dilated carotid artery, which produces a partial Horner's syndrome. Usually the same side is involved during a cluster of attacks.

Attacks last from 30 min to 2 hours (mean 45 min); occasional mild attacks may last only 10 minutes. The attacks range in frequency from six per day to one per week during a cluster; and they tend to occur

Table 76.6
Interval Therapy of Migrainous Attacks—Prescribing Information [a]

Drug	Tablet Size(s)	Daily Dose Range	Commonest Side Effects
Ergonovine	0.2 mg	0.4–2.0 mg	Nausea, abdominal pain, leg "tiredness"
Amitriptyline	10, 25, 50 mg	10–175 mg	Sedation, dry mouth
Propranolol	10, 20, 40, 80 mg	40–320 mg	Lethargy, insomnia, constipation, lightheadedness
Papaverine	150, 300 mg	300–900 mg	Nausea
Cyproheptadine	4 mg	12–32 mg	Sedation, weight gain
Ergotamine-phenobarbital-belladonna	tabs	1–4 tablets	Nausea, sedation
Phenelzine	15 mg	15–75 mg	Insomnia, lightheadedness, constipation
Methysergide	2 mg	2–8 mg	Nausea, abdominal pain, muscle cramps, insomnia, weight gain, edema, peripheral vasoconstriction

[a] From N. H. Raskin and O. Appenzeller: *Headache.* W. B. Saunders, Philadelphia, 1980.

at the same time each day, mostly commonly in the evening just after the patient has gone to bed. In some patients, alcohol may be a particularly potent trigger factor; nitrates and vasodilator drugs may also induce attacks. Therefore there should be a full inquiry about the use of drugs in evaluating these patients.

These characteristics describe the typical syndrome of cluster headache. Some individuals have less well-defined episodes, whereas other patients may have almost daily attacks of pain for a number of years, a syndrome known as "chronic paroxysmal hemicrania" (9).

Except during an attack, when the unilateral findings described above are present, the physical examination in patients with cluster headache is unremarkable.

Differential diagnosis. Cluster headache must be carefully distinguished from tic douloureux (see below); acute glaucoma (by the presence of miosis, normal tonometry, no lasting visual impairment); sinusitis (by lack of history of upper respiratory infection, lack of purulent rhinorrhea or sinus tenderness, and by negative X-rays); from periapical dental abscess (by the absence of tenderness on tooth percussion); and from atypical facial neuralgia (see below).

TREATMENT

Because attacks are relatively short in duration and very distressing, they should be treated with a drug with rapid onset of action and high likelihood of efficacy. Ergotamine administered by inhaler or sublingually is the drug which best meets these criteria. The dose is one or two puffs from an inhaler or one sublingual tablet (see Table 76.4 for available preparations). When administered by aerosol, this drug is effective in about 80% of attacks (14). Codeine, 60 mg, or Demerol, 50 to 100 mg, can also be utilized.

The best approach to management during an episode of cluster headache is *short term prophylaxis.* Ergotamine 1 to 2 mg orally 3 times daily for a total of 6 weeks, is a reasonable regimen. When the duration of prophylactic treatment is strictly limited and the risks of daily ergotamine are explained carefully to the patient, the hazards associated with chronic ergotamine adminstrations can be avoided. Because of the incapacitating nature of cluster headaches, most patients will choose to try prophylaxis after the risks have been carefully explained. The principal hazard is ischemia due to peripheral vasoconstriction. This problem chiefly affects the lower extremities; it can lead to gangrene (ergotism) if not identified early. The early symptoms of ischemia are distal coolness and paresthesias, and at times claudication. If a patient is instructed to discontinue the drug promptly and to report these symptoms, there is very little risk of gangrene.

There are anecdotal reports of effective prophylaxis for cluster headache by treatment with propranolol, amitriptyline, and cyproheptadine, in doses similar to those used in migraine (see Table 76.6). In addition, for the rare patient who suffers from almost daily cluster headache (chronic paroxysmal hemicrania), indomethacin (Indocin), in doses of 25 to 150 mg daily, has been very effective (9). Indomethacin may be useful in the prophylaxis of ordinary cluster headaches.

The patient in whom neither treatment nor prophylaxis with the above regimens helps should be referred to a neurologist or to an internist with wide experience in headache management.

Sinus Headache

The pain of *acute sinusitis* may be described by the patient as headache. The diagnosis is based upon the other manifestations of acute sinusitis and on the reproduction of the patient's "headache" by applying pressure to affected sinuses (see Chapter 27 for a full account).

Chronic sinusitis is often cited by patients as the reason for their headaches; it is actually a relatively uncommon cause for chronic intercurrent headache. Chronic sinusitis can present diagnostic difficulties, particularly when it involves the sphenoid sinus (causing a dull boring pain behind the eyes). The physician's suspicions should be aroused if there is a history of preceding acute sinusitis, especially if there is not a long history of headache. The diagnosis and management of chronic sinusitis are discussed in Chapter 27.

Acute Exertional Headache (Orgasmic Headache, Cough Headache, Sneeze Headache) (12)

The features of acute exertional headache are (a) that it is of sudden (or almost instantaneous) onset and (b) that it is directly related to exertion of some kind (orgasm, coughing, sneezing, straining, bending, running, lifting, etc.). It may last from minutes to half an hour, rarely longer. In 90% of patients the headache is presumably due to intracranial-spinal pressure dissociations and the course is benign. In 10% of patients significant organic disease has been found (Arnold-Chiari malformation, hydrocephalus, tumor, and subarachnoid hemorrhage).

Exertional headache must be differentiated chiefly from the headache of *subarachnoid hemorrhage.* The headaches of major subarachnoid hemorrhages are usually far more persistent and are usually associated with fever, stiff neck, progressive clouding of consciousness, and focal neurologic signs. Exertional headaches may be quite severe, but they are brief and they recur with the trigger activity. Because it may be impossible to distinguish the first episode of exertional headache from a minor subarachnoid hemorrhage, and because of the 10% risk of another organic basis for the headache, computerized tomography (CT) on an up-to-date machine (with and without contrast, because of the possibility of tumor or arteriovenous malformation; see "Patient Experience," Chapter 75). should be considered when patients initially report the problem.

If CT findings are normal, the benign nature of the condition should be explained to the patient. The patient will usually find ways to avoid some of the activities which produce headache. If desired, propranolol, 40 mg to 80 mg twice per day, or indomethacin, 25 mg 3 times daily, can be tried for prophylaxis.

Temporomandibular Joint (TMJ) Syndrome

On history and examination, some patients complaining of headache will have the stigmata of this common syndrome—pain brought on by motion of the jaw and tenderness of the temporomandibular joint. The epidemiology, course, and management of this syndrome are described in Chapter 98.

Headache Due to Drugs

Headache is listed as an occasional side effect of many drugs. Among those commonly used drugs for which headache is more than an occasional side effect are indomethacin (Indocin), nalidixic acid (NegGram), trimethoprim-sulfamethoxazole (Bactrim, Septra), oral contraceptives, and vasodilators. Therefore, as noted earlier, it is important to ask the patient routinely about new drugs when evaluating a headache of recent onset. Clearly whenever it seems likely that a drug side effect is causing headache, temporary discontinuation of the drug (and selection of an alternative drug if necessary) will establish the role of the drug. Some patients, reassured that the headache is only a drug side effect, will prefer to continue taking the drug.

A throbbing vascular-type headache frequently occurs shortly after initiation of treatment (or a dose increase) with a *vasodilator drug*. The most common offenders are the short and long acting nitrates and the vasodilators used to treat hypertension (hydralazine and minoxidil). The management of this problem depends upon the importance of the drug and the severity of the headache. Some patients, if informed in advance of the possibility of headache, will choose to take the drug anyway; this is particularly true of sublingual nitrates administered for angina. For the long acting nitrates, dose reduction may effectively reduce headache for some patients, while alternate antianginal treatment will be needed for others (see Chapter 54). The headache associated with antihypertensive vasodilators can usually be prevented by treating the patient with a beta blocker before the vasodilator is added (see Chapter 59).

Headache in Acute Febrile Illnesses

Acute febrile illnesses may cause vascular-type throbbing headaches which remit when the illness resolves. A febrile patient in whom the headache is the major symptom and in whom nuchal rigidity is present requires a cerebrospinal fluid examination to exclude meningitis.

Giant Cell Arteritis and Polymyalgia Rheumatica (3, 4)

Giant cell arteritis (GCA) is a vasculitis which affects large arteries throughout the body. Clinical manifestations, however, are usually due to involvement of branches of the internal carotid artery and the most common syndrome is headache. GCA has also been called temporal arteritis (TA) because temporal headaches and a positive temporal artery biopsy are the findings which are most typical of the disease. The etiology of GCA is unknown.

Polymyalgia rheumatica (PR), a debilitating condition which presents with stiffness and aching of the neck and shoulder muscles, occurs in about 50% of patients with GCA. PR may also occur in patients who do not have GCA.

EPIDEMIOLOGY

GCA is almost exclusively a disease of persons over the age of 50; the average age of onset is 65. It is very uncommon in black individuals. It is somewhat more common in women than in men. In the single reported community study of GCA, it was found that the yearly incidence in persons over 50 was approximately 17 per 100,000 and the prevalence, 130 per 100,000 (4).

MANIFESTATIONS

Giant Cell Arteritis. The *headache* of GCA does not have specific features which distinguish it clearly from other headaches. It is temporal in over one-half of patients; however, it may be frontal, occipital, parietal, or holocephalic. The patient usually reports that it involves the surface and is not intracranial. It may be made worse by hair-brushing, resting the head on a pillow, and, at times, by exposure to cold. It is usually not described as throbbing. It is often described as being worse at night, and building up gradually over a number of hours. Because these symptoms are not specific, the most important factors in suggesting the diagnosis of GCA are a number of associated findings, listed in Table 76.7. It is important to inquire specifically about pain (claudication) associated with chewing, swallowing, and arm or tongue motion, as these symptoms are highly suggestive of GCA. The combination of one or more of the findings listed in Table 76.7 with a *new* headache in an older individual is sufficient to suspect GCA.

Polymyalgia Rheumatica (PR). This condition is insidious in onset. The chief complaints are aching and stiffness of the shoulder girdle; and, less commonly, of the thigh muscles. These symptoms may make it particularly hard for the patient to get up in the morning. Associated low grade fever, weight loss, and anorexia are common. On physical examination, there may be some tenderness of the shoulder and neck muscles, but there is no significant loss of muscle strength.

Table 76.7
Clinical Features of Giant Cell Arteritis[a]

Common Features (% of Patients with Feature at Initial Evaluation)		Less Common but Characteristic Features
Headache	(85)	Raynaud's phenomenon of limbs or tongue
Temporal artery tenderness	(70)	Tender scalp nodules
Jaw claudication	(65)	Thick, tender occipital arteries
Lingual, limb or swallowing claudication	(20)	Necrotic lesions of scalp, tongue
Brachiocephalic bruits	(50)	Carotid artery tenderness
Thickened or nodular temporal artery	(45)	Swelling of the hands
		Taste, smell disturbances
Pulseless temporal artery	(40)	
Visual symptoms	(40)	Distended, beaded retinal veins
Fixed blindness, partial or complete	(15)	Diminished or absent radial artery pulses
Polymyalgia rheumatica	(40)	Mononeuropathy—median, peroneal, cervical root
Weight loss > 6 kg	(35)	
Erythrocyte sedimentation rate:		
>50 mm/hr	(95)	
>100 mm/hr	(60)	
Fever (>37.7°C)	(20)	
Abnormal liver function	(50)	
Anemia (hematocrit < 35%)	(50)	

[a] Adapted from N. H. Raskin and O. Appenzeller: *Headache.* W. B. Saunders, Philadelphia, 1980.

DIAGNOSIS

Whenever GCA or PR is suspected, the erythrocyte sedimentation rate (ESR) measured by the Westergren method is the most useful screening test. The majority of patients will have a markedly elevated ESR (often 100 or greater). Since the upper limit of normal for persons over 60 may be as high as 40, an ESR 40 to 60 is less informative than is a very high rate. *Definitive diagnosis of GCA* is made with a temporal artery biopsy. Because the typical histologic changes (inflammatory cells, edema, and giant cells) are patchy in distribution, examination of serial sections of the resected segment of artery is essential; in occasional patients with GCA, even extensive sampling of one temporal artery does not yield a positive biopsy and the other artery must be biopsied also.

Patient Experience. A temporal artery biopsy can be done in an ambulatory surgery facility (by a general surgeon, vascular surgeon, plastic surgeon, or a neurosurgeon). The scalp hair is shaved, the skin is anesthetized with xylocaine, and the segment of artery (4 to 6 cm) is excised. The entire procedure requires about half an hour. There are no serious sequelae.

The *diagnosis of polymyalgia rheumatica* is based on the combination of the typical symptoms, a high ESR, and exclusion of other explanations for the patient's symptoms. If a patient with typical PR has manifestations suggesting GCA (see Table 76.7), a temporal artery biopsy is indicated, since the recommended treatment for the two conditions is different.

COURSE AND TREATMENT

Both GCA and PR are self-limited conditions, lasting up to 2 years. Treatment with corticosteroids produces dramatic symptomatic relief in patients with both conditions. More important, treatment appears to prevent almost entirely the most serious complication of GCA, blindness due to ischemic optic neuropathy. In untreated persons with GCA, unilateral or bilateral blindness occurs in 20 to 30% of patients.

If the diagnosis of GCA is strongly suspected, treatment should be initiated immediately and the temporal artery biopsy should be obtained within 3 to 4 days. The initial treatment is high dose prednisone (60 to 80 mg daily) for 4 to 6 weeks. During this time, symptoms usually remit entirely and there is a significant decrease in the ESR. After this initial period, the prednisone should be tapered weekly by about 10% until a dose of 10 to 15 mg daily has been reached. This dose should be continued for about 2 years, being discontinued by gradual tapering at the end of the second year (see Chapter 71 for details regarding long term steroid therapy).

If the patient has isolated PR, the treatment is 10 to 15 mg of prednisone daily, from the outset. Treatment is also continued for approximately 2 years, with gradual discontinuation at the end of that time. The symptoms of PR, and the ESR, respond to this regimen within a few days to a week.

Although the symptoms of both GCA and PR may respond to aspirin and other nonsteroidal anti-inflammatory agents, these agents have not been shown to prevent the progressive vasculitis in GCA which may lead to blindness in this condition. The evidence for the efficacy of prednisone therapy in preventing blindness is based not upon controlled trials but upon the dramatic difference in the occurrence of blindness in untreated patients before prednisone was used (20 to 30% of patients) and in prednisone-treated patients (little or no occurrence of blindness).

The diagnosis and treatment of typical cases of GCA and PR can be accomplished readily by the generalist in the ambulatory setting. Whenever there is some question about the diagnosis or an unsatisfactory response to treatment, the opinion of an experienced rheumatologist should be obtained.

Benign Intracranial Hypertension (Pseudotumor Cerebri) (10, 17)

Benign intracranial hypertension is thought to result from idiopathic swelling of the brain tissue and/or an increase in brain vascular volume. The net result of either of these processes is a generalized increase in intracranial pressure. Headache in this condition is presumably due to stretching of the dura and perhaps the large vessels. Papilledema is a direct result of the increased pressure; and the paucity of focal neurologic symptoms and signs is due to the generalized nature of the pressure increase. Those focal signs which do appear (for example, sixth nerve palsies producing horizontal diplopia) are probably related to stretching of the involved structure.

This condition may occcur de novo or may appear in association with a number of purported contributing factors (obesity, menstrual irregularity, steroid therapy or steroid withdrawal, oral contraceptives, nalidixic acid, vitamin A intoxication).

MANIFESTATIONS

The prototypical patient is an obese young woman who develops progressively more severe headaches, nausea, vomiting, dizzinesss, and blurred vision. In approximately one-half of patients, onset is abrupt, while the rest develop symptoms progressively over several weeks or months. The headache always precedes visual symptoms. It is usually generalized, constant or throbbing, and episodic; it is often more severe in the morning and is aggravated by coughing, straining, or position change. The diagnosis is suggested strongly by these historical characteristics coupled with a physical examination which shows papilledema (plus retinal hemorrhages in about one-forth of patients) without focal neurologic signs.

The diagnosis of pseudotumor is always one of exclusion, as its name implies. The most important considerations in the differential diagnosis are intracranial mass lesion, hydrocephalus, and hypertensive encephalopathy. To exclude an intracranial mass or hydrocephalus, a contrast CT scan (see "Patient experience," Chapter 75) should be obtained; in pseudotumor, the scan typically shows small ventricles and no evidence of a mass lesion. Following a negative scan, a lumbar puncture should be performed; in pseudotumor, the cerebrospinal fluid (CSF) pressure is high (200 to 400 mm H_2O or more) and the content of CSF protein is normal or low. The diagnosis of hypertensive encephalopathy should be made if the patient has the typical clinical features of pseudotumor, severe diastolic hypertension (equal to or greater than 120 mm Hg), and a negative CT scan. In a very obese woman, with a history of amenorrhea for many months, it is also important to consider pregnancy-induced hypertension (toxemia), which is ruled out by a negative pregnancy test (see Chapter 90).

For less clear-cut cases, such as a typical clinical presentation in an older male patient, more exhaustive investigations may be indicated; after initial workup, such patients should therefore be referred to a neurologist.

TREATMENT AND COURSE

Most patients recover completely from pseudotumor within several weeks or months. Because the disease itself is self-limited, it is difficult to assess the role of treatment in recovery. One standard treatment is elimination of any associated contributing factor and decompression of the subarachnoid space by repeat lumbar punctures. Initially, a lumbar puncture should be performed twice per week, than at longer intervals until symptoms have remitted entirely. The objective is to remove enough fluid (usually 5 to 30 ml) to reduce the CSF pressure to less than 200 mm H_2O. If marked symptoms persist after several weeks of lumbar punctures, steroid therapy or other modalities (including shunting procedures) should be considered (some physicians, in fact, treat with steroids at the time of initial presentation).

The majority of patients recover from pseudotumor without sequelae. Resolution of papilledema, however, may not occur for a number of months after symptoms have remitted. A small proportion of patients have recurrent episodes or permanent blindness due to optic atrophy.

Post-Traumatic (Postconcussive) Headache

MANIFESTATIONS

Head trauma, which may or may not have been severe enough to cause loss of consciousness, may be followed by a number of symptoms which have been collectively entitled the postconcussive syndrome: headache, vertigo (often positional, see Chapter 78), light-headedness or giddiness, poor concentration and memory, lack of energy, irritability, and anxiety. There is convincing evidence that these varied symptoms may be organic consequences of the injury, even though their exact causal mechanism are not understood. Raskin and Appenzeller (see "General References") provide an excellent review of the syndrome with the focus on headache.

Headache is the most frequent and often the most troubling manifestation of this syndrome. It typically begins with 24 hours of the trauma, as a dull, constant generalized aching or cephalic discomfort which may wax and wane through the day, or become concentrated at different points on the head (bifrontal or unilateral). During exacerbations, the pain typically becomes more vascular, with a throbbing quality. Headache may be worsened by sneezing, coughing, stooping, straining, or rapid head motions and changes in body position; it may be accompanied by nausea and vomiting.

Typically, these headaches worsen over days to weeks, then resolve over weeks or months; in some patients (roughly 15%) headache and other postconcussive symptoms continue for more than a year.

DIFFERENTIAL DIAGNOSIS

Subdural hematoma and other expanding mass lesions: Although postconcussive syndrome is a far more likely explanation of post-traumatic headache and ill-defined intellectual impairments than subdural hematoma, the seriousness of this possibility and the ease of ruling it out with CT scan make it an important consideration.

Post-traumatic dysautonomic cephalgia: Predominantly vascular (throbbing) headache pain associated with sweating of one side of the face, pupillary dilation, and sometimes, carotid bifurcation tenderness, may represent a lesion of the carotid sympathetic plexus produced by whiplash-like injury (15). This condition may respond well to propranolol.

Preexisting *migraine* or chronic *tension headaches* will have to be excluded by history; furthermore, post-traumatic headaches may make a preexisting headache condition temporarily worse.

Cervical spine injury: See Chapter 61.

OBJECTIVE TESTS

In addition to the neurologic history and examination, a number of currently available objective tests may be helpful for confirming the diagnosis of postconcussive syndrome: electroencephalography; vestibular function tests; electronystagmography; and auditory and visual evoked potentials. These tests, when positive, may be helpful medically and medicolegally. Because the abnormalities in these patients may be below the threshold of detectability, negative test results do not exclude an organic explanation of the patient's symptoms.

TREATMENT

For some patients with postconcussive headache, treatment similar to that used for migraine, with ergotamine and other agents, (see p. 815) may occasionally be successful. In most patients, the course of the illness is self-limited even though fairly lengthy.

Characteristics of Headache Due to a Mass Lesion

For both the headache sufferer and the physician, concern about the possibility of a brain tumor often dominates the situation. A number of clinical clues suggest that one is *not* dealing with a benign process; the most important clue to the presence of an intracranial lesion in a headache sufferer is the simultaneous onset of headache and focal neurologic signs/symptoms or a change in mental status. In a person over the age of 50, the onset of persistent headache for the first time, especially in the absence of psychosocial stress, is also very worrisome.

A number of other features, none of them specific, may be clues to the presence of an intracranial mass lesion:

1. Although the headache associated with a mass lesion can initially be intermittent, mild, and responsive to mild analgesics, typically it becomes more continuous and intense and, at the same time, less responsive to analgesics.

2. The headache may wake the patient from sleep or be present on waking every day. The value of these characteristics is somewhat diminished by the comparatively larger number of patients with chronic tension headache, migraine, and cluster headache

who are also awakened by or wake up with headache. True sinus headache may also be worse in the morning due to lack of postural drainage during the night.

3. Coughing, sneezing, and straining may aggravate a persistent headache due to mass lesion, presumably by transiently increasing intracranial pressure and accentuating the stretching of pain-sensitive structures. Again, however, migraine headache can show the same features.

4. Anorexia, nausea, and vomiting may accompany the headache, but these symptoms are not distinguishable from those caused by severe migraine headache. Projectile vomiting is rarely seen in adults with intracranial masses.

Except when there are focal neurologic signs or symptoms, the decision to evaluate a patient for a mass lesion will usually be made after an initial period of observation and a trial of analgesics. A CT scan (see "Patient Experience," Chapter 75) is the diagnostic procedure of choice when the decision is made to evaluate for a mass lesion. Because of its safety, high sensitivity, and moderate specificity, this procedure is the only screening test usually needed in the search for a mass lesion. When the CT scan is positive for intracranial disease, the patient should be referred to a neurologist or a neurosurgeon for definitive care.

FACIAL PAIN SYNDROMES

Idiopathic Trigeminal Neuralgia (Tic Douloureux)

MANIFESTATIONS

Trigeminal neuralgia is a problem seen almost exclusively in patients over the age of 40, most of them elderly. It has several distinguishing features: the pain is severe, paroxysmal, and lancinating; it lasts only a few seconds to a minute. The patient's face usually contorts with the pain, and the patient may find it impossible to control his emotional response. Between attacks the patient is usually pain-free although some patients may have a dull ache in the area. The interval between paroxysms is usually at least 2 or 3 minutes. The frequency of paroxysms is highly variable; some individuals have hundreds each day.

The pain is usually felt in those structures innervated by the second and third divisions of the trigeminal nerve (lips, gums, cheek, chin). There is a slightly greater tendency for tic to affect the right side of the face than the left. The pain is typically unilateral in a single attack, and in 95% of patients it remains unilateral. It is exceedingly uncommon for attacks to involve both sides of the face simultaneously.

The patient frequently can identify trigger points on the face or in the mouth, which, when touched (even by contact with a gust of cold air) or moved, precipitate pain.

A few patients with idiopathic trigeminal neuralgia

will have some areas of slightly decreased sensation which may be difficult to distinguish from normal; however, there is generally no objective decrease in sensation (in men, no more decrease than would normally be observed over the beard area).

DIFFERENTIAL DIAGNOSIS

A syndrome identical to or similar to idiopathic trigeminal neuralgia can be produced by a number of known conditions (secondary trigeminal neuralgia), e.g., multiple sclerosis, acoustic neuroma, aneurysms, trigeminal neuromas, meningiomas, and others. These conditions should be considered, particularly if the patient is under 40 years, and has any of the following: pain predominantly in the upper division of the trigeminal nerve (forehead and eye); bilateral pain; or evidence of bilateral sensory loss or associated motor signs (e.g., weak jaw, facial weakness, swallowing difficulty).

In a patient with a typical clinical presentation, medical therapy (see below) can be initiated without further workup. If medical therapy is ineffective, or if there are any atypical features, referral to a neurologist is appropriate. He will usually request X-ray views helpful in evaluating the divisions of the trigeminal nerve which are clinically most involved (for the first division, the superior orbital fissure; for the second division, the foramen rotunda; for the third division, the foramen ovale). A contrast CT scan (see "Patient Experience," Chapter 75) may also be obtained to check for a neuroma or a meningioma involving the trigeminal or other nerves.

TREATMENT

Advances in drug therapy have made the treatment of idiopathic trigeminal neuralgia relatively easy. The patient should initially be given carbamazepine (Tegretol, 200-mg tablets) one-half tablet (100 mg) twice daily, with meals, increasing every 2 to 3 days to a 3 times daily schedule and a total dose of 300 to 600 mg. An occasional patient may need doses as high as 1200 mg per day; in these cases, blood levels should be monitored to confirm the adequacy of the drug trial. Sixty-seventy percent of patients can expect excellent to satisfactory relief with carbamazepine. Benign side effects of the drug include nausea, vomiting, ataxia, vertigo, and transient leukopenia. The most serious side effects seem to be either allergic or idiosyncratic, including persistent leukopenia and aplastic anemia. Patients must be informed of these possible risks, the incidence of which is unknown but which appears to be quite low. Because of these risks, patients should have serial hemograms performed, weekly for the first 3 months, and monthly thereafter. Because trigeminal neuralgia may remit spontaneously after 6 months to a year, cautious withdrawal from drug therapy should be attempted at periodic intervals (some recommend attempted withdrawal every few weeks).

If the patient fails to improve with carbamazepine or fails to tolerate the drug, he should be referred to a neurosurgeon for percutaneous radiofrequency treatment of the trigeminal ganglia on the affected side. This procedure has essentially no morbidity or mortality. It can be repeated if pain relief is not achieved or if pain recurs.

Atypical Facial Pain

"Atypical facial pain" is a collective term for a variety of painful facial symptoms which do not meet the diagnostic criteria for any recognized entity (16). If untreated, most patients with this problem continue to complain of it for many years. The management of these patients involves excluding all reasonable possibilities; a one-time referral to a dentist and to an otolaryngologist should be part of this evaluation.

Most of these patients whose workup is negative have psychosocial problems and may improve with psychotherapy, provided either by the general physician or a psychiatrist. For additional details, see the discussion of the patient with chronic pain in Chapter 11.

References

General

Caviness, VA and O'Brien, P: Current concepts—headache. *NEJM* 302:446, 1980.
> A succinct review of several types of headache and recent therapeutic modalities.

Delassio, DJ (ed): *Wolff's Headache and Other Head Pain*, Ed. 4. Oxford University Press, New York, 1980.
> The most recent edition of the classic reference work on headache.

Diamond, S and Delessio, DJ: *The Practicing Physician's Approach to Headache*, Ed. 2. Williams & Wilkins, Baltimore, 1978.
> A good general reference by two authorities in the field.

Diamond, S and Medina, JL: Review article: current thoughts on migraine. *Headache* 20: 208, 1980.
> A practical and up to date review.

Raskin, NH and Appenzeller, O: *Headache*. W.B. Saunders, Philadelphia, 1980.
> Extensively referenced book on selected headache syndromes (migraine, tension headache, cluster headache, post-traumatic headache, giant cell arteritis).

Saper, JR: Migraine; I. Classification and pathogenesis. *JAMA* 239: 2380, 1978; Migraine; II. Treatment. *JAMA* 239: 2480, 1978.
> An extensive review of migraine and its treatment.

Specific

1. Dhopesh, V, Anwar, R and Herring, C: A retrospective assessment of emergency department patients with complaint of headache. *Headache* 19: 37, 1979.
2. Friedman, AP, von Storch, TJC and Merritt, HH: Migraine and tension headaches: a clinical study of 2,000 cases. *Neurology* 4: 773, 1954.
3. Hamilton, CR, Jr, Shelley, WM and Tumulty, PA: Giant cell arteritis: including temporal arteritis and polymyalgia rheumatica. *Medicine* 50: 1, 1971.
4. Huston, KA, Hunder, GG, Lie, JT, Kennedy, RH and Elveback, LF: Temporal arteritis: a 25-year epidemiologic, clinical and pathologic study. *Ann Intern Med* 88: 162, 1978.
5. Lance, JW, Curran, DA and Anthony, J: Investigations into the mechanism and treatment of chronic headache. *Med J Aust* 2: 909, 1965.
6. Markush, RE, Karp, HR, Heyman, A and O'Fallon, WM: Epi-

demiologic study of migraine symptoms in young women. *Neurology* 25: 430, 1975.

7. Medina, JL and Diamond, S: The clinical link between migraine and cluster headaches. *Arch Neurol 34:* 470, 1977.
8. Packard, RC: What does the headache patient want? *Headache 19:* 370, 1979.
9. Price, RW and Posner, JB: Chronic paroxsymal hemicrania: a disabling headache syndrome responding to indomethacin. *Ann Neurol 3:* 183, 1978.
10. Johnston, I and Patterson, A: Benign intracranial hypertension. *Brain 97:* 289, 1975.
11. Raskin, NH and Schwartz, RK: Interval therapy of migraine: long-term results. *Headache 20:* 336, 1980.
12. Rooke, ED: Benign exertional headache. *Med Clin North Am 52:* 801, 1968.

13. Schnarch, DM and Hunter, JE: Migraine incidence in clinical versus nonclinical populations. *Psychosomatics 21:* 314, 1980.
14. Speed, WB: Ergotamine tartrate inhalation: a new approach to the management of recurrent vascular headaches. *Am J Med Sci 240:* 327, 1960.
15. Vijayan, N and Dreyfus, PM: Posttraumatic dysautonomic cephalalgia. *Arch Neurol 32:* 649, 1975.
16. Weedington, WW and Blazer, D: Atypical facial pain and trigeminal neuralgia: a comparison study. *Psychosomatics 20:* 348, 1979.
17. Weisburg, LA: Benign intracranial hypertension. *Medicine 54:* 197, 1975.
18. Ziegler, DK, Hassasein, RW and Cough, JR: Characteristics of life headache histories in a nonclinic population. *Neurology 27:* 265, 1977.

CHAPTER SEVENTY-SEVEN

Seizure Disorders

ROBERT S. FISHER, M.D., Ph.D.

Approximately 1% of the United States population, 2 million Americans, are considered to be epileptic. Many additional patients who do not carry the diagnosis of epilepsy present to their personal physicians or to emergency rooms for evaluation and management of seizures. Convulsive disorders are estimated to account for about 5% of visits to all physicians in private practice, and 20% of visits to neurologists (16). Because seizures are so common and the potential consequences of the disease which they cause are so serious, all physicians should be familiar with the basic principles of their diagnosis and management.

DEFINITION AND MECHANISM OF SEIZURES

The precise definition of a "seizure" is not easy, in part because no single behavior or laboratory result is pathognomonic. One approach is to define a seizure as an episode, with a clear start and finish, which affects motor control, sensation, speech or consciousness, and which is associated with certain characteristic electrical abnormalities of the brain. Most patients are relatively normal during the period between seizures (the interictal period), and their electroencephalograms may be normal as well.

The term "*epilepsy*" describes the condition of recurrent seizures due to primary (and persisting) nervous system disease. Therefore, single or even multiple seizures which occur as a result of temporally limited circumstances (such as high fever) should not be labeled "epilepsy."

Although many predisposing factors are known, the basic mechanisms of seizures are still uncertain. Until a clear understanding of these mechanisms emerges, all classification schemes must be empirical. A widely accepted, clinically relevant scheme is shown in Table 77.1 (9).

Table 77.1
Classification of the Epilepsies

PRIMARY GENERALIZED EPILEPSY
  Grand mal
  Petit mal
  Myoclonic
  Infantile spasms, akinetic, other
    pediatric syndromes
PARTIAL (FOCAL) EPILEPSY
  With elementary symptomatology:
    Focal motor
    Focal sensory
    Mixed focal motor and sensory
  With complex symptomatology: partial
    complex epilepsy
  Secondarily generalized
UNCLASSIFIABLE

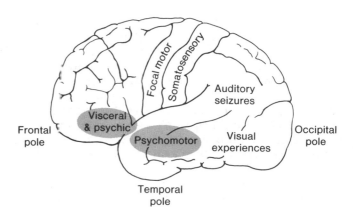

Figure 77.1 Relation of local seizure phenomena to brain topography.

About 75% of all epileptic patients can easily be classified according to this scheme. About 22% of classifiable epileptic patients over the age of 15 have generalized epilepsy and 78% have partial epilepsy. Complex partial seizures, labeled in the past "temporal lobe epilepsy," "psychomotor epilepsy," or "limbic seizures," are the most common form of seizures in adults. Specific causes for these different categories of seizures are considered below.

CLINICAL PRESENTATIONS OF THE EPILEPSIES

The clinical manifestations of a seizure depend upon several factors: the degree of maturity of the nervous system, the location of the initial abnormal electrical discharges, and the manner in which these discharges spread. A seizure focus in the motor cortex will produce jerking of those parts of the body normally governed by the region of the focus; a seizure in a "sensory region" of the brain will generate abnormal sensation; a seizure in the so-called areas of "higher function" leads to complex cognitive and behavioral manifestations (see Fig. 77.1). Certain types of seizures present with sudden changes in consciousness rather than with focal motor or sensory signs or symptoms.

Grand Mal

In patients with grand mal epilepsy seizure discharges present nearly synchronously in widespread regions of the cortex. The term "grand mal" should not be applied to seizures having focal onset and *secondary* generalization. These latter events should be called "generalized seizures" or "major motor seizures" instead of "grand mal," because the latter connotes *initial* generalization of seizure activity, and the two situations have very different etiologies.

Grand mal seizures typically begin with an arrest of activity and sudden loss of consciousness, followed by trembling, tonic stiffening of the upper and lower extremities, then clonic rhythmical jerking of the limbs, followed by waxing and waning to a state of flaccidity. The usual duration of the sequence is 2 to 5 min. After a seizure, patients may remain stuporous for minutes to hours. During the seizure loss of consciousness is invariable; consequently, production of speech, purposeful eye movements, or subsequent recall for events during the seizure are features which rule out the diagnosis of grand mal epilepsy. Although a general sensation of unease may warn of an impending grand mal attack, a definite sensory, motor, or psychologic aura should raise strong suspicion of a partial (focal) seizure, which has become secondarily generalized. Common associated findings during both grand mal or secondary major motor seizures include incontinence, sweating, tachycardia, and minor cardiac arrhythmias.

The electroencephalogram (EEG) recorded during a grand mal seizure is abnormal, but interictal recordings may be normal in up to 20% of cases.

Grand mal seizures may first develop at any age, though onset is rare after about age 35. Frequency may range from one seizure in an entire lifetime to several seizures per day.

Petit Mal

Petit mal is another example of primary generalized epilepsy. It comprises about 10% of seizures but it is primarily a disease of children, with onset usually between 4 and 12 years of age. The clinical presentation of petit mal seizures is quite distinct from grand mal. Petit mal is an entity in its own right, and not a "little grand mal." Similarly, the use of the term "petit mal" to describe any brief lapse of consciousness or attention is a misnomer and an invitation to inappropriate therapy. Petit mal seizures present with absence attacks (*i.e.*, lapses of consciousness), lasting about 3 to 30 sec. There is no tonic/clonic phase, nor loss of posture. Slight rhythmic twitching of the mouth or periorbital musculature may be observed. After the seizure, recovery of awareness occurs within seconds, but amnesia for events during the seizure is lasting. Petit mal seizures can occur over 100 times per day: children who suffer such frequent seizures may be labeled daydreamers or slow learners, until a correct diagnosis is made.

The EEG during a petit mal seizure shows a characteristic three per second spike-wave pattern. Interictal EEGs in children with petit mal epilepsy are often normal. Sometimes hyperventilation or stimulation with regularly flashing lights may bring out abnormalities. Both clinical and EEG findings should be used to secure a diagnosis of petit mal epilepsy; neither alone is diagnostic.

About three out of four children outgrow petit mal by age 20, but up to 50% may later develop grand mal seizures.

Myoclonic Seizures

Myoclonus consists of involuntary nonrhythmic jerking of limbs, trunk, or head, which is usually not fully synchronous (i.e., all parts do not move at the same time). When a series of frequent myoclonic jerks occur in a limited period of time—exact criteria are arbitrary—the term "myoclonic seizure" is sometimes applied. Myoclonus is encountered by general physicians as a consequence of diffuse cortical injury from such causes as anoxia, hypoglycemia, severe renal or hepatic failure, or drug toxicity. In these conditions myoclonic seizures are often self-limited, and resolve as the underlying illness stabilizes. Primary neurologic disease e.g., viral encephalitis, Jakob-Creutzfeldt disease, Huntington's chorea, or Wilson's disease also may present in part with myoclonus.

Cases of familial myoclonus with associated neurologic symptoms may be parceled into several different syndromes. These patients are generally managed in consultation with a neurologist.

Partial (Focal) Elementary Seizures

Focal motor or sensory seizures may present at any age. The clinical manifestations depend upon the site of the brain in which the seizure originates.

The motor cortex is the most common site of origin for focal seizures: as the seizure discharge spreads across the motor strip, clonus (alternating contraction and relaxation) may "march" across the limb and face. Sensory seizures most often begin from a focus in the postcentral gyrus, and are manifest by numbness in the face or fingers. Sensory seizures can also involve areas of special sensation. A focus in or near the visual cortex may cause perception of spots and lights, similar to the experience of patients suffering from classic migraine. Buzzing or ringing may be generated from a focus in the superior temporal lobe. Gustatory and olfactory sensations are components of partial complex (temporal lobe) seizures. Seizures dominated by vestibular symptoms are rare.

Retention of awareness is characteristic of focal seizures, so that patients may walk, talk, and think normally during a seizure—accomplishments which would be impossible during a generalized seizure. However, a large focus in the dominant hemisphere may generate seizures which blunt awareness.

After a focal motor seizure, there may be weakness of the body parts which have been involved. This so-called "Todd's paralysis" usually resolves within a few hours or, in unusual cases, after a few days. Distinction between cerebrovascular ischemic events with associated seizures and seizures with Todd's paralysis may be impossible without clues from the past history. Presence of a Todd's paralysis has localizing value, and is good evidence that a seizure was focal.

Electroencephalography will not necessarily reveal a seizure focus, especially if it is small, particularly during the interictal stage.

Partial (Psychomotor) Complex Seizures

"Partial complex epilepsy" may be considered synonymous with "temporal lobe epilepsy," "psychomotor epilepsy," and "limbic epilepsy." This category of seizures is important for several reasons: the condition is common in the adult population; psychomotor seizures are often misdiagnosed; and correct diagnosis leads to a search for potentially correctable lesions and to effective therapy. Complex partial epilepsy is classified as a focal epilepsy because of clinical evidence linking these seizures with foci in or near the temporal lobe.

The presentation of partial complex epilepsy is more varied than are the other forms of epilepsy, and may include autonomic, psychic, visceral, sensory, or motor symptoms. Warning of an impending seizure may be signaled by an "aura." The classic aura of olfactory or gustatory hallucination is actually less common than is an aura of nondescript unpleasant visceral sensations or a sense of unease. There is, in general, no clear boundary between the aura and the seizure itself, particularly when seizures feature distorted visual or auditory sensations, or vertigo or general disequilibrium. Arrest of motor activity, rigid posturing of the head and eyes, and slow repetitive limb movements may occur and are easily distinguished in most cases from the tonic-clonic sequence of major motor attacks. Autonomic instability, such as fluctuating heart rate or blood pressure, flushing, sweating, salivating, alterations in pupillary reactions, or incontinence of urine or feces have all been described in patients with temporal lobe seizures. The term "psychomotor epilepsy" derived from the frequent mental changes which characterize this form of epilepsy: patients often say that they felt strange, in a "dream," or experienced inappropriate emotions such as intense dread or strange serenity. During the seizure, consciousness is impaired to a variable extent; if they can talk, patients may portray what appears to be a primarily psychiatric illness. The distinction between partial complex epilepsy and psychosis may be obscured further in patients whose interictal personality is abnormal. Such individuals can easily be misdiagnosed as schizophrenics.

In a condition whose presentation may range from apparent appendicitis to apparent schizophrenia the physician must make special efforts to elicit a detailed history of a "spell," and, when possible, to observe one personally. Complex partial seizures should have a definite start and finish; they should be associated with some impairment in ability to register and process information during the seizure; and they should be relatively stereotyped from episode to episode. Observations of automatic behavior, such as repetitive mouth-smacking, raising and lowering the arm, buttoning and unbuttoning a shirt over and over, or pacing in circles may secure the diagnosis of a partial complex seizure disorder, for such "automatisms" are common in psychomotor epilepsy and uncommon in other forms of seizures (excluding the minor stereotypical behavior in petit mal or in psychiatric illness).

The standard EEG is abnormal in only about half of patients with partial complex seizures. The yield may be increased to 80 to 90% by recording EEGs during sleep, and by using special electrodes positioned close to the undersurface of the temporal lobe.

Although partial complex seizures may begin at any age, the majority begin before age 20. Adult onset of temporal lobe epilepsy carries the same significance as does a new onset of any focal seizure: a significant structural lesion must be ruled out. Patients with onset of temporal lobe seizures, who come to surgery or to postmortem, may show either no pathology or may have tumors, infarcts, granulomas, or infections, or more often a generalized gliosis of the mesial temporal lobe ("mesial temporal sclerosis"). It is not known whether gliosis causes temporal lobe seizures or follows from them.

Prognosis for spontaneous remission of complex partial seizures is not as favorable as it is for grand mal seizures.

Secondarily Generalized Seizures

Secondarily generalized seizures begin clinically as focal seizures (including those beginning as partial complex seizures) and then generalize to seizures indistinguishable from grand mal attacks. The focal onset can be as fleeting as a few tremors in an arm, numbness of the hand or one side of the face, or marked conjugate deviation of the eyes or head. Sensory or visceral auras are also evidence of focal onset, as is preservation of consciousness during the early part of a seizure.

Complex electrophysiological mechanisms govern whether seizure discharges remain in a local focus, spread along certain prescribed anatomical pathways, or generalize to much of the brain. A focal seizure may generalize when conditions of overall brain excitability are "right." Conversely, anticonvulsive therapy may convert a secondarily general-

ized seizure into a focal seizure. It is not known how often grand mal attacks are actually secondarily generalized seizures with occult primary origins.

The treatments for secondarily generalized seizures are the same as those for grand mal seizures (see pp. 834–837), except for the need to treat, if possible, any structural lesions responsible for the focal origins.

Unclassifiable Seizures

With an adequate history, most seizures should be classifiable by the scheme given above. Unfortunately, the history is sometimes lacking, as when observers report "falling down and shaking" or "stopping and starting," but cannot describe the full sequence of events. In these instances it is best to list the seizure as "unclassifiable," or to use nondescript terms such as "major motor attack" (if there was apparent tonic/clonic activity) or an "absence attack" (if there was a brief lapse of consciousness), until the specific seizure type becomes evident.

ETIOLOGY OF SEIZURES

General Comments

Classification of seizures, as given above, depends upon clinical and EEG observation of the patient. A seizure represents a symptom: once the presence of a seizure has been established and the seizure classified, an etiology must be sought. How likely this search is to be successful is difficult to ascertain from the medical literature, because of serious biases in selecting populations for study.

Epilepsy secondary to identified causes is sometimes called "symptomatic" as opposed to "essential" or "idiopathic" epilepsy. It is agreed that most cases of primary generalized epilepsy are idiopathic, so that a child presenting with typical petit mal or grand mal seizures, in the context of a normal examination, normal screening laboratory tests, and a positive family history for similar seizures, would not warrant an extensive search for underlying causes. The yield is higher from investigation of partial or atypical generalized seizures; without a computerized tomography (CT) scan a lesion can be demonstrated about 50% of the time (4, 6, 22, 28), with a CT scan, about 65 to 70% of the time (8, 17).

Table 77.2 lists specific etiologies which should be considered for different types of seizures at various ages; the diagnoses are listed from top to bottom roughly in the order of their frequency (except that "idiopathic" is placed at the end of each list because it is a diagnosis of exclusion). It is worth emphasizing that all of the partial epilepsies can become secondarily generalized, and that the focal onset may be obscured. Therefore, the clinician should give some thought to "focal etiologies" even in apparently generalized seizures.

Special issues are raised by seizures that are man-

Table 77.2
Etiological Factors for Seizures with Onset at Various Ages[a]

Adolescent (12–21 yr)	Adult (21–65 yr)	Elderly (65+ yr)
Common Causes		
Genetic (g)	Alcohol withdrawal (g)	Cerebrovascular (m)
Mesial temporal sclerosis (f)	Toxins or drugs (g)	Thrombotic
Infection (m)	Drug withdrawal (g)	Embolic
Meningitis	Tumor (f)	Hemorrhagic
Viral encephalitis	Trauma (f)	Cardiac arrhythmia
Abscess	Scar	Trauma (f)
TORCHS[b]	Subdural hematoma	Scar
Parasites	Mesial temporal sclerosis (f)	Subdural hematoma
Hysteria/factitious (m)	Genetic (g)	Tumor (f)
Toxins or drugs (g)	Hysteria/factitious (m)	Infection (m)
Drug withdrawal (g)	Infection (m)	Meningitis
	Meningitis	Viral encephalitis
	Viral encephalitis	Abscess
	Abscess	Syphilis
	Syphilis	Parasites
	Parasites	
Occasional Causes		
Metabolic (g)	Metabolic (g)	ETOH withdrawal (g)
Hypoglycemia	Hypoglycemia	Toxins or drugs (g)
Hyponatremia	Hyponatremia	Drug withdrawal (g)
Hypocalcemia	Hypocalcemia	Hypoxia (g)
Porphyria	Hypomagnesemia	Metabolic (g)
Trauma (f)	Hypoxia (g)	Hypoglycemia
Scar	Cerebrovascular (m)	Hyponatremia
Subdural hematoma	Thrombotic	Hypocalcemia
Tumor (f)	Embolic	
Arteriovenous malformation (f)	Hemorrhagic	
Subarachnoid hemorrhage (m)	Cardiac arrhythmia	
Eclampsia (m)	Renal failure (g)	
Renal Failure (g)	Eclampsia (m)	
Rare Causes		
Collagen disease (m)	Collagen disease (m)	Hypertensive encephalopathy (m)
Hepatic failure (g)	Hypertensive encephalopathy (m)	Hyperosmolar (m)
Multiple sclerosis (f)	Hyperosmolar (m)	Renal failure (g)
	Multiple sclerosis (f)	Hepatic failure (g)
	Degenerative (m)	Degenerative (g)
		Factitious (m)
Idiopathic	Idiopathic	Idiopathic

[a] f = usually focal; g = usually generalized; m = often mixed.
[b] TORCHS = toxoplasmosis, rubella, cytomegalovirus, herpes, syphilis.

ifest for the first time in the elderly. First, they are comparatively rare. Second, cerebrovascular disease accounts for 30 to 60% of all new seizures in this population (26). Tumors, the major cause of focal seizures in the middle-aged, cause 2 to 30% (26) of seizures in the elderly; however, brain tumors in this age group are very likely to be malignant. Infection, trauma, metabolic disease, hypertensive encephalopathy, and degenerative conditions are all documented causes of seizures in the geriatric population; however, a cause is not found to explain seizures in half or more of this group. When an elderly patient presents with seizures, a special effort should be made to rule out treatable conditions—carotid artery occlusions, cardiac arrhythmias, infection, and toxic-metabolic derangements.

Particular Etiologies

Some classes of seizures are so commonly encountered by the primary physician that detailed consideration of them is warranted.

POST-TRAUMATIC SEIZURES

According to the National Head and Spinal Cord Injury Survey of the National Institutes of Health (1) 422,000 patients were hospitalized in 1974 for head injuries, 200 per 100,000 U.S. population. Four to five times that number of head injuries are sustained by people who are not hospitalized but who still have a significant risk of brain damage (5). The incidence of post-traumatic epilepsy depends upon several factors: the population under study, the severity of the injury, the duration of follow-up, and the criteria used to label a seizure as a manifestation of epilepsy. In patients with a mild injury (brief unconsciousness or amnesia) risk of later epilepsy is not increased significantly above baseline, whereas severe injuries (intracranial hematomas, focal neurologic signs, unconsciousness for more than 24 hours) result in epilepsy in 7% of patients after 1 year and in 11.5% after 5 years (2). Moderately severe injuries (skull fractures or unconsciousness for 30 min to 24 hours) impose an intermediate risk. Injuries over the vertex are more epileptogenic, and tend to produce secondarily generalized motor seizures, in contrast with temporo-occipital lesions which tend to produce psychomotor seizures, or with frontal injuries which tend to produce a picture of "pseudo-grand mal" (21).

The value of prophylactic therapy in preventing post-traumatic seizures has not been firmly established although there are retrospective studies which suggest that it is useful (23, 31). Until more data become available, a reasonable approach for clinicians includes the following elements: patients with minor scalp lacerations or brief loss of consciousness should not be considered to have a significantly increased risk of epilepsy. A single seizure occurring during the first 2 weeks after head injury, or while the patient is still suffering from the acute effects of injury, should not be an indication for long term therapy. A second seizure in this setting might be grounds for treatment. Patients with brain injuries should be given a 2- to 4-year course of prophylactic phenytoin (unless there are particular contraindications to chronic medication), especially if consciousness has been lost for more than 24 hours, if the dura has been penetrated (by trauma or by surgery), or if the vertex has been involved. If a patient has a "spontaneous" seizure more than 2 weeks after a head injury, he should be evaluated and treated as would any other patient with a new onset of seizure disorder—assignation of the seizure to a recent or remote episode of head trauma should not be made until other treatable causes of seizures have been ruled out.

ALCOHOL–RELATED SEIZURES

Alcohol withdrawal is a very common cause of seizures; almost all of them occur within the first 48 hours of abstinence and most of them are generalized. In some series up to 25% of seizures may be focal, presumably because of a concomitant old cortical scar from trauma, infection, or vascular disease. If a known alcoholic has had a prior withdrawal seizure, presents a typical picture of a generalized seizure without focal features, has a normal examination and no complications, then investigations may be limited. More often, the history is imprecise and findings are equivocal or the patient has a fever or an elevated leukocyte count. In these instances lumbar puncture, EEG, and continued observation are indicated.

Treatment of alcohol withdrawal seizures is controversial, because the majority of patients (approximately 95%) in a state of withdrawal do not have seizures, or have them only once or twice (13). Many of the standard medications, such as chlordiazepoxide, which are used to treat the abstinence syndrome, have anticonvulsant activities as well, although the value of these medications (or of phenytoin) in the prevention of seizures is uncertain (13). Alcoholics with no prior seizure history should not be given prophylactic phenytoin during withdrawal. If a patient who is entering alcohol withdrawal gives a history of prior seizures, then a 5-day course of phenytoin (300 mg/day) may prevent the occasional seizure with its attendant risks of aspiration pneumonias and falls. Long term therapy with anticonvulsants is not recommended.

Alcohol abusers are sometimes poly-drug abusers. Withdrawal from barbiturates or tranquilizers at the same time as withdrawal from alcohol may cause fulminant seizures.

For the alcoholic, ability to abstain is the principal determinant of seizure frequency. There is a strong relationship in this population between drinking and seizure frequency. On the other hand, nonalcoholic epileptics can usually tolerate occasional alcohol, and should be permitted to do so unless they have seizures more often when they drink.

SEIZURES AND BRAIN TUMORS

Brain tumor is a relatively uncommon cause of epilepsy, but epilepsy is a common symptom of brain tumors. About one-third of intracranial and one-half of intrahemispheric tumors are associated with seizures. Slow growing tumors appear to be more epileptogenic: seizures occur in 90% of patients with oligodendrogliomas, 69% of patients with astrocytomas, 34% of patients with glioblastomas, 37% of patients with meningiomas, and 41% of patients with metastases to the brain (19).

The prevalence of brain tumors among epileptic patients varies from 2 to 12% (25) depending upon the population studied and on the type of seizures. Young and middle-aged adults with new onset of focal seizures have the greatest chance of harboring a tumor, with rates quoted from 35% (28) to 62% (15). The following features suggest that seizures may be associated with a brain tumor: onset after 20 years of age, presence of focal neurologic signs, increased intracranial pressure, focal unilateral δ waves on the EEG, asymmetry of β wave activity on the EEG, and inducibility by hyperventilation (30). If a tumor is suspected, a computerized tomographic scan, with and without contrast, is the test of choice.

SEIZURES AND CEREBROVASCULAR DISEASE

Cerebrovascular disease is the most common, and epilepsy the second most common, of the serious neurologic illnesses. The two conditions are found together fairly often. It is generally assumed in such patients that ischemia leaves a damaged area of brain, which then somehow "matures" into an epileptic focus. One series (14) reported an overall incidence of seizures of about 8% in patients with stroke, 4% in those with bland infarction, and 10% in those with hemorrhage. The seizures are more likely to be focal (60%) than generalized (40%). In 40% of the patients, seizures occur at the onset of the deficit or within the first 2 weeks: only a few of these patients later develop recurrent epilepsy. However, most patients who have seizures after the second week do develop epilepsy. Consequently, early seizures after stroke do not mandate the use of anticonvulsants, but late seizures should be treated as epilepsy.

As discussed above (p. 828), seizures in the elderly should raise the suspicion of cerebrovascular disease, and may be the first clue to the presence of transient ischemia or of impending stroke. In young patients, cerebral vascular disease is uncommon, but a seizure may lead to a diagnosis of an arteriovenous malformation, an aneurysm, collagen vascular disease, or a rare case of cortical thrombophlebitis.

SEIZURES AND INFECTIONS

A seizure may be one of the first manifestations of bacterial meningitis, particularly in the very young and in the very old patient in whom the classic signs of meningitis may be lacking. Less fulminant forms of meningitis, such as cryptococcal or tuberculous meningitis, have been known to produce seizures which recur over weeks or months. Viral encephalitides—for example, herpes simplex encephalitis—may also produce seizures. Meningoencephalitis can scar the cortex, so that an epileptic focus is established which remains symptomatic years after the infection is eradicated.

For reasons which are poorly understood, systemic infections may trigger seizures in epileptic patients, even if the infection does not directly involve the central nervous system. However, when a patient presents with a seizure and signs of infection, especially if the seizure is focal or if focal signs are detected on neurologic examination, the possibility of brain abscess must be explored.

EVALUATION OF THE PATIENT WITH SEIZURES

When a physician evaluates a patient for a possible seizure disorder, three questions must be answered: First, was the event a seizure? Second, if so, what type of seizure was it? Third, are there clues in the history, physical examination, or laboratory tests which point to an etiology of the seizure?

Because the answers to these questions are derived from the standard history and physical, initial data should be gathered by the primary physician. In certain instances referral to a neurologist for a consulting opinion may be warranted. Threshold for referral will depend upon the practitioner's own desires and experiences, but many obtain neurologic consultation before performing lumbar puncture or a CT scan, or initiating long term therapy in all but the most straightforward of cases. This is particularly

true if there is uncertainty about the nature of the "seizure," its etiology, and the need for special diagnostic tests, or if the examination or EEG have focal features (see p. 831 and Table 77.4).

Differential Diagnosis of Seizure-like Behavior

Determination of the nature of a seizure-like episode may be difficult (Table 77.3). Unless the physician has been fortunate enough to observe an attack, the patient and surrogate observers must specify whether or not it represented an episode "punched out in time" with specific signs of neurologic dysfunction. The features which are most helpful in confirming that a seizure has occurred include tonic-clonic sequences, with or without tongue-biting and incontinence; rhythmic jerking of a limb or of the face; and speech and motor arrest followed by automatisms. The differential diagnosis is dependent upon the character of the attack. Loss of consciousness raises the possibility of syncope (see Chapter 78): if a careful observer can specify sudden loss of consciousness and tone with no abnormal motor activity, syncope is a much more likely diagnosis than is seizure. Transient numbness, weakness, speech or vision problems, or dizziness may occur as part of a cerebrovascular syndrome (see Chapter 80), including transient ischemic attacks, stroke, bleeding from an arteriovenous malformation or from an aneurysm, or a classic migraine. Context may help to distinguish seizure from cerebrovascular disease, but particularly in the elderly, where the two conditions are linked, a firm diagnosis may have to be deferred.

Narcolepsy (see Chapter 82) is a relatively uncommon disorder in which people suddenly drop into "REM" (rapid eye movement) sleep with associated inhibition of muscle tone ("cataplexy"). These patients can be aroused from their sleep, will often report that they dreamed during the attack and will deny postictal confusion. A waxing and waning organic mental syndrome (see Chapter 16) with occasional motor manifestations, such as might be produced by renal failure or by a drug intoxication, may superficially resemble a seizure but the episode will usually lack both the stereotypical aspects of a seizure and its clear start and finish.

Vertigo, from disease of the inner ear, can present paroxysmally, and may be confused with epilepsy

Table 77.3
Differential Diagnosis of Seizure-like Behavior

Syncope
Cerebrovascular
Narcolepsy
Organic mental syndrome
Paroxysmal vertigo
Breath-holding spells (children)
Tics
Functional episodes
Hysteria

(see Chapter 78). Certain adults have *tics*, which, unlike a true seizure, may be brought in part under voluntary control, and often occur at predictable times.

In an ambulatory setting, the most common problem in seizure diagnosis is making a distinction between a *functional spell* and a true seizure. Anxiety attacks can produce recurrent, fulminant, and moderately stereotyped symptomatology, all of which may be seen in partial complex seizures. Since seizures may have emotional concomitants (for example, an aura of extreme fear) and may be triggered by stressful situations, it is evident how difficult the differential diagnosis may be. If a diagnosis of functional problems can be supported on other grounds, if the attacks are strongly linked to preceding anxiety, and if automatisms are lacking, then a functional spell becomes more likely.

Hysterical seizures represent extreme cases in the spectrum of functional seizure-like behavior. Unlike a malingerer, the patient with hysterical pseudoseizure has no clear awareness of "faking" a spell. Observation of a generalized attack may reveal features unlikely to be part of physiologic seizures—for example, retention of protective reflexes such as blink reflex or struggling to breathe when the airway is briefly occluded, or speech, or directed eye movements. The motor activity may lack the organized tonic-clonic stages seen with grand mal epilepsy, unless the patient is sophisticated and has observed seizures before (unfortunately, this is often the case). Hysterical psychomotor spells may be the most difficult to diagnose. As a general rule, purposeful, goal-directed behavior, such as driving, shopping, talking in full sentences, or committing acts of specific violence should not be considered to be part of the seizure unless there is strong supporting evidence. As with simple functional spells, positive features suggestive of hysteria—presence of secondary gain, "la belle indifference," inappropriate reactions to stress—may contribute to a correct diagnosis. Consultation among primary physician, neurologist, and psychiatrist may be required for proper diagnosis and management (see also Chapter 11).

Classifying the Seizure

In actual practice, classifying a seizure (see p. 825) goes hand-in-hand with establishing that a seizure has in fact occurred. Emphasis should be placed on a careful description of the start of the episode, because a fleeting focal onset or an aura may be the only indication that a seizure was a secondarily generalized rather than a grand mal seizure.

Establishing an Etiology

The history is the main clue to the etiology of a seizure. Careful note should be taken of any birth trauma or perinatal illness, febrile convulsions, past head trauma, prior stroke or intracranial hemorrhage, previous encephalitis or meningitis, cancers, and any prior seizures. A family history of seizures is pertinent, because there is increased risk, particularly with primary generalized epilepsies, for seizures in relatives of epileptics. Use of alcohol and/or barbiturates and of seizurogenic drugs, such as amphetamines, phenothiazines, tricyclic antidepressants, anticholinergics, or aminophylline must be ascertained. Many patients know of factors that precipitate their attacks. Most commonly, visual flashing at a rate of about 10 per sec is a precipitant, but a few percent of epileptics have idiosyncratic precipitants such as touch of certain regions of skin, loud sounds, or even complex activities such as reading, calculating, laughing, eating, or listening to music. These so-called "reflex seizures" may be aborted in some instances by avoiding the offending stimuli.

Physical examination will reveal whether a seizure patient is neurologically normal. Subtle asymmetries on the neurologic examination may lead to diagnosis of a structural lesion which is generating the seizures. Furthermore, the general physical examination may give clues to an underlying cause (Table 77.4). A physician should be wary of findings occurring in the immediate wake of a seizure, and should take the opportunity to recheck them in a few hours or a few days.

LABORATORY DIAGNOSIS OF SEIZURES

Laboratory tests are not very helpful in determining whether or not a seizure has taken place, but may be useful in establishing an etiology and in patient management.

Routine Laboratory Tests

The data base should include a hematocrit value, a white blood cell and differential count, a measurement of blood urea nitrogen or of serum creatinine and serum glucose. Other tests (for example, measurement of serum electrolytes including serum calcium, of blood gases, and of liver function) should be ordered only if there is some suspicion that they may be abnormal. A number of striking abnormalities (metabolic acidosis, marked leukocytosis) may develop transiently immediately after an attack. A baseline electrocardiogram is useful, although immediately after a seizure it may show ST-T wave changes or arrhythmias which are quite transient and which are results of, rather than causes of, seizure activity.

Electroencephalography

The EEG is the most useful of the laboratory studies in the diagnosis of seizure disorders. An EEG may show generalized or focal epileptiform activity or, even in the absence of such activity, may demonstrate asymmetries of basic rhythms, focal δ waves or diffuse slowing, all of which may give direction to further investigation. In general, the experienced clinician does not rely on the EEG to make a diagnosis

Table 77.4
General Physical Signs Suggesting Causes of Epilepsy[a]

System	Signs	Disease
Skin and membrane	Petechiae	Subacute bacterial endocarditis (SBE), blood dyscrasias, leukemia, thrombocytopenic purpura, fat emboli
	Cyanosis	Cyanotic congenital heart disease, pulmonary disease
	Icterus	Liver disease, sickle cell disease, thrombotic thrombocytopenic purpura (Moschowitz)
	Malar skin rash	Systemic lupus erythematosus
	Facial port wine stain	Sturge-Weber-Dimitri disease
	Café au lait spots	Neurofibromatosis
	Depigmented spots	Tuberous sclerosis
Head	Head circumference ↑ or ↓	Hydrocephalus, macrocephaly, microcephaly
	Bruit	Arteriovenous malformation
Fundi	Papilledema	↑ Intracranial pressure—brain tumor, hemorrhage
	Hemorrhage	Subarachnoid hemorrhage, hypertension, systemic bleeding tendency
	Exudate	SBE, diabetes mellitus, hypertension
	Retinal lesions	Intrauterine infections, tuberous sclerosis
Neck	Meningeal signs—stiff neck	Meningitis, subarachnoid hemorrhage, fractured odontoid, herniated cerebellar tonsils
	↓ Carotid pulses or bruit	Cerebrovascular disease
Circulation	Hypertension	Renal disease, cardiovascular disease, coarctation of aorta, collagen disease
	Arrhythmia	Cardiac disease—congenital, rheumatic, arteriosclerotic heart disease
Abdomen	Organomegaly	Liver disease, neoplasm, hematologic disease
	Mass	Neoplasm
Bones and joints	Clubbing	Lung carcinoma, cyanotic congenital heart disease

[a] Printed with permission from G. E. Solomon and F. Plum: *Clinical Management of Seizures.* W. B. Saunders, Philadelphia, 1976.

of a seizure, but uses it for confirmation of a clinical impression derived from the history. When history and EEG are at variance, primacy should go to the history. Patients should not be treated for epilepsy because of an abnormal EEG alone, because interictal epileptiform discharges may be seen in 0.4% of the healthy population, in 2.2% of patients with nonepileptic neurologic disease, and in 3.5% of asymptomatic relatives of epileptics (10). On the other hand, a clinician should not be dissuaded from a clear impression of a seizure disorder just because the EEG is negative. Interictal EEGs are usually normal in children with petit mal epilepsy, and may be normal in from 10 to 50% of individuals with grand mal or partial elementary or partial complex seizures, depending upon the conditions of recording, the duration of recording, and the vagaries of any sampling process (7, 19). Where EEG confirmation of seizure activity is needed (for example, when the history is equivocal) repeated studies, 24-hour monitoring of tracings with concomitant observation of behavior, recordings after sleep deprivation, stimulatory techniques such as hyperventilation or flash, or use of nasopharyngeal or sphenopalatine leads may be indicated. Since EEGs can remain abnormal for a few weeks after a major seizure, any findings should be confirmed with repeat studies. An EEG is without risk, unless there are consequences from an injudicious interpretation (see "Patient Experience," Chapter 75).

Lumbar Puncture

Certain conditions which lead to seizures may require examination of cerebrospinal fluid to secure a diagnosis: chronic meningitis is an example. Data are not available from the medical literature on the yield of lumbar puncture in investigation of patients with various types of seizures; consequently, it is not possible to be dogmatic about whether this test is a requirement for all patients with seizures. The context of the seizure often resolves the issue. A normal child with classic petit mal epilepsy probably does not need a lumbar puncture. A patient with a strongly suspected mass lesion should not have a routine spinal tap, until other studies have given information on the risk of brainstem herniation. Most other patients, with focal or generalized seizures of uncertain etiology, should have their spinal fluid analyzed.

After prolonged generalized seizures the cerebrospinal fluid may show a pleocytosis up to about 100 cells for several days, presumably from a transient breakdown of the blood-brain barrier (24). Clearly, however, infection must be the diagnosis of first concern in this setting.

Computerized Tomographic Scans

Scans (see "Patient Experience," Chapter 75) of patients with primary generalized seizures are normal or show nonspecific atrophy in over 90% of instances. Scans of individuals with focal or secondarily generalized seizures are abnormal about 65% of the time (8, 17). If the neurologic examination reveals even mildly focal signs the CT scan is especially likely to be positive.

The following recommendations seem reasonable: all patients with focal or secondarily generalized seizures or with an abnormal neurologic examination should have a CT scan with (unless there is a contraindication) and without contrast injection. Patients with generalized seizures and normal examinations have no more than about a 2% chance of showing a treatable abnormality on a CT scan. In this group of patients, the decision to perform a scan should be individualized; often a scan done without contrast injection can be justified. Lastly, CT scanning may be indicated when a stable pattern of seizures deteriorates.

Other Diagnostic Tests

"Traditional" neuroradiologic studies—skull X-rays, radionuclide brain scan, pneumoencephalography, and arteriography—have to a great extent been supplanted by CT scanning in the initial evaluation of a seizure disorder, but each still has its own special indications which will be pointed out when appropriate by the consulting neurologist.

TREATMENT OF EPILEPSY

Except in unusual instances, epilepsy cannot be "cured." In about three of four patients it can, however, be controlled so that patients experience no seizures or only a very rare seizure. Most attention in the medical literature has been focused on details of pharmacologic management for seizures, but the importance of a comprehensive approach cannot be overemphasized: an individual who is seizure-free, but so toxic from medicines that employment is impossible, is at best a dubious success. Employment problems and other social aspects of managing epilepsy are considered below. General measures of therapy should not be neglected: removal of precipitating factors for seizures, reduction of stress, provision for adequate amounts of rest, and attention to proper diet can all be important in control of epilepsy.

General Principles of Drug Therapy

It has been said that half of those having generalized seizures monthly or more frequently are probably undertreated. In contrast, other patients are maintained on unnecessary or improper regimens of anticonvulsants. To achieve the ideal goal of seizure control without toxicity, clinicians should follow the general principles enumerated in Table 77.5.

In deciding whether to treat a first seizure, the physician should recall that a single seizure does not necessarily mandate a diagnosis of epilepsy nor a need for chronic therapy. As noted previously, early seizures after head trauma or stroke, or seizures in association with some clear precipitant should in general be treated conservatively. The more difficult decision involves the patient with a single

Table 77.5
Principles of Drug Therapy

Decide whether to treat
Select the proper drug for the particular form of epilepsy
Start drugs slowly, build up levels gradually, to avoid toxicity
Start with one drug, and use it to effect or toxicity before adding another
Choose the simplest regimen possible
Suspect compliance problems in treatment failures
Monitor blood levels in problem cases
Withdraw medications gradually
Decide how long to treat

"idiopathic" convulsion, because the risk of having a second seizure cannot be determined (the few studies on the natural history of epilepsy have usually begun analysis after the second seizure). Some patients are so frightened of the possibility of having another seizure, with potential repercussions for employment, social relations, and license to drive, that they are willing to accept the inconvenience and morbidity of chronic medication. Other patients would prefer not to be medicated until they have another seizure. Clearly, the decision to treat after a first seizure must be individualized. At a second attack, most physicians would initiate therapy.

To treat the patient appropriately, the physician must know the type of seizure under consideration. Not only are the drugs of choice different for the different categories of epilepsy (Table 77.6), but incorrect medication—for example, use of phenytoin for petit mal—may actually make the patient worse. In several instances, more than one drug may be considered the "drug of choice" in terms of efficacy, in which case the selection can be made on the basis of personal familiarity with the drug or on the relative risk of side effects.

Drugs should be initiated at one-quarter or one-half of the anticipated maintenance dosage (except for phenytoin and phenobarbital—see below), and the dosage should be built up over several weeks, in order to avoid significant early toxicity which might discourage the patient from continuing with treatment. Since some of the medications remain in the blood for some time, it may take several days before the effects of a dosage adjustment are manifest.

There is a long and deplorable tradition of treating epilepsy with polypharmacy, stemming from times when most epileptics were started automatically on phenytoin, 100 mg, and phenobarbital, 32 mg, each 3 times a day. There is no evidence that two drugs in subtherapeutic doses are better tolerated or more effective than one drug in full dose. Shorvon and colleagues (27) argued that about 90% of new-onset seizures can be controlled with one drug (in their study, phenytoin or carbamazepine), and that, when one drug is unsuccessful, addition of a second helps in only 36% of cases.

Table 77.6
Drugs of Choice

Seizure Category	Drugs of Choice	Alternates
Grand mal	Phenytoin Phenobarbital	Carbamaze- pine Primidone Valproic acid
Petit mal	Ethosuximide	Valproic acid
Myoclonus	Clonazepam	Diazepam Valproic acid
Partial elementary	Phenytoin	Carbamazepine Phenobarbital
Partial complex	Carbamazepine Primidone	Phenytoin Phenobarbital Valproic acid

Compliance is a major factor in success of drug therapy for epilepsy (also see Chapter 4). Every effort should be made to simplify the dosage regimen. Phenytoin has a half-life of about 20 hours, so except for difficult cases with uncontrolled attacks, or with brands of the medicine for which bioavailability is substandard, the usual 3 times a day schedule is unnecessarily complex. This is even more true for phenobarbital which has a half-life of 3 days. Therefore, medicines such as carbamazepine, primidone, and valproic acid, which must be given in divided doses, should be employed only when there is an identifiable advantage over phenytoin or phenobarbital. At each visit a patient (or the responsible person) should be asked to report on the exact medication regimen; all too often the answer indicates a need for better spoken and written communication with the patient. Physicians should have some familiarity with cost of medicines because patients may be hesitant to purchase an expensive medicine, unless the need is clearly explained. In general, poor compliance is the most common cause of treatment failure: when in doubt, the serum levels of drugs should be measured.

The optimum dose of an anticonvulsant medication may vary severalfold among different patients. Determination of serum levels of medicines (Table 77.7) is now a reliable way to measure how much medication is circulating, but such measurements should not be ordered indiscriminately. If a patient has a good response and little toxicity from a drug regimen, measurement of a serum level is wasteful, and might even encourage the physician to alter a successful regimen. If control is not optimal, drug levels can document inadequate compliance or absorption, or highlight the occasional case where drug toxicity is manifest by increased seizures. The levels can also provide guidance for patients with symptoms which might or might not be due to drug intoxication. Practitioners should be aware that drug dose and drug level are not linearly related: a saturation point is reached above which minor increments in daily dose (for example, increasing phenytoin from 400 to 500 mg a day) may lead to major increases in serum level and in side effects. A level is most informative if measured in the "steady state" (see Table 77.7), which requires a stable dosage for about four or five half-lives of the medicine before measurement.

Medication should be withdrawn over periods of weeks or months, because sudden withdrawal of even relatively ineffective medications may precipitate seizures. Phenobarbital is particularly treacherous in this respect.

The determination of how long to maintain treatment with anticonvulsants is a difficult issue, because freedom from seizures may or may not be due to the medicine. Before the development of anticonvulsant medication the spontaneous remission rate for all types of seizures was about 10 to 32% (20). A recent longitudinal study of patients with seizures (3) found that there was a 70% possibility of being in remission, defined as 5 years seizure-free, at 20 years after diagnosis. Patients with primary generalized seizures had more than an 80% chance of a remission, assessed at 20 years; and only half of the patients were continuing to take medication. The remission rate at 20 years for patients with partial complex seizures was slightly lower, 65%; and 65% of these patients were continuing to take medication. The question of "how long to treat?" must be set in the context of this good prognosis.

About one-half to two-thirds of patients will be entirely seizure-free for 2 years of therapy. If an adult patient is seizure-free for about 5 years on medication, and stops treatment by gradual tapering, there is a 40% chance of relapse in the next 5 years (11). About 90% of the relapses are registered within the first 2 years after discontinuing medication (12). As with the decision to initiate therapy, the decision to terminate anticonvulsant therapy must be individualized. A patient who was very difficult to control initially, who has an underlying structural lesion, or a persistently abnormal EEG may benefit from lifelong therapy. In contrast, a patient with idiopathic epilepsy who has been well and seizure-free for 2 to 5 years, and who is willing to accept an increased risk of seizure, may be a candidate for drug withdrawal. If more than one drug has been prescribed, the medications should be tapered one at a time, each over a period of several months, and reinstated rapidly if problems arise.

Specific Medications

The literature on anticonvulsive medication is vast, but surprisingly few studies exist to establish firmly the value of one drug over another. Table 77.5 represents a general, but not unanimous, consensus of opinion on drugs of choice and alternates for the main forms of epilepsy. Dosages, half-lives, serum levels, and main potential side effects of the drugs are given in Table 77.7.

PHENYTOIN (DIPHENYLHYDANTOIN, DPH, DILANTIN)

Since its introduction in 1938, phenytoin has been one of the two major drugs used to treat seizures. It

Table 77.7
Major Antiseizure Medications

Medication (Brand Name)	Typical Adult Dose and Range[a]	Half-life (hr)	Levels (μg/ml)	Major Side Effects
Phenytoin (Diphenylhydantoin DPH) (Dilantin)	300 mg q.d.[b] or 100 mg t.i.d. (200–500 mg)	22	10–20	Ataxia Cosmetic chanes Rash Rare blood changes Osteomalacia Peripheral neuropathy
Phenobarbital (Luminal)	100 mg q.h.s. (60–200 mg)	72	15–40	Sedation Hyperactivity Confusion
Primidone (Mysoline)	250 mg q.i.d. (500–1500 mg)	3–12[c] 72[d]	6–12[c] 15–40[d]	Sedation
Carbamazepine (Tegretol)	200 mg q.i.d. (400–1200 mg)	10–25	4–12	Gastrointestinal (GI) distress Ataxia Blood changes
Ethosuximide (Zarontin)	250 mg q.i.d. (500–1500 mg)	30–55	40–70	GI distress Sedation Headache Dizziness Rare blood changes
Valproic acid (Depakene)	250 mg q.i.d. (750–2000 mg)	8–12	50–150	GI upset Drowsiness Ataxia Alopecia Tremor Rare liver toxicity Rare pancreatitis
Clonazepam (Clonopin)	2 mg t.i.d. (4–10 mg)	20–40	0.05–0.7	Drowsiness Ataxia Behavior change Dizziness Hypotonia

[a] These doses are usually attained gradually over days to weeks. The ranges are relatively rough guidelines: because absorption varies, serum levels are better guides to dosage.
[b] Only for Dilantin capsules.
[c] For primidone.
[d] For phenobarbital.

is most useful in grand mal epilepsy, partial elementary epilepsy, and secondarily generalized epilepsy. Although it is often used for partial complex seizures, and may keep the seizures from becoming generalized, it is not as effective as carbamazepine for psychomotor spells. Phenytoin may make petit mal worse.

Phenytoin is absorbed from the gastrointestinal tract in 4 to 8 hours. Without a loading dose, a full week is required to reach therapeutic levels, but a load of 3 times the daily maintenance, given in the first day, will achieve immediate therapeutic levels. The mean half-life is 22 hours, with a range from 7 to 42 hours. Phenytoin is 90% protein-bound, so that low serum albumin can lead to an increased concentration of the free agent and to increased toxicity. The drug is metabolized in the liver and is not excreted by the kidney: dosage should only be lowered in renal failure to compensate for a severe decrease in serum proteins, and then about a 25% reduction usually suffices (note that serum levels may register

artifactually low when more drug is unbound). Uremic patients may in fact bind more of the drug than normals do, reducing the therapeutic effect. Phenytoin is partially removed by hemodialysis.

The usual starting dose of phenytoin is 300 mg per day. This medication can be given once a day if it is given as Dilantin capsules, for this preparation is manufactured in a slow-release form. All other preparations are fast-release capsules and must be given in divided doses (i.e., 100 mg 3 times a day). The therapeutic level is generally between 10 to 20 μg per ml; the toxic range is usually over 20 μg per ml but patients show fairly wide individual susceptibility to side effects. The lethal dose may range from 2 to 20 g. Several drugs elevate phenytoin plasma levels: disulfiram and isoniazid, commonly; coumadin, chloramphenicol, methylphenidate, phenothiazines, benzodiazepines, and propoxyphene, less often.

There are many potentially untoward effects of phenytoin. Nystagmus is seen at therapeutic levels of 10 to 20 μg per ml, ataxia at 10 to 30 μg per ml, lethargy and paradoxical tendency to increased seizures at 30 to 40 μg per ml. Cosmetic side effects can be vexing in young women. Gum hypertrophy occurs in about 30%; it may be forestalled by good oral hygiene, but once established may regress only partially; hirsutism is seen in 5% overall, but in 30% of young women. Even more disconcerting are facial changes due to thickening of subcutaneous tissue about the nose and eyes, the so-called "leonine faces." Skin rash occurs in 2 to 10% of users, with a peak incidence about 2 weeks into the course. A few patients develop a full Stevens-Johnson syndrome. Lymphadenopathy occurs in 2 to 5%, sometimes in association with fever, arthralgia, eosinophilia, and hepatosplenomegaly, presenting a picture of "pseudolymphoma," and, very rarely, true lymphoma. Hepatitis and a variety of blood dyscrasias have been reported. Megaloblastic anemias occur, and respond to folate. Many patients develop measurable antinuclear antibodies in the serum: a minority of this group progresses to clinical systemic lupus erythematosus. Peripheral neuropathy with loss of muscle stretch reflexes can be documented in about 20% of chronic users. Occasional pulmonary infiltrates and fibrosis have given rise to the term "Dilantin lung." Phenytoin can induce liver enzymes, thereby secondarily affecting metabolism of numerous hormones and drugs. Induced inactivation of vitamin D leads to radiologic or biochemical evidence of bone disease in one of every three chronically treated patients. Teratogenic effects of phenytoin are strongly suspected (see later, p. 839).

PHENOBARBITAL

Phenobarbital competes with phenytoin as the drug of choice for major motor seizures: it is particularly useful in the pediatric age group, where its side effects may be better tolerated than those of phenytoin.

Phenobarbital is a long-lasting drug. The gastrointestinal absorption is slow so that levels reach a peak in 10 to 12 hours after an oral dose, compared to 20 min after an intravenous dose. The drug is detoxified by the liver and excreted by the kidney, but the dosage need be only slightly reduced in renal failure. The serum half-life is about 72 hours, ranging from 37 to 96 hours. Therapeutic levels are 15 to 40 μg per ml. Phenobarbital is a potent inducer of liver enzymes, and leads to rapid tolerance, as well as to alteration of kinetics of numerous other medications. The dose of phenobarbital is 1 to 3 mg per kg per day, or about 100 mg per day for the average adult. Little justification can be made for giving it in divided doses.

The main side effect of phenobarbital in adults is sedation. In elderly patients phenobarbital can cause confusion and respiratory depression. Ataxia and nystagmus are common in all patients at high doses. Occasionally, there is idiosyncratic allergy, with accompanying dermatitis or gastrointestinal symptoms.

Phenobarbital must not be administered to potential drug-abusers or to unreliable patients, who might precipitously discontinue their medicine.

PRIMIDONE (MYSOLINE)

Primidone is a barbiturate which is used for treatment of partial complex seizures (usually as a second choice after carbamazepine—see below). It has also been used in place of phenobarbital for treatment of grand mal or focal seizures, when the latter drug has failed; but it should not be a drug of first choice for these conditions. Primidone is excreted in part unchanged, and is in part metabolized to phenobarbital and to phenylethyl malonic acid (PEMA). Primidone and PEMA are cleared in a matter of hours, whereas the phenobarbital persists for days. Serum levels of primidone and PEMA can be ascertained, but it often suffices just to confirm that a therapeutic steady-state level of phenobarbital is present. In order to benefit from the short-lived primidone and PEMA, each of which has some anticonvulsant action, primidone must be given in 3 or 4 divided doses. A therapeutic dose is usually around 250 mg orally 3 or 4 times a day, but the initial doses should be much lower to avoid inducing extreme sedation. It is reasonable to start with 125 to 250 mg total per day, and then to increase by 250 mg daily, with increments each week, until therapeutic effect, therapeutic levels, unacceptable sedation, or the maximum dose of 2 g per day is reached. The dosage should be reduced by about half in patients with significant renal failure.

Side effects of primidone parallel those of phenobarbital, except that primidone tends to be more sedating.

CARBAMAZEPINE (TEGRETOL)

Carbamazepine is the second newest of the major anticonvulsants used in the United States, but over a decade of use for seizures and for treatment of chronic neuropathic pains has proven it to be a safe and effective medicine. Carbamazepine is the drug of choice in partial complex epilepsy. It has efficacy probably equal to that of phenytoin in the treatment of focal and of generalized seizures. The adult dose is 400 to 1200 mg per day. Tablets come in 200-mg sizes, and it is advisable to initiate therapy with no more than 1 or 2 tablets per day, building up to the full dose over a week or two. The half-life is about 10 to 25 hours, and dosage should be divided into t.i.d. or q.i.d. regimens (if compliance is a problem, sometimes a b.i.d. dosage will suffice). Therapeutic serum levels are about 4 to 12 μg per ml.

The side effects of carbamazepine include fatigue (although it is not very sedating); nystagmus; diplopia; dizziness; ataxia; dysarthria; rash, including a rare Stevens-Johnson syndrome; inappropriate secretion of antidiuretic hormone; occasionally abnormal liver function tests; and an infrequent lupoid syndrome. Gastrointestinal distress is the most common side effect, particularly if the medication is initiated too rapidly. Reversible leukopenia or thrombocytopenia is seen in 5–10% of patients, so that blood counts should be monitored weekly at the start of therapy, and then every few months. This drug has had a reputation for causing aplastic anemia, based largely on six cases of this complication that were reported in the 1960s (even though a causal relation to carbamazepine was not established). The actual incidence of aplastic anemia is not known, but it is thought to be very rare.

ETHOSUXIMIDE (ZARONTIN)

Ethosuximide is the drug of choice for treatment of petit mal epilepsy or absence spells in children. It has little efficacy in other types of seizures.

VALPROIC ACID (VALPROATE, DEPAKENE)

Valproic acid is the most recent addition to the list of drugs used to treat seizures. Its effectiveness is quite broad, but it is thought to be particularly valuable for petit mal or absence attacks in children. As a second-line agent, it may be of use in major motor seizures or in myoclonus, though it is not approved formally for use in these conditions. Valproic acid is a fatty acid, structurally dissimilar from all other common anticonvulsants. It comes in 250-mg capsules and as an elixir. Peak serum levels are reached in 1 to 4 hours after ingestion, and the half-life is about 8 to 12 hours. The drug is metabolized in the liver and excreted in the urine in modified form. Serum levels may be measured, but at present have limited utility. The approximate therapeutic range is 50 to 150 μg per ml. The manufacturer suggests initiation of therapy with a dose of about 10 to 15 mg/kg/day, to be increased at weekly intervals by about 5 to 10 mg per day to a maximum dose of 60 mg per kg per day. A common final regimen is approximately 250 mg orally, 3 or 4 times per day.

In studies on several thousands of patients abroad, before the release of the drug in the United States in 1978, valproic acid proved to be quite safe. About one in five patients had significant side effects—commonly gastrointestinal upset, drowsiness, rash, reversible hair loss, anorexia, ataxia, tremor, or hyperactivity. Valproic acid inhibits platelet aggregation and may prolong the bleeding time. Less commonly, it may produce frank thrombocytopenia. After release in this country, there have been about a dozen filed cases of liver toxicity in association with administration of valproic acid. About five patients have developed serious cases of pancreatitis. Because of these recently discovered toxicities, and because of high cost, valproic acid has not yet replaced ethosuximide as the drug of choice for petit mal epilepsy.

CLONAZEPAM (CLONOPIN)

Clonazepam is a benzodiazepine drug, closely related to diazepam, and is used principally for treatment of myoclonus. It is not approved for treatment of motor or psychomotor seizures, but has been used effectively for these conditions in Europe. Clonazepam is an oral medicine, with a serum half-life of 20 to 40 hours. Serum levels vary from 5 to 70 ng per ml, and correlate only very roughly with clinical effect. Because of the sedative effect of the medicine, therapy is usually initiated very gradually, beginning with 0.01 to 0.15 mg per kg, increased each 3rd day to clinical effect or to maintenance at 0.1 to 0.2 mg per kg per day. In adults the daily maximum dose is 20 mg. Clonazepam commonly produces drowsiness, ataxia and behavioral changes, and can also cause dizziness and decreased muscle tone.

OTHER ANTICONVULSANTS

No attempt has been made to catalog all the agents used as anticonvulsants; only the major drugs of choice for the common types of seizures have been discussed. Ineffectiveness of the standard agents, when applied in accordance with the general therapeutic principles given previously, is certainly an indication for specialty referral, and for possible trials of the more unusual therapies. Practitioners frequently use diazepam or chlordiazepoxide to treat seizures, and although these drugs do have some efficacy, this practice cannot be condoned, except in special cases such as ethanol withdrawal or status epilepticus. Benzodiazepines (other than clonazepam) have drawbacks for chronic therapy: anticonvulsant effects tend to diminish as sedative effects accumulate.

When to Refer Patients

The use of a neurologist for help with therapy of the epileptic depends upon the experience of the primary physician. There are a number of common management problems for which referral may be helpful (Table 77.8). Patients often present for adjustment of a complex polypharmaceutical regimen. This can be accomplished best in conjunction with a neurologist. Consultation should be requested in most instances in which a patient does not respond to, or experience significant side effects from, the "drug-of-choice" for a seizure type. A neurologist's advice also may be helpful in the management of a pregnant epileptic and when an attempt is to be made to taper the medication dose. Lastly, change in the frequency or type of seizure may dictate referral to a consultant.

When to Hospitalize the Patient

Few general statements can be made about the need for hospital admission of seizure patients, because availability of monitoring systems, emergency room "holding rooms," and availability of inpatient beds vary from locale to locale. Nonetheless, a set of reasonable guidelines is shown in Table 77.8. Individuals brought to offices or emergency rooms after a first seizure are usually admitted, in order to facilitate the diagnostic workup, and to observe the patient in case a serious underlying cause—for example, men-

Table 77.8
When to Refer or to Hospitalize the Patient with Seizures

DIAGNOSTIC ISSUES
  Question about whether a seizure took place
  Abnormal physical examination
  Questionable focal findings
  Focal seizures
  Focality on the EEG
  Need for special diagnostics (lumbar puncture, CT scan)
  Uncertainty about etiology
THERAPEUTIC ISSUES
  Adjustment of an existing drug regimen which is complex
  Patient does not respond to a drug-of-choice
  Patient has significant medication side effects
  Patient wishes to become pregnant
  Patient wishes to taper off medication
  Significant change in the pattern of seizures
WHEN TO HOSPITALIZE
  Most new-onset seizures
  New focal signs on examination
  Obtunded or prolonged "postictal" patients
  Febrile patients
  Crescendo pattern of seizures
  All cases of status epilepticus
  Barbiturate withdrawal seizures
  Possibility of rapidly expanding mass lesion
  Seizures after recent head trauma
  Need for special inpatient studies
  Consideration for neurosurgery
  Monitoring of compliance

ingitis or subdural hematoma—is present. This principle has exceptions: a young patient, with a normal examination, positive family history for epilepsy, and a reliable family may be evaluated in an ambulatory setting. Any patient with new focal signs on examination should be admitted, as should obtunded patients, febrile patients, or those whose postictal lethargy persists for over half an hour. A crescendo pattern of seizures, with several in one day, especially if major-motor in character, calls for inpatient management. Status epilepticus, where continuous or back-to-back seizures occur without intervening return of consciousness, is a true medical emergency, and is an absolute indication for hospitalization. Barbiturate-withdrawal seizures may become fulminant; patients having seizures in this setting therefore should be admitted. If the possibility exists of a rapidly expanding mass lesion—tumor, abscess, or possible hematoma after head trauma—admission should not be delayed. Legitimate reasons for elective admissions include a need for special inpatient studies (arteriography, continuous monitoring), for evaluation for possible neurosurgical procedures in cases of intractable epilepsy, and lastly, for trials of supervised drug management to rule out noncompliance as a factor in treatment failure.

As a general rule-of-thumb, the physician need not admit those patients who are known to be epileptic, whose pattern of seizures is stable, whose etiology is established or is thought to be idiopathic on the basis

of a prior thorough workup, who are fully recovered from their seizures, who have normal examinations (or static documented old deficits), and who are reliable enough to present for ambulatory follow-up.

SOCIAL ISSUES

Once a serious underlying etiology has been ruled out, the physician tends to view epilepsy as a benign disease. From the viewpoint of the patient, this is often far from the case. Seizures are distressing even to the experienced patient, whereas for the unsophisticated they may be horrifying. Fear of having a seizure can cause epileptics to withdraw from society, and those who are willing to compete may be faced with nearly insurmountable discrimination.

The Commission for the Control of Epilepsy and Its Consequences (1977) found that the unemployment rate among those with epilepsy is twice the national average, and the underemployment rate even higher. Suspension of a driver's license may make it nearly impossible to get to work. Children may be denied participation in sports or moved unnecessarily to "special sections" in school. Epileptics marry less often than matched nonepileptic cohorts; a significant fraction of the public believes that an epileptic is likely to be physically unattractive. Because of the social stigma associated with epilepsy, the physician caring for these individuals must take special efforts to focus on the patient's overall social setting, rather than simply on seizure control. The patient and family should be counseled regularly to address those concerns which limit an epileptic's full participation in society.

Patients should be told that epilepsy is a medical illness, for too many carry notions, passed down from centuries of medical unenlightenment, that it is a punishment for some past abuse. Whereas a single seizure should not be labeled as "epilepsy," definite epilepsy should not be mislabeled as something else, to avoid facing the correct diagnosis. The patient should know that individual seizures do not cause measurable brain damage, and that the condition does not lead to mental deterioration: several great historical figures (Julius Caesar, Emperor Charles V, Dostoevski, and possibly the prophet Mohammed) achieved high stations while suffering from frequent seizures. The prognosis of epilepsy is excellent.

Restrictions of Activity

Patients often ask for guidelines about what they can and cannot do. Maximal activity consistent with avoidance of personal injury should be the goal. The specifics must be formulated by a physician familiar with the individual patient and his pattern of seizures. Patients with nocturnal seizures need not be restricted during the day. Contact sports are safe for people with infrequent seizures. Common sense dictates limits on activities during which a seizure could be fatal, for example, rock climbing, hang gliding, or scuba diving. Some potentially hazardous activities, such as swimming, are acceptable if provisions can be made for proper supervision. Seizures are not contraindications to strenuous activities, including sex. Alcohol consumption (in moderation) can be enjoyed by most epileptics with impunity (see earlier).

Driving

The issue of driving is complex. The number of traffic accidents caused by epileptics is low (estimated at 1 per 10,000 by van der Lugt) (29); nonetheless, seizures at the wheel do occur and can represent both personal and public dangers. Some states require that physicians directly report epileptics to the Department of Motor Vehicles; others require only documentation in the medical record that the patient has been informed of the risks for traffic accidents, and has been instructed to contact the Department for a hearing. Patients and physicians should be honest in their communications: both are potentially liable for consequences of inaccurate or incomplete information. In general, the physician should address the medical facts of a case and leave the final determination of licensing to the state authorities. Often, if an applicant has regular lapses of consciousness, the license will be suspended until a period of 1 to 2 seizure-free years has lapsed.

Employment

It is now illegal to discriminate against handicapped individuals, including epileptics, in the job marketplace. If an epileptic patient is unemployed or dissatisfied with work, the primary physician should be quick to refer the case to a local rehabilitation agency for possible retraining, patient and employer education, or advice on legal action. The Epilepsy Foundation of America (1828 L Street NW, Washington, DC 20036) is a central nonprofit organization which can serve as a source for information and action on social aspects of epilepsy; at least one chapter exists in each state. Their training and placement service ("TAPS") has been effective in training seizure patients for work and in finding them employment, either in the general work pool or in sheltered workshops. The same local organizations may further aid patients and physicians with regular group counseling for epileptics who cannot live independently, or in providing for regular home visits by visiting nurses and other medical personnel.

Pregnancy

Special problems are raised by the pregnant epileptic or the epileptic who wishes to become pregnant. About 0.4% of all pregnancies occur in mothers with seizures. Epileptics are a high risk group for childbearing and have an above-average incidence of toxemia, vaginal hemorrhage, and complicated labor. The rate of premature births and perinatal deaths is elevated. Seizures become more difficult to control during pregnancy in about 50% of cases, easier to control in about 10%, and unchanged in the rest.

Rarely, pregnancy can induce a new onset of recurring idiopathic seizures. Antiepileptic medication—phenytoin, carbamazepine, valproic acid, and to a lesser extent all of the other agents—are believed to be teratogenic. Studies suggest that the incidence of congenital abnormalities, particularly cleft lip, cleft palate, and cardiac defects, are 2 to 6 times more common in offspring of drug-treated epileptic mothers than in babies of nonepileptic or epileptic nontreated mothers. Unfortunately, no study has yet been able to specify the relative contribution of medication and of epilepsy itself to this increased incidence. Authorities agree that major motor seizures can produce anoxic, ischemic, or traumatic damage to a fetus, and that this risk must be balanced against the teratogenic potential of medication. The best solution to the above dilemma is careful advance planning. Physicians should not only ask their patients to plan pregnancies, but to alert them months in advance. Prior to pregnancy special efforts can be made to taper medications or to switch to phenobarbital, which may be less teratogenic than phenytoin or carbamazepine. Brief psychomotor or absence seizures pose no known risk to a fetus, and a decision may be made that the patient should tolerate them during pregnancy. If pregnancy is unexpected, an ongoing successful regimen of anticonvulsants should probably be continued, to avoid the possibility of fulminant withdrawal seizures during a critical obstetrical stage. Ultimately, all these relative risks must be discussed among primary and specialist physicians, patient and husband, so that a mutually satisfactory plan can be derived. The problems of childbearing are increased for epileptic mothers, but not greatly, and only the severely disabled epileptic woman should be flatly discouraged from having children.

Mothers taking anticonvulsants who wish to breastfeed may do so, because antiepileptic medications are excreted in breast milk only to a minor degree.

Potential parents wonder about the likelihood that their child will be epileptic if they or a previous child have epilepsy. Although there are methodological problems in performing these studies, it can generally be said (18) that there is about a 1 in 40 risk of transmitting idiopathic epilepsy (the risk is primarily from the mother, not the father), and that a positive family history increases the risk 2- to 4-fold. When seizures result from head trauma, tumor, drug withdrawal, or other identified causes, then the hereditary risk is not above baseline.

Family Counseling

Families must be told how to behave during a seizure; too often, frantic efforts to "treat" the seizure result in extreme anxiety and broken teeth. Seizures should be allowed to run their course; unless convulsions become nearly continuous (status epilepticus) they are not dangerous, and no first aid can shorten them. The mouth should not be forced open so that matchbooks, pencils, or other objects can be pushed in. The family should be informed that it is impossible to swallow the tongue. It is advisable to move the individual undergoing a seizure away from sharp corners and heights, and to turn him on his side to decrease the risk of aspiration. Forcible restraint during a tonic-clonic phase is of no value, and during the automatisms of partial complex seizures restraints may increase agitation. There is little need to fear the behavior of epileptics during automatisms, because directed violence is extremely rare.

Concerned family members are "resources" to the physician who may be used to improve seizure control. A doctor must ask them about compliance, about the cost of a medicine regimen, and about how the seizures and drug toxicities affect school, work, and social relations. Intelligent patients may wish to keep a log of their seizures, medication times, side effects, and possible precipitating stresses. Perfect control of epilepsy with no toxicity is an ideal attained in only a minority of cases; in the remainder, patient, family, and physician can decide in concert how to balance the inconvenience of seizures against the unpleasant effects of medication, and thereby achieve the best possible therapeutic results.

References

General

Anonymous: Drugs for epilepsy. *Med Lett* 21: 25, 1979.
Tabular summary of antiseizure medicines.
Epilepsy Foundation of America: *Basic Statistics on the Epilepsies.* F.A. Davis, Philadelphia, 1975.
Epidemiologic sourcebook.
Niedermeyer, E: *Compendium of the Epilepsies.* Charles C Thomas, Springfield, Ill., 1974.
A succinct overview of diagnosis and treatment of epilepsy.
Penry, JK and Newmark, ME: The use of antiepileptic drugs. *Ann Intern Med* 90: 207, 1979.
A review of antiseizure medication, written for practicing physicians.
Schmidt, RP and Wilder, BJ: *Epilepsy.* F. A. Davis, Philadelphia, 1968.
A well-referenced basic and clinical review of epilepsy, circa 1968.
So, EL and Penry, JK: Epilepsy in adults. *Ann Neurol* 9: 3, 1981.
An excellent, well-referenced review.
Solomon, GE and Plum, F: *Clinical Management of Seizures: A Guide for the Physician.* W. B. Saunders, Philadelphia, 1976.
Pithy summary of seizure therapeutics.
Temkin, O: *The Falling Sickness: A History of Epilepsy from the Greeks to the Beginnings of Modern Neurology.* The Johns Hopkins Press, Baltimore, 1971.
The definitive history of epilepsy from ancient to modern times.

Specific

1. Anderson, DW and McLawsin, RL: The national head and spinal cord injury survey. *J Neurosurg* 53: 51, 1980.
2. Annegers, JF, Grabow, JD, Groover, RV, Lawn, ER, Jr, Elveibach, LR and Kurland, LT: Seizures after head trauma: a population study. *Neurology* 30: 683, 1980.
3. Annegers, JF, Hauser, WA, Elvebach, LR and Kurland, LT: Remission and relapse of seizures in epilepsy. In *Advances in Epileptology: The Xth Epilepsy International Symposium,* edited by JA Woda and JK Penry. Raven Press, New York, 1980.
4. Bergamini, L, Bergamasco, B, Benna, P and Gilli, M: Acquired etiological factors in 1,785 epileptic subjects: clinical-anamnestic research. *Epilepsia* 18: 437, 1977.
5. Caveness, WF: Epilepsy, a product of trauma in our time. *Epilepsia* 17: 207, 1976.
6. Daly, DD: Focal seizures. *Proc Mayo Clin* 33: 480, 1978.
7. Delgado-Escueta, AV: Epileptogenic paroxysms: modern approaches and clinical correlations. *Neurology* 29: 1014, 1979.
8. Gastaut, H and Gastaut, JL: Computerized transverse axial tomography in epilepsy. *Epilepsia* 17: 325, 1976.
9. Gastaut, H, Gastaut, JL, Gonçalves e Silva, GE and Fernandez Sanchez, GR: Relative frequency of different types of epilepsy: a study employing the classification of the International League Against Epilepsy. *Epilepsia* 16: 457, 1975.
10. Gastaut, H and Tassinari, CA: Epilepsies. In *Handbook of EEG and Clinical Neurophysiology, Vol. 13,* Part A, edited by A Remand. Elsevier, Amsterdam, 1975.
11. Janz, D and Sommer-Burkhardt, EM: Discontinuation of antiepileptic drug in patients with epilepsy who have been seizure free for more than 2 years. In *Epileptology: Proceedings of the 7th International Symposium on Epilepsy,* edited by D Janz. PSG Publishing, Littleton, Mass., 1976.
12. Juul-Jensen, P: Frequency of recurrence after discontinuance of anticonvulsant therapy in patients with epileptic seizures: a new follow-up study after 5 years. *Epilepsia* 9: 11, 1968.
13. Kaim, SC, Klett, CJ and Rothfeld, B: Treatment of the acute alcohol withdrawal state: a comparison of four drugs. *Am J Psychiatry* 125: 1640, 1969.
14. Louis, S and McDowell, F: Epileptic seizures in nonembolic cerebral infarction. *Arch Neurol* 17: 414, 1967.
15. Martin, HL and McDowell, F: Evaluation of seizures in the adult. *Arch Neurol Psychiatry* 71: 101, 1954.
16. Masland, RL: Commission for the control of epilepsy. *Neurology* 28: 861, 1978.
17. McGahan, JP, Dublin, AB and Hill, RP: The evaluation of seizure disorders by computerized tomography. *J Neurosurg* 50: 328, 1979.
18. Metrakos, JD and Metrakos, K: Genetics of convulsive disorders; II. Genetic and electroencephalographic studies in centrencephalic epilepsy. *Neurology* 11: 474, 1961.
19. Niedermeyer, E: *Compendium of the Epilepsies.* Charles C Thomas, Springfield, Ill., 1974.
20. Okuma, T and Kumashiro, H: Natural history and prognosis of epilepsy. In *Advances in Epileptology: The Xth Epilepsy International Symposium,* edited by JA Wada and JK Penry. Raven Press, New York, 1980.
21. Paillas, JE, Paillas, N and Bureau, M: Post-traumatic epilepsy: introduction and clinical observations. *Epilepsia* 11: 5, 1970.
22. Ramamurthi, B: Focal fits. *Arch Neurol* 13: 545, 1965.
23. Rapport, RL, II and Penry, JK: Pharmacologic prophylaxis of post-traumatic epilepsy; a review. *Epilepsia* 13: 295, 1972.
24. Schmidley, JW and Simon, RP: Postictal pleocytosis. *Ann Neurol* 9: 81, 1981.
25. Schmidt, RP and Wilder, BJ: *Epilepsy.* F.A. Davis, Philadelphia, 1968.
26. Schold, C, Yarnell, PR and Earnest, MP: Origin of seizures in elderly patients. *JAMA* 238: 1177, 1977.
27. Shorvon, SD, Chadwick, D, Galbraith, AW and Reynolds, EH: One drug for epilepsy. *Br Med J* 1: 474, 1978.
28. Sumi, SM and Teasdall, RD: Focal seizures; a review of 150 cases. *Neurology* 13: 582, 1963.
29. van der Lugt, PJ: Traffic accidents caused by epilepsy. *Epilepsia* 16: 747, 1975.
30. Vignaendra, V, Ng, KK, Lim, CL and Loh, TG: Clinical and electroencephalographic data indicative of brain tumors in a seizure population. *Postgrad Med J* 54: 1, 1978.
31. Young, B, Rapp, R, Brooks, WH, Madauss, W and Norton, JA: Post-traumatic epilepsy prophylaxis. *Epilepsia* 20: 671, 1979.

CHAPTER SEVENTY-EIGHT

Dizziness (Vertigo, Motion Sickness, Near-Syncope, Syncope, and Disequilibrium)

L. RANDOL BARKER, M.D., BARRY GORDON, M.D., Ph.D.,
and HAMILTON MOSES III, M.D.

In health surveys of the general population, about 10% of adults report that they have "dizziness" (18). A large proportion of persons with dizziness probably do not seek medical attention for it; however, in the 1975 National Ambulatory Care Survey, dizziness was the reason given by the patient for 1.5% and 2.3% of office visits to general/family physicians and to internists, respectively (see Tables 1.4 and 1.3, Chapter 1). The purpose of this chapter is to provide a practical approach to the common conditions which patients describe as dizziness and to two related problems, motion sickness and frank syncope.

DELINEATING THE MECHANISM FOR A PATIENT'S DIZZINESS

Patients complaining of dizziness usually mean that they are uncertain of their position or their motion in relation to the environment—they are spatially disoriented. A large number of terms may be used to describe this sensation (see Table 78.1). Sometimes the "dizzy" patient is not even referring to spatial disorientation but to fatigue, dysphoric mood, and other subjective states. Drachman and Hart (5) have pointed out that dizziness due to spatial disorientation may be related to one of the following three mechanisms: (a) the illusion that the patient or the environment is moving or rotating (vertigo), (b) a sensation of impending faint or loss of consciousness (near-syncope, syncope), and (c) disequilibrium or loss of balance without vertigo or near-syncope (cerebellar ataxia, multiple sensory deficits, and miscellaneous other causes). These authors also point out that there are patients with ill-defined "light-headedness" other than vertigo, presyncope, or disequilibrium and that the basis for their complaint may be impossible to establish. They emphasize that as many as 25% of patients with chronic dizziness have it on the basis of hyperventilation, which may produce a typical presyncopal pattern or may present as ill-defined dizziness.

In taking a history from the patient with dizziness, the first objective should be to determine the probable mechanism for the complaint. In most patients, the history will determine this initial step in diagnosis. After this step, questions about associated fea-

Table 78.1
Terms Which Patients May Use to Describe Spatial Disorientation

Dizziness	Blurred vision	Staggering
Vertigo	Whoozy	Weaving
Unsteadiness	Poor equilibrium	Moving
Imbalance	Drunk feeling	Blackout
Spinning	Haziness	Passing out
Floating	Weird feeling	Tilting
Fainting	Fuzzy-headed	Listing
Light-headed	Bouncing	Rocking
Swaying	Falling	Rolling
Twisting	Swimming	

tures will help to classify the patient's problem more specifically (peripheral *vs.* central vertigo, metabolic *vs.* vascular presyncope, etc.). In obtaining the patient's history, the patient should be asked to use words more specific than "dizziness," and he should be encouraged to describe the most recent episode of dizziness. If the patient's brief account does not point to the probable mechanism, the following questions, directed also to the most recent episode, may help:

1. (Positive response favors vertigo). Is there actually the sensation of movement or rotation of your head or your body?

2. (Positive response favors presyncope). Is it like the sensation you might get if you stand up too quickly after resting? A sensation as if you might black-out?

3. (Positive response favors dysequilibrium). Is it a sensation of unsteadiness on your feet? A sensation that you are not sure where your hand or body is and that you cannot quite catch your balance and might fall?

For patients whose history does not establish the probable mechanism asking *if he can reproduce his symptoms* may be more efficient than exhaustive questioning.

The patient who says that he is dizzy "right now" while sitting before the physician should:

1. Be checked for hypotension, while seated.

2. Be observed for hyperventilation (slow, hyperpneic breathing, not overt tachypnea); if hyperventilation seems likely, he should be instructed to control his breathing and then to hyperventilate (see description Chapter 11).

3. Be examined for nystagmus (see below).

A patient who produces "dizziness" by turning his head should then be asked to elaborate on his symptoms; vertigo (positional) and presyncope (due to compromise of cerebral blood flow) are the two problems most likely to be described.

If the patient reports typical dizziness on rising from his chair, orthostatic hypotension is likely; this can be confirmed by measuring the blood pressure before and after he stands up. If the patient demonstrates gait ataxia (see Chapter 75) or reports dizziness as he turns while walking, the problem may be dysequilibrium rather than vertigo.

As part of this preliminary inquiry, it is important to ask the patient whether his dizziness has interfered with his usual activities. This information will be important in the management of the patient, regardless of the mechanism of dizziness.

VERTIGO

It has been estimated that somewhat less than half of the patients who visit physicians for dizziness have vertigo (5). Most vertigo is due to conditions affecting labyrinthine structures or the vestibular nerve (peripheral vertigo); although these conditions are distressing and at times disabling, they are usually self-limited.* In some patients, however, vertigo is a manifestation of progressive disease of the central nervous system (central vertigo) or is a secondary manifestation of a systemic condition. The major causes of vertigo in these three categories are listed in Table 78.2.

Vestibular Reflexes

In evaluating the patient with vertigo, it is helpful to have an understanding of the principal reflexes involved in vestibular function. The vestibular system functions through the vestibulospinal and vestibulo-ocular reflexes. The *vestibulospinal reflex* uses information from the sensory structures contained in the bony labyrinth (semicircular canals, utricle, and saccule) to determine the orientation of the head with respect to the ground and to promote appropriate postural adjustments to keep the body upright. The *vestibulo-ocular reflex* uses information from these sensory structures to detect rotational movements of the head and to generate appropriate compensatory eye movements which are exactly equal and opposite to head movements. This reflex permits maintenance of ocular fixation during head movements. All reflex arcs between the vestibular sensory structures and the central nervous system utilize the vestibular branch of the eighth cranial nerve and the four vestibular nuclei of the brainstem.

In these reflex systems there is a tonic discharge from each vestibular sensory organ that elicits a perfectly balanced motor response in the central nervous system. When the head is moved in any direction, the labyrinthine output from one side increases while the output from the other decreases; this temporary imbalance of sensory input elicits the compensatory motor commands for vestibulospinal and vestibulo-ocular reflexes. If the input from the labyrinths or its central processing becomes disordered, abnormal subjective states (*i.e.*, vertigo) and motor responses (*i.e.*, nystagmus and loss of balance) occur.

Approach to the Patient

INITIAL OFFICE EVALUATION

A systematic approach to the history and physical examination should be utilized for all patients with vertigo. Even when a working diagnosis of a self-

* See Fig. 93.1 (anatomy of the ear and the eighth cranial nerve).

Table 78.2
Major Causes of Vertigo[a]

PERIPHERAL CAUSES OF VERTIGO
"Benign" positional vertigo
Post-traumatic vertigo
Peripheral vestibulopathy (labyrinthitis, vestibular neuron-
itis, acute and recurrent peripheral vestibulopathy)
Vestibulotoxic drug-induced vertigo (aminoglycosides)
Ménière's syndrome (endolymphatic hydrops)
Luetic labyrinthitis
Other focal peripheral disease (acute and chronic otitis
media, cholesteatoma, tumor, fistula, genetic anom-
alies, rarely focal ischemia and others)
CENTRAL CAUSES OF VERTIGO
Brainstem ischemia and infarction
Cerebellopontine angle tumor (acoustic neuroma, menin-
gioma, metastatic tumor, etc.)
Demyelinating disease (multiple sclerosis, postinfectious
demyelination, remote effect of carcinoma)
Cranial neuropathy with focal involvement of eighth nerve
Intrinsic brainstem lesions (tumor, arteriovenous malfor-
mation, trauma, etc.)
Other posterior fossa lesions (primarily other intrinsic or
extra-axial masses of the posterior fossa such as
meatoma, metastatic tumor, and cerebellar infarc-
tion)
Seizure disorder (temporal lobe epilepsy)
Migraine
Heredofamilial disorders (spinocerebellar degenerations:
Friedreich's ataxia, olivopontocerebellar atrophy,
etc.)
SYSTEMIC CAUSES OF VERTIGO AND DIZZINESS
Drugs (anticonvulsants, hypnotics, antihypertensives, alcohol, analgesics, tranquilizers)
Infectious disease (viral and bacterial meningitis, and
systemic infection)
Endocrine disease (diabetes and hypothyroidism partic-
ularly)
Vasculitis (collagen vascular disease, giant cell arteritis,
and drug-induced vasculitis)
Other systemic conditions (polycythemia, anemia, dysproteinemia, Paget's disease of the bone, sarcoidosis,
granulomatous disease, and systemic toxins)

[a] Adapted from: B. T. Troost: *Current Concepts of Cerebrovascular Disease, 14:* 21, 1979.

limited peripheral type of vertigo is made, follow-up
is needed for confirmation, since there is significant
overlap in the symptoms and signs produced by
peripheral and central vertigo. The following information should be obtained in the initial office evaluation of the patient (the presentation and course of
the major causes of vertigo are described on subsequent pages):

History:

1. Symptoms constant or strictly episodic?
2. Symptoms severe, moderate, or mild?
3. Symptoms occur only with certain motions or
   positions of the head (positional vertigo) or
   occur spontaneously?
4. Hearing impairment or tinnitus present?

5. History of recent ear infection, otorrhea, ear
   surgery, or barotrauma?
6. Recent symptoms of viral illness?
7. Recent head or neck trauma?
8. Symptoms suggesting brainstem disease
   (diplopia, dysarthria, dysphagia, motor
   clumsiness or weakness, facial numbness)?
9. Any drugs associated with the onset of
   symptoms (especially history of recent
   aminoglycoside treatment)?

Examination:

1. Inspection of external auditory canal and tympanic membrane (see Chapter 93).
2. Simple office assessment for hearing impairment (see Chapter 93).
3. Observation for spontaneous nystagmus (see below).
4. Tests for positional vertigo and positional nystagmus (see below).
5. Selective neurologic and neurovascular examination (cranial nerves, particularly 5 and 7; cerebellar tests, gait testing, Romberg test; motor
   testing—see Chapter 75 for recommended brief
   neurologic and neurovascular examination).

Laboratory Tests:

Because luetic labyrinthitis and hypothyroidism
can cause peripheral vertigo, a serologic test for syphilis and a T4 level should be obtained on patients
with peripheral vertigo. There are no other routinely
indicated laboratory tests in the initial office evaluation of vertigo. Several tests of vestibular function
may be utilized by a consulting otolaryngologist,
however (see below, p. 848). With the exception of
hypothyroidism, most of the systemic causes of vertigo listed in Table 78.2 will present with other symptoms in addition to the vertigo; rarely, vertigo and
decreased hearing may be the only symptoms described by a hypothyroid patient.

EVALUATION OF NYSTAGMUS

Nystagmus is rhythmic movement of the eyes.
When it is *pendular* (to and fro movements about
equal in amplitude and speed), it is usually due to
disturbance of central vision. *Jerk nystagmus* (having
a slow and a quick component) is typically, but not
exclusively, a sign of vestibular disease; every patient
complaining of vertigo should be checked for this
type of nystagmus. It is important to know how to
recognize and test for jerk nystagmus since it is the
only objective indicator of vestibular dysfunction.

Spontaneous Nystagmus. In patients with peripheral or central vestibular dysfunction, jerk nystagmus
may be present with the eyes in midposition or in
any direction of gaze. The nystagmus may be detected even when the patient is not experiencing
vertigo. During an episode of acute vertigo, there
should usually be accompanying nystagmus if the
vertigo is due to organic disease; absence of nystag-

mus suggests that one of the other mechanisms for dizziness described above is present. Spontaneous nystagmus should be sought in five positions of gaze: frontal, right, left, up, and down. The patient should be instructed to turn his eyes only about 30° from midline, since extreme lateral gaze may produce a few physiologic jerks in normal individuals. Visual fixation tends to suppress the spontaneous nystagmus of peripheral vestibular disease. Therefore, if spontaneous nystagmus is not observed, the patient should close his eyes (to eliminate visual fixation) and be observed for nystagmus through the eyelids. Alternatively, he can be examined, with eyes open, through Frenzel lenses, which distort the patient's view, making fixation impossible. If spontaneous nystagmus is present with the eyes open, the patient should be asked to fixate on a nearby object; *suppression of nystagmus with fixation favors peripheral vestibular disease* while persistence or enhancement of the nystagmus is typical of central disease.

Features which distinguish peripheral from central spontaneous nystagmus are summarized in Table 78.3.

Testing for Positional Vertigo/Nystagmus. Positional vertigo/nystagmus is that which is produced by a sudden change in head or body position. The patient with positional vertigo usually gives a history of symptoms brought on by such changes as lying back in bed, turning the head while lying, arising from bed, or bending over, but usually not occurring when the body is erect or when the head is not in motion. The purposes of provocative testing are (a) to replicate the patient's symptoms, (b) to demonstrate nystagmus as objective evidence for vestibular impairment, and (c) to determine whether the nystagmus is fatigable.

The test utilized to detect positional vertigo was described by Bárány in 1921 (2), and is illustrated in Figure 78.1. The patient sits close enough to one end of the examining table so that his head would be over the edge if he were lying down. He is asked to keep

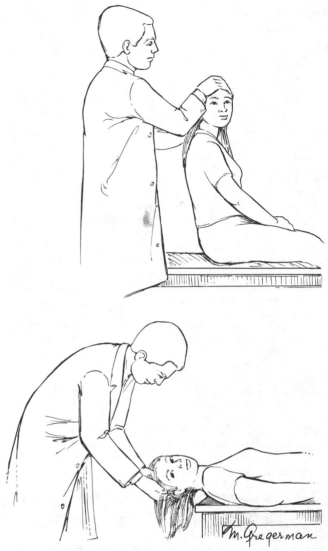

Figure 78.1   Bárány maneuver for testing a patient for positional vertigo and nystagmus.

his eyes open during the maneuver and to report any sensations (vertigo, nausea, etc.) that he experiences. The patient is asked to turn his head to one side. Then, while the examiner supports the head and shoulders, the patient is quickly brought to a reclining position with his head still rotated to one side and hanging over the end of the table. This position should be maintained for 20 to 30 sec. In addition to listening to the patient's symptoms, the examiner should observe his eyes for nystagmus. If nystagmus appears, the examiner should note its time of onset (relative to the start of the maneuver), the direction of eye motion (horizontal, vertical, rotatory, or mixed), the nature of associated symptoms, the adaptability of nystagmus (does it disappear despite maintaining the same head position?), and its fatigability on repeated testing. The maneuver should then be repeated with the head turned in the opposite direction. In particular, if nystagmus was present in

Table 78.3
Features of Spontaneous Nystagmus

Feature	Peripheral	Central
Direction	Usually horizontal-rotatory Never purely vertical	Any direction May be purely vertical
Direction of fast component (when side of disease is known)	Away from side with disease	Toward side with disease (or variable)
Effect of visual fixation	Suppressed	Not suppressed (may be enhanced)
Usual anatomic location of problem	Labyrinth or vestibular nerve	Brainstem or cerebellum

one position, the physician should pay careful attention to any change in its direction or amplitude when tested in the opposite direction.

Features which distinguish peripheral from central positional nystagmus are summarized in Table 78.4.

Peripheral Causes of Vertigo

IDIOPATHIC BENIGN POSITIONAL VERTIGO (BPV)

This is probably the most common type of vertigo seen in adult patients. It occurs in all age groups but is most common after the fourth decade and in persons with recent head trauma. The pathologic basis for idiopathic BPV is not known. The differentiation of BPV from endolymphatic hydrops and vertebral-basilar insufficiency is often the principal challenge for the physician.

Symptoms are first noted when the head is turned either (a) as the patient is assuming a recumbent position or (b) when the patient is already recumbent. The episodes of vertigo are short-lived (usually lasting less than 1 min), and they are always brought on with a change in head position. If the vertigo is related to trauma (see below), it may begin immediately after the trauma or days to weeks later. Typically, patients with BPV do not complain of tinnitus or of hearing impairment. They may, however, have nausea during episodes of vertigo.

On examination, spontaneous nystagmus (see above) is not present. The provocation of positional vertigo/nystagmus with peripheral features (see above), and the absence of other otologic or neurologic findings supports the working diagnosis of idiopathic BPV.

BPV is usually self-limited; however, symptoms may persist for weeks or months and episodes may recur in later years. Because positional vertigo is observed in other conditions besides BPV, it is important to re-evaluate the patient serially, following the systematic approach utilized initially and looking for ancillary evidence for one of the other causes of vertigo listed in Table 78.2. Any patient whose course is atypical should be seen in consultation by an otolaryngologist.

There is no specific treatment for BPV. Since positional vertigo is usually not evoked when the patient is erect, most patients will not have to modify activities such as driving. Each patient learns to avoid the position changes which cause symptoms; individual patients may have to curtail some regular activities until symptoms have abated significantly. Symptomatic treatment may be helpful (see below, p. 848).

POST-TRAUMATIC VERTIGO (8)

Vertigo is very common after both blunt head trauma and whiplash (flexion-extension) injury to the neck. The basis for the vertigo may be disruption of the utricular otolithic membrane (so-called "cupulolithiasis"), hemorrhage into the endolymph or into the eighth nerve, or fracture of the temporal bone causing damage to the nerve.* Clinically, it may be impossible to determine which of these mechanisms is responsible for a patient's symptoms. However, there are two typical patterns which are thought to suggest the dominant problem.

The first pattern is *immediate* post-traumatic vertigo, with associated spontaneous nystagmus (beating away from the side of injury), nausea and vomiting, positional nystagmus, and either conductive or sensorineural hearing loss. This pattern suggests temporal bone fracture and is typical of moderately severe trauma to the temporal bone or occiput. A history of brief unconsciousness, the presence of Battle's sign (postauricular hematoma), and bleeding in the external auditory canal are other findings which suggest this diagnosis. Polytomograms of the temporal bone are needed to detect the fracture. Because there is the possibility of finding surgically correctable damage, these patients should always be evaluated immediately by an otolaryngologist; based upon this evaluation an exploratory tympanotomy may be recommended.

In the majority of patients with immediate post-traumatic vertigo, the vestibular symptoms usually improve rapidly over the first few days and they are gone entirely within 6 to 12 weeks. Symptomatic treatment (see below) may be helpful.

The second common pattern is that of *delayed onset* (latent period of days to weeks) of post-traumatic vertigo, which presents in the same way as idiopathic BPV does (see above). This pattern is more typical of minor head or whiplash injury and is thought to be due to cupulolithiasis. BPV, without spontaneous vertigo or nystagmus and without hearing deficit, is the typical finding on physical examination. The course is similar to that of idiopathic BPV. The patient may benefit from symptomatic treatment (see p. 848).

Table 78.4
Features of Positional Nystagmus Elicited by the Bárány Maneuver

Feature	Peripheral	Central
Time to onset after quick position change	3–45 sec	Immediate
Duration	Less than 1 min (often only a few seconds)	Persists longer than 1 min
Fatiguability	Marked (may not be present on immediate repetition)	None
Subjective vertigo	Often marked	Often minimal or absent
Nystagmus direction	Fixed irrespective of head position	Changing with change in head position
Usual anatomic location of problem	Labyrinth or vestibular nerve	Brainstem or cerebellum

*See Fig. 93.1 for relevant anatomy.

Some patients with post-traumatic vertigo may have a combination of the features of these two typical patterns. After systematic examination, these patients should be managed symptomatically since it is likely that their vertigo will be self-limited.

PERIPHERAL VESTIBULOPATHY (ACUTE LABYRINTHITIS AND VESTIBULAR NEURONITIS)

The collective term "peripheral vestibulopathy" has been suggested by Drachman and Hart (5) for a number of benign conditions for which the pathologic basis is chiefly conjectural. Because these conditions often follow viral upper respiratory or gastrointestinal infections, they are thought to be due to inflammation of the vestibular end organ (labyrinthitis) or of the vestibular nerve (neuronitis). They are most common in the third to the fifth decade but may occur at any age. Occasionally, a cluster of cases occurs (epidemic vertigo). Like BPV, the working diagnosis of peripheral vestibulopathy is based on typical clinical features which are not pathognomonic; therefore, consideration of one of the progressive causes of central vertigo listed in Table 78.2 must be kept in mind in follow-up evaluation.

Typically, there is a sudden onset of moderate to severe spontaneous vertigo. Often there is accompanying nausea and vomiting and symptoms are made worse by any position change. The initial symptoms usually persist for several days, during which they may be incapacitating. A patient may describe tinnitus but there is usually no complaint of hearing loss. There may be a tendency for the patient to fall when he tries to walk.

On systematic examination spontaneous nystagmus with peripheral features (see above) is present. Since involvement is often unilateral, there may be a typical nystagmus pattern in which (a) the fast component is away from the side of the lesion when the subject is asked to look away from the lesion and (b) the nystagmus may lessen or cease when the subject looks toward the side of the lesion. Caloric testing (see below) shows an absence of the normal response on the affected side, but this test is not needed routinely. Positional testing (if performed) may produce a markedly positive response with peripheral characteristics (see Table 78.4). There is usually no hearing loss, and the neurologic and neurovascular examinations are unremarkable.

The vertigo of peripheral vestibulopathy usually resolves within 6 weeks, although nystagmus may be demonstrated for several months, especially if electronystagmography (ENG) is performed (see below). In occasional patients, the vertigo may also persist for more than 6 weeks. Such patients should be systematically re-examined for evidence of a central cause of vertigo, in particular acoustic neuroma and brainstem or inferior cerebellar infarction (see below).

There is no specific treatment. Patients should be told that the worst symptoms will last only a few days, that all symptoms will resolve within 1 month to 6 weeks, and that they should adjust their usual activities according to how they feel (during the first few days, many patients will require strict bed rest for symptomatic relief). Antivertigo drugs may be helpful (see p. 848). Diazepam (Valium) 2.5 to 5 mg, 3 times daily, may also be useful in patients with peripheral vestibulopathy.

VERTIGO DUE TO VESTIBULOTOXIC DRUGS (9)

Ototoxicity is an occasional complication of aminoglycoside antibiotics, salicylates, and potent diuretics (ethacrynic acid and furosemide). Most of these drugs are cochleotoxic and produce sensorineural hearing loss and tinnitus (see Chapter 93). Two aminoglycosides, streptomycin and gentamicin, are vestibulotoxic. The basis for aminoglycoside ototoxicity seems to be that these drugs are concentrated in the inner ear. Pathologically, there is destruction of the sensory hair cells of either the cochlea or the labyrinth. Ototoxicity due to aminoglycoside can usually be prevented by avoiding serum concentrations above the therapeutic range and by limiting the duration of therapy.

In office practice, vestibular toxicity due to an aminoglycoside may appear shortly after the patient has been treated with an aminoglycoside drug while in hospital. Because these drugs produce bilateral, symmetric damage, the patient will usually not describe frank vertigo, but will have unsteadiness and intolerance to motion. The pathologic changes produced by aminoglycosides are permanent, and the symptoms may persist indefinitely. Fortunately, most patients with vestibular toxicity are able to adjust to their problem, and hearing aids may help those with cochlear toxicity.

Mild vertigo or dysequilibrium may occur as a side effect of a number of drugs (Table 78.2) which do not produce permanent pathologic damage; these side effects remit promptly after stopping the drug.

MÉNIÈRE'S SYNDROME (ENDOLYMPHATIC HYDROPS)

This condition is described in Chapter 93. Ménière's syndrome should always be considered in the differential diagnosis of a patient with the acute onset of severe vertigo with peripheral characteristics. The features which distinguish it from other causes of vertigo are the spontaneous onset of attacks, the limited duration of symptoms during each discrete attack (minutes to hours, not one or more days as seen with peripheral vestibulopathy), the associated sensorineural hearing loss found in most patients, and normal brainstem and cerebellar function. At times, Ménière's syndrome may present initially with only vertigo (isolated hydrops of the labyrinth) or only hearing loss (isolated hydrops of the cochlea). Serial observation is therefore important. In clinically suspected cases of isolated hydrops, a trial of diuretic treatment may be helpful.

LUETIC LABYRINTHITIS

Labyrinthitis may occur, although rarely, as a manifestation of secondary or tertiary syphilis. It is always important to consider this etiology, as it may mimic other forms of peripheral vertigo and it requires antibiotic treatment.

Typically, the patient has a combination of (a) sensorineural hearing loss, which may be unilateral or bilateral and fluctuating or sudden, and (b) peripheral-type vertigo which is not positional. As noted earlier, this problem should be sought by sending a serologic test for syphilis (STS) routinely in every patient with new peripheral-type vertigo. If the STS is positive, the patient should have a cerebrospinal fluid STS determination and be treated according to the stage of the disease (see Chapter 29).

Central Causes of Vertigo

Table 78.2 lists the principal central causes of vertigo. Most are uncommon. The important clues to the presence of one of these conditions are the finding of associated neurologic signs and symptoms, the presence of nystagmus with central characteristics (see Tables 78.3 and 78.4), or deviation of the patient's presentation and course from that expected for the common peripheral causes of vertigo. Whenever a central cause for vertigo is suspected, the patient should be referred for evaluation to a neurologist or an otolaryngologist. When the onset of symptoms is acute or there is evidence of rapidly progressive neurologic symptoms, the patient should be hospitalized.

The principal manifestations of the two types of central vertigo which a generalist is most likely to see (tumor and vascular disease) are described here.

CEREBELLOPONTINE (CP) ANGLE TUMOR

Acoustic neuroma, the commonest CP angle tumor, is described in Chapter 93. The usual manifestations of these tumors are due to compression of the auditory component of the eighth nerve (sensorineural hearing loss) and, much later, to compression of adjacent structures (the fifth and seventh cranial nerves in particular). Frank vertigo and nystagmus are present in a minority of patients. A vague complaint of unsteadiness, however, is present in almost half the patients when they are first seen; and ENG may demonstrate nystagmus when simple office observation does not (see below). The symptoms of CP angle tumor typically are insidious in onset (usually confined to sensorineural hearing loss for a prolonged interval), constant, and progressive. This time course distinguishes them from the periodic or severe symptoms typical of most peripheral vertigo and of the central vertigo of transient ischemia.

As pointed out elsewhere (Chapter 93), consultation with an otolaryngologist is the most appropriate plan for a patient who may have a CP angle tumor. The consultant should determine which of a large variety of otoneurologic tests is appropriate in pursuing this diagnosis (7).

VERTEBROBASILAR ARTERIAL DISEASE

Cerebrovascular ischemia may cause vertigo. When this symptom is due to atherosclerosis, there are almost always symptoms or signs of other brainstem involvement, in particular clumsiness or weakness, loss of vision, diplopia, perioral numbness, ataxia, drop attack (sudden loss of motor tone in the lower extremities, without loss of consciousness), or dysarthria.

When these symptoms are *transient*, they may be due (a) to a transient ischemic attack (TIA) (see Chapter 80), (b) to mechanical compromise of the vertebrobasilar circulation (see Fig. 78.2) brought on by rotation of the neck (detected either in the history or by having the patient replicate his symptoms in the office), or (c) to diversion of blood from the brainstem to an arm during use of that arm—the subclavian steal syndrome (suspected on the basis of history and of the finding of a subclavian artery bruit or a decreased blood pressure in the symptom-provoking arm). When the symptoms are abrupt in onset and *persistent*, they may be due to infarction of the brainstem or cerebellum. Insidious onset of persistent symptoms would be more suggestive of tumor. Acute cerebellar infarction in the distal territory of the posterior inferior cerebellar artery (PICA), a relatively uncommon problem, may initially mimic acute vestibulopathy, presenting as sudden marked vertigo, nausea, and vomiting. Usually infarction due to PICA

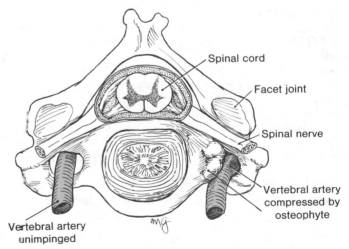

Figure 78.2 Anatomic relationship of the vertebral artery in a transverse foramen. The artery lies alongside the uncinate portion of the vertebra, the most common site of degenerative changes due to cervical spondylosis with osteophyte formation. (From S. Sheehan, R. B. Bauer and J. S. Meyer: Vertebral artery compression in cervical spondylosis. *Neurology, 10:* 968, 1960.)

occlusion will involve the brainstem, so that other neurologic signs will be present (ipsilateral loss of pain and temperature sense of the face and contralateral loss of these sensations in the rest of the body, cerebellar ataxia, or ipsilateral Horner's syndrome).

Sudden vertigo and unilateral hearing loss may occur due to *selective occlusion of the internal auditory artery*; in such patients, a condition affecting small arteries (syphilitic arteritis or other vasculitides, or microembolism) is a more likely cause than atherosclerosis.

Symptomatic Treatment of Vertigo

When the working diagnosis is peripheral vertigo of any type, treatment with one of the *"antivertigo" antihistamines* may provide symptomatic relief. There have been no systematic studies to evaluate the efficacy of these drugs. It is hypothesized that these agents work both by suppressing the vestibular end organ receptors and by inhibiting activation of vagal responses. Commonly recommended drugs in this group are listed in Table 78.5, with appropriate doses and schedules. Because peripheral vertigo from common causes is usually self-limited, the patient should be instructed to take an antivertigo agent only for a few weeks and then to try discontinuing the drug. The major side effects of these drugs are dry mouth and sedation.

When nausea and vomiting are pronounced, in either peripheral or central vertigo, an *antiemetic* can be tried. It is hypothesized that these agents work by suppressing central vestibular pathways which activate vagal responses. Commonly recommended antiemetic drugs are listed in Table 78.5. The major side effect occurring with short term use is sedation; with the phenothiazine antiemetic, prochlorperazine, acute dystonias may occur in occasional patients (see Chapter 15 for a full discussion of phenothiazine side effects).

Patients with persistent and disabling vertigo should be referred to an otolaryngologist for definitive evaluation and management. For permanent relief of symptoms, some persons will require *surgery* which may consist of sectioning of the singular nerve (a branch of the vestibular nerve) or eighth nerve, repair of an inner ear fistula, or labyrinthectomy).

Several of these procedures produce unilateral deafness.

Tests Utilized in Evaluation of Vertigo

When a patient with vertigo which is difficult to diagnose is referred to a neurologist or an otolaryngologist, one or more of the studies listed in Table 78.6 will usually be conducted. A combination of results from two or more tests will support the diagnosis or exclusion of a number of the causes of vertigo.

AUDIOMETRY (15)

A number of audiologic tests are usually performed in evaluating vertigo (*i.e.*, pure tone audiometry, speech audiometry, tone decay testing, acoustic reflex testing, and others). Typically, there is no audiometric abnormality in the most common forms of peripheral vertigo (BPV and peripheral vestibulopathy), while there are typical patterns of hearing loss in Ménière's syndrome (low frequency hearing loss), acoustic neuroma (high frequency hearing loss), and a variety of middle ear disorders.

Patient Experience. These tests are performed in a small sound-proof testing room. There is no significant discomfort for the patient. Complete testing may take up to 1 hour.

CALORIC STIMULATION (13)

This is the only test which enables the consultant to evaluate individually the vestibular end organs on each side of the head. The test is based upon the fact that the intact labyrinth responds to caloric stimulation with a typical pattern, *i.e.*, warm water induces horizontal nystagmus with the slow phase away from the stimulated ear, and cool water produces nystagmus in the opposite direction. Vertigo may be induced with both hot and cold stimulation. Under certain circumstances, ENG is utilized (see below) in addition to direct observation during caloric stimulation. Ideally, the water temperatures are set at 30°C and 44°C; these are equidistant from normal body temperature, constitute equal stimuli, and produce less distress than more extreme temperatures. Absence of the normal caloric response or deviation from the normal response may be helpful in diagnosis. Vestibular neu-

Table 78.5
Drugs for Symptomatic Treatment of Vertigo

Type of Action	Generic (Trade Name)	Available Preparation	Dose and Schedule
Labyrinthine Suppressants (Antihistamines)	Meclizine (Antivert, Bonine)	12.5 and 25-mg tablets	12.5–25 mg t.i.d. or q.i.d.
	Dimenhydrinate (Dramamine)	50-mg tablets	50 mg t.i.d. or q.i.d.
Antiemetics	Prochlorperazine (Compazine)	5-, 10-mg tablets 10- and 25-mg suppositories	5–10 mg q4h p.r.n. 10 mg q.i.d. or 25 mg b.i.d.
	Trimethobenzamide (Tigan)	250-mg capsule 200-mg suppository	t.i.d.—q.i.d. t.i.d.—q.i.d.

Table 78.6
Tests Used in the Evaluation of Vertigo

Audiometry (pure tone, speech, tone decay,
  brainstem evoked potentials, etc.)
Caloric tests
Electronystagmography
Skull X-rays
Mastoid X-rays
Polytomogram of temporal bone and internal
  auditory canal
CT scan
Air contrast myelogram, with CT scan

ronitis, acoustic neuroma, and Ménière's syndrome
are examples of conditions in which the normal response to caloric stimulation is absent or decreased
on the involved side.

Patient Experience. The patient lies on his side with the
head positioned comfortably at an angle of about 30°.
Flowing water is introduced into the external auditory
canal for 30 sec. For optimal testing, there should be about
a 30-min wait between irrigations. During caloric stimulation, the patient will experience vertigo. An absent caloric
response signifies vestibular disease.

ELECTRONYSTAGMOGRAPHY (ENG) (16)

ENG records changes in the electrical potential
between the cornea and the retina; when the eye
moves, characteristic changes in electrical potential
can be picked up (and recorded with a penwriter) in
the skin adjacent to the eye. ENG has two advantages
over direct inspection in detecting nystagmus. First,
it is more sensitive than simple inspection and can
confirm the presence of nystagmus when simple inspection is equivocal (often because the patient fix-
ates and suppresses nystagmus under these conditions). Second, it can provide serial tracings which
permit comparison of a patient's nystagmus pattern
over time. The disadvantages of ENG are that it
requires considerable cooperation from the patient
and skill from the operator both for correct conduction of the test and proper interpretation. The principal value of ENG is in picking up subtle spontaneous nystagmus and in differentiating peripheral
from central nystagmus, usually by caloric stimulation.

Patient Experience. The patient is recumbent. Small
electrodes are taped to the skin on either side of the eye.
Nystagmus is measured under a number of conditions,
including caloric stimulation (see above), optokinetic testing (the patient is asked to follow the stripes on a rotating
drum), and others. The entire procedure may take up to 1
hour. The major discomfort is that associated with caloric
stimulation.

MOTION SICKNESS

Motion sickness is experienced by almost 100% of
normal persons when they are exposed to conditions

analogous to those at sea in severe storm conditions.
About one-third of people experience symptoms
when exposed to the equivalent of moderate sea
conditions such as may occur with automobile travel
and air travel, as well as boating. Normal vestibular
function is necessary for an individual to experience
motion sickness. Visual stimuli are contributory, but
not necessary for the experience of motion sickness
(for example, looking out of the window of a vehicle
on a curving or undulating road).

Manifestations

The symptoms of motion sickness vary from person to person, but an individual usually experiences
the same symptoms each time. Malaise and nausea
are always present, and vomiting is common. Other
symptoms may include drowsiness, salivation, swallowing, hyperventilation, headache, flushing, and
diaphoresis. There is a major psychologic component
in motion sickness; for example, some persons develop their typical symptoms in anticipation of an air
flight or a boat ride. Vertigo is usually not present.

Most people adapt fairly rapidly to motion. After
the first few days of a sea voyage, for example, they
are able to tolerate the motion which made them ill
at the beginning of the voyage.

Treatment (19)

In tests simulating sea conditions, a number of
drugs have been shown to be quite effective in preventing motion sickness. These drugs are much less
effective if taken after the onset of symptoms. Because all drugs which prevent motion sickness are
sedating, individuals should not operate cars, boats,
planes, or potentially dangerous machines while taking these drugs.

ANTIHISTAMINES

Either meclizine (Antivert, Bonine), 25 to 50 mg, or
dimenhydrinate (Dramamine), 50 to 100 mg, can be
used. For persons who routinely get moderate or
marked motion symptoms, taking one of these drugs
about 1 hour before embarking in a car, plane, or
boat may be very helpful. The protective effect from
meclizine lasts from 12 to 24 hours, while that from
dimenhydrinate lasts only 4 hours. The principal side
effect is drowsiness; because this is more prominent
with dimenhydrinate, meclizine is the better choice
for persons who wish to remain alert during travel;
others may prefer the greater sedating property of
dimenhydrinate.

SCOPOLAMINE

The anticholinergic drug scopolamine prevents severe motion sickness in a high percentage of persons
known to suffer from this problem. Scopolamine is
available in tablet form and in the form of a plastic
disc for continuous administration through the skin.
A 0.4-mg tablet can be taken 1 hour before travel or
boating. Alternatively, the button-sized disc (Trans-

derm-V) can be applied behind the ear. The disc works optimally when applied a number of hours before travel or boating. Dry mouth, sedation, and impaired visual accommodation may occur, probably more frequently with the oral preparation. Known closed-angle glaucoma and benign prostate hypertrophy are relative contraindications to the use of this anticholinergic drug.

SYNCOPE AND NEAR-SYNCOPE

Definitions and Normal Physiology

Syncope is a loss of consciousness which begins abruptly and lasts for a finite length of time (usually less than 5 min). A prodrome or aura may or may not be present and if recalled is usually quite short. Similarly, full recovery, though often abrupt, may be prolonged under certain circumstances described below. Syncope must be distinguished from delirium, where the content of consciousness is altered but the person is awake; from stupor, where the person appears asleep but can be aroused; and from coma, where the person appears asleep and cannot be aroused by simple maneuvers. Several conditions which may present with brief episodes resembling syncope (hysterical fainting, drop attacks, and narcolepsy) are discussed in more detail below (p. 858).

Near-syncope, or impending syncope, is a state of transient dizziness caused by any of the conditions which can cause frank syncope. Near-syncope is far more common than syncope; and most persons (for example, those with transient orthostatic light-headedness) probably do not report the problem to their physicians. The physiologic changes leading to the two problems are identical; they are simply shorter in duration or less severe in the person who becomes dizzy without actually losing consciousness. Since episodes of near-syncope often predate frank syncope, the potentially devastating consequences of syncope can often be prevented by early diagnosis and treatment of the underlying cause of a patient's dizziness.

Normal wakefulness requires the proper functioning of one, but not necessarily both, cerebral hemispheres and of the ascending reticular formation of the brainstem. Unconsciousness, therefore, implies that either both cerebral hemispheres are impaired or that critical structures in the brainstem have failed. Syncope (or near-syncope) occurs when there is *temporary* impairment of the reticular formation or of both hemispheres.

Causes

The causes of syncope and near-syncope can be divided into failure of the systemic circulation, cardiac disease, metabolic derangements, and primary intracranial conditions (see Table 78.7).

Based on reports of large numbers of syncopal patients, it is estimated that failure of the circulation is the cause in about 70% of patients, heart disease in about 10%, intracranial disease in about 10%, and metabolic disorders in about 5%. In the remaining 5% of patients presenting with syncope, no cause can be discerned. The single most common cause of syncope is the common faint or vasovagal episode. Orthostatic hypotension due to diverse causes is also very common. Mobilization after bed rest, postmicturition and tussive syncope, and carotid sinus hypersensivity are the other common causes of circulatory syncope. Cardiac arrhythmias, aortic stenosis, and syncope associated with angina or with myocardial infarction are the common causes of cardiogenic syncope. Epilepsy and cerebrovascular disease account for most transient loss of consciousness due to intracranial disease. Only hypocapnia (due to hyperventilation) is a common metabolic cause of syncope; hypoglycemia rarely leads to unconsciousness, although it frequently causes the cerebral symptoms of impending syncope.

The management and prognosis of the patient with a history of syncope or near-syncope depends upon correct identification of the underlying cause. The following discussion focuses chiefly upon the *diagnostic evaluation* of the syncopal/near-syncopal patient. *Appropriate management* for most of the common causes of these problems is discussed elsewhere in the book, as indicated by cross-referencing.

General Approach to the Patient

Most patients who come to a physician after an episode of syncope or near-syncope do so after their symptoms have resolved. The physician should obtain the history both from the patient and from anyone who observed the episode. The inquiry should focus upon the events immediately preceding and following the attack; upon associated problems which may have been present for days to weeks before the episode; and upon evidence of significant trauma, neurologic deficit, or aspiration complicating the current episode of syncope. The objectives of these initial steps are (a) to reach a working diagnosis or decide what further evaluation is needed to do so and (b) to decide upon the appropriate initial management for the patient. Appropriate management may range from reassurance (for example, the patient with vasovagal syncope) to volume expansion (for example, the patient with a diarrheal illness) to hospital admission for observation, prompt diagnostic testing, and necessary treatment (for example, the patient with a history suggesting recurrent life-threatening arrhythmias or the patient with a fracture or an aspiration pneumonia complicating syncope).

HISTORY

Current Episode. The patient should always be questioned about what position he was in immediately before the attack. Syncope from most causes does not occur unless the patient is in the upright position. If the attack occurred when the patient first stood up, orthostatic hypotension due to venous pool-

Table 78.7
Causes of Syncope/Near-Syncope

FAILURE OF THE SYSTEMIC CIRCULATION	CARDIAC DISEASE
Simple faint (vasovagal syncope)	*Arrhythmia (heart block, brady- and tachyarrhythmias)*
Autonomic impairment	*Outflow obstruction*
1. Drugs:	1. Aortic stenosis
Antihypertensives	2. Idiopathic hypertrophic subaortic stenosis
Neuroleptics	3. Aortic dissection
Tricyclics and monoamine oxidase (MAO) inhibitors	4. Myxoma
Levodopa	*Acute myocardial infarction*
Nitroglycerine preparations	*Mitral valve prolapse*
Cholinergic agents	*Cyanotic congenital heart disease*
2. Autonomic neuropathy:	*Cardiac tamponade*
Peripheral neuropathy	METABOLIC CONDITIONS
Postsympathectomy	*Hypoglycemia*
Tabes dorsalis and diabetic psuedotabes	1. Exogenous insulin
Parkinsonism	2. Feactive
Idiopathic	3. Starvation (islet cell tumor)
Decreased blood volume	4. Dumping syndrome
1. Hemorrhage	*Hypocapnia (hyperventilation)*
2. Salt and water deficit (diarrhea, vomiting, perspiration, diuretics, hyperglycemia)	*Hypoxia*
3. Fasting	1. Anemia
4. Adrenal insufficiency	2. Airway obstruction
5. Hypoalbuminemia	3. Carbon monoxide
Venous pooling	*Hyperviscosity*
1. Prolonged immobility while standing	*Electrolyte derangements (hyponatremia, hypokalemia, hypocalcemia, hyperglycemia)*
2. Severe varicose veins	*Drug overdose*
3. Late pregnancy	1. Sedatives and ethanol (venous pooling)
4. After exercise	2. All drugs causing autonomic impairment (see above)
Mobilization after bed rest	INTRACRANIAL CONDITIONS
Orthostasis of aging	*Seizure disorder*
Valsalva maneuver	*Subarachnoid hemorrhage*
1. Tussive	*Cerebral embolism or thrombosis*
2. Micturition	*Migraine*
3. Defecation (with straining)	*Acutely increased intracranial pressure*
4. Intermittent positive pressure breathing	1. Tumor
Compromise of cerebral blood flow due to cervical osteoarthritis or subclavian steal	2. Trauma
Carotid sinus hypersensitivity	3. Ventricular obstruction
Pulmonary embolism	4. Hypertensive encephalopathy
Severe pain of visceral origin	*Brainstem compression*
	1 Cervical or odontoid fractures
	2. Metastasis
	3. Cysts or anomalies of the posterior fossa
	4. Platybasia

ing, loss of intravascular volume, or autonomic failure should be considered. If exercise preceded the attack, a number of cardiopulmonary abnormalities are likely, including aortic stenosis, idiopathic hypertrophic subaortic stenosis, arrhythmia, or pulmonary hypertension. If syncope was associated with micturition, cough, or passing stool, this suggests diminished venous return due to a Valsalva maneuver. If there was psychologic stress (e.g., an argument, fear associated with a medical or other procedure, etc.), vasovagal syncope is highly likely. In each case, the patient will usually recall feeling dizzy, that events were moving very slowly and that he was distant from them, that his limbs became heavy, and his vision dimmed or objects lost their color and seemed tinted just before loss of consciousness. Nausea, usually without vomiting, is quite characteristic of va-

sovagal syncope, syncope associated with bradyarrhythmias, and of syncope associated with loss of intravascular volume.

Syncope which occurs when the patient is *seated or recumbent* should suggest hypoglycemia, carotid sinus hypersensitivity, cardiac arrhythmia, hyperventilation, a seizure, or hysteria. Syncope or dizziness occurring with position change while recumbent should always be distinguished from benign positional vertigo, which occurs most frequently in the recumbent position (see above, p. 845).

Other manifestations just before syncope may suggest the diagnosis. Hunger may indicate hypoglycemia. Headache or characteristic visual disturbances may precede migrainous syncope. Hemiparasis, paraparesis, diplopia, dysarthria, or other neurologic abnormalities may precede syncope/near-syncope due to transient occlusion of the basilar artery or to vasospasm associated with migraine.

The physician should always take advantage of *observations made by others* who witnessed the period of unconsciousness. Particular attention should be paid to the duration of the spell, whether a convulsion occurred, if incontinence was noted, the sequence of events, and how the patient seemed during the period of recovery. In general, recovery of consciousness is swift. Slow recovery of clear consciousness (recovery after more than 5 min) should raise suspicion of a seizure, hypoglycemia, or of an occluded intracranial vessel.

Associated Recent History. Information about the patient during the hours, days, or weeks preceding syncope/near-syncope is often very helpful in the differential diagnosis.

A large proportion of patients will give a history of episodic near-syncope. The patient will usually use the word "dizziness" or one of the other terms listed in Table 78.1. The circumstances surrounding these episodes may support a working diagnosis for a current episode of frank syncope. For example, the patient may have started, or increased the dose of, a drug known to cause orthostatic hypotension (see Table 78.7); or there may be a history of a problem leading to volume deficit, e.g., diarrhea, heat exposure, diuretic use; increased polyuria (in a diabetic), or melena. A patient convalescing from recent illness may relate his symptoms to beginning to be up and around after bed rest. An insulin-using diabetic or a patient with reactive or starvation hypoglycemia may describe episodic hypoglycemic symptoms, successfully aborted with carbohydrate intake, during the week(s) prior to frank syncope. In the absence of any relevant changes in the patient's circumstances, a history of recent near-syncopal episodes is suggestive of arrhythmia, transient cerebral ischemia, or chronic idiopathic orthostatic hypotension.

A second group of patients will describe prior episodes of frank syncope, without prodromal near-syncope. Most often, these will be patients with a history, often long-standing, of syncope due to vasovagal attack brought on by psychologic or physical stress. A history of recurrent syncope without near-syncopal episodes and without the features of vasovagal attacks is most suggestive of arrhythmia, transient cerebrovascular occlusion, or a seizure disorder.

PHYSICAL EXAMINATION

General Examination. The physical examination after an attack should include a systematic search for abnormalities in the blood pressure, heart and great vessels, abdomen, and the central and peripheral nervous system. In particular, the blood pressure should be measured after the patient has been recumbent for several minutes, again after he is seated, and finally while he is standing. The character, volume, and timing of the carotid pulses should be appraised, and any bruits should be noted. The pulse should be palpated for 1 to 2 min to look for irregularities. The heart should be carefully examined for murmurs, systolic clicks, or gallop rhythms. Abdominal examination may reveal a large bladder or signs of a visceral catastrophe. If unexplained orthostatic hypotension has been found, a rectal examination should be performed to check the stool for occult or gross blood.

Neurologic Examination. A brief examination of the major components of the nervous system (see Chapter 75) may reveal evidence of either preexisting neurologic disease or of an acute insult related to the current episode of syncope/near-syncope. Orientation, speech, memory for the event itself as well as for general information, and judgment should be noted. The fundi may reveal microemboli or subhyaloid hemorrhages (a sign of subarachnoid hemorrhage). Nystagmus, ophthalmoplegia, or abnormalities of the pupils, facial movement and sensation, the corneal reflexes, speech, or movement of the palate or tongue indicate involvement of the midbrain, pons, or medulla. Weakness, sensory abnormalities, and pathologic reflexes found in a general neurologic examination may indicate a lesion elsewhere in the central nervous system. Any neurologic abnormalities should raise the suspicion of cerebrovascular disease, a mass causing an epileptic focus, subarachnoid hemorrhage, or central nervous system infection. If trauma has occurred in the recent past or if a fall was sustained during the syncopal episode, subdural or epidural hemorrhage should be considered.

Significance of Seizures and Neurologic Deficits. Seizure activity may occur after syncope due to any of the common causes, including the simple faint, hyperventilation, orthostatic hypotension, or venous pooling. This is not surprising since unconsciousness signifies a major disruption in normal brain function. In particular, a single tonic convulsion is quite common; less often a focal seizure or a generalized convulsion may occur. In all three of these instances, the patient's evaluation should include routine tests for a seizure focus (see Chapter 77).

Minor neurological signs such as slight focal weakness, reflex asymmetries, or pathologic reflexes may also occur following syncope from any cause. These findings may be present particularly if the patient is examined immediately after recovering consciousness, and they rarely persist for more than a few minutes. If such signs persist longer, are more profound, or occur in a constellation which suggests a particular anatomic lesion, they warrant further pursuit. However, one should not be surprised if a source is not found even after a thorough search is completed, since neurologic abnormalities are deceptively common after general ischemic or metabolic insults to the brain.

LABORATORY TESTS

No laboratory test is indicated routinely in the evaluation of syncope/near-syncope although an electrocardiogram will often be indicated if the cause of the patient's problem is not obvious. Noble (14) estimates that the carefully taken history with a screening physical examination, plus an electrocardiogram will lead to the correct diagnosis in most patients. The indications for other laboratory tests are cited in the discussion of specific problems which follows.

Features of Common Causes of Syncope/Near-Syncope

FAILURE OF SYSTEMIC CIRCULATION

Because of autoregulation, cerebral blood flow is protected over a wide range of systemic blood pressure. In normal persons, a critical decrease in CNS blood flow (clinically producing near-syncope or syncope) does not occur until the mean blood pressure is below 50 mm Hg. Under a number of circumstances (e.g., sympatholytic drug treatment, cerebrovascular disease, aging), however, the minimum tolerated blood pressure may not be this low. Therefore, symptomatic failure of the systemic circulation may occur over a relatively wide range of blood pressures.

Simple Faint

The simple faint (vasovagal episode) has long been known to afflict young people; it is particularly apt to occur in the setting of anxiety, tension, fatigue, or during venipuncture or other painful procedures. The simple faint is not just a disease of the young but can occur in older patients in identical settings. Early theories suggested that bradycardia due to vagal overactivity was the initial event; but it is now known that venous pooling due to peripheral arterial constriction with venous dilation occurs in the first phase, with a vagal phase (bradycardia) occurring only after the faint itself. Vasovagal attacks nearly always occur while the patient is upright, but may occur while he is seated; and consciousness is nearly always regained promptly when the patient becomes recumbent. Typically there is a prodromal warning period, at times lasting 3 to 5 min, during which the patient feels dizzy, light-headed, and flushed and has palpitations, often with a tightness in his throat or mild nausea. If the subject assumes a recumbent position during this stage, he may avoid loss of consciousness. An observer will note cold hands, pale skin, and tachycardia just before the patient loses consciousness. After the faint, when the patient is usually recumbent, a flush replaces the pallor and a bradycardia replaces the tachycardia. If the patient is unable to lie flat, recovery may be prolonged; and an occasional death has been noted, as in a faint occurring in a telephone booth or if the person is held upright during the spell. Bradycardia may persist for up to ½ hour after a simple faint. During this time the patient should remain in a recumbent position. The examination is otherwise normal unless there has been trauma or aspiration.

Autonomic Impairment

Syncope/near-syncope due to autonomic impairment is always associated with orthostatic hypotension. To document this problem, blood pressure must be taken while the patient is supine, seated, and standing. In some patients, exercise while standing (walking for a few minutes for example) may be required for a significant orthostatic drop (20 mm systolic) to occur.

The most common cause of this problem nowadays is antihypertensive drug use; most syncope due to these drugs is preventable if these drugs are prescribed cautiously and the standing blood pressure, after exercise, is monitored routinely. Other drugs may also produce orthostatic symptoms (see Table 78.7). The initial management of drug-induced orthostasis is described in Chapter 59; definitive management requires discontinuation or reduced dose of the offending drug.

Orthostatic hypotension can also be due to autonomic neuropathy. In patients suspected of having this problem, the integrity of the autonomic nervous system can be tested by noting the size and reaction of the pupils, the distribution of sweating, and the response to a Valsalva maneuver (6, 10, 11). The Valsalva maneuver is performed by having the patient expire against a closed glottis for 20 to 30 sec, then release air from the chest (see Table 78.8). This maneuver creates a sudden reduction in cardiac output, stimulating vagal (afferent) and sympathetic (efferent) responses. Absence of the reflex tachycardia (phase II) and/or absence of the blood pressure overshoot and reflex bradycardia (phase IV) indicate autonomic impairment.

Table 78.8
Four Phases of a Normal Valsalva Maneuver

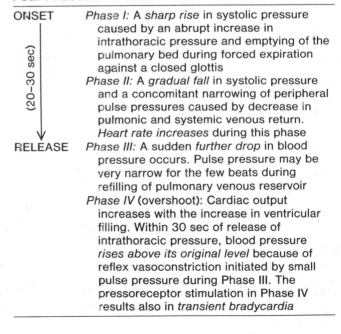

ONSET (20-30 sec) RELEASE

Phase I: A *sharp rise* in systolic pressure caused by an abrupt increase in intrathoracic pressure and emptying of the pulmonary bed during forced expiration against a closed glottis
Phase II: A *gradual fall* in systolic pressure and a concomitant narrowing of peripheral pulse pressures caused by decrease in pulmonic and systemic venous return. *Heart rate increases* during this phase
Phase III: A sudden *further drop* in blood pressure occurs. Pulse pressure may be very narrow for the few beats during refilling of pulmonary venous reservoir
Phase IV (overshoot): Cardiac output increases with the increase in ventricular filling. Within 30 sec of release of intrathoracic pressure, blood pressure *rises above its original level* because of reflex vasoconstriction initiated by small pulse pressure during Phase III. The pressoreceptor stimulation in Phase IV results also in *transient bradycardia*

Sympathetic failure commonly occurs late in diabetic peripheral neuropathy (Chapter 69), but may be the presenting feature of amyloidosis or the neuropathy associated with various neoplasms. Idiopathic orthostatic hypotension, a disease due to the failure of certain central autonomic neurons, occurs in late life and is characterized by faints, pupillary abnormalities, constipation, and impotence (1). A similar mechanism accounts for fainting in patients with idiopathic parkinsonism. Sympathectomy, particularly when done bilaterally or in the lumbar segments, may be followed immediately by orthostatic hypotension and syncope, though usually venous tone recovers several weeks after the operation. Tabes dorsalis and more commonly diabetic pseudotabes may present with lighting pains and autonomic failure. The management of orthostasis due to autonomic neuropathy is symptomatic; it is summarized in Chapter 81.

Decreased Intravascular Volume

Decreased intravascular volume due to hemorrhage or to salt and water loss (e.g., of gastroenteritis, heat exposure, diuretics, etc.) is recognized by the combination of orthostatic hypotension and an associated basis for the volume deficit. Hot weather and exercise predispose to volume depletion and thereby to syncope, particularly after vigorous exercise. Prolonged fasting, as in anorexia nervosa or with fad diets, also may produce syncope through volume depletion. Adrenal insufficiency due to pituitary or primary adrenal disease may produce syncope, due to the combination of chronic volume deficit and the loss of vascular tone; the syncope is often precipitated by an intercurrent illness which would not produce syncope in a healthy person. Hypoalbuminemia due to liver disease, enteropathies, or chronic disease can also lead to syncope/presyncope due to intravascular volume deficit. Volume expansion, either by increased salt and water ingestion or by intravenous fluids, is the initial treatment; the choice of ambulatory or hospital management and the planning of definitive treatment depends upon the severity and the primary cause for the volume deficit.

Venous Pooling

Venous pooling prevents return of blood to the heart, lowering cardiac output, at times sufficiently to produce near-syncope or syncope. Symptoms may occur after prolonged standing in one position, particularly after exercise, as in recruits standing at attention. Severe dependent varicose veins or the compression of pelvic veins by a fetus or a large abdominal mass may produce symptoms due to a similar mechanism. Syncope 15 to 30 min after exercise has been attributed to dilation of the splanchnic circulation before blood flow to the skeletal muscles has completely returned to normal. Management of patients with these conditions is chiefly by avoidance of the precipitating circumstances after an initial episode. Supportive elastic stockings may be helpful for patients with marked pooling due to varicose veins (see Chapter 85).

Orthostatic Syncope/Near-Syncope after Bed Rest

This problem is due to the combined effects of venous pooling, relative hypovolemia, and probably to some degree of lowered sensitivity of the baroreceptor system. It is a very common occurrence, and should be anticipated in any person who has been at bed rest for more than a few days, in the hospital or at home; moreover, it may persist for 1 or 2 weeks, occasionally longer, after mobilization begins. Orthostatic symptoms may be minimized or prevented by having the patient gradually stand only after several minutes of sitting on the bed with his legs dependent. Practical exercises which may help convalescing patients in overcoming postural weakness and hypotension are illustrated in Figure 78.3.

Orthostasis of Aging

Transient orthostatic symptoms are relatively common among older persons. An orthostatic fall of 30 mm Hg in systolic pressure is found in approximately 10% of healthy older persons (4). The physiologic basis for this problem is not established, although studies of small numbers of elderly persons have shown an impaired Valsalva response (11), indicating autonomic dysfunction. This often asymptomatic condition is important insofar as it increases the risk associated with drugs and conditions which may cause orthostatic hypotension. Clearly, older persons should have their standing blood pressure checked whenever they complain of even mild orthostatic symptoms and should be monitored similarly whenever a drug in one of the groups listed in Table 78.7 is prescribed. Those who are troubled by orthostatic symptoms should be advised to follow the steps recommended above for patients convalescing from bed rest.

Other Forms of Syncope Related to Systemic Circulation

Tussive syncope may follow a prolonged bout of coughing in otherwise normal individuals; in these persons, the syncope is thought to be due to the Valsalva mechanism. Tussive syncope may also occur after only a slight cough in persons with obstructive airways disease; abnormalities of pulmonary and pleural vagal receptors in such individuals may aggravate their tendency to faint. Syncope during *positive pressure breathing* occurs by similar mechanisms. *Micturition syncope* often occurs in young men who awaken with a full bladder in the middle of the night, walk to the bathroom and void without difficulty, only to faint while returning to bed. Both the Valsalva mechanism and direct vagal stimulation have been hypothesized as the basis for this form of syncope. Alcohol predisposes to faints after voiding by provoking volume loss and venous pooling. Older

LEG EXERCISES

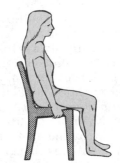

Starting position: Sitting in
chair, exercise one leg at
a time

Raise leg up and down.
Repeat 10 times

Keeping knee bent, raise
leg up and down

ARM EXERCISES: To increase effectiveness, hold a soup can in each hand for weight

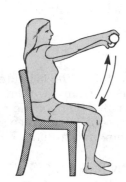

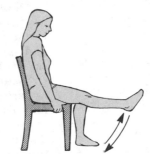

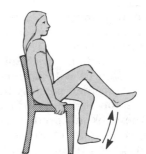

Start with arms straight out in front.
Raise arms up and down, only to
chin level. Repeat 10 times

Start with arms straight out in front. Swing
arms out to sides and return to front. Repeat
10 times

RISING EXERCISE

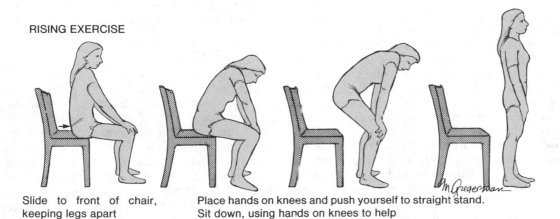

Slide to front of chair,
keeping legs apart

Place hands on knees and push yourself to straight stand.
Sit down, using hands on knees to help

Repeat 3–5 times using hands less and legs more each
time. Repeat exercise without using hands to help

Figure 78.3 Exercise for weakness and orthostatic hypotension after prolonged bed rest. Patient must be out of bed 2 hr a day, morning, afternoon, and evening (for meals). Exercises are done 3 times a day. (Courtesy of Ms. Karen Ryder, Registered Occupational Therapist.)

men may faint while voiding if they have some urinary obstruction. Persons with recurrent micturition syncope should be advised to sit while urinating and to remain seated for a minute after urination.

Hypersensitivity of the carotid sinus is a controversial entity and probably an uncommon cause of syncope. Stimulation of the baroreceptors in the carotid sinus may provoke sympathetic relaxation and lead to hypotension with a normal heart rate; it may increase vagal activity leading to bradycardia without hypotension; or it may provoke abnormalities in the brainstem which lead to syncope without a change in circulatory dynamics. These mechanisms have been invoked in patients with long-standing and severe hypertension or with coronary or carotid arteriosclerosis. Older men wearing tight collars, women with cumbersome necklaces, or patients having large masses in the neck are predisposed to the problem. In some patients thought to have carotid sinus hypersensitivity, compression of the common or internal carotid arteries (or the external carotid, an important collateral in the case of a carotid occlusion) may lead to the symptoms of cerebral ischemia if the contralateral artery is not fully patent. While some authorities recommend provoking syncope by unilateral or bilateral carotid massage, this may be a dangerous maneuver and should be performed only with intravenous fluid running, ECG monitoring, and atropine at hand.

Syncope with *pulmonary embolism* is estimated to occur in 15 to 20% of cases (17). It may lead to prolonged unconsciousness, at times lasting for 10 to 15 min and often accompanied by a small seizure, and it may be followed by minor neurologic abnormalities, even when paradoxical embolization has not occurred.

Severe pain arising from any site may be followed immediately by a faint, occurring probably by a vasovagal mechanism.

CARDIAC ABNORMALITIES

Rhythm Disturbances

Heart block may reflect ischemic, infiltrative, or neoplastic lesions of the heart and may lead to syncope when the heart rate falls below 40 per min or if ineffective ventricular contraction occurs. Likewise, brady- or tachyarrhythmias without block may lead to cerebral symptoms or to syncope. Cardiac arrhythmias should be strongly considered in older patients or when unconsciousness occurs nocturnally or while seated or recumbent. A number of drugs may cause arrhythmias (e.g., quinidine, digitalis, tricyclic antidepressants, neuroleptics). Though premonitory warnings may be recalled (particularly gray-outs, sweating, mild nausea, and fear) palpitations are notoriously unreliable and should not be used to substantiate or refute the diagnosis of a cardiac arrhythmia. Most patients with cerebral symptoms due to cardiac arrhythmias have normal resting ECGs, or at most minor PR or QT prolongations (12). Therefore, 24-hour cardiac monitoring is usually essential in confirming this diagnosis. Particular attention should be paid to sustained tachycardia, bradycardia, paroxysmal blocks, and spells of asystole. Details regarding the diagnosis and management of patients with these problems are found in Chapter 56.

Outflow Obstruction

An obstruction to ventricular outflow due to rheumatic or calcific *aortic stenosis* may lead to syncope in older individuals. It nearly always follows exertion and is usually associated with chest pain. Unconsciousness may be prolonged and may be followed by neurological abnormalities. Similarly, idiopathic *hypertrophic subaortic stenosis* in patients of any age may lead to syncope by outlet obstruction after exercise or due to an arrhythmia at any time. The diagnostic approach to patients thought to have outflow obstruction from these causes is described in Chapter 57. *A left atrial myxoma* (very rare) may cause syncope by obstruction of blood flow when a patient leans over or exerts himself. *Cyanotic congenital heart disease* also leads to syncope after exercise or, rarely, during an airplane flight. Hypoxia and increased blood viscosity are contributing factors.

Myocardial Infarction

Acute myocardial infarction may present with syncope which may result from arrhythmia, low cardiac output, or severe pain. Embolization from a mural thrombus should be considered when syncope occurs during recovery from myocardial infarction.

METABOLIC ABNORMALITIES

Since some metabolic derangements (e.g., hypoglycemia or hypoxia) may lead to lasting damage, the physician should be very alert to the possibility of these problems in patients with syncope who have features or abnormalities characteristic of these derangements in their history or examination.

Hypoglycemia

Hypoglycemic syncope may occur in the adult when the blood glucose level is below 40 mg/100 ml. Hunger, palpitations, sweating, and anxiety nearly always occur 5 to 15 min before the patient loses consciousness. As the brain can survive for only about 10 min with a blood glucose of 20 mg/100 ml, the prophylactic administration of glucose is warranted in anyone who remains unconscious long enough for the physician to prepare the solution. Convulsions and incontinence commonly accompany hypoglycemic coma. The evaluation and management of hypoglycemia due to *exogenous insulin* is described in Chapter 69. *Reactive* hypoglycemia and *starvation* hypoglycemia (which may be due to insulinoma) usually produce near-syncope but not unconsciousness. These problems are described in Chapter 71. Mild hypoglycemic symptoms may also occur postprandially in patients who have had ulcer surgery, as part of the *dumping syndrome* (see Chapter 33).

Hypocapnia

Hyocapnia due to *hyperventilation* leads to syncope/near-syncope by decreasing cerebral blood flow through vasoconstriction of small arterioles throughout the brain. A pCO_2 of 25 mm Hg is sufficient to lower cerebral blood flow to levels at which symptoms occur; such a value may be produced in some persons by a few very deep breaths. Athletes preparing to race, musicians playing wind instruments, or anyone who is fearful or anxious may develop transient symptoms in this way. Tetany or carpopedal spasm may or may not precede the cerebral symptoms. Recovery is prompt if ventilation is slowed. The diagnosis and management of hyperventilation related to anxiety, the commonest cause of this problem, is described in Chapter 11.

Hypoxemia

Hypoxemia due to any primary cause may cause syncope/near-syncope. *Severe anemia* (see Chapter 46) may sufficiently deprive the brain of oxygen to lead to syncope after exercise; it may also predispose to syncope from any other cause. Asphyxiation due to *obstruction of the upper airway* should be considered in small children, patients with bad teeth, or in patients with masses about the neck. The "cafe coronary" due to laryngeal aspiration of food is usually betrayed by sudden collapse at the table. Patients with esophageal diverticula, however, may choke hours after a meal. Poisoning with *carbon monoxide* is suggested by a history of intentional or unintentional exposure to products of combustion (e.g., poorly ventilated space heaters, gas-burning engines in closed spaces). Manifestations may include prodromal headache and confusion plus bright pink color and prolonged unconsciousness.

Seizures are very common in patients with acute hypoxemia, and neurologic sequelae are the rule after unconsciousness lasting more than 1 or 2 min. The management of hypoxemic syncope depends entirely on prompt and accurate diagnosis in order to prevent recurrence or worsening of the primary cause of hypoxemia.

Drug Overdose

Overdose of some drugs may cause syncope/near-syncope due to orthostatic hypotension. These drugs include sedatives, which may produce venous pooling (particularly chloral hydrate, paraldehyde, and ethanol, and less often benzodiazepines and barbiturates) and all of the drugs listed as potential causes of autonomic impairment in Table 78.7. Stupor or coma due to the sedating effects of drug overdose are more common than transient cerebral symptoms (syncope/near-syncope) due to acute orthostatic hypotension.

INTRACRANIAL ABNORMALITIES

Seizure

A seizure may occur with or without warning in any position and may be the primary event leading to an episode of syncope. The diagnosis and management of seizure disorders is described in detail in Chapter 77.

Subarachnoid Hemorrhage

A brief period of unconsciousness at the beginning of subarachnoid hemorrhage is the rule. This diagnosis is strongly suggested when the constellation of headache, confusion, and neck stiffness follow shortly after a syncopal episode. Any patient who is confused and who develops headache during initial evaluation demands more scrutiny, even if meningismus has not yet developed. Such patients should be admitted for observation and evaluation.

Embolism or Thrombosis

Cerebral embolism or thrombosis may cause brief (TIA) or prolonged (CVA) unconsciousness if the basilar artery is affected. Rarely, a carotid occlusion may cause unconsciousness initially, even if the remaining vessels are patent. A carotid occlusion likewise may cause syncope or coma if the contralateral carotid is already occluded; in this instance, the period of unconsciousness is usually prolonged and seizures may occur; neurologic symptoms and signs nearly always are present simultaneously (near-syncope) or after the patient awakens (syncope). The ambulatory diagnosis and management of cerebrovascular disease is described in detail in Chapter 80.

Migraine

Migraine (see Chapter 76) may produce syncope/near-syncope, albeit rarely, due to spasm of the basilar artery or of the posterior cerebral arteries. Syncope which occurs with migraine is more often due to hyperventilation or to a vasovagal mechanism than to a central abnormality.

Increased Intracranial Pressure

Increased intracranial pressure, whether due to a brain tumor, trauma, or an obstruction to the ventricular system may result in syncope when a Valsalva maneuver is performed such as during straining at stool or bending over. The hallmarks are preexisting symptoms, papilledema, or neurologic signs.

Brainstem Compression

Rarely, brainstem compression due to a displaced fracture of C1 or of the odontoid process or to metastatic tumors or cystic anomalies of the posterior fossa may lead to syncope with movement of the neck which causes transient compression of critical structures of the brainstem. Associated neurologic abnormalities are the rule. The diagnosis and management of patients thought to have this problem require prompt hospital admission.

Selected Conditions which May Mimic Syncope

HYSTERICAL FAINT

Hysterical faints were common during Victorian times. Today they occur less commonly but are often more complex. Dramatic fainting usually occurs in a manner that avoids injury; the patient crumples to the ground, often on a carpet or in soft surroundings, the body becomes limp and respirations are shallow. The period of unconsciousness is variable but recovery is quite abrupt, with full consciousness occurring usually immediately as the eyes open. The period of unconsciousness with an hysterical faint may be embellished with movements resembling seizures, incontinence, tongue-biting, prolonged "twilight states," or paralyses, all of which may be diagnostically vexing. Often those patients will betray their state by having complete or partial memory of the spell, by showing purposeful movements during the episode, or by reproducing the spell when coaxed or when asked to hyperventilate. Chapter 11 provides additional detail regarding the evaluation and management of such patients, whose physical symptoms are invariably due to psychosocial stress.

DROP ATTACK

Drop attacks occur because of an abrupt loss of tone in the extensor muscles of the legs and trunk. These changes are produced by ischemia to the central midbrain or pons causing an abrupt and transitory ischemia of the descending pyramidal motor tracts. The precise pathophysiology of the spells is unclear. Drop attacks are frequently stereotyped and very brief. The patient is usually older, at risk for arteriosclerotic disease, and is often hypertensive. He describes a sudden loss of muscle power so that he crumples to the ground but recovers immediately. Incontinence is rare. These attacks are distinguished from syncope because loss of consciousness does not occur. The patient can, in fact, give a vivid account of the details of each spell. Such patients should be managed identically to those with transient ischemic attacks occurring in the posterior circulation (see Chapter 80).

NARCOLEPSY AND CATAPLEXY

Narcolepsy (see Chapter 82) causes sleeplike unconsciousness at unpredictable times during the day. An incomplete form of narcolepsy may exist, in which a person feels irresistibly sleepy without actually falling asleep. Attacks of *cataplexy* (spells causing the patient to fall to the ground due to a loss of muscle tone but without loss of consciousness) are often associated with narcolepsy. They are often triggered by laughing, sneezing, or a sudden startle.

Sleep paralysis (paralysis of the limbs for a minute or two upon awakening) and peculiar visual hallucinations on awakening or before falling asleep may also accompany narcolepsy. (See Chapter 82 for additional details.)

Overall Prognosis

The overall prognosis of syncope and near-syncope depends ultimately on the underlying disorder and upon any trauma or other morbidity which may have occurred as a consequence of losing consciousness. The simple faint, hyperventilation, venous pooling, or syncope with a Valsalva maneuver may occur repeatedly when the patient finds himself in the same circumstance and can be prevented if he avoids it. Drug-provoked syncope/near-syncope can be eliminated by discontinuating or decreasing the dose of the offending drug; and syncope due to intravascular volume deficit is usually amenable to therapy. While limiting exercise may prevent syncope due to cardiac outflow obstruction, surgical therapy is usually needed (particularly for aortic stenosis), and the prognosis depends on the outcome of the surgery. Cerebral symptoms due to cardiac arrhythmias can usually be eradicated by pacemaker or antiarrhythmic treatment. Similarly, most symptoms due to common metabolic or intracranial abnormalities are amenable to treatment.

DISEQUILIBRIUM OF MISCELLANEOUS ORIGINS

Some patients with relatively persistent "dizziness" do not have manifestations which make it possible to classify their problem as vertigo or near-syncope. Most of these persons have disequilibrium, or a sense of imbalance, which may be due to one of the following problems: cerebellar ataxia (see Chapter 75 for physical findings); multiple sensory deficits (3) (e.g., partial hearing, visual, and proprioceptive impairment); lower extremity weakness (e.g., from an old stroke or from disuse after a fracture or after a period of bedrest); pain in a weight-bearing joint; recently initiated drugs, especially sedatives; or the onset of a progressive central nervous system disease such as parkinsonism (see Chapter 79), normal pressure hydrocephalus (see Chapter 16), or CP angle tumor (see Chapter 93). These problems often occur in older persons, in debilitated persons (particularly chronic alcoholics), or in patients with long-standing diabetes. In these persons, cerebrovascular disease or autonomic neuropathy may cause periodic vertigo and near-syncope to be superimposed on their day-to-day problem with imbalance.

The evaluation of persons describing imbalance consists chiefly of obtaining a history of the duration, progression, and day-to-day characteristics of the problem, focusing upon the limitations imposed upon the usual activities and upon any falls or near accidents which may have occurred. In the physical examination, it is important to determine which of the many problems listed above may be contributing to the patient's symptoms.

Depending upon the individual patient, management by the generalist may include (a) referring the patient for correction of deafness or cataract (see Chapters 93 and 94); (b) obtaining a consultant's opinion whenever unexplained progressive symptoms are found (for example, cerebellar ataxia in a relatively healthy person); (c) obtaining the help of a physical therapist if weakness or the need for selecting a cane or a walker is apparent; (d) discontinuing any drugs which may be contributing to the patient's symptoms and avoiding drugs which may worsen symptoms (see Tables 78.2 and 78.7); and (e) assuring that the patient's home environment is as safe as possible and that others in the household are aware of the risks which should be avoided (these objectives may be most effectively accomplished by having the patient evaluated in his home by a physical therapist or a nurse from a home health agency, see Chapter 3).

References

General

Lee, JE, Killip, T and Plum, F: Episodic unconsciousness. In *Diagnostic Approaches to Presenting Syndromes*, edited by JA Barondess. Williams & Wilkins, Baltimore, 1971.
   A detailed discussion of normal physiology and specific causes of syncope.
Troost, BT: Dizziness and vertigo in vertebrovasilar disease: I. Peripheral and systemic causes of dizziness, II. Central causes and vertebrobasilar disease. *Curr Concents Cerebrovasc Dis* 14: 21, 25, 1979.
   Excellent brief review of vertigo.
Wayne, HH: Syncope—physiological considerations and an analysis of the clinical characteristics in 510 patients. *Am J Med 30*: 418, 1961.
   A retrospective compilation of consecutive cases in one hospital.

Wolfson, RJ: Symposium on vertigo. *Otolargynol Clin North Am* 6: No. 1, 1973.
   Excellent coverage of all aspects of vertigo.

Specific

1. Bannister, R: Chronic autonomic failure with postural hypotension. *Lancet* 2: 404, 1979.
2. Barany, R: Diagnosis of disease of the otolith apparatus. *J Laryngol Otol* 36: 229, 1921.
3. Brandt, T and Daroff, RB: The multisensory physiological and pathological vertigo syndromes. *Ann Neurol* 7: 195, 1980.
4. Caird, FI, Andrews, GR and Kennedy, RD: Effect of posture on blood pressure in the elderly. *Br Heart J* 35: 527, 1973.
5. Drachman, DA and Hart, CW: An approach to the dizzy patient. *Neurology* 22: 323, 1972.
6. Ewing, DJ, Campbell, IW and Clarke, BF: Assessment of cardiovascular effects in diabetic autonomic neuropathy and prognostic implications. *Ann Intern Med* 92: 308, 1980.
7. Glassock, ME, III and Hayes, JW: Pitfalls in the diagnosis of acoustic and other cerebellopontine angle tumors. *Laryngoscope* 83: 1038, 1973.
8. Hart, CW: Evaluation of post-traumatic vertigo. *Otolaryngol Clin North Am* 6: 157, 1973.
9. Hybels, RL: Drug toxicity of the inner ear. *Med Clin North Am* 63: 309, 1979.
10. Ibrahim, MM: Localization of lesion in patients with idiopathic orthostatic hypotension. *Br Heart J* 37: 868, 1975.
11. Johnson, RJ, Smith, AC, Spalding, JMK and Wollner, L: Effect of posture on blood-pressure in elderly patients. *Lancet* 1: 731, 1965.
12. Jonas, S, Klein, I and Dimant, J: Importance of Holter monitoring in patients with periodic cerebral symptoms. *Ann Neurol* 1: 470, 1977.
13. Jongkees, LBW: The caloric test and its value in evaluation of the patient with vertigo. *Otolaryngol Clin North Am* 6: 73, 1973.
14. Noble, RJ: The patient with syncope. *JAMA* 237: 1372, 1977.
15. Page, JM: Audiologic tests in the differential diagnosis of vertigo. *Otolaryngol Clin North Am* 6: 53, 1973.
16. Rubin, W: Electronystagmography and its value in the diagnosis of vertigo. *Otolaryngol Clin North Am* 6: 95, 1973.
17. Thames, MD, Alpert, JS and Dalen, JE: Syncope in patients with pulmonary embolism. *JAMA* 238: 2509, 1977.
18. Weiss, NS: Relation of high blood pressure to headache, epistaxis, and selected other symptoms. *N Engl J Med* 287: 631, 1972.
19. Wood, CD and Graybiel, A: The antimotion sickness drugs. *Otolaryngol Clin North Am* 6: 301, 1973.

CHAPTER SEVENTY-NINE

Common Disorders of Movement: Tremor and Parkinson's Syndrome

BARRY GORDON, M.D., Ph.D., and L. RANDOL BARKER, M.D

TREMOR

Definition and Classification

Tremor is the involuntary rhythmic or semi-rhythmic motion of antagonistic muscle groups.

Clinically, there are three major types of tremor—resting, postural, and intention (see Table 79.1)—which can be identified readily by history and examination. Each type of tremor points to a group of specific underlying conditions (Table 79.2).

Evaluation of the Patient with Tremor

HISTORY

The history is useful both in assessing the significance of the tremor to the patient and in classifying the type of tremor.The following questions may be particularly useful:

1. How long ago did the tremor begin? How did it begin (slowly and insidiously, or suddenly, which suggests a drug-induced tremor or a vascular event)? Where did the tremor begin? Where did it spread to, and over what time period?
2. What part(s) of the body is affected by the tremor, and under what circumstances (rest, motion, active reaching)?
3. Has the tremor interfered with activities such as eating, dressing, or handwriting? Has it caused the patient to modify significantly his usual activities, especially socially valued activities such as playing cards, engaging in sports, or going to social gatherings?
4. What medication(s) is the patient taking currently and what is the temporal relationship to the onset of the tremor?

Almost all tremors are made worse by anxiety, so that this is not an important historical point in differentiating the type of tremor.

EXAMINATION

The classification of tremors is based chiefly upon findings in the physical examination, specifically upon the character of the tremor in the resting state and during voluntary motion.

Examination for Resting Tremor. The patient should sit with his hands resting on his lap and his head unsupported. Often it is best to have the subject distracted by conversation. Under these conditions, relatively slow (3 to 5 per sec) flexion-extension tremor of the metacarpophalangeal joints ("pill-rolling" tremor), pronation-supination of the forearm, or flexion-extension of the wrists or feet may be seen. If the patient becomes too relaxed, the tremor may lessen or disappear; typically, it disappears during sleep. Resting tremor is typical of Parkinson's syndrome (see below, p. 863) and other conditions affecting the basal ganglia.

Examination for Postural Tremor. The patient should hold his hands outstretched, with eyes closed, and the physician should observe whether there is any tremor in the hands, arms, or head. A relatively rapid (6 to 12 per sec) medium to high amplitude remor is abnormal. Some degree of hand or finger tremor is normal. Postural tremor is typical of exaggerated physiologic and essential tremor. A side-to-side tremor of the head (titubation) may also be noted; usually this is an expression of essential (senile) but not physiologic tremor.

Examination for Intention Tremor. The patient should reach for the examiner's finger with his hands (finger-nose-finger testing) or feet (toe-to-finger testing). Normal subjects frequently have a very fine lateral tremor of the distal limb during purposeful motion. Exaggeration of this tremor, with worsening as greater precision is demanded and often with continuation for a fraction of a second after the action is completed, is characteristic of an intention tremor. The combination of intention tremor and

Table 79.1
Principal Features of Common Tremors

Feature	Three Major Types of Tremor		
	Resting	Postural	Intention
Situation(s) in which the tremor is present	Resting posture, in awake patient; extinguished or decreased with purposeful movement; absent during sleep	Posture involving effort against gravity (e.g., outstretched arms, holding an object); not present in resting limb	Purposeful movement of extremity from one point to another
Frequency of tremor	3–12/sec (usually 3–5)	6–12/sec	3–5/sec
Clinical conditions	Parkinsonian syndrome	Exaggerated physiologic tremor Essential tremor	Cerebellar dysfunction

Table 79.2
Conditions Associated with the Three Major Types of Tremor[a]

RESTING TREMOR
  Parkinson's disease
  Secondary parkinsonism: postencephalitic, toxic (phenothiazines, reserpine, carbon monoxide, manganese, carbon disulfide), tumor, trauma, vascular, metabolic (hypoparathyroidism, chronic hepatocerebral degeneration)
  Heterogeneous disorders with parkinsonian features: striatonigral degeneration, olivopontocerebellar atrophy, progressive supranuclear palsy, Wilson's disease, Huntington's disease, normal pressure hydrocephalus
POSTURAL TREMOR
  Exaggerated physiologic tremor
    Stress-induced: anxiety, fright, fatigue
    Endocrine: thyrotoxicosis, hypoglycemia, pheochromocytoma
    Drugs: any sympathomimetics, caffeine, theophylline, levodopa, lithium, tricyclic antidepressants, phenothiazines, butyrophenones, thyroid hormone, hypoglycemic agents, withdrawal from alcohol and sedative-hypnotic drugs
  Essential tremor
    Familial (may be autosomal dominant)
    Sporadic
    Senile
    With other movement disorders: parkinsonism, torsion dystonia, spasmodic torticollis
INTENTION TREMOR (CEREBELLAR DYSFUNCTION)
  Cerebellar degeneration, atrophy, infarction
  Multiple sclerosis
  Wilson's disease
  Drugs—toxins: phenytoin, barbiturates, lithium, alcohol, mercury, 5-fluorouracil
  Miscellaneous cerebellar and cerebellofugal lesions

[a] Adapted from J. Jankovic and S. Fahn: Physiologic and pathologic tremors. *Annals of Internal Medicine, 93:* 460, 1980.

dysmetria (inaccuracy in actually touching a point at the termination of a voluntary movement) is typical of cerebellar disease and related problems.

Common Conditions Presenting as Tremor

PARKINSON'S SYNDROME

The typical resting tremor of Parkinson's syndrome is discussed on page 864.

PHYSIOLOGIC AND EXAGGERATED PHYSIOLOGIC TREMOR

Normally, some people have a barely perceptible postural tremor that may be best appreciated by placing a piece of paper over their outstretched hands. Exaggeration of this physiologic tremor is usually due to a transient condition; it occurs most commonly under stress, after ingestion of caffeine or another stimulant, in withdrawal from alcohol or other sedating drugs (where an underlying essential tremor may also be unmasked), and as part of a variety of generalized metabolic or systemic illnesses (see Table 79.2). With severe disease, this kind of tremor becomes generalized, and there is widespread hyperexcitability. Other manifestations of this central excitatory state include myoclonic jerks, delirium, hallucinations, and seizures. A florid example of this state is delirium tremens; less extreme forms are very common.

Treatment. The major step in management is identification and removal of the offending cause; resolution of the tremor confirms the diagnosis of exaggerated physiologic tremor. Discontinuation of tremor-producing drugs usually leads to prompt resolution of the problem. With severe metabolic disturbances, it may take 1 to 2 weeks for the tremulousness to subside, even after the underlying abnormalities have been corrected. If the underlying condition cannot be eliminated, propranolol (see dosage information below) usually abolishes the tremor; in fact, if it does not do so, the tremor is probably misclassified. For persons subject to situational anxiety, manifested as exaggerated physiologic tremor and/or heightened perception of cardiac activity, prophylactic treatment with propranolol before an anxiety-producing situation (for example a public address) may be helpful (see Chapter 12).

ESSENTIAL TREMOR (SENILE TREMOR, FAMILIAL TREMOR)

In its prototypical form, this is a marked postural tremor in the hands, which also may involve the head (typically with side-to-side rotatory tremor). This tremor resembles an exaggerated physiologic tremor, and a common mechanism may underlie the two tremors. A major difference is that essential tremor is a relatively constant problem while exaggerated physiologic tremor is usually related to a transient condition. Frequently, intention tremor (see below) is present as well.

Essential tremor is quite common; in various forms, it has been reported in up to 8% of a normal population. The family history is positive in 25 to 50% of cases, and many families show autosomal dominant transmission. Onset is insidious, starting anywhere from childhood (familial) to old age (senile). There is a wide spectrum of severity; some patients show a mild, almost unnoticeable, exaggeration of physiologic tremor; in other patients, the tremor is totally disabling, making self-care and feeding impossible so that the patient becomes a social embarrassment. When the tremor has had its onset in late middle life, its progression is typically quite slow, and years pass before deterioration becomes apparent. With aging, the frequency of the tremor may diminish while the amplitude increases. When the condition begins earlier, an accurate prognosis is difficult; however, when there is a family history of essential tremor, the experience of others in the family is helpful in anticipating a patient's course.

Many patients report that alcohol markedly reduces the amplitude of their tremor within 15 to 30 min (10). Some patients use alcohol as a method of treatment without consulting a physician; this may lead to alcohol addiction and should be considered in the evaluation of alcoholic patients.

As with most tremors, anxiety and situational stress markedly enhance the symptom. Essential tremor can occur in association with tics, dystonic motions of the head or feet, choreiform movements, and even resting tremors (4).

Some older patients with essential tremor, especially those who may have had a prior stroke or other incapacitating illness, are mistakenly thought to have Parkinson's syndrome. In fact, essential tremor may be seen in 5 to 10% of patients with Parkinson's syndrome; furthermore, L-dopa may cause exaggerated physiologic tremor as a side effect. However, the patient with essential tremor can usually be distinguished readily from a patient with Parkinson's syndrome, by checking for other distinctive features of extrapyramidal disease (see below).

Treatment. When essential tremor is asymptomatic, no treatment is needed. If the problem is mild, reassurance and treatment of transient situation-specific anxiety with agents such as diazepam (Valium), 2.5 to 5 mg once or twice daily, may be sufficient. Used judiciously, small amounts of alcohol (e.g., one glass of wine) can be quite helpful in many of the situations where tremor would be particularly bothersome (10).

If the condition is significantly symptomatic, propranolol is usually quite effective in reducing the amplitude of the tremor to the point where it no longer interferes with writing, eating, drinking, and other daily activities (20). It is best to begin with a small initial dose (10 mg, 2 or 3 times daily), increasing to a maximum of 300 to 400 mg daily while monitoring benefits and side effects. For patients intolerant of propranolol, the β_1 selective blocker, metaprolol (Lopressor) may be a suitable substitute. Precautions and additional information about the use of these two β-blocking agents is found in Chapter 59.

When essential tremor is extremely severe or disabling and is not responsive to symptomatic therapy, referral to a neurologist is indicated. For selected patients, stereotactic surgery has been used with some success.

TREMOR DUE TO CEREBELLAR DYSFUNCTION

The finding of intention tremor points to cerebellar or cerebellar-related disease. Conditions which superficially may mimic this aspect of cerebellar disease are marked physiologic tremor or essential tremor (which may impair purposeful movements) and proprioceptive sensory neuropathy. Careful assessment of all of the patient's signs and symptoms usually enables the physician to distinguish these conditions from cerebellar dysfunction (see Table 79.3 which compares cerebellar and posterior column incoordination). Some patients with cerebellar-related disease have a low frequency (3 to 5 per sec) postural tremor as well as a typical intention tremor.

Unilateral intention tremor in a hand and/or leg points to ipsilateral disease of the cerebellar hemisphere; infarction is the most frequent cause. When tremor is bilateral, it may reflect more generalized

Table 79.3
Characteristics of Cerebellar and Sensory Posterior Column Incoordination

Observation or Examination	Cerebellar	Sensory and/or Posterior Column
Influence of vision	Elimination of visual aid (night, eyes closed) does not affect symptoms or signs	Symptoms and signs markedly increased by eliminating visual aid
Sensation	No necessary sensory problems (although may be superimposed, as in alcoholic cerebellar degeneration and sensory neuropathy)	Impaired position and vibration sense is *sine qua non* for diagnosis
Finger-nose-finger and/or toe-finger testing of coordination	Could be marked intention tremor and dysmetria (inaccuracy); affected limbs depend upon site of lesion(s)	Marked intention tremor and dysmetria (inaccuracy), usually most marked in legs
Gait	Wide-based, asynchronous limb movements (depending upon nature of the lesion)	Wide-based, high-stepping, foot-slapping (steppage) gait (often due to foot drop from motor neuropathy)
Romberg testing	Patient equally unsteady with eyes open or closed (uninterpretable Romberg)	Patient can find a stable position with eyes open, but becomes markedly unsteady with eyes closed (positive Romberg)

cerebellar degeneration (carcinomatous, drug-induced) or reversible drug effect (particularly phenytoin (Dilantin)). Disease of the anterior midline cerebellum more typically presents as gait ataxia (common etiologies in adults are alcoholic cerebellar degeneration and carcinomatous cerebellar degeneration); and disorders of the inferior midline cerebellum present typically as posture imbalance (in adults, infarcts involving the posterior inferior cerebellar artery are the most common causes).

With the exception of drug-induced cerebellar dysfunction (see Table 79.2), which should be managed by discontinuation or dose reduction of the drug, a patient with newly diagnosed cerebellar disease should be referred promptly to a neurologist for help in obtaining an accurate diagnosis and prognosis. Most of the diseases producing cerebellar dysfunction are not amenable to treatment, and there is little that can be done to treat the coordination problems symptomatically.

PARKINSON'S SYNDROME

Definition

Parkinson's syndrome consists of a resting tremor, rigidity on passive motion of the extremities, bradykinesia (slowing of voluntary movements), and abnormalities of posture and gait. It can result from any process which affects the basal ganglia of the brain (see Table 79.2).

Parkinson's disease is a specific clinical and neuropathologic entity and the most common cause of chronic Parkinson's syndrome. It is a sporadic disease of unknown etiology. Neuropathologically, there is degeneration of brain structures, including, but not limited to, the subtantia nigra, which normally sends dopaminergic projections to the nuclei of the basal ganglia. In most patients, the disease begins after the age of 40, with the peak incidence in the sixth and seventh decade. The approximate prevalence of Parkinson's disease in persons over 50 is 1%. The problem is equally common in men and women.

Postencephalitic Parkinson's syndrome was seen in a large number of victims of the global epidemic of encephalitis following World War I. Members of this cohort no longer account for newly diagnosed cases of Parkinson's syndrome, although presumably some new cases are due to sporadic encephalitides which have occurred since the epidemic.

Drug-induced parkinsonism is very common in persons taking neuroleptic antipsychotic drugs. This problem is usually transient and reversible. It is described in Chapter 15.

Differential Diagnosis of Parkinson's Syndrome

PARKINSON'S DISEASE

The diagnosis of Parkinson's disease is based entirely on the clinical evaluation of the patient. If slowly progressive tremor, rigidity, and bradykinesia are present in a person over 50, the diagnosis is simple to make. When antiparkinsonian drugs are initiated, prompt improvement helps to confirm the diagnosis of idiopathic Parkinson's disease.

DRUG-INDUCED PARKINSONISM (see Chapter 15)

The diagnosis of neuroleptic-induced parkinsonism is not difficult. This problem usually commences within 1 to 4 weeks of initiating or increasing the dose of a neuroleptic antipsychotic drug. A similar problem was seen in the past in psychotic patients treated with high doses of reserpine, a practice which has been virtually discontinued.

OTHER CONDITIONS

Any disease process that affects the basal ganglia and/or their connections can produce manifestations of Parkinson's syndrome; and a number of other central nervous system diseases may have features which mimic parkinsonism. In any patient with presumed Parkinson's disease in whom the disorder is atypical (e.g., very early or very late age of onset, striking predominance of one of the principal manifestations of parkinsonism, rapid onset, marked asymmetry or prominent neurologic findings in addition to extrapyramidal manifestations), another condition should be considered. Because accurate diagnosis is essential to both prognosis and management, these atypical patients should always be referred to a neurologist for evaluation. For most of the conditions causing or resembling parkinsonism other clinical clues may be noted on initial evaluation.

Wilson's Disease (Hepatolenticular Degeneration)

This is an autosomal recessive condition. It is due to ceruloplasmin deficiency which leads to copper accumlation throughout the body, expressed clinically in the liver, the eyes, and the central nervous system. Parkinsonian features in a patient under the age of 40, particularly under the age of 30, should prompt an investigation for this condition. Chronic liver disease may be present at the onset of neurologic symptoms. Kayser-Fleischer rings (green or golden deposits of copper in Descemet's membrane of the cornea), blood ceruloplasmin level less than 20 mg/100 ml, and urine copper in excess of 100 μg per day are the usual criteria for this diagnosis.

Degenerative Diseases

Huntington's chorea. This autosomal dominant condition is due to degeneration of the caudate, putamen, and cerebral cortex. It usually begins in midlife with symptoms of dementia and with abnormal movements (tics, chorea, athetosis), but it may begin with or include prominent rigidity.

Alzheimer's disease. This disorder can present at times with a parkinsonian-like rigidity, immobility, and dementia evolving over many months to several years. However, usually tremor is not present; the rigidity is actually a "gegenhalten" (i.e., resistance to passive motion is present in all directions but varies with the force and speed applied by the examiner); and intellectual deterioration is extremely marked. It is important to note that this diagnosis does not exclude coexisting Parkinson's disease, since, as noted below, Alzheimer's and Parkinson's disease frequently occur in the same patient.

Atypical degenerative conditions involving the basal ganglia, such as progressive supranuclear palsy, pallidal atrophy, and some atypical spinal-cerebellar syndromes may present as a parkinsonian syndrome. These conditions often have other clinical features, a positive family history, or complete unresponsiveness to L-dopa, which should alert the clinician to the possibility of an alternate diagnosis.

Hydrocephalus, and Normal Pressure Hydrocephalus. Frontal lobe-like apathetic and immobile behavior, apraxic gait, and rigidity have sometimes led to the mistaken diagnosis of Parkinson's disease in patients with these conditions.

Subdural Hematomas and Multiple Cerebral Infarctions

Sometimes the demented, immobile, and spastic/rigid state resulting from these conditions can mimic Parkinson's disease. The presence of pyramidal tract signs is an important clue to the presence of one of these conditions.

Metabolic Disorders

Subacute metabolic encephalopathies (hepatic, pulmonary, or renal) can produce symptoms which superficially resemble Parkinson's syndrome. The metabolic abnormality underlying the patient's neurologic manifestations should easily be recognized in these patients. Some patients with severe hepatic failure, especially patients with portocaval shunts, may have degeneration of the basal ganglia, producing a parkinsonian picture (hepatocerebral degneration).

Manifestations of Parkinson's Disease

The onset of symptoms is insidious; the patient usually cannot specify a beginning of his disease and is often not initially fully aware of its extent. Most of the time, the earliest presentation of symptoms is asymmetric or even clearly unilateral. The patient may notice, for example, tremor and rigidity of only one limb; the physician, on closer examination, may discover mild signs on the contralateral side to confirm the diagnosis. As the disease progresses, these asymmetries may or may not be maintained. Many patients, even with advanced disease, recognize that one side is worse than the other.

RESTING TREMOR

Tremor is the initial complaint in 70% of patients with Parkinson's disease. It is a relatively slow tremor with a 3 to 5 per sec rate, usually most prominent in the hands as a "pill-rolling" (metacarpal-phalangeal flexion and extension) or in the arms, as forearm pronation and supination. Sometimes it involves the lips and tongue, but it is relatively uncommon for it to involve the whole head. The latter feature, plus the fact that it is present at rest and usually decreases or disappears when the limb is used, distinguishes the parkinsonian tremor from essential tremor (see above, p. 861). The tremor is accentuated when the patient becomes excited or uses the opposite limb. There is frequently an intention tremor superimposed on the resting tremor.

RIGIDITY

Rigidity is abnormal resistance to passive movement, which is typically present throughout the whole range of motion, in both extensor and flexor muscle groups. Therefore, the limb gives the examiner a feeling of a plastic or lead pipe resistance. "Cog-wheel rigidity" is the ratcheting sensation often superimposed on this type of rigidity; it is not an expression of the resting tremor (a common misconception), but instead seems to be a separate kind of tremor, perhaps an exaggeration of physiologic tremor brought out by the rigidity itself. "Cog-wheeling" is not specific for Parkinson's disease; it may coexist with rigidity of any cause.

BRADYKINESIA

Patients with Parkinson's disease have difficulty initiating movements and their movements are slow. In contrast to the almost unconscious way that normal persons utilize their limbs, the Parkinson's patient consciously must force the limb to move; and what movements do occur are usually quite slow (bradykinetic). Speech gradually becomes soft and slow and is delivered in a monotone. Even automatic movements such as blinking and facial expression are suppressed. When bradykinesia is extreme, the patient may sit helplessly immobile for hours, expressionless and unblinking.

Since rigidity and bradykinesia can occur independently of each other, bradykinesia cannot be a consequence of rigidity (although this is a common misconception). This becomes apparent when treatment markedly decreases a patient's rigidity but has no effect on his bradykinesia.

POSTURAL ABNORMALITIES

Patients with Parkinson's disease sit and stand with a stooped, flexed posture of the head, trunk, arms, and legs. Tone abnormalities may produce an ulnar flexion deformity of the fingers, distinguished from that of rheumatoid arthritis by the lack of demonstrable joint and synovial disease.

GAIT ABNORMALITIES

Parkinsonian patients may have a great deal of difficulty initiating gait, related to their general bradykinesia. They may be unable to rise from a chair or, once standing, be unable to initiate stepping motions (apraxia of gait). For a variety of reasons, they have poor control of balance with a tendency to fall forward and backward; typically, they will be aware of beginning to fall but will be unable to make corrective movements to prevent the fall. When the patient with Parkinson's disease does begin to walk, his steps are short and shuffling. The tendency to fall forward and the partial attempt to prevent this, may lead to a festinating ("hurrying") propulsive gait. Even after walking is initiated, the patient may suddenly freeze while going through doorways or while attempting to make a turn. A common pattern is to have difficulty initiating gait, but then be capable of making short shuffling steps which lengthen into a normal stride—only to freeze again upon reaching a doorway. This transient freezing may throw the patient completely off balance.

OTHER ASSOCIATED SYMPTOMS OR SIGNS

Seborrhea and *excessive perspiration* are both common; the former may be due to hypothalamic release of excess sebotrophic hormone and the latter to disordered central temperature regulation.

Constipation is quite prominent in many patients, representing both inactivity and the side effects of anticholinergic drugs. Constipation can progress to obstipation, large bowel obstruction, megacolon, and volvulus of the sigmoid.

Dysphagia is a common complaint in Parkinson's disease. Some patients become completely incapable of swallowing. This problem may be due to incoordination of the inferior pharyngeal constrictors and perhaps of the other muscles involved in swallowing.

Sialorrhea (increased salivation) is probably explained by hypokinesia of swallowing, rather than by overproduction of saliva.

Urinary hesitancy/urinary retention may be due to the disease itself but it may also be due to other urinary problems which afflict older patients (such as prostatic hypertrophy) and which are aggravated by immobility and by anticholinergic drugs.

Orthostatic hypotension is common and may be caused by the disease itself or by levodopa therapy (see below). The degenerative process in Parkinson's disease affects not only the substantia nigra but also other regions of the brainstem and spinal cord, including the intermediolateral sympathetic cell column of the spinal cord. In this respect, Parkinson's disease might be included on a continuum of orthostatic conditions along with the Shy-Drager syndrome and idiopathic orthostatic hypotension. The Shy-Drager syndrome (17) begins with evidence of autonomic dysfunction (*i.e.*, episodes of hypo- and/or hypertension or impotence). It progresses after several years to show many of the features of Parkinson's disease, particularly rigidity, which may respond to levodopa. The intermediolateral cell column and the basal ganglia show pathologic changes. In patients with isolated idiopathic orthostatic hypoten-

sion, often only the intermediolateral cell column is found to be diseased (2).

Sensory Symptoms. Many patients with Parkinson's disease complain of a tightness or a pulling sensation in their affected extremities without objective sensory deficit. The basis for these symptoms is not clear, but treatment of the disease often alleviates them.

Two *abnormal reflexes* are usually found in parkinsonian patients: (a) the palmomental reflex (contraction of the ipsilateral mentalis muscle, producing wrinkling of the chin, elicited by stroking the palm near the base of the thumb), and (b) an exaggerated glabellar reflex (contraction of the orbicularis oculi muscles after repeatedly tapping the frontal bone superior to the bony septum of the nose; in a normal person, this reflex fatigues afters repeated tapping). Neither of these reflexes is specific for Parkinson's syndrome.

Depression (14). A large proportion of parkinsonian patients develop a depressive illness having either predominantly endogenous or reactive features (see Chapter 14). Some studies have found a close correlation between the severity of depression and the severity of physical impairment; others have found these two manifestations to be independent of each other.

Dementia (16). Up to 30% of patients with Parkinson's disease will develop an irreversible dementia syndrome. The dementia in many patients seems to be due to typical Alzheimer's disease, which for some reason occurs with a higher than expected frequency with Parkinson's disease (11). A parkinsonian patient who develops dementia should be evaluated like any other demented patient, in order to rule out potentially treatable conditions (see Chapter 16). The relationship of cognitive deterioration to antiparkinsonian drugs should always be considered, as the problem may be reversible (see below, p. 869). Delirium, as discussed below, is seen occasionally in patients with Parkinson's disease—but as a drug side effect, not as a manifestation of the disease itself.

Course of Parkinson's Disease

The course of Parkinson's disease varies substantially among individual patients. This variation is due to a combination of the temporal progression of the disease itself; the variable impact of treatment on individual symptoms (see below); the patient's mental adaptation to his illness (as distinct from those mental changes which may be part of the disease); the amount of social and rehabilitative support the patient receives; the complications of bradykinesia, especially falls and prolonged bed rest; and drug side effects.

Table 79.4 divides the "typical" course of Parkinson's disease into five stages, indicating for each stage the principal manifestations of the disease and the impact on the patient's overall function. These stages of parkinsonism occur eventually in most patients, usually over a time span of 5 to 15 years. As discussed in the following section, drug treatment and supportive therapy can significantly modify the course of Parkinson's disease; however, neuronal degeneration progresses despite treatment, and the patient's symptoms ultimately fail to respond to treatment.

A rough indication of the prognosis of "untreated" patients with Parkinson's disease comes from a study of patients followed before the L-dopa era (3). In this study, the average survival after diagnosis was 9 years; the prognosis was best when tremor was the major manifestation at the time of diagnosis. Twenty-five percent of patients were severely disabled or dead 5 years after the diagnosis; 66% after 10 years; 80% after 15 years. There was a small, very atypical group, still ambulatory 20 years after the diagnosis of Parkinson's disease. Deaths are generally due to bronchopneumonia, urinary tract infection, thromboembolism, or severe malnutrition.

Pharmacologic Management

OVERVIEW

The current pharmacotherapy of Parkinson's disease is based upon what is known of neurotransmission in the basal ganglia of the brain. The two major neurotransmitters found in these regions are dopamine and acetylcholine. It is hypothesized that the smooth control of voluntary movements depends upon a delicate balance between dopaminergic and cholinergic activity. Imbalance in these transmitter systems is the apparent basis for some movement disorders. Parkinson's disease, in which dopamine depletion follows damage to the source of dopamine (the substantia nigra), is attributed to a deficiency of dopamine and a relative excess of cholinergic activity.

The antiparkinsonian drugs currently used are either *anticholinergic* or *dopaminergic*; the fact that drugs in these two groups ameliorate the symptoms of Parkinson's disease supports the pathophysiologic concept of neurotransmitter imbalance.

To obtain the best results with drug therapy for Parkinson's disease, *the approach to each patient must be individualized.* Systematic monitoring for the benefits and side effects of treatment and careful (often frequent) adjustment of the medical regimen are the mainstays of this approach. Combination treatment with dopaminergic and anticholinergic agents is needed for optimal results in most patients with moderately advanced symptoms. Even the most skillfully tailored regimen rarely controls all symptoms of Parkinson's disease, and it is important to explain this to the patient and his family from the outset. Eventually, all patients with Parkinson's disease can be expected to become unresponsive to medical therapy.

There is evidence that L-dopa, the most effective of the available drugs for Parkinson's disease, becomes much less effective after 3 or 4 years of use (8), although some investigators have disagreed with this view (13). The progressive loss of effectiveness seems to be further complicated by increasing sensitivity to the side effects of this drug. Therefore, it seems prudent to limit the initial use of L-dopa, reserving this drug for a time when the patient's disease begins

Table 79.4
Five Stages of "Typical" Parkinson's Disease[a]

Stage	Principal Manifestations	Overall Functional Status
1	Unilateral involvement, blank facies, affected arm in semiflexed position with tremor and diminished swing, patient leans to affected side. Gait slightly affected or normal	Patient can continue most activities as usual except those requiring quick motor responses (playing tennis, for example). Social embarrassment may be a problem
2	(Usually within 1 to 2 years of Stage 1.) Bilateral involvement with early postural changes (stooped); slow shuffling gait with decreased excursion of legs; executes turns slowly and deliberately	Patient usually must retire, if still working. High risk of becoming withdrawn (reactive depression) and abandoning valued social and recreational activities (although physical impairment may not prohibit them)
3	Pronounced gait disturbance with postural instability and tendency to fall	Patient begins to need assistance with some tasks because of slowness in accomplishing them (*e.g.*, dressing, packing a suitcase)
4	Significant disability; ambulation limited and only with assistance because of marked difficulty in standing and tendency to fall	Patient needs almost constant supervision and requires assistance in completing most activities of daily living
5	Complete invalidism; confined to bed or chair; unable to stand or walk even with assistance; head becomes flexed on trunk; speech barely audible; face expressionless and blinking infrequent	Patient requires total care; death from aspiration or other form of infection related to immobilization

[a] Adapted from R. Duvoisin: Parkinsonism. In *Clinical Symposia, Vol. 28*, No. 1, published by CIBA Pharmaceutical Co., Summit, N.J., 1976.

to interfere appreciably with his life. Since many patients (or their families) will have heard about L-dopa and will expect it to be prescribed from the onset of treatment, it is essential for the physician to explain to the patient and the patient's family the sequence of drug therapy which will be tried.

Table 79.5 summarizes a *stepwise approach to medical management* which most authorities would recommend; and Table 79.6 summarizes practical information about currently available drugs. For persons who are minimally affected at the time of diagnosis, it may be reasonable to delay medical treatment and to encourage the patient to decide when symptoms are interfering with valued activities; however, only a small proportion of patients are likely to

be in this category at the time of diagnosis, as most will wait until their symptoms are troublesome before consulting their physician. Once the symptoms of Parkinson's disease begin to interfere with valued activities, drug treatment should be initiated. At this point, individual consideration is essential in deciding whether to use L-dopa from the outset. For most persons, a trial of anticholinergics should be the first step in treatment. In situations where prompt control of symptoms is essential, e.g., for public figures, technical workers who depend on fine manual skills, or persons threatened with job loss due due to their impairment, initial therapy with L-dopa (as carbidopa/levodopa, Sinemet, see below) is appropriate.

It is impossible to predict with certainty the degree

Table 79.5
Recommended Steps in Drug Therapy for Parkinson's Disease

Step	Patient Status	Treatment
1	Very mild symptoms which do not interfere with usual activities	None (explain rationale to patient)
2	Neurologic symptoms are troublesome but do not threaten income, psychological well-being, or social activities	Anticholinergic agent (substitute or add amantidine if patient unable to tolerate anticholinergic or if patient's symptoms transiently worse)
3	Disease advanced at the time of diagnosis; control inadequate with Step 2 strategy; or symptoms threaten employment or valued social activities	Add Sinemet to Step 2 regimen (and attempt to decrease dose of anticholinergic) or begin Sinemet alone
4	Initial response to Sinemet inadequate or diminished after good response (usually after 2 or more years)	Consider adding bromocriptine. Consultation with a neurologist advised

Table 79.6
Drugs Used for Parkinson's Disease

Drug	Available Preparation (mg)	Schedule	Starting Dose (mg)	Usual Daily Dosage Range (mg)
ANTICHOLINERGIC AGENTS				
Trihexyphenidyl (Artane)	Scored tablets—2, 5 Elixir—2/5 ml Time release capsule—5	t.i.d.–q.i.d. (after meals and bedtime) q.d. (after breakfast)	2 (Substitute for tablets, same total amount, after appropriate dose found)	1–10
Benztropine mesylate (Cogentin)	Tablets—0.5, 1, 2	q.d. (bedtime)	1	1–2 (0.5–6)
Procyclidine (Kemadrin)	Scored tablets—2, 5	t.i.d. (after meals)	2	1–10
Biperiden (Akineton)	Scored tablets—2	t.i.d.–q.i.d.	1	1–10
Cycrimine (Pagitane)	Tablets—1.25, 2.5	t.i.d.	1.25	1.25–10
Diphenhydramine hydrochloride (Benadryl)	Capsules—25, 50 Elixir—12.5/5 ml	t.i.d.–q.i.d.	50	50–200
DOPAMINERGIC AGENTS				
Levodopa (Larodopa, Dopar)	Tablets, capsules—100, 250, 500	q.i.d. with meals	100	1500–6000
Carbidopa/levodopa (Sinemet)	Scored tablets—10/100, 25/250, 25/100	t.i.d.–q.i.d. with meals (more often in selected patients)	10/100	40–200 carbidopa/ 400–2000 levodopa
Bromocriptine (Parlodel)	Tablets—2.5	t.i.d.	2.5	25–50
Amantidine (Symmetrel)	Capsule—100	b.i.d.	100	200–400

and duration of amelioration of symptoms which an individual patient can expect. Overall, however, most patients should have significant improvement in tremor, rigidity, and bradykinesia (in this order) and in activities affected by these symptoms. Anticholinergic therapy is effective in this respect in about one-half of patients while L-dopa produces good results in approximately 80%. Apart from reactive depression, mental deterioration usually does not respond to antiparkinsonian drugs. Depression which persists despite physical improvement, however, may respond to tricyclic antidepressants (1). (See Chapter 14.)

Carefully planned treatment of Parkinson's disease usually adds 3 or more functional years to the patient's life—a considerable benefit in otherwise active persons who acquire the disease relatively late in life.

ANTICHOLINERGIC DRUGS

Practical information about commonly prescribed drugs in this category is contained in Table 79.6. All of these agents cross the blood-brain barrier and are thought to work by blunting the cholinergic activity of the basal ganglia. The first five drugs listed in the table belong to the antimuscarinic class of anticholinergic agents. None of these five drugs is known to be superior to the others in the management of Parkinson's disease. They differ principally in the schedules recommended; two of them, Cogentin tablets and Artane sustained action capsules, offer the advantage of once daily administration. A patient who shows little response to one anticholinergic may respond to another. Therefore, a 2- to 4-week trial of several of these agents is reasonable in a patient with mild disease. In general, these drugs may be tested at the starting dose and increased every few days until the maximum recommended dose is reached or until the patient shows a response or unacceptable side effects. The maximum recommended doses are shown in the table. Some patients do not develop therapeutic anticholinergic levels and improvement in extrapyramidal symptoms until they are taking a relatively high dose; patients with neuroleptic-induced parkinsonism (see Chapter 15), in particular, should be given a trial of high dose anticholinergic treatment (19).

The antihistamine-anticholinergic diphenhydramine (Benadryl) has the least antiparkinsonian effect; it may be useful, however, because of its sedating property, in patients who are agitated and in patients who cannot tolerate the more pronounced side effects of the antimuscarinic drugs.

When L-dopa or amantidine is added to anticholinergic therapy, it is advisable to try to reduce the total daily dose of anticholinergic; usually this step will not alter the effect on parkinsonian symptoms, but it will decrease the risk of mental confusion, a side effect which may attend all the antiparkinsonian drugs.

The common *side effects* of anticholinergic drugs include dry mouth (which may be an advantage if the patient has marked sialorrhea), blurred vision, urinary retention, constipation, confusion, and agitation. The risk of these problems is increased if the patient is taking other drugs with anticholinergic properties, such as antihistamines, tricyclic antidepressants, or antispasmodics. As noted earlier, the patient should be questioned routinely about side effects with each increase in dose of anticholinergic drugs. Because other options are available, these drugs should be discontinued or the dose reduced whenever side effects add to the patient's distress. Angle closure glaucoma is an absolute contraindication to antimuscarinic agents.

Compared to other antiparkinson drugs (see below), the anticholinergics are relatively inexpensive (less than $10 per 100 tablets, capsules).

L-DOPA AND CARBIDOPA/L-DOPA (SINEMET)

Levodopa (L-dopa) penetrates the blood-brain barrier and is decarboxylated to dopamine, the neurotransmitter which is deficient in Parkinson's disease. When L-dopa alone is given, most of the drug is converted by enzymes outside the central nervous system into metabolites which are responsible for many of the "peripheral" side effects of the drug. Carbidopa is a peripheral decarboxylase inhibitor which is combined with L-dopa (usually in a 1:10 ratio) in Sinemet. Seventy to 100 mg of carbidopa per day will effectively saturate the extracerebral decarboxylating enzymes, thereby decreasing the severity of the peripheral side effects of L-dopa and permitting more of the administered dose of L-dopa to reach the brain. Because of these advantages, Sinemet is recommended when a patient requires L-dopa treatment. The principal disadvantage of Sinemet is the greater cost of this drug to the patient (in the range of $25 per 100 tablets, as compared to approximately $10 per 100 tablets of L-dopa).

Initiation and Adjustment of Treatment

Sinemet is available in scored tablets containing carbidopa/L-dopa (in milligrams) in the following ratios: 10/100, 25/250, and 25/100. The usual starting dose is 10/100, 3 times daily. The dosage of Sinemet should be increased until side effects appear or until the patient shows a satisfactory response. The daily dose should be increased no more frequently than every 3 days, since it may take several days for full clinical improvement to be seen or for side effects to be fully evident. Elderly patients or patients felt to be potentially more sensitive to the side effects of the drug should have their dose increased less often. Dosage can be increased to a total of six 10/100 tablets daily; at that point Sinemet 25/250 can be substituted, and increments of one-half to one tablet per day can be added, if needed, every 3 days until a satisfactory response or the usual maximum dose (eight tablets) is reached. The increased dose should be given at the time of day when the patient reports that his symptoms are worst.

For patients being *converted from L-dopa to Sinemet*, the L-dopa must be discontinued at least 8 hours before initiation of Sinemet, as the decarboxylase inhibitor will significantly potentiate the effects of any L-dopa remaining from the last dose. Usually the transfer is best accomplished by having the patient take an evening dose of L-dopa and then begin therapy with the combination tablet on the following morning. The starting dose of Sinemet (in 1:10 ratio) should contain approximately 25% of the previous L-dopa dose. After this transfer, the usual plan for increasing Sinemet should be followed.

A variety of problems and side effects are associated with the use of L-dopa; most patients will experience some of them.

Perpheral Side Effects

Nausea, vomiting, anorexia, and cardiac arrhythmia are side effects which seem to be mediated principally outside of the central nervous system by L-dopa and its metabolites. They occur early in L-dopa treatment. They can be largely prevented or greatly reduced by using Sinemet because peripheral metabolism is impeded. Since approximately 100 mg per day of carbidopa is needed to block peripheral decarboxylation of L-dopa, the 25/100 preparation of Sinemet may be useful in a patient who responds to a relatively small dose of L-dopa. The peripheral side effects can be minimized also by having the patient take the drug with meals or with a snack; and by temporarily reducing the total dose of Sinemet if side effects become a problem. Eventually, patients become tolerant to most of the peripheral side effects.

Orthostatic hypotension is an important side effect which appears to be partly due to peripheral actions and partly due to central actions of L-dopa; it may be reduced but not eliminated by the use of Sinemet. It is critical to measure the patient's standing blood pressure before initiating L-dopa, as orthostatic hypotension may also occur as part of the parkinsonian syndrome in some patients. Whether disease or drug-induced, orthostatic hypotension should be managed by having the patient always change position from lying to standing gradually; by avoiding other drugs which may exacerbate hypotension; by recommending increased salt intake and use of elastic stockings; and, if necessary, by prescribing fluorocortisone 0.1 mg to 1 mg daily (see Chapter 81, Table 81.8).

Central Side Effects

In general, the centrally mediated side effects occur after the patient has taken L-dopa at relatively high doses for 2 or more years. They occur with both L-dopa alone and with Sinemet.

Dyskinesias (involuntary movements of the limbs, hands, trunk, and lingual-buccal-facial musculature) occur in 40 to 90% of treated patients. Their occurrence and severity seem related to the total duration of therapy and/or disease, and they become progressively worse with time. The longer they have been present, the smaller is the dose of L-dopa needed to produce them; this observation suggests that they are due to a denervation hypersensitivity of dopamine receptor sites. Dyskinesias improve with a reduction of the total daily L-dopa dose, but this also diminishes the antiparkinsonian effect.

When dyskinesias first appear, it is important to determine whether they show a stereotyped relationship to each dose of drug (15). Some patients may report the following sequence after taking the drug: (a) initial improvement in parkinsonian symptoms, (b) dyskinesias, and (c) resolution of the dyskinesia but continued antiparkinsonian effect. In this instance, the total daily dose of L-dopa should be taken on a more frequent schedule, avoiding the peak doses which apparently provoked the dyskinesia. A less common sequence is (a) dyskinesia immediately after taking a dose, (b) resolution of dyskinesia as antiparkinsonian effect occurs, and (c) return of dyskinesia as the drug level falls. In this situation, a higher total daily dose may preserve the clinical effect and eliminate the dyskinesia.

Mental Disturbances. L-Dopa is contraindicated in schizophrenic patients, as it will predictably cause psychotic deterioration in these persons. At times, a patient with no psychiatric history may develop a florid schizophreniform psychosis, usually after an increase in the dose of L-dopa. Confusion, bizarre dreams, hallucinations, delirium, and paranoid ideation may also occur as dose-related side effects. These problems may be produced either by L-dopa alone or by the combined effect of L-dopa and any of the other antiparkinsonian agents, usually after a small increment in the dose of any of these drugs. The patient's family should always be forewarned that psychiatric disturbances may occur, particularly after the patient has received medical therapy for 2 or more years. Management consists of prompt reduction, but not discontinuation, of L-dopa, followed by either careful redistribution of the previous dose in more frequent, smaller doses or prescription of a smaller daily dose. Disruptive behavior can be treated with diphenhydramine (Benadryl) or thioridazine (Mellaril) for 1 or 2 days while awaiting resolution of the side effect.

Fluctuations in Response to L-Dopa

At least two distinct patterns of transient worsening of symptoms may occur during L-dopa therapy.

1. *"Wearing off"* refers to a loss of effect several hours after taking a dose. If a patient reports a pattern of recurring symptoms 3 or 4 hours after a dose of L-dopa, the problem can be eliminated usually by redistributing the total daily amount of drug (e.g., converting from every 8 to every 6 hours, etc.).

2. The *"on-off effect"* refers to distressing episodes of sudden freezing or bradykinesia, lasting minutes to hours and not occurring in a predictable temporal relationship to a prior dose of L-dopa. This side effect is usually first seen after several years of therapy. At

times, fluctuating dose levels may play a role, and the problem may be eliminated by more frequent doses, again keeping the daily dose unchanged (7); in addition, amantadine or bromocriptine (see below) may ameliorate the problem in some patients. Transient freezing may, however, be unresponsive to treatment and may in some patients represent progression of the parkinsonian state.

Interaction with Other Drugs

Coadministration of a number of drugs may diminish the antiparkinsonian effect of L-dopa (see Table 79.7), either by decreasing absorption, by antagonizing its effects in the central nervous system, or by other mechanisms. Apart from the neuroleptic drugs, the other drugs listed can be given with L-dopa and the dose can be adjusted as necessary. MAO inhibitors should not be given with L-dopa, as this can precipitate a hypertensive crisis. Potential drug interactions which may exacerbate the side effects of L-dopa have been mentioned above.

Progressive Loss of Responsiveness

After several years of disease and/or L-dopa treatment, the symptoms of Parkinson's disease become less responsive to medication, and side effects often increase at a dose that was previously tolerated. This seems to represent not only progression of the disease but also a change in the patient's responses to medicine (12). For optimal medical management at this stage, consultation with a neurologist well-versed in the handling of Parkinson's disease is advisable. Some patients who reach a plateau or show deterioration in their response to L-dopa may regain responsiveness to the drug after a gradual reduction in their daily dose or after a 5- to 10-day "drug holiday" (5). This latter maneuver must be undertaken in the hospital under the supervision of a physician acquainted with the technique; for the patient temporarily becomes immobilized by severe parkinsonism and requires excellent supportive care and judicious reinstitution of L-dopa therapy.

AMANTIDINE (SYMMETREL) (18)

This drug was developed as an antiviral (A-2 influenza) agent and was found to have antiparkinsonian

Table 79.7
Drugs which May Diminish the Antiparkinsonian Effect of L-Dopa

Drug	Probable Mechanism
Anticholinergics	Decreased levodopa absorption
Antidepressants, tricyclic	Decreased levodopa absorption
Clonidine	Not established
Methionine	Not established
Papaverine	Not established
Neuroleptics	Inhibition of dopamine uptake
Phenytoin	Not established
Pyridoxine[a]	Enhancement of decarboxylation of levodopa at periphery

[a] Not a problem if patient taking Sinemet.

properties. It is thought to promote dopamine release from intact dopaminergic terminals remaining in the nigrostriatum. Overall, it is somewhat more effective initially than the anticholinergic drugs. Amantidine is useful chiefly as an adjunct to either anticholinergic or L-dopa treatment. This is because its effects are self-limited; patients improve within a few days, but show a loss of responsiveness after about 2 months. Therefore, it may be useful periodically for a few weeks in a patient who appears to be transiently worsening on his usual regimen. Amantidine is also useful for short term management of neuroleptic-induced parkinsonian in patients who cannot tolerate anticholinergics (6). (See additional details Chapter 15.)

Amantidine is available in 100-mg capsules. It should be given as 100 mg daily for the first 1 or 2 weeks, then increased to 100 mg twice daily for 1 week and to 200 mg twice daily if needed. Side effects include depression, orthostatic hypotension, and urinary retention. As noted earlier, it must be used carefully with anticholinergics, as both groups of drugs may produce mental confusion. Like Sinemet, this is a relatively expensive drug (approximately $20 per hundred capsules).

BROMOCRIPTINE (PARLODEL) (9)

This drug is an ergot derivative which was developed for use in the amenorrhea-galactorrhea syndrome; it also acts as a dopamine agonist. In Parkinson's disease, it is useful chiefly as an adjunct in patients whose symptoms are not adequately controlled with L-dopa. Fifty percent of patients show initial improvements in a variety of symptoms (tremor, bradykinesia, rigidity, freezing) although only about one-third of patients show sustained improvement. There is a very high incidence of side effects (approximately 70% of patients), which are similar to the peripheral and central side effects of L-dopa described above. This greatly limits the usefulness of the drug.

Bromocriptine is available in 2.5-mg tablets. Therapy should be initiated with a test dose of one-half a tablet because occasionally orthostatic hypotension with this drug can be quite severe. If the test dose is tolerated, treatment is initiated at 2.5 mg, 3 times daily, increasing every 4 to 5 days up to a dose of 25 to 50 mg. The dose of L-dopa can usually be decreased concomitantly with increases in bromocriptine.

Other Aspects of Management

GENERAL MANAGEMENT

The patient's physician, aware of the prognosis of Parkinson's disease, can provide much helpful advice to prevent the patient from withdrawing from valued activities and to ensure that the patient avoids unsafe activities.

Physical activities should be encouraged, particularly activities which require walking. However, activities which can be dangerous if balance is imperfect or motor response is delayed should be avoided (e.g., skiing, bicycling, driving in heavy traffic, using electric tools, etc.)

Weak or *slow speech and poverty of facial expression* can produce the impression of lack of interest during a conversation. Therefore, the patient should be advised tactfully to make a conscious effort to let others know that he is interested, despite his lack of facial expression. Having the patient practice speech by reading aloud and by recording and listening to his voice may help to overcome his reticence to speak.

Fear of falling is experienced by virtually all parkinsonian patients. Walking with hands clasped behind the back or using a walker (but not a cane) may improve stability. The patient's living environment should be free of obstacles which may cause him to stumble and he should avoid walking in places where he is apt to encounter obstacles (rocky terrain, for example).

When the patient becomes progressively disabled, the *assistance of others* is necessary to avoid as much as possible the complications of bradykinesia and of sedentary living. Such assistance includes periodic change in the patient's position to avoid skin breakdown, passive range of motion of the limbs and digits to avoid flexion contractures, and as much mobility and social or intellectual stimulation as possible.

GENERAL SURGERY

Special considerations in the parkinsonian patient who must undergo surgery are discussed in Chapter 83.

STEREOTACTIC SURGERY

Twenty percent of patients with Parkinson's disease do not respond significantly to L-dopa from the outset. In others, L-dopa and other therapy ameliorates only some of their symptoms. In some of these patients, stereotactic surgery can be considered. This approach seems especially useful in the relatively uncommon patient in whom uncontrollable parkinsonian tremor alone is disabling; surgery does not seem to be useful for bradykinesia or rigidity. While it may be transiently useful, surgery carries a risk of significant morbidity without definite lasting benefit in most patients. Consultation with a neurologist or a neurosurgeon should be obtained in patients who may meet the criteria for consideration of surgery.

References

General

TREMOR

Jankovic, J and Fahn, S: Physiologic and pathologic tremors: diagnosis, mechanism, and management. *Ann Intern Med 93:* 460, 1980.
    Useful review article.

PARKINSON'S DISEASE

Bianchine, JR: Drug therapy of parkinsonism. *N Engl J Med 295:* 814, 1976.
    Useful review of antiparkinsonian drugs.
Boshes, B: Sinemet and the treatment of parkinsonism. *Ann Intern Med 94:* 364, 1981.
    Critical and practical review of Sinemet.
Duvoisin, R: Parkinsonism. In *Clinical Symposia,* published by CIBA Pharmaceutical Co., Summit, N.J., 1976
    Well-illustrated account of clinical and physiologic aspects of parkinsonism.
Pallis, CA: Parkinsonism: natural history and clinical features. *Br Med J 3:* 683, 1971.
    Extensively referenced review of clinical features of parkinsonism; includes useful information about conditions which mimic parkinsonism.

Specific

1. Andersen, J, Aabro, E, Gulmann, N, Hjelmsted, A and Pedersen HE: Anti-depressive treatment in Parkinson's disease: a controlled trial of the effect of nortriptyline in patients with Parkinson's disease treated with L-dopa. *Acta Neurol Scandinav 62:* 210, 1980.
2. Bannister, R and Oppenheimer, R: Degenerative diseases of the nervous system associated with autonomic failure. *Brain 95:* 457, 1972.
3. Barbeau, A: Six years of high-level levodopa therapy in severely akinetic parkinsonian patients. *Arch Neurol 33:* 33, 1976.
4. Critchley, E: Clinical manifestations of essential tremor. *J Neurol Neurosurg Psychiatry 35:* 365, 1972.
5. Direnfeld, LK, Feldman, RG, Alexander, MP and Kelly-Hayes, M: Is L-dopa drug holiday useful? *Neurology 30:* 785, 1980.
6. DiMascio, A, Bernardo, DL, Greenblatt, DJ and Marder, JE: A controlled trial of amantadine in drug-induced extrapyramidal disorders. *Arch Gen Psychiatry 33:* 599, 1976.
7. Fahn, S: "On-off" phenomenon with levodopa therapy in parkinsonism. *Neurology 24:* 431, 1974.
8. Fahn, S and Calne, DB: Considerations in the management of parkinsonism. *Neurology 28:* 5, 1978.
9. Fahn, S, Cote, LJ, Snider, SR, Barrett, RE and Isgreen, WP: The role of bromocriptine in the treatment of parkinsonism. *Neurology 29:* 1077, 1979.
10. Growdon, JH, Shahani, BT and Young, RR: The effect of alcohol on essential tremor. *Neurology 25:* 259, 1975.
11. Hakim, AM and Mathieson, G: Dementia in Parkinson disease: a neuropathologic study. *Neurology 29:* 1209, 1979.
12. Lesser, RP, Fahn, S, Snider, SR, Cote, LJ, Isgreen, WP and Barrett, RE: Analysis of the clinical problems in parkinsonism and the complications of long-term levodopa therapy. *Neurology 29:* 1253, 1979.
13. Markham, CH and Diamond SG: Evidence to support early levodopa therapy in Parkinson's disease. *Neurology 31:* 125, 1981.
14. Mindham, RHS: Psychiatric aspects of Parkinson's disease. *Br J Hosp Med* p. 411, March 1974.
15. Muenter, MD, Sharpless, NS, Tyce, GM and Darley, FL: Patterns of dystonia ("I-D-I" and "D-I-D") in response to L-dopa therapy for Parkinson's disease. *Mayo Clin Proc 52:* 163, 1977.
16. Pollock, M and Hornabrook, RW: The prevalence, natural history and dementia of Parkinson's disease. *Brain 89:* 429, 1966.
17. Shy, GM and Drager, GA: A neurological syndrome associated with orthostatic hypotension: a clinical-pathologic study. *Arch Neurol 2:* 511, 1960.
18. Timberlake, WH and Vance, MA: Four-year treatment of patients with parkinsonism using amantadine alone or with levodopa. *Ann Neurol 3:* 119, 1978.
19. Tune, LE, McHugh, PR and Coyle, JT: Management of extrapyramidal side effects induced by neuroleptics. *Johns Hopkins Med J 148:* 149, 1981.
20. Winkler, GF and Young, RR: Efficacy of chronic propranolol therapy in action tremors of the familial, senile or essential varieties. *N Engl J Med 290:* 984, 1974.

CHAPTER EIGHTY

Cerebrovascular Disease

ALFRED C. SERVER, M.D., Ph.D., and L. RANDOL BARKER, M.D.

OVERVIEW

Cerebrovascular disease is a major cause of disability and the third leading cause of death in the United States. The impact on society is far-reaching with an estimated annual cost of greater than 7.3 billion dollars. According to a recent survey (27), the *annual incidence* of first stroke is 150 per 100,000 population; about 80% of these are due to thrombotic or embolic cerebral infarction, 12% to cerebral hemorrhage, and 8% to subarachnoid hemorrhage. As shown in Table 80.1, approximately 75% of strokes occur in individuals who are 65 or older. The *annual death rate* from stroke is 75 per 100,000 population with a disproportionately greater number of early deaths among patients with hemorrhage as compared to patients with infarction. Data on *the prevalence of stroke* suggest that in a population of 100,000 there are approximately 500 stroke survivors at any particular time.

The incidence of stroke declined by almost 50% in one population (Rochester, Minnesota) during the 5-year period 1970 to 1974 compared to the 5-year period 1945 to 1949 (16). The decline was found for all age groups. It is not yet known whether this trend has occurred nationwide, nor is the explanation for the trend known, although more aggressive treatment of hypertension may be a major factor.

Cerebrovascular disease presents *two major challenges in ambulatory practice*: First, the prevention of stroke in the large number of individuals with risk factors which make them stroke-prone; and second, the optimal care of the many stroke survivors in each community.

RISK FACTORS

A major goal of patient evaluation in ambulatory practice is the identification of the individual with an increased risk of stroke. Patients who have previously suffered a stroke constitute an important subgroup of this high risk population. A community-based study of the natural history of stroke in Rochester, Minnesota, has shown that the first year recurrence rate among survivors of a first stroke was 10% and that the 5-year recurrence rate was 20% (31). In addition to a previous history of stroke, other factors predispose a patient to stroke. Epidemiologic data indicate that the incidence of stroke and the associated death rate increase markedly with age. Three other factors, all amenable to therapy, have also been found to correlate strongly with stroke occurrence: transient episodes of focal cerebral dysfunction of vascular origin called transient ischemic attacks (TIA), hypertension, and certain types of cardiac disorders.

TIA

The etiology, natural history, and treatment of TIA are discussed in detail later in this chapter (pp. 880–882). Suffice it to say that approximately one-third of patients with a TIA subsequently develop a stroke and that the TIA provides a significant warning of impending infarction.

Hypertension

Data accumulated during the Framingham study indicate that the risk of both nonhemorrhagic and hemorrhagic stroke are strongly related to *hypertension*. Atherothrombotic brain infarction occurred in

Table 80.1
Percentage Distribution of Stroke Occurrence by Age Group[a]

		Percent of Total Persons in Each Age Group[b]						
	All ages	Under 35	35–44	45–54	55–64	65–74	75–84	84+
U.S. population	100.0	58.3	10.4	11.4	9.5	6.6	3.3	1.0
Stroke patients	100.0	1.2	2.0	6.8	15.6	28.3	33.4	12.7

[a] Source: National Survey of Stroke, U.S. DHEW, Public Health Service National Institutes of Health, NIH Pub. No. 80-2069, January 1980.
[b] Note that while the age group 65 years and older constitutes only 10.9% of the population, approximately three-fourths (74.4%) of all strokes occur in this age group.

hypertensive subjects (blood pressure greater than 160/95) four times more often than in normotensive subjects (25). Moreover, the available evidence suggests that stroke risk is significantly reduced by the treatment of hypertension in all patients including those with a history of cerebrovascular disease (3, 7, 40, 41) (see below p. 880). The evaluation and long term management of hypertension is discussed in detail in Chapter 59.

Cardiac Impairment

The last major factor which clearly predisposes to stroke is *cardiac impairment*. It has long been known that the heart is often the source of emboli that lodge in cerebral vessels leading to infarction. However, this type of stroke is thought to be relatively uncommon, constituting only 3 to 8% of all cerebral infarctions. Data from the Framingham study have identified cardiac impairment as a significant risk factor in the occurrence of the more frequently encountered nonembolic atherothrombotic brain infarction (ABI) (43). Subjects with electrocardiographic evidence of left ventricular hypertrophy (LVH) were 9 times more likely to develop ABI than individuals without this abnormality. Patients with coronary artery disease (CAD) had 5 times the risk of ABI and those with radiographic evidence of cardiomegaly had 3 times the risk. When the contribution of concomitant hypertension was eliminated, LVH and CAD were each associated with a 3-fold increase in the risk of ABI; the contribution of cardiomegaly on X-ray was not found to be significant when other variables were controlled. On the basis of these findings it was concluded that cardiac impairment, especially if associated with hypertension, significantly heightens the risk of stroke occurrence. It is not clear that cardiac abnormalities, once established, can be modified so that the risk of subsequent stroke is reduced.

Other Factors

A number of other factors have been associated with an increased incidence of stroke: family history of vascular disease, elevated serum glucose, elevated serum lipids, cigarette smoking, elevated blood hemoglobin and hematocrit, and the presence of a cervical bruit. To date, it is not known whether modification of any of these risk factors reduces the like-

lihood of stroke, and each requires some qualification. Data on *family history* are incomplete although the available evidence suggests that the parents of stroke patients have a higher mortality from vascular disease. With regard to *diabetes mellitus*, prospective data from the Framingham study indicated an increased risk of cerebral infarction in subjects with even a modest abnormality of glucose tolerance (23). This study also demonstrated that *elevated serum lipids* were associated with increased stroke risk, but only in subjects under the age of 50. The contribution of *cigarette smoking* to the risk of stroke occurrence remains controversial. However, in the Framingham study male cigarette smokers had a 3-fold greater risk of cerebral infarction than nonsmokers. The data on female smokers was too limited to draw a valid conclusion. *Elevated blood hemoglobin and hematocrit* have also been implicated as possible risk factors, but a cause and effect relationship has not been established (24, 39). *Oral contraceptive use* is associated with a 5- to 10-fold increase in risk of vascular diseases, including stroke (see details in Chapter 90). Finally, it is generally accepted that the presence of an *asymptomatic cervical bruit* correlates with an increased incidence of subsequent stroke, but there is controversy regarding the appropriate management of patients with this finding (see below, p. 882).

CLASSIFICATION OF CEREBROVASCULAR EVENTS

Type of Event

Symptoms and signs of vascular origin are characterized by their relatively rapid onset. The following classification has been developed based upon their duration.

A *transient ischemic attack* (TIA) is defined as a transient episode of focal cerebral dysfunction, rapid in onset (from no to maximal symptoms in less than 5 min) that usually lasts from 2 to 15 min but always resolves completely within 24 hours.

A *reversible ischemic neurologic deficit* (RIND) is defined as an episode of focal cerebral dysfunction that lasts longer than 24 hours but resolves completely within 3 weeks.

A *completed stroke* is defined as an episode of focal cerebral dysfunction that has stabilized and may have improved but has not resolved completely after 3 weeks. The term "stroke in evolution" is used to describe a vascular syndrome which is acute in onset and worsens during the period of observation.

Vascular Territory

Cerebrovascular events are also classified on the basis of the vascular territory involved. Symptoms and signs referable to the two major vascular territories are listed in Table 80.2. There is some overlap in the symptom complexes, making the distinction between carotid and vertebrobasilar disease difficult at times. However, frequently the history alone provides the physician with the evidence necessary to diagnose a cerebrovascular episode and to identify the arterial territory involved.

Another group of ischemic events, presenting as *lacunar syndromes*, is due to occlusion of penetrating nonanastamosing branches of the major cerebral arteries. The pathology of the involved vessels has been characterized; occlusion is due either to miniature atherosclerotic plaques at the origin of vessels 400 to 1,000 μ in diameter or, more commonly, to a degenerative process called lipohyalinosis affecting vessels 200 μ or less. These changes correlate strongly with the presence of hypertension. There are several lacunar syndromes which usually, but not invariably, result from ischemic infarcts in the deep substance of the brain (13, 34):

Pure motor hemiparesis (internal capsule or pons): hemiplegia or hemiparesis involving the face, arm, and leg without sensory deficit, dysphasia, or hemianopsia.

Pure sensory stroke (thalamus): numbness of the face, arm, and leg on one side without weakness or hemianopsia.

Homolateral ataxia and crural paresis (pons): cerebellar ataxia, weakness, and pyramidal signs involving the limbs on the same side, the leg more than the arm.

The *dysarthria-clumsy hand syndrome* (pons): dys-

Table 80.2
Clinical Features of Ischemia Involving the Major Vascular Territories

CAROTID ARTERIAL DISEASE
  Paresis (mono- or hemi-)
  Sensory loss or paresthesias (mono- or hemi-)
  Speech or language disturbances
  Loss of vision in one eye or part of one eye (amaurosis fugax)
  Homonymous hemianopsia
VERTEBROBASILAR ARTERIAL DISEASE
  Vertigo, diplopia, dysphagia, or dysarthria when two occur together or when one occurs with any of the following:
  Paresis (any combination of the extremities)
  Sensory loss or paresthesias (any combination of the extremities)
  Ataxia
  Homonymous hemianopsia (unilateral or bilateral)

arthria, facial weakness, clumsiness of the hand with little or no weakness, a slight imbalance, and a Babinski sign on the affected side.

COMPLETED STROKE

Any occlusive arterial disease may lead to a completed stroke. The vast majority of strokes are due to atherosclerosis, lipohyalinosis, or emboli from the heart. A number of conditions may produce a syndrome resembling a completed stroke, RIND, or TIA. These are summarized in the discussion of the differential diagnosis of TIA (see below, p. 881).

Both the diagnostic evaluation and initial care of the patient with a new stroke should be accomplished in the hospital. This includes patients with lacunar syndromes, which vary as to their etiology and their appropriate treatment (34). Following hospital discharge, ambulatory or home care for the stroke survivor requires the colloboration of the patient, the family, the physician, and other professionals, as explained below.

Natural History

The major studies on the natural history of stroke differ with regard to two important variables: the type of stroke patient studied and the treatment available to the study population. The few studies which attempted to restrict the variables under consideration were performed before the advent of cerebral computed tomography (CT scanning) and were therefore marred by a significant degree of diagnostic inaccuracy. Despite these criticisms, the extensive body of literature on the "natural history" of stroke provides useful information.

EARLY PROGNOSIS

There is general agreement that *age* influences greatly the early prognosis for the patient who sustains a stroke, regardless of the type. The older the patient, the less likely he is to survive (see Table 80.3). Studies which classify strokes on the basis of *etiology* indicate that the early prognosis is much better for thrombotic or embolic disease than for hemorrhage. During the interval 1955 to 1969, 82% of stroke patients from the Mayo Clinic with a clinical diagnosis of cerebral thrombosis and 67% of those with cerebral embolism were alive 30 days after the acute episode (31). These values compare favorably with the 1-month survival of 48% observed for subarachnoid hemorrhage and 16% observed for intracerebral hemorrhage.

MORBIDITY IN STROKE SURVIVORS

A number of studies have evaluated stroke survivors on the basis of the degree of neurologic, functional, and psychosocial impairment.

Table 80.4 shows the spectrum and frequency of *neurologic impairments* found in stroke survivors in the Framingham study (18). It is notable that half of

Table 80.3
Percentage Distribution of Stroke Survivors by Age Group[a]

| Age Group | Percent Surviving | | | | | | | | | |
| | | Days | | | | Years | | | | |
	Onset	30	60	90	180	1	2	3	4	5
Under 65	100.0	73.7	71.1	69.4	65.9	63.2	57.6	57.6	52.0	49.2
65–74	100.0	75.6	69.5	65.2	63.1	59.4	52.9	46.1	42.7	34.5
75–84	100.0	68.1	62.1	57.6	52.4	45.7	37.2	30.0	23.1	21.9
85+	100.0	52.4	45.8	37.2	33.0	27.8	20.7	15.1	9.2	7.4

[a] Source: National Survey of Stroke, U.S. DHEW, Public Health Service National Institutes of Health, NIH Pub. No. 80-2069, January 1980.

Table 80.4
Prevalence of Neurologic Deficits in the 123 Survivors of Completed Stroke, Framingham Study (1972 to 1974)[a]

| Type of Peripheral Motor Deficit | Survivors | No. Surviving with: | | | |
		Sensory deficit	Hemi-anopsia	Dysar-thria	Dys-phasia
No motor deficit	63	3	5	2	10
Left hemiparesis	28	13	6	3	2
Right hemiparesis	27	10	5	13	9
Bilateral motor deficit	4	4	3	2	1
No data	1	1	1	1	1
Total survivors	123	31	20	21	23

[a] From G. E. Gresham et al.: New England Journal of Medicine, 293: 954, 1975 (18).

Table 80.5
Prevalence of Four Types of Functional Disability in 119 Survivors of Completed Stroke and in 119 Controls, Framingham Study (1972 to 1974)[a]

| Type of Disability | Survivors | | Matched Controls[b] | | P Value |
	No.	%	No.	%	
All persons examined for functional disability	119	100	119	100	—
Dependent in activities of daily living	37	31	9	8	<0.0001
Dependent in mobility	24	20	6	5	<0.0001
Decrease in level of vocational function[c]	85	71	49	41	<0.0001
Decrease in socialization outside home	74	62	37	31	<0.0001

[a] From G. E. Gresham et al.: New England Journal of Medicine, 293: 954, 1975 (18).
[b] Matched for age and sex.
[c] Either stopped working or incomplete resumption of homemaking activities.

these individuals (63 of 123) had no motor deficit. These community-based data are probably representative of the situation in other communities.

In an extensive study of *overall function*, Katz et al. (26) found that, of the patients who survive a stroke, approximately 50% regain independence within 2 years and are able to ambulate and perform activities of daily living with minimal or no assistance. Spontaneous improvement is most rapid in the first few months after the stroke and is rarely noted after 2 years. Only a small percentage of stroke survivors remain bedridden and completely dependent. These findings are supported by results from the Mayo Clinic where only 4% of the survivors of a stroke required total care at 6 months; 36% had some degree of neurologic deficit, yet were able to work; and 29% were functioning normally (31). On the basis of the authors' assessment, 54% of their patients may have benefited from rehabilitative care, including the 10% who were aphasic.

The Framingham study provided information on the equally important *social and psychological sequelae* of stroke (18). A significant decrease in the levels of vocational function and socialization outside the home was noted among stroke survivors as compared to age and sex-matched controls (see Table 80.5), and the decrease exceeded that anticipated based on the levels of neurologic deficit. In a more recent study in Monroe County, New York, the social

and psychologic difficulties facing the stroke survivor were evaluated prospectively (12). Within the first 6 months after hospital discharge, 37% of the patients demonstrated moderate or severe depression, 32% anger and/or anxiety, 56% social isolation, 43% reduction in community involvement, 46% economic strain causing life-style alteration, and 52% disruption of normal family functioning. Recognition and treatment of the psychosocial problems of the stroke patient and his family are discussed below.

MORTALITY IN STROKE SURVIVORS

The death rate among stroke survivors is significantly greater than that expected for the general population matched for age and sex. The 5-year cumulative mortality is approximately 50 to 60%, with the greatest number of deaths occurring in the first year. With time, however, the mortality rate approaches that of the general population and in at least one study the accelerated rate of death following a stroke subsided completely after 24 to 30 months (26). There is evidence to suggest that the etiology of a stroke (occlusive vs. hemorrhagic) is a less reliable predictor of late prognosis than early prognosis. Eisenberg et al. (9) reported that while cerebral hemorrhage was more lethal acutely than cerebral thrombosis, those cerebral hemorrhage victims who lived 1 month had a 5-year survival equal to or better than cerebral thrombosis victims. The leading cause of death in stroke survivors is cardiovascular disease, with cardiac related deaths exceeding deaths attributed to cerebrovascular disease by a factor of 2 to 1. Thorough evaluation and management of cardiac disease is, therefore, of great importance in the care of stroke survivors.

Management

Management of the patient who has survived a stroke involves the evaluation and treatment of any physical and psychosocial sequelae and the selection of appropriate therapy to lessen the risk of stroke recurrence. Once the patient has been discharged from the hospital, his personal physician plays a critical role in coordinating his care. Reduction in a patient's disability and dependency frequently requires the concerted efforts of the patient's family; physical, occupational, and speech therapists; and occasionally a psychiatrist. It is the responsibility of the primary physician to recognize the particular needs of his patient and to coordinate efforts to meet these needs.

ROLE OF THE FAMILY

At the time of discharge from the hospital, the physician should devote time to the education of the stroke survivor and his family. It is during this period that the patient is confronted with the full extent of his functional loss and that the actions of well-meaning but uninformed family members can increase the patient's feeling of inadequacy. The physician must dispel myths regarding stroke and supplant them with accurate and useful information. The American Heart Association (AHA) has produced a series of invaluable booklets which discuss stroke and its sequelae in lay terms and provide guidelines for the home management of the stroke patient. The titles of these publications are listed in Table 80.6. Table 80.7 shows, as an example, the table of contents of *Up and Around*, a booklet designed to assist in restoration of mobility. The AHA booklet entitled *Strokes— A Guide for the Family* provides the following general suggestions for the family of a stroke patient with residual disability:

Divide duties so that the full burden of care does not fall on one person.

Help the patient take responsibility for doing his exercises regularly.

Allow the patient to take on responsibilities for self-care and other activities gradually and by easy steps. It calls for fine judgement to encourage independence and still not to frustrate a patient with over-difficult tasks; to

Table 80.6
Booklets Published by the American Heart Association[a]

Strokes: A Guide for the Family—a brief overview of the mechanisms causing strokes and general suggestions for care of the patient at home

Strike Back at Stroke—a well illustrated booklet prepared for the physician, the patient, and the patient's family demonstrating the following aspects of home care of the stroke patient: position of the patient in bed, passive exercises which must be done for the patient, active exercises which the patient can do, methods for getting out of bed, standing, use of a sling, and walking with the assistance of a cane or other devices

Up and Around—an extensively illustrated booklet written for the physician, the patient, and the patient's family, on ways in which the patient can regain activities of daily living (see "Table of Contents" in Table 80.7)

Do it Yourself Again—well illustrated booklet on self-help devices for eating, grooming, dressing, using the bathroom, reading, writing, telephoning, preparing food, cleaning, sewing, walking, and selecting and using a wheelchair

Stroke: Why Do They Behave that Way?—a detailed booklet providing recommendations for the care of the patient who has completed most of his spontaneous recovery of higher functions and has major residual deficits (see "Summary of Recommendations" in Table 80.8)

Aphasia and the Family—explains many of the problems in aphasia and suggests practical ways in which the family can help the aphasic patient

[a] Available without charge from local AHA chapters.

stimulate progress and still not to encourage unrealistic expectations.

Praise any successful efforts that he makes, don't be discouraged by failures. Recovery from a severe stroke is a slow process.

Have him participate in as many family activities and as much family planning as he can. Feeling useful is a tremendous morale builder.

Help him keep in contact with the world he has known.

Don't relegate him to the side lines and leave him with only television and radio to occupy himself. Encourage him to develop a hobby. Spend time with him... Encourage visitors if his condition warrants it. Make him feel wanted and a part of the social picture.

Check with the doctor regularly. Get in touch with him if things are not going as you think they should.

ROLE OF REHABILITATION

Success in stroke rehabilitation is often dependent upon the extent of permanent central nervous system damage and the patient's ability to utilize alternative methods of function to compensate for fixed deficits. As noted above, spontaneous improvement in the stroke survivor may continue to occur for the first 6 to 12 months after the stroke, yet the mechanisms underlying such gains remain obscure. Lehmann and his colleagues (28) have studied the important question of whether or not an intensive program of reha-

Table 80.7
Table of Contents of U.S. Public Health Service Publication Entitled *Up and Around—A Booklet to Aid the Stroke Patient in Activities of Daily Living* **(Available from American Heart Association)**

bilitation will result in functional gains after the period of spontaneous improvement. They found that even among significantly impaired patients admitted to a rehabilitation program 12 months after a stroke, marked improvement was attainable in dressing skills, bladder and bowel function, and walking. These findings formed the basis for their conclusion that a program of rehabilitation does improve the outcome of the stroke survivor. Furthermore, they estimated that the savings derived in returning a patient to his family or to independent living more than equaled the costs of rehabilitation.

It is clear that not all patients in a rehabilitation program show significant functional improvement. A number of patient characteristics correlate with poor rehabilitation results, including: bowel and bladder incontinence, low self-care status on admission, right hemispheric involvement, intellectual and perceptual deficits, heart failure, signs of generalized arteriosclerosis, and lower educational levels (4, 29). However, since none of these factors correlates strongly with poor outcome, the best approach is to offer rehabilitation services whenever possible to each stroke survivor with significant functional impairments.

It is generally agreed that, except for patients with evidence of subarachnoid bleeding, for whom bed rest and mild sedation are indicated, a program of functional rehabilitation should begin as soon as possible after a stroke occurs. *There are several reasons for the early initiation of a program of rehabilitation:* First, it is generally accepted that patients who are provided with rehabilitation services early are likely to experience greater long term functional improvement. Second, early transfer from bed to chair coupled with physical therapy reduces the complications that can develop in the immobile bedridden patient and that can subsequently limit the extent of functional recovery. Stretching of tight muscles, passive range of motion, and active or resistive exercises minimize the degree of muscle atrophy and prevent the development of contractures. In addition, even limited mobility of the patient will reduce the risk of circulatory complications such as thrombophlebitis, postural hypotension, and pressure sores. Third, early rehabilitation is of particular benefit to the patient who demonstrates an impaired ability to communicate due either to dysphasia or to dysarthria. Approximately one-third of stroke patients exhibit some form of communication disorder and many of these remain severely impaired beyond the period of spontaneous recovery (38). Such patients may feel desparately isolated because of their sudden loss of ability to communicate. Therapists who specialize in speech and hearing are skilled in the evaluation and management of these problems and play an integral role in daily interactions with the patient and in recommending appropriate strategies to the patient's family and physician.

Everyone involved in the rehabilitation process must appreciate the significance of the functional losses sustained by the patient and to do so, the losses must be viewed from the patient's perspective. This requires an *awareness of the patient's usual activities before the stroke;* this essential information should be obtained in conjunction with a social worker who can evaluate the patient's role at home prior to the stroke and can project how the stroke will alter that role when the patient returns to his home.

Ideally, the *rehabilitation initiated in the hospital is continued* in the patient's home or in ambulatory care facilities. Many communities have physical, occupational, and speech therapists available for both home and ambulatory follow-up. The patient, his family, and the patient's personal physician should be acquainted with the goals and plans for rehabilitation before discharge to home or to a rehabilitation facility. The comprehensive text of Licht (see "General References") provides details about the many individualized approaches available for rehabilitation.

MANAGEMENT OF PSYCHOLOGIC AND BEHAVIORAL SEQUELAE

The high incidence of psychologic and behavioral problems among stroke survivors has been noted above. These problems often hinder rehabilitation efforts. Fear of a second stroke and depression due to loss of functional ability are readily understandable in the context of the patient's predicament. Appropriate counseling (as outlined above) of the patient and his family, coupled with participation in an active rehabilitation program, are the best ways to minimize these problems.

A number of stroke survivors experience *disturbances of mood* which do not correlate with the level of functional disability. Folstein *et al.* (14), who addressed this issue, concluded that for many patients the mood disorder is a specific complication of cerebral damage rather than simply a reaction to functional loss. This hypothesis is supported by earlier results which suggest that the type of mood disorder is dependent upon the side of the brain affected by the stroke. Gainotti (15) reported that behavior denoting a catastrophic reaction (see Chapter 16) and anxious depressive orientation of mood (anxiety reactions, bursts of tears, provocative utterances, depressed renouncements, or sharp refusals to go on with the examinations) are more frequent among patients with left (dominant) hemisphere damage. Symptoms denoting an opposite emotional reaction (denial of illness, minimization, indifference reactions, and tendency to joke) and expressions of hate toward the paralyzed limbs are more frequent among patients suffering from a lesion of the right (minor) hemisphere. A number of theories have been advanced to explain the observed lateralization of mood disorder, ranging from the psychodynamic to the pharmacologic. Most authorities agree, however, that both psychologic and physiologic factors contribute to the development of mood disorders following strokes. Management of these problems is discussed in Chapter 16. The AHA booklet *Stroke: Why Do They Behave That Way?* (1974) is particularly helpful for the family and for health care professionals caring for the patient who has survived a major stroke involving the cerebral cortex. Table 80.8 contains summaries of the recommendations for dealing with permanent behavioral problems in these patients.

MANAGEMENT OF LATE COMPLICATIONS

The interaction between physician and stroke survivor is often extended over several years, and this requires that the physician be aware of late complications that can occur.

Shoulder Problems

The *painful shoulder* is one of the most frequent and most disturbing complications encountered in the stroke patient with a residual hemiparesis. Shoulder pain is frequently caused by increased traction on the shoulder capsule secondary to abnormal positioning of the paralyzed arm. The normal alignment of the joint can be restored through the use of a sling and proper positioning of the arm at night. Physical therapy, following initial symptomatic treatment with analgesics and the application of heat, can limit the extent of permanent structural damage (see Chapter 60, for additional detail).

The *shoulder hand syndrome*, also called reflex sympathetic dystrophy, occurs in approximately 5% of stroke patients. It is characterized by the occurrence of a painful shoulder associated with stiffness and swelling of the hand and fingers. Onset is acute or subacute, (developing over a 3- to 6-month period), and may involve the hand and shoulder simultaneously or one followed by the other. While a number of conditions can result in shoulder discomfort, the dystrophic changes in the hand are characteristic of the shoulder hand syndrome. There is swelling below the wrist but no pitting edema, and the skin of the hand is warm and pink. With time, the intrinsic muscles of the hand atrophy and extension deformities in the metacarpophalangeal joints develop. At this stage radiographic examination of the hand often shows spotty demineralization of the carpal bones. The severe pain associated with this condition greatly hinders rehabilitation efforts. Therefore, early recognition and treatment are important. Ross and Chipman (36) offer the following plan for the management of this condition. Begin treatment with analgesics and with heat to the shoulder; then carefully initiate and gradually increase abduction and external rotation exercises of the arm (described in Chapter 60). If there is no significant improvement after 1 month, stellate ganglion blocks should be used, followed by a course of oral steroids if symptoms persist.

Complications of Inactivity

The partially paralyzed stroke survivor often leads a sedentary existence. This life-style is conducive to the development of vascular complications such as *thrombophlebitis* and *pressure sores*. Appropriate use of elastic stockings and frequent repositioning of the

Table 80.8
Recommendations for Dealing with Behavioral Problems Associated with Permanent Loss of Higher Functions in Stroke Patients[a]

LEFT HEMISPHERE DAMAGE

Right hemiplegics will often have difficulties with speech and language. They also tend to be somewhat cautious, anxious, and disorganized when attempting a new task. Keep in mind the following suggestions:

1. Do not underestimate the patient's ability to learn and communicate even if he cannot use speech
2. If he cannot use speech, try other forms of communication. Pantomime and demonstration are often useful
3. Do not overestimate his understanding of speech and overload him with "static"
4. Do not shout. Keep messages simple and brief
5. Do not use special voices
6. Divide tasks into simple steps
7. Give much feedback and many indications of progress

RIGHT HEMISPHERE DAMAGE

If the patient is having difficulty with self-care activities, you can expect spatial-perceptual deficits. He will tend to talk better than he can actually perform. He may be impulsive or careless. Remember, when working with the patient who has significant spatial-perceptual deficits:

1. Do not overestimate his abilities. Spatial-perceptual difficulties are easy to miss
2. Use verbal cues if he has difficulty with demonstration
3. Break tasks into small steps and give much feedback
4. Watch to see what he can do safely rather than taking his word for it
5. Minimize clutter around him
6. Avoid rapid movement around the patient
7. Highlight visual reference points

ONE-SIDED NEGLECT

One-sided neglect is a problem which involves more than a simple visual field cut or hearing loss. It can occur in both right and left hemiplegics but seems to be more common and more persistent among left hemiplegics. When dealing with a neglect problem, you should:

1. Keep the unimpaired side toward the action unless specifically working with neglected side
2. Avoid trapping the patient in an unnecessarily confined environment
3. Avoid nagging but give frequent cues to aid orientation
4. Provide reminders of the neglected side
5. Arrange the environment to maximize performance

MEMORY PROBLEMS

Some memory problems can be expected in most stroke patients. When working with memory deficits, you can often increase the patient's ability to perform if you:

1. Establish a fixed routine whenever possible
2. Keep messages short to fit his retention span
3. Present new information one step at a time
4. Allow the patient to finish one step before proceeding to the next
5. Give frequent indications of effective progress; he may forget his past "successes"
6. Train in settings that resemble, as much as possible, the setting in which the behavior is to be practiced
7. Use memory aides such as appointment books, written notes, and schedule cards whenever possible
8. Use familiar objects and old associations when teaching new tasks

[a] Adapted from *Stroke: Why Do They Behave That Way?* American Heart Association

---

immobile patient by an informed family member will minimize these problems.

Neurologic Complications

Prolonged pressure on a paralyzed limb may lead to a *peripheral nerve lesion* which may be difficult to recognize when superimposed on brain damage resulting from the stroke. An awareness of this potential complication can expedite its recognition and electrodiagnostic studies can confirm the lower motor neuron damage (see Chapter 81). Once a diagnosis is made, prompt initiation of physical therapy will limit the degree of functional loss resulting from this usually reversible lesion.

Approximately 2.5 to 5% of stroke survivors develop *focal or generalized recurrent seizures* (epilepsy), as a late complication. Patients with damage to their sensorimotor cortex are the most likely to develop epilepsy, with the first seizure usually occuring 6 to 12 months after the stroke (30, 35). Transient neurologic dysfunction following a seizure in a stroke survivor is often attributed to a second stroke. The rapid resolution of symptoms and electroencephalogram (EEG) evidence of an epileptogenic focus point to seizure activity rather than ischemia as the cause. Recurrent seizures in the stroke survivor confirm the diagnosis of epilepsy. Seizure control can

usually be achieved through the use of anticonvulsant medication (see Chapter 77).

Finally, *stroke-related deficits may transiently worsen* when the patient develops a major intercurrent illness such as pneumonia or myocardial infarction. In this instance, neurologic status returns to baseline after resolution of the intercurrent illness. (See discussion of upper motor neuron symptoms in Chapter 75.)

General Surgery

The approach to general surgery in the stroke patient is discussed in Chapter 83.

PREVENTION OF STROKE RECURRENCE

The selection of appropriate therapy to lessen the risk of stroke recurrence is based on the pathophysiology of the initial stroke. Many of the recommendations for the management of stroke survivors are controversial and a critical review of this topic is beyond the scope of the chapter. In this section only the most frequently advocated treatment modalities are discussed.

Antihypertensive Therapy

In a prospective randomized clinical trial, Carter (7) assessed the efficacy of antihypertensive therapy in the treatment of hypertensive patients who had sustained a nonembolic ischemic stroke. He reported that 44% of the untreated patients as compared to 20% of the treated patients suffered another major stroke. At the end of a 2- to 5-year follow-up period 46% of the untreated patients and 26% of the treated patients had died. While the number of recurrent strokes was too small to allow a valid comparison, the difference in mortality was statistically significant in favor of the treated group at the 0.05 level. Moreover, no treated patient sustained a major neurologic complication as a result of a documented hypotensive episode.

Two subsequent studies of the effect of antihypertensive treatment on stroke recurrence included patients with hemorrhagic as well as ischemic strokes. Beevers et al. (3) noted that the stroke recurrence rate varied inversely with success in controlling blood pressure. In patients with good, fair, and poor control of hypertension, the recurrence rates were 16%, 32%, and 55%, respectively. In contrast, the Hypertension-Stroke Cooperative Study Group (21) failed to demonstrate a significant reduction in stroke recurrence in the treated as compared to control patients, although the incidence of congestive heart failure was reduced among the treated patients. In comparing their results to those reported by Beevers et al., the Study Group noted that their patients were less hypertensive. They suggested that "... when stroke survivors with blood pressures considerably higher than those that prevailed in our study are given antihypertensive therapy, a beneficial effect on stroke recurrence can be obtained."

In summary, despite the differences in the studies cited above, critical assessment of the data yields the conclusions that antihypertensive medication can be safely administered to hypertensive stroke survivors and that it is indicated for these patients to reduce cerebrovascular and cardiovascular sequelae. (See Chapter 59 for details on the treatment of hypertension.)

Anticoagulant and Antiplatelet Agents

Anticoagulant and antiplatelet agents have been extensively evaluated for their efficacy in the prevention of stroke recurrence. There is evidence from noncontrolled studies that patients with ischemic infarcts due to emboli from the heart will benefit from long term anticoagulation with Coumadin (8). However, for the large majority of stroke survivors, those with completed strokes due to atherothrombotic cerebrovascular disease, anticoagulation does not result in a significant reduction in the incidence of stroke recurrence or death and is frequently associated with hemorrhagic complications (17).

Data on the antiplatelet agents are somewhat more encouraging. In the Canadian randomized trial of antiplatelet treatment there was a significant decrease in the risk of recurrent stroke or death in aspirin-treated men with TIAs or partial completed ischemic strokes (6). However, the benefit was not seen in women or men with a history of myocardial infarction and it was concluded that the administration of aspirin, 650 mg twice daily, is only indicated for a select group of patients at risk for initial or recurrent stroke (6). Additional studies of platelet-inhibiting drugs are currently in progress and it is hoped that certain of these medications, alone or in combination, will prove useful for a larger patient population. At present, many investigators have recommended the use of antiplatelet agents for both men and women based on the documented efficacy of these agents for a selected patient population, the potential for their use in combination, and their limited toxicity (32, 37).

Carotid Artery Surgery

Based upon careful analysis of a number of studies, Byer and Easton (see "General References") concluded that carotid artery surgery may benefit a carefully selected group of patients with a completed stroke. According to these authors, carotid endarterectomy can be recommended to patients with a small infarct in the carotid system who have surgically correctable arterial lesions appropriate to the deficit (e.g., a large ulcerated plaque or stenosis of greater than 60%) and who are otherwise in good health and neurologically stable. Angiography and surgery should only be performed by a team of specialists with a record of documented success in the evaluation and treatment of occlusive cerebrovascular disease.

TRANSIENT ISCHEMIC ATTACK (TIA)

As noted earlier, TIAs are defined as transient episodes of focal cerebral dysfunction, rapid in onset (no to maximal symptoms in less than 5 min), with symptoms referable to the carotid or vertebrobasilar arterial territory (see Table 80.2), which resolve completely within 24 hours.

Early studies on the pathophysiology of TIAs suggested that they are primarily caused by vasospasm or hypotension. However, according to Barnett (2) "subsequent observations have led to the firm conviction that these ischemic events result from a variety of conditions, including hemodynamic factors, cardiac emboli, extracranial mechanical interference with arteries, altered coagulability, thrombocytosis, nonarteriosclerotic vasculopathies, lacunar infarction, and artery to artery emboli." Artery to artery emboli resulting from atherosclerotic disease of intra- and extracranial cerebral vessels are currently considered the most common cause of TIAs (2).

Differential Diagnosis

Before the diagnosis of TIA is made, other conditions which can produce transient neurologic dysfunction must be considered. Epileptic *seizures* (see Chapter 77) can result in transient neurologic symptoms, but the history of either a grand mal seizure with loss of consciousness, clonic movement of a subsequently weakened limb, or a rapid march of sensory symptoms will aid in reaching the correct diagnosis. *Migraine* attacks (see Chapter 76) are occasionally associated with sensory or motor symptoms which resemble TIAs. With migraine, however, the patients are usually younger, headache is almost invariably present, and the spread of symptoms often occurs with a characteristic march over minutes to hours. Disorder of a *vestibular end organ* (see Chapter 78) can lead to dizziness or vertigo suggestive of the brainstem ischemia of a vertebrobasilar TIA. However, as noted earlier, brainstem ischemia usually results in additional symptoms such as diplopia, dysphagia, dysarthria, weakness, sensory changes, ataxia, or loss of vision. A *mass lesion* such as a tumor or subdural hematoma will occasionally present with recurrent transient neurological symptoms. A careful examination of the patient may reveal mild persisting neurological signs which progress over time, and the lesion can often be detected by CT scan (see "Patient Experience," Chapter 75). *Hypoglycemia* can lead to transient neurologic symptoms, which may be focal if the hypoglycemia is superimposed on existing occlusive cerebrovascular disease. Finally, transient neurologic abnormalities may be present for a short interval *following syncope due to any cause* (see Chapter 78).

Natural History

The natural history of TIAs has long been debated. In a recent review of 27 articles on this subject Brust (5) concluded that "differences in definition, patient selection, therapy, duration of follow-ups, patient age, socioeconomic status, associated disease and other factors, leave considerable uncertainty about the natural history of TIA". Despite this variability in the published reports, the available data indicate that TIAs represent a significant warning of impending stroke, with between 25% and 40% of patients experiencing a cerebral infarction within 5 years of their first TIA (33). The 15-year experience (1955 to 1969) of the Mayo Clinic perhaps provides the best information on natural history. During this period the average annual incidence of first TIA in Rochester, Minnesota, was 31/100,000 population with the rate increasing with age (42). While long term survival after the first TIA was not significantly different from that anticipated for the general population matched for age and sex, the risk of stroke occurrence was markedly increased. Specifically, 36% of patients with TIAs experienced a stroke over an average follow-up of 7.5 years; this was an incidence 9 times greater than the incidence in subjects without a history of TIAs. A large percentage of the strokes occurred in the first few months after the onset of TIAs

indicating that this was a particularly high risk period. The risk was similar for TIAs in the carotid and vertebrobasilar territories.

Evaluation and Management

The patient who experiences an episode of transient focal neurologic dysfunction should be hospitalized for observation and evaluation. A detailed personal and medical history is essential to identify risk factors for cerebrovascular disease and to classify the presenting symptoms (see above). During the general physical and neurologic examination the physician should seek evidence of hypotension, hypertension, cardiac disease, peripheral vascular disease, and persisting neurologic disability. Auscultation of the head and neck should be performed to detect the presence of a bruit. The patient should also have a careful fundoscopic evaluation to assess the status of the retinal vessels and to detect emboli which suggest atherothrombotic carotid occlusive disease or cardiac valve disease. (See detailed description of the neurovascular exam in chapter 75.)

Selected patients with TIA should have a noninvasive carotid evaluation (ophthalmodynamometry or Doppler—see "Patient Experience," Chapter 75) to detect evidence of a stenotic and hemodynamically significant arterial lesion (1). Laboratory evaluation should routinely include a complete blood count, prothrombin time, erythrocyte sedimentation rate, serum glucose and lipid profile, serological test for syphilis, serum creatinine, and urinalysis. In selected patients, valuable information may be provided by additional studies such as EEG, cerebral CT scan, vestibular and auditory function tests, and 24-hour ECG monitoring.

The data generated in the initial workup are often sufficient to allow an accurate diagnosis of the disorder underlying the transient neurologic symptoms. Although the most common type of TIA results from artery to artery emboli, optimal treatment for this condition remains controversial. Despite the extensive data generated on this subject, the proponents of the use of anticoagulants, antiplatelet agents, and surgery continue to disagree. The following guidelines are based on recommendations by Sandok *et al.* (37) and McDowell *et al.* (32).

Patients with a diagnosis of artery to artery embolic TIA who demonstrate evidence of an active process (*i.e.,* multiple recurrent events) should be started on intravenous heparin therapy, if there are no contraindications, while their evaluation proceeds.

Those patients with typical symptoms referable to the distribution of the carotid artery, who would accept surgery and who have a low surgical risk (see Chapter 83), should have *angiography* to determine whether there is a localized, extracranial, surgically accessible lesion of the artery. Angiography should also be considered for patients with less typical symptoms who have markedly positive carotid noninvasive studies. Carotid endarterectomy followed by long term antiplatelet therapy can be recommended to those patients whose angiogram shows a significant arterial lesion.

Patient Experience. The patient can expect the following experience when admitted for four-vessel carotid angiography. He is allowed nothing by mouth for 12 hours before the study and will usually receive premedication consisting of either an analgesic or an anxiolytic drug before going to the radiology suite. After local anesthesia, a catheter-containing needle is inserted percutaneously into a femoral artery. Substantial time is devoted to the positioning of catheters, under fluoroscopic guidance. Dye is injected into both vertebral and both carotid arteries; also into the aortic arch when an arch study is included. For about 30 sec after each dye injection the patient feels intense warmth in a location adjacent to the injection (the neck, the face, or the substernal area). Nausea may also occur. Throughout the procedure, the patient is supine and his head is immobilized in a soft mold. Total time in the radiology suite is about 1½ hours. The reported incidence of neurologic complications from angiography in TIA or stroke patients varies from 1% to 12%; a small proportion of these complications may leave permanent deficits (10, 11).

Patients who are not candidates for surgery must be managed medically. Those initially placed on heparin should be switched to coumadin and continued on this oral anticoagulant, with close follow-up, for a period of 1½ to 3 months. Thereafter, they should be maintained indefinitely on aspirin, 650 mg twice daily, or a combination of aspirin and another antiplatelet agent. Patients with a single TIA who do not require anticoagulants or those for whom these medications are contraindicated should be placed directly on aspirin or other antiplatelet agents (see Chapter 48).

These guidelines for the management of patients with TIAs due to artery to artery emboli are not comprehensive and the reader is referred to the excellent review by Sandok *et al.* (37). Treatment must be individualized to meet the unique needs of each patient. Decisions regarding management, especially in an area as controversial as this, often require input from a neurologist who specializes in the field of cerebrovascular disease.

ASYMPTOMATIC CERVICAL BRUIT

The asymptomatic patient with a cervical bruit is encountered commonly in ambulatory practice. For example, 4.4% of subjects over the age of 45 had asymptomatic cervical bruits in a population-based study in Evans County, Georgia, and the majority of the bruits were heard anteriorly in the neck over the location of the carotid artery (19). Although atherosclerosis probably accounts for most of these bruits, a number of other mechanisms are possible (see Table 80.9).

Table 80.9
Possible Causes of Cervical Bruit

Physiologic murmur
Venous hum
Transmitted cardiac murmur
Atherosclerosis of carotid, vertebral, subclavian, or innominate artery
Loops, kinks, inflammation, fibromuscular dysplasia of carotid artery
Arteriovenous fistula
Angiomatous malformation
Intracranial neoplasm
Paget's disease of the skull

Natural History

Prospective studies of asymptomatic patients with an anterior cervical bruit have demonstrated an increased risk of cerebrovascular disease. There is disagreement, however, as to (a) whether the intial neurologic deficit in the patient who becomes symptomatic is more likely to be transient or permanent and (b) whether the side of the bruit is of any predictive value in determining the location of the initial neurologic event. At one exteme is the view that the initial deficit is often permanent and is most likely to occur in the vascular territory distal to the carotid artery with the bruit. At the other extreme is the belief that the initial event is almost invariably transient and can occur with equal frequency in the distribution of the affected or contralateral carotid artery. It is clear from a review of the available data that further studies are required to resolve these critical issues which bear directly on the need for aggressive management of these asymptomatic patients.

Evaluation and Management

The physical examination of the neurovascular system is described in detail in Chapter 75. At times, the auscultatory characteristics of a cervical bruit can help to estimate its importance (see Fig. 75.3).

The evaluation and treatment of the asymptomatic patient with an anterior cervical bruit is highly controversial. Many authorities believe that there is no role for cerebral angiography and surgical intervention in the management of these patients (19), while others feel that for certain "high risk" patients these invasive procedures may be indicated (20). According to the latter view, a patient whose bruit is in the location of the carotid bifurcation (near the angle of the jaw) should have a careful funduscopic examination as well as a noninvasive carotid evaluation (ophthalmodynamometry and Doppler study; see "Patient Experience," Chapter 75). Angiography should be considered for those patients with markedly positive noninvasive studies, those with retinal emboli seen on funduscopic examination, or those scheduled for major vascular surgery in the thorax or abdomen which might result in transient intra- or postoperative hypotension. Implicit in any recommendation for angiography is the absence of absolute contraindications to surgery and the availability of a team of skilled radiologists and surgeons. If angiography reveals a large ulcerative or severely stenotic lesion of the internal carotid artery, surgical intervention should be considered.

There is general agreement that patients who do not undergo surgery must be followed closely for any change in the character of their bruit suggestive of progressive disease and for the occurrence of symptoms referable to an underlying arterial lesion. It is reasonable to prescribe antiplatelet drugs, alone or in combination, for these patients, although to date no study has assessed the role of these agents in this situation. Because serial angiographic studies have suggested that the rate of atheromatous change at the carotid bifurcation is directly related to hypertension (22), antihypertensive treatment is important in patients with asymptomatic bruits and high blood pressure; in these patients, it is particularly important to avoid the orthostatic hypotension which may accompany use of any antihypertensive drug.

References

General

Benton, AL (editor): Behavioral Changes in Cerebrovascular Disease. Harper & Row, New York, 1970.
   A detailed account of psychological problems complicating stroke.
Byer, JA and Easton, JD: Therapy of ischemic cerebrovascular disease. Ann Intern Med 93: 742, 1980.
   Thorough review of the subject, extensively referenced.
Licht, S (editor): Stroke and Its Rehabilitation. Williams & Wilkins, Baltimore, 1975.
   A detailed, well-illustrated, and extensively referenced resource on all aspects of the rehabilitation of stroke patients.
Sessler, GJ: Stroke—How to Prevent It/How to Survive It. Prentice-Hall, Englewood Cliffs, N.J., 1982.
   A comprehensive discussion of stroke and its prevention for the physician and potential patient.

Specific

1. Ackerman, RH: Non-invasive carotid evaluation. Stroke 11: 675, 1980.
2. Barnett, HJM: The pathophysiology of transient cerebral ischemic attacks. Therapy with platelet antiaggregants. Med Clin North Am 63: 649, 1979.
3. Beevers, DG, Fairman, MJ, Hamilton, M and Harpur, JE: Antihypertensive treatment and the course of established cerebrovascular disease. Lancet 1: 1407, 1973.
4. Bourestom, NC: Predictors of long term recovery in cerebrovascular disease. Arch Phys Med Rehabil 48: 415, 1967.
5. Brust, JCM: Transient ischemic attacks: natural history and anticoagulation. Neurology 27: 701, 1977.
6. Canadian Cooperative Study Group: A randomized trial of aspirin and sulfinpyrazone in threatened stroke. N Engl J Med 299: 53, 1978.
7. Carter, AB: Hypertensive therapy in stroke survivors. Lancet 1: 485, 1970.
8. Easton, JD and Sherman, DG: Management of cerebral embolism of cardiac origin. Stroke 11: 433, 1980.
9. Eisenberg, H, Morrison, JT, Sullivan, P and Foote, FM: Cere-

brovascular accidents: incidence and survival rates in a defined population. Middelsex County, Connecticut. JAMA 189: 883, 1964.
10. Eisenberg, RL, Bank, WO and Hedgcock, MW: Neurologic complications of angiography for cerebrovascular disease. Neurology 30: 895, 1980.
11. Faught, E, Trader, SD and Hanna, GR: Cerebral complications of angiography for transient ischemia and stroke: prediction of risk. Neurology 29: 4, 1979.
12. Feibel, JH, Berk, S and Joynt, RJ: The unmet needs of stroke survivors. Neurology 29: 592, 1979.
13. Fisher, CM: Cerebral ischemia—less familiar types. Clin Neurosurg 18: 267, 1971.
14. Folstein, MF, Maiberger, R and McHugh, PR: Mood disorders as a specific complication of stroke. J Neurol Neurosurg Psychiatry 40: 1018, 1977.
15. Gainotti, G: Emotional behavior and hemispheric side of the lesion. Cortex 8: 41, 1972.
16. Garraway, MW, Whisnant, JP, Fulan, AJ, Phillips, LH, Kurland, LT and O'Fallon, WM: The declining incidence of stroke. N Engl J Med 300: 449, 1979.
17. Genton, E, Barnett, JHM, Fields, MD, Gent, M and Hoak, JC: XIV. Cerebral ischemia: the role of thrombosis and of antithrombotic therapy. Stroke 8: 147, 1977.
18. Gresham, GE, Fitzpatrick, TE, Wolf, PA, McNamara, PM, Kannel, WB and Dawber, TR: Residual disability in survivors of stroke—The Framingham Study. N Engl J Med 293: 594, 1975.
19. Heyman, A, Wilkinson, WE, Heyden, S, Helms, JM, Bartel, AG, Karp, HR, Tyroler, HA and Hames, CG: Risk of stroke in asymptomatic persons with cervical arterial bruits: a population study in Evans County, Georgia. N Engl J Med 302: 838, 1980.
20. Hurst, JW, Hopkins, LC and Smith, RB: Noises in the neck. N Engl J Med 302: 862, 1980.
21. Hypertensive-Stroke Cooperative Study Group: Effects of antihypertensive treatment on stroke recurrence. JAMA 229: 409, 1974.
22. Javid, H, Ostermiller, WE, Hengesh, JW, Dye, WS, Hunter, JA, Najafi, H and Julian, CC: Natural history of carotid bifurcation atheroma. Surgery 67: 80, 1970.
23. Kannel, WB: Current status of the epidemiology of brain infarction associated with occlusive arterial disease. Stroke 2: 295, 1971.
24. Kannel, WB, Gordon, T, Wolf, PA and McNamara, P: Hemoglobin and the risk of cerebral infarction: the Framingham study. Stroke 3: 409, 1972.
25. Kannel, WB, Wolf, PA, Verter, J and McNamara, PM: Epidemiologic assessment of the role of blood pressure in stroke. JAMA 214: 301, 1970.
26. Katz, S, Ford, AB, Chinn, AB and Newill, VA: Prognosis after strokes; II. Long term course of 159 patients. Medicine 45: 236, 1966.
27. Kurtzke, JF: Epidemiology of cerebrovascular disease. In Cerebrovascular Survey Report edited by RG Siekert. Whiting Press, Rochester, Minn., 1980.
28. Lehmann, JF, DeLateur, BJ, Fowler, RS, Warren, CG, Arnhold, R, Schertzer, G, Hurka, R, Whitmore, JJ, Masock, AJ and Chambers, KH: Stroke: does rehabilitation affect outcome? Arch Phys Med Rehabil 56: 375, 1975.
29. Lehmann, JF, Delateur, BJ, Fowler, RS, Warren, CG, Arnhold, R, Schertzer, G, Hurka, R, Whitmore, JJ, Masock, AJ and Chambers, KH: Stroke rehabilitation: outcome and prediction. Arch Phys Med Rehabil 56: 383, 1975.
30. Louis, S and McDowell, F: Epileptic seizures in nonembolic cerebral infarction. Arch Neurol 17: 414, 1967.
31. Matsumoto, N, Whisnant, JP, Kurland, LT and Okazaki, H: Natural history of stroke in Rochester, Minnesota, 1955 through 1969: an extension of a previous study, 1945 through 1954. Stroke 4: 20, 1973.
32. McDowell, FH, Millikan, CH and Goldstein, M: Treatment of impending stroke. Stroke 11: 1, 1980.

33. Millikan, C: The transient ischemic attack. *Adv Neurol 25:* 135, 1979.
34. Nelson, RF, Pullicino, P, Kendall, BE and Marshal, J: Computed tomography in patients presenting with lacunar syndromes. *Stroke 11:* 256, 1980.
35. Richardson, EP, Jr and Dodge, PR: Epilepsy in cerebral vascular disease: a study of the incidence and nature of seizures in 104 consecutive autopsy proven cases of cerebral infarction and hemorrhage. *Epilepsia 3:* 49, 1954.
36. Ross, GS and Chipman, M: The neuralgias. In *Clinical Neurology,* Vol. 3, edited by AB Baker and LH Baker. Harper & Row, Hagerstown, 1974.
37. Sandok, BA, Furlan, AJ, Whisnant, JP and Sundt, TM, Jr.: Guidelines for the management of transient ischemic attacks. *Mayo Clin Proc 53:* 665, 1978.
38. Sarno, MT: Disorders of communication in stroke. In *Stroke and Its Rehabilitation,* edited by S Licht. Williams & Wilkins, Baltimore, 1975.
39. Tohgi, H, Yamanouchi, H, Murakami, M and Kameyama, M: Importance of the hematocrit as a risk factor in cerebral infarction. *Stroke 9:* 369, 1978.
40. Veterans Administration Cooperative Study Group on Anti-hypertensive Agents: Effects of treatment on morbidity in hypertension. Results in patients with diastolic blood pressures averaging 115 through 129 mm Hg. *JAMA 202:* 1028, 1967.
41. Veterans Administration Cooperative Study Group on Anti-hypertensive Agents: Effects of treatment on morbidity in hypertension; II. Results in patients with diastolic blood pressure averaging 90 through 114 mm Hg. *JAMA 213:* 1143, 1970.
42. Whisnant, JP, Matsumoto, N and Elveback, LR: Transient cerebral ischemic attack in a community. *Mayo Clin Proc 48:* 194, 1973.
43. Wolf, PA, Kannel, WB, McNamara, PM and Gordon, T: The role of impaired cardiac function in atherothrombotic brain infarction: the Framingham study. *Am J Public Health 63:* 52, 1973.

CHAPTER EIGHTY-ONE

Peripheral Neuropathy

LORRAINE F. JOSIFEK, M.D., and BARRY GORDON, M.D., Ph.D.

DEFINITIONS AND PATHOPHYSIOLOGY

A peripheral nerve is a bundle of fibers called *axons;* the large and medium sized axons are normally covered with an insulating layer of myelin. Most peripheral nerves are mixed nerves carrying both incoming sensory information (afferent fibers) and outgoing motor and autonomic impulses (efferent fibers). Large diameter afferent fibers convey information about position and vibration; large diameter efferent fibers innervate the muscles themselves. Small diameter, often unmyelinated, fibers convey pain and temperature sensation, as well as autonomic information.

Peripheral neuropathies result from disease processes which involve nerve axons or their myelin encasements. *Axonal neuropathies* are the result of processes which primarily affect the cell body and axon, whereas *demyelinating neuropathies* result from processes which primarily affect the myelin sheath. Often, especially in chronic disorders such as diabetes, irrespective of the initial type of pathologic process, the interdependence between axon and myelin produces secondary changes which, on biopsy, reveal a mixed pathologic picture. The etiologic diagnosis of peripheral neuropathies, therefore, usually depends upon their clinical features and on other supportive laboratory findings.

The three major patterns of peripheral nerve disease may be distinguished by clinical presentation:

mononeuropathy, mononeuropathy multiplex, and polyneuropathy. *Mononeuropathies* are lesions of the individual nerve roots or peripheral nerves; they usually are due to local causes such as trauma or entrapment (compression of a nerve by adjacent structures). *Mononeuropathy multiplex* refers to involvement of two or more discrete nerves, usually asymmetrically and not contiguously, either at the same time or sequentially. This less common pattern is usually caused by systemic diseases such as polyarteritis nodosa or diabetes which may affect several nerves focally. *Polyneuropathy* is the result of a generalized disease process. In general, in both axonal and demyelinating diseases, the longer axons (longer nerves) tend to be affected earlier and more severely than the shorter ones. In demyelinating neuropathies, this is because the longer axons have more potential sites for demyelination; in the axonal neuropathies, the longer axons require more metabolic support and are therefore more susceptible to curtailment of this support. Therefore, symptoms of both types of neuropathies tend to appear first in the distal feet followed by symptoms in the distal hands. Most polyneuropathies indiscriminately affect both the sensory and the motor nerve fibers (mixed polyneuropathies or sensory-motor neuropathies). However, clinically (and occasionally pathologically), in some patients there will be a predilection for either the sensory nerves (sensory polyneuropathies) or motor nerves (motor polyneuropathies).

APPROACH TO THE PATIENT

History and Physical Examination

Symptoms of peripheral neuropathy include weakness, muscle cramps, loss of sensation (sometimes accompanied by pain), and symptoms of autonomic dysfunction (impotence; urinary retention or overflow incontinence; constipation or diarrhea; and orthostatic hypotension). In polyneuropathies, the sensory loss begins distally and is usually noticed first in the feet: the patient complains of cold feet, diminished ability to distinguish carpeting from other flooring, and of stumbling in the dark (sensory ataxia). This is sometimes associated with sensations of pins and needles (paresthesias). The paresthesias and pain are often made worse by light touch (from bed sheets, for example) or by heat, and they may be somewhat relieved by pacing the floor, by firm massage, or by cold (*e.g.*, leaving the legs outside the covers at night).

The major *signs* of peripheral neuropathy are weakness, muscle atrophy, sensory loss, diminished or absent tendon reflexes, and trophic changes in the skin. In polyneuropathies, the weakness is most often distal, affecting dorsiflexion of the feet (causing the patient to stumble) and less often the small muscles of the hands. In acutely evolving neuropathies, weakness precedes atrophy by approximately 2 to 3

Table 81.1
Common Causes of Neuropathy

MONONEUROPATHY
  Trauma—direct (occupational, recreational) (*e.g.*, ulnar nerve), compression and entrapment (carpal tunnel, root compression, etc.)
  Infection—herpes zoster
  Toxins (*e.g.*, penicillin injection into a sciatic nerve)
  Vascular—vasculitis, diabetes mellitus
  Neoplasm—lymphoma, neurofibroma
MONONEUROPATHY MULTIPLEX
  Diabetes mellitus
  Vasculitis
POLYNEUROPATHY
  Multiple etiologies (see Table 81.2)

weeks. Eventually the shin may appear prominent because of atrophy of the tibialis anterior muscle and there may be striking wasting of the small hand muscles ("skeletal hand"). The skin of the lower extremities often appears shiny, scaling, and atrophic. Marked loss of proprioception in the feet may be manifest as unsteadiness, ataxia, or a positive Romberg test (see Chapter 75 for additional details about neurologic signs).

Distinctive Features

While a limited number of conditions produce mononeuropathy and mononeuropathy multiplex (Table 81.1), there are many etiologies of polyneuropathy (Table 81.2). Diagnosis often depends on obtaining a thorough history (for example of alcoholism or of occupational exposure to toxins) or on finding a relevant systemic condition (for example, diabetes). Therefore, the physician must be alert to distinctive features in the history or on the physical examination that suggest a specific diagnosis. Table 81.3 summarizes the distinctive clinical features of a number of polyneuropathies.

TIME COURSE

Compression neuropathies and other mononeuropathies are often acute in onset. The most common of the acute polyneuropathies is the Guillain-Barré syndrome (p. 889) but other processes—metabolic, infectious, or toxic—may cause severe neurologic dysfunction rapidly, sometimes within hours. Most toxic neuropathies (lead poisoning, for example) develop somewhat more slowly—within weeks—as do neuropathies associated with malnutrition (*e.g.*, thiamine deficiency). The most common of the chronic neuropathies are associated with diabetes mellitus (p. 889) and with alcoholism (p. 889); and, in an unselected population, these are the most common of the polyneuropathies in general.

Patients with *hereditary neuropathies* sometimes may be unaware that they suffer from a long-standing progressive disorder. A history of a lack of athletic prowess in school or in the military or of problems

Table 81.2
Distinctive Features, by Etiology, of the Polyneuropathies

Etiology	Dominant Pathology	Involvement	Typical Distribution	Typical Time Course	Treatment and Response
METABOLIC DEFI-CIENCY					
Diabetes mellitus:					
Polyneuropathy	Axonal	Sensory	Distal symmetric	Chronic	Multivitamin, supportive treatment—slowly progressive course
Mononeuropathy	Ischemic	Sensory-motor	Mononeuropathy (femoral, cranial)	Acute or subacute	Recovery good over months
Autonomic	Ganglion cell	Autonomic	Bladder, gastrointestinal, peripheral vessels	Chronic	Supportive treatment, slowly progressive
Alcoholism and vitamin deficiency	Axonal	Sensory-motor Autonomic	Distal, symmetric	Chronic/subacute	No alcohol, multivitamins, may improve with treatment
Uremia	Axonal	Sensory-motor	Distal, symmetric	Chronic/subacute	May improve with dialysis or transplant
Hypothyroidism	Demyelination	Sensory > motor	Distal, symmetric, Carpal tunnel	Subacute/chronic	Improves with thyroid replacement
Porphyria	Axonal	Motor > sensory	Proximal	Acute	Pyridoxine, treatment for porphyria—slow recovery
Toxin:					
Lead	(?) Axonal	Motor	Asymmetrical, radial wrist drop	Subacute	Chelation
Most other toxins	Axonal	Sensory-motor	Distal	Subacute	May improve when toxin withdrawn
INFECTION					
Diphtheria	Demyelination	Motor	Bulbar and distal	Acute 30–50 days following pharyngitis	Supportive, antitoxin—recovery in 15–30 days
Leprosy	Demyelination	Sensory	Distal, temperature areas	Chronic	Treat infection, supportive—slowly effective, relapses
INFLAMMATORY					
Guillain-Barré	Demyelination	Motor	Ascending proximal, bulbar	Acute	Supportive, in hospital with monitoring
Recurrent inflammatory polyneuropathy	Demyelination	Motor	Proximal	Relapsing	Supportive, steroids
COLLAGEN VASCULAR					
Systemic lupus erythematosus, Polyarteritis nodosa	Ischemic	Sensory-motor	Mononeuropathy multiplex	Acute/subacute	Treat underlying condition
TUMOR					
Carcinomatous, sensory	Ganglion cell	Sensory painful	Distal	Subacute	Treat cancer, neuropathy remains progressive
Carcinomatous, sensory-motor	Axonal	Sensory-motor	Distal	Subacute	May reach plateau with treatment of cancer
Myeloma, paraproteinemia	Axonal	Sensory-motor	Distal	Chronic	Mild course
HEREDITARY					
Charcot-Marie-Tooth	Axonal or demyelinating	Motor	Distal	Very chronic	Supportive functional aids
Interstitial hypertrophic (Dejeurine-Sottas)	Demyelinating, hypertrophic	Sensory-motor	Distal	Very chronic	Supportive
Amyloidosis	Compressive, axonal, ischemic	Sensory-motor, autonomic	Distal or entrapment	Chronic	Slowly progressive

fitting shoes may be a useful clue in that regard. High arched feet and hammertoes reflect long-standing disease and may point to the diagnosis of one of these hereditary processes.

PATTERNS OF INVOLVEMENT

Mononeuropathy usually produces both motor and sensory involvement in the distribution of the af-

Table 81.3
Differential Diagnosis of Polyneuropathies[a, b]

COURSE	Tabes dorsalis
Acute (days):	Dissociated loss of pain sensibility:
Guillain-Barré syndrome	*Diabetes* (small fiber type)
Porphyric neuropathy	Amyloidosis
Diphtheritic neuropathy	Hereditary sensory neuropathies
Some toxins (*e.g.*, tri-orthocresyl phosphate)	Lepromatous leprosy
Subacute (weeks):	Dissociated loss of joint position and vibration sensibility:
Many toxins	Subacute combined degeneration
Nutritional neuropathies	Friedreich's ataxia
Carcinomatous neuropathies	Autonomic neuropathy:
Uremic neuropathy	*Diabetes*
Relapsing:	*Amyloid*
Relapsing inflammatory neuropathy	Acute, chronic, and relapsing pandysautonomia
Refsum's disease	Dysautonomia (Riley-Day)
Chronic (many months or years):	DISTRIBUTION[d]
Diabetic motor-sensory neuropathy	Proximal weakness:
Alcoholic neuropathy	Guillain-Barré
Chronic inflammatory neuropathies	Porphyria
Very chronic (childhood onset):	Carcinomatous neuropathy with proximal weakness
Heritable motor-sensory neuropathies (*e.g.*, Charcot-	("carcinomatous neuromyopathy")
Marie-Tooth disease)	Spinal muscular atrophies
SELECTIVE FUNCTIONAL INVOLVEMENT[c]	Proximal sensory loss:
Predominately motor:	Porphyria
Guillain-Barré syndrome	Tangier disease (analphalipoproteinemia)
Relapsing and chronic inflammatory neuropathy	Temperature-related distribution:
Acute intermittent porphyria	Lepromatous leprosy
Lead neuropathy	AGE
Heritable motor-sensory neuropathies (Charcot-Marie-	Childhood:
Tooth)	*"Steroid dependent"* inflammatory neuropathies
Diphtheritic neuropathy	Giant axonal neuropathy
Predominately sensory:	Krabbe's disease
Diabetes	Metachromatic leukodystrophy
Carcinomatous sensory neuropathy (*ganglioradiculitis*)	Neuroaxonal dystrophy
Paraproteinemic and cryoglobulinemic neuropathy	Heritable sensorimotor neuropathy (Dejerine-Sottas)

[a] From JW Griffen: Peripheral neuropathies. In *Principles and Practice of Medicine*, Ed. 20, edited by AM Harvey, RJ Johns, VA McKusick, AH Owens and RS Ross. Appleton-Century-Crofts, New York, 1980.
[b] The most common etiologies are set in *italic*.
[c] Most polyneuropathies produce sensory and motor disturbances.
[d] Most polyneuropathies produce distal involvement.

fected nerve root or peripheral nerve (see below, p. 892).

In polyneuropathy, *predominantly sensory* involvement suggests diabetes, carcinoma, amyloidosis, dysproteinemia, and alcoholism. Occasionally, sensory loss is *dissociated*, with diminished appreciation of pain and temperature but preserved appreciation of light touch and joint position. When pain sensation is preserved but position sense is lost, vitamin B_{12} deficiency (usually pernicious anemia) and, much more rarely, Friedreich's ataxia should be considered.

In polyneuropathy, *predominantly motor* involvement suggests the Guillain-Barré syndrome, hereditary neuropathies, lead intoxication, and acute intermittent porphyria. Weakness due to polyneuropathy is usually distal and symmetrical.

Proximal involvement suggests the Guillain-Barré syndrome, porphyria, or brachial plexus injury. Predominant involvement of the *upper extremity* (partic-

ularly wrist drop due to radial nerve involvement) suggests a toxin (*e.g.*, lead).

Predominantly autonomic involvement suggests diabetes, amyloidosis, alcoholism, dysautonomia, and dysproteinemia.

INVESTIGATIONS

Laboratory

It is important to identify the cause of a peripheral neuropathy because often neurologic dysfunction will persist unless the underlying disease can be treated. The common causes of polyneuropathy (shown in italics in Table 81.3) are usually obvious to the physician; but sometimes, even these require direct questioning (concerning alcoholism, for example) or specific laboratory tests (for example, measurement of serum glucose or of thyroid function) before they are appreciated. If the cause of the neuropathy is not obvious, routine screening tests should include erythrocyte sedementation rate, fasting blood glucose, serum urea nitrogen or serum creatinine, thyroxine (T_4), a complete blood count (CBC), a chest X-ray, and, in men over the age of 40, a serum protein electrophoresis. It is obvious that there are many relatively unusual conditions that may be associated with neuropathy, but an extensive screening program to rule out all of these processes would be expensive and almost always unrewarding *unless there is some clue in the history or physical examination to warrant a particular test* (for example, measurement of blood lead in a patient with a history of occupational exposure). If, after the general physician has evaluated a patient with neuropathy, no cause of the process has been identified, consultation with a neurologist is indicated.

Nerve Conduction Studies

The measurement of nerve conduction velocity is only occasionally helpful in the diagnosis of peripheral neuropathy. It is useful mainly in documenting that neuropathy exists in situations where there is some question about the diagnosis (for example, polyneuropathy vs. myopathy or an entrapment neuropathy vs. nerve root compression). Although there are laboratories that will perform nerve conduction studies upon demand, the general physician would be wise to let a neurologist decide about the usefulness and the interpretation of the procedure.

Motor nerve conduction velocities (NCVs) are obtained by electrically stimulating a peripheral nerve at two separate points, and using the difference in muscle response times as an indication of the conduction velocity of the nerve segment between the two points of stimulation. Sensory conduction velocities are obtained by stimulating a peripheral nerve at one point and then recording the evoked action potential over the nerve at another point.

The procedure has several limitations: First, NCVs only test directly that portion of the nerve between the two sites; they generally do not detect damage more distal than (e.g., muscle) or more proximal to (e.g., nerve root) the segment tested. So the standard test is not really applicable to such common clinical situations as spondylosis or lumbar or cervical disc disease (see Chapters 61 and 62). (More specialized testing—F-wave velocities—can measure conduction velocity in the proximal segment, but is not routinely done.)

Second, NCVs measure the speed of conduction in the largest and fastest conducting fibers of peripheral nerves. Therefore, nerve conduction studies are only sensitive to diseases which involve such fibers.

NCV measurements are most useful in the detection of demyelinating neuropathies. They are less likely to be slowed by axonal neuropathies. Furthermore, NCVs will not reveal an abnormality of small fibers, which is the basis of many painful peripheral neuropathies.

It is important for the clinician to be able to specify as precisely as possible which nerves need to be tested; stating only "numbness in the upper extremities" or "test nerves in lower extremities" without any specific guidance is likely to be both unpleasant for the patient and unproductive for the physician.

Patient Experience. With the patient lying down a paste is applied over the sites to be tested and electrodes are taped over the appropriate muscles and nerves. The shocks are usually mildly unpleasant, but occasionally are painful. For accurate results, the shocks may have to be repeated rapidly. Usually the nerves on both sides of the body are compared. Testing takes approximately 20 to 60 minutes.

Electromyography (Table 81.4)

Electromyography (EMG) is not often helpful in the diagnosis of peripheral neuropathy; the sensitivity and specificity of the procedure are relatively low. It is useful primarily in situations in which the distinction between neuropathy and myopathy is difficult (polyneuropathy *vs.* polymyositis, for example) and in confirming the diagnosis of a denervation syndrome (see below). Since EMG is unpleasant, the physician should consider carefully whether the information to be gained from it is likely to benefit the patient. Consultation with a neurologist is advised in helping to make this decision.

EMG involves the insertion of needles within a muscle to record electrical activity directly. During *complete rest*, no electrical activity should be observed. Spontaneous *fibrillation* potentials are the action potentials of single fibers that are twitching spontaneously in the absence of innervation. Fibrillation potentials are usually, but not invariably, a good indication of primary denervation (they also occur in polymositis and more rarely in other myopathic processes). *Fasciculations* are the spontaneous firings of whole motor units (all of the muscle fibers innervated by a single nerve fiber). Fasciculations and bizarre (polyphasic) fasciculations may be seen in normal individuals, although they are more frequent and likely to be more bizarre in states of denervation. Therefore, the presence of fasciculations is only moderately useful in diagnosing denervation.

Muscle action potentials are examined individually by asking the patient to move only slightly. Large amplitude, long duration polyphasic potentials suggest a denervating process. Small amplitude, short duration polyphasic potentials are associated with myopathic processes.

The *interference pattern* is the pattern produced when the subject is asked to contract the muscle fully. A "full" interference pattern is normal. Anything less may indicate less than maximal effort (hysteria, malingering), poor conduction of nerve impulses to the muscle (denervation), or poor ability of the muscle to respond (myopathy).

Table 81.4
Electromyography

Disorder	Insertion Activity	Complete Rest	Action Potentials	Interference Patterns
Denervation[a]	May be increased	Positive denervation potentials, fibrillations, or fasciculations	High amplitude, long duration, poly-phasic	Incomplete
Myopathy[b]	May be increased	May be normal or show fibrillations	Low amplitude, usually short duration, may be polyphasic	Reduced in amplitude, may be incomplete

[a] Neuropathy, radiculopathy, disc disease.
[b] Dystrophy, polymyositis.

The highest yield of useful information with EMG is from moderately affected muscles. The physician should expect a low yield from muscles that are clinically normal or only minimally involved and should anticipate uninterpretable results from muscles that are severely involved, as end stage muscle disease of almost any cause ultimately presents the same EMG picture.

The physician should remember that the EMG electrodes damage and inflame the muscles into which they have been inserted. Thus if there is a possibility that a muscle biopsy will be required, the muscle that may be biopsied should not be tested by EMG.

Patient Experience. There is usually considerable pain with the initial insertion of the needles and also during movement of the muscles when the needles are in place. As the needles are very thin and only penetrate skin and muscle, the risks of infection or hemorrhage are almost nil. The procedure takes 30 to 90 minutes.

Nerve Biopsy

Nerve biopsy should be reserved for those patients in whom a specific histologic diagnosis is a possibility (for example, amyloidosis or vasculitis). In general the procedure has limited usefulness, since the pathology is usually nonspecific; also the nerve biopsied is usually a sensory nerve (the sural) and may not reflect a disease process which has affected the motor nerves. The biopsy may lead to painful sequelae in the distribution of the biopsied nerve. If the nerve biopsy is done, it must be specially processed for maximum information at centers which are familiar with nerve pathology. Consultation with a neurologist will be helpful in deciding whether or not a nerve biopsy is indicated.

COMMON PROBLEMS

Guillain-Barré Syndrome (7)

Most cases of the Guillain-Barré syndrome follow a mild viral illness (by 10 to 12 days); the syndrome is also associated with pregnancy, the postoperative period, and recent influenza vaccination. There is rapid progression of motor weakness (usually moving from the lower extremities to the upper extremities) accompanied by loss of deep tendon reflexes. Although pain or paresthesias may be prominant early symptoms, objective evidence of sensory loss is minimal. Cranial nerve weakness may be present, with bilateral facial nerve palsy, in 40% of patients. Nerve conduction velocities may be abnormal, and the cerebrospinal fluid may show increased protein with normal cell counts (cyto-albumin dissociation). Because of rapid progression of the disease patients suspected of the disorder should be admitted to the hospital for close monitoring for potential respiratory distress and autonomic disturbances (hypotension, hypertension, cardiac arrhythmias, hyperpyrexia) which are often part of the course. Recovery is complete in about half the patients (although it may take 6 to 18 months); most of the remainder have only mild deficits; but 10% have severe permanent disability. The differential diagnosis includes diphtheria, botulism, and porphyria.

Diabetic Neuropathy (4, 11)

Reliable figures for the prevalence of diabetic neuropathy are not available, but it is clearly one of the more common neuropathies. The problem is discussed in detail in Chapter 69, "Diabetes Mellitus."

Alcoholic Neuropathy (2)

Neuropathies associated with alcoholism and with associated vitamin deficiences usually occur in the fourth to seventh decade with a slow onset over a period of months. The presenting symptoms are varied, but they often reflect a distal, motor and sensory, symmetric polyneuropathy with pain and paresthesias in the feet and legs. Autonomic features including impotence, bladder dysfunction, and orthostatic hypotension may also be seen. Malnutrition and vitamin deficiencies (particularly thiamine deficiency), probably make a major contribution to the neuropathy, although there is evidence that alcohol has a direct toxic effect on peripheral nerves.

Treatment is aimed toward nutrition and vitamin replacement as well as toward decreased alcoholic consumption (see Chapter 20). Since alcoholism is so difficult to treat successfully, the neuropathic process often persists.

Carcinomatous Neuropathy

There are several patterns of carcinomatous neuropathy (excluding nerve damage from direct invasion of nerves by tumor); they occur most commonly in association with cancer of the lung, sometimes years before the tumor has been diagnosed (12).

DISTAL SENSORY—MOTOR NEUROPATHY

This is primarily an axonal process. It develops over weeks or months, and often becomes stationary, or, if the underlying cancer responds to treatment, it may improve.

CARCINOMATOUS SENSORY NEUROPATHY

This has the uncommon but distinctive picture of a progressive sensory neuropathy beginning in adulthood. The neuopathy usually begins distally and asymmetrically, and over many weeks spreads more proximally with the development of profound sensory loss, sometimes accompanied by pain and pseudoathetosis (seemingly purposeless movements that, in reality, are due to loss of position sense). Proprioceptive loss may become generalized so that the patient may be unable to stand or walk unassisted. The face is seldom involved. NCV may show normal motor potentials but unobtainable sensory potentials. The neuropathy is usually irreversible, even if an underlying malignancy is successfully treated.

Toxic Neuropathy

Toxic neuropathies are becoming increasingly more frequent. They are important to recognize since they are potentially reversible if the toxin can be identified. At times the diagnosis may be easily made if a history of drug exposure (e.g., isoniazid, hydralazine, vincristine) or of industrial exposure (e.g., lead, organophosphates—see also Chapter 7) is known. If the history of toxic exposure is not obtained, these neuropathies have no distinguishing features on routine history or on physical examination. Therefore a detailed history of exposure to drugs, and the patients

Table 81.5
Toxins Associated with Peripheral Neuropathies

INDUSTRIAL (see Chapter 7 for a more detailed list)
  Pesticides—organophosphates, dichlorophenyoxyacetate (2, 4-D), Vacor rodenticide
  Metal work—lead, arsenic
  Plastics, synthetic fabrics—n-hexane, methyl n-butyl ketone, acrylamide, carbon disulfide
EUPHORIANTS
  Glue sniffing—n-hexane, solvents
  Nitrous oxide inhalation—whipped cream dispensers, dental offices
PHARMACOTHERAPEUTIC AGENTS
  Antimicrobial—isoniazid, nitrofurantoin, metronidazole (Flagyl)
  Cardiovascular—hydralazine, procainamide
  Other—phenytoin, disulfiram (Antabuse)

occupation and recreational habits is important (see Table 81.5).

Compression and Entrapment Neuropathies (9)

When a peripheral neurologic abnormality occurs in one upper or lower extremity, the abnormality is usually due to a nerve entrapment or compression, although a polyneuropathy may present initially as a focal deficit in one extremity. With careful evaluation, it is usually possible to determine whether the patient's problem is due to nerve root damage or to damage to a peripheral nerve or one of it branches. Tables 81.6 and 81.7 and Figures 81.1 and 82.2 summarize the information needed to make this distinction, i.e., distribution of sensory, motor, and reflex deficits; common causative lesions; and critical anatomic relationships.

Several commonly encountered problems due to entrapment or compression are discussed here. Root compression symptoms due to cervical and lumbar spine disease are discussed in Chapters 61 ("Neck Pain"), 62 ("Low Back Pain"), and 65 ("Degenerative Joint Disease").

CARPAL TUNNEL SYNDROME

Median nerve entrapment at the wrist is often accompanied by nocturnal discomfort and sensory loss in the median distribution (palmar surface of the thumb, index, middle, and radial half of the ring fingers). There may be retrograde pain of the arm to the shoulder, weakness and atrophy of the thenar eminence (weak thumb opposition and abduction). Light percussion of the nerve at the wrist may cause paresthesias in the distribution of the pain (Tinel's sign). Forced wrist flexion (Phanlan sign) or, less commonly, forced extension, may also reproduce the symptoms. The most common associated causes are pregnancy, old fractures, diabetes mellitus, rheumatoid arthritis, hypothyroidism, gout, and amyloidosis; occupational trauma (e.g., scrubbing) also may play a role.

Nerve conduction studies (see p. 888) are important to support the clinical diagnosis by revealing slowing over the segment that is clinically involved. *Sensory nerve conduction is the most sensitive indicator of a lesion*, showing both reduced amplitude and prolonged latencies in the distal segment in virtually all patients with carpal tunnel compression. *Motor nerve conduction is less frequently abnormal* (60 to 80%). Nerve conduction studies may also be useful to evaluate other areas (e.g., legs), for evidence of a more generalized neuropathic process.

Treatment. For self-limited conditions (e.g., pregnancy), or others when there is no evidence of denervation, symptoms may be relieved by a night splint (cock-up splint which maintains the wrist in extension, especially useful in pregnancy). A steroid injection into the tunnel, adjacent to the nerve, often relieves the painful symptoms of the syndrome, but

Table 81.6
Comparative Data on Root and Nerve Lesions in the Arm[a]

Roots[b]	C5	C6	C7	C8	D1
Sensory supply	Lateral border upper arm	Lateral forearm including thumb	Over triceps, mid-forearm and middle finger	Medial forearm to include little finger	Axilla down to the olecranon
Sensory loss	As above	As above	Middle fingers	As above	As above
Area of pain	As above and medial scapula border	As above, especially thumb and index finger	As above and medial scapula border	As above	Deep aching in shoulder and axilla to olecranon
Reflex arc	Biceps jerk	Supinator jerk	Triceps jerk	Finger jerk	None
Motor deficit	Deltoid Supraspinatus Infraspinatus Rhomboids	Biceps Brachioradialis Brachialis (Pronators and supinators of forearm)	Latissimus dors. Pectoralis majo. Triceps Wrist extensors Wrist flexors	Finger flexors Finger extensors Flexor carpi ulnaris (thenar muscles in some patients)	All small hand muscles (in some thenar muscles via C8)
Causative lesions	Brachial neuritis Cervical spondylosis[c] Upper plexus avulsion	Cervical spondylosis[c] Acute disc lesions	Acute disc lesions Cervical spondylosis[c]	Rare in disc lesions or spondylosis[c]	Cervical rib Outlet syndromes Pancoast tumor Metastatic carcinoma in deep cervical nodes

Nerves	Axillary	Musculocutaneous	Radial	Median	Ulnar
Sensory supply	Over deltoid	Lateral forearm to wrist	Lateral dorsal forearm and back of thumb and index finger	Lateral palm and lateral fingers	Medial palm and 5th and medial half ring finger
Sensory loss	Small area over deltoid	Lateral forearm	Dorsum of thumb and index (if any)	As above	As above but often none at all
Area of pain	Across shoulder tip	Lateral forearm	Dorsum of thumb and index	Thumb, index and middle finger. Often spreads up forearm	Ulnar supplied fingers and palm distal to wrist. Pain occasionally along course of nerve
Reflex arc	Nil	Biceps jerk	Triceps jerk and supinator jerk	Finger jerks (flexor digitorum sublimis)	Nil
Motor deficit	Deltoid (Teres minor cannot be evaluated)	Biceps Brachialis (coracobrachialis weakness not detectable)	Triceps Wrist extensors Finger extensors Brachioradialis Supinator of forearm	Wrist flexors Long finger flexors (thumb, index and middle finger) Pronators of forearm. Abductor pollicis brevis	All small hand muscles excluding abductor pollicis brevis. Flexor carpi ulnaris. Long flexors of ring and little finger
Causative lesions	Fractured neck of humerus. Dislocated shoulder. Deep i.m. injections	Very rarely damaged	Crutch palsy. Saturday night palsy. Fractured humerus. In supinator muscle	Carpal tunnel syndrome Direct trauma to wrist	Elbow: trauma, bed rest, fractured olecranon Wrist: local trauma, ganglion of wrist joint

[a] From J. Patten: *Neurological Differential Diagnosis*, Springer-Verlag, New York, 1977.
[b] See also dermatome map, Figure 75.2.
[c] See details in Chapters 61 and 65.

the response is usually transient. When symptoms and signs persist or when denervation is present, surgical release of the flexor retinaculum is indicated. These procedures should be performed by an orthopaedic, plastic, or neurologic surgeon experienced in hand surgery.

ULNAR NERVE ENTRAPMENTS

The ulnar nerve is most commonly compressed at the elbow, usually as a result of repeated occupational/recreational trauma or entrapment due to a chronic deformity or arthritis involving the ulnar aspect of the elbow. Sensory symptoms (numbness and tingling of the ulnar border of the hand, and of the 5th finger and the ulnar side of the 4th finger) are more prominent than motor symptoms (weakness of finger abduction and adduction, and of distal phalangeal extension).

If the ulnar nerve is compressed in the wrist, hand sensation and fifth finger abduction strength are maintained, but there is weakness of index finger abduction. This is most often caused by a ganglion, but can also be caused by rheumatoid arthritis and by trauma (such as long distance bicycling).

Nerve conduction studies can localize the site of ulnar nerve entrapment or damage. When the prob-

Table 81.7
Comparative Data on Root and Nerve Lesions in the Leg[a]

Roots[b]	L2	L3	L4	L5	S1
Sensory supply	Across upper thigh	Across lower thigh	Across knee to medial malleolus	Side of leg to dorsum and sole of foot	Behind lateral malleolus to lateral foot
Sensory loss	Often none	Often none	Medial leg	Dorsum of foot	Behind lateral malleolus
Area of pain	Across thigh	Across thigh	Down to medial malleolus	Back of thigh, lateral calf—dorsum of foot	Back of thigh, back of calf—lateral foot
Reflex arc	None	Adductor reflex	Knee jerk	None	Ankle jerk
Motor deficit	Hip flexion	Knee extension Adduction of thigh	Inversion of the foot	Dorsiflexion of toes and foot (latter L4 also)	Plantar flexion and eversion of foot

	L2 – L4			L5 – S1	
Causative lesions (in order of frequency)	Neurofibroma Meningioma Neoplastic disease Disc lesions very rare (except L4 < 5% *all*)			Disc lesions[c] Metastatic malignancy Neurofibromas Meningioma	

				Sciatic Nerve	
Nerves	Obturator	Femoral	Peroneal Division	Tibial Division	
Sensory supply	Medial surface of thigh	Antero medial surface of thigh and leg to medial malleolus	Anterior leg, dorsum of ankle and foot	Posterior leg, sole and lateral border of foot	
Sensory loss	Often none	Usually anatomical	Often just dorsum of foot	Sole of foot	
Area of pain	Medial thigh	Anterior thigh and medial leg	Often painless	Often painless	
Reflex arc	Adductor reflex	Knee jerk	None	Ankle jerk	
Motor deficit	Adduction of thigh	Extension of knee	Dorsiflexion, inversion and eversion of the foot (+ lateral hamstrings)	Plantar flexion and inversion of foot (+ medial hamstrings)	
Causative lesions	Pelvic neoplasm Pregnancy	Diabetes Femoral hernia Femoral artery aneurysm Posterior abdominal neoplasm Psoas abscess	Pressure palsy at fibula neck Hip fracture/dislocation Penetrating trauma to buttock Misplaced injection	Very rarely injured even in buttock Peroneal division more sensitive to damage	

[a] From J. Patten: *Neurological Differential Diagnosis*, Springer-Verlag, New York, 1977.
[b] See also dermatome map, Figure 75.2.
[c] See details in Chapter 61 and 65.

lem appears to be entrapment, surgical decompression may restore function to normal.

LATERAL FEMORAL CUTANEOUS NERVE SYNDROME (NEURALGIA PARESTHETICA)

This nerve may be compressed or stretched at the anterior superior iliac spine at the lateral end of the inguinal canal, causing burning pain, paresthesia, and decreased sensation over the lateral thigh. The sensory involvement is more lateral than that in femoral neuropathy, and there is no motor involvement or loss of patellar reflex. Common causes include pelvic tilt, acute abdominal enlargement (ascites, pregnancy), external mechanical trauma (girdle, utility belt), and diabetes. Pain may respond to medical management (see below, p. 894). If the pain is severe, local injection of an anesthetic may provide relief for long periods; sectioning of the ligament over the canal is only rarely needed.

Bell's Palsy

Paralysis of the facial muscles due to inflammation and swelling of the seventh (the facial) cranial nerve (Bell's palsy) is seen occasionally in a general medical practice. One large series reported an incidence of 23 cases per 100,000 population per year (6). There is no predilection for a particular sex, age group, or race. The cause of the condition is unknown. Although involvement of the facial nerve results in the predominant signs and symptoms, the process is actually a polyneuropathy that affects, subclinically, other cranial nerves as well. Usually patients will note the sudden onset, within hours, of a unilateral paralysis of a facial nerve: the eyebrow sags; the eye cannot be closed; the nasolabial fold disappears; and the mouth appears drawn to the unaffected side. Less commonly, there is loss of taste on the anterior two-thirds of the tongue; and there is hyperacusis (an accentuation of loud sounds) in the affected ear. Most patients recover spontaneously within weeks to a few months; approximately 15% recover incompletely, but severe residual weakness is rare (6). There is, in incomplete responders, a considerable risk of synkinesis, a contraction of all of the facial muscles on the affected side when the patient attempts to move just one or a few of them.

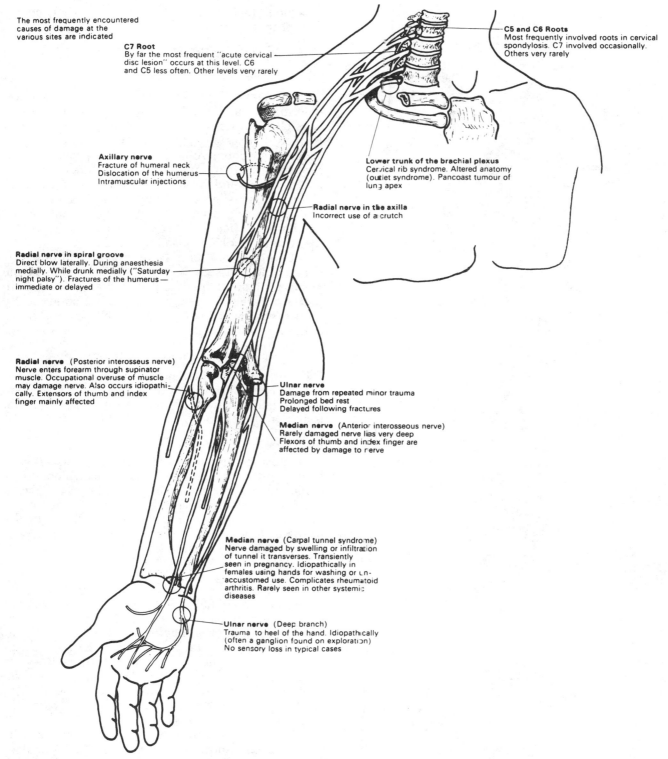

The most frequently encountered causes of damage at the various sites are indicated

C7 Root
By far the most frequent "acute cervical disc lesion" occurs at this level. C6 and C5 less often. Other levels very rarely

C5 and C6 Roots
Most frequently involved roots in cervical spondylosis. C7 involved occasionally. Others very rarely

Axillary nerve
Fracture of humeral neck
Dislocation of the humerus
Intramuscular injections

Lower trunk of the brachial plexus
Cervical rib syndrome. Altered anatomy (outlet syndrome). Pancoast tumour of lung apex

Radial nerve in the axilla
Incorrect use of a crutch

Radial nerve in spiral groove
Direct blow laterally. During anaesthesia medially. While drunk medially ("Saturday night palsy"). Fractures of the humerus— immediate or delayed

Radial nerve (Posterior interosseus nerve)
Nerve enters forearm through supinator muscle. Occupational overuse of muscle may damage nerve. Also occurs idiopathically. Extensors of thumb and index finger mainly affected

Ulnar nerve
Damage from repeated minor trauma
Prolonged bed rest
Delayed following fractures

Median nerve (Anterior interosseous nerve)
Rarely damaged nerve lies very deep
Flexors of thumb and index finger are affected by damage to nerve

Median nerve (Carpal tunnel syndrome)
Nerve damaged by swelling or infiltration of tunnel it transverses. Transiently seen in pregnancy. Idiopathically in females using hands for washing or unaccustomed use. Complicates rheumatoid arthritis. Rarely seen in other systemic diseases

Ulnar nerve (Deep branch)
Trauma to heel of the hand. Idiopathically (often a ganglion found on exploration) No sensory loss in typical cases

Figure 81.1 Clinically relevant anatomy of the nerve supply to the arm. (From J. Patten: *Neurological Differential Diagnosis*, Springer-Verlag, New York, 1977.)

Corticosteroids appear to reduce somewhat the incidence of incomplete recovery (1, 13) of patients in Bell's palsy. Thus, it is reasonable to administer prednisone for 9 days after diagnosis—60 mg for 3 days, and then tapered by 10 mg a day. Some advocate early surgical decompression of the facial nerve in patients who demonstrate by electromyography complete or nearly complete denervation (5), but

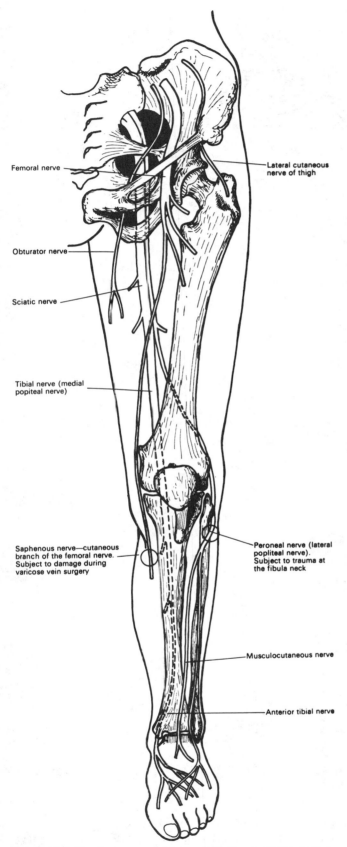

Figure 81.2 Course and bony relations of the nerve supply of the leg. (From J. Patten: *Neurological Dif-*

most neurologists believe that the data do not support this more radical approach.

THERAPEUTIC PRINCIPLES

General

Treatment of peripheral neuropathies first requires determining and treating any underlying cause if possible. Efforts should be made also to prevent further damage: e.g., patients with an underlying generalized polyneropathy are more prone to pressure palsies and it is important to educate them about habits that could be injurious (such as leaning on elbows or crossing legs). The daily administration of multivitamins is prudent to prevent any contributing nutritional deficiencies. Avoidance of potential toxins such as alcohol is also important.

For *entrapment and compression* neuropathies, eliminating pressure on the affected nerve is the primary mode of treatment. For deficits which are partial or recent in onset, recovery of function usually occurs within about 6 weeks of eliminating nerve entrapment or compression.

Symptomatic Treatment

Unfortunately, polyneuropathy is often irreversible (and progressive), even if the cause is known. Symptomatic therapy to maintain the best function is all that the physician can offer these patients.

MOTOR

In most polyneuropathies, weakness usually affects dorsiflexion of the feet early (causing foot drop); ambulation can be greatly improved by a rigid plastic splint worn in the shoe or by a spring-loaded brace attached to the shoe. Fine motor weakness in the hands can be aided by built-up tools and other devices provided by occupational therapists.

SENSORY

Anesthetic limbs are vulnerable to repeated, unrecognized trauma. The patient should always check the temperature of bath water, pot handles, etc., with parts of his body that have normal sensation. Small hard objects (keys, faucet handles) can be built up with soft materials. Occupational therapists can make useful suggestions along these lines. Meticulous care should be given to feet and toenails (see Chapter 99). Moisturizing cream for dry, insensitive, skin will reduce serious abrasions.

Pain associated with sensory neuropathies is usually a difficult and chronic problem. Simple analgesics (aspirin), whirlpool, and massage may help relieve relatively mild pain. Narcotics are to be avoided, because of the potential for addiction. Phenytoin (Dilantin) 300 to 500 mg per day to yield a serum level of 15 to 20 μg/ml may provide relief of refractory

ferential Diagnosis, Springer-Verlag, New York, 1977.)

pain and thus is worth a therapeutic trial. If phenytoin has been maintained in the therapeutic range for 2 weeks, and still proves unsuccessful, it may be followed with a trial of carbamazepine (Tegretol) 200 to 1000 mg/day in divided doses (2 or 3 times a day). This is started at 100 mg twice a day and must be increased slowly (200 mg every 4 days in divided doses), as intolerance (with ataxia, drowsiness and nausea) is especially likely in the older patient. Hematologic values and liver function tests must be checked pariodically (see Chapter 77). Tricyclic antidepressants (such as amitriptyline 25 to 75 mg at bedtime) may also be tried.

AUTONOMIC

Autonomic dysfunctions should also be approached symptomatically. The hypotonic bladder may be treated by drugs that increase bladder tone (urecholine, 10 to 25 mg every 8 hours) or with surgery to decrease resistance to bladder emptying. (A urologic consultation is important in both diagnosis and therapy of this condition.) Sexual impotence cannot be helped directly, although penile prostheses have been tried with variable success (see Chapter 17). The knowledge that the dysfunction is on a neurologic basis may relieve the anxiety which accompanies the problem. A thorough search for medications which may be contributing to impotence is important (see Chapter 17).

Orthostatic hypotension (see also Chapter 78) may be treated with a volume-expanding mineralocorticoid (fluorocortisone 0.1 mg daily) and sometimes salt supplementation in patients without congestive heart failure. Most patients tolerate support stockings (e.g., Jobst) poorly, but learning to arise slowly, maintaining active ambulation, and sleeping with head raised (to stimulate renin release) may help. Table 81.8 summarizes the various practical ways to manage patients with this vexing problem.

Table 81.8
Management of Patients with Orthostatic Hypotension

Avoid sudden changes in position
Avoid excessive intake of alcohol
Avoid excessive diuresis
Correct hypovolemia (see text)
Discontinue or reduce the dosage of drugs known to cause orthostatic hypotension:
   Antihypertensive drugs
   Nitroglycerine
   Diuretics
   Neuroleptics
   Tricyclic antidepressants
   CNS depressants (opiates, alcohol)
   Levodopa
Tilt up the head of the bed
Use elastic support stockings

OTHER CONDITIONS

Restless Legs Syndrome

This is a common syndrome and an important cause of insomnia (see Chapter 82), which is often unrecognized or attributed to "hysteria" or "malingering." Patients complain of cold, unpleasant, sometimes painful crawling sensations in their legs at rest or in the early stages of sleep. The sensations are usually bilateral, symmetrical, and most frequently in the lower leg; they are described as "deep inside" the muscles or bones. Movement of the limbs provides some relief; affected patients usually find it impossible to keep their limbs still.

Five percent of a group of otherwise healthy subjects had recognizable symptoms of this syndrome (3). The syndrome has been related in some patients to a mild neuropathy; it can be seen in diabetes, after gastrectomy, and in uremia. Sometimes the condition seems hereditary, in that it is present in several family members. It is possible that those patients have hereditary mild neuropathy or motor neuron disease. There seems to be a relationship between anemia and restless legs in some patients. In a series of 77 unselected, typical cases of the syndrome, one-fourth had definitely decreased serum iron levels, whereas in a series of patients with iron deficiency anemia one-fourth had restless legs (3). Correction of an iron deficiency state improved symptoms in these patients.

In some patients diazepam and clonazepam may relieve the restless legs syndrome.

Muscle Cramps

Cramps are localized involuntary painful contractions of skeletal muscles and produce a visibly and palpably hard and bulging muscle. They must be distinguished from the *sensory* experience of cramp, such as that of intermittent claudication.

Ordinary muscle cramps are common and may be stopped by stretching the affected muscles. Cramps are associated with fatiguing exercises, salt depletion, dehydration, pregnancy, hypothyroidism, uremia, hypomagnesemia, myopathy, or denervation. Patients with frequent daytime cramps, usually healthy adults, should be evaluated for the rare muscle enzymatic defects (e.g., phosphorylase, phosphofructokinase, or carnitine palmatyl transferase deficiency). If no associated condition exists, these patients may be given a therapeutic trial of phenytoin, carbamazepine, or amitriptyline (see above for dosages).

Nocturnal cramps occur in 15% of healthy young adults and are more common in the elderly. Two drugs have proven effective in a double blind trial against placebo: quinine sulfate, 200 mg at bedtime, and chloroquine phosphate, 250 mg a day. Relief occurred in 1 to 3 weeks and often lasted several months after treatment ended (8, 10).

References

General

Asbury, A and Johnson, P: *Pathology of Peripheral Nerve.* W. B. Saunders, Philadelphia, 1978.
  A standard reference.
Dyck, P, Thomas, PK and Lambert, EH (editors): *Peripheral Neuropathy.* W. B. Saunders, Philadelphia, 1978.
  An excellent comprehensive review—probably the first general source for clinicians.

Specific

1. Adour, KK, Wingerd, J, Bell, DN, Manning, JJ and Hurley, JP: Prednisone treatment for idiopathic facial paralysis (Bell's palsy). *N Engl J Med 287:* 1268, 1972.
2. Behse, F and Buchthal, F : Alcoholic neuropathy: clinical, electrophysiological and biopsy findings. *Ann Neurol 2:* 95, 1977.
3. Ekbom, KA: Restless legs. In *Handbook of Clinical Neurology,* Vol. 6, p. 311, edited by PJ Vinken and GW Bruyn. American Elsevier, New York, 1970.
4. Ellenberg, M: Diabetic neuropathy: clinical aspects. *Metabolism 25:* 1627, 1976.
5. Fisch, U: Surgery for Bell's palsy. *Arch Otolaryngol 107:* 1, 1981.
6. Hauser, WA, Karnes, WE, Annis, J and Kurland, LT: Incidence and prognosis of Bell's palsy in the population of Rochester, Minnesota. *Mayo Clin Proc 46:* 258, 1971.
7. Kennedy, RH, Danielson, MA, Mulder, DW, *et al.*: Guillain-Barré syndrome: a 42-year epidemiologic and clinical study. *Mayo Clin Proc 53:* 93, 1978.
8. Moss HK and Herrman, LG: Night cramps in human extremities. A clinical study of the physiologic action of quinine and prostigmine upon the spontaneous contractions of resting muscles. *Am Heart J 35:* 403, 1948.
9. Nakano, KK: The entrapment neuropathies. *Muscle Nerve 1:* 264, 1978.
10. Parrow, A and Samuelsson, SM: Use of chloroquine phosphate. A new treatment for spontaneous leg cramps. *Acta Med Scand 181:* 237, 1967.
11. Spritz, N: Nerve disease in diabetes mellitus. *Med Clin North Am 62:* 787, 1978.
12. Wilkinson, M, Croft, PB and Urich, H: The remote effects of cancer on the nervous system. *Proc R Soc Med 60:* 683, 1967.
13. Wolf, SM, Wagner, JH, Davidson, S and Forsythe, A: Treatment of Bell's palsy with prednisone: a prospective, randomized study. *Neurology 28:* 158, 1978.

CHAPTER EIGHTY-TWO

Sleep Disorders

RICHARD P. ALLEN, Ph.D.

EPIDEMIOLOGY AND CLASSIFICATION

Recent population studies indicate that, within a given year, approximately one in three adults in America has trouble sleeping. Of these, about one in six actually reports the problem to his physician. Four percent of adults use prescription sleep medication at some time each year, and 1% of these report using prescription sleep medication on consecutive nights for 2 months or more (2, 13).

The sleep-related problems described by patients should be regarded as symptoms rather than diagnoses *per se*. In recent years, a classification of sleep disorders has been developed which enables physicians to formulate and to manage their patients' sleep problems appropriately (1). The four major categories in this classification are: (a) disorders of initiating and maintaining sleep—DIMS (the insomnias), (b) disorders of excessive somnolence—DOES (the hypersomnias), (c) disorders of the sleep-wake cycle, and (d) parasomnias (sleepwalking, sleep terrors, enuresis, etc.). A number of discrete entitites have been identified within each of these categories.

PHYSIOLOGIC PATTERNS OF NORMAL SLEEP

Normal sleep can be separated physiologically into two fundamental categories: rapid eye motion (REM) sleep and nonrapid eye movement (NREM) sleep. Initially, sleep consists of the four successively "deeper" stages of NREM sleep. The pre-sleep wake stage and each sleep stage has distinctive clinical and electroencephalographic (EEG) characteristics:

Pre-Sleep Wake. As the patient begins to fall asleep eye blinks, limb movements, and moderate tone in skeletal muscles are accompanied by either low voltage, mixed frequency EEG or the characteristic alpha pattern (basic posterior rhythm).

Stage 1. This is a light sleep with slow rolling eye movements (pursuit eye movements). Alpha pattern disappears with lower frequency and usually higher voltage than the wake EEG. Sudden limb jerks may occur episodically particularly during early Stage 1 sleep.

Stage 2. Eye movements become infrequent or absent and muscle tone is usually reduced. The EEG shows characteristic occasional sleep spindle bursts, vertex sharp waves, K complexes and some slow wave forms.

Stages 3 and 4. Muscle tone is variable. The EEG high voltage, slow wave activity predominates. Arousal is difficult from these deeper sleep stages.

At 1 to 2 hours after sleep onset, the first period of REM sleep occurs with a characteristic marked decrease in muscle tone and bursts of rapid (saccadic) eye movements. During REM sleep there is a partial paralysis of the limbs except for occasional episodes of muscle twitches.

On a typical night, a subject passes through 3 to 5 cycles of NREM and REM sleep. Typical sleep patterns for young healthy adults and for healthy elderly adults are shown in Figure 82.1. The major differences between the two age groups are the greater frequency and longer intervals of REM sleep in young adults and the decreased frequency of Stage 4 sleep plus more frequent awakenings and decreased total sleep time in elderly subjects. As discussed later in this chapter, deviations from these normal sleep patterns are helpful at times in establishing the correct diagnosis for a sleep disorder.

GENERAL APPROACH TO DIAGNOSIS AND MANAGEMENT OF SLEEP DISORDERS

Although patients with significant sleep disorders or relatives of such patients will usually report the problem to the physician, it is important for physicians to inquire at least briefly about sleep in taking the medical history of any patient. Four questions will detect the presence of most significant sleep disorders:

1 Do you have any trouble sleeping; either falling asleep, staying asleep, or getting enough sleep? (Positive response suggests a DIMS.)

2. Do you or others notice that you are disturbed by excessive sleepiness when engaged in your usual daytime activities? (Positive response in a patient reporting no difficulty initiating or maintaining sleep suggests a DOES.)

3. Do you or your bed partner notice that you have any problem with unusual movement at night? (Positive response suggests sleep disorder, especially if

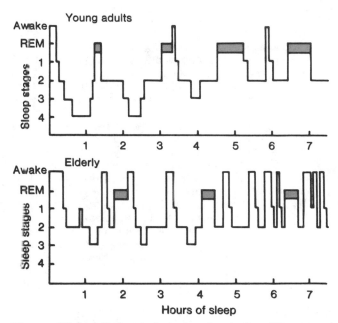

Figure 82.1 Normal sleep cycles in healthy young and elderly subjects. Darkened area indicates REM sleep. (Adapted from A. Kales and J. D. Kales: *New England Journal of Medicine, 290:* 487, 1974.)

there is daytime sleepiness, insomnia, or parasomnia.)

4. Do you snore very much? (Positive response raises the possibility of sleep-induced respiratory impairment and further questions should be asked, especially about excessive daytime sleepiness.)

It is very important at the outset *to distinguish genuine sleepiness from other problems* perceived by the patient as "sleepiness." Sleepiness by definition involves the need to fall asleep, and the patient usually reports some relief of the symptom after sleeping. Muscle weakness, loss of interest in usual activities, exertional dyspnea, postural dizziness, and other symptoms may be referred to as sleepiness, tiredness, or fatigue. By having the patient describe concrete circumstances in which the symptom occurs, these problems can usually be distinguished from true sleepiness.

A number of strategies are helpful in assuring

Table 82.1
Strategies which may be useful for patients with sleep disorders

1. Sleep in the same room consistently, preferably not a room utilized for most wake-time activities
2. Develop a regular bedtime, with lights out or dimmed and a regular waking time, and avoid sleeping longer than usual except occasionally
3. Adjust total sleep time to fit your needs—may be as little as 4 hours or as much as 9 hours.
4. Avoid routine daytime naps
5. Plan regular daily exercise, preferably in the evenings and preferably exercising leg and arm muscles; no exercise for 30 minutes before bed
6. Sleep in a cool room, avoiding temperature extremes
7. Avoid heavy meals within 2 hours of bedtime; however, a light snack such as milk, cheese, crackers at bedtime may be soporific
8. Take no more than one alcoholic drink (equivalent of 2 oz, 90 proof) after dinner
9. Avoid stimulants, particularly within 8 hours of bedtime (e.g., no coffee, cola drinks, tea, cocoa, chocolates, etc.)
10. For poor sleep onset, do not stay awake in bed for more than 30 min. Instead, get out of bed, read or engage in another quiet but productive activity. Try sleep again in an hour; if still unable to sleep, repeat this cycle
11. For troublesome recurrent thoughts disturbing sleep onset: write them down with a possible plan of action. Try to start thinking about simpler, less troubling matters
12. Accept occasional nights with sleeplessness—it is a normal, healthy bodily adjustment to various conditions and provides extra time for hobbies, work, etc.
13. Use sleep medications, including bedtime alcohol, only rarely and never for more than 4 days out of a week or for more than 2 consecutive weeks without consulting your doctor.
14. Do *not* complain to others about being tired on having had a bad night's sleep; and, unless you are unable to stay awake, do not alter your daily activities because you feel tired. You may think you are less alert than others do

effective sleep for most people. These are summarized in Table 82.1. Counseling about the value of such strategies is often helpful for patients with insomnia whose history shows poor sleep habits.

Patients with excessive waketime sleepiness should be cautioned against driving a car, operating heavy machinery, and working in high places or other activities where decreased attention or sleepiness could be dangerous.

SLEEP CENTER REFERRAL

For a number of the problems discussed in this chapter, referral for expert evaluation and management is recommended. Referral can be made to individual physicians expert in managing sleep disorders or, ideally, to a regional sleep disorder center. Table 82.2 lists the accredited sleep disorder centers active in 1981. Because access to the centers is limited by their geographic distribution, discussion about particular patients by telephone may be extremely valuable.

Patient Experience. When a patient is evaluated at a sleep center, he undergoes a careful historical review of his sleep problem, a general physical examination, and, in addition, he may have one or more polysomnograms. A *polysomnogram* is a noninvasive technique permitting simultaneous measurements of a number of physiologic activities during sleep: eye movements, brain activity by EEG, submental and anterior tibialis muscle activity, respiratory air flow, respiratory effort indicated by chest and diaphragm movement, cardiac rhythm by electrocardiogram, and continuous blood oxygen level by ear oximeter or another noninvasive technique. Sometimes additional parameters are recorded such as rectal temperature, esophageal pH, and penile circumference. These records are interpreted by a certified polysomnographer at the sleep center.

DISORDERS OF INITIATING AND MAINTAINING SLEEP (DIMS) (Insomnia)

Patients with DIMS have *difficulty getting to sleep, intermittent disruption of sleep, or early waking with difficulty going back to sleep.* Insomnia is usually secondary to an underlying psychologic or medical condition.

Transient Psychophysiologic Insomnia

This is the most common sleep disorder in our society. The majority of affected persons probably do not seek medical help for it. By definition, the symptoms of transient psychophysiologic insomnia last less than 3 weeks. Symptoms characteristically have an abrupt onset, with an identifiable precipitating event (usually a domestic or occupational problem). Since these patients recover spontaneously, treatment is needed only when the symptoms are severe or when the patient appears vulnerable to recurrence. Treatment includes short term counseling

Table 82.2
Sleep Disorder Centers, 1981[a]

State	Location
FULLY OR PROVISIONALLY ACCREDITED	
California:	Holy Cross Hospital, Mission Hills, (213) 365-8051 (ext. 1497)
	Univ. of Calif. Irvine Medical Center, Orange, (714) 634-5777
	Stanford Univ. Medical Center, Stanford, (415) 497-7458
Florida:	Mt. Sinai Medical Center, Miami Beach, (305) 674-2613
Illinois:	Rush-Presbyterian-St. Luke's, Chicago, (312) 942-5440
	Northwestern Memorial Hospital, Chicago, (312) 649-2650
Louisiana:	Tulane Medical School, New Orleans, (504) 588-5236
Maryland:	Baltimore City Hospital, Baltimore, (301) 396-8603
Massachusetts:	Univ. of Massachusetts Medical Center, Worcester, (617) 856-3081
Michigan:	Henry Ford Hospital, Detroit, (313) 876-2233
Minnesota:	Hennepin County Medical Center, Minneapolis, (612) 347-2430
New Hampshire:	Dartmouth Medical School, Hanover, (603) 646-2043
New York:	Montefiore Hospital, Bronx, (212) 920-4841
	SUNY at Stony Brook, Stony Brook, (516) 246-2561
Ohio:	Univ. of Cincinnati Hospital, Cincinnati, (513) 872-5087
	Ohio State University, Columbus, (614) 422-5982
	Mt. Sinai Hospital, Cleveland, (216) 795-6000 (ext. 531)
Oklahoma:	Presbyterian Hospital, Oklahoma City, (405) 271-6312
Pennsylvania:	Western Psychiatric Institute, Pittsburgh, (412) 624-2246
	Crozer-Chester Medical Center, Upland-Chester, (215) 847-1184
Tennessee:	Baptist Memorial Hospital, Memphis, (901) 522-5651
Texas:	Baylor College of Medicine, Houston, (713) 790-4886
	Metropolitan Medical Center, San Antonio, (512) 223-4057
UNDER DEVELOPMENT	
Alabama:	University of Alabama, Birmingham, (205) 934-3421
Arkansas:	Univ. of Arkansas Medical Center, Little Rock, (501) 661-5525
Arizona:	Good Samaritan Hospital, Phoenix, (602) 257-2000
California:	UCLA School of Medicine, Los Angeles, (213) 825-9555
Connecticut:	The Griffin Hospital, Derby, (203) 735-7421
Colorado:	National Jewish Hospital, Denver, (303) 388-4461
Massachusetts:	Boston Children's Hospital, Boston, (617) 735-6242
	Beth Israel Hospital, Boston, (617) 735-2000
Missouri:	755 W. Big Beaver Road, Suite 2009, Troy, (313) 362-2610
Minnesota:	Mayo Clinic, Rochester, (507) 284-8403
New Jersey:	New Jersey Medical School, Newark, (201) 456-4300
	Rutgers Medical Center, Piscataway, (201) 463-4416
New York:	VA Medical Center, Syracuse, (315) 476-7461
Ohio:	St. Luke's Hospital, Cleveland, (216) 368-7000
Texas:	Shoal Creek Hospital, Austin, (512) 452-0361
Utah:	Utah Neurological Clinic, Provo, (801) 226-2300

[a] For further information, including location of new centers accredited after 1981, contact: Association of Sleep Disorders Center, c/o Stanford Sleep Center, Stanford University Medical Center, Stanford, CA 94305.

focused upon the precipitating event (see Chapter 10), sleep hygiene advice (Table 82.1), and judicious use of hypnotic-sedative medications (see below).

Frequent recurrent episodes of transient insomnia suggest an underlying personality or depressive disorder, which should be more clearly delineated and then managed appropriately as discussed in Chapters 13 and 14.

Another cause of transient insomnia is discontinuation of alcohol, antianxiety drugs, or cigarettes by patients habituated to one of these substances. In mild cases only transient insomnia occurs, but in more severe cases insomnia may become a persistent disorder-sometimes not diagnosed. These problems are discussed in Chapters 19, 20, and 21.

Persistent Insomnia

By definition, these patients have insomnia lasting more than 3 weeks. This problem may be seen in a number of situations.

PSYCHOLOGIC PROBLEMS

These constitute the commonest reasons for persistent insomnia. The sleep-related symptoms usually decrease as the primary psychologic problem improves.

Psychophysiologic insomnia can become persistent but otherwise, like the transient DIMS noted above, has an abrupt onset, a precipitating event, and usually a good response to short term counseling (see Chapter 10). A sedative-hypnotic should be used cautiously since dependence is likely to develop; difficult cases should be referred for evaluation by a mental health specialist.

Affective disorders (see Chapter 14) often present initially with insomnia. Patients with unipolar depressions have less difficulty with sleep onset than with repeated awakenings and difficulty returning to sleep after awakening; patients with bipolar depressions commonly have episodic hypersomnia with complaints of awakening tired. In manic states there is a profound inability to fall asleep, but even brief periods of sleep seem to restore fully alert wakefulness. Depression secondary to other medical or psychiatric conditions (reactive or neurotic depression) may also present with premature arousals and some sleep onset problems; these patients, however, show distinctive REM sleep characteristics on a polysomnogram. There may also be periods of excessive daytime sleepiness. In some patients, a polysomnogram may be helpful in establishing the diagnosis of depression (5). Management of persistent insomnia should include improvement in sleep habits (Table 82.1) in addition to the appropriate management of the affective disorder.

Patients with *personality problems* (see Chapter 13), particularly those with obsessive thoughts and phobias, frequently have insomnia associated with excessive ruminating thoughts at sleep onset. These patients usually require psychotherapy. Hypnotics should be avoided, because of their abuse potential in these patients; judicious use of 25 to 50 mg of amitriptyline (Elavil) may be effective (see below, p. 908).

Some patients will describe *anxiety only at the onset of sleep* and not in relation to other life events. The patient becomes afraid that he will not sleep and becomes too conscious of trying to sleep, noting every few minutes that he is still awake. Such patients may be very sleepy and even fall asleep in their chair watching television; but when they get into bed, they suddenly become wide awake as if conditioned not to sleep in bed. Many have poor sleep hygiene (see Table 82.1). Some patients show minor depression. Generally, these patients are helped by problem-oriented, short term counseling (see Chapter 10). If minor depression is suspected, low dose (25 to 75 mg) amitriptyline (Elavil) 2 hours before bed can be tried, (see below, p. 898). Benzodiazepines, barbiturates, and related medications should be used cautiously because of the possibility of serious dependence with prolonged use of these drugs.

CHRONIC SEDATIVE-HYPNOTIC USE

Protracted use of sedative-hypnotic medication paradoxically may lead to poor sleep onset with repeated premature awakenings (9). This condition may develop both in patients with transient insomnia who continue to use medication and in patients with persistent insomnia due to a psychologic problem. Diagnosis is based on a history of prolonged sedative-hypnotic use, with the development of worsening insomnia while taking the drug. Treatment is often difficult. At the outset of treatment, the patient should be told his sleep disorder is caused at least in part by the medication, that it will get worse transiently while the medication is being withdrawn, and that overall improvement may not occur until several weeks after the drug has been stopped. The patient should be reassured that, if his problem continues thereafter (*i.e.*, it is not due solely to sedative abuse), the appropriate diagnosis and treatment can be accomplished after withdrawal. It is generally advised that the medication be stabilized at a fixed dosage and then *gradually* reduced, by one therapeutic dose per week. Support and reassurance needed during withdrawal should be provided by brief contacts with the physician, such as weekly office visits or telephone calls. Supportive psychotherapy (Chapter 10) may be necessary in more difficult cases. It is essential for the physician to get the idea across to the patient that he has the internal strength to deal successfully with this problem.

SLEEP APNEA AND SLEEP-INDUCED RESPIRATORY IMPAIRMENT

This disturbance of respiration during sleep usually presents with hypersomnia and is discussed under DOES below (p. 902). However, some patients with persistent insomnia, especially those with short sleep onset but frequent awakenings, may have this condition. As noted below, this condition will be exacerbated if treated with hypnotics, sometimes with serious complications (7).

MEDICAL CONDITIONS

Patients with most symptomatic medical conditions may describe persistent insomnia related to the condition. Insomnia may occasionally be the presenting symptom, but generally the medical condition will be identified first by its more specific manifestations other than insomnia. The sleep disturbance, while probably related to the pathophysiology of the disease in some conditions, is due to nonspecific psychologic or physical distress in most situations. The insomnia generally improves or worsens with the course of the associated medical condition. Sedative-hypnotic drugs may be of value (see below, p. 906) in these patients, particularly those whose insomnia is due to distress associated with their illness.

SLEEP-RELATED MYOCLONUS

This diagnosis is suggested if the patient reports repeated nocturnal awakenings, very active sleep, disturbing the bed sheets during sleep, or if a bed partner reports that the patient moves excessively in sleep, kicking his legs frequently. The movements are characterized as rhythmic, stereotyped leg kicks or arm jerks occurring every 20 to 40 sec for much of the sleeping time. They start *after* sleep onset; they may appear intermittently for several minutes any time during sleep or, in severe cases, persist throughout sleep. The movements typically involve flexion at the ankle and knee (occasionally also at the hip) with extension of the big toe. Arm movements are less common.

The etiology, prevalence, and course of this condition are unknown, but it appears to persist once established.

Differential diagnosis includes normal twitches, sleep-onset leg kicks which stop after sleep is well-established, and epileptic seizure activity during sleep. Diagnosis of sleep-related myoclonus requires a polysomnogram (10). When the diagnosis is suspected, telephone consultation with a sleep specialist may be helpful.

Treatment, which should be planned in consultation with a sleep disorder specialist, usually involves exercise and moderate doses of clonazepam, (Clonopin), oxazepam (Serax), or baclofen (Lioresal) before bed. This treatment is usually quite effective, and tolerance is not a major problem.

"*Restless legs*" (see Chapter 81) is a wake-time disorder; almost all patients also have sleep-related myoclonus (although most patients with myoclonus do not have daytime restless legs). The patient reports deep, unpleasant sensations in the leg muscles resolved by moving the legs. Inactivity and tiredness exacerbate the problem. This condition has a strong familial incidence and generally becomes progressively worse with age. Treatment of the sleep-related myoclonus is important here to reduce daytime tiredness, but care should be taken to watch for morning or wake-time drowsiness (produced by the drug used to treat the myoclonus) which will exacerbate the wake-time restlessness.

Sleep Disorders which Mimic DIMS

Disorders of excessive somnolence or DOES (see details below) may present commonly with disturbed nocturnal sleep and are frequently misdiagnosed as DIMS. This problem is exacerbated by the patient's tendency to minimize wake-time sleepiness and to emphasize disturbances of night time sleep. When there is a history of napping, particularly with an irresistible need to nap, DOES must be considered as the primary diagnosis.

Sleep-wake schedule disturbance (see details below) can also be confused with DIMS. Again, the significant information comes first from looking at wake-time functioning. If the patient reports marked drowsiness and impaired functioning in a particular part of the day, along with difficulty related principally to sleep onset, then a sleep-wake schedule disturbance should be considered.

Natural short sleepers may also present with DIMS symptoms. Again, the significant information relates to wake-time functioning. The amount of sleep needed by any person varies considerably, with recorded examples of patients who sleep very little and appear to function without difficulty (8). A short sleeper awakens refreshed with little difficulty functioning in the day. He generally has short sleep latency with few awakenings during sleep. The short sleep period is constant over weekends and holidays and has been stable since late adolescence. The patient will usually come to the physician because others have convinced him that his sleep is abnormal and might cause medical problems; or because he has trouble using his wake-time when others are asleep.

Since his sleep restores wakefulness, he can be reassured that he has no sleep problem and can be advised to use his extra wake-time constructively.

DISORDERS OF EXCESSIVE SOMNOLENCE (DOES) (HYPERSOMNIA)

Diagnostic Evaluation

Symptoms of hypersomnia, unlike symptoms of insomnia, are often hard to elicit with certainty from the patient (4). Once reported, either by the patient or a reliable observer, the symptoms deserve very careful attention, for they may indicate the presence of life-threatening sleep apnea. To assess symptom severity, behavior must be observed and recorded systematically. This is done by having either an observer or the patient himself complete for 1 or 2 days an hourly check of alertness using a scale such as that used in the Hopkins Alertness Report (see Fig. 82.2). Excessive wake-time sleepiness is present when the *patient reports no decrease in the amount of sleep he gets but has periods of very low alertness, significant sleepiness, and even takes naps during wake-time.* The patient's prior sleep history serves as the baseline for his "normal" amount of sleep, as there are no established sleep-time norms that can be applied to patients generally. In severe cases, there may be a history of accidents that can be attributed to the excessive sleepiness. Wake-time activities that may

Behavior	1	2	3	4	5	6	7	8	9	10	11	12 (Noon)	1	2	3	4	5	6	7	8	9	10	11	12 (Mid-night)
6. *Wide Awake: Alert* — Active, moving a lot, talking, listening, interacting, actively working—continually									√	√	√	√	√		√	√	√							
5. *Awake: Quiet* — Sitting, resting or leaning. Not participating in conversation or activities—only listening or watching. Working some—but not all the time (less than 50%)								√										√	√		√			
4. *Awake: Inattentive* — Not listening or following conversation or activity. Not working (more than 15% of time) Staring, lack of facial expression. Decreased body movements							√							√										
3. *Possibly dozing* 10% of time. — Head dropping, eyes closing momentarily (less than 1 min) during 10–20% of time																				√				
2. *Definitely dozing* 20% of time. — Head drops, eyes close for brief *naps* (less than 5 min) during at least 20% of time																					√			
1. *Asleep-Napping:* 20–50% time. — Total nap time at least 12 min (20% of hr) or one nap of more than 5 min																								
0. *Asleep* for at least 50% of time	√	√	√	√	√	√																		√

HOPKINS ALERTNESS REPORT   Patient Name: John Doe   Date: 1/10/81

Figure 82.2. Example of an alertness report which can be completed by a patient being evaluated for a sleep disorder. The example shows a normal sleep-wake pattern. (Source: Baltimore Regional Sleep Disorder Center of Johns Hopkins University School of Medicine, located at Baltimore City Hospital, with permission.)

lead to sleepiness in most individuals lead to even more sleepiness for individuals with these disorders. These activities include watching television, riding in or driving a car, reading, sitting in a conference, waiting to be seen at a physician's office, and relaxing shortly after a large meal.

Definitive assessment of excessive somnolence requires observation such as that provided in a sleep disorder center (see above, p. 898). Because specialized centers are limited in number, telephone consultation with the nearest center is often the most practical plan; this is essential when the diagnosis of sleep apnea or narcolepsy is entertained.

Transient Hypersomnia

Excessive daytime somnolence lasting less than 3 weeks is usually due to a psychologic response to stress. Onset is abrupt, symptoms are generally persistent fatigue and loss of energy, behavior is characterized by long periods of time in bed, and a precipitating event is usually identified. In contrast to other patients with DOES, these patients spend excessive time in bed and generally do not express significant drive or effort to leave the bed. The condition should improve simultaneously with improvement in the psychologic problem; if the patient's sleep problem persists beyond this point, an alternate diagnosis should be considered. Drug abusers may present with DOES symptoms in trying to obtain stimulant medication; therefore, physicians must use judgment in treating patients complaining of hypersomnolence who are not well known to them.

Persistent Hypersomnia

By definition, persistent hypersomnia is present when symptoms last longer than 3 weeks.

SLEEP APNEA AND SLEEP-INDUCED
RESPIRATORY IMPAIRMENTS (6)

Definitions. These are by far the most serious sleep disorders. They are characterized by respiratory problems occurring during sleep. These problems vary from reduction to complete cessation of air flow at the nose and mouth for at least 10 sec (hypopnea and apnea, respectively). The sleep apneas are divided into *central* (cessation of respiratory effort with no blockage of airway) and *obstructive* (blockage of air flow in the upper airway both on inhalation and exhalation). Mixed apneas (central apnea at the onset of a predominantly obstructive apnea episode) are essentially equivalent to obstructive apnea. Isolated central apneas are usually associated with coexisting symptoms of insomnia; obstructive apneas present typically with symptoms of excessive wake-time somnolence and no complaint of insomnia.

Epidemiology. Sleep apnea may occur at any age. In adults onset is generally after age 40. Prevalence is not well established, as the syndrome is not yet widely appreciated; however, obstructive sleep apnea

is more common in middle-aged men while central sleep apnea is more common in infants and in persons over 65. For obstructive apnea in adults, the male:female ratio is 30:1.

Manifestations and Course. Loud, intermittent snoring is almost always present and is a major indicator of the disorder. Although obesity is commonly associated with this disorder, only about 5% of cases have morbid obesity (Pickwickian), and many are not overweight. However, patients with short, fat necks are commonly seen. Pulmonary function tests are usually normal, although resistance to air flow may be increased in the upper airway. Abnormalities which compromise the upper airway, such as tonsillar hypertrophy, goiter, micrognathia, and reduced airway size (on CT scan) may be found. Evaluation for evidence of brainstem neurologic dysfunction, seizures, or hypothyroidism should be made. In many cases, however, the etiology is unknown.

The *course of sleep apnea* appears to be chronic and progressive. Onset of excessive somnolence is usually preceded by a history of snoring and other nocturnal sleep disturbances, including complaints of insomnia. After onset the following sequence of events may occur: slowly worsening hypertension, headaches on awakening, dry mouth on awakening, increased abnormal movements at night, decreased wake-time alertness with progressive deterioration of cognitive and social functioning, and, eventually, right-sided heart failure. Sudden death may occur from myocardial infarction or arrhythmias; therefore, a 24-hour electrocardiogram may be indicated to look for the life-threatening arrhythmias which may occur during apneic episodes.

Sleep-induced hypoventilation occurs in association with the development of sleep apnea, in certain medical conditions such as myotonic dystrophy, and in most patients with chronic obstructive pulmonary disease (COPD) (14). Probably most COPD patients with a wake-time pO_2 of less than 55 mm Hg should be questioned about both insomnia and wake-time sleepiness, particularly when they have associated morbid obesity (12).

Diagnosis. A *working diagnosis* of sleep apnea or hypopnea can be made by direct observation of the patient during sleep, either at home or in a general hospital. Definitive diagnosis requires a polysomnogram (see above, p. 898). The cessation of, or marked decrease of, airflow for intervals of 10 sec or longer at rates greater than seven per hour in a sleep condition, including REM sleep, confirms the diagnosis.

Management. Since treatment of these patients is complex, they should be managed in consultation with a specialist at a sleep disorder center (see above). The prognosis in the treated patient appears to be good, with improved or normal wake-time functioning and resolution of congestive failure and hypertension.

The *medical management of obstructive sleep apnea* includes avoiding sedatives, weight reduction, and treatment with medroxyprogesterone (Provera) or with the tricyclic agent, protriptyline (Vivactil). Progesterone causes increased minute ventilation in normal individuals, but its efficacy in sleep apnea is not well established.

The *surgical management of obstructive sleep apnea* consists of correction of anatomic airway abnormalities, surgical enlargement of the airway by a uvulopalatopharyngoplasty or, in extreme cases, tracheotomy with a tracheal button allowing closure by the patient during wake-time.

The *management of central sleep apnea* is less well understood. This problem is probably associated with the sudden infant death syndrome, and children at risk are usually placed on alarms. Central apnea occurs commonly in the elderly, whose principal presenting complaint may be wake-time sleepiness and sometimes poor sleep at night. Management of such persons emphasizes good sleep habits and avoiding sedative-hypnotics and alcohol since these may cause suppression of respiration.

NARCOLEPSY AND IDIOPATHIC HYPERSOMNOLENCE (16)

These are perhaps the best recognized primary disorders of excessive somnolence. Nonetheless, they remain difficult to diagnose. These disorders are characterized by irresistible need for wake-time naps. The naps vary in duration from 30 sec to 15 min. The subject awakens refreshed only to become somnolent again 2 to 3 hours later. Most patients with these disorders will report frequent near-accidents and socially embarrassing situations related to their uncontrollable hypersomnolence.

Narcolepsy

The approximate prevalence of narcolepsy is 4 per 10,000 population. It is equally common for both sexes and usually develops in the second decade of life. Symptoms are relatively stable once the wake-time sleepiness has developed fully. There is a strong familial tendency. The precise pathogenesis is unknown, but centers on an abnormality in the control of REM sleep.

In narcolepsy, excessive wake-time sleepiness is usually accompanied by one or more of the following symptoms: (a) *cataplexy:* a transitory sudden loss of muscle tone, sometimes involving falling to the ground without loss of consciousness and usually precipitated by an emotional response such as laughing, crying, or anger; (b) *sleep paralysis:* awakening with a transitory inability to move or speak, sometimes associated with dreamlike hallucinations. (This symptom is different from the *sleep palsies* experienced occasionally by most people—transient sensorimotor palsies of the ulnar, radial, and peroneal nerves which, owing to their superficial locations, are subject to prolonged compression during deep sleep); (c) *hypnagogic hallucinations:* dream-like, usually visual, hallucinations occurring at the transition from wakefulness to sleep; and (d) *disturbed nocturnal sleep:* frequent brief awakening during a night's sleep. In some narcoleptic patients, these four symptoms may occur before the development of wake-time sleep attacks; in others they may never occur.

Conditions which may be found in association with narcolepsy include: sleep apnea (see above), sleep-related myoclonus (see above), and automatic behaviors. These all occur more commonly in narcoleptics than in the general population.

A *working diagnosis* of narcolepsy can be made on the basis of the history given by the patient and other observers. The definitive diagnosis is based upon characteristic findings in the polysomnogram with napping tests (see above, p. 898).

Treatment of narcolepsy focuses on reducing symptoms by medication and environmental management. Before initiating treatment, the patient's usual pattern of daytime hypersomnolence should be documented, giving a baseline against which treatment results can be evaluated. Any of three stimulant drugs—magnesium pemoline (Cylert), methylphenidate (Ritalin), dextroamphetamine (Dexedrine)- and one tricyclic—protriptyline (Vivactil)—will provide relief from the wake-time sleepiness. Tolerance is a major problem for all stimulants, and weekend drug "holidays" are advised. Doses should start at the minimally effective dose and be gradually increased until symptom relief or side effects occur (see Table 82.3). Environmental management centers on diet and planned wake-time naps. Dietary management emphasizes avoiding large meals when the patient desires to stay awake and avoiding the use of alcohol altogether. The tricyclics, imipramine (Tofranil), and protriptyline (Vivactil) are used to reduce the frequency of cataplectic attacks (see Table 82.3). A regimen which has been effective in one large group of patients with sleep attacks plus cataplexy is treatment with imipramine 25 mg and methylphenidate 5 to 10 mg 3 times daily (16). However, desipramine (Norpramin) may be more effective than imipramine for reducing cataplexy with less sedation (see Chapter 14 for additional details about tricyclic antidepressants).

Idiopathic Hypersomnolence

This disorder does not center on REM sleep abnormalities. These patients often present as being more *chronically tired* during wake-time. About 12 to 15% of all patients with DOES have this problem. This condition does not generally respond well to stimulants, although in some cases they may help, and naps are not always beneficial in restoring full wakefulness. There are isolated reports of successful treatment with methysergide (Sansert), which is not helpful in narcolepsy.

Table 82.3
Drugs for Narcolepsy

Drug	Available Strengths (mg)	Minimum Effective Dose (mg)	Maximum Effective Dose (mg)	Time for Dose Effect
FOR HYPERSOMNOLENCE				
Dextroamphetamine (Dexedrine, generics)	5, 10, 15	5 q.d.	20 t.i.d.	3 days
Magnesium pemoline (Cylert)	18.75, 37.5	37.5 q.d.	112.5 q.d.	1 week
Methylphenidate (Ritalin, generics)	10, 20	10 b.i.d.	30 t.i.d. and q.i.d.	3 days
FOR CATAPLEXY				
Protriptyline (Vivactil)[a, b]	5, 10	5 b.i.d.	10 q.i.d.	1 week
Imipramine (Tofranil, generics)[b]	25	25 b.i.d.	25 q.i.d.	1 week
Desipramine (Norpromin, Pertofrane)[b]	25, 50	25 b.i.d.	50 b.i.d.	1 week

[a] May also help reduce wake-time sleepiness.
[b] For details on the use of tricyclics, see Chapter 14.

In light of the difficult diagnosis, the variable response to treatment, and the significant risk of a false historic report by a patient seeking stimulant medications, patients with suspected narcolepsy or idiopathic hypersomnolence should be discussed with a specialist in sleep disorders (see Table 82.2).

MEDICAL AND ENVIRONMENTAL CAUSES (15)

Causes for hypersomnia not due to a specific sleep disorder are varied and usually result in persistent wake-time sleepiness. The more common *medical conditions* which should be considered are: hypothyroidism (or apathetic hyperthyroidism in the elderly), hypoglycemia, anemia, uremia, hypercapnia, hypercalcemia, liver failure, and a number of neurologic abnormalities (epilepsy, post-traumatic hypersomnia, encephalitis, neurosyphilis, multiple sclerosis, chronic brain syndrome, brain tumors involving the brainstem and 3rd ventricle, and progressive hydrocephalus from any cause). Progressive hydrocephalus may present initially as excessive somnolence without localizing findings; and sleepiness after head trauma may not develop until 6 to 18 months after the trauma.

Iatrogenic hypersomnia may accompany the use of a number of drugs with sedating side effects including, in particular, centrally acting antihypertensives (reserpine, methyldopa, clonidine, β-blockers), antihistamines, anxiolytic agents, tricyclic antidepressants, neuroleptics, sedative-hypnotic drugs, and barbiturates used in epilepsy.

Physical confinement and reduced environmental stimulation may lead to excessive somnolence. In the elderly, a natural tendency toward wake-time sleepiness plus some restrictions on activities may combine to promote excessive somnolence.

In each of these conditions, improvement in hypersomnolence depends largely upon improving the primary conditions. Thus, discontinuation or adjustment of sedating medications is a particularly important responsibility of the physician.

PSYCHOLOGIC CONDITIONS

Psychosocial stress, affective disorders, and schizophrenia may present with persistent wake-time sleepiness. Patients of this type will usually report precipitating stressful events or will have symptoms of severe depression. The wake-time status also often involves a feeling of general fatigue and loss of energy, without need for sleep to restore wakefulness. These patients require management with a combination of psychotherapy and appropriate medications (see Chapters 11, 14, and 15).

OTHER SLEEP DISORDERS WHICH MIMIC DOES

Sleep-wake schedule disturbance (see below) may be incorrectly diagnosed as hypersomnia since these patients sleep late in the day and report inability to stay awake for a large part of society's normal work day. In sever cases, the patient may have occasional reversal of the sleep-wake cycle with very long periods of sleep, short periods of wakefulness, and a complaint of never feeling very much awake.

Sleep-related myoclonus (see above, p. 900) often presents with wake-time sleepiness and in extreme cases may be confused with narcolepsy, although it also may accompany narcolepsy.

Insufficient sleep may occur for cultural or environmental reasons and may be forced on a long or even a normal sleeper. Minor symptoms generally associated with DIMS (insomnia) or DOES are present in wake-time, e.g., morning malaise, minor eye irritations, diplopia, irritability, and multiple somatic complaints. Unlike DIMS there is no problem initiating and maintaining sleep. A successful treatment trial with a prolonged single sleep period confirms the diagnosis.

Natural long sleepers also complain of excessive somnolence, sometimes because they have insufficient sleep owing to requirements of daily living, but more often because they feel they need too much sleep. Total sleep time required by a small subgroup of individuals (less than 2% of the adult population) is greater than 9 hours. When not under pressure, these individuals may sleep as much as 12 to 14 hours per day. This trend develops by early adolescence and remains stable throughout life. When sleep time increases significantly later in adult life, it should not be attributed to this condition. Adequate protracted sleep, in one sleep period each day, serves as both the diagnostic test and treatment for natural long sleepers. In difficult cases, sleep center referral should be considered to evaluate the patient for one of the causes of DOES.

DISORDERS OF THE SLEEP-WAKE SCHEDULE

Definition and Manifestations. Although transient "jet lag" has long been recognized as a sleep-wake problem with travelers and shift workers, persistent disruption of the normal sleep-wake cycle, somewhat like living with perpetual jet lag, has only in recent years been recognized as a biologically based sleep disorder. This disorder may begin in childhood but usually begins in young adult life following some change in living schedule. Prevalence is unknown since the disorder has only been recognized recently.

Circadian rhythms have a major influence upon sleep. In an environment free of all time cues (e.g., prolonged living in a cave without reference to any kind of standard), the circadian rhythm for man runs slightly longer than 24 hours (about 24.5 to 25.5 hours). Under normal circumstances, the internal clock in each individual is reset slightly every 24 hours in response to external cues. For reasons which are not clear, some people fail to entrain their internal cycle to the socially prescribed 24-hour clock. They either lose a stable cycle (*progressive* sleep-cycle delay) or the cycle becomes *fixed*, unhappily out of phase with social demands. In the former case, the patient's sleep period changes rapidly, with occasional periods of prolonged sleepiness. In the latter case, the patient tries to sleep when he is physiologically most active and therefore finds sleep difficult to establish; he also attempts to stay awake when he is physiologically ready for sleep. Thus he may complain about both insomnia and daytime sleepiness.

These patients report normal, good quality sleep when they are allowed to sleep on their own schedule (such as on nonworking days). Most report a nearly fixed delay in sleep onset several hours after the expected bedtime, with an ability to sleep late, feeling refreshed on the late awakening. Less commonly the patients report the following cycle in their sleep disturbance: a period of insomnia with wake-time sleepiness; then a period of premature sleepiness with premature awakenings; then a period of normal sleep; and then back again to insomnia with wake-time sleepiness. Compared to the fixed sleep-cycle delay, this progressive sleep-cycle delay is a very unusual condition.

Diagnosis. A sleep-wake log (see Fig. 82.2) and a temperature record assist in the diagnosis. For 2 consecutive days, the patient is instructed to keep an oral temperature record for every 2 hours when not asleep. The temperature should not be taken within 10 min of consuming hot or cold beverages or food nor within 30 min after physical exercise. Body temperature fluctuates 1 to 2°F (about 0.5 to 1°C) during

the day, reaching a peak during the time of greatest alertness and dropping off just before sleep onset. A temperature record showing no relative decrease before the planned bedtime supports the diagnosis.

Differential Diagnosis. This disorder is commonly misdiagnosed as insomnia or as a problem of excessive somnolence. Both of these are excluded if, during extended sleep, the patient sleeps well with good restoration of wakefulness. In some psychologic disturbances, particularly manic-type bipolar affective disorders and neurotic depression (see Chapter 14), sleep onset is delayed for a few hours; in these patients, the total sleep time is usually markedly reduced.

Schizophrenic decompensation may present with a sleep cycle delay which resembles this disorder, but requires treatment directed at the schizophrenia. Some patients seen for chronic sedative-hypnotic (or stimulant) use may, in fact, have a primary disturbance in the sleep-wake cycle, a diagnosis which becomes apparent once the sleep-wake medication has been discontinued.

Treatment. Patients with the working diagnosis of fixed sleep-wake cycle delay can be placed on "chronotherapy". The first night the patient sleeps at the time suited for his internal clock. Each consecutive day the bedtime and waketime are advanced to 2 hours later, until after 8 to 10 days the desired bedtime is reached. Good sleep habits (Table 82.1) are then recommended to maintain the desired bedtime. Use of sedative-hypnotics or stimulants in this group of patients will not reset the sleep cycle and will seriously complicate the treatment. Chronotherapy is not effective in patients with the progressive sleep-cycle delays; in these uncommon patients, the best plan is referral to a sleep center (see Table 82.2) for diagnosis and individualized environmental management without medication.

DYSFUNCTIONS ASSOCIATED WITH SLEEP (PARASOMNIAS)

There are a number of miscellaneous problems associated with sleep, including three major disorders associated with *incomplete arousal, usually from deep sleep.* These incomplete arousals are increased by stress and tend to co-occur in the same person, who is often seen as a "deep" sleeper. There is a familial tendency for these disorders, and they occur most often in childhood.

Sleepwalking

Sleepwalking occurs in the first third of the sleep period with partial or total amnesia for the event on awakening. It is most common between ages 6 and 12, and although in these cases the problem sometimes lasts for several years, it stops before age 20. In adults, there is usually a history of some sleepwalking in childhood with a complete remission until a recurrence in the late 20s or 30s when it may persist for several years. During sleepwalking, arousal from sleep can be difficult and sometimes almost impossible. The disorder is complicated by the fact that sleepwalking is clumsy and accidents may occur. Measures should therefore be taken to reduce the risks of accidents (e.g., ensure closed lower windows, restricted access to stairways, and cleared floor areas). Parents can be reassured that sleepwalking is otherwise of no great concern even though they may report that it is worse during stress. In adults, however, there is usually an associated psychologic problem requiring evaluation and appropriate psychotherapy. The possibility of sleep-induced seizures—particularly temporal lobe seizures in the REM stage of sleep—should be ruled out (see Chapter 77).

Sleep Terrors (3)

Sleep terrors occur in childhood as loud and uncontrollable screaming during the first third of the sleep period and occasionally repeated later in sleep. During an episode the child is generally uncontrollable until shortly before he returns to sleep. Fortunately, there is complete amnesia for the event. The behavior is very disturbing to the family, but not to the child. Adults also experience sleep terrors, usually with a sudden awakening in the first third of the night accompanied by a profound sense of dread but without the loud scream. Marked autonomic activity (tachycardia, diaphoresis) occurs in both children and adults. Sleep terrors occur in 1 to 4% of children, usually starting between ages 4 and 12 and ceasing by early adolescence. Adult onset is less common but does occur in the 20s or 30s but almost never after 40. Treatment of children involves reassurance of the family that the condition is benign. When the problem is very disrupting, a low dose anxiolytic agent, such as 2 to 5 mg of diazepam (Valium), at bedtime usually provides complete remission. Treatment for adults includes psychotherapy and a short course of treatment with a benzodiazepine agent before bed. Adults may have some memory of the attacks, and they may have some cognitive content to their fears. Counseling should focus upon this and upon the benign nature of this disorder. Bedtime doses of tricyclic antidepressants and neuroleptics may exacerbate sleep terrors. The differential diagnosis includes sleep apnea, sleep-related epilepsy, and dream anxiety attacks. When sleep terrors persist in adults, sleep center referral (see above, p. 898) should be considered to ensure correct diagnosis. For children, a referral should be considered if the condition is extreme and persistent.

Sleep-related Enuresis (3)

Sleep-related enuresis is relatively common in childhood, occurring at age 5 in 15% of boys and 10% of girls. By puberty the problem usually remits. Unless the sleep-related enuresis is associated with other problems, persists beyond puberty, or recurs after remission of several months, it can be considered

benign. For adult onset or for recurring enuresis, the most important possibilities in the differential diagnosis are epilepsy, psychologic disturbance, neurogenic bladder, dementia, and sleep apnea.

SLEEP MEDICATIONS

Sedative-Hypnotic Drugs

As noted in previous sections, sedative-hypnotic drugs may be useful in dealing with a number of sleep disorders. The benefits from these medications may be very significant, but on the average the effects are a 10- to 30-min reduction in sleep onset time and a 20- to 40-min increase in total sleep time (13). The most important contraindication for sedative-hypnotic drug use is any symptom or sign of unexplained respiratory problems at night, including a history of heavy snoring or significant wake-time sleepiness, as these may indicate sleep apnea (see above, p. 902).

SELECTION AND USE

The sedative-hypnotics of first choice are the *benzodiazepines*. Table 82.4 summarizes available tablet sizes and recommended doses for drugs in this group. There is very little reason to select barbiturates or other sedative-hypnotics.

Since tolerance develops to all sedative-hypnotics, the daily use of any of these drugs should be limited to 2 to 4 weeks, except for rare situations where at least weekend drug-free periods can be assured. It is best to start at the minimum effective dose (see Table 82.4) and to increase the dose if necessary every 3 to 4 days until the effective dose is found or the usual maximum dose is reached. Most patients can follow directions to titrate their own dose for symptom relief. Except in unusual circumstances the dose should not be increased once tolerance to an effective dose develops. Even in the most unusual case, increasing doses more than twice is likely to create a new problem of drug dependence and does little to solve the patient's sleep problem.

In adjusting dosage, particular attention should be given to wake-time function. Several of the popular benzodiazepines (flurazepam, diazepam, chlordiazepoxide) and their active metabolites have long half-lives and may produce a hangover effect even after one dose. When taken daily, they may have cumulative effects, so that in some cases wake-time drowsiness develops after a few days of consecutive or alternate-day use. Whenever wake-time drowsiness develops, the dosage should be decreased. For the longer acting benzodiazepines, such as flurazepam (Dalmane), diazepam (Valium), and chlordiazepoxide (Librium), weekend drug-free intervals should be recommended; alternatively the shorter acting benzodiazepines, clonazepam (Clonopin), oxazepam (Serax), lorazepam (Ativan), and temazepam (Restoril) may be considered. Very short acting benzodiazepines such as triazolam (Halcion) are available in Europe and may be available soon in this country.

Table 82.4
Sedative-Hypnotic Benzodiazepine Drugs (in Order by Increasing Duration of Action)

Drug	Available Strengths (mg)	Minimum Effective Dose (mg)	Maximum Effective Dose (mg)
SHORT ACTING			
Midazalam[a]	5, 10	N/A	N/A
Triazolam (Halcion)[a]	0.25, 0.5	0.25	0.5
Brotizolam[a]	0.25, 0.5	0.25	0.5
INTERMEDIATE ACTING (half-lives usually 10–20 hr)			
Oxazepam (Serax)	10, 15, 30	10	30
Lorazepam (Ativan)	0.5, 1, 2	0.5	4
Estazolam[a]	1, 2	1.0	2.0
Temazepam (Restoril)	15, 30	15	30
Clonazepam (Clonopin)	0.5, 1, 2	0.5	1.5
LONG ACTING			
Diazepam (Valium)	2, 5, 10	2	15
Chlordiazepoxide (Librium)	5, 10, 25	5	25
Flurazepam (Dalmane)	15, 30	15	30

[a] These medications were not available in the U.S. market at the time this table was prepared.

The *barbiturate* sedative-hypnotics have three distinct disadvantages in comparison with the benzodiazepines: the frequent occurrence of hangover after only one dose, the development of physiologic dependence with the accompanying risk of a severe withdrawal reaction, and the potential for committing suicide with a relatively small number of tablets. A number of *other sedative-hypnotics* (chloral hydrate, glutethimide, meprobamate, methaqualone, and methyprylon) have been shown to be effective. Each has the potential for physiologic dependence and lethal respiratory depression with overdose; therefore, there is little reason to select one of these agents or a barbiturate instead of a benzodiazepine. Of the entire group, chloral hydrate (500 to 1000 mg) is perhaps the safest if an alternative to the benzodiazepines is needed.

INFORMATION TO PATIENTS

When prescribing a sedative-hypnotic medication, the physician should recommend taking the medication 15 to 30 min before bedtime. He should also warn the patient of the following: (a) the risk of tolerance and dependence with later withdrawal problems (especially with barbiturates and the short acting benzodiazepines) and the risk of developing the "sleeping pill habit" and never adequately resolving the sleep problem; (b) potential problems of interaction with other drugs, particularly alcohol (alcohol abstinence, particularly after dinner, is essential and the patient should generally not take more than one sedating medication in the same day; (c) hangover effects and the possibility of becoming sleepy while driving, especially after the first few days on the longer acting benzodiazepines or barbiturates; and (d) the uncertain knowledge about effects on pregnancy, meaning that the medication should be used by women of child-bearing age only when they know they are not pregnant.

SEDATIVE-HYPNOTIC WITHDRAWAL

For patients taking too much sleeping medication, the medication should be withdrawn gradually, particularly if the patient has been taking it for 3 months or longer. A patient in this category may be one who reports worsening insomnia due to chronic use of the medication (see above, p. 900) or one who has developed physiologic dependence and risks serious withdrawal symptoms. The patient should be informed that he may get worse for a short period during withdrawal but will then get better. The dose of the medication should be reduced by one therapeutic dose per week. If more than one medication is involved, one medication at a time should be reduced. The patient should stay in close contact with the physician during this trying experience. Difficult but motivated patients may need expert assistance from a psychotherapist with broad experience in managing withdrawal from drugs (see Chapter 21).

Over-the-Counter Medications and Antihistamines

Over-the-counter (OTC) medications and antihistamines clearly are effective for many patients with transient insomnia and may be as effective as low doses of the commonly prescribed sedative-hypnotics. The *OTC medications* contain low dose antihistamines (see Table 82.5). The effects of these medications, when taken at therapeutic doses, are mild. Tolerance apparently develops quickly and continued use can be habit-forming.

The *prescription sedative-antihistamines* include diphenhydramine (Benadryl) 25 mg to 50 mg and hydroxyzine (Vistaril and Atarax) 25 mg and 50 mg. These drugs are more potent sedatives than the OTC sleeping medications. They may be particularly useful in patients with chronic obstructive pulmonary disease, for whom benzodiazepines are hazardous because they can suppress respiration.

Table 82.5
Constituents of Commonly Used Over-the-Counter Sleep Remedies

Product Name	Constituent	
Miles Nervine[a]		
Sleep-Eze	Pyrilamine maleate[b]	25 mg
Sominex[c]		
Nytol		
Unisom Night-time Sleep Aid	Doxylamine succinate[d]	25 mg

[a] This product no longer contains bromine.
[b] Antihistamine of the ethylene diamine class.
[c] This product no longer contains scopolamine.
[d] Antihistamine of the ethanolamine class.

Tricyclic Antidepressants

The most sedating of the tricyclic antidepressants, such as amitriptyline (Elavil) and imipramine (Tofranil), are useful in low doses for the management of persistent insomnia associated with those psychologic conditions in which there is a depressive or obsessive-compulsive component. These medications are particularly effective either when sleep onset is disturbed by anxiety or ruminating thoughts or when sleep is interrupted in the latter part of the sleep period by dreams characterized by anxiety. Under these conditions, the tricyclics are preferable to sedative-hypnotics both because of better efficacy and the lesser probability of dependence. Usual dose is 25 to 75 mg about 1 to 2 hours before bed. At this dose, the side effects are usually minimal. Additional information about tricyclics is found in Chapter 14.

References

General

Hauri, P: *The Sleep Disorders, Current Concepts.* Upjohn Co., Kalamazoo, Mich., 1977.

A useful general introductory work to sleep, sleep disorders, and their treatment (the Upjohn Company provides copies of this small booklet).

Kales, A and Kales, JD: Sleep disorders: recent findings in the diagnosis and treatment of disturbed sleep. *N Engl J Med 290:* 487, 1974.

Good general review article, with emphasis on the actions of sedative-hypnotic drugs.

William, RL and Karacan, I (editors): *Sleep Disorders: Diagnosis and Treatment.* John Wiley, New York, 1978.

Excellent general reference on sleep disorders.

Specific

1. Association of Sleep Disorders Centers: Diagnostic classification of sleep and arousal disorders. *Sleep 2:* 1, 1979.
2. Bixler, EO, Kales, A, Soldatos, CR, Kales, JD, and Healey, S: Prevalence of sleep disorders in the Los Angeles metropolitan area. *Am J Psychiatry 136:* 1257, 1979.
3. Broughton, R: Sleep disorders: disorders of arousal? *Science 159:* 1070, 1978.
4. Dement, WC, Carskadon, MA and Richardson, G: Excessive daytime sleepiness in the sleep apnea syndrome. In *Sleep Apnea Syndromes,* p. 23, edited by C Guilleminault and WC Dement. Alan R. Liss, New York, 1978.
5. Gilin, JC, Duncan, W, Pettigew, KD, Frenkel, BL and Snyder, F: Successful separation of depressed, normal and insomniac subjects by EEG sleep data. *Arch Gen Psychiatry 36:* 85, 1979.
6. Guilleminault, C and Dement, WC: Sleep apnea syndromes and related sleep disorders. In *Sleep Disorders: Diagnosis and Treatment,* p. 9, edited by RL Williams and I Karacan. J Wiley, New York, 1978.
7. Guilleminault, C, Eldridge, FL and Dement, WC: Insomnia with sleep apnea: a new syndrome. *Science 181:* 856, 1973.
8. Jones, H and Oswald, I: Two cases of healthy insomnia. *Electroencephalogr Clin Neurophysiol 24:* 378, 1968.
9. Kales, A, Bixler, EO, Tan, TL, et al.: Chronic hypnotic drug use: ineffectiveness, drug withdrawal insomnia and hypnotic drug dependence. *JAMA 227:* 513, 1974.
10. Lugaresi, E, Coccagna, G, Gambi, D, Berticeroni, G and Poppi, M: Symond's nocturnal myoclonus. *Electroencephalogr Clin Neurophysiol 23:* 289, 1967.
11. National Center for Health Statistics: Selected symptoms of psychological distress. U.S. Public Health Service Publication 1000, Series II, No. 37, Washington, D.C., U.S. Department of Health, Education and Welfare, August 1970.
12. Rochester, DF and Enson, Y: Current concepts in the pathogenesis of the obesity-hypoventilation syndrome. *Am J Med 57:* 402, 1974.
13. Solomon, F, White, CC, Parron, DL and Mendelson, WB: Special report: sleeping pills, insomnia and medical practice, from the Institute of Medicine of the National Academy of Sciences. *N Engl J Med 300:* 803, 1979.
14. Wayne, JW, Block, AJ and Boysen, Jr. PG: Oxygen desaturation in sleep: sleep apnea and COPD. *Hosp Pract,* p. 77, October 1980.
15. Williams, RL: Sleep disorders in various medical and surgical conditions. In *Sleep Disorders,* p. 285, edited by RL Williams and I Karacan. John Wiley, New York, 1978.
16. Zarcone, V: Narcolepsy. *N Engl J Med 288:* 1156, 1973.

SECTION 12

Selected General Surgical Problems

CHAPTER EIGHTY-THREE

Preoperative Planning for Ambulatory Patients

RICHARD J. GROSS, M.D., EVERETT K. SPEES, M.D., Ph.D., and
L. RANDOL BARKER, M.D.

PREOPERATIVE PLANNING: OVERVIEW

The general physician often invests substantial time and effort in preoperative planning for a patient with a problem amenable to surgery. He schedules tests to confirm the diagnosis, discusses the findings with the patient and the patient's family, proposes consultation with a surgeon, and consults on the care of the patient's medical problems in the perioperative period. Most preoperative planning can be done in the ambulatory setting. Moreover, increasingly large proportions of operations are performed in ambulatory surgery units.

In general, the surgeon expects the referring physician to have made an independent assessment of the need for surgery *and of the patient's general fitness for surgery*. Although the surgeon obtains the actual consent for the surgical procedure, the patient's expectations and assumptions are often based upon the counseling provided by his personal physician. The referral itself is usually understood by the patient and his family as an endorsement of the importance of a surgical opinion and of the competence of the consulting surgeon. For these reasons, the general physician should know the place of surgery in the management of a broad array of conditions (or should discuss the possibility of surgery with a surgeon whenever he is uncertain) and should be aware of the competence of the surgeon whom he selects. Two recently published books which summarize the probability of success and failure in a large variety of surgical procedures are especially useful (7, 8).

In counseling the patient and his family, the general physician, as well as the surgeon, should explain clearly the objective and the expected outcome of the operation. This is especially important for surgical procedures which are undertaken for asymptomatic conditions (such as elective cholecystectomy) and for procedures which may be disfiguring (such as mastectomy or amputation). Preoperative counseling should be documented in the patient's record, and this documentation should always include any special issues raised by the patient and how they were resolved (such as obtaining additional consultations or providing supportive counseling).

Approximately 50% of adults who undergo surgery are ostensibly in good general health; the other 50% have various medical problems (the percentages vary depending upon the age of the population). In perhaps 5 to 10% of patients, new medical problems will be identified during preoperative evaluation, a small proportion of which will have implications for the planning of surgery. For every patient, the general physician should complete an appropriate preoperative evaluation (see below) and should assure that existing medical conditions which may affect the outcome of surgery are optimally controlled. These steps should be taken before admission for surgery, and specific recommendations should be communicated to the surgeon regarding the care of the patient's medical problem(s) during the perioperative period. This chapter provides guidelines for these steps in the management of patients with a number of common medical problems.

GENERAL PREOPERATIVE EVALUATION

There is no consensus on the makeup of a general preoperative evaluation. For adult patients undergoing general or spinal anesthesia, most physicians currently perform a history and physical examination and order a number of routine laboratory tests (e.g.,

chest X-ray and electrocardiogram in patients over 40; and complete blood count, tests of hemostasis, electrolytes, glucose, measurement of blood urea nitrogen or creatinine, and urinalysis in all adults). This complete workup has been criticized for having a low yield and for being unnecessarily costly (19).

The large number of factors that influence the preoperative evaluation make a consensus unlikely. The patient's age, the nature of the planned surgery (major or minor), the type of anesthesia to be used (general, spinal, regional, or local), and the interval since the patient's last comprehensive evaluation are all relevant in the preoperative evaluation of every patient. In addition, one or more of the following considerations is often pertinent: estimating operative risk, establishing a baseline for expected postoperative changes or possible complications, avoiding harm to other patients or medical personnel (e.g., hepatitis, tuberculosis), documenting selected information for medicolegal reasons, determining drug dosage, and detecting rare but potentially catastrophic circumstances (e.g., thrombocytopenia in a patient scheduled for a craniotomy). A practical approach for the individual patient is to select one of the two general types of preoperative evaluation as summarized in Table 83.1 *i.e., a limited or a comprehensive workup*. Guidelines for choosing between these alternatives are summarized in Table 83.2. Selected screening tests should be added to either workup in order to avoid potential catastrophes associated with certain high risk situations (see Table 83.3).

CURRENT MEDICATIONS AND KNOWN ALLERGIES

All drugs which a patient is taking and any known drug allergies should be specified at the time of referral for surgery. Planning should be initiated at that time, for the following reasons: to avoid possible interactions with anesthetic agents and possible complications during surgery; to manage the patient when an essential drug cannot be administered orally during the perioperative period; and to avoid exposure to drugs to which the patient is allergic. The patient should be asked specifically about nonprescription drug use, which, although very common, is often not mentioned spontaneously (particularly aspirin-containing compounds, which may potentiate postoperative bleeding; and sedatives which may interact with anesthetic drugs); about prior allergic reactions to drugs (especially penicillin and other antibiotics which may be indicated postoperatively at a time when a patient is unable to provide information); about use of corticosteroids within the past year (particularly patients with obstructive airways disease or seasonal allergy); and about current use of recreational substances which may affect the patient's course during or after surgery (alcohol, tobacco, illicit drugs).

Table 83.1
Two Types of General Preoperative Evaluation

Component of Workup	Limited Workup[a]	Comprehensive Workup[a]
History	Heart, lungs, hemostasis, medications, allergies, and new symptoms (especially upper respiratory infection)	Brief review of all systems, medications, allergies, past operations
Physical examination	Vital signs, oral cavity, chest, heart, and abdomen	Vital signs, eyes, oral cavity, neck, chest, breast, heart, peripheral pulses, abdomen, nervous system
Laboratory[a]	Hematocrit value, urinalysis, pregnancy test[b]	Chest X-ray, ECG (>age 40), complete blood count, serum electrolytes, blood urea nitrogen or serum creatinine, serum glucose, urinalysis, pregnancy test[b]

[a] Basic evaluation for screening and baseline data. Other tests may be added to evaluate known disease in a patient or to follow-up findings in the preoperative history and physical.
[b] Women in child-bearing age group.

For patients taking one or more drugs regularly, preoperative office management consists of adjusting some drugs before hospitalization and of communicating to the surgeon specific recommendations regarding the patient's medications during the perioperative period (see Table 83.4). Most medications have a duration of action between 6 and 12 hours, and omission of one or more doses may precipitate symptoms. For patients who are expected to be awake and to be able to take oral medications within this time span, it is appropriate to recommend giving a dose, with a small amount of water (1 ounce or less) just before the induction of anesthesia and resuming the medication orally 6 to 12 hours later. When oral medications cannot be continued throughout the perioperative period, alternate medications or routes of administration should be recommended.

THE PATIENT WITH CARDIOVASCULAR DISEASE

Overview

Most forms of general anesthesia may cause cardiovascular stresses (decreased myocardial contractility, arrhythmias, hypotension); and spinal or epidural anesthesia may cause hypotension. These factors and the stresses associated with surgery itself probably account for the greatly increased risk of surgery for patients with underlying cardiovascular disease. Knowledge of the risks of surgery and of the appropriate preoperative management for patients with established cardiovascular disease is needed frequently by the general physician.

Table 83.2
Guidelines for Selecting the General Preoperative Evaluation

Limited Workup	Comprehensive Workup
Age < 40	Age > 40 (especially > 60)
Local, regional, or spinal anesthesia	General anesthesia
Minor procedure	Major procedure (especially thoracic, abdominal, neurosurgical)
Well patient	Patient with moderate-severe major organ disease
	No, old, or inadequate data base

Table 83.3
Additional Preoperative Screening Tests for Common High Risk Situations

High Risk Situation	Screening Tests
Patient undergoing neurosurgical, cardiac, vascular, or major abdominal procedure	Tests of hemostasis: platelet count, prothrombin time, partial thromboplastin time
Patient with increased risk of chronic pulmonary disease (e.g., smoker with ≥10 pack years) who is undergoing general anesthesia	Pulmonary function tests (see Table 83.12)
Patient with increased risk of active liver disease (e.g., alcoholism, drug addiction, homosexuality, dialysis patient) who is undergoing general or spinal anesthesia	Liver function tests: serum transaminases, alkaline phosphatase, bilirubin
Patient with increased risk of tuberculosis (e.g., known exposure, underprivileged population)	Chest X-ray, PPD
Patient with increased risk of coronary artery disease (i.e., smoker, hypertensive, strong family history, diabetic, hyperlipidemia)	ECG

Ischemic Heart Disease

SIZE OF THE RISK (21)

Ischemic heart disease poses two major risks perioperatively in the patient undergoing general anesthesia: myocardial infarction and death. These risks depend upon the patient's preoperative status. Overall, the risks for patients with arteriosclerotic heart disease are 2 or 3 times those of patients of the same age without cardiac disease.

The increased risk posed by ischemic heart disease is dependent on preoperative cardiac status (see Table 83.5). *Stable angina pectoris* represents only a small increase in risk. The risk attending *severe* or *unstable angina* cannot be estimated accurately because of varying definitions and the small number of patients reported in the medical literature; but there is a significantly increased risk. *A myocardial infarction within 6 months* before surgery represents a very high risk, particularly in the 3 months following infarction. Even 6 months after an infarction, the risk of a perioperative myocardial infarction is considerably larger than the risk in a control population.

Table 83.4
Management of Drugs in the Surgical Patient[a]

Drug Class	Anticipated Problems	Recommendations to Surgeon for Perioperative Period
CARDIOVASCULAR		
Antihypertensives[b]	Interaction with anesthetics, hypotension	Inform anesthesiologist of use
	Inability to give orally	Plan postoperative regimen with alternative agents if needed
Antiarrhythmics[b]	Inability to give orally	ECG monitor in operating room and postoperatively, use alternative parenteral agents
β-Blockers[b]	Myocardial depression, bradycardia	Continue intravenously (propranolol, 1–2 mg every 6 hr), taper to lower dose, or discontinue depending on circumstances
Digitalis[b]	Toxicity	Obtain serum levels preoperatively
	Inability to give orally	Give 75% of daily oral dose of digoxin intravenously each day
GASTROINTESTINAL		
Antacids[b]	Inability to give orally	Intravenous cimetidine, nasogastric suction (if patient has active peptic ulcer disease)
ANTIBIOTICS		
Tetracycline	Risk of renal failure if given with methoxyflurane	Use alternative antibiotic or anesthetic
CORTICOSTEROIDS[b]	Adrenal insufficiency	Plan coverage (with intravenous corticosteroids) adequate for the stress of surgery
	Poor wound healing	Discuss with surgeon
NEUROLOGIC		
Levodopa/Carbidopa[b]	Interaction with anesthetics (hypertension or hypotension), inability to give orally	Inform anesthesiologist of use. Resume orally as soon as possible after surgery
Barbiturates	Increased CNS depression by anesthesia, inability to give orally	Inform anesthesiologist of use. Give daily dose intramuscularly
Dilantin	Inability to give orally	Give daily dose slowly intravenously (or substitute phenobarbital before admitting patient for surgery)
BRONCHODILATORS		
Theophylline[b]	Inability to give orally	Switch to intravenous aminophylline
β₂-Sympathomimetics[b]	Inability to give orally	Switch to aerosolized β₂-agent
PSYCHIATRIC		
Antidepressants[b]	Hypotension or hypertension, arrhythmias	Inform anesthesiologist of use; withhold MAO inhibitors 1–2 weeks preoperatively; withhold other agents 24 hours preoperatively.
Neuroleptics (i.e. phenothiazines and haloperidol)[b]	Arrhythmias, enhancement of neuromuscular blocking agents, hypotension	Inform anesthesiologist of use; withhold 24 hours preoperatively
Benzodiazepines	Increased CNS depression by anesthesia	Inform anesthesiologist of use
Lithium[b]	Myocardial depression, hypernatremia	Inform anesthesiologist of use; determine blood levels; withhold 24 hours preoperatively; avoid diuretics and nonsteroidal anti-inflammatory agents
ANALGESICS		
Narcotics	Decreased cough reflex, increased CNS depression by anesthesia, hypotension	Inform anesthesiologist of use
Aspirin compounds[b]	Increased bleeding	Discontinue 1 week before surgery
ANTICOAGULANTS		
Warfarin[b]	Increased bleeding	Discontinue 48 hr before surgery, vitamin K₁ if needed, check prothrombin time before operation
DIURETICS	Electrolyte abnormalities, hypotension, inability to give orally	Obtain electrolytes and check blood pressure (lying, standing) within 24 hr preoperatively, use intravenous furosemide if needed
GOUT		
Benemid, allopurinol	Inability to give orally	Observe, treat acute gout with intravenous colchicine
DIABETES		
Oral hypoglycemics[b]	Inability to give orally	Switch to insulin preoperatively in selected patients
Insulin[b]	Risk of hyper- or hypoglycemia	Give one-third to one-half of usual dose preoperatively
THYROID THERAPY		
Thyroid hormone[b]	Inability to give orally	Usually can be discontinued for up to 7–10 days
Antithyroid drugs[b]	Inability to give orally	Use parenteral iodides or propranolol if necessary
TOPICAL DRUGS FOR GLAUCOMA		
Timolol	Systemic β-blockage	Notify anesthesiologist preoperatively
Phospholine iodide	Prolonged muscle relaxant activity	Discontinue 7–10 days preoperatively
RECREATIONAL DRUGS		
Alcohol	Affect drug metabolism, drug interactions, withdrawal syndrome, impaired respiratory function	If possible, have patient discontinue use 1 or more weeks before admission for surgery, inform anesthesiologist and surgeon of recent use
Illicit drugs		
Tobacco[b]		

[a] If the patient will be able to take medication orally within 12 hr postoperatively, most maintenance drugs can be given at that time. If a shorter interval is crucial, a maintenance drug can be given with less than 1 ounce of water, before anesthesia, and the drug can be resumed orally after surgery.

[b] See additional details in subsequent section of this chapter.

In addition to a recent myocardial infarction, a number of factors contribute to the risk of perioperative cardiac complications or mortality. The most important of these factors are decompensated congestive heart failure, arrhythmias, and significant chronic obstructive lung disease. These and other factors have been incorporated into a *cardiac risk index* (Tables 83.6 and 83.7) (10). Until this cardiac risk index is validated in other studies, it should not be used as an absolute classification; however, it provides helpful guidelines for assessing the significance of multiple risk factors.

Table 83.5
Approximate Cardiovascular Risk in Relation to Preoperative Cardiac Status

Patient Preoperative Status	Approximate Risk of Postoperative Myocardial Infarction (%)	Approximate Mortality Risk (%)
No "cardiac" disease	0.2–2[a]	3[a]
"Cardiac disease" present	6	5
Angina (stable)	3	3–10
Post myocardial infarction		
<6 months	25	18–20
<3 months	30–35	25–40
3–6 months	15–20	10–20
>6 months	5	No data

[a] Risk varies with age of population studied.

Table 83.6
Cardiac Risk Factors in Surgical Patients[a]

Risk Factors	Points for Cardiac Risk Index (see Table 83.7)
HISTORY	
Myocardial infarction in past 6 months	10
Age >70	5
PHYSICAL	
S3 gallop or jugular venous distention	11
Significant aortic stenosis	3
ECG	
Rhythm other than sinus or premature atrial contractions on last preoperative ECG	7
>5 premature ventricular contractions/min any time preoperatively	7
OTHER ORGAN SYSTEMS	
$pO_2 < 60$, $pCO_2 > 50$	
$K < 3.0$, $HCO_3 < 20$ mEq/dl	
BUN > 50, CR > 3.0 mg/dl	
Signs of chronic liver disease or abnormal SGOT	3 (each factor)
Bedridden from noncardiac causes	
OPERATION	
Intraperitoneal or intrathoracic	3
Emergency	4
TOTAL POSSIBLE	53

[a] Adapted from L. Goldman *et al.*: *New England Journal of Medicine*, *297:* 845, 1977 (10).

Table 83.7
Cardiac Risk Index (Based on a Prospective Study of Patients at the Massachusetts General Hospital)[a]

Class	Point Total[b]	No or Moderate Complication ($N = 943$)[c] (%)	Life-threatening Complication ($N = 39$)[d] (%)	Cardiac Deaths ($N = 19$)[e] (%)
I	0–5	99	0.7	0.2
II	6–12	93	5	2
III	13–25	86	11	2
IV	≥26	22	22	56

[a] Adapted from L. Goldman *et al.*: *New England Journal of Medicine, 297:* 845, 1977 (10).
[b] See Table 83.6.
[c] New or worsened heart failure without pulmonary edema, supraventricular tachyarrhythmia, or intraoperative or postoperative ischemia (as indicated by chest pain or ECG changes) without documented myocardial infarction.
[d] Documented intraoperative or postoperative myocardial infarction, pulmonary edema, or ventricular tachycardia without progression to cardiac death.
[e] Deaths due to arrhythmia or to low output heart failure.

PREOPERATIVE PLANNING

Office Evaluation. Patients with established ischemic heart disease should have a comprehensive preoperative evaluation (see Table 83.1). Noninvasive tests of cardiac function including echocardiography, nuclear scanning, and stress tests should be reserved for situations where the existence or severity of cardiovascular disease is questioned.

Based upon the preoperative evaluation, the risk of general anesthesia and surgery should be estimated for each patient. For patients with recent myocardial infarction (within less than 6 months), with unstable angina, or with less severe coronary artery disease and multiple other risk factors (see Table 83.6), only urgent life-saving surgery should be undertaken. Surgery may be done 3 months after infarction when the risk of waiting the additional 3 months is thought to be significant (*e.g.*, recurrent cholecystitis). Patients with stable angina or uncomplicated recovery from myocardial infarction more than 6 months previously have an increased risk which does not decline further with time; thus necessary operations need not be postponed.

Coronary artery bypass surgery should be considered before elective noncardiac surgery, in consultation with a cardiologist, only in patients who have other indications for bypass surgery (see Chapter 54).

Recommendations to the Surgeon. A baseline ECG should be obtained before surgery for all patients with known coronary artery disease and for all patients over age 40. Routine postoperative ECGs should be obtained only in high risk patients, since the yield of useful information from them is low.

For patients taking a long acting oral nitrate for angina, the drug should be administered until midnight prior to surgery. While the patient is unable to take medications orally, Nitrol paste should be substituted; because there is no simple way to determine the paste dose equivalent to an oral nitrate, an intermediate dose (1 to 2 inches every 4 to 6 hours) should be recommended.

For patients taking a β-blocking agent for angina, intravenous small doses of propranolol (i.e., 1 to 2 mg every 6 hours) should be substituted, given by a physician, while the patient is unable to take medications by mouth. This should protect the patient from the risk of acute cardiac ischemia which occasionally follows abrupt cessation of a beta blocking agent. Patients able to resume oral intake within 12 to 24 hours usually can be observed without intravenous propranolol.

Intensive intraoperative monitoring, using Swan-Ganz and radial artery catheters should be considered for patients who are very sensitive to volume changes, such as those in congestive heart failure (see below) and for operations where loss and replacement of large volumes of fluid are expected (e.g., aneurysm repair).

Hypertension

SIZE OF THE RISK

Controversy still exists about whether mild to moderate hypertension (diastolic ≤110 mg Hg) increases anesthetic and surgical risks. The only prospective study showed no correlation between uncontrolled diastolic pressures in this range and the risk of perioperative cardiac, renal, or cerebrovascular events (9). Patients in this study often had other cardiac risk factors which did correlate with the incidence of perioperative cardiac morbidity (see Table 83.6 and 83.8).

Too few patients have been studied to define adequately the risk for persons operated on when their diastolic pressure exceeds 110 mm Hg, but there is probably an increased risk (18).

PREOPERATIVE PLANNING

Office Evaluation. The basic preoperative evaluation in the hypertensive patient should determine whether there is end organ damage (renal: serum creatinine concentration and urinalysis; cerebrovascular: history, neurologic and neurovascular examination; and cardiovascular: history, cardiac examination, chest X-ray, and ECG). Blood pressure and pulse measurements should be made with the patient sitting and standing (after brief exercise, to identify the maximum orthostatic fall in patients taking antihypertensive drugs); the preoperative status of blood pressure control may then be classified as untreated, hypertensive despite therapy, or controlled.

Patients who are controlled, or patients who are partially controlled and have diastolic pressures ≤ 110 mm Hg should be continued on their prescribed antihypertensive medication. Two exceptions to this rule are guanethidine and monoamine oxidase inhibitors. A patient taking either of these should be switched to a different drug as both of these drugs may cause markedly labile blood pressure during anesthesia.

Untreated patients with diastolic pressures ≤ 110 mm Hg may undergo surgery, with institution of antihypertensive therapy after convalescence from surgery.

Individual judgments must be made about patients with diastolic pressures ≥ 110 mm Hg, depending on the severity and duration of hypertension, the presence of end organ damage, and the extent of planned surgery. Patients with severe hypertension (i.e., diastolic ≥ 120 mm Hg) should have their blood pressure at least partly controlled before admission for nonurgent surgery (18), although there are no studies proving that such control modifies risks. Attempts to control blood pressure too rapidly (for example, rapid increases in diuretic treatment over several days), may result in volume depletion, hypokalemia, or hy-

Table 83.8
Risk of Perioperative Cardiac Complications in Patients with Mild to Moderate Hypertension[a]

Preoperative Characteristics	Mean Point Total[b] (± SEM)	Patients with No Cardiac Complication (%)	Patients with Minor Complications Only (%)	Patients with Major Nonfatal Complications (%)	Patients with Cardiac Death (%)
Normal blood pressure No history of hypertension	4.3 ± .3	89	9	2	0.2
Hypertension controlled Taking antihypertensive drug(s)	6.9 ± .6	76	15	8	1
Hypertensive Taking antihypertensive drug(s)	4.4 ± .5	93	8	—	1
Hypertensive Not taking antihypertensive drug(s)	5.5 ± .6	88	9	1	1

[a] Adapted from L. Goldman and D. L. Caldera: *Anesthesiology,* 50: 285, 1979 (9).
[b] See Table 83.6 for risk factor index.

potension at the time of surgery. Therefore, these patients should have their blood pressure stabilized during 1 to 2 weeks before admission for surgery.

Recommendations to the Surgeon. For all hypertensive patients it is important to advise the surgeon to avoid significant intravascular volume expansion or contraction, as these conditions may either cause a significant rise in blood pressure (volume expansion) or fall in blood pressure (volume contraction, especially in the patient who is taking antihypertensive drugs).

Current antihypertensive medications should be continued until midnight before surgery and resumed postoperatively when the patient is stable and can take oral medications. Because of bed rest and inactivity during convalescence, some patients will require less antihypertensive medication during the first few weeks following major surgery.

Omission of one or more doses of some sympatholytic antihypertensives (clonidine, methyldopa, β-blockers) is occasionally (<1%) followed, 12 to 48 hours after the last dose, by rebound hypertension accompanied by manifestations of increased sympathetic activity (tachycardia, diaphoresis, headache). Therefore, patients who must miss scheduled doses of any of these drugs should be observed carefully during the first 48 hours after surgery. If they develop signs of the rebound state, they should be treated with either intravenous propranolol (1 to 2 mg every 6 hours) or methyldopa (250 to 500 mg every 4 to 6 hours) until they are able to take their usual medication orally.

Valvular Heart Disease

SIZE OF THE RISK

The risk of surgery in the patient with valvular heart disease varies with the valve affected (aortic vs. mitral), the nature (stenosis vs. insufficiency), and the severity of the lesion. The severity of valvular lesions as judged clinically by New York Heart Association (NYHA) classification (see Table 58.3, Chapter 58) provides a reasonable indication of surgical risk, with the exception of aortic stenosis.

Valvular heart disease poses two major surgical risks: cardiac death and congestive heart failure. The presence of aortic stenosis of any degree of hemodynamic significance (*i.e.*, NYHA class 2 to 4) poses a high risk of surgical mortality. Mild to moderate mitral lesions or aortic insufficiency represent only slightly increased risks of cardiac death; however, hemodynamically severe valvular disease (*i.e.*, NYHA class 3 or 4) due to these lesions creates major risks. In addition to increasing the risk of perioperative mortality, significant valvular disease poses an increased risk of decompensated heart failure.

No specific information exists regarding the risks associated with prolapsed mitral valve or with idiopathic hypertrophic subaortic stenosis (IHSS). It is reasonable to assume that the risk in patients with prolapsed mitral valve depends upon the degree of mitral regurgitation. Patients with IHSS may be very sensitive to volume contraction, and are probably best managed with a Swan-Ganz catheter in place during major procedures associated with rapid volume changes.

Patients with artificial heart valves, patients with any evidence of valvular heart disease (including mitral prolapse and IHSS), and patients with congenital structural defects (e.g., patent ductus arteriosis, ventricular septal defect) have a small but definite risk of acquiring bacterial endocarditis when they undergo procedures in the oral cavity, and upper respiratory, gastrointestinal, or genitourinary tracts.

PREOPERATIVE PLANNING

Office Evaluation. The basic cardiac evaluation should delineate the nature and severity of the valvular disease and should identify any associated cardiac conditions. The uses of echocardiography and cardiac catheterization to evaluate valvular heart disease are described in Chapter 57. Patients with severe valvular disease should have corrective cardiac surgery followed by a period of convalescence before they undergo major noncardiac operations.

Recommendations to the Surgeon. Patients undergoing procedures attended by a risk of endocarditis should receive antimicrobial prophylaxis as summarized in Table 83.9.

The preoperative management of congestive heart failure, arrhythmia, or anticoagulant therapy (in patients with artificial valves) is described in subsequent sections of this chapter.

Congestive Heart Failure

SIZE OF THE RISK

Information on the risk of developing congestive heart failure (CHF) perioperatively is limited because of the few studies available. However, the best prospective study (11) closely corresponds to general clinical experience. The most significant risk factors for postoperative CHF are decompensated failure preoperatively and, to a lesser extent, prior CHF which is clinically stable preoperatively (Table 83.10). However, only 40% of patients who develop perioperative CHF have had prior failure. The best predictors for the other 60% of patients are age greater than 60, major surgery (especially abdominal aortic aneurysm repair or major abdominal surgery), and nonspecific electrocardiographic abnormalities.

Patients with postoperative pulmonary edema have a high total mortality (20–57%), most of which is cardiac. Patients who develop less severe postoperative CHF do not have an increased risk of postoperative cardiac death, although the overall mortality for all causes is increased. Most postoperative CHF occurs during or within several hours of surgery.

Table 83.9
Prevention of Bacterial Endocarditis in Patients with Valvular Heart Disease, Prosthetic Heart Valves, and Other Abnormalities[a] of the Cardiovascular System[b]

Antibiotic and Route	Dose	Schedule
DENTAL AND UPPER RESPIRATORY PROCEDURES[c]		
Parenteral[d]		
Aqueous penicillin G	1 to 2 million units i.m. or i.v.	30 min to 1 hr before procedure
plus Procaine penicillin G	600,000 units i.m.[e]	
then Penicillin V	500 mg p.o. q6h	For 4–8 doses
Penicillin allergy:		
Vancomycin	1 g i.v.	Infused over 30 min beginning 1 hr before procedure
then Erythromycin	500 mg p.o. q6h	For 4–8 doses
Oral[d]		
Penicillin V	2 g p.o.	30 min to 2 hr before procedure
then Penicillin V	500 mg p.o. q6h	For 4–8 doses
Penicillin allergy:		
Erythromycin	500 mg p.o.	30 min to 2 hr before procedure
then Erythromycin	500 mg p.o. q6h	For 4–8 doses
GASTROINTESTINAL AND GENITOURINARY PROCEDURES[c]		
Aqueous penicillin G	2 million units i.m. or i.v.	30 min to 1 hr before procedure
or Ampicillin	1–2 g i.m. or i.v.	
plus Gentamicin	1.5 mg/kg i.m.	30 min to 1 hr before procedure
then repeat both	As above	Every 8 hr for 2 more doses
Penicillin allergy:		
Vancomycin	1 g i.v.	Infused over 30 min beginning 1 hr before procedure
plus Gentamicin	1.5 mg/kg i.m.	30 min to 1 hr before procedure
then repeat both	As above	Once 12 hr later

[a] Most forms of congenital heart disease (but not uncomplicated secundum atrial septal defect), idiopathic hypertrophic subaortic stenosis, and mitral valve prolapse syndrome with mitral insufficiency murmur.
[b] Source: *The Medical Letter*, *23:* 92, 1981.
[c] Data are limited on the risk of endocarditis with a particular procedure. (For a review of the risk of bacteremia with various procedures, see E. D. Everett and J. V. Hirschmann: *Medicine*, *56:* 61, 1977.)
[d] *In vitro* data and animal studies suggest that the parenteral regimens are more likely to be effective; they are recommended especially for patients with prosthetic valves or those taking continuous oral penicillin for rheumatic fever prophylaxis.
[e] Some *Medical Letter* consultants would also give streptomycin 1 g i.m., especially for patients with prosthetic heart valves or those taking continuous oral penicillin for rheumatic fever prophylaxis.

PREOPERATIVE PLANNING

Office Evaluation. Patients with compensated CHF, should have a comprehensive preoperative evaluation (see Table 83.1). This evaluation should include a meticulous assessment of volume status (lying and standing blood pressures, inspection of neck veins, determination if edema is present) and examination for cardiac gallops and for rales. Laboratory data should include a digoxin level if that drug is being administered. Noninvasive methods for assessing left ventricular function (see Chapter 58) may be useful when the degree of cardiac dysfunction is uncertain.

Although there are no definitive studies in this regard, it is prudent to *digitalize* patients with a confirmed history of moderate or severe CHF, ideally during the week before admission. Most controversy about preoperative digitalization has concerned the patient who has a past history of no or minimal CHF, but a "risk" of developing CHF because of an enlarged heart or because the surgery will involve major volume shifts. Although data are lacking, it is likely that digitalis does not help the latter type of patient

and that the risk of digitalis toxicity is not warranted (6).

Patients with decompensated CHF should have all but life-saving surgery postponed until the failure is controlled, either in the office or in the hospital.

Recommendations to the Surgeon. Patients with controlled CHF should be maintained on their usual oral regimen until midnight before surgery and maintained with intravenous diuretics and digoxin (75% of the oral dose) during the immediate postoperative period.

Arrhythmias

The arrhythmias which are encountered most frequently in ambulatory patients are described in detail in Chapter 56.

SIZE OF THE RISK

Patients with arrhythmias before surgery have significantly increased risks of cardiac morbidity and death. These risks have not been quantified for subgroups of patients with specific arrhythmias, except as indicated in the cardiac risk index shown in Tables

**Table 83.10
Risks of Developing Congestive Failure (CHF) in
Perioperative Period**[a, b]

Patient Characteristics	Size of Risk	
	All CHF (%)	Pulmonary edema (%)
No prior CHF	4	2
Past CHF:		
All—now compensated	16	6
Past pulmonary edema (regardless of current status)	32	23
Decompensated CHF preoperatively	21	16
Preoperative physical findings:		
S3 gallop	47	35
Jugular venous distention	35	30
NYHA Class preoperatively (see Table 58.3)		
1	5	3
2	7	7
3	18	6
4	31	25

[a] Adapted from L. Goldman et al.: *Medicine*, 57: 357, 1978 (11).

[b] Based upon 1,001 consecutive patients undergoing general surgery, orthopaedic surgery, or urologic surgery (transurethral resection of the prostate omitted because of existing evidence of its safety even in elderly patients).

83.6 and 83.7. Patients with complete heart block, Mobitz Type II second degree block, and sick sinus syndrome have a significant risk of complications during anesthesia if a pacemaker is not inserted. On the other hand, there is little or no increased risk associated with bi- or trifascicular block on ECG in patients who are asymptomatic.

Arrhythmias do occur in approximately 20% or more of adult patients during general anesthesia; however, most of these patients do not have preoperative arrhythmias. Most intraoperative arrhythmias are supraventricular, transient, related to specific anesthesic or surgical manipulation, and do not require specific therapies. The number of arrhythmias that are detected clinically, without the use of continuous monitoring, is lower: supraventricular arrhythmias are detected clinically in 4% of patients and other arrhythmias in 11% (11).

PREOPERATIVE PLANNING

Office Evaluation. Patients with arrhythmias should have the comprehensive preoperative evaluation (Table 83.1) expanded in several ways. The probable etiology of the arrhythmia should be delineated (see Chapter 56). If the arrhythmia is intermittent or control is not certain, 24-hour Holter monitoring should be done. Drug levels of antiarrhythmic drugs that are being administered should be obtained. In general, this entire evaluation should be accomplished before admission for surgery.

Patients with *supraventricular arrhythmias* should have their ventricular rates controlled or should be converted to more stable rhythms. Except for atrial fibrillation, this usually means conversion either to normal sinus rhythm or to atrial fibrillation, since other supraventricular arrhythmias are either hemodynamically unstable or give an unpredictable ventricular response even with appropriate drug therapy. Patients with atrial fibrillation should have their rates slowed but should be able to accelerate their heart rate under stress as indicated by their ability to raise their pulse rate more than 10 points by mild exercise.

Established indications for *preoperative digitalization* in patients with arrhythmias are control of rate in atrial fibrillation and prophylaxis of supraventricular arrhythmias in selected patients (e.g., patients with past histories of supraventricular arrhythmias, especially atrial fibrillation or flutter, who remain at high risk for recurrence; and patients with significant mitral stenosis).

Patients with *premature ventricular contractions* (PVCs) or other ventricular arrhythmias should be treated according to the criteria outlined in Chapter 56.

Recommendations to the Surgeon. Antiarrhythmic drugs should be continued orally until midnight before surgery after which the following intravenous treatment should be substituted until the patient is able to take oral medications again: intravenous digoxin (75% of the oral dose) for patients on digoxin, and intravenous lidocaine or procainamide, for patients taking quinidine or disopyramide for ventricular arrhythmias.

There is general agreement that patients undergoing general anesthesia should have a *prophylactic or therapeutic pacemaker* inserted for the following conditions:

1. Symptomatic or significant dysfunction of the sinoatrial node.

2. Idioventricular rhythm.

3. Current or past history of third degree or second degree (Mobitz Type II) atrioventricular (AV) block.

4. Some instances of second degree (Mobitz Type I) AV block.

5. Some instances of trifascicular block (RBBB plus LAH plus first degree AV block; alternating LBBB and RBBB; or LBBB and first degree AV block) especially in the presence of severe valvular disease, ischemic disease, or congestive failure.

6. A history of Stokes-Adams attacks.

Patients with findings suggesting bradyarrhythmias, (especially a history of syncope or near-syncope, and an underlying ECG abnormality) probably should have a temporary pacemaker recommended if a full workup to evaluate the etiology of the symptoms cannot be performed preoperatively or is not revealing. Isolated conditions for which a pacemaker is more controversial, but probably not indicated, include bifascicular block, bundle branch block, first degree AV block, and sinus bradycardia which is asymptomatic.

Table 83.11
Nonpulmonary Factors which Increase Pulmonary Risks During General Surgery (in Approximate Order of Importance)

Age over 60
Upper abdominal or thoracic operation
Repeat operations within 1 yr
General anesthesia lasting more than 3 hr
Obesity
Abnormal ECG
Poor patient effort/cooperation
Narcotic analgesics
Minor upper respiratory illness

THE PATIENT WITH PULMONARY DISEASE (26)
Overview

Patients with significant pulmonary disease have an increased mortality and morbidity during surgery. The increased risks are due chiefly to the following physiologic changes produced by the effects of anesthesia, sedatives, and analgesics: (a) abnormalities of pulmonary gas exchange, causing hypoxemia; and (b) depression of the cough reflex, decrease in clearance of respiratory secretions, and loss of sighing and normal lung inflation—each of which increases the risk of atelectasis and pneumonia. In addition, normal breathing and voluntary coughing are decreased after surgery because of pain and discomfort, especially after upper abdominal and thoracic surgery. Optimal preoperative treatment of pulmonary disease can reduce perioperative morbidity and mortality.

Chronic Obstructive Pulmonary Disease (COPD)
SIZE OF THE RISK

The precise risk of perioperative death from pulmonary causes for patients with COPD is not known because of the lack of information regarding patients with mild lung disease. Men with clinically moderate to severe COPD have an overall perioperative mortality of approximately 10% following general anesthesia (vs. 2% for comparable men without COPD); women with COPD seem to have a lower risk of perioperative mortality (24).

The presence of a smoking history, dyspnea, cough, or of abnormal spirometry increases the risk of minor postoperative pulmonary complications (i.e., atelectasis or infection without significant respiratory compromise). The risk of respiratory failure requiring vigorous postoperative respiratory therapy is increased in patients with an FEV-1 (forced expiratory volume in 1 sec) less than 1.5 liters. A FEV-1 less than 1.0 liter, or a pCO_2 greater than 45 mm Hg defines a high risk group with a marked increase in perioperative pulmonary mortality and with a 30 to 40% incidence of postoperative respiratory failure requiring prolonged mechanical ventilation.

A number of *nonpulmonary factors* are helpful in predicting postoperative pulmonary complications in patients with COPD (see Table 83.11). The greatest risks are in patients who are older than 60, who undergo upper abdominal and thoracic operations or

operations under general anesthesia lasting more than 3 hours, or who have repeat operations within 1 year. A much lower risk is posed by operations on the extremities, back, breast, and central nervous system. Lower abdominal surgery represents an intermediate risk. Combining these factors with the pulmonary factors listed above increases the physician's ability to predict operative morbidity.

The *type of anesthesia* may affect the risk of pulmonary complications. Local anesthesia creates very little risk; if the patient is heavily sedated, however, there may be temporary deterioration in respiratory control and there may be a suppression of the cough reflex. Spinal anesthesia has had a low mortality in patients with COPD (24) in some studies. Because of the simultaneous use of sedatives and because the patient must ventilate in the supine position, spinal anesthesia creates a substantial risk of intraoperative and postoperative respiratory complications; this is especially true of obese patients with chronic pulmonary disease. Because of these problems, general anesthesia, which permits control of ventilation and clearance of secretions, is preferable to spinal anesthesia in patients with moderate or severe COPD.

PREOPERATIVE PLANNING

Office Evaluation. Patients with known COPD should have a comprehensive preoperative evaluation (see Table 83.1) and if they are taking aminophylline, measurement and adjustment of the serum aminophylline concentration. Any history of smoking, chronic or intermittent sputum production, recent upper respiratory infection, dyspnea on effort or concomitant cardiovascular disease is particularly pertinent. Ideally smokers should stop smoking 2 weeks before admission for surgery to be performed under general or spinal anesthesia, and patients with upper respiratory infections should have surgery postponed at least 2 weeks, regardless of how minor the episode.

Table 83.12 summarizes for patients undergoing general or spinal anesthesia the principal indications for preadmission spirometry alone (forced vital ca-

Table 83.12
Indications for Evaluation of Patients with Pulmonary Disease

SPIROMETRY ONLY (FEV_1 and FVC)
  Smokers (>10 pack years)
  Any pulmonary symptoms (e.g., dyspnea, wheezing, cough, or sputum production)
  Upper abdominal surgery
  Age > 60
  Repeat surgery within 1 yr
  Multiple other risk factors (obesity, recent upper respiratory infections, narcotics abuse, abnormal ECG)
COMPLETE PULMONARY FUNCTION TESTS[a] AND ARTERIAL BLOOD GASES
  Thoracic surgery
  Upper abdominal surgery and any pulmonary disease
  Patients with restrictive lung disease
  Patients with COPD with FEV_1 < 1.5 liters

[a] Spirometry and lung volumes.

pacity (FVC) and FEV_1)) or for complete pulmonary function tests (spirometry plus lung volumes) and arterial blood gases. Unfortunately, operations are often performed without pulmonary function testing, but even experienced clinicians sometimes misjudge the severity of obstructive lung disease. Spirometry will clarify the presence and severity in questionable cases.

Pulmonary consultation should be obtained for patients whose FEV_1 is less than 1.0 liter and for patients with less severe pulmonary disease who are being evaluated for thoracic or upper abdominal surgery.

Recommendations to the Surgeon. After admission to the hospital, the patient should be instructed preoperatively about coughing and deep breathing exercises; as well as the use of devices such as an incentive spirometer that will be used postoperatively. Patients already taking bronchodilators should continue their regimen through midnight before surgery; patients who have a history of intermittent airways obstruction should also be started on a theophylline compound after admission. In order to prevent bronchospasm, especially in the immediate postoperative period, inhaled specific β_2-sympathomimetics and intravenous aminophylline should be administered, and the serum aminophylline level should be kept in the therapeutic range (10–20 mg/liter), during the time that the patient cannot take oral medications. Patients who have received corticosteroids for more than 2 weeks during the year before surgery should be appropriately covered for stress with parenteral steroids (see below, p. 921). Patients with chronic purulent sputum production should receive a 5- to 7-day course of broad spectrum antibiotics (tetracycline, ampicillin, or trimethoprim-sulfamethoxazole) to decrease the quantity and purulence of secretions. Finally, arterial blood gases should be checked in all patients with moderate to severe COPD just before and just after surgery. There is some dispute about the efficacy of most of these individual measures. However, controlled trials combining bronchodilators, antibiotics, lung expansion, and mobilization of secretions have been shown consistently to decrease the number of perioperative complications (22, 24).

LUNG RESECTION AND COPD (12)

Overall mortality rates for lung resection are about 5% for lobectomy and about 15% for total pneumonectomy. The mortality and morbidity rates for lung surgery vary widely depending upon patient factors (particularly age and pulmonary function), type of operation (pneumonectomy, lobectomy, segmental resection), and experience and skill of the surgical team.

Assessment of pulmonary function in the patient with COPD who has an indication for lung resection (usually a tumor) can be performed in the ambulatory setting. Use of the following criteria to select candidates for lung resection has reduced mortality for patients with COPD.

For pneumonectomy, the major criteria for operability are $FEV_1 \geq 2$ liters and FVC $\geq$ 50% of predicted. Patients with an FEV_1 less than 2 liters should have quantitative lung scanning to determine the FEV_1 which can be expected following pneumonectomy (e.g., if 30% of ventilation and perfusion goes to the affected lung, the patient's pulmonary function will be decreased by approximately 30% postoperatively). Those with a predicted postoperative remaining FEV_1 greater than 0.8 to 1 liter by quantitative lung scanning can undergo pneumonectomy, although their mortality risk is probably increased.

Patients not meeting the criteria for pneumonectomy may tolerate lobectomy or segmental resection. Most patients with a preoperative $FEV_1 \geq 1.5$ liters can tolerate a lobectomy. The patient may undergo resection if removal of the segment or lobe will leave him with an FEV_1 greater than 0.8 to 1 liter.

Other measures in the preoperative planning for the patient with COPD undergoing pulmonary resection are similar to those described for such patients in the preceding section.

Asthma

SIZE OF THE RISK

Asthma affects approximately 3% of Americans, which makes it one of the most common pulmonary diseases (see Chapter 52). It is difficult to give a firm estimate of the operative risks posed by asthma because in most reports data on asthma are pooled with results for other types of obstructive airways disease. The most dangerous period for the asthmatic is not usually the period during general anesthesia, since the anesthetic may be an effective bronchodilator, but the immediate postoperative period. The major risks are severe bronchospasm and inspissation of thick secretions.

PREOPERATIVE PLANNING

Office Evaluation. The asthmatic patient should have a comprehensive evaluation (see Table 83.1) in the office before admission for surgery. This allows adequate time for changes in chronic management prior to admission. The patient should stop smoking 2 weeks before surgery.

Recommendations to the Surgeon. Spirometry (FEV_1 and FVC) should be performed in all asthmatic patients the day before the operation. Arterial blood gases should be measured in patients who are not in their stable baseline state or who have significant abnormalities in FEV_1. β_2-Sympathomimetics can be continued, as inhaled aerosols, until the induction of anesthesia, and can be resumed in the recovery room. The concentration of aminophylline in the serum should be measured in all patients preoperatively because of the large number who have subtherapeutic or toxic levels on standard doses; planning for the immediate preoperative period should include continuation of oral bronchodilators until midnight the night before surgery and scheduling of surgery early in the day to avoid the need for preoperative intravenous aminophylline. In very severe asthmatics, a constant infusion of aminophylline should be recommended for the preoperative period and for the period when the patient is unable to take medicine by mouth; other patients are adequately managed by resuming aminophylline, intravenously, in the recovery room. Patients taking maintenance corticosteroids or who have been taking systemic corticosteroids for more than 2 weeks during the previous year should receive doses of parenteral steroids sufficient to cover the stress of surgery (see below).

THE PATIENT WITH RENAL DISEASE

SIZE OF THE RISK

The size of the operative risk for patients with chronic renal disease depends upon the severity of their disease (see Chapter 44). Overall, the surgical mortality for major surgery in patients with severe renal disease (i.e., creatinine clearance less than 10 to 15 ml/min) including patients on dialysis, is about 2 to 4% when these patients are managed carefully. In patients not requiring dialysis, postoperative acute renal failure is the gravest complication, as it carries a high mortality (4).

The major complications associated with surgery in the patient with moderate to severe renal disease are electrolyte disturbances (especially acidosis and hyperkalemia), volume contraction, volume overload, toxicity due to agents which are nephrotoxic or which are excreted by the kidneys, and bleeding. Volume contraction, with the risk of ischemic cerebral, cardiac, or renal damage, is a particular risk in patients with the nephrotic syndrome; these patients usually have a slightly contracted intravascular volume at baseline and are at risk of hypovolemia if an effort is made to decrease their edema with potent diuretics preoperatively. Toxic renal damage may follow the use of two agents which are frequently used in the perioperative period: radiocontrast agents and aminoglycoside antibiotics.

PREOPERATIVE PLANNING

Office Evaluation. Before admission for surgery, patients with chronic renal failure should have the comprehensive evaluation outlined in Table 83.1, and current volume status should be documented. Radiocontrast studies should be avoided, if at all possible, in the preoperative workup of patients with serum creatinine concentrations greater than 4.5 mg%, since the subsequent risk of acute renal failure is about 30% (27).

Recommendations to the Surgeon. The most important consideration in perioperative management of patients who do not require dialysis is avoidance of fluid imbalance. When the surgery carries a risk of significant volume shifts, Swan-Ganz catheterization should be considered to assure close monitoring of the intravascular volume. Administration of drugs such as antihypertensives should follow the guidelines stated elsewhere in this chapter. Adjustments in the doses of drugs should be appropriate for

the patient's degree of renal insufficiency (2). The concentration of electrolytes and creatinine in the serum should be monitored carefully before and after surgery, to detect particularly hyperkalemia and deterioration of renal function. Patients with renal failure frequently have a metabolic acidosis compensated by hyperventilation; postoperatively continued appropriate hyperventilation will be necessary to avoid a potential precipitous fall in arterial pH. Preoperative prophylactic dialysis is not generally recommended. Furthermore, patients with a chronic anemia secondary to renal failure usually are well compensated and do not require preoperative transfusion unless they are symptomatic from the anemia or a large blood loss is expected during surgery.

In general, the nephrologist caring for patients on chronic dialysis should coordinate the medical management of these patients throughout the surgical episode. Although these patients have a very high postoperative complication rate (due to hyperkalemia, bleeding, arteriovenous fistula thrombosis, pneumonia, wound infection, and arrhythmias), their risk of dying due to surgery remains in the 2 to 4% range if they are carefully managed (3).

THE PATIENT WITH ENDOCRINE DISEASE
Diabetes
SIZE OF THE RISK (28)

Total surgical mortality for all diabetic patients is about 4%; and approximately 0.3% die as a result of poor control of their diabetes. About 14% of diabetics have postoperative complications which may be related to diabetes, particularly wound infection.

PREOPERATIVE PLANNING

Office Evaluation. Each diabetic patient should have the comprehensive preoperative evaluation outlined in Table 83.1. Patients controlled with diet alone or with oral agents may be hospitalized the day before surgery if their diabetes is mild or if the planned procedure is minor. Otherwise they should be admitted earlier so that adequate time is allowed for switching to insulin. In general, insulin-dependent diabetics should be admitted 2 days before surgery in order to assure satisfactory preoperative control of their diabetes.

Recommendations to the Surgeon. Fasting blood sugars should be obtained on all diabetics on the day before and on the day of surgery, and their state of hydration should be evaluated to assure that they are not significantly volume-contracted. Elective surgery should not be undertaken until diabetes is at least reasonably controlled (i.e., fasting blood sugar of 250 mg/100 ml or less for 2 or more days).

The appropriate perioperative treatment of diabetes depends upon the type of surgical procedure planned and upon the preadmission regimen, as summarized in Table 83.13.

Diabetics who are controlled by diet can be monitored with daily fasting blood sugars throughout the

Table 83.13
Management of Diabetes on Day of Surgery

Surgical Procedure	Treatment Required to Control Glucose Preoperatively		
	Diet only	Oral hypoglycemic agent	Insulin
Minor	Observe	Withhold until after procedure	Withhold until after procedure or use "major" protocol
Major	Observe	Change to long acting insulin (achieve control with insulin before operation)	Preferred regimen: One-half to two-thirds of total long acting insulin dose preoperatively; regular insulin only if needed OR One-third of total long acting insulin dose preoperatively; one-third postoperatively; regular insulin only if needed OR Continuous low dose infusion of regular insulin OR Regular insulin in each liter of dextrose 5% in water (D_5W)

operative episode and treated with insulin if unacceptable rises in glucose occur.

Management of *patients taking oral agents* varies because they represent a heterogeneous group. Patients with mild elevations of glucose who are undergoing minor procedures that will allow them to eat the same day can take their hypoglycemic drug on the day *before* surgery and resume it when they begin eating on the day of surgery. The exception is the patient taking chlorpropamide (Diabinese) which should be withheld on the day before surgery because of its long half-life. If the patient is to undergo a major procedure, oral agents should be discontinued because they have long half-lives, control is less predictable, and the drugs cannot be given parenterally. Therefore, such a patient should be switched to management by diet only or to insulin.

For the patient who is *taking insulin before surgery*, one of several strategies is recommended for the preoperative period (see Table 83.13). Because of its simplicity and the small risk of hypoglycemia, the first regimen (giving one-half to two-thirds of the usual total daily dose of long acting insulin preoperatively) is the preferred regimen. Postoperative management should consist of resuming the patient's usual daily insulin dose and monitoring afternoon and morning (fasting) blood sugars to determine whether adjustments in the regimen are needed.

Adrenal Insufficiency and Chronic Steroid Therapy (28)

SIZE OF THE RISK

Too few patients have been adequately studied to estimate the increased surgical risks or the risk of precipitating an Addisonian crisis in patients who are currently taking or who have recently taken corticosteroids. It is generally agreed that patients who are currently taking a *pharmacologic dose* of corticosteroids (i.e., more than the equivalent of 20 to 30 mg of hydrocortisone daily) or who have taken corticosteroids at a pharmacologic dose in the past year require additional steroid coverage for surgery. Patients who are receiving *replacement doses* for adrenal insufficiency also require additional coverage, as these patients cannot produce the extra steroids needed during the stress of surgery (see Chapter 71 for additional details).

PREOPERATIVE PLANNING

Office Evaluation. These patients should have a comprehensive evaluation before admission (see Table 83.1). For patients with adrenal insufficiency, the evaluation should include particular attention to factors which may reflect the adequacy of corticosteroid replacement (i.e., lying and standing blood pressure, concentration of serum urea nitrogen and/or serum creatinine, glucose, and electrolytes). Some authorities suggest adrenocorticotropic hormone (ACTH) stimulation or insulin-hypoglycemia testing to determine the need for steroid coverage in patients who are no longer receiving steroids, but who have received large doses of steroids in the past; however, these tests cannot be recommended for routine use since adequate evidence that a normal response precludes the need for steroid coverage during surgery is lacking.

Recommendations to the Surgeon. The patient may receive his usual steroid dose by mouth the day before surgery. On the day of surgery, the patient should be given hydrocortisone, 100 mg intravenously, at 6:00 a.m.; a second 100 mg is infused continuously during surgery; then a 100-mg dose is given intravenously every 6 hours for the first 24 hours following surgery followed by 50 mg every 6 hours for the second 24 hours after surgery, and 25 mg every 6 hours for the third 24-hour period. The patient may then return to his preoperative medical regimen.

There are two exceptions to these guidelines. First, the regimen is based on the assumption that there is no prolonged stress after surgery; if this occurs, higher doses of steroids must be continued for a longer time postoperatively. Second, for minor procedures, the patient may return to his usual dose within 24 to 48 hours postoperatively.

Hypothyroidism (28)

SIZE OF THE RISK

The major potential complications of surgery in hypothyroid patients are increased sensitivity to and prolonged half-life of anesthetic agents, hypoventilation and respiratory arrest in the immediate postoperative period, hyponatremia due to decreased free water clearance, and myxedema coma.

PREOPERATIVE PLANNING

Office Evaluation. Hypothyroid patients should be evaluated carefully before admission for surgery. The patient should have the comprehensive evaluation outlined in Table 83.1 and the thyroxine (T_4) level should be checked (unless a value from the past 2 months is available). The serum thyroid-stimulating hormone (TSH) concentration should be obtained in newly hypothyroid patients and in patients in whom there is a question about the adequacy of their replacement dose of thyroid hormone (see Chapter 70 for details).

Recommendations to the Surgeon. Specific recommendations for preoperative management depend upon the status of the patient's hypothyroidism. Patients with previously known and adequately treated hypothyroidism can undergo surgery. The half-life of administered thyroxine is about 7 days. Therefore, oral thyroxine can usually be discontinued before surgery and resumed when the patient is able to take oral medication. The stress of major surgery or of severe infection may accelerate the turnover of thyroxine, necessitating daily treatment with intravenous thyroxine (one-half the oral dose) in patients in either of these situations.

For patients with diagnosed but inadequately treated hypothyroidism, there are several options. If the hypothyroidism has been effectively treated for a long period (as indicated by only minor symptoms or only a slightly decreased level of T_4), the patient can usually tolerate surgery and thyroid replacement can be adjusted postoperatively. For hypothyroid patients who have not been treated or who remain significantly hypothyroid because of inadequate replacement therapy surgery should be postponed because of the risks listed above. Such patients should receive adequate thyroid replacement for a minimum of 1 to 2 months before elective surgery (4 to 6 months for patients with profound myxedema). Surgery required before this period (especially minor surgery under local anesthesia) may be performed, if the patient can be started on a total replacement dose immediately and if there is prompt improvement in signs and symptoms of hypothyroidism (see Chapter 70 for additional details).

When a patient with previously undiagnosed hypothyroidism requires immediate major surgery, an endocrinologist should be consulted regarding perioperative treatment and monitoring.

Hyperthyroidism (28)

SIZE OF THE RISK

The major risk of operation in patients with uncontrolled hyperthyroidism is thyroid storm. In one series, there were only 25 episodes of thyroid storm after 1,383 operations on thyrotoxic patients (16). However, surgery accounts for up to one-third of the cases of thyroid storm reported.

PREOPERATIVE PLANNING

Office Evaluation. The patient with known hyperthyroidism should be reassessed clinically and with thyroid function tests before admission for surgery. In previously undiagnosed patients, the usual approach should be used in diagnosis (see Chapter 70).

Recommendations to the Surgeon. The treatment of the hyperthyroid patient during surgery depends on his current thyroid status. Patients previously diagnosed and adequately treated should take their current treatment until midnight the night before surgery and should resume treatment when they can take substances by mouth again. Patients with new, known, or recurrent hyperthyroidism who are not euthyroid should be brought to a euthyroid state with thyroid blocking agents and/or iodides (see Chapter 70). Ideally, surgery should be postponed for several months in these patients until a consistent euthyroid state is attained.

An endocrinologist should be consulted regarding the treatment and monitoring of any patient with uncontrolled hyperthyroidism who requires urgent surgery.

THE OBESE PATIENT

SIZE OF THE RISK

Massive obesity significantly increases the mortality risk associated with surgery. In one study, for example, women undergoing surgery for adenocarcinoma of the uterus had a 20% operative mortality if they weighed more than 300 lb (136 kg), compared to a 1.5% mortality for obese women weighing between 200 and 240 lb (91 and 110 kg) (23). Less severe obesity probably does not increase mortality risks.

Moderate or massive obesity also increases the risk of a number of perioperative problems, including difficult intubation, difficulty in ventilating the patient during anesthesia, the need for a large amount of anesthetic during induction, potential delay in anesthesia washout because of slow release of anesthetic agents from adipose tissue, postoperative atelectasis and pneumonia, difficult postoperative mobilization when the patient is unable to help himself, nosocomial wound infection (particularly when there is increased moisture due to pannus adjacent to the surgical incision), wound dehiscence, and late incisional hernia.

PREOPERATIVE PLANNING

Office Evaluation. For massively obese persons, a program of gradual weight reduction (see Chapter 73) should be planned before any elective operation; this may require up to 6 months. When prompt surgery is needed, these patients should have a comprehensive evaluation (see Table 83.1). In particular these patients should be checked for uncontrolled diabetes and significant hypoventilation, two common complications of obesity which increase the risk of surgery. Either of these two problems should be managed preoperatively as discussed above.

Recommendations to the Surgeon. Massively obese patients should be given preoperative instruction in deep breathing and in the use of the incentive spirometer or of other devices designed to prevent pulmonary complications postoperatively. Other recommendations for perioperative management depend upon the obesity-associated conditions, such as diabetes, which the patient may have.

THE PATIENT WITH GASTROINTESTINAL DISEASE

Peptic Ulcer Disease

SIZE OF THE RISK

Data are lacking on the risk and the management of surgery in patients with active peptic ulcer disease.

PREOPERATIVE PLANNING

Office Evaluation. Patients with active ulcer disease should have elective non-ulcer surgery postponed until the ulcer heals. The average time required for the healing of uncomplicated ulcers is 4 to 6 weeks for duodenal ulcer and 6 weeks for gastric ulcer (see Chapter 33). There is no consistent relationship between disappearance of ulcer symptoms, ulcer healing, and recurrence. Therefore, it is best to wait several weeks after all symptoms have disappeared and 2 to 3 months from the beginning of an episode before admission for elective non-ulcer surgery. If surgery cannot be deferred this long or if ulcer recurrence is suspected, endoscopy should be performed preoperatively. Before admission, these patients should also have the comprehensive medical evaluation summarized in Table 83.1, and multiple stool samples should be checked to exclude active bleeding.

There are no empirical data to confirm these guidelines, nor to indicate whether surgery can be done safely as soon as an ulcer has healed as shown endoscopically. If abdominal surgery must be performed in a patient with active ulcer disease, consideration should be given to surgical treatment for the ulcer as well (see detailed discussion of indications for and types of surgery, Chapter 33).

Recommendations to the Surgeon. Patients with remote or inactive ulcer disease require no special therapy preoperatively or postoperatively.

Patients with recently active ulcer disease should continue their current therapy until midnight the day before surgery. Because cimetidine can be given intravenously (300 mg every 6 hours), it should be utilized throughout the period when the patient cannot take medicines by mouth; nasogastric suctioning should also be recommended during this period.

Hepatitis

SIZE OF THE RISK

General anesthesia and surgery during acute hepatitis are associated with a high mortality and morbidity (13). The major problem accounting for these risks is postoperative hepatic encephalopathy and its complications. The catabolic effects of surgery, hypotension during anesthesia, and hepatic toxicity from anesthetic agents are the principal factors which may precipitate hepatic encephalopathy.

PREOPERATIVE PLANNING

Office Evaluation. Patients with a history of acute hepatitis should have a comprehensive evaluation (see Table 83.1) and liver function tests (serum transaminases, bilirubin, alkaline phosphatase, albumin, globulin, and prothrombin time) obtained before admission for surgery. Tests for hepatitis B antigen should also be performed (see Chapter 39). Liver biopsy is only necessary if the diagnosis or activity of the disease is uncertain.

Ideally, surgery should be postponed for a minimum of 6 to 12 months after all laboratory evidence of active liver disease has returned to normal. This cautious approach is advised because there is a risk of exacerbating hepatic injury if surgery is performed earlier. Only urgent, life-saving surgery should be performed during the acute phase of hepatitis whatever its etiology.

Recommendations to the Surgeon. Anticipation of postoperative complications (particularly bleeding and encephalopathy) is important in the patient with active hepatitis who must undergo surgery. For the patient with an abnormal prothrombin time (less than 50% of normal), fresh frozen plasma should be given throughout the immediate perioperative period. When immunologic tests or epidemiologic information indicates infectious hepatitis (see Chapter 39), the surgical team should be notified in order to minimize the risk of spreading infection.

Cirrhosis

SIZE OF THE RISK

Most of the quantitative data regarding the risks of surgery in the cirrhotic patient have been collected in trials of portal-systemic shunts; therefore, these data may not accurately reflect the risks of surgery unrelated to the liver. The most widely used measure of the mortality risk from shunt procedures is Child's index which incorporates measurements of serum bilirubin, albumin, ascites, encephalopathy, and nutrition (see Table 83.14). The perioperative complications encountered in these patients are those associated with chronic cirrhosis: encephalopathy, jaundice, gastrointestinal hemorrhage, infection, and hepatorenal syndrome.

Regional and spinal anesthesia do not entirely eliminate the risks of complications in cirrhotic patients. For example, increased morbidity and mortality due to liver disease have been associated even with hernia repair under local anesthesia in some patients (1). The stress of the procedure itself and complications such as hypotension and wound infection may worsen hepatic function, even in the absence of toxic general anesthetics.

PREOPERATIVE PLANNING

Office Evaluation. In addition to a comprehensive preoperative evaluation (see Table 83.1), patients with cirrhosis should have liver function tests (serum transaminase, bilirubin, alkaline phosphatase, albumin, and prothrombin time). Liver biopsy is indicated in selected patients to establish the presence of cirrhosis, to provide an additional indicator of the severity of liver damage, or to exclude active hepatitis. Liver scan is only occasionally needed to exclude other causes of hepatomegaly. In the history and physical examination, a careful search should be made for complications of cirrhosis, especially encephalopathy, bleeding, and ascites.

The expected benefits of surgery must be weighed carefully against the risks in patients with cirrhosis. In general, risks are higher and only essential surgery should be performed. There are stable patients with mild cirrhosis, however, who have no ongoing injury (e.g., due to removal of a toxin or to discontinuation of alcohol) and in whom standards may be liberalized.

Recommendations to the Surgeon. A number of precautions should be emphasized in the cirrhotic patient who does require surgery. Local (or, as a second choice, spinal) anesthesia may be safer than general anesthesia, although data are lacking. Therapy to prevent complications of liver disease, such as postoperative bleeding (fresh frozen plasma for the patient with an abnormal prothrombin time or partial thromboplastin time) and encephalopathy (see Chapter 39), should be established and maintained throughout the operative period and the patient should be repeatedly checked for evidence of these two problems. The occasional patient who is taking chronic steroid therapy for liver disease should have his steroids increased during the perioperative period as described above, p. 921.

THE PATIENT WITH AN IATROGENIC IMPAIRMENT OF HEMOSTASIS

All anticoagulants increase the risk of intraoperative and postoperative bleeding and should be discontinued before any type of surgery. Patients receiving anticoagulants should have a comprehensive preoperative evaluation (see Table 83.1) before admission for surgery, and an appropriate plan for perioperative management of anticoagulation should be communicated to the surgeon.

Coumadin

A reasonable protocol for discontinuing anticoagulation with coumarin derivatives is to stop treatment 48 hours preoperatively for most patients, including those with artificial heart valves (25). If there is less time or if the prothrombin time does not return rapidly enough to normal or near normal (less than 1½ times normal), vitamin K₁ (Aquamephyton), 10 mg can be given orally or intravenously over 10 to 15 min; the prothrombin time will usually return to normal within 24 to 36 hours. Where there is a particularly high risk of clotting, such as in patients with artificial heart valves who have developed emboli in the past, anticoagulation can be stopped 24 to 36 hours before surgery, followed by intravenous vitamin K₁; when the prothrombin time becomes subtherapeutic (usually within 12 hours), full anticoagulation should be resumed with heparin and continued until 6 hours before surgery. In all of these situations, the prothrombin time (and if heparin is given, the clotting time and the partial thromboplastin time) should be normal before surgery.

Warfarin (coumadin) ordinarily can be resumed 24 hours after surgery, at the preoperative dose. Patients who have undergone intracranial, spinal, or ophthalmologic operations probably should not be anticoagulated for 48 to 72 hours after surgery. For patients with a high risk of thromboembolism (artificial mitral valves, active venous thromboembolic disease), heparin can be reinstituted 12 to 24 hours postoperatively, if the surgeon is confident hemostasis is assured, and continued until full anticoagulation with warfarin has been re-established. After the administration of vitamin K₁, the patient may be relatively refractory to the administration of warfarin for a week or more.

Aspirin

Aspirin prolongs the bleeding time and may increase blood loss during and after operation in some patients. Generally, if aspirin is not being used as a critical therapy, it should be discontinued 1 week

Table 83.14
Child's Classification of Operative Risk in the Cirrhotic Patient[a]

	Group		
	"A" Minimal	"B" Moderate	"C"Advanced
Bilirubin (mg/100 ml)	<2.0	2.0–3.0	>3.0
Serum albumin (g/100 ml)	>3.5	3.0–3.5	<3.0
Ascites	None	Controlled	Poorly controlled
Encephalopathy	None	Minimal	Coma
Nutrition	Excellent	Good	Poor "wasted"
Operative mortality	0%	9%	53%

[a] Source: A. D. Siefkin and R. J. Bolt: Preoperative evaluation of the patient with gastrointestinal or liver disease. *Medical Clinics of North America, 63:* 1309, 1979.

preoperatively since aspirin continues to affect platelets for this period of time.

THE PATIENT WITH CHRONIC BACTERIAL INFECTION

Two types of chronic bacterial infection pose risks to the patient and to others in the operating room and therefore require appropriate management before surgery—staphylococcal skin infections and pulmonary tuberculosis.

Skin Infections

Chronic bacterial skin infections (usually due to staphylococci) pose a high risk for wound sepsis and may be the source of infections in other patients (15). Therefore, they should be suppressed or eradicated prior to admission of the patient for an elective operation. Chapter 24 describes the antibiotic treatment of the various types of staphylococcal skin infection.

Tuberculosis

Active pulmonary tuberculosis poses a problem for the surgical patient because of the general debilitation it causes. It also creates the risk of infection for others in the operating room. Therefore, adult patients with a history of unexplained chronic cough or with a prior history of tuberculosis should be evaluated for active tuberculosis before admission for surgery. Patients with active pulmonary tuberculosis should be stable and sputum-negative before admission for elective surgery. The ambulatory treatment of tuberculosis is described in Chapter 28.

THE PATIENT WITH NEUROPSYCHIATRIC DISEASE

Neuropsychiatric problems present ill-defined risks during surgery and the postsurgical period. The major concerns are worsening of mental status due both to metabolic changes and to psychologic stresses. The patient with psychiatric disease may decompensate postoperatively, making care difficult and jeopardizing wound healing.

Cerebrovascular Accident

SIZE OF THE RISK

Patients with recent strokes have a significant risk of worsening focal deficits during carotid artery surgery, but this cannot necessarily be extrapolated to other types of surgery. Patients with recent strokes (less than 6 weeks duration) also have a risk of deterioration in their general mental status, regardless of the status of their focal deficits, if they undergo major surgery; but firm data are lacking on the size of this risk.

PREOPERATIVE PLANNING

Patients with recent strokes should have a comprehensive preoperative evaluation (see Table 83.1), emphasizing documentation of the preoperative neurologic impairment. The data regarding the course of the patient's stroke should be reviewed and additional testing (see Chapter 80) should be performed if necessary to exclude a treatable etiology.

No specific perioperative therapy for the patient with a stable completed stroke is needed.

Asymptomatic Cervical Bruit

SIZE OF THE RISK

Cervical bruits are present in about 4% of persons over the age of 45 (14). These bruits may be due to a number of processes (see Table 80.9, Chapter 80) including common or internal carotid stenosis. In the patient with asymptomatic cervical bruit, there is slight or no increased risk of a cerebrovascular accident during surgery (5).

PREOPERATIVE PLANNING

Apart from a careful history and physical examination to exclude evidence of a prior stroke or a transient ischemic attack (TIA) related to the cervical bruit, there is no special approach needed for these patients. The patient with a history of symptoms possibly related to the bruit should be evaluated as described in Chapter 80.

Parkinson's Disease

SIZE OF THE RISK

The perioperative risks in patients with Parkinson's disease derive from their rigidity, which may impair voluntary postoperative ventilation and mobilization. The rigidity of patients taking antiparkinson's medication may recur after the patient has missed several doses. Despite this potential problem, most patients with Parkinson's disease do tolerate anesthesia and temporary omission of medications (17).

PREOPERATIVE PLANNING

The patient should have a comprehensive preoperative evaluation (see Table 83.1) and the antiparkinsonian regimen should be tailored to provide the best possible relief of his symptoms (see Chapter 79). For patients taking an anticholinergic agent, the drug may be continued until midnight before surgery and resumed when the patient is able to take oral medications. L-Dopa or Sinemet (L-dopa/carbidopa), should be continued up until induction of anesthesia and the drug should be resumed as soon as possible after surgery.

Dementia and Organic Brain Syndrome

SIZE OF THE RISK

Patients with dementia have an increased risk of mortality and morbidity during surgery. The increase in mortality is due to lack of cooperation (e.g., with postoperative respiratory care). Much of the morbidity is related to worsening mental status due to anesthesia and surgical stress. Because surgery is always a difficult process for a demented patient and because the degree of increased risk is ill-defined, the potential benefits of surgery should be carefully reviewed before the final decision to operate is made.

PREOPERATIVE PLANNING

The patient should have a comprehensive evaluation (see Table 83.1) before admission for surgery. A careful search for metabolic abnormalities that may worsen cerebral function should be made before admission, just before surgery, and throughout the postoperative period. Emphasis should be placed on detecting and correcting hypovolemia, electrolyte abnormalities, and hypoxia.

For patients undergoing major procedures, constant observation is recommended for the first 24 to 48 hours after surgery.

Psychiatric Problems

SIZE OF THE RISK

The major problems associated with general surgery in psychiatric patients are lack of cooperation with postoperative care, postoperative psychosis, and interactions between psychotropic medications and anesthetic agents. The degree of cooperation that can be expected postoperatively can generally but not always be predicted on the basis of the patient's past behavior and his preoperative mental status.

PREOPERATIVE PLANNING

Office Evaluation. A careful history of past psychiatric illness should be obtained. The patient's mental status should be documented preoperatively (see Chapter 9) so that it can be compared to postoperative changes. A psychiatric consultation should be obtained in all patients with psychosis or with other severe psychiatric problems. Additional issues that must be dealt with by the patient's personal physician and surgeon are the ability of the patient to give informed consent (see Chapter 9) and the effect of the patient's psychiatric state on the surgical evaluation (such as evaluating symptoms in a patient with hysteria or evaluating the need for cosmetic surgery).

Careful explanation of the operation is especially crucial to management of patients with psychiatric disorders or with anticipated stress reactions to surgery. The procedure should be explained in language the patient can understand. After the explanation, the patient should be asked to express any concerns which he has about the planned surgery and his comprehension of the planned surgery should be assessed. The need to ventilate about anxiety associated with disfiguring surgery (e.g., mastectomy, amputation, etc.) and with the fear of "not waking up" is particularly common in both anxiety-prone patients and in persons who are usually free of anxiety.

Patients with severe psychosis should be in a stable, manageable state before admission for elective surgery; this should be accomplished through close collaboration between the primary physician, the surgeon, and a psychiatrist.

Patients with mild to moderate anxiety or depression can be managed by supportive counseling, use of support by family members, selective use of antidepressants or minor tranquilizers, and by careful explanation of the procedure to the patient. These interventions should be initiated before hospital admission, not at the last minute before surgery.

Recommendations to the Surgeon. The principal recommendation for the perioperative period is that the patient's use of psychotropic drugs should be communicated to the anesthesiologist.

Neuroleptics and tricyclic antidepressants can interact with anesthetics to cause increased sedation, hypo- or hypertension, and arrhythmias. Small to moderate doses of phenothiazines, haloperidol, and tricyclic antidepressants should be continued until about 12 hours before surgery. In the occasional patient taking very high doses of these agents, it is recommended that the drug be stopped about 24 hours before surgery, except in patients who have severely decompensated in the past when their medication has been changed.

The dose of benzodiazepines does not need to be changed unless it is very high.

Lithium carbonate can prolong the action of muscle relaxants, and cause myocardial depression and hypernatremia. Lithium should be discontinued 24 hours preoperatively; however, the anesthesiologist should be aware that it has been administered recently, and a blood lithium level should be obtained before surgery as a guideline. Additional information about lithium is found in Chapter 14.

Monoamine oxidase (MAO) inhibitor antidepressants can lead to an enhancement of the effect of sympathomimetic agents, to enhanced sympathetic responses to anesthesia, and to a decrease in the rate of elimination of certain anesthetic agents. Because of these problems, MAO inhibitors should be discontinued at least 1 to 2 weeks before surgery, and the anesthesiologist must be informed of their recent administration.

PROBLEMS FOLLOWING DISCHARGE

Miscellaneous Problems

During the weeks and months after surgery, patients will often have questions about incisional pain, about various symptoms in the system which was operated on, and about restrictions of activity. These questions are best answered by the surgeon. In addition, patients who have major surgery will often complain of postoperative fatigue, a problem which can usually be handled by the patient's regular physician or by the surgeon.

Postoperative Fatigue

Patients with postoperative fatigue may describe any of a number of symptoms: the need for increased sleep, weakness of the arms and legs when resuming usual activity, symptoms of orthostatic hypotension, and loss of interest in resuming usual activities (20). The physiologic changes responsible for these symptoms have not been well defined.

Although the symptoms of postoperative fatigue often last for 1 or more months, it is important to evaluate each symptom carefully in order to identify drugs or underlying medical problems which may be contributing to the problem. Sleepiness may be related to sedatives, tranquilizers, or analgesics prescribed at the time of discharge and may improve with discontinuation of these drugs. The patient with orthostatic symptoms may have had a drug prescribed which can produce this problem (diuretics, antihypertensives, long acting nitrates, antidepressants); because bed rest alone may cause orthostasis, it is important to resume these drugs cautiously in a patient who has had recent major surgery and to try discontinuing the drug or reducing the dose whenever the patient complains of orthostatic symptoms. Loss of interest may also be secondary to drugs prescribed after surgery (see list of drugs producing dysphoria, Table 11.1, Chapter 11). Alternatively, this symptom may represent a minor mood disturbance in a patient who has had similar problems at previous times of stress (see Chapter 11); or it may represent a reactive depression, similar to a grief reaction (see Chapter 18), which is related to disfiguring surgery.

When evaluation of postoperative fatigue does not disclose contributing factors which can be treated, the patient should be reassured that the problem will gradually resolve; he should also be given a rough timetable for a return to regular activities which is realistic both in terms of the surgical procedure and of the fact that postoperative fatigue may take a number of months to resolve entirely. Simple exercises for patients convalescing from bedrest are illustrated in Figure 78.4, Chapter 78. For selected patients, these or similar exercises can be recommended during the period of recovery from postoperative fatigue.

References

General

Corman, LC and Bolt, RJ (editors): Symposium on medical evaluation of the preoperative patient. *Med Clin North Am 63:* 1129, 1979 (entire issue).
  Reviews many common medical conditions in the preoperative patient.
Smith, NT, Miller, RD and Corbascio, AN (editors): *Drug Interactions in Anesthesia.* Lea & Febiger, Philadelphia, 1981.
  Detailed account of interactions of commonly prescribed drugs with anesthethic agents.
Vandam, LD (editor): *To Make the Patient Ready for Anesthesia: Medical Care of the Surgical Patient.* Addison-Wesley, Publishing Company, 1980.
  Brief, practical recommendations for preoperative management of most common medical problems.

Specific

1. Baron, HC: Umbilical hernia secondary to cirrhosis of the liver. *N Engl J Med 263:* 824, 1960.
2. Bennett, WM, Muther, RS, Parker, RA, Freg, P, Morrison, G, Golper, TA and Singer, I: Drug Therapy in renal failure; dosing guidelines for adults. Part 1 and Part 2. *Ann Intern Med 93:* 62 and 286, 1980.
3. Brencwitz, JB, Williams, CD and Edwards, WS: Major surgery in patients with chronic renal failure. *Am J Surg 134:* 765, 1977.
4. Burke, GR and Gulyassy, PF; Surgery in the patient with renal disease and related electrolyte disorders. *Med Clin North Am 63:* 1191, 1979.
5. Corman, LC: The preoperative patient with an asymptomatic cervical bruit. *Med Clin North Am 63:* 1335, 1979.
6. Deutsch, S and Daten, JE: Indication for prophylactic digitalization. *Anesthesiology 30:* 648, 1969.
7. Eisman, B (ed): *Prognosis of Surgical Disease.* W. B. Saunders, Philadelphia, 1980.
8. Eisman, B and Watkins, RS (editors): *Surgical Decision Making.* W. B. Saunders, Philadelphia, 1978.
9. Goldman, L and Caldera, DL: Risks of general anesthesia and elective operation in the hypertensive patient. *Anesthesiology 50* 285, 1979.
10. Goldman, L, Caldera, DL, Nussbaum, SR, Southwick, FS, Krogstad, D, Murray, B, Burke, DS, O'Malley, TA, Goroll, AH, Caplan, CH, Nolan, J, Carabello, B and Slater, EE: Multifactorial index of cardiac risk in noncardiac surgical procedures. *N Engl J Med 297:* 845, 1977.
11. Goldman, L, Caldera, DL, Southwick, FS, Nussbaum, SR, Murray, B, O'Malley, TA, Goroll, AH, Caplan, CH, Nolan, J, Burke, DS, Krogstad, D, Carabello, B and Slater, EE: Cardiac risk factors and complications in non-cardiac surgery. *Medicine 57:* 357, 1978.
12. Harman, E and Lillington, G: Pulmonary risk factors in surgery. *Med Clin North Am 63:* 1289, 1979.
13. Harville, DD and Summerskill, WHJ: Surgery in acute hepatitis. *JAMA 184:* 257, 1963.
14. Heyman, A, Wilkinson, WE, Heyden, S, Helms, MJ, Bartel, AG, Karp, HR, Tyroler, HA and Hames, CG: Risk of stroke in asymptomatic persons with cervical arterial bruits: A population study in Evans County, Georgia. *N Engl J Med 302:* 838, 1980.
15. Hirai, D: Nasal staphylococcus aureus and postoperative infection. *Am Surg 46:* 310, 1980.
16. McArthur, JW, Rawson, RW, Means, JH and Cope, O: Thyrotoxic crisis: an analysis of the thirty-six cases seen at the Massachusetts General Hospital during the past twenty-five years. *JAMA 134:* 868, 1947.
17. Ngai, SH: Medical intelligence: parkinsonism, levodopa, and anesthesia. *Anesthesiology 37:* 344, 1972.
18. Prys-Roberts, C: Hypertension and anesthesia-fifty years on. *Anesthesiology 50:* 281, 1979.
19. Robbins, JA and Mushlin, AI: Preoperative evaluation of the healthy patient. *Med Clin North Am 63:* 1145, 1979.
20. Rose, EA and King, TC: Understanding postoperative fatigue. *Surg Gynecol Obstet 147:* 97, 1978.
21. Rose, SD, Courman, LC and Mason, DT: Cardiac risk factors in patients undergoing noncardiac surgery. *Med Clin North Am 63:* 1271, 1979.
22. Stein, M and Cassara, EL: Preoperative pulmonary evaluation and therapy for surgery patients. *JAMA 211:* 787, 1970.
23. Strauss, RJ and Wise, L: Operative risks of obesity. *Surg Gynecol Obstet 146:* 286, 1978.
24. Tarhan, S, Moffitt, ED, Sessler, AD, Douglas, WW and Taylor, WF: Risk of anesthesia and surgery in patients with chronic bronchitis and chronic obstructive pulmonary disease. *Surgery 74:* 720, 1973.
25. Tinker, JH and Tanhan, S: Discontinuing anticoagulant therapy in surgical patients with cardiac valve prostheses. *JAMA 239:* 738, 1978.
26. Tisi, GM: Preoperative evaluation of pulmonary function; validity, indications, and benefits. *Am Rev Respir Dis 119:* 293, 1979.
27. Van Zee, BE, Hoy, WE, Talley, T and Jaenike, JR: Renal injury associated with intravenous pyelography in nondiabetic and diabetic patients. *Ann Intern Med 89:* 51, 1978.
28. White, VA and Kumager, LF; Preoperative endocrine and metabolic considerations. *Med Clin North Am 63:* 1321, 1979.

CHAPTER EIGHTY-FOUR

Peripheral Vascular Disease and Arterial Aneurysms

CALVIN B. ERNST, M.D.

Most people, if they live long enough, develop arterial disease. Each specific disease entity is only an isolated clinical manifestation of a generalized atherosclerotic process, and evaluation and management of specific problems of arterial disease must be viewed in this context. Quality and quantity of life may be improved by recognition, thorough evaluation, and appropriate therapy of peripheral arterial diseases. The purpose of this chapter is to provide guidelines for recognition and management of the more commonly encountered arterial problems: acute and chronic occlusive disease and abdominal and peripheral aneurysms.

ACUTE ARTERIAL OCCLUSION OF LOWER EXTREMITIES

Acute ischemia of the legs demands immediate recognition and management since late recognition and treatment may eventuate in loss of limb or loss of life. If collateral circulation is not well developed, muscle necrosis and irreversible changes may occur as early as 4 to 6 hours following acute arterial occlusion.

The two major causes of acute arterial occlusion are emboli and thromboses. Since surgical management of these two entities may be quite different, it is important to distinguish between them. Embolism demands immediate operation because preexisting collaterals are scanty, and relief of ischemia is easily accomplished by a simple operation involving extraction of the clot using local anesthesia. Thrombosis usually can be managed under less emergent conditions than embolus because preexisting collateral channels stimulated by chronic underlying occlusive arterial disease provide marginal but adequate blood flow. Furthermore, management of ischemia secondary to thrombosis requires complex reconstructive surgical procedures which are best performed under elective conditions after adequate evaluation, which includes arteriographic study. Attempted thrombectomy of a badly diseased artery is doomed to failure and may preclude subsequent reconstructive procedures. However, faced with a nonviable extremity, immediate operation for thrombosis is mandatory.

Over 90% of the time, acute embolic occlusion may be distinguished from acute thrombotic occlusion on clinical grounds alone (see below). In instances in which doubt exists about the etiology, arteriography is key in distinguishing embolus from thrombosis (see below, "Laboratory and X-ray Studies").

Etiology

The majority of arterial emboli originate in the heart. In a series of 338 patients, Fogarty ascribed 94% of emboli to cardiac disease (9). Whereas several years ago a preponderance of patients had rheumatic heart disease, in recent years peripheral embolization associated with the sequelae of arteriosclerotic cardiac disease has predominated (2). Arrhythmias secondary to coronary insufficiency, recent myocardial infarction with mural thrombosis, or old myocardial infarction with ventricular aneurysm are sources of emboli. Less common sources include proximal arterial lesions such as aortic aneurysms or large thromboulcerative mural aortic plaques. Such lesions cause arterio-arterial emboli. Left atrial myxomas, debris from prosthetic heart valves, paradoxical emboli (venous clots passing through a congenital cardiac defect into the arterial circulation), and foreign body emboli, although quite rare, all have been implicated in sudden arterial occlusion.

Although most acute arterial occlusions follow emboli, *in situ* thrombosis of an arteriosclerotic lesion accounts for approximately 25% of acute occlusive events. Such thrombotic complications are most likely to occur in segments of severe stenosis such as the aortic bifurcation, iliac bifurcation, common femoral bifurcation, and superficial femoral artery just above the knee. Concomitant problems such as hypovolemia from volume depletion or hemorrhage, congestive heart failure, polycythemia, or trauma all have profound influences on management.

Clinical Manifestations

Emboli lodge at arterial bifurcations: abdominal aortic (saddle embolus), 14%; iliac, 18%; common femoral, 46%; popliteal, 11% (Fig. 84.1). The brachial artery in the antecubital fossa is the most common site of embolism in the upper body. Approximately 20% of upper body emboli go to the cerebral circulation.

Ten percent travel to the abdominal viscera. Multiple emboli result from a "shower discharge" of clots from the heart. Recurrent embolic episodes, during the same hospitalization, may affect 15% of patients. Therefore, although the legs are affected most often, there may be symptoms and signs of ischemia elsewhere.

Clinical manifestations vary depending on the adequacy of preexisting collateral circulation and on the site of occlusion in the lower extremities. If preexisting collateral vessels, stimulated by underlying occlusive arterial disease, are present, acute ischemic symptoms may be mild; however, total arterial occlusion of a previously normal arterial tree causes severe symptoms. Cardinal features include the six "P's" of arterial occlusion: pulselessness, pallor, poikilothermia, pain, paralysis, and paresthesias. The latter three P's reflect neurophysiologic sequelae of ischemia, while the former three result from mechanical occlusion of an artery. Three-quarters of patients complain of pain, but 20% note numbness as the first manifes-

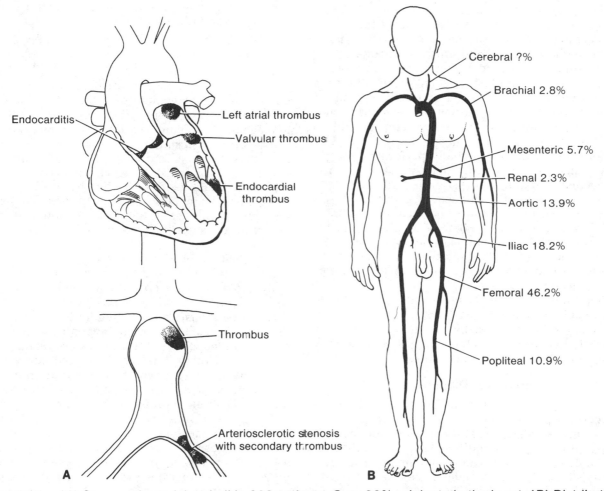

Figure 84.1   (*A*) Source of arterial emboli in 338 patients. Over 90% originate in the heart. (*B*) Distribution of arterial emboli in the same group. Over 90% impact in the distal aorta or lower extremities. (Adapted from: R. B. Rutherford (editor): *Vascular Surgery*, W. B. Saunders Co., Philadelphia, 1977.)

tation of sudden arterial occlusion. Initially, pain may be mild; but as the ischemic process progresses, pain worsens only to subside late in the course of the disease as anesthesia and paralysis develop.

Additional findings other than the six "P's" include poor capillary filling and collapsed or severely sunken veins on the dorsum of the foot. Although pedal edema rarely, if ever, accompanies embolic occlusion, it may be noted among individuals with thrombotic occlusion who have had nocturnal ischemic rest pain and who attempt to gain relief by sleeping sitting or by dangling their leg over the edge of the bed.

Cardiac examination may reveal atrial fibrillation, a diastolic rumble or the opening snap of mitral stenosis, or a gallop associated with congestive failure. Recent history of chest pain or electrocardiographic evidence of myocardial infarction implicates a cardiac origin of acute leg ischemia.

Laboratory and X-ray Studies

Laboratory studies usually are not helpful in making the diagnosis of acute arterial ischemia of the lower extremities. Arterial blood gases and pH should be obtained to serve as baseline studies for subsequent comparative measurement as well as to identify metabolic acidosis from muscle ischemia which might require correction prior to operation. Hyperkalemia may be manifest, particularly if advanced muscle ischemia has occurred. A roentgenogram of the chest may document cardiac enlargement or congestive heart failure. All of these studies should be obtained after the patient is hospitalized.

Arteriography is not routinely performed except, occasionally, in instances of modest ischemia when it is needed to distinguish between thrombosis and embolus (see below). Evidence of generalized and severe arteriosclerosis, tapered occlusions of arteries, and of well developed collateral vessels indicates acute thrombotic occlusion. Normal appearing arteries with scanty collateral circulation and an occlusion with an inverted meniscus configuration indicate embolic occlusion.

Other studies, such as Doppler ultrasonic velocity detection of peripheral blood flow, plethysmography studies, and other noninvasive evaluation procedures serve only to confirm the clinical impression already evident and therefore are not required.

Differential Diagnosis

The most important differential, because surgical management depends upon it, is to distinguish embolus from thrombosis. History is often quite helpful in separating these two entities. History of intermittent claudication or rest pain would implicate arterial thrombosis as the acute ischemic event. Complete lack of history of intermittent claudication usually indicates embolus. However, approximately 25% of patients who suffer acute superficial femoral arterial occlusion secondary to thrombosis have never had symptoms of intermittent claudication prior to the sudden occlusive event. On physical examination classic findings of chronic ischemia such as loss of hair on the toes and dorsum of the foot and the shin, along with nail, skin, and muscle atrophy may be noted. Such findings also suggest arterial thrombosis rather than embolus. A pulsatile abdominal mass diagnostic of abdominal aortic aneurysm from which mural thrombus may have discharged to the distal arterial tree might be evident. Finally, if the acute ischemic episode involves only one leg, palpating the popliteal and femoral arteries may detect an aneurysm. If the contralateral vessel is vigorously pulsating and aneurysmal, a thrombosis of an aneurysm on the side of the ischemia may have occurred. This is indicative of acute ischemia secondary to popliteal aneurysm thrombosis.

An acute dissecting thoracic aortic aneurysm may present as unilateral lower extremity ischemia. Under these circumstances, patients will relate a history of severe, searing, ripping thoracic back pain and provide a history of long-standing hypertension. Also, among such patients a murmur of aortic insufficiency may be present and chest roentgenograms document a widened mediastinal silhouette.

Treatment

Evaluation and therapy must proceed simultaneously in the management of acute arterial ischemia of the lower extremities. The cornerstone of early management of acute arterial occlusions is administration of heparin sodium. When diagnosis of sudden arterial ischemia is first made, 100 to 150 units/kg of heparin sodium must be given intravenously. This injection should be given in the physician's office, if there are no major contraindications (see Chapter 48). Patients should then be hospitalized immediately and an urgent consultation obtained with a vascular surgeon.

Introduction of the balloon-tipped embolectomy catheter by Fogarty and his co-workers in 1963 revolutionized management of acute embolic occlusion (10). Adoption of the balloon-tipped catheter converted a previously complex undertaking to a simple operative procedure which invariably can be performed under local anesthesia. Consequently, since introduction of this device, improved survival and limb salvage rates have been reported from many centers. Practically any patient, no matter how ill, may be operated upon using this device.

The surgeon must be knowledgeable of vascular reconstructive techniques so that, should acute arterial thrombosis be encountered rather than acute arterial embolus, definitive treatment may be employed which will usually require arterial reconstruction. In a critically ill patient in whom sufficient time has not been available for proper preoperative preparation, because the acutely ischemic limb mandates immediate management, aortofemoral bypass reconstruction may carry prohibitive operative risks. Under such circumstances, extra-anatomic arterial reconstructive procedures such as axillofemoral, axillobifemoral, or femoral-femoral bypass may be warranted.

Following discharge from the hosptial, patients must be maintained on therapeutic levels of oral anticoagulants for the rest of their lives (see Chapter 48). Furthermore, they must be evaluated several times a year in order to maintain optimal cardiac function and for continued evaluation of their peripheral circulation.

Results

In spite of improved diagnosis, preoperative care, operative management, and postoperative support, mortality from acute lower extremity ischemia continues to be discouraging. Prior to 1963 mortality following arterial embolectomy ranged between 34 and 63%. Mortality since 1963 has remained high and ranges between 10 and 40% (13, 18). Death associated with acute arterial occlusion of the lower extremities has been unrelated to surgical intervention. Virtually all deaths are related to complications of cardiovascular disease (11). Such findings reinforce the contention that recognition and correction of causes of embolism or thrombosis represent an important aspect in the management of such patients.

If the patient does not succumb to complications secondary to diffuse arteriosclerosis, limb salvage exceeds 95% in most series. Likelihood of successful limb salvage is directly related to time between arterial occlusion and restoration of blood flow. Therefore, it is improbable that a 100% limb salvage rate will ever be achieved.

CHRONIC ARTERIAL OCCLUSIVE DISEASE OF LOWER EXTREMITIES

In contrast to the management schema for acute arterial occlusion, which requires emergent or urgent treatment, chronic arterial occlusive disease, manifest by symptoms covering the spectrum from mild intermittent claudication to rest pain and gangrene, almost never requires emergent treatment. By virtue of development of collateral channels which bypass slowly developing atherosclerotic lesions, chronic arterial occlusive disease may be approached in an unhurried and organized fashion, often by nonoperative management. Thorough knowledge of the natural history of chronic arterial occlusive disease is key to proper management of patients suffering such problems. In an era of vascular surgery when practically any arterial circuit may be successfully reconstructed, and sophisticated diagnostic procedures offer objective data confirming clinical impressions and results of treatment, perspectives are occasionally distorted and operative management is enthusiastically overadopted.

Etiology and Pathophysiology

Atherosclerosis is the cause of chronic arterial occlusive disease affecting the legs in the vast majority of affected individuals. The symptoms and signs of the disease are unusual before the 5th decade. The disease process is influenced significantly and adversely by the presence of diabetes mellitus, hypertension, hyperlipoproteinemia, use of tobacco, factors affecting blood viscosity such as polycythemia, and by reduction in cardiac output. Furthermore, symptoms of arterial insufficiency of the legs are only regional manifestations of a generalized disease process.

Although atherosclerosis is a generalized disease, it has a remarkably segmental distribution. Arteriosclerosis is prone to develop at major arterial bifurcations, in areas of arterial fixation, and at points of marked arterial angulation such as the distal superficial femoral artery as it enters Hunter's canal, the bifurcation of the common femoral artery, the aorta distal to the renal arteries and, most commonly, at its bifurcation, and the common iliac bifurcations.

With gradual development of such lesions, the formation of collateral vessels compensates for segmental obstructive processes, and in many instances collaterals are sufficient to provide adequate blood flow even during moderate exercise. On the other hand, sudden occlusion of a previously unobstructed vessel may not be compensated by immediate collateral blood flow so that tissue necrosis and gangrene ensue. When collateral channels are adequate, no or only minimal symptoms may be present. However, as progressive main arterial involvement occurs, collateral channels may be progressively lost, and symptoms of severe and significant exercise ischemia (intermittent claudication) occur which may progress to gradual development of rest pain and tissue necrosis. The spectrum, then, of symptomatic arterial occlusive disease to the legs extends from mild exercise ischemia to severe rest pain and frank gangrene of the toes and forefoot or to ulceration of the ankle (see Chapter 85).

Diabetes mellitus (see Chapter 69) has a unique influence on the pathogenesis of atherosclerosis. Diabetic patients manifest atherosclerosis of a more severe degree and at an earlier age than nondiabetic individuals. Furthermore, distribution of the atherosclerotic process in the lower extremity of a diabetic compared to a nondiabetic is different in that distal vessels such as popliteal, peroneal, and tibial arteries are more commonly involved than are aortoiliac segments. Microangiopathy also affects peripheral nerves as well as nutrient vessels to skin and muscle which may result in insensitivity and progressive ischemia and in lack of natural protective mechanisms in the diabetic foot. Breakdown of skin and entry of bacteria with subsequent infection may cause extensive damage, since normal sensation is lost and significant symptoms may be obscured. Diabetic neuropathy (Chapter 69) also involves the sympathetic nervous system, and many of these patients have undergone autosympathectomy at the time they are initially seen by a clinician.

Buerger's disease, thromboangiitis obliterans, is a severe chronic panarteritis leading to fibrosis and obliteration of small vessels at the tibial and pedal levels. It is an infrequent cause of lower extremity arterial insufficiency in the United States. This entity affects young men in their 20s and 30s and is almost always associated with severe tobacco addiction. Successful management hinges on cessation of use of all forms of tobacco.

Natural History

The studies of Boyd, Imparato and co-workers, and Juergens and co-workers, are remarkably similar in documenting the natural history of occlusive arterial disease, in particular, intermittent claudication (1, 14, 15). These investigators concluded that intermittent claudication is a relatively benign condition; approximately one-third of patients with claudication improve; one-third remain stable and tolerate their symptoms; and one-third deteriorate and require operation. Relentless deterioration of the lower extremity associated with intermittent claudication is unlikely in most nondiabetic patients, particularly if use of all tobacco products is discontinued. The chance for amputation occurring among individuals initially seen with intermittent claudication is approximately 1% per year. Patients with ischemic rest pain or gangrene, however, are at very high risk for amputation if surgical management is not employed.

The overall 5-year survival rate among individuals with intermittent claudication approximates 70%. The 10-year survival rate is approximately 40%. Of note is that of those individuals dying, three-quarters succumb to complications of coronary artery disease.

Clinical Manifestations

Symptoms among individuals suffering occlusive arterial disease to the legs range from mild pain in the calves on exercise to severe rest pain and gangrene. Such individuals should be carefully questioned for symptoms involving other arterial circuits such as transient cerebral ischemic attacks. The distance a patient walks before developing claudication should be documented. Men should be questioned specifically about impotence. Patients with rest pain will often note that they can alleviate their pain by dangling their legs over the side of a bed or a chair.

On *physical examination,* in the mildest form of the disease, only a diminution in intensity of peripheral pulses may be noted. Complete vascular examination should be performed noting locations of bruits, blood pressure measurements in both upper extremities, and the recording of all peripheral pulses. Among individuals with mild intermittent claudication, skin of the feet may appear normal; there may

be hair growth on toes; nails may appear normal; and there may even be faintly palpable dorsalis pedis and posterior tibial pulses. With progressive arterial involvement, however, trophic changes may involve the lower extremities with loss of hair on toes and anterior tibial areas. Poor skin nutrition is reflected by thin parchment-like skin. Lack of pulses below the inguinal ligaments, blanching and pallor with elevation of the extremity, and dependent rubor all indicate advanced ischemia. Gangrenous areas may be evident involving digits. The typical locations of ischemic ulcers are over the calcaneus, the lateral malleolus, and the dorsum of the foot (see Chapter 85).

Laboratory and X-ray Studies

The distribution and severity of peripheral arterial disease can be determined objectively by noninvasive Doppler flow studies. These studies are performed by the consulting vascular surgeon. A sphygmomanometer cuff is placed immediately above the malleoli and the cuff is inflated to above systolic pressure. As it is slowly deflated, with the Doppler velocity detector placed over the dorsalis pedis or the posterior tibial artery, pulsatile sounds will occur at systolic opening pressure. The highest pressure recorded is utilized to compare with brachial arterial systolic pressure and the ankle/arm pressure index is determined. Normal individuals have a mean index of over 1; for individuals suffering intermittent claudication the mean index is 0.59; for those with rest pain, 0.26; and patients suffering impending gangrene have a mean ankle/arm blood pressure index of 0.05 (22).

A Doppler study of lower extremity blood flow, although important, is not needed in evaluating all patients with lower extremity arterial occlusive disease. However, noninvasive testing is very helpful in distinguishing vascular insufficiency from other causes of leg pain (e.g., neurogenic claudication secondary to cauda equina compression from spinal stenosis). In the latter, Doppler ankle/arm indices are normal and, of particular note, remain normal after exercise. Noninvasive studies can also provide data which objectively document whether or not nonoperative therapy is effective in management or if deterioration of circulation is progressive. In addition, comparison of preoperative and postoperative noninvasive data are useful in documenting effectiveness of operative therapy.

The most important laboratory study, if it is determined the patient is a candidate for operation, is arteriography (see below). Although risks are very small in experienced hands, arteriography is utilized only when operation is indicated and agreed to by the patient.

Treatment and Results

Treatment for arterial insufficiency of the legs may be either operative or nonoperative. Knowing the natural history of the occlusive process aids significantly in determining whether or not the patient's symptoms warrant operative intervention in light of associated risk factors and life expectancy. Except for very poor surgical candidates, individuals with ischemic rest pain, pregangrenous changes, or gangrene, always require operative intervention.

There are patients, however, who are not, and probably never will become, candidates for operation. This group includes individuals whose symptoms are not severe enough to warrant operation and those whose symptoms, although they may be severe, are of such recent onset that sufficient time has not elapsed to determine whether or not development of collateral circulation will cause symptoms to lessen or significantly abate. Indications for operation are shown in Table 84.1. Patients should be managed by nonoperative therapy unless one of these indications is present.

Much can be recommended to control or improve symptoms; and an itemized list of recommendations, written in layman's language, is often very helpful in managing such individuals. Such recommendations should first be reviewed with the patient, after which the patient should be given the list for ready reference (Table 84.2). Many of these recommendations pertain to protection of the feet. It should be emphasized that avoidance of trauma to the feet from ill fitting shoes and avoidance of extremes of temperature are very important in the management program. If the patient finds that his feet are cold, particularly at night, he should be told not to use heating pads or hot water bottles since these may cause tissue breakdown and ulceration. A warm pair of socks or a muffler is advised. Patients should bathe their feet at least once a day in lukewarm water (tested by the hand) and thereafter apply lanolin or hand cream to the skin to keep it soft and pliable, thereby avoiding cracking and fissuring, particularly between the toes, which might lead to skin breakdown.

Other measures that significantly affect outcome include improving cardiac output, if congestive heart failure is present, by administration of digitalis and diuretics (being cautious to avoid volume depletion) and controlling diabetes mellitus. Very important, the patient should be advised to *exercise* to tolerance every day to stimulate collateral channel development. Exercise tolerance can be improved in up to two-thirds of individuals in this way. Also, it is most important to urge strongly the cessation of use of all tobacco products. It must be emphasized to patients that smoking accelerates atherogenesis, causes further hypoxia because of carbon monoxide poisoning,

Table 84.1
Indications for Operation

Claudication that is intolerable because of occupation
Rest pain in good risk patient
Impending gangrene in good risk patient

Table 84.2
Advice which Should Be Given to Patients with Arterial Insufficiency

QUIT SMOKING—Use NO tobacco in ANY form
If overweight—lose weight
Exercise (walk) to the point of discomfort or at least 2 miles a day
Keep feet very clean. Bathe at least daily in LUKEWARM water
Gently apply lanolin or mild hand cream to feet after bathing
Use a night light to avoid hitting toes or shins
Wear clean, preferably cotton, socks daily (cotton does not retain moisture)
Avoid injury to feet. Wear proper fitting shoes to prevent calluses, corns, blisters
Place lamb's wool (available from pharmacies) between over-riding toes
Avoid extremes of temperature. Do not put feet in hot water or use heating pads on lower extremities. In cold weather, wear socks to bed to warm feet. Do not get feet cold or wet
If feet hurt at night, raise head of bed 6–10 inches (15 to 25 cm) on blocks
For any sudden change in symptoms such as prolonged pain, numbness or tingling, or inability to move foot or leg, consult your physician *immediately*

and causes vasospasm secondary to nicotine which may last up to 1 hour after each cigarette. Patients must be admonished that nicotine in any form is absorbed through the buccal mucosa, be it pipe, or cigarette smoke, or tobacco juice.

Management of coexistent hypertension is sometimes challenging because among such patients, if blood pressure is too well controlled, symptoms may increase. Therefore, when managing hypertension in such individuals, one often must settle for less than ideal blood pressure control.

There is little objective evidence to suggest that *vasodilating drugs* offer significant benefits to patients with symptomatic peripheral arterial insufficiency. Since all systemic vessels may be dilated by these drugs, blood flow to the involved extremity may actually decrease and vasodilators may have the paradoxical effect of causing further ischemia. Furthermore, ischemia probably produces more effective and complete local vasodilation than can be achieved by drugs. Therefore, vasodilator therapy should not be used in the treatment of patients with occlusive vascular disease.

Similarly, except for heparin anticoagulation in hospital among patients who suffer acute deterioration of their peripheral circulation, long term anticoagulation with oral agents has not been shown to have any beneficial effect on retardation of atherosclerosis or on improving symptoms. Oral anticoagulants in elderly, forgetful, and unreliable individuals may pose significant hazards from complications of anticoagulation therapy (see Chapter 48). Platelet-inhibiting agents have not been shown to be effective in management of lower extremity arterial occlusive disease (see Chapter 48).

OPERATIVE INTERVENTION

It is only upon failure of nonoperative therapy or among individuals with clear indications for operation that arteriographic studies are obtained. Occasionally arteriography documents distribution of arterial involvement which is either too extensive or too peripheral to permit reconstruction. Under these circumstances, nonoperative therapy usually is recommended; but if ischemic rest pain and tissue necrosis are present, both patient and family are informed that when an operation is required, amputation is all that may be offered.

Indications for operation among patients with intermittent claudication relate mainly to rehabilitation to retain or gain employment. Trivial claudication and even mild ischemic rest pain, controlled by nonnarcotic analgesics, are not indications for operation, particularly in high risk individuals. A trial of conservative management is particularly important if other risk factors, such as recent myocardial infarction, are present (see Chapter 83 on Preoperative Planning).

When it is determined that the condition of the patient warrants operative intervention and when arteriography documents repairable vessels, a number of options for arterial reconstruction are open to the vascular surgeon. Procedures employed include bypass reconstruction by use of a prosthetic graft and endarterectomy. In the past decade definite preference for bypass reconstructive procedures over endarterectomy has become apparent, and endarterectomy is rarely used at the present time. Reconstructive procedures include aortofemoral bypass, femoral-popliteal bypass and femoral-tibial bypass. Recently, there has been enthusiasm for extra-anatomic reconstruction, bypassing the diseased aorto-iliac arterial tree, particularly among individuals deemed to be at great risk from a major intra-abdominal procedure. Such extra-anatomic reconstructive procedures include axillounifemoral bypass, axillo-bifemoral bypass, and femoral-femoral bypass.

RESULTS OF THERAPY

It is not appropriate to compare results between various treatment modalities and various patient populations because of variability among patient groups. As a generalization, however, operative mortality for aortofemoral bypass reconstruction is approximately 5%. The patency rate for aortofemoral bypass reconstruction using grafts as well as endarterectomy is approximately 80 to 90% at 5 years. Operative mortality rates for extra-anatomic reconstruction are slightly less than aortofemoral reconstruction but graft patency rates are significantly worse.

Operative mortality for autogenous vein femoral-popliteal bypass procedures ranges from 0.5 to 1%

depending on the general condition of the patient. Five-year patency rates for such procedures vary between 60 and 70%, but it should be emphasized that patency varies directly with the extent of the disease in the vessel being reconstructed.

In general, in contrast to arterial reconstruction for aneurysmal disease, arterial reconstruction for occlusive disease is at best palliative and does not significantly increase the patient's life expectancy because most individuals have significant coincident coronary artery disease. However, the quality of life is vastly improved, particularly among those individuals who would have undergone amputation if successful arterial reconstruction had not been feasible.

Patients with aortofemoral arterial occlusive disease, but without coronary artery disease or diabetes, have survival rates that equal those of the normal age- and sex-adjusted population. Observed differences in life expectancy between "normal" populations and those undergoing arterial reconstructive procedures are usually due to the high prevalence of associated coronary artery disease and diabetes mellitus. It appears that the presence of coronary artery disease reduces life expectancy approximately 10 years, and the presence of diabetes mellitus reduces life expectancy by an additional 15 years (16).

ABDOMINAL AORTIC ANEURYSMS

Abdominal aortic aneurysm is the most commonly encountered aneurysm of the arterial tree. It is encountered two to three times more often than popliteal arterial aneurysm, the second most common aneurysm. Abdominal aortic aneurysms have been found in almost 2% of consecutive post mortem studies (3).

Men are affected by aneurysmal disease ten times more often than women. Occurrence of abdominal aortic aneurysms increases with age.

Although it is not possible to implicate precisely a single etiology of abdominal aortic aneurysm, most are arteriosclerotic in origin. The infrarenal abdominal aorta is more susceptible to aneurysmal degeneration than are other arterial segments, although the reasons for this are unknown. Only about 5% of abdominal aortic aneurysms encroach upon visceral vessels, most commonly the renal arteries.

The *natural history* of untreated abdominal aortic aneurysms was unknown until the report of Estes in 1950 which documented, for the first time, the grave consequences of this disease (8). Five-year survival of patients with untreated aneurysms approximates only 20%. Forty to fifty percent of patients with untreated abdominal aortic aneurysms die of rupture; and 30% die of other causes, usually from complications of diffuse arteriosclerosis, most notably myocardial infarction. In recent years, multiple groups have presented corroborating data emphasizing the improved life expectancy following surgical treatment of this condition (4, 5, 12, 20) (see below).

Clinical Manifestations

HISTORY

The presentation of an abdominal aortic aneurysm depends upon whether or not complications have occurred. Over 50% of abdominal aortic aneurysms are asymptomatic when first discovered. Asymptomatic aneurysms may be noted during routine examination by a physician for another problem or may be found by the patient. Occasionally, patients complain of a "second heart" in the abdomen after they palpate a pulsatile epigastric mass.

The patient may complain of abdominal, flank, or back pain as the aneurysm expands and becomes symptomatic. Such symptoms are a harbinger of disaster because rupture may follow at an unpredictable time after onset of symptoms.

Rupture. Most aneurysms rupture into the retroperitoneal space, affording life-saving tamponade after blood pressure falls sufficiently. Under these circumstances, the patient presents with a history of syncope, flank, or back pain, and in a hypovolemic-hypotensive state. Most patients suffering intraperitoneal rupture of abdominal aortic aneurysms are dead by the time medical therapy is available. However, a few do present for treatment; such individuals are profoundly hypotensive and require immediate operative intervention, in spite of seemingly lethal coincidental problems. Aneurysms may rupture also into an adjacent vein, causing a large arteriovenous fistula (such as an aortocaval or aortorenal fistula); or they may rupture into the gastrointestinal tract, usually duodenum, causing an aortoenteric fistula.

Other Complications. If aneurysms are large enough, they may compress adjacent structures, such as ureter, duodenum, vena cava, or vertebral column, with production of appropriate symptoms (for example, symptoms of gastric outlet obstruction in patients with duodenal compression).

Dislodgement of laminated clots from the wall of the aneurysm may cause peripheral embolization to femoral, popliteal, or distal vessels. When emboli occur, patients may complain of symptoms of sudden leg ischemia as the first indication of an abdominal aortic aneurysm (see below). If embolic bits of debris are small and distal vessels are patent, patients may complain of small areas of tissue necrosis such as digital gangrene of the tip of a toe, or small punctate pretibial ischemic lesions.

Finally, aneurysms which suddenly thrombose may present with abrupt ischemia of a lower extremity that can be confused with the presentation resulting from cardiac or from arterial emboli.

Although the incidence of the various complications (other than rupture) is not known, they do underscore the pessimistic natural history of untreated abdominal aortic aneurysms. After seeking specific historical information regarding the aneurysm itself, it is important to question the patient regarding other symptoms of arteriosclerosis so that an estimate of the extent of involvement is obtained; this information will frequently influence recommendations for or against surgical therapy (see Chapter 83). Symptoms of transient cerebral ischemia or previous stroke, angina pectoris or previous myocardial infarction, or symptoms of cardiac decompensation such as significant severe shortness of breath, ankle edema, orthopnea, and paroxysmal nocturnal dyspnea all are especially important in determining the risks in this group of patients.

PHYSICAL EXAMINATION

Physical examination is the single most valuable source of information in the diagnosis of infrarenal abdominal aortic aneurysms and has been reported to be accurate in almost 90% of cases (8). Depending on the clinical presentation, either complicated or uncomplicated, physical examination will vary. As noted, most patients present with asymptomatic abdominal aortic aneurysms which are discovered on routine physical examination during evaluation for other problems. Under these circumstances, an epigastric pulsatile mass usually is felt. However, in extremely obese individuals or in those with very small aneurysms, a mass may not be palpable. Among these individuals asymptomatic aneurysms may be discovered when X-rays are obtained for other intra-abdominal conditions such as peptic ulcer or renal or colonic disease.

It is important to palpate the epigastrium since the bifurcation of the abdominal aorta is at the level of the umbilicus. Only rarely when palpating inferior to the umbilicus will one identify an abdominal aortic aneurysm unless both common iliac arteries are also greatly aneurysmal. The laterally pulsatile nature of an abdominal aortic aneurysm is key to differentiating it from a mass which might feel pulsatile because it overlies the aorta. Lesions confused with abdominal aortic aneurysm include pancreatic neoplasms, pancreatic pseudocyst, horseshoe kidneys, neoplasms of the stomach or transverse colon, and retroperitoneal soft tissue tumors. Not uncommonly, a normal but prominently pulsatile abdominal aorta in a healthy individual is confused with an abdominal aortic aneurysm. Furthermore, in elderly patients an undilated but tortuous aorta may simulate an abdominal aortic aneurysm. In this curcumstance, the pulsatile mass is felt to the left of the midline but not to the right. One should palpate the abdomen by approaching the midline both from the right and from the left to identify the laterally pulsatile characteristic of an aneurysm.

Risk of rupture correlates best with the size of the aneurysm (see below). Estimation of the size by physical examination alone, however, is so variable that it is completely unreliable.

One-quarter to one-third of patients have significant associated occlusive arterial disease as well as the abdominal aortic aneurysm; therefore, a systematic evaluation of all peripheral pulses should be performed. Systemic blood pressure in *both* arms should be measured because many patients with aortic aneurysms have hypertension. By listening with a stethoscope (the bell is most efficient) over the carotid bifurcations the physician may determine if concomitant carotid arterial occlusive disease is present. When examining the lower extremities, particular attention should be directed to the character of the femoral, popliteal, and pedal pulses. In a small percentage of patients (probably less than 10%) there may be coexistent peripheral aneurysms involving the popliteal or femoral arteries.

Laboratory and X-ray Studies

It is particularly important that the suspicion, on physical examination, of an abdominal aortic aneurysm be confirmed by roentgenography. Confirmation is readily accomplished by use of standard X-ray techniques since approximately 70 to 80% of abdominal aortic aneurysms are calcified. Anteroposterior and cross table lateral films of the abdomen document abdominal aortic aneurysms in such individuals (Fig. 84.2). If anteroposterior, cross table lateral, or oblique abdominal X-rays do not substantiate an aneurysm, ultrasonic B-mode scanning may prove helpful. The accuracy of ultrasonic diagnosis of ab-

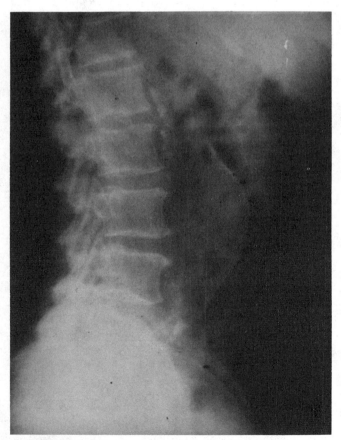

Figure 84.2 Cross table lateral abdominal X-ray documenting calcified abdominal aortic aneurysm.

dominal aortic aneurysms approaches 98% (17, 21). Since the size of the aneurysm may affect therapy, particularly in asymptomatic and in very poor risk individuals, reliance on accurate ultrasonography or on X-ray assumes great importance. Although there are certain pitfalls in ultrasonography (e.g., the size of the aneurysm is often underestimated), it is an excellent technique, not only for detection of abdominal aortic aneurysms but for following patients who are not candidates for operation; repeated studies every 3 to 6 months are helpful in monitoring the size of the aneurysm.

It is useful, also, to have an objective measurement of peripheral pulses in the lower extremities to gauge the results of therapy or to follow the progression of coexistent occlusive arterial disease. This measurement is best made by the vascular surgeon by use of a Doppler blood velocity detection device.

Treatment and Results

Once the presence of an abdominal aortic aneurysm has been verified by either plain abdominal X-rays or ultrasound, a decision regarding therapy must be made. The risk of catastrophic rupture among patients with aneurysms greater than 6 cm in transverse diameter is so great that almost all such individuals must be considered candidates for operation. Aneurysms less than 6 cm in transverse diameter (small aneurysms) are less prone to rupture than aneurysms greater than 6 cm (large aneurysms). However, small aneurysms grow and, if thin walled, also may rupture. If patients have significant life-limiting concurrent disease and small asymptomatic abdominal aortic aneurysms, a close follow-up program can be instituted. Operative candidates should, of course, be referred to a vascular surgeon; the general physician might, in patients that he thinks are not operative candidates, profit from telephone consultation with a vascular surgeon.

The natural history of abdominal aortic aneurysms dictates that even patients with small aneurysms should be treated surgically unless the risk is prohibitive. Szilagyi and co-workers classic study (20) comparing nonoperative *vs.* operative therapy is summarized in Figure 84.3. Even with the worst operative mortality (13%), survival following surgical management of small aneurysms is better than nonsurgical management. As operative mortality declines, the disparity becomes greater. When dealing with large aneurysms, even assuming an operative mortality rate of 13%, surgical therapy is clearly superior to nonsurgical therapy. Over the last two decades, operative mortality has declined to between 2 and 5% for elective aneurysmectomy (4, 7). Should operation be delayed until the aneurysm ruptures, operative mortality increases to a formidable 60 to 80%, particularly if the patient arrives at the hospital in hypovolemic shock. Even when such patients can be resuscitated adequately prior to operation, operative mortality remains approximately 50%.

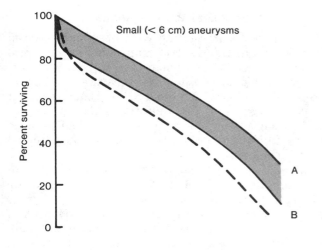

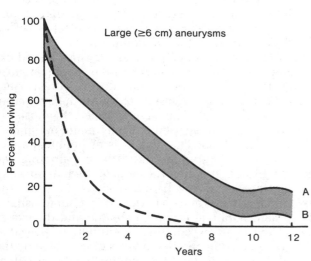

Figure 84.3 Survival curves for surgical and non-surgical patients with large and small aortic aneurysms. The dashed lines represent mortality rates in the nonsurgical groups; the bands, in the surgical groups (the top of the bands (*A*) assumed no operative mortality; the bottom (*B*), a 13% operative mortality). (Modified by Rutherford from data provided by Szilagyi). Even with 13% operative mortality, surgical treatment is better than nonsurgical treatment (Adapted from R. B. Rutherford (editor): *Vascular Surgery*, W. B. Saunders Co., Philadelphia, 1977.)

Age in itself is not a determinant of indication for operation. Elective aneurysmectomy can be performed in a very elderly individual with an operative mortality rate comparable to a similar operation in younger individuals, provided the patient is a satisfactory operative candidate. Furthermore, as a group patients with major complications of their aneurysm (see above) do better with surgical therapy than they do without surgical therapy (19).

Therefore, it is generally advised that aneurysmectomy be performed in all individuals with a reason-

able life expectancy who, in the judgment of the physician and surgeon, would tolerate the operative procedure with an operative mortality of less than 5%. Clearly, operation is mandatory for any individuals who have complications of their aneurysms (see above).

Controversy exists regarding routine use of preoperative aortography among patients with abdominal aortic aneurysms. Although some surgeons routinely recommend aortography, the majority employ aortographic studies selectively. One thing is clear—aortography should neither be used to confirm the diagnosis of an abdominal aortic aneurysm nor to make the diagnosis. Because of laminated clots within the aneurysmal sac, abdominal aortography may actually be misleading, giving an impression of an aneurysm which is actually smaller than it is or even giving the impression that an aneurysm is not present.

Under certain circumstances, abdominal aortographic studies are helpful and even mandatory. Indications for aortography include the possibility of the involvement of other blood vessels, either by the aneurysm itself encroaching upon the renal arteries or by concomitant occlusive arterial disease involving inferior mesenteric, superior mesenteric, or celiac vessels. It is important to determine the extent of reconstruction necessary so that these occlusive lesions do not go untreated and thereby jeopardize the over-all result following aneurysmectomy. Drug-resistant hypertension, possibly on a renovascular basis, is another indication for aortography to document renal arterial involvement which might be correctable during abdominal aortic aneurysmectomy. Also, if aneurysmal disease is associated with extensive involvement of the iliac vessels, aortography is indicated. If there is suspicion of congenital arterial anomalies or other congenital defects such as horseshoe kidneys, abdominal aortography is helpful to delineate variances in blood supply associated with such abnormalities and to facilitate operative correction.

It is essential to inform the patient and family of various risks of operative *vs.* nonoperative therapy. Equally important is explaining what complications may occur in the postoperative period. Although this is primarily the responsibility of the operating surgeon, it is appropriate for the primary physician to discuss with the patient what is likely to occur. The patient should know that a Dacron or Teflon prosthesis will be used to replace the abdominal aorta and that such arterial grafts are durable and, in general, never need to be replaced. Complications, fortunately, are very rare and in aggregate probably occur less than 2 to 3% of the time. Such complications include paraplegia from spinal cord ischemia, renal failure, loss of one or both legs, graft infection, ischemic colitis, and aortoenteric fistula development. In addition, approximately a quarter of male patients may develop impotence following abdominal aortic reconstruction. It should be stressed to the patient and family that postoperative complications of abdominal aortic aneurysmectomy are magnified by the urgency of the operative procedure.

If, for any reason, operation is not recommended or accepted, patients should be evaluated at 3- to 6-month intervals for progression of disease or for improvement of coincidental problems, either of which might mandate operation. Since abdominal aortic aneurysms do not dissect, symptoms mimicking dissecting thoracic aneurysms, such as pain shooting into the legs, do not occur. Most commonly, a patient with a rupturing or symptomatic aneurysm will complain of steady, dull abdominal, flank, or back pain. If such pain occurs or if a change in existing symptoms is noted in a patient being followed with an abdominal aortic aneurysm, he and his family should be instructed to seek surgical attention promptly.

PERIPHERAL ARTERIAL ANEURYSMS

Peripheral arterial aneurysms may involve the carotid, subclavian, brachial, iliac, femoral, and popliteal arteries. Over 90% of peripheral aneurysms involve either popliteal or femoral arteries. Popliteal arterial aneurysms predominate. More commonly, tortuous vessels presenting as serpiginous pulsations under the skin, are mistaken for peripheral aneurysms. The most noted example of this is a tortuous subclavian or common carotid artery in an elderly, hypertensive individual which may be confused with a carotid or subclavian artery aneurysm.

Most peripheral arterial aneurysms are arteriosclerotic in origin although mycotic, traumatic, and syphilitic aneurysms are seen occasionally. Peripheral arteriosclerotic aneurysms are localized manifestations of a generalized disease process. This is underscored by noting that, among patients who have femoral arterial aneurysms, 95% have another aneurysm elsewhere; and, more important, 92% have abdominal aortic aneurysms (6). Almost 60% of femoral arterial aneurysms are bilateral. Similarly, among individuals with popliteal arterial aneurysms, almost 80% have another aneurysm elsewhere; two-thirds have abdominal aortic aneurysms; and about half have another popliteal arterial aneurysm (6). Therefore, upon identifying a peripheral arterial aneurysm, the physician should routinely look for a potentially lethal abdominal aortic aneurysm.

Femoral and, particularly, popliteal arterial aneurysms are associated with a very high incidence of distal thromboembolism and of eventual limb loss. Untreated peripheral aneurysms may eventuate in limb loss approximately 75% of the time from either distal embolization or acute thrombosis. On the other hand, rupture with exsanguinating hemorrhage from femoral or popliteal arterial aneurysm is not a major risk.

Clinical Manifestations

Most patients presenting with peripheral arterial aneurysms are elderly, and many may be asymptomatic. Femoral arterial aneurysms usually are quite evident, particularly when they measure 4 or 5 cm in diameter. Similarly, popliteal arterial aneurysms, if they are large, are easily identified. However, popliteal arterial aneurysms may be overlooked because many clinicians do not routinely palpate the popliteal fossa during a physical examination.

Clinical manifestations depend upon whether or not complications are associated with peripheral aneurysms. Patients may present with sudden acute ischemia of an extremity because of thrombosis of the popliteal or femoral arterial aneurysm and manifest any of the six "P's" of acute arterial ischemia: pallor, pulselessness, poikilothermia, pain, paresthesia, or paralysis. Among individuals in whom complications of peripheral aneurysms develop, successful limb salvage is significantly less likely than among patients in whom surgical therapy is offered before the development of such complications.

Similar to abdominal aortic aneurysms, lateral expansileness of a prominent femoral or popliteal pulse makes the diagnosis of a femoral or popliteal aneurysm. A bruit may be associated with the aneurysm but it is of no clinical significance. Diagnosis of femoral arterial aneurysm is easily made on clinical examination alone. The diagnosis of popliteal aneurysm may be more difficult. When palpating the popliteal fossa, it is helpful to have the patient relax his leg in a passively flexed position to allow the examiner's fingers access to the fossa. If an unusually prominent popliteal fossa is palpated and the examiner suspects aneurysm, the patient may be placed in the prone position and the lower leg supported by the examiner's arm to facilitate popliteal arterial palpation. If diagnosis of politeal arterial aneurysm is in doubt, X-rays of the popliteal region may be obtained since approximately 25 to 30% of popliteal arterial aneurysms are calcified and may be identified on standard X-ray films. B-mode ultrasonography may be a helpful adjunct but is required only rarely. Occasionally, the only manifestations of a popliteal arterial aneurysm are small punctate necrotic areas of skin over the anterior tibial region or small gangreous areas of the tips of toes. This "blue toe syndrome" is a result of microemboli from the aneurysm that have showered to the periphery.

Once the diagnosis of a peripheral arterial aneurysm is made, the patient should be referred to a vascular surgeon. Although arteriography is not required, but is highly recommended in management of abdominal aortic aneurysms (see above), arteriography is mandatory in management of peripheral aneurysms and in particular, of popliteal arterial aneurysms. The arteriogram is used not so much to make the diagnosis but to document patency of arteries distal to the aneurysm, information which is critical to the vascular surgeon in planning arterial reconstruction.

Treatment and Results

Treatment of peripheral aneurysms is indicated in all instances in which it is the physician's estimate that the patient has a reasonable life expectancy. Since the natural history of peripheral aneurysms is one of eventual limb loss, it is important to offer surgical therapy to maintain or improve quality of life by avoiding amputation. If however, patients have concurrent significant disease or are bedridden for other reasons, operation is not justified. Surgical correction includes replacement of femoral arterial aneurysms with Dacron grafts or with segments of reversed autogenous saphenous vein. Similarly, popliteal arterial aneurysms are managed by bypassing the diseased segment, preferably with autogenous saphenous vein but, if vein is not available, with any suitable prosthetic material.

Operative mortality for management of peripheral aneurysms approximates 1 to 3%. Limb salvage is obtained in over 90% of cases and is related to the degree of arterial involvement peripheral to the aneurysm. In almost all series reporting repair of popliteal arterial aneurysms, amputations in the postoperative period have been associated with severe occlusive arterial disease manifest by gangrene and rest pain preoperatively.

References

General

Boyd, AM: The natural course of arteriosclerosis of the lower extremities *Angiology* 11: 10, 1960.

> *This study of 1,440 patients with intermittent claudication, carefully evaluated and followed over an interval of 15 years, for the first time documented the natural history of intermittent claudication. This study provides the control data base against which results of surgical and nonsurgical therapy are judged.*

Crawford, ES, Saleh, SA, Babb, JW, III, Glaeser, DH, Vaccaro, PS and Silvers, A: Infrarenal abdominal aortic aneurysm; factors influencing survival after operation performed over a 25-year period. *Ann Surg* 193: 699, 1981.

> *Experience of an outstanding vascular surgeon evaluating 920 consecutive patients operated upon for abdominal aortic aneurysm. This paper will become the "gold standard" by which others will measure results.*

Dent, TL, Lindenauer, SM, Ernst, CB and Fry, WJ: Multiple arteriosclerotic arterial aneurysms. *Arch Surg* 105: 338, 1972.

> *Evaluation of 57 patients with peripheral aneurysms among 1,488 having aneurysmal disease. Importance of coincidental multiple aneurysms when encountering patients with aneurysmal disease stresses need for thorough vascular evaluation.*

Rutherford, RB (editor): *Vascular Surgery.* W. B. Saunders, Philadelphia, 1977.

> *The first comprehensive text of vascular surgery. Specific disease entities are extensively discussed including nonoperative as well as operative aspects. Basic pathophysiologic concepts are lucidly presented. This work should be in the library of all interested in vascular diseases.*

Specific

1. Boyd, AM: The natural course of arteriosclerosis of the lower extremities. *Angiology* 11: 10, 1960.
2. Campbell, HC, Hubbard, SG and Ernst, CB: Continuous heparin anticoagulation in patients with arteriosclerosis and arterial emboli. *Surg Gynecol Obstet* 150: 54, 1980.
3. Carlsson, J and Sternby, NH: Aortic aneurysms. *Acta Chir Scand* 127: 466, 1964.
4. Crawford, ES, Saleh, SA, Babb, JW, III, Glaeser, DH, Vaccaro, PS and Silvers, A: Infrarenal abdominal aortic aneurysm; factors influencing survival after operation performed over a 25-year period. *Ann Surg* 193: 699, 1981.
5. DeBakey, ME, Crawford, ES, Cooley, DA and Morris GC, Jr: Aneurysm of the abdominal aorta; analysis of results of graft replacement therapy 1 to 11 years after operation. *Ann Surg* 160: 622, 1964.
6. Dent, TL, Lindenauer, SM, Ernst, CB and Fry, WJ: Multiple arteriosclerotic arterial aneurysms. *Arch Surg* 105: 338, 1972.
7. DeWeese, JA, Blaisdell, FW and Foster, JH: Optimal resources for vascular surgery. *Arch Surg* 105: 948, 1972.
8. Estes, JE: Abdominal aortic aneurysm. A study of 102 cases. *Circulation* 2: 258, 1950.
9. Fogarty, TJ and Buch, WS: The management of embolic and thrombotic arterial occlusion. In *Vascular Surgery*, p. 423, edited by RB Rutherford. W. B. Saunders, Philadelphia, 1977.
10. Fogarty, TJ, Cranley, JJ, Krause, RT, Strasser, ES and Hafner, CD: A method for extraction of arterial emboli and thrombi. *Surg Gynecol Obstet* 116: 241, 1963.
11. Fogarty, TJ, Daily, PO, Shumway, NE and Krippaehne, W: Experience with balloon catheter technique for arterial embolectomy. *Am J Surg* 122: 231, 1971.
12. Foster, JH, Bolasny, BL, Gobbel, WG, Jr and Scott, HW, Jr: Comparative study of elective resection and expectant treatment of abdominal aortic aneurysm. *Surg Gynecol Obstet* 129: 1, 1969.
13. Hardin, CA and Hendren, TH: Arterial embolism. *Vasc Dis* 2: 11, 1965.
14. Imparato, AM, Kim, G-E, Davidson, T and Crowley, JG: Intermittent claudication; its natural course. *Surgery* 78: 795, 1975.
15. Juergens, JC, Barker, NW and Hines, EA: Arteriosclerosis obliterans. Review of 520 cases with special reference to pathogenic and prognostic factors. *Circulation* 21: 188, 1960.
16. Malone, JM, Moore, WS and Goldstone, J: Life expectancy following aortofemoral arterial grafting. *Surgery* 81: 551, 1977.
17. Nusbaum, JW, Freimans, AK and Thomford, NR: Echography in the diagnosis of abdominal aortic aneurysm. *Arch Surg* 102: 385, 1971.
18. Satiani, B, Gross, WS and Evans, WE: Improved limb salvage after arterial embolectomy. *Ann Surg* 188: 153, 1978.
19. Szilagyi, DE, Elliott, JP and Smith, RF: Clinical fate of the patient with asymptomatic abdominal aortic aneurysm and unfit for surgical treatment. *Arch Surg* 104: 600, 1972.
20. Szilagyi, DE, Smith, RF, DeRusso, FJ, Elliott, JP and Sherrin, FW: Contribution of abdominal aortic aneurysmectomy to prolongation of life. *Ann Surg* 164: 678, 1966.
21. Winsberg, G, Cole-Beuglet, C and Mulder, DS: Continuous ultrasound "B" scanning of abdominal aortic aneurysms. *AJR* 121: 626, 1974.
22. Yao, JST: Hemodynamic studies in peripheral arterial disease. *Br J Surg* 57: 561, 1970.

CHAPTER EIGHTY-FIVE

Leg Ulcers and Varicose Veins

ANDREW MUNSTER, M.D., and CALVIN B. ERNST, M.D.

LEG ULCERS

Ulceration of a lower extremity is a common and important problem in ambulatory medical practice. Accurate diagnosis is based mainly on history and physical examination and is essential for appropriate treatment. Often the management of various types of leg ulcers is completely different so that inappropriate therapy can lead to the loss of a toe or even of a limb. Generally it is necessary for the physician (a) to give detailed instructions to the patient and (b) to have a great deal of patience.

History

In addition to a complete general medical history, specific attention should be paid to the following: duration of ulceration, symptoms of peripheral arteriosclerotic vascular disease such as intermittent calf claudication, intermittent thigh or gluteal claudication, impotence, rest pain, and feelings of coldness and tingling in the legs. It is also important to ask if there has been a history of previous ulceration or of injury to the lower extremities; if the patient feels that his footwear are uncomfortable; if there has been a history of chronic swelling; and, in particular, if swelling has occurred, whether it has been alleviated by lying down.

Rest pain is usually a symptom of advanced arteriosclerotic vascular disease, and it is characteristically alleviated if the patient dangles his feet over the edge of the bed, or sits in a chair when awakened at night by ischemic pain. In contrast, the common nocturnal leg cramps that occur in many individuals with no evidence of peripheral vascular disease are usually accompanied by palpable hardening of the calf muscles, and by involuntary muscle contraction of the extensor muscles of the toes. The cramps usually are relieved if the patient gets out of bed and walks around. Examination of the extremities in these patients (see below) is usually normal.

Physical Examination

A thorough physical examination of the patient should be undertaken in conjunction with the examination of the lower extremities, particularly searching for abdominal aneurysm and other intra-abdominal masses, as well as for signs of hypertension, cardiac disease, lymphatic masses in the groin, and for other stigmata of vascular disease.

EXAMINATION OF THE LOWER EXTREMITIES

The patient should be undressed and both lower extremities should be bared. Initial examination is performed while the patient is supine. Both legs are examined and compared. Particular points to be noted are: (a) the presence of either pitting or nonpitting edema. Pitting edema is a sign of chronic venous obstruction or of an acute inflammatory process. Nonpitting edema is a sign of lymphatic obstruction. If edema is present, it is important to note whether it is unilateral, and if it is bilateral, whether it is asymmetrical or symmetrical; (b) the presence of hemosiderin deposited in the skin of the ankles (a sign of venous insufficiency); (c) the general appearance and quality of the skin, including hair growth (hair loss may signify arterial insufficiency); (d) evidence of fungal infection (scaling, apparently pruritic lesions); and (e) the status of the nails.

Following inspection of the feet and legs, a vascular examination of the lower extremities should be conducted. Femoral, popliteal, dorsalis pedis, and posterior tibial pulses should be palpated and the capillary refill time following pressure on the toes should be observed (normally less than 10 sec). Auscultation from the midabdomen down to the popliteal regions should be performed to detect bruits that are produced by narrowed atherosclerotic arteries. The temperature of the legs should be felt with the dorsum of the hand, both descending from the thigh to the foot and symmetrically from side to side, comparing one side to the other. Evidence of varicose veins is best sought with the patient standing.

INSPECTION OF ULCER OR ULCERS

Ulcerated areas on the legs are often very tender, and palpation, although necessary, should be done gently, with the gloved hand.

Site. An accurate description of the site of the ulcer, preferably with reference to some immovable anatomic landmark—e.g., the medial or the lateral malleolus—should be made, and the findings should be recorded.

Size. The size of the ulcer must be documented, and the vertical and horizontal diameter in centimeters should be noted in the patient's record for future reference.

Shape. It should be noted whether the ulcer is regular or irregular in outline, whether the edges are undermined, whether the base is clean or covered with exudate, and what type of tissue is at the base of the ulcer (clean fascia, granulation tissue, dirty exudate, debris, etc.).

Mobility. With the gloved hand, an attempt should be made to move the ulcer over the underlying tissue. It is important to know whether the ulcer is attached to the deep fascia of the leg and particularly to the bone, or whether it moves freely with its surrounding skin over the underlying structures.

Examination of Edge of Ulcer. It should be noted whether the edges are raised, heaped, everted, or flat and whether there is any evidence of epithelial ingrowth from the edge of the ulcer towards the center—i.e., healing.

Tenderness. If the ulcer is tender, it should be determined whether it is *very* tender such as in an acute inflammatory process or only mildly tender as in a neuropathy with loss of superficial sensation.

Changes in Adjoining Skin. It should be noted whether there are fluctuant areas of purulence near the ulcer, particularly on the sole of the foot, whether there are any callosities surrounding the ulcer, and whether there is a heavy deposition of pigment near the ulcer.

When this examination is complete, the patient should stand, preferably on a stool, and face the examiner. Edema should now be looked for together with the appearance of varicose veins along the course of the short and long saphenous veins on the front and back of the leg (see Fig. 85.1). In particular, the appearance of perforator varicosities (see below, p. 946) should be noted, usually above the medial malleolus, and the relationship of these perforators to ulcerated areas should be sought.

Types and Characteristics of Leg Ulcers

The principal characteristics of common ulcers are shown in Table 85.1.

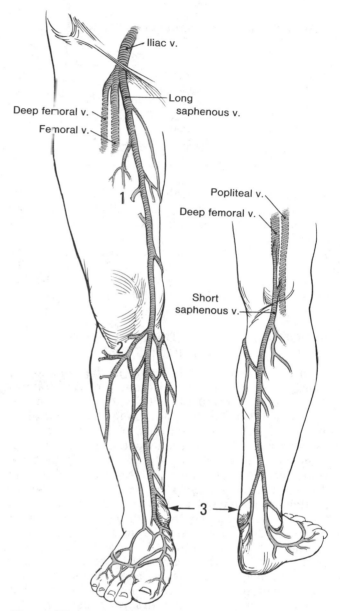

Figure 85.1 Venous circulation of the lower extremity. *1*, Hunter's canal perforator; *2*, anterior communicating vein of the leg; and *3*, ankle perforators.

VENOUS—ASSOCIATED WITH VARICOSE VEINS (see pp. 945–947)

Ulcers associated with varicose veins characteristically occur in the presence of advanced varicose veins, usually affecting the long saphenous system (Fig. 85.1). Such varicosities should be apparent when the patient has stood for a few minutes. Ulcerations associated with varicose veins occur where the deep perforators meet the long saphenous or the accessory long saphenous system just above, or 3 or 4 cm higher, than the medial malleolus. Edema and hemosiderin deposition are usually absent or minimal and there are no signs of peripheral arterial insufficiency. The

Table 85.1
Characteristics of Common Leg Ulcers

Type of Ulcer	Usual Location	Edema	Pigmentation	Evidence of Arterial Insufficiency
Varicose	Medial leg	0 to +	0 to +	0
Stasis	Medial leg	+ + to + + + +	+ + +	0 to +
Arterial	Lateral leg, foot	0 to +	0	+ + + +
Dystrophic	Sole, tip of toe	+ +	0	0
Traumatic	Midleg, toe	0	0	0 to + + + +
Diabetic	Toes, dorsum of foot	+ +	0	+ to + + +
Factitious	Anywhere	+	0	0

ulcers are characteristically fairly shallow, regular, and tender; they are usually initiated by minor trauma. They move with the skin and fascia over the underlying tissues. The edges are not undermined. There may be evidence of varicose veins on the nonulcerated side of the extremity. The patient will complain that the ulcer hurts and that he has a feeling of heaviness in his legs. Claudication and chronic edema are usually absent.

VENOUS—ASSOCIATED WITH CHRONIC VENOUS INSUFFICIENCY ("STASIS")

Chronic venous insufficiency is the commonest cause of leg ulcers. The disorder probably follows deep venous thrombophlebitis with destruction of valves in the deep venous system and reversal of normal superficial-to-deep flow of blood in the perforating veins. The muscular action of the calf becomes ineffective and blood flows to the superficial veins instead of in the usual centripetal direction through the deep venous system. Valves in the superficial (saphenous) system become incompetent, thereby raising the hydrostatic venous pressure at the ankle. As a result, small venous capillaries rupture and an extravasation of red cells takes place; hemoglobin from these red cells is processed locally by macrophages and is deposited in the tissues, causing pigment deposition (hemosiderosis). The pigment acts as an irritant to the tissues, causing further collagen deposition which results in strangulation of the nutrient arteriolar circulation to the skin. Both venous stasis and arterial capillary nutrient insufficiency therefore relate eventually to ulceration.

The patient usually gives a history of long-standing swelling of the affected leg. Often, there is a history of minor trauma at the site of the ulcer. The physical examination reveals edema, hemosiderin deposition, and ulceration, usually in line with the long saphenous vein, the short saphenous vein, or over a medial ankle perforator (Fig. 85.1). Arterial circulation in the leg may be entirely normal. Varicosities may or may not be present. The ulcer is usually fairly superficial and involves the skin, with irregular margins and with exudate covering the floor of the ulcer. The ulcer is usually moveable with the skin and is tender. In grossly neglected cases, the ulceration may be massive and may involve most of the circumference of the leg. Occasionally, cellulitis may be evident,

with erythema, tenderness, and fever secondary to superimposed bacterial infection.

ULCERATION ASSOCIATED WITH ARTERIAL INSUFFICIENCY

Arterial insufficiency is the second most common cause of leg ulcers and, with the ulcer of venous insufficiency, accounts for the great majority of leg ulcers. Ulcers associated with peripheral arterial occlusive disease usually begin with trauma and therefore appear at sites which are most subject to trauma—i.e., on toes, over the lateral or medial malleolus, at the base of the fifth metatarsal, at the head of the first metatarsal, on the heel or the ball of the foot, and in the distal pretibial region. However, occasionally, ulceration occurs in the untraumatized leg, in which case it is more likely to involve the lateral rather than the medial malleolar region, the common site of venous ulceration. Ulcers secondary to occlusive arterial disease are characteristically quite painful, and may be surrounded by cellulitis. Edema is usually absent. The foot may appear atrophic with shiny, fragile transparent hairless skin; the nails are often hypertrophied and deformed. Other hallmarks of arterial insufficiency—e.g., pulselessness and coolness—may be present. Because some patients are relieved of rest pain when they dangle the ulcerated leg, dependent edema may be present.

DYSTROPHIC ULCERS

A neuropathic or dystrophic ulcer is usually associated with somatic or sympathetic neurologic dysfunction. The precise pathogenesis of these ulcers is not known. Perhaps sympathetic dysfunction causes a reduction of arterial blood flow to local areas of skin resulting in ulceration, or hypesthesia or anesthesia renders the patient more susceptible to trauma. Dystrophic ulcers are most commonly associated with the neuropathies of congenital or acquired disease of the spine, such as Friedreich's ataxia, syringomyelia, or multiple sclerosis. Peripheral neuropathies due to vitamin deficiency or to injuries may also result in ulcers. Ulceration almost always occurs in areas of pressure. The patient may complain of pain in the ulcer, but the ulcer is usually insensitive to light touch. There may be deformity in the foot associated with the neuropathy (talipes calcaneovalgus or equinus) or there may be a back deformity or a surgical scar as might occur in a patient with a meningomyelocele. Usually, neurologic examination of the lower extremity will be abnormal, revealing decreased proprioception, decreased cutaneous sensation, and perhaps impaired movement. The ulcer may be undermined and there may be subcutaneous tracking of infected material into adjacent tissues which, on pressure, will exude loculated pus from the undermined border of the ulcer. If the neuropathy is severe, the patient may be ambulating without pain, yet show quite advanced ulceration of the sole of the foot.

POST-TRAUMATIC ULCERS

Post-traumatic ulcers are common and usually are associated with impairment in nerve or vascular supply of the leg. Minor injury to the toe of a patient with arteriosclerotic occlusive vascular disease, or a leg injury in an individual with chronic venous insufficiency, may lead to ulceration. However, such ulcers may develop in the legs of otherwise healthy individuals, particularly after major injuries, such as fractures, which involve areas where vascular supply is normally marginal. The most susceptible site is the junction of the middle and lower third of the subcutaneous surface of the tibia. In this situation, most traumatic ulcers, even in healthy youngsters, heal with some difficulty, and in older patients and in those with even minimal arterial insufficiency, injury at this site resolves with great difficulty. Post-traumatic ulcers may be accompanied by problems of chronic infection and present with tenderness and local cellulitis.

A specific instance of a post-traumatic ulcer is the brown recluse spider bite, common in the southeastern United States. The poison of the brown recluse spider contains a necrotizing enzyme which causes a rounded sloughing ulcer of approximately 3 to 4 cm with an indurated edge. The patient may not be aware that he has been bitten by a spider. These ulcers are refractory to healing by use of conservative measures, and should be surgically excised and closed.

DIABETIC ULCERS

Diabetic ulcers have features of dystrophic, traumatic, and arterial ulcers since all three factors contribute to their development. The characteristic location of such an ulcer is in an area of pressure such as a corn or a callosity. The ulcer is fairly insensitive, often heavily infected, with undermined edges, and tracks under the plantar fascia or proximally on the dorsum of the foot. Although usually patients are aware that they are diabetic, some are not, and a thorough evaluation upon suspicion of diabetes is mandatory since control of the ulcer will depend to a large extent on control of the diabetes. Radiologic examination is important, for the bone underlying the ulcer may be the site of chronic osteomyelitis that will necessitate surgical intervention.

FACTITIOUS ULCERS

Factitious ulcers commonly occur in the legs of addicts who inject drugs into slightly varicose leg veins. Perhaps the most common drug in this regard is pentazocine (Talwin) which, when either extravasated or injected in the suspension form, which the patient makes by emptying the capsule into some water, is a strongly thrombogenic agent causing widespread skin necrosis. The distribution of these ulcers is usually bizarre. They may be multiple and bilateral; and, if the history can be obtained, the diagnosis is easily made. Factitious ulcers may also occur in patients with poor hygiene or who have disorders associated with itching, such as scabies, which has led to excoriation.

NEOPLASTIC ULCERS

Neoplastic ulcers of the leg are rare; but when they do occur, they are usually either basal cell or squamous cell carcinomas and have the usual characteristics of these tumors. They have elevated or rolled edges, are anesthetic, and are usually attached to deeper tissue. Margolins' ulcer, a rare form of squamous epithelioma occurring in healed burn scars, also may be seen on the legs.

MISCELLANEOUS

Ulceration of the legs may occur in sickle cell disease, in polyarteritis nodosa and other collagen diseases, and in other systemic conditions (e.g., ulcerative colitis). In these instances, the diagnosis depends on making the diagnosis of the systemic disorder.

In the tropics, ulceration of the foot and leg may occur from local mycoses such as maduromycosis; these conditions should be kept in mind when an individual is returning from a prolonged sojourn in a tropical climate.

Laboratory Aids in Diagnosis

BACTERIOLOGY

Leg ulcers are often infected and almost invariably contaminated, usually with enteric organisms. Infections are particularly hazardous in the diabetic and in the patient with chronic arterial insufficiency. Cultures of the ulcer bed are useful, and cultures of obviously purulent ulcers are mandatory since antibiotic therapy is an important part of management (see Chapter 24). If fungal infection is suspected (unusual degree of scaling and of excoriation), unless the physician is experienced in the scraping of lesions and in the microscopic identification of fungi, dermatologic consultation is indicated.

BIOPSY

Biopsy, by a surgeon or a dermatologist, is indicated if neoplastic or obscure fungal disease is suspected. Biopsy may be performed in the office under local anesthesia, and should include a wedge-shaped section of the edge and floor of the ulcer.

LABORATORY TESTS FOR SYSTEMIC DISEASE

These tests are performed as dictated by the clinical diagnosis, when the ulcer is suspected to be part of a systemic disorder—e.g., diabetes, polyarteritis nodosa, sickle cell disease, etc.

NONINVASIVE VASCULAR TESTING

When ulceration is noted in a patient with occlusive arterial disease, he should be referred to a vascular laboratory for testing. This is more fully discussed in Chapter 84.

Natural History and Management

VENOUS ULCERS ASSOCIATED WITH VARICOSE VEINS

These lesions will invariably heal with elevation and appropriate elastic compression to counteract the increased hydrostatic pressure in the varicose venous system. If the patient is at home, he should be at bed rest for a period of 2 weeks with only bathroom privileges. A Telfa gauze pad is placed over the ulcer and the leg is carefully wrapped in Ace bandages. Alternatively the leg may be wrapped in gauze impregnated with a zinc-gelatin dressing (Unna boot). If an Unna boot is used (the impregnated gauze is commercially available), it should be removed within 48 hours to ascertain that the compression is adequate, since either too tight or too loose compression will result in treatment failure. The bandage may then be reapplied and changed weekly, and healing will usually result. If the ulcer is grossly infected, a Unna boot should not be used. Following adequate bacteriologic cultures, it is best to treat an infected ulcer with a suitable topical antibacterial preparation such as Bacitracin-Neomycin cream, a Telfa pad on the ulcer, and Ace bandage compression. The dressing should be reapplied twice a day. It is important *never to apply a Unna bandage to a leg when peripheral arteriosclerotic vascular disease is suspected or cannot be excluded.*

The patient should be followed at twice weekly intervals in the physician's office. After healing of the ulcer, the patient should be referred for surgical opinion about whether stripping and ligation of the long saphenous vein and ligation of the incompetent perforators are indicated to prevent recurrence. If the ulcerations do not heal in 2 to 3 weeks, hospitalization and surgical consultation are indicated.

ULCERATION OF CHRONIC VENOUS INSUFFICIENCY ("STASIS" ULCER)

There is probably no other form of ulcer which taxes the patient or the physician as much as stasis ulcer. The mainstays of therapy are elimination of infection, and reduction of edema by elevation and compression. The patient should be at bed rest, and the ulcer should be treated with dressings and with topical antibacterial agents, if appropriate (see Chapter 24). The patient should be instructed to change the dressing twice a day. Resolution of the edema usually can be accelerated with the use of diuretics even when no element of cardiac or renal failure exists; but, to avoid the danger of volume depletion, elastic stockings should be tried first. If the edema can be controlled, the ulcers usually can be healed, although several weeks to months may be required. Following healing, the patient must be advised to wear some form of elastic compression permanently: preferably, a made to measure, elastic support garment such as a Jobst stocking or Sigvaris.

If, with the above measures, the ulcer still fails to heal, then skin grafting may be required along with venous ligation and stripping. This will require surgical consultation and hospitalization.

ARTERIAL ULCERS

Arterial ulcers are almost impossible to heal unless a surgical procedure can improve blood flow to the area. Therefore, if there is any suspicion of arterial insufficiency, the patient should be referred for surgical evaluation. If the patient's lesion is unsuitable for surgical correction, or the patient has already had an operation but ulceration persists, the ulcer can sometimes be healed with painstaking debridements every 2 or 3 days. This treatment, however, requires expertise; in case of doubt, surgical referral should be made. A pair of sharp scissors is used to remove the necrotic edges of the ulcer carefully without causing bleeding, and wet to dry dressings are then applied, using a topical antibiotic solution such as Polymixin-Bacitracin 5% aqueous suspension to set the bandages. The patient is instructed to apply the bandage wet with antibiotic solution, in the morning, and remove it in the evening after it has been allowed to dry. This has the effect of debriding the ulcer, and allowing the delicate epithelial edges the best chance for ingrowth.

If there is a great deal of debris in the ulcer bed, twice daily application of a debriding agent such as Travase, Debrisan, or Elastase applied for a few days will usually help to clear the thick debris from the ulcer. In conjunction with these measures, meticulously compulsive foot protection, soft footwear, elevation of the extremity, and avoidance of weight-bearing are mandatory.

DYSTROPHIC ULCERS

Dystrophic ulcers are a real threat to the limb because infection will often advance unnoticed by the patient until there is considerable spread of pus around and under the ulcer. Treatment consists of bed rest, appropriate antibiotic therapy as indicated following culture (see Chapter 24), debridement of necrotic skin edges (which can be done without anesthesia in the office), and wet to dry dressings as described above. Dystrophic ulcers probably take the longest of all to heal, perhaps several months. If, despite office measures and adequate bed rest at home, no progress seems to be made, the patient should be hospitalized in a setting where debridement can be performed once or twice a day by a skilled individual.

TRAUMATIC ULCERS

Traumatic ulcers will usually heal by avoidance of weight-bearing, elevation, appropriate topical antibiotic therapy, and protection of the ulcer by dressings. If no progress is made within 2 to 3 weeks, the patient should be seen by a surgeon for possible operative debridement and surgical closure of the wound.

DIABETIC ULCERS

An ulcer in the diabetic foot imposes such serious risk of limb loss that the majority of these patients should be hospitalized.

In the hospital, diabetes can be more meticulously regulated; any pockets of suppuration can be drained, and treatment of osteomyelitis in the metatarsals, and proper debridement can be carried out.

FACTITIOUS ULCERS

Factitious ulcers will usually heal if the cause can be found and controlled.

NEOPLASTIC AND OTHER ULCERS

Neoplastic and other unusual ulcers, such as the previously mentioned brown recluse spider bite, are a surgical problem; and these patients should be referred promptly for consultation.

Prevention and General Foot Care in Susceptible Patients (see Chapter 99)

Foot and leg ulcers from any cause often recur after healing, since, with the exception of varicose veins and factitious ulcers, the underlying disease is difficult to reverse. It is therefore mandatory to be familiar with the principles of foot care, and patients must understand and carry out instructions aimed at minimizing exposure to trauma. Patients with peripheral arterial disease or diabetes should wear very comfortable footwear, even if it is not fashionable. The front of the shoe should be broad so that the toes can spread. Areas of pressure caused by foot deformities should be corrected by orthopaedic shoes with appropriate fittings—e.g., insoles, or metatarsal bars; these problems should be referred to an orthopaedic surgeon or to a podiatrist. Patients should be instructed to keep their feet very clean—i.e., at least once daily showers or footbaths in tepid water; nails should be very carefully trimmed, preferably with clippers; under no circumstances should sharp scissors be used to trim the sides of nails, as they may cause injury to the delicate nail fold and become a portal of entry for infection and consequent ulceration. Patients can protect their toes during walking by the insertion of small, fluffy pieces of cotton wool

between them. Lanolin or other emollient creams are useful in preventing cracking of hardened areas of skin, and in keeping the skin soft and supple. Patients should avoid extremes of temperature, and reduce exposure to trauma (e.g., a night light in the bedroom to avoid "stubbing" a toe). With attention to these small details, recurring trouble can often be prevented.

VARICOSE VEINS

Causes

Varicose (dilated) veins of the lower extremities are common, affecting females more often than males, and usually become symptomatic between the ages of 20 and 40. They are due to an incompetence of the valves of the long or short saphenous veins (see Fig. 85.1), permitting retrograde or downward flow of blood, or simply stagnation of the normal centripetal flow. In the perforator system, which is a system of veins communicating between the deep and the superficial veins, destruction of valves interferes with the unidirectional movement of blood from superficial to deep.

The disorder is aggravated, indeed may be caused, by conditions elevating intra-abdominal pressure, such as pregnancy, large intra-abdominal tumors, conditions causing chronic straining—e.g., prostatic obstruction, carcinoma of the sigmoid colon, and occasionally, by mechanical interference with venous return in the venous system itself such as thrombosis of the pelvic veins.

Symptoms

The symptoms of uncomplicated varicose veins usually consist of heaviness and aching in the area of the veins or in the calves. The patient may complain of mild edema at the end of a long day's work. Occasionally, patients will complain of varicose veins for cosmetic reasons and desire treatment. Patients with uncomplicated varicose veins do not complain of intermittent claudication or severe pain; in the presence of these symptoms, other causes must be carefully sought. Occasionally, thrombophlebitis will supervene in a varicose vein and can cause severe pain; the culpable vein is then palpable as an inflamed cord. Following bed rest, elevation, application of local heat, and appropriate anti-inflammatory therapy (e.g., aspirin), thrombophlebitis in the varicose veins will result in cure of that particular varix.

Physical Examination

It is useful to have some idea of the anatomy of the venous system of the leg (Fig. 85.1). This will enable the clinician to judge the patient's symptoms on the basis of an anatomical abnormality detected by physical examination. There are several types of varicose veins which conform to the underlying anatomic arrangement of these veins.

SUBCUTANEOUS VARICOSE VEINS ("SUNBURST" VARICES)

These are not, in the true sense of the word, varicose veins, but rather dilations of intracutaneous venous plexuses which have a spiderlike arrangement and an unsightly purple color. These veins are quite frequently the object of cosmetic complaints by patients. Otherwise, they are essentially asymptomatic.

VARICOSITIES OF LONG SAPHENOUS SYSTEM

These are the most common type of varicose veins. The long saphenous vein begins anterior to the medial malleolus at the ankle, courses superficially to the medial side of the knee and then curves upwards to enter the deep system just below the inguinal ligament medial to the femoral artery. The vein has several tributaries in the calf and in the thigh which are superficial, and it is also joined by several perforating veins from the deep venous system which can become incompetent and cause varicosities at a point of junction (Fig. 85.1). There are three or four consistent perforators—three above the medial malleolus at a distance separated by approximately 3 cm, and a fourth just above the knee joint. If varicosities appear in this situation, then the perforator system is almost certainly incompetent. Otherwise, varicosity of the long saphenous vein is clearly visible with the patient standing.

VARICOSITIES OF SHORT SAPHENOUS SYSTEM

The short saphenous vein arises behind the lateral malleolus and courses upward behind the calf to join the popliteal vein in the popliteal space (Fig. 85.1). Varicosities of this system are best seen with the patient standing with his back to the examiner.

PERFORATOR VARICOSITIES

As mentioned above, perforator incompetence is usually noticed in the long saphenous vein where the ankle perforators and the above-the-knee perforator join the vein; however, perforators join other superficial veins which in turn, join the long and short saphenous system. Examination may reveal that there is no incompetence of the short or long saphenous veins, only of the perforators.

Clinical Testing to Determine Level of Incompetence

One or two easy clinical tests can be performed in the office which will aid in the determination of the severity of the problem and in the selection of appropriate treatment.

TRENDELENBURG'S TEST

The patient lies on his back and raises his leg to empty the veins. A venous tourniquet is applied just below the saphenous opening about 3 inches (7.7 cm) below the inguinal ligament and the patient then stands up. Constriction is released; if the saphenofemoral valve is incompetent, the veins will fill immediately from above; if not, the veins fill slowly from below. If the veins fill rapidly from above *before* the release of the tourniquet, this indicates an incompetent valve at the entry of the long saphenous vein into the femoral vein and signifies major long saphenous incompetence. This test is now repeated at successively lower levels in the leg; and thereby, the location of incompetence may be mapped.

PERTHES' TEST

This is a test for deep venous thrombosis in association with varicose veins. A tourniquet is lightly applied below the inquinal ligament as in Trendelenburg's test and the patient is instructed to walk in place. If varicose veins are accompanied by a thrombosed deep femoral system, the varicose veins will become very prominent after this exercise.

Treatment

SUBCUTANEOUS VARICOSITIES ASYMPTOMATIC EXCEPT FOR COSMETIC APPEARANCE

If the offending venous plexus is deemed large enough to accommodate a 25 gauge needle, a sclerosing solution may be injected. The technique is described below. Other treatments such as freezing with carbon dioxide snow, cautery under local anesthesia, and even laser therapy have been advocated, but their use requires a great deal of skill, and unnecessary skin scarring may result which is, in the end, more unsightly than the original vein. Probably the safest treatment of this kind of vein is the use of masking cosmetic creams, together with reassurance.

LOCALIZED SMALL VARICOSITIES NOT ACCOMPANIED BY MAJOR LONG SAPHENOUS OR SHORT SAPHENOUS INCOMPETENCE

These veins are suitable for treatment by a sclerosing injection and compression therapy. The procedure can easily be performed in the office by anyone skilled with a needle; however, the patient should be warned that several sittings may be required for complete elimination of the veins.

Technique. The patient stands with a light tourniquet around the thigh, just enough to make the vein prominent. The area of the vein is lightly prepped with a suitable antiseptic and 0.5 ml of sclerosing solution is injected by use of a 2-ml syringe, following initial aspiration to make sure the needle is in the vein. Immediately after the end of the injection, the needle is withdrawn; and the vein is gently compressed with a 2- × 2-inch gauze for 3 min, after which the tourniquet is released and compression continued for 2 min more. The patient now wears an Ace bandage on the area for approximately 4 hours. The sclerosant produces an inflammatory reaction in the intima which obliterates the vein by phlebitis.

Failure to use a tourniquet may release an unnecessarily large amount of sclerosant into the major veins of the leg and cause undesirable thrombosis at distant sites. The patient should be warned that extravasation of the sclerosant is a possibility and may cause a small skin slough. There are several commercially available sclerosant solutions, morrhuate sodium and sodium tetradecyl sulfate (Soltradecal) which are suitable for injection.

MAJOR LONG OR SHORT SAPHENOUS VARICOSITIES, OR PERFORATOR VARICOSITIES IN SYMPTOMATIC PATIENTS

Symptomatic patients should be referred for surgical consultation. Attempts to inject and compress veins associated with clear-cut varicosities of the major superficial systems are doomed to failure without surgical intervention.

If an operation has been performed on either the long or short saphenous system or both, there are often residual varicosities of a minor degree requiring additional injection therapy which may be performed in the office. The recurrence rate of major varicosities after operation is only approximately 10%.

Varicose veins should *not be treated* in individuals who have an underlying cause associated with increased intra-abdominal pressure, until the primary cause has been removed. The wearing of elastic stockings may, however, give comfort during this time. Such stockings may be advisable for support in any individual with varicose veins in whom other treatment is either undesirable or contraindicated.

References

Bailey, L: Leg ulcers. Nurs Time 72: 1752, 1976.
   Primarily directed to nurses, it carries some practical suggestions on equipment and on dressing techniques for dealing with leg ulcers in the office.
Beninson, J: Medical management of the peripheral vascular ulcer. Angiology 30: 48, 1979.
   A simple, sensible description of management by a physician who has over 30 years experience running a major leg ulcer clinic. Some very practical suggestions on basic advice to the patient with leg ulcers.
Litchfield, R, Wolfson, P, Haspel, L and Dunlap, S: Differential diagnosis of leg ulcers. JAOA 78: 204, 1978.
   An excellent series of photographs showing various types of ulceration and a good description of the clinical features of the more common ulcers.
Robson, MC and Edstrom, LE: Conservative management of the ulcerated diabetic foot. Plast Reconstr Surg 59: 551, 1977.
   An article on a currently controversial subject, the management of diabetic ulcer. It points out the disastrous complications of mismanagement, and the excellent results that can be obtained from meticulous conservative therapy.
Young, JR: Differential diagnosis of ulcers on legs of vascular cause. J Dermatol Surg Oncol 4: 687, 1978.
   A useful discussion of vascular ulceration.

CHAPTER EIGHTY-SIX

Diseases of the Breast

ROBERT M. QUINLAN, M.D., and CALVIN B. ERNST, M.D.

A mass is the most common symptom of breast disease that causes women to seek help from their physician. Although the majority of these masses are benign, 90% of breast cancers are discovered by the patient. No mass, therefore, is too trivial to be investigated.

One in every 13 women develops breast cancer; it is the leading cause of cancer death in women, claiming 34,000 lives in this country each year. Approximately one-third of the 90,000 new cases each year present at an advanced stage, often because of delays by either patients or physicians. The primary physician must have a rational approach to the diagnosis and treatment of breast masses and to other, nonspecific, complaints referred to the breast. A surgeon usually enters into the diagnostic and treatment plan since the most definitive diagnostic test for a breast mass is biopsy and histologic review. A reassuring patient-doctor relationship is critical in dealing with this emotionally charged area, and although this relationship should be shared by all of the physicians involved in the case, the role of the primary physician is critical.

NORMAL ANATOMY AND PHYSIOLOGY OF THE BREAST

The breast is a modified sweat gland, situated in a fascial envelope on the anterior chest wall. There is an extension of breast tissue reaching toward the axilla. There are 12 to 20 acini arranged like a bunch of grapes with draining ducts emptying into openings on the nipple. These ducts are lined by two layers of epithelium, one of which serves as a basement membrane and source of epithelial cell reproduction. It is this "reverse layer" which can proliferate in certain pathologic conditions (16). Surrounding each duct is a specialized periductal fibrous layer, which is under hormonal influence.

Only ducts are present at birth. At puberty, under stimulation of estrogen and progesterone, these ducts branch into surrounding stroma and acini bud from them. With each menstrual cycle, a fall in hormonal activity at the menses results in the desquamation of duct lining, which proliferates again at the cessation of menses. Increases in periductal vascularity and lymphocytic infiltration accompany this proliferation. During pregnancy, with prolonged hormonal stimulation, the ducts and acini proliferate maximally, often never returning to normal in the postpartum period. In many parts of the breast the glandular hypertrophy will remain until it involutes at menopause. At that time there is a loss of parenchyma and an increase in fat, especially in the periductal region. The lobular anatomy slowly disappears. It is thought that variations in hormonal balance can result in various benign pathologic conditions occurring during the active menstrual childbearing years and at menopause. It is important to realize that anatomic changes associated with normal hormonal fluctuations during a menstrual cycle do not all occur to the same degree in all areas of the breast. This accounts for the asymmetric palpatory findings in the normal breast, which is often very "lumpy."

SCREENING PROCEDURES

A major report (11) has documented decreased mortality from breast cancer in women over the age of 50 who were involved in a screening program (physical examination and mammography), but there has been no demonstrated survival benefit from screening in women less than 50 years of age. It is important to remember these facts when considering how to advise women about screening and to consider as well the possible drawbacks of screening procedures: increased anxiety, unnecessary biopsies, false reassurance, and radiologically induced cancer. However, it is important to stress to the patient the possible reduction in morbidity if lesions are detected earlier so that treatment is less deforming (6).

Self-examination

There has been no definitive evidence that breast self-examination (BSE) decreases the mortality from breast cancer (7). However, since the procedure imposes no risk, it is worthwhile encouraging women to perform it. There is, however, a major problem of patient compliance with BSE which limits its effectiveness. It is well known that twice as many women will practice BSE if it is taught by a physician or his designee.

The premenopausal woman should be instructed to examine her breasts approximately 7 to 10 days after her menses. The menopausal or postmenopausal woman should examine her breasts on a convenient day once a month, such as the first calendar day. BSE should be done both in the sitting or standing and in the supine positions. Instructions (15) should be kept simple: for example, "palpate the breast in a clockwise fashion." The physician should perform the initial instructional self-examination with the patient so that he can answer questions which might arise concerning the normal "lumpy" character of the breast.

Mammography

The controversy surrounding screening with mammography (X-rays of the breast) stems from concern about radiologically induced breast cancer. It has been estimated that the risk from radiation is equivalent to six cases of breast cancer for each one million women irradiated with 1 rad each (14). With increased technologic improvements, the standard two mammographic views can now be obtained with good quality images using less than 1 rad for both exposures. The physician should be aware of how his radiology consultants accomplish mammography. The American Cancer Society and National Cancer Institute have suggested the following guidelines for mammography screening for breast cancer:

1. Women over age 50 should have routine annual mammograms for screening purposes.

2. Women ages 40 to 49 should have routine mam-

mography screening if *they* have a prior history of breast cancer or if their *mothers* or *sisters* had breast cancer.

3. Women ages 35 to 39 should have routine mammography screening if *they* have a prior history of breast cancer.

4. Women less than 30 should not have routine mammography screening.

5. Women ages 35 to 50 may have *baseline* mammography screening regardless of medical history.

In summary, screening for breast cancer should include BSE monthly, mammography (according to the guidelines listed above), and annual breast examination by a qualified medical professional. More frequent examinations by a physician might be suggested for patients at increased risk of developing breast cancer (9) (see below, p. 951).

CLINICAL CHARACTERISTICS OF COMMON DISEASES OF THE BREAST

Benign Tumors

FIBROADENOMA

Fibroadenoma is the most common unilateral discrete mass in the 15- to 35-year-old age group. The peak incidence is from 21 to 25 years of age. In 10 to 15% of cases, there will be multiple tumors. Rapid growth during pregnancy, just prior to menopause, and in animals given estrogens, all support a concept that fibroadenomas are under hormonal control.

The patient with a fibroadenoma usually complains only of the mass and denies pain, nipple discharge, or other breast changes. On physical examination, the lesion is usually firm, but not rock hard; it is smooth and well circumscribed, nontender, and easily movable. It often rolls about in the breast, mimicking a very large marble. In some adolescents, giant fibroadenomas can be confused with virginal hypertrophy; despite the adenoma's size, however, it is usually more discrete than is diffuse hypertrophy.

A fibroadenoma has both fibrous and epithelial components. The tumor probably arises from terminal ducts and lobules, and the rare finding of lobular carcinoma rather than intraductal carcinoma within or in the vicinity of a fibroadenoma (5) is consistent with such an origin.

Although no definite evidence exists, there is suspicion that *cystosarcoma phylloides,* a noncarcinomatous neoplasm of the breast, arises from fibroadenomas (13). The overgrowth of stroma in cystosarcoma is the main difference between it and a fibroadenoma. The best estimates suggest a malignancy rate of between 20 and 30% in cystosarcomas; only 2 to 3% of these tumors will metastasize. Nevertheless, there is a high rate of local recurrence even with the benign type of cystosarcoma. The rate of local recurrence increases with increasing tumor pleomorphism regardless of the extent of surgical excision. Cur-

rently, wide local excision would be favored for benign cystosarcoma and modified radical mastectomy for the malignant tumor. In tumors of questionable histology, the more extensive procedure would be appropriate. The criteria of malignancy in this disease are often difficult for the pathologist to define.

The natural history of fibroadenoma is of a tumor growing old with the patient, perhaps calcifying in the postmenopausal woman, and rapidly growing in the pregnant patient. Because of the rare possibility of simultaneous lobular carcinoma or of progression to cystosarcoma phylloides and the inability to exclude definitively carcinoma in a breast mass, the physician should recommend excisional biopsy (see p. 953).

INTRADUCTAL PAPILLOMAS

These often present with serosanguinous, spontaneous, recurrent or persistent nipple discharge from a single duct. These small tumors are not palpable, but their location can usually be determined by applying pressure on various quadrants of the areolocutaneous margin and noting which quadrant produces the discharge. An intraductal papillary cancer is a possibility that must be excluded. Surgical exploration and excision are performed by removing a small pie-shaped segment in the area producing the discharge.

Fibrocystic Disease

Cystic and proliferative changes in the breasts are common: autopsy studies have revealed them in 4 to 90% of women, depending on the criteria that are applied. The incidence of fibrocystic disease, like that of breast cancer, increases between the ages of 30 and 50. It is reasonable to assume that approximately 50% of women will be affected during their reproductive years. After menopause fibrocystic disease usually disappears, as the disproportionately increased fibroepithelial tissue is replaced by fat.

The disease is usually bilateral, and frequently multiple lesions are found in each breast; however, unilateral discrete lesions are seen occasionally. Diffuse lesions (5 cm or more) are more easily distinguished from cancer than are discrete lesions (less than 5 cm).

The patient with fibrocystic disease usually complains about dull, aching pain in the area of most pronounced nodularity; and this pain is often more prominent just before menses. It is possible that much of the pain related to fibrocystic disease is due to cancer phobia, and it does often lessen with improvement in the doctor-patient relationship (10). Some patients will not have pain and will complain only of a mass or of nipple discharge. Many patients are only first aware of a fibronodular mass in their breast after being examined for another reason. At other times, when patients are asked about the "lumps" in their breasts, they reassure the doctor that they have been present for many years.

The cause of fibrocystic disease is unknown, but is suspected to be linked to changes in the activity of female sex hormones. The great majority of lesions appear benign when examined histologically, but occasionally epithelial hyperplasia or cellular atypia is seen which causes the pathologist and the clinician to worry about the potential for malignant transformation. And, although a continuation from fibrocystic disease to carcinoma has never been established, there is a 2½ times greater risk of breast cancer developing eventually in women who have biopsy-proved fibrocystic disease. This relationship and the inability to exclude cancer in a discrete unilateral fibrocystic lesion are the reasons why biopsies are performed so commonly in women with this condition. A general surgeon interested in breast disease will biopsy 10 to 20 benign lesions for every malignant one. Often clinical examination is consistent with fibrocystic disease (bilateral, upper outer quadrant, diffuse, tender, easily movable masses), but the patient has a persistent *localized* symptom of pain or unilateral discharge. In these patients, if there is a family history of breast cancer or a suspicious area on a mammogram, a biopsy is often recommended. In addition to excluding carcinoma, the physician will be able better to evaluate the epithelial component of the fibrocystic change and thereby plan more appropriate follow-up with clinical examination and mammography.

Sometimes fibrocystic disease is associated with *duct ectasia*, usually heralded by spontaneous discharge of thick, gray-green fluid from multiple dilated ducts. At other times duct ectasia may be present in the absence of palpable fibrocystic lesions. In the first instance, a biopsy should be done to rule out carcinoma; in the second, the administration of estrogen may stop the discharge. If it does, mammography should be performed and then a biopsy should be considered.

Cancer

Unfortunately, one-third of patients with breast cancer present with advanced disease. Their case histories are often replete with multiple risk factors; and physical findings are unmistakable (for example, nipple retraction; marked skin changes; mass fixation to the chest wall; hard, matted axillary nodes). Other patients (85% of the remainder) will present with a painless, hard, irregular mass, less than 5 cm in size, frequently (37%) located in the upper outer quadrant. Again it is this latter group who can be confused with patients with the discrete type of fibrocystic disease (see above). The patient with a carcinoma will often have subtle skin dimpling or nipple retraction even with a mass less than 5 cm.

A lesion which mimics the rock hard texture of a carcinoma, although generally more mobile, is *traumatic fat necrosis*. This lesion can be even more

worrisome on mammography where the small microcalcifications of fat necrosis are similar to those found in carcinoma.

Because surgical intervention is so common, the natural history of breast cancer is not known. A report from the Middlesex Hospital in England demonstrated a median survival of 2.7 years from the first symptom in 250 untreated patients seen between 1805 and 1933. Five percent of patients died from causes other than breast cancer, and the last death did not occur for almost 20 years (Fig. 86.1) (2). These patients were not staged according to extent of disease. Prognosis with current treatment modalities is dependent upon the stage of disease at the time of diagnosis.

The American Joint Committee on Cancer Staging has devised a clinical staging for breast cancer based on tumor size, nodal status, and the presence or absence of metastases (Table 86.1). In addition, histologic evaluation of removed axillary lymph nodes provides the most precise data on survival and is independent of tumor size.

Despite this elaborate clinical and histologic staging there are qualitative differences in biologic potential of breast cancers in similar stages. Bloom (1) in a study of 1250 patients, matched for stage, noted a decrease in 5-year survival with patient delay of up to 6 months prior to consulting a physician; yet with delays greater than 6 months, there were smaller adverse effects on survival. Patients delaying more than a year had results as good as those seeking prompt therapy. This would imply more and less aggressive types of tumors. Currently, these distinctions are not made in reporting end results of treated patients.

Premature Hyperplasia

A concentric swelling can occur unilaterally beneath the nipple before puberty in girls. This com-

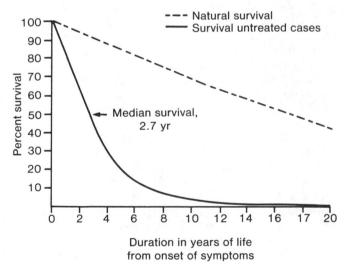

Figure 86.1 Survival of untreated beast cancer, Middlesex Hospital, 1805–1933 (250 cases). (Adapted from H. J. G. Bloom *et al.*: *British Medical Journal, 2:* 213, 1962 (2).

Table 86.1
Survival of Patients with Breast Cancer Relative to Clinical and Histologic Stage[a]

Clinical Staging (American Joint Committee)	Crude 5-Year Survival (%)	Range of Survival (%)
STAGE I	85	82–94
Tumor <2 cm in diameter		
Nodes, if present, not felt to contain metastases		
Without distant metastases		
STAGE II	66	47–74
Tumor <5 cm in diameter		
Nodes, if palpable, not fixed		
Without distant metastases		
STAGE III	41	7–80
Tumor >5 cm or,		
Tumor any size with invasion of skin or attached to chest wall		
Nodes in supraclavicular area		
Without distant metastases		
STAGE IV	10	—
With distant metastases		

Histologic Staging (NSABP[b])	Crude Survival (%) 5-Year	Crude Survival (%) 10-Year	5-Year Disease-free Survival (%)
All patients	63.5	45.9	60.3
Negative axillary lymph nodes	78.1	64.9	82.3
Positive axillary lymph nodes	46.5	24.9	34.9
1–3 positive axillary lymph nodes	62.2	37.5	50.0
>4 positive axillary lymph nodes	32.0	13.4	21.1

[a] From I. C. Henderson and G. P. Canellos: *New England Journal of Medicine, 302:* 17, 1980.
[b] National Surgical Adjuvant Breast Project.

monly occurs during ages 7 to 9. The lump can be 1 to 2 cm in diameter and is usually nontender. Within a year, a contralateral lump will appear and often both lumps remain static until puberty. A biopsy is *contraindicated* and would be equivalent to total mastectomy.

Gynecomastia (see Chapter 74)

The main differential in male breast masses lies between gynecomastia and male breast cancer. The latter is extremely rare, accounting for approximately 1% of all breast cancers. Although gynecomastia has many causes, its physical characteristics are usually unvaried. Gynecomastia presents as a breast mass beneath the areola, is usually slightly tender, and is easily movable. It is never associated with ulceration or nipple retraction. If gynecomastia is ruled out, a breast mass in a male should be biopsied.

EVALUATION OF A BREAST MASS

History: Risk Factors (Table 86.2) and Symptoms

A *family history* of breast cancer increases a woman's risk of developing breast cancer when compared to the general population. This risk varies from 0.8 times higher in mothers of daughters who have had breast cancer to 4 to 5 times higher in daughters

Table 86.2
Risk Factors for Carcinoma of the Breast

Factors	Relative Risk
Positive family history	1–5 (see text)
Early menarche and late menopause (cyclic ovarian activity greater than 30 years)	Slight
Nulliparity	3
Previous breast cancer	5
Benign disease of the breast	2½–3
Radiation	Dependent on dose

of mothers who have had breast cancer. The risk is lower for daughters if the mother was postmenopausal at the time of diagnosis.

A detailed past medical history of *previous breast problems* should be obtained. It should include details of previous symptoms, masses, mammograms, biopsies, other operations, and any known pathologic findings. A previous breast cancer will increase a woman's risk 5-fold of developing cancer in the contralateral breast. Likewise, certain proliferative ductal changes of fibrocystic disease found on previous biopsy place the patient in a higher risk category for breast cancer (see p. 949).

The *menstrual and reproductive history* is also important. Early menarche and late menopause (i.e., prolonged duration of cyclic ovarian activity—greater than 30 years) have been associated with a slightly increased risk of developing breast cancer. Surgical menopause (bilateral oophorectomy) before age 40 reduces the risk of breast cancer by 75%. The risk of breast cancer is increased 3-fold in nulliparous women, while a full term pregnancy before age 25 offers some protective benefit.

The patient should be asked about the presence of other *symptoms* (pain, discharge) related to a breast mass, the duration of those symptoms if present, and if the discovery of the mass or onset of the other symptoms was associated with changes in the menses, injury to the breast, pregnancy, or to changes in medication.

Nipple discharge is the second most frequent symptom of breast cancer. Nonlactational nipple discharge can be unilateral or bilateral, spontaneous or evoked only by pressure and massage, and persistent or recurrent. If the discharge is associated with a mass on physical examination, then the mass should be the primary concern.

Nipple discharge in women over 50 years old must be viewed with more suspicion than in younger women, regardless of its presentation.

Discharge evoked only by trauma, massage, or pressure has no clinical importance. Spontaneous, recurrent, or persistent discharge from one or two ducts not associated with a mass requires surgical exploration of the duct to differentiate benign papilloma (see p. 949) from intraductal papillary carcinoma. Both are possible without a presenting mass lesion. The character of the discharge cannot help in distinguishing benign from malignant conditions.

Physical Examination

The patient should be seated undressed to the waist on an examining table, in a warm, well-lit room. Inspection and palpation of the nodal drainage areas (supraclavicular, infraclavicular, and axillary) should be performed. Inspection and palpation of nipples, areolae, and breasts are next done. While the patient is sitting, her arm on the side being examined can be raised by the physician to allow palpation high into the axilla. The examination should then be repeated with the patient in the supine position with her arm raised over her head so that the breast flattens on the chest wall.

If the clinician cannot appreciate a mass noted by the patient, it is critical to allow the patient sufficient time to find the lesion herself rather than to dismiss the complaint. If both the patient and the physician cannot locate the mass, the patient should be reassured that benign fibrous masses often disappear spontaneously.

Initial Management

The three most common masses producing lesions in the breast are fibroadenoma, fibrocystic disease, and carcinoma. Each of these common lesions has a peak incidence at different ages; yet there is a high degree of overlap. It is because of this overlap and the clinician's inability to distinguish with certainty the lesions clinically that a biopy is usually the only definitive test to rule out carcinoma.

AGES 15 TO 30

An easily movable, nontender, smooth, marble-like mass in a woman less than 30 years of age is most likely to be a fibroadenoma. The mass should be electively excised. In a teenager, excision can be delayed several months until a school vacation if the mass is not growing rapidly and if there are no other risk factors.

A mammogram should not be obtained in the evaluation of a discrete mass in this age group. In all likelihood, the mass will be excised regardless of mammographic findings. If carcinoma, rather than fibroadenoma, is found on histologic examination, mammography to search for multicentric or contralateral nonpalpable lesions can be easily obtained. Even in the absence of a palpable mass, but with symptoms referred to the breast (pain, tenderness, nipple discharge), mammography is rarely indicated in patients less than 30 years of age. Perhaps a young obese patient with very large pendulous breasts which are difficult to examine, a persistent symptom (3 months duration) but no mass, and a strong family history of breast cancer (mother) deserves a mammogram.

AGES 30 TO 50

If a discrete mass is noted during the reproductive years and is clinically suspicious for fibrocystic disease, a watch-and-wait policy through one or two menstrual periods might be justified. Significant risk factors for developing breast cancer would make such a policy unreasonable (see Table 86.2). Mammography would be appropriate if the patient had previous benign breast biopsies unless a mammogram had been obtained within the previous year. If a previous biopsy had revealed high risk epithelial changes, the patient should be referred to a surgeon for possible repeat biopsy. If the previous biopsy was benign without epithelial changes or if a mammogram at that time revealed no worrisome changes, it would be reasonable to follow the lesion through one or two menstrual cycles.

Any patient with a persistent (1 to 3 months duration) discrete mass, compatible with fibrocystic disease, which has never been biopsied should be referred for surgical consultation. A mammogram need not be obtained before this consultation for evaluation of a breast mass. If the patient presents with complaints related to the breast not associated with a mass and any one of the following conditions exists, a mammogram is appropriate before consultation: (a) risk factors for breast cancer; (b) large, pendulous, breasts that are difficult to examine; or (c) absence of a baseline mammogram in a patient over 35 years old. Mammography, however, should not be obtained within a year of a previous study, regardless of presentation.

AGES 50 AND OVER

A patient with a mass very suspicious for breast cancer should be referred to a surgeon as soon as possible. Mammography is not necessary since a suspicious discrete mass will be biopsied, after which mammography can be obtained to search for multicentric or contralateral disease. A possible exception is the patient who desires biopsy and simultaneous definitive treatment based on the results of frozen section if the mass is malignant.

ALL AGES

In summary, the preferred treatment of discrete breast masses in the absence of a recent (less than 2-year interval) previous benign breast biopsy is excision of the mass under *local* anesthesia. If the mass is too large (greater than 2 cm in diameter) to be easily excised *in toto*, incisional biopsy is appropriate. A Tru-cut needle biopsy is obtained of the mass which is highly suspicious for malignancy. This type of biopsy results in less tumor spill and does not interfere as much as does open biopsy with planning the definitive mastectomy incision. A needle biopsy is *only* definitive if carcinoma is found. If malignancy is not found on the frozen section of the needle biopsy, formal excisional or incisional biopsy should be performed. Tumor tissue must be submitted at some time for estrogen receptor analysis (cancers with estrogen receptor sites respond better to hormonal manipulation) and if this is not done at the time of needle biopsy, some of the excised surgical specimen must be saved.

Simultaneous biopsy, frozen section, and mastectomy should be discouraged. Not only is frozen section analysis of breast tumors sometimes difficult, but many patients require time to deal with the realization that they have breast cancer. Problems with self-esteem, body image, and dependence are especially common at this time. By helping the patient take an active role in carefully weighing all the options of treatment, once a diagnosis of carcinoma is established on permanent section, her acceptance of recommended therapy is facilitated.

Needle Aspiration

The primary physician should not attempt needle aspiration of discrete breast masses. Even with extensive clinical experience, it is often difficult to distinguish solid and cystic breast masses. Ultrasound is being used increasingly (12) to help in this differential diagnosis. If the surgeon decides the mass is cystic, based on clinical or sonographic examination, he will attempt needle aspiration. This is accomplished in the surgeon's office by sterile technique, under local anesthesia. If fluid is obtained and the mass disappears, the patient will be requested to return in 2 to 3 weeks.

Before aspiration is attempted, the patient must understand that if the mass is solid, if it does not completely disappear following aspiration, if aspirated fluid is bloody, or if the mass recurs within 2 weeks, formal biopsy will be required.

Surgical Biopsy

It is important not only for the referring physician to inform the patient of the plan for surgical consultation, but also for the physician to state clearly the likelihood of the need for a minor surgical procedure. The patient will often ask questions about the biopsy before any firm decision has been made; yet she will be somewhat reassured to hear some initial information from her personal physician.

Preparation. Most biopsies can be carried out on an outpatient, ambulatory surgery schedule. Either local (preferred) or general anesthesia can be used. The patient should not eat or drink after 12 midnight on the night before operation.

Operation. Local anesthetic is infiltrated into the skin around the tumor, causing mild to moderate transient burning. Accompanying sedation can be given intravenously. A 1- to 3-inch (2.5 to 7.5 cm) incision is used to allow an adequate biopsy to be made and to be cosmetically satisfactory. The biopsy may remove the entire mass or only a segment of it. This should be explained to the patient, along with

reassurance that there is no ultimate difference to her health. In addition to the possible residual mass, there is often a ridge of tissue secondary to sutures and scar remaining after the operation. Removal of a large mass might necessitate a small drain, which is withdrawn in the office 1 or 2 days following the biopsy.

Follow-up. Ecchymoses or hematoma (5% of patients) and wound infection (1 to 2% of patients) are the two main complications of breast biopsy. A large hematoma may require evacuation, but this usually can be done in the office. Exercise and strenuous activities should be avoided for 2 to 3 weeks following a breast biopsy to guard against late bleeding.

The long term sequelae of breast biopsy are minimal; the only one worth noting is a residual mass secondary to chronic scar formation, which may cause some difficulty with follow-up examinations and mammograms. Detailed descriptions of this biopsy site must be noted in the chart by all physicians on follow-up, and details of the previous biopsy should be conveyed to the radiologist responsible for reading future mammograms.

FOLLOW-UP MANAGEMENT OF A BREAST MASS

Fibroadenoma

After excision of a fibroadenoma, the patient should have routine yearly follow-up, but should be seen more often if there are high risk factors for developing breast cancer. The patient should be reassured there is no increased risk of malignancy because of the fibroadenoma.

Fibrocystic Disease

Pathologists should be requested to determine the presence or absence of hyperplastic epithelial changes in any fibrocystic tissue. If there are no epithelial changes of concern, then the patient should be reassured that no special follow-up is necessary. Whether a patient will be told of the only slight increase in the risk of breast cancer associated with hyperplastic epithelial changes will depend on her personal physician. The physician, however, should at least stress the importance of breast self-examination *monthly*, a physician examination *twice* yearly, and periodic mammography according to specified guidelines. The likelihood of a breast cancer developing is remote; yet many patients aware of a slightly increased risk feel more comfortable having some control over their future health maintenance.

As mentioned above (p. 949), the pain associated with fibrocystic disease is often ameliorated once a cancer has been excluded. If pain continues, the patient should be advised to wear a brassiere both day and night. Many patients will try this on their own. A number of different drugs have been suggested to be helpful in the treatment of fibrocystic

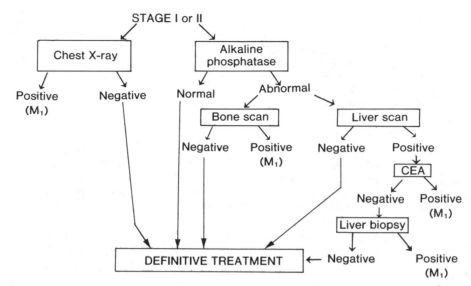

Figure 86.2 Clinical assessment of patients with stage I and II breast cancer. Negative = no evidence of metastases, positive = evidence of metastases, M_1 = distant metastases, CEA = carcinoembryonic antigen. (Adapted from R. B. Baker: Preoperative assessment of the patient with breast cancer. *Surgical Clinics of North America, 58:* 689, 1978.)

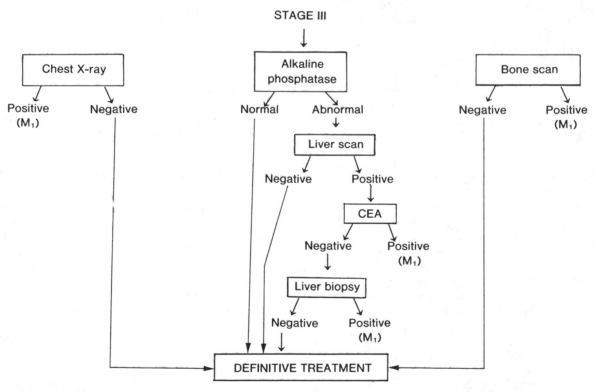

Figure 86.3 Clinical assessment of patients with stage III breast cancer. See Figure 86.2 for definitions. (Adapted from R. B. Baker: Preoperative assessment of the patient with breast cancer. *Surgical Clinics of North America, 58:* 689, 1978.)

disease (antihistamines, anabolic steroids, for example), but none has been shown to be clearly beneficial.

Cancer

If the biopsy is consistent with carcinoma, definitive staging and treatment should be instituted within 1 to 2 weeks. Once clinical staging (Table 86.1) is complete, appropriate studies are obtained. Bilateral mammography is necessary to identify multicentric or contralateral nonpalpable lesions. In addition, certain other studies are useful (Figs 86.2 and 86.3). It has been well documented that bone scans or liver scans in the absence of symptoms or of abnormal liver function tests are not useful in stage I or II of breast cancer. Although a bone scan is routinely recommended in stage III patients, liver scan is not.

The definitive treatment of operable breast cancer is variable; however, certain statements can be made regarding therapy.

1. Modified radical mastectomy (pectoral muscle remains) including axillary dissection yields similar 5- and 10-year survival data when compared with radical mastectomy.

2. The necessity of removing the entire breast vs. only the tumor-bearing segment is currently being evaluated in the National Surgical Adjuvant Breast Project. Because of the importance of staging, axillary node dissection is included in each protocol (Fig. 86.4). It is hoped that this study will determine the importance of multicentric lesions and the value of radiation in comparison to mastectomy in the treatment of patients with breast cancer.

3. Knowledge of nodal involvement is the best prognosticator of tumor recurrence (Table 86.1) and aids the oncologist in planning possible adjuvant therapy. Axillary nodal dissection is included with modified radical mastectomy since clinical evaluation of axillary lymph nodes is unreliable 20 to 30% of the time.

4. In the elderly patient (older than 70 years) with operable breast cancer, most surgeons would recommend total mastectomy without axillary dissection unless the axillary nodes are grossly involved but resectable. These patients are often at risk from other diseases, and estimates of tumor recurrence are not critical. In addition, postmenopausal adjuvant therapy has not been proven to be of definite benefit.

5. Inflammatory carcinoma of the breast is inoperable.

6. There is evidence that radiotherapy may be as effective as operation in the primary treatment of breast cancer (8). The physician may wish to advise his patient of this option, especially if she is extremely fearful of operation and of disfigurement. After radiation, the normal breast tissue does gradually atrophy, but, because the process is slow, patients have more time to adapt to the change.

MODIFIED RADICAL MASTECTOMY AND AXILLARY DISSECTION

The operation requires general anesthesia, and hospitalization varies from 1 to 2 weeks. Most patients are ambulating and eating normally within 24 hours of the operation. Rarely, early postoperative bleeding will necessitate reoperation (less than 1%). Skin necrosis at the wound edge and prolonged serous drainage are more common complications but still occur in less than 5% of patients. Limited skin necrosis requires minimal wound debridement by the surgeon and wet to dry dressings at home by the patient. Secondary healing occurs in 3 to 6 weeks. Serous fluid may accumulate under the skin flaps even after drains are removed, and may require aspiration under sterile conditions. Aspirations may be done in the surgical office and the patient suffers no long term sequelae.

In the early postoperative period the patient may be inconvenienced with arm and shoulder discomfort, but is able to use the arm normally within 2 to 3 weeks.

Since local recurrence (varies from 2 to 4% depending on site, size, and nodal involvement of the pri-

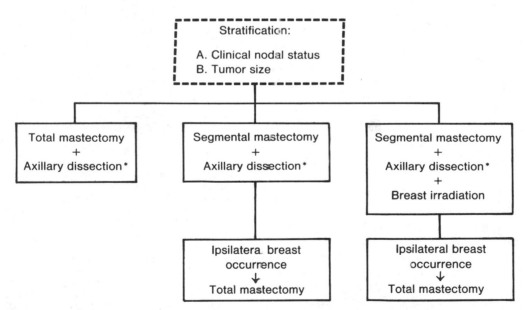

Figure 86.4   National Surgical Project for Breast Cancers schema. [*All patients with histologically positive nodes receive chemotherapy.] (Adapted from B. Fisher, C. Redmond, and E. R. Fisher: Clinical trials and the surgical treatment of breast cancer. *Surgical Clinics of North America, 58:* 723, 1978.)

mary) usually occurs within the first few years, close follow-up with physical examination is recommended every 3 to 6 months for the first several years. Chest X-ray, contralateral mammogram, and liver function tests are obtained yearly. Bone scan should be added for stage III patients or if symptoms occur. Liver and brain scans are obtained only for appropriate symptoms or signs.

Within 3 to 6 weeks of operation, most patients can be fitted with a breast form if skin healing is complete. These forms can be obtained in retail stores. Most hospitals have a representative from the American Cancer Society's Reach for Recovery program who is of considerable assistance in this regard. Breast reconstruction with subcutaneous implants is becoming increasingly popular. There is no contraindication to this procedure other than inadequate chest wall tissue to ensure a satisfactory result. However, the authors prefer not to recommend reconstruction at the time of mastectomy, but advise waiting a year, especially in stage II and III patients.

In 30% of patients following radical mastectomy and in 10% following modified radical mastectomy, lymphedema (pitting or nonpitting) of the ipsilateral upper extremity develops. Usually swelling is minimal in the mornings and increases during the course of the day. Typically, the degree of swelling becomes worse gradually over several years. Management (4) can usually be restricted to the following measures:

1. The patient should be instructed to sleep with her arm propped up on a pillow and to take special care not to sleep with her arm under her head.

2. When sitting, and as often as possible otherwise, the arm should not be allowed to hang down.

3. The patient and the physician should take care to avoid trauma to the arm. With respect to the physician, this includes avoidance of the use of a tourniquet or a blood pressure cuff on the affected arm.

4. An infection of the arm, no matter how minimal, should be seen as soon as possible by the physician and treated aggressively (see Chapter 24). (Cellulitis is the major complication of lymphedema.)

5. If the degree of swelling is great enough to be unsightly or uncomfortable, the patient should be fitted with a Jobst sleeve (available in Jobst outlets in most cities), which should be worn during waking hours.

FOLLOW-UP OF PATIENTS WITH DISEASE BEYOND THE BREAST

Metastases to Regional Nodes. Adjuvant cytotoxic chemotherapy, administered after mastectomy, prolongs survival of premenopausal women who have axillary node metastases. The treatment of postmenopausal women with adjuvant drugs is controversial (3) and is still being evaluated. Patients who have negative nodes have an excellent prognosis and have, for the most part, not been studied in this regard.

Treatment, which is usually given for 12 months, should be administered only by a medical or surgical oncologist.

Metastases Beyond Regional Nodes. Patients with metastases beyond the regional nodes present complicated problems and should be evaluated and treated by an oncologist. The role of the primary physician in the care of such patients is discussed in Chapter 8.

References

General

Bonnadonna, G and Veronesi, U (editors): Breast cancer. *Semin Oncol 5:* No. 4, 1978.
    An excellent up-to-date review.
Cooperman, AM and Esselstyn, CB, Jr (editors): Breast cancer. *Surg Clin North Am 58:* No. 4, 1978.
    A well-referenced series of monographs covering all aspects of breast cancer.
Donegan, WL and Spratt, JS: *Cancer of the Breast,* Ed. 2. W. B. Saunders, Philadelphia, 1979.
    An up-to-date in-depth review of breast cancer problem. Covers benign breast disease very well.
Henderson, IC and Canellos, GP: Cancer of the breast; the past decade. N Engl J Med 302: 17 and 78, 1980.
    A recent excellent critical review.
Townsend, CM: Breast lumps. *Ciba Clinical Symposia,* 32: 3–32, 1980.
    Concise review of the subject.

Specific

1. Bloom, HJG: The influence of delay on the natural history and prognosis of breast cancer; a study of cases followed for five to twenty years. Br J Cancer 19: 228, 1965.
2. Bloom, HJG, Richardson, WW and Harries, EJ: Natural history of untreated breast cancer (1805–1933). Comparison of untreated and treated cases according to histologic grade of malignancy. Br Med J 2: 213, 1962.
3. Bonnadonna, G, Valagussa, P. Rossi, A, Zucali, R, Tancini, G, Bajetta, E, Brambilla, C, DeLena, M, Di Fronzo, G, Banfi, A, Rilke, F and Veronesi, U: Are surgical adjuvant trials altering the course of breast cancer? Semin Oncol 5: 450, 1978.
4. Grabois, M: Rehabilitation of the postmastectomy patient with lymphedema. CA 26: 75, 1976.
5. Fondo, EY, Rosen, PP, Fracchia, AA and Urban, JA: The problem of carcinoma developing in a fibroadenoma; recent experience at Memorial Hospital Cancer 43: 563, 1979.
6. Foster, RS, Lang, SP, Costanza, MC, Worden, JK, Haines, CR and Yates, JW: Breast self-examination practices and breast-cancer stage. N Engl J Med 299: 265, 1978.
7. Greenwald, P, Nasca, PC, Lawrence, CE, Horton, J, McGarrah, RP, Gabriele, T and Carlton, K: Estimated effect of breast self-examination and routine physician examinations on breast-cancer mortality. N Engl J Med 299: 271, 1978.
8. Harris, JR, Levene, MB and Hellman, S: The role of radiation therapy in the primary treatment of carcinoma of the breast. Semin Oncol. 5: 403, 1978.
9. Mahoney, LJ, Bird, BL and Cooke, GM: Annual clinical examination; the best available screening test for breast cancer. N Engl J Med 301: 315, 1979.
10. Peacock, EE Jr: Management of benign disease of the breast. Am Surg 44: 626, 1978.
11. Shapiro, S: Evidence on screening for breast cancer from a randomized trial. Cancer 39: (6 Suppl) 2772, 1977.
12. Teixidor, HS: The use of ultrasonography in the management of masses of the breast. Surg Gynecol Obstet 150: 486, 1980.
13. Treves, N: A study of cystosarcoma phylloides. Ann NY Acad Sci 114: 922, 1964.
14. Upton, AC, Beebe, GW, Brown, JM, et al.: Report of the N.C.I.

Ad Hoc Working group on the risks associated with mammography in mass screening for the detection of breast cancer. DHEW Publication No. (NIH) 77-1400, March 1977.
15. Venet, L.: Self-examination and clinical examination of the

breast. *Cancer 46:* 930, 1980.
16. Wilson, RE: The breast. in *Davis-Christopher Textbook of Surgery,* ed. 11, edited by DC Sabiston. W. B. Saunders, Philadelphia, 1977.

CHAPTER EIGHTY-SEVEN

Diseases of the Biliary Tract

ROBERT M. QUINLAN, M.D., and CALVIN B. ERNST, M.D.

Diseases of the biliary tract are encountered commonly in ambulatory practice. Many patients will be discovered to have asymptomatic gallstones during the course of evaluation of another condition; others will be found to have symptomatic chronic cholecystitis. Less commonly, patients will present with an acute illness due to acute cholecystitis or to common bile duct obstruction. This chapter describes the cause, diagnosis, and treatment of these various conditions.

CHOLELITHIASIS

Epidemiology

It is estimated from autopsy studies that there are 10 to 15 million people with gallstones in the United States, but only about 2 to 3 million (20%) are recognized to have cholelithiasis—either incidentally or because they are symptomatic—during their lives. About 300,000 individuals, 2 to 3% of the total population with gallstones, undergo a cholecystectomy each year.

Ninety percent of gallstones found in patients in this country are cholesterol gallstones; 10% are pigment (bilirubinate) stones. The prevalence of gallstones is greater in women than in men and increases with age. In the United States 10% of men and 20% of women between the ages of 55 and 65 are affected (3). The prevalence of cholesterol gallstones is particularly high in the Southwest Indians of the United

States; for example, 70% of Pima women over age 25 have cholelithiasis (11).

Gallstone Formation

Bile is produced in the liver and excreted into the duodenum. Bile contains bile acids (primarily cholic, deoxycholic, and chenodeoxycholic acid), phospholipids (primarily lecithin), and cholesterol. The solubility of cholesterol depends on its incorporation with bile and phospholipids into a micelle. In the intestinal tract, bile salts are necessary for the absorption of dietary fats; they solubilize fatty acids and monoglycerides into micellar solutions. The fatty acids are absorbed in the jejunum, while the bile salts are absorbed in the ileum and enter an enterohepatic circulation.

There are three major types of gallstones that form in human bile: cholesterol stones (>70% cholesterol), mixed stones (50 to 70% cholesterol), and pigment stones (12% cholesterol). These stones probably develop in three stages: first, the formation of a supersaturated bile; second, the crystallization or initiation of stone formation; and third, the growth of the stone to a certain detectable size before crystals in the bile are expelled into the intestine. It is likely, but not clearly established, that one of these stages is more important in the formation of certain types of stones than in others. The formation of pigment or bilirubinate stones may depend more on crystallization and growth and cholesterol stones more on supersaturation.

CHOLESTEROL STONES

An alteration of the critical relationship between bile salts, phospholipids, and cholesterol can produce bile which is supersaturated with cholesterol and therefore predisposed to the development of cholesterol stones (10). At a low rate of bile flow, the ratio of cholesterol to bile salts and phospholipids increases, favoring supersaturation. Bile flow can decrease because of (a) excess loss of bile salts from the body (after ileal resection or bypass); (b) inability to synthesize normal amounts of bile acids in the liver (*i.e.*, the rare disease of cerebrotendinous xanthomatosis—characterized by xanthomatous deposits in the tendons, lung, and brain); or (c) from a faulty regulatory system which does not increase bile acid production in the liver appropriately when there is a decrease in the enterohepatic circulation of bile salts. If the enteroheptic feedback system is faulty, a diseased gallbladder which does not empty appropriately may trap bile salts and prevent them from participating in the enterohepatic circulation.

Once supersaturated bile is present in the gallbladder, desquamated mucosal cells, bacteria, parasites, foreign bodies, or other random crystals may provide a nidus for crystallization of gallstones. Growth of these stones may then occur, especially in a dyskinetic gallbladder, one in which contraction is impaired—such as in diabetes, celiac disease, or pregnancy. However, if there is normal enterohepatic regulation of bile flow, even with a sluggish gallbladder, bile salt excretion will increase with an eventual increase in the total bile acid pool and, consequently, less lithogenic bile.

PIGMENT STONES

Formation of pigment stones is probably initiated by supersaturation of unconjugated bilirubin in the gallbladder and common bile duct. Unconjugated bilirubin, like cholesterol, is relatively insoluble in water. An increased concentration of unconjugated bilirubin in bile results either from formation of unconjugated bilirubin from conjugated bilirubin in the biliary tree through the action of a glucuronidase (perhaps of bacterial origin, in patients with infected bile, see below) or from increased production of unconjugated bilirubin by the liver (*e.g.*, in patients with hemolytic anemia). Unlike the formation of cholesterol stones, a diseased gallbladder is probably not a factor in the formation of pigment stones.

Risk Factors

Since most patients with cholelithiasis are asymptomatic, it is difficult to evaluate risk factors precisely. Known risk factors for the development of cholesterol and pigment stones are listed in Table 87.1 (1).

CHOLESTEROL STONES

The demography of cholesterol stones probably reflects, in part, a genetic predisposition and, in part, nongenetic ethnic characteristics. For example, it is known that obese people, and nonobese people who eat a high calorie diet, secrete relatively more cholesterol into their bile than does the average person. Therefore, populations in whom obesity is common (*e.g.*, the Indians of the American Southwest) or who consume high calorie diets (occidental societies in general) are more susceptible to cholelithiasis.

Table 87.1
Risk Factors for Gallstones[a]

CHOLESTEROL STONES
  Demography: Northern Europe, North and South America more than the Orient; American Indians; probably familial predisposition
  Obesity
  High caloric diet
  Drugs used in the treatment of hyperlipidemia: clofibrate, cholestyramine, and colestipol
  Gastrointestinal disorders involving major malabsorption of bile acids; ileal disease, resection or bypass; cystic fibrosis, with pancreatic insufficiency
  Female sex hormones: women more at risk than men, use of oral contraceptives and other estrogenic medications
  Age, especially among men
  Probable but not well-established: pregnancy, diabetes mellitus, and polyunsaturated fats
PIGMENT STONES
  Demography: oriental more than occidental; rural more than urban
  Chronic hemolysis
  Alcoholic cirrhosis
  Biliary infection
  Age

[a] After L. J. Bennion and S. M. Grundy: *New England Journal of Medicine, 299:* 1161, 1978 (1).

The reasons for the increasing incidence of gallstones in middle-aged and elderly people are unknown but may be related to the time that elapses, first, between formation of supersaturated bile and formation of stones, and second, between formation of stones and recognition of them.

The influence of estrogens on the secretion of cholesterol in bile is reflected in the increased prevalence of gallstones in women (between puberty and menopause) compared to men (see above, p. 957) and in women who take estrogenic preparations compared to women who do not (see Chapter 90).

Finally, there are a number of ways by which the concentration of bile acids in bile is reduced, favoring the formation of gallstones: drugs utilized to treat hyperlipidemia such as clofibrate, cholestyramine, and colestipol (see Chapter 72) decrease bile acid secretion; and certain disorders of the gastrointestinal tract (ileal resection, Crohn's disease of the ileum, pancreatic insufficiency) reduce bile acid reabsorption.

PIGMENT STONES

The demography of pigment stones is entirely different from that of cholesterol stones. The propensity of orientals to develop pigment stones is not entirely understood, but it may be attributable to the higher prevalence of bacterial infection of the bile (usually *Escherichia coli* infections), and of *Ascaris* infestation, in the Orient compared to the Occident. In the United States, patients with pigment gallstones do not usually have infected or infested bile. The recognized risk factors in this country-hemolysis and alcoholic cirrhosis—are unexplained. Like cholesterol stones, pigment stones are more common with advancing age; and for the same reasons that may pertain to cholesterol stones (see above). Unlike cholesterol stones, endogenous and exogenous estrogens or obesity have no influence on the development of pigment stones.

Natural History

Many attempts have been made to study the natural history of gallstones among the 2 to 3 million people in this country known to harbor them. Thirty percent of these people are asymptomatic, having had gallstones discovered incidentally on abdominal film (10 to 15% are radiopaque) or during celiotomy for treatment of another condition. The other 70% are symptomatic: i.e., gallstones are discovered during evaluation of the typical or atypical abdominal pain of cholecystitis (see below).

It has been estimated that between 30 and 50% of individuals with "silent" stones will develop symptoms and 20% will develop complications of biliary tract disease: acute cholecystitis, pancreatitis, or jaundice (15). The risk of developing complications is unrelated to the severity of symptoms but does increase with the length of time symptoms have been present. Most complications occur only among symptomatic patients. However, 20% of the time acute cholecystitis is the first indication of cholelithiasis. If complications occur, they usually occur within 5 years of the discovery of gallstones. Common causes of death among patients not having cholecystectomy are acute cholecystitis, cholangitis with liver abscess, necrotizing pancreatitis, gallbladder carcinoma, and gallstone ileus with mechanical small bowel obstruction. In Lund's study of the natural history of cholelithiasis, 2.7% of the deaths among patients not operated upon were attributed to gallbladder disease (6).

The Asymptomatic Patient

It cannot be predicted, on the basis of the size, number of stones, sex, or age of the patient, which asymptomatic patients are likely to become symptomatic (14). Whether or not asymptomatic patients should undergo elective cholecystectomy, therefore, depends largely on the bias of the general physician and of the consulting surgeon. About 30% of patients become symptomatic (see above), sometimes at a point in their lives when operation is more dangerous because of age, intercurrent illness, or the presence of acute cholecystitis. The risk of complications of cholelithiasis, other than acute cholecystitis, is negligible in the asymptomatic patient. Carcinoma of the gallbladder is more common among people with gallstones but the risk—0.3 to 1% over a lifetime—is approximately the same as is the operative mortality from cholecystectomy. If the gallbladder is calcified,

risk of cancer is markedly increased, however, and cholecystectomy should be performed.

Over the past several years bile acids have been available—first chenodeoxycholic acid and then ursodeoxycholic acid—which reduce the concentration of cholesterol in bile and ultimately dissolve gallstones (4). Depending on the size of the stones, dissolution takes 1 to 2 years during which time 12 to 15 mg/kg of chenodeoxycholic acid or 8 to 10 mg/kg of ursodeoxycholic acid must be taken by mouth each day. These agents, although widely available, are not yet approved for general use. Ultimately they may become the treatment of choice for asymptomatic or mildly symptomatic patients who, because of their age or physical condition, are poor operative risks. Patients with cholecystitis (see below) do not respond to treatment with bile acids because the diseased gallbladder does not concentrate the acid sufficiently. Chenodeoxycholic acid, but not ursodeoxycholic acid causes diarrhea in approximately 10% of patients. Neither agent has been found to be hepatotoxic.

CHOLECYSTITIS

The hallmark of cholecystitis is abdominal pain, often epigastric at onset, but localizing within a few hours to the right upper quadrant. The pain is characteristically, but not always, severe and unremitting with only slight variations in intensity. Use of the term "biliary colic," therefore, is not precise because colic is defined as pain that waxes and wanes. Some patients describe the pain as heavy and aching; some, as knifelike. Occasionally it radiates into the right side of the back or, less often, into other parts of the abdomen. The pain usually begins abruptly, within 1 to 3 hours of eating a meal. Patients may also complain of being awakened in the middle of the night. Pain is often accompanied by slight nausea. A typical attack subsides spontaneously within 2 to 3 hours. The frequency of such attacks is extremely variable, from every few days to once or twice a year.

A patient who presents this history is very likely to have gallstones. However, the degree of inflammation of the gallbladder often cannot be determined from the history: there may be gallstones without any inflammation at all; there may be acute inflammation; or there may be chronic inflammation with fibrosis. The severity of the symptoms and the presence or absence of signs of inflammation and/or of biliary obstruction determine the physician's response (see below).

Acute Cholecystitis

PATHOPHYSIOLOGY

Acute cholecystitis is caused over 90% of the time by a gallstone which obstructs the cystic duct. Acalculous cholecystitis occurs primarily in patients who have sustained major trauma, including major operations, or in patients with emphysematous cholecystitis due to infection with gas-forming bacteria. Inflammation of the gallbladder in early acute cholecystitis is probably due to irritation by concentrated static bile. In some cases, as the process progresses, infection may play a role; bile cultures are positive in only 20 to 30% of patients during the first few days of an attack but, by 7 to 10 days, almost 80% of biliary cultures are positive. In certain patients, e.g., diabetics, mural ischemia might also play a role.

The difference between the presentation of acute and chronic cholecystitis (see below) is probably due to the length of time the cystic duct has been totally obstructed and to the intensity of the inflammation.

SIGNS AND SYMPTOMS

The pain of classical acute cholecystitis is severe and persistent. It is usually accompanied by nausea and fever (99 to 102°F; 37 to 39°C) and less often, by vomiting. Unless treated, the symptoms are likely to persist for up to a week.

The severity and persistence of the pain will usually cause the patient to call or see his physician (see Chapter 32 for a general discussion of abdominal pain). On examination, the patient is restless. There is considerable right upper quadrant abdominal tenderness, associated with involuntary guarding of the abdominal wall. This guarding, indicative of early peritoneal inflammation, is particularly important to recognize. It is not a feature of less acute disease (see below). *Murphy's sign*, the sudden involuntary arrest of inspiration (because of pain), when the examiner palpates the right upper quadrant during inspiration, is caused by the abutment of the inflamed gallbladder against the examiner's fingers as it moves downward with expansion of the chest cavity. This sign is more often elicited after several days of inflammation. In one-third of the patients, the gallbladder is palpable during an attack of acute cholecystitis, if the physician probes the right upper quadrant very gently. Occasionally patients are mildly jaundiced (see below).

LABORATORY TESTS

Leukocytosis (12,000 to 15,000 WBC/mm^3) due to a neutrophilic granulocytosis is common. Serum amylase activity may be increased, in the absence of other evidence of acute pancreatitis. Often, serum transaminase activity (SGOT and SGPT) is slightly increased as well. Twenty percent of patients have mild hyperbilirubinemia (< 4 mg/100 ml).

A TcHIDA or PIPIDA radioisotopic study is the test of choice in the diagnosis of acute cholecystitis. The study requires injection of isotope intravenously and evaluation of uptake of the isotope by the gallbladder. If the cystic duct is obstructed, because of acute inflammation, or because of a common duct stone, uptake does not occur. The test is performed in the nuclear medicine department of a hospital and takes 1 to 4 hours to complete. A positive study shows isotope in the biliary tree and in the duodenum but not in the gallbladder. A negative study shows isotope in the gallbladder as well. If isotope is not excreted, the test is uninterpretable.

DIFFERENTIAL DIAGNOSIS

The differential diagnosis must include those disorders which might cause severe right upper quadrant abdominal pain and, usually, leukocytosis and slightly abnormal hepatic function: acute pancreatitis, appendicitis, hepatitis, hepatic abscess, a perforated or penetrated peptic ulcer, acute pyelonephritis, myocardial infarction, and right lower lobe pneumonia or pleuritis. Because of the severity of the illness, these distinctions should be made in the hospital.

TREATMENT

The patient suspected of having acute cholecystitis should be hospitalized for observation, hydration, and further diagnostic procedures (see below, p. 961, and Chapter 32 for a discussion of these procedures as they pertain to ambulatory patients). If the pain is intolerable, the physician can administer morphine or meperidine parenterally. Since these drugs increase biliary pressure by causing spasm of the sphincter of Oddi, it is reasonable to administer 0.6 mg of atropine along with the narcotic to prevent that effect. The patient should be told that he will be fed intravenously, rather than by mouth, and that a nasogastric tube will be passed. Antibiotics may be administered, depending on the severity of the inflammatory response. If the temperature, white blood count, and pulse rate increase further and if abdominal tenderness and guarding increase as well, emergency operation will be required to prevent acute gangrenous cholecystitis and perforation. This progression of signs and symptoms occurs in 30 to 40% of patients. On the other hand, if the patient improves and the diagnosis is confirmed, elective cholecystectomy may be performed within a few days. A recent randomized prospective study which compared early and delayed cholecystectomy for acute cholecystitis concluded that the duration of hospitalization and the duration of disability were significantly reduced by early operation (5). Because of an increased likelihood of rapid progression of the disease to gangrene and perforation in elderly or diabetic patients (8, 9), cholecystectomy should be performed in these patients as soon as they can be prepared for it (assuming that they are considered able to tolerate an operation). Similarly, the presence of emphysematous cholecystitis due to gas-forming bacterial infection dictates emergency operation (air bubbles in the right upper quadrant on a plain film of the abdomen indicate the diagnosis).

A discussion of biliary surgical therapy and of the results and complications of operation is provided below (p. 963 and p. 964).

CHRONIC CHOLECYSTITIS

PATHOPHYSIOLOGY

Symptomatic chronic cholecystitis is associated with gallstones over 95% of the time; the remaining cases are due to other diseases of the gallbladder such as cholesterolosis (the appearance of macrophages laden with cholesterol crystals in the wall of the gallbladder—often without stones). Recurring attacks of relatively mild acute cholecystitis cause eventual fibrosis so that the gallbladder empties poorly. The symptoms of chronic disease, like those of acute cholecystitis, are due to obstruction by a gallstone of the cystic duct. In chronic recurrent cholecystitis obstruction of the cystic duct is relatively short (probably no more than a few hours) compared to the length of time of obstruction in acute cholecystitis, and therefore, inflammation is less intense. Chronicity of symptoms may also be related to gallbladder dyskinesia secondary to mural fibrosis.

SIGNS AND SYMPTOMS

Many patients who complain of biliary pain for the first time probably already have chronic gallbladder inflammation. The character and location of the pain are identical to those of acute cholecystitis. Pain is variably associated with nausea and, occasionally, vomiting. Unlike classical acute cholecystitis, fever is unusual with chronic disease. Typically, pain follows eating, beginning 1 to 6 hours after a meal (see above)—and lasts for 2 to 3 hours. Nonspecific symptoms—vague postprandial pain, bloating, belching, flatulence, so-called fatty food intolerance—thought by many to suggest gallbladder disease, are extremely common in the general population and therefore are not helpful diagnostically.

The patient with chronic cholecystitis usually seeks the physician less urgently than does the patient with acute cholecystitis. On examination during the attack, although there is tenderness to deep palpation in the right upper quadrant of the abdomen, there is no muscle guarding as there is in patients with acute inflammation. *Murphy's sign* (see above) is absent, the gallbladder is rarely palpable, and jaundice usually is not present. Between attacks, there is no abdominal tenderness.

LABORATORY TESTS

The white blood count, serum amylase, serum transaminases, and serum bilirubin are usually normal.

Unlike patients with acute cholecystitis, patients with symptoms due to chronic cholecystitis can be evaluated further in an ambulatory setting.

Oral Cholecystogram. The oral cholecystogram (OCG) is the mainstay in the diagnosis of gallbladder disease. The patient is given 3 g of iopanoic acid (Telepaque) in the evening after dinner and is instructed not to eat overnight; films of the abdomen are taken the following morning. If the gallbladder

fails to visualize, the patient is given another 3 g of Telepaque and X-rays are repeated the following day. The patient should be warned that he may experience mild diarrhea for up to a day after the ingestion of the Telepaque.

Approximately 75% of gallbladders are visible on the first dose and another 15% will become visible on the second dose. The test is 96% accurate in diagnosing biliary tract disease if either radiolucent stones are present in an opacified gallbladder or if the gallbladder fails to concentrate contrast material after the second Telepaque dose. Although, as stated above, 10–15% of gallstones are radiopaque and can be seen on plain film, confirmation of their location in the gallbladder should be obtained by OCG. The OCG is reliable only if the Telepaque is ingested at the proper time, retained in the gastrointestinal tract, absorbed from the small bowel, transported to the liver, esterified to glucuronide, and excreted by the liver into the bile. Therefore, gastrointestinal or hepatic disease may cause a false positive study.

Ultrasound. The detection rate for gallstones 3 mm or greater in diameter is between 89 to 96% by ultrasound with 93 to 97% specificity (3 to 7% false positive) (2). In a fasting patient, failure to identify the gallbladder by ultrasonography also suggests gallbladder disease. The advantages of ultrasound are that it exposes the patient to no radiation; it is much quicker (5 to 10 min); and it has no side effects. It also is not influenced by associated gastrointestinal or hepatic disease. Because of familiarity with the technique, however, and its lower cost, most surgeons still prefer OCG as the initial diagnostic test except in patients who are pregnant or who have concomitant gastrointestinal or hepatic disease. It is reasonable to perform ultrasonography in patients whose gallbladders fail to opacify by OCG and in patients with typical symptoms of gallbladder disease who have a normal OCG.

CT Scan. Computerized tomography accurately identifies gallstones 80% of the time. Currently, it has no advantages over OCG and ultrasonography in the diagnosis of gallbladder disease. CT scans might be useful occasionally, however, if both the oral cholecystogram and ultrasound are equivocal.

Upper Gastrointestinal Series (UGI). Many patients are evaluated with a UGI series in addition to an oral cholecystogram, especially if symptoms are atypical of biliary tract disease. Max and Polk (7) reported 250 patients who underwent cholecystectomy, 145 of whom had a UGI and 105 of whom did not. Of the 145 patients selectively chosen for UGI only 39 had positive findings. In only 7 of these patients was an associated gastroduodenal operation done at the time of cholecystectomy. Of these 7, only 3 patients had any new information added by UGI. Based on these data, Max and Polk suggested guidelines for selectively choosing patients who might benefit from a UGI (Table 87.2).

Duodenal Drainage. Patients with symptoms

Table 87.2
Suggested Indications for Upper Gastrointestinal Series in Patients with Documented Biliary Tract Disease[a]

Older patients (> 50 years)
Men
Previous gastroduodenal operations
Previously documented upper gastrointestinal disease
History of pancreatitis
History or presence of jaundice
Long atypical history

[a] After M. H. Max and H. C. Polk: *Surgery, 82:* 334, 1977 (7).

suggestive of biliary tract disease who have a normal OCG, a normal abdominal sonogram, and a normal abdominal CT scan may have biliary sludge or stones too small to be detected. In such patients, duodenal drainage, ordinarily done by a consulting gastroenterologist, may prove useful by identifying cholesterol crystals or bilirubin granules in the bile indicative of supersaturation. The test is performed by having the patient swallow a plastic tube with a double lumen weighted at the end by a mercury-filled bag. There are holes in the tube above the bag. When the bag has passed into the second portion of the duodenum (documented by fluoroscopy), magnesium sulfate is injected into one lumen of the tube to stimulate contraction of the gallbladder. Duodenal contents are then aspirated and the sediment is separated by centrifugation, and examined under a microscope. In the absence of hepatic disease (which may produce abnormal bile even though the gallbladder is normal), a positive duodenal drainage is highly suggestive of gallbladder disease.

TcHIDA or PIPIDA Scan. Radioisotopic imaging of the gallbladder (see p. 960) is useful in the diagnosis of symptomatic chronic cholecystitis if the patient is experiencing pain at the time of the study (*i.e.,* if there is acute inflammation of the gallbladder or obstruction of the cystic duct).

TREATMENT

The treatment of choice of chronic cholecystitis is elective cholecystectomy (see below). Patients who cannot tolerate an operation are candidates for therapy with bile acids to dissolve the gallstones (see above, "The Asymptomatic Patient"). Such treatment has not been approved by the FDA. Risks of not treating, surgically or medically, patients with chronic cholecystitis include gangrene and perforation of the gallbladder, choledocholithiasis (see below), pancreatitis, and, rarely, gallstone ileus (the obstruction of the small bowel by a large gallstone passed through an acute fistula which has formed between the gallbladder and the duodenum).

CHOLEDOCHOLITHIASIS

Epidemiology

Common duct stones occur in approximately 15% of patients with chronic cholecystitis, either before or after cholecystectomy. The incidence increases with age and length of time symptoms of gallbladder disease have been present. There are three categories of common duct stones: (a) concomitant gallbladder stones and common duct stones; (b) retained stones found in the common duct soon after cholecystectomy and/or common duct exploration; and (c) common duct stones identified long after cholecystectomy and/or common duct exploration. The incidence of common duct stones decreases exponentially in the first year after cholecystectomy only to rise again, reaching a peak at 3 years. In one study 26% of symptomatic common duct stones occurred 10 or more years after cholecystectomy (12). Also, patients with congenital agenesis of the gallbladder have a 20% incidence of common duct stones. These observations support the concept that common duct stones originate either in the gallbladder or in the intrahepatic or common bile duct.

Signs and Symptoms

Approximately 6% of patients with common duct stones are asymptomatic. More typically patients develop severe colicky right upper quadrant pain, often associated with jaundice, mild fever, and nausea and vomiting. The pain usually begins abruptly and lasts up to an hour. If nothing is done, attacks recur at variable periods of time. Eventually cholangitis will develop, manifest by persistent malaise and anorexia and intermittent fever, chills, and jaundice—associated with persistently high serum alkaline phosphatase activity. Suppurative ascending cholangitis characterized by right upper quadrant pain, high fever, shaking chills, and jaundice (Charcot's triad) is life-threatening and constitutes a surgical emergency.

On physical examination, if the patient is asymptomatic, no abnormal signs are elicited. If the patient is symptomatic, right upper quadrant abdominal tenderness and muscle guarding are usually present—similar to the findings in patients with acute cholecystitis. The patient is usually mildly to moderately jaundiced.

Laboratory Tests

Because of the acute onset of symptoms and the severity of pain in patients with choledocholithiasis, laboratory studies in the ambulatory setting are usually not appropriate. If such studies are done, leukocytosis and increases in serum alkaline phosphatase activity, serum bilirubin, serum transaminase activity, and serum amylase activity are likely to be observed.

Treatment

If common duct stones are discovered during cholecystectomy, they are removed. If the patient presents to the physician with severe right upper quadrant pain, tenderness, guarding, and/or jaundice, he should be hospitalized for further diagnostic studies and for treatment. If sonography or CT scan shows a dilated biliary tree, cholangiography should be performed. The patient should be aware that percutaneous transhepatic cholangiography is the likely procedure unless the serum bilirubin concentration is under 3 mg/100 ml, in which case intravenous cholangiography is possible. The patient experience during transhepatic cholangiography is essentially the same as it is during liver biopsy (see Chapter 39), except that the former procedure is done in the radiology department. Common duct stones must be removed, either by operation (see below), or, if possible, by endoscopic retrograde cholangiopancreatography (ERCP). (ERCP is performed only in the hospital, usually in the radiology department since fluoroscopy and X-rays of the cannulated duct are required. The patient experience during the procedure is essentially the same as it is during other kinds of upper endoscopy (see Chapter 32), except that ERCP usually lasts for 30 to 60 min and may be complicated 5 to 10% of the time by postendoscopic infection, especially if the common duct is manipulated, and by pancreatitis.)

BILIARY TRACT OPERATIONS

The general physician should be aware of the mechanics of biliary surgical procedures so that he can inform and reassure the patient who is to be referred to a surgeon.

Cholecystectomy

Elective cholecystectomy has a mortality rate of 0.5% or less. Urgent or emergency operation for acute cholecystitis associated with common duct stones in an elderly patient with cardiac and/or pulmonary disease has a mortality rate of 10%. The morbidity of cholecystectomy primarily relates to superficial wound infection (< 5 to 7%). Wound infection is more common if the operation lasts longer than 2 hours, if the patient is obese or diabetic, and if the patient has acute, rather than chronic cholecystitis. Other possible but rare (<1%) immediate complications of cholecystectomy are postoperative bleeding, postoperative bile leak, injury to biliary ducts (common hepatic or common bile duct), and overlooked common duct stones. A drain may be left in place for 24 to 48 hours after operation.

Cholecystostomy

This operation may be required in the patient who is critically ill from acute cholecystitis and who has associated severe cardiac, pulmonary, or renal disease which contraindicates the use of general anesthesia. Another less often cited indication for cholecystostomy is inability to detect normal biliary anatomy because of a severe inflammatory process near the main bile ducts. Rather than risk possible injury to structures in the porta hepatis, a cholecystostomy may be performed.

A cholecystostomy can be done through a small incision in the right upper quadrant under local anesthesia. A large drainage tube is inserted into the gallbladder through a stab wound in the fundus. The tube is brought through the abdominal wall and allowed to drain freely. An attempt should be made to empty the gallbladder of stones before placing the tube. If a stone is impacted at the cystic duct, future cholecystectomy will be necessary or a mucous fistula will persist after the tube is removed. If, however, *all* stones are removed, only 30 to 50% of patients will develop recurrent symptoms of cholelithiasis within 2 years after the tube is removed. The operative mortality is very high from cholecystostomy, not because of the operation, but because of the patient's critical condition.

Choledochotomy

Common duct exploration or choledochotomy, whether combined with a gallbladder operaton or as an isolated operation, has a higher morbidity and mortality rate than does simple cholecystectomy. The operation takes longer than cholecystectomy and patients are generally older, two factors very important in determining morbidity and mortality. Generally the patient will be hospitalized 3 to 5 days longer for common duct exploration than for cholecystectomy alone (see below).

COURSE AFTER OPERATION

Normal Course

The patient is usually discharged 5 to 10 days following an uncomplicated biliary tract operation. Skin sutures will have been removed and the patient will be allowed to bathe. Usually patients are requested to avoid driving and sexual relations for 2 to 3 weeks from the day of discharge. Patients are also advised to avoid heavy (approximately 15 lbs (7 kg) or more) lifting for 6 weeks. The incidence of incisional hernia (see Chapter 88) is very low following a right subcostal oblique incision, slightly higher with a vertical midline incision, and highest with vertical paramedian incisions. The patient returns to the surgeon's office for evaluation at 3 to 6 weeks after operation. The drain site and wound should be healed unless there has been wound infection. The patient should have been able to resume an unrestricted regular diet within a few days of operation without

Table 87.3
Frequency of Postcholecystectomy Syndrome (PCS) and Distribution of its Etiology[a]

	Bodvall and Oevergaard (1967)	Stefanini et al. (1974)	Hess (1977)	Brandstatter et al. (1976)
Number of patients with cholecystectomy	1930	800	919	—
PCS total	764(40%)	249(31%)	241(26%)	—
Mild PCS	660(35%)	317(27%)	—	—
Severe PCS	104(5%)	32(4%)	—	—
Etiology:				
Organic total	—	—	58%	66%
Organic biliary	9%	14%	4.5%	43%
Organic extrabiliary	—	—	53.5%	23%
Nonorganic total	—	—	42%	34%

[a] After P. Tondelli, et al.: *Clinics in Gastroenterology, 8:* 487, 1979 (13).

difficulty. Stools should be at preoperative frequency, and of normal color.

The patient should be expected to complain about pulling sensations in the area of the incision since the right rectus muscle has been divided and resutured. If the subcostal incision has made close to the costal margin, the patient will often complain also about discomfort on bending or sitting. The area just below a right subcostal incision is apt to be numb for several months because of interruption of a cutaneous sensory nerve to this area. Sensitivity does return, however, in the majority of cases. It is not surprising to find patients gaining weight after cholecystectomy, especially if they had lost weight preoperatively.

Postcholecystectomy Syndrome

About 90% of patients operated upon for symptomatic biliary tract disease become asymptomatic or have relatively trivial symptoms (occasional dyspepsia, for example). The other 10% may continue to be symptomatic either because they were treated for the wrong disease or because they have developed a postoperative complication. In the former category are patients who had gallstones but whose symptoms actually emanated from another disease (e.g., recurrent pancreatitis, peptic ulcer disease, angina, reflux esophagitis, or hiatus hernia).

Postoperative problems associated with the operation itself include retained common duct stones, an excessively long cystic duct remnant, and common duct injury with eventual bile duct stricture and recurrent pancreatitis.

Tondelli et al. (13) have collated data from a number of series on the incidence and cause of the postcholecystectomy syndrome (PCS) (Table 87.3). Mild PCS refers to symptoms of dyspepsia, constipation, diarrhea, and intolerance to certain foods. Severe PCS refers to severe upper abdominal pain, cholangitis, or biliary fistula. Organic biliary etiologies include retained common duct stones, papillary stenosis, bile duct stricture, cystic duct remnant, chronic

pancreatitis, or bile duct tumor. Organic extrabiliary etiologies include esophagitis, ulcer disease, pancreatitis, liver disease, heart disease, colon or urinary tract disease, and adhesions. Nonorganic disease includes irritable bowel syndrome and psychiatric or metabolic disease.

References

1. Bennion, LJ and Grundy, SM: Risk factors for the development of cholelithiasis in man. *N Engl J Med 299:* 1161, 1978.
2. Ferruci, JT: Body ultrasonography. *N Engl J Med 300:* 538 and 590, 1979.
3. Friedman, GD, Kannel, WB and Dawber, TR: The epidemiology of gallbladder disease; observations in the Framingham study. *J Chronic Dis 19:* 273, 1966.
4. Hofman, AF: The medical treatment of cholesterol gallstones. A major advance in preventive gastroenterology. *Am J Med 69:* 4, 1980.
5. Järvinen, HJ and Hastbacka, J: Early cholecystectomy for acute cholecystitis; a prospective randomized study. *Ann Surg 191:* 501, 1980.
6. Lund, J: Surgical indications in cholelithiasis; prophylactic cholecystectomy elucidated on the basis of long-term follow-up on 526 nonoperated cases. *Ann Surg 151:* 153, 1960.
7. Max, MH and Polk, HC: Routine preoperative upper gastrointestinal series (UGIS) in patients with biliary tract disease; a plea for more selectivity. *Surgery 82:* 334, 1977.
8. Morrow, DJ, Thompson, J and Wilson, SE: Acute cholecystitis in the elderly, a surgical emergency. *Arch Surg 113:* 1149, 1978.
9. Mundth, ED: Cholecystitis and diabetes mellitus. *N Engl J Med 267:* 642, 1962.
10. Small, DM and Rapo, S: Source of abnormal bile in patients with cholesterol gallstones. *N Engl J Med 283:* 53, 1970.
11. Thistle, JL and Schoenfield, LJ: Lithogenic bile among young Indian women; lithogenic potential decreased with chenodeoxycholic acid. *N Engl J Med 284:* 177, 1971.
12. Thurston, OG and McDougall, RM: The effect of hepatic bile on retained common duct stones. *Surg Gynecol Obstet 143:* 625, 1976.
13. Tondelli, P, Gyr, K, Stalder, GA and Allgöwer, M: The biliary tract. Part I. Cholecystectomy. *Clin Gastroenterol 8:* 487, 1979.
14. Way, LW and Sleisenger, MH: Cholelithiasis and chronic cholecystitis. In *Gastrointestinal Disease. Pathophysiology, Diagnosis, Management*, Ed. 2, edited by MH Sleisenger and JS Fordtran. W. B. Saunders, Philadelphia, 1978.
15. Wenchert, A and Robertson, B: The natural course of gallstone disease. Eleven year review of 781 nonoperated cases. *Gastroenterology 50:* 376, 1966.

CHAPTER EIGHTY-EIGHT

Abdominal Hernias

W. ROBERT ROUT, M.D., and CALVIN B. ERNST, M.D.

DEFINITIONS

A hernia is a protrusion of any part of the body from the compartment which ordinarily contains it. Most commonly, the term is applied to a protrusion from the abdominal cavity. The site at which the protrusion occurs defines the hernia further: epigastric, umbilical, incisional, inguinal, femoral, etc. If the protrusion can be pushed back into the abdominal cavity, the hernia is said to be *reducible*: if it cannot, it is said to be *irreducible* or *incarcerated*. If the blood supply to the herniated part is occluded, the hernia is said to be *strangulated* (all strangulated hernias are incarcerated).

This chapter describes the more common types of hernias and discusses the role of the general physician in their diagnosis and treatment.

HERNIAS OF THE GROIN

Inguinal Hernias

Inguinal hernias (Fig. 88.,1, *A* and *B*) are classified either as direct or indirect; the great majority (over two-thirds) are indirect. Direct hernias are portions of the bowel and/or omentum which protrude directly through Hesselbach's triangle (the triangle formed by the inguinal ligament inferiorly, the lateral border of the rectus muscle medially, and the inferior epigastric vessels laterally) to emerge at the external inguinal ring (Fig. 88.2). Indirect hernias enter the inguinal canal through its internal ring, lateral to the inferior epigastric vessels (the lateral boundary of Hesselbach's triangle), traverse the canal, and emerge also at the external inguinal ring (Fig. 88.2)

EPIDEMIOLOGY AND ETIOLOGY

Inguinal hernia is a common problem in ambulatory practice: it accounts for approximately 75% of all abdominal hernias. Approximately 85% of inguinal hernias are in men. At some time in their lives, about 5 to 10% of men in the United States will develop an inguinal hernia. Even in women, inguinal hernia accounts for more than half of the abdominal hernias. Although femoral hernias (see below) are much more common in women than in men, the most common groin hernia in women is an indirect inguinal hernia. Less than 10% of inguinal hernias in adults are bilateral when the patient is first seen. The chance of later developing a contralateral hernia is the same whichever side is affected first.

All *indirect inguinal hernias* are due to a congenital defect in which the processus vaginalis remains patent. Under such circumstances, a tract lined with peritoneum extends from the abdominal cavity into the scrotum. With time this may enlarge, and abdominal contents may herniate into it. Occasionally, however, only intra-abdominal fluid may gravitate into the scrotum, causing scrotal swelling while the patient is erect but draining back into the abdominal cavity when the patient is supine. Such a lesion is termed a *communicating hydrocele* and is more commonly seen in children than adults. The severity of the combination of a congenital abnormality and a predisposing acquired condition which increases intra-abdominal pressure (such as obesity, chronic obstructive airway disease, ascites, chronic constipation with straining at stool, prostatism with straining at urination, and hard physical labor) determine when an inguinal hernia develops.

Direct inguinal hernias are acquired lesions and are not only influenced by changes in intra-abdominal pressure but also by progressive attenuation of the inguinal structures as part of the normal aging process. Occasionally, inherited defects in collagen synthesis (*e.g.*, Marfan's syndrome) provide an obvious explanation for accelerated weakening of these structures.

Direct hernias are for the most part problems of the middle-aged and elderly; they are unusual before the age of 40. Indirect hernias, since they are associated with a congenital defect, are more likely to develop in younger people but these too increase in incidence with advancing age and are about 4 to 5 times more common after the age of 50 than before.

HISTORY

Most patients complain of a dull ache in the groin and of a bulge, either localized to the groin or extend-

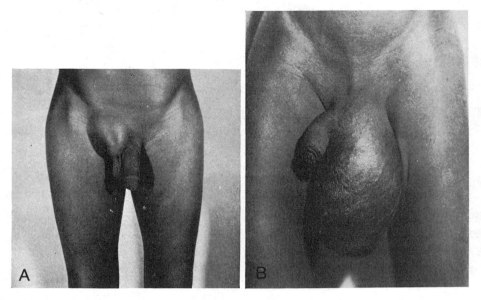

Figure 88.1 (*A*) Right inguinal hernia in young adult male and (*B*) left scrotal hernia. (Reproduced from L. M. Zimmerman and B. J. Anson: *Anatomy and Surgery of Hernia*, Ed. 2, p. 152, Williams & Wilkins, Baltimore, 1967.

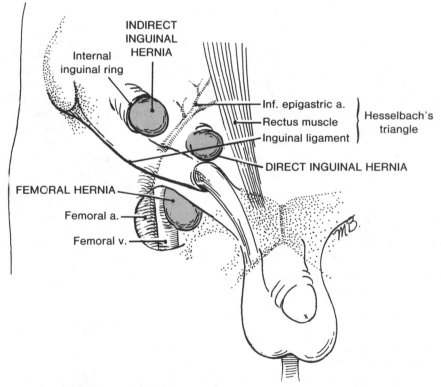

Figure 88.2 Artist's rendition of groin region illustrating femoral hernia and indirect and direct inguinal hernias. (Modified from J. E. Dunphy and T. W. Botsford: *Physical Examination of the Surgical Patient*, Ed. 3, p. 118, W. B. Saunders Co., Philadelphia, 1964.)

ing into the scrotum (in women, the labia are the anatomic counterpart of the scrotum). Sometimes pain precedes discovery of the mass by some months (perhaps because a piece of omentum has become pinched in the canal before the bowel has followed

it). Occasionally a patient will recall a short burning pain during straining, which represents the initial herniation. Often the patient, or the physician, notices the herniated mass, but no pain has been experienced. If the hernia becomes large enough, it may cause a dragging sensation when the patient walks. Small reducible indirect hernias may be noticed intermittently, at times of increased intra-abdominal pressure.

If a hernia incarcerates, it may become more painful, although many patients with chronically incarcerated hernias are pain-free. Indirect hernias have an approximately 10% chance of incarcerating; direct hernias incarcerate less often, although the risk seems to be greater than was originally thought. Strangulated hernias are always symptomatic: the hernia becomes extremely painful and tender; and nausea, vomiting, and fever (with granulocytosis) are common.

PHYSICAL EXAMINATION

The patient should first be examined while he is standing. An indirect hernia sometimes can be distinguished from a direct hernia by inspection: an indirect hernia, once it has entered the inguinal canal presents as an elliptical swelling descending toward or even into the scrotum (Fig. 88.3). A direct hernia presents as an isolated oval swelling near the pubis; it rarely is found in the scrotum (Fig. 88.4). If the hernia is visible, an attempt should be made to push it back into the abdominal cavity. If the hernia cannot be reduced, the patient should be asked to lie down and another attempt should be made to reduce it. Approximately 10% of inguinal hernias will be incarcerated when they are first diagnosed.

If the hernia is not visible, the physician's finger should be placed at the base of the scrotum and then gently advanced cephalad and laterally into the inguinal canal (Fig. 88.5). The external ring can be

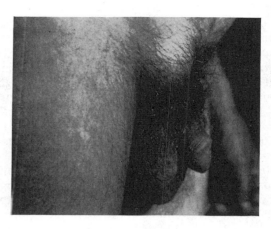

Figure 88.4   Direct inguinal hernia. Note medially situated globular swelling. (Reproduced from L. M. Zimmerman and B. J. Anson: *Anatomy and Surgery of Hernia*, Ed. 2, p. 154, Williams & Wilkins, Baltimore, 1967.)

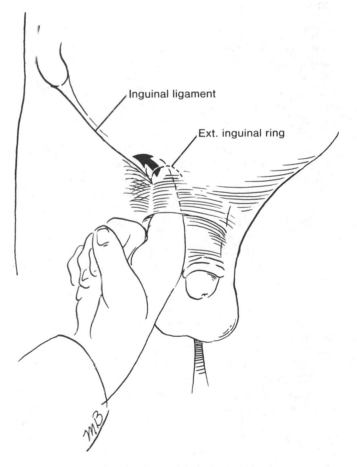

Figure 88.5   Examination of the inguinal canal. The examining finger gently invaginates the scrotum into the inguinal canal. (Modified from J. E. Dunphy and T. W. Botsford: *Physical Examination of the Surgical Patient*, Ed. 3, p. 116, W. B. Saunders Co., Philadelphia, 1964.)

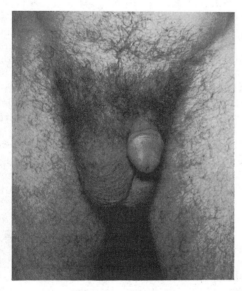

Figure 88.3   Indirect inguinal hernia. Swelling is oblique, cylindrical and extends into scrotum. (Reproduced from L. M. Zimmerman and B. J. Anson: *Anatomy and Surgery of Hernia*, Ed. 2, p. 155, Williams & Wilkins, Baltimore, 1967.)

examined without causing the patient a great deal of discomfort. The size of the ring, in itself, does not predict the presence of a hernia or the propensity to develop one because the external ring is an opening in the external abdominal oblique aponeurosis which does not contribute to the integrity of the inguinal floor. Further palpation will identify the crest of the pubic bone, the fibers of the external inguinal ring, the spermatic cord, and weakness in the posterior inguinal canal. When the examining finger has been directed through the external ring, having the patient increase intra-abdominal pressure by coughing or straining will cause a hernia to protrude and to be felt as an impulse or bulge at the tip of the examining finger.

Occasionally, contents of the hernia sac may be determined by physical examination: omentum may feel nodular and pliant; intestine, smooth and tense. Occasionally intestinal gas can be palpated as it moves through the bowel; also, a gas-filled loop of bowel may be tympanitic and on auscultation, bowel sounds may be heard within it.

DIFFERENTIAL DIAGNOSIS

An incarcerated scrotal hernia must be distinguished from other scrotal lesions (Fig. 88.6). One of the most common of these is a *hydrocele*, a tense, slightly fluctuant mass which can be distinguished from a hernia and from solid masses by transillumination (the mass is made tense between examining fingers and, with the room darkened, a flashlight is pressed into the side of it; light passes through the hydrocele, but not through other masses).

Another common scrotal mass is a *varicocele*, an enlarged venous plexus which on palpation feels soft and wormlike and which extends from the testicle up toward the spermatic cord. It does not transilluminate and, when the patient lies down, it collapses. If a varicocele is of recent onset in the adult, occurs on the left, and does not disappear in the supine position, one must suspect obstruction of the left spermatic vein (which enters the left renal vein) by retroperitoneal neoplasm or renal tumor.

A *spermatocele* is a localized but vaguely circumscribed mass which also does not transilluminate and which persists when the patient lies down.

Apart from distinguishing a hernia from another kind of scrotal mass, an important component of the physical examination is the examination of the testicle and its surrounding structures. In that way epididymal cysts, epididymitis, orchitis, testicular torsion, and testicular tumors can be detected. *Epididymal cysts* may be in any portion of the epididymis and may be smooth or lobulated; some of them transilluminate; they are innocuous and require no treatment. *Epididymitis* presents as a tender, swollen epididymis. The inflammation, if untreated, may spread to the testicle (orchitis); see Chapter 26 for a discussion of this problem. Frequently, elevation and immobilization of the scrotum will relieve the pain

associated with an inflammatory process. In contrast, the pain produced by *torsion of the testicle* is unremitting. Sudden onset of testicular pain in an otherwise healthy person is characteristic of this problem. On examination, the testicle is enlarged and exquisitely tender. The patient should be referred immediately to a general surgeon or to a urologist. *Testicular tumors* can involve the entire testicle or simply protrude as a small nodule from the testicular surface. These masses are more indurated than the common benign scrotal masses and usually lack the slight tenderness of the normal testicle. Patients with suspected tumors should be referred as soon as possible to a urologist.

MANAGEMENT AND COURSE

Almost all inguinal hernias should be repaired. Severe coexistent illness is the only real contraindication to herniorrhaphy (see Chapter 83 for a discussion of anesthesia/surgery risks in patients with coexistent medical conditions). Nonoperative therapy should be discouraged; the wearing of a truss is potentially dangerous and does not guarantee that a hernia will remain reduced. Also, the pressure of the truss on the margin of a large defect will eventually lead to atrophy of the fascial and aponeurotic (broad tendinous) layers causing the hernia to enlarge. Subsequent repair will be more difficult and, therefore, will carry a greater risk of recurrence.

Elective herniorrhaphy precludes acute incarceration (and strangulation) and the necessity to perform an emergency operation. If the hernia is chronically incarcerated and there are no symptoms of strangulation (strangulation is primarily a risk in acutely incarcerated, relatively small hernias), repair may still be scheduled electively. If the hernia has incarcerated acutely, the patient must be hospitalized and attempts made to reduce the hernia before operation. If the hernia is strangulated, an operation must be performed immediately.

If there are bilateral hernias, depending on their size, the type of repair required, the age of the patient, and coexistent problems, they may be repaired as staged procedures or at one operation. If the patient is elderly, and the hernias are large and require complex repair, herniorrhaphies should be staged, 4 to 6 weeks apart. Bilateral repairs of indirect inguinal hernias in children or young adults are routinely done at one operation.

One concern of the patient with a hernia is the type of anesthesia that will be administered. Currently, general, spinal, or local anesthesia is used, depending on the preference of the surgeon. Local anesthesia is becoming more popular; the patient is rarely uncomfortable during the procedure, and usually can leave the hospital within 48 hours (see below). Also, postoperative complications (atelectasis, for example) are less likely.

No matter which anesthesia is employed, certain *complications of herniorrhaphy* are possible (in about

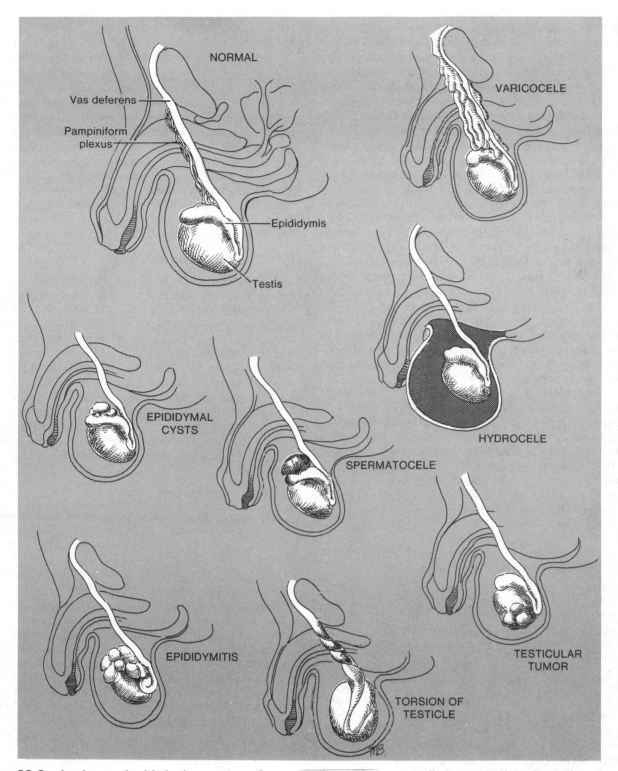

Figure 88.6 Lesions palpable in the scrotum. A correct diagnosis can usually be made if the normal anatomical relationships of the contents of the scrotum are borne in mind. (Modified from J. E. Dunphy and T. W. Botsford: *Physical Examination of the Surgical Patient*, Ed. 3, p. 111, W. B. Saunders Co., Philadelphia, 1964.)

7% of patients): urinary retention, wound infection, hydrocele formation, femoral neuritis, and, rarely, unilateral testicular atrophy. The general physician and the surgeon should discuss these complications with the patient before the operation and assure him that, if they do occur, they are usually treatable or transient problems.

When the patient is discharged from the hospital,

he is ambulatory and usually requires no more than codeine for relief of pain. The time of discharge is determined by the patient's response to pain and by his ability to ambulate. For the first 2 to 4 weeks, he is told to avoid lifting or straining and to use a stool softener and a mild laxative (see Chapter 35). The patient can return to light work (and light activity such as long walks) within another 2 weeks, but an occupation that requires heavy lifting or considerable exertion requires a total convalescence of about 6 weeks. Driving a car during this time should be discouraged, not because it is a form of strenuous activity, but because the patient, fearing pain or injury, may not react to crisis situations such as stepping on the brake vigorously enough or soon enough to avoid a collision. Sexual activity should be avoided for about 4 weeks. Resumption of normal recreational and work activities requires common sense. Most patients are fully rehabilitated and working 2 months following herniorrhaphy. Since recurrence may be related to premature untoward exertion, patients must be cautioned to avoid strenuous activity for 2 to 3 months. However, most episodes of recurrence result from wound infection or from operations performed with poor technique.

Approximately 1 to 7% of indirect and 4 to 10% of direct inguinal hernias recur. Over 50% of the recurrences will occur within 5 years of the initial repair. Unfortunately, the recurrence rate after repair of a recurrent hernia is very high, ranging from 5 to 35%. Apart from advising patients with a recurrent hernia which has been repaired to avoid straining and heavy lifting and to lose weight if they are obese, there is no special advice that these patients can be given.

Femoral Hernias

EPIDEMIOLOGY AND ETIOLOGY

A femoral hernia is a protrusion of omentum and/or bowel through the femoral canal (Fig. 88.2). It is the second most common type of abdominal hernia, accounting for 10% of all abdominal hernias. It is much more common in women than in men; 33% of abdominal hernias in women, but only 3% of abdominal hernias in men, are femoral hernias. The incidence increases with increasing age, presumably again because of the degradation of collagen and tissue attenuation that accompanies aging (see above, "Inguinal Hernia"). It is likely, however, that a contributing cause of a femoral hernia is a congenitally large femoral ring. Preperitoneal fat, forced through the large ring, enlarges it further. Increased pressure produced by straining or by pregnancy undoubtedly contributes to femoral herniation.

HISTORY

The primary symptom of a femoral hernia is a bulge in the groin. A dull pain may be experienced, but less commonly than in patients with an inguinal hernia. About 20% of femoral hernias incarcerate

(twice the rate of indirect inguinal hernias). The symptoms of incarceration and of strangulation are the same as they are in patients with inguinal hernias.

PHYSICAL EXAMINATION

A mass is often palpable, medial to the femoral vessels and inferior to the inguinal ligament. The mass is usually reducible, and occasionally it is tender. Despite careful examination, the hernia frequently is difficult to detect, especially in obese women, even if it is incarcerated or strangulated. Therefore, women who present with signs and symptoms of unexplained intestinal obstruction should be examined carefully for evidence of a femoral hernia which has strangulated.

DIFFERENTIAL DIAGNOSIS

A femoral hernia must be distinguished from an enlarged lymph node, a lipoma, a saphenous varix, and a direct inguinal hernia. The first three of these possibilities are not reducible. A lymph node or lipoma may not transmit an impulse to the examiner's finger when the patient coughs. A saphenous varix may simulate a hernia impulse, however, since increased venous pressure induced by the Valsalva maneuver is transmitted to the varix. A lymph node or a lipoma is more movable than a hernia; and a varix can be collapsed by compression of the saphenous vein. The distinction between a femoral and other groin hernias sometimes can be made only at operation.

MANAGEMENT AND COURSE

Femoral hernias should be repaired unless the patient is unable to tolerate an operation. The operative and postoperative considerations of inguinal hernia (see above) apply to femoral hernias as well. From 1 to 7% of femoral hernias recur; and, like inguinal hernias, 5 to 35% of repaired recurrent hernias also recur.

INCISIONAL HERNIAS

An incisional hernia is the protrusion of omentum and/or bowel through a surgical incision. Unlike the other types of abdominal hernia, a congenital weakness of the abdominal wall does not contribute to the development of the hernia. Any abdominal incision may be the site of a hernia. The major risk factors leading to the development of an incisional hernia are poor surgical technique, wound infection, and obesity.

The hernia usually presents as a bulge through the incision which may enlarge if neglected (Fig. 88.7) and may even lead to intestinal obstruction. It should be repaired soon after the diagnosis is made, to avoid the development of a larger defect which will complicate repair and will be more likely to recur. If possible, an obese patient should lose weight before the operation (see Chapter 73).

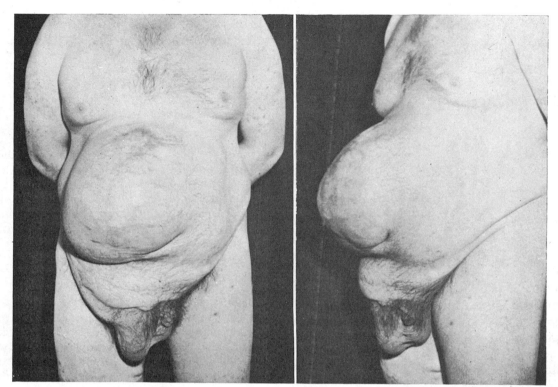

Figure 88.7   Large postoperative hernia after cholecystectomy. (Reproduced from L. M. Zimmerman and B. J. Anson: *Anatomy and Surgery of Hernia*, Ed. 2, p. 287, Williams & Wilkins, Baltimore, 1967.)

UMBILICAL HERNIAS

An umbilical hernia is a protrusion of omentum and/or bowel through the umbilical ring. These hernias are probably due to congenital defects. Among adults, they appear most often in middle-aged multiparous women, in patients with cirrhosis of the liver and ascites, and in old, malnourished, chronically ill people.

Most umbilical hernias are obvious as an enlargement of the umbilical ring with protrusion of intraabdominal contents through it. However, a few patients present with only the complaint of vague intermittent pain and tenderness in the region of the umbilicus. On examination, a small defect is usually found which contains a small piece of omentum, preperitoneal fat, or a knuckle of bowel. If the patient is placed in the supine position and is asked to raise his head and cough, the hernia can be palpated.

The most common complication of umbilical hernia is incarceration with or without strangulation. For that reason, unless the patient simply cannot tolerate an operation, all umbilical hernias should be repaired. Morbidity and mortality from such an operation are much lower if it can be done electively rather than in response to acute incarceration or strangulation.

EPIGASTRIC HERNIAS

An epigastric hernia is a protrusion of fat or omentum through the linea alba between the umbilicus and the xiphoid cartilage. A congential defect in the linea alba is probably the major disposing factor. Epigastric hernias most commonly appear between the ages of 20 and 50 and are 3 times more common in men than in women.

Most patients complain of a small painless subcutaneous mass, most often just to the left of the midline. Usually the hernia consists of preperitoneal fat or of fat of the falciform ligament. Larger defects also contain omentum and, sometimes, small bowel.

Complications are more common in patients with small hernias, because these are more likely to incarcerate. When this happens, there is usually local pain and tenderness and, less often, deep epigastric pain, abdominal distention, and nausea and vomiting.

Treatment must be individualized. Small asymptomatic hernias require no treatment; an asymptomatic hernia greater than 1.5 cm in diameter should be repaired. Incarceration of a small hernia is an indication for operation. The recurrence rate following epigastric herniorrhaphy is approximately 10% and usually can be attributed to failure to appreciate multiple defects in the linea alba at the time of the initial operation.

Reference

Nyhus, LM and Condon, RE (editors): *Hernia*. J. B. Lippincott, Philadelphia, 1978.
   The definitive text but directed primarily to a surgical audience.

CHAPTER EIGHTY-NINE

Benign Conditions of the Anus and Rectum

W. ROBERT ROUT, M.D., and CALVIN B. ERNST, M.D.

Anorectal disorders are often encountered in ambulatory practice. This chapter describes four particularly common problems—pruritis ani, anal fissure, hemorrhoidal disease, and perirectal abscess. Also included, because of their importance to the general physician, are somewhat less common problems such as proctalgia fugux and rectal prolapse. Cutaneous disorders that affect the perianal area, such as psoriasis, are discussed in Chapter 97 (Common Problems of the Skin). Venereal diseases as they affect the anus and the rectum are discussed in Chapter 26 (Genitourinary Infections) and in Chapter 29 (Syphilis). Inflammatory conditions of the rectum are discussed in Chapter 25 (Acute Gastroenteritis and Associated Conditions) and in Chapter 35 (Constipation and Diarrhea).

PRURITUS ANI

Definition

Pruritus ani, a distressing perianal itch, is a very common complaint, particularly in men. The intensity of the symptom is variable, but is usually greatest at night. Often the itching abates spontaneously only to recur after widely variable asymptomatic periods.

Etiology

Although the cause of pruritis ani is often unknown (50 to 75% of the time), the symptoms may be the manifestation of many anorectal disorders (Table 89.1). Whatever the cause, the itching is frequently associated with fecal contamination of moist macerated skin, often complicated by excoriation and secondary infection.

Diagnosis

Whenever a patient complains of perianal itching, the physician should obtain specified historical information and make several observations to aid in establishing a diagnosis.

HISTORY

A limited dietary history is important since an excess intake of milk, coffee, tea, alcohol, cola, and spices (especially tomato ketchup), may be associated with pruritus ani. It is important to review the drugs the patient is taking since medication, such as laxatives or colchicine, which cause gastrointestinal irritation, may be associated with perianal itching.

GENERAL EXAMINATION

The physician should examine the patient for the presence of a dermatologic problem such as psoriasis, scabies, or fungal infection (Table 89.1) which may be associated with pruritus ani. In addition, in women, a pelvic examination should be performed because of the occasional association of vaginal infection (see Chapter 91) with pruritus ani.

Table 89.1
Common Problems Associated With Pruritus Ani

DERMATOLOGIC DISORDERS
  Psoriasis
  Atopic dermatitis
  Contact dermatitis
  Lichen planus
  Condylomata
  Venereal warts
  Herpes simplex
  Tumors
DIARRHEA
FISSURES
FISTULAS
INFECTION
  Fungi and yeast (especially in diabetic patients) (see
    Chapter 97, Common Problems of the Skin)
  Erythrasma
  Scabies (see Chapter 97, "Common Problems of the
    Skin")
  Pinworm infestation—more common in children—*Enterobius vermicularis*
  Vaginal infections (see Chapter 91, "Benign Vulvovaginal
    Disorders")
OBESITY
POOR ANAL HYGIENE
RECTAL PROLAPSE
PROLAPSED HEMORRHOIDS (most often hemorrhoids are
  not associated with pruritus and other causes should
  be sought)

RECTAL EXAMINATION

With the patient in the lateral decubitus or the knee-chest position and with the buttocks separated, the physician should inspect the perianal area. During the inspection the patient should be asked to strain, a maneuver which may demonstrate prolapse or fecal or flatal incontinence.

Digital rectal examination should always be accomplished using a well-lubricated gloved finger. Evaluation must be gentle in order to avoid spasm of the anal sphincter which will preclude adequate examination. At initiation of the examination, the patient should be asked to bear down, which will minimize discomfort. Excessive pain should alert the physician to the presence of an anal fissure (see below). All structures of the anal canal within the limits of the reach of the finger should be assessed (the anus, the distal rectum, the prostate gland, the cervix.)

ANOSCOPY

After rectal examination, and without laxative or enema preparation, an anoscopy (with the use of an instrument that permits a side or oblique view) should be performed. A well-lubricated anoscope should be inserted gently, while the patient bears down to minimize discomfort. The instrument should be inserted slowly as deeply as possible. Then, after removal of the obturator, the rectum should be inspected using adequate light. Visualization is possible only through the side or oblique aspect of the instrument as it is withdrawn gradually. It is important to avoid rotation of the anoscope which will be uncomfortable and which may actually tear the anal mucosa. For adequate inspection of all quadrants of the anal canal, the instrument must be reinserted and withdrawn three or four times.

If skin lesions are identified, appropriate evaluation (such as a KOH preparation) to establish a diagnosis (such as *Tinea* or *Candida*) should be done in order to initiate definitive therapy (see Chapter 97). If no lesions are visualized, or if only excoriated skin or hemorrhoids are seen, the evaluation should include a series of three to five cellophane tape preparations in an attempt to demonstrate the ova of pinworms.

CELLOPHANE TAPE EXAMINATION FOR PINWORMS

This is easily accomplished by the patient at home or by the physician in the office. Swabs are commercially available (Pinworm Diagnostic Tapes; Parke-Davis), but they are also easily made by folding clear cellophane tape, sticky side out, over a tongue blade. Pinworms migrate from the anal canal to the perianal area at night where they deposit eggs. Therefore, the swab should be obtained first thing upon arising and before a bowel movement or before the perianal area is cleansed. The swab is placed at the anal verge and then the tape is stuck to a glass microscopic slide. A specimen obtained in this way will keep for several days. The slides should be examined under the low power ($\times$ 10) objective of the microscope searching for the typical ova of pinworm (Fig. 89.1).

Treatment

GENERAL MEASURES

Most patients with pruritus ani can be diagnosed and treated adequately by the general physician. Even when the evaluation is inconclusive, except for the identification of excoriation, symptoms can be controlled by relatively simple measures:

Tepid sitz baths for 15 to 20 min provide excellent temporary relief (for example, at bedtime). If used several times daily at the outset of symptoms, sitz baths may be sufficient to control pruritus ani. However, often the patient will find frequent sitz baths impractical.

Anal cleanliness is mandatory. After a bowel movement the anus should be cleaned with soft white nonperfumed toilet tissue (colored or perfumed tissue is potentially allergenic or irritative and should be avoided). If paper is too irritating, cotton swabs moistened with warm water or with glycerin may be used (cotton fiber is less irritating than paper fiber). Glycerin-witch hazel wipes (Tucks, available without

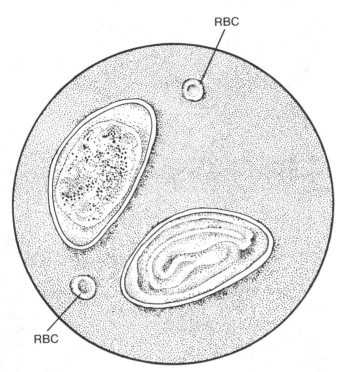

Figure 89.1 Appearance of the eggs of *Enterobius vermicularis* (pinworm). The egg is approximately 20–50 μm and typically has one relatively flattened side.

prescription) are helpful to cleanse the anal area. The patient should discontinue the use of these preparations if he notices intense burning, and use plain glycerin (available without prescription) instead.

The anal area should be cleaned once or twice a day with plain soap such as Ivory or Purpose or plain shaving cream and should be kept dry between times by the application of plain talc (such as Johnson's Baby Powder); cornstarch is not a good substitute as it may promote the growth of microorganisms which could compound the problem. At night, zinc oxide paste (available without prescription) may be substituted for talc. This should be applied thickly to the anal area and will absorb moisture and provide comfort. In the morning it may be removed with soap and water, mineral oil, glycerin, or with Tucks, or it may be reapplied in the morning and after each bowel movement.

The patient should use *cotton underwear* to provide better ventilation and avoid polyester clothing. Prolonged sitting, especially on synthetic materials (such as vinyl automobile seats) which prevent proper ventilation, should be avoided.

SPECIFIC MEASURES

If a rectal problem is identified during the initial evaluation of a patient with pruritus ani (Table 89.1), it must be treated (see below or the chapters on dermatology (Chapter 97) and on benign vulvovaginal disorders (Chapter 91) or the section on gastrointestinal problems (Section 4)).

When the pruritis is severe, commonly at night, the patient may gain relief by the temporary application of a minimal amount of *hydrocortisone cream*, 0.5% (available without prescription) or 1% (requires a prescription). Chronic use of fluorinated steroids should be avoided because of their tendency to cause atrophy and telangiectasias. Topical steroids will help the patient *avoid scratching* the anal area, reducing trauma and subsequent injury.

The diet, when found to contain foods thought to be associated with pruritus ani (see above), may be modified, at least on a trial basis. If a food is incriminated, the patient may find that symptoms will not resolve for 1 or 2 weeks after the diet is appropriately modified. Morever, the patient will note recurrence of symptoms usually within 24 to 48 hours after the reinstitution of an offending food.

Diarrhea and/or constipation should be controlled (see Chapter 35); stool softeners such as psyllium (Effersyllium or Metamucil), which are not irritating and which absorb mucus, a possible irritant to the sensitve perianal tissue, are preferred.

Occasionally these relatively simple measures do not provide adequate relief and it may be necessary to acidify the stool. There is evidence that in some patients with pruritus ani the stool pH is alkaline (pH 9 to 10) instead of slightly acid (pH 6 to 7) as it is normally. The stool pH may be measured in the office by using litmus paper or a urine dipstick after mixing some water with the stool specimen. If the pH is high, therapeutic acidification of the stool is indicated. Acidification may be accomplished with *Lactobacillus acidophilus* (such as Acidophilus, Bacid or DoFus, all available without prescription), 1 to 2 capsules 3 times/day or with malt soup extract (Maltsupex) available without prescription in powder, liquid, or tablet form.

Occasionally antipruritic sedatives such as diphenhydramine (Benadryl), 25 to 15 mg, or trimeprazine (Temaril), 2 to 5 mg, taken before bed may be helpful in controlling nocturnal symptoms.

Referral

Should a patient with idiopathic pruritus ani not be responsive to these therapies, he should be referred to a dermatologist or gastroenterologist.

Enterobius vermicularis (Pinworms)

Because the infestation is passed via the fecal-oral route and because the ova may remain alive on bed clothing for up to 3 weeks, dissemination of the disorder within families readily occurs. Once the problem is identified, all members of the household should be evaluated with the cellophane tape test.

The drug of choice to eradicate this infestation is pyrantel pamoate (Antiminth). It is available as an oral suspension (50 mg/ml) and is given as a single oral dose (11 mg/kg, not to exceed a total dose of 1 g). An alternative drug, mebendazole (Vermox), 100 mg, is given as a single oral dose; it should not be used in infants or in pregnant women. These agents approach 100% effectiveness in killing the worms and symptoms usually subside within 48 hours. The patient is no longer infective once the deposited eggs are removed from the perinal area and clothing by cleaning. Both drugs are well tolerated but may be occasionally associated with mild, transient gastrointestinal distress. Pyrantel pamoate may occasionally be associated with transient elevation of liver enzymes and its use should be avoided in patients with known liver disease.

Patients who have been identified to have pinworm infection should launder their clothing and bed linens with detergent and hot water on the same day that they have received oral treatment. All infected members of the household should be treated simultaneously. Reinfection is common and re-evaluation is appropriate whenever symptoms recur. Retreatment is necessary with recurring infestation.

ANAL FISSURE

Definition

An anal fissure is a painful elliptical tear, usually located in the posterior portion of the anal canal where the mucosa is relatively fixed. The problem is very common and is observed with equal frequency in men and women. Fissures can extend to the pectinate line (Fig. 89.2) from their origin at the anal verge. A primary fissure represents a tear in the mucosa which occurs because of trauma associated with the passage of a hard stool or with another similar insult.

Secondary fissures are much less common; they result from inflammatory bowel disease, infections such as syphilis, gonorrhea, or tuberculosis, or an anatomical anal abnormality, such as scarring that may occur after a hemorrhoidectomy.

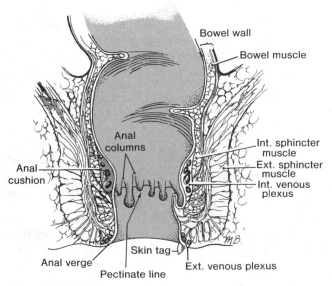

Figure 89.2   Important structures of the anal area.

Presentation

An acute anal fissure presents with the sudden onset of sharp rectal *pain*, especially during defecation and often is followed by a more dull *discomfort* which may persist for several hours (a symptom thought to be due to contraction of the internal anal sphincter (8)). A fissure may be associated with *spotty bleeding* usually noticed as red staining of the toilet tissue or as blood on the surface of the stool. Occasionally, *pruritus ani* is the major symptom associated with a fissure, in which case a mucus discharge is almost always present.

If the buttocks are gently retracted, thereby everting the anal mucosa, many anal fissures can be readily visualized, usually at the posterior margin of the anal verge. During this examination it is important to avoid inducing pain which will result in spasm of the anal sphincter, increasing discomfort and masking the findings. Occasionally anoscopy (using a side view instrument) will be required to identify the fissure.

If an anal fissure is identified, and if it is necessary to perform a rectal examination despite the presence of such a fissure (e.g., if a rectal cancer is suspected), a cotton pledget saturated with Xylocaine gel may be placed over the fissure before the examination. During digital rectal examination the examining finger should be pressed away from the fissure. If anoscopy is required, abundant Xylocaine gel should be used.

A chronic fissure, less common than an acute fissure, may be recognized by its indurated edges and especially by a collection of redundant tissue at the outer lip (the sentinel pile). If anal intercourse has been practiced, a venereal disease should be considered (see Chapter 29, "Syphilis," and Chapter 26, "Genitourinary Infections").

Either acute or chronic fissures may be associated with development of a perianal abscess, readily recognized as an area of intense inflammation and fluctuation.

Treatment

Many patients with an acute anal fissure can be made comfortable within a day or two and cured within 3 weeks by use of conservative therapy. Bulk laxatives such as Effersyllium or Metamucil should be taken as necessary to provide a soft stool. Irritant cartharties such as Dulcolax, magnesia, and cascara should be avoided as they exacerbate the problem. Once the fissure has healed, it is important for the patient to continue ingesting a high fiber diet and to continue using a stool softener as necessary.

Anal discomfort may be relieved by the use of showers or sitz baths for 15 to 20 min 2 to 3 times/day, followed by the application of 1% hydrocortisone cream or by the use of topical anesthetics such as Nupercainal cream, ointment, or suppositories or Perifoam aerosol (both available without prescription). Anesthetic agents may occasionally be associated with a contact allergy and should be immediately discontinued should the patient notice intensification of symptoms or a rash after their use. Topical steroids and anesthetics should be used only on a temporary basis (i.e., 2 to 3 weeks).

If after 3 or 4 weeks of therapy the ulcer has not improved or if initially the ulcer appears to be chronic (see above), the patient should be referred to a surgeon, because in these instances conservative therapy is not likely to be successful.

If the problem is found to be primary, the surgeon may perform an internal sphincterotomy often without having to remove the actual fissure. This procedure requires a 1- to 3-day hospitalization, is well-tolerated, and quite successful. After this procedure, patients generally return to work within a week, although minimal discomfort may persist for 2 to 3 weeks. Postoperative discomfort is controlled by oral analgesics and sitz baths. In approximately 70% of patients who undergo this procedure, there is a transient problem controlling flatus and some patients have mild mucus soiling. After internal sphincterotomy, there is less than a 3% chance of a recurrence of a primary fissure (6).

HEMORRHOIDAL DISEASE

Definition

A precise characterization of hemorrhoidal disease is not possible since the pathogenesis has never been elucidated. To define a hemorrhoid as a varicosity of the rectal venous plexus is too simplistic.

Hemorrhoidal veins provide one of the normal communications between the systemic and portal venous systems. These veins have the tendency to dilate and develop into a tortuous plexus. Anal cushions are part of the normal anatomy of the anal canal (Fig. 89.2). These cushions, which consist of hemorrhoidal venous and arterial plexuses, smooth muscle, and connective tissue, lie under the mucosa. The cushions apparently permit the passage of variable sized stools without disruption of the rectal mucosa. Hemorrhoidal disease is thought to be the result of displacement of these vascular anal cushions. The three cushions that are most likely to be involved are found in the right anterior, right posterior, and the left lateral portions of the anal canal (Fig. 89.3). Venous drainage from these cushions is into the portal venous system.

Many physicians classify hemorrhoids as being external or internal; most of the time the diagnosis of external hemorrhoids is incorrect. Often the term is being used to describe redundant skin tags at the anal verge (Fig. 89.2). A small plexus of veins at the anal verge communicates with the systemic venous system. Dilation of these veins is uncommon and is usually associated with an internal hemorrhoid; isolated thrombosis may occur, and it usually causes only minor discomfort.

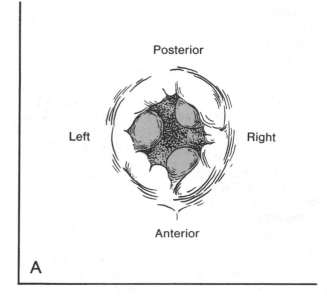

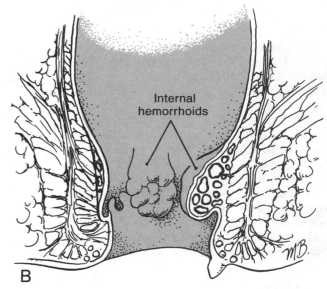

Figure 89.3 (A) Common sites of hemorrhoids and (B) protrusion of anal cushions.

A classification of hemorrhoidal disease is outlined in Table 89.2.

Pathogenesis

Internal hemorrhoidal disease (or piles) occurs when an anovascular cushion prolapses through the anal canal and becomes entrapped and congested by the internal anal sphincter. Prolapse is believed to be initiated by a shearing force produced by the passage of a large firm stool, from urgent defecation that may occur with explosive diarrhea, or with some form of partial obstruction of the anal canal. Increased portal or systemic venous pressure may predispose to development of hemorrhoids. This increase in pressure might occur from congestive heart failure, pregnancy,

Table 89.2
Classification of Hemorrhoids

EXTERNAL SKIN TAGS: Small discrete skin tags arising from the anal verge

EXTERNAL HEMORRHOIDS: Hemorrhoids arising from the inferior hemorrhoidal plexus exterior to the anal verge, covered by pain-sensitive skin

INTERNAL HEMORRHOIDS: Hemorrhoids arising from the vascular cushions, normal structures, lying above the anal verge, covered by pain-insensitive mucosa. Internal hemorrhoids may be classified further:

First degree. Hemorrhoids bulging into the lumen of the anal canal producing bleeding

Second degree. Hemorrhoids that prolapse during defecation but which reduce spontaneously

Third degree. Prolapsed hemorrhoids that require manual reduction

Fourth degree. Hemorrhoids that are irreducibly prolapsed

THROMBOSED HEMORRHOIDS. An internal hemorrhoid may prolapse and strangulate which leads to thrombosis, an excruciatingly painful condition. If swelling progresses, gangrene of the hemorrhoids with ulceration, local infection, or pylephlebitis (septic phlebitis of the portal venous system) may result

portal hypertension, or pelvic inflammatory or neoplastic disease. Straining at micturation because of urethral or bladder outlet obstruction or straining that occurs with lifting or defecation has been implicated in causing hemorrhoids. Carcinoma of the rectum may be associated with hemorrhoidal development because of straining with bowel movements and local obstruction of venous outflow.

Epidemiology

Asymptomatic hemorrhoids are present in half of the population over age 50, but are uncommon in individuals under the age of 25 to 30 except in women who have been pregnant. A more precise definition of hemorrhoids—one in which *symptoms* are associated with these normal vascular plexuses—reduces the prevalence to approximately 5% of the population over age 50.

Presentation

Asymptomatic "hemorrhoids" noticed incidentally during an examination should not be considered a problem and should not be treated. Symptomatic hemorrhoids result in pain, bleeding, and prolapse. Symptoms that follow persistent prolapse such as fecal soilage, mucus production, or pruritus ani, symptoms of localized infection or rarely portal venous infection (pylephlebitis) may also occur.

EXTERNAL HEMORRHOIDS

External hemorrhoids are covered by pain-sensitive skin. The most common manifestation, therefore, is pain, which results from thrombosis in the external

venous plexus. Pain is perianal in location and can be exacerbated by defecation. The patient may be aware of a tender perianal lump.

INTERNAL HEMORRHOIDS

Internal hemorrhoids are covered by pain-insensitive mucosa, produce symptoms primarily from bleeding or prolapse, and are only painful in the event of thrombosis or strangulation (ischemia caused by constriction of a prolapsed hemorrhoid) with or without associated ulceration and infection.

Bleeding. Characteristically the bleeding from hemorrhoids is intermittent, bright red, and spots toilet tissue or the surface of the stool. Occasionally it may be sustained and described as a dripping of blood. Rarely, massive hemorrhage may occur, particularly among patients with portal hypertension. Bleeding may also be occult; but because of their common occurrence, hemorrhoids should never be considered the cause of occult bleeding until other causes of gastrointestinal blood loss have been ruled out by appropriate evaluation. Gastrointestinal bleeding is fully discussed in Chapter 34.

Prolapse. Prolapse of internal hemorrhoids produces the sensation of fullness in the anal canal, especially after defecation. Usually prolapsed hemorrhoids will reduce spontaneously. Occasionally prolapse is more severe and manual reduction may be necessary. When reduction is not possible, prolapse may be associated with fecal soilage, mucus accumulation, and the development of pruritus ani.

Pain. Pain from internal hemorrhoids suggests thrombosis or strangulation and referral to a surgeon is necessary. Thrombosis and strangulation occur when prolapse of a hemorrhoid through the anal canal is followed by increasing congestion created by spasm of the entrapping anal sphincter. If the hemorrhoid strangulates, it may ulcerate and cause infection, which is usually localized or which rarely may spread through the portal venous plexus resulting in pylephlebitis.

Examination

Hemorrhoids are readily visualized by observing the anal canal in good light after the patient gently retracts his buttocks and strains as if having a bowel movement. This maneuver produces slight eversion of the anal canal and enables the examiner to see the internal hemorrhoidal plexus.

An external hemorrhoid will be seen as a mass just outside the anal verge and will usually be tender.

If the patient is in severe pain from thrombosis, strangulation, or ulceration, no further evaluation is necessary and urgent referral to a surgeon is appropriate (see below). If the patient is not in severe pain, a more thorough evaluation of the anal canal should be accomplished by anoscopy (using a side view instrument). It is important that this procedure be done carefully as described above (p. 973). Anoscopy is the definitive diagnostic procedure for establishing the diagnosis of internal hemorrhoids.

Sigmoidoscopy should be performed in patients with recent onset of symptomatic hemorrhoidal disease because of the possibility that sigmoid or rectal carcinoma has caused the development of hemorrhoids. The need for additional evaluation of the colon by barium enema, air contrast barium enema, or by colonoscopy must be determined on an individual basis; it is mandatory if there has been significant or repeated bleeding (see Chapter 34).

Differential Diagnosis

Several problems may be confused with hemorrhoidal disease:

Hypertrophied anal papilla (sentinel pile) occurs along the pectinate line (Fig. 89.2) in association with an anal fissure (see above), Crohn's disease, or without obvious cause. These papillae usually are asymptomatic and require no therapy unless they have become particularly large, eroded, or infected, or unless they bleed. Sentinel piles are easily differentiated from hemorrhoids by their location and by the absence of a vascular swelling.

Anal skin tags are very common. They appear as small projections of redundant skin external to the anal verge. They may be remnants of previously active external hemorrhoidal disease, associated with internal hemorrhoidal disease, or with Crohn's disease. They are of no consequence unless they are very large, bleed, or become infected or excoriated.

Prolapse of rectal mucosa is a problem affecting the elderly and probably results from similar pathogenetic mechanisms to those responsible for internal hemorrhoids, except that the anal cushions are small. Prolapse is identified by the abnormal downward displacement of rectal mucosa without evidence of localized venous swelling (see below).

Protruding tumors such as rectal polyps, anal carcinoma, or, in women, endometriosis can be confused with hemorrhoids. If there is suspicion about the diagnosis, referral to a surgeon or a gastroenterologist for evaluation and biopsy is appropriate.

Course

Without treatment, symptoms due to hemorrhoids usually resolve spontaneously within several days to several weeks even when thrombosis is present. Most patients, however, develop recurrent symptoms although the intervals between symptoms may be long.

Treatment

The aim of treatment is to relieve symptoms while permitting spontaneous healing; treatment does not necessarily reduce venous bulges although not infrequently they regress spontaneously. Most patients respond to conservative therapy:

Avoidance of direct pressure is essential in the relief of pain due to hemorrhoids. The patient will usually find a position which gives him relief. For persons who must sit (doing desk work, for example) a donut-shaped inflatable ring is usually helpful in preventing pressure on a symptomatic hemorrhoid.

Sitz baths or showers 2 to 3 times a day for 15 to 20 min on each occasion provide comfort.

Stool softeners are mandatory, if stools are hard, to reduce straining with defecation and to prevent evacuation of hard stools which may prolapse the mucosa. Bran-containing breakfast cereal and/or whole wheat bread help maintain soft stools. An alternative is daily ingestion of a bulk laxative-stool softener such as Effersyllium, Metamucil, Colace, or Peri-Colace (see also Chapter 35). Instructing the patient to increase fluid consumption, especially water, facilitates effectiveness of stool softeners. Use of stool softeners should continue even after the resolution of the acute problem as it may help prevent recurrence.

Topical preparations may provide relief of pain or pruritis. *Hydrocortisone-containing rectal preparations* such as Anusol-HC cream, Protofoam-HC aerosol, or Wyanoids-HC ointment (all require prescription) used 3 to 4 times a day may provide symptomatic relief. Cream, foam, or ointment are preferred to suppositories, which tend to be expelled or drawn up in the rectum, and therefore, have less local effect. One-half percent (available without prescription) or 1% (requires a prescription) hydrocortisone cream (generic) is also useful, but a rectal applicator may not be provided with these, as it is with the other preparations.

Analgesic rectal preparations are also useful when pain is prominent, but they may occasionally result in contact allergy. Preparations such as Nupercainal (available without prescription) or Xylocaine 2.5% ointment (requires a prescription) used 3 to 4 times a day may provide relief of rectal discomfort, particularly over the first several days when the discomfort tends to be most intense.

There is no acceptable evidence that Preparation H, which contains the antiseptic phenylmercuric nitrate, 3% shark liver oil, and "live yeast cell derivative" can shrink hemorrhoids, reduce inflammation, or heal injured tissue (9).

Bed rest for several days may help reduce prolapse and will avoid the exacerbation of discomfort associated with "upright" daily activities.

Systemic analgesics such as meperidine (Demerol), 50 to 100 mg every 4 to 6 hours, may occasionally be necessary for pain associated with hemorrhoids. Severe pain is usually associated with thrombosis, which may be more effectively treated by a surgeon by thrombectomy (instant relief of pain) as compared to conservative therapy (4 to 5 days before pain is relieved). Systemic analgesics such as codeine or meperidine may be associated with constipation; therefore, they should be used in conjunction with laxatives.

When to Refer

Patients should be referred to a surgeon for evaluation whenever there is doubt about the diagnosis (see above), if the patient does not respond within 1 or 2 weeks to conservative therapy, if pain is severe as may occur with thrombosis, or if there is evidence of strangulation, ulceration, or perianal infection. When uncomplicated hemorrhoids are recurrently symptomatic, the patient should be referred to a surgeon for definitive treatment.

The surgeon will evaluate the patient, confirm the diagnosis, and then consider several therapeutic options which are not normally provided by general physicians (10):

INJECTION OF SCLEROSING AGENTS (1)

The submucosal injection of a symptomatic hemorrhoid with several milliliters of a sclerosing solution causes fibrosis and retraction of the hemorrhoid. This procedure is ideal therapy for small internal hemorrhoids; it is simple, requires no anesthesia, and can easily be performed in the office (requires only a few minutes). There may be a period of several days during which the patient experiences a sensation of anal fullness. This symptom is usually well-tolerated or is easily controlled by use of sitz baths or showers 3 to 4 times/day and by mild analgesics such as acetaminophen or aspirin. After this procedure the patient usually requires no recovery period and can return to work immediately.

It is important that the physician peforming this procedure be experienced with its use. If the solution is improperly injected, severe pain, necrosis, and rectal stenosis may occur. Sclerotherapy is rarely associated with the development of infection, an oleoma, or an oil embolus. Injection of sclerosing agents generally provides temporary relief, but does not prevent the development of subsequent hemorrhoids. The procedure may be repeated several times. However, it produces an area of fibrosis and if repetitively used, may result in rectal stenosis.

RUBBERBAND LIGATION (11)

Rubberband ligation of hemorrhoids is a relatively simple office procedure used primarily for the treatment of mild hemorrhoids that have not responded to conservative therapy. The patient requires no special preparation and usually the only discomfort results from anoscopy required during the procedure. No anesthesia is necessary, although some surgeons administer a local analgesic before "banding." With use of an anoscope and a special instrument one or two rubberbands are applied near the base of one or two and occasionally three hemorrhoids which are at least 0.5 cm above the pectinate line. Constriction by the rubberband results in ischemic necrosis of the hemorrhoid, which eventually sloughs and is passed in the stool. Sloughing usually occurs between the 5th and the 10th day after banding and is associated with passage of a small amount of blood. Occasionally, bleeding may be massive and urgent reassessment by the surgeon is necessary to control the bleeding by electrocautery or by ligation.

Usually, following rubberband ligation of hemorrhoids, the patient is not disabled and has only minimal discomfort characterized by a sensation of rectal fullness, a symptom which is usually well-controlled by the use of sitz baths and/or mild oral analgesics such as acetaminophen or aspirin. If the rubberband is improperly placed below the pectinate line, the patient may experience considerable pain in which case reassessment by the surgeon is appropriate.

Following rubberband ligation the patient should suppress having a bowel movement for 12 hours. A bulk-forming stool softener such as Effersyllium or Metamucil should be prescribed to prevent straining. This will be necessary for several weeks and should be continued as long term therapy to prevent straining, which may predispose to the subsequent development of new hemorrhoids.

Complete healing after this procedure occurs within 4 to 6 weeks, after which the patient may be treated with further rubberband ligations if there are other symptomatic hemorrhoids. Banding provides good temporary relief of hemorrhoidal disease approximately 70 to 90% of the time. Mild symptoms may recur in as many as 60 to 70% of patients. Should there be recurrence, the general physician may treat the hemorrhoidal symptoms conservatively (see above) and if this is unsuccessful, rereferral to a surgeon may be necessary.

MANUAL DILATION OF THE ANUS (7)

This procedure is predicated on the belief that hemorrhoids result from partial anal canal obstruction necessitating increased pressure for evacuation of the bowel. The pressure is transmitted to the anal vascular cushion resulting in the development of hemorrhoids. Dilation is used occasionally in the United States and is popular in England. The patient requires general anesthesia with good muscle relaxation. The dilation is performed in an ambulatory surgery center or in a hospital. In the latter instance hospitalization is usually limited to 1 or 2 days. The surgeon manually dilates the anus up to the size of six to eight fingers. This disrupts the muscular fibers and relieves the partial obstruction. The procedure is well tolerated with only minimal discomfort of rectal fullness for several days following the procedure. Frequently there is a 2- to 4-day period of incontinence of flatus and occasionally of stool. After dilation the patient is required to perform anal dilation using a special device daily for at least 2 weeks and then occasionally for as long as 6 months.

Despite reports of 75 to 85% initial satisfactory results with anal dilation, the procedure has not been widely accepted. Complications occur because the dilation is not well-controlled and may be excessive, causing long term anal sphincter incontinence. Up to 25% of patients develop incontinence of flatus following dilation. Chronic postoperative incontinence tends to be highest in the elderly, especially in females with atrophy of the perineum. Rectal mucosal prolapse can occur. Recurrence of hemorrhoids, despite claims to the contrary, is quite common. If the anal sphincter is excessively disrupted, anal stenosis may occur secondary to scarring.

PARTIAL INTERNAL SPHINCTEROTOMY (2)

This procedure is based on the same logic as manual anal dilation: that relief of partial anal sphincter obstruction, which leads to increased straining during defecation thus causing the development of hemorrhoids, will cure the hemorrhoids. This procedure may be performed under local or general anesthesia and usually requires only 1 or 2 days of hospitalization. The surgeon divides portions of the internal anal sphincter. Following this procedure the patient is usually able to return to his usual activities within a few days and the associated local discomfort is usually short-lived and easily controlled by sitz baths and oral analgesics. The major complication of this relatively simple procedure is incontinence, which may occur in up to 25% of patients, but is usually minimal or transient.

Recurrence of hemorrhoids following this procedure is high and the procedure is inferior to rubber-band ligation in the relief of symptoms in patients with first and second degree hemorrhoids.

CRYOTHERAPY (1, 4)

This procedure is practiced in the United States by only a few surgeons. A freezing probe destroys the hemorrhoid, which in time sloughs off. Usually the procedure is done in a surgeon's office without anesthesia. After the procedure there is often an uncomfortable, profuse, foul smelling anal discharge which persists until the necrotic hemorrhoid sloughs off, which usually occurs on about the 14th day. At this time bleeding may occur and is usually minor. However in an occasional patient bleeding can be marked and will require re-evaluation with subsequent cauterization or ligation. After this procedure the patient is unable to return to his usual activities for a period of 2 to 3 weeks, primarily because of the anal discharge. Healing generally is complete by 6 weeks. Postoperatively, the patient is required only to take sitz baths and oral analgesics in addition to stool softeners.

HEMORRHOIDECTOMY

Hemorrhoidectomy is usually performed for treatment of moderate or large hemorrhoids. This procedure requires general or spinal anesthesia and the patient is usually hospitalized for 4 to 5 days. The patient is prepared for the procedure by taking stool softeners for approximately a week before the pro-

cedure and is given a laxative the evening before the operation. The purpose of the operation is to remove hemorrhoidal tissue and to appose the skin and mucus membrane. Usually postoperative discomfort is not severe and is easily controlled by sitz baths, oral analgesics, and stool softeners.

Following hemorrhoidectomy there is a recovery period of 3 to 4 weeks before the patient is able to return to his usual activities.

When hemorrhoidectomy is performed by an experienced surgeon, the complications of infection, fistula formation, fissure development, significant bleeding, or acute thrombosis of an external hemorrhoid occur only rarely (less than 1%). Minor bleeding is more common but is usually present during the first 2 weeks. Acute urinary retention following hemorrhoidectomy occurs in about 10% of individuals and may require the short term use of an indwelling catheter. Late complications of incontinence or of anal stenosis are quite rare. Skin tags are usually excised with the hemorrhoid although small ones may develop after hemorrhoidectomy and are usually of no consequence (see above).

Following hemorrhoidectomy the surgeon will usually evaluate the patient weekly for two to three visits until healing is complete and before the patient returns to work. The patient is seen 6 months following hemorrhoidectomy to be examined for the presence of additional hemorrhoids, stenosis, stricture, or skin tags.

Hemorrhoidectomy offers the best chance of long term control with less than a 5% late recurrence rate. Its use is limited because of the associated short term morbidity and the observation that many hemorrhoids can be eliminated by less traumatic procedures.

Special Considerations

Because of an increased rate of complications associated with operative procedures in individuals with severe congestive *heart failure or debilitating disease*, the treatment of hemorrhoids in these patients should be as conservative as possible. Patients who have *portal hypertension* present a special risk because of the frequent association of a coagulopathy and because operative hemorroidectomy in a few instances can diminish shunting between the portal and systemic systems and result in a rise in portal pressure which on occasion may be associated with esophageal or gastric variceal bleeding.

Hemorrhoids are very common in *pregnancy* and are best managed conservatively. They frequently resolve spontaneously after delivery. Occasionally, development of strangulated hemorrhoids requires surgical evaluation during the pregnancy. Patients with *inflammatory bowel disease* and hemorrhoidal disease should be managed in consultation with a gastroenterologist and a surgeon.

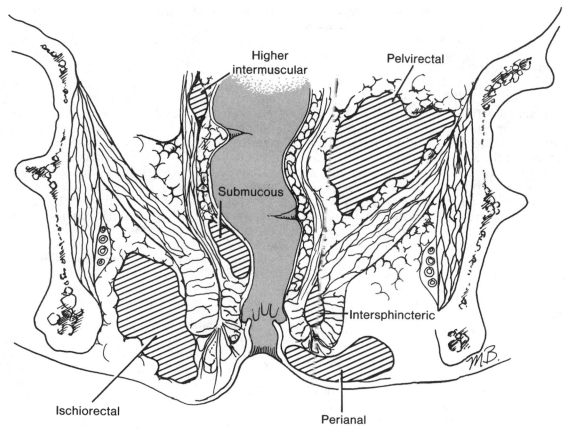

Figure 89.4   Anatomic classification of common anorectal abscesses.

ANORECTAL ABSCESSES AND ANORECTAL FISTULA

Definition

An anorectal abscess is an abscess involving the perineum and perianal structures. Abscesses are classified by their anatomic location (Fig. 89.4). *Low intramuscular or perianal abscesses* are located in the subcutaneous tissue immediately surrounding the anus, which is the site of 50 to 75% of all anorectal abscesses. An *ischiorectal abscess* is located in the ischiorectal fossa, a fat-filled space present between the levator ani (external anal sphincter) and the ischial tuberosity, and accounts for 20 to 40% of anorectal abscesses. *Intersphincteric, high intermuscular, pelvirectal,* and *submucosal abscesses* are far less common and account for about 10% of all abscesses. Anorectal abscesses are common, and the general physician should be familiar with presentation of such an abscess so that patients suspected of having this problem are promptly referred to a surgeon. Most anorectal abscesses are associated with anal fistulas. Occasionally, anorectal abscesses occur in association with other anal and perianal disorders (Table 89.3).

An *anal fistula* (fistula-in-ano) is a tract lined by

Table 89.3
Secondary Causes of Anorectal Abscess and Fistula-in-Ano

INFLAMMATORY BOWEL DISEASE
CHRONIC SPECIFIC INFECTIONS (uncommon)
   Actinomycosis
   Tuberculosis
   Lymphogranuloma venereum
   Schistosomiasis (rare)
   Amebiasis (rare)
INFECTION ANATOMICALLY ADJACENT TO THE RECTAL
   AREA AND PRESENTING AS ANORECTAL ABSCESS
   OR FISTULA-IN-ANO
   In women:
      Pelvic inflammatory disease
      Bartholin gland abscess
   In men:
      Infections of a Cowper gland (small periurethral glands)
      Pilonidal sinus (occasionally occurs in females)
FOREIGN BODY (*e.g.,* an ingested bone or a penetrating
   wooden splinter)
TRAUMA
   Surgery (*e.g.,* hemorrhoidectomy or prostatectomy)
   Radiation
   Laceration (*e.g.,* from an enema)
ABNORMALITIES OF HOST DEFENSE (*e.g.,* bone marrow
   aplasia, leukemia or lymphoma, diabetes)
CARCINOMA OF ANUS OR RECTUM

granulation tissue having an internal opening in the anal canal and an external opening in the perianal skin. The internal opening is usually located in one of the anal crypts. If only one opening is identifiable, it is termed an *anorectal sinus*.

Etiology

Anorectal abscesses are more common in men. Most often they represent a primary bacterial infection of anal glands and ducts. Anal glands, thought to be diverticula of the anal canal mucosa, are located along the pectinate line. Many of these glands pass through the internal sphincter into the intersphincteric space. Muscle tone in the internal sphincter prevents discharge from the glands causing stasis, dilation, and eventual infection. Bacterial cultures from the abscesses frequently isolate *Staphylococcus aureus*, *Escherichia coli*, *Bacteroids* species, *Proteus* species, *Streptococcus* species, or a mixed flora. Since anal glands in the adult are concentrated more in the anterior and posterior walls of the anus, abscesses and fistulas tend to occur in these areas also. The majority of abscesses are located in the posterior rectal wall.

Most anal fistulas result from abscess formation and drainage through the perianal skin. Therefore, bacterial flora of fistulas are similar to those of abscesses. Some fistulas are not pyogenic in origin and are associated with inflammatory bowel disease or tuberculosis. Fistulas that do not originate in anal crypts may result from diverticular disease, neoplastic disease, or trauma.

Diagnosis

HISTORY

Most commonly, a patient with an anorectal abscess will describe an abrupt onset of perianal pain described as full or throbbing and often intensified by sitting, walking, coughing, or defecating. Systemic symptoms are frequently present and include malaise, chills, and fever. Most patients will have a marked leukocytosis. If the abscess has opened, the patient may complain of a mucopurulent discharge and/or a small amount of blood staining the stool and toilet paper.

An uncomplicated anal fistula may create only minor complaints. The most common symptom is painful perianal swelling. The swelling is frequently intermittent and intensity of the discomfort is variable. Often the patient complains of purulent anal discharge. A high intrasmuscular fistula can cause tenesmus or pain during defecation. An anterior fistula in a female can cause dyspareunia.

RECTAL EXAMINATION

A perianal abscess is easily recognized as a warm, tender, subcutaneous swelling located adjacent to the anus. An ischiorectal abscess may be identified by fluctuation in the ischiorectal fossa felt only on digital rectal examination. Often there is only tenderness detected by pressure to the skin overlying the ischiorectal fossa or the lateral wall of the anal canal during a rectal examination. Higher anorectal abscesses may present few or no findings on perianal examination. However, many of these individuals will complain of severe pain, pyrexia, and exhibit a marked leukocytosis. Under such circumstances, digital examination of the anal canal usually reveals a high, exquisitely tender, posterior rectal wall mass.

The diagnosis of a rectal fistula is established by inspection and palpation of the perianal area and performance of a digital rectal examination. Frequently the external opening of the fistula in the perianal area can be seen. Digital examination of the rectum may enable identification of the indurated tract of the fistula as it transverses to its internal opening. Anoscopy is required to identify the internal opening.

Treatment

Identification or suspicion of an anorectal abscess with or without a fistula-in-ano should lead the physician to arrange for an urgent referral to a surgeon. If there is a history of inflammatory bowel disease, a gastroenterologist should also be consulted because of the complexity in the management of these patients.

Without adequate drainage an abscess will progress, cause systemic infection, and can rupture spontaneously either externally or internally into deeper areas of the pelvis. An anorectal abscess may also be associated with a rapidly spreading necrotizing infection destroying large areas of skin, subcutaneous tissue, and fascia. Patients with coincident diabetes mellitus are particularly vulnerable to complicated extensive perirectal involvement.

If possible, the surgeon will open and remove the fistulous tract during the drainage procedure. If simple incision and drainage of an anorectal abscess are performed, greater than 50% of patients will present postoperatively with a fistula-in-ano. If a fistulectomy is performed at the time of drainage, recurrence is uncommon. In the unusual event of a recurrence, referral to the surgeon is again appropriate. Most fistulas require excision. Both internal and external openings must be excised and the tract must be converted into an open wound and the granulation tissue excised or curetted.

The average hospital stay after drainage of an abscess and/or fistulectomy is 6 days; however, the wound can take 5 to 12 weeks to heal.

PROCTALGIA FUGAX

Occasionally healthy young adults develop the sudden onset of severe rectal pain, variably intermittent and generally lasting less than 30 min to 1 hour—proctalgia fugax. It frequently will awaken a patient at night. In women it can occur after sexual intercourse. The pain is described usually as a spasm or a cramp. The problem is not associated with systemic illness and the etiology is uncertain. Proctalgia fugax is thought to result from spasm of a portion of the levator ani muscle (3). Patients with proctalgia fugax may obtain relief by taking a hot sitz bath or by applying pressure in the perianal area near the site of the discomfort. Occasionally if the attacks are severe and frequent, the patient may find relief by the use of sublingual or cutaneous nitrates. The problem usually persists for many years but then disappears in later life.

RECTAL PROLAPSE (5)

Definition

This problem is occasionally encountered by the general physician who should be able to recognize it and evaluate the need for referral to a surgeon. Prolapse is a protrusion of the rectum through the anus. The protrusion can contain only mucosa, a mucosal prolapse, or it may contain all layers of the bowel wall, a full thickness prolapse (procidentia).

Etiology

Prolapse is more prevalent in women (approximately 80% of the cases) with a peak incidence between the ages of 60 and 80. In men the peak incidence occurs at about the age of 40. The exact pathogenic mechanism of this disease is not known. Factors that are associated with this disease are multiple. Weakening of fascial attachments of the rectum, attenuated muscles in the perirectal area and pelvic diaphragm, straining due to chronic constipation, and even congenital fascial defects all lead to the development of rectal prolapse. Prolapse is often observed after severe chronic diarrhea.

Diagnosis

HISTORY

Patients have variable symptoms, depending upon the degree of prolapse. There is always some incontinence; at first it is intermittent and consists only of liquid stool. Incontinence is associated with increased intra-abdominal pressure associated with coughing or sneezing. Prolapse will always progress and eventually the incontinence will become continuous. The patient may complain of a sensation of displaced tissue at the time of defecation. Since prolapse is often intermittent, most patients learn to reduce the prolapsed tissues. The patient often may complain of a sensation of inadequate evacuation of the bowel. With more profound prolapse the patient may complain of tenesmus and also develop a continuous mucous discharge. The prolapsed rectum will almost always become excoriated and ulcerated, leading many patients to complain of bleeding. In instances of advanced degree of prolapse the patient may suffer

urinary incontinence and in the female there may be associated uterine prolapse. Patients with increasing degrees of prolapse suffer from considerable embarrassment and subsequently will avoid social contact.

EXAMINATION

The physician will best recognize rectal prolapse by inspecting the anus when the patient strains in a squatting position. It is usually best to anticipate incontinence with this maneuver. If the prolapse is full thickness (procidentia), concentric folds of the rectal mucosa will be seen, while if there is only mucosal prolapse, only radial folds are seen. Digital examination will almost always reveal a patulous and relaxed anal sphincter which often will admit two to four fingers. Palpation of the protruding tissue between the examiner's fingers will provide the sensation of only mucosa in mucosal prolapse and a double layer of bowel wall in full thickness prolapse. The rectal examination in patients with prolapse is usually associated with minimal if any discomfort.

Occasionally prolapsed hemorrhoids may be confused with rectal prolapse, but absence of concentric or radial folds of mucosa and the prominent location of prolapsed hemorrhoids in the left lateral or right anterior or right posterior edges of the anus suggest the proper diagnosis (Fig. 89.3, p. 976). On occasion a prolapse may be associated with a rectal tumor. For that reason a sigmoidoscopy should be performed on any patient with rectal prolapse.

Treatment

When the prolapse is small and limited to the mucosa, the patient may benefit from the use of stool softeners and by use of an irritant rectal suppository (see Chapter 35) to initiate defecation and thereby avoid straining at stool. If prolapse progresses despite this treatment or if extensive mucosal prolapse is noted, it is appropriate to refer the patient to a surgeon. Redundant tissue may be treated either by banding or sclerosis. Both procedures can usually be performed in the surgeon's office under local anesthesia and are usually successful in preventing progressive degrees of rectal mucosal prolapse.

When procidentia (full thickness prolapse) is present, only operative treatment will be effective. Several procedures are available for restoration of anal continence and reduction of prolapse. All surgical procedures require hospitalization and general anesthesia. All procedures are successful, with a recurrence rate of less than 4%. One important factor to consider before operation is whether incontinence will be improved. In some centers rectal manometric studies are advocated before surgical intervention. In most instances where the gastroenterologist and surgeon feel that incontinence will not be improved, it may be best to provide the patient with an end colostomy rather than to perform an abdominal proctopexy. All operative procedures for full thickness rectal prolapse require an abdominal proctopexy in which the rectum is secured to presacral fascia either by primary suture or the use of synthetic mesh. Complications associated with surgical repair of prolapse are those of fecal impaction, presacral hemorrhage, stricture, infection, fistula formation, pelvic abscesses, and intestinal obstruction. The complication rate is less than 1 to 3%. Fecal impaction, however, can occur in up to 6 to 10% of the patients after operative repair. It is important to follow the patient carefully during this period so that this problem may be recognized early and treated appropriately.

References

General

Goldberg SM, Gordon, PH and Wivatvongs, S: *Essentials of Anorectal Surgery.* J. P. Lippincott, Philadelphia, 1980.
    This excellent monograph provides a thorough and well illustrated discussion of the medical as well as the surgical aspects of anorectal problems

Specific

1. Alexander-Williams, J and Crapp, A R: Conservative management of haemorrhoids; Part I. Injection, freezing and ligation. *Clin Gastroenterol 4:* 595, 1975.
2. Arabi, Y, Gatehouse, J, Alexander-Williams, J and Keighley, MRB: Rubber band ligation or lateral subcutaneous sphincterotomy for treatment of haemorrhoids. *Br J Surg 64:* 1737, 1977.
3. Douthwaite, AH: Proctalgia fugax. *Br Med J 3:* 164, 1962.
4. Goligher, JC: Cryosurgery for hemorrhoids. *Dis Colon Rectum 19:* 213, 1976.
5. Henry, MM: Rectal disease. Rectal prolapse. *Br J Hosp Med 24:* 302, 1980.
6. Hoffmann, DC and Goligher, JC: Lateral subcutaneous internal sphincterotomy in treatment of anal fissure. *Br Med J 3:* 673, 1970.
7. Hood, TR and Williams, JA: Anal dilatation versus rubber band ligation for internal hemorrhoids. *Am J Surg 122:* 545, 1971.
8. Nothmann, BJ and Schuster, MM: Internal anal sphincter derangement with anal fissures. *Gastroenterology 67:* 216, 1974.
9. *The Medical Letter,* Vol. 17, 1975.
10. Thomson, H: Rectal disease. Nonsurgical treatment of haemorrhoids. *Br J Hosp Med 24:* 298, 1980.
11. Wrobleski, DE, Corman, MI, Veidenheimer, MC and Coller, JA: Long-term evaluation of rubber ring ligation in hemorrhoidal disease. *Dis Colon Rectum 23:* 478, 1980.

SECTION 13

Gynecologic Problems

CHAPTER NINETY

Birth Control

J. COURTLAND ROBINSON, M.D.

INTRODUCTION

The avoidance of an unplanned or unwanted pregnancy is the decision of the patient and of her partner. In consultation with the physician, she (or they) acquires knowledge of the available contraceptive methods and then is helped in carrying out a satisfactory program.

There are many contraceptive methods. It is important for the physician to understand the limits and risks of all of them to be able to educate his patient fully about her options. The physician must be prepared to deal with patients who have varying knowledge and experience about contraception. Table 90.1 lists the current percentage distribution of use of contraceptive methods by married women in the United States.

Figure 90.1 shows the risks of using various methods of contraception. The figure is similar to that inserted in all the oral contraceptive packages that are sold to patients. There is a low mortality rate associated with all methods in patients under 30 so that younger women have a wide choice. On the other hand, a patient who is over 35 years of age has a greater risk with some contraceptives and the physician must inform his patients of these risks.

The theoretical and actual effectiveness of various methods of contraception is shown in Table 90.2. *Theoretical effectiveness* is determined in very carefully controlled studies in which a method is used exactly as it was designed to be used. *Actual effectiveness* is a measure of what is found when a method is used by large numbers of people in a less controlled manner. Clearly there is very little difference between the theoretical and actual effectiveness of some methods, while others show a considerable difference. This information should be used in helping to educate the patient.

In the physician's office, most often the discussion

concerning fertility control will be initiated by the patient, and often it will be the main reason for the visit. However, the physician, as part of a routine health plan, should inquire about the method of con-

Table 90.1
Contraceptive Use among Married Women at Risk [a]

Contraceptive Status	U.S. Women Aged 15–44 (N = 4,766)
TYPE USED	89.8
Oral contraceptive	29.5
IUD	8.1
Female sterilization	12.7
Male sterilization	12.8
Condom	9.5
Withdrawal	2.6
Diaphragm/cap	3.8
Other	10.6
NONE USED	10.2
TOTAL	100.0

[a] Percentage distribution of contraceptive use among married women at risk of pregnancy (including the contraceptively sterilized), arranged by method, United States, 1976. (Adapted from R. Ford: Contraceptive use in the United States. *Family Planning Perspectives, 10:* 264, 1978.)

traception that the patient uses, and offer help in understanding it and in monitoring any possible side effects. While pregnant patients with every kind of serious health condition have been carried successfully to term, there may be an increased risk (16) for the patient or the fetus. Therefore, the physician is responsible for ascertaining that patients, who, because of an underlying health problem, do not want the added risk of pregnancy, are educated about the various options for birth control.

Once it is established that fertility regulation is desired by the patient, a careful medical history should be obtained, including information about past pregnancies, menstruation, and fluctuations in weight. A physical examination with special emphasis on the pelvic examination is important. A cancer detection smear and a gonorrhea culture of the cervix are suggested. After this evaluation, the physician and patient are ready to discuss the various contraceptive methods and to develop a satisfactory plan.

Although fertility declines with increasing age and eventually is lost, protection is necessary until menopause (see Chapter 74). The uncertainty about pregnancy is further compounded by the increasing rate of abnormal menstrual cycles, and in particular episodes

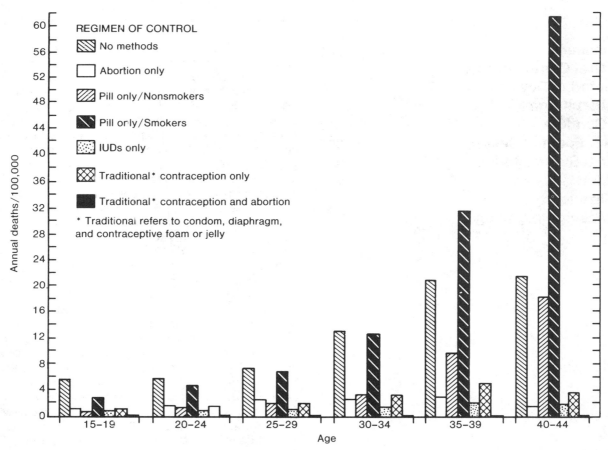

Figure 90.1   Death risk of various methods of contraception. (Data from C. Tietze and S. Lewit: Life risks associated with reversible methods of fertility regulation. *International Journal of Gynaecology and Obstetrics, 16:* 456, 1979.)

Table 90.2
Method Effectiveness: Theoretical and Actual Use Rates [a]

Method	Used Correctly and Consistently: Theoretical Effectiveness	Average U.S. Experience among 100 Women Who Wanted No More Children: Actual Effectiveness
Abortion	0	0+
Abstinence	0	?
Hysterectomy	0.0001	0.0001
Tubal ligation	0.04	0.04
Vasectomy	0.15	0.15+
Oral contraceptive	0.34	4–10
Condom + spermicide	Less than 1	5
IUD	1–3	5
Condom	3	10
Diaphragm (with spermicide)	3	17
Spermicidal foam or suppository	3	20–25
Coitus interruptus	9	20–25
Rhythm (calendar)	13	21
Lactation for 12 months	15	40
Chance (sexually active)	90	90
Douche	?	40

[a] Number of pregnancies during the first year of use per 100 nonsterile women initiating method. (Adapted from R. A. Hatcher: *Contraceptive Technology, 1980–81*, Irving Publishers, New York.

Table 90.3
Oral Contraceptive Preparations and Dosage Schedules [a]

Preparation	Schedule
Combination:	
Contains a fixed ratio of estrogen to progestogen	Daily on cycle days 5 to 26
Progestogen only:	
Each tablet contains progestogen only	Daily—including during menstruation

[a] Adapted and reproduced with permission from J. L. Durand, and R. Bressler: Clinical pharmacology of the steroidal oral contraceptives, in G. H. Stollerman, *et al.* (eds.): *Advances in Internal Medicine*, Volume 24. Copyright © 1979 by Year Book Medical Publishers, Inc., Chicago.

of amenorrhea, as a woman gets older. Missing a period is very disturbing to a woman in the perimenopause unless a very reliable method of contraception is being used.

The *postpartum patient* needs help in getting back on a contraceptive program, and usually her obstetrician will have given her advice in this regard. In general, all methods are suitable for the healthy patient except for the breast-feeding mother who should avoid the oral contraceptives. Also, the patient wishing to use an intrauterine device (IUD) will need to wait for involution of the uterus and, therefore, is at risk for pregnancy until the IUD is inserted at her first postpartum menses.

THE ORAL CONTRACEPTIVE
Mechanism of Action

Oral contraceptives prevent ovulation by inhibition of gonadotropin-releasing factors in the hypothalamus. The principal effect of this inhibition appears to be a suppression of the surge in activity of luteinizing hormone at midcycle, thereby removing a major stimulus to ovulation. In addition, oral contraceptives make cervical mucus more viscid and therefore less easily traversed by sperm and have a direct effect on endometrial development, making the uterus less receptive to implantation of the fertilized ovum (2).

Preparations and Dosage Schedules

There are two basic types of preparations of oral contraceptives currently available (another type—the sequential preparation—is no longer marketed). The dosage schedule depends on which type is administered (Table 90.3). The preparations containing fixed combinations of estrogen and progestin are by far the more commonly used and should be recommended by the practitioner in most cases to patients wishing hormonal contraception. The progestogen-only preparations do not inhibit ovulation, and unwanted pregnancy is 3 to 5 times more likely than it is with the oral contraceptives which contain estrogen and progestin. They should be prescribed, therefore, only for patients who cannot be given estrogen (e.g., those with a history of thromboembolism) and who prefer an oral hormone to another method of birth control. Many of the currently available oral contraceptive preparations are listed in Table 90.4. Because lower doses of estrogen are associated with fewer side effects, a combination preparation containing 35 μg of estrogen and 1 mg of progestin (see Table 90.4) is selected most often for the initial cycle. Occasionally, it will be necessary to change to a higher dose of estrogen in order to control breakthrough bleeding (see below).

In order to suppress ovulation and yet allow periodic bleeding the combination tablet is taken every day for 3 weeks beginning before the development in the ovary of the next follicle. This cycle is accomplished by packaging the tablets for use during either a 21- or 28-day period and having the patient start the medication on the 5th day of her cycle, counting the first day of menstrual bleeding as day one. An alternative is to start it on the first Sunday which occurs after the onset of a menstrual period. This latter practice allows the packaging of the tablets to provide for the user a minicalendar which minimizes missing a dose. The tablets are arranged in either circles or rows making it easier to use them regularly. The 21-day formulation and the 28-day formulation are packaging techniques to improve compliance. In all 28-day preparations the last seven tablets have no hormonal effect and are there only to keep the patient on schedule. The drop in hormone level after 21 days produces withdrawal bleeding just as it does normally when fertilization has not taken place.

Table 90.4
Some Currently Available Oral Contraceptives

Estrogen	Progestin	Trade Name	Manufacturer
60 μg mestranol	10 mg norethindrone	Ortho-Novum	Ortho
80 μg mestranol	1 mg norethindrone	Ortho-Novum 1/80	Ortho
50 μg mestranol	1 mg norethindrone	Ortho-Novum 1/50	Ortho
35 μg mestranol	1 mg norethindrone	Ortho-Novum 1/35	Ortho
80 μg mestranol	1 mg norethindrone	Norinyl 1/80	Syntex
50 μg mestranol	1 mg norethindrone	Norinyl 1/50	Syntex
35 μg mestranol	1 mg norethindrone	Norinyl 1/35	Syntex
35 μg ethinyl estradiol	0.5 mg norethindrone	Brevicon	Syntex
75 μg mestranol	5 mg norethynodrel	Enovid 5 mg	Searle
100 μg mestranol	2.5 mg norethynodrel	Enovid-E	Searle
100 μg mestranol	1 mg ethynodiol acetate	Ovulen	Searle
50 μg ethinyl estradiol	1 mg ethynodiol acetate	Demulen	Searle
50 μg ethinyl estradiol	0.5 mg norgestrel	Ovral	Wyeth
30 μg ethinyl estradiol	0.3 mg norgestrel	Lo/Ovral	Wyeth
35 μg ethinyl estradiol	0.4 mg norethindrone	Ovcon-35	Mead Johnson
50 μg ethinyl estradiol	1 mg norethindrone acetate	Norlestrin 1/50	Parke-Davis
30 μg ethinyl estradiol	1.5 mg norethindrone acetate	Loestrin 1.5/30	Parke Davis
20 μg ethinyl estradiol	1 mg norethindrone acetate	Loestrin 1/20	Parke-Davis
	0.35 mg norethindrone	Micronor	Ortho
	0.35 mg norethindrone	Nor-Q.D.	Syntex
	0.075 mg norgestrel	Ovrette	Wyeth

When a postpartum woman selects an oral contraceptive for contraception, it is initiated within a few days of delivery. However, oral contraceptives are usually avoided in women who are breast-feeding as the medication appears in the milk; and also full time breast-feeding delays onset of ovulation.

Benefits

Oral contraceptives, used correctly, are very effective methods of contraception (Table 90.2). In addition, they significantly lower the incidence of dysmenorrhea and, by reducing menstrual flow, of anemia due to blood loss. Furthermore, patients on oral contraceptives have a reduced incidence of ovarian cysts, benign tumors of the breast, and possibly have some degree of protection against endometrial cancer (6).

Risks

Oral contraceptives should not be used by women with any of the conditions listed in Table 90.5.

THROMBOEMBOLIC DISEASE (11)

There is an increased risk of both venous and arterial thrombosis (and of hemorrhagic stroke) in women taking oral contraceptives. The magnitude of the risk is approximately 5 to 10 times that of the general population. The risk is even greater after the age of 35 and is compounded further by the smoking of cigarettes (10). Women who are over 40 or who smoke more than 15 cigarettes a day should be strongly advised to use another contraceptive method. A history of venous or arterial thrombosis or evidence on examination of thrombotic disease is an absolute contraindication to the administration of

Table 90.5
Absolute Contraindications to Oral Contraceptions

Thrombophlebitis or thromboembolic disorders (current or remote)
Cerebral vascular or coronary artery disease (current or remote)
Known or suspected carcinoma of the breast
Known or suspected estrogen-dependent neoplasia
Undiagnosed, abnormal genital bleeding
Known or suspected pregnancy

oral contraceptives. Also, because of the risk of thromboembolism, it is wise to discontinue the use of oral contraceptives for 1 to 2 months before elective surgery and in any patients immobilized for prolonged periods of time (for example, patients in long leg casts). In such cases an alternate contraceptive method should be recommended.

HYPERTENSION (7)

The risk of developing high blood pressure is increased in women who use oral contraceptives, especially after several years of use. At the end of 5 years it has been shown that the prevalence of hypertension is three times the level shown after initial exposure. Women with preexisting hypertension, or with a family or personal history of hypertension are probably more likely to develop high blood pressure when they take oral contraceptive hormones. Nevertheless oral contraceptives can be used by these patients who are at greater risk if their physician measures their blood pressure (or teaches them to do so) every few months. If hypertension increases or develops, it is best to find another contraceptive method (see Chapter 59).

NEOPLASIA

There is no evidence that *cancer* is more common in women who use an oral contraceptive preparation. On the contrary, the careful monitoring of women who use this method of contraception may have resulted in earlier detection and easier management of cervical and uterine cancer.

Benign hepatic adenomas have been reported rarely in patients using oral contraceptives (3). Sometimes the tumors are first detected, on physical examination, as masses in the right upper quadrant of the abdomen. At other times, women present with severe abdominal pain and shock because the adenomas have ruptured (most likely at the time of menstruation). In such instances, the physician who is aware of the association between use of oral contraceptives and these tumors will be able to diagnose and deal with the problem more quickly.

The incidence of *benign breast tumors* and of fibrocystic disease is reduced by administration of oral contraceptive hormones (12). Unfortunately the epithelial atypia associated with the type of fibrocystic disease that is a risk factor for the development of breast cancer is not influenced by oral contraceptives (8) (see Chapter 86).

ALTERED METABOLISM OF GLUCOSE OR OF LIPIDS

A *reduced glucose tolerance* may be seen in women who take oral contraceptives, for reasons that are not known. Diabetics should be followed particularly closely for this effect. Similarly, *triglyceride levels may increase*, but it is unlikely that this imposes a significant risk.

GALLBLADDER DISEASE

There is a 2-fold increase in the incidence of gallbladder disease requiring surgery within the first 1 to 2 years of oral contraceptive use (12). An estrogen-associated increase in the concentration of cholesterol in the bile has been demonstrated.

HEADACHES

Headaches, especially migraine headaches, are more common in women who use oral contraceptives. The development of severe recurrent headaches is a reason for the physician to recommend another contraceptive method.

BIRTH DEFECTS

There is an increased risk of congenital abnormalities in fetuses exposed to exogenous estrogen or progestogen. Therefore, patients contemplating pregnancy after using oral contraceptive hormones should be told to use a barrier form of contraception for 2 to 3 months after discontinuing the oral contraceptive, before attempting to become pregnant. This prevents any risk of congenital abnormality from oral contraceptive agents.

OTHER SIDE EFFECTS

In general, minor side effects occur early in the course of taking oral contraceptives and may be transient. Thorough education by the physician will increase the likelihood that the patient will tolerate these effects and continue taking the medication.

Nausea. Nausea occurs in approximately 5% of patients but can almost always be eliminated by taking the contraceptive at bedtime.

Fatigue. Increased fatigability is occasionally described by patients but usually is of short duration.

Change in Menstrual Flow. The most typical pattern is a reduction in the amount and duration of menstrual flow, and this is usually welcomed by the patient. On occaison, there will be no bleeding; and if the patient has taken the oral contraceptive regularly (so that pregnancy is not likely), she can be advised to continue it for another cycle. If she is again amenorrheic, a pregnancy test (see below) should be done. Whether positive or negative, an obstetrician/gynecologist should then be consulted, at least by telephone. If pregnancy is ruled out, the patient can either select another contraceptive method or can be placed temporarily on a preparation with a slightly higher estrogen content which results in more menstrual bleeding.

Breakthrough Bleeding. Breakthrough bleeding is most common in the early cycles after initiation of an oral contraceptive. It is of no concern as long as the patient has not missed a dose. Failure to take daily doses increases the chance of breakthrough bleeding, particularly in the early part of the cycle. If a dose or two has been forgotten early in the cycle, the patient should catch up and continue the normal regimen together with temporary use of a barrier form of protection. If breakthrough bleeding continues for several cycles, referral to a gynecologist is indicated to rule out an organic cause and to consider using a higher dose estrogen.

Weight Gain. About 5% of patients will show some weight gain, sometimes associated with fluid retention.

Vaginitis. It has been difficult to document a close relationship between oral contraceptives and vaginitis. The hormones do alter the vaginal milieu but only in a small proportion of patients will vaginitis develop. Standard diagnostic methods and subsequent therapy (see Chapter 91) will allow the vast majority of patients to continue to use the oral contraceptive.

Skin Changes. Some patients, especially dark skinned individuals, will note chloasma (yellowish brown discoloration of the skin) and a change in hair texture. Chloasma is unlikely to resolve with continued administration of the oral contraceptive and is, therefore, a reason to discontinue it if the cosmetic effect is unacceptable.

Emotional changes. Some women have become depressed while taking oral contraceptives. Therefore patients who have a history of depression should be followed especially carefully. If depression develops, the medication should be discontinued.

Effects on Laboratory Tests. Oral contraceptives can alter the results of a number of laboratory tests (13). The alterations reflect physiologic changes in the patient in most instances but rarely signify clinically significant disease. Table 90.6 lists alteration in selected laboratory tests.

Drug Interactions. Oral contraceptives may alter the effectiveness of a number of other drugs; and, conversely, a number of other drugs may alter the effectiveness of oral contraceptives. Physicians should investigate the possibility of drug interaction before prescribing any other medication to a patient using an oral contraceptive preparation. Table 90.7 lists drugs which may interact with oral contraceptives (4, 17).

Monitoring

A patient taking oral contraceptives should see a physician twice a year for an interim history (including a menstrual history), an interim physical examination and any tests warranted by this review. Any possible change in family planning should be discussed at that time. Once a year, the pelvic examination should be done, which should include a cervical smear for cytology and a cervical culture for gonorrhea.

THE INTRAUTERINE DEVICE (14)

The mechanism of action of the intrauterine device (IUD) is not known, but it is thought to cause a local inflammatory reaction and, in essence, to prevent uterine implantation of the fertilized ovum. The de-

Table 90.6
Effects of Oral Contraceptives on Selected Laboratory Tests[a]

Laboratory Test	Effects	Probably Mechanism
SERUM, PLASMA, BLOOD		
Albumin	Slightly decreased	Decreased hepatic synthesis
Aldosterone	Increased	Activates renin-angiotension system
Amylase	Slightly increased (common)	Not established
	Markedly increased (rare)	Pancreatitis
Antinuclear antibodies	Become detectable	Not established
Bilirubin	Increased (rare)	Reduced secretion into bile
Coagulation factors	Increased II, VII, IX, X	Increased synthesis
Cortisol	Increased	Increased cortisol-binding globulin
		Urinary free cortisol unchanged
Folate	Decreased or no change	Decreased folate absorption
Haptoglobin	Decreased	Decreased hepatic synthesis
High density lipoprotein cholesterol	Increased with estrogens and decreased with progestins	Not established
Iron-binding capacity	Increased	Increased transferrin levels
Magnesium	Decreased or no change	Decreased bone resorption
Phosphatase, alkaline	Increased (rare)	Altered secretion in bile
Platelets	Slightly increased	Not established
Prolactin	Increased	Not established
Renin activity	Increased	Increased synthesis of renin substrate
Thyroxine (total)	Increased	Increased thyroxine binding globulin
Transaminases	Slightly increased	Not established
Triiodothyronine resin uptake	Decreased	Increased thyroxine binding globulin
Vitamin B_{12}	Decreased	Not established
URINE		
δ-Aminolevulinic acid	Increased	Increased hepatic synthesis
Calcium	Decreased	Decreased bone resorption
Porphyrins	Increased (may precipitate porphyria in susceptible patients)	Increased delta-aminolevulinic acid synthetase
17-Hydroxycorticosteroids	Slightly decreased or no change	Increased binding proteins
17-Ketosteroids	Slightly decreased or no change	Increased binding proteins

[a] Adapted from *The Medical Letter on Drugs and Therapeutics*, 21: 54, 1979 (13).

Table 90.7
Selected Drugs Which May Interact with Oral Contraceptive Preparations (OCP)

Drugs which may decrease the effectiveness of OCP resulting in breakthrough bleeding, pregnancy, or both:
A. Well established relatively commonly occurring drug interactions
  1. *Anticonvulsants*—Barbiturates, phenytoin (Dilantin), or primidone (Mysoline)
  2. *Antimicrobials*—Rifampicin
B. Reported instances of possible drug interactions
  1. *Antimicrobials*
    a. *(Breakthrough bleeding only)—Neomycin, nitrofurantoin, phenoxymethylpenicillin (penicillin V)*
    b. *(Breakthrough bleeding and pregnancy)—Ampicillin, chloramphenicol, sulfamethoxypridazine (Kynex, Midicel)*
  2. *Others*—Chlordiazepoxide (Librium), meprobamate, phenacetin, and phenylbutazone (Butazolidin)
Drugs whose effectiveness may be altered by OCP:
A. *Anticoagulants*—The effect of anticoagulants may be reduced by the simultaneous administration of OCP
B. *Clofibrate (Atromid-S)*—Control of cholesterol and triglyceride levels may be lost when OCP were simultaneously administered with clofibrate.
C. *Thyroid hormone in patients without functioning thyroid gland*—Mostly a theoretical concern; however, there may be a need for an increased dose of thyroid hormone in patients without a functioning thyroid gland.
D. *Tricyclic antidepressants*—Higher doses of estrogen may inhibit effect of antidepressants, and tricyclic toxicity may be increased.

vice may also interfere with sperm and/or ovum transport. Devices which contain copper or progesterone are more effective in interfering with implantation.

The IUD is 95 to 99% effective when properly inserted and monitored.

Types

The Lippes loop is the most popular IUD in current use. It is a plastic device which straightens out for insertion. It may remain inserted until not needed and may, therefore, remain in place for years. The Cu 7 and Copper T are IUDs containing plastic and copper; they are smaller than the Lippes loop, but the copper increases their effectiveness. They must, however, be replaced every 3 years. The progesterone-containing IUDs are quite large and, therefore, need more careful insertion. Furthermore, they last only 1 year. All IUDs come in individual, sterile packages which also contain instructions for insertion and important educational material for patients.

Use and Insertion

If the physician is not experienced in IUD insertion, it is wise to refer the patient to a gynecologist. The IUD is best inserted at the time of a menstrual period (the usual small amount of bleeding associated with insertion becomes a part of the normal menstrual flow). The patient thereafter will usually notice some increased bleeding with her periods, possibly some increased cramping and a certain amount of vaginal discharge.

Patient Experience. Most often the patient experiences minimal or no discomfort when the IUD is inserted. However, occasionally some cramps are experienced which often subside in a few hours or days but which rarely may be so severe as to necessitate removal of the device.

The effectiveness of the IUD will be increased if the patient learns to feel for the string which protudes from the cervix and to report when she cannot feel it.

Benefits

The IUD is highly effective in preventing pregnancy. In contrast to oral contraceptives it has no systemic effects and requires relatively little participation on the part of the user.

Risks

Absolute and relative contraindications to the use of an IUD are shown in Tables 90.8 and 90.9. The most common serious side effects is the 1 to 3-fold increased incidence of *pelvic inflammatory disease* (1) The patient must be instructed to report any fever, pelvic pain, or discomfort promptly. She must also report any missed menstrual periods since they will indicate that she must be evaluated for pregnancy. Removing the IUD from a pregnant woman will result in an *abortion* in about 25% of patients. If the IUD is in place throughout pregnancy, an abortion will occur in about 50% of patients; however, there is an increased risk of septic abortion in this population. The patient who has missed a menstrual period must be evaluated also for *ectopic pregnancy* since the IUD prevents only intrauterine pregnancy. *Uterine perforation*, a rare complication, is most likely to occur at the time of insertion. Finally, the use of the intrauterine device by a young nulliparous patient who has multiple sex partners is associated with an increased incidence of uterine infection.

Monitoring

Follow-up should be annual and should include a review of any problems, a pelvic examination including a cervical cancer smear, a gonorrhea culture, and detection of the device. The follow-up is best done by a gynecologist.

The IUD is easily removed by gentle traction on the string at or around the time of a menstrual period. Removal at this time allows the bleeding associated with removal to be part of the menstrual period.

As with oral contraceptives, if a patient terminates this form of contraception other than to attempt

Table 90.8
Absolute Contraindications to the IUD

Acute or subacute pelvic inflammatory disease
Pregnancy
Recurrent pelvic infection
Acute cervicitis
History of ectopic pregnancy
Abnormal cancer detection smear
A single episode of pelvic inflammatory disease in a
patient who has not had a child

Table 90.9
Relative Contraindications to the IUD

Patients with severe dysmenorrhea (In the case of
dysmenorrhea and hyperplasia of a mild type the
progestin-containing IUD has been thought to have
a beneficial effect.)
Patients with heavy menstrual flow
Patients with dysfunctional uterine bleeding
Congenital anomalies of the uterus such as bicornate
uterus
Patients with a history of endometrial hyperplasia

pregnancy, she will need help in choosing another
form of contraception.

THE DIAPHRAGM

The diaphragm is a dome-shaped rubber device
which is held open by a metallic band or spring. It is
filled with a spermicidal cream or jelly before each
use and placed in the vagina over the cervix to
prevent sperm deposited during ejaculation from
reaching the cervical os. As seen in Table 90.2, the
theoretical effectiveness is much better than actual
effectiveness, as is true of all barrier methods.

The diaphragm is fitted by a physician or his
assistant. The device fits in the posterior fornix and
tucks up behind the symphysis. The largest device
which is comfortable is the proper one to use. The
manufacturers of diaphragms have excellent booklets
which are useful in helping a patient acquire the skill
necessary for comfortable use of this form of contraception. For better effectiveness, the patient should
be asked to insert the diaphragm and have the physician or assistant check its placement.

The patient will apply the spermicidal jelly to the
inside of the dome and insert it in the vagina. She
may insert it as long as 4 hours before intercourse.
She should check for position with her finger and
allow the device to remain in place for at least 6 to 8
hours following coitus. Repeat intercourse within 6
to 8 hours requires additional jelly without removal.
The failure rate increases rapidly when an attempt is
made to combine the diaphragm with the rhythm
method of contraception.

With care a diaphragm should last 2 years. The
patient will need a new fitting if she gains or loses
significant weight, has a baby, or has pelvic surgery.

A modification of the diaphragm is *the cap*. This is
similar in shape to the diaphragm but smaller and is
designed to be placed over the cervix and remain in
place until menstruation when it is temporarily removed. Preliminary clinical trials in this country have
not yet defined its limits, although international studies have suggested some women may be able to keep
it in place for only 3 or 4 days at a time. This device
will require Federal Drug Administration approval
before it is commercially available in the United
States.

Benefits

The diaphragm is a low cost device that has no real
risks other than the higher risk of unwanted pregnancy compared to oral contraceptives or to the IUD.

Risks

Contraindications to the use of the diaphragm are
sensitivity to the rubber or to the spermicidal material. Alterations in pelvic shape may also preclude
the proper fitting of the different diaphragms available. It is not suited for individuals who will not or
cannot touch their vagina as, for example, in patients
who are very obese or who have a musculoskeletal
disorder.

Some women may report discomfort during the
time the diaphragm is in place. This discomfort is
most often related to a wrong design or to improper
fitting, and re-evaluation usually resolves the problem.

THE CONDOM

The condom is a latex sheath which is phallus-
shaped and is placed over the erect penis and thus
prevents the sperm from remaining in the vagina
after intercourse. Its effectiveness can be enhanced
if combined with application of spermicidal jelly or
foam in the vagina. Some care is needed when the
penis is withdrawn as the condom may come off.
The condom is available in a number of different
colors and shapes, and it is the only device advocated
as a way of increasing sexual pleasure for the female
partner. Its only side effect is sensitivity to the material. It requires male involvement and so is a good
choice for couples who wish to share the responsibility of avoiding a pregnancy. It also is effective in
reducing the spread of sexually transmitted disease.
Condoms are available at most pharmacies.

BARRIER FOAM OR JELLY (15)

A number of preparations are readily available
without prescription which contain a spermicidal
material combined with either a cream, jelly, or aerosol. The cream or jelly is inserted with an applicator
just before intercourse and creates a barrier around
the cervical os which theoretically prevents the
sperm from entering. The foam material is more

likely to remain dispersed and thus to provide better protection.

VAGINAL SUPPOSITORIES (15)

Vaginal spermicidal suppositories are put in place at least 10 to 15 min before intercourse. This form of contraception may be obtained without a prescription and is especially useful when additional protection is desired at midcycle with the condom or to increase the effectiveness of the diaphragm when repeated intercourse occurs. It is also useful as a temporary aid to contraception when an IUD string is noted to be missing or when the patient is postpartum or has discontinued the contraceptive pill. The only problems with its use are sensitivity to the material and a somewhat lower theoretical effectiveness.

RHYTHM

With the discovery of the point of ovulation in the menstrual cycle and the knowledge that sperm have a limited life expectancy, the development of a method of contraception which avoids intercourse at the fertile time was logical. Three methods have been developed:

1. The *calendar method* attempts to establish that portion of the cycle when intercourse is safe. The patient keeps a careful record of the duration of each cycle and then subtracts 18 days from the shortest cycle and 11 days from the longest cycle. This will then give her the beginning and end of the fertile time. Obviously, the more regular she is, the shorter will be this interval and the better the protection. For example, if the shortest cycle is 27 days; and the longest, 33 days, then she is possibly fertile from day 9 until day 22 or an interval of 12 days. On the other hand, if she is very regular and bleeds every 28 days, her fertile period will be 7 days in duration.

2. The *basal body temperature method* takes advantage of the slight drop in body temperature associated with ovulation, followed by a rise in temperature. The woman takes her temperature each morning from day 3 of the cycle until it has remained elevated for 72 hours, indicating that she is postovulatory and can resume coitus (the ovum must be fertilized within 24 or 48 hours).

3. The *cervical mucus method* requires the patient to learn, over a number of cycles, those changes which indicate ovulation. She is taught to examine her cervical mucus for clarity. She learns to identify abdominal discomfort associated with ovulation and then to use this information to avoid intercourse when conception is possible. This method requires effort and regular cycles but has been used effectively by many women.

The rhythm method is the only method of birth control approved by the Roman Catholic Church and other religious organizations who oppose contraception. The risk of pregnancy in women who use this method of contraception is relatively high (Table 90.2).

STERILIZATION (5)

Simple methods of permanent contraception are available to both men and women. At present in the United States sterilization is the most popular method of contraception in persons over 30. The total number of sterilizations is rising, and at present the rate of elective sterilization is about equal for both sexes.

Patients considering sterilization need very careful education so that they understand its nature and risks. Informed consent is required for these procedures.

Vasectomy

For the male, *vasectomy* is the most popular method and when properly performed has a failure rate of only 1/1000. The complication rate is approximately 4/1000; and, for the most part, complications are minor. They include infection, hematoma, epididimytis, and granuloma formation. Long term serious side effects have not been reported among the very large numbers of men who have had the procedure performed. Antibodies to sperm have been reported to occur in some men, but the significance of this is not yet known.

Patient Experience. This procedure is done under local anesthesia and there is minimal operative discomfort. Postoperatively there may be some discomfort but this is controlled by the use of a mild analgesic such as acetaminophen. Vigorous physical activity and sexual activity are restricted for 5 to 7 days until the wound has healed. Follow-up visits are necessary so that sperm counts can be performed and it is usual to require 4 to 6 weeks for the ejaculate to become free of sperm. Because of sperm stored in the prostate gland, it is important that the patient or his partner use another form of contraception until the ejaculate has been found to be sperm-free.

Reanastomosis of the vas deferens may be accomplished surgically and results in potency in approximately 60% of patients. Vasectomy should, nevertheless, not be undertaken unless the patient genuinely wants permanent sterilization.

Tubal Ligation

For the female *tubal ligation* by either the minilaparotomy or with the laparoscope is the method of choice (hysterectomy has too high a risk/benefit ratio to make it a satisfactory contraceptive method). The procedure in the female may be carried out either in the immedite postpartum or at some later time. The overall failure rate is approximately 2 to 3/1000 and is largely a function of the experience of the surgeon. The complications are bleeding, infection, and the additional risk of general anesthesia. Laparoscopy under local anesthesia is usually a completely satisfactory way to perform tubal ligation.

Patient Experience. Uncomplicated tubal ligation is generally very well tolerated. Mild abdominal discomfort when present lasts usually only for a few days and rarely for a few weeks. Mild analgesics such as acetaminophen provide relief. Sterilization is immediate and intercourse is permitted as soon as the wound is no longer painful. Tubal ligation is performed in the first half of the hormonal cycle before ovulation has occurred. This avoids the possibility of fertilization of an ovum occurring a day or two before the surgical procedure. If the woman is using effective contraception, tubal ligation may be performed at any time.

Reanastomosis of the fallopian tubes can be accomplished surgically and results in a significant chance of fertility. Nevertheless, a woman should not undergo tubal ligation unless she genuinely desires permanent sterilization.

There is some evidence to suggest a "post-tubal syndrome" (9). The syndrome has been characterized by heavier menstrual bleeding, more pelvic pain, and more discomfort than are found in the unsterilized population. However, the vast majority of properly counseled patients are very satisfied with the results of tubal ligation.

DIAGNOSING PREGNANCY

For the patient who on the basis of a history and examination is suspected to be pregnant, immediate confirmation in the office can be done utilizing one of several urine slide immunologic tests for the presence of human chorionic gonadotropin (for example, the Pregnosticon Dri-Dot Test). Six weeks after the first day of the last menstrual period (*i.e.*, 4 weeks after the onset of pregnancy) these tests are highly reliable. Chorionic gonadotropin in urine specimens can also be measured in the office by more sensitive tube tests (*e.g.*, Sensi-Tex) but they require more time. They may be used when early pregnancy is suspected and the slide test is negative. These more sensitive tests have been positive as early as 9 days after ovulation. Both the slide and tube test kits are supplied with detailed instructions as well as a description of any limits of the test. In addition, highly sensitive and highly specific serum radioimmunoassay tests for measuring chorionic gonadotropin are

available from many commercial laboratories. These tests may be used if a physician does not have an office kit, if delay for a day or two in obtaining results is not a concern, or if there is some concern about the validity of the urine test kit (e.g., proteinuria is present).

References

General

Hatcher, RA, Stewart, GK, Stewart, F, Guest, F, Schwartz, DW and Jones, SA: *Contraception Technology, 1980–81,* 10th Rev. Ed. Irvington Publishers, New York.
   A regularly updated text covering all aspects of contraception. It is highly recommended.

Specific

1. Burkman, RT and The Woman's Health Study: *Association between intrauterine device and pelvic inflammatory disease.* Obstet Gynecol 57: 269, 1981.
2. Durand, JL, and Bressler, R: Clinical pharmacology of the steroidal oral contraceptives. *Adv Intern Med 24:* 97, 1979.
3. Edmondson, HA, Henderson, B and Benton, B: Liver-cell adenomas associated with use of oral contraceptives. *N Engl J Med 294:* 470, 1976.
4. Hansten, PD: *Drug Interactions,* Ed. 4. Lea & Febiger, Philadelphia, 1979.
5. Hulka, JF: Current status of elective sterilization in the United States. *Fertil Steril 28:* 515, 1977.
6. Kaufman, DW, Shapiro, S, Slone, D, Rosenberg, L, Miettmen, OS, Stolley, PD, Knapp, RC, Leavitt, T, Jr, Watring, WG, Rosenshein, NB, Lewis, JL, Jr, Schottenfeld, D and Engle, RL, Jr: Decreased risk of endometrial cancer among oral-contraceptive users. *N Engl J Med 303:* 1045, 1980.
7. Laragh, JH: Oral contraceptives—induced hypertension—nine years later. *Am J Obstet Gynecol 126:* 141, 1976.
8. LiVolsi, VA, Stadel, BV, Kelsey, JL, Holford, TR and White, C: Fibrocystic breast disease in oral-contraceptive users. *N Engl J Med 299:* 381, 1978.
9. Neil, JR, Noble, AD, Hammond, GT, Rushton, L and Letchworth, AT: Late complications of sterilization by laparoscopy and tubal ligation. A controlled study. *Lancet 2:* 699, 1975.
10. Royal College of General Practitioners: Oral contraception study—mortality among oral-contraceptive users. *Lancet 2:* 727, 1977.
11. Stadel, BV: Oral contraceptives and cardiovascular disease (two parts). *N Engl J Med 305:* 612 and 672, 1981.
12. The Boston Collaborative Drug Surveillance Programme: Oral contraceptives and venous thromboembolic disease, surgically confirmed gallbladder disease and breast tumours. *Lancet 1:* 1399, 1973.
13. *The Medical Letter on Drugs and Therapeutics: 21:* 54, 1979.
14. The Medical Letter on Drugs and Therapeutics: 22: 86, 1980.
15. The Medical Letter on Drugs and Therapeutics: 22: 90, 1980.
16. Tyson, LE (guest editor): Symposium on pregnancy. *Med Clin North Am 61:* 1, 1977.
17. Westerholm, B: Hormonal contraceptives. In *Meyler's Side Effects of Drugs,* Ed. 9, edited by MNQ. Dukes. Excerpta Medica, Amsterdam, 1980.

CHAPTER NINETY-ONE

Benign Vulvovaginal Disorders

J. COURTLAND ROBINSON, M.D.

INTRODUCTION

Vulvovaginal complaints are very common. The probable anatomic location of the problems underlying these complaints can be appreciated from the report from one facility that of 1000 consecutive patients with vulvovaginal problems, 78% had a cutaneous vulvar disorder, 19% had a significant vaginal component (vulvovaginitis), and less than 3% could not be classified (11) (see Table 91.1).

Anatomy and Physiology (see Fig. 91.1)

The *vulva*, sometimes called the pudendum, consists of the labia majora, labia minora, clitoris, mons, perineal body, and prepuce. Bartholin's glands, vestigial lubricating organs, are located bilaterally on the posterior portion of the fourchette. With certain exceptions, the vulva is really specialized skin. It differs from ordinary integument in that it has an increased concentration of sweat and sebaceous glands and of hair follicles. It has a rich blood supply and an extensive venous plexus; this vasculature engorges the vulva under sexual stimulation. Along with this vascular supply there is also an abundant criss-crossing lymphatic system which provides a rational explanation for the finding that diseases which affect the vulva are almost always bilateral. There is also an extensive nerve plexus which has abundant sensory as well as sympathetic endings, and accounts for the increased sensitivity of the area.

The *vaginal mucosa* is composed of a stratified epithelium, the morphology of which changes when stimulated by estrogen. Determining the ratio of mature cells to less mature cells and the ratio of less mature to basal cells, gives a reasonably accurate indication of the amount of estrogen present (see "Maturation Index," p. 1004). The vaginal mucosa contains no secretory glands but under stimulation by estrogen increases the amount of material that is desquamated which then will allow leukocytes to pass and thus produce a normal vaginal "secretion." The cervix and its glands also contribute to the production of this "secretion."

Bacteriology

The vulva, vagina, and cervix are exposed to the external environment. The cervical canal is the main barrier of the female reproductive system to the external environment. Above this point, the organs are normally sterile. In the vagina, there are on the average four to five aerobic and a similar number of anaerobic species of bacteria. No organisms are consistently present, except for Döderlein bacilli, which are almost always found (7), and which seem to have a role in maintaining the normal low vaginal pH. Occasionally, even pathogenic organisms, such as *Clostridium welchii*, are present in healthy women, and the healthy vagina will occasionally also be found to contain fungi.

APPROACH TO DISORDERS OF THE VULVOVAGINAL AREA

General Considerations

It is important that the physician educate his patients about the normal variations in the vulvovaginal "secretions," the consistency and amount of which will be influenced by menstrual flow, oral contraceptive hormones, antibiotics, and even clothing. Other-

Table 91.1
Causes of Vulvovaginal Problems[a]

CUTANEOUS VULVAR DISORDERS (78%)
  Primary cutaneous disorders (70.3%)
   1. Inflammation (10.5%)
    Intertrigo, contact dermatitis, neurotic excoriation, etc.
   2. Infection (35.3)%
    Bacterial, viral, mycotic, and parasitic
   3. Disorders of pigmentation (3.8%)
   4. Vulvar dystrophy (22.3%)
   5. Neoplasms (28.2%)
  Secondary cutaneous vulvar disorders (7.7%)
  Generalized skin inflammation or infections
VULVOVAGINAL DISORDERS (19.4%)
  Nonspecific vaginitis, candidiasis, trichomoniasis, and senescent vaginitis.
UNDETERMINED DISORDERS (2.6%)

[a] Based on experience with 1000 consecutive patients. (Adapted from H. M. Tovell and H. J. Young, Jr.: *Clinical Obstetrics and Gynecology, 21:* 955, 1978 (11).)

wise women may become needlessly concerned about changes that have no real significance.

HYGIENE

Cleansing during a bath or a shower is all that is needed to maintain proper hygiene of the vulva. Routine douching of the vagina is unnecessary; however, some women will wish to douche after intercourse or menstruation. In such circumstances a tepid solution of vinegar (2 tablespoons of white vinegar to 1 quart of water) should be used. Many preparations are available at pharmacies also, but they offer no real advantage. Women should be especially cautioned about excessive douching as this usually results in increased irritation and increased vaginal discharge.

MENSTRUATION

At the time of menstruation either vaginal tampons, absorbent pads, or both provide acceptable

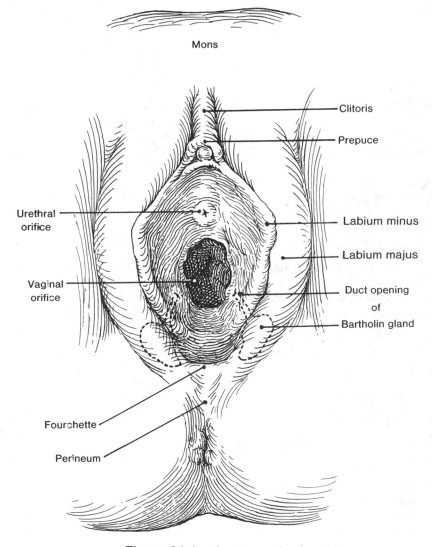

Figure 91.1   Anatomy of vulva.

ways to absorb the menstrual flow. However, a rare "toxic-shock" syndrome has been observed in menstruating women, apparently with increasing frequency; the syndrome is associated with staphylococcal bacteremia and a significant mortality (10 to 15%) (5). There is a correlation between the use of highly absorbent tampons and the development of this syndrome. The assumption is that the tampons favor the development of the infection. Therefore, women who use tampons should be advised to change them at least every 8 hours and to interrupt their use by substituting pads at night.

History

A patient with a benign vulvovaginal disorder rarely has systemic symptoms such as a fever, weight loss, or malaise. The symptoms almost always are restricted to the vulvovaginal region. The most common complaints, reflecting an inflammatory process are itching, burning of the region, often associated with a bad odor, an increased vaginal discharge, or dysuria. The history should include a description of the onset, duration, and character of the symptoms and of their relationship to bowel, bladder, menstrual, and sexual activity. It is important also to question the patient about her general health, medications she is taking or has recently taken, her method of contraception, her vulvovaginal hygiene (frequency of bathing, use of douches, deodorants, tampons, etc.), and the wearing of tight clothing (jeans, for example, which might irritate the vulva). If a physician is precise in taking a history, a specific etiology may be suggested. For example, intense itching which began after the patient was given an antibiotic suggests a fungal infection (see p. 1000).

Physical Examination

The extent of the general physical examination of a patient with vulvovaginal symptoms depends on the nature of the complaints and on the time that has passed since the last comprehensive evaluation. However, the *abdomen* should always be examined to assess especially for the presence or absence of tenderness or of a suprapubic mass. During this phase of the examination, the inguinal nodes should also be evaluated.

PELVIC EXAMINATION

The patient is then assisted to the lithotomy position and properly draped. A careful *inspection* of the vulva under a good light (such as a gooseneck lamp with a 100-watt bulb) is performed first. The labia are then gently separated to allow a complete examination. It is important to inspect the pubic hair for evidence of folliculitis, not uncommonly restricted to one follicle. The physician should note whether the vulva appears inflamed—more red than normal, tender, edematous, denuded, or excoriated—and the

distribution (local or bilateral) of the process. The appearance of any discharge should be noted.

After the external examination, the next step is the insertion of a dry warm *speculum*. If the speculum does not readily pass, it may be moistened with warm water, but lubricant will interfere with the interpretation of a cancer detection smear as well as with growth of microorganisms if a culture is taken. Gentleness is mandatory, especially when there is inflammation. The vaginal wall is inspected and should have a moist pink appearance and there may be a small amount of "secretion" present which is usually pooled in the apex of the vagina.

A *Pap smear* can be obtained at this time if needed for screening for cancer (see Chapter 92); it is not reliable in the diagnosis of specific infection (with the exception of Herpes simplex infection where the finding of multinucleated giant cells may be helpful, see below).

A *gonococcal culture* should be obtained routinely in sexually active women since gonorrhea is often asymptomatic or associated with a nonspecific vaginal discharge. The culture should be obtained from the cervical os after removal of the mucus plug, if one is present. The swab should be placed in the end of the cervical canal (leaving the swab in the canal for a moment to absorb bacteria) and immediately plated (by rolling the swab) on a warmed gonococcal transport medium (Transgrow). The medium may be warmed to approximate body temperture by holding the container for several minutes in the hand or axilla. The transport medium supports the gonococcus for at least 48 hours, and transportation to the bacteriologic laboratory should be accomplished within this time. A single culture obtained under ideal circumstances will be accurate 90% of the time (1). If gonorrhea is strongly suspected, the diagnostic accuracy will be even greater if a rectal gonococcal culture is obtained at the same time. The swab should be introduced approximately 2 to 3 cm into the anal opening; if the swab, when withdrawn, is visibly contaminated with feces it must be discarded and the test repeated.

Following the gonococcal culture, a specimen of the secretion from the posterior fornix should be obtained and placed on a slide containing a drop of physiologic saline and on another slide containing a drop of 10% potassium hydroxide (KOH). After the completion of the pelvic examination the slides should be examined microscopically for *Trichomonas* and *Gardnerella vaginalis* (physiologic saline) and *Candida* (KOH). After the "secretions" have been obtained, the cervix is inspected for evidence of inflammation, nodularity, etc.

Cultures of the cervical or vaginal "secretions," except for gonorrhea, are not very satisfactory, and various bacterial species (such as *G. vaginalis*) may be normal inhabitants of the region; finding them on culture is not proof that they are the cause of inflammation. Culture for herpes simplex, type II, is important in the pregnant patient (where the disease is more severe and may affect the neonate); but in the nonpregnant patient, the signs and symptoms are usually sufficient to establish the diagnosis (see below).

A bimanual examination is then carried out to determine the consistency of the cervix and the size, shape, and position of the uterus. The adnexa are next examined for size, shape, and tenderness. This portion of the examination is usually less useful with respect to the primary complaint, but it is necessary to rule out any other problem.

The *rectal examination* is last; the anus should be inspected to be certain there is no involvement from the vulvar process and palpated to determine the degree of posterior vaginal wall relaxation. If fecal material is present, a screening test for occult blood should be performed.

HERPES SIMPLEX

Manifestations

Herpetic infection is probably the most common of the vulvovaginal disorders. It is sexually transmitted and is associated with significant pain and tenderness of the vulvar area. Occasionally, the patient may develop urinary retention because of the intense pain she experiences when she voids and the urine passes over the lesions.

Herpes simplex infection is characterized by single or multiple vesicles, 1 to 10 mm in size and approximately 1 mm deep. Vesicles are most commonly found on the labia minora and the labia majora and around the clitoris. The lesions may be in clumps or, on occasion, they may be arranged in linear formation and in this instance are diagnostic (Fig. 91.2). With extensive disease the entire vulvovaginal area and cervix may be involved. When there is vaginal and cervical involvement, a white thick exudate may be present which may mimic gonorrhea. Mucosal vesicles ulcerate early; those on the skin remain intact longer but eventually break and become secondarily infected. Often, in patients who are infected for the first time and who have no protective antiviral antibodies, there is an intense inflammatory reaction with vulvar edema, lymphadenopathy and, rarely, fever. Patients with recurrent disease, who have developed antibodies to the virus usually have less inflammation and consequently are less symptomatic.

This infection is due to type II herpes simplex virus in 95% of cases; occasionally type I virus, ordinarily found in the mouth, may be incriminated because the patient has participated in oral-genital sexual activity. However, it is rarely possible or necessary for the general physician to arrange for viral cultures in his office so that the diagnosis of herpetic infection is almost always established by the appearance of the lesions and by cytology. In this regard a Pap smear of the vaginal wall and also of the base of an ulcer

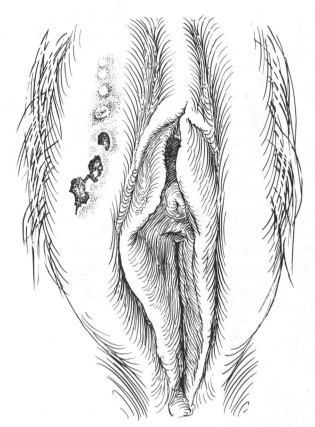

Figure 91.2   Herpes simplex.

often reveals changes characteristic of herpes simplex (multinucleated giant cells and eosinophilic internuclear inclusions); and the cytologist, therefore, should be alerted to the possibility of the diagnosis. The measurement of titers of serum antibodies to herpes virus is generally not helpful in diagnosing herpetic infection because of lack of specificity of the findings.

The *differential diagnosis* in patients who present with herpetic vulvovaginitis includes other sexually transmitted diseases (chancroid and syphilis), vulvar or cervical cancer, and other diseases associated with ulceration; e.g. Behçet's syndrome (a vasculitis which is manifest by oral and genital ulcers, uveitis, and systemic symptoms) and herpes zoster infection. If any of these disorders is suspected, appropriate smears, cultures, or biopsies should be performed; often consultation with a gynecologist will be useful at this juncture.

Treatment

There is no cure for herpes vaginitis, but local and systemic medication will provide symptomatic relief. The infection usually lasts 5 or 6 days, rarely more than 10 days. During that time, soothing solutions such as boric acid or witch hazel (Tucks—cream, ointment, or wipes) which may be gently applied by the patient to the painful area every 4 hours are helpful, as is local heat (sitz baths). Analgesics such as aspirin, 600 mg, 4 times a day, or codeine 30 mg, 3 to 4 times a day, may be necessary to control pain.

Sexual activity often must be temporarily stopped or drastically curtailed because of the pain associated with it; but if it is continued, the sexual partner should use a condom until the ulcers are healed to reduce the risk of reinfection of the patient. Bacterial superinfection is common (manifested with the appearance of exudate and crusting of the ulcers), and if it occurs, the application of an antibiotic cream such as Neosporin or Chloromycetin 1% applied 3 or 4 times a day will control the secondary infection. Dysuria is frequently improved by the use of sitz baths or by phenazopyridine (Pyridium), 100 to 200 mg, 3 to 4 times a day for 3 or 4 days. Acylovir, a topical antiviral agent approved in 1982, is discussed on p. 1054.

Prognosis

Recurrent infections are common. They seem to be milder than the initial infection (see above) and generally become less frequent as time goes on. However, after 1 year some patients still have recurrent problems and, in these situations, a gynecologic consultation is suggested. It has been suggested that herpes simplex virus is associated with the development of cervical cancer. This possibility is currently under debate (8). However, there is no reason to perform more frequent Pap smears for early cancer detection (see Chapter 92) in patients who have had herpetic vulvovaginitis.

MOLLUSCUM CONTAGIOSUM

This benign lesion is caused probably by a pox virus and transmitted by contact including sexual intercourse. The patient characteristically sees a physician because of a painless new growth in the vulva, perineal area, or thighs. The lesions have a typical appearance, permitting diagnosis by inspection in most instances (Fig. 91.3). The individual lesions are wartlike papules varying from 1 to 10 mm in size. They have a smooth surface and a central umbilical depression which contains a mass of keratin. There may be as many as 20 separate lesions; but, occasionally, the lesions will coalesce. If there is any doubt about the diagnosis, the central cheeselike core may be expressed onto a slide, and examined under a microscope. Characteristically large inclusion bodies which occupy most of the cytoplasm of cells will be identified. Occasionally, the lesion resembles bacterial infection such as folliculitis or furunculosis; but in these instances, the expression of pus from the lesion permits differentiation. If doubt remains regarding the diagnosis, the patient should be referred to a dermatologist or gynecologist for confirmation or for consideration of a biopsy of the lesion.

The problem is contagious, and because resolution may take many months or even 2 or 3 years, treatment should be given. *Therapy*, which accelerates healing, consists of scraping open the papule (with a

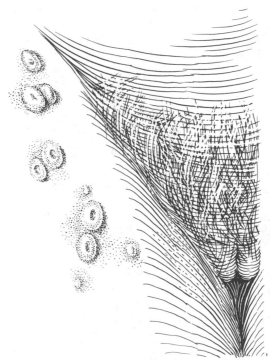

Figure 91.3 Molluscum contagiosum.

scalpel blade), evacuating its contents, and curetting the base. It is *not* necessary to apply irritating chemicals to the lesions (large lesions may need to be anaesthetized before they are opened or curetted). The patient should be seen in 1 week for retreatment of any resistant or new lesions. The patient should be reassured that healing is inevitable.

The patient's sexual partner should be evaluated, if possible, as occasionally lesions are found on the penis. If the sexual partner is not available or is a casual partner other venereal disease may have been acquired and should be assessed. Even if other venereal disease is not found, a culture for gonorrhea (see above) and a serologic test for syphilis should be obtained and the latter repeated in 1 month if initially negative.

CONDYLOMATA ACUMINATA (VENEREAL WARTS)

This common disorder is caused by a papovavirus and is transmitted sexually. It occurs usually during the reproductive years and is most commonly seen in association with other vulvovaginal infections (including candidiasis but also trichomoniasis, G. vaginalis infection, gonorrhea, or syphilis). It occurs more frequently in pregnancy and has a more active course in pregnant women.

The patient most often complains of a new growth on her vulva, perineum, or anus; and there is often associated itching and a vaginal discharge. These symptoms may be part of an associated vaginal infection or may represent infection in the crevices of the wart. Often there will be a history of warts on the penis of the sexual partner, who should also be evaluated.

The examination is characteristic and almost always diagnostic. A wart of 1 to 2 cm usually first appears on the labia, frequently about the posterior introitus, but then spreads, with discrete or congruent lesions appearing on the perineum, anus, vagina, and cervix. They may coalesce into a cauliflower-like lesion which may become huge (Fig. 91.4).

Treatment

Treatment should simultaneously be directed at eradication of other associated infections, if present, such as candidiasis or trichomoniasis (see below); as well as the warts themselves. Treatment of the warts is best accomplished by careful application (usually for 3 to 5 min) to the surface of the wart of a 20% tincture of podophyllum in benzoin. Ample time (2 to 3 min) should be permitted for the solution to dry on the lesions before contact is permitted with other areas of skin or with clothing. The solution may be applied with a cotton-tipped applicator to the wart surface. The material is very irritating to normal skin and mucosa and it should be applied carefully. Should any contamination of normal tissue occur, the solution should be removed with alcohol and then with water. Also, because an intense tissue

reaction may occur after the application of the podophyllin, pain and discomfort are common. The patient should be seen every 5 to 7 days for reapplication of podophyllin until healing occurs. Her sexual partner should be treated simultaneously if he has warts, and he should use a condom to prevent reinfection until the healing is complete. The podophyllin should be left on for 8 to 12 hours, then removed with soap and water. There should be no sexual intercourse until the podophyllin is removed. Should burning of normal tissue occur, the patient should sponge off the podophyllin with soap and water.

Podophyllin is not suitable for eradication of large warts (greater than 2 to 2.5 cm), and its use is not indicated in that situation. Also, podophyllin has been reported to cause fetal abnormalities and should not be used during pregnancy. In these instances, referral to a dermatologist or gynecologist is suggested for evaluation and for consideration of treatment using other modalities such as electrocautery or surgery.

CANDIDIASIS (MONILIASIS)

Candidiasis is a common vulvovaginal fungal infection that is seen more commonly in women who are in their reproductive years except for women with diabetes and/or immunologic deficiencies (such as patients receiving corticosteroids or cytotoxic chemotherapy). The infection is caused by the yeast *Candida albicans* which has no true mycelial form; because of this, it is properly referred to as candidiasis rather than moniliasis which implies infection by true mycelia. The incidence of candidiasis approaches 8% of women in the reproductive period, but as many as 25% of infected women are asymptomatic (2).

The sources of the organism are not precisely known. It is likely that most organisms derive from the gastrointestinal tract where they are normal inhabitants. The organism may be cultured from the feces very often if the patient has been taking broad spectrum antibiotics. During intercourse infection may be passed to the male who may harbor it asymptomatically and thus may reinfect his partner or other women with whom he is sexually intimate.

While infection may occur *de novo*, there is a predisposition to infection in women who are being treated with broad spectrum antibiotics (especially tetracycline or with corticosteroids), those who are pregnant, or those who have diabetes mellitus—all of which change the vaginal milieu. Whether or not oral contraceptives predispose patients to vaginal candidiasis is controversial (3).

Symptoms

Patients complain typically of vaginal burning and itching, and of a thick vaginal discharge that, however, may be less voluminous than it is in tricho-

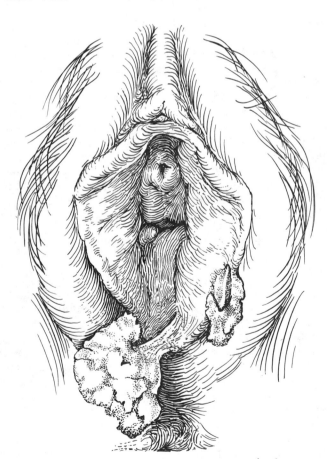

Figure 91.4 Condylomata acuminata.

monas infection (see below). Painful intercourse may be particularly disturbing.

Physical Examination

Examination may reveal an inflamed vulva, especially in older individuals. When vulvitis is present, red vesicular lesions spreading out from the vulva may also be seen. These may appear intertriginous and should be differentiated from this condition (see Chapter 97). The vaginal walls are often intensely inflamed and covered with a curdlike thick adhesive material. Occasionally, the actual discharge may be thin but the thick curdlike material will be seen adhering to the intensely inflamed vaginal wall.

Laboratory Examination

The diagnosis is established by identification of the infectious agent on direct smear with the use of KOH. Budding spores and pseudohyphi will be identified (Fig. 91.5). Cultures are not usually necessary and will not differentiate between pathogenic and nonpathogenic species of fungi.

Treatment

Treatment is aimed at eradication of the infection and requires attention to predisposing factors. Antibiotics may have to be stopped or changed to an agent with a less broad spectrum; diabetes mellitus should be controlled (see Chapter 69); and glucocorticosteroids may need to be withdrawn or reduced in dose if possible. When vaginal candidiasis occurs in pregnancy, an obstetrician/gynecologist should be consulted. If there are no predisposing factors or if they cannot be controlled, specific antifungal agents are usually very effective.

The patient is instructed to administer the contents of one vaginal applicator of miconazole nitrate (Monistat) daily at bedtime for 7 days. Monistat is very effective (4). Clotrimozole (Gyne-Lotrimin), one ap-

plicator of cream or a vaginal tablet used daily at bedtime for 3 to 7 days, is an effective alternative. Nystatin (e.g., Mycostatin or Nilstat) vaginal tablets, one tablet twice daily, are also effective but require 2 weeks of use. Combination preparations containing an antifungal, antibacterial, and a steroid agent (such as Mycolog) are not recommended and, in fact, the application of any potent steroid in areas of skinfolds may lead to serious cutaneous atrophy.

If there is a great deal of pain or if pruritus is intense, nonspecific therapy to control these symptoms is an important part of the initial treatment. The patient may benefit from tepid baths or from compresses of water and oatmeal (e.g., Aveeno) or of witch hazel. The use of daily vaginal douches with vinegar water (see p. 996) and the application of plain talc (e.g., Johnson's Baby Powder) may help also. If pain and itching are not controlled, excoriation and secondary bacterial infection may seriously complicate the situation. The patient should avoid the use of moisture-retaining underwear such as nylon and use more porous cotton materials. The sexual partner should use a condom until the infection is eradicated so that he does not become an asymptomatic reservoir for reinfection of the patient.

Because of the significant amount of itching associated with candidiasis, most patients will telephone their physician immediately if the condition recurs to ask for a renewal of the prescription for antifungal medication. A single renewal in this manner is acceptable; but if symptoms again recur, the patient should be seen by the physician and evaluated. The frequent use of vaginal antifungal agents may result in a secondary irritative vaginitis. Resistance to eradication should raise suspicion of diabetes mellitus, and a fasting blood sugar should be obtained. Furthermore, the patient may become reinfected either from her sexual partner or from her gut or urinary tract, or both. Since it is difficult to prove any of these situations, a reasonable approach in resistant cases is to treat both the patient and her sexual partner with oral nystatin (such as Mycostatin) suspension or tablets, 500,000 units, 3 times a day until the infection has been eradicated (which may require 2 to 3 weeks). Sometimes resistance to treatment results because of a mixed infection; this occurs most often when trichomoniasis (see below) emerges after control of candidiasis (which frequently overgrows and camouflages *Trichomonas* infection initially).

If a *Candida* infection cannot be eradicated, referral to a gynecologist is recommended. If the gynecologist confirms the diagnosis, he may consider the application of 1% gentian violet solution which is very effective, but causes considerable staining and requires some experience in application.

TRICHOMONIASIS

Trichomoniasis is an extremely common infection, second only to herpetic infection as a cause of vul-

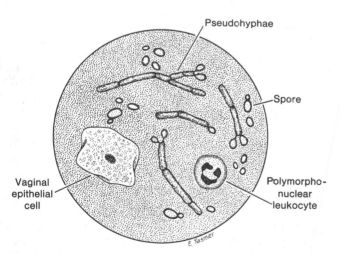

Figure 91.5 KOH preparation, showing yeast and pseudohyphi.

vovaginitis; it is the most common vulvovaginal infection associated with a discharge. The protozoan flagellate, *Trichomonas vaginalis* grows best in an environment which is slightly more alkaline than the normal vagina, but it will grow sometimes at a lower pH. The source of infection is not clear. The organism can exist in the vagina without causing symptoms; when the vaginal environment favors its growth, it multiplies and produces the discomfort which brings the patient to the physician. Men can harbor the organism, and treatment of the sexual partner is, therefore, important. The trichomonad has been implicated as a factor in the development of cervical dysplasia, but the significance of this is unknown.

Symptoms

The patient complains usually of a copious discharge, vaginal burning, discomfort and, often of a musty odor. Itching is less common than it is in patients with candidiasis. Occasionally, minor vaginal bleeding will occur. Some patients will describe symptoms of urethral irritation—dysuria, frequency, and urgency, while others will experience pelvic discomfort. Dyspareunia is very common.

Physical Examination

Examination of the patient reveals a vaginal discharge which may be very profuse and may have a slightly dry musty odor. The discharge is usually greenish and frothy but there is a wide variation. The mucosal surfaces appear moist but are only moderately inflamed. The cervix, in about 10% of patients, will show a pathognomonic "strawberry" pattern (reddish coloration with punctation).

A sample of the discharge should be examined under the microscope with physiological saline as a diluent; the motile protozoan will be identified under a lower power objective (Fig. 91.6). The preparation should be thin so that the pathogens are not obscured.

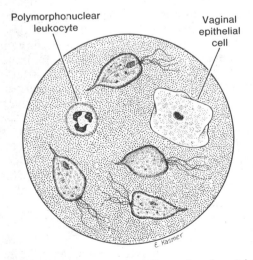

Figure 91.6 Saline preparation showing trichomonads.

It is important to use saline rather than water as a diluent as water causes swelling and immobilization of the organism, making diagnosis very difficult. Also, if the saline is too cold, it may inhibit the motility of the organisms. Staining of the slides is of little use, and a culture (using special media) also is rarely necessary and is probably best left to a gynecologist. Dead trichomonads can be seen on a Pap smear, but such a finding does not correlate very well with clinical symptoms.

Treatment

The therapy for this condition is metronidazole (Flagyl). This compound is readily absorbed from the intestinal tract. Its use topically in the vagina is not very effective and is not recommended. There have been disturbing reports of carcinogenic and mutagenic activity of Flagyl in animal and bacterial models (10). The use of the drug in pregnant women is, therefore, controversial; it is definitely contraindicated in the first 12 to 14 weeks of pregnancy. However, after 30 weeks, if there is significant discomfort and because of a suspected role of trichomonad in premature rupture of membranes, it is reasonable to prescribe Flagyl in consultation with the gynecologist-obstetrician.

Flagyl is given in a dose of either 2 g once by mouth or 250 mg, 3 times a day for 5 days, along with a similar regimen for the sexual partner. Patients are to be cautioned to avoid alcohol because the combination frequently results in nausea and vomiting. The response to Flagyl is dramatic and often is permanent. The patient should avoid synthetic underwear that results in a more moist vulvar environment and should use cotton materials. The sexual partner should use a condom until the infection has been eradicated.

Initial symptomatic relief and eradication of trichomoniasis can be obtained with acid douches twice daily for 2 or 3 days (2 tablespoons of white vinegar in 1 quart of warm water). Commercial douches are more expensive, may be more irritating, and are not recommended.

Since no immunity develops, *recurrences* are common, especially in women with multiple sexual partners. When there is inadequate initial response to treatment (10% of patients do not respond to Flagyl) or when there is reinfection and only a single sexual partner, there may be an associated nonspecific vaginitis which should be confirmed and treated.

"NONSPECIFIC VAGINITIS" (GARDNERELLA VAGINALIS)

Evidence over the past several years has accumulated indicating that *Gardnerella vaginalis* (formally called *Haemophilus vaginalis* or *Corynebacterium vaginale*) either alone or in combination with an anaerobic organism causes most, if not all, cases of "nonspecific vaginitis" (6). *G. vaginalis* is a very small nonmotile Gram-negative rod. The infectious agent may be transmitted by contact with contaminated objects such as towels or toilet seats, but the major route is by sexual intercourse. To flourish, the organism requires an estrogen-enriched vaginal environment and for this reason, infection is seen almost exclusively in women who are in their reproductive years.

Infection with *G. vaginalis* is found in up to 20% of women in the reproductive period, but less than 25% of these individuals have symptoms.

The infection is limited to the vaginal surface, and *symptoms* are usually less prominent than they are in candidiasis or trichomoniasis. The patient may describe slight burning and pruritus, but usually the major complaint is of a discharge which characteristically is grayish and has an unpleasant odor.

Examination may show redness or some tenderness of the vagina, but often no abnormalities are seen. The discharge may be minimal, or it is a thick sticky flourlike paste, adhering to the vaginal wall.

The *diagnosis* is made by preparing and examining saline wet mounts and KOH preparations. Candidiasis and trichomoniasis will be ruled out by this method, and the saline preparation may show the short rods. In addition, under the low power objective and with reduced light, *clue cells* (stippled epithelial cells) may be seen (Fig. 91.7); they are due to the bacteria adhering to the cell surface. This finding in a typical discharge may be considered diagnostic. If these cells are not seen, a Gram stain should be done in an attempt to differentiate Gram-negative pleomorphic rods. Culture is usually not necessary.

Treatment

Treatment (when the diagnosis is confirmed by clinical and microscopic criteria) is best accomplished with metronidazole (Flagyl), 250 mg, 3 times daily for 5 days (9). An alternative is ampicillin, 500 mg, four times per day for 7 days. The patient should use cotton underwear. A gentle douch with vinegar

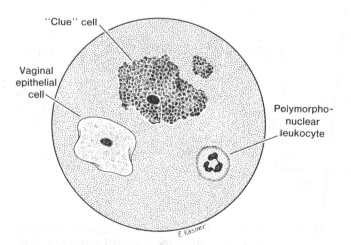

Vaginal epithelial cell
"Clue" cell
Polymorphonuclear leukocyte

Figure 91.7   "Clue" cells.

(1 tablespoon of white vinegar in 1 quart of warm water) once or twice a day for 1 to 2 days will help control symptoms if they are particularly uncomfortable. The sexual partner should use a condom until the infection has been eradicated.

The infection may recur; if it does, it usually can be controlled by once or twice weekly vaginal douching with vinegar water (see above) or with povidone (Betadine or Femidine). However, if douches are not successful, a gynecologic consultation is appropriate.

Simultaneous infection with *Trichomonas* and overgrowth with *Candida* after the use of antibiotics can also be reasons for recurrent symptoms, and these conditions should be especially looked for and appropriately treated.

Occasionally the physician will suspect (after ruling out trichomoniasis and candidiasis) the diagnosis of nonspecific vaginitis, but is unable to identify clue cells or Gram-negative pleomorphic rods and the diagnosis cannot, therefore, be established. In this situation, the discharge may be *increased normal "secretion"* and there is a danger of overmedicating the patient. The patient should, therefore, be reassured that there is no true infection and advised to use cleansing douches (see above) daily for 2 or 3 days if the discharge is distressing. If symptoms do not improve, consultation with a gynecologist should be requested.

GONOCOCCAL INFECTION

Gonococcal infection is quite common in women, particularly those with multiple sex partners. Infected patients may have no symptoms, symptoms due to direct inoculation of organisms (vaginal, rectal, or pharyngeal), or symptoms due to local or distant spread of infection. Transmission of gonorrhea from infected men to uninfected women or to other men (homosexuals) is efficient and occurs in 90% of exposures; transmission from infected women to uninfected men is somewhat less efficient, occurring in about 20 to 50% of exposures (the diagnosis and management of gonorrhea in male patients are discussed in Chapter 26).

In the majority of women the infection remains asymptomatic, so that routine screening for all women is important. In some 10 to 20%, for unknown reasons, the organism spreads, usually after a menstrual period, to the fallopian tubes and initiates acute salpingitis and acute pelvic inflammatory disease (PID). Early consultation and prompt therapy will significantly reduce the serious sequelae of this condition, i.e., ectopic pregnancy and sterility. A single mild episode of acute salpingitis will cause infertility in approximately 5% of patients. This figure rises to almost 100% with severe and/or repeated episodes of PID. Other forms of dissemination (arthritis-dermatitis, endocarditis) are uncommon.

Clinical Manifestations

When clinical manifestations of gonococcal infection occur in women, they do so within 3 to 7 days of exposure. They include vaginal symptoms (onset or increase in vaginal discharge, vaginal itching, dyspareunia, dysuria, vague lower abdominal pain), anorectal symptoms (pruritus, painful defecation, rectal fullness), and pharyngeal symptoms (see description of this entity, Chapter 27). PID usually begins shortly after a menstrual period and is characterized by fever, nausea, abdominal pain and tenderness, and marked tenderness of the pelvic organs to touch or motion. In addition, there may be a cervical discharge, alteration in the menstrual pattern, elevation of the white blood cell count, and evidence of enlarged adnexa. Symptoms and signs of the arthritis-dermatitis syndrome (polyarthralgia, tenosynovitis of elbows, wrists, or knees; skin lesions which begin as tiny red papules or petechiae, then either disappear or evolve through vesicular and pustular stages to develop a gray necrotic center; and, occasionally, purulent monoarthritis) usually develop 1 or more weeks after the initial infection.

Diagnosis

Cervical culture for gonorrhea should be obtained as described above (p. 997) in all women with or without symptoms. When the disease is suspected strongly because of new symptoms, the addition of a rectal culture will increase detection by about 10%. The value of routine culture of the rectum in asymptomatic patients is less certain. Gram stain of the cervical material, when properly done, is highly reliable and may be used as a basis for diagnosis and treatment before the results of culture are obtained. In most states the physician is required to report a positive smear even if the culture is negative. Pharyngeal cultures are indicated in those who give a history of oral-genital sexual activity.

Management

The management plans appropriate for the various forms of gonococcal infection are summarized in Table 91.2. Follow-up cultures should be done 1 week after treatment is completed. Women being treated for gonorrhea should either abstain from sexual intercourse or assure that their partner(s) uses a condom until the result of the 1-week "proof of cure" culture is known. Furthermore, the partner(s) should be treated for presumed infection (see Chapter 26 for treatment of male partners).

A significant proportion of nongonococcal PID is polymicrobial in etiology and may not respond to treatment for gonorrhea. Any woman whose culture does not show gonococci should therefore be evaluated by a gynecologist if she does not respond promptly to therapy.

Whenever gonorrhea is confirmed, the patient should be reported to the local health department so that sexual contacts will receive appropriate evaluation and treatment.

FOREIGN BODY

Another occasional cause of vaginal discharge in adults, although it is much more common in children, is a foreign body. Lost tampons, forgotten diaphragms, and other smaller objects will be easily found by examination. Symptoms will improve after removal of the foreign body and, because secondary bacterial infection is also present, a triple sulfa cream (Sultrin), twice daily for 3 to 4 days or povidone (such as Betadine or Femidine) douch once daily for 3 to 4 days may accelerate healing.

ATROPHIC VAGINITIS

This condition is very common and is caused by estrogen lack. It is primarily a problem of older, postmenopausal women, but may be seen in younger women who are postoophorectomy or who have been intensely breast-feeding for a long period.

Estrogen deficiency results in a thinning of the vaginal vulvar epithelium, a loss of capillary network, and a decrease or loss of vaginal "secretions" as well as a rise in the pH of the vagina.

Patients with this problem complain of dyspareunia, dryness of their genitalia, and occasionally of some vaginal mucoid discharge which may be blood-streaked. Symptoms are more prominent than are signs.

Examination reveals atrophy of the vulva and of the vagina, loss of the subcutaneous fat, and a reduction in the size of the clitoris. The vulvar skin and vaginal mucosa appear dry and pale and adhesions may develop. There may be superficial erosions on the vaginal wall, and uterine atrophy is noted on bimanual examination.

Diagnosis is established by the history and physical examination and by ruling out an associated infection (if a discharge is prominent) by obtaining a wet mount and a KOH preparation. If there is some doubt about the diagnosis, determination of the *maturation index* may be helpful in confirming it. This technique takes advantage of the effect of estrogens and progesterone on the vaginal epithelium and is an index of the percent of basal, intermediate, and superficial cells. A scraping of the vaginal wall is fixed on a slide with Pap smear fixative and sent to a cytologist. In atrophic vaginitis a typical report would be approximately 80-20-0, respectively, of basal-intermediate-superficial cells; in contrast, a well estrogenized vagina would show the percentage of cells as approximately 0-20-80.

Treatment

Atrophic vaginitis is treated with vaginal estrogens to improve vaginal epithelization. An estrogen-containing cream (such as Dienestrol or Premarin) should

Table 91.2
Management of Gonococcal Infection

UNCOMPLICATED INFECTION (asymptomatic, cervicovaginal, or anorectal symptoms; pharyngitis)
1. a. Procaine penicillin, 4.8 million units i.m. plus 1.0 g of probenecid p.o. 30 min before injection
   or
   b. Ampicillin, 3.5 g p.o. in a single dose plus 1.0 g of probenecid p.o.
   or
   c. Tetracycline, 500 mg p.o. q.i.d. for 5 days Tetracycline should not be used in pregnant women because of potential toxic effects for mother and fetus,
   or
   d. Spectinomycin, 2.0 g i.m. (single dose) for penicillin-resistant gonococci, or for patients allergic to penicillin who are pregnant, or are intolerant of tetracycline
2. Treat partner(s) appropriately
3. Follow-up culture 1 week after completing treatment
4. Report to local health department

PELVIC INFLAMMATORY DISEASE
1. Ambulatory treatment
   a. Tetracycline, 500 mg p.o. q.i.d. for 10 days
      or
      Procaine penicillin or ampicillin as above followed by ampicillin, 500 mg p.o. q.i.d. for 10 days
   b. Daily contact or observation to assure improvement
2. Indications for hospitalization
   a. Diagnosis uncertain (to exclude appendicitis, ectopic pregnancy, nongonococcal PID, pelvic abscess)
   b. Diagnosis is certain but patient is toxic or unable to follow ambulatory treatment reliably
   c. Patient does not respond promptly to ambulatory treatment

ARTHRITIS-DERMATITIS SYNDROME
1. In patients without known allergy to penicillin or probenecid
   a. Hospitalize: Aqueous crystalline penicillin G, 10 million units intravenously per day for 3 days or until there is significant clinical improvement. This may be followed with ampicillin, 500 mg, four times a day orally to complete 7 days of antibiotic treatment
   or
   b. Hospital or ambulatory treatment: Ampicillin, 3.5 g orally, plus probenecid 1 g, followed by ampicillin, 500 mg, four times a day orally for at least 7 days (may be given to an ambulatory patient who is not toxic, is reliable, and is contacted/examined daily)
2. In patients allergic to penicillin and/or probenecid
   a. Tetracycline, 500 mg four times a day orally for at least 7 days (avoid in pregnancy, see above),
   or
   b. Erythromycin, 500 mg orally four times a day for 7 days,
   or
   c. Spectinomycin 2.0 g i.m. twice a day for 3 days

be prescribed, one or two applicators full every night for 2 to 3 weeks until symptoms have improved, and then the dose is gradually tapered, omitting one dose per week every 1 or 2 weeks until the patient is administering only one dose per week; and it is continued then at this level as long as necessary (usually as long as sexual activity continues). The estrogen present in vaginal creams is readily absorbed into the circulation and, therefore, precautions should be taken just as they are with the continued use of oral estrogens (see Chapter 74).

If the problem is mild the patient may be able to relieve dyspareunia by using a water-soluble lubricant such as K-Y jelly, available at pharmacies, just before sexual intercourse.

The symptoms of atrophic vaginitis may alternatively be controlled by the oral administration of cyclic low dose estrogen and progestin as described in Chapter 74.

URETHRAL SYNDROME

This syndrome includes dysuria, frequency, and urgency, but "significant" bacterial infection is not identified. It has many causes but vulvar, vaginal, or cervical inflammation accounts for a significant proportion of cases. This syndrome is discussed fully in Chapter 26.

CUTANEOUS VULVAR LESIONS

There are a large number of cutaneous vulvar lesions which may cause the patient to seek medical advice. In these situations, the *history* is very informative. There is usually a variable degree of itching, and often the patient says she has a feeling that her genitalia feel "different."

The history should include information about perineal hygiene, the use of perineal perfumes or recently acquired undergarments, medications, and general health. The *objective data base is developed* by a careful examination of the pelvis, cancer smears when needed, and in certain cases, biopsies of suspicious lesions (performed by the general physician if he is experienced or, if not, by a gynecologist or a dermatologist).

Cutaneous vulvar lesions can best be divided into five primary disorders on the basis of their etiology (Table 91.1, p. 996): inflammation, infection, neoplasia, dystrophy, and altered pigmentation (11).

Inflammation

Intertrigo and contact dermatitis are the most common noninfectious problems of the vulva that are associated with inflammation.

INTERTRIGO

Intertrigo is an eruption that occurs on body surfaces where the skin rubs together. It is especially common in the vulva and inguinal area of obese patients. It appears as an erythematous sharply defined area, often with secondary excoriations. Infectious diseases such as candidiasis which may also have satellite lesions, tinea, or erythrasma should be ruled out by scraping the margin of the lesion and making a KOH preparation for the microscopic diagnosis of fungal infection or by showing coral red fluorescence using a Wood's lamp (an inexpensive lamp available from physician supply stores) for the diagnosis of erythrasma (caused by a *Corynebacterium* species) as discussed in Chapter 97.

Noninfectious causes of intertrigo such as psoriasis and seborrheic dermatitis also should be considered, and a search for other areas of involvement should be made (see Chapter 97). If there remains doubt about the diagnosis, a dermatologist should be consulted.

The treatment of various forms of intertrigo is discussed in detail in Chapter 97.

CONTACT DERMATITIS

Contact dermatitis located in the vulva and perineum is quite common and may be either primary irritant or allergic in type. Soaps and detergents are common irritants; and perfumes (such as in cosmetics, soaps, or toilet tissue), dyes, rubber (in clothing), drugs, and nickel (in jewelry) are common allergens.

In acute contact dermatitis the eruption begins in the area of contact and is characterized by erythema, edema, and the formation of vesicles or bullae. Often, secondary excoriations and infections are present. In chronic cases, the diagnosis is more difficult and the changes are more indurated and less vesicular and edematous.

The management of contact dermatitis is discussed in Chapter 97.

Infection/Infestations

Vulvovaginal infections are sometimes limited to the cutaneous vulvar area; but they are managed in the same way as the more widespread vulvovaginal infections discussed above. In addition to the causative agents already discussed, parasitic infestation should be considered. Pediculosis and scabies are common and are usually associated with severe pruritus and often the former simultaneously involves the umbilicus and breast. The diagnosis and management of these parasitic infestations are discussed fully in Chapter 97.

Miscellaneous Conditions

BARTHOLIN CYSTS

These are common swellings of the vulva. The Bartholin glands are located posteriorly on either side of the fourchette (see Fig. 91.1) and open onto the vaginal wall. They may become infected with a variety of organisms including *E. coli*, *Gonococcus*, *Trichomonas*, as well as staphylococci and streptococci. Where there is intense infection or abscess formation, the patient should be referred urgently to a gynecologist for evaluation and possibly marsupialization of the abscess under local anaesthesia. The

gynecologist will probably use systemic antibiotics. If the patient is seen after resolution of the acute inflammation the symptoms are not dramatic and often the swelling is episodic. The location of the lesion is diagnostic. Sitz baths several times a day may provide temporary relief, but recurrence is likely, and when the cyst is large, the patient should be referred to a gynecologist for consideration for marsupialization or removal.

SEBACEOUS CYSTS, LIPOMATA, AND FIBROMATA

All of these conditions may occur in the vulvar area. When they are distressing to the patient or when there is doubt about their nature, referral to a gynecologist or dermatologist for evaluation and for consideration for removal is suggested.

Malignant disease of the vulvar area is rare and affects primarily postmenopausal women. Nevertheless, early detection may remarkably improve survival and since vulvar malignancies have a precancerous phase, early detection is the responsibility of the physician performing the annual health maintenance assessment (see Chapter 92). Any abnormal appearing tissues such as leukoplakia or Bowen's disease (which is observed as a superficially ulcerating red plaque often appearing granular and occasionally secondarily infected) should raise concern, and the patient should be referred to a gynecologist for evaluation and, usually, biopsy.

Vulvar Dystrophy

Vulvar dystrophy is a condition best managed by a gynecologist or dermatologist because it is chronic and very difficult to eradicate. Patients are older and usually complain of persistent itching and soreness, and examination reveals whitish, thickened skin and excoriated, often atrophic areas.

A biopsy of these lesions is necessary for proper classification.

PSYCHOSEXUAL ASPECTS OF VULVOVAGINAL COMPLAINTS

Because of the normal variation in vaginal "secretions" and the normal physiologic variations in the vulvovaginal region, a physician should not suggest treatment for an organic vulvovaginal disorder unless its diagnosis is confirmed. The vulvovaginal region is often the focus of symptoms of an emotional disorder. For example, sexual contact with a new partner often produces vulvovaginal symptoms in which the findings are normal and a sense of guilt is the real etiology. Also patients may develop persistent symptoms due to an unverbalized desire to avoid sexual intercourse. A psychologic problem may affect a woman of any age; the diagnosis should be considered when the patient seeks appointments with the physician and no organic cause can be identified.

The psychiatric section (Section 2) of this book deals in detail with diagnosis and management of psychologic disorders.

References

General

Gordner, L and Kauman, RH: *Benign Diseases of the Vulva and Vagina,* Ed. 2. G. K. Hall Medical Publisher, Boston, 1981.
    This extensively illustrated textbook is a valuable resource covering diagnosis and treatment of common disorders of the vulva and vagina.
Ridley, CM: *The Vulva.* W. B. Saunders, Philadelphia, 1975.
    This short monograph is a well written review of dermatologic conditions encountered in the vulvar area. It covers all aspects of diagnoses and treatment.

Specific

1. Caldwell, JG, *et al.*: Sensitivity and reproducibility of Thayer Martin culture media in diagnosing gonorrhea in women. *Am J Obstet Gynecol 109:* 463, 1971.
2. Davis, BA: Vaginal moniliasis in private practice. *Obstet Gynecol 34:* 40, 1969.
3. Duddle, AW: Oral contraceptive medications and vulvo-vaginal conditions. *Obstet Gynecol 34:* 373, 1969.
4. Eliot, BW, Howat, RC and Mack, AE: Comparison between effects of nystatin, clotrimazole and Miconazole on vaginal candidiasis. *Br J Obstet Gynecol 86:* 573, 1979.
5. Glasgow, LA: Staphylococcal infection in toxic shock syndrome. *N Engl J Med 303:* 1473, 1980.
6. Kaufman, RH: The origin and diagnosis of "non-specific vaginitis." *N Engl J Med 303:* 637, 1980.
7. Larsen, B and Galask, RP: Vaginal microbial flora; practical and theoretic relevance. *Obstet Gynecol 55:* 1005, 1980.
8. Lauke, A: Herpes virus—cancer of the cervix. In: *Viruses Associated with Human Cancer,* edited by LA Phillips. Marcell-Derker, New York, 1982.
9. Pheifer, TA, Forsyth, PS, Durfee, MA, Pollock, HM and Holmer, KK: Non-specific vaginitis; role of *Haemophilus vaginalis* and treatment with metronidazole. *N Engl J Med 298:* 1429, 1978.
10. *The Medical Letter, 17:* 53, June 20, 1975.
11. Tovell, HM and Young HJ, Jr: Classification of vulvar diseases. *Clin Obstet Gynecol 21:* 955, 1978.

CHAPTER NINETY-TWO

Early Detection of Gynecological Malignancy

J. COURTLAND ROBINSON, M.D.

PREVENTIVE GYNECOLOGY

The benefits of preventive medicine are especially applicable in office gynecology. Ambulatory care provides an ideal setting in which preventive measures can be carried out, particularly with respect to the early detection of cancer of the organs of reproduction.

The female organs of reproduction are important sites for the development of malignancies. Twenty percent of cancers found in women involve the genital organs (8). Overall 5-year cure rates are in the range of 55 to 60% and are related to the stage of the disease upon discovery. A most impressive event in the past 30 years has been the decline in mortality of cancer of the cervix and uterus, attributable primarily to earlier detection (6). As with the breast, having the patient herself take responsibility for looking for abnormalities in a regular and systematic manner and, equally important, the annual examination by a trained person, have resulted in the diagnosis of a higher proportion of lesions at early stages, at which time cures are much more likely (3).

DETECTION OF VULVAR LESIONS

The vulva, like the skin, has a premalignant phase in the development of epidermal carcinoma. Lesions of the vulva represent about 4% of all cancers of the pelvic organs. The invasive stage is seen primarily, but not exclusively, in postmenopausal women. *Intraepithelial carcinoma of the vulva* is the term now used to include diseases that were once called Bowen's disease, erythroplasia of Queyrat, squamous cell carcinoma *in situ,* and Paget's disease. While intraepithelial lesions can be distinguished by microscopic examination, they often appear to the physician to be well-defined innocent lesions of the vulva or mucous membranes. They may be red, raised, granular, or velvety lesions, or simple white patches; or a mixture of these, with or without superimposed ulceration and crusting. The lesions are often asymptomatic but may be associated with itching or soreness. The physician should be suspicious when anything is seen other than well-developed intact skin and mucous membrane and especially if the lesions are chronic and unresponsive to topical treatment. At that point he should refer the patient to a gynecologist for consultation, biopsy and treatment. Intraepithelial carcinoma is managed either by surgery or locally applied 5-fluorouracil and a gynecologist should follow the patients regularly to evaluate for a recurrence.

Prevention of advanced disease requires that the patient be taught to examine her vulva periodically by use of a mirror, and to report to her physician any changes in the external genitalia. It is important that the physician examine the patient promptly if a change is noted and that an annual examination be performed when there are no complaints. Special care must be taken in older women who are often reluctant to complain of a vaginal or vulvar problem. Examination by both patient and physician requires a good light and separation of the labia majora and labia minora.

DETECTION OF CERVICAL LESIONS

Invasive *epidermoid carcinoma* of the cervix is the second most common malignancy of the reproductive organs (endometrial cancer is the first) (8); there are 16,000 new cases in the United States every year. Significant reduction in mortality and morbidity has been achieved by vigorous promotion and acceptance of the annual pelvic examination in combination with the cancer detection smear (Pap smear) (6).

The incidence of *preinvasive cervical cancer* (i.e., *in situ* cancer) seems to be increasing among younger patients (1). The etiology of this condition is still not settled, but at present, herpes simplex virus Type II is thought to be a factor. The major risk factors are onset of sexual activity at a young age, early childbearing, and multiple sexual partners. The malignancy involves the squamocolumnar junction which is exposed in the young patient to an acid milieu resulting from estrogen stimulation, to foreign material secondary to intercourse, and to the trauma of childbearing (1). All these are common events for most women; therefore, the reason why less than 1% of women develop invasive or preinvasive neoplasia of the cervix is still a mystery. *Metaplasia* in the cervix is a normal response; but in 2 to 6% of women *dysplasia* occurs; and it is in this group with an atypical cellular process that neoplasia may arise. It is in this situation that cytologic screening becomes important since the changes are not visible to the naked eye.

The cancer detection smear, when properly obtained, is from 80 to 90% effective in identifying a problem (1). Proper technique requires an appropriately shaped plastic or wooden stick which abuts the cervical os and permits the squamocolumnar junction to be scraped. The anatomic relationship of this junc-

tion varies in the adolescent, the sexually active woman, and the postmenopausal woman (see Fig. 92.1). When the junction is not seen (e.g., in an atrophic cervix), a cotton-tipped stick should be used. If no inflammation is present, secretion in the posterior fornix may be submitted along with the material from the squamocolumular junction. Vaginal bleeding within 24 hours, douching, or vaginal medication are relative contraindications to obtaining a Pap smear since the vast majority will be technically unsatisfactory and will necessitate a repeat examination. Also, since lubricant will interfere with the reading of the smear, its use should be avoided, if possible. In patients with atrophic vaginitis, where lubricant may be necessary, it should be used sparingly to avoid contaminating the smear. The physician should select a cytology laboratory that has satisfactory quality control, use the proper fixative techniques required by the laboratory, and learn the systems of reporting. It is important for the physician to provide the laboratory the patient's age, the date of her last menstrual period, and to comment on the presence or absence of infection. The laboratory report should state whether the sample was satisfactory or unsatisfactory. An unsatisfactory slide must be repeated. There is disagreement about whether the cytologic sample must contain endocervical cells to be satisfactory (1).

The cytologist's report usually will describe the results as negative (with or without inflammation) or as showing atypia, dysplasia, or changes suggestive of cancer; these findings may be quantitated as mild, moderate, or severe. The presence of yeast or trichomonads may be noted also.

Patients with *significant dysplasia* or with *moderate* or *severe atypia* should be referred for further evaluation of the cervix. The *colposcope* (Fig. 92.2) is an optical system which permits the magnification by 10 to 20 times of the appearance of the cervix and the squamocolumnar junction (Fig. 92.3). During colposcopy the woman is in the lithotomy position with a vaginal speculum in place; the procedure requires 5 to 10 min. Colposcopy, in addition to the Pap smear, is very important in helping the gynecologist to decide the site from which abnormal cells have arisen and to guide the location of a cervical biopsy.

Patients with *mild dysplasia* or *mild atypia* with inflammation (such as trichomoniasis) can be managed by local treatment of the infection (see Chapter 91), but a follow-up smear should be taken in 3 months. If infection is not present or if it was present and has now healed, the patient should be followed closely with a follow-up smear at 6-month intervals for 2 years. If on follow-up examination the smear continues to show persistent mild dysplasia or mild atypia, the patient should be referred to a gynecologist for colposcopic examination. Patients who are asymptomatic, who have only a normal discharge, and in whom the report indicates only inflammation, need not undergo colposcopic examination. Also,

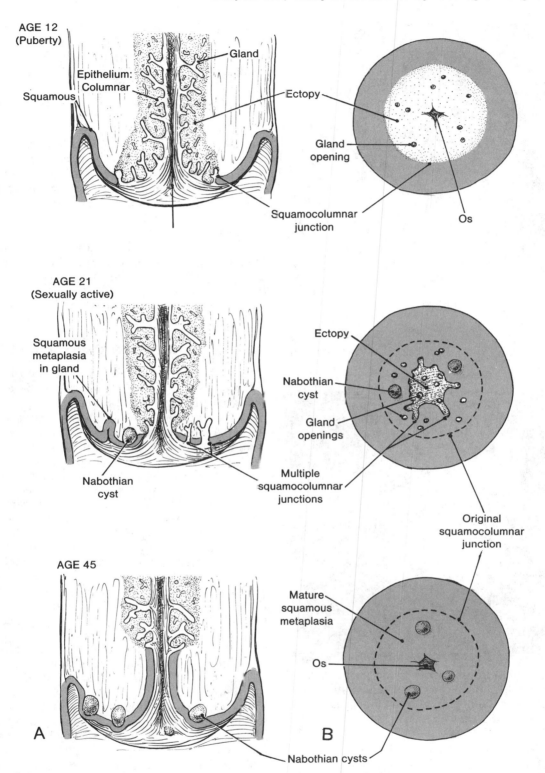

Figure 92.1   The uterine cervix in women of various ages. (*A*) Coronal section of the cervix and vaginal vault. (*B*) Vaginal view of the cervix. (Redrawn with permission from R. M. Briggs: *Obstetrical and Gynecological Survey, 34:* 70, 1980.)

asymptomatic patients with a report indicating the presence of a few yeast or trichomonad cells do not require therapy.

The suggested *frequency* of obtaining a cancer de-tection smear in controversial (2, 5); it depends in part on the patient's virginity and age. Pap smears are not necessary until sexual activity begins (except for adolescent and young women who have been

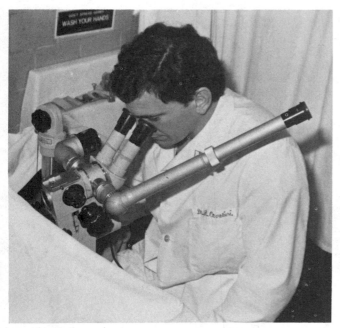

Figure 92.2   Use of the colposcope in examination of the cervix.

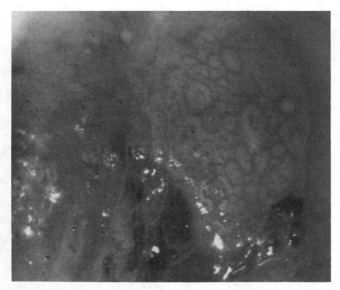

Figure 92.3   Photograph taken through the colposcope showing the mosaic pattern associated with dysplasia of the cervix. (Taken from the files of the late Dr. Rafael Garcia-Bunuel.)

exposed to diethylstilbestrol in utero). Also, a woman who has had three negative smears taken at least a year apart after the age of 60 is at a very low risk of developing invasive cancer of the cervix and need not have routine smears obtained thereafter.

The appropriate frequency of Pap smears in women who are in their reproductive years is uncertain. Many argue that the current decline in the incidence of invasive cervical cancer is a direct result of the practice of yearly monitoring, and that that

practice should be continued. Others point out that invasive neoplastic changes in the cervix take years to develop; they argue that smears at 5-year intervals are adequate and that the cost of more frequent Pap smears is not justified. Perhaps a reasonable compromise is to obtain a smear at 2 to 3-year intervals in women in the reproductive years unless suspicious changes in the cervix are seen at the time of the annual pelvic examination or unless the patient feels more satisfied with a yearly smear. Since an annual pelvic examination is suggested to detect other lesions, such as gonorrhea or ovarian cancer, the additional cost of the Pap smear at the time of the pelvic examination is relatively low. There is no reason to obtain a smear every 6 months if previous specimens have been negative. Also, if a woman has had a total hysterectomy (cervix removed) there is no need for a Pap smear unless the surgery was for cervical dysplasia or cancer, in which case a regular smear from the apex of the vagina should be obtained every year.

DETECTION OF ENDOMETRIAL LESIONS

Adenocarcinoma of the endometrium is the most common cancer of the genital organs; there are 38,000 new cases in the United States every year. The disease is associated with a relative excess of estrogen and a lack of progesterone. This hormone pattern is found in the postmenopausal period, when 75% of these cancers occur (8). There is an increased risk of endometrial cancer in infertile patients, obese patients, patients with dysfunctional bleeding, women with a history of prolonged estrogen therapy, patients who do not ovulate regularly, patients with a history of adenomatous hyperplasia, and possibly patients with diabetes mellitus. Bleeding is the major symptom, and early detection requires patients to be educated to report abnormal bleeding when they are approaching the perimenopausal period and when they are postmenopausal (see Chapter 74). With abnormal bleeding at these times, the physician should strongly suspect endometrial cancer and refer the patient to a gynecologist for endometrial biopsy and/or for dilation and curettage. A pelvic examination is not helpful in the early detection of malignancy of the endometrium.

The cancer detection smear is of use only in detecting endometrial cancer when, by chance, malignant cells from the endometrium have passed into the vaginal pool.

Therefore, attempts have been made to design a method of obtaining cells from the endometrium by uterine aspiration cytology (only fair accuracy) and by aspirational biopsy (reasonable accuracy) (7). Most lesions which are precursors of endometrial carcinoma are present during the perimenopausal period, and they are recognizable by examination of material from an aspirational curettage, an office procedure usually done with minimal discomfort.

Therefore, it is reasonable that patients who have an increased risk of endometrial cancer (see above) and who are at the menopause be referred to a gynecologist for suction endometrial biopsy (4); the benefit of this approach to early detection will require time to confirm.

DETECTION OF OVARIAN CANCER

Malignancies of the ovary are silent until they are sufficiently large to produce symptoms or until they have spread to other organs. Early detection depends upon the annual pelvic and rectal examination; unfortunately, most ovarian cancers are advanced when diagnosed, and the cure rate is low (8, 9). On very rare occasions, a malignant ovarian tumor will be found in the premenarchal patient; but it is important that the incidence increases with age. The genesis of ovarian cancer is unknown, and little progress has been made in identifying the patient at risk, in early detection, or in improving the survival rate (9).

Except for the relatively uncommon functioning ovarian tumors, symptoms from cancer of the ovary are minimal in the early stages, and the symptoms which develop later are largely a function of the size and location of the tumor. Symptoms of abdominal enlargement, a sense of fullness in the pelvis, changes in bowel function, or evidence in the lower extremities of venous or lymphatic obstruction all occur late. Sudden discomfort raising suspicion of an acute abdominal catastrophe may be experienced if a tumor undergoes torsion, necrosis, hemorrhage, rupture, or infection. Signs of ascites, nodules in the cul-de-sac, and either venous or lymphatic obstruction all suggest that a malignant disease is present.

The examination of the patient with ovarian cancer reveals that the ovary is enlarged, but it must be remembered that during the reproductive years some enlargement may be physiologic. The normal ovary is about $1 \times 2 \times 3$ cm in size and is found lateral to the dome of the uterus. When the uterus is retroverted, the ovaries may not be palpable. When the ovaries are compressed by the examining finger an uncomfortable sensation is noted by the patient. Functional ovarian (follicle or corpus luteum) cysts are common; they may enlarge up to 4 to 5 cm and may be detected during a pelvic examination. Functional cysts should be soft, cystic, and no larger than 4 to 5 cm in diameter; and after an observation period of 8 to 10 weeks, they should disappear. If there is any doubt about the nature of the cyst and follow-up of 8 to 10 weeks is not desired, physiologic cysts may be shown to be functional by suppressing the pituitary hormones; this can be accomplished by prescribing an oral contraceptive preparation such as Demulin, Norlestrin 1/50, or Ortho-Novum 1/50 daily for 6 weeks. Functional cysts regress, but tumors do not. When there is question about the presence of a cyst, a sonographic study of the pelvis may be helpful, especially in obese patients. A sonogram can detect a cyst which is 1 to 4 cm or greater in diameter; cysts that are less than 4 cm in the ovulating woman are usually functional and can be followed (see above). All patients found to have hard or firm adnexal masses and all cystic tumors larger than 4 to 5 cm regardless of the age of the patient should be evaluated by a gynecologist.

Based on the idea that the ovary shrinks in the menopause, there are those who feel that any ovary which can be felt in a menopausal woman should be investigated. While there is controversy about this, it is reasonable to evaluate those patients in which the ovary feels enlarged or is observed to be enlarging on annual examination.

References

General

Jones, HW, Jr and Jones, GS (editors): *Novak's Textbook of Gynecology*, Ed. 10. Williams & Wilkins, Baltimore, 1981.

> This text is a valuable resource to the general physician and covers all aspects of pertinent gynecology. It is heavily illustrated and very readable.

Specific

1. Briggs, RM: Dysplasia and early neoplasia of the uterine cervix. A review. *Obstet Gynecol Survey* 34: 70, 1980.
2. Consensus—more of less—on the Pap smear: *Science* 209: 672, 1980.
3. Cramer, DW: The role of cervical cytology in the declining morbidity and mortality of cervical cancer. *Cancer* 34: 2018, 1974.
4. Gusberg, SB: An approach to the control of carcinoma of the endometrium. *Ca-A Cancer J Clin* 30: 16, 1980.
5. Guidelines for the cancer-related check-up: *Ca-A Cancer J Clin* 30: 194, 1980.
6. Guzick, DS: Efficacy of screening for cervical cancer; a review. *Am J Public Health* 68: 125, 1978.
7. Kwada, CY and An-Foraker, SH: Screening for endometrial cancer. *Clin Obstet Gynecol* 22: 713, 1979.
8. Silverberg, E: Cancer statistics, 1980. *Ca-A Cancer J Clin* 30: 23, 1980.
9. Woodruff, JD: The pathogenesis of ovarian neoplasia. *Johns Hopkins Med J* 144: 117, 1979.

SECTION 14

Problems of the Eyes and Ears

CHAPTER 93

Hearing Loss and Associated Ear Problems

L. RANDOL BARKER, M.D., and EDWARD S. COHN, M.D.

A 1971 report from the National Health Survey estimated that 13.2 million persons in the United States had significant bilateral hearing impairment; of these, 5.5 million were over 65 years of age (1). The survey also indicated that a large proportion of symptomatic adults go directly to a hearing aid dealer rather than to a physician and/or audiologist for initial evaluation. Many patients, however, will present the problem of hearing loss to their physician. This chapter provides an approach to hearing loss and associated ear problems which is appropriate in an ambulatory setting. The fundamental steps are classification of the severity, mechanism, and probable etiology of hearing loss; management of the problem either by treatment and follow-up in the office or by referral; and prognostication regarding the long term expectations for the patient.

EAR STRUCTURE AND FUNCTION

In order to classify the mechanism of hearing impairment (conductive or sensorineural), the structure and function of the components of the ear must be understood (see Fig. 93.1).

The *external ear* is composed of the auricle, the auditory meatus, and the external auditory canal. The outer portion of the canal is cartilaginous and is covered by thick skin which contains hair follicles and the cerumen-secreting glands. Cerumen protects the epithelium and captures foreign particles entering the canal. The inner portion of the canal is bony and

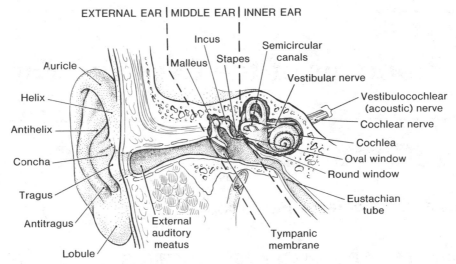

EXTERNAL EAR | MIDDLE EAR | INNER EAR

Figure 93.1   Normal structures of the ear.

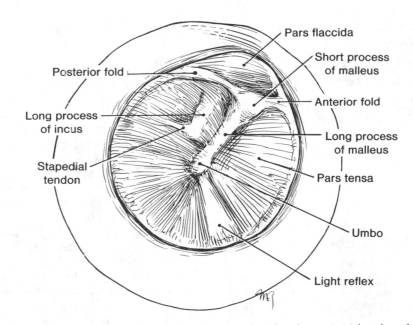

Figure 93.2   Right tympanic membrane, showing important landmarks.

is covered by thin skin without hair follicles or cerumen glands.

The *middle ear* consists of the tympanic membrane, the air space behind it, and the three linked ossicles (malleus, incus, and stapes). The malleus is attached to the tympanic membrane, while the stapes makes contact with the inner ear via the bony stapes footplate at the oval window. The landmarks seen on inspection of the tympanic membrane are shown in Figure 93.2. The lining of the middle ear is a mucus-secreting epithelium similar to that which lines the nose. The middle ear communicates with the nose via the eustachian tube, which enters the lateral nasopharynx; patency of the eustachian tube assures equal pressure on either side of the tympanic membrane, a condition which is critical for transmission of sound via the middle ear.

The *inner ear* is encased in very hard bone (the otic capsule) and is fluid-filled. It consists of a sensory organ for hearing (cochlea) and the sensory organ for balance (labyrinth). Nerves from the cochlea and labyrinth unite to form the acoustic nerve, which runs through the bony internal auditory canal in the temporal bone to the brainstem.

The *conductive system* of the ear includes the external auditory canal, the tympanic membrane, the middle ear, and the ossicles. Hearing loss due to defects in this portion of the ear is termed *conductive hearing loss*. The *sensorineural system* of the ear consists of the cochlea, the auditory nerve, and the

Table 93.1
A Practical Method for Assessing Severity of Hearing Loss in the Office[a]

Severity of Hearing Loss	Social Difficulty	Office Voice Test	Pure Tone Audiogram
Normal hearing	None	18 ft or more using normal voice	No loss over 10 dB[b]
Slight hearing loss	Long distance speech	Not over 12 ft using normal voice	10–30 dB loss
Moderate hearing loss	Short distance speech	Not over 3 ft using normal voice	Up to 60 dB loss
Severe hearing loss	All unamplified voices	Raised voice at meatus	Over 60 dB loss
Total hearing loss	Voices never heard	All speech and sound	Over 90 dB loss

[a] Adapted from S. R. Mawson: *Diseases of the Ear*, Williams & Wilkins, Baltimore, 1974.
[b] dB, decibel.

brainstem auditory pathways projecting to the auditory cortex. In these structures, sound waves delivered by the conductive system are transformed into nerve impulses. Hearing loss due to defects in this portion of the ear is termed *sensorineural hearing loss*, which may be localized as cochlear or retrocochlear.

DETERMINING SEVERITY AND MECHANISM OF HEARING LOSS

Office Testing

Regardless of the specific cause of hearing loss, the severity of the impairment and the probable mechanism (conductive or sensorineural) can be determined in the office. This determination can be made from a combination of the history, the patient's ability to hear the spoken voice in the office, and testing with a tuning fork and a ticking watch.

A practical method for evaluating the *severity of hearing impairment* includes an estimate of the social problems that have accrued due to difficulty in hearing and an assessment of response to voice testing in the office; these two findings can be equated with various levels of abnormality in the audiogram (see Table 93.1). *Slight* impairment indicates difficulty in hearing long distance speech; for example, at small group meetings, social gatherings, or the theater. *Moderate* impairment includes some difficulty with short distance speech and conversation. *Severe* impairment indicates no understanding of the conversational voice but understanding of the amplified voice. Amplification may be achieved by raising the voice or electronically by use of a hearing aid (see below, p. 1016). *Total* impairment indicates inability to hear and understand the spoken voice despite maximum amplification.

In the patient with significant hearing impairment, the *frequency range* which is involved can also be approximated in the office by testing recognition of the sounds "ah" (low frequency, vowel sound) and "ss" (high frequency, consonant) when these sounds are spoken about 2 feet behind the ear being tested, with the other ear covered. A ticking watch, held a few inches from the ear, also tests hearing at high frequencies, while tuning forks test relatively low frequency hearing.

The *mechanism* of hearing impairment can be classified tentatively as conductive or sensorineural by the use of *tuning fork tests* (Rinne and Weber). A 512 cycle per second (cps) tuning fork is preferable to very low frequency tuning forks (the sound from 128 cps or 256 cps tuning forks may be masked by ambient noise; also low frequency stimuli may be felt even though they are not heard). The interpretation of tuning fork tests is summarized in Table 93.2.

RINNE TEST

This test is used to evaluate hearing loss in one ear. It is important to mask the hearing in the other ear by rubbing paper over that ear to create a rustling sound. The tuning fork is struck against a firm surface; then it is held against the mastoid bone until the patient no longer hears the sound; then it is held about 1 inch from the canal until the patient no longer hears the sound. The patient with normal hearing should hear the sound twice as long by air as by bone conduction. A modified Rinne is simply to have the patient compare the loudness of bone and air conduction; air conduction should definitely be louder.

Table 93.2
Classification of Probable Mechanism of Hearing Loss Using Tuning Fork Tests

Classification	Rinne Test	Weber Test
NORMAL HEARING		
Both ears	AC>BC[a]	Not lateralized
CONDUCTIVE LOSS[b]		
Right ear	Right ear—BC>AC	Lateralized to right ear
	Left ear—AC>BC	
Left ear	Right ear—AC>BC	Lateralized to left ear
	Left ear—BC>AC	
Both ears	Right ear—BC>AC	Lateralized to poorer ear
	Left ear—BC>AC	
SENSORINEURAL LOSS		
Right ear	AC>BC bilaterally	Lateralized to left ear
Left ear	AC>BC bilaterally	Lateralized to right ear
Both ears	AC>BC bilaterally	Lateralized to better ear

[a] AC, air conduction; BC, bone conduction.
[b] Because sound transmission by air is much more efficient than by bone, air conduction may remain greater than bone conduction in early or minimal conductive hearing loss.

WEBER TEST

This test is performed by placing the tuning fork on the forehead and asking the patient if the sound is louder on one side. The reason for lateralization to the side with conductive loss is that environmental noise is masked on this side, increasing the efficiency of cochlear detection of sound created by stimulating adjacent bone.

Audiometry

When the patient is referred to an otolaryngologist for evaluation of hearing loss, *pure tone audiometry* is utilized to characterize the extent of impairment. Both air conduction and bone conduction measurements are made for sounds of varying intensity (decibels) and frequency (cps). The usual frequencies tested are 250, 500, 1000, 2000, 3000, 4000, 6000, and 8000 cps (the range 500 to 3500 is most important for understanding speech). The results are plotted on a graph called an audiogram. The vertical axis shows hearing loss in decibels and the horizontal axis shows the frequency of the stimulus. Examples of audiograms showing normal hearing, conductive hearing loss, and sensorineural hearing loss are reproduced in Figure 93.3. Speech audiometry, which measures the subject's ability to hear *and* understand the spoken voice, is also done as part of a formal hearing evaluation.

GENERAL APPROACH TO CHRONIC HEARING LOSS

Assessment and care for moderate or severe chronic hearing loss usually require the assistance of a consulting otolaryngologist. For many patients, little can be done to reverse the primary process, and care consists of compensating for existing hearing loss and preventing further loss.

Communication

Counseling of the family and others who speak to the patient with moderate to severe hearing loss should emphasize two principles:

1. Facilitate communication by consistently using the following adjuncts to speech: face the patient; obtain his attention before speaking; speak slowly; utilize gestures; and speak louder if the patient says that it helps.

2. Expect some difficulty in discriminating consonants (the high frequency hearing loss typical of most sensorineural deafness particularly affects this type of discrimination; for example, the word "yes" may be understood as "yet, get, less, mess," etc.).

For the patient with *total hearing loss*, the principle governing all communication is that the message must be *seen* by the patient. Most patients will let the physician know the mode of communication they prefer: lipreading or writing. Whenever there is any question about the effectiveness of lipreading, written exchange of information should be utilized. This can be facilitated by assuring that paper and a pen or pencil are always available to the patient. In large communities, a translator who can communicate in American Sign Language may be available to assist patients who know sign language.

Hearing Aids

Hearing aids (miniature microphone-amplifier-loudspeaker units) can assist the patient with sensorineural hearing loss (and some patients with irreversible conductive loss). These aids can increase the intensity of a sound by up to 70 decibels. Thus, a sound of about 60 decibels (the level of average conversational speech) passing through an aid may enter the ear at a level of 130 decibels. This represents the maximum usable gain of an aid since sounds above this level become painful. Only trial and ad-

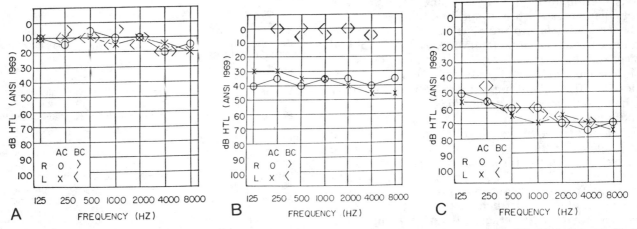

Figure 93.3 Examples of audiograms. (*A*) Audiogram in a person with normal hearing. (*B*) Bilateral conductive hearing loss (moderate). (*C*) Bilateral sensorineural hearing loss (severe). (From L. Price and R. Snider: *Clinical Aspects of Aging*, edited by W. Reichel. Williams & Wilkins, Baltimore, 1978 (5).)

Table 93.3
Major Causes of Hearing Loss in Adults

Causes	Mechanism[a]	Onset Rapid (Hours to Days) or Gradual (Months to Years)	Bilateral or Unilateral
EXTERNAL AUDITORY CANAL			
Cerumen impaction	C	Either	Usually unilateral
Foreign body	C	Rapid	Unilateral
Otitis externa	C	Rapid	Unilateral
New growth	C	Gradual	Unilateral
MIDDLE EAR			
Serous otitis media	C	Either	Either
Acute otitis media	C	Rapid	Unilateral
Barotrauma	C or SN	Rapid	Unilateral
Traumatic perforation of tympanic membrane	C	Rapid	Unilateral
Chronic otitis media	C	Gradual	Unilateral
Ossicular chain problems:			
Adhesive otitis media	C	Gradual	Unilateral
Tympanosclerosis	C	Gradual	Either
Traumatic injury	C or SN	Rapid	Unilateral
Otosclerosis	C	Gradual	Bilateral
New growths	C or SN	Gradual	Unilateral
INNER EAR			
Presbycusis	SN	Gradual	Bilateral
Acoustic trauma	SN	Gradual	Bilateral
Drug-induced	SN	Either	Bilateral
Ménière's syndrome	SN	Rapid	Either
Central nervous system infection:			
Meningitis	SN	Rapid	Either
Syphilis	SN	Either	Either
Tuberculosis	SN	Either	Either
Acoustic neuroma	SN	Gradual	Unilateral
ATRAUMATIC SUDDEN SENSORINEURAL HEARING LOSS	SN	Rapid	Unilateral

[a] C, conductive; SN, sensorineural.

justment will determine whether an individual patient will benefit from a hearing aid. The cost to the patient is usually between $300.00 and $500.00. Under federal law, a patient now has 30 days to decide whether he wishes to keep a hearing aid.

A patient may mention certain specific *problems with the hearing aid* to his personal physician. There may be irritation of the conchal cartilage or even infection in the external canal. A poorly fitted hearing aid mold can cause pressure sores on the external ear (a particular hazard in the diabetic). Patients may also note an increase in cerumen accumulation in the aided ear. In each of these situations use of the aid should be discontinued until the process resolves. A better fitting mold will be needed to avoid recurrence in some patients. Others may do well by removing the aid periodically during the day.

CAUSES OF HEARING LOSS

The major causes of hearing loss in adults are listed in Table 93.3. For each condition, the table indicates mechanism, onset (rapid or gradual), and whether the condition is unilateral or bilateral. The guidelines that follow will enable the general physician to reach

a working diagnosis in most instances and to choose between primary treatment and referral for care by a specialist.

CONDITIONS OF THE EXTERNAL AUDITORY CANAL

A number of conditions may cause hearing impairment by blocking the external canal.

Cerumen Impaction

The patient will usually complain of intermittent fullness and hearing impairment on the affected side and may give a history of prior episodes. These symptoms may increase after showering, as moisture may cause cerumen to swell. Diagnosis is made by otoscopy.

If the cerumen appears to be soft, it may be removed by irrigation with use of a rubber-bulb syringe and warm tap water (close to body temperature), directing the water upwards and backwards against the wall of the canal. If the cerumen is impacted and difficult to remove, a few drops of hydrogen peroxide should be instilled twice daily for 1 week before removal. Alternatively, a cerumenolytic agent (Cerumenex) may be utilized. In general cerumenolytic agents should be used only in the office, as casual use by the patient at home increases the risk of allergic dermatitis (seen in about 1% of users). The following steps are taken: with the patient's head tilted laterally at 45° the ear is filled with cerumenolytic drops; a cotton plug is inserted for 15 to 20 min; the ear is then irrigated with lukewarm water and use of a soft rubber syringe. After irrigation, the tympanic membrane will usually show some injection around the handle of the malleus. In certain situations, cerumen removal should be done by an otolaryngologist: (a) in the patient with a known tympanic membrane perforation or a history of mastoidectomy, irrigation is contraindicated; wax removal must be done by suction-tip aspiration; (b) in the occasional patient with an impaction which does not respond to the usual measures described above; in this instance, removal of cerumen is accomplished by aspiration or by the use of an operating microscope.

Hearing impairment will usually be relieved immediately after removal of cerumen: occasionally after removal of a large impaction, complete return of hearing may take 1 or 2 days.

An impaction often follows vigorous efforts by the patient to remove wax with a cotton-tipped applicator. The patient should be reminded that ear wax is secreted to protect the lining of the canal and that the applicator should be used only to remove cerumen in the outer portion of the canal, for cosmetic purposes. Patients who have had recurrent impactions, often due to excess secretion of cerumen, may prevent recurrences by gently syringing their ears once or twice monthly, by using a soft rubber bulb and warm water.

Foreign Body

Usually the history discloses accidental insertion of a foreign body or entrance of an insect, which is followed by fullness and hearing impairment. Foreign bodies can be removed by use of fine forceps or a wax spoon. Removal by irrigation should be avoided if the foreign body is a vegetable, as water will cause further swelling. Insects should first be killed by instillation of mineral oil. Hearing impairment resolves promptly after removal of a foreign body.

Otitis Externa (Swimmer's Ear)

This condition is most common in the summer months, when heat and humidity, plus moisture introduced by swimming or perspiration, promote swelling and maceration of the stratum corneum of the skin; in the external canal, this process may cause pruritus. The patient will give a history of having scratched his ear for a few days, which is followed by exudation and pain; the pain is aggravated by movement of the external ear or the jaw. Hearing impairment will occur in those patients who present with swelling or debris which occludes the canal. The characteristics of the skin of the canal and of the exudate usually provide adequate clues to etiology, and cultures are needed only for patients who do not respond promptly to topical treatment. Copious or greenish exudate suggests *Pseudomonas*, the bacteria most frequently seen in otitis externa. Yellow crusting in the midst of a purulent exudate suggests *Staphylococcus aureus*. Canal skin that is scaling, cracked, and weeping indicates eczema (the history usually indicates that the condition is chronic). Fluffy material resembling bread mold, varying in color from white to black, suggests a fungal etiology (*Aspergillus* or *Candida*).

There are two general *principles of treatment* for all types of otitis externa: meticulous removal of all infected debris (with the use of a cotton applicator with a tightly rolled fresh cotton bud and a suction cannula if available) and instillation of an appropriate topical medication: for bacterial infections—an antibiotic-steroid combination, 3 or 4 drops, 3 to 4 times daily (e.g., Cortisporin Otic Suspension, containing polymyxin B-neomycin-hydrocortisone); for fungal infections—Burow's solution or 2% nonaqueous acetic acid (e.g., VoSol Otic Solution) 3 to 4 drops, 3 to 4 times daily; for eczema without superimposed infection—a topical steroid cream or solution applied 3 to 4 times daily (e.g., triamcinolone 0.1%). In some patients, the canal may be so swollen that topical medication does not enter the canal efficiently. In this case, a cylindrical cotton wick (or a commercially available sponge wick, such as Otowick), approximately the length of the ear canal (1 inch in adults), should be saturated with the desired medication and worked by gentle twisting into the canal until only the end is visible. The patient may then apply several drops of the medication to the wick 3 to 4 times daily, and the wick will carry it into the canal. The wick can usually be removed after 48 to 72 hours, and treatment can be completed as stated above.

Most episodes of otitis externa resolve completely after 5 to 7 days, and it is important to terminate topical treatment at this time. The ear cannot return to a normal physiologic state as long as a foreign substance (topical medicine) is constantly introduced into it; persistent treatment may lead to dermatitis medicamentosa. As a precaution against overtreatment, the prescription for ear drops should be nonrefillable, and only a small amount (10 ml) should be dispensed.

During treatment of otitis externa, moisture should be strictly avoided. During bathing, the ear should be plugged with cotton impregnated with petroleum jelly. To prevent recurrence, the patient should be warned against meddling with the ear (particularly frequent cleansing with cotton-tipped applicators, a common inciting cause).

Hearing impairment due to otitis externa should resolve promptly when swelling recedes.

In the following two situations the patient with otitis externa requires prompt referral to an otolaryngologist: (a) the patient whose findings suggest *mastoiditis* (these include slow response of the otitis externa to treatment plus persistent tenderness of the mastoid process); and (b) patients with the findings of "*malignant otitis externa*," usually diabetics or severely debilitated patients. This process is actually an osteitis of the bone underlying the external auditory canal caused by *Pseudomonas*. The distinguishing features are fever, excruciating pain, and the presence of friable granulation tissue in the area of apparent otitis externa. Because of the propensity for rapid spread to contiguous structures, this condition is an emergency, requiring hospital admission for debridement and intravenous antibiotics.

New Growth

Occasionally, unilateral, gradual onset hearing impairment may be due to a benign or malignant growth seen in the canal. Such patients must be referred for diagnosis and surgical excision of the growth.

CONDITIONS OF THE MIDDLE EAR

Most conductive hearing loss is due to conditions of the middle ear. In addition to history, evaluation of the middle ear includes assessment of eustachian tube function by air insufflation (pneumatic otoscopy), inspection for signs of acute inflammation (erythema, discharge, or bulging of the tympanic membrane), and inspection for changes in the tympanic membrane not due to acute inflammation (fluid level, retraction, scarring, distortion of normal structures, perforation).

Serous Otitis Media

This problem is very common in childhood and relatively common in adults. The patient usually complains of fullness and decreased hearing in one or both ears with minimal or no pain. There is often a history of a recent viral upper respiratory infection (see Chapter 27) or exacerbation of allergic or vasomotor rhinitis (see Chapter 22). On physical examination the patient is afebrile, and there may be evidence of eustachian tube closure—retraction of the tympanic membrane, failure of the membrane to move on pneumatic otoscopy (a crude test of eustachian tube patency, not always abnormal in serous otitis), or a fluid level behind the membrane. Even when none of these signs is present, the presumptive diagnosis of serous otitis can be made in patients with typical symptoms and conductive hearing loss.

The objective of *medical treatment* is to relieve obstruction of the eustachian tube. This is accomplished by the use of topical or oral decongestants. The quickest relief is obtained with *topical decongestants*. Nasal sprays containing the decongestant phenylephrine (Neo-Synephrine Nasal Spray 0.25%

or 0.50% or other over-the-counter preparations) are the simplest to use. The patient administers two puffs to each nostril followed 5 to 10 min later by two more puffs, 4 times daily. Alternatively, a phenylephrine-containing nasal solution (Neo-Synephrine 0.25% or 0.50%, also over-the-counter) can be instilled by dropper 4 times daily. The head is hyperextended, 3 or 4 drops are instilled in each nostril to open the nasal passages; the head is then turned to the lateral position with the involved ear down, and 3 to 4 more drops are instilled into the nostril. After 2 or 3 days of topical treatment, rebound nasal mucosal hyperemia may occur. Therefore, when topical treatment is initiated for prompt relief, the patient should be instructed to switch to an *oral decongestant* after 1 or 2 days. Oral treatment consists of pseudoephedrine (Sudafed 30 mg over-the-counter or 60 mg by prescription 4 times daily or Sudafed S.A. a long acting preparation, every 12 hours). At a dose of 60 mg, this drug has been shown objectively to increase nasal air flow in patients with nonsuppurative nasal congestion (6). If there is a history of allergic rhinitis, a decongestant-antihistamine combination may be more effective (see Chapter 22). In addition to medications, patients should be instructed to promote eustachian tube patency by blowing the nose against closed nostrils with the mouth closed (Valsalva maneuver) every few hours during the day; this should not be recommended, however, to the patient while he still has a purulent nasal discharge.

All patients should be re-evaluated after 4 to 6 weeks of continuous medical therapy. If conductive hearing loss persists beyond 6 weeks, the patient should be referred to an otolaryngologist. He will confirm and quantify the degree of conductive hearing loss, using an instrument known as an impedance audiometer. Some patients will require myringotomy with aspiration of fluid from the middle ear to restore hearing. Patients with persistent unilateral serous otitis should be examined by an experienced otolaryngologist to exclude eustachian tube obstruction by an enlarged lymph node, nasopharyngeal tumor, or other mass lesion.

Even with optimal treatment serous otitis media may recur in susceptible individuals.

Acute Otitis Media

All patients with this condition will complain of marked pain in the inner ear; most will give a history of a recent upper respiratory infection with or without drainage of purulent material from the ear (indicating tympanic membrane perforation); and many will describe unilateral hearing impairment. On examination, there is injection and loss of luster of the tympanic membrane, grayish pink coloration of the entire membrane, and, eventually, bulging of the membrane and loss of landmarks. There may be tenderness to palpation of the mastoid bone, since the mucosa lining the mastoid cells is continuous with that of the middle ear. Evidence of otitis externa is usually not present. The most common etiologic agents are *Streptococcus pneumoniae* (pneumococcus), *Haemophilus influenzae*, *Staphylococcus aureus*, and β-hemolytic streptococcus. An unknown proportion of cases are due to viral pathogens; since clinical distinction of these cases from those with bacterial infection is not possible, treatment should be the same for all patients with acute otitis media.

Medical treatment consists of systemic antibiotics for 10 days. Amoxicillin or ampicillin, 500 mg, 4 times daily, is the best regimen. For penicillin-allergic persons, trimethoprim-sulfamethoxazole, 2 tablets every 12 hours, is appropriate. Decongestants should be used to promote eustachian tube patency as described above. Aspirin, 600 mg, every 4 to 6 hours, should be recommended for pain; if needed, codeine, 30 mg, can be given with the aspirin.

If perforation with purulent discharge occurs, hydrogen peroxide may be applied, as described under "Otitis Externa" above, to help remove debris from the external canal. If the tympanic membrane is bulging with pus and pain is very severe, myringotomy by an otolaryngologist is indicated.

Recovery from the pain of acute otitis media is usually prompt. Within 1 to 4 weeks, hearing impairment resolves, and the tympanic membrane returns to normal appearance. Serous otitis may be present after other signs or symptoms of acute otitis have resolved.

In the patient who is worse after several days of treatment or who is not well after 10 days, smoldering mastoiditis may be present, and referral to an otolaryngologist is therefore indicated. Failure of serous otitis to resolve, persistence of a tympanic membrane perforation, or significant persistent hearing loss after 3 weeks are also indications for referral.

Barotrauma

Barotrauma refers to symptoms and signs produced by a sudden pressure differential between the middle ear and the surrounding atmosphere. The patient gives a history of fullness, pain, and decreased hearing in one or both ears, usually associated with flying or diving. All patients with symptoms which are severe or which persist for more than a day should be examined. The findings on otoscopy vary from mild tympanic membrane retraction to hemotympanum with or without perforation. There may be conductive or neurosensory hearing loss. Any patient with moderate or severe unilateral hearing loss should be referred to an otolaryngologist because of the possibility of a surgically treatable fistula of the round window.

For patients with mild symptoms, treatment and outcome are similar to those described above for serous otitis media.

Prophylaxis against barotrauma consists of use of the Valsalva maneuver and chewing of gum or swallowing during descent in airplanes.

Traumatic Perforation of Tympanic Membrane

Traumatic rupture, affecting the pars tensa of the tympanic membrane (see Fig. 93.2), may be caused by solids (deliberate introduction of a cotton-tipped applicator or other object for removing wax, foreign bodies entering during an accident, etc.); liquids (forcefully directed jet of water used in syringing the ear); and air (blast waves resulting from detonation of high explosives). Symptoms are decreased hearing, tinnitus, pain, and, at times, bleeding.

The *objectives of treatment* are repair of the defect and prevention of infection. Linear tears and small perforations of the membrane will often heal spontaneously in 1 to 2 weeks without any residual loss of function. Large perforations may require fascia grafting by an otolaryngologist (myringoplasty). If there is a strong possibility that the middle ear has been contaminated at the time of injury (*i.e.*, by syringing), antibiotics (ampicillin or erythromycin, 250 mg, 4 times daily for 1 week) are indicated. In addition, it is essential to guard against the subsequent entry of organisms as long as the perforation persists. Thus the patient should prevent water or other contaminants from entering the ear. Before bathing, the patient should insert a petroleum jelly-covered cotton plug. Swimming should be avoided altogether. Patients whose perforation was self-inflicted should be warned against future syringing and probing to remove cerumen.

After spontaneous closure (takes 2 to 3 weeks) or myringoplasty, the hearing loss due to perforation usually resolves completely.

Chronic Otitis Media

Chronic otitis media implies discharge from the middle ear, either persistent or recurrent, with perforation of the tympanic membrane, and usually some degree of conductive hearing loss. The management of this problem has two objectives: eradication of infection and restoration of hearing. When chronic otitis media is initially recognized, the patient should be referred to an otolaryngologist for evaluation. An appreciation of the major clinical characteristics, the treatment principles, and the long term expectations for these patients is, however, important to the patient's primary physician.

Chronic otitis media can be divided into *two major subgroups, benign and dangerous*. The clinical characteristics of these two groups are summarized in Table 93.4. The fundamental difference in the dangerous subgroup is the presence of, or potential for, bone destruction due to invasion by squamous epithelium (keratoma, formerly known as "cholesteatoma"). *Keratoma* occurs either when the squamous epithelium of the auditory canal invades the middle ear through a preexisting perforation (secondary ac-

Table 93.4
Chronic Otitis Media: Features Distinguishing Benign and Dangerous Forms

Feature	Benign	Dangerous (Keratoma)
Discharge	Mucoid or mucopurulent	Purulent, foul
Location of pathology	Middle ear; eustachian tube	Middle ear, attic, antrum, any part of temporal bone
Tympanic membrane perforation	Pars tensa (central)[a]	Pars flaccida[a] or marginal
Middle ear mucosa	Mucous membrane	Stratified squamous epithelium
X-rays	Normal; clouding of mastoid cells	Underdevelopment and sclerosis of mastoid cells; bone destruction
Keratoma (cholesteatoma) formation	No	Yes
Bone erosion	No	Yes
Treatment of infection	Medical	Surgical

[a] See Figure 93.2.

quired keratoma) or when squamous epithelium spontaneously replaces the columnar epithelium of the middle ear, leading to perforation (primary acquired keratoma). The keratoma is the mass of whitish debris which accumulates at the site of invasion of squamous epithelium. As this mass enlarges, it has the potential to erode bone and promote chronic infection.

The commonly performed surgical procedures for chronic otitis media are the following.

Mastoidectomy. In this operation, the mastoid cells are exteriorized so that they form a common cavity with the external auditory canal, draining and eradicating infection due to keratoma.

Mastoid Obliteration. After infection is eradicated by mastoidectomy, the cavity which has been created is obliterated with the use of muscle or other tissue graft. The purpose of this procedure is to restore normal anatomic contour and avoid the after care which a mastoid cavity requires.

Myringoplasty. The tympanic membrane perforation is closed by use of a tissue graft.

Tympanoplasty. Reconstruction of parts of the hearing mechanism, including tympanic membrane and ossicular chain, which have been disrupted by chronic infection.

Complications of Otitis Media

Acute or chronic suppurative otitis media may become complicated by extension of infection beyond the confines of the middle ear into bone and other surrounding structures. The patient's primary physician should be aware that *symptoms not attributable to the typical course* of acute or chronic otitis media may signify the presence of one of these complications. They are uncommon and usually occur in compromised hosts (diabetics, immunosuppressed patients, etc.) and in patients who have neglected pronounced symptoms of acute or chronic otitis media. All require immediate referral and hospitalization. They are: mastoiditis, facial nerve paralysis, petrositis (inflammation of petrous portion of the sphenoid), labyrinthitis, brain abscess, extradural abscess, subdural abscess, lateral sinus thrombophlebitis, meningitis, and otitic hydrocephalus.

Ossicular Chain Problems

A number of chronic conditions affect the ossicular chain. These may be recognized by the combination of conductive hearing loss (usually chronic, either unilateral or bilateral), the absence of evidence for active otitis media, and, in some cases, typical findings on otoscopy. Each of these conditions requires referral to an otolaryngologist for consideration of surgical management.

ADHESIVE OTITIS MEDIA

There is a history of prior ear infection, and the tympanic membrane is retracted, thickened, and atrophic in areas of healed perforations. This is usually a late complication seen in patients who have been inadequately followed up after treatment for repeated acute otitis or serous otitis and who have had persistent middle ear inflammation. Hearing aids are helpful for some of these patients. Surgical results are far from ideal.

TYMPANOSCLEROSIS

There is a history of prior infection, often bilateral. There is usually, but not always, a tympanic membrane perforation and discrete plaques of whitish material may be seen in the middle ear. In selected patients, surgical removal of the plaques restores lost hearing. In others, ossicular reconstruction is necessary to improve hearing.

TRAUMATIC OSSICULAR INJURY

There is a history of external trauma (such as basal skull fracture and those causes of traumatic perforation listed above) followed by unilateral hearing loss which may be conductive or mixed. The tympanic membrane may be normal in appearance or there may be blood behind the membrane. Hearing status after surgery depends upon the type of injury found at surgery.

OTOSCLEROSIS

This is a disease of the labyrinthine capsule in which a vascular type of spongy bone is laid down, causing fixation of the stapes and conductive hearing loss, usually bilateral. The history discloses slowly progressive hearing loss beginning in the second or third decade, usually bilateral, more commonly in females, and frequently accelerated after pregnancy. Examination of the tympanic membrane is usually normal. This is the most common cause of progressive conductive hearing loss in young adults. Since the results of surgery, consisting of stapedectomy and prosthetic replacement, are excellent, it is particularly important to detect and refer these patients.

New Growths of Middle Ear

A number of benign and malignant growths may be seen on inspection of the tympanic membrane of patients with progressive unilateral conductive hearing loss. Malignant tumors most commonly present with a history of chronic discharge, occasionally bloody.

CHRONIC SENSORINEURAL HEARING LOSS

Presbycusis ("the Hearing of the Old")

A certain amount of hearing loss, beginning in the high frequency range, is virtually universal among elderly people; and approximately 1 in 5 people over 65 will develop moderate to severe hearing loss. The majority do not complain of deafness, and often a family member mentions the problem to the patient's physician. When hearing deficits are objectively evaluated in older persons, the deficits of the "complainers" and "noncomplainers" overlap considerably (5). Clearly, social and psychologic factors are important in determining the seriousness of hearing loss reported by the individual patient.

Periodically, the primary physician should make a practical assessment of the hearing status of each of his patients over 65 (see Table 93.1). When an older patient is first found to have hearing loss, the patient and his family should be counseled as outlined above (p. 1016), and the patient should be offered a referral for evaluation by an otolaryngologist.

Acoustic Trauma

This form of sensorineural hearing loss is found commonly in individuals employed in high noise industries or exposed to extremely loud, electrically amplified music. Like presbycusis, it is initially a high frequency hearing loss, eventually spreading to lower frequencies. Personal prevention by wearing earplugs in high noise settings and environmental prevention by reducing noise level are the best ways to prevent acoustic trauma. Established hearing loss due to noise is usually irreversible, but progressive hearing loss can be prevented.

Drug-induced Hearing Loss

A number of drugs may produce bilateral sensorineural hearing loss (Table 93.5), and the patient's personal physician will often be the first to learn of this problem. (Example: a patient will be seen in the office following hospitalization for an illness which was treated with aminoglycoside antibiotics or with intravenous diuretics and will complain of hearing loss.) For most drugs, ototoxicity is dose-related; how-

Table 93.5
Drugs which May Cause Hearing Loss

ANTIBIOTICS	DIURECTICS
Streptomycin	Ethacrynic acid
Neomycin	Furosemide
Gentamycin	
Tobramycin	OTHER DRUGS
Chloramphenicol	Salicylates
Kanamycin	Quinidine
Vancomycin	Quinine
Polymixin B	

ever, hearing impairment may occur even at therapeutic doses. A recent study showed that objective mild hearing loss (15 to 30 decibels at high frequencies) occurs in as many as 10% of individuals whose serum levels of gentamycin and tobramycin are maintained within the therapeutic range (7).

The prognosis for drug-induced hearing loss varies according to the drug. Salicylates and quinine usually produce temporary, high frequency deafness; but permanent deafness has been reported in patients surviving salicylate poisoning and in infants of mothers who received quinine during pregnancy. Aminoglycoside ototoxicity may occur suddenly after a few doses, may be permanent, and may progress after discontinuation of the drug. Diuretic-induced ototoxicity may be seen after extremely high doses, usually in patients with renal insufficiency. Its onset may be sudden, following intravenous or (in a few reported cases) oral administration, and the hearing deficit may be permanent. Fortunately, this is a rare complication of ethacrynic acid therapy and an extremely rare complication of furosemide therapy.

Ménière's Syndrome

This benign but temporarily disabling condition will be seen one or more times per year in a typical practice. It is present in any age group, but is most common in the 4th to 6th decade. Symptoms are due to endolymphatic hydrops, (excess fluid and pressure in the cochlea and the labyrinth).

The individual attack consists of a sudden temporary failure of vestibular function (vertigo) combined with fluctuating hearing loss, tinnitus, and nausea; an attack lasts from minutes to hours. During the attack, spontaneous nystagmus will be present; the nystagmus will not be affected by position change. Between attacks, tinnitus and sensorineural hearing loss may persist. Symptoms are unilateral in approximately 70% of cases. In about half of the cases vestibular and cochlear symptoms appear at the same time; in approximately 25%, deafness and/or tinnitus precedes the onset of vertigo; and in 25% vertigo precedes deafness (3). The vertigo is accompanied by nausea and vomiting, probably due to a spread of nervous impulses from the vestibular nerve to the vagal nuclei in the brainstem. In severe cases, other vagal symptoms may occur (abdominal pain, bradycardia, pallor, and sweating). Audiometry demonstrates sensorineural hearing loss, greater for lower frequencies in the early stage of the disease.

An attack may occur spontaneously at any time. Attacks may occur singly, with an interval of months or years between, or there may be a series of attacks over a period of weeks, followed by a long period of complete remission.

The *differential diagnosis* of Ménière's syndrome includes a number of conditions which may present with hearing loss and vertigo unrelated to position change: viral labyrinthitis, acoustic neuroma, syphilitic vertigo, labyrinthine fistula, vestibular granuloma, temporal bone fracture, or multiple sclerosis. Additional information regarding the assessment of the patient with vertigo is found in Chapter 78.

Treatment. Patients with suspected Ménière's syndrome should be referred promptly to an otolaryngologist to confirm the diagnosis and to initiate treatment. All patients will be treated with diuretics (25 to 50 mg of hydrochlorothiazide daily or its equivalent). Bed rest is recommended when the patient is having recurrent severe symptoms; bed rest does not prevent the periodic vertigo but prevents exacerbation due to position change. The antihistamine meclizine (Antivert or Bonine) can be tried in a dose of 25 mg, 3 to 4 times daily. For nausea, the patient should take the antiemetic prochlorperazine (Compazine) either as a 5- or 10-mg capsule, 4 times daily, or as a 25-mg suppository twice daily. After the acute attack has subsided, the patient should continue diuretic treatment; after 1 year without recurrence, diuretic treatment can be stopped. For the occasional patient with severe recurrent Ménière's syndrome refractory to medical treatment, one of a number of surgical procedures can be performed, selectively decompressing or destroying the vestibular labyrinth.

Acoustic Neuroma

This uncommon, benign tumor may arise from either the cochlear or vestibular fibers of the eighth cranial nerve. It grows slowly, expanding within the internal auditory meatus until large enough to extend into the posterior fossa and cause damage to adjacent structures. Onset of symptoms is generally between the ages of 30 and 50. Essentially all patients will present with symptoms of eighth nerve impairment: unilateral hearing loss is found in the majority of patients and chronic, usually mild, positional vertigo or sense of imbalance occurs in many patients. Audiometry usually demonstrates significant sensorineural hearing loss with poor discrimination. Neurologic examination shows involvement of the following neurologic structures, in decreasing order of frequency: nerve VII, nerve V, nerve VI, and cerebellum (ataxia, with a tendency to fall toward the side of the lesion).

Referral to an otolaryngologist for evaluation is essential whenever unilateral sensorineural hearing loss is initially found. Diagnosis of acoustic neuroma is based on a characteristic audiogram and on computerized tomography. The results of surgical treatment generally permit the patient to resume his or her usual activity, but with permanent unilateral hearing loss (4).

SUDDEN SENSORINEURAL HEARING LOSS

This condition, usually unilateral, is an otologic emergency. The etiology is often difficult to ascertain and includes: viral cochleitis, end artery occlusion (in patients with other evidence of arterial occlusive disease such as embolic transient ischemic attacks), inner ear fistula, sudden expansion of a cerebellopontine angle tumor, temporal bone fracture, and noise trauma (gunshot, for example). The symptoms, which occur over a matter of minutes to hours, are either tinnitus or hearing loss. After prompt evaluation for conductive hearing loss (including simple cerumen impaction), these patients should be referred immediately for evaluation by an otolaryngologist. A number of empirical medical therapies have been tried. For patients with inner ear fistulas, surgical closure is possible.

The majority of patients will have permanent, severe unilateral hearing loss, and they and their families should be instructed regarding hearing safety (adequate noise protection for the other ear, preferential seating for optimal use of the good ear, precautions when driving in heavy traffic).

TINNITUS

Tinnitus ("ringing") refers to the perception of sounds in the absence of a normal external stimulus.

Subjective Tinnitus

The term *subjective tinnitus* is used when the subject complains of noises which cannot be heard by the observer. Subjective tinnitus may be subdivided into two types:

Tympanic. This usually arises as a result of a conductive lesion (all of the causes of conductive hearing loss). It is thought to be due to removal of the normal masking effect of ambient noise, with emergence of otherwise subaudible tympanic, vascular, and muscular noises. The patient will often describe the tinnitus as pulsating.

Petrous. This is due to conditions affecting the cochlea or eighth nerve (all of the conditions leading to sensorineural hearing loss). It is attributed to cerebral recognition of auditory stimuli produced by mechanical cochlear deformation or by hyperirritability of the acoustic nerve. It may be intermittent or continuous with varying intensity.

After the patient's primary otologic problem has

been defined, the most important requirement in dealing with tinnitus is reassurance (many patients believe that their tinnitus signifies the presence of a serious intracranial condition). Bedtime sedation to assure adequate sleep is important. Some patients will also find that the sound of a radio helps them to get to sleep by competing with the more distressing sound due to tinnitus. For patients with severe tinnitus, masking treatment by the consulting otolaryngologist may be helpful.

Objective Tinnitus

This is a noise audible to the examiner, sometimes inaudible to the patient, and originating from the region of the patient's ear. Causes include aneurysm of the internal carotid artery, temporomandibular joint problems, and myoclonus of palatal muscles.

VERTIGO

The problem of vertigo is discussed in depth in Chapter 78.

References

General

Paparella, MM and Shumrick, DA: *Orolaryngology, Vol. 2. Ear.* W. B. Saunders, Philadelphia, 1980.
Exhaustive textbook.

Specific

1. Bailey, HAT, Jr, Pappas, JJ, Graham, S and Winston, ME: Total hearing rehabilitation. *Arch Otolaryngol 102:* 323, 1976.
2. Department of Health, Education and Welfare: A report on hearing aid health care. U.S. Printing Office, Washington, DC, 1974.
3. Mawson, ST: *Diseases of the Ear,* Chapter 17. Williams & Wilkins, Baltimore, 1974.
4. Ojemann, RG, Montgomery, WW and Weiss, AD: Evaluation and surgical treatment of acoustic neuroma. *N Engl J Med 287:* 895, 1972.
5. Price, LL and Snider, RM: The geriatric patient; ear, nose and throat problems. In *Clinical Aspects of Aging,* edited by W Reichel. Williams & Wilkins, Baltimore, 1978.
6. Roth, RP, Cantekin, EI, Welch, RM, Bluestone, CD and Cho, YW: Nasal decongestant activity of pseudoephendrine. *Ann Otol Rhinol Laryngol 86:* 235, 1977.
7. Smith, CR, Lipsky, JJ, Laskin, OL, Hellmann, DB, Mellits, ED, Longstreth, J and Lietman, PS: Double-blind comparison of the nephrotoxicity and auditory toxicity of gentamicin and tobramycin. *N Engl J Med 302:* 1106, 1980.

CHAPTER NINETY-FOUR

Cataracts

EARL D. R. KIDWELL, Jr., M.D.

A cataract is an opacification of the lens of the eye or of its capsule. Ninety-six percent of individuals over 60 years of age will have some opacification of the lens, but most often these opacities are of no importance. A *significant cataract* results in interference with visual acuity. In the United States cataracts are a very common cause of diminished vision. Cataracts are usually bilateral and the progression is slow and may vary between eyes. The rate of progression is not individually predictable, and there is no treatment which will retard the progression. When the cataract is advanced the only therapy is surgery.

This chapter will provide a review of the anatomy and physiology of the lens as well as a review of cataracts to help the general physician advise and follow his patients appropriately.

ANATOMY AND PHYSIOLOGY

The lens is derived entirely from the evagination of surface ectoderm in the fetus. It is located immediately posterior to the iris and is suspended there by radially attached zonular fibers from the ciliary body (see Fig. 95.1, p. 1029). It is a biconvex uniquely transparent structure with an elastic capsule whose shape may be altered by ciliary body contraction permitting images to be brought into sharp focus on the retina. The lens is acellular and avascular and lacks innervation. Nourishment is provided from the surrounding aqueous and vitreous humor, and metabolic by-products are removed by diffusion into the aqueous humor. The continued transparency of the lens requires the active metabolism of the elastic capsular epithelium so that any insult to the epithelium may result in lenticular opacities. Also, new lenticular fibers are produced throughout life; and, since none are lost increasing density of the fibers of the lens develops with age, which contributes to cataract formation.

ETIOLOGY

There are many causes of cataracts (Table 94.1). While senescent cataracts—the result of the aging phenomena described above—account for the vast majority of cataracts, the general physician will occasionally see patients with congenital or traumatic lens opacities as well. The mechanism of opacification in all these instances is thought to be due to interference with the metabolic activity of the capsular epithelium and with continued fiber production.

Many of these various types of cataracts have a destinctive appearance. The ophthalmologist may therefore suggest to the general physician the possibility of an underlying disorder such as hypoparathyroidism (punctate opacities in anterior and posterior lens cortex) or Wilson's disease ("sunflower" cataract).

SYMPTOMS AND EXAMINATION

The primary symptom of cataract is impaired vision; usually patients describe a constant fog over the

Table 94.1
Etiology of Cataracts

CONGENITAL
  Autosomal dominant inheritance—25% of congenital cataracts
  Maternal malnutrition
  Maternal infections—*e.g.,* rubella, syphilis
  Maternal metabolic disease—*e.g.,* diabetes mellitus
  Maternal medication—corticosteroids
  Prematurity
TRAUMATIC
SENESCENT
SECONDARY (Examples)
  Drug therapy—corticosteroids
  Degenerative eye disease—severe myopia
  Retinal dystrophy
  Essential iris atrophy
  Retinal detachment
  Glaucoma
  Intraocular neoplasia
  Ocular ischemia (*e.g.,* Takayasu's disease)
ASSOCIATED WITH METABOLIC DISEASE
  Diabetes mellitus
  Wilson's disease
  Hypoparathyroidism

eye. They may also see rings or halos around lights and objects. The color that objects appear change, particularly, toward blue and yellow. Not infrequently, with immature cataract formation, distant vision is impaired and near vision is preserved.

The location of the cataract within the lens determines the extent of the visual loss. Central opacities cause noticeable loss of vision and a distinct glare when the patient is in bright light which will constrict the pupil so that the dense portion of the lens occludes and diffuses light. For this reason the patient who has central opacities finds his vision is better in low light when his pupil is open. Peripheral opacities will cause noticeable loss of vision only late in the development of the cataract.

Cataracts are easily identified by illuminating the lens with a slit lamp, but most general physicians will find that they can see a cataract easily through the plus 4–10 lens of their direct ophthalmoscope. The lens appears cloudy. Similarly, a light from a small flashlight may be reflected off the opacity in the lens. Visual acuity should be tested in both eyes when cataracts are suspected. If the patient describes any visual symptoms or if the physician measures an impairment in visual acuity, the patient should be referred to an ophthalmologist. In individuals who are over 60 years of age screening for cataracts is best done by a visual acuity examination with use of a Snellen chart.

CATARACT SURGERY

Indications

Even before surgery is indicated, glasses may improve the vision of patients with cataracts. The decision to remove a cataract is determined by the visual needs of the patient, as well as by the degree of capsular involvement and of any other ocular abnormalities. The ophthalmologist will perform a complete ocular assessment (see Chapter 95) before advising the patient about surgery.

Each patient must determine his own visual need based on his daily activities. The ability to read, drive, cross streets safely, and to perform a daily routine is clearly of prime importance. For example, a patient usually requires visual acuity of at least 20/40 in the better eye to operate a motor vehicle safely or to continue moderately active daily life.

Surgery

Cataract surgery should not be done without considerable deliberation as there are a number of complications which might occur (see below), and vision after cataract extraction may be a major problem (see below). The general physician and the ophthalmologist should plan cataract surgery together. Cataract extraction is an elective procedure, and the patient should be in the best possible condition at the time of operation.

Approximately 400,000 cataract extractions are performed in the United States every year; surgery involves the removal of the opacified lens from the eye. The extraction may be intracapsular, involving complete removal of the lens, or extracapsular, leaving the posterior capsule of the lens intact. Microsurgical techniques have greatly improved the immediate outcome of surgery and have significantly shortened the period of disability. Usually only one lens is extracted at a time so that the patient will have vision in the nonoperated side when the eye that has been operated upon is covered by a patch for a few days after surgery.

Patient Experience. Cataract surgery is performed most often by use of local anesthesia supplemented with intravenous analgesia and sedation. The patient experiences moderate discomfort, but it lasts only a day or so and is controlled with analgesics. A hyperosmotic agent (such as glycerin or mannitol) may be employed to dehydrate and to soften the eye in preparation for surgery. Following surgery the patient will remain hospitalized 1 to 4 days to assure that the occasional complications of postoperative intraocular infection or of acute rise in intraocular pressure are promptly recognized and treated.

After discharge from the hospital a patient must restrict his activities for several weeks to avoid complications. These restrictions are listed in Table 94.2. There are no permanent restrictions; however, caution with steps or when walking and working with machinery may be necessary if perception is seriously altered using aphakic spectacles (see below).

Complications

Complications occur in approximately 5% of patients who have had cataract extraction, and 1 of every 5000 eyes operated upon is lost because of complications. Knowledge of the possible complications following cataract surgery will aid the general

Table 94.2
Temporary Restrictions following Cataract Surgery[a]

Wear eye shield during sleep and wear glasses at other times—shields are usually worn for 1 month and then discontinued
Absolutely no bending or stooping for 3 or 4 weeks
Do not sleep on side of operated eye for 3 or 4 weeks
Do not wash hair for 2 weeks
No showers for 2 weeks although a bath is allowed (but with assistance to prevent a fall)
No strenuous or excessive physical activity for 4 weeks and then only after approval of the ophthalmologist
Do not lift objects that weigh over 5 pounds for 3 or 4 weeks

[a] These are suggested to prevent inadvertent injury to the eye, to diminish disruptive pressure on the wound, to avoid sudden rise in ocular pressure, and to diminish the chance of infection.

physician in educating his patients. Because of the potential for complications, the general physician must be sure that the patient keeps his scheduled postoperative appointments with the ophthalmologist.

GLAUCOMA (see Chapter 95)

This secondary form of glaucoma is due to several factors leading to angle closure: the effect of the proteolytic agent, chymotrypsin, on the angular structures at the time of operation; scarring due to postoperative inflammation; or the misdirection into and subsequent trapping of the aqueous in the vitreous body. Glaucoma may develop within a few days of surgery and may occur in as many as 20% of patients depending on the technique and whether chymotrypsin is used. Early glaucoma is usually transient but it may become chronic. Also, glaucoma may appear as late as 1 to 2 years after surgery in 0.6 to 5% of patients depending on the type of surgery. The patient who has developed secondary glaucoma will usually complain of redness, tenderness, and pain in the eye. Further, if the patient has been fitted with a temporary spectacle, he will notice decreased visual acuity due to corneal edema. A postoperative patient suspected of having glaucoma should be seen by an ophthalmologist immediately.

INFLAMMATION AND INFECTION

All postoperative patients have some degree of traumatic intraocular inflammation. This is usually controlled effectively with topical corticosteroids. Bacterial endophthalmitis is a dangerous postoperative inflammation that must be recognized early before it devastates the eye. If a patient complains of pain, discharge and redness, endophthalmitis may be present and the patient should be seen immediately by an ophthalmologist. Most infections occur within a few days of surgery; however, an operated eye is predisposed to infection from systemic infection and therefore a patient with an acute red eye occurring at any time after eye surgery should be seen urgently by an opthalmologist.

HEMORRHAGE

The sudden occurrence of hemorrhage in the uveal tract can adversely influence the final visual outcome. Although this complication is usually seen intraoperatively, rarely it may occur postoperatively. The event is characterized by a painless but precipitous change in visual acuity. Postoperative hemorrhage from the iris or from an inadequately closed scleral wound is, however, more common than is vitreous hemorrhage. In all instances of hemorrhage, urgent referral to an ophthalmologist is indicated.

RETINAL DETACHMENT

The incidence of retinal detachment following cataract surgery is approximately 1 to 3%. Retinal detachment is characterized by suddenly decreased visual acuity, flashes of light, and the development of floaters, veils, and/or curtains in the visual field. These patients should be seen immediately by an ophthalmologist so that surgical reattachment of the retina may be accomplished. The success of reattachment is excellent provided that it can be done expeditiously.

Newer Approaches to Cataract Extraction

Phacoemulsification is an innovative procedure in which a cataract is emulsified by ultrasound. A metal probe is inserted into the cataract and then it is vibrated (40,000 cycles/sec) causing dissolution of the lens nucleus, which is then aspirated. In theory, this procedure requires a much smaller incision and reduces the recuperative period. The posterior lens capsule is left intact and this is thought, though not proven, to reduce the chance of retinal detachment. Unfortunately, this procedure solves none of the optical problems that occur following lens removal.

Intraocular lens implantation is discussed below.

OPTICAL CORRECTION AFTER CATARACT EXTRACTION

The removal of a cataract improves the transmission of light to retina, but vision remains blurred without corrective lenses, and these may present problems. With aphakic spectacles there is a narrower field of vision, as well as considerable distortion of images which appear rounded and 3 to 5 times larger than when the lens is present in the eye. Also, there are peripheral ring scotomata and loss of some depth perception. Even modern aphakic spectacles are heavy and thick so that a patient frequently will have considerable initial difficulty adjusting to them and will need support, understanding, and encouragement from family members. With experience, however, most patients will be able to function acceptably and perform all of their necessary daily activities.

The use of contact lenses after cataract extraction provides considerable improvement over spectacles. There is, especially, improvement in distortion and

expansion of the field of vision. The patient, however, must be motivated to use contact lenses, and this motivation must be considered before surgery is undertaken. Often elderly patients are concerned about being agile enough to insert contact lenses. The patient must also be fitted with a pair of spectacles with one lens missing so that he may see to place one contact lens. A regular set of spectacles is also necessary as a backup to the contact lens.

A unilateral cataract extraction results in a pronounced disparity in image size if an aphakic spectacle is used postoperatively; therefore, unilateral surgery is generally not advised unless the patient will be able to use a contact lens or is a candidate for an intraocular lens implantation. Under certain circumstances, however (such as when glaucoma or diabetic retinopathy is present in addition to cataract), monolenticular extraction may be indicated to permit the ophthalmologist to follow the course of these ocular diseases.

Because of the visual handicap experienced after cataract extraction, *implantable plastic lenses* have been developed. These devices hold promise, and long term study is underway. Intraocular lens implants are often used as the first choice in elderly individuals, especially those with physical handicaps (such as tremors) that make the use of contact lenses or aphakic spectacles difficult. Some ophthalmologists feel almost all patients should receive implants, while others are more conservative and await the results of long term follow-up studies. The insertion of intraocular implants adds approximately 15 to 20 min to the operative time beyond that required for lens extraction.

References

Bellows, JG (editor): *Cataract and Abnormalities of the Lens.* Grune & Stratton, New York, 1975.
   This comprehensive multiauthored monograph provides in-depth information about all aspects of cataracts.
Emery, JM and Jacobson AC (editors): *Current Concepts in Cataract Surgery.* C. V. Mosby, St Louis, 1980.
   A series of review articles on all aspects of cataract surgery.
Havener, WN: *Synopsis of Ophthalmology.* C. V. Mosby, St. Louis, 1975.
   A concise, practical text for the generalist with excellent section dealing with patient's experience with some problems and ophthalmologic procedures.

CHAPTER NINETY-FIVE

Glaucoma

EARL D. R. KIDWELL, Jr., M.D.

Glaucoma is a common disorder characterized by an increase in intraocular pressure sufficient to cause damage to the optic nerve and retina. The glaucomas are classified into primary and secondary groups (Table 95.1). The primary group accounts for 95% of all patients with glaucoma in the United States.

Patients with glaucoma will usually be followed by an ophthalmologist. However, the general physician will need to be familiar with the techniques of screening for and diagnosing glaucoma and with the long term care of patients who are found to have glaucoma.

ANATOMY AND PHYSIOLOGY (see Fig. 95.1)

The aqueous humor maintains the shape of the eye and the correct relationship among the refractile elements of the eye; it provides also the nutrition of the avascular intraocular structures such as the lens. There is continuous production and removal of the aqueous humor. In most cases of glaucoma, an obstruction to the outflow of aqueous humor appears to be the basis for the increased intraocular pressure.

The aqueous humor is a clear ultrafiltrate of the blood and occupies part of the posterior and anterior chambers of the eye. It is produced by the ciliary epithelium of the ciliary body which is a portion of the uveal tract of the eye. It appears most likely that the aqueous is formed partially by secretion and partially by a process of ultrafiltration. At least two enzymes have been implicated in aqueous formation: sodium/potassium-activated ATPase and carbonic anhydrase. Antagonists of these enzymes reduce the rate of aqueous formation and thereby lower intraocular pressure. Acetazolamide (Diamox), a carbonic anhydrase inhibitor, has in this manner proved clinically important in the treatment of glaucoma. Once produced, the aqueous humor circulates from the posterior chamber into the anterior chamber of the eye. The trabecular meshwork, an intricate system of connective tissue fibers, is located in the periphery of the anterior chamber. The aqueous percolates through this meshwork to be reunited with the venous blood via Schlemm's canal.

TYPES OF GLAUCOMA

Table 95.1 outlines the major types and causes of glaucoma. However, only primary open-angle and primary angle-closure are discussed in this chapter since they are the only types of glaucoma likely to be seen with any frequency by the general physician. Open-angle glaucoma takes its name from the relatively normal appearing anterior chamber angle as shown in Figure 95.2, a contrast to the narrow angle of angle-closure glaucoma.

Primary Open-Angle Glaucoma

PREVALENCE AND RISK FACTORS

This form of glaucoma is by far the most common cause of glaucoma in the United States; the prevalence increases after the age of 40 years and approaches 3% of individuals over 75 years of age (3). Primary open-angle glaucoma causes 15 to 20% of all blindness in this country. Men and women are affected equally; but blacks are affected at an earlier age, and open-angle glaucoma is the leading cause of blindness in black Americans. Open-angle glaucoma is familial, but the pattern of inheritance is not yet known with certainty. In patients who have a positive family history of glaucoma, there is an association between glaucoma and leukocyte antigen HLA B12 (6). It has been proposed that there is an association between open-angle glaucoma and both diabetes mellitus and elevated blood pressure, but these hypotheses are controversial (3) and more research will be necessary to define or negate such relationships. Patients who have high degrees of myopia (defective distant vision) are often said to have a higher risk of open-angle glaucoma, but there remains some controversy about this hypothesis as well (3).

DIAGNOSIS

In primary open-angle glaucoma, ocular hypertension results from resistance in the trabecular meshwork to aqueous outflow. The elevation of the intraocular pressure is roughly related to the degree of obstruction. The disease has no associated symptoms in its early stages. When symptoms do occur, neural damage is present and may be substantial. Macular (central) vision and the ability to recognize forms on a vision test chart are preserved until very late. For this reason testing of visual acuity is not a reliable method to screen for glaucoma. Occasionally a patient with open-angle glaucoma may notice halos around lights and blurring of vision if there is a sudden rise in intraocular pressure such as might occur with rapid ingestion of a large quantity of fluid (e.g., 1 liter). Patients with this history should be referred urgently to an ophthalmologist regardless of the intraocular pressure. Patients only rarely complain of headache that can be attributed to increased intraocular pressure. The ocular pressure may be elevated for years, however, before any change in the optic disc is noted. The change will be revealed by increasing excavation of the central physiological disc cup, visible on fundoscopic examination (Fig. 95.3). This is most easily seen by use of the red filter of the direct ophthalmoscope. Over years the pink

Table 95.1
Types of Glaucoma

PRIMARY
    Open-angle—90% of patients
    Angle-closure—5% of patients
    Congenital—Infant and juvenile onset
SECONDARY
    Open-angle—Results from topical or systemic steroids, ocular inflammation, or obstructed venous return from the eye (e.g., carotid cavernous sinus fistula)
    Angle-closure—Results from trauma, neovascular change of the iris postoperatively, ocular neoplasia, cataracts, and iris degenerations from various causes

color of the disc fades and becomes pale, and vessels coursing over the disc show a sharp bend at the rim.

In evaluating the patient with increased intraocular pressure the ophthalmologist will perform tonometry, gonioscopy (see below), fundoscopy, and visual field examinations. Characteristic visual field changes called "nerve fiber bundle defects" are seen in glaucoma.

SCREENING FOR OPEN-ANGLE GLAUCOMA

Screening (4) for primary open-angle glaucoma is warranted for several reasons: (a) the disease is silent until permanent ocular damage has occurred, (b) screening is relatively simple and without significant risk, (c) treatment can prevent eye damage, and (d) this form of glaucoma is common, especially in older individuals. Screening in theory could be accomplished in one or more of three ways: tonometry (4), fundoscopic assessment of the optic cup (1), and visual field assessment (5). Ophthalmologists generally do all three evaluations, but this is not practical for the general physician. While there are advocates for each of these three techniques, the most practical and reliable screening method for the general physician is tonometry with the use of the Schiötz tonometer (Fig. 95.4).

This tonometer measures the weight required to indent the anesthetized cornea of the eye. If the ocular pressure is elevated, an increased weight is

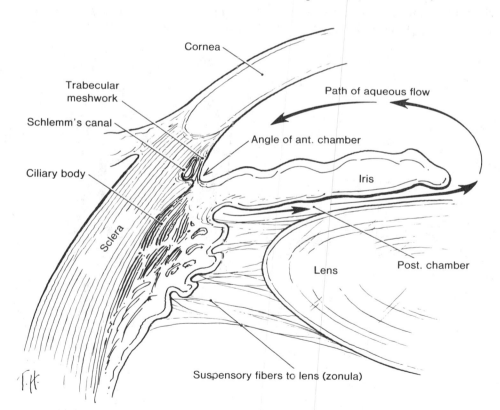

Figure 95.1   Anatomy of eye. (From J. V. Basmajian: *Grant's Method of Anatomy*, Ed. 8, p. 543. Williams & Wilkins, Baltimore, 1971.)

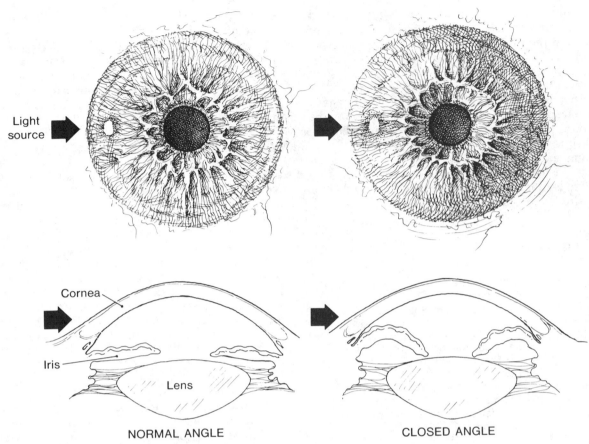

Figure 95.2 Illustration showing a shadow cast on the iris resultant from the bowed iris in angle-closure glaucoma. In open-angle glaucoma, the iris is not bowed and the shadow, therefore, is not cast.

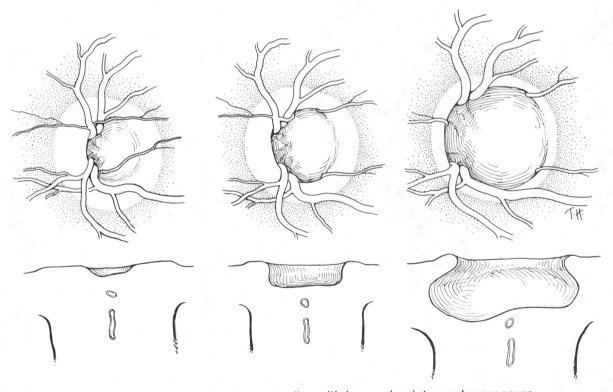

Figure 95.3 Changes in the optic disc with increasing intraocular pressure.

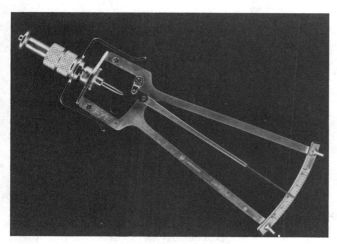

Figure 95.4   Schiötz tonometer.

necessary to cause indentation. The ocular pressure is less than 20 mm Hg in 95% of normal individuals. Patients found to have pressures in one or both eyes equal to or greater than 20 mm Hg should be referred to an ophthalmologist. Should the physician also notice an enlarged physiological cup (greater than 30% of the disc diameter, see Fig. 95.3), prompt referral to an ophthalmologist is indicated. Complications of tonometry include corneal abrasion, sensitivity reaction to the anesthetic, or infection. These complications are all quite rare and occur in less than 1% of examinations.

With practice, the general physician can perform ocular tonometry in 2 min (4). This, therefore, can be done at the time of a general physical examination or at the time of periodic health assessment. Tonometry can be performed with accuracy by technicians and office personnel under a physician's supervision. If the physician is unfamiliar with the use of the Schiötz tonometer or is unwilling to take the time to perform the test, patients should be encouraged to have periodic glaucoma screening by an ophthalmologist.

Since open-angle glaucoma is a disease of older individuals, routine tonometry should be performed in individuals over 45 years of age. An initial assessment at the time of a general physical examination in these individuals is appropriate, with periodic follow-up at 5-year intervals until age 75 when the frequency of assessment should be increased to 1-year intervals in parallel with the increasing incidence of glaucoma.

Patients referred to an ophthalmologist because their intraocular pressure is equal to or greater than 20 mm Hg will generally have an evaluation consisting of: *repeat assessment of the intraocular pressure by applanation tonometry*, by use of a complex piece of equipment and requiring only a drop of topical anesthetic; *fundoscopic assessment of the optic disc and retina*; *formal visual field assessment and gonioscopic examination* which permits the ophthalmologist to visualize the angle of the anterior chamber by using an instrument containing a contact lens and

mirror. The patient usually experiences minimal or no discomfort during any of these procedures.

Approximately one-third of patients referred to an ophthalmologist because of the finding of asymptomatic increased intraocular pressure will be found to have glaucoma. Of the remaining two-thirds, approximately 30% may be found not to have elevated pressures on reassessment, while about 25% will have ocular hypertension without glaucoma (4).This latter group should be followed yearly by the ophthalmologist; some of these patients may, over a period of time, develop glaucoma.

Rarely, patients may have normal pressure glaucoma, but the general physician will not be able to detect these patients unless an enlarged physiologic optic cup is noticed, after which an ophthalmological consultation is indicated.

TREATMENT

When the ophthalmologist establishes the diagnosis of open-angle glaucoma, he will prescribe treatment based on the level of intraocular pressure (although a pressure of greater than 30 mm Hg is an absolute indication for treatment), the degree of visual field loss, and the amount of optic nerve damage.

The treatment of open-angle glaucoma is largely medical, with use of agents that facilitate the outflow or reduce the amount of production of aqueous humor. The aim of therapy is to maintain the intraocular pressure below 20 mm Hg. Patients are usually prescribed a mild miotic such as carbachol or pilocarpine. Other agents such as carbonic anhydrase inhibitors and stronger miotics are added or replace the milder agents as necessary. Also the β-adrenergic receptor blocking agent timolol maleate (*e.g.*, Timoptic Ophthalmic Solution) will reduce ocular pressure and has the advantage of producing little or no effect on pupil size or visual acuity. For this reason decreased, blurred, or impaired night vision is not the problem with timolol that it is with miotic agents. However, systemic effects of the β-blocker may occur.

Frequently, early in the course, treatment may need to be changed by the ophthalmologist since tolerance is not uncommon and side effects may occur. Once the decresed ocular pressure has been attained, the ophthalmologist should examine the patient approximately 3 times per year for assessment of visual fields, measurement of intraocular pressure, fundoscopic examination, and gonioscopy.

Surgery in primary open-angle glaucoma is designed to construct outflow channels for the aqueous humor or to freeze the ciliary body and destroy the site of aqueous production. This surgical procedure is reserved for patients in whom medical management fails. Medications may still be required after surgery.

MONITORING

The primary physician should ensure that the patient with diagnosed open-angle glaucoma is receiving regular ophthalmologic follow-up. Further, he should be alert to any side effects from the drugs prescribed by the ophthalmologist.

There has been particular concern about systemic medications which have anticholinergic (atropine-like), adrenergic, vasodilator, or corticosteroid properties (2) and which may adversely affect ocular pressure. However, there are few data that would contraindicate the use of these agents in patients with open-angle glaucoma. Only if an anticholinergic drug paralyzes accommodation (noticeable as blurriness when the eyes are used for close work as in reading) should there be concern about it causing increased ocular pressure, in which situation the drug should be withdrawn; or if its use is mandatory, an ophthalmologist should be consulted. Systemic corticosteroids and, in particular corticosteroids applied to the eye in the absence of intraocular inflammation may make the control of open-angle glaucoma more difficult. There is no evidence that vasodilator or adrenergic drugs affect the course of glaucoma.

Primary Angle-Closure Glaucoma

While this form of glaucoma is far less common than open-angle glaucoma it is important that the general physician be aware of it because an attack may be precipitated by the use of mydriatics, and if this occurs urgent recognition and treatment are mandatory to prevent damage to the eye. Patients frequently have a positive family history and women are affected more than men.

The basic defect in primary angle-closure glaucoma is the inability of aqueous humor to reach the filtration apparatus. There is a blockage of the trabecular meshwork by the peripheral iris. When the pupil is mid-dilated, the iris is bowed forward which blocks the outflow of aqueous humor (see Fig. 95.2).

Individuals who have narrow anterior ocular chambers are predisposed to primary angle closure glaucoma. Moreover, the lens may be of such size that there is encroachment of the aqueous-filtering trabecular meshwork. Individuals with these predispositions often have acute attacks of increased intraocular pressure when the eye is dilated, occluding outflow, as might occur in the dark or when mydriatic is placed in the eye for fundoscopic examination.

DIAGNOSIS

Early diagnosis of this problem is critical because virtually every case is surgically curable. Cure is increasingly less likely if repeated attacks have occurred and have resulted in scarring of the trabecular meshwork at the angle of the anterior chamber. The acute attack frequently is unilateral and often is precipitated by emotion. The classical symptoms are episodes of ocular pain (usually located in the periocular or supraocular region), episodes of blurred vision, and halos around lights at night. These symptoms occur because of corneal epithelial edema which has developed as a result of the increased

intraocular pressure. Often patients find relief in well-lighted rooms or out-of-doors where daylight causes constriction of the pupil and opening of the angle of the anterior chamber.

Examination during an acute attack usually reveals marked elevation of intraocular pressure, to 60 to 90 mm Hg. However, chronic obstruction may compromise the circulation to the ciliary body and result in a fall in aqueous production and subsequently reduce ocular pressure. However, there is considerable individual tolerance of the vascular supply of the ciliary body to the increased pressure.

In patients predisposed to angle-closure glaucoma, the anterior chamber is shallow. This may be seen by illuminating the eye with a flashlight from the side and showing a shadow over the nasal portion of the eye resulting from the bowed iris (Fig. 95.2). Ophthalmoscopic examination may reveal scarring of the trabecular meshwork—peripheral anterior synechia. Corneal edema will be present during an acute attack, and the anterior chamber may appear cloudy due to inflammation.

If the diagnosis of acute angle-closure glaucoma is suspected, immediate administration of acetazolamide (Diamox), 250 mg orally, and instillation of two drops of a miotic—such as pilocarpine, 4% every 15 min—is indicated; and the patient should see an ophthalmologist within 6 hours. In severe cases, the ingesting of hyperosmotic glycerol—1 ml per kg mixed as a 50% solution with chilled juice—almost always will interrupt an acute attack. Physicians who use mydriatics for fundoscopic examination or patients who have narrow anterior ocular chambers and who do not have immediate access to an ophthalmologist should have an "angle closure kit" consisting of pilocarpine, glycerol, and acetazolamide (Diamox) for use with an acute attack. Patients found to have a shallow anterior chamber even if they have not had a symptomatic attack of glaucoma should be referred to an ophthalmologist for evaluation, for education regarding specific manifestations of an acute attack, and for their initial treatment as well as for consideration for prophylactic iridectomy.

DIFFERENTIAL DIAGNOSIS

The patient who has acute angle-closure glaucoma may come with an acute red eye to a general physician. Initially the physician will want to differentiate angle-closure glaucoma from acute iritis, acute conjunctivitis, and iridocyclitis. Chapter 96 discusses this differential diagnosis.

COURSE WITHOUT TREATMENT

Severe attacks of angle-closure glaucoma may cause blindness in 2 to 3 days depending on the level of intraocular pressure and on the sensitivity of the ciliary body and optic nerve to ischemia. In some instances, ciliary ischemia stops aqueous production before blindness occurs; but repeated attacks are the rule, and these will eventually result in scarring of the trabecular meshwork. The frequency and rapidity of recurrences are unpredictable. An examination between attacks usually will reveal only a shallow anterior chamber (Fig. 95.2) and normal intraocular pressure. Peripheral anterior synechia and segmental iris atrophy may be seen depending on the frequency and severity of previous attacks. A history of an acute attack, an actual acute attack, or the demonstration of a shallow anterior chamber should lead to an ophthalmological consultation.

TREATMENT

The treatment of primary angle-closure glaucoma is essentially surgical. If the diagnosis is made early enough in the course of the disease, a peripheral iridectomy can be done to prevent the attacks of increased intraocular pressure and the development of scarring. Surgical peripheral iridectomy under local anesthesia has little risk and results in cure. Iridectomy may also be done by using a laser beam. The eye involved in an acute attack is operated upon as soon as the attack is controlled (see above). Generally, the other eye is operated upon prohylactically a week or so later. Follow-up care by the ophthalmologist after surgery is necessary. If pressure control has not been achieved, medical therapy (see above) may be necessary. This, however, is unusual if surgery is performed early.

When the physican is aware that a patient has a narrow anterior chamber or is under treatment for angle-closure glaucoma, there should be concern about the use of certain medications. Systemic anticholinergics or adrenergic drugs may precipitate an acute attack by causing dilation of the pupils. Corticosteroids or vasodilating drugs are not contraindicated in patients with angle-closure glaucoma (2).

References

General

Schwartz, B: Current concepts in ophthalmology. The glaucomas. N Engl J Med 299: 182 1978.
  A brief, helpful review of the glaucomas.

Specific

1. Graham, PA and Hollows, FC: A critical review of detecting glaucoma. In *Glaucoma: Epidemiology, Early Diagnosis and Some Aspects of Treatment* edited by LB Hunt. Livingstone, Edinburgh, 1966.
2. Grant, WG: Systemic drugs and adverse influence on ocular pressure. In *Symposium on Ocular Therapy, Vol. 3,* edited by IH Leopold. C.V. Mosby, St. Louis, 1968.
3. Leske, MC and Rosenthal, J: Epidemiologic aspects of open-angle glaucoma. *Am J Epidemiol 109:* 250, 1979.
4. Robertson, D: Tonometry screening on the medical service. *Arch Intern Med 137:* 443, 1977.
5. Rock, WJ, Drance, SM and Morgen, RW: Visual field screening in glaucoma; an evaluation of the Armaly technique for screening glaucomatus visual fields. *Arch Ophthalmol 89:* 287, 1973.
6. Rosenthal, AR and Payne, R: Association of HLA antigens and primary Open-angle glaucoma. *Am J Ophthalmol 88:* 479, 1979.

CHAPTER NINETY-SIX

The Red Eye

EARL D. R. KIDWELL, Jr., M.D.

The patient with a red eye is frequently encountered in an ambulatory practice. The problem is usually caused by an infection, and most often is self-limited; however, there are serious considerations in the differential diagnosis which the general physician must recognize so that he can initiate urgent ophthalmologic consultation if necessary. This chapter provides a framework for recognizing conditions which require consultation and provides a discussion of conditions which may be managed by the general physician. Figure 96.1 illustrates the important structures and landmarks of the external eye.

DIFFERENTIAL DIAGNOSIS (Table 96.1)

Conditions which Require Referral

The conditions requiring urgent ophthalmologic consultation can be recognized by the general physician if he pays attention to several important features of the history and physical examination. The patient should be asked specifically whether he has been treated for an ocular disorder or whether he has recently experienced pain in one or both of his eyes. When the eyes are examined, it is essential to evaluate the following features: visual acuity, the nature of the discharge, the appearance of the cornea, the size and reactivity of the pupil, and the extent of the redness. In selected patients special tests, such as measurement of ocular tension or inspection of the eye after fluorescein staining, are necessary. Table 96.2 (p. 1037) shows how this information may suggest a specific diagnosis.

SPECIFIC CONDITIONS

Acute glaucoma is discussed in Chapter 95.

Iritis may be due to a specific problem such as trauma or infection, but often a specific etiology cannot be identified. In this condition failure to initiate proper treatment may result in permanent scarring which will affect pupillary movement and may cause glaucoma.

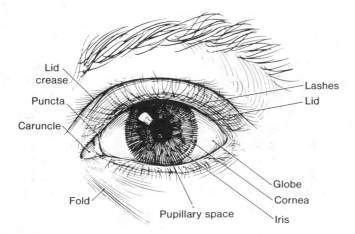

Figure 96.1 External landmarks of the eye.

Table 96.1
Major Causes of a Red Eye

CONDITIONS WHICH REQUIRE REFERRAL
  Acute glaucoma
  Acute iritis
  Acute corneal tear or infection
  Acute scleritis and/or episcleritis
CONDITIONS WHICH USUALLY CAN BE MANAGED BY THE GENERAL PHYSICIAN
  Bacterial conjunctivitis—hyperacute, acute, and chronic
  Viral conjunctivitis
  Inclusion conjunctivitis
  Allergic conjunctivitis
  Chemical conjunctivitis
  Foreign body
  Subconjunctival hemorrhage

Iritis can usually be recognized by the general physician because it is a painful eye condition which characteristically is associated with photophobia. Often vision is blurred as well. Occasionally, the pupil of the involved eye is small and fixed compared to the contralateral one. Typically the redness in iritis surrounds the cornea.

Corneal injury is usually recognized easily because of intense pain localized to the cornea following an injury and because of identification of a corneal lesion. If the injury is secondary to minor trauma (corneal abrasion) from a foreign body, the eye may be irrigated with a sterile eyewash (such as Collyrium) and a patch placed over it for 24 hours (see below, "Foreign Body"). If, on the other hand, an extensive epithelial defect (as revealed by fluorescein staining) is present, urgent ophthalmologic referral is indicated.

Fluorescein staining is easily accomplished by moistening a sterile fluorescein strip in the lower conjunctival sac and waiting a moment for the fluorescein to diffuse into the tears. The eye is then irrigated with physiologic saline or eyewash and the epithelial defect will remain stained a brilliant green. A corneal ulcer will also stain with fluorescein, but staining will appear to be deeper indicating subepithelial corneal involvement. Patients with this latter problem should see an ophthalmologist urgently.

Scleritis is often associated with iritis and usually is seen in association with a systemic disorder (such as collagen vascular disease). The deep vessels of the sclera are dilated and this may be demonstrated by the instillation of a drop of Neo-Synephrine 5 or 10% which will constrict the superficial, but not the deep vessels. The patient usually complains of a discomfort in the eye, and sometimes of severe pain, which is intensified if the eye is moved.

Episcleritis is a relatively common problem characterized by pain caused by a characteristically sharply localized area of inflammation of the superficial layer of the sclera. The etiology is unknown but it is occasionally associated with a systemic disorder such as collagen vascular disease or a specific infec-

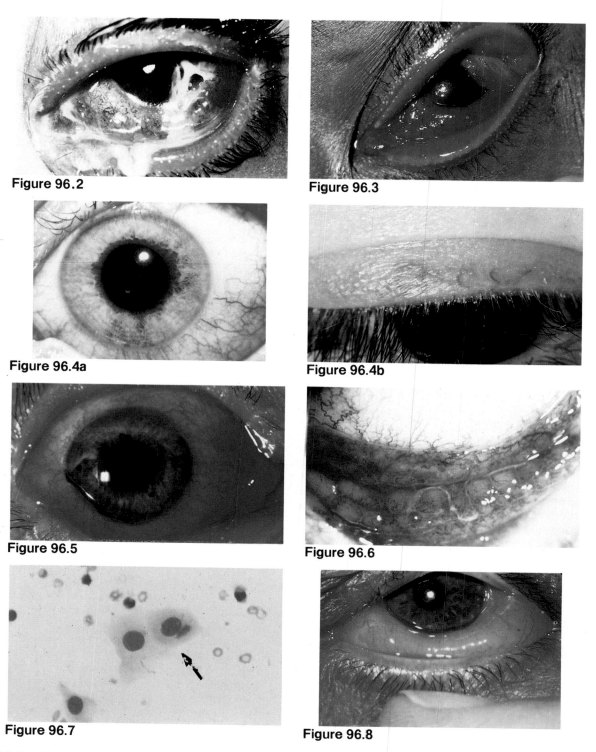

Figure 96.2

Figure 96.3

Figure 96.4a

Figure 96.4b

Figure 96.5

Figure 96.6

Figure 96.7

Figure 96.8

Figure 96.2 Hyperacute bacterial conjunctivitis. Note the severe degree of infection, swelling and pustular discharge.

Figure 96.3 Acute bacterial conjunctivitis. Note the severe erythema and edema.

Figure 96.4 Chronic bacterial conjunctivitis: (a) injected conjunctiva and erythema of lid margins; (b) telangiectasia of upper lid and debris in the lashes.

Figure 96.5 Viral conjunctivitis. Note the redness as well as the edema of the lid and conjunctiva.

Figure 96.6 Inclusion conjunctivitis. Note the conjunctival follicular hypertrophy.

Figure 96.7 Scraping of conjunctiva from a patient with inclusion conjunctivitis showing inclusion body (*arrow*) (Giemsa stain).

Figure 96.8 Allergic conjunctivitis. Note the conjunctival edema.

tion such as herpes zoster or tuberculosis. A few patients will have an associated iritis, which is usually mild. The palpebral conjunctiva is not involved and there is no discharge; these two observations help to differentiate this problem from conjunctivitis. Episcleritis is short-lived but is frequently recurrent; for this reason, ophthalmologic consultation is indicated.

Conditions which Usually Can Be Managed by the General Physician

Conjunctival infections, allergies, and irritation are the commonest causes of red or irritated eyes and are discussed in detail below. Almost always a general physician can manage these problems without consulting with an ophthalmologist.

CONJUNCTIVITIS

General Considerations

The diagnosis and management of conjunctivitis can be confusing, considering the variety of ocular infections. Most cases are not absolute emergencies, and, frequently, they are self-limited. Conjunctivitis may, however, cause serious complications such as corneal scarring, lid damage, or, in cases in which the patient has had antecedent intraocular surgery, endophthalmitis.

Conjunctival Flora

Under normal conditions the conjunctival sac has a bacterial flora composed of several species (1). The most commonly encountered organism is *Staphylococcus albus*, followed by *Corynebacteria*, *Staphylococcus aureus*, and *Streptococcus* species. This complex flora complicates the establishment of a specific etiology in a patient with infectious conjunctivitis.

Presentation

Conjunctivitis is usually not painful, but often there is mild discomfort, burning, discharge, tearing, itching, and lid swelling. Vision is well preserved. Most often, infectious conjunctivitis is bilateral.

Laboratory Diagnosis

Whenever there is doubt about the diagnosis, a simple culture and/or staining of the conjunctival material will help in determining the cause and subsequent management of the condition. Most often, however, the appearance of the conjunctivitis will be adequate for diagnosis.

CULTURE

Specimens for culture should be obtained with a sterile cotton swab by everting the eye lid and wiping the conjunctival sac. This material must be obtained without topical anesthesia because the preservatives in the anesthetic solution might inhibit the growth of organisms. The specimen must be transferred immediately into transport media or delivered immediately to the laboratory for culturing. Whenever a culture is considered necessary, both eyes should be cultured separately, even if there is only monocular involvement, so that the apparently uninfected eye will provide information about the nature of the normal flora.

SCRAPING

Following culture, a topical anesthetic (such as Ophthaine) should be instilled, and scrapings of the conjunctiva, well away from the cornea, should be obtained. A sterile platinum *spatula* (available from physician supply stores) or the dull side of a sterile scalpel *blade* can be used to scrape the conjunctiva. The material obtained by this method is smeared on a glass slide and is stained with Gram stain and/or Giemsa stain. The appearance of the cells found in these scrapings is helpful in determining the diagnosis and, therefore, scraping is recommended in the evaluation of patients with conjunctivitis when the diagnosis is uncertain. The differential findings are discussed below and listed in Table 96.3.

Specific Types

HYPERACUTE BACTERIAL CONJUNCTIVITIS

The name of this condition reflects its onset and the very thick exudate associated with it (Fig. 96.2). Typically, the discharge is so copious that it accumulates in the lashes or runs down the patient's cheek. One eye is usually involved before the other, but within several days the second eye becomes involved through autoinoculation. The infection quickly involves the surrounding structures and is associated with aching discomfort, swelling of the lid, and tenderness of the eye. Enlarged preauricular lymph nodes are often present. Early in the infection the cornea is not involved, but as the conjunctival swelling and reaction increase, a peripheral corneal ring ulcer may develop due to the compression of the peripheral corneal circulation.

Neisseria gonorrhoeae or *Niesseria meningitidis* is usually implicated in this infection. Inoculation is a result of fomite spread or through autoinoculation from infected genitalia. The gonococcus has the ability to penetrate the intact corneal epithelium so that central corneal ulceration and endophthalmitis also may occur. Meningococcal conjunctivitis is indistinguishable from gonococcal conjunctivitis, although the former occurs more frequently in younger individuals, may be bilateral at the onset, and can proceed to metastatic meningitis or meningococcemia.

Conjunctival scrapings reveal an overwhelming number of polymorphonuclear leukocytes and intracellular Gram-negative diplococci. Culture should be obtained on Thayer-Martin selective medium or be sent to the laboratory on Transgrow medium. The

Table 96.2
Important Observations in Evaluation of a Patient with a Red Eye

	Glaucoma	Iritis	Corneal Injury	Scleritis	Episcleritis	Bacterial Conjunctivitis	Inclusion Conjunctivitis	Viral Conjunctivitis
History of previous ocular disorder or condition predisposing to an ocular disorder	+	+/−	−	+	−	−	−	−
Pain	+	+ Photophobia	+	+	+	Mild discomfort or burning	Mild discomfort or burning	Mild discomfort or burning
Visual acuity	Diminished and blurred	Blurred	Usually diminished	Normal	Normal	Normal	Occasionally blurred, if chronic	Normal
Discharge	None	None	Usually some	None	None	Present: thick or thin	None or mucopurulent	None
Appearance of cornea	May be hazy	Normal	May be streaky	Normal	Normal	Normal	Normal except if late when superior dots or streaking may be seen	Normal
Pupil	Often dilated, mid-dilated, or fixed	Small and different from opposite side	Normal	Normal	Normal	Normal	Normal except if late when it may be small and different from other side	Normal
Redness	Around cornea	Around cornea	Localized or diffuse	Localized or diffuse	Localized	Diffuse	Diffuse (variable)	Segmental or diffuse
Selected evaluations	Ocular pressure in eye is high (see Chapter 95)[a]	Normal	Fluorescein stain[b] shows epithelial defect as brilliant green	A drop of Neo-Synephrine 5 or 10% in conjunctiva will constrict superficial but not deep vessels (see text)	None	None	None	None

[a] Should not be measured if a discharge is present or if a corneal ulceration is seen.
[b] Use individually packaged sterile fluorescein strips.

Table 96.3
Diagnosis Based on Cells in Material Scraped from Conjunctiva

Cells	Significance
Polymorphonuclear leukocytes	Bacteria, fungus, chlamydia (inclusion conjunctivitis), trachoma, Stevens-Johnson syndrome.
Mononuclear cells	Viral
Eosinophils	Allergy, ocular pemphigoid
Epithelial metaplasia (atypical, large cells)	Chlamydia, herpes simplex

differentiation between gonococcus and meningococcus requires special bacteriologic studies.

Therapy of hyperacute conjunctivitis must be prompt to avoid corneal damage or systemic spread and should include the administration of both systemic and topical antibiotics (Table 96.4). Institution of appropriate antibiotics should result in the disappearance of the discharge within 24 to 48 hours, although lid swelling and conjunctival reaction do not abate for several days. If a corneal ulcer occurs, it is slow to heal; and if the cornea has been scarred or if endophthalmitis has developed, visual acuity may be affected. Therefore, whenever there is evidence of impaired vision, an ophthalmologist should be consulted immediately.

ACUTE BACTERIAL CONJUNCTIVITIS

This condition, like hyperacute bacterial conjunctivitis, has an abrupt onset but is characterized by a less thick, often mucopurulent, discharge. This form of conjunctivitis is often called *catarrhal or pink eye* (Fig. 96.3); it is seen at all ages and at any time of year. The most common cause of the condition is *Staphylococcus aureus* infection. *Pneumococcus* and *Haemophilus* species also cause the problem, but infections with these organisms have a more restricted geographic distribution than do staphylococcal infections; pneumococcal infections occur primarily in the northern states during the colder months, and haemophilus infections occur more commonly in the warmer regions of the United States throughout the year. Also, pneumococcal or haemophilus conjunctivitis is more common in younger individuals than is staphylococcal conjunctivitis. Rarely, other bacteria, such as *Moraxella lacunata*, *Escherichia coli*, or *Proteus* species, cause this form of conjunctivitis.

Patients complain of eye irritation and watering and typically the eyelids stick together after sleep. The infection starts unilaterally; but very often, because of autoinoculation, the contralateral eye becomes involved in 1 or 2 days. Examination reveals hyperemia of the palpebra; bulbar conjunctival petechiae, characteristic of haemophilus infection, may be seen.

These infections are self-limited and generally last 7 to 14 days, although haemophilus infections may last somewhat longer.

The diagnosis is suspected by the examination; however, wherever there is doubt, diagnosis should be confirmed by examination of the scrapings of the conjunctiva and by culturing the exudate.

Topical treatment usually results in the resolution of symptoms in a day or two. The preferred therapy is with sodium sulfacetamide (Sulamyd-10%)—either the solution, 2 drops in the eye every 3 hours while awake, or the ointment, a small amount applied to the lower conjunctival sac four times a day and at bedtime. If there is an allergy to sulfa drugs, a 1% chloramphenicol ointment (Chloromycetin ophthalmic ointment), four times a day and at bedtime, may be used. This agent is particularly efficacious against *Haemophilus* and *Moraxella*.

CHRONIC BACTERIAL CONJUNCTIVITIS

Staphylococcus aureus causes most cases of chronic bacterial conjunctivitis; but occasionally it is caused by other agents, such as *Staphylococcus epidermidis*, *Moraxella lacunata*, *Corynebacterium diptheriae*, or *Streptococcus pyogenes*. *S. aureus* colonizes the margin of the eyelid and the follicles containing the eyelashes. Both *S. aureus* and *S. epidermidis* elaborate an exotoxin which injures the conjunctiva and cornea, and it is this toxin which is responsible for the chronic inflammation.

Patients with this problem complain of a sensation of a foreign body in the eye as well as of redness and itching; frequently the eyelids stick together after sleep. There is often a history of recurrent styes and

Table 96.4
Antimicrobials which May Be Used in Treatment of Hyperacute Conjunctivitis (Both a Systemic and Topical Agent should Be Used)

SYSTEMIC
Procaine penicillin G 4.8 million units intramuscularly preceded by 1 g of probenicid administered orally
or
Ampicillin, 3.5 g and probenicid 1 g administered orally, simultaneously
or, if penicillin-sensitive:
Spectinomycin, 4 g intramuscularly at initial visit given in 2 injections
or
Tetracycline 1.5 g orally as an initial dose followed by 0.5 g, 4 times a day for 4 days
TOPICAL
Gentamicin ophthalmic in the involved eye every 2 hr for 5 days, then 4 times a day for 7–10 days.
or
Chloramphenicol 0.5% ophthalmic, in the involved eye every 2 hr for 2 days then 4 times a day for 7–10 days.
or
Bacitracin ointment 500 units per g, in the involved eye every 2 hr for 2 days then 4 times a day for 7–10 days

of loss of eyelashes. Examination shows erythema of the lid margin and, sometimes, a minimal exudate is present. Occasionally, mucous strands may be found in the conjunctival fornices, and the eyelids may appear thickened and red (Fig. 96.4).

The lid margins, surrounding skin, conjuctiva, and cornea may be involved singly or collectively. The skin may also show changes of seborrheic dermatitis or it may be excoriated and macerated, especially at the lateral canthal margin. Crusting is noted at the bases of the eyelashes. The conjunctiva may show changes of papillary hyperplasia (multiple conjunctival mounds with a central single vessel). Corneal changes occur after months of inflammation and are manifest as fine discrete inferior defects. There may also be ulceration, clouding, and vascularization of the margins of the cornea.

The diagnosis is made by examination and, in cases in doubt, by scraping the conjunctivae as well as the margins of the eyelids and by culturing the exudate.

Usually, gentamicin solution or ointment (Garamycin ophthalmic drops or ointment), 1 or 2 drops or a small amount of ointment every 4 hours while awake, or erythromycin ointment (Ilotycin ophthalmic ointment), every 4 hours while awake, will be effective. Treatment should be continued for 2 weeks. Daily cleansing of the eyelashes with a neutral soap (such as Johnsons Baby Shampoo) followed by the application of an antibiotic ointment (such as gentamicin or erythromycin) to the eyelashes 4 times a day for several weeks will reduce the bacterial count, cleanse the lids, and prevent recurrences.

VIRAL CONJUNCTIVITIS

Viral conjunctivitis is also known as *acute follicular conjunctivitis* and it quite common. It is caused by a variety of viral agents. The onset is abrupt and unilateral, but contralateral involvement from autoinoculation is frequent in a day or two. Excessive tearing is often a major complaint, but there is no purulent discharge. The conjunctiva nearly always shows hyperemia, which may be diffuse or segmental (see Fig. 96.5). Viral conjunctivitis may be accompanied by tender preauricular lymphadenopathy. Frequently, the lymphoid tissue of the eyelid enlarges in response to the infection and may appear as elevated palpebral as well as bulbar conjunctival lesions (Fig. 96.5). In cases where there is doubt about the diagnosis, examination of the conjunctival scrapings shows mononuclear cells.

The disease is self-limited, lasting only a few days; and treatment is therefore supportive. Astringent drops containing naphazoline (such as over-the-counter agents—Albalon, Naphcon-A, or Vasocon-A) are very helpful in relieving conjunctival congestion and hyperemia, and cool compresses also provide relief. Sulfacetamide (Sulamyd) or erythromycin (Ilotycin) may be used if symptoms have not been controlled in 1 or 2 days with astringent drops, as in this instance bacterial conjunctivitis may have developed.

Rarely, corneal inflammation may develop and cause an opacity in the cornea. When this complication is noted, an ophthalmologist should be consulted urgently because loss of vision may occur.

INCLUSION CONJUNCTIVITIS (INCLUSION-BLENNORRHEA)

This problem is seen frequently in sexually active young adults. The disease is caused by a species of *Chlamydia* and is a result of contamination of the eye from the urethra after a sexual contact.

The problem is characterized, usually, by the abrupt onset of eye discomfort with varying degrees of diffuse conjunctival hyperemia and sometimes with mucopurulent discharge which may result in matting of the eyelashes. The eyelids appear swollen and inspection of the palpebral conjunctiva, especially of the lower lid, shows many small follicles (raised pale mounds of varying size) (Fig. 96.6). Occasionally, preauricular lymphadenopathy develops. Without treatment, the disease becomes chronic and remitting and, in 2 or 3 weeks, a superficial corneal inflammation (keratitis) may appear. This may be identified with the naked eye as dots or cloudy streaks on the superior portion of the cornea. Also at this stage, there may be an associated iritis manifest by photophobia and blurring of vision.

This syndrome may occur in association with urethritis in the male or cervicitis and a vaginal discharge in the female. Most often, however, there are no genitourinary symptoms although *Chlamydia* species can be cultured (by using special techniques) from the urethra in men or the endocervical canal in women. In some cases, Reiter's syndrome will be present (see Chapter 68).

The diagnosis is suggested by the history and appearance but, if there is doubt, it may be confirmed (especially in younger individuals) by examination of the material obtained from conjunctival scraping. This material when stained with Giemsa stain shows large basophilic cytoplasmic inclusion bodies (Fig. 96.7). Gram stain will not reveal these bodies but will show many polymorphonuclear leukocytes. The diagnosis can also be confirmed by demonstrating a rising complement fixation titer to chlamydia group antigen.

Therapy is effective, but must be systemic. Oral tetracycline, 250 mg, 4 times daily for 21 days, is the preferable regimen; but where tetracycline cannot be given, good results will be achieved with erythromycin, 250 mg, 4 times a day for 21 days or sulfonamide (Gantrisin), 500 mg, 4 times a day for 21 days. It may take several months for the follicular hyperplasia to resolve, but the patient should experience symptomatic improvement within several days. The application of cool compresses for 20 min several times a day will also provide comfort in the first few days of treatment.

Since the disease must be assumed to be sexually transmitted, the sexual partner should be similarly treated; other venereal diseases should be looked for, and the male should use a condom until therapy has been completed.

ALLERGIC CONJUNCTIVITIS

This is a common and mild conjunctivitis frequently encountered in patients with allergic rhinitis (see Chapter 22). Often the patient describes a history of allergy to grasses and pollens as well as to other agents and usually complains of itching and tearing. Frequently, there is marked swelling of the conjunctiva (Fig. 96.8) and slight to moderate redness of the eye, and at times there is serous crusting in the morning.

Whenever there is doubt about the diagnosis, conjunctival scrapings may be examined. A finding of many eosinophils is diagnostic. When conjunctivitis is associated with allergic rhinitis, it usually parallels the rhinitis in severity and duration. When it occurs as an isolated problem, it is short-lived, and treatment is symptomatic. A topical astringent solution (Albalon, Naphcon-A, or Vasocon-A) and cool compresses are very effective. Occasionally, symptoms are severe and oral antihistamines may relieve itching.

Corticosteroid eyedrops are very effective for this condition but they must be used cautiously because their use is associated with corneal ulceration and perforation in the presence of herpes simplex infection, the development of fungal infection, and when used chronically, with the development in some individuals of open-angle glaucoma and, rarely, cataract formation. For these reasons, topical corticosteroids are not recommended without at least telephone consultation with an ophthalmologist.

CHEMICAL CONJUNCTIVITIS

Many agents may enter the conjunctiva and produce inflammation. Irritation from agents such as smoke, smog, sprays, chlorinated water, hair spray, makeup, or industrial dust occurs frequently. It is the history of the exposure that makes the diagnosis obvious. The patient should thoroughly rinse the conjunctival sac with water as soon as contamination with a chemical has occurred. The patient will also benefit from cool compresses for 15 to 20 min several times a day and occasionally the use of a topical astringent solution (Albalon, Naphcon-A, or Vasocon-A) will be necessary.

In the case of an injury from an acid or alkali, serious permanent damage may occur and this problem is a true ophthalmologic emergency. Patients should be advised to irrigate the conjunctival sac with copious amounts of water and to see an ophthalmologist immediately.

FOREIGN BODY

Foreign bodies frequently lodge in the conjunctiva or cornea. Most often they can be visualized with the naked eye; but, if not, sterile fluorescein staining (see p. 1034) will outline the area of epithelial damage. Foreign bodies may be removed by irrigation of the conjunctival sac with a sterile solution of physiologic saline or eyewash. If they are not rinsed away, mechanical removal is indicated. This may be accomplished, when the object is in the cornea, by placing in the eye a drop of topical anesthetic (such as Ophthaine) and removing the foreign body with a sterile needle held carefully with the physician's arm braced. A cotton swab should not be used to remove a foreign body from the cornea since frequently it is very irritating to the structure and thus delays healing. If the foreign body is not on the cornea, removal is easier and usually does not require anesthesia. After removal, it is wise to instill a drop of antibiotic (such as Sulamyd or Bacitracin) and the eye should be covered by a patch for 24 hours. The patch should be applied tightly enough to prevent the eyelids from moving. If the patch falls off before the 24-hour period is up, the patient should not try to reapply it, as often this may cause more irritation.

If the offending material is a piece of metal, rust rings surrounding the area of the epithelial defect may be observed. These rings are not harmful *per se* and only the foreign body should be removed.

In any instance where the foreign body is not easily removed, an ophthalmologist should see the patient urgently.

SUBCONJUNCTIVAL HEMORRHAGE

Subconjunctival hemorrhage is a common condition which very often is alarming to the patient. A small blood vessel ruptures in the conjunctival tissue after the patient coughs or strains and a painless wedge-shaped hemorrhage develops. Often the patient will have no memory of the coughing or straining, but incidentally notices the red eye. Occasionally, viral conjunctivitis may be manifest only by the appearance of a subconjunctival hemorrhage (Fig. 96.5). Isolated subconjunctival hemorrhage requires no treatment and should resolve within several days. If the problem becomes recurrent and/or multiple an abnormality of hemostasis should be considered.

References

General

Havener, WH: *Synopsis of Ophthalmology,* Ed. 4. C. V. Mosbey, St. Louis, 1975.
  A very well written short textbook which provides an overview of many eye problems, including the differential diagnosis of the red eye and of the different forms of conjunctivitis.

Specific

1. Fahmy, JA: The conjunctival flora of 499 patients on no therapy. *Acta Ophthalmol* 53: 485, 1975.

SECTION 15

Miscellaneous Problems

CHAPTER NINETY-SEVEN

Common Problems of the Skin

STANFORD I. LAMBERG, M.D.

One-third of all patients with a primary dermatologic complaint consult a general physician or an internist rather than a dermatologist, according to a 1979 survey of dermatologic care, conducted by the American Academy of Dermatology (14). Some 10 diseases, listed in order of frequency in Table 97.1, account for 70% of all skin diseases seen by dermatologists in their practices.

This chapter provides assistance in diagnosing and managing these disorders. In addition, because they

Table 97.1
The Ten Most Common Skin Problems

1. Acne
2. Fungal infections
3. Seborrheic dermatitis
4. Atopic dermatitis/eczema
5. Warts
6. Tumors—benign and malignant
7. Psoriasis
8. Hair disorders
9. Vitiligo
10. Herpes simplex

are common, contact dermatitis, herpes zoster, pityriasis rosea, and scabies are discussed. For maximal usefulness, specific rather than general treatment plans are outlined.

ACNE

Definition

Acne vulgaris is a chronic disorder of the sebaceous glands, particularly those on the face, chest, and back, where they are the largest and most dense. Sebum from sebaceous glands reaches the surface by emptying into the hair follicle and flowing along the hair shaft, the two skin appendages forming the pilosebaceous unit. The earliest lesions of acne is the *comedone*, due to impaction of the opening of the pilosebaceous duct by horny material and dried sebum. The plugs are visible as closed comedones ("whiteheads") and, if the surface is darkened, open comedones ("blackheads"), black, not due to dirt, but to oxidation of melanin and sebum in the plugs. Comedones become inflamed as nonpathogenic bacteria, normal residents within the duct and gland, especially *Staphylococcus epidermidis* and an anaerobic diptheroid, *Corynebacterium acnes*, proliferate within the obstructed glands and produce erythematous tender papules. As inflammation progresses, these papules may become pustular and, in severe cases, cystic. Cysts are presumed to be due to abscess formation deep in the dermis. Various manifestations of the disorder usually are present in the same patient.

Epidemiology

Acne occurs primarily in adolescents; there is an equal incidence in males and females, although the eruption often is worse in males. Almost all teenagers have acne to some degree, but only a minority require treatment. In most, the lesions resolve by age 20. Sometimes acne may persist into adulthood or develop for the first time in adults, especially women, usually those using cosmetics (so-called acne cosmetica).

Acne can be produced or exacerbated by drugs, including corticosteroids, androgenic steroids, phenytoin, iodides, and lithium and by external irritants such as creosote, tar, and industrial cutting oils (chloracne). Pomade acne is acne near the hair line, especially common in blacks, caused by the use of hair pomades.

Pathogenesis

The underlying cause of acne is unclear, but several events participate in its development. These include: proliferation of sebaceous glands and increased production of sebum by sebaceous glands under the stimulation of androgens as puberty occurs; obstruction of the sebaceous glands with proliferation of bacteria, followed by the development of inflammation and characteristic lesions of acne. The precise reasons why some individuals develop severe disease while most have mild disease is not known, although severe acne often is hereditary.

Evaluation

The following information should be recorded before planning therapy:

1. *Topical medications used*, past and present, including prescription and nonprescription preparations. Many of the patients will have initiated therapy themselves and the preparations they used may be irritating. Response or failure to previously used antibiotics is particularly important information.

2. *Face care* including soap used, scrubbing technique, use of skin machine, and cosmetics (brand and type). Information about the use of foundations, cold creams, and astringents also is important. These preparations or techniques may be irritating or actually acnegenic.

3. *Factors that improve or worsen the acne*, including menses, diet, and stress, should be explored. Diet is not an important factor, although patients who believe that certain foods lead to flare-ups may avoid those foods.

4. *Other medical conditions and current medications* including oral contraceptive agents, corticosteroids, etc. (see above).

A table should be prepared for the patient's record for use in selecting and following therapy (Table 97.2). These data allow the physician to evaluate progress objectively.

Table 97.2
Data to Be Recorded in Evaluation and Follow-up of Patients with Acne

	Face	Back	Chest
Comedones	( )	( )	( )
Papules	( )	( )	( )
Pustules	( )	( )	( )
Cysts	( )	( )	( )

0 = none
1+ = few
2+ = moderate
3+ = many
4+ = extensive

Therapy

No single treatment is effective for all patients with acne. The overall goal is to reverse and prevent plugging of the sebaceous ducts as well as to reduce and prevent inflammation of the sebaceous glands and surrounding tissue (17). Patients should be told that a delay of 4 to 8 weeks before obvious improvement is common with any treatment of acne. If there is no improvement after 8 weeks or if lesions are cystic or deep and inflammatory with scarring, referral to a dermatologist is appropriate.

COMEDONES

If only comedones are present, a desquamating agent such as 5% benzoyl peroxide lotion, gel, or cream (such as Desquam-X 5 Gel, Oxy-5 lotion, Persadox lotion or cream, Xerac BP5 gel) should be prescribed. Initially the agent should be applied only at bedtime as it may cause intense inflammation if used excessively. After a few weeks, if treatment is tolerated, the end point being slight erythema and dryness, the frequency of use may be increased to twice a day and then the concentration increased to 10% (such as Desquam-X 10 Gel, Oxy-10 lotion, Persadox HP cream or lotion, or Xerac BP10 gel). Some of these agents are available without prescription such as Oxy-5, Oxy-10, Persadox, and Persadox HP.

Patients who do not respond to benzoyl peroxide within 4 to 8 weeks should be given topical vitamin A acid. The 0.01% gel (Retin-A gel, requires a prescription) seems to be least irritating and easiest to use. This agent appears to interfere with keratinization of the follicular duct thereby decreasing the comedone plug. Because vitamin A acid is quite irritating, it too should be started at a low concentration at bedtime, applied to the entire face, increasing the dose to 0.025% gel or 0.05% solution gradually over 2 to 3 months. The patient need not experience discomfort and peeling for the drug to be effective. The drug should be avoided in blacks as it may darken their skin. Experiments in mice have shown an increased incidence of skin cancer when vitamin A acid was used with high doses of ultraviolet light. Therefore, patients should be told to stop using the medication if they intend to be in the sun.

INFLAMMATORY LESIONS (PAPULES OR PUSTULES)

If inflammatory lesions are present, the initial therapy differs depending on the sex of the patient (1, 18).

Females. (a) Topical clindamycin (Cleocin-T) should be applied to the entire face morning and afternoon after washing with plain soap (such as Ivory, Camay, Purpose, or Basis). This should be continued for 2 months before alternative topical antibiotics or a systemic antibiotic is prescribed. Oral tetracycline (see below) generally should be avoided in women because of the common complication of vaginitis. However, if the lesions are pustular or cystic, systemic antibiotics will be necessary, at least initially. The dose schedule given for males (see below) may be followed. Tetracycline must not be used if the patient is pregnant. (b) In addition to the antibiotic, a topical desquamating agent will be needed: Benzoyl peroxide or vitamin A acid should be used as for comedone acne (see above). (c) The physician should also educate the patient to: STOP hard scrubbing, including the use of skin machines; STOP use of antibacterial soaps because nonpathogenic bacteria are reduced and replaced by pathogens. Instead, substitute a plain soap such as Ivory, Camay, Purpose, or Basis; STOP use of oil-based cosmetics (ingredients of cosmetics are listed on the labels) as they obstruct the sebaceous duct. Water-based and oil-free makeup may be safe for some, but it is best to avoid all foundations. Blusher and eye shadow do not seem to cause acne.

Males. (a) The physician should prescribe oral tetracycline, 250 mg 3 times daily. However, if the acne is severe, 500 mg 3 times daily should be prescribed. The medication should be taken 1 to 2 hours before or after meals to maximize absorption. The starting dose should be continued for 6 weeks or until there is clear improvement, then slowly decreased by 1 capsule daily each month. At the point that the acne recurs or flares up, the dose should be increased to the level that had maintained clearing and left at that level for several months. The lowest dose that is effective should be used. The usual maintenance level of tetracycline is 250 mg twice a day; no complications need be anticipated at this dose. (b) In addition to the antibiotics, a topical desquamating agent will be needed: Benzoyl peroxide or vitamin A acid should be used as for comedone acne (see above). (c) The physician should also educate the patient to: STOP hard scrubbing, including the use of skin machines; STOP use of antibacterial soaps because nonpathogenic bacteria are reduced and replaced by pathogens. Instead, substitute a plain soap such as Ivory, Camay, Purpose, or Basis.

Both men and women should wash their hair frequently and should not apply oil to the scalp.

Prognosis

Acne in the adolescent may require treatment until age 20 or so. Persistent acne in middle aged women usually is due to excessive use of occlusive cosmetics and moisturizers. Clearing may not occur until such cosmetics are stopped. Good results from the treatment outlined above can be anticipated in 80%. About 15% will require alternative therapies such as high doses of alternative antibiotics or specialized techniques such as cryotherapy, intradermal steroid injections, or acne surgery performed by a dermatologist. The remaining 5% will not respond well to any therapy; stabilization will be the goal. Dermabrasion, the superficial abrasion of the skin to reduce scars, may be useful for some patients, although most scars flatten and become less noticeable with time.

ATOPIC DERMATITIS (ATOPIC ECZEMA)

Atopic dermatitis is a chronic, pruritic inflammation of the skin with a characteristic course and pattern and with an associated personal and family history of allergy (3).

Etiology

Although still debated, the cause appears to be immunologic with both cellular and humoral mechanisms at fault (see Chapter 22). Severe cases often have an elevated serum IgE level and about 30% have a personal history of allergic rhinitis or asthma. In addition, 60% have a family history of atopy with cutaneous and/or respiratory symptoms. However, more than the immune system may be involved as signs of decreased production of eccrine sweat and increased vasoconstriction of small blood vessels also are often evident.

Presentation

Onset may be as early as the second month after birth. The major distress is due to the chronic and pruritic nature of the condition. Sleep is difficult; the discomfort may make the individual appear nervous and demanding. Other manifestations of atopy, or hypersensitivity, also may develop, including hay fever, rhinitis, or asthma. Early cataracts are a complication in a small percentage of severe cases, but general health is otherwise unaffected. A parent with atopic dermatitis may need to be told that the disorder is inherited and that about half their children are likely to be affected to some degree.

Although the entire skin seems "dry" with fine flaky scaling, dermatitis with eczematous lichenified plaques tends to involve certain regions and the distribution depends on age. During infancy, the disorder involves the extensor and exposed parts, and only later does it take on the adult distribution in flexoral folds including the antecubital, popliteals, wrists, and sides of the neck (Fig. 97.1). Itching is generalized but worse in the lichenified plaques, which sometimes become suprainfected. Many patients will have an extra crease below the margin of the lower eyelids (Dennie or Morgan fold).

Itching may be triggered by low humidity, high temperature, sweating, environmental allergens such as irritating or occlusive medications, wool clothing, greases, and detergents. Dietary factors do not appear to be important and control cannot be achieved through manipulation of the diet. Many cases improve during infancy and about half the cases have cleared by puberty. Some will remain clear but in many the dermatitis will recur. Many atopic patients have exacerbations throughout life, often when under physical or emotional stress. In most cases itching improves during the summer although skin infections may be more common then.

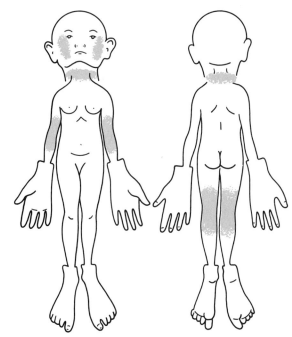

Figure 97.1   Lichenified pruritic areas in flexual regions and on the face are typical locations for adult atopic dermatitis.

Differential Diagnosis

Seborrheic dermatitis, psoriasis, and contact dermatitis may be confused with atopic dermatitis (see below).

Therapy

TOPICAL

Bathing and Lubrication. The patient must avoid soap on the inflamed areas of skin. If a shower/tub combination is available, the patient should first soap and shower areas such as axilla, groin, and buttocks using a mild soap such as Ivory, Dove, Purpose, or Basis. The soapy water should be drained out and a few inches of lukewarm water drawn into the tub. The patient should add 15 to 30 ml of bath oil (such as Domol or Alpha-Keri) and use this water for sponge bathing. Unlike soap, the oil will cleanse but will not "dry out" the skin. The tub will be slippery and the patient should be careful. After the sponge bath and while the skin is still damp, a lubricating cream such as Eucerin, Aquaphor, or Shepard's should be applied and repeated as desired. Perfume in emollients should be avoided as they are potentially sensitizing. In general the patient should not bathe more than twice a week. The house should be humidified (see Chapter 22) during the winter.

Topical Corticosteroids. Triamcinolone ointment 0.1% (prescribed as generic) is the mainstay of topical therapy and will control most cases. The ointment is better absorbed than the cream and is less drying.

However, the cream may be used when the eruption is subacute with oozing. A large quantity of topical steroids must be dispensed. The physician should calculate the amount to prescribe based upon the fact that at least 30 g of ointment are needed for a single total body application to an adult. At that rate, a typical application to the thighs and legs might be about 10 g. If the medication is to be used 3 times daily for 2 weeks, almost 1 lb (10 g × 3 = 30 g × 14 days = 420 g) should be dispensed. Topical steroids are expensive—1 lb may cost up to $50—and treatment plans have to take the cost into account. Absorption of topical steroids does occur but is not a significant problem unless the steroids are applied to large areas of dermatitic skin, particularly under occlusion. Topical steroids may produce atrophy of the skin when used in intertriginous areas; the patient should not use any additional steroid if the skin can be controlled with lubrication alone.

Because potent topical steroids can induce vascular dilation which may become permanent, nothing stronger than 1% hydrocortisone cream should be used on the face.

SYSTEMIC

Systemic antibiotics should be prescribed at the first sign of pyoderma—oozing, crusting, and odor. Erythromycin, 250 mg 4 times daily for 7 days for an adult usually is sufficient. Dicloxacillin 500 mg twice daily may be used as an alternative. Cultures generally are not needed unless abscesses develop; they are particularly important, however, if abscesses develop while the patient is taking antibiotics.

A rare complication, but a serious one, is infection with herpex simplex or varicella with multiple blisters, particularly at the site of active dermatitis. This is called eczema herpeticum. Vaccinia is no longer a problem as smallpox vaccinations are not given. Those affected are toxic and the complication is life-threatening. Hospitalization usually is required.

There is still a debate about whether antihistamines help beyond the side effect of sedation that normally accompanies their use. A trial for a week with 50 mg 3 times a day of diphenhydramine (Benadryl), 10 mg 3 times a day of hydroxyzine (Atarax, Cartrax, Vistrax) or an equivalent dose of others (see Chapter 22) may be appropriate if the patient has marked pruritus and is restless. The dose may be increased at bedtime to help with sleep.

THERAPY FOR RESISTANT CASES

Systemic corticosteroids occasionally are necessary for severe flare-ups of atopic dermatitis. A suggested starting schedule is 40 mg of prednisone in a single daily morning dose, reduced by 5 to 10 mg a day as soon as improvement is seen and tapered completely off within 2 to 3 weeks. Patients may obtain such relief from the systemic steroids that the physician may not be able to persuade them to stop the drug; however, since atopic dermatitis may be lifelong, eventual difficulties from continuous systemic corticosteroids are bound to ensue. Situations that justify courses of steroids are few; if there is doubt, referral to a dermatologist may be appropriate.

When To Refer

Consideration should be given for referral to a dermatologist if the diagnosis is uncertain, if the patient is unresponsive to initial therapy, or if the condition is so severe that frequent short courses of systemic corticosteroids are required. The dermatologist has several other therapies, including the application of tar preparations and ultraviolet (UV) light, sometimes combined with oral psoralens, which are not available therapies for most general physicians. Occasionally, hospitalization is necessary.

CONTACT DERMATITIS

Definition

Contact dermatitis is a cutaneous reaction to an external substance and may be either irritant or allergic. An irritant reaction affects most individuals exposed and generally produces discomfort immediately after the exposure. Allergic contact dermatitis affects only individuals previously sensitized to the contactant. The reaction is delayed until the cascade of cellular immunity is completed, requiring up to several hours. Both in industry and in the home, irritant reactions are more frequent than allergic reactions (8).

Irritant contact dermatitis is due to direct injury of the skin as, for example, that caused by detergents, solvents, or alkaline abrasives, including cement. If the irritant is a mild one, repeated or prolonged exposure, or exposure combined with abrasion may be necessary to produce a reaction. In allergic contact dermatitis, lymphocytes, previously exposed to antigen which has been processed through the macrophage or Langerhan's cell system, react selectively to subsequent exposure with initiation of inflammation. Genetic predisposition, frequency of exposure to the antigen, and coexisting dermatitis are among the factors that affect the development of sensitization. Allergic sensitivity is usually a more difficult problem than irritation because sensitized individuals may respond to only minute quantities of the offending substance.

Characteristics

An eruption with an asymmetric or restricted distribution, such as a rash limited to the axillae or ear lobes, or a rash only in exposed areas such as the face, "V" of the neck, lower arms, and hands, probably is contact in origin. The deeper skinfolds protected from external contactants tend to remain clear, while an intrinsic dermatitis, such as seborrheic dermatitis, will involve the entire area, including the skinfolds. Involvement of the palms or soles or of the mucous membranes, both ordinarily resistant to chemicals, is evidence against a contactant. Irritant and allergic dermatitides may be identical in appearance; distinction depends upon the history of exposure and response to patch testing.

Allergic reactions to systemic medications are usually central and are worse on the trunk than on exposed peripheral parts. The major exceptions are reactions to drugs that induce photosensitization to ultraviolet light. Tetracycline, sulfonamides, and thiazides are known photosensitizers, leading to exaggerated sunburn reaction or eczematous dermatitis.

Common Contactants

PLANT DERMATITIS

Poison ivy, oak, and sumac, the most common of the plant contactants, produce eczematous or even blistering eruptions, usually restricted to exposed parts and often with bizarrely shaped angular lesions, the result of contact with a plant resin (oleoresin). Contrary to popular belief, leakage of blister fluid does not "spread" the rash to other sites; however, lesions often are delayed in appearance because of the continuing unintentional exposure to the resin which may persist on the patient's clothing, tools, or sports equipment or on the fur of the family pet. Sensitive individuals will continue to develop new lesions for up to the 3 weeks that is required for the resin to evaporate.

METAL ALLERGY

Nickel contact allergy is common, particularly in women, where it may be seen near hooks, zippers, or jewelry, such as on the ear lobe and the wrist. Dermatitis under a gold ring could be due to metal allergy but is more often due to irritating soap residue. The eruption of metal allergy tends to be mild and chronic with scaling, pigmentation, and pruritus. A simple and convincing patch test can be performed to confirm the diagnosis of nickel allergy: a moistened 5-cent piece should be taped to the upper inner arm with an occlusive tape (such as Blenderm) and left on for 48 hours. The patient should remove the patch earlier if itching develops. Individuals allergic to nickel will develop dermatitis under the nickel; the area should be examined by the patient for several days, as patch test reactions occasionally may be delayed.

TOPICAL MEDICATIONS

Allergy to topical medications is frequent, probably due to the loss of the protective barrier of dermatitic skin. Common culprits include neomycin, anesthetics (such as benzocaine or tetracaine), and preservatives, such as parabens and merthiolate. The original eruption may appear to persist but the difficulty may be due to the imposition of a new contact allergy from the medication. The situation becomes even more confusing if corticosteroids are in the medication, thus partly masking the dermatitis.

COSMETICS

Following 1977 Food and Drug Administration guidelines, ingredients of cosmetics are now listed on the label. Manufacturers will make these substances available to the physician for patch-testing. However, many of the reactions to cosmetics are caused by the perfume; the chemical composition of perfumes may not be known, even to the manufacturer. The physician should suggest discontinuing or changing the cosmetic, a step the patient probably would have taken on her own, and using 1% hydrocortisone cream sparingly until the reaction subsides. More potent topical corticosteroids are to be avoided on the face, since long use may lead to telangiectases. It should be recognized that cosmetic reactions may take several weeks to regress; a change to another brand for a few days is not enough. If changing cosmetics does not provide relief, referral to a dermatologist is appropriate since patch-testing may be necessary to identify the allergen; alternatively, another dermatitis, such as seborrheic dermatitis, may be present.

Therapy

PLANT DERMATITIS

Immediately after exposure, the patient should wash the exposed parts thoroughly and wash or clean items that were in contact with the irritant or allergen and, in the case of plant dermatitis, isolate items not washable in a ventilated area for 3 weeks. Also in this instance the family pet should be bathed if it could have come into contact with the plants.

If acute dermatitis does develop, the patient should start cooling compresses with saline (1 teaspoon of salt/pint of tap water) or Burow's solution (1 tablet or packet/pint of tap water) for 20 min every 2 or 3 hours. An antihistamine, such as diphenhydramine (Benadryl) 50 mg, or chlorpheniramine (Chlor-Trimeton), 4 mg, every 4 to 6 hours, as well as a topical lotion, such as calamine, or a corticosteroid cream, such as triamcinolone 0.1%, may be used. If the reaction is particularly extensive, or is located on the face and is acute with edema and blisters, or if the patient is known to have had severe reactions to the same antigen in the past, systemic corticosteroids may be necessary. A substantial dose of prednisone should be given for acute contact dermatitis; low doses are not effective. The average sized adult patient should start with 60 mg each day in three divided doses until relief is produced, and continue for a total of 2 or 3 weeks, decreasing the dosage as the condition subsides. It should be kept in mind that systemic steroids will reduce the dermatitis only partially if the irritant or antigen remains in the environment. Secondary bacterial infection requires treatment with systemic antibiotics, such as erythromycin, 250 mg 4 times a day for a week. Currently available preparations for hyposensitization treatment of poison ivy, oak, or sumac cannot be recommended except in unusual situations (such as a very sensitive forestry worker) and in these situations referral to a dermatologist or allergist is appropriate.

OTHER CONTACTANTS

To be effective, therapy must include the identification and elimination of the irritant or allergen. If the contactant cannot be eliminated from the environment, protection while in the work place may suffice. For dermatitis of the hands, vinyl gloves, best worn with separate thin white cotton liners that can be removed and washed when needed, provide protection. Low grade exposure may be kept under control with topical corticosteroid ointments, such as triamcinolone 0.1% or fluocinonide (Lidex, Topsyn), while the source of antigen is being investigated.

In the case of jewelry (nickel) sensitivity the patient may still be able to use the jewelry provided that it is painted with a clear acrylic paint or colorless nail polish to prevent the metal from coming into contact with the skin.

When to Refer

After the dermatitis has subsided and suspicious irritants and antigens have been removed from the patient's environment, it is important to prove that the patient did have a specific allergy so that the substance can be avoided in the future. The relationship is proven with patch-tests. A kit to perform patch tests may be obtained from the American Academy of Dermatology, 820 Davis Street, Evanston, Illinois 60201. However, patch-testing is time-consuming and experience is needed to interpret the test results properly; therefore, patients are more appropriately referred to a dermatologist or allergist for this testing. In the case of a possible cosmetic contact dermatitis, extensive investigation may be necessary before the cause can be determined; it is estimated that the average woman applies 13 cosmetic products including deodorants and shampoos to herself each day and that Americans are exposed to 30,000 chemicals during the year.

GROIN DERMATITIS
General Considerations

Rashes in the groin are common and most are due to one of four causes: candidiasis, tinea infections, intertrigo, and erythrasma. Less common causes of groin dermatitis are contact dermatitis, psoriasis, and seborrheic dermatitis. Rarely Bowen's disease and extramammary Paget's disease, forms of squamous cell carcinomas, must be considered, particularly if the lesions do not respond to topical therapy. Because of the moist environment, dermatitides of the groin have some similarities in appearance regardless of cause. Most cases show erythema, scale, oozing (if severe), and manifest some degree of pruritus. Table 97.3 provides criteria for the diagnosis of the four major causes of groin dermatitis. The proper evaluation of groin dermatitis requires a KOH preparation and an inspection with use of a Wood's lamp; both are easily performed.

KOH PREPARATION

Scrape the edge of the lesion with a sterile No. 10 or 15 scalpel blade and transfer the scale to a microscope slide. If the blade is moistened with a drop of water the scales will adhere to it and this will make collection easier. Add a drop or two of 15% potassium hydroxide, apply a coverslip, and heat gently to dissolve epidermoid cells. KOH does not dissolve fungal hyphae. Boiling may "bubble" the scales off the slide and should be avoided. The preparation should be examined with the low powered ($\times$10) objective with the light turned low and the condenser racked down to increase contrast between hyphae and cell borders. Hyphae are thin, branching, double-walled filaments that can be distinguished from cell borders by their double-walled smooth appearance often several cell diameters long (Fig. 97.2). The high dry ($\times$40) objective can be used to confirm the observation.

WOOD'S LIGHT EXAMINATION

An inexpensive "black light" can be obtained from physician supply stores or hobby shops. The examining room must be completely dark and the light placed close to the patients skin since the light output usually is low. The physician should look for a coral-red or salmon colored fluorescence in erythrasma. The light also will be useful for examination of patients with tinea versicolor and vitiligo (see below).

Table 97.3
Diagnostic Criteria for Four Major Causes of Groin Dermatitis

	Moist	Sharp Border	Pustules at Edge	KOH[a]	Wood's light[a]	More Pain than Itch	More Itch than Pain
Candidiasis	Yes	No	Yes	+	−	Yes	
Tinea cruris	No	Yes	No	+	−		Yes
Intertrigo	Yes	No	Maybe	−	−	Yes	
Erythrasma	No	Yes	No	−	+		Yes

[a] See text for description.

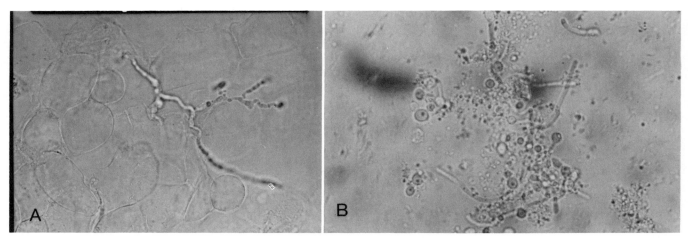

Figure 97.2 (*A*) Hyphae of tinea (KOH preparation, ×400). (*B*) Pseudohyphae of candida (KOH preparation, ×400; photograph (*B*) courtesy of William G. Merz, Ph.D.).

Candidiasis

DEFINITION

Candidiasis is a yeast infection almost always restricted to mucous surfaces and moist intertriginous areas of the skin (19).

THERAPY

For inflammation with oozing and discomfort, often associated with candidiasis, the patient should apply cool compresses of either saline (1 tsp salt/pint of water) or Burow's solution (1 tablet or packet/pint of water) for 20 min 3 times daily. Compresses are not soaks; compressing is done by immersing a soft cloth in the solution, wringing it out so that it is sodden but not dripping, and then applying the dressing to the dermatitic area. It should be left on for 5 min, removed, redipped, wrung out, and reapplied. The effect of the compress is to cool and gently to debride the area. The patient should, after compressing, thoroughly dry the area of dermatitis with a towel or fan and apply topical nystatin (Mycostatin) cream. If the area is moist, nystatin powder may be used instead. Alternatives to nystatin are miconazole cream (MicaTin) and clotrimazole cream (Lotrimin, Mycelex) twice a day. These alternatives have the advantage that, in contrast to nystatin, they also are active in tinea infections (*i.e.*, a true fungal infection as opposed to yeast infections) and may be used if there is uncertainty about the diagnosis.

In severe cases, where there is considerable oozing, the patient may layer zinc oxide paste (available without a prescription) thickly over the area at bedtime, to be removed with mineral oil-soaked cotton balls in the morning. Compresses usually are not needed for longer than 3 days. The antifungal agent, however will need to be continued for 2 weeks. Distinct improvement should be apparent within 7 days of initiating therapy.

EVALUATION AND THERAPY FOR RESISTANT CASES

A number of factors account for apparent clinical resistance and these need to be considered if there has been no improvement within 7 days of initiating therapy. Local factors, such as polyester clothing that encourage sweat retention and maintain the infection, should be modified. Loose, nonocclusive cotton clothes are preferred. Other skinfolds, such as the axilla, under the breasts, and about the neck and abdomen, should be examined for candidiasis. Candidiasis is likely to be present in the vagina and in the gut; organisms from these sites may be reinfecting the area (see Chapter 91). Reinfection is common and the sexual partner should be examined for the presence of candidiasis. A KOH smear to search for pseudohyphae and spores is more practical than culture as results are immediate and are not invalidated by overgrowth of contaminants (Fig 97.2*B*). Among the *Candida* species, only *Candida albicans* is a common pathogen, so that there is no advantage in subclassification.

In resistant cases in women, the physician should prescribe miconazole vaginal cream (Monostat 7), clotrimazole vaginal cream or tablets (Gyne-Lotrimin or Mycelex-G), or nystatin (Mycostatin) vaginal suppositories to be used daily for 2 weeks to control the vaginal candidiasis. Also for women with resistant cases, the gut may be the source of reinfection and a 5-day course of oral nystatin suspension (100,000 units/ml) at a dose of 5 ml (1 tsp) 4 times a day should be prescribed. Furthermore, diabetes mellitus predisposes patients to candidiasis; however, if diabetes mellitus is a true causal factor, glucosuria will be present.

Tinea Cruris

DEFINITION

Tinea cruris, as the name defines, is a fungal infection of the groin. Tinea cruris is common in males and rare in females and does not occur in childhood; it tends to recur during the summer months (19).

THERAPY

A topical antifungal agent such as miconazole cream (MicaTin), haloprogin cream (Halotex), or clotrimazole cream (Lotrimin, Mycelex) should be applied to the rash sparingly twice a day for 3 weeks. The patient should try to decrease moisture in the area of the rash by using plain talc (such as Johnson's Baby Powder) and cotton underwear. If acute with oozing and discomfort, compresses for 2 or 3 days (see above) followed by the short term application (e.g., 1 week) of a topical corticosteroid (such as triamcinolone cream 0.1%) may be necessary before topical antifungal medications are begun.

If the lesions are extensive or involve other parts of the body as well, oral griseofulvin-UF (generic by prescription), 250 mg 3 times daily for 30 days with food should be given. On occasion, griseofulvin may be the initial therapy with topical antifungal agents used to maintain the clearing. Griseofulvin generally is devoid of serious side effects; headaches and gastrointestinal distress develop when high doses are used and, rarely, photosensitivity can occur. Griseofulvin can reduce the effects of anticoagulants by increasing the rate of liver metabolism.

Intertrigo

DEFINITION

Intertrigo is a moist, brightly erythematous and irritating dermatitis occurring in occluded body folds, generally in obese individuals. Excessive moisture, heat, and maceration produce conditions conducive to superficial infection with mixed bacterial flora.

THERAPY

Therapy is directed at reducing heat and maceration by wearing light absorbent clothing (i.e., cotton rather than polyester), by frequent drying of the skin, and by the frequent use of plain talc (such as Johnson's Baby Powder). Cornstarch, which may encourage fungal and bacterial growth, should be avoided. Following the drying measures, a corticosteroid containing cream (such as Vioform-Hydrocortisone cream) should be applied 3 times daily. Vioform is mildly antibacterial and antifungal. The patient should be warned that Vioform may permanently stain white clothing slightly yellow. Plain talc should be used over the cream during the day and a thick layer of zinc oxide paste can be applied at bedtime, as with candidiasis, to absorb moisture. Improvement should be evident within a few days.

Treatment of obesity is important to prevent recurrences (see Chapter 22).

Erythrasma

DEFINITION

Erythrasma is a dry, slightly scaly, mildly inflammatory dermatitis limited to the intertriginous areas and can easily be mistaken for tinea infection (13). Moisture and maceration are frequent underlying conditions. It is due to an infection by a bacteria, *Corynebacterium minutissimum*. The bacteria produce porphyrins which fluoresce a salmon-red color when exposed to a Wood's light (see above).

THERAPY

Treatment with erythromycin, 250 mg 3 times daily for 2 weeks or with 2% erythromycin topically for 2 weeks generally is successful. Recurrences are frequent; there is no effective method of avoidance but the disease generally is not passed between family members.

HAIR

The medical advantage of hair seems so slight that the physician, particularly the nonbalding one, may not share the concern of the patient when problems develop. Yet the social and sexual impact of hair is so great that the mention of hair loss should be received sympathetically and informed advice provided. Hair density varies substantially among individuals so that the patient's estimate of hair loss should be taken seriously and recorded. A substantial amount of hair, perhaps 20%, can be lost before the person notices the change; about 50% of the hair is lost before others notice thinning as well.

Pathophysiology

To understand hair problems better, a brief review of the physiology of hair growth is necessary. The change from immature vellus hair of children to the coarse dark terminal hair of adults is under androgenic control, but is modified by genetic factors. Sebaceous glands are almost always associated with hair follicles, the two are referred to as a pilosebaceous unit. Thick hairs such as in the scalp are associated with large sebaceous glands.

Hair growth in man is cyclical, not continuous. The period of active growth is called anagen and the resting phase, telogen. Growing and resting hairs are intermingled and not synchronized so that, unlike molting in animals, no obvious thickening and thinning cycle occurs. At any one time about 80% of the scalp hairs are in anagen and 20% are in telogen. Once hairs have entered telogen they do not restart their growth. Instead, as the hair follicle reenters the growing phase, a new hair forms below the resting hair and eventually the resting hair is pushed up and out and is shed (much like the shedding of primary teeth). It takes about 3 months for hair to enter the resting phase and be shed by newly formed hair from below. Shedding is quite normal and involves 25 to 100 hairs every day. A very high level of metabolic activity is maintained in anagen hair follicles: About 1 cm of hair emerges every month from a follicle that is no thicker than this page.

Patterns of Hair Loss

The physician must first decide whether the hair loss is diffuse or patchy (thinned in regions). For example, the usual male pattern balding is patchy. The second important observation which will be useful in the classification of alopecia is the appearance of the scalp (11).

DIFFUSE ALOPECIA WITH NORMAL APPEARING SCALP

It is important to determine whether the hair loss has been recent (weeks or months). If so, the cause was usually a precipitating event that took place within 3 months of the time hair began to fall out. Patchy alopecia is not caused by such events. Events which cause hair loss include the use of many drugs (most frequently oral contraceptives, see below), pregnancy or traumatic events such as surgery, crash diets, severe accidents, a high fever, or severe illness. Hair follicles are susceptible to conversion from anagen to telogen from such events and, when the hair follicle restarts its growth, the resting telogen hairs are shed.

This hair loss is not seen at the time of the reversion from anagen to telogen but rather when growth resumes, generally 1 to 3 months later. This type of hair loss is called *telogen effluvium*. The hair eventually returns to its previous appearance. However, occasionally the thinned hair is not restored. In such individuals, mostly women, the hair loss apparently triggers a form of balding, female pattern baldness, that would have been delayed until a later age. Female pattern baldness is no more reversible than is male pattern baldness.

Drug-induced Hair Loss. Hair thinning has been associated with numerous medications; the mechanism generally is that of telogen effluvium with excessive conversion of anagen hair follicles into telogen. Thinning of hair on the scalp is noticed anytime between about 3 months after beginning the drug and about 3 months after stopping it. Besides oral contraceptive preparations, other medications that may produce this effect include heparin, coumarin, high dose vitamin A, allopurinol, amphetamines, iodine, thiouracil, and trimethadione.

Cytotoxic medications cause another type of hair thinning which is usually quite dramatic. The cytotoxic drugs have their greatest effect on rapidly growing cells; therefore, the disturbance is in the anagen rather than in the telogen follicle. It is easy to understand why the hair loss is dramatic—80% of hairs are in anagen and all of these may be damaged simultaneously. The result is a hair fall that is sudden and extensive. Fortunately, hair almost always regrows normally when treatment is concluded; in some patients hair grows back more profusely and darker than it was. The hair loss can be reduced in some instances by temporary reduction of the circulation to the scalp with a tight tourniquet about the head or cooling the scalp with icebags. This is practical only if perfusion of the scalp is not necessary for therapy and when the drug is given intravenously and has a short half-life in the circulation.

General debility due to many severe endocrine, nutritional, or systemic disorders also can lead to hair loss, developing gradually over weeks, months, or even years. The scalp usually does not appear abnormal or inflamed. If caused by a general medical disorder, the hair loss is usually a minor sign with the medical problem overwhelming the picture. However, either hypo- or hyperthyroidism and iron deficiency anemia may present as hair loss without obvious signs or symptoms; both should be ruled out by appropriate laboratory tests (see Chapters 46 and 70).

Intrinsic Hair Shaft Disorders. Additional causes of diffuse hair loss, usually developing over months or years, are intrinsic disorders of the hair shaft. These disorders can be congenital, with scalp hair never having grown normally, or more commonly, are acquired. Acquired forms are usually due to trauma, such as harsh chemicals or excessive brushing. The diagnosis may be evident on low power (×10) microscopic examination of the hair shaft. This usually requires some experience. The most common intrinsic hair shaft weakness developing in adulthood is trichorrhexis nodosa. In this disorder, the hair grows at a normal rate but breaks easily due to the development of clumps or nodes along the hair shaft, appearing as bristles under the microscope.

DIFFUSE ALOPECIA WITH INFLAMED AND/OR SCALY SCALP

The most common dermatitic conditions of the scalp are psoriasis and seborrheic dermatitis, but these, by themselves, do not cause hair thinning. However, trauma from intense scratching or harsh "treatment" may break the hair and produce temporary and partial alopecia. Psoriasis tends to be restricted to the scalp, up to the margins, like a helmet, while seborrheic dermatitis tends to extend over the ears, forehead, and central part of the face. Seborrheic dermatitis and psoriasis of the scalp are best diagnosed by finding the condition elsewhere on the body (see pp. 1056 and 1059). Psoriasis may be limited to the scalp and in those cases the diagnosis is more difficult. Dermatologists distinguish between dandruff and seborrheic dermatitis; dandruff has scale and mild itching but lacks the inflamed and erythematous component of seborrheic dermatitis.

Treatment. The physician should follow the treatment outlined for psoriasis and seborrheic dermatitis of the scalp. If unresponsive after 1 month of care, the patient should be referred to a dermatologist.

PATCHY ALOPECIA WITH A NORMAL APPEARING SCALP

The usual cause is *alopecia areata*, particularly if the patches appeared during the previous few days or weeks or have been recurrent. The patches of hair loss in alopecia areata tend to be sharply demarcated from the surrounding normal scalp and are nearly or entirely devoid of hair. The patches may be single or multiple. A striking feature is the lack of inflammation; the scalp is not reddened or scaly. A history of severe emotional or physical trauma preceding the hair loss is common but the underlying cause of alopecia areata is not known. Currently, the suspicion is that the fault is immunologic since antiepithelial and antithyroid antibodies have been found in many of the cases studied. Trichotillomania, compulsive hair pulling, is an important diagnostic alternative but patches in this disorder are not completely bald; apparently the patient cannot pull the hair out until it regrows long enough to grab again.

Spontaneous resolution of alopecia areata is the rule. Most cases will have regrowth of all hair within several months and almost all will resolve within 2 years. Alopecia areata does not cause scarring and the potential for hair regrowth always remains. Unfortunately, one-third of the patients will have recurrences. A severe course with recurrences is more likely if the patches appear at the nuchal hair line and are multiple or if they began appearing in childhood.

Treatment. Moderate tugging of the hair at the margins of the patch with the fingertips is a useful test of activity of the process. If the hairs come out easily, the process is still active and the patch is going to continue to expand. Topical or intralesional corticosteroids may slow or reverse progression. High potency topical steroids such as those used for acne keloid (see below) may be gently rubbed into the bald patch 3 times a day. Absorption can be increased by asking the patient to wear a plastic shower cap to bed. If hair does not appear in 1 month, intradermal injections of long acting repository corticosteroids, such as triamcinolone acetonide 10 mg/ml (Kenalog-10), may be tried. Excessive concentrations of intradermal steroids can produce local atrophy. To prevent this, the physician should dilute the 10 mg/ml triamcinolone to 4 mg/ml by mixing 0.4 ml Kenalog-10 with 0.6 ml sterile physiologic saline in a tuberculin syringe and injecting 0.05 to 0.1 ml into sites about 1 cm apart with a 25 gauge needle. No more than 1 to 2 ml should be injected at each visit. Monthly repeated injections may be needed. In most cases, hair regrowth will be stimulated at the injection sites although several weeks will pass before new hair growth becomes visible. The newly appearing hair often is light in color but it will eventually darken to the patient's normal hair color. The hair produced by the injections usually is retained.

When to Refer. Referral to confirm the diagnosis and to outline therapy often is warranted. For severe cases, systemic steroids may be needed but new hairs often are shed when the steroids are discontinued. Newer therapies, including primary sensitization to

antigens followed by repeated challenges at the bald sites, appear beneficial in some cases and are being investigated.

PATCHY ALOPECIA WITH SORE, INFLAMED, SCALY AND/OR LUMPY SCALP

This is most often caused by an infection, either fungal or bacterial.

Fungal Infection

Preadolescents with an infection of the scalp most frequently have a fungal ("ringworm") infection, due to either *Microsporum* or *Trichophyton* species. Infections of scalp hair due to *Microsporum* species are not usually inflammatory or symptomatic and show a typical apple green fluorescence when viewed with a Wood's lamp. However, infections due to trichophyton infections are becoming increasingly common. Here, inflammation often is severe with pustulation and discomfort. If the inflammation becomes sufficiently severe, a boggy swelling, a kerion, will develop which can lead to scarring of hair follicles and permanent hair loss. To diagnose either, several hairs should be plucked, allowed to soak for 15 min in a drop of KOH on a microscope slide, and examined with the high dry objective to look for spores and hyphae in and on the hair shaft. Hair also should be submitted for fungal culture. The physician should submit hair or scale in a sterile tube without medium; fungi withstand transport well and the laboratory personnel can choose appropriate media depending upon the site and clinical diagnosis.

Treatment. If it seems likely that a fungal infection is present, ultrafine griseofulvin (generic by prescription) should be started, generally before cultures have been identified, which may take weeks, at the dose of 500 mg twice daily for adults. The drug is best absorbed when taken with food. It is best to treat *Microsporum* species for 3 weeks and *Trichophyton* species for 6 weeks and then to continue griseofulvin in both for 4 additional weeks after apparent cure.

Bacterial Infection

The scalp is generally resistant to bacterial infection because of its rich blood supply; but, pyodermas, with pustules and bogginess of the scalp and with discomfort and adenopathy, can develop, usually secondary to an underlying dermatitis. It is important to look carefully for live larvae and nits of *Pediculus humanus* var. *capitis*, sometimes difficult to find if bacterial suprainfection has overshadowed the evidence of infestation. The characteristic findings of infestation are pinhead-sized, firmly attached egg cases on the hair shaft (Fig. 97.3) and these can be confirmed as nits under the low powered objective. As the eggs are deposited at scalp level and as hair grows at the rate of about 1 cm per month, an estimate of the length of time since infection can be made by

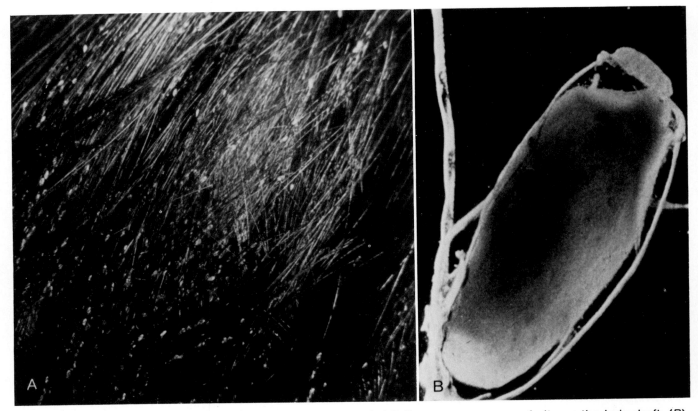

Figure 97.3 *Pediculus humanus var. capitis* (head louse). (*A*) Gross appearance of nits on the hair shaft. (*B*) Microscopic appearance (×100; photograph (*B*) courtesy of Reed & Carnrick, Kenilworth, N.J.).

measuring the length of hair between the nits and the scalp.

Treatment. As for other cutaneous pyodermas, erythromycin, 250 mg 4 times a day for a week, usually is sufficient. It is best to obtain a culture at the time the erythromycin is begun so that an alternative, such as dicloxacillin, can be chosen if sensitivity is confirmed and if the scalp pyoderma proves unresponsive to erythromycin. The scalp should be cleansed by shampooing with a mild soap (such as Johnson's Baby Shampoo) up to 4 times a day. Pediculosis should be treated with Kwell Shampoo, leaving the shampoo on for 5 min, and then combing out the nits with a fine toothed comb (see below). The shampoo treatment should be repeated 4 days later.

Acne Keloid

Acne keloid resembles a bacterial infection of the scalp with pustules and abscesses scattered among firm papules. Permanent hair loss can result from the scarring that develops. The condition usually is limited to the occipital part of the scalp and the back of the neck and is seen primarily in black males. It is a granulomatous and inflammatory foreign body reaction due to disordered and incurving ingrown hairs, perhaps first induced by barber clipping.

Treatment. Therapy tends to be disappointing. However, partial relief may be achieved by long courses of systemic antibiotics, such as tetracycline

or erythromycin 250 mg 3 times a day for 2 months; or topical high potency corticosteroids such as triamcinolone cream 0.5% (Kenalog-HP), betamethasone cream (Valisone), or fluocinonide cream (Lidex, Topsyn). Intradermal injections of long acting steroids, such as triamcinolone acetonide (Kenalog-10) diluted to 4 mg/ml with physiologic saline (see above), may be tried next if a satisfactory response has not been achieved. The physician may inject up to 1 ml in 0.1-ml amounts intradermally and sublesionally using a tuberculin syringe with a 25 gauge needle. The patient usually gets relief which may last 1 or 2 months from this treatment. If treatment response is inadequate, referral to a dermatologist is appropriate. In resistant severe cases, epilation with X-ray may be tried which often gives relief that persists when the hair regrows.

PATCHY ALOPECIA WITH LUMPS AND WITHOUT DERMATITIS

In this instance the hair loss is restricted to the scalp over the lumps. Nodules or tumors, benign or malignant, may lead to hair loss from either excessive underlying pressure or from infiltration of hair-bearing skin by tumor.

Epidermal Inclusion Cysts

General Considerations. Epidermal inclusion cysts are the most common underlying lesion. Patients often have signs of severe acne, past or present, as well. These cysts are firm to soft and usually are painless. The scalp surface appears normal without erythema or scale, but the hair is thinned or absent.

Treatment. Surgical removal is not necessary unless there is discomfort or hair loss. A nonsurgical approach that often succeeds is an injection, into and just below the sac, of 0.5 ml full strength triamcinolone acetonide 10 mg/ml (Kenalog-10) with a tuberculin syringe and 25 gauge needle. A month may elapse before the cyst flattens or disappears. If the scalp lump is hard or has appeared suddenly, a biopsy should be obtained to rule out malignancy.

PATCHY "PATTERN" ALOPECIA PROGRESSIVE OVER YEARS WITHOUT DERMATITIS

The normal rate of hair growth may slow and then stop in many or all of the follicles due to the aging process. It follows a rate and distribution that we have come to regard as typical. This thinning and baldness accompanying aging is called *pattern baldness.* It is the most common cause of alopecia. If plugs of scalp containing viable hairs are transplanted into bald regions of the scalp, the newly planted hairs will follow the intrinsic growth pattern of the area the plugs came from rather than the bald area to which the plugs are placed. The hair follicles seem to have an intrinsic "clock." Underlying scalp vasculature has nothing to do with this clock; scalp massage has nothing to do with decreasing baldness. Only the absence of hormones before puberty prevents the clock from being set, as in the case of male eunuchs castrated before puberty who never become bald. Graying of the hair also is dependent on this "clock," which, like balding, is modified by family inheritance patterns. The cause of graying is unknown.

The onset and rate of thinning varies with each individual due to complex genetic factors. It is often not appreciated that women as well as men develop thinning. The pattern in most women who develop thinning is not that seen in men but rather a diffuse thinning over the crown. It is obvious that the balding process starts earlier in men than in women.

Treatment. There is no medical treatment for balding. No product sold to cure or treat balding is of any benefit and some may do harm. However, it is important to treat any inflammatory scalp conditions (see below, "Psoriasis" and "Seborrheic Dermatitis").

The portion of the scalp at the back of the head is likely to retain hair into very old age. Surgical procedures that involve the transplantation of plugs or strips of hair from that region to bald areas do work and are of value; however, hundreds of plugs may be needed for good coverage and many months may be necessary for placement; the process is painful and expensive. The physician should advise against implantation of artificial hair into the scalp; the technique simply does not work; the fibers act like foreign bodies and their rejection is accompanied with infection and pain. It is particularly important to convey to patients the utter waste of money spent on hair growth products. The FDA may restrict all advertising of such products as none have been shown to be of any value. Most men learn to accept their appearance but, for those sufficiently motivated, referral to a dermatologic surgeon or plastic surgeon may be justified for consideration of hair transplants.

HERPES SIMPLEX

General Considerations

Herpex simplex, caused by *Herpesvirus hominis* is of two subtypes. One type appears in extragenital sites and is caused by type 1 virus, while the type 2 strain causes most genital herpes infections. The initial or primary herpes simplex infection, due to type 1, usually occurs in childhood, while type 2 is spread by sexual contact, with most primary infections involving persons beyond the age of puberty. On occasion, type 1 virus will be found to be the cause of genital herpes and type 2 of the extragenital case; this reversed situation usually is the result of sexual activities.

After primary infection, the virus remains latent within regional nerve root ganglia. Patients who suffer recurrent blisters do so because of periodic reactivation of the virus which reaches the skin via nerve fibers and replicates.

Presentation

Cutaneous herpes simplex infection in the adult most commonly presents as a localized group of pinhead- to rice grain-sized blisters usually recurring at intervals and at the same site.

Primary infection, particularly type 1, usually is associated with severe systemic symptoms including fever, malaise, and localized tender adenopathy. The primary infection resolves in 1 to 3 weeks without a scar. Primary herpes simplex infections of neonates is serious and may be fatal; therefore, a pregnant woman with active vaginal or vulvar herpes should be delivered by cesarean section. Primary ophthalmic herpes simplex may lead to corneal ulcerations, scarring, and blindness. Such lesions are quite painful. Patients should be directly referred to an ophthalmologist for diagnosis and therapy.

Patients with atopic dermatitis may develop a generalized herpes infection, eczema herpeticum, with the worst lesions in the areas of preexisting dermatitis. Patients who are immunosuppressed, either due to an inherent disorder or acquired due to malignancy or drug therapy, may become seriously ill from herpes simplex and fatalities may occur.

More frequent and quite troublesome are recurrent lesions, particularly if recurrences are frequent. Recurrent lesions usually are preceded by several hours to a day of a prodrome consisting of local burning or tingling. This is followed by the appearance of multiple small vesicles appearing at or near the site of previous episodes. The most common location for type 1 recurrences is about the mouth and is the usual cause of the "cold sore." The genitals and buttocks are the sites where type 2 infections appear.

The episode lasts 3 to 7 days and may recur almost immediately or not for a year or more. However, recurrence every month to every few months is more typical. Eventually the tendency for recurrence diminishes. The lesions are not scarring. Recurrences are more likely to develop following febrile episodes, systemic illness, or local trauma such as sunburn or intercourse (9).

The diagnosis of a herpes infection can be confirmed with a Tzanck smear, or the finding of rising levels of viral antibodies, or a positive viral culture, if the latter two specialized techniques are available.

TZANCK (CYTOLOGY) SMEAR

The purpose of a Tzanck smear is to identify multinucleated giant cells and intranuclear inclusion bodies in cells obtained from the base of the blister. For the smear to be reliable, an early intact blister must be examined. The technique involves removing the blister roof with a scalpel or scissors and gently scraping the floor of the vesicle with a No. 10 or No. 15 blade to obtain cells. The examiner should make a thin smear on a glass slide, immerse the slide in methanol or 95% ethanol for 1 min, air dry, and stain with Wright's or Giemsa as for blood smears. Blisters due to herpes simplex, herpes zoster, and varicella show identical abnormal cells and inclusions (Fig. 97.4).

Differential Diagnosis

Primary herpes simplex, particularly in an unusual location, may be misdiagnosed as cellulitis or acute contact dermatitis. A common example is the her-

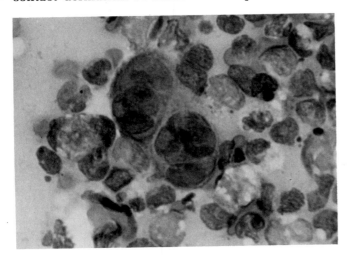

Figure 97.4 Tzanck smear: Gentle scraping from the base of a vesicle and stained with Wright's or Giemsa stain. Multinucleated cells from herpes simplex are shown (×400).

petic whitlow, a herpes infection of the fingertip sometimes acquired by a nurse while providing mouth care to a patient. As herpes type 2 generally is acquired through sexual contact, other venereal diseases may have been transmitted at the same time and should be considered. A urethral or vaginal smear and culture for gonorrhea and a serological test for syphilis (STS) at the initial examination, with the latter repeated 2 months later, is advisable.

The grouped vesicles seen in recurrent herpes zoster closely resemble those of herpes simplex, but the two conditions can usually be distinguished by the tendency for herpes zoster to involve a more extensive area following a dermatomal distribution. Zoster is only rarely recurrent so that the history of repeated episodes of blisters, particularly if they are at the same site, also strongly favors a diagnosis of herpes simplex. The Tzanck smear will be useful to rule out other blistering disorders including impetigo, erythema multiforme, and pemphigus.

Erythema multiforme, an acute blistering eruption with target-like lesions and mucosal erosions, appears to be a hypersensitivity reaction and may resemble herpes simplex, particularly as patients frequently give a history of an antecedent "cold sore." Erythema multiforme often follows herpes simplex infections although it also follows drug and bacterial or nonsimplex viral exposure (see also Chapter 98).

Therapy

Therapy of the primary infection is aimed at relieving the discomfort by using analgesia, both systemic, with salicylates or mild opiates, and topical (Dyclone, Xylocaine), especially if mucosal surfaces are involved. The area should be kept cleansed and, if the lesions are extensive, the patient should be supported by hospitalization for fluid replacement if necessary.

Some patients seem to have a decrease in the severity and length of an episode from topical idoxuridine solution (Herplex, Stoxil), an analog of thymidine available as an ophthalmic solution by prescription. A drop should be applied to the site hourly during the first 12 hours of a prodrome. There is no apparent beneficial effect after vesicles have appeared.

Acyclovir ointment (Zovirax, 15 g, by prescription) was approved in 1982 for use in patients with genital herpes or in immunocompromised patients. It may prove useful for recurrent herpes as well. The drug decreases pain and viral shedding and speeds healing. It is used every 3 to 4 hours during the day for up to 7 days.

Corticosteroids applied to the skin may decrease inflammation after vesicles have developed. Any full strength cream, such as triamcinolone 0.1%, may be used, 4 times a day, but the periorbital region should be avoided to prevent steroids from entering the eye. Secondary bacterial infection of herpes lesions is not common and lesions heal at the same rate whether antibiotics are used or not.

The contagious nature of the infection must be stressed. Herpes simplex can be transmitted from either primary or recurrent lesions. Crusts as well as blister fluid contain infectious virus.

HERPES ZOSTER (SHINGLES)

General Considerations

Two weeks following primary infection with zoster-varicella virus, clinical lesions of chicken pox appear and, in most patients, clear without complication during the next 2 weeks. However, in many or perhaps all individuals who have had chicken pox, the virus continues to reside in a latent state within dorsal root or cranial nerve ganglia. Latent virus does not replicate and can only be identified with specialized culture or antibody techniques. The clinical signs of zoster are due to the reactivation of the virus and its emanation from the ganglia to peripheral nerve endings.

Zoster is more likely to appear when mechanisms limiting reactivation of the virus are blunted. Conditions associated with reactivation include old age, acute systemic illness, injuries to or neoplasia of cranial nerves or the spinal column, and disorders associated with diminished immunocompetency, including lymphoma-leukemia and immunosuppressive therapy. In support of the premise that reactivation of virus rather than new infection is the cause of zoster, epidemiologic studies have shown that patients with zoster have not been exposed to recent active cases of chicken pox and do not have an increased likelihood of acquiring zoster during epidemics of chicken pox.

Presentation

A prodrome of 1 to 4 days, but occasionally up to 10, is characterized by tingling, tenderness, or itch restricted to the nerve segment involved. Patients with a severe prodrome may present with acute chest or abdominal pain or acute sciatica or joint pain. Cutaneous tenderness can be demonstrated by finding increased unilateral sensitivity to pinprick.

Very occasionally, zoster manifests only with localized pain, in which case establishing the diagnosis requires the demonstration of a rising antibody titer. Usually, however, there is a typical skin lesion; a patch of grouped vesicles on an erythematous base, each vesicle having a central dell. The eruption is almost always strikingly demarcated at the midline. However, the earliest lesions will present closest to the ganglia and the dermatomal distribution may not be obvious. Before lesions are visible, hypesthesia, dysesthesia, or more commonly hyperesthesia will be evident in the dermatome so that a sensory neurologic examination of the area may provide early confirmation of the diagnosis. A Tzanck test may be performed (see above for technique) to confirm the presence of multinucleated giant cells and intranuclear inclusions. Like herpes simplex and varicella,

zoster can present a serious danger to immunosuppressed patients who may get severe clinical chicken pox and pneumonia; patients with zoster must be isolated.

Differential Diagnosis

Difficulties with diagnosis are more likely in the early stages before the blistering becomes evident. Patients may be considered to have cellulitis, contact dermatitis, neuralgia, arthritis, or a chest or abdominal disorder. Herpes simplex may present in a linear pattern but will cause less local discomfort and dysesthesia than zoster.

A history and physical examination should be performed in patients with herpes zoster and, if there is any suspicion of an underlying malignancy, further workup including at least a blood count and differential and an X-ray of the involved spinal column segment should be made.

Therapy

As there is no specific anti-zoster-varicella drug, treatment is symptomatic. The pain may be excruciating and often requires mild opiates such as codeine at the dose of 30 to 60 mg every 3 or 4 hours as well as night time sedation such as with diphenhydramine (Benadryl), 50 to 100 mg. A thick coat of zinc oxide paste or ointment (available without prescription) reduces the tendency of serum from the denuded blisters from sticking to clothing and decreases discomfort by providing an air-tissue barrier. The zinc oxide may be removed with cotton balls moistened with mineral oil and reapplied morning and bed time.

Controlled studies support the use of systemic corticosteroids during the acute phase for the subsequent reduction of postherpetic neuralgia, a severe and peristent pain in the involved nerve root and dermatome that may continue for years, particularly common and severe in the elderly (7). The mechanism of the pain probably is fibrosis and scarring of the nerve, a complication that may be reduced by corticosteroids. The steroids should be started during the acute phase, but administration may safely be delayed until new blisters are no longer appearing. The dose is 60 mg of prednisone in a single morning dose daily for 1 week, 30 mg daily for the second week, and 15 mg for the third. Corticosteroids should not be used if there is an overriding medical contraindication such as bacterial infection, tuberculosis, or active peptic ulceration.

If the eye is involved, urgent ophthalmologic consultation is necessary. High risk patients, such as those with leukemia-lymphoma or who are immunosuppressed, and who have had an exposure to varicella or zoster within the previous 72 hours, should receive zoster-immune globulin (ZIG), obtainable from local state health departments or the Communicable Disease Center, Atlanta, Georgia.

PITYRIASIS ROSEA

Pityriasis rosea (PR) is common, particularly during ages 15 to 35. Although the cause is not known, PR acts like an infectious disease with seasonal increases and mini-epidemics (4). Efforts to isolate an agent have been unsuccessful. There is no specific histopathology or diagnostic test.

Presentation

The initial lesion, the "herald patch," is a 2- to 6-cm round scaly plaque that, in about half the patients, appears on the trunk. Several days later, 1- to 2-cm, pale, red, round-to-oval macular and papular scaly lesions appear on the trunk and proximal parts of the extremities, forming a fern-like pattern (Fig. 97.5). New lesions develop on more distal parts, while others clear centrally. The face is involved infrequently and less often in whites than in blacks. The eruption usually is pruritic and, at times, intensely so, but it may be asymptomatic. PR runs its course in 6 to 8 weeks.

The eruption mimics secondary syphilis; an STS should be obtained in all sexually active patients suspected of having PR. The STS is always positive in secondary syphilis.

Therapy

If the lesions are not itchy, no treatment is needed. It is important, however, for the physician to explain the disease and describe the anticipated course. If pruritus is mild, diphenhydramine (Benadryl) 25 to

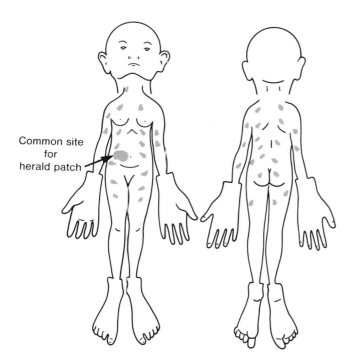

Common site for herald patch

Figure 97.5   Pityriasis rosea typically starts with a "herald patch" followed by oval patches in a fern-like pattern.

50 mg 3 times a day and a topical antipruritic suspension, such as calamine lotion with menthol or phenol added, may be prescribed.

Occasionally, pruritus is so severe that the patient cannot work or sleep. In that case, prednisone may be necessary to control the symptoms. The physician should prescribe 40 mg daily in four divided doses until the patient is comfortable, usually a few days, then taper the prednisone over a 3-week period by prescribing one pill less every third day. The patient does not require isolation and may attend school or work.

PSORIASIS

This genetic and usually lifelong disease affects 1 to 3% of the population. Psoriasis may first appear in childhood, especially in those instances that prove to be severe, but usually psoriasis begins during the 20s. In most instances, it remains throughout adulthood, improving in the summer and during pregnancies and becoming worse with emotional and physical stress. The disease affects males and females equally. Most patients have only mild pruritus but the scaly patches are unsightly and often interfere with work, social relationships, and self-image.

Certain histocompatibility antigens (HLA) are associated with the disorder, supporting the theory that psoriasis is inherited, but the underlying cause of psoriasis still is unknown. Vastly increased epidermal proliferation explains the histologic alterations of elongation of epidermal ridges and increased numbers of mitotic cells; epidermal turnover rates may be increased up to 10-fold over normal. This epidermal proliferation is reflected clinically as overproduction of scale, the characteristic sign of the disease.

Presentation

The typical lesion is an erythematous, circumscribed plaque covered by loosely adherent, silvery scales appearing most often on the elbows, knees, and scalp; the external genitalia and the region over the coccyx frequently are involved as well (Fig. 97.6). Peeling of the scale often produces minute bleeding points that reflect the proximity of underlying dilated capillaries. These dilated capillaries, rather than inflammation, are the cause of the plaque's redness. Nails may show pitting (Fig. 97.7) or, when more severely involved, a large volume of subungual keratotic debris leading to separation of the nail from the nail bed.

The diagnosis is not always obvious; the patient may present with severe "dandruff," with nail dystrophy, an apparent drug eruption, or arthritis and a rash. Seborrheic dermatitis (see below), fungal infection (see above), a psoriasiform drug eruption, or even a contact dermatitis to the therapy being used to treat the psoriasis must be considered.

Severe types of psoriasis are exfoliative with generalized erythema, scale, and shivering; and pustular

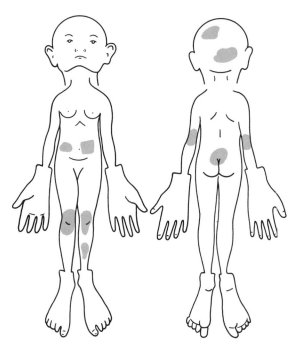

Figure 97.6   Psoriasis tends to be found on extensor surfaces and areas of repeated trauma, such as the waistline.

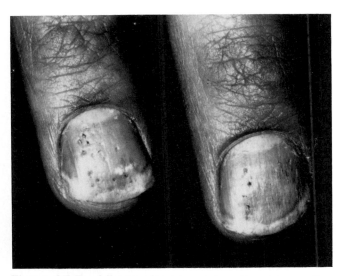

Figure 97.7   Minute pits are commonly seen on the surface of nails in patients with psoriasis.

with toxicity, fever, and denuded areas. These situations usually require hospitalization. Arthritis, typically involving the terminal interphalangeal joints and sacroiliac joints, may be associated with psoriasis, particularly if the patient does not demonstrate a positive rheumatoid factor.

Therapy

SKIN

Because fluorinated corticosteroids applied topically are clean, odorless, and rapidly suppress scale and pruritus, they are the first step in the topical therapy of psoriasis (5). However, topical steroids do not produce complete remissions; within a few days of discontinuing the medication, psoriasis returns to its pretreatment appearance.

Steroid ointments are preferred to creams for scaly chronic skin disorders; ointments are better absorbed and are less drying than creams or lotions. It is important to keep in mind the area to be treated and frequency of application; topical steroids are expensive (see example under "Atopic Dermatitis"). Ointments should be applied sparingly 2 or 3 times a day.

The effectiveness of topical steroids can be increased by applying them at bedtime and then wrapping the area with any kitchen plastic wrap (Glad, Saran, etc.). When applied this way, only the cream should be used; the occluded ointment may lead to folliculitis. The wrap should be held in place with socks, hose, an undershirt, etc., rather than tape, which may be irritating. Occlusion increases absorption and therapeutic effect so that daytime application may no longer be necessary.

Long term relief for psoriasis of the glabrous skin often can be achieved through the addition of tar preparations including Alphosyl, Estar Tar Gel, or Psorigel—all of which are available without prescription. All of these have a slight tar odor and tint, they should be applied sparingly, only to the patch, and generally only at bedtime. If steroids with occlusion by wrapping are being used at bedtime (see above), the two therapies can be used on alternate nights.

Further benefits may result from the use at home of ultraviolet light. The patient should choose a floor model (if the unit is too small the patient will become frustrated by the long time that the therapy requires) with a timer (an absolute necessity) and can expect to pay approximately $100. The patient should follow the instructions with the unit to determine the initial exposure as this time will vary among models. Treatments should be every other day, with increasing exposure each time until slight redness is still visible 24 hours after the UV light exposure. The patient can increase the dose when the persistent erythema no longer develops. Tanning will deepen after several weeks of UV light. The morning following the nighttime application of a tar preparation is the best time to use UV light, but the tar appears to be effective if left on for as short a time as 2 hours prior to the light. The psoriasis-suppressing effect of natural sunlight appears to be more effective than artificial UV light and should be utilized when it is available. Little evidence for late skin cancers has ever appeared in psoriatics exposed to UV light and tars.

SCALP

The patient should shampoo daily or as desired. Frequent shampooing may be all that is needed in mild cases. Although a number of shampoos containing tars (Ionil T, Sebutone, Zetar), selenium sulfate

(Exsel, Iosel, Selsun), and zinc compounds (Danex, Head and Shoulders, Zincon) often are prescribed, very little medication will be left on the scalp after shampooing, so that medicated shampoos alone will help only those patients with minimal involvement.

If shampooing is not sufficient, the physician may prescribe a topical steroid solution or lotion (Diprosone lotion, Valisone lotion, Synalar solution) rubbed into the scaly plaques with the fingertips immediately following shampooing and while the scalp is still moist. Ointments and creams are difficult to use in hairy parts. If scales are too thick to be loosened by shampoos alone, the patient may apply phenol/saline lotion (Baker's P&S liquid, available without prescription) to the scalp at bedtime before the morning shampooing. A stronger, but messier, preparation is a mixture of sulfur, salicylic acid, and tar (Pragmatar cream, available without prescription), which may be used if the phenol/saline lotion does not produce resolution of the thick scale within a month of use. Both preparations are used in the same way. Wearing a showercap at night may be advised to protect bed linens.

NAILS

No consistently effective and easy treatment exists. On occasion, dermatologists inject nailfolds with steroids, but the treatment is painful and relief is temporary.

When to Refer

It usually is beneficial to refer patients with extensive psoriasis, and cases not satisfactorily controlled with simple topical therapies, to a dermatologist. Other therapies considered effective include psoralen with long wave ultraviolet light (PUVA) and systemic antimetabolites (methotrexate, hydroxyurea). Patients with very extensive psoriasis may need to be hospitalized for tar and UV light treatment, the Goeckerman regimen.

SCABIES

Presentation

Scabies is an infestation caused by a mite, *Sarcoptes scabiei* var. *hominis*. Scabies seems to run in cycles; there has been a dramatic upswing in cases since the 1970s. Most of the signs and symptoms of scabies are due to sensitization to the mite and mite products rather than to the physical effects of the mite itself. Hence, there is delayed appearance of the rash until approximately 14 days after exposure and delayed clearing following effective therapy. Because of the sensitization, symptoms start sooner with recurrent infection. Only a few mites usually are present, generally fewer than 10, even though the signs and symptoms can be extensive. The distribution of the mite does not correspond closely with the distribution of the rash (Fig. 97.8). Untreated scabies continues to progress; it is not self-healing.

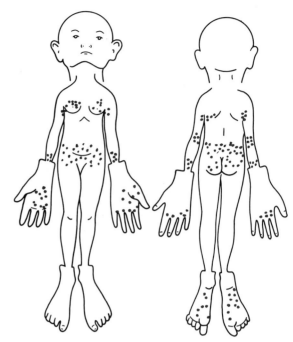

Figure 97.8 Pruritic papules are most prevalent about the waist, pelvis, elbows, and hands and feet in scabies.

The overwhelming symptom is severe itching, typically worse at night. The lesions appear as excoriated, inflamed rice- to pea-sized papules, some with a burrow. Sites most involved are the fingerwebs, wrists, antecubital fossae, elbows, areolae, umbilicus, lower abdomen, genitalia, and gluteal cleft. Superimposed excoriations and eczematous dermatitis are common. Findings may be minimal in scrupulously clean individuals. Family members and sexual partners almost invariably are involved and should be treated. Transmission requires close contact, such as sleeping in the same bed or living in the same house; scabies usually is not transmitted casually, as between schoolmates. If the patient is sexually active, it is important to look for other venereal disease by obtaining an STS and doing a pelvic and urethral examination to obtaining a gonococcal culture.

A diagnosis of scabies should be considered in any patient who has a pruritic eruption with excoriated papules, especially if family members or close friends also are experiencing itching. Scabies can be proven by finding the mite microscopically. This is accomplished by placing a drop of glycerol or mineral oil, preferably sterile, on the papule to keep the scales and scrapings in place, and scraping through the oil with a blade or syringe needle to the point of just drawing blood. The mite or its eggs must be sought using the ×10 microscope objective. The mite is an ugly bristled ectoparasite about 0.4 mm long with 4 pairs of legs. It is hard to find; even experts may be unable to confirm the diagnosis. Therefore, it is appropriate to treat on strong clinical suspicion.

Scabies is hard to diagnose and may be confused,

even by the experienced clinician, with a variety of cutaneous disorders. Atypical presentations account for delayed treatment and provide opportunities for spread. Further confusion often is generated by the use of topical corticosteroids than can partially suppress the eruption.

Therapy

Two topical scabicides are in general use, gamma benzene hexachloride, GBH (Lindane, Gamene, Kwell), and crotamiton (Eurax). Either is effective but GBH should not be used in children under 6 or in pregnant women because of the potential to cause neurotoxicity (15).

GBH

The patient should apply lotion to all crevices of the entire body from the chin down and leave on for 12 hours, then remove it by thorough washing. It should be applied when the skin is dry, not immediately after bathing, as toxicity may be increased because of the increased absorption through damp skin. One treatment is probably sufficient but, since GBH is not ovicidal, retreatment 1 week later is appropriate to destroy later hatching larvae. Recently used clothing should be thoroughly washed or dry cleaned and linens and towels changed and laundered. For practical purposes, scabies is not transmissible after the first day of therapy. There is no need to suggest extermination procedures as the lifespan of the mite on clothing and bedding is short. All family members should be treated at the same time. The physician should prescribe enough to apply 30 ml to each person for each of the two treatments and should not allow refills; extensive repeated use of GBH may cause irritation and pruritus which may be confused with the original symptoms.

CROTAMITON

Crotamiton is an effective alternative to GBH. It is applied from the chin down and to all body folds and creases in the same way as GBH, but it is reapplied 24 hours later. Clothing and linen should be changed the first morning after treatment. The medication should be left on for a total of 48 hours, after which patients should take a cleansing bath. Crotamiton is antipruritic and appears to be safe for use in children and pregnant women.

FOLLOW-UP

If the initial therapy did not appear to work, there are several points to consider: First, it must be kept in mind that itching often persists for a week or two following effective antiscabicide treatment, usually as a result of slow subsiding of hypersensitivity to the mite and mite products, although sometimes due to irritation from GBH or to reinfection. An antihistamine, such as diphenhydramine (Benadryl, a 25- or 50-mg capsule, 3 or 4 times a day), a topical steroid ointment, such as triamcinolone 0.1%, or, if severe,

systemic steroids, such as prednisone, 30 mg per day in three divided doses and tapered over 2 weeks, may be needed to provide relief. Second, if symptoms persist beyond 2 weeks or recur when the antipruritics are stopped, the patient should be re-examined for persistent infestation or reinfestation. If there are signs of secondary infection, a 7-day course of an antibiotic, such as erythromycin 250 mg 4 times a day, is indicated. The pruritic papules frequently accompanying scabies may require weeks to clear. Animal scabies is different from human scabies; therefore, pets are not a reservoir and do not have to be treated.

SEBORRHEIC DERMATITIS

Presentation

Seborrheic dermatitis takes its name because it is found in regions where sebaceous glands are in greatest density, i.e., the scalp, eyebrows, ear canals, midface and midchest area (Fig. 97.9). The main features are erythema and a yellow, greasy scaling. Itching is mild but troublesome. Typically, the severity fluctuates so that patients recall months of relative clearing and months of relative worsening.

Onset of seborrheic dermatitis is generally at puberty when it appears concomitantly with acne; the condition continues in its fluctuating course for years or decades without a decrease in old age. Both sexes are equally affected. Seborrheic dermatitis is worsened in patients with Parkinson's disease, syringomyelia, emotional stress, and at the time of an acute stroke or myocardial infarction.

Although occurring in regions of dense sebaceous

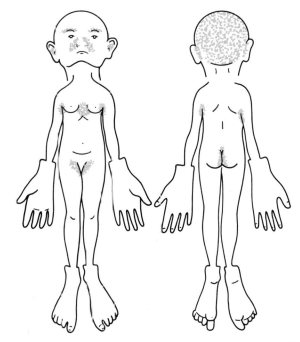

Figure 97.9 Usual location of erythema and scale in seborrheic dermatitis.

glands and having a greasy appearance, seborrheic dermatitis does not appear to be a disorder of the sebaceous glands. Other possible causes of seborrheic dermatitis have been sought, including differences in bacteria and sebum, but none have been found (6).

Differential Diagnosis

The common scalp condition, dandruff, is distinguished from seborrheic dermatitis by the absence of erythema and the lack of involvement in other regions. The most frequent confusion is with psoriasis, as both conditions are erythematous, scaly, and chronic. Psoriasis, however, tends to involve the extensor surfaces, particularly the elbows and knees; a search for such lesions in patients with severe scalp dermatitis may be helpful. Psoriasis of the scalp often stops at the hairline, seborrheic dermatitis does not. The differential diagnosis also includes contact dermatitis, scaly drug eruptions, tinea corporis, and tinea versicolor. Lupus erythematosus, photo-induced dermatoses, and a number of uncommon diseases such as Darier's disease should be considered.

These alternative diagnostic possibilities should especially be considered when the response to therapy for seborrheic dermatitis is not satisfactory.

Therapy

The patient should understand that only relief, not cure, is possible. A fluctuating course is expected and therapy will need to be modified with exacerbations. If the patient does not understand this, the result will be disappointing. The treatment depends on the site of involvement.

SCALP

If mild, control with shampoos (see above, "Psoriasis") may be sufficient. Frequent, even daily, shampooing is not harmful and does not cause hair loss.

If the condition is severe or unresponsive to simple shampooing, the physician should prescribe a topical corticosteroid to be applied after shampooing, while the scalp is still damp. A lotion, such as betamethasone (Diprosone or Valisone lotion), a solution such as fluocinolone (Synalar solution), or a gel such as fluocinonide (Topsyn gel) must be used since creams and ointments are difficult to use in hairy parts. If the scales are thick, the phenol/saline or tar preparations (see above, "Psoriasis") may be used at bedtime, followed by the steroid preparation after shampooing in the morning. If the condition proves resistant to intensive therapy, psoriasis is more likely to be the diagnosis than seborrheic dermatitis.

SKIN

The patient should apply 1% hydrocortisone cream (prescribed as generic) to the face and any potent fluorinated corticosteroid cream or lotion (see "Psoriasis") elsewhere twice a day until clear, then as needed to maintain clearing, usually two or three times a week, generally in the morning. Fluorinated steroids should not be used on the face for *any* chronic condition as permanent redness and telangiectasias may result from long term use. Potent steroids may lead to atrophy if used chronically in occluded body folds, such as the axilla and groin. One percent hydrocortisone is safer in those regions. The addition of 3% iodochlorhydroxyquin, which is slightly antibacterial, to the steroid (Vioform-Hydrocortisone cream, requires a prescription) for resistant areas is often helpful but is best used only at bedtime, as it permanently stains clothing yellow. If there is much oiliness, a sulfur-resorcinol preparation (Sulforcin, available without prescription) should be added at bedtime, applied with the fingertips to the entire area of the face, back, or chest.

If, after a 3-week trial, the initial therapy proves insufficient, tetracycline, 250 mg twice daily, an hour before or 2 hours after meals, should be prescribed. Tetracycline generally will be necessary for extensive, severe, and recalcitrant cases. The physician should plan on a 2-month course at the initial dose and then should taper slowly by going to 250 mg twice a day alternating with once a day for a month and then 250 mg a day for an additional month. Although this may seem homeopathic, tetracycline is concentrated in sebaceous glands and exerts a therapeutic effect at such doses. The possibility of psoriasis should be considered if the dermatitis seems especially resistant to treatment.

EYELIDS

Seborrheic marginal blepharitis is chronic scaling at the lid margins without signs of conjunctivitis or globe discomfort. It can be controlled by gentle scrubbing each morning with baby shampoo (e.g. Johnson's), diluted one to one with water, using a cotton-tipped applicator to cleanse the lids. If not sufficiently controlled, a mild topical steroid such as 1% hydrocortisone cream may be used. However, long use of potent fluorinated topical steroids can lead to glaucoma, is dangerous in the presence of herpes infection and should not be used. Hydrocortisone is safer and can be tried alone (1% hydrocortisone ophthalmic ointment) or in combination with antibiotics, such as neomycin (Cortisporin, Neo-Cortef ophthalmic ointment) or tetracycline (Terra-Cortril ophthalmic ointment). The patient should apply the ointment with a clean fingertip just to the lid margins twice daily. Treatment should continue at this frequency only until the condition has cleared, after which the patient should decrease the frequency of application to two or three times a week for an additional 2 weeks and then stop therapy. Like seborrheic dermatitis elsewhere, the condition tends to recur. Since therapy can be restarted when needed, the medication should not be continued when the eyelids are clear.

Contact dermatitis to mascara or eye shadow can manifest as blepharitis and both these agents should be discontinued for at least a month to determine if either are related to the dermatitis. The patient should be referred to an ophthalmologist if unresponsive or if the onset was abrupt, particularly if accompanied by conjunctivitis and/or cornea or globe discomfort.

DERMATITIS OF FEET

The most common dermatologic disorders of the feet are: (a) tinea infection, (b) dyshidrosis, (c) contact allergy, (d) essential hyperhidrosis, and (e) erythrasma. The most important diagnostic clues are location (Fig. 97.10) and appearance; all of these disorders, except hyperhidrosis, are pruritic.

Tinea

PRESENTATION

Tinea pedis, or superficial fungal infection of the feet, occurs in about 20% of the population, a problem related to the common use of closed shoes which retain generated heat and moisture, conditions perfect for fungal growth. Summer exacerbations are typical. This infection presents as scales, itching, and slight redness between the toes and on the soles, especially at the instep. In acute stages, blistering can develop, usually involving the instep rather than the thick keratin on the balls of the feet. Secondary infection and lymphangitis may be superimposed on tinea pedis. Yellow crumbly toenails infected with

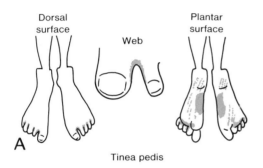

A — Tinea pedis

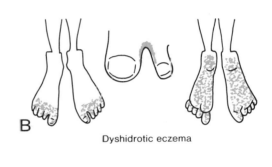

B — Dyshidrotic eczema

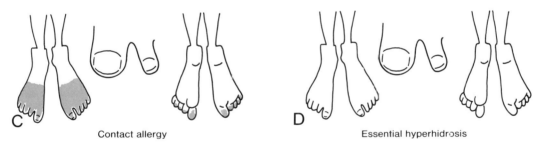

C — Contact allergy

D — Essential hyperhidrosis

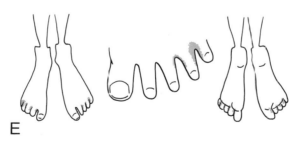

E — Erythrasma

Figure 97.10 Distribution of lesions is useful to distinguish among causes of dermatitis of the feet. (*A*) Tinea pedis—moisture, scale, and pruritus confined to the plantar surface (especially the instep) and between the toes. (*B*) Dyshidrotic eczema—vesicles and severe pruritus on the plantar as well as the dorsal surface and between the toes. (*C*) Contact allergy—the dorsum of the feet and underside of toes may be involved while the plantar surface and webs are clear. (*D*) Essential hyperhidrosis—sodden soles but no dermatitis. (*E*) Erythrasma—mild erythema and scale limited to the toe webs, especially the fourth to fifth.

fungi, onychomycosis, often are associated with chronic tinea pedis and serve as a source of continuing reinfection. A scraping of the scale or debris under the nail incubated on a slide with KOH for 10 min will reveal hyphae (see KOH technique, p. 1047). Culture usually is not necessary.

THERAPY

The patient should be instructed to dry the toe webs thoroughly after bathing and to use talc freely. Footwear should be nonocclusive (ventilated leather shoes or sandals are best; vinyl footwear or sneakers should be avoided). The patient should use cotton socks (dark or light) and avoid wool and synthetic fibers which absorb moisture poorly. If the lesions are dry and pruritic, the physician should prescribe a topical antifungal agent such as miconazole cream (MicaTin), haloprogin cream (Halotex), or clotrimazole cream (Lotrimin, Mycelex) to be applied to the feet sparingly each morning and evening. When the feet are particularly scaly and sweaty, a keratolytic in an insoluble ointment base (half-strength Whitfield's ointment, available without prescription) applied each morning, alternating with an antifungal cream at bedtime may be needed. If the lesions are moist and acute, they should be treated with compresses of Burow's solution (Domeboro, available without prescription), made with one packet or tablet dissolved in a pint of lukewarm water, for 20 min 3 times a day for 3 days before starting topical antifungals.

If initial therapy does not work, a 30-day course of griseofulvin, ultrafine (generic, by prescription), 250 mg 3 times a day with meals usually will be effective. The topical antifungals should be continued, when the griseofulvin is discontinued, to maintain clearing. If accompanied by hyperhidrosis, 6% aluminum chloride in absolute ethanol (Xerac-AC, requires a prescription) applied to the feet each morning will induce dryness; the patient should continue with the topical antifungals at bedtime until clear, then continue them for an additional month and reinstitute the therapy only upon recurrence.

Onychomycosis responds involving the toenails poorly to any therapy, including griseofulvin.

Dyshidrosis

PRESENTATION

Dyshidrosis is the second most common dermatosis of the feet and the most difficult of the common disorders to diagnose and treat; it affects both sexes with equal frequency. The cause of dyshidrosis is uncertain but many patients have flare-ups following nonspecific irritation. The physician should inquire about causes, including contact allergens, especially from occupational, household, and hobby sources, exposures to nonspecific irritants, and a history of atopy. The eruption also occurs on the hands where

it is particularly common in cooks, beauticians, and housewives. It often resembles a combination of tinea infection and contact allergy. Dyshidrosis starts as minute, intraepidermal blisters on the sides of the palms and/or soles and between the fingers and/or toes. Scale and erythema accompanied by severe pruritus usually are present. Unlike tinea pedis, involvement of the dorsum of the foot is common. Dyshidrosis frequently is accompanied by hyperhidrosis (see below), but there is no disorder of the sweat mechanism, despite the misleading name given to the condition. Recurrences, are typical. The KOH examination will be negative.

THERAPY

During the blistering phase, the patient should use compresses for 20 min 3 times a day with Burow's solution (Domeboro, available without prescription), made with one packet or tablet dissolved in a pint of lukewarm water, followed by any potent full strength topical corticosteroid cream (such as triamcinolone 0.1%). At bedtime, in order to absorb serous fluid, a thick coating of zinc oxide ointment (available without prescription) should be applied and cotton socks used to keep the paste in place. In the morning, the patient should wipe off the paste with simple mineral oil on cotton balls and reapply the steroid. During the acute phase, an antihistamine (such as Benadryl, a 25- or 50-mg capsule 3 to 4 times a day) for sedation will be useful. As the dermatitis becomes less acute, the compressing should be stopped and a steroid ointment, instead of cream, used 3 times a day.

If initial therapy does not work within 2 weeks, a short course of systemic steroids may be necessary. Prednisone, 40 mg/day for the average adult, is prescribed, continued until relief is obtained and then tapered by giving 20 mg/day for a week and then 10 mg/day for an additional 2 weeks after which it is discontinued. Dyshidrosis is notoriously difficult to treat; it is a bane, even to the dermatologist. However, the dermatologist or allergist is able to perform contact allergy patch tests which may be of help in locating the cause; the physician should not hesitate to refer patients with this problem.

Contact Allergy (see also above, "Contact Dermatitis")

PRESENTATION

As implied in the name, contact allergy as a cause of dermatitis of the feet is an allergic reaction to a footwear product, usually leather, tanning compounds, metals, dyes, adhesives, or foot medications. It is less common than tinea pedis but should be considered, particularly when the dorsum of the feet and toes rather than the interdigital areas are involved with show erythema, scale, and pruritus. Sometimes, blisters may appear. Unlike tinea pedis, the toewebs, protected from direct exposure, and the soles, protected by thick keratin, are not involved.

THERAPY

Topical or even systemic corticosteroids do not fully suppress contact dermatitis if exposure to the antigen continues. Therefore, if the patient is able to connect the outbreak with any particular footwear, it should be avoided. If the dermatitis is severe, bedrest, compresses, and systemic antibiotics may be needed, while efforts to locate the source of the allergy are initiated. Referral to an allergist or dermatologist is suggested, as either will have access to specialized patch-testing materials as well as knowledge of sock and shoe components, and sources of less antigenic substitutes.

HYPERHIDROSIS

PRESENTATION

This is a common disorder with excessive sweating of the soles, frequently accompanied by excess palmar sweating (12). It can be severe, with sweat dripping from the fingers and toes, interfering with the patient's occupation and social life. Pruritus or scale are not present. The increased moisture on the feet may lead to fissuring and infection and the odor may be objectionable.

THERAPY

Six percent aluminum chloride solution (Xerac-AC or Drysol requires a prescription) applied nightly until the condition has improved (usually by 48 hours) and then as needed, is very effective. It appears to work by causing the sweat duct to leak sweat back into the dermis rather than transporting it to the surface. In severe cases, surgical sympathectomy has been used with fair success.

Erythrasma

PRESENTATION

Erythrasma is a superficial skin infection presenting on the feet with scale and erythema, particularly between the fourth and fifth toes. It is due to a bacterium, *Corynebacterium minutissimum*, which produces a porphyrin, recognized by a salmon red fluorescence on exposure to Wood's light (see p. 1047). Although not a common cause of foot dermatitis, erythrasma should be considered when a scaly foot dermatitis does not respond to topical antifungal medications. A KOH examination (see p. 1047) will be negative.

THERAPY

Erythrasma is successfully treated with erythromycin, 250 mg 3 times daily for 2 weeks or with 2% erythromycin topically for 2 weeks. Recurrences are frequent; there is no effective method of avoidance.

The disease generally is not passed among family members.

TINEA VERSICOLOR

Presentation

Tinea versicolor is a superficial fungal infection due to an organism not easily cultured, *Malassezia furfur* (20). It appears as desquamating macular patches found primarily on the trunk, below the chin and above the waist. The rash may be mildly itchy. The varied colors of the rash, from red to pink to brown, gives the eruption its name. Tinea versicolor is common, particularly in hot humid environments.

The fungus interferes with normal pigmentation, so that the patches become more noticeable during the summer when the skin under the patches does not tan as well as the rest of the skin. This effect is seen in blacks as well as whites. The infection does not seem to be contagious; marital partners usually are not both affected. However, individuals, who have had tinea versicolor seem prone to have recurrences.

An examination with KOH shows short hyphae and spores ("spaghetti and meat balls") (Fig. 97.11). The physician should search under the high dry objective (×40); the low power objective (×10) is too low to reveal the fungal structures. The organism cannot be cultured on usual office media. A Wood's light examination (see p. 1047) is useful as it reveals the extent of the infection better than does room light.

Differential Diagnosis

Because of the pigment disruption, vitiligo must be considered. However, vitiligo is never scaly and a KOH examination will be negative. The pigment loss in tinea versicolor is partial; the pigment loss in

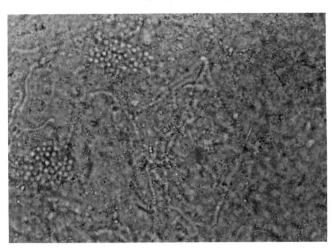

Figure 97.11   Short hypae and spores of *Malassezia furfur* seen in tinea versicolor (KOH preparation, ×400).

vitiligo is complete. Other disorders to consider are seborrheic dermatitis (see above), pityriasis rosea (see above), and infection due to other tinea species. Seborrheic dermatitis most commonly involves the face and scalp, but tinea versicolor almost never goes above the chin; pityriasis rosea may be worse on the upper trunk but usually extends below the waist and the KOH examination will be negative; a KOH examination of the other tinea that affects man causing tinea cruris and corporis ("ringworm" of the groin and body) reveals long hyphae without spores, not short hyphae with spores.

Therapy

Numerous therapies work, but recurrences are common. An irritating soap applied at bedtime and showered off in the morning usually is sufficient. Selenium sulfide suspension (Exsel, 2.5%, requires a prescription or Selsun Blue, 1%, available without prescription) or a peeling soap (Fostex cream, available without prescription) should be used for 4 consecutive nights or until the skin shows irritation. The patient should apply the material from neck to wrists to waist. The use of 25% sodium thiosulfate (generic or Tinver, a prescription is required) twice a day for an additional 10 days assures resolution but should be used only after work and at bedtime as it has an unpleasant smell. Prescription antifungal agents, such as miconazole, clotrimazole, and haloprogin, are effective but too expensive to apply to the large surface area usually involved.

After the initial therapy, the patient may expect the lesions to be cleared of fungi; a return visit is not needed. However, the patient must be warned that the lightened patches will remain until retanned naturally through normal melanocytic processes. Otherwise, the patient may consider the treatment to be a failure. Pigmentation will take several weeks, although the process can be speeded up by activating the melanocytes through exposure of the skin to tanning doses of ultraviolet light. Patients also should be told that recurrences are common and advised to repeat therapy if needed, which is generally once each spring or summer. Only the unusual case, such as a patient with uncontrolled diabetes mellitus or Cushing's syndrome, is not cleared with the initial therapy.

VITILIGO

Presentation

When melanocytes stop producing melanin and, later, completely disappear from the site, the skin turns nearly ivory in color, regardless of background racial coloration. The patches have sharp borders without evidence of erythema or inflammation. They are most frequent over bony prominences and around orifices such as the mouth and eyes (Fig. 97.12). The patches reflect light and appear bright white under a

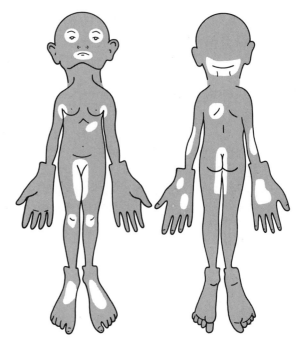

Figure 97.12 Depigmented macules of vitiligo occur most commonly at orifices, extensor surfaces, and at areas of repeated trauma.

Wood's lamp (see p. 1047), an examination which may be useful in revealing additional patches of vitiligo, especially if the patient is light complexioned. Vitiligo may be inherited. Unfortunately, its course is unpredictable.

Differential Diagnosis

The usual confusion is caused by postinflammatory hypopigmentation. In this case there is typically a history of a preceding inflammatory or traumatic condition as well as a persistence of at least some pigment, so that the patches are not ivory white as they are in vitiligo. Phenolic compounds, ingredients of some industrial janitorial products, may destroy melanocytes and lead to permanent depigmentation. The depigmentation may be indistinguishable from vitiligo, except by distribution, as the patches induced by phenol tend to be restricted to the region of contact, notably the hands and arms.

Tinea versicolor also may be confused with vitiligo (see above). Vitiligo is more frequent in patients with thyroid disease, Addison's disease, pernicious anemia, and alopecia areata.

Therapy

For initial lesions that are not extensive, the treatment is cosmetic. There is no early medical therapy for vitiligo that will affect its course. In addition, if new vitiliginous patches are appearing or extending, it is best to wait for the depigmentation to stabilize before embarking on more drastic treatments. Several products are available that hide the lesions, with various degrees of success. They are either stains, including Dy-O-Derm (Owens Lab) and Vitadye (Elder Co.), or cosmetics, such as Covermark (Lydia O'Leary Co.) and Erase (Max Factor); all these preparations are available without prescription. The proper shading and use of Covermark needs to be taught; the Lydia O'Leary Co. (New York, NY 10022) will provide the names of local cosmetologists trained in the use of their products. One advantage of cosmetics over stains is that they provide a barrier to sunlight; the patches of vitiligo are easily sunburned since there are no melanocytes to produce tanning.

Nonprescription sun-blockers now are labeled with a Skin Protective Factor (SPF) number, indicating the multiple of time that an individual using the product can be exposed to ultraviolet light without burning, compared to the time for the same person not using the product. Patients with vitiligo should be advised always to use a sunblocker (such as Eclipse-Total, PreSun-15, or Super Shade) with an SPF of 15 or more before any sun exposure. Not only will sunburning of the patches of vitiligo be minimized but normal skin will not tan, thus minimizing the contrast between the light and dark areas.

When to Refer

Further therapy necessitates referral to a dermatologist. There, the options are either repigmentation with psoralen and long wave ultraviolet light (PUVA), or bleaching residual dark skin with hydroquinone. Both procedures generally are beyond the scope (and equipment) of the generalist; further, both are time-consuming and potentially dangerous; PUVA can lead to severe ultraviolet light burns and, perhaps, late skin cancer; and hydroquinone is irritating and a contact sensitizer. Only about half the patients will respond to PUVA and up to a year may be required for repigmentation to be "adequate." Bleaching dark skin white will not be acceptable to all patients.

WARTS

Presentation

There are several types of warts, generally classified on the basis of their location or their clinical appearance. Warts generally breed true to type. These clinical types were once thought to be caused by the same virus but are known now to be due to a family of DNA papovaviruses of different antigenic subtypes (16). Warts are all mildly contagious and have an incubation period, after inoculation, of 1 to several months. They are frequent in immunosuppressed individuals in whom they may be nearly impossible to eradicate. However, in normal individuals, spontaneous involution is common; half will clear in 1 year.

The major types of warts are vulgaris, plantar, flat, and venereal.

Verruca Vulgaris (Common Wart)

PRESENTATION

Common warts start as minute papules and grow over many weeks or months to raised, rough, cauliflower-like papules. They are most common on the extremities but may be found on any part of the body in persons of all ages. The physician should consider the source of the virus; a friend or the entire family may need treatment.

DIFFERENTIAL DIAGNOSIS

It is important to consider molluscum contagiosum in children and young adults; seborrheic keratoses or cutaneous horns in the elderly.

THERAPY

The treatment of warts usually proceeds in definite order, based on ease of use (Table 97.4). A most convenient, painless and frequently effective office treatment is salicylic acid and lactic acid in flexible collodion (Duofilm, requires a prescription), which works by softening the keratin in which the wart is growing, thereby allowing the wart to be pared away. It is particularly useful for warts around the nail as the medication seeps under the nail. The patient should follow the directions in the package insert, which suggests soaking the wart, at bedtime, in warm water for 5 min and then applying a small drop of medication to the wart with the applicator or a toothpick; the surrounding skin should be avoided to reduce irritation. The solution dries quickly. The patient should reapply 3 more drops allowing each to dry before applying the next one. Excess dead tissue should be pared the next morning. The therapy should be stopped for a day or two if the area becomes sore. The patient should continue treatment for 5 days, after which the wart usually is tender; at that time the patient should stop treatment to allow the inflammation to subside, and repeat the course every 2 weeks until clear. If the wart has not been eradicated after three courses, the patient should change the manner of Duofilm use. The patient should apply a single drop of Duofilm to each wart at bedtime, allow the medication to dry, then cover it overnight with an occlusive tape (such as Blen-

Table 97.4
Treatment of Warts in Order of Ease of Use

1. Salicylic acid/lactic acid in collodion (Duofilm) (podophyllin for venereal warts)
2. Liquid nitrogen
3. Electrodesiccation and curettage
4. Surgical excision

derm). The patient should pare the wart each morning and continue nightly application of medication unless the area becomes tender.

The most common alternative initial therapy is liquid nitrogen, but a large number of patients with warts must be treated to justify the expense of the material. Nitrogen is a liquid at normal atmospheric pressures at −200°C, and maintains that temperature only through steady evaporative loss. Special storage vessels are available (costing approximately $300) so that only monthly replenishment (from a gas-medical supplier, listed as such in the telephone directory) is necessary. If liquid nitrogen is available, warts may be treated by freezing for 20 sec by using a thick cotton swab pulled to a narrow point. The aim is to get full freezing of the wart as well as 2 to 3 mm beyond. It is important to avoid the lateral sides of the fingers as the digital nerves are subject to damage. The digital nerve is located at the tip of the crease made when the finger is flexed. Liquid nitrogen freezing is painful; the area will hurt for several hours. A blister usually develops 2 to 3 days later. If the blister becomes inconveniently large, the patient can be allowed to puncture it with a clean needle to drain the contents, but it need not be deroofed. An 80% cure rate is usual. The patient should return in 1 month for retreatment if not clear.

If initial therapy did not work and if facilities are available, the next best alternative is electrodesiccation and curettage; otherwise, referral to a dermatologist is appropriate. The physician should consider underlying immunosuppression such as Hodgkin's disease, diabetes mellitus, or drug abuse if the warts are extensive and resistant.

Plantar Warts (see also Chapter 99)

PRESENTATION

Plantar warts can be troublesome in that they tend to be persistent and painful. They are not raised from the surface like other warts but extend into the horny layer. They may be distinguished from corns and calluses by paring them down with a scalpel blade. Warts show a speckled surface due to blood in dilated capillaries, while a shiny smooth surface is typical of corns. Corns and calluses are likely to be bilateral and over pressure points, especially the metatarsal heads, while warts may develop at any site.

THERAPY

The goal of treatment is to destroy the wart without producing a scar, as such scars may be permanently painful. The best way to avoid scars is to avoid the use of surgical or electrodesiccation techniques in therapy. Surgical procedures may be justified if the wart proves untreatable by chemical means, but surgery is not appropriate initially. X-ray therapy is infrequently used as it may produce late scarring and discomfort.

For initial therapy, the patient may use salicylic acid and lactic acid in flexible collodion (Duofilm) in the same way as suggested for verruca vulgaris. A single drop covered by an occlusive tape, as described, seems to work better than does the open technique. Salicylic acid plaster (such as Duke—available in rolls from a physician supply store or pharmacy or Scholls—available in individual plasters; both available without prescription) also may be used at bedtime under occlusive tape, followed by paring each morning.

Freezing with liquid nitrogen does not work as well on the sole as elsewhere because of the thickness of the plantar surface.

Treatment of plantar warts can be frustrating; the physician should therefore not hesitate to refer a patient to a dermatologist or podiatrist if the warts are resistant or extensive.

Flat Warts

PRESENTATION

Flat warts are much smaller individually than verruca vulgaris, usually only 2 to 3 mm in size and are barely raised above the surface. Although always superficial, flat warts are troublesome because they usually are numerous and affect exposed parts, such as the face, neck, or legs. Flat warts often are spread by nicking the skin during shaving and implanting the virus.

THERAPY

For a small number of flat warts, use of liquid nitrogen, salicylic acid/lactic acid in flexible collodion (Duofilm—see above), or gentle electrodesiccation may be satisfactory. If numerous, the physician should prescribe 10% salicylic acid cream, prepared by the pharmacist, or 0.025% vitamin A acid gel (Retin-A gel, requires a prescription) once or twice daily. To prevent scarring, it is important to avoid aggressive procedures. An electric razor or depilatory may be used to decrease spreading of the warts through nicks and autoinoculation. Spread to other family members is unlikely.

Flat warts take a long time to cure, perhaps months. It is therefore important for the physician to be aware of this or he should refer the patient to a dermatologist.

Venereal Warts

PRESENTATION

Also called moist warts, accuminate warts, or condyloma accuminata, these primarily affect the anogenital area and usually are acquired through sexual contact. They seem to be more contagious than other types of warts. Patients may not be aware of intraurethral, anal, or intravaginal warts and must be properly examined. The physician should suspect homosexuality in a male with anal or perianal warts. An STS and smear and culture for gonorrhea should be obtained on all patients with venereal warts as other venereal diseases may have been contracted. Venereal warts are also discussed in Chapter 91.

DIFFERENTIAL DIAGNOSIS

Condyloma of secondary syphilis (the STS always is positive in secondary syphilis) and malignancies, such as Bowen's disease or extramammary Paget's disease, must be considered (see Chapter 92).

THERAPY

The mainstay of treatment is 20 to 25% podophyllin, an extract of the mandrake plant, in compound tincture of benzoin. Podophyllin is a poison and should never be dispensed to the patient. It works only for moist verrucous warts; less well on dry warts located on the shaft of the penis or on the scrotum. Podophyllin should be applied carefully with a wooden stick just to the wart; it is quite irritating to normal skin. The benzoin should dry for a few minutes before allowing the patient to dress. The medication should be thoroughly washed off in 4 hours. If this initial treatment has not been too irritating, the medication may be left on longer after the next application. It is important not to apply podophyllin to large areas at one time if the warts are extensive because it may be quite irritating. The patient should return weekly for retreatment, until cured. Usually at least four treatments are necessary. Podophyllin should not be used in pregnant women as it is potentially cytotoxic to the fetus (see also Chapter 91).

After several treatments, a nubbin of the warts may remain. As the wart is now dry, it may not resolve further with podophyllin; liquid nitrogen or electrodesiccation may be needed for final cure.

If initial therapy does not work, a surgical procedure such as electrodesiccation may be necessary. If the warts are vaginal or urethral, referral to a gynecologist or urologist is appropriate. If cutaneous warts recur or prove recalcitrant to therapy, a biopsy or referral to a dermatologist for diagnosis and further therapy is warranted.

XEROSIS (DRY SKIN)

Presentation

"Dry," itchy, and scaly skin is common, increasing in frequency and degree in the elderly. Although usually generalized, xerosis is most frequent and severe on the legs. The cause is not fully understood, but it seems most likely to be due to a diminished epidermal lipid barrier, allowing loss of normally retained moisture from the stratum corneum. For that reason, dry skin is exacerbated by excessive soapy bathing and relieved somewhat by lubricating creams. Xerosis is worse in the winter when the humidity of warm air in the house in lowest. As the skin becomes desiccated, scaling, chapping, and pruritus develop, sometimes leading to dermatitis with erythema and scale.

Differential Diagnosis

A generalized itchy dermatitis, especially in the elderly, may be associated with underlying renal or hepatic insufficiency, diabetes mellitus, thyroid and other endocrine diseases, or lymphoma. Xerosis, to varying degrees, is present in all patients with atopic dermatitis or in patients with an atopic diathesis such as eczema, hayfever, or asthma. If present in the young or present since an early age, the physician should consider congenital ichthyosis.

Therapy

The patient should use soap only in the axillae, groin, and buttocks followed by careful rinsing away of the soap. This is easier in a shower/tub combination, but can be done if only a bathtub is available. A fat-based soap, such as Ivory, Camay, or Basis is preferred to one containing a chemical detergent, such as Zest or Dial. The patient should allow the soapy water to drain out. Next, the patient should fill the tub with a few inches of lukewarm water and add about ½ ounce (⅓ jigger or 2 capfuls) of any nonperfumed bath oil (such as Alpha-Keri or Domol). Mineral oil will not work as it will not mix with water. The patient should use the oily water to sponge bathe. Surfactants in the bath oil will cleanse well enough without extracting the lipid barrier. It is important for the patient to understand that soap and bath oil do not mix and must be used separately. The tub will be slippery and the patient should be careful. After drying, but while the skin is still damp, the patient should apply an emollient cream such as Eucerin, Keri, Shepard's, or a nonperfumed store brand. The patient should limit bathing to no more than twice a week. Topical steroids are not necessary, unless dermatitis is present. Antihistamines merely sedate and should be avoided for simple xerosis. The house or, at least, the sitting and sleeping rooms should be humidified. Successful treatment requires persistent care.

The patient should be much improved after the first visit; if not relieved, the physician should consider underlying disease and obtain appropriate laboratory studies (see above).

TUMORS

New growths on the skin are common, particularly in later life; it is important to be on the lookout for lesions during the physical examination and to distinguish benign from premalignant and/or malignant new growths. Two references (2, 10) provide resource information on skin tumors.

Seborrheic Keratoses

These are common and practically universal, characterized by an irregular, rather than smooth, surface which feels waxy on being rubbed. These keratoses are superficial and they feel "stuck on" the skin rather than implanted or growing into the skin. They vary in color from beige or dark brown to black, to the point of resembling malignant melanoma. However, seborrheic keratoses never become malignant. Examples of seborrheic keratoses are shown in Figure 97.13.

The usual reason for their removal is bothersome irritation from clothing, belts, or straps but, on occasion, their appearance is unacceptable to the patient and removal for cosmetic reasons may be justified. The simplest usually effective therapy for seborrheic keratoses is to paint them with 75% trichloroacetic acid (obtainable from a pharmacy for office use but too caustic to be dispensed to the patient). The compound should be kept in the refrigerator. The keratoses should be lightly painted, taking care to avoid normal skin. After a few moments, the lesion will turn white and the patient will notice mild burning, which will subside shortly. During the next week, the lesion will form a crust and fall away; however, thick lesions may require two or three monthly applications. One drop of trichloroacetic acid in the wrong place can cause great damage; therefore, the physician should take care not to hold the bottle or the applicator near the patient's eyes. If the lesions are thick or irritated, they may be lightly curetted after local anesthesia. Hemostasis may be obtained by fulguration or application of Monsel's solution (usually available from a large pharmacy) with a cotton-tipped applicator.

Angiomas

These common lesions are 1- to 3-mm bright red, cherry-colored, nonblanching, shiny papules usually located on the trunk and known as cherry angiomas (Fig. 97.14). These are benign and not premalignant. Because of their small size and lack of bleeding tendencies, therapy usually is not warranted.

Other Benign Lesions

NEVI

Although nevi usually are benign, they must be examined with care. Quite often even a specialist is uncertain. If the patient believes the lesion recently has changed, or if the lesion has been bleeding, has irregular or dark pigment, or is large, removal is justified. However, less than half of all malignant melanomas come from preexisting nevi and the average adult has 20 pigmented nevi; prophylactic removal of all moles is practically impossible and certainly unjustified. If the primary reason for removal is cosmetic, without evidence of recent change or suspicious signs, and if the mole is in a site visible to the patient, such as the face, the mole can be shaved with a scalpel blade to reduce it to the level of the skin surface. Hemostasis is achieved as with seborrheic keratosis removal (see above). The portion removed should be preserved in formaldehyde and sent for pathological examination. The cosmetic results of this "shave removal" are better than with excision, and surgery is not thought to increase the likelihood that the nevus will evolve into a melanoma. On the other hand, if there have been recent changes or suspicious signs, the lesion should be excised by a surgeon in its entirety and with adequate margins.

ACTINIC KERATOSES

These appear as red, scaly, nonhealing crusty lesions, predominantly restricted to light-exposed areas such as the face, nape and back of the hands (Fig. 97.15). These keratoses are most common in light complexioned individuals who have worked outdoors or otherwise have spent a lot of time in the sun. These lesions, although benign, are premalignant and should be dealt with by local destruction using any one of several methods, usually desiccation and curettage, with local anesthesia or freezing with liquid nitrogen. 5-Fluorouracil (Fluoroplex, Efudex, requires prescription) is useful for patients with more than a dozen or so keratoses and has the advantage that early, premalignant lesions will be destroyed as well. The medication is applied twice daily until irritation develops, normally in 2 weeks, and then continued for an additional 2 weeks. The patient should expect discomfort, redness, and peeling. A topical corticosteroid cream (such as triamcinolone 0.1%) can be applied 4 times a day for a week once the reaction has reached its peak. The keratoses will be cleared, but new ones will appear eventually as the tendency for their development has not been altered. Any lesion still present after the course of therapy should be biopsied and destroyed or removed.

Individuals with actinic keratoses usually have multiple lesions with a tendency to develop new ones with time and such patients should be examined twice yearly. Therapy of these lesions may be beyond the scope of general office practice; such patients are most often treated and followed by dermatologists.

KERATOACANTHOMA

Keratoacanthoma is a rapidly growing tumor with a hard keratotic center (Fig. 97.16). It is not malignant but acts aggressively; local surgery is curative. As it may be confused with squamous cell carcinoma, early biopsy is mandatory.

A myriad of other benign or potentially malignant lesions can appear on the skin; biopsy followed by reassurance or definitive surgery is the usual technique of care.

Malignant Lesions

The most common malignant lesions are *basal cell epithelioma* and *squamous cell epithelioma*, both most frequently occurring in sun-exposed areas but, especially in the case of squamous cell epithelioma, not restricted to those regions. Basal cell epithelioma

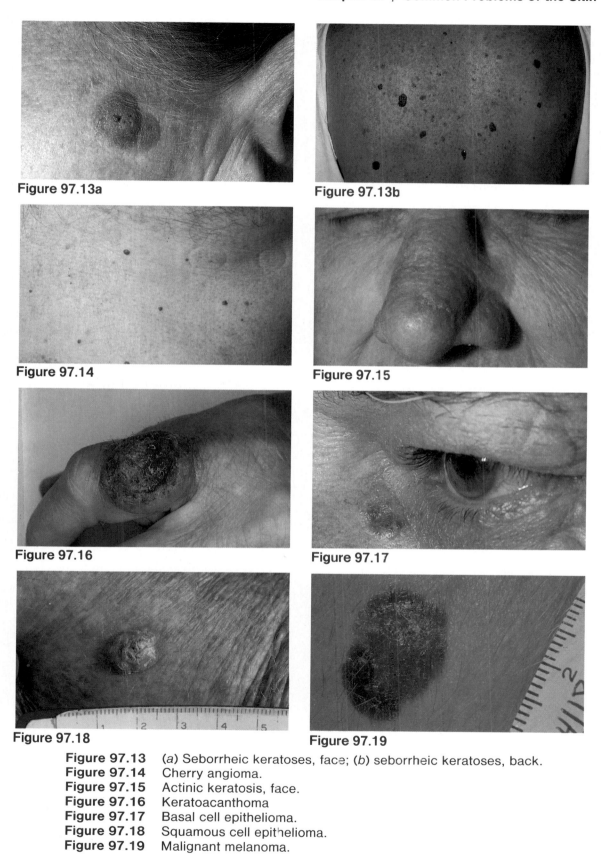

Figure 97.13a

Figure 97.13b

Figure 97.14

Figure 97.15

Figure 97.16

Figure 97.17

Figure 97.18

Figure 97.19

Figure 97.13 (*a*) Seborrheic keratoses, face; (*b*) seborrheic keratoses, back.
Figure 97.14 Cherry angioma.
Figure 97.15 Actinic keratosis, face.
Figure 97.16 Keratoacanthoma
Figure 97.17 Basal cell epithelioma.
Figure 97.18 Squamous cell epithelioma.
Figure 97.19 Malignant melanoma.

typically has a smooth surface often with an area of central atrophy; occasionally the nodule is pigmented (Fig. 97.17). Squamous cell epithelioma is usually a painless, firm, irregular lesion with a smooth or an irregular surface which is often scaling and erythematous (Fig. 97.18). Both are locally destructive and potentially fatal and patients suspected of having either lesion should be referred to a dermatologist or surgeon.

Perhaps as a result of increasing sun exposure in the population, the frequency of malignant melanoma has been on the rise. *Malignant melanoma* (see above, "Nevi") can be rapidly fatal with early metastases and patients suspected of having a malignant melanoma should be referred urgently to a dermatologist or a surgeon. The physician should suspect malignancy in a pigmented lesion if there is variegation of color (blue, red, white, pink, purple, or gray mixed in with the usual brown or tan) or if the border is irregular. Recent growth of a mole or the presence of a halo around a mole also are observations suggestive of malignancy; inspection of suspicious skin lesions by using a hand lens and a good light source is helpful to the physician. An example of a malignant melanoma is shown in Fig. 97.19. Other malignant lesions are less common but there should be little hesitation in referring the patient to a dermatologist or surgeon for biopsy and therapy or primary excision.

References

General

Arndt, KA: *Manual of Dermatologic Therapeutics*, Ed. 2. Little, Brown, Boston, 1978.
　Handbook of therapy including details of usage, tradenames and prices.
Epstein, E: *Common Skin Disorders*. Medical Economics Co., Oradell, N.J., 1979.
　Practical advice including tear-sheets for the patient.
Fitzpatrick, TB, Eisen, AZ, Wolff, K, Freedberg, IM and Austen, KF: *Dermatology in General Medicine*, Ed. 2. McGraw-Hill, New York, 1979.
　Complete reference for the specialist. Does not deal with specifics of therapy.

Specific

1. Ad Hoc Committee Report: Systemic antibiotics for the treatment of acne vulgaris. *Arch Dermatol 111:* 1630, 1975.
2. Belisario, JV: *Cancer of the Skin*. Butterworths, London, 1959.
3. Blalock, WK: Atopic dermatitis; diagnosis and pathobiology. *J Allergy Clin Immunol 57:* 62, 1976.
4. Bjornberg, A and Hellgren, I: Pityriasis rosea. *Acta dermatol venereol 42:* 1, 1962.
5. Champion, RH: Psoriasis and its treatment. *Br Med J 282:* 343, 1981.
6. Editorial: Seborrheic dermatitis. *Br Med J 1:* 436, 1973.
7. Eaglstein, W, Katz, R and Brown, JA: The effects of early corticosteroid therapy in skin eruptions and pain in Herpes zoster. *JAMA 211:* 1681, 1970.
8. Fisher, AA: *Contact Dermatitis*, Ed. 2. Lea & Febiger, Philadelphia, 1973.
9. Knight, V and Noall, NW: Recurrent herpes. *N Engl J Med 294:* 337, 1976.
10. Lever, WF and Schaumburg-Lever, G: *Histopathology of the Skin*, Ed. 5. Lippincott, Philadelphia, 1975.
11. Muller, SA: Alopecia; syndromes of genetic significance. *J Invest Dermatol 60:* 475, 1973.
12. Munro, DD, Vernov, JL, O'Gorman, DJ and Viver, AD: Axillary hyperhidrosis. *Br J Dermatol 90:* 325, 1974.
13. Noble, WC (editor): Microbial skin disease. *Br J Dermatol* (Suppl 8) 1972.
14. Odland, GF and Kraning, KK: Prevalence, morbidity and cost of dermatological diseases. *J Invest Dermatol 73:* 395, 1979.
15. Orkin, M, Epstein, E and Maibach, HI: Treatment of today's scabies and pediculosis. *JAMA 236:* 1136, 1976.
16. Pass, F: Warts, biology and current therapy. *Minn Med 57:* 844, 1974.
17. Plewig, G and Kligman, AM: *Acne Morphogenesis and Treatment*. Springer-Verlag, New York, 1975.
18. Resh, W and Stoughton, RB: Topically applied antibiotics in acne vulgaris. *Arch Dermatol 112:* 182, 1976.
19. Rippon, JW: *Medical Mycology*. W. B. Saunders, Philadelphia, 1974.
20. Roberts, SOB: Tinea versicolor; a clinical and mycological investigation. *Br J Dermatol 81:* 315, 1969.

CHAPTER NINETY-EIGHT

Common Problems of the Teeth and Oral Cavity

DOUGLAS K. MacLEOD, D.M.D.

The purpose of this chapter is twofold: first, to provide the physician with sufficient knowledge to recognize, to treat, and to properly refer patients with acute dental and oral problems; and second, to increase the physician's awareness of chronic dental and oral problems which may require referral and treatment. These types of problems are often neglected by the patient because of fear or ignorance about possible corrective treatment, because of anticipated pain from the procedure, or because of the anticipated cost of treatment.

THE ORAL EXAMINATION

The clinician should examine the oral cavity in a systematic manner. The examination should include lips, cheeks (buccal mucosa), hard and soft palate, salivary ducts (parotid duct orifice in the buccal mucosa opposite the upper second molars and submandibular duct orifice beside the lingual frenulum), tonsillar area, tongue, floor of the mouth, gingiva, and teeth, noting the normal structures and any deviations from normal.

A dental examination includes an evaluation of the number (20 in the primary dentition and 32 in the permanent dentition—see Fig. 98.1), position, and arrangement of the teeth, and a check for caries (see below), erosions, abrasions, and fractures. It is important to examine the gingiva completely. The normal healthy gingiva is firm, pink, free of pain, and does not bleed on palpation. The parts of a tooth and its adjacent structures are shown in Figure 98.2, *A* and *B*.

ACUTE DENTAL AND ORAL PROBLEMS

Toothaches (Pulpitis)

PRESENTATION

Patients with toothache present with a large carious lesion (see "Dental caries", p. 1078), a large restoration (filling), or a combination of both. In the early stages, there is inflammation involving a portion of the pulp tissue (the central portion of the tooth containing vital soft tissue—see Fig. 98.2A). There is relatively severe pain in response to thermal stimuli, particularly to cold, and this pain persists for longer than 15 sec after the stimulus is removed. As the area of inflammation increases, the pain becomes more severe; it may radiate to the suborbital area, to the side of the face, or to the ear. When total necrosis occurs, sensitivity to thermal stimuli is lost. If at this point the inflammatory exudate cannot escape into the oral cavity, the pressure is released via the root apex; and there is exquisite sensitivity to percussion of the crown of the tooth. The signs and symptoms of pulpitis may be confused with pericoronitis (painful wisdom teeth, see below) or periodontitis (see below), and without further diagnostic aids (*i.e.*, dental radiographs) it may be difficult to differentiate between these conditions.

If pulpitis is not treated, *complications* may occur, ranging from a localized alveolar abscess (an abscess of the bony supporting structure of the teeth) to facial cellulitis. The rate and type of complication depend upon the location of the affected tooth, host resistance, and the virulence of the bacteria present.

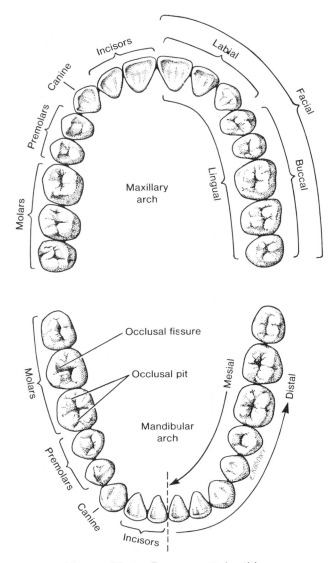

Figure 98.1 Permanent dentition.

TREATMENT

Depending upon the situation when the patient is seen, the physician has three options. For patients who are afebrile and have no extraoral swelling (a swelling producing facial asymmetry) or intraoral swelling (swelling causing disruption of the supporting alveolar bone and soft tissue), analgesics (aspirin 600 mg and codeine 30 mg every 4 hours) and referral within 24 hours are indicated. When either slight extraoral or intraoral swelling, or a low grade temperature elevation is present, antibiotics (penicillin V 250 mg or, for patients allergic to penicillin, erythromycin 250 mg, every 6 hours) should be added, and the patient should be seen by a dentist within 12 to 24 hours. Patients with temperatures greater than 101°F (38.5°C) with intraoral and/or extraoral swelling causing facial asymmetry need immediate consultation and treatment by a dentist. Treatment of these types of problems varies from extraction of the affected tooth, root canal therapy (endodontics), or incision and drainage, to hospital admission for intravenous antibiotics for facial cellulitis.

Pericoronitis (Third Molar or Wisdom Tooth Pain)

PRESENTATION

Pericoronitis is acute inflammation of the tissue around the crown of a partially erupted tooth. Patients presenting with pericoronitis are usually between the ages of 15 and 25 and may give a history of previous subacute episodes of pain of the gingiva partially covering the crown of an incompletely erupted tooth. The tooth most often affected is the mandibular third molar (wisdom tooth). The space between the crown of the tooth and the overyling gingival flap is an ideal area for the accumulation of food and bacteria; this leads to inflammation. The flap is traumatized by contact with the tooth in the opposing jaw, usually the maxillary third molar, and the inflammation is aggravated (see Fig. 98.3A).

The patient describes pain which radiates to the ear, the throat, and the floor of the mouth. He complains of a foul taste, and there is swelling of the affected area so that he cannot close the jaw properly. In severe cases, pain spreading to the oropharynx and base of the tongue make it difficult to swallow. The gingival tissue is markedly red, swollen, and tender. Occasionally, tender lymphadenopathy and

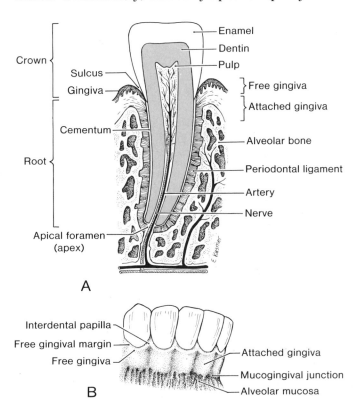

Figure 98.2 Structure of normal teeth and gingiva. (*A*) A tooth and its parts. (*B*) Teeth and gingiva (shows lower incisors and canines).

systemic manifestations (fever, leukocytosis, and malaise) are present. Peritonsillar abscess, cellulitis, and Ludwig's angina (cellulitis of the floor of the mouth) are possible complications.

TREATMENT

In afebrile patients the physician needs only to make a dental referral and to prescribe analgesics. Febrile patients should be treated with antibiotics (penicillin V, 250 mg or, for patients allergic to penicillin, erythromycin 250 mg, every 6 hours) and moderate analgesics (aspirin, 600 mg, and codeine, 30 mg, every 4 to 6 hours). All patients should be seen by a dentist within 24 hours. Depending upon many factors, the dentist will either excise or debride the flap or remove the partially erupted lower tooth. The preferred treatment for third molars which are erupting in a position that produces poor occlusion is to remove the traumatizing maxillary third molar tooth and to allow the infected flap to heal. The mandibular tooth is then removed 7 to 10 days later, after the acute infection has resolved. When pericoronitis involves eruption of third molars which are in good position for occlusion, the inflamed gingival flap is removed and the teeth are left in place.

Acute Necrotizing Ulcerative Gingivitis (ANUG, Vincent's Infection, Trench Mouth)

Acute necrotizing ulcerative gingivitis, or ANUG, may occur at any age, but is more common among young to middle aged adults.

PRESENTATION

ANUG has a sudden onset and is usually associated with a debilitating illness or an acute respiratory infection. Often there is a history of a change in the patient's life; for example, protracted work without rest or recent psychologic stress. There is a fetid mouth odor and the patient describes a foul metallic taste, increased salivation, spontaneous gingival hemorrhage, and pronounced bleeding upon the slightest stimulation. The lesions are extremely sensitive to touch; pain is constant, gnawing, and is intensified by hot or spicy foods. The oral findings are punched out crater-like depressions at the crest of the interdental papillae and/or marginal gingiva. The surface of the gingiva is covered by gray pseudomembranous slough which is demarcated from the gingiva by a pronounced linear erythema (Fig. 98.3B). Patients usually have submandibular lymphadenopathy and slight elevation in temperature; in severe cases, high fever, tachycardia, leukocytosis, loss of appetite, and malaise are seen.

Most investigators believe ANUG is caused by two agents which are normal oral flora: a fusiform bacillus and *Borrelia vincentii*, a spirochete. Histologically, the stratified squamous epithelium of the gingiva is ulcerated and replaced by a thick fibrinous exudate containing many polymorphonuclear leukocytes and microorganisms.

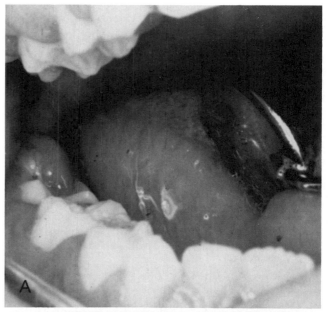

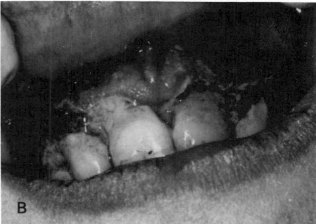

Figure 98.3 (A) Pericoronitis of the mandibular third molar; (B) acute necrotizing ulcerative gingivitis (ANUG).

Complications include destruction of the gingiva and underlying supporting tissues. In rare cases, severe sequelae such as noma (rapid spreading gangrene of oral and facial tissue that occurs in the debilitated and nutritionally deficient patient), fusospirochetal meningitis, peritonitis, pneumonia, bacteremia, and brain abscess have been reported.

TREATMENT

Patients with severe ANUG need immediate hospital admission, intravenous antibiotics, and supportive care (analgesics, hydrogen peroxide mouthwashes) until systemic symptoms subside. Patients with less severe ANUG need immediate attention by a dentist. At this visit, after treatment with a topical anesthetic, a cotton pellet and glyoxide (an oxygenating and foaming agent) are used to remove the pseudomembrane and surface debris. After irrigating with warm water, the superficial calculus is removed. Patients are instructed to avoid tobacco and alcohol, rinse with warm water and 3% hydrogen peroxide every 2 hours, and confine tooth-brushing to the removal of surface debris. When these instructions are followed after effective removal of all irritants by the dentist, a patient usually improves markedly within 5 days. If after the acute phase the patient does not continue periodic dental care, ANUG may recur and lead to eventual tooth loss.

Aphthous Stomatitis (Canker Sore) (4)

Aphthous ulcers occur at some time in 20 to 50% of the adult population, are slightly more common in females, have familial tendencies, and occur most frequently during the winter and spring months.

PRESENTATION

Aphthous stomatitis is characterized by superficial ulcerations on the mucous membranes of the lips, cheek, tongue, floor of the mouth, palate, and gingiva. This condition begins with discrete vesicles that are approximately 2 to 5 mm in diameter and are painful; after 2 days, they rupture and form saucer-like ulcers which consist of a red or grayish-red central portion and an elevated rimlike periphery. There may be a single lesion or multiple ulcers; the etiology is unknown.

The lesions heal spontaneously within 7 to 10 days. As a rule the lesions are larger than those seen in acute herpetic gingivostomatitis (see below) and do not exhibit the diffuse gingival involvement or systemic symptoms seen in that condition.

Aphthous stomatitis occurs in the following forms:
1. *Occasional aphthae* (a single lesion, at intervals from months to years, healing uneventfully).
2. *Acute multiple aphthae* (acute episode persisting for weeks, with lesions rotating to different sites in the mouth, often associated with acute gastrointestinal disorders).
3. *Chronic recurrent aphthae* (one or more lesions always present for a period of years).

TREATMENT

Treatment of aphthae is symptomatic. A mouthwash containing equal parts of Benadryl suspension and Kaopectate is helpful in reducing the pain as is viscous Xylocaine applied by cotton-tip applicator to painful lesions. In more severe cases, tetracycline has been successful in decreasing pain and duration of the ulcers; the patient should be instructed to empty a 250-mg capsule in 50 ml of water and to use this as a rinse followed by swallowing, 3 or 4 times a day for 5 to 7 days. The patient should be encouraged to take sufficient amounts of nonirritating liquids or soft food to maintain hydration and nutrition. Intake may be facilitated by using a straw to prevent contact with the painful ulcers.

Acute Herpetic Gingivostomatitis

Acute herpetic gingivostomatitis occurs most frequently in infants and children below the age of 6 years, and it is observed with equal frequency in males and females. It occasionally occurs in adolescents and adults. Most adults have developed immunity to herpes simplex virus as a result of childhood infection, usually inapparent. Although recurrent acute herpetic gingivostomatitis has been reported, it does not usually recur unless immunity has been altered by a debilitating systemic disease.

PRESENTATION

Acute herpetic gingivostomatitis is an infection of the oral cavity caused by herpes simplex virus. It appears as a diffuse, erythematous, shiny involvement of the gingiva and the adjacent oral mucosa with varying degrees of edema and gingival bleeding. In the initial stage it is characterized by the presence of discrete spherical gray vesicles which may occur on the gingiva, the labial and buccal mucosa, the soft palate, the pharynx, the sublingual mucosa, and the tongue. Within 24 hours the vesicles rupture and form small painful ulcers with a red elevated halo-like margin and a depressed yellowish or grayish white central portion. Regional lymphadenopathy, fever as high as 105°F (40.5°C), and generalized malaise are common. The course is limited to 7 to 10 days and the ulcers heal without scarring.

TREATMENT

There is no specific treatment for herpetic gingivostomatitis. The symptomatic treatments (Benadryl-Kaopectate mouthwash and viscous Xylocaine) and advice regarding nutrition for aphthous stomatitis, summarized in the preceding section, are also useful for herpetic gingivostomatitis.

Herpes Simplex Labialis

Recurrent herpes simplex infections of the lips or perioral area occur in 20 to 40% of the adult population.

PRESENTATION

The natural history of this problem has been well delineated (8). Most affected subjects have several episodes during an average year. In approximately 60% of episodes, there is prodromal tingling for a number of hours before the appearance of the first vesicles. Pain is moderate to severe during the first 24 hours after appearance of vesicles and then rapidly diminishes. After 48 hours, vesicles are usually replaced by ulcer crusts. The process usually resolves after 7 to 9 days, but lesions may persist as long as 2 weeks.

The therapy of this condition is discussed in Chapter 97, "Common Problems of the Skin."

Sialadenitis

PRESENTATION

Sialadenitis is an inflammatory condition of the salivary gland. Patients with either form of sialadenitis (bacterial or obstructive) present with pain and enlargement of the affected gland. In *bacterial* sialadenitis, the pain and swelling are not related to eating. The overlying skin may be red and tense; and the affected gland will yield a purulent discharge at the duct oriface. Bacterial sialadenitis is more common in children than in adults. *Obstructive* sialadenitis is more common than the bacterial condition and is associated with salivary stones or a mucous plug. It occurs most frequently in middle aged males. The involved gland is enlarged and painful, and the symptoms are more prominent before, during, and soon after eating. The submandibular gland is most often affected (75% of cases), whereas the parotid (20% of cases) and major sublingual glands (5% of cases) are less often involved.

TREATMENT

Treatment of bacterial sialadenitis consists of heat application, (external moist heat packs to affected gland for 15 to 20 min and intraoral warm rinses), analgesics (aspirin, 600 mg, and codeine, 30 mg, every 4 to 6 hours), antibiotics (penicillin V, 250 mg or, for patients allergic to penicillin, to erythromycin, 250 mg, every 6 hours for 10 days), and a liquid diet for the first 2 to 3 days.

The management of obstructive sialadenitis is more complex. When this diagnosis is suspected the patient should be referred to a dentist or otolaryngologist. In cases where the stone is lodged in the duct, the acute phase is managed as is the bacterial type after which a sialagram is obtained to determine the extent of the problem. Surgical removal of the stone from the duct is eventually performed to prevent recurrence. In chronic obstructive sialadenitis, surgical excision of the gland is often necessary.

Temporomandibular Joint Pain

Several studies of healthy populations have shown that symptoms of temporomandibular joint (TMJ) disorders are present at some time in 25 to 50% of people, but are not considered a serious problem by most (3). The vast majority (70 to 90%) of patients who present with these symptoms are women between the ages of 24 and 40. Multiple factors may lead to TMJ pain; there may be a history of emotional tension, bruxism (grinding of teeth), external blows to the jaws, or whiplash injury. TMJ pain may be present at some point in 20% of patients with rheumatoid arthritis (5). Patients with osteoarthritis of other joints may complain of TMJ clicking and snapping, but pain is usually absent.

PRESENTATION

Temporomandibular joint disorders are characterized by pain and tenderness in the muscles of mastication and in the TMJ, crepitus when the joint is moved, and a decrease in range of motion. Examination may show malocclusion due to teeth which interfere with the normal movement of the mandible or tenderness of the muscles of mastication.

TREATMENT

Patients with acute TMJ pain should be managed with moderate analgesics (aspirin 600 mg and codeine 30 mg, every 4 to 6 hours) and referral to a dentist within 24 to 48 hours to begin therapy. The dentist's goal will be to make the patient aware of the etiology of his problem through education. Depending upon the severity of symptoms and the state of the patient's dentition, the dentist will prescribe one or a combination of the following: avoidance of excessive jaw motion; moist heat to affected muscles; soft diet; disengagement of upper and lower jaws with a night guard (similar to the mouth guard worn for contact sports); therapeutic exercises; and vapocoolant spray (ethylchloride to decrease muscle pain). In atypical cases, trigger point injections of Xylocaine may be utilized to distinguish TMJ symptoms from trigeminal neuralgia (see Chapter 76). Once the acute episode has subsided (in about 7 to 14 days) the dentist can detect and eliminate any occlusal interferences and rule out any degenerative joint disease which may have predisposed the patient to TMJ symptoms. In the past, injections of sclerosing agents into the TMJ and condylectomy were tried, but with very poor success.

In a 10-year study, 97 of 100 patients treated conservatively improved. Of these, 83 had permanent improvement. Of the 3 patients who had intractable, severe symptoms, 2 required prolonged psychotherapy and 1 developed systemic arteritis (1).

CHRONIC DENTAL AND ORAL PROBLEMS

Periodontal Disease (Pyorrhea)
(Figs. 98.4 and 98.5)

Periodontal disease is a general term used to describe diseases which destroy the gingival and bony structure which support the teeth. Periodontal disease is usually subdivided into *gingivitis* and *periodontitis*. The major difference between the two is that in periodontitis there is loss of the supporting bony apparatus of the teeth.

Two-thirds of young adults, 80% of middle aged adults, and 90% of people in the United States over 65 suffer from periodontal disease (10). Poor oral hygiene, which permits plaque to accumulate on the teeth, is the major etiologic factor. Most periodontal disease, and therefore most loss of teeth, is preventable. Prevention consists of routine plaque control (see below).

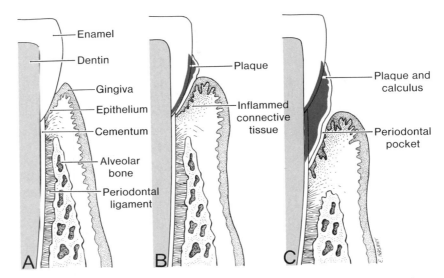

Figure 98.4   Dentogingival junction in health (*A*), gingivitis (*B*), and periodontitis (*C*).

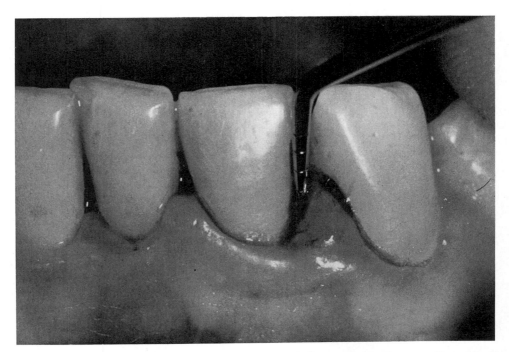

Figure 98.5   Clinical signs of chronic inflammatory periodontal disease including swelling, blunting of interdental papillae, color change, and bleeding upon gentle probing. The patient is a 55-year-old woman with periodontitis. (Reproduced from R. L. Braham and M. E. Morris: *Textbook of Pediatric Dentistry.* Williams & Wilkins, Baltimore, 1980.)

Gingivitis

PRESENTATION

Gingivitis is usually seen in one of four forms: *acute*, a painful condition which has a rapid onset and is of short duration; *subacute*, which is less severe than the acute condition; *recurrent*, which reappears after being eliminated by treatment or after disappearing spontaneously; and *chronic*, the most common form, which has a slow onset, is of a long duration, and is usually painless unless complicated by acute exacerbations (see Fig. 98.5).

The early signs of inflammation of the gingiva which precede frank gingivitis are increased gingival fluid secretions and bleeding from the gingival sulcus upon gentle probing (7). Healthy gingiva is usually "coral pink" whereas in gingivitis the gingiva becomes "bright red" secondary to increased vascularity and a decrease in keratinization. These changes start in the interdental papillae and free gingiva and spread to the attached gingiva. Both acute and chronic forms produce changes in the normally firm, resilient consistency of the gingiva. In acute gingivitis the gingiva has a diffuse edematous appearance, whereas in the chronic form the tissue has a fibrous appearance that pits on pressure.

The development of gingivitis is a consequence of supragingival and subgingival *plaque formation* (see Fig. 98.4). Plaque is a transparent deposit which is composed primarily of bacteria and their by-products. Gram-positive filamentous rods, mainly *Actinomyces*, appear to be of major significance. Small amounts of plaque are not visible unless they are stained. As plaque accumulates, it becomes visible as a mass that varies in color from gray to yellowish gray to yellow. Measurable amounts of plaque may form within 1 hour after a thorough cleaning of the teeth with maximum accumulation in 30 days or less (9). Bacterial plaque, if left undisturbed, will mineralize and form *calculus* (tartar), as shown in Figure 98.4C. This process usually starts between the 1st and 14th day after plaque formation. Calculus is always covered by plaque. When calculus is present, the gingival tissues are unhealthy by definition.

The major *complication* of untreated gingivitis is periodontitis, that is, the extension of the inflammation to the supporting bony structures of the teeth (see below and Fig. 98.4C).

TREATMENT

Patients presenting with any one of the four forms of gingivitis usually require one to three dental visits (spread over a 4-week period) for treatment. The mechanical removal of plaque and calculus from the affected areas of the teeth and gingiva is achieved with the appropriate instruments. After all the plaque and calculus have been removed by the dentist, the disease process is explained to the patient, who is then instructed in proper *plaque control measures,* i.e., effective tooth brushing (a soft bristled tooth brush which facilitates cleansing of the gingiva and the teeth without laceration should be recommended) and effective flossing (the floss should be rubbed vertically up and down 3 to 5 times in each interdental space, once daily). Maintenance of the disease-free state is only possible by continued effective plaque control measures by the patient and by professional cleaning every 6 to 12 months (to remove plaque and calculus that may be missed by brushing and flossing).

Factors which usually result in recurrence are (a) incomplete removal of plaque and calculus, (b) inadequate plaque control because of insufficient patient instruction, (c) premature dismissal of the patient before he demonstrates competence, and (d) lack of patient cooperation.

Periodontitis (see Fig. 98.4C)

PRESENTATION

A patient with periodontitis has red and bleeding gums and an unpleasant taste in his mouth, but he is usually free of pain unless there is an acute infection superimposed upon the underlying chronic process. The principal physical findings are the signs of inflammation of the gingiva described above and periodontal pockets around the teeth from which pus may often be expressed upon gentle pressure. As periodontitis advances, the teeth loosen and spread apart, creating unattractive spaces and exposing the roots of the teeth as the bony support is lost. Mastication is impaired, and spontaneous pain and acute abscess may occur.

The most important consequence of periodontitis is the destruction of the alveolar bone which deprives the teeth of their support and is responsible for the loss of the teeth. The essential steps leading to destruction of bone are gingivitis, degeneration of collagen bundles of the periodontal ligament, and conversion of the shallow (≤3mm) physiologic gingival sulcus to a deepened periodontal pocket (>3mm). As this pocket deepens, more debris accumulates in it; inflammation progresses further inward; and the gums recede permanently. The apically progressing inflammation eventually reaches the alveolar crest, and bone resorption begins. This process continues, resulting in continued destruction of the alveolar bone.

TREATMENT

Most periodontitis can be treated, provided that the diagnosis is made before a significant amount of supporting alveolar bone is lost. The aims of treatment are to preserve the teeth by eliminating the disease, to restore effective function, and to prevent recurrence. When treated in the early stages, the major consequence of periodontitis (loss of bone support for the teeth) can be prevented. If proper treatment is postponed, there may be insufficient bone support once treatment is undertaken and the natural teeth may eventually be lost. Some patients are not concerned with this problem, but are ultimately disappointed when their dentures do not function efficiently.

Treatment of periodontitis is divided into two phases. *Phase I* is similar to the treatment of gingivitis described above—i.e., removal of local irritant (plaque and calculus) and the institution of effective plaque control (continual removal of the plaque). This treatment allows resolution of the inflammation. The success of this phase of therapy depends largely upon the patient's ability to maintain plaque-free teeth (see above under gingivitis). *Phase II* is the surgical phase in which the goal is to improve the gingival architecture which remains in spite of the disease. Experience has shown that patients have difficulty in preventing inflammation in periodontal pockets greater than 5 mm. Surgical treatment is therefore designed to decrease the depths of the pockets.

Denture Problems

Twenty million American adults are missing all of their teeth. Of these, many have obtained dentures. In addition, a large portion of the edentulous population have managed well without teeth, are content to remain as they are, and, regardless of the quality of dentures constructed, are unwilling and/or unable to adapt to using dentures.

PRESENTATION

Often the physician will be confronted with a patient who, although he has had dentures for years, upon specific questioning by the physician indicates that the dentures are not as satisfactory as the patient would wish. The most common denture problems are looseness and discomfort. If the patient is followed at least yearly by his dentist, the physician can generally assume the present situation is the best that can be achieved. On the other hand, if the patient has tolerated the same set of loose or uncomfortable dentures without seeking help for a number of years, he should be encouraged to seek care promptly. Failure to remove dentures at night is the reason for denture problems in some patients. This practice can cause (a) bony erosion with loss of conformity of the dentures to the supporting structures, (b) mucosal ulceration, and (c) oral candidiasis.

TREATMENT

Depending upon the condition of the patient's oral cavity, the present dentures, and the edentulous ridges, a number of treatment modalities are available, including rebasing or relining the existing dentures (5 to 7 days), making a new set of dentures (2 to 5 weeks), and pre-prosthetic correction of soft and hard tissue (4 to 6 weeks healing), followed by relining, rebasing, or remaking of dentures.

Dental Caries

Dental caries is a disease of the calcified tissues of the teeth characterized by demineralization of the inorganic portion (enamel and dentin—see Fig. 98.2*A* of the tooth).

Dental caries is one of the most common diseases of man. It affects all persons regardless of race, location, or economic stratum and it can occur at any age. Poor oral hygiene and a diet high in fermentable carbohydrates promotes caries, whereas routine oral hygiene and raw, coarse foods tend to reduce caries. Ingestion of fluorides in drinking water reduces susceptibility to caries. The form of the tooth affects caries; i.e., the deep pits and fissures on molars and premolars especially predispose these teeth to the disorder.

PRESENTATION

Dental caries usually presents as a nonpainful, white, brown, or black spot on the enamel of a tooth. The most common location is the occlusal surface in conjunction with the pits and fissures of the tooth. Other locations include the mesial and distal smooth surface where the teeth come into contact with each other. Without the aid of special equipment (radiographs and hand instruments) and expertise of dental personnel, the best indicator of dental caries is the presence of brown or black spots in areas associated with lost portions of the tooth.

When caries progresses rapidly to involve the pulp, as in children, the term *acute* caries is used. Slowly progressing caries seen in adults is referred to as *chronic* caries. Occasionally a carious lesion may cease to progress (*arrested* caries). This is due to breakage of enamel walls, thereby exposing the lesion to the cleaning action of the toothbrush, saliva, and mastication. The term *recurrent* caries is used for carious lesions that begin around the margins of defective restorations.

A carious lesion usually develops after bacterial plaque (see above) forms on the tooth surface. The primary bacteria involved in this process are *Streptococcus mutans* and *Lactobacillus acidophilus*. These bacteria metabolize dietary fructose to produce lactic acid, which results in decalcification of the enamel. The rate of development of caries depends upon the susceptibility of the enamel.

TREATMENT

The treatment for most carious lesions is their removal, followed by a restoration (filling) which replaces the lost portions of the tooth. The goals are to remove the lesion, to protect the pulp from irritants, and to restore the tooth to function. In those cases when caries involves a tooth already significantly affected by peridontal disease, the tooth must be removed.

The major *complication* which results from delaying treatment is acute pulpitis and its complications (see above, p. 1071). In addition, delaying of treatment may result in a more difficult restoration or possible loss of the involved tooth. In those cases where the existing decay process is very close to the pulp the heat generated by the rotary instruments used to prepare the restoration may result in a transient pulpal inflammation. This inflammation results in a dull ache in the tooth for 2 to 3 days, which is usually relieved by aspirin. When the restoration process leaves only a paper-thin layer of dentin covering the pulp tissue, the transient pulpitis may be converted to acute pulpitis (irreversible) which then requires either tooth extraction or root canal therapy for relief of pain. Root canal therapy consists of three parts. The removal of the infected nerve tissue, the debridement and preparation of the nerve canal space, and obturation (filling) of the canal space with a biologically inert material.

Angular Cheilosis

PRESENTATION

Angular cheilosis occurs in children but more frequently in adults and is characterized by a feeling of dryness and a burning sensation at the corners of the mouth. The epithelium at the commissures appears wrinkled and macerated. In time, the wrinkles deepen to fissures which appear ulcerated but do not bleed, although a crust may form. These lesions stop at the junction of the mucous membranes. They show a tendency for spontaneous improvement; only rarely do the lesions completely disappear.

There are several etiologies for cheilosis. A number of microorganisms may cause it in otherwise healthy people: *Candida albicans, staphylococci,* and *streptococci.* In addition, angular cheilosis due to overclosure of the jaws may be seen in edentulous patients. Overclosure causes a fold to be produced at the corners of the mouth in which saliva tends to collect, inviting the growth of microorganisms. Angular cheilosis is also seen in riboflavin deficiency, which usually occurs in patients with multiple vitamin deficiencies. The lips show fissures, painful cracks, and scaling; these changes become severe at the corners of the mouth and are similar in appearance to angular cheilosis due to overclosure of the manidible.

TREATMENT

Edentulous patients troubled by angular cheilosis should be referred to a dentist who will evaluate them for mandibular overclosure, as correction of this problem (making or remaking of dentures) may lead to remission. Treatment is otherwise symptomatic and consists of applying petrolatum-containing ointment (e.g., Vaseline, Chapstick) to the scaling area to minimize discomfort.

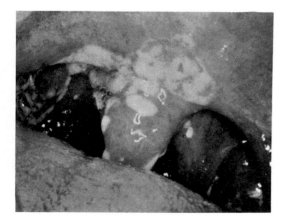

Figure 98.6 Candidiasis (thrush) of soft palate and uvula. The white plaques resemble milk curds. (Reproduced from R. L. Braham and M. E. Morris: *Textbook of Pediatric Dentistry.* Williams & Wilkins, Baltimore, 1980.)

Thrush (Oral Candidiasis)

PRESENTATION (Fig. 98.6)

The typical lesions of oral candidiasis are white, curd-like plaques on an erythematous mucosa. These plaques are loosely attached and may be scraped off of the oral mucosa. They begin as pinpoint spots. Involvement may include the corners of the mouth, as noted in the previous section. The tongue is often reddened and the patient describes a burning sensation.

Thrush may occur chronically in patients with poor oral hygiene and poor nutrition. It may also be brought on or exacerbated by debilitating systemic illness, antibiotic therapy, use of steroids or antimetabolites, or dental extraction. Thrush does not appear to be more common in diabetics.

The white plaques of thrush may suggest hyperkeratosis or leukoplakia. In these instances, a scraping will reveal hyphae and blastospores when the condition is candidiasis.

TREATMENT

The patient should be advised to follow good oral hygiene practices. Specific treatment consists of nystatin oral suspension, 4 to 6 ml held in the mouth for several minutes before swallowing, 4 times daily. Thrush usually resolves entirely after 1 to 2 weeks of treatment. Treatment should be continued for several days after visible lesions have disappeared.

Halitosis

PRESENTATION

Halitosis is a foul or offensive odor emanating from the oral cavity. Mouth odors originate from local or remote sites. The local causes can be retention of odoriferous food particles on or between the teeth, acute necrotizing ulcerative gingivitis, dehydration, caries, chronic periodontal disease, dentures, tobacco smoking, and healing of surgical or extraction wounds. Extraoral causes of halitosis include infection in adjacent structures (rhinitis, sinusitis, tonsillitis), pulmonary infections, alcoholic breath, the acetone odor of the diabetic, or the uremic breath associated with renal failure.

TREATMENT

Local causes of this condition are treated by improvement in oral hygiene and by specific treatment of the underlying conditions. If these measures are unsuccessful, pleasant smelling mouthwashes or breath fresheners used frequently (every 2 to 4 hours) may greatly reduce the problem. Halitosis due to remote factors may be masked with mouthwashes and fresheners until the remote problem has been resolved.

Common Tongue Conditions

GEOGRAPHIC TONGUE (Fig. 98.7A).

Benign migratory glossitis or geographic tongue is an asymptomatic inflammatory condition consisting

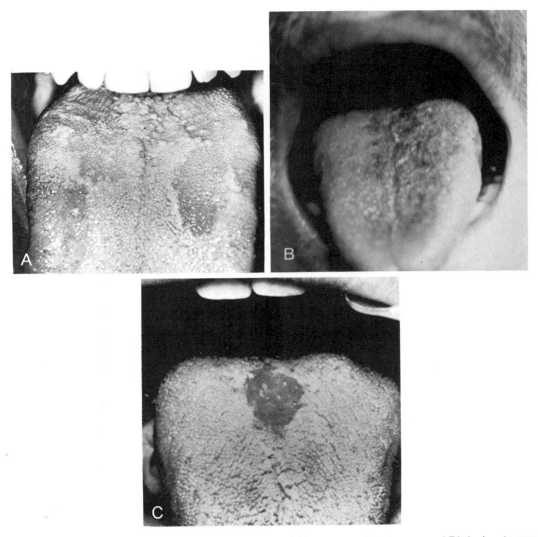

Figure 98.7 Common benign problems of the tongue: (*A*) geographic tongue, (*B*) hairy tongue, and (*C*) median rhomboid glossitis.

of multiple areas of desquamation of the filiform papillae of the tongue in an irregular pattern. The central portion of an affected area is usually denuded, while the border may be outlined by a thin yellowish white line or band. The fungiform papillae persist in the desquamated area as small elevated red dots. The areas of desquamation remain for a short time in one location, then heal and reappear in other locations. The condition may persist for weeks or months and then regress, only to recur at a later date. Women are affected twice as often as men and there is no racial difference. Since the etiology is unknown and the condition is benign, management consists of reassurance. Large doses of vitamins are not effective.

HAIRY TONGUE (98.7*B*)

Hairy tongue is a condition characterized by hypertrophy of the filiform papillae of the tongue due to the lack of normal desquamation of the keratin layer. This results in a thick, matted layer on the dorsum of the tongue. The color of the papillae varies

from yellowish white to brown or even black depending upon their staining by extrinsic factors (tobacco, foods, or medications). The hypertrophied tissue may touch the palate and produce gagging in some patients. The majority of patients with hairy tongue are heavy smokers, but the etiology is unknown. Treatment of this benign condition is to brush the tongue with a tongue blade or toothbrush to promote desquamation and remove debris.

MEDIAN RHOMBOID GLOSSITIS (Fig. 98.7*C*)

Median rhomboid glossitis is a congenital abnormality of the tongue which appears clinically as an ovoid, diamond, or rhomboid shaped reddish patch on the dorsal surface of the tongue. On examination, there is a slightly raised or flat area which is distinctive because there are no filiform papillae. Despite its name, this abnormality is not inflammatory; it is due to failure of the tuberculum impar to retract before fusion of the lateral halves of the tongue, so that a structure free of papillae is interposed. The prevalence of the abnormality is less than 1% and there are no sex or racial differences. The only clinical significance of this innocuous condition is that it is occasionally mistaken for a carcinoma; differentiation from cancer is aided by a history of the presence of the lesion since childhood and by the fact that a carcinoma rarely develops on the dorsum of the tongue.

Leukoplakia and Erythroplakia

PRESENTATION

Leukoplakia and erythroplakia are asymptomatic conditions of the oral mucosa which may become malignant.

Leukoplakia varies in appearance from a grayish white flattened scaly lesion to a thick, irregularly shaped plaque (see Fig. 98.8). Histologically, there is hyperkeratosis, acanthosis, and some degree of dyskeratosis. It is commonly associated with underlying inflammation due to a chronic irritant (tobacco, alcohol, poorly constructed dentures). Leukoplakia may be found anywhere in the oral cavity but most frequently it is found in the buccal mucosa, followed, in descending order, by the alveolar mucosa, tongue, lip, hard and soft palates, floor of mouth, and gingiva.

Erythroplakia refers to a lesion which is velvety red in appearance, small (2 cm or less), and with or without a hyperkeratotic component. It is found in the floor of the mouth, soft palate, and ventrolateral border of the tongue.

The significance of these lesions has been delineated in a longitudinal study of mucosal lesions (6). Of 200 white lesions biopsied only 4 were malignant. In the same study, an erythroplastic component was present in 90% of the 158 asymptomatic malignant squamous cell lesions which were found, suggesting, but not proving, that erythroplakia may be an important precusor of squamous cell cancer.

TREATMENT

It is impossible to determine which lesion showing leukoplakia or erythroplakia will undergo malignant transformation. Discontinuance of chronic irritants is recommended, followed by a 14-day observation period to allow inflammatory lesions to heal. If the lesion persists, referral to a dental surgeon for a biopsy is indicated. The biopsy procedure is as simple as having a restoration (filling) or a tooth extraction.

Other conditions which may resemble leukoplakia or erythroplakia are lichen planus, chemical burns, moniliasis, psoriasis, lupus erythematosus, and syphilitic mucous patches. Each of these has characteristic histologic features.

Squamous Cell Carcinoma (see Fig. 98.9)

Squamous cell carcinoma represents over 90% of all malignant tumors of the oral cavity. It is 4 times more common in men than women and is most common after the fourth decade. In the United States oral cancer is the 8th most common form of cancer in men and 12th in women. Fifteen thousand new cases are found each year, and about 7500 patients die of this disease annually. Of lip carcinomas, 95% occur on the lower lip and appear as an ulcer, wart, sore, or scale. This lesion is more frequent in fair skinned individuals. Of the intraoral carcinomas, 50% occur on the tongue (usually ventrolateral border) and 16% on the floor of the mouth; the remaining 34% are equally distributed between the gingival mucosa, palate, and buccal mucosa. Sixty percent of intraoral

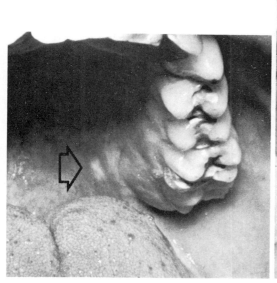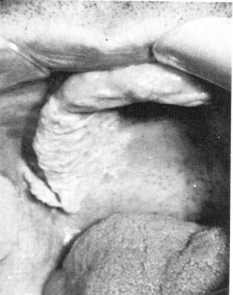

Figure 98.8 Leukoplakia. (*Left*) Small, discrete area on palate in a pipe smoker, resulting from smoke and heat emitted at this area. (*Right*) Diffuse leukoplakia of an edentulous dental ridge in 45-year-old man who smokes 15 cigars per day. (Reprinted from J. Giunta: *Oral Pathology*. Williams & Wilkins, Baltimore, 1975.)

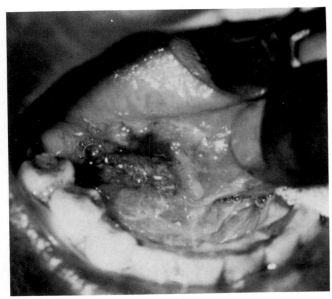

Figure 98.9   Squamous cell carcinoma of the floor of the mouth.

carcinomas present as ulcers, 30% as growths, and the remaining 10% as white lesions or other abnormalities of the mucosa (2). Carcinoma of the tongue and floor of the mouth metastasizes early and carries a very poor prognosis.

The etiology of oral carcinoma is unknown. Ill-fitting dentures, actinic radiation, smoking, jagged teeth, syphilitic glossitis, and alcoholism are believed to play a role.

PRESENTATION AND EVALUATION

Patients usually give a history of knowledge of the sore for 6 to 18 months when they first present; for many reasons they have not sought evaluation. All patients with suspicious lesions should be referred promptly to a dental surgeon for biopsy. Biopsy is a simple procedure, not very different from having a restoration or tooth extraction; usually it is done under local anesthesia. Definitive surgery is a team effort between the otolaryngologist and the dentist. The dentist's role is to evaluate, for long term prognosis, any of the teeth which are *not* to be removed in the surgical field and to remove any of these teeth that are affected with untreatable periodontitis; this

is done to avoid later osteoradionecrosis, a condition seen in the postradiation patient in whom the socket of an extracted tooth fails to heal as the result of diminished blood supply.

TREATMENT

The definitive treatment for oral carcinomas is excision, with or without radiotherapy. Lip tumors have the highest success rate (10-year cure rate between 80 and 92%), while only one-fifth of patients with tongue cancer live longer than 5 years.

Reference

General

Bhaskar SN: *Synopsis of Oral Pathology*, Ed. 4, C. V. Mosby, St. Louis, 1973.
    Valuable reference text of oral pathology.
Carronza, FA (editor): *Glickman's Clinical Periodontology*, Ed. 5. W.B. Saunders, Philadelphia 1979.
    Excellent text for discussion of periodontal disease and related problems.

Specific

1. Apfelberg, DB, Lavey, E, Janetos, G, Maser, MR and Lash, H: Temporomandibular joint disease: results of a ten year study. *Postgrad Med 65:* 167, 1979.
2. Bhaskar, SN: *Synopsis of Oral Pathology*, Ed 4, p. 463. C. V. Mosby, St. Louis, 1973.
3. Franks, AS: The social character of temporomandibular joint dysfunction. *Dent Pract Dent Rec 15:* 94, 1964.
4. Graykowski, EA, Barile, MF, Lee, WB and Stanley, HR, Jr: Recurrent aphthous stomatitis; clinical, therapeutic, histopathologic, and hypersensitivity aspects. *JAMA 196:* 637, 1966.
5. Helkimo, M: Epidemiological surveys of dysfunction of the mastication system. In *Oral Sciences Reviews: Temporomandibular Joint Function and Dysfunction III*, edited by AH Meicher and GA Zarb. Munksgaard, Copenhagen, 1976.
6. Mashberg, A, Morrissey, JB and Garfinkel, L: A study of the appearance of early asymptomatic oral squamous cell carcinoma. *Cancer 32:* 1436, 1973.
7. Mühlemann, HR and Son, S: Gingival sulcus bleeding—a leading symptom in initial gingivitis. *Helv Odentol Acta 15:* 107, 1971.
8. Spruance, SL, Overall, JC, Kern, ER, Krueger, GG, Plaim, V and Miller, W: The natural history of recurrent herpes simplex labialis; implications for antiviral therapy. *N Engl J Med 297:* 69, 1977.
9. Thenard, JC, Hefflin, CM and Steinberg, AI: Neuraminidase activity in mixed culture supernatant fluids of human oral bacteria. *J Bacteriol 89:* 924, 1965.
10. United States Department of Health, Education and Welfare, Public Health Service: *Research Explores Pyorrhea and Other Gum Diseases: Periodontal Disease*, (PHS Publication 1482). Government Printing Office, Washington, D.C., 1970.

CHAPTER NINETY-NINE

Common Problems of the Feet

BRUCE S. LEBOWITZ, D.P.M.

The internist or family physician is often called upon to treat patients who complain of problems with their feet, either as a primary care provider or in conjunction with a podiatrist. Although disorders of the feet are not life-threatening, they should not be taken lightly. Any patient with a painful foot will attest that his pain can and does take the joy out of living.

STRUCTURE AND FUNCTION

The abnormal foot cannot be understood unless the structure of the foot and its function during gait are understood.

Normal Gait (see Fig. 99.1, *A* and *B*)

The bones and joints of the feet facilitate walking and running in an upright position. The foot and leg function together to allow a smooth, even transfer of weight as one extremity moves ahead of the other. During gait, the foot first adjusts to a variable terrain, and then acts to propel the body's weight forward.

In the *first stage of gait*, the heel strikes the ground and body weight begins to move distally over the lateral aspect of the foot. The foot is in a *pronated* position, meaning that the arch is relatively flattened. In effect, the foot resembles a "loose bag of bones" during this stage, permitting it to adapt to the terrain and to act as a shock absorber when body weight strikes the ground.

In the *second stage of gait*, as weight moves distally to the ball of the foot and the body is propelled forward, the foot must convert to a rigid lever. This conversion, or *supination*, takes place in the subtalar and midtarsal joints. Supination serves to heighten the arch, pushing the bones and joints of the foot together rigidly enough to propel body weight forward efficiently.

For the lower extremity to function normally, certain structural criteria must be met; if they are not met, compensation will occur. Ideally, the leg should be in a plane perpendicular to the foot and ground, as in a stick figure drawing. The forefoot should be in a plane parallel to the rearfoot; but various congenital factors may act to prevent this normal angulation. A varus (toward the midline or inverted) or valgus (away from midline or everted) position of the forefoot or hindfoot are the most common of these congenital factors.

Excessive Pronation

Excessive pronation—pronation extended through too much of the gait cycle—is the most common compensating mechanism when structural abnormalities are present. When the foot remains pronated during gait, and does not resupinate in time, or at all, the condition known as "flatfoot" exists. The degree of this flatfoot position reflects the degree of pronation that is present. A number of problems may evolve from excessive pronation during gait—among them bunions, calluses, and hammertoes. As pointed out in the discussion of these conditions which follows, assessment of the mechanical basis for the condition is important in planning appropriate treatment for it.

Shoe Gear

Shoe gear clearly plays a role in the way feet function. Shoes protect feet from the elements, cushion the effect of walking on hard, flat surfaces, and provide some support to the bones and ligaments. Unfortunately, many individuals favor short, narrow shoes, high heels, and pointed toes. Obviously, squeezing a basically rectangular foot into a triangular shoe with the feet elevated from 2 to 5 inches creates significant stress for the foot. Most of the disorders of the foot discussed in this chapter are intensified by these demands of fashion.

Most people, in fitting themselves for shoes, do not take into account the variations in their foot size

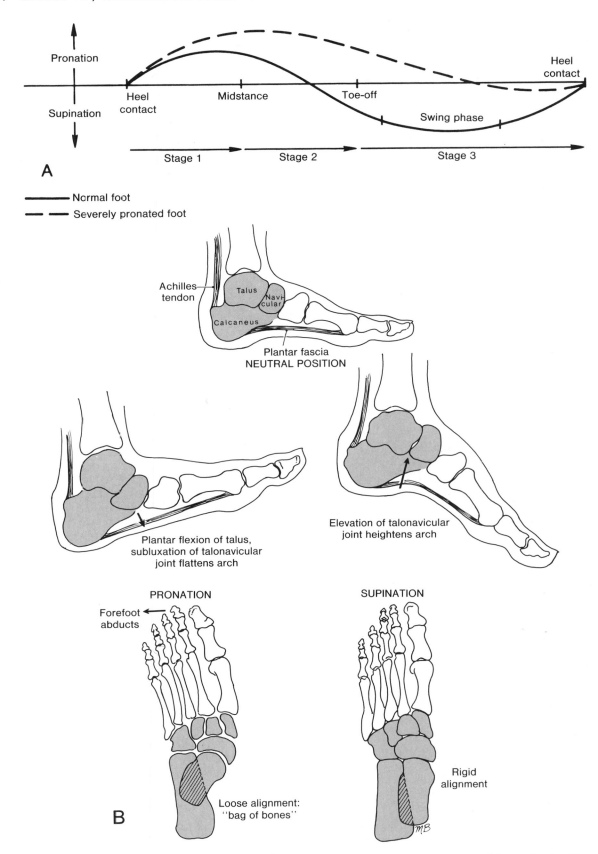

Figure 99.1 (*A*) Schematic representation of the gait cycle for a normal foot and for a foot with excessive pronation. (*B*) Schematic illustration of foot structure during pronation and supination.

throughout the day and the variation in shoe size from manufacturer to manufacturer. Therefore, the following advice is often helpful: buy shoes in the late afternoon when any swelling that might occur is already present; try to buy shoes in stores that also have an active trade in infant shoes, as shoe fitters for infants are experienced in fitting the shoe to the foot and not vice versa; light weight shoes are preferable to heavy ones; and, finally, leather, because it is more porous, is preferable to synthetic materials in shoe construction.

Interest in *shoe gear related to sports*, especially to jogging and running, has escalated in recent years. Sneakers or running shoes should be well-fitted and firm enough to prevent excessive splaying of the foot during activity. For shock absorption, the shoes should have studded soles; and there should be a raised, resilient heel wedge. The midsole should be flexible to help prevent Achilles tendon stress, and there should be a well-molded Achilles pad to prevent irritation of the tendon. The tongue should be well-padded to prevent irritation of the dorsum of the foot. These features are illustrated in Figure 99.2.

It is a misconception that wearing sneakers excessively will harm the feet. Actually, the better running shoes available today are so supportive and well-padded that they may be prescribed for numerous painful foot conditions. For example, highly arched feet (which are supinated and may pronate only slightly) lack shock-absorbing qualities; and constant impact on the ground can cause severe metatarsal, heel, and arch pain. For patients with this condition, the support and resiliency provided by a modern running shoe is ideal. Likewise, a flat or pronated foot may be very well supported by the built-in arch supports of well-made running shoes.

Running magnifies the problems associated with excessive pronation, and the long term management of runners with this condition requires the selection of shoes which provide good support. The use of well-designed running shoes is important in preventing most exercise-related injuries of the lower extremity as explained in Chapter 64, "Exercise-related Musculoskeletal Syndromes."

PREVENTIVE FOOT CARE FOR PATIENTS WITH DIABETES AND ARTERIAL INSUFFICIENCY

Prevention and early detection of problems on the surface of the foot are particularly important in patients with these conditions. This requires periodic examination by the physician and routine examination by the patient. The single most important advice that can be impressed upon the patient is to look at his feet every day. When obesity or lack of visual acuity is a problem, someone else should examine the patient's feet every day. Irritations, abrasions, and calluses which usually produce pain must be identified visually when there are sensory abnormalities in the feet. Advice about selection of shoe gear (see above) should be provided routinely to patients with diabetes and vascular insufficiency. By following these procedures, most serious foot ulcers and infections can be prevented.

These patients should also be advised not to utilize over-the-counter corn and ingrown toenail remedies. Such commercial preparations include acids and tanning agents which can seriously injure the tender skin of these patients. Normal toenails should be allowed to grow past the end of the fleshy part of the toe; thick nails are best handled by a podiatrist as are corns and calluses (see below). Soft cotton should be worn between toes which tend to rub each other, and talcum powder should be used to prevent interdigital moisture and maceration.

BUNIONS (see Fig. 99.3, *A–D*)

Definition and Pathogenesis

Bunion (literally "turnip") is a term used by laymen and physicians to describe the collective deformities of the first metatarsophalangeal joint. These deformities include enlargement of the medial, medial-dorsal, or dorsal aspect of the first metatarsophalangeal joint and lateral deviation of the great toe. The enlargement of the joint may consist of bone, or soft tissue, or a combination of the two.

For many years, tight fitting shoes were mistakenly considered to be the cause of bunions. It is known now that, while the pressure of tight shoes on an existing bunion can certainly result in pain which calls attention to the problem, bunions are not caused by poorly fitted shoes. The chief cause of the deformity is a hypermobile first metatarsal bone most often related to excessive pronation (see above). The first metatarsal and great toe, which help propel body weight forward, should be quite stable during the final stage of gait when a tight, rigid bony structure

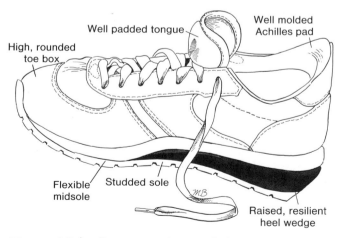

Figure 99.2 Features of a well-designed running shoe.

High, rounded toe box

Well padded tongue

Well molded Achilles pad

Flexible midsole

Studded sole

Raised, resilient heel wedge

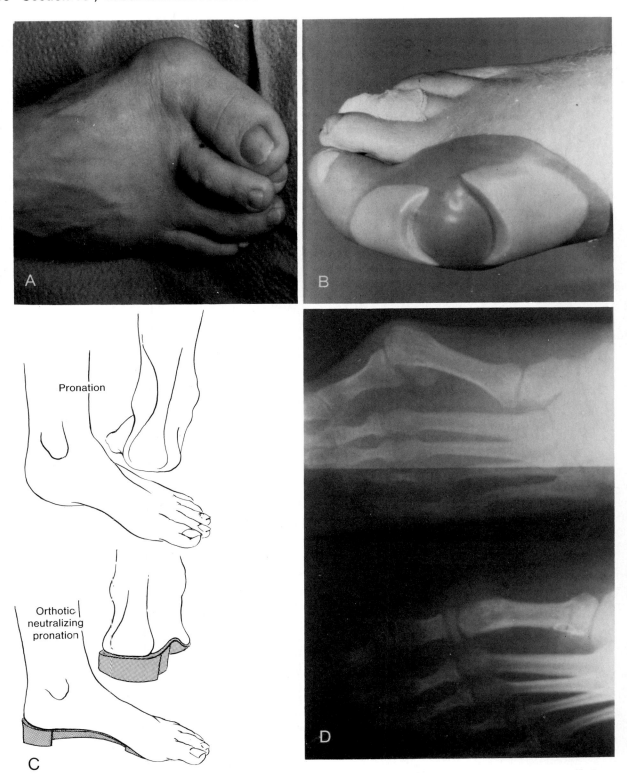

Figure 99.3   Bunions: appearance, orthotic compensation, and surgical repair. (A) Bunion deformity, (B) bunion protected by latex shield, (C) leather orthotic arch support, and (D) bunion deformity shown radiologically before and after surgical correction.

is needed. The intrinsic and extrinsic musculature should help to hold the metatarsal tight at this point. When there is excessive pronation, the entire foot remains loose and relatively unstable. One result of

such laxity in this stage of gait is the hypermobility of the first metatarsal and the "buckling" of the first toe: intrinsic and extrinsic muscles cause the first metatarsal to deviate medially and the great toe to deviate laterally. The combined deformity is called *hallux abducto valgus.* Eventually, arthritic hypertrophy of the head of the first metatarsal bone develops.

Symptoms

The presenting complaint of a patient with a bunion is pain localized to the first metatarsophalangeal joint. Pressure of the shoe on the enlarged metatarsal head, with or without pressure on adventitious bursa, can cause pain that is severe and even disabling; pain can also result from the joint motion itself. Often, crepitus can be felt within the joint. Sometimes the patient seeks help, not because of pain, but because he is unable to wear shoes as a result of the deformity.

In evaluating a patient, the physician must be certain that the symptoms are a result of the bunion alone. Gout (see Chapter 66) may not only produce acute pain in the first metatarsophalangeal joint, but may also aggravate a chronically painful joint. Therefore, gout should always be considered, especially in patients with bilateral bunion deformity and acute monoarticular pain in a foot.

Management

Acute symptoms due to a bunion should be managed with rest, elimination of pressure on the bunion, soaks in warm water, and systemic anti-inflammatory medication such as aspirin, 600 mg every 4 to 6 hours. After the acute symptoms have subsided, the patient should be started on a program of long term management.

Conservative long term management of a bunion involves accommodating the deformity and attempting to arrest its progress. This is achieved by the use of molds and protective shields (see Fig. 99.3, *B* and *C*). A mold, usually referred to as an arch support, may be made from various types of materials to accommodate the plantar aspect of the foot. Protective shields are made of latex rubber.

Full foot molds or protective shields made by a podiatrist from a plaster impression are preferable to commercially made devices found in pharmacies and shoe stores. Commercial devices are manufactured to fit average shoe and foot sizes and do not take into account the shape of the individual patient's foot. The mold should be in place during the fitting of all new shoes. Occasionally, if the mold makes conventional shoes too tight, a specially built shoe, called an extra depth-inlay shoe, may be used. These enlarged shoes have a removable insole, for which one may substitute the patient's mold. The mold and shoes should minimize pressures against the bunion. In addition, the mold acts to reduce excessive pronation, thereby reducing the deforming forces in the forefoot.

Patients whose bunion symptoms are not adequately controlled with conservative measures should be considered for surgery. The *surgical management* of a bunion must be individually planned for each patient, and in fact, for each foot, to correct the specific deformity (3). Correction might involve resection of the bony protuberance of the first metatarsal head only. In occasional patients with severe degenerative joint disease surgical management involves removal of all or part of the joint and insertion of a silastic joint replacement (see Fig. 99.3 *D*). Depending on locale, referral for surgical correction of a bunion may be made to a general, orthopaedic, or podiatric surgeon. A patient should expect to return to most of his preoperative activities within 6 to 8 weeks following bunion surgery; the interval may be somewhat longer after bilateral surgery. A tendency for the foot to swell postoperatively may persist for many months, however. Excessive pronation, the primary cause for bunion, persists after surgery. Therefore a major determinant of the long term results of surgery is follow-up foot care with orthotic appliances such as those described above.

Prevention

The annoying symptoms of bunion deformity may be prevented altogether if the physician recognizes the deformity early (usually in the second or third decade) and refers the patient for conservative management by a podiatrist.

CALLUSES AND CORNS (see Fig. 99.4)

Definition and Pathogenesis

A *callus* is a thickening of the epidermis as a result of chronic intermittent trauma. When there is intermittent irritation of an area of skin, the initial response is vasodilation; this is followed by increased production of corneum and hyperkeratosis. This process is normal and protective to skin and underlying tissue. When the process continues until there is build up of excessive or highly concentrated callus, resulting in a *corn*, problems may develop. Skin lines may remain visible in callused tissue, but they usually do not pass through the highly concentrated center of a corn. Corns are most frequently located overlying the proximal interphalangeal joints of the lesser toes and centrally within plantar calluses. A number of processes not related to chronic trauma can produce focal calluses as well, namely *verruca plantaris* (plantar wart), foreign body granuloma, and *porokeratosis plantaris discreta.* These lesions are discussed below (p. 1089).

The primary cause for most symptomatic calluses is excessive pronation (see above, p. 1083) and not restrictive shoes or walking on unyielding surfaces. During excessive pronation, the long flexor and extensor tendons pull on the distal phalanges, the toes appear to "hammer," and a retrograde force pushes down on the metatarsal heads, increasing pressure on the plantar skin. Other conditions which may promote this increased pressure are excessive supination (highly arched foot) and imbalance of the peroneal and tibial muscles due to weakness, arthritis, or other conditions affecting one or both legs.

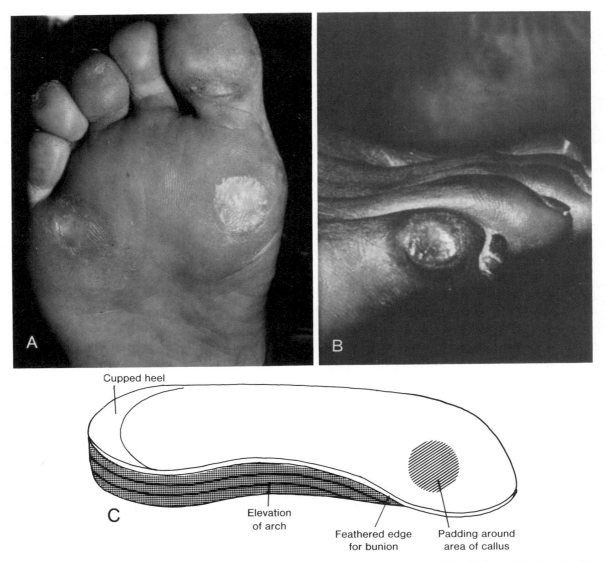

Figure 99.4 Calluses and corns. (*A*) Typical plantar callus, (*B*) corn on the fifth digit, and (*C*) orthotic device designed to shift weight from area of callus formation. (Photographs courtesy of Max Weisfeld, D.P.M.)

Symptoms

Diffuse callus is usually asymptomatic and easily controlled by the patient with pumice stones and cleansing agents readily available in pharmacies. Both calluses and corns produce pain. Thick accumulation of callus tends to cause a burning sensation in the foot. A corn located within a plantar callus gives the sensation of walking on a sharp pebble. Corns which occur dorsolaterally on fifth toes (Fig. 99.4*B*) often cause exquisite pain, especially with tight fitting shoes. Such corns often have adventitious bursae associated with them and may produce symptoms due both to bursitis and to the discomfort of the corn pressing down on subcutaneous tissues.

While corns and calluses can cause discomfort for the average person, they can cause serious morbidity in a *diabetic patient*. If hyperkeratotic lesions on an extremity are added to a diabetic's lowered resistance to infection, circulatory impairment, and decreased perception of pain, there is a clear potential for serious problems. A discrete lesion on the foot produces constant pressure on the underlying dermis. It is not unusual for this pressure, in a diabetic, to result in local breakdown of tissues, ulceration, and infection. Diabetics have the additional medical and mechanical problem of neurotrophic joints. In patients with the tendency to develop hammertoe and plantar flexed metatarsal heads, these changes (and the calluses and corns which accompany them) may be accelerated by the loss of normal proprioception and pain sensation of a neurotrophic joint.

Corns and calluses can be a serious problem also for patients with conditions other than diabetes which impair arterial circulation to the lower extremities (see Chapter 84).

Treatment

Treatment of corns and calluses depends upon the location, severity, and type of lesion and upon the physical condition of the patient.

The physician will occasionally see patients who complain of severely painful corns and calluses. Dramatic relief may be obtained from the simple debridement of these very painful lesions, using a sterile No. 10 or No. 15 scalpel blade. If the blade is kept nearly parallel to the skin, injury to the underlying healthy dermis can be avoided. There is no need to debride the entire callus; any reduction in the thickness of the lesion will bring relief to the patient.

Conservative long term management of corns and calluses in the feet of otherwise healthy people requires the control of the source of the problem, namely excessive pronation. If excessive pronation is neutralized with orthotic devices (see above), foot function is improved, pathologic forces are decreased, and lesions may regress. Lesions which have been present for a year or longer usually indicate that there have already been structural changes in the bones and joints, as well as histopathologic changes in the skin.

For patients whose symptoms are not controlled with conservative treatment, *surgery* may be very helpful. A number of surgical procedures may be used to realign metatarsal heads, or to reduce hammertoe deformities. Often it is necessary to combine the surgical reconstruction of affected areas with control of pronation in order to achieve lasting resolution of symptoms. This may mean 6 to 8 weeks of convalescence after foot surgery and the continued use of orthotics in shoes. The end result, however, is greater foot health and comfort.

For the patient with *diabetes or peripheral vascular disease*, conservative treatment involves frequent debridement of the hyperkeratotic areas, padding for protection, and the fabrication of molds (by a podiatrist or orthopaedist) to shift weight away from problem areas and to accommodate deformities (see Fig. 99.4C). Extra depth shoes are often prescribed in conjunction with such appliances. When refractory infection or ulceration occurs despite conservative management, surgical procedures may be performed to eliminate a bony prominence. Surgery may return a bedridden patient to his feet or eliminate the need for future amputation. The management of this type of patient requires close collaboration between the patient's physician and the consultant.

OTHER HYPERKERATOTIC LESIONS (see Fig. 99.5, *A* and *B*)

Other discrete hyperkeratotic lesions commonly found on the foot include *verruca plantaris, porokeratosis plantaris discreta,* and *foreign body granuloma.*

Verruca plantaris, or plantar warts, occur on the plantar aspect of the foot, usually on weight-bearing surfaces (Fig. 99.5A). They are discussed also in Chapter 97, "Common Problems of the Skin," but a

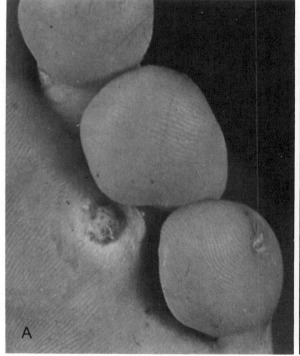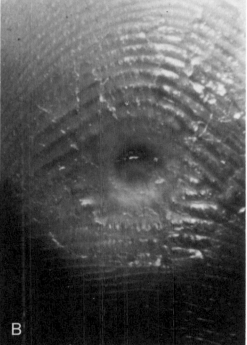

Figure 99.5 Hyperkeratotic lesions not due to chronic trauma. (*A*) Plantar wart and (*B*) porokeratosis. (Photographs courtesy of Max Weisfeld, D.P.M.)

brief account is provided here because of the importance of differentiating them from corns, calluses, and other hyperkeratotic lesions. Plantar warts can be asymptomatic or extremely painful. They are caused by a papilloma virus for which there is no specific treatment or prevention. Because they are benign and often resolve spontaneously, aggressive or untried therapies should be avoided.

The appearance of a verrucous lesion is illustrated in Figure 99.5A. They may vary in size from 1 mm to 1 cm. The lesions can be differentiated from hyperkeratotic corns in several ways: warts usually have rough surfaces, are painful with both surface and lateral pressure, and bleed upon debriding because of their capillary supply; corns are usually smooth surfaced, most painful with surface pressure, and do not bleed upon debridement.

The treatment of plantar warts is discussed in Chapter 97, "Common Problems of the Skin."

A *porokeratotic lesion* is a circumscribed, discrete hyperkeratotic lesion on the plantar aspect of the foot which develops as a result of keratin occluding a sweat duct in the skin (see Fig. 99.5B). The obstruction and resultant backup create a reaction in the skin similar to a deep, large corn. This lesion need not be under a weight-bearing surface. It is usually very painful, and after debridement there is characteristically even more distress. Treatment by the dermatologist or podiatrist is usually by local curettage.

Foreign bodies in the plantar surface of the foot can generate a local inflammatory reaction and thus create a hyperkeratotic lesion. One of the most common offending substances is hair (animal or human). For example, a dog hair, trapped in a carpet long enough to have dried out, can penetrate the skin rather easily. This lesion, while grossly resembling a simple callus, will, upon examination with a magnifying glass, have a small aperture (entry wound) near the center. The local reaction may or may not include infection. Treatment is simple excision of the foreign body.

NAIL CONDITIONS

There are only two nail conditions which are frequently brought to medical attention: onychomycosis (fungal infection) and ingrown toenails, with or without concomitant inflammation (paronychia).

Onychomycosis (2) (see Fig. 99.6)

ETIOLOGY AND FINDINGS

The typical fungal infection of a toenail begins distally at the tip of the toe and moves proximally, subungually, and through the nail plate itself. Etiologic agents are *Trichophyton mentagrophytes, Trichophyton rubrum,* or *Candida albicans.* The fungus produces yellowish discoloration and longitudinal striations in the nails and in the epidermis; the accompanying local inflammatory reaction stimu-

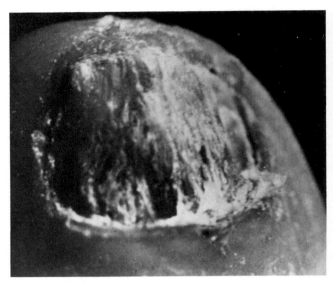

Figure 99.6 Mycotic toenail.

lates hyperkeratosis under the nail. This hyperkeratotic accumulation tends to lift the nail up from the epidermis, facilitating further progression of the fungus. Eventually, the nail becomes brownish yellow, mottled, thickened, and powdery. Usually these infections are asymptomatic; patients are most concerned about the appearance of their nails, the possibility of spread of infection, and sometimes the inability to wear shoes when severe thickening of the nail plate is present.

TREATMENT

Fungus infections of toenails are difficult to eradicate medically. There are no topical medications that have been shown to be effective. Only the griseofulvin group of medications, taken orally, may eliminate the infection. Griseofulvin treatment is prolonged (1 to 2 years) and carries the small but real risk of bone marrow suppression. There is also the possibility that, following such a regimen, the infection will recur. Therefore, simple debridement or radical removal of the nail are the treatments of choice for this problem.

When nail thickening is regarded as a problem by the patient, he can be instructed to control the process by regular and thorough *debridement.* Debridement by a dermatologist or podiatrist is recommended for patients with diabetes and peripheral vascular disease in whom the thickness of the nails could lead to pressure ulcerations and hazardous infections of underlying skin.

Another treatment is *permanent removal* of the nail, including matrixectomy. Since toenails serve no useful function, their absence causes no functional impairment. Surgical correction should be reserved, however, for those patients whose nails are painful or for whom the appearance of the feet is a significant factor. The most frequent type of surgical correction of toenails performed by dermatologists, podiatrists, or surgeons is nail excision, followed by chemical destruction of matrix tissue and nailbed with 88% phenol. After a sterile dressing is applied to the toe, the patient may continue his normal routine. He needs only to change bandages and soak his feet daily until healing is complete in 2 to 3 weeks. Skin formerly below the nail plate thickens. Women can disguise the fact that their nails have been removed by applying nail polish to this thickened skin.

Ingrown Toenails (see Figs. 99.7 and 99.8)

ETIOLOGY AND FINDINGS

Ingrown toenail, a painful condition in which the medial or lateral border of a toenail penetrates the flesh, is a common problem. Ingrown toenails have been attributed to factors such as improper trimming, heredity, bony pathology, improper shoe fit, tight socks, obesity, and trauma. However, there is no clear-cut etiology, and there are probably many contributing causes. The nail of a great toe is almost always involved, and the problem can be identified by inspection and by the finding of point tenderness upon pressing the margin of the toenail.

TREATMENT

There is a popular misconception among many people that cutting a "V" in the center of a toenail will cause the lateral borders to grow toward the center, thereby relieving the ingrown condition. This

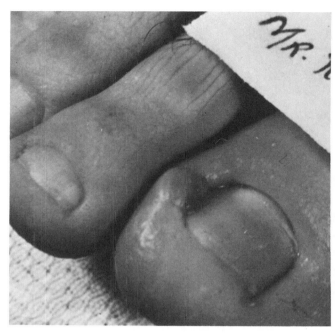

Figure 99.8   Infected ingrown toenail (paronychia).

belief has no basis in fact, since the nail plate is merely hornified keratin—nonliving, fixed tissue in which growth no longer occurs.

Initial treatment of ingrown toenail depends upon whether the patient's toe is infected (paronychia) or is chronically painful but not infected when the patient seeks care. The patient with an ingrown toenail will often seek help after attempting to excise the offending edge of toenail with whatever instruments are available; most of the nail edge may be removed in this way by the patient, but a small, sharp piece of nail usually remains which pierces the skin with each step and promotes infection: the toe is red, swollen, and exquisitely tender. The most vigorous soaking and the use of local and systemic antibiotics will not arrest such an infection as long as a nail spicule continues to penetrate the flesh. Therefore, the patient should be referred (to a dermatologist, podiatrist, or surgeon) for excision of the offending border of the nail; this procedure is done under local anesthesia. Systemic antibiotics are rarely necessary.

Definitive treatment of the ingrown nail itself, as in the case of corns and calluses, varies according to the condition and needs of the patient.

For *otherwise healthy patients*, the procedure described above for removal of the entire toenail and for matrix destruction can also be utilized to eradicate permanently an ingrown border. Following local anesthesia, the offending edge of toenail is excised; then phenol and alcohol are applied to cauterize the matrix tissue. This procedure, followed by 2 to 3 weeks for complete healing, will usually eliminate permanently this painful and sometimes dangerous condition.

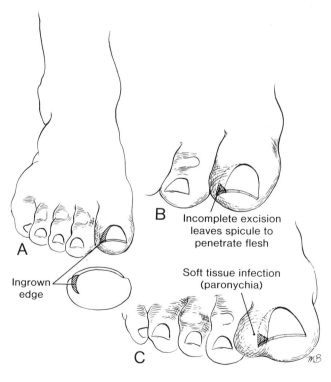

Figure 99.7   Schematic illustration of an ingrown toenail and complications which may occur.

Management of *diabetics* and patients with arterial insufficiency must be conservative, as wound healing may be poor after surgical removal of the nail. In these patients, frequent and thorough debridement of ingrown borders is effective and safe. Treatment by a podiatrist or other practitioner who is skilled in this procedure, may be needed every 3 to 4 weeks to prevent complicating soft tissue infection.

HEEL PAIN (1)

Heel pain is a common complaint. The pain is localized to the medial plantar aspect of the heel. Characteristically, the first step in the morning is particularly painful. After 5 to 10 min of walking the pain eases, but during the course of the day's activities it becomes progressively worse. The reason that these symptoms appear, disappear, and reappear is not understood.

Examination of the foot reveals a tender area of the heel approximately 4.5 cm from the posterior margin of the plantar surface, corresponding to the medial condyle of the calcaneus. X-rays frequently reveal a calcaneal exostosis or spur at the point of tenderness (see Fig. 99.9). These spurs are commonly found on X-rays of asymptomatic heels and they are not the cause of the pain in symptomatic heels. Since the attachment of the plantar fascia coincides with the point of greatest tenderness, it is felt that pain is due to *plantar fasciitis*. One can picture the plantar

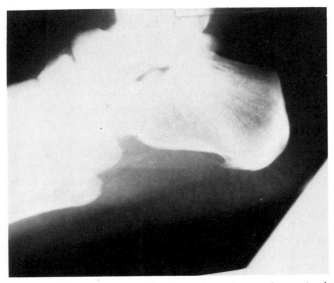

Figure 99.9 Radiologic view of a calcaneal exostosis (spur). (Photograph courtesy of Max Weisfeld, D.P.M.)

fascia as an extension of the Achilles tendon, with the calcaneus acting as a fulcrum between fascia and tendon (see Fig. 99.1B). Any condition which increases stress on the Achilles tendon may also stress the plantar fascia, e.g., overuse in running or jogging (especially with shoes having inflexible midsoles), excessive pronation (see above, p. 1083), or a sudden change to flat shoes after wearing high heels for prolonged periods. Heel pain may also be a manifestation of gout and this diagnosis should always be considered when evaluating such a patient.

Treatment

Treatment should be aimed both at the local inflammatory process and the underlying mechanical problem. Initial treatment would include use of an oral anti-inflammatory medication (aspirin, 600 mg every 4 to 6 hours), rest, and soaking in warm water. An injection of a corticosteroid and Xylocaine into the tender area from the medial aspect of the heel will usually bring dramatic relief from pain which has not responded to other measures.

Recurrent symptoms can be prevented by having the patient use a ¼-inch felt heel pad. When this is inserted into the shoes, it decreases tension on the Achilles tendon, and, consequently, tension on the plantar fascia is also reduced. The increased angulation of the foot shifts weight away from the heel to the forefoot. Felt—rather than foam, which is too compressible—is available from medical and surgical supply houses. When a simple heel pad is not sufficient, consultation with an orthopaedist or podiatrist is indicated. The consultant will fabricate an appropriate orthotic to minimize pronation, raise the heel, and protect the painful area. Rarely, a painful heel will require surgical intervention.

References

General

Ashur, M: *Principles and Practices of Podiatry*, edited by F Weinstein. Lea & Febiger, Philadelphia, 1968.
   A useful text for basic understanding of podiatric medicine.
Jamits, MH: *Cutaneous Lesions of the Lower Extremity*, J.B. Lippincott, Philadelphia, 1971.
   Well-illustrated text covering dermatologic conditions of the foot.

Specific

1. Cailliet, R: *Foot and Ankle Pain*, pp. 108–116. F.A. Davis, Philadelphia, 1968.
2. Lurdeen, G: Onychomycosis: Its classification, pathophysiology and etiology. *J Am Podiatry Assoc* 68: 395, 1978.
3. Mercado, OA: *The Surgical Treatment of Hallux Abducto Valgus*, edited by M Fielding. Futura Publishing Co., New York, 1973.

Index